Psychiatric & Mental Health Nursing

for Canadian Practice

Psychiatric & Mental Health Nursing

for Canadian Practice

THIRD EDITION

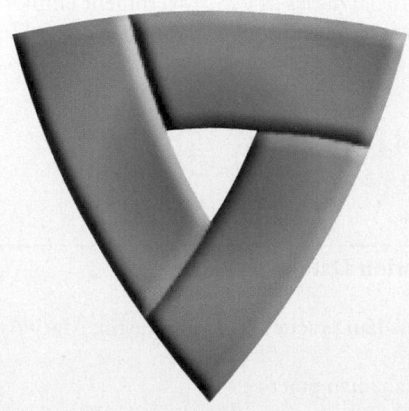

Wendy Austin, RN, BScN, MEd (Counselling), PhD

Professor Emeritus
University of Alberta
Edmonton, Alberta, Canada

Mary Ann Boyd, PhD, DNS, APRN, BC

Professor Emeritus
Southern Illinois University Edwardsville
Edwardsville, Illinois

. Wolters Kluwer

Philadelphia • Baltimore • New York • London
Buenos Aires • Hong Kong • Sydney • Tokyo

Acquisitions Editor: Patrick Barbera
Product Development Editor: Katherine Burland
Editorial Assistant: Dan Reilly
Production Project Manager: Marian Bellus
Design Coordinator: Holly McLaughlin
Illustration Coordinator: Jen Clements
Manufacturing Coordinator: Karin Duffield
Prepress Vendor: SPi Global

3rd edition

9 8 7 6 5 4 3 2 1

Printed in the United States of America

Library of Congress Cataloging-in-Publication Data
Austin, Wendy, 1947- author.
   Psychiatric & mental health nursing for Canadian practice / Wendy Austin, Mary Ann Boyd. — Third edition.
     p. ; cm.
   Psychiatric and mental health nursing for Canadian practice
   Includes bibliographical references and index.
   ISBN 978-1-4511-9087-8 (hardback)
  I. Boyd, M. (Mary Ann), author. II. Title. III. Title: Psychiatric and mental health nursing for Canadian practice.
  [DNLM: 1. Psychiatric Nursing—methods—Canada. 2. Mental Disorders—nursing—Canada. WY 160]
  RC440
  616.89'0231—dc23
                                               2014014231

This book is dedicated to individuals living with a mental health problem or mental disorder and their families. May you always receive competent, compassionate, and ethical nursing care that supports recovery.

In Memorium
Ginette Pagé

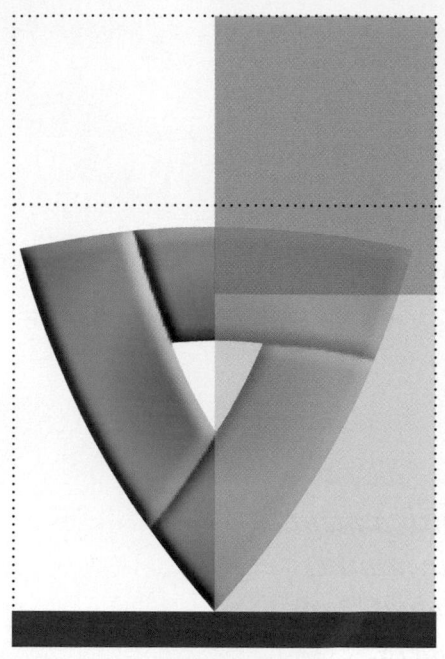

Canadian Contributors

Current Edition

Geertje Boschma, RN, PhD
Associate Professor
School of Nursing
University of British Columbia
Vancouver, British Columbia, Canada

Diana Clarke, RN, PhD
Associate Professor and Associate Dean (Research)
College of Nursing
Faculty of Health Sciences
University of Manitoba
Winnipeg, Manitoba, Canada

Anne Marie Creamer, RN, MSN, PhD
Nurse Practitioner Primary Health Care
Saint Joseph's Community Health Centre
Horizon Health Network
Saint John, New Brunswick, Canada

Christine Davis, BScN, MEd, MN, CPMHN(C)
Coordinator
Collaborative BScN Program
St. Lawrence College
Laurentian University
Brockville, Ontario, Canada

Charl Els, MBChB, FCPsych, MMedPsych, ABAM, MROCC
Associate Clinical Professor
School of Public Health, Faculty of Medicine
    and Dentistry, and the John Dossetor Health
    Ethics Centre
University of Alberta
Edmonton, Alberta, Canada

Carol Ewashen, RN, PhD
Associate Professor
Faculty of Nursing
University of Calgary
Calgary, Alberta, Canada

Lorelei Faulkner-Gibson, RN, BSN, MN, CPMHN(C)
Professional Practice Leader—Nursing
BC Children's Hospital
Vancouver, British Columbia, Canada

Dorothy Forbes, RN, PhD
Professor
Faculty of Nursing
University of Alberta
Edmonton, Alberta, Canada

Cheryl Forchuk, RN, PhD
Distinguished University Professor
Arthur Labatt Family School of Nursing
Faculty of Health Sciences
University of Western Ontario
London, Ontario, Canada

Marlee Groening, RN, MSN
Lecturer
School of Nursing
University of British Columbia
Vancouver, British Columbia, Canada

Jane Hamilton Wilson, BScN, MHSc, PhD
Professor
McMaster Mohawk Conestoga BScN Program
Conestoga College Institute of Technology and
    Advanced Learning
Kitchener, Ontario, Canada

Yvonne M. Hayne, RN, PhD
Senior Instructor
Faculty of Nursing
University of Calgary
Calgary, Alberta, Canada

Kathleen Hegadoren, RN, BScN, MSc, PhD
Professor
Canada Research Chair in Stress Disorders in
    Women
Faculty of Nursing
University of Alberta
Edmonton, Alberta, Canada

**Arlene Kent-Wilkinson, RN, BSN, MN,
CPMHN(C), PhD**
Associate Professor
College of Nursing
University of Saskatchewan
Saskatoon, Saskatchewan, Canada

Diane Kunyk, RN, BScN, MN, PhD
Assistant Professor
Faculty of Nursing and the John Dossetor Health Ethics
    Centre
University of Alberta
Edmonton, Alberta, Canada

**Gerri Lasiuk, RPN, RN, BA(Hons), MN, PhD,
CPMHN(C)**
Associate Professor and Director, Nursing Simulation
    Centre
Faculty of Nursing
University of Alberta
Edmonton, Alberta, Canada

D. Stewart MacLennan, MN, NP
Faculty Lecturer
Faculty of Nursing
University of Alberta
Edmonton, Alberta, Canada

Elizabeth A. McCay, RN, PhD
Associate Professor and Research Chair in Urban Health
Daphne Cockwell School of Nursing
Ryerson University
Toronto, Ontario, Canada

Sharon L. Moore, RN, BA, MEd, PhD
Professor
Centre for Nursing and Health Studies
Athabasca University
Athabasca, Alberta, Canada

B. Lee Murray, RN, BSN, MN, PhD
Clinical Nurse Specialist
Associate Professor
College of Nursing
University of Saskatchewan
Saskatoon, Saskatchewan, Canada

Margaret Osborne, RN, PhD
Instructor (retired)
Centre for Nursing and Health Studies
Athabasca University
Athabasca, Alberta, Canada

Cindy Peternelj-Taylor, RN, MSc, PhD(c), DF-IAFN
Professor
College of Nursing
University of Saskatchewan
Saskatoon, Saskatchewan, Canada

Cheryl Pollard, PN, RN, BScN, MN, PhD
Assistant Professor
Faculty of Health & Community Studies
MacEwan University
Edmonton, Alberta, Canada

Yvonne Savard, RPN, RN, BScN, MAED/CI
Instructor/Year 3 Coordinator
Faculty of Health Sciences
Department of Psychiatric Nursing
Douglas College
Coquitlam, British Columbia, Canada

Peggy (Margaret) Simpson, RN, PhD
Clinical Nurse Specialist Psychiatric Consultation Liaison
Providence Health Care—St. Paul's Hospital
Adjunct Professor
School of Nursing
University of British Columbia
Vancouver, British Columbia, Canada

Nicole Snow, RN, CPMHN(C), PhD(c)
Assistant Professor
School of Nursing
Memorial University of Newfoundland
St. John's, Newfoundland and Labrador, Canada

Michel A. Tarko, RPN, PhD
President and CEO
Justice Institute of British Columbia
New Westminster, British Columbia, Canada

Kathryn Weaver, BN, MN, PhD
Professor
Faculty of Nursing
University of New Brunswick
Fredericton, New Brunswick, Canada

Kimberly Wong, RN, BSN, MBA, CPMHN(C)
Clinical Nurse Educator
Children and Women's Mental Health
BC Mental Health and Substance Use Services
Vancouver, British Columbia, Canada

Previous Editions

Freida S. Chavez, RN, BScN, MHSc, CHE
Senior Lecturer
Faculty of Nursing
University of Toronto
Toronto, Ontario, Canada

Julia Gajewski-Noel, RN, BA, MN
Certificate in Mental Health Nursing
Senior Teaching Associate—Retired 2009
Faculty of Nursing
University of New Brunswick
Fredericton, New Brunswick, Canada

Ruth Gallop, RN, PhD
Professor Emerita
Faculty of Nursing
University of Toronto
Toronto, Ontario, Canada

Mary Haase, RPN, RN, BScN, PhD
Faculty Member
BScN Program
MacEwan University
Edmonton, Alberta, Canada

Brad Hagen, RN, R. Psych, PhD (Nsg)
Associate Professor
Faculty School of Health Sciences
University of Lethbridge
Lethbridge, Alberta, Canada

Sandy Harper-Jaques, RN, MN, RMFT
Clinical Nurse Specialist
Adult Mental Health
CHR South Calgary Health Centre
Calgary, Alberta, Canada

Marion Healey-Ogden, RN, RCC, BSN, MEd, MA, PhD
Assistant Professor
Faculty of Nursing
Thompson Rivers University
Kamloops, British Columbia, Canada

L. Elizabeth Hood, RN, MSN, PhD
Clinical Nurse Specialist (Mental Health)
Regional Mental Health Program
Alberta Hospital Edmonton
Edmonton, Alberta, Canada

Jean Robinson Hughes, RN, PhD
Associate Professor
School of Nursing
Dalhousie University
Halifax, Nova Scotia, Canada

Annette M. Lane, RN, PhD
Assistant Professor
Faculty of Nursing
University of Calgary
Calgary, Alberta, Canada

Lori Houger Limacher, RN, PhD, RMFT
Private Practice
Calgary, Alberta, Canada

Ginette Pagé, RN, PhD
Clinical Nurse Specialist, Consultant in
    Nursing
Private Practice
Dunham, Québec, Canada

Hélène Provencher, RN, PhD
Professor
Faculty of Nursing
Laval University
Québec City, Québec, Canada

Tracey Tully, RN, PhD
Clinical Nurse Specialist
Sunnybrook and Women's College Health Sciences
  Centre
Toronto, Ontario, Canada

Stephen VanSlyke, RN, BN, MN
Senior Teaching Associate
Faculty of Nursing
University of New Brunswick
Fredericton, New Brunswick, Canada

Olive Yonge, RN, PhD, R Psych
Professor
Faculty of Nursing
Vice Provost (Academic Programs)
University of Alberta
Edmonton, Alberta, Canada

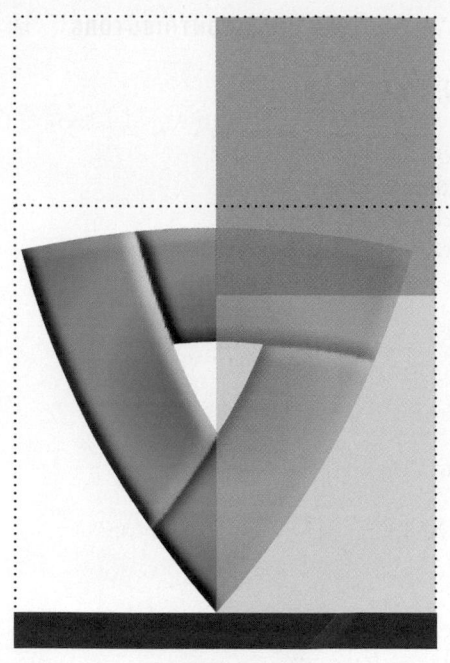

American Contributors to Previous Editions

Marjorie Baier, PhD, RN
Associate Professor
School of Nursing
Southern Illinois University Edwardsville
Edwardsville, Illinois

Doris E. Bell, PhD, APRN, BC
Professor of Nursing
Southern Illinois University Edwardsville
Edwardsville, Illinois

Ann R. Bland, PhD, APRN, BC
Associate Professor
Department of Baccalaureate & Graduate Nursing
Eastern Kentucky University
Richmond, Kentucky

Andrea C. Bostrom, PhD, RN, APRN, BC
Associate Professor and Dean of Academic Programs
Kirkhof College of Nursing
Grand Valley State University
Allendale, Michigan

Mary R. Boyd, PhD, RN
Associate Professor
College of Nursing
University of South Carolina
Columbia, South Carolina

Stephanie Burgess, PhD, APN-BC
Clinical Professor and Associate Dean for Nursing
    Practice
College of Nursing
University of South Carolina
Columbia, South Carolina

Rita Canfield, RN, MSN, DNSc
School of Nursing
Southern Illinois University Edwardsville
Edwardsville, Illinois

Jeanne A. Clement, EdD, APRN, BC, FAAN
Associate Professor and Director of Graduate Specialty
    Program in Psychiatric-Mental Health Nursing
College of Nursing
The Ohio State University
Columbus, Ohio

Harvey Davis, RN, PhD, CARN, PHN
School of Nursing
San Francisco State University
San Francisco, California

Catherine Gray Deering, PhD, RN, APRN, BC
Professor
Clayton State College
Morrow, Georgia

Peggy El-Mallakh, PhD, RN
Post-Doctoral Scholar
Chandler Medical Center
College of Nursing
University of Kentucky
Lexington, Kentucky

Barbara G. Faltz
Clinical Nurse Specialist
Addiction Treatment Services, Veterans Administration
Palo Alto Healthcare System
Palo Alto, California

Judith E. Forker, PhD, APRN, BC
Associate Dean for Academic Affairs
School of Nursing
Adelphi University
Garden City, New York

Denise M. Gibson, MSN, APRN, BC
Instructor
Southern Illinois University School of Nursing
    Edwardsville
Edwardsville, Illinois

Vanya Hamrin, RN, MS, APRN, BC
Assistant Professor
School of Nursing
Yale University
New Haven, Connecticut

Beverly Gilliam Hart, RN, PhD
Associate Professor of Baccalaureate and Graduate
    Nursing
Eastern Kentucky University
Richmond, Kentucky

Emily J. Hauenstein, PhD, APRN, LCP, BC
Professor
School of Nursing
University of Virginia
Charlottesville, Virginia

Nancy Anne Hilliker, MA, RN, ANP, CS
Nurse Practitioner
Barnes-Jewish Hospital
St. Louis, Missouri

Gail L. Kongable, MSN, RN, FNP
Associate Professor
Neurological Surgery
University of Virginia Health Systems
Charlottesville, Virginia

Kathy Lee, MS, RN, APRN, BC
Associate Professor and Psychiatric Mental Health
    Nurse Practitioner
School of Nursing—SNSN
Oregon Health & Science University
Center for Women's Health
Portland, Oregon

Susan McCabe, EdD, APRN, BC
Associate Professor
College of Nursing
East Tennessee State University
Johnson City, Tennessee

**Ruth Beckmann Murray, MSN, EdD, N-NAP,
FAAN**
Professor Emerita
School of Nursing
Doisy College of Health Sciences
St. Louis University
St. Louis, Missouri

Robert B. Noud, MS, APRN, BC
Adjunct Faculty Staff
University of Missouri St. Louis
St. Louis University Hospital
St. Louis, Missouri

Maryellen C. Pachler, MSN, APRN
Child Psychiatric Nurse Practitioner
Child Study Center
School of Medicine
Yale University
New Haven, Connecticut

Nan Roberts, MS, APRN, BC
Director of Clinical Trials
Advent Research Institute
St. Peters, Missouri

Lawrence Scahill, PhD, MSN, FAAN
Professor of Nursing and Child Psychiatry
Child Study Center
Yale University
New Haven, Connecticut

Victoria Soltis-Jarrett, PhD, APRN-BC
Clinical Associate Professor and MSN Coordinator,
    Psychiatric Mental Health
Family Psychiatric Nurse Practitioner and Clinical
    Nurse Specialist
School of Nursing
University of North Carolina at Chapel Hill
Chapel Hill, North Carolina

Mickey Stanley, PhD, RN
Associate Professor
School of Nursing
Southern Illinois University Edwardsville
Edwardsville, Illinois

Roberta Stock, MS, APRN, BC
Advanced Practice Nurse
Comtrea, Inc.
Festus, Missouri

Sandra P. Thomas, PhD, RN, FAAN
Professor and Director, PhD Program
College of Nursing
The University of Tennessee
Knoxville, Tennessee

Barbara Jones Warren, PhD, APRN, BC
Associate Clinical Professor
College of Nursing
The Ohio State University
Executive Nurse
Ohio Department of Mental Health
Columbus, Ohio

Jane White, PhD, DNSc, APRN, BC
Vera E. Bender Professor of Nursing
Associate Dean for Research and Graduate Programs
Adelphi University
Garden City, New York

Lorraine D. Williams, RN, PhD, APRN, BC
Associate Professor
School of Nursing
Southern Illinois University Edwardsville
Edwardsville, Illinois

Rhonda Kay Wilson, RN, BSN, MS
Quality Manager
Chester Mental Health Center
Chester, Illinois

Richard Yakimo, PhD, APRN, BC
Assistant Professor
School of Nursing
Southern Illinois University Edwardsville
Edwardsville, Illinois

Reviewers

Leigh Blaney, MA, BScN, RN, CFMHN(c)
Professor
Bachelor of Science in Nursing Program
Vancouver Island University
Nanaimo, British Columbia, Canada

Sharon Chin, MHScN, RN, CPMHN(c)
Professor
Collaborative BScN Program
Canadore College/Nipissing University
North Bay, Ontario, Canada

Elizabeth Harris, MEd, BScN
Professor
Department of Nursing
Algonquin College
Ottawa, Ontario, Canada

Melodie Hull, MEd, MSC, BA, RPN
Nursing Faculty
College of the Rockies
Cranbrook, British Columbia, Canada
Open Learning Faculty
Thompson Rivers University
Kamloops, British Columbia, Canada

Sonya Jakubec, MN, BHScN, RN, PhD(c)
Associate Professor
School of Nursing & Midwifery
Mount Royal University
Calgary, Alberta, Canada

Christa MacLean, MN, BSN, RN
Faculty/Curriculum Coordinator
Saskatchewan Collaborative BScN
Saskatchewan Institute of Applied Science and
    Technology
Regina, Saskatchewan, Canada

Cindy Pallister, MScN, BScN, RN
Nursing Professor
St. Clair College—Thames Campus
Chatham, Ontario, Canada

Cheryl Pollard, PN, RN, BScN, MN, PhD
Assistant Professor
Faculty of Health & Community Studies
MacEwan University
Edmonton, Alberta, Canada

Wilma Schroeder, MMFT, BN, RN
Nursing Faculty
Red River College
Winnipeg, Manitoba, Canada

Wendy Stanyon, EdD, MAEd, BN, RN
Associate Professor
University of Ontario Institution of Technology
Oshawa, Ontario, Canada

John Stone, MA, BScN, RN, BA, CPMHN(c)
Program Coordinator
Practical Nursing Program
Humber I.T.A.L.
Toronto, Ontario, Canada

Mary Jean Thompson, MHS, MPC, BN, RN
Nursing Faculty
Division of Health Studies
Medicine Hat College
Medicine Hat, Alberta, Canada

Wendy M. Wheeler, MN, RN
Nursing Instructor
Red Deer College
Red Deer, Alberta, Canada

Bernadine Wojtowicz, MScN, RN
NESA BN Programs Co-Chair
Theory Courses Coordinator
Faculty of Health Sciences
University of Lethbridge
Lethbridge, Alberta, Canada

Preface

This third edition of *Psychiatric & Mental Health Nursing for Canadian Practice* reflects the myriad changes in mental health care that are occurring in Canada and around the world. The global recognition that "there is no health without mental health" informs the World Health Organization's *Mental Health Action Plan 2013–2020*. In Canada, the enactment of *Changing Directions, Changing Lives: The Mental Health Strategy for Canada* is creating significant transformation in the ways that mental health is fostered and the manner in which our mental health care system supports recovery and well-being. The need for the active voice and engagement of individuals and families who use the system has become evident. There is now a national framework for child and youth mental health care, *Evergreen*. Further, the implications of the distinct circumstances, rights, and cultures of First Nations, Inuit, and Métis peoples in meeting their mental health care needs have been acknowledged. The stigma of mental illness is being actively addressed; the mental health literacy of Canadians has increased; training in mental health first aid is offered; and the importance of mental health in addressing disaster events is recognized. A "housing first" approach to homelessness of persons living with mental illness has been proven successful, both economically and in terms of recovery. And Canada is the only nation to date that has national psychological health and safety guidelines for the workplace. Ensuring that these significant changes in mental health care are reflected in this textbook has been a necessary and exciting challenge, given that nurses are key players in this concerted effort to ensure quality mental health care across our country.

This textbook also encompasses changes to the way in which mental health and mental disorders are conceptualized in North America, based on the fifth edition of the American Psychiatric Association's *Diagnostic and Statistical Manual*, the *DSM-5*, which was released May 2013. There is one completely new chapter in this edition: *Sleep-Wake Disorders*. Nurses encounter individuals with sleep–wake issues in all practice settings, and, as many nurses are shift workers, they face their own potential problems in this area. Understanding sleep and its promotion is necessary to nursing practice and to nurses' own health and well-being. In this edition of the textbook, the standards of practice and ethical codes of registered psychiatric nurses have been acknowledged, psychiatric advance directives discussed, and attention to gender paid when appropriate. A lifespan focus has been maintained.

As in the previous editions, the terminology used to identify individual recipients of nursing care—patient, client, or consumer—has been left to the preference of the chapter contributors. The many pedagogical features of the previous editions have been retained, as well, but some will now appear on thePoint. The move of **Web Links** to thePoint will allow links to be kept current. The **Movies and Other Things** feature, now on thePoint, has evolved to include TED Talks, novels, and biographies. See below for a listing of features and information about the teaching–learning package.

▮▮ FEATURES

- Chapters open with **Learning Objectives**, **Key Terms**, and **Key Concepts** that cue students to the material they will encounter.
- **Summary of Key Points** encapsulates core chapter content to facilitate assimilation and review.
- **Critical Thinking Challenges** are grounded in chapter content and aimed at stimulating both analytical and reflective thinking about it on the part of students.
- **Research Boxes** focus on specific studies, primarily Canadian, which contribute to improving PMH nursing practice. The selected studies reflect the broad range of research methods used to inform practice, from systematic reviews, through quantitative and qualitative empirical research projects, to philosophical inquiry.
- **Study Notes** are suggestions regarding important areas of preparation for examinations.
- The **In a Life** feature illustrates the way the topic of the chapter has shaped or been played out in a particular person's life.
- **Therapeutic Dialogue Boxes** encourage the comparison of therapeutic and nontherapeutic communication by giving relevant examples of both.
- **Clinical Vignette Boxes** present reality-based clinical portraits of persons with symptoms of interest to the chapter topic. Questions are posed to help students consider solutions to issues presented.
- **Drug Profile Boxes** present a profile of specific psychotropic medication, commonly prescribed in the treatment of mental disorders.
- **Psychoeducation Checklists** identify content areas for the education of persons with specific disorders and their families.
- **Line art, photos, scan images, and flow charts** illustrate the interrelationship of the biologic, psychological, social, and spiritual domains of mental health and illness.

▮▮ TEACHING–LEARNING PACKAGE

Student Resources

Online student resources for this book include:

- *Web Links* that are listed to direct students to excellent sources of supplemental information.
- *Movies and Other Things*, which has suggestions regarding movies, documentaries, TED Talks, and books that can help students further explore some of the complex ideas or issues related to PMH nursing practice. Points to consider are offered. Students can use the suggested works to stimulate discussion with their family and friends, as well as their classmates and teachers.
- *Movie Viewing Guides* that highlight films depicting individuals with mental health disorders and provide students the opportunity to approach nursing care related to mental health illness in a novel way.
- *Clinical Simulations* on schizophrenia, depression, and the acutely manic phase that walk students through case studies and put them in real-life situations.

These and other valuable student resources are also available on thePoint.

Instructor Resources

The Instructor Resources on thePoint include additional information and activities that will help you engage your students from the semester's beginning to its end, including:

- PowerPoint slides
- Assignments
- Case Studies
- Image Bank
- Test Generator
- WebCT, Blackboard, and Angel-Ready Material

Wendy Austin
RN, BScN, MEd (Counselling), PhD
Professor Emeritus
University of Alberta

Contents

Canadian Contributors   vi
American Contributors to Previous Editions   x
Reviewers   xiii
Preface   xv

UNIT 1   **Contemporary Canadian Mental Health Care   1**

1   Psychiatric and Mental Health Nursing: From Past to Present   2
Geertje Boschma and Marlee Groening
Early Forms of Institutional Care   2
A Revolutionary Idea: Humane Treatment   3
The 19th and Early 20th Centuries: An Era of Asylum
   Building   4
Modern Thinking   8
The Late 20th and Early 21st Century   11

2   Mental Health, Mental Disorder, Recovery, and Well-Being   17
Wendy Austin
Mental Health   17
Well-Being   18
Mental Illness   19
Recovery   21

The Mental Health of Canadians   22
Research-Based Care   23

3   The Context of Mental Health Care: Cultural, Socioeconomic, and Legal   25
Arlene Kent-Wilkinson
Cultural Context of Mental Health Care   25
Aboriginal People of Canada   27
Religion as a Culture System   29
Stereotyping, Prejudice, Discrimination,
   and Stigma   29
Cultural Competence and Cultural Safety   32
Socioeconomic Context of Mental Health Care   33
Geographic Location and Access to Mental
   Health Services   35
The Legal Context of Mental Health
   Care   36
Research and the Context of Mental Health
   Care   39

4   The Continuum of Psychiatric and Mental Health Care   42
Cheryl Pollard
Primary Health Care Approach   42
Defining the Continuum of Care   43
Comprehensive Mental Health System: Core
   Programs and Services   45

UNIT 2 Foundations of Psychiatric and Mental Health Nursing Practice 53

5 Contemporary Psychiatric and Mental Health Nursing Practice 54
Wendy Austin and Margaret Osborne
The Bio/Psycho/Social/Spiritual Model of PMH Nursing 54
Standards of Professional Practice 57
Key Components of PMH Nursing Practice 58
Challenges of PMH Nursing 61
PMH Nursing in a Global Community 62

6 Communication and the Therapeutic Relationship 64
Cheryl Forchuk
Self-Awareness 64
The Bio/Psycho/Social/Spiritual Self 65
Understanding Personal Feelings and Beliefs, and Changing Behaviour 65
Communication 65
Using Verbal Communication 66
Using Nonverbal Communication 69
Recognizing Empathic Linkages 70
Selecting Communication Techniques 70
Applying Communication Concepts 71
Analyzing Interactions 74
The Nurse–Client Relationship 76
Nontherapeutic Relationships 79
Strategies Within the Therapeutic Relationship 79

7 Ethical Practice 82
Wendy Austin
What Is Ethics? 82
Codes of Ethics for Nurses 83
Approaches to Ethics 84
Ethical Practice Environments 88
Moral Dilemmas and Moral Distress 88
Some Ethical Issues in PMH Settings 89

8 Theoretic Basis of Psychiatric and Mental Health Nursing 96
Wendy Austin
Nursing Theories 96
Biologic Theories 101
Psychological Theories 101
Social Theories 109
Spiritual Theories 110
Recovery as a Framework for Mental Health Care 111
Theories as Maps 111

9 Biologic Basis of Practice 114
Anne Marie Creamer
Foundational Concepts 114

Current Research Approaches and Advances 117
Neuroanatomy of the Central Nervous System 122
Neurophysiology of the Central Nervous System 130
New Fields of Study 139
Diagnostic Approaches 141
Integration of the Biologic, Psychologic, Social, and Spiritual Domains 143

UNIT 3 Interventions in Psychiatric and Mental Health Nursing Practice 147

10 The Assessment Process 148
Gerri Lasiuk and Kathleen Hegadoren
Assessment as a Process 148
Bio/Psycho/Social/Spiritual Psychiatric/Mental Health Nursing Assessment 154

11 Diagnosis, Intervention, and Outcomes in Psychiatric and Mental Health Nursing 165
Nicole Snow and Christine Davis
A Commitment to Collaboration and Client Centredness 167
Evolution of Nursing Diagnosis and Individual Outcomes 167
Deriving a Nursing Diagnosis 168
Developing Individual Outcomes 169
Nursing Interventions and PMH Nursing 171
Evaluation of Outcomes 183

12 Psychopharmacology and Other Biologic Treatments 186
Kathleen Hegadoren and Gerri Lasiuk
Pharmacodynamics 187
Pharmacokinetics: How Drugs Move Through the Body 193
Phases of Drug Treatment 198
Antipsychotic Medications 200
Mood Stabilizers (Antimania Medications) 209
Antidepressant Medications 213
Antianxiety and Sedative–Hypnotic Medications 218
Stimulants 221
New Medications 223
Other Biologic Treatments 223
Psychosocial Issues in Biologic Treatments 226

13 Cognitive–Behavioural Techniques 232
Wendy Austin
The Cognitive Model 233
Levels of Cognition 234

Principles of Cognitive–Behavioural Therapy   235
Treatment Strategies   238
Mindfulness-Based CBT   242
Conclusion   242

14   Interventions With Groups   244
Carol Ewashen
Group: Definitions and Concepts   244
Group Leadership   250
Types of Groups   254
Common Nursing Intervention Groups   255
Self-Care Groups   256

**15   Family Assessment and
        Interventions   259**
Peggy (Margaret) Simpson
Characteristics of Canadian Families   259
Family Caregivers   260
Contextual Issues to Consider When Working With
    Families   261
Family Assessment   261
Family Assessment in the Bio/Psycho/Social/Spiritual
    Domains   264
The Pyramid of Family Care Framework   270
Family Interventions   270

**16   Psychological Health and Safety
        in the Workplace   275**
Wendy Austin
Work   276
Healthy Workplaces   277
Threats to Workplace Psychological Health and
    Safety   280
Mental Health Problems and Disorders in the
    Workplace   281
Nurses and Workplace Psychological Health and
    Safety   283

**UNIT 4   Challenges to Mental
             Health   287**

**17   Trauma- and Stressor-Related
        Disorders, Crisis, and Response
        to Disaster   288**
*Gerri Lasiuk, Kathleen Hegadoren, and
Wendy Austin*
Stress   288
Crisis   302

18   Anger, Aggression, and Violence   317
Yvonne Savard
Anger   318
Aggression and Violence   319
Models of Anger, Aggression, and
    Violence   320

19   Self-Harm and Suicidal Behaviour   340
B. Lee Murray and Wendy Austin
Canada's Suicide Prevention Strategy   341
Epidemiology of Suicidal Behaviour   341
Aetiology of Suicidal Behaviour   346
Effects of Suicide   351
Suicide and the Law   351
Nursing Assessment and Interventions   353

**UNIT 5   Care and Recovery of Persons
             With a Psychiatric Disorder   365**

20   Schizophrenia   366
Jane Hamilton Wilson
Clinical Course   367
Epidemiology   372
Aetiology   374
Interdisciplinary Treatment   379
Priority Care Issues   380
Family Response to Disorder   380

**21   Schizoaffective, Delusional, and Other
        Psychotic Disorders   415**
Diana Clarke
Schizoaffective Disorder   415
Delusional Disorder   427
Other Psychotic Disorders   434

22   Mood Disorders   439
Yvonne M. Hayne
Depressive Disorders   440
Bipolar Disorders (Manic–Depressive
    Disorders)   457

**23   Anxiety and Obsessive–Compulsive
        Disorders   480**
Kathleen Hegadoren and Gerri Lasiuk
Normal Versus Abnormal Anxiety Response   481
Overview of Anxiety Disorders   481
Aetiologic Theories of Anxiety Disorders   487
Evaluation and Treatment Outcomes   497
Continuum of Care   497
Assessment and Treatment Issues Specific to
    Obsessive–Compulsive Disorder   499

**24   Somatic Symptom and Related
        Disorders   505**
D. Stewart MacLennan
Somatization   506
Somatic Symptom Disorder   506
Other Somatic Symptom and Related
    Disorders   517
Psychological Factors Affecting Other Medical
    Conditions   520
Factitious Disorders   520

25 **Feeding and Eating Disorders** 523
Kathryn Weaver
Anorexia Nervosa 524
Bulimia Nervosa 549
Binge-Eating Disorder 557
Prevention of Eating Disorders 563
Future Directions in Eating Disorder
    Knowledge 564

26 **Substance-Related and Addictive
Disorders** 572
Diane Kunyk and Charl Els
Neurobiology 573
Diagnostic Criteria 573
Epidemiology 575
Aetiologic Theories 576
Interdisciplinary Treatment 578
Nursing Interventions for Specific
    Substance-Related Disorders 586
Special Populations and Situations 598
The Nurse as Health Advocate 601

27 **Personality and Disruptive, Impulse-
Control, and Conduct Disorders** 605
Wendy Austin
Personality Disorders (PD) 606
Cluster A Disorders 610
Cluster B Disorders 612
Cluster C Disorders 636
Other Personality Disorders 637
Disruptive, Impulse-Control, and Conduct
    Disorders 637

28 **Sleep–Wake Disorders** 642
Anne Marie Creamer
Historical Perspectives on Sleep and
    Dreams 642
What Is Sleep? 643
Dreaming 645
Biologic Processes 647
Epidemiology: Canadian Sleep Habits 650
Overview of Sleep–Wake Disorders 651
Comorbid Mental Illnesses and Mental Health
    Problems 656
Insomnia 657
Obstructive Sleep Apnea 662
Common Circadian Rhythm Sleep–Wake
    Disorders 663

UNIT
6 **Mental Health Across the
Lifespan** 667

29 **Mental Health Promotion With
Children and Adolescents** 668
Lorelei Faulkner-Gibson and Kimberly Wong
Childhood and Adolescent Mental Health 668

Common Childhood Stressors 669
Development of Child Psychopathology 676
Mental Illness Among Children and
    Adolescents 683
Approaches to Addressing Childhood
    Trauma 683
New Directions in Community-Based Mental Health
    Promotion 686

30 **Mental Health Assessment of Children
and Adolescents** 691
Lorelei Faulkner-Gibson and Kimberly Wong
Assessing the Mental Health of Children and
    Adolescents 692
Collection of Assessment Data 693
Bio/Psycho/Social/Spiritual Psychiatric Nursing
    Assessment of Children and Adolescents 702

31 **Psychiatric Disorders Diagnosed in
Children and Adolescents** 718
*Lorelei Faulkner-Gibson, Kimberly Wong, and
Wendy Austin*
Schizophrenia Spectrum and Other Psychotic
    Disorders 720
Disorders of Mood and Anxiety 721
Anxiety Disorders 721
Trauma- and Stressor-Related Disorders 725
Gender Dysphoria 728
Neurodevelopmental Disorders of
    Childhood 729
Disruptive Impulse Control and Conduct
    Disorders 734
Elimination Disorders 746

32 **Mental Health Promotion With Older
Persons** 752
Sharon L. Moore
Mental Health of the Older Adult 752
Healthy Aging: The Example of Sexual
    Health 757
Risk Factors for Geriatric Psychopathology 758
Mental Illness Prevention and Mental Health
    Promotion 759

33 **Mental Health Assessment
of Older Persons** 765
Sharon L. Moore
Techniques of Data Collection 766
Bio/Psycho/Social/Spiritual Geriatric Mental Health
    Nursing Assessment 766

34 **Neurocognitive Disorders: Delirium
and Dementia** 780
Dorothy Forbes and Wendy Austin
Delirium 781
Dementia 791
Alzheimer's Disease 791
Other Major NCDs (Dementias) 813

UNIT 7 Care of Persons With Additional Vulnerabilities   821

35 Care of Persons With Concurrent Substance-Related, Addictive, and Other Mental Disorders   822
Charl Els and Diane Kunyk

Epidemiology of Concurrent Disorders   823
Aetiologic Theories: Development of Concurrent Disorders   824
The Effects of Alcohol, Tobacco, and Other Substances on Mental Health   825
Assessment Approaches Specific to Concurrent Disorders   825
Care and Treatment Approaches Specific to Concurrent Disorders   825
Implementing Interventions for Specific Concurrent Disorders   826
Nursing Management: Summary   828
Where Do We Go From Here?   829

36 Care of Medically Compromised Persons   831
Michel A. Tarko

Psychological Illness Related to Specific Physiologic Disorders   832
Psychological Impact of Pain   832
Psychopathologic Complications of AIDS   839
Psychological Illness Related to Trauma   841
Psychological Illness Related to CNS Disorders   843
Psychological Illness Related to Acute and Chronic Mental Illness   846
Intervening in Mental and Medical Illnesses   849

37 Care of Persons With a History of Abuse   853
Elizabeth A. McCay

Types of Abuse   854
Theories of Abuse   860
Survivors of Abuse: Human Responses to Trauma   865

Nursing Management: Human Response to Abuse   872
Evaluation and Treatment Outcomes   883

38 Care of Persons Under Forensic Purview   891
Cindy Peternelj-Taylor

Criminalization of the Mentally Ill   892
The Paradox of Custody and Caring   892
Forensic Nursing: A Model for Care   893
Societal Norms   902

Appendix A
Brief Psychiatric Rating Scale   907

Appendix B
Simpson-Angus Rating Scale   908

Appendix C
Abnormal Involuntary Movement Scale (AIMS)   910

Appendix D
Simplified Diagnoses for Tardive Dyskinesia (SD-TD)   912

Appendix E
Hamilton Rating Scale for Depression   914

Appendix F
Clinical Institute Withdrawal Assessment of Alcohol Scale, Revised (CIWA-Ar)   915

Glossary   917

Index   933

Contemporary Canadian Mental Health Care

UNIT
1

1

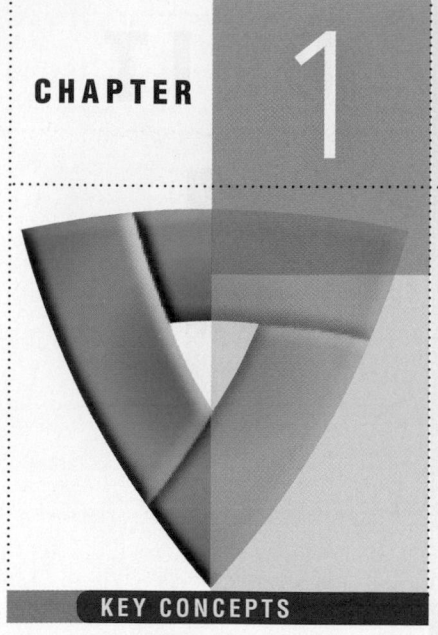

1 Psychiatric and Mental Health Nursing

From Past to Present

Geertje Boschma and Marlee Groening

Adapted from the chapter "Psychiatric and Mental Health Nursing: From Past to Present" by Mary Ann Boyd

LEARNING OBJECTIVES

After studying this chapter, you will be able to:

- Identify the historical influences and social changes that affect the delivery of mental health care.
- Relate the concept of social change to the history of psychiatric and mental health care.
- Discuss the history of psychiatric and mental health (PMH) nursing and its place within nursing history.
- Analyze the theoretical arguments that shaped the development of contemporary scientific thought about PMH nursing practice.
- Summarize the impact of current social, economic, and political forces on the delivery of mental health services.

KEY CONCEPTS

- historical context
- social change

KEY TERMS

- biologic view • community mental health nursing
- deinstitutionalization • moral treatment • psychiatric and mental health nursing education • psychiatric hospitals • psychiatric pluralism
- psychoanalytic movement • psychosocial theory

Until the 19th century, mentally ill people mainly were kept at home and cared for by their families. Sometimes their legal guardians boarded them with other families for a fee, as part of a broader poor-relief system. Only the most seriously afflicted people, whose behaviour was severely disturbing or who were considered a danger to themselves, their families, or other citizens, were locked in, often in prison or a poorhouse. Indigent mentally ill people were grouped with old, sick, orphaned, or convicted people, and the circumstances in these scanty public facilities were most basic and often harsh. For those who could afford it, privately maintained institutions emerged as well (Boschma, 2003; Shorter, 1997).

EARLY FORMS OF INSTITUTIONAL CARE

Around the turn of the 15th century—the beginning of the European Renaissance—some towns in Europe established small-scale asylums as charitable enterprises, each one initially housing about 10 people. Most often they were civilian, charitable initiatives in which neither the church nor doctors were involved. London's Bethlehem Hospital (famously known as "Bedlam") (Fig. 1-1), founded in 1371, and the Reinier van Arkel asylum, founded in 1442 in the Dutch town of Den Bosch, are early examples of the insane asylums or "mad houses" that would over the next centuries spread throughout

FIGURE 1-1. Interior of Bethlehem Asylum ("Bedlam"), London, as depicted by William Hogarth in his series *A Rake's Progress*. (From U.S. National Library of Medicine. Images from the history of medicine. National Institutes of Health, Department of Health and Human Services.)

Europe and, in the wake of colonialism, other parts of the world. These asylums were managed as large households, like other guesthouses or poorhouses, and administered by a board of noted citizens, with a steward and matron, often a married couple, taking charge of day-to-day management with the assistance of a few servants. With the social and economic changes of the 18th and 19th centuries, these homes grew into larger institutions (Boschma, 2003).

Religious orders, often under the protection or authority of the church, also involved themselves with charitable work and poor relief. Roman Catholic orders, for example, reemerged in 17th-century France during the Counter-Reformation, and many of them managed the care in small-scale, premodern hospitals. The orders themselves sometimes owned the houses. Influential cases in point were the male order of the Congregation of Lazarists and the female congregation of the Sisters of Mercy (or Daughters of Charity), founded by Vincent de Paul in 1625 and 1633, respectively (Jones, 1989). These orders produced early models for nursing work as a socially respectable endeavour at a time when medical care had barely developed and was scarcely available (Nelson, 1999, 2001; Porter, 1993). In the Americas, one of the first institutions that took in mentally ill people was San Hipólito in Mexico City, which opened in 1589 as a hospital for the insane, under the auspices of the Roman Catholic Church. It was run by the brothers of the order of La Caridad y San Hipólito, who, vowing poverty and charity, relied on alms to support themselves and worked as attendants in the institution (Leiby, 1992). The earliest forms of institutional treatment in Canada date back to the 19th century.

Diverse beliefs and approaches to deal with mental illness or attempts to treat it have been employed and must be understood in their historical context. Spiritual, biologic, and social explanations commonly were intertwined in popular perceptions of causes of mental illness. Evil spirits, sin, demonic possession, contagious environments, or brain disturbances have figured in explanations of mental disorders and accordingly shaped people's responses and medical treatment. The various ways of caring for mentally ill people typically depended on such views and on a community's perceived notions and fears of those with mental disorders as well as on community resources.

History reflects that, generally, social fears and tolerance for what is deemed deviant behaviour are related to social stability and availability of resources. In periods of relative social stability, individuals with mental disorders often have a better chance to live safely within their communities. During periods of rapid social change and instability, there are more general anxieties and fears and, subsequently, more intolerance and ill-treatment of people with mental disorders. As industrialization and urbanization increased during the 18th and 19th centuries, the rising middle class became concerned about a growing number of poor and deviant people who were not able to work and sustain themselves. At the same time, under the influence of ideas associated with the Enlightenment, medical and social ideas about mental illness changed, and medical concern with the treatment of mental illness increased. The insight gained ground that, rather than being afflicted by loss of reason, mentally ill people were rational beings with a human nature common to all human beings. The idea that spirits or demons kept the insane in a bestial stage—which legitimized the use of restraints or enchainment—was rejected in favour of the view that mentally afflicted people should be treated humanely. The idea of a moral, pedagogical treatment thus emerged that would help the suffering restore their innate capacity for self-control (Boschma, 2003; D'Antonio, 2006).

KEY CONCEPTS **Social change**, the structural and cultural evolution of society, is constant but often erratic. Psychiatric and mental health care has evolved within a **historical context** of social, economic, and political influences and cannot be separated from such realities.

A REVOLUTIONARY IDEA: HUMANE TREATMENT

By the height of the French Revolution in 1792, **moral treatment** became an influential idea that altered the care of the mentally ill and gave rise to important initiatives in which reform-minded physicians had an influential role. During this time, Philippe Pinel (1745–1826) was appointed physician to Bicetre, a hospital for men, which had a very poor reputation. Pinel, influenced by

Enlightenment ideas, believed that the insane were sick patients who needed humane treatment, and he ordered the removal of the chains, stopped the abuses of drugging and bloodletting, and introduced more appropriate medical care. Three years later, the same standards were extended to Salpetrière, the asylum for female patients. At about the same time in England, William Tuke (1732–1822), a Quaker tea merchant in York and a member of the Society of Friends, raised funds for a retreat for mentally ill members of his Quaker community. The York Retreat, which opened in 1796, became another influential example for reform initiatives (Fig. 1-2). Tuke also introduced a regimen of humane, moral treatment, a

PERSPECTIVE VIEW of the NORTH FRONT of the RETREAT near YORK.

FIGURE 1-2. The perspective view of the north front of the retreat near York. (From U.S. National Library of Medicine. Images from the history of medicine. National Institutes of Health, Department of Health and Human Services.)

pedagogical approach of kind supervision, proper medical treatment, and meaningful activities and distractions. Those reformers believed that a purposefully designed asylum provided a proper environment to indeed cure the mentally ill (D'Antonio, 2006; Tomes, 1994).

Based on these influential examples, initiatives emerged throughout the Western world to establish purposefully designed asylums that provided sympathetic care in quiet, pleasant surroundings with some form of industrial occupation such as weaving or farming. In the United States, the Quaker Friends Asylum was proposed in 1811 and opened 6 years later in Frankford, Pennsylvania (now Philadelphia), to become the second asylum in the United States. The humane and supportive rehabilitative attitude of the Quakers was seen as an extremely important influence in changing techniques of caring for those with mental disorders (D'Antonio, 2006).

■ THE 19TH AND EARLY 20TH CENTURIES: AN ERA OF ASYLUM BUILDING

In Canada, New Brunswick was the first of the old British North American provinces to open a mental institution. In 1835, a committee was appointed to prepare a petition to the provincial legislature proposing the establishment of a provincial lunatic asylum. Until that time, counties had carried the responsibility under the Poor Laws system to confine indigent insane who could no longer be managed within the family, in local jails, or in poorhouses. As the population increased in the early 1800s, so did the number of mentally ill people in need of publicly provided care. In that same year, the provincial government approved the conversion of a building in Saint John, formerly a hospital for cholera patients, to a Provincial

---

IN A LIFE

Boarding Mentally Ill People with Families
(12th to 19th Centuries)
The Geel Lunatic Colony, Belgium
The Legend of Saint Dymphna
According to legend, Dymphna, an Irish princess, came to Geel in the 6th century. Her father, the king of Ireland, disappointed that she was not a son, had left her and her mother in the care of a priest who converted them to Christianity. After Dymphna's mother died, the king became filled with grief and wanted another woman just like his former wife. His advisors decided that only his own daughter could match the queen. However, when her pagan father wanted to marry Dymphna, she fled out of fear with her priest and came to Geel. When the Irish king eventually found Dymphna and the priest, he beheaded both. In some sources, the legend tells that several lunatics witnessing this frightful scene suddenly became cured. Symbolic for her resistance to the spirit of evil, Dymphna became patron of lunatics, and the site of her death a place of miraculous healing. Some sources tell how the Saint Dymphna Guesthouse and chapel were built at this place, becoming a place of pilgrimage.

A Powerful Example of Family Care in Geel, Belgium
Since the Middle Ages (1286), the Saint Dymphna Guesthouse and chapel have existed in Geel, Belgium, eventually with a separate sick room for lunatic pilgrims. Chronically mentally ill patients who came to the Guesthouse as pilgrims seeking healing were often boarded out to families, and the Geel Lunatic Colony came into being. In the 19th century, the place became a formal institution with a strong emphasis on boarding outpatients with foster families, which became a model for many countries to follow. The legend of Saint Dymphna illustrates mythical and religious beliefs, explanations, and practices that have lost their meaning today. However, the cultural heritage of the Geel Colony demonstrates how powerful past ideas and beliefs can be in structuring creative and humane solutions to the care of mentally ill people.

Compiled from Parry-Jones, W. L. L. (1981). The model of the Geel Lunatic Colony and its influence on the nineteenth-century asylum system in Britain. In A. Scull (Ed.), *Madhouses, mad-doctors, and madmen. The social history of psychiatry in the Victorian Era* (pp. 201–217). London, UK: The Athlone Press; Boschma, G. (2003). *The rise of mental health nursing: A history of psychiatric care in Dutch asylum, 1890–1920.* Amsterdam, NL: Amsterdam University Press; and Goldstein, J. L., & Godemont, M. M. L. (2003). The legend and lessons of Geel: A 1500-year-old legend, a 21st-century model. *Community Mental Health Journal, 39*(5), 441–458.

During the latter half of the 19th century and beginning of the 20th century, each Canadian province established an asylum (Table 1-1). Involuntary confinement and institutional care became the dominant treatment modality for mentally ill people, replacing older forms of familial care and Poor Law–based approaches (Moran, 2000; Moran & Wright, 2006). In-depth historical analyses of admission patterns, one of the Ontario-based Homewood Retreat, for example, showed that gender differences were reflective of the social situation of the time (Warsh, 1989). Another analysis of the British Columbia psychiatric system revealed that many Aboriginal patients died soon after being admitted to the asylum, often from tuberculosis (Menzies & Palys, 2006).

The Legal Basis for Mental Health Care

Following the terms established by the British North America Act of 1867, the organization of mental health care in Canada became provincially based and each province developed its own legislation to deal with problems created by mental illness. In the late 19th century, all provinces passed legislation, most often called an Insanity Act, to provide a legal basis to publicly supported confinement of the mentally ill. In the course of the 20th century, the legislation had been changed and updated several times and eventually renamed a provincial Mental Health Act, reflecting changing views and a stronger medical influence on the care and treatment of people

FIGURE 1-3. Canada's first hospital for the mentally ill, Saint John, New Brunswick, ca. 1885. (From Provincial Archives of New Brunswick, Saint John Stereographs—P86-67.)

Lunatic Asylum until a new facility could be built. By 1848, this new facility was ready for use (Fig. 1-3) (Hurd, 1973/1916–17; Sussman, 1998).

Table 1-1		The First Asylums in British North America and Canada

Province	Date	Notes
Quebec	1845	• Beauport, or the Quebec Lunatic Asylum, was opened.
		• A small dwelling for 12 mentally ill women was erected by Bishop St. Vallier.
	1714	• The Hotel Dieu cared for indigents, the crippled, and "idiots."
New Brunswick	1848	• The Provincial Lunatic Asylum was erected.
	1835	• Canada's first mental hospital opened in a small wooden building, a former cholera hospital, and was used as a temporary asylum.
Ontario	1850	• The Provincial Lunatic Asylum in Toronto admitted patients.
	1841	• Mentally ill people were placed in county jails until 1841, after which the Old York Jail served as a temporary asylum.
Newfoundland	1854	• An asylum for mentally ill patients was erected and admitted its first patients.
Nova Scotia	1857	• The first patients were admitted to the Provincial Hospital for the Insane.
British Columbia	1872	• A remodelled provincial general hospital (the old Royal Hospital) was opened as the Asylum for the Insane in British Columbia.
Prince Edward Island	1877	• The Prince Edward Island Hospital for the Insane was built.
Manitoba	1886	• The Selkirk Lunatic Asylum was opened.
Saskatchewan	1914	• The Saskatchewan Provincial Hospital admitted the first patients.
Alberta	1911	• The Provincial Asylum for the Insane opened in Ponoka.
Yukon and Northwest Territories		• These districts had no asylums in the early 20th century. The Royal North West Mounted Police assisted in transporting mentally ill patients to asylums in neighbouring provinces.

Adapted from Sussman, S. (1998). The first asylums in Canada: A response to neglectful community care and current trends. *Canadian Journal of Psychiatry, 43*, 260–264; Hurd, H. M. (Ed.). (1973, originally printed 1916–1917). *The institutional care of the insane in the United States and Canada (Vol. IV)*. New York, NY: Arno Press.

with mental illness. In the beginning of institutional psychiatric care in Canada, all patients admitted to public institutions were certified patients. Today, patients are being admitted to an institutional facility on either a voluntary or a certified basis. A carefully designed legal process has to be followed for patients admitted as certified patients under the terms of a mental health act, although criteria may differ between provinces. In several provinces, the use of community treatment orders is a new development under the mental health act (see Chapter 3 for the current legal context of mental health care).

A Social Reformer: Dorothea Lynde Dix

An ardent advocate for this new form of state-supported, public care was Dorothea Lynde Dix (1802–1887). Her crusade for more humane treatment generated much of the reform of mental health care systems in North America in the 19th century (Fig. 1-4). Almost 40 years of age, Dix, a retired school teacher living in Massachusetts, was solicited by a young theology student to help in preparing a Sunday school class for women inmates at the East Cambridge jail. Dix herself led the class and was shocked by living conditions in the jail. She was particularly struck by the treatment of inmates with mental disorders. It was the dead of winter, and the jail was providing no heat. When she questioned the jailer about this, his answer was that "the insane need no heat." The prevailing myth was that the insane were insensible to extremes of temperature. Dix's outrage initiated a long struggle in care reform (Lightner, 1999).

Influenced by a wider social reform movement that had a strong cultural influence throughout the Western world, drawing men and women into a wide range of reform activities, Dix followed the pattern of new women's activism that were also employed by social reformers such as Elizabeth Fry in prison reform and Josephine Butler in protecting women against prostitution (Van Drenth & De Haan, 1999). Dix diligently investigated

FIGURE 1-4. Dorothea Lynde Dix. (From U.S. National Library of Medicine. Images from the history of medicine. National Institutes of Health, Department of Health and Human Services.)

the conditions of jails and the plight of mentally ill people, while promoting the building of mental hospitals. In Canada, she was instrumental in advocating for mental institutions in Halifax and St. John's (Hurd, 1973/1916–17; Lightner, 1999). Dix eventually expanded her work into Great Britain and other parts of Europe.

Life Within Early Institutions

Despite the good intentions of early reformers, the approach inside the institution was one of custodial care and practical management, and treatment rarely occurred. The major concern was the management of a large number of people, many of whom exhibited disruptive behaviours. Patient numbers grew rapidly after provinces became legally responsible for financing care of the mentally ill. Institutions soon experienced severe overcrowding and had little more to offer than food, clothing, pleasant surroundings, and perhaps some means of employment and exercise. Limited resources made life in these institutions difficult. Although they were typically under the direction of a medical superintendent, overcrowding and resource shortages created rowdy, dangerous, and often unbearable situations. Quiet patients were involved in work as institutions grew into self-contained communities that produced their own food and made their own clothing. Day-to-day care was in the hands of lay personnel who shared with patients the routines of eating, sleeping, and working. Once admitted, many patients remained cut off from society.

Ontario psychiatrist Charles K. Clarke (1857–1924) had an influential role in bringing about new models of care to change this situation. As superintendent of various Ontario psychiatric hospitals (e.g., Rockwood Hospital, 1881–1905), he was aware of the enormous problems that asylums experienced (Brown, 2000). The asylums under his direction saw continuous improvements, including the introduction of nurse training for asylum personnel. To find better treatments and approaches, he sought to start an urban centre for the treatment of acute mental illness under the best possible conditions and supported by university-based scientific research. His dream was eventually realized with the establishment in 1925 of the Toronto Psychiatric Hospital. Clarke's name was commemorated when the hospital became the Clarke Institute of Psychiatry in 1966 (Greenland, 1996). Following a merger with other Ontario institutions, the Clarke Institute would become part of the Centre for Addiction & Mental Health.

The deplorable state of large mental institutions soon gave rise to public commotion. In 1908, the American Clifford Beers (1876–1943) published an autobiography, *A Mind That Found Itself*, depicting his 3-year experience in three different types of hospitals: a private for-profit hospital, a private nonprofit hospital, and a state institution. He reported that in each facility, he had been beaten; choked; imprisoned for long periods in dark, dank, padded cells; and for many days had been confined in a straitjacket. He became an ardent advocate of the reform of psychiatric care. Beers' cause was supported by a prominent neuropathologist, Adolf Meyer (1866–1950), who suggested the term "mental hygiene" for bringing about improvement of people's mental health in a manner similar to other public health initiatives. By 1909, Beers had helped form a National Committee for Mental Hygiene, through whose efforts there developed child guidance clinics, prison clinics, and industrial mental health approaches. Beers and Meyer found a close Canadian ally in Clarence Hincks, a leading Toronto psychiatrist who was instrumental in founding the Canadian National Committee for Mental Hygiene (CNCMH) in 1918, together with his colleague Charles Clarke.

The appalling situation of Canadian provincial mental hospitals triggered particular political concern following World War I, when returning veterans suffering from shell shock had to rely on existing psychiatric facilities in their home provinces. A new belief gained ground in scientific approaches and reliance on expert knowledge in the prevention of mental illness. These views were intertwined with class-based concern about an alleged weak-mindedness among lower social classes and the need for betterment of the human race, influenced by eugenic ideas of the time. This context of change provided a climate for expanding professionalism of many groups, including psychiatrists, psychologists, and nurses. The CNCMH clearly promoted improvement of mental hospitals. Introducing a trained nursing staff was part of this strategy. Voluntary admission controlled by physicians was supported, thus advancing the view that mental illness was similar to any physical illness.

Development of Psychiatric and Mental Health Nursing

Early Developments

In its many surveys of institutional facilities, the CNCMH promoted the introduction of training schools for mental nurses, later called psychiatric nurses, similar to nurse training schools in general hospitals (Boschma, Yonge, & Mychajlunow, 2005; Tipliski, 2004). During his tenure as superintendent of Rockwood Mental Hospital (1881–1905), Charles Clarke was instrumental in establishing one of the first nurse training schools for female personnel at this hospital and then at the Provincial Hospital in Toronto (Brown, 2000). Well-educated women with a sense of order and compassion had been essential in the introduction of training schools in general hospitals. In their efforts to model **psychiatric hospitals** after the general hospitals, psychiatrists took that ideal and geared the training of mental nurses toward women. The trained nurses provided them with the assistance they needed for new therapies and enhanced the hospital's reputation

BOX 1-1 Highlights From Psychiatric Mental Health Nursing History

1888	The first mental nurse training school established at Kingston's Rockwood Asylum
1918	Foundation of the Canadian National Committee of Mental Hygiene
1920	First psychiatric nursing text published, *Nursing Mental Diseases*, by Harriet Bailey
1922	First Registration of Nurses Act passed in Ontario including nurse training schools at the mental hospitals
1930s	Mental hospitals in western Canada established schools for mental nurses and attendants
1950	Psychiatric Nurses Association of Canada (PNAC) founded
1952	Publication of Hildegard E. Peplau's *Interpersonal Relations in Nursing*
1963	*Perspectives in Psychiatric Care* and *Journal of Psychiatric Nursing* first issued
1979	PNAC working paper on Standards of Practice for Psychiatric Nurses published
1986	The Canadian Nurses Association establishes a national certification program for specialty nursing practice
1988	Canadian Federation of Mental Health Nurses (CFMHN) founded
1995	CFMHN *Standards of Psychiatric and Mental Health Nursing Practice* published
2006	*Canadian Standards for Psychiatric-Mental Health Nursing*, 3rd edition published

(Boschma, 2003; Brown, 2000; Connor, 1996), as it was thought that women had the right moral, feminine characteristics for good patient care. Whereas in general hospitals, the care of male patients was put in the hands of female nurses assisted by male orderlies, in psychiatry this shift was less easily made, owing to the nature of difficult patient behaviour. Male attendants retained a prominent place in the care of the mentally ill, but their training obtained a lower status, or, in the Ontario mental hospitals, they initially did not receive any training at all (Tipliski, 2002). See Box 1-1 for historical highlights.

Regional Influences

In western Canada, which had a stronger orientation to British traditions of institutional care, the introduction of mental nurse training schools did not occur until the 1930s, by which time men were also being trained. In Alberta, for example, in 1932, the Department of Health hired psychiatrist Charles A. Barager, initially as acting superintendent and soon as commissioner of mental health service, to implement reform. Barager came from Manitoba, where he had introduced a nurse training school as superintendent at the Brandon Asylum (Dooley, 2004). He had a strong belief in the ability of female compassion: "The nursing of mental patients requires women of finer personality, of wider sympathies, greater self-control and higher intelligence than even the nursing of those who are physically ill" (Tipliski, 2002, p. 95).

Barager's term in Alberta was short-lived (he died in 1936), but the training for nurses and attendants that he initiated in the Alberta Hospital at Ponoka had a lasting influence. Despite opposition to his ideas from the Registered Nurses Association in Alberta, which had controlled the registration of nurses since 1916, he was able to secure approval for a new diploma in mental nursing through the Alberta Department of Health. He also established arrangements with general hospitals so that, after 2 years of training in the mental hospital, female nurse students could undertake an additional 18 months of training at a general hospital and take licensing exams for registered nurses, after which they would return to the mental hospital. For male attendants, a 3-year certificate course was implemented, leading to a diploma in mental nursing. Male graduates did not obtain registered nursing status, reflective of the gendered context in which mental nurse training emerged. Skilled nursing was essential for new therapies, such as electroshock and insulin coma therapy introduced in the 1940s. Alberta Hospital at Ponoka also had a large infirmary with many frail and sick elderly patients (Boschma et al., 2005).

This climate of change created many new opportunities for working- and middle-class men and women to pursue careers as psychiatric nurses, and nurses began to articulate nursing knowledge in nursing textbooks. The first psychiatric and mental health (PMH) nursing textbook that appeared in North America was *Nursing Mental Diseases*, written by Bailey (1920). The content of the book reflected an understanding of mental disorders of the times and set forth nursing care in terms of appropriate procedures.

MODERN THINKING

As PMH nursing began to develop as a profession in the early 20th century, it incorporated new perspectives on mental illness that were emerging, particularly ideas on prevention as well as biologic views on mental illness. These new theories would profoundly shape the future of mental health care for all practitioners. Chapter 8 examines the underlying ideologies, but it is important to understand their development within the social and historical context to appreciate fully their impact on treatment approaches.

Evolution of Scientific Thought

In the early 1900s, there were two opposing views of mental illness: the belief that mental disorders had biologic origins and the belief that the problems were attributed to environmental and social stresses. **Psychosocially oriented ideas** proposed that mental disorders resulted from environmental and social deprivation. Moral treatment grew out of this idea, and the notion of prevention advocated by the mental hygiene movement also reflected a psychosocial orientation. The **biologic view** held that mental illnesses had a biologic cause and could be treated with physical interventions. However, biologic approaches and physical treatments such as bed rest, wet packs—which entailed wrapping patients in wet sheets—and prolonged baths became popular as new treatments around 1900 as part of the rise of scientific psychiatry. They were grounded in the idea that overstrained nerves should obtain rest. Such treatments turned out to be largely ineffective.

Meyer and Psychiatric Pluralism

Adolf Meyer bridged the ideologic gap between the two approaches by introducing the concept of **psychiatric pluralism**, an integration of human biologic functions with the environment. He focused on investigating how organic functions related to the person and how the person, constituted of these organs, related to the environment (Neill, 1980). Unfortunately, this included the surgical treatment of psychosis by one of his disciples, Henry Cotton, who believed infection caused insanity and attempted to cure patients by removing sites of sepsis such as the teeth, tonsils, and colon (Scull, 2005). Meyer's ideas had little chance to evolve and flourish as the emerging psychoanalytic theories would soon dominate the psychiatric world in North America for a long time to come. It was not until after World War II, when a new emphasis on community-based care evolved, that environmental views and psychosocial approaches gained renewed prominence with the application of psychosocial rehabilitation models for people living with severe and persistent mental illness (Shephard, Boardman, & Slade, 2008).

Freud and Psychoanalytic Theory

Sigmund Freud (1856–1939) and the **psychoanalytic movement** of the early 1900s promised a radically new approach to PMH care. Trained as a neuropathologist, Freud developed a personality theory based on unconscious motivations for behaviour, or drives. Using a new technique, psychoanalysis, he delved into the patient's feelings and emotions regarding past experiences, particularly early childhood and adolescent memories, to explain the basis of aberrant behaviour. He showed that symptoms of hysteria could be produced and made to disappear while patients were in a subconscious state of hypnosis.

According to the Freudian model, normal development occurred in stages, with the first three—oral, anal, and genital—being the most important. The infant progressed through the oral stage, experiencing the world through symbolic oral ingestion; into the anal stage, in which the toddler developed a sense of autonomy through withholding; and on to the genital stage, in which a beginning sense of sexuality emerged within the framework of the oedipal relationship. Freud posited that any interference in this normal development, such as psychological trauma, would give rise to neurosis or psychosis.

Primary causes of mental illnesses were now viewed as psychological, and any physical manifestations or social influences were considered secondary (Malamud, 1944). Psychoanalysts believed that mental illnesses originated from disturbed personality development and faulty parenting. They categorized mental illnesses either as a psychosis (severe) or as a neurosis (less severe). A psychosis impaired daily functioning because of breaks in contact with reality. A neurosis was less severe, but individuals were often distressed about their problems. The terms psychosis and neurosis entered common, everyday language and added credibility to Freud's conceptualization of mental disorders. Freud's ideas would soon represent the forefront of psychiatric thought, and they shaped society's view of mental health care. Freudian ideology dominated psychiatry well into the 1970s. Intensive psychoanalysis, aimed at repairing the trauma of the original psychological injury, was the treatment of choice. Psychoanalysis was costly and time consuming and required lengthy training; few could perform it, and as a result, thousands of patients in state institutions with severe mental illnesses were essentially ignored.

Integration of Biologic Theories into Psychosocial Treatment

Until the 1940s, the biologic understanding of mental illness was unsophisticated and did not result in effective treatment. Early somatic treatments based on these views often were unsuccessful because of the lack of understanding and knowledge of the biologic basis of mental disorders. As discussed, the use of hydrotherapy, or baths, was an established procedure in mental institutions. The use of warm baths and, in some instances, ice cold baths were thought to produce calming effects for patients with mental disorders. However, the treatment's success was ascribed to its effectiveness as a form of restraint because the physiologic responses that hydrotherapy produced were not understood. Baths often ended up as a form of restraint rather than as a therapeutic practice. During the 1930s and 1940s, other biologic treatments emerged, which sparked new hope that they would result in effective treatment, such as insulin coma therapy and electroconvulsive therapy (ECT) (Shorter & Healy, 2007; Kneeland & Warren, 2002). Yet, often these biologic procedures were applied either indiscriminately or inappropriately with substantial side-effects including psychosurgery and ECT (see Chapter 13). ECT, the application of a short (1 to 2 seconds) electrical current to the brain in order to generate a convulsion for an allegedly healing effect, was first used around 1940. Unlike the original procedure, contemporary ECT is modified by being applied under anesthesia. Psychosurgical treatment, direct surgical intervention in lobes of the brain, also called lobotomy,

began to be applied as of the late 1940s. Results from such brain therapies were mixed, and by the 1970s, the use of lobotomy became increasingly controversial; the use of ECT as treatment across a broad range of disorders was also questioned, but it remained widely used for the treatment of depression (Kneeland & Warren, 2002; Pressman, 2002; Tomes, 1994). Recent insights resulting from brain research and new technologic advancements such as electromagnetic brain-stimulating techniques have generated a renewed interest in biologic treatments, offering new possibilities for treatment of depression and other neurophysiologic disorders (George, 2003). Thanks to modern technology and improved methods, neurosurgical techniques, such as deep brain stimulation, as well as ECT and transcranial magnetic stimulation can now be applied more humanely with positive therapeutic outcomes for some psychiatric disorders (George, 2003; Rai, Kivisalu, Rabheru, & Kang, 2010; Sadowsky, 2006).

Support for the biologic approaches received an important boost in the early 1950s as successful symptom management with psychopharmacologic agents became a more widespread possibility. Psychopharmacology revolutionized the treatment of mental illness and led to an increased number of patients discharged into the community, and the eventual focus on the brain became a key to understanding psychiatric disorders. Chlorpromazine was an early neuroleptic drug that became widely used. Profound behavioural changes observed as a result of this medication in long-term mentally ill patients created an enormous enthusiasm about the potential of new medications. Understanding of the working of these drugs was in infancy, however, and their side effects soon became serious drawbacks. As knowledge increased and the management of side effects improved, psychopharmacotherapeutics obtained a central place in the treatment of mental illness. The introduction of lithium in the early 1970s brought a lasting change in the treatment of bipolar disorder, as did antidepressants in the treatment of mood disorders (LaJeunesse, 2000). Nurses obtained an essential role in administering medications, monitoring their effects, and teaching patients about their effects.

New Trends in Post–World War II Mental Health Care

Following the experiences of World War II, insight grew among governments, as well as health professionals, that psychiatric services had to be placed on a new footing. By the end of the 1940s, patients in overcrowded and isolated psychiatric hospitals outnumbered the number of patients in other health care facilities, including general hospitals. Increased federal funding for health services and training of health care personnel created new opportunities. The implementation of universal health insurance for hospital care and medical services during the 1950s and 1960s, based on a 50/50 cost sharing between federal and provincial governments, generated funding for the establishment of psychiatric departments in general hospitals, shifting the focus of services away from large provincial institutions (Ostry, 2009).

The Canadian Mental Health Association (CMHA), renamed from the earlier CNCMH, had an instrumental role in policy development for integrated services in general hospitals and the community. In its influential 1963 report, *More for the Mind*, the CMHA argued that mental illness had to be dealt with in ways similar to those of physical illness, and it argued for the application of multiple perspectives—medical, social, and familial—in multidisciplinary services and community treatment. A broader movement of social critique also emerged, protesting the poor circumstances in large mental hospitals and the lack of patient rights. Psychiatry became the target of fierce debate and antipsychiatric critique in the 1970s (Crossley, 2006). Power relationships and the dominance of the medical model were questioned, and an emerging patient movement obtained a new voice and presence in mental health. Improving support and resources for people with mental illness within the community was a key target (Fingard & Rutherford, 2011).

A shift in mental health policy resulted in **deinstitutionalization**, the downsizing of the large provincial psychiatric hospitals, and a new orientation on community-based services to support people with mental illness within their own communities (Boschma, 2011; Dyck, 2011). Services and treatments diversified. Biologic approaches, such as use of psychopharmacology and safer application of ECT, were complemented by new rehabilitative services, the use of group therapy and other psychotherapies, as well as the provision of day treatment. In the 1950s, mental hospitals began to reduce their size and, over the course of the next decades, many closed, or changed their focus—a process that in Canada would last until the end of the 20th century. In British Columbia, for example, the provincial mental hospital Riverview closed its doors permanently in 2012 (Hall, 2012). During the second half of the 20th century, funding for mental health care became part of the larger health care system, with a stronger emphasis on general hospital–based psychiatric care and community-based care. Nurses had an essential role in this transformation in the emerging field of **community mental health nursing** (Boschma, 2012).

In the late 1970s, the federal government shifted to a new funding structure for health care, reducing its share in the cost. Provinces developed different models and strategies to fund specialized services such as alcohol- and substance-abuse treatment programs, which following World War II were pressing mental health care needs. To address the needs of different population groups, subspecialties also emerged, such as child psychiatry, forensic, and geriatric services. The perception of health care as a human right enhanced consumer and volunteer involvement, as well as public education on mental illness, and it increased the demand for patient autonomy.

Continued Evolution of Psychiatric and Mental Health Nursing

The new multidisciplinary approaches and services generated a pressing need for more and better trained mental health care personnel, including nurses. The changes created a context for new developments in **PMH nursing education**. Organized responses of provincial professional nurses' organizations, as well as efforts of hospital administrators and psychiatrists to continue staffing psychiatric hospitals through hospital-based nurse training programs, resulted in a diverse pattern of PMH nurse education. As of the 1950s, Canada entertained two models of education for PMH nursing, resulting in the preparation of two different professional nursing groups for nursing care in mental health services. Regional influences played a large role in the generation of the two models. On the one hand, general hospital–based schools of nursing, especially in eastern Canada, began to integrate psychiatric nursing into their curriculum. In Ontario, for example, under the influence of the mental hygiene movement, as of the 1930s, general hospital training schools began to include care of mentally ill patients into their training. Student nurses attended the provincial psychiatric hospitals for a brief period of training, called an affiliation program. Conversely, mental nurse trainees, mostly women, from the psychiatric hospital–based nurse training programs opted for an affiliation to the general hospital, resulting in both groups' obtaining the title of registered nurse. After World War II, the provincial government and the provincial association of registered nurses in Ontario formalized this pattern into a permanent structure. Gradually, the psychiatric hospital–based programs decreased in number and size, and the registered nurse became the main nursing care provider in mental health services (Tipliski, 2004).

In the less densely populated western Canadian provinces, the pattern emerged of general hospital nurse trainees choosing affiliation experiences at the psychiatric hospitals, but the bulk of nursing care in the provincial hospitals continued to be provided by nurses and attendants graduated from psychiatric hospital–based nurse training programs. As noted previously of Alberta Hospital in Ponoka, some western provinces established an affiliation program for female mental nurse trainees, and its graduates obtained the title of registered nurse. The program was limited in size, however, and many women worked in the institution as untrained attendants until the 1960s. Male trainees received a diploma in mental nursing. In British Columbia, a training school for mental nurses, later called psychiatric nurses, was established in 1930 at Essondale, which eventually became Riverview Hospital (Fig. 1-5).

FIGURE 1-5. Graduation ceremony, School of Psychiatric Nursing, Essondale (Riverview Hospital), ca. 1950s. (From Historical collection, Riverview Hospital Historical Society, Coquitlam, BC.)

In the western provinces, the government had less control over nurse training than in neighbouring Ontario. Provincial associations of registered nurses in western provinces failed to support affiliation for psychiatric hospital–based nurse trainees, while medical superintendents of psychiatric hospitals retained much of their influence over psychiatric nurse education (Boschma et al., 2005; Tipliski, 2004).

Around 1950, attendants in the province of Saskatchewan took the lead in obtaining political support for a different pattern of nurse education that would lead to a separate Psychiatric Nurses Act and subsequent training acts independent of provincial registered nurse practice acts. In Saskatchewan, registered nurses had never successfully integrated into the mental hospitals. Although the psychiatric training program that had existed for Saskatchewan asylum attendants since the 1930s was expanded after World War II to address the new need for psychiatric expertise, it never resulted in registration as a nurse. Dissatisfied with their exclusion from any professionally recognized nursing title, provincial hospital attendants, who in Saskatchewan had obtained the right to unionize after the election of the new Co-operative Commonwealth Federation government in 1944, became instrumental in generating union support, as well as backing from the new government, for legislation of a separate psychiatric nurses act, which passed Parliament in 1948. In 1950, the Psychiatric Nurses Association of Canada was formed. Their action resulted in a distinct professional group of psychiatric nurses (Dickinson, 1989; Tipliski, 2002, 2004). During the 1950s, all four western Canadian provinces passed acts that entitled graduates of western Canadian psychiatric hospital–based nurse training programs to receive the title of psychiatric nurse. The two separate models of psychiatric nursing education still exist today and have over past decades been integrated into the regular education system, resulting in baccalaureate education programs in generic and psychiatric nursing education.

THE LATE 20TH AND EARLY 21ST CENTURY

In the post–World War II era, nurses continued their work in facilitating the therapeutic climate within psychiatric hospitals (Fig. 1-6). The shift to community mental health and deinstitutionalization generated many new functions for PMH nurses (Boschma et al., 2005; Church, 1987). Nurses obtained a central role in supporting large numbers of discharged patients in their transition to living in the community. In the psychiatric hospitals and general hospital units, nurses obtained new therapeutic roles in group therapies, and their work in community mental health services expanded (Boschma, 2012). New theoretical models became available that emphasized building therapeutic nurse-patient relationships and holistic nursing approaches. Hildegard Peplau, who in recent scholarship has been considered the most important psychiatric nurse of the 20th century, proved to be a strong leader in the development of these new frameworks for psychiatric nursing (Boschma et al., 2005; Calaway, 2002).

Expansion of Holistic Nursing Care

In 1952, Peplau published the landmark work *Interpersonal Relations in Nursing*. It introduced PMH nursing practice to the concepts of interpersonal relations and the importance of the therapeutic relationship. In fact, the nurse-patient relationship was defined as the very essence of PMH nursing and supported a holistic perspective on patient care (see Chapters 5, 6, and 7). These new frameworks underscored a new professional and disciplinary independence for nurses.

By 1963, two U.S.-based nursing journals, the *Journal of Psychiatric Nursing* (now the *Journal of Psychosocial Nursing and Mental Health Services*) and *Perspectives in Psychiatric Care*, as well as the *Canadian Journal of*

FIGURE 1-6. Sports Day on Riverview Hospital grounds, nurses and patients, 1966. (From Historical collection, Riverview Hospital Historical Society, Coquitlam, BC.)

Psychiatric Nursing (1975–1990), focused on psychiatric nursing. Also, the *Canadian Journal for Nursing Research* began to publish PMH nursing research. During the 1980s, the Canadian Federation of Mental Health Nurses (CFMHN) formed as an interest group of the Canadian Nurses Association with a view to promoting the interests of mental health nurses and bringing matters of mental health nursing interest and psychiatric patient care to the attention of the public at large. In 1995, this group published the Canadian Standards of Psychiatric and Mental Health Nursing Practice. Based on the influential work of Patricia Benner (1984), the standards were written within a framework of "domains of practice." This promoted a holistic perspective on nursing care, with PMH nurses practicing in a variety of settings with a variety of clientele. The emphasis was on activities ranging from health promotion to health restoration. The standards reflected the belief that PMH nursing should be research-driven, continually incorporating new findings into nursing practice. Relying on these standards, the Canadian Nurses Association created the opportunity to become certified in mental health nursing as part of their larger certification program of specialty nursing areas established during the 1980s. The CFMHN updated its standards in 2006 and again in 2014 to incorporate the most recent perspectives on PMH care. The 2006 revisions to the standards were unique in that input was sought for the first time from mental health care consumers (Beal et al., 2007).

Contemporary Issues

During the 1980s, wrinkles in the social fabric of mental health care emerged. The mixed results of deinstitutionalization became apparent and generated a series of government-commissioned reports in all provinces to improve mental health services. Enormous variation existed among provinces in the extent and timing in which they implemented deinstitutionalization policies. People with mental disorders were discharged into communities that were often ill prepared to offer sufficient support in the way of community support programs, housing, or vocational opportunities. Communities were sometimes hesitant in accepting people with persistent mental illness in their midst, and stigma remained attached to mental health services (Hector, 2001; Sealy & Whitehead, 2004). The 1981 Charter of Rights and Freedoms reflected a public statement intended to counter such responses (Greenland, Griffin, & Hoffman, 2001).

Self-help groups and family and consumer organizations, such as the Schizophrenia Society of Canada and the Mood Disorder Society of Canada, have become active participants in mental health care services during the past decades. Outreach and mobile crisis response teams emerged to address problems people with severe mental illness experienced in the community. A new category of "revolving door" patients signified that long-term, severe mental illness remained a persistent problem, with patients continuously moving in and out of the acute care system. Also, the interconnected issues of severe mental illness, substance dependency, and inadequate community resources and housing have resulted in a growing number of homeless people with mental illness, as well as a large population of mentally ill winding up in the criminal justice systems. Within these groups, the specific mental health needs of women remain poorly addressed. Likewise, there exists a growing awareness that diverse cultural populations have distinctive mental health needs and experience inequity in the social and mental health pressures placed upon them. Aboriginal mental health is a critical issue in Canada because Aboriginal communities experience disproportionate rates of both physical and mental illness due to an unbalanced health care system that has not been adaptive to the specific health needs of Aboriginal peoples (see Chapter 3). Today, mental health services are still fragmented and not sufficiently developed to meet the need. Millions of adults and children are disabled by mental illness every year. When compared with all other diseases, mental illness ranks first in terms of causing disability in North America and Western Europe (Hart Wasekeesikaw, 2006; Morrow, 2002; World Health Organization, 2001).

The New Era of Health Care Reform

Both public and private expenditures for health care services have increased in North America. Financial and social barriers continue to affect the overall funding for mental health. Now, large networks of public and private organizations share responsibility for mental health care, with the state remaining as the major decision maker for resource allocation. The emphasis is on reducing expensive institutional care and increasing the resources devoted to community-based care for the mentally ill, such as those in clinics, homes, schools, and treatment centres. With so many organizations involved in mental health services, the voice of mental health care remains fragmented. It became clear during the 1990s that new federal initiatives in mental health policy were urgently needed. In 1998, the Canadian Alliance on Mental Illness and Mental Health (CAMIMH) was formed as a conjoint initiative of the Canadian Psychiatric Association, the CMHA, the Mood Disorder Association of Canada, the National Network for Mental Health, and the Schizophrenia Society of Canada. Consumers and service providers jointly began to lobby the federal government to come to an action plan and a new national agenda for mental health care (Beauséjour, 2001). Two years later, the CAMIMH joined the Canadian Collaborative Mental Health Initiative, which was formed to focus specifically on the improvement of mental health care in the primary health care setting. Consumers and caregivers were actively involved in this collaborative initiative (see Chapters 7 and 11).

In 2002, the CAMIMH published its first report, a collation of the latest Canadian data on mental illness, with assistance from Health Canada (Health Canada, 2002). Among other aspects of mental health care, the report revealed that 86% of hospitalizations for mental illness in Canada occurred in general hospitals. This profound change from traditional institutional care to general hospital care underscored the need for additional and improved acute and community-based mental health services. A senate-commissioned review of the Canadian health care system led to another influential report urging the need for better service: *Out of the Shadows at Last: Transforming Mental Health, Mental Illness and Addiction Services in Canada* (Kirby & Keon, 2006) highlighted the fragmented mental health care for Canadians and in particular the disparate services provided across the provinces. Woven throughout the report are stories of Canadians suffering from mental illness, illustrating the complex issues of stigmatization and discrimination. The report also drew attention to the far-reaching social, economic, and policy effects on health, health care, housing, employment, social welfare, as well as the justice system for Canadians with mental health concerns (Kirby & Keon, 2006). Also highlighted were disparities in access to care between urban and rural Canada, which are further complicated by unique regional multicultural needs. Regional discrepancy has been blamed on the lack of a nationwide mental health strategy and the inconsistency between provincial jurisdictions that determine mental health policies and the allocation and delivery of services for Canadians. While the report has been embraced by many mental health care consumers and caregivers, some critics noticed a lack of emphasis on "preventative determinants" and a lack of recognition of the depth of disability caused by mental illness (Arboleda-Flórez, 2005). Some women's advocate groups challenged the report's "silence" on the disparities between mental health and addiction services for men and women, while others critiqued the report's alleged neutrality to ongoing erosion of the publically funded health care system (Canadian Women's Health Network, 2006). The data from the CAMIMH and Kirby reports laid bare the need for continued, integrated mental health policy development across Canada, for all Canadians. The need to develop a national mental health strategy became the impetus for the establishment in 2007 of the Mental Health Commission of Canada.

● STUDY NOTE

Current mental health policy's focus on community-based care and integration aims at moving away from older, more stigmatizing approaches of long-term institutionalization and custodial care.

Developing a National Mental Health Strategy

Canada's national health strategy was first adopted in 1984 through the Canada Health Act, which set out the values, principles, and guidelines for health care. While to some degree mental health care principles are ensconced in the overall Act, there continued to be significant gaps and inconsistencies in mental health care across the country, and Canada continued to be the only one of the eight wealthiest nations without a national mental health strategy (Kirby, 2009).

To address these gaps, Health Canada funded the Mental Health Commission of Canada, a 10-year initiative. While the MHCC was established outside the federal health mandate, the federal government continues to contribute funding to support the commission's work, and the commission's structure mirrors inclusive intentions (Goldbloom & Bradley, 2012). For example, its membership consists of all levels of government and a wide range of stakeholders, from health care professionals to individuals living with mental illness and their family members.

The MHCC was originally assigned three primary objectives: to develop a mental health strategy for Canada, begin an anti-stigma campaign, and create a knowledge exchange centre to promote research and build capacity and opportunities in evidence-based mental health strategies. Several additional objectives and initiatives have been added since its inception (Box 1-2). We highlight two of these initiatives. The *At Home/Chez Soi* initiative

---

BOX 1-2 The Mental Health Commission of Canada Initiatives and Projects

The original goals of the commission have expanded to include six key initiatives and projects:

- Opening Minds addresses stigma as a barrier to seeking help. Antistigma initiatives have focused on health care provider education, early intervention for youth aged 12 to 18, mental health awareness in the workforce, and decreasing negative stereotypes in media.
- Mental Health First Aid parallels the training for physical emergencies with the need to train Canadians for mental health emergencies.
- Mental Health Strategy for Canada addresses the need for change to ensure equitable care of Canadians with mental health concerns.
- Knowledge Exchange Centre is intended to ensure access, sharing, and exchanging of mental health knowledge for all.
- At Home addresses the social determinant of housing as a fundamental component of mental health for Canadians.
- Peer Project is the latest initiative to address the importance of peer support for individuals with mental health concerns.

From Mental Health Commission of Canada. (2012). *Changing Directions, Changing Lives: The Mental Health Strategy for Canada.* Retrieved from http://www.mentalhealthcommission.ca/English/Pages/default.aspx

constitutes a large federally funded ($110 million) mental health research project examining housing for mentally ill individuals in five large urban settings. It explores the effectiveness of providing housing to individuals with mental health and addictions without also requiring them to be in treatment or sober, while providing a range of supportive health and social services (Hwang, Stergiopoulos, O'Campo, & Gozdzik, 2012). Another initiative addresses Mental Health First Aid and involves provision of training to the public on how to identify the early signs and symptoms of mental illness and suitable interventions for the unique needs of youth or adults. Educating first-aid trainers for the workplace, including teachers and health care providers, plays an essential role in disseminating awareness of mental health issues and the importance of early intervention to minimize long-term harm.

The work of the MHCC in the past 5 years has been prolific and received with much enthusiasm. Many insights have been gained through the MHCC initiatives, which resulted in the 2012 release of a comprehensive set of guidelines with six key strategic directions to address mental health needs for Canadians (Box 1-3). As some of the research initiatives are coming to an end, however, a note of caution is also warranted. A significant source of concern is that financial support for continuation of the projects will not be maintained once the research is completed. An example of this is the *At Home/Chez Soi* project, which comes to an end in 2013, and at the time of this writing, the financial sustainment of this novel approach is unclear (Goldbloom & Bradley, 2012). This

brings to the fore concern that the lack of continuity of promising initiatives might constrain resources and as a consequence cause further harm for this population.

Such fundamental and persistent challenges stay on the policy agenda, and the priority of continued community-based care for Canadians with mental health concerns, and their families, remains. While we come to the end of an era of mental illness invisibility, we still need more ways to provide permanent and persistent support for the most vulnerable populations. These challenges are not unique to Canada. They have been recognized at a global level by the World Health Organization. Accepted by the World Health Assembly in May 2013, the Comprehensive Mental Health Action Plan 2013–2020 has four major objectives:

• Strengthen effective leadership and governance for mental health
• Provide comprehensive, integrated, and responsive mental health and social care services in community-based settings
• Implement strategies for promotion and prevention in mental health
• Strengthen information systems, evidence, and research for mental health.

This plan promotes and guides a transformative worldwide mental health agenda (WHO, 2013).

The challenge before Canadian nurses at this time is to strive to address these national and global goals. We must work with a view to include mental health around the world while working within existing constraints to provide cost-effective services. To address pressing mental health care needs in the 21st century, nurses must continue to participate in devising and implementing a continuum of mental health services that provides access for all and to develop appropriate partnerships with other health professionals and consumer groups.

BOX 1-3 Changing Directions, Changing Lives: The Mental Health Strategy for Canada (May 2012)

Six key strategic directions to address the mental health needs for Canadians.
• Promote mental health across the life span in homes, schools, and workplaces, and prevent mental illness and suicide wherever possible.
• Foster recovery and well-being for people of all ages living with mental health problems and illnesses, and uphold their rights.
• Provide access to the appropriate combination of services, treatments, and supports, when and where people need them.
• Reduce disparities in risk factors and access to mental health services, and strengthen the response to the needs of diverse communities and Northerners.
• Work with First Nations, Inuit, and Métis to address their mental health needs, acknowledging their distinct circumstances, rights, and cultures.
• Mobilize leadership, improve knowledge, and foster collaboration at all levels.

From Mental Health Commission of Canada. (2012). *Changing Directions, Changing Lives: The Mental Health Strategy for Canada.* Retrieved from http://strategy.mentalhealthcommission.ca/pdf/strategy-text-en.pdf

---

SUMMARY OF KEY POINTS

■ Throughout history, attitudes and treatment toward those with mental disorders have drastically changed as a result of the changing socioeconomic backdrop of our society and the development of new theories and study by key individuals and groups.

■ During the 1800s, as mental illness began to be viewed as an illness, more humane and moral treatments began to develop.

■ Social reformers such as Dorothea Dix, Charles Clarke, Clifford Beers, and Clarence Hincks dedicated their efforts to raising society's awareness and advocating public responsibility for the proper treatment of persons with mental illness. At the turn of the

19th century, mental hospitals started implementing Schools of Nursing to build psychiatric nursing capacity and quality within the hospitals.

■ Theoretic arguments characterized the evolution of scientific thought and psychiatric practice. Gradually, the importance of the biologic aspect of mental disorders was recognized while psychosocial approaches were also developed. After the 1950s, the discipline of nursing began to add to the theoretical basis of mental health practice, adding holistic and interpersonal frameworks of psychiatric nursing.

■ Although the need for PMH nursing was recognized near the end of the 19th century, initially there was resistance to training attendants for the care of the insane. At the initiative of Charles Clarke, medical superintendent of Rockwood Hospital (1881–1905), the first Training School for Mental Nurses was established in 1888.

■ All provinces gradually adapted to education for PMH nurses. By the 1930s, all provinces had established training schools for asylum attendants and nurses. In the era following World War II, provinces started to downsize mental hospitals in a process of deinstitutionalization and a shift to community-based care. Two models of education for psychiatric nurses emerged, leading to two distinct professional groups.

■ Key federal and provincial initiatives generated political support and funding for mental health services, but these remain inadequate to many pressing mental health issues.

■ Initiatives such as the CAMIMH, the Canadian Collaborative Mental Health Initiative, and reports such as *Out of the Shadows at Last: Transforming Mental Health, Mental Illness and Addiction Services in Canada* (Kirby & Keon, 2006) highlight the importance of a national mental health strategy.

CRITICAL THINKING CHALLENGES

1 Compare the ideas of psychiatric care during the 1800s with those of the 1990s and 2000s and identify some major political and economic forces that influenced care.
2 Analyze the social, political, and economic changes that influenced the transition to community mental health.
3 Explain how training and education of nurses became essential in psychiatric care.
4 Present an argument for the need to develop alternatives to large mental hospitals.
5 Trace the history of biologic psychiatry and highlight major ideas and treatments.
6 Identify the strengths and challenges of accessible community-based care.

REFERENCES

Arboleda-Flórez, J. (2005). The epidemiology of mental illness in Canada. *Canadian Public Policy: Analyse de Politique, 31*(s1), 13–16.
Bailey, H. (1920). *Nursing mental diseases.* New York, NY: Macmillan.
Beal, G., Chan, A., Chapman, S., Edgar, J., McInnis-Perry, G., Osborne, M., & Mina, E. S. (2007). Consumer input into standards revisions: Changing practice. *Journal of Psychiatric and Mental Health Nursing, 14*, 13–20.
Beauséjour, P. (2001). Advocacy and misadventures in Canadian Psychiatry. In Q. Rae-Grant (Ed.), *Psychiatry in Canada: 50 years, 1951–2000* (pp. 137–148). Ottawa, ON: Canadian Psychiatric Association.
Beers, C. (1908). *A mind that found itself.* New York, NY: Longmans, Green, & Co.
Benner, P. (1984). *From novice to expert: Excellence and power in clinical nursing practice.* Menlo Park, CA: Addison-Wesley.
Boschma, G. (2003). *The rise of mental health nursing: A history of psychiatric care in Dutch asylum, 1890–1920.* Amsterdam, NL: Amsterdam University Press.
Boschma, G. (2011). Deinstitutionalization reconsidered: Geographic and demographic changes in mental health care in British Columbia and Alberta, 1950–1980. *Histoire Sociale/Social History, 44*(88), 223–256.
Boschma, G. (2012). Community mental health nursing in Alberta, Canada: An oral history. *Nursing History Review, 20*, 103–135.
Boschma, G., Yonge, O., & Mychajlunow, L. (2005). Gender and professional identity in psychiatric nursing practice in Alberta, Canada, 1930–1975. *Nursing Inquiry, 12*(4), 243–255.
Brown, W. H. (2000). Dr. C. K. Clarke and the Training School for Nurses. In E. Hudson (Ed.), *The provincial asylum in Toronto: Reflections on social and architectural history* (pp. 167–180). Toronto, Canada: Toronto Region Architectural Conservancy.
Calaway, B. J. (2002). *Hildegard Peplau: Psychiatric nurse of the century.* New York, NY: Springer.
Canadian Women's Health Network. (2006). *Women, mental health, mental illness and addiction in Canada. Response to Out of the Shadows at Last.* Retrieved from http://www.cwhn.ca/resources/cwhm/mentalHealth.html
Church, O. (1987). From custody to community in psychiatric nursing. *Nursing Research, 36*(1), 48–55.
Connor, P. J. (1996). "Neither courage nor perseverance enough": Attendants at the Asylum for the Insane, Kingston, 1877–1905. *Ontario History, 88*(4), 251–272.
Crossley, M. L. (2006). *Contesting psychiatry: Social movements in mental health.* New York, NY: Routledge.
D'Antonio, P. (2006). *Founding friends: Families, staff, and patients at the Friends Asylum in early nineteenth century Philadelphia.* Bethlehem, PA: Lehigh University Press.
Dickinson, H. D. (1989). *The two psychiatries: The transformation of psychiatric work in Saskatchewan, 1905–1984.* Regina, SK: University of Regina Canadian Plains Research Centre.
Dooley, C. (2004). "They gave their care, but we gave loving care": Defining and defending boundaries of skill and craft in the nursing service of a Manitoba Mental Hospital during the Great Depression. *Canadian Bulletin of Medical History, 21*(2), 229–251.
Dyck, E. (2011). Dismantling the asylum and charting new pathways into the community: Mental health care in twentieth-century Canada. *Histoire Sociale/Social History, 44*(88), 181–196.
Fingard, J., & Rutherford, J. (2011). Deinstitutionalization and vocational rehabilitation for mental health consumers in Nova Scotia since the 1950s. *Histoire Sociale/Social History 44*(88), 385–408.
George, M. S. (2003). Stimulating the brain: The emerging new science of electrical brain stimulation. *Scientific American, 289*(3), 66–73.
Goldbloom, D., & Bradley, L. (2012). The Mental Health Commission of Canada: the first five years. *Mental Health Review Journal, 17*(4), 221–228.
Goldstein, J. L., & Godemont, M. M. L. (2003). The legend and lessons of Geel: A 1500-year-old legend, a 21st-century model. *Community Mental Health Journal, 39*(5), 441–458.
Greenland, C. (1996). Origins of the Toronto Psychiatric Hospital. In E. Shorter (Ed.), *TPH: History and memories of the Toronto Psychiatric Hospital, 1925–1966.* Toronto, Canada: Wall & Emerson.
Greenland, C., Griffin, J., & Hoffman, B. F. (2001). Psychiatry in Canada from 1951–2000. In Q. Rae-Grant (Ed.), *Psychiatry in Canada: 50 years, 1951–2001* (pp. 1–16). Ottawa, ON: Canadian Psychiatric Association.
Hall, N. (2012). Closure of Riverview Hospital marks end of era in mental health treatment. *Vancouver Sun* Retrieved from http://www.vancouver-sun.com/index.html
Hart Wasekeesikaw, F. (2006). Challenges for the new millennium: Nursing in First Nations. In M. McIntyre, E. Thomlinson, & C. McDonald (Eds.), *Realities of Canadian nursing: Professional, practice and power issues* (pp. 415–433). Philadelphia, PA: Lippincott Williams & Wilkins.

Health Canada. (2002). *A report on mental illnesses in Canada*. Ottawa, ON: Author.

Hector, I. (2001). Changing funding patterns and the effect on mental health care in Canada. In Q. Rae-Grant (Ed.), *Psychiatry in Canada: 50 years, 1951–2001* (pp. 59–76). Ottawa, ON: Canadian Psychiatric Association.

Hurd, H. M. (Ed.). (1973, originally printed 1916–17). *The institutional care of the insane in the United States and Canada, (Vol. IV)*. New York, NY: Arno Press.

Hwang, S. W., Stergiopoulos, V., O'Campo, P., & Gozdzik, A. (2012). Ending homelessness among people with mental illness: the *At Home/Chez Soi* randomized trial of a Housing First intervention in Toronto. *BMC Public Health, 12*(1),787–802.

Jones, C. (1989). *The charitable imperative: Hospitals and nursing in ancien régime and revolutionary France*. London, UK: Routledge.

Kirby, M. (2009). *Key note address*. Halifax, NS: Mental Health Commission of Canada National Child and Youth Mental Health Day.

Kirby, M. J. L., & Keon, W. J. (2006). Out of the shadows at last: Transforming mental health, mental illness and addiction services in Canada. Retrieved from Parliament of Canada website: http://www.parl.gc.ca/39/1/parlbus/commbus/senate/com-e/soci-e/rep-e/rep02may06-e.htm

Kneeland, T. W., & Warren, C. A. B. (2002). *Pushbutton psychiatry: A history of electroshock in America*. Westport, CT: Praeger.

LaJeunesse, R. A. (2000). *Political asylums*. Edmonton, AB: Muttart Foundation.

Leiby, J. S. (1992). San Hipólito's treatment of the mentally ill in Mexico City, 1589–1650. *The Historian, 54*(3), 491–498.

Lightner, D. L. (Ed.). (1999). *Asylum, prison, and poorhouse: The writings and reform work of Dorothea Dix in Illinois*. Carbondale and Edwardsville, IL: Southern Illinois University Press.

Malamud, W. (1944). The history of psychiatric therapies. In J. K. Hall, G. Zilboorg, & H. Bunker (Eds.), *One hundred years of American psychiatry* (pp. 273–323). New York, NY: Columbia University Press.

Menzies, R., & Palys, T. (2006). Turbulent spirits: Aboriginal patients in the British Columbia psychiatric system, 1879–1950. In J. E. Moran & D. Wright (Eds.), *Mental health and Canadian society: Historical Perspectives* (pp. 149–175). Montreal and Kingston, Canada: McGill-Queen's University Press.

Moran, J. E. (2000). *Committed to the state asylum: Insanity and society in nineteenth-century Quebec and Ontario*. Montreal and Kingston, Canada: McGill-Queen's University Press.

Moran, J. E., & Wright, D. (Eds.). (2006). *Mental health and Canadian society: Historical perspectives*. Montreal and Kingston, Canada: McGill-Queen's University Press.

Morrow, M. (2002). *Violence and trauma in the lives of women with serious mental illness: Current practices in service provision in British Columbia*. Vancouver, Canada: Centre of Excellence for Women's Health.

Neill, J. (1980). Adolf Meyer and American psychiatry today. *American Journal of Psychiatry, 137*(4), 460–464.

Nelson, S. (1999). Entering the professional domain: The making of the modern nurse in 17th century France. *Nursing History Review, 7,* 171–187.

Nelson, S. (2001). *Say little, do much: Nursing, nuns, and hospitals in the nineteenth century*. Philadelphia, PA: University of Pennsylvania Press.

Ostry, A. (2009). The foundations of national public hospital insurance. *Canadian Bulletin of Medical History, 26*(2), 261–282.

Parry-Jones, W. L. L. (1981). The model of the Geel Lunatic Colony and its influence on the nineteenth-century asylum system in Britain. In A. Scull (Ed.), *Madhouses, mad-doctors, and madmen. The social history of psychiatry in the Victorian Era.* (pp. 201–217) London, UK: The Athlone Press.

Peplau, H. (1952). *Interpersonal relations in nursing*. New York, NY: Putnam.

Porter, R. (1993). *Disease, medicine and society in England 1550–1860*. Houndmills, UK: Macmillan Education.

Pressman, J. D. (2002). *Psychosurgery and the limits of medicine*. Cambridge, MA: Cambridge University Press.

Rai, S., Kivisalu, T., Rabheru, K., & Kang, N. (2010). Electroconvulsive therapy clinical database: A standardized approach in tertiary care psychiatry. *Journal of Electro-Convulsion-Therapy (ECT), 26*(4), 304–309.

Sadowsky, J. (2006). Beyond the metaphor of the pendulum: Electroconvulsive therapy, psychoanalysis, and the styles of American psychiatry. *Journal of the History of Medicine, 61,* 1–25.

Scull, A. (2005). *Madhouse: A tragic tale of megalomania and modern medicine*. New Haven, CT: Yale University Press.

Sealy, P., & Whitehead, P. C. (2004). Forty years of deinstitutionalization of psychiatric services in Canada: An empirical assessment. *Canadian Journal of Psychiatry, 49,* 249–257.

Shepherd, G., Boardman, J., & Slade, M. (2008). *Making recovery a reality*. Available at http://www.centreformentalhealth.org.uk/publications/making_recovery_a_reality.aspx?ID=578

Shorter, E. (1997). *A history of psychiatry: From the era of the asylum to the age of Prozac*. New York, NY: John Wiley & Sons.

Shorter, E., & Healy, D. (Eds.). (2007). *Shock therapy: A history of electroconvulsive treatment in mental illness*. Toronto, Canada: University of Toronto Press.

Sussman, S. (1998). The first asylums in Canada: A response to neglectful community care and current trends. *Canadian Journal of Psychiatry, 43,* 260–264.

Tipliski, V. M. (2004). Parting at the crossroads: The emergence of education for psychiatric nursing in three Canadian provinces, 1909–1955. *Canadian Bulletin of Medical History, 21*(2), 253–279.

Tipliski, V. M. (2002). Parting at the crossroads: The development of education for psychiatric nursing in three Canadian provinces, 1909–1955. Ph.D. thesis, University of Manitoba.

Tomes, N. (1994). *The art of asylum-keeping: Thomas Story Kirkbride and the origins of American psychiatry*. Philadelphia, PA: University of Pennsylvania Press.

Van Drenth, A., & De Haan, F. (1999). *The rise of caring power: Elizabeth Fry and Josephine Butler in Britain and the Netherlands*. Amsterdam, NL: Amsterdam University Press.

Warsh, C. K. (1989). *Moments of unreason: The practice of Canadian psychiatry and the Homewood Retreat, 1883–1923*. Montreal and Kingston, Canada: McGill-Queen's University Press.

World Health Organization. (2001). The world health report: Mental health 2001. In: *Mental health: New understanding, new hope*. Geneva, IL: Author.

World Health Organization. (2013). *Comprehensive mental health action plan 2013–2020*. Retrieved from http://www.who.int/mental_health/action_plan_2013/en/

2 Mental Health, Mental Disorder, Recovery, and Well-Being

Wendy Austin
Adapted from the chapters "Mental Health and Mental Illness"
by Marion Healey Ogden and by Mary Ann Boyd

KEY CONCEPTS

- mental disorder
- mental health
- recovery
- well-being

LEARNING OBJECTIVES

After studying this chapter, you will be able to:

- Recognize the integral relationship between mental and physical health.
- Define mental health and mental illness.
- Explain the concepts of recovery and well-being.
- Discuss the strategic directions of Canada's national mental health strategy.
- Describe the classification of mental disorders used in North America, in accordance with the criteria of the *Diagnostic and Statistical Manual of Mental Disorders* (5th ed.).
- Discuss Canada's strategy on mental health.
- Identify the role of research in psychiatric and mental health nursing.

KEY TERMS

- Canadian Index of Wellbeing (CIW) • Classification and Measurement System of Functional Health (CLAMES) • gender differences • Gross National Happiness (GNH) index • mental health literacy • Social Progress Index (SPI)

This chapter presents and explores concepts foundational to psychiatric and mental health (PMH) nursing practice. While these key concepts may appear to be straightforward and even obvious at first glance, their meaning continues to evolve. For instance, nurses, other health care professionals, and the public have for some time viewed "recovery" as the restoration of health. However, as a cornerstone of Canada's strategy on mental health and the World Health Organization's (WHO) mental health action plan, the concept embraces more. Recovery is envisioned as gaining hope and purpose, understanding one's abilities, disabilities, rights and resources, and living a meaningful, satisfying life even with mental health problems or illnesses (Mental Health Commission of Canada, 2009; WHO, 2013). It is

important that nurses have a deep understanding of these basic terms, as such knowledge will implicitly and explicitly shape their practice.

MENTAL HEALTH

Mental health, as defined by the Mental Health Commission of Canada (MHCC, 2013), is "a state of well-being in which the individual realizes his or her own potential, can cope with the normal stresses of life, can work productively and fruitfully, and is able to make a contribution to his or her own community" (p. 3). Mental health is not the polar opposite of mental illness. In fact, one can experience mental health while one is living with a severe mental disorder. Imagine mental health and mental illness as existing on two separate and simultaneously occurring continua (Epp, 1988). Optimal mental health and minimal mental health represent the extremes on one continuum, while maximal mental disorder and absence of mental disorder represent the extremes on the other continuum (Fig. 2-1). It is possible that a person with a mental disorder can experience optimal mental health, and a person without a mental disorder can experience minimal mental health. This situation is similar to that of a person with diabetes who, using diet, exercise, and medication, is healthy and symptom free, and a person without a diagnosable medical condition who, eating a diet of "fast food," avoiding exercise, and smoking a pack of cigarettes daily, can be unhealthy. Both the level of mental health and the severity of a person's mental disorder can vary over his or her lifetime.

Mental health and physical health are integrated, not distinct. Nevertheless, many health professionals and health care systems behave otherwise. The reality is that mental health has been excluded too often from key global health policies and strategies (e.g., there is no millennium development goal explicit to mental health). This has happened even though, at its beginnings, the WHO's first Director-General, Dr. Brock Chisholm, a Canadian psychiatrist, stipulated that without mental health, there could be no true physical health (Kolappa, Henderson, & Kishore, 2013). "There is no health without mental health," has once again become a WHO slogan (WHO, 2010a). The WHO and the World Association of Family Doctors (2008) are currently working with nations to enable them to integrate mental health into general health care at the primary care level and to educate and support health care workers to implement and sustain this integration. The International Council of Nurses' (2008) position is that all nurses must have knowledge and skills to respond to mental health needs, including their own.

KEY CONCEPT Mental health is a state of well-being in which the individual realizes self-potential, copes with life stresses, and is able to work productively and contribute to his or her society. It is integral to general health and can be possessed even in the presence of mental illness.

WELL-BEING

Mental health is considered a state of well-being, but what does "well-being" mean? The Oxford English Dictionary (OED Online, 2014) defines well-being as "the state of being or doing well in life; happy, healthy, or prosperous condition; moral or physical welfare (of a person or community)." A Canadian phenomenological study reveals that well-being is not purposeful but that it lies on the journey through life events and is experienced when the individual is self-forgetful about how she or he is supposed to live and, instead, engages in living well. It is experienced as coming home to self where the notion of home is critical (Healey-Ogden & Austin, 2011). It is noteworthy that one of the exemplars of well-being in this study was terminally ill.

Psychological well-being is understood in the nation of Bhutan as the way people evaluate their lives. Bhutan is noted for its unusual approach to national assessment as, rather than focusing on overall economic activity [such as that measured by Gross Domestic Product (GDP)], Bhutan looks to its population's happiness and well-being, measured by the **Gross National Happiness (GNH) index**. The GNH has nine domains: psychological well-being, health, education, time use, cultural diversity and resilience, good governance, community vitality, ecological diversity and resilience, and living standards (Ura, Alkere, Zangno, & Wangdi, 2012). (See Web Links on thePoint to connect to the research on the GNH.)

Canadian Index of Wellbeing

There is a **Canadian Index of Wellbeing (CIW)** that is used as a measure of our quality of life. With data primarily from Statistics Canada, the CIW is calculated using 64 indicators across eight interconnected quality-of-life domains: community vitality, democratic engagement, education, environment, healthy populations, leisure and culture, living standards, and time use (CIW, 2012). The 2012 CIW report states that, from 1994 to 2010, Canada's Gross Domestic Product (GDP) grew by 28.9% but quality of life only improved by 5.7%. The gap between the

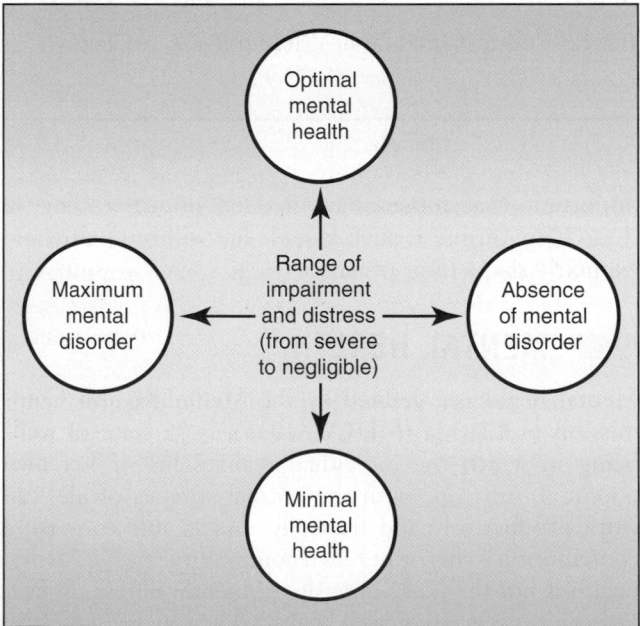

FIGURE 2-1. Diagram of mental health and mental disorder continua. (Adapted from Epp, J. (1988). *Mental health for Canadians: Striking a balance* (p. 9). [Cat. H39-128/1988E]. Ottawa, ON: Supply and Service Canada.)

richest and the poorest in our society continues to grow, a cause for concern as poor health and well-being outcomes, even for the wealthy, are associated with societies with greater inequality.

Using measures like the CIW to examine our national status is important. The GDP provides a measurement of national income, but growth in the GDP is affected by all goods and service activities (including smoking, hiring more police when crime is on the upswing, overharvesting our forests, increasing use of fossil fuels): it is like a giant calculator with an addition but no subtraction button (Johnston, 2012). The CIW allows a broader depth of understanding that, when used with GDP, will allow Canadians to move towards a society with a quality of life that we may all enjoy.

Social Progress Index

In 2014, based on the **Social Progress Index (SPI)**, Canada was ranked the seventh most socially advanced country of 132 nations, leading all the G8 countries (Social Progress Imperative, 2014). The SPI measures national progress in delivering social and environmental value. It was created to complement the GDP index to give a more holistic picture of a country's overall performance. (Canada's 2014 GDP = ninth highest globally.) **Social progress** is defined as "the capacity of a society to meet the basic human needs of its citizens, establish the building blocks that allow citizens to improve their lives, and create the conditions for individuals and communities to meet their full potential" (Porter & Stern with Green, 2014, p.5). The SPI components are basic human needs (i.e., nutrition and basic medical care, water and sanitation, shelter, personal safety), foundations of well-being (i.e., access to basic knowledge, access to information and communication, health and wellness, ecosystem sustainability), and opportunity (i.e., personal rights, personal freedom and choice, tolerance and inclusion, access to advance education) (Porter & Stern with Green, 2014). Canada performs well across the SPI components, but particularly for "tolerance and inclusion" due to tolerance towards religious minorities and immigrants. The challenges for Canada appear to lie in the areas of ecosystem sustainability (rated 51st) and obesity (almost one in four Canadians are classified as obese).

> **KEY CONCEPT Well-being** is "a person's state of being well, content, and able to make the most of his or her abilities" (CNA, 2008, p. 28).

■ MENTAL ILLNESS

Each year, one in five Canadians will be living with a mental health problem or illness; this translates to nearly seven million people (MHCC, 2013). The annual cost of mental health problems and disorders is estimated at $50 billion (MHCC). **Mental disorder** is the medical term for mental illness and refers to a diagnosable health condition based on an accepted classification system with criteria related to alterations in mood and affect, behaviour, and thinking and cognition. These alterations are beyond the parameters of psychological states such as sadness and grief encountered in a life. Cultural definitions of responses must be considered: when a particular culture sees a certain behaviour as normal, its members do not view the behaviour as a symptom of a mental disorder. For example, it is common in some religious groups to "speak in tongues." To an observer, it may appear that the individuals are experiencing hallucinations (see Chapter 10), a psychiatric symptom, but this behaviour is usual for this group within a particular setting.

> **KEY CONCEPT Mental disorders** are health conditions characterized by alteration in a variety of factors that include mood and affect, behaviour, and thinking and cognition. The disorders are associated with various degrees of distress and impaired functioning.

Diagnosing Mental Disorders

Classification systems for medical diagnoses identify the criteria required for a particular condition to be diagnosed and provide a common language for health care professionals to use. The two most accepted psychiatric classifications are the Mental and Behavioural Disorders Section of the WHO's *International Statistical Classification of Diseases and Related Health Problems (ICD)*, currently in its 10th revision (*ICD-10*) (WHO, 2010b), and the American Psychiatric Association's (2013) *Diagnostic and Statistical Manual of Mental Disorders* (*DSM*). The fifth edition of the *DSM*, the *DSM-5*, was released in May 2013. In North America, the *DSM* classification is most commonly used. Efforts have been made by those revising these two classifications to harmonize them as much as possible. For instance, unlike the previous version, the *DSM-IV-TR*, the *DSM-5* does not have a multiaxial system but rather a structure similar to the *ICD-10*, and it includes the equivalent *ICD-10* Codes for reference. Although there remain differences between these systems, they are not grounded in scientific disagreements but rather differences in historical and committee processes (APA, 2013).

The DSM-5

The *DSM-5* has three sections: (I) an introduction and explanation of its use, including a caution regarding its forensic use; (II) the diagnostic criteria and codes; and (III) emerging measures (assessment) and models (e.g., cultural formulation), an alternative model for personality disorders, and conditions for further study (e.g., Internet

BOX 2-1 *DSM-5* Diagnostic Categories

Neurodevelopmental Disorders
Schizophrenia Spectrum and Other Psychotic Disorders
Bipolar and Related Disorders
Depressive Disorders
Anxiety Disorders
Obsessive–Compulsive and Related Disorders
Trauma- and Stressor-Related Disorders
Dissociative Disorders
Somatic Symptom and Related Disorders
Feeding and Eating Disorders
Sleep–Wake Disorders
Sexual Dysfunctions
Gender Dysphoria
Disruptive, Impulse Control, and Conduct Disorders
Substance-Related and Addictive Disorders
Neurocognitive Disorders
Personality Disorders
Paraphilic Disorders
Other Mental Disorders
Medication-Induced Movement Disorders
Other Adverse Effects of Medication

Source: American Psychiatric Association. (2013). *Diagnostic and statistical manual of mental disorders* (5th ed.). Arlington, VA: Author.

gaming disorder). For clinical utility, the *DSM-5* is organized along development and life span lines (e.g., diagnoses reflecting developmental processes appearing early in life are at the beginning). Mental disorders are delineated in a way such that cultural, social, and familial norms and values can be recognized as influencing the expression and experience of symptoms, signs, and behaviours addressed in the criteria (APA, 2013). See Box 2-1 for *DSM-5* diagnostic categories and Box 2.2 for other conditions that may be a focus of clinical attention or may affect diagnosis, course, prognosis, or treatment.

BOX 2-2 *DSM-5* and Other Conditions That May Be a Focus of Clinical Attention or May Affect Diagnosis, Course, Prognosis, or Treatment

Relationship Problems
Abuse and Neglect
Educational and Occupational Problems
Housing and Economic Problems
Other Problems Related to Social Environment (e.g., phase of life problem, problems related to living alone)
Problems Related to Crime or Interaction With the Legal System
Other Health Service Encounters for Counselling and Medical Advice
Problems Related to Other Psychosocial, Personal, and Environmental Circumstances (e.g., unwanted pregnancy, experience with war, victim of torture)
Other Circumstances of Personal History (e.g., self-harm, nonadherence to medical treatment)

Source: American Psychiatric Association. (2013). *Diagnostic and statistical manual of mental disorders* (5th ed.). Arlington, VA: Author.

Gender Differences

The *DSM-5* notes gender differences (or the lack thereof) for several disorders. **Gender differences** are defined in the *DSM-5* as "variations that result from biological sex as well as an individual's self-representation that includes the psychological, behavioral, and social consequences of one's perceived gender" (APA, 2013, p. 15). The variations may result from only biologic sex differences, self-representation of gender, or both. Gender influences illnesses in several ways, including risk for a disorder, symptom presentation, and willingness to endorse symptoms (which impacts willingness to seek help for them). Events related to reproductive life cycle (e.g., postpartum period) affect risk and symptom expression.

Culture and the *DSM-5*

The *DSM-5* uses three concepts to point to ways culture influences the illness experience, including symptom presentation, help-seeking behaviours, expectations of and response to treatment, and adaptation to living with the illness (APA, 2013). These concepts are *cultural syndrome*, *cultural idiom of distress*, and *cultural explanation or perceived cause* (APA, 2013, p. 14). Box 2-3 offers a perspective on

BOX 2-3 "Saving Normal": An Alternative Approach to Some Psychiatric Symptoms

Frances, A. (2013). *Saving normal: An insider's revolt against out-of-control psychiatric diagnosis, DSM-5, big pharma, and the medicalization of ordinary life.* New York, NY: HarperCollins.

Allen Frances, the Chair of the *DSM-IV* Task Force, has serious reservations about the *DSM-5*. In his book, he outlines concerns about the influences on psychiatric diagnosis in general, as well as some specific concerns about the *DSM-5* changes to it. He wants to "save normal" in that he finds aspects of everyday life are being transformed into illness. For instance, he suggests that grief is becoming "medicalized," reducing the dignity of grief's pain, interfering with processing the loss, and reducing the use of rituals that can console. The grieving person, he argues, may be put at risk if prescribed unnecessary medication. Frances is concerned that "Big Pharma's" marketing of their products means that "psychiatric illness" also gets marketed. Shyness readily becomes "social phobia"; ardent interest in something (chocolate, the Internet, working, running, texting, shopping, television, etc.) becomes an addiction. If criteria for a mental disorder are too broad, it means the incidence of misdiagnosis can drastically increase. He points to the field trials for the *DSM-5* that found one in six cancer and coronary disease patients met the criteria for the *DSM-5*'s "somatic symptom disorder."

A Different Approach: For symptoms that do not clearly indicate a serious known disorder, Frances recommends a stepped approach, beginning with gathering baseline data, continued assessment, and moving to minimal intervention (e.g., education, self-help therapy) and brief therapy before a definitive diagnosis is made and substantive treatment begun. This would, he believes, help psychiatry to stay within appropriate bounds.

how changes to *DSM* criteria and a growing global pharmaceutical industry affect cultural practices and behaviours through medicalizing the "ordinary." See Chapter 3 for a discussion of culture and mental illness, including culture and the *DSM-5*.

Diagnosis as Labelling

Receiving a diagnosis can be a relief for an individual and his or her family if it allows for better understanding of symptoms, signs, and behaviour and means that treatment can begin (Hayne, 2001). As a way of labelling a particular person's illness, however, diagnosis can have negative consequences, such as the loss of personal identity if the labelled person becomes viewed as the disease and experiences stigma associated with mental illness. To avoid labelling a person, refer to individuals using person-first language. For example, refer to someone with diabetes mellitus as a "person with diabetes" rather than as a "diabetic." Likewise, someone with a mental disorder should be referred to as a "person with schizophrenia" or as a "person with bipolar disorder" rather than as "schizophrenic" or as "bipolar." Understanding labelling processes can facilitate conceptualization and implementation of stigma reduction strategies (Yang et al., 2012). It is particularly important that nurses and other health care professionals avoid the pitfalls of negative labelling and stigmatization (Austin, 2000; Kirby & Keon, 2006).

Health States and Mental Illness

An overview of how living with a specific mental illness can affect everyday quality of life is available from the Health Analysis Division of Statistics Canada: *Health State Descriptions for Canadians: Mental Illnesses* (Langlois, Samokhvalov, Rehm, Spence, & Connor Gorber, 2012). This document is part of a series describing health states related to the diseases classified in Canadian Population Health Impact of diseases research. Using the **Classification and Measurement System of Functional Health (CLAMES)** in which 11 attributes (each with 4 to 5 levels) are used to indicate daily functioning, aspects of living with a particular disorder are described (see Box 2-4). As well, there is a brief review of the disorder, including prevalence and treatment. For example, living with agoraphobia at moderate and severe levels is portrayed.

Mental Health Literacy

The Canadian Alliance on Mental Illness and Mental Health (CAMIMH) was funded by the Public Health Agency of Canada to examine Canadians' **mental health literacy**, defined as "the knowledge and skills that enable people to access, understand, and apply information for mental health" (CAMIMH, 2008, p. 2). Unfortunately,

---

BOX 2-4 Attributes of the Classification and Measurement System of Functional Health (CLAMES)

Core	Supplementary
Pain or discomfort	Anxiety
Physical functioning	Speech
Emotional state	Hearing
Fatigue	Vision
Memory and thinking	Use of hands and fingers
Social relationships	

From Langlois, K. A., Samokhvalov, A. V., Rehm, J., Spence, S. T., Connor Gorber, S. K. (2012). *Health state descriptions for Canadians: Mental illnesses.* Statistics Canada, catalogue no. 82-619MIE2005002. Ottawa, ON: Statistics Canada.

---

it was found that stigma and discrimination are negatively influencing Canadians' responses to people with mental illnesses, especially serious mental illnesses. Also affected is Canadians' willingness to disclose having a mental illness, especially in the workplace. In the CAMIMH project, focus group participants pointed to a variety of sources of stigmatization, including that by health professionals. Mental health literacy is especially important in its power to positively influence awareness and acceptance of mental illness and, ultimately, the mental health of Canadians (CAMIMH).

■ RECOVERY

Recovery, viewed as an active process unique to each individual, is a cornerstone of Canada's approach to mental health care (Kirby & Keon, 2006). Conceptually, this process is broader than clinical recovery (i.e., remission or cure) and, although persons with mental illness certainly can experience clinical recovery, recovery is viewed as being about having a satisfying and hopeful life, even with mental health problems or illness. A recovery orientation for nurses and other health care professionals means that engagement with those in their care involves a focus on those persons' strengths, resources, and rights and is shaped by culturally safe and competent practices. This orientation requires a less medically centred approach and a wider perspective on what constitutes positive outcome measures (see Chapter 8).

> **KEY CONCEPT Recovery** related to mental illness means "gaining and retaining hope, understanding of one's abilities and disabilities, engagement in an active life, personal autonomy, social identity, meaning and purpose in life and a positive sense of self." It is not synonymous with "cure" (WHO, 2013, p. 39).

Austin Albert Mardon (1962–)
Mental Health Advocate

Public Persona

Austin Mardon (PhD, LLD, CM) is a Canadian author, researcher, and mental health activist who has been awarded the United States Antarctic Service Medal, obtained a doctorate in geography from Greenwich University, Australia, and published in both *Science* and *Nature*. An international fellow of the Explorer's Club, he is a corresponding member of the International Academy of Astronautics. He has authored over 120 scholarly articles and edited, translated, and authored 50 books. A well-known mental health activist in Canada and abroad, Austin Mardon's advocacy work addresses mental health issues at both the front-line and policy levels. He has received numerous awards for this work, including the Order of Canada, Queen Elizabeth II Golden Jubilee Medal, the Alberta Centennial Medial, and the Flag of Hope Award.

Personal Realities

At age 24, Mardon was a promising young geographer and a junior field member with the International Meteorite Recovery Expedition to Antarctica, surviving a fall into a deep crevasse. In the years immediately following his Antarctic journey, he developed schizophrenia and his promising career was abruptly cut short. With his wife, Catherine Newman, he has established and endowed an annual award at the University of Alberta (UA) to support students who have schizophrenia or who have close family members with the illness. Austin Mardon hopes "to see the day when schizophrenia is treated like any other disease and is finally detached from the stigma that makes a difficult burden to bear even worse." He is currently an adjunct professor with the Dossetor Health Ethics Centre, UA.

THE MENTAL HEALTH OF CANADIANS

Nurses need to be engaged in the national strategy that guides Canada's approach to addressing the mental health of Canadians. The six key directions of the strategy (see Chapter 1, Box 1-3) involve promoting mental health across the life span, including in the workplace; fostering recovery and well-being for those living with mental health problems and illnesses and upholding their rights; providing appropriate services and reducing disparities in access to them; working with First Nations, Inuit, and Métis people to address their needs; and mobilizing collaboration and leadership at all levels. The MHCC plays a catalytic role in the strategy's enactment: promoting positive change through knowledge exchange, sponsoring major initiatives such as *Opening Minds* (i.e., antistigma), *At Home*, *Chez Soi* (i.e., housing-first), psychological health and safety in the workplace, mental health first aid, and others (Goldbloom & Bradley, 2012).

The growth of Canadians' knowledge of mental health and mental illness is increasingly apparent. It is revealed in the greater media promotion of mental health awareness and acceptance, the business community's more informed approach to the well-being of workers,

the partnerships with law enforcement (e.g., the *Police Project* and the *National Trajectory Project* [related to persons declared "not criminally responsible"]) and the more informed attention given to protecting the rights of all people, including persons with disabilities.

Homelessness and Mental Illness: *At Home/Chez Soi*

Homelessness is a national public health problem: an estimated 300,000 people live in shelters and on the streets in Canada every year, costing taxpayers $1.4 billion in health,

BOX 2-5 Research for Best Practice

AT HOME/CHEZ SOI: ADDRESSING HOMELESSNESS OF PERSONS LIVING WITH MENTAL ILLNESS

Goering, P., Veldhuizen, S., Watson, A., Adair, C., Kopp, B. M., Latimer, E., ... Aubry, T. (2014). National At Home/Chez soi final report. Calgary, AB: MHCC.

Question: Does the "housing first" (HF) approach work in Canadian cities? In which environments? For whom? At what cost?

Method: A mixed-method study, it involved randomized control trials (RCTs) and qualitative inquiry (e.g., life histories, focus groups). Five cities were project sites, each with a particular focus: Vancouver (people who also had problematic substance use), Winnipeg (urban Aboriginal population), Toronto (ethnoracialized populations, including new immigrants without English), Montréal (included a vocational study), Moncton (services in smaller community). Participants were recruited from shelters and the streets; $n = 1158$ for HF intervention group; $n = 990$ in the "treatment-as-usual" (TAU) control group. The typical participants were males and in their 40s; however, there were females (32%), Aboriginal persons (22%), and persons from other ethnic groups (25%). The average length of homelessness experienced by a participant was over 5 years. Almost all were in extreme poverty at the time of the study; nearly 90% had at least one chronic health problem. Their life histories often included childhood trauma with many leaving home to escape abuse. Two kinds of support services were offered: Assertive Community Treatment for those with high needs; and Intensive Case Management for those with moderate needs. Quality of life, community funding, recovery, employment, and related outcomes were measured. Assessment of program fidelity was done to document quality of the HF interventions being carried out.

Findings: HF works in Canadian cities with different population size and composition. It rapidly reduces homelessness. Participants in the HF intervention used and retained housing at a rate significantly higher than the control (TAU) group. It proved to be a sound investment. For every $10 invested, $960 was saved for persons with higher needs and $342 for persons with moderate needs. It led beyond housing to other positive, symptom-related outcomes for participants.

Implications: HF is an effective, pragmatic, and humane intervention for homelessness of persons living with mental illness in Canada. It can contain costs, but requires meaningful collaboration among governments, communities, and service users. Training and technical support are necessary to success.

justice, and social services (Picard, 2013). Homelessness is costly not only to people's health but also to their society's budget. While only some homeless persons are living with addictions and other mental illnesses (usually untreated), deinstitutionalization, lack of long-term treatment beds, and insufficient mental health services have created a serious public health crisis. Some of our most vulnerable citizens, those living with mental health problems and disorders, have no shelter or no place to call home. In fact, "prisons and shelters have become the asylums of the 21st century" (Kirby & Keon, 2006).

In addressing this critical situation, the federal government allocated funds ($110 million) to the MHCC for a demonstration project addressing mental illness and homelessness. The MHCC implemented a project, *At Home/Chez Soi*, based on the principles of "Housing First (HF)" that turns on its head the notion that treatment must come first before housing issues can be addressed. Instead, this approach requires immediate access (without readiness conditions) to permanent housing along with community-based supports. Other HF principles include consumer choice and self-determination, recovery orientation, individualized and person-driven supports, and social and community integration (Goering et al., 2014). The *At Home/Chez Soi* project has been highly successful, revealing that this approach can work in Canadian cities of different sizes and ethnoracial and cultural composition, that it rapidly ends homelessness, and that it is a sound investment (Goering et al., 2014). (See Box 2-5 for research for best practice.) Based on the demonstrated success of this intervention, the MHCC has developed a toolkit for communities interested in implementing HF projects, as well as developed training programs and technical supports necessary to such projects' success.

RESEARCH-BASED CARE

In the urgent quest to improve the lives of Canadians living with a mental health problem or illness, research will be a major tool. Nurses are challenged to generate evidence for best care interventions, to use methods of inquiry that allow a better understanding of the experiences of mental health, mental illness, recovery and well-being, and to translate new knowledge into better care. For instance, the science related to decreasing the use of seclusion and restraint or that which underscored the need to determine an individual's trauma-related experiences when diagnosing as well as research showing the efficacy of new approaches to mental health community services are transforming care in positive ways. In most chapters of this textbook, "Research for Best Practice" is featured. As well as noting the implications research findings have for practice, attention should be paid to the various research methods that are being utilized, from RCTs to philosophical inquiry.

The need to improve mental health care is a global one, requiring shared efforts, as indicated by the fourth global

target of the WHO Action Plan (2013): "to strengthen information systems, evidence, and research for mental health" (p. 22). An example of such shared efforts is the formal agreement between the MHCC and the National Mental Health Commission of Australia to share knowledge and best practices in mental health research. These kinds of agreements should foster better care for the millions living with mental health problems and disorders.

SUMMARY OF KEY POINTS

■ Four complex concepts are the cornerstone of Canada's mental health strategy and fundamental to psychiatric and mental health nursing practice: *mental health*, *well-being*, *mental illness*, and *recovery*.

■ "There is no health without mental health." Mental health needs to be integrated into general health in all areas of practice and around the world.

■ ICN and CNA take the position that all registered nurses must have the knowledge and skills to respond to mental health needs, including their own.

■ Measures used to explore well-being include the GNH index, the CIW, and the SPI.

■ The medical term for mental illness is mental disorder. In Canada, the *DSM* is the most commonly used classification of mental disorders. Its fifth edition was released in 2013, the *DSM-5*. The Mental and Behavioural Disorders section of the ICD classification of the WHO is an alternative system that can also be used.

■ Diagnosis can be used in a way that increases negative labelling of persons living with mental health problems or illnesses. It is important not to use language such as "She is a schizophrenic," but rather say "She has schizophrenia."

■ Health Canada describes health states related to specific diseases using the CLAMES, which indicates daily functioning attributes of living with that disease or disorder.

■ Nurses need to play a role in increasing the mental health literacy of Canadians.

■ The six strategic directions of our national mental health strategy guide the Canadian approach to mental health and mental health care.

CRITICAL THINKING CHALLENGES

1 Distinguish between the concepts of *mental health*, *mental illness*, and *mental disorder*.

2 In what way is *recovery*, viewed as more than restoration of health, influencing practice in psychiatric and mental health settings? What are the facilitators and barriers to this change in perspective in such settings?

3 Consider your own well-being. Are you a good role model for the public in terms of living and being well? If not, what change would need to occur for you to be a good example to others?

4 Examine the *DSM-5* classification system. What are the advantages of using this type of system in PMH nursing? The disadvantages?

5 Monitor the language that nurses in your practicum areas use to identify a person with a mental disorder. Is calling a patient "a schizophrenic," "a depressive," "a borderline," etc. still common? If so, how might you respond when such language is used?

6 What are you doing to increase mental health literacy in your community?

REFERENCES

American Psychological Association. (2013). *Diagnostic and statistical manual of mental disorders* (5th ed.). Arlington, VA: Author.

Austin, W. (2000). Ethics and the stigma of mental illness. *In Touch: The Provincial Health Ethics Network, 2*(12), 1–2.

Canadian Alliance on Mental Illness and Mental Health (CAMIMH). (2008). *National integrated framework for enhancing mental health literacy in Canada: Final report.* Available at www.camimh.ca

Canadian Index of Wellbeing. (2012). *How are Canadians really doing? The 2012 Canadian Index of Wellbeing report.* Waterloo, ON: Canadian Index of Wellbeing & University of Waterloo.

Canadian Nurses Association (CNA). (2008). *Code of ethics for registered nurses.* Ottawa: Author.

Epp, J. (1988). *Mental health for Canadians: Striking a balance.* (Cat.H39-128/1988E). Ottawa, ON: Supply and Services Canada.

Frances, A. (2013). *Saving normal: An insider's revolt against out-of-control psychiatric diagnosis, DSM-5, Big Pharma, and the medicalization of ordinary life.* New York, NY: HarperCollins.

Goering, P., Veldhuizen, S., Watson, A., Adair, C., Kopp, B., Latimer, E. … Aubry, T. (2014). *National At Home/Chez Soi final report.* Calgary, AB: MHCC.

Goldbloom, D. & Bradley, L. (2012). The Mental Health Commission of Canada: the first five years. *Mental Health Review Journal, 17*(4), 221–228.

Hayne, Y. M. (2001). *To be diagnosed: The experience of presenting with chronic mental illness* (unpublished doctoral thesis). University of Alberta, Canada.

Healey-Ogden, M. & Austin, W. (2011). Uncovering the lived experience of well-being. *Qualitative Health Research, 21*, 85–98.

International Council of Nurses. (2008). Position statement: Mental health. Available at http://www.icn.ch/publications/position-statements/

Johnston, D. (2012). Wellbeing in Canada. In Canadian Index of Wellbeing (2012). *How are Canadians really doing? The 2012 Canadian Index of Wellbeing report.* Waterloo, ON: Canadian Index of Wellbeing & University of Waterloo.

Kirby, M. J. & Keon, W. J. (2006). *Out of the shadows at last: Highlights and recommendations.* Ottawa, ON: The Standing Committee on Social Affairs, Science and Technology.

Kolappa, K., Henderson, D., & Kishore, S. P. (2013). No physical health without mental health: Lessons unlearned? *Bulletin of the World Health Organization, 91*(1):3–3A.

Langlois, K. A., Samokhvalov, A. V., Rehm, J., Spence, S. T., & Connor Gorber, S. K. (2012). *Health state descriptions for Canadians: Mental illnesses.* Statistics Canada, catalogue no. 82-619 MIE2005002. Ottawa, ON: Statistics Canada.

Mental Health Commission of Canada. (2009). *Toward recovery & well-being: A framework for a Mental Health Strategy for Canada.* Available at http://www.mentalhealthcommission.ca/English/document/241/toward-recovery-and-well-being

Mental Health Commission of Canada. (2013). *Making the case for investing in mental health in Canada.* Available at http://www.mentalhealthcommission.ca/English/node/5020

OED Online 2014. "well-being, n.". Oxford University Press. Retrieved from http://www.oed.com.login.ezproxy.library.ualberta.ca/view/Entry/227050?redirectedFrom=well-being

Picard, A. (2013, Tuesday, October 29). Lessons on homelessness from Vancouver. Second Opinion, *The Globe and Mail*, p. L8.

Porter, M. E. & Stern, S., with Green, M. (2014). Executive Summary, *Social Progress Index 2014.* Available at http://www.socialprogressimperative.org/

Social Progress Imperative. (2014). News release: "Canada ranks world's 7th most socially advanced country: Social Progress Index launched to enable better understanding of worldwide progress and growth." Available at socialprogressimperative.org

Ura, K., Alkere, S., Zangno, T., & Wangdi, K. (2012). *An extensive analysis of GNH Index.* Thimphu, Bhutan: Centre for Bhutan Studies. Available at www.grossnationalhappiness.com

World Health Organization & World Association of Family Doctors. (2008). *Integrating mental health into primary care: A global perspective.* Geneva, Switzerland: WHO.

World Health Organization. (2010a). Mental health: Strengthening our response. Fact sheet No. 220. Retrieved from http://www.who.int/mediacentre/factsheets/fs220/en/

World Health Organization. (2010b). *International statistical classification of diseases and related health problems (10th rev.) (ICD-10).* Geneva, Switzerland: Author.

World Health Organization. (2013). *Mental health action plan 2013–2020.* Geneva, Switzerland: Author.

Yang, L. H., Lo, G., WonPat-Borja, A. J., Singla, D. R., Link, B. G., & Phillips, M. R. (2012). Effects of labeling and interpersonal conflict upon attitudes towards schizophrenia: Implications for reducing mental illness stigma in urban China. *Social Psychiatry and Psychiatric Epidemiology, 47*(9), 1459–1473.

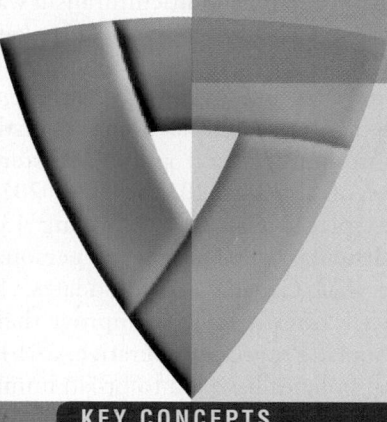

3 The Context of Mental Health Care

Cultural, Socioeconomic, and Legal

Arlene Kent-Wilkinson

Adapted from the chapter "The Context of Mental Health Care" by Mary Ann Boyd

KEY CONCEPTS

- culture
- cultural competence
- cultural safety
- Mental Health Act
- poverty
- stigma

LEARNING OBJECTIVES

After studying this chapter, you will be able to:

- Explore the cultural roots of mental illness and its relationship to beliefs of religion and spirituality.
- Relate the concepts of cultural competence and cultural safety to the role of the psychiatric and mental health (PMH) nurse.
- Consider the unique culture of Aboriginal people in Canada and their mental health beliefs.
- Identify the influence of socioeconomic factors (poverty, geographic) on the mental health of Canadians.
- Describe the mental health care delivery issues related to providing services to culturally diverse populations, including new immigrants and refugees in Canada's many geographic areas.
- Identify and explain the mental health legislation enacted to help protect, promote, and improve the lives and mental well-being of Canadians.

KEY TERMS

- Aboriginal health • assimilation • best interests • colonialism
- community treatment order • competence • discrimination
- ethnocentrism • historical trauma • mandatory outpatient treatment • prejudice • religion • spirituality • stereotyping
- substitute decision maker • telehealth

Health, including the mental health, of any human population is the product of a complex web of cultural, environmental, historical, physiologic, psychological, spiritual, socioeconomic, and legislative factors. This chapter examines three contexts of mental health and illness in Canada: *cultural, socioeconomic,* and *legal.* Culture will be examined with regards to cultural roots, spirituality, and religion. The unique culture of Canada's indigenous people will be a focus, along with the concepts of stigma of mental disorders and the need for cultural competence and cultural safety. Socioeconomic factors that influence mental health (poverty, geographic access to services) will then be explored. Finally, international agreements and Canadian legislation enacted to protect, promote, and improve the lives and mental well-being of citizens will be discussed, in addition to the research context.

CULTURAL CONTEXT OF MENTAL HEALTH CARE

All people have a culture. It reflects the basic values and biases through which we interpret the world around us and make decisions about our own behaviour and our relationships with others. Our culture shapes our perceptions and attitudes, from our personal space comfort zones to our attitudes towards mental health and mental illness. Canada's mental health strategy has emphatically asserted that in service and treatment of mental health, culture counts (Mental Health Commission of Canada [MHCC], 2012).

Culture

Humans have been described as animals who have spun "webs of significance" for themselves (Geertz, 1973). These webs are culture. Understanding mental health and culture is not about finding its "laws" but about interpreting its meaning. The metaphor of a complex web is strong, as webs show intricacy and interconnectedness, creativity, and skill that can only be seen close-up. Each individual thread contributes to the strength of the web.

"Culture is commonly understood as learned traditions and unconscious rules of engagement that people use to interpret experience and to generate social behaviour" (Srivastava, 2007, p. 324). Individuals, organizations including professions and religious denominations, and countries all have culture (Alexander, 2008). "Culture is the lens through which the world is viewed and approached. It influences decisions made, actions taken, and personal relations" (Alexander, 2008, p. 420). Members of a culture, however, rarely have insight into their own culturally learned ideas and values regarding normal and abnormal behaviours; typically, these values are seen as correct and proper for everyone. This is termed **ethnocentrism**.

> ▼ **KEY CONCEPT Culture** is not only a way of life for people who identify or associate with one another on the basis of some common purpose, need, or similarity of background; it is also the totality of learned, socially transmitted beliefs, values, and behaviours that emerge from its members' interpersonal transactions.

Cultural Diversity in Canada

According to the most recent census data, the racial, ethnic, linguistic, and religious diversity of the Canadian population is growing and will continue to do so in the near future. As diversity increases, so too do the needs of the population, which presents unique challenges to social institutions and governments (Citizenship and Immigration Canada, 2010).

Canadian Multiculturalism Policies

Canada has always been a culturally diverse nation. Even prior to European settlement, it was highly diverse. Today, the majority of Canadians are descendents of immigrants or are immigrants themselves. Moreover, Canadians view cultural diversity and immigration as a national asset (Government of Canada, 2012a). In 1971, Canada became the first country to adopt a policy of multiculturalism. The 1971 *Multiculturalism Policy of Canada* affirmed the rights, dignity, and value of all Canadians

regardless of ethnic, linguistic, or religious background. The policy also confirmed the rights of indigenous people in Canada as well as recognized Canada's two official languages (Government of Canada, 2012b).

In 1982, the value of Canadian multiculturalism was reaffirmed in the *Canadian Charter of Rights and Freedoms* (Government of Canada, 2012a). In 1997, a new multiculturalism program was announced (Government of Canada, 2012b). Recent research has found Canada to be one of the most multicultural among Western nations (Government of Canada, 2012b). The 2014 Social Progress Index placed Canada 7th among 132 nations, citing in particular the amount of personal freedom and choice that Canada accommodates, as well as the opportunity it offers people to improve their position in society (Social Progress Imperative, 2014). Canada's multicultural policies have led to broad immigration. Many immigrants choose to come to Canada because there is no pressure to assimilate. Moreover, upon arrival, they may freely choose to self-identify with their culture of origin or not. In all cases, their individual rights are protected and they have the right to fully participate in the democratic process (Government of Canada, 2012a).

Culturally Diverse Populations

Cultural diversity differs by region in Canada and is considered the variation of "cultural factors" that appears between people and groups (Registered Nurses' Association of Ontario [RNAO], 2007), particularly differences from the dominant culture or the assumed norm (Srivastava, 2007). In health care, "understanding complexities of culture from the perspective of providers and recipients of care is critical because culture pervades all

---

BOX 3-1 Culturally Sensitive Mental Health Services

There are numerous clinics across Canada offering culturally sensitive mental health services. Listed here are a few outstanding examples and their Websites.

Vancouver
Native Health Society — vnhs.net/

Edmonton
Boyle Street Co-op, "Street Works" — Professionals: streetworks.ca/pro/aswstaff.html
Clients: streetworks.ca/client/contactinfo.html

Regina
Four Directions Community Health Centre — rqhealth.ca/programs/comm_hlth_centres/four_directions/4directions.shtml

Toronto
Inner City Health Program at St. Michaels Hospital — stmichaelshospital.com/programs/ich/index.php
CMHA
Use the map of Canada to locate facilities in each province and territory — cmha.ca/get-involved/find-your-cmha/

aspects of health care and all aspects of life" (Alexander, 2008, p. 416). Acceptance and respect are essential for integrated cultural diversity (International Council of Nurses, 2007). See Box 3-1 for links to examples of culturally sensitive mental health services in Canada.

Cultural Roots of Mental Health and Illness

The experience of mental illness is influenced by culture. Symptoms of a disorder that are prominent in one culture may be insignificant or absent in another and may even be interpreted as normal in a third. Some mental disorders may be a recent development in response to cultural change. The *totally discouraged syndrome* (depression, alcoholism, lack of social responsibility, neglect of family, suicidal behaviour), described for the Sioux, may be such a disorder (Johnson & Johnson, 1965). *Residential school syndrome* as discussed by Brasfield (2001) suggests that this syndrome is similar to posttraumatic stress disorder (see Chapter 17) yet different due to its cultural impact. Symptoms of *residential school syndrome* present in a variety of ways through social and psychological issues. Addressing these requires cultural understanding and awareness of culturally sensitive approaches to healing.

Diagnostic Cultural Formulations

The American Psychiatric Association (APA) *Diagnostic and Statistical Manual of Mental Disorders* (DSM) is used to set the boundaries, conditions, and criteria for psychiatric diagnosis throughout North America. The *DSM* is the manual used by clinicians and researchers to diagnose and classify mental disorders. Culture was not specifically addressed until the manual's fourth edition (*DSM-IV*) (APA, 1994). After exploring different ways of facilitating the application of a cultural perspective to the process of clinical interviewing, a cultural formulation outline was adopted. However, it was relegated to the back of the book, in the ninth appendix along with a glossary of cultural terms and idioms of distress. This was a problematic solution for many who believed that culture must be more central to the process of clinical evaluation and treatment (Austin, Gallop, McCay, Peternelj-Taylor, & Bayer, 1999). Psychiatric researchers, focused on a biologic model of mental disorders, tend to ignore cultural factors. For instance, in a review of psychiatric drug studies, it was found that only 8% of patient subjects were from minority groups (Vedantam, 2005).

In 2013, the APA published the *DSM-5* after a 14-year revision process (APA, 2013b). The fifth edition explicitly seeks to provide culturally appropriate diagnosis by incorporating cultural sensitivity throughout the manual. One significant change is that it no longer lists culture-bound syndromes. Instead, it provides criteria reflecting cross-cultural variation, outlines cultural concepts of distress, and provides an interview tool (APA, 2013a). The *DSM-5* has also worked to make its criteria universally valid across different cultures. For example, "offending

others" has been added to the criteria for social anxiety disorder in order to better reflect the appearance of social anxiety disorder in Japan, where avoiding harm to others is of greater concern than avoiding harm to oneself (APA, 2013a).

The Impact of Cultural Difference

Because symptoms manifest and are understood differently across cultures, clinicians must attend to relevant aspects of a patient's context when making a diagnosis. For instance, depending on the patient's culture, panic attacks may manifest as uncontrollable crying and headaches or as difficulty breathing. Understanding these cultural differences will allow for more accurate diagnoses and more effective treatment (APA, 2013a).

Health and Culture

Every culture has a conception of what constitutes health and illness and how illness should be treated (Brascoupé & Waters, 2009). Culture is strongly linked to identity; the suppression or marginalization of one's cultural identity has a negative impact on self-worth. However, if a culture is valued and supported, individuals and communities self-identifying with that culture will experience a sense of belonging and value. Shared cultural beliefs, practices, and language create social cohesion in communities, which can positively influence the health of individuals. When cultural practices and language are denied to communities, as historically occurred with many Aboriginal communities in Canada, social cohesion and health are negatively affected (Brascoupé & Waters, 2009).

■■■ ABORIGINAL PEOPLE OF CANADA

Canadian psychiatric and mental health (PMH) nurses recognize the importance of understanding Aboriginal culture and knowledge (Austin et al., 1999). According to the 2011 Canadian census, 1,400,685 people in Canada (4.3% of the total population) self-identify as First Nation, Métis, or Inuit (Statistics Canada, 2013a). At present, there are nearly 600 recognized First Nations governments or bands in Canada (Statistics Canada, 2013a). Section 35(2) of Canada's *Constitution Act, 1982*, defines "Aboriginal people" as Indian (First Nations), Inuit, and Métis people. The term "Indian" along with "Eskimo" (the name formerly given to the Inuit) are no longer used in Canada, as they are considered pejorative. While government documents tend to use the term "Aboriginal," many Aboriginal people prefer the term "Indigenous." Although often treated as a single group, there are many indigenous cultures in Canada, each having a unique heritage, language, set of cultural practices, and spiritual beliefs (Statistics Canada, 2013a). See Box 3-2 for definitions of the three groups of Aboriginal people in Canada: First Nations, Inuit, and Métis.

BOX 3-2 Aboriginal People of Canada

First Nation

The term *First Nation* replaces the term *Indian* (Royal Commission on Aboriginal Peoples, 1996). *First Nation* began to be used in the 1970s as a substitute for *Indians*, which fell into disfavour with Aboriginal people. The term does not mean the same as *Aboriginal people* or *First People* because it does not include Inuit and Métis (Public Health Agency of Canada, 2006). *Indian Band Member* or *First Nation* refers to those people who reported being a member of an Indian band or a First Nation of Canada (Statistics Canada, 2013a).

Inuit

The term *Inuit* replaces the term *Eskimo* (Royal Commission on Aboriginal Peoples, 1996). The Inuit are Aboriginal people in northern Canada who live above the tree line in Nunavut, the Northwest Territories, Northern Quebec, and Labrador. The word means *people* in the Inuit language—*Inuktitut*. The singular of Inuit is Inuk (Aboriginal Health Glossary, 2004).

Métis

The term *Métis* refers to Aboriginal people of mixed First Nation and European ancestry. Métis people self-identify as Métis, as distinct from First Nations people, Inuit, or non-Aboriginal people with mixed background. The Métis have a unique culture that draws on their diverse ancestral origins, such as Scottish, French, Ojibway, and Cree (Government of Saskatchewan, 2003).

Cultural Diversity Among Aboriginal People of Canada

Of the 596 First Nations bands and 2,284 reserves, 40% of Aboriginal people in Canada live on reserve, while 60% reside in nonreserve areas (54% urban, 6% rural; Statistics Canada, 2013a). The cultural and linguistic differences among Aboriginal groups are greater than the differences that divide European nations. In addition to intergroup social, cultural, and environmental differences, there is an enormous diversity of values, lifestyles, and perspectives within any community or urban Aboriginal population (Kirmayer, Brass, & Tait, 2000).

Aboriginal Mental Health

"Aboriginal health is influenced by the rich diversity of social, economic, and political circumstances that give rise to a variety of health problems and healing strategies in Aboriginal communities" (Waldram, Herring, & Young, 2006, p. 3). Many Aboriginal people are raised to believe the body is governed by four elements comprising the spiritual, emotional, mental, and physical. Traditionally, Aboriginal people have a holistic view of health, wherein mental health is considered a part.

The traditional Aboriginal healing systems encompass a holistic view of manifestations of illness in an individual. There is little evidence of a clear distinction between what science would call somatic disorders and disorders of the psyche. The mind, body, and spirit are seen as an integrated whole. Notions of *sanity* and *insanity* and of *personality disorders* are not strictly defined, as in the case of the Western biomedical tradition. The Western approach, in contrast, separates the body from the mind and spirit, and the emphasis is on the physical disease and treatment (Waldram, 2004). To understand the mental health problems or disorders of an Aboriginal person, it is necessary to recognize the historical, socioeconomic, and political circumstances of Aboriginal people in Canada, because the mental health issues arising may relate to these circumstances.

Mental Health Services to Aboriginal Populations

In the early 1990s, it was noted that less than 1% of health care workers in Canada were of Aboriginal ancestry, and this was affecting the provision of health services to this population (Royal Commission of Aboriginal People [RCAP], 1996). In response to the RCAP (1996) recommendation that the number of Aboriginal health care workers be increased, federal and provincial initiatives were implemented. The Romanow Report of 2002 recognized that social problems among Aboriginal people are a legacy of history—a result of the repeated assaults on their culture and identity (Standing Senate Committee on Social Affairs, Science and Technology, 2006). The foundation of Aboriginal society has been weakened and has resulted in the alienation that drives some to self-destruction and antisocial behaviour (Health Canada, 2009). Abuse of alcohol and drugs, family violence, youth crime, poverty, suicide, and sexual abuse are all public health issues that require attention when promoting the mental health of Aboriginal people.

Colonialism, Assimilation, and Historical Intergenerational Trauma

Colonialism is the institutionalized political domination of one nation over another. There is direct political administration by the colonial power, control of all economic relationships, and a systematic attempt to transform the culture. Before Confederation and up through the first half of the 20th century, the strategy of the Government of Canada towards First Nations was a colonial one. Assimilation was the government policy to "Canadianize" Aboriginal people to the extent that they would abandon their own culture and adopt the dominant culture (i.e., French or British Canadian) and religion (i.e., Protestant or Catholic) (Thira, 2005). Aboriginal populations have been subjected to historical trauma, which is the cumulative effect of maltreatment across generations and which results in the reproduction of maladaptive social and cultural patterns with each generation.

Canada's official policy of assimilation directly resulted in social and health disparities. These have been perpetuated through ongoing government policies, including the residential school system and the "60's Scoop," whereby Aboriginal cultures, traditions, and languages were systematically undermined and children taken from their families (Aboriginal Affairs and Northern

Development Canada, 2013). It has been suggested that "poorer socioeconomic circumstances and social exclusion can entrench feelings of helplessness, hopelessness, alienation, and mistrust among vulnerable populations and can increase the likelihood of adopting unhealthy or risky behaviours" (Statistics Canada, 2013b, para 12).

Residential Schools

From first contact, European missionaries sought to convert local indigenous people. It is out of this history that the Indian Residential School (IRS) system arose. In 1874, the federal government began to develop and administer the IRS (Health Canada, 2013). Residential schools were located in every province and territory except Newfoundland (where the entire indigenous population had been decimated), New Brunswick, and Prince Edward Island. The majority of federally run residential schools had ceased operations by the mid-70s, with the last closing in 1996. An estimated 80,000 people alive today attended residential schools in Canada (Health Canada, 2013).

The IRS system has had a traumatic legacy. Students were often forcibly removed from their families, denied their native language and culture, and often subjected to physical, sexual, and emotional abuse (Health Canada, 2013). In 2007, the Indian Residential Schools Settlement Agreement (IRS SA) was implemented. As part of this agreement, Health Canada and Aboriginal Affairs and Northern Development Canada developed a series of services to support IRS survivors and their families (Health Canada, 2013). The Indian Residential Schools Resolution Health Support Program offers counselling and support services to all IRS survivors and their families (Health Canada, 2013).

In 2009, the Truth and Reconciliation Commission of Canada began a 5-year process of gathering statements from former students and their families about the effects of the Indian Residential School System. The purpose was to make Canadian society at large aware of what happened in the IRS, to shed light on the long-term impact of the IRS, to create a permanent record of students' experiences, and to encourage reconciliation between Aboriginal people and Canadian society. A National Research Centre on Indian Residential Schools, situated at the University of Manitoba, will house the statements, documents, and other materials collected by the Commission in order that its work and spirit may continue.

■■■ RELIGION AS A CULTURE SYSTEM

Religion can be seen as a cultural system, in that it is a system of meanings that shapes our experience. (*Religion* comes from the Latin *religare*, to bind together). People who have shared common experiences, including religious experiences, over time develop commonalities of culture. Family traditions are a commonality that develops over a generation or two. Religion is a commonality that develops over a longer period of time among larger groups of people. Prior to the advent of modern Western medicine, the provision of care was often inexorably linked with spirituality or faith (Skip Knox, 2004). Often, there was little that could be done about a medical condition except to pray or give offerings (Srivastava, 2007).

Religious Beliefs and Approaches to Mental Illness

Religious beliefs often define an individual's relationship within a family and community. Many different religions are practised throughout the world. Although Judeo-Christian beliefs tend to dominate Western societies and other religions such as Islam, Hinduism, and Buddhism dominate Eastern and Middle Eastern cultures, it is likely that all religions are represented among Canadians. (See Web Links on the thePoint for religions in Canada.)

Beliefs about mental illness are intimately linked with concepts of religion, social values, norms, and ideals of human relationships. These shared beliefs determine the nature of traditional medicine and provide the framework for interpreting symptoms and guiding action in response to them. Western medicine and psychiatry are premised on the belief that mental illness is caused by biologic and experiential events; many other cultures ascribe a metaphysical or spiritual cause as well.

Aboriginal Spirituality and Culture

Spirituality is an important aspect in Aboriginal culture. Traditional medical practices of Aboriginal people are closely related to other aspects of the culture, especially their spirituality (Waldram et al., 2006). For some, there is no distinction between spiritual life and cultural life. Getting in touch with one's own spirituality is identified as a key to recovery or healing. Spirituality is linked to a sense of life purpose and personal identity and is seen as a key element for individuals to find their place in the world. To most Aboriginal people, the concept of spirituality refers to a sense of direction: it is not a religion but a way of life.

Though the rites have been modified throughout the years, Aboriginal spirituality remains alive and continues to be practised. Interest in Aboriginal spirituality has grown in recent years, attracting both Aboriginal and non-Aboriginal followers. Many people admire the holistic aspect of Aboriginal spirituality and are drawn to this expression of faith, seeking inner peace and wellness. This renewed interest has created a unique opportunity for the preservation of Aboriginal spirituality and culture.

■■■ STEREOTYPING, PREJUDICE, DISCRIMINATION, AND STIGMA

It is often difficult for one cultural group to understand the values, beliefs, and patterns of accepted behaviour of a different cultural group. This is especially true in regards to mental illness—some cultures view it as a condition for which the ill person must be punished, banished, or ostracized from society, whereas other cultures are more tolerant and believe that family and community members are key to the care and treatment of the mentally ill.

Mental illness not only affects those individual suffering from it, it also impacts families, communities, and health care systems (Smetanin et al., 2011). In fact, mental illness indirectly affects all Canadians through family members, friends, or colleagues. Arboleda-Florez (2005) notes that families may also become casualties under the stress of caring for acutely mentally ill relatives, especially within a rejecting community. The concepts of stereotyping, prejudice, discrimination, and stigma are important in understanding the life of people with mental disorders, their families, and cultural groups.

Stereotyping is an ongoing issue with mental illness. Stereotyping is expecting individuals to act in a characteristic manner that conforms to a usually negative perception of their cultural group. Individual characteristics are not considered. Stereotyping occurs because of lack of exposure to enough people in a particular group. "Health professionals who make unsubstantiated assumptions and have stereotypical attitudes about those who differ from themselves not only place the health and well-being of their patients at risk, they also seriously impair service delivery" (Richardson, 2008, p. 40). For instance, despite the fact that only 5% to 7% of violent crimes are committed by individuals with some form of mental illness, the most prevalent misconception about mental illness is the belief that persons with a mental disorder are dangerous (Arboleda-Florez, 2003) or are typically violent. In fact, rather than committing these acts of violence, persons with mental illness are more likely to be the victims (MHCC, 2013a). Media representations of people with mental illness (e.g., movies, television, magazines, newspapers) help perpetuate this negative stereotype.

Prejudice is a hostile attitude towards others simply because they belong to a particular group that is considered to have objectionable characteristics. Srivastava (2007) notes that everyone has some biases and prejudices, but that health care providers need to acknowledge and examine their biases in preparation for competent, sensitive care for all patients and families. If health care providers do not address their biases in a meaningful way, their ability to form trusting, healing relationships will be affected.

Discrimination is the differential treatment of others because they are members of a particular group or identified as being negatively different. It can include ignoring, derogatory name-calling, denying services, and threatening. Discrimination arises from a lack of understanding and appreciation of differences among people, but it can be overcome.

Nurses, too, can experience subtle discrimination from patients and families: patients may express a desire to have a nurse "more like them" assigned to their care. Alberta Pasco's (2004) study of Filipino Canadians'

experience of hospital care found that her participants initially desired nurses who were "one of us" (*hindi ibang tao*). However, non-Filipino nurses became "one of us" as the patient came to know the nurse as a caring person who was kind, respectful, and trustworthy.

Because cultural, socioeconomic, and political issues are intertwined, the Canadian Nurses Association (CNA) (2010) has determined that social justice is central to its mandate and insists that nurses not discriminate on the basis of a person's culture.

Stigma is the mark of a spoiled identity. In ancient Greece, stigma was literally a sign cut or burnt into a person's body to indicate low moral status (Goffman, 1963). People with mental illnesses or mental health problems often are stigmatized by the society in which they live, a phenomenon that has occurred throughout history (see Chapter 1). In his work *Madness and Civilization*, Foucault (1967) argues that in the Middle Ages, madness came to occupy the position leprosy once held. Individuals deemed mad were excluded from society as lepers had been. "Stigma is a form of prejudice that spreads fear and misinformation, labels individuals, and perpetuates stereotypes" (MHCC, 2013a, para 1). It often prevents people with mental health concerns from seeking help, denying them access to treatment and support services (MHCC, 2013a).

> **KEY CONCEPT** According to the Mental Health Commission of Canada (MHCC, 2013a), **stigma** is the "negative, unfavourable attitudes and the behaviour they produce" (para 1) associated with a particular trait displayed by or activity engaged in by an individual or group.

The Stigma of Mental Illness and Interventions

Stigma can be a barrier to all aspects of life; it limits access to employment opportunities, housing, education, and health care. It can also adversely affect people's relationships with family and friends. When someone begins to internalize the negative views held by others, defined as self-stigma, it can also affect their self-image (MHCC, 2013a). Persons with mental health issues have reported experiencing stigma from a wide range of sources: family and friends, the general public, coworkers, and even the health professionals they encounter in search of mental health services (MHCC, 2012, p. 16). Often, the stigma of mental illness has a greater negative impact on an individual than the illness itself.

Out of the Shadows at Last (2006)

This government report found that the stigma of mental illness has pervaded all levels of Canadian society today (Standing Senate Committee on Social Affairs, Science and

Technology, 2006). In response, stigma has increasingly been addressed as an issue in government reports.

The Mental Health Commission of Canada (MHCC) has had much to say on stigma. Despite the fact that mental illness affects an estimated one in five Canadians, widespread stigma of mental illness still occurs (MHCC, 2013a). The MHCC claims that, as a result, 60% of people with a mental health problem will not seek help for fear of being labelled (MHCC, 2013a). This indicates that stigma is a major obstacle when it comes to an individual's recovery and that stigma results in unfair treatment for people with mental disorders as well as their families.

Opening Minds Initiative (2009)

In response to the widespread recognition of the effects of stigma, the *Opening Minds* program was initiated by the MHCC in 2009 (MHCC, 2012). Its goal was to change Canadians' behaviours and attitudes towards mental illness so that people living with mental health issues felt comfortable seeking treatment and support (MHCC, 2013c). The 10-year-long antistigma and antidiscrimination campaign is the largest systematic effort to reduce the stigma of mental illness in Canadian history. "Instead of creating one program to reach the entire Canadian population, *Opening Minds* is taking a targeted approach. Its initial target groups are youth, health care providers, the workforce, and news media, with other groups to be added in future years" (MHCC, 2012, p. 33).

Often under pressure to see patients quickly, health care providers may not have the time or training to address mental health issues properly. Youth were also targeted, because due to the high incidence of symptoms occurring before an individual reaches the age of 18, early intervention has the potential to create a positive, long-term impact in their lives. The workforce in general was chosen because many people with mental health issues choose to go untreated rather than the risk being labelled by coworkers. Lastly, the news media were identified due to the considerable influence they have in shaping public opinion (MHCC, 2012).

Opening Minds promotes *contact-based education*, which the international literature has identified as one of the most promising practices for reducing stigma. It involves individuals with lived experience of mental illness sharing their personal stories of illness, stigma, and recovery" (MHCC, 2012, p. 33). Whenever possible, *Opening Minds* builds on already-existing programs. "The goal is to replicate successful programs, sharing toolkits and resources with other organizations across the country" (MHCC, 2012, p. 33). *Opening Minds* evaluates projects and identifies those most effective at reducing stigma, in order to identify best practices that can be adopted in antistigma resources (MHCC, 2013c).

Position Statement on Depression and Stigma by Beyondblue (2012)

This document, issued by the Australian government–supported advocacy group Beyondblue, identifies different types of stigma associated with mental illness: personal stigma, perceived stigma, self-stigma, and structural stigma. Beyondblue notes how vital it is to educate about all stigmas associated with mental disorders and promotes research on how to reduce discrimination. It outlines three major approaches: educational approaches, contact approaches, and protest approaches (Beyondblue, 2012).

Needs Assessment of Programs and Services of Mentally Disordered Offenders (MDOs) in Saskatchewan (2012)

In 2012, the *Mental Health Strategy for Corrections in Canada* pointed out the double stigmatization of being mental ill and being an offender (Correctional Service Canada, Federal–Provincial/Territorial Partnership, 2012). In Saskatchewan, a province-wide needs assessment of MDO was conducted to identify and understand the complex needs of the MDO population (Kent-Wilkinson et al., 2012a). Data were collected through online surveys and interviews. Interviews with family members of offenders alluded to the stigmatization of Aboriginals in the correctional systems. As one woman stated, "My son has not been recognized in the court system. The judge looks blankly at him: 'Just another Indian, just one of those.' They don't understand...." (p. 8). A thematic analysis of findings from the *Needs Assessment* in Saskatchewan showed a triple stigmatization regarding individuals who are offenders, mentally ill, and Aboriginal (in terms of racial description) (Kent-Wilkinson et al., 2012a). Families of offenders spoke to a further stigmatization of being poor: "It's hard enough being First Nations—but there's lots of poor bashing on the outside—we're bums, trouble makers. They get no skills on the inside, we need sensitivity training in this area for social services, police, and officers that deal with the mentally ill" (Kent-Wilkinson et al., 2012a, p. 8). The qualitative interview data were not only rich with statements describing the issues but also revealed what interventions were needed (Kent-Wilkinson et al., 2012a).

The Canadian Community Health Survey: Mental Health (2012)

The *Mental Health Stigma and Discrimination Report* of this large community health survey found that 4 out of 10 people who had had unmet mental health treatment needs preferred to manage things on their own. The reason may lie in the stigma still associated with mental health problems (Statistics Canada, 2013c). Statistics Canada is conducting a test of new survey modules on mental health stigma and discrimination.

CULTURAL COMPETENCE AND CULTURAL SAFETY

Cultural competence in the workplace can be viewed as "a set of congruent behaviours, attitudes, and policies that come together in a system, agency, or among professionals, and enables…[them] to work effectively in cross-cultural situations" (RNAO, 2007, p. 19). It embraces the values of inclusivity, respect, the valuing of differences, equity, and commitment (RNAO, 2007, p. 19). It is both process and outcome oriented (Alexander, 2008). Obtaining cultural competence, however, is an ongoing, lifelong process, not an end point (Campinha-Bacote, 2011). Cultural competence is considered an entry-to-practice competence that is evident in quality practice environments and improves health outcomes. According to the CNA (2010), cultural competence and cultural safety are prerequisites for working effectively in global health.

> **KEY CONCEPT** The CNA believes that **cultural competence** is the application of knowledge, skills, attitudes, and personal attributes required by nurses to maximize respectful relationships with diverse populations of patients (patients may be individuals, families, groups, or populations) and coworkers. "Underlying values for cultural competence are inclusivity, respect, valuing differences, equity and commitment" (CNA, 2010; RNAO, 2007, p. 19).

Responsibilities of Health Care Professionals for Providing Culturally Competent Care

Canadian nurses provide care for a multicultural group of patients whose needs and expectations are diverse. The CNA (2010) expects nurses to use their knowledge and skills to maximize respectful relationships with all patients. Accommodating cultural differences, particularly in terms of how mental illness is understood and conceived, requires skill and sensitivity. Effective communication and developing understanding can result in the creation of appropriate treatment plans that will improve adherence and, thus, more positive health outcomes (CNA, 2010).

It is imperative that a nurse is culturally competent whether he or she is caring for a patient with cancer or a patient with suicidal behaviour disorder (Kersey-Matusiak, 2012). Cultural competence is an ongoing process and requires continuous skill development, self-evaluation, and growing knowledge about different cultural groups (Kersey-Matusiak, 2012). In order to determine someone's cultural competence, one cultural competency model directs nurses to ask themselves questions based on a series of five constructs that form the acronym ASKED: awareness, skill, knowledge, encounters, and desire (Kersey-Matusiak, 2012). First, nurses must be aware of their own cultural biases, knowledge, and skills. Next, there needs to be a willingness to encounter culturally diverse groups. Finally, nurses must have the desire to be culturally competent. It has been shown that better nurse–patient communication and adherence to treatment have been attributed to being culturally competent (Kersey-Matusiak, 2012).

Nurses must strive to understand the way people of various cultures think, feel, behave, and respond when it comes to matters of health. This can be especially difficult because the cultural face of Canada continues to change, and we have a larger range of ethnicity, language, and country of origin than ever before (CNA, 2010).

Becoming culturally competent requires "continuous self-evaluation, skill development, and knowledge building about culturally diverse groups" (Kersey-Matusiak, 2012, p. 34). The quality of the nurse–patient relationship may even determine whether a patient returns for care in the future. "Evidence shows that having cultural competency skills promotes better nurse–patient communication" (Kersey-Matusiak, 2012), and for the nurse it can be the difference between treatment of mental illness or the ignorance of a mental condition due to a limited nursing relationship.

> **● STUDY NOTE**
> Cultural competence of the nurse impacts many aspects of care, including assessment and communicating the meaning of signs and symptoms to patients and families.

Cultural Safety

Cultural safety is comprised of three components: cultural awareness, cultural sensitivity and cultural competence (CNA, 2010; RNAO, 2007). While cultural competence is an important concept, it cannot necessarily account for systemic barriers, which makes it inadequate to fully address health care inequities. Cultural safety, however, "promotes greater equity in health and health care as it addresses the root causes of health inequities" (CNA, 2010). See Boxes 3-3 and 3-4 for research on cultural safety and research on the integration of cultural competence skills into educational curricula.

> **KEY CONCEPT** **Cultural safety** is both a process and an outcome whose goal is greater equity. It focuses on root causes of "power imbalances and inequitable social relationships in health care" (Aboriginal Nurses Association et al., 2009; Kirkham & Browne, 2006, as cited in Browne et al., 2009, p. 168).

BOX
3-3 **Research for Best Practice**

CULTURAL SAFETY

Josewski, V. (2012). Analysing 'cultural safety' in mental health policy reform: Lessons from British Columbia, Canada. Critical Public Health, 22(2), 223–234.

The Question: How can culturally safe mental health policy and practices be fostered in the political realm?

Method: Drawing on a critical policy review and ethnographic interviews with four community-based Aboriginal organizations and one health authority, cultural safety is used as a critical lens to discuss emerging tensions within the context of regional Aboriginal mental health care reform in British Columbia.

Findings: The results of this study draw attention to the intersecting ways that dominant sociohistorical and political ideologies undermine cultural safety in decision-making and funding practices. Situations of cultural risk are thereby created for Aboriginal people working within the area of Aboriginal mental health and, by extension, for Aboriginal people who are seeking mental health and addiction care. The insights gained from this research contribute to the ongoing dialogue regarding how to foster culturally safe mental health policy and practice and for action in the political realm (Josewski, 2012, p. 223).

Implications: In response to the mental health disparities experienced by Aboriginal people and related inequities regarding the accessibility to appropriate mental health care, there has been a shift in health policy to endorse "By Indigenous for Indigenous" health care delivery models (Josewski, 2012, p. 223). In Canada, this has resulted in the creation of new mechanisms for Aboriginal participation in health care planning by health authorities, with the goal of fostering culturally safe mental health and addiction care. Yet, there is a growing concern about the effects of neoliberal cost concerns in health policy on the effective implementation of such progressive reform ideas (Josewski, 2012, p. 223).

BOX
3-4 **Research for Best Practice**

INTEGRATING CULTURAL COMPETENCE INTO THE NURSING CURRICULUM

Chircop, A., Edgecombe, N., Hayward, K., Ducey-Gilbert, C., & Sheppard-LeMoine, D. (2013). Evaluating the integration of cultural competence skills into health and physical assessment tools: A survey of Canadian schools of nursing. Journal of Transcultural Nursing, 24(2), 195–203.

The Question: Are cultural competence skills being integrated effectively by the use of audiovisual (AV) teaching tools in teaching health and physical assessment?

Method: To understand the current approach to teaching health and physical assessment, it was necessary to identify commonly used AV teaching tools and then evaluate each tool. This study used a two-part descriptive quantitative method design: (1) Survey of schools of nursing across Canada and (2) the identified AV teaching tools were evaluated for content and modelling of cultural competence.

Findings: The reviewed AV teaching tools did not contain any learning objectives that promoted cross-cultural skills, such as asking permission before performing physical exams, using an interpreter, or asking questions regarding sexual orientation. The failure to include cultural competency components in teaching materials affects learning and risks marginalizing diverse groups. Any identification of culturally specific examples given during the videos was superficial and did not provide students with a comprehensive understanding of necessary culturally competent skills.

Implications: A culturally competent health care workforce remains needed. To educate such a workforce, health educators need appropriate teaching tools that effectively integrate cultural competence into all aspects of curricula.

SOCIOECONOMIC CONTEXT OF MENTAL HEALTH CARE

The determinants of health, factors that influence our health status, are greatly affected by sociocultural and socioeconomic circumstances. Factors such as income and social status, social support networks, education, employment, and working conditions, physical environment, and health services affect one's well-being. Although Canada consistently ranks in the top five on the United Nations (UN) Human Development Index, Canadian Aboriginal children rank 78th (PovNet, 2006).

What Makes Us Healthy?

In 2013, the Canadian Medical Association conducted wide-ranging consultations through a series of town hall meetings to gather input on Canadians' views on the social determinants of health. The process sought to identify what factors, beyond the health care system, influenced health, what mitigated against the negative determinants, what government and heath care providers could do, and how equal access could be achieved (CMA, 2013). Four main social determinants of health were identified: income, housing, nutrition and food security, and early childhood development. One key finding was that mental health issues were "the elephant in the room," and they underlie many of the social determinants of health (CMA, 2013). Addressing the problems underlying the social determinants of health was seen as the collective responsibility of government, health professionals, and society at large.

Poverty in Canada

Poverty changes a population's ability to make choices. **Poverty** is the lack of income necessary to meet the basic necessities of life as defined by the society in which one lives (Williamson & Reutter, 1999). A broader definition of poverty used by the Policy Research Initiative, a research institute providing advice to Human Resources and Social Development Canada (Canadian Mental Health Association [CMHA], 2007), is as follows: "Nationally and internationally, there is growing recognition that poverty involves more than just income deprivation. It can also extend to (or result from) exclusion from essential goods and services, meaningful employment and decent earnings, adequate and affordable housing, safe neighbourhoods with public amenities, health and well-being, social networks, and basic human rights" (CMHA, 2007).

Poverty and Mental Health

People with mental illness often live in chronic poverty. Moreover, poverty can be a significant risk factor for poor physical and mental health. The relationship between poverty and mental illness is both straightforward and complex. Understanding this relationship is key to addressing poverty, promoting mental health, and supporting the recovery of persons with mental illness (CMHA, 2007). For persons who are poor and predisposed to developing a mental illness, a loss of income, employment, and housing can increase the chance of their developing a mental illness or, if recovered, of relapsing (CMHA, 2007). Conversely, people with serious mental illness encounter many barriers, not the least of which is the fact that discrimination against persons with mental illness can prevent them from securing education, housing, and employment (CMHA, 2007). Further, developing a mental illness can seriously interrupt a person's education or career path, which leads to fewer and less secure employment opportunities and, correspondingly, a lower income. As a result, some people, particularly those with a recurrent mental illness, drift into poverty (CMHA, 2007). See Chapter 2 for information on homelessness and the mentally ill in Canada.

> **KEY CONCEPT Poverty** is the lack of income and access to essential goods and services, housing, and employment required to meet the basic necessities of life relative to one's society.

● **STUDY NOTE**
Mental illness puts a person at greater risk for poverty and homelessness, which, in turn, places serious constraints on regaining and maintaining health. While addressing poverty and homelessness is outside the realm of health care systems, nurses should be aware of the impact of poverty and homelessness on mental health and be able to identify relevant policy changes that could be enacted in both public and private spheres (MHCC, 2012).

Needed: A Federal Action Plan to Eradicate Child and Family Poverty in Canada (2012)

This document called on the federal government to take the lead in reducing child and family poverty. The report offers a range of policy recommendations to all political parties (Campaign 2000, 2012). Currently, one out of six Canadian children lives in poverty, and this figure does not

include the First Nations communities, where one in every four children grows up in poverty (Campaign 2000, 2006).

Making the Case for Investing in Mental Health in Canada (2010)

The purpose of this study by the Mental Health Commission of Canada (MHCC, 2013b) was to determine the number of Canadians living with mental health problems and the associated costs. Using a unique model based on a wide range of existing studies in Canada and internationally, the study identified effective interventions and key reasons why governments should invest in mental health (MHCC, 2013b). For instance, the study effectively argued that investing in mental health contributes to Canada's economy and improves the sustainability of the health care system. Each year, 20% of Canadians experience a mental health problem or illness at the cost of over $50 billion to the economy. This represents 2.8% of the 2011 Gross Domestic Product (MHCC, 2013b, 2013d; Smetanin et al., 2011). Increased attention to mental health programming in Canada would reduce limitations caused by mental disorders and prevent early problems from developing into larger problems and ultimately improve overall quality of life (MHCC, 2013b).

The Life and Economic Impact of Major Mental Illnesses in Canada: 2011 to 2041

The objective of this study was to determine the economic impact of major mental illnesses in Canada, beginning in 2011 and annually over the next three decades (Smetanin et al., 2011). For 2011, the cost of mental illness was $42.3 billion in direct costs and $6.3 billion in indirect costs. Over the next 30 years, the impact will be magnified due to the expected increase in the number of people living with mental illness (due to aging and population growth). Within a generation, more than 8.9 million Canadians will have a mental illness (Smetanin et al., 2011).

Socioeconomic Influences on Aboriginal Mental Health

Although Canada is considered to have one of the finest publicly funded health care systems, Aboriginal populations continue to exhibit morbidity and mortality rates in some dimensions in excess of some Third World countries. According to the United Nations Human Development Index, Canada's indigenous population ranks low in comparison with the country as a whole (Mikkonen & Raphael, 2010). The gap in life expectancy between First Nations individuals and other Canadians is 7 years less for First Nations men and 5 years less for First Nations women. In 2010, the average life expectancy of a Canadian was 79 years for men and 83 years for women. Among the Aboriginal population, the Inuit have the lowest life expectancy of 64 years for men and 73 years for women (Health Canada, 2010a).

Socioeconomic Status and the Criminal Justice System

There has long been a connection between socioeconomic status and involvement with the criminal justice system, in which Aboriginal people are overrepresented. The prevalence of mental disorder among those in the criminal justice system is significantly higher than is found in the general population (Correctional Service Canada, 2009; Office of the Correctional Investigator, 2013). The Aboriginal incarceration rate is 10 times higher than the national average. Although Aboriginal people represent about 4% of the Canadian population, 22% of the total federal inmate population is of Aboriginal ancestry. Current sentencing trends combined with a growing and youthful demographic indicate that the overrepresentation of Aboriginal people in Canada's correctional system is likely to grow (OCI, 2013; Statistics Canada, 2013a). Findings of a needs assessment by Kent-Wilkinson and colleagues (2012b) revealed that family and frontline respondents saw a lack of culturally relevant forensic programming as a factor in the criminality or recidivism of Aboriginal offenders. Family members believed that the presence of cultural programs made a positive difference during incarceration. Continued focus on cultural elements for indigenous offenders is needed to reduce recidivism (Kent-Wilkinson et al., 2012b). Cultural programming, ongoing support, and involvement of elders, Aboriginal liaison officers, community representatives, and Aboriginal organizations is essential for closing the outcome gaps for First Nations, Métis, and Inuit offenders (OCI, 2006).

Disparities in Health Outcomes

The disparities in health outcomes between Aboriginal and other Canadians are stark. Many First Nation and Inuit communities have higher unemployment, lower income, lower levels of education, overcrowded houses, and higher poverty in comparison with the rest of Canada (Statistics Canada, 2013a). Aboriginal people have higher rates of premature deaths—no small concern in the only group in Canada having a natural population increase (Statistics Canada, 2013a). They also experience higher disease rates, including HIV/AIDS (Public Health Agency of Canada [PHAC], 2010). Aboriginal youth are at much higher risk of contracting HIV than non-Aboriginal youth, and Aboriginal women in particular are overrepresented in the HIV/AIDS population. From 1998 to 2008, "women represented 48.8% of all positive HIV test reports among Aboriginal people as compared with 20.6% of reports among those of other ethnicities" (PHAC, 2010).

Aboriginal people also have significantly higher rates of mental health problems and suicide compared with the general population (Health Canada, 2010a). The rate of suicide among Aboriginals is 2.1 times the national rate. For First Nations youth and adults (up to age 44 years), suicide and self-inflicted injuries are the leading causes of death. For Inuit youth, suicide rates "are among the highest in the world, at 11 times the national average" (Health Canada, 2010a).

GEOGRAPHIC LOCATION AND ACCESS TO MENTAL HEALTH SERVICES

Although comprehensiveness, universality, portability, and accessibility are key components of the *Canada Health Act* (Government of Canada, 2013; Health Canada, 2010a), getting mental health services to rural and isolated communities continues to be a challenge. Most mental health services are located in urban areas, with access for people in the far North being very different from that of people living in the more highly populated areas of Canada. All age groups in rural areas have limited access to health care, but the lack of resources is particularly problematic for children and elderly people, who have specialized needs.

According to the 2011 census, 80% of Canadians live in urban areas (Statistics Canada, 2013d). Transportation is a major barrier to the receipt of health services in rural areas. For instance, past reports of the Office of the Auditor General (2008) have noted that 121 First Nations communities have no road access, and an additional 75 communities with road access were more than 90 km from the nearest physician. Costs of travel and accommodation for patients and families can be high, in dollars and energy. Services should be delivered in communities where possible, but the small population of some rural communities can be a deterrent. As well, specialized services are located in large urban centres (Office of the Auditor General of Canada, 2008). Mobile service delivery and specialist circuits are one option used to address this issue (Statistics Canada, 2013d).

Telehealth has been effective. Telehealth is the use of electronic information and communication technologies to support health care services over distance. It ranges from the retrieval of laboratory results or other health records posted on a network to the assessment of a person by a psychiatrist through videoconferencing.

The Role of Nurses in Rural and Remote Areas and in the North

The role of nurses takes on new dimensions in rural and remote areas or in Canada's north, where they are often the only or the most accessible health care professionals, and thus the primary health care providers. Nurses in these regions often practise in expanded roles, acting as the first point of contact in the health system. These nurses may be advocates, collaborators, or mediators in encouraging the development of public policies and resources for their region. Furthermore, nurse practitioners are increasingly recognized as serving a unique role in meeting the needs of people living in rural and remote areas and in the north.

■ THE LEGAL CONTEXT OF MENTAL HEALTH CARE

Every society needs laws to achieve its objectives. According to the WHO (2005a), the fundamental aim of mental health legislation is to protect, promote, and improve the lives and mental well-being of citizens.

Human Rights and Mental Illness

In accordance with the objectives of the *UN Charter* and international agreements, a fundamental basis for mental health legislation is human rights. Key rights and principles include equality and nondiscrimination, the right to privacy and individual autonomy, freedom from inhuman and degrading treatment, the principle of the least restrictive environment, and the rights to information and participation.

In 2010, Canada ratified the United Nations' *Convention on the Rights of Persons With Disabilities (CRPD)*. This provided a new touchstone for legislation, policies, and regulations affecting people living with mental health problems. "The CRPD is rooted in a social model of disability, a 'paradigm shift' in which disability is understood to arise from the ways in which external environments interact with people, and not just as a result of a person's condition" (MHCC, 2012, p. 33). As a signatory of the Convention, Canada committed to ensuring the promotion and protection of the human rights of all persons with disabilities. According to the Convention, these protections need to be implemented on a daily basis in order "to eliminate barriers to the full participation of people living with mental health problems and illnesses in schools, workplaces, and other sectors, as well as in communities in general" (MHCC, 2012, p. 33).

Around the world, persons with disabilities face discrimination, violence, and abuse. In many cases, policies and laws reinforce human rights violations (WHO, 2013). The WHO's MiNDbank, the online platform that brings together international and national resources, policies, strategies, laws, and standards for mental health and disability, promotes dialogue, debate, and research for the purposes of achieving national reforms that conform to international human rights and best practice standards (WHO, 2013).

International Agreements

There are many significant international agreements to help protect people with mental illness. The most significant are listed in Box 3-5. The rights of persons with mental illnesses and mental health principles adopted by the United Nations in 1991 (UN, 1991) are outlined in Box 3-6. See Web Links on the thePoint for information regarding national and international advocacy organizations.

Mental Health Legislation

Mental health legislation is a powerful tool for codifying and consolidating fundamental values and principles, for protecting the rights of people with mental

---

BOX 3-5 Canadian and International Agreements Relevant to Culture and to Mental Health

1948	Universal Declaration of Human Rights (United Nations, 1948)
1957	The Indigenous and Tribal Populations Convention, 1957 (No. 107)
1965	The International Convention on the Elimination of All Forms of Racial Discrimination (Canadian ratification in 1969)
1966	The International Covenant on Economic, Social, and Cultural Rights (ICESCR; Canadian ratification in 1976)
1966	The International Covenant on Civil and Political Rights (Canadian ratification in 1976)
1971	Multiculturalism policy (Canada) (Government of Canada, 2012a)
1976	International Covenant on Economic, Social, and Cultural Rights (ICESCR)
1982	Canadian Charter of Rights and Freedoms (Government of Canada, Department of Justice, 2013)
1984	Canada Health Act (Government of Canada, 2013; Health Canada, 2010b)
1886	Canada Employment Equity Act
1988	Multiculturalism Act (Canada) (Government of Canada, 2012b)
1989	Indigenous and Tribal (People Populations) Convention (Revised)
1990	Declaration of Caracas (WHO, 1990)
1991	Principles of Protection of Persons With Mental Illness (United Nations, 1991)
1997	Renewed Multiculturalism Program in Canada (Government of Canada, 2012b)
2001	Immigration and Refugee Protection Act (IRPA, 2001)
2012	Mental Health Strategy for Canada (MHCC, 2012)
2012	Mental Health Strategy for Corrections in Canada (Correctional Service Canada, Federal–Provincial/Territorial Partnership, 2012, June).

---

disorders, and for promoting the mental health of populations. It offers an important mechanism to ensure adequate and appropriate care and treatment. Being unable to access treatment and care is an infringement of a person's right to health and right to access mental health care (WHO, 2005b).

BOX 3-6 Rights of Persons With Mental Illness

- Right to medical care (Principle 1.1)
- Right to be treated with humanity and respect (Principle 1.2)
- Equal protection right (Principle 1.4)
- Right to be cared for in the community (Principle 7)
- Right to provide informed consent before receiving any treatment (Principle 11)
- Right to privacy (Principle 13)
- Freedom of communication (Principle 13)
- Freedom of religion (Principle 13)
- Right to voluntary admission (Principles 15 and 16)
- Right to judicial guarantees (Principle 17)

From United Nations. (1991). *Principles for the protection of persons with mental illness and the improvement of mental health care.* Adopted by General Assembly resolution 46/119 of 17 December 1991, Office of the United Nations High Commissioner for Human Rights. Retrieved from http://www.unhchr.ch/html/menu3/b/68.htm

Mental Health Acts in Canada

Legislation in Canada strongly influences the context of our mental health care. Each province and territory is guided by its own *Mental Health Act*. Each act must be congruent with the rights stipulated under the *1982 Charter of Rights and Freedoms* (Government of Canada, Department of Justice, 2013) and the resources to enforce the Act must be in place. See Box 3-7 for Internet access information on the various mental health acts.

Gray and O'Reilly (2001) reviewed the Mental Health Act provisions in all Canadian jurisdictions. They found significant differences among the provinces and territories and raised a concern that some provisions might prevent people from receiving appropriate care. See Box 3-8 for an overview, based on their work, of basic criteria for involuntary admission in the various jurisdictions. It is the responsibility of PMH nurses to understand the Mental Health Act of their province or territory. Nurses need to be able to explain the act's basic provisions to people with mental illness and their families.

Mental Health Acts within Canada may allow involuntary treatment of a person admitted under such an Act if the person is not considered competent to make decisions regarding treatment. **Competence**, in this respect, means being able to understand (at a basic level) matters relevant to the decision and to understand the consequences of the decision. Competence is not a fixed capacity; it changes over time. There are specific provisions within mental health acts regarding the evaluation of competency and what action may be taken if a person is deemed not competent. When a person is unable to consent to treatment, consent from a **substitute decision maker** may be sought. Depending on the jurisdiction, these substitute decision makers can be state appointed, appointed by the person when competent, or be a guardian or relative. There are different criteria to guide substitute decision making: **best interests** (e.g., treatment will make the person less ill, the person will get more ill without treatment, the benefits outweigh any risks), *capable wishes* (what the person expressed while capable, even if not in current best interests), and *modified best interests* (follow expressed wishes except if they would endanger the person or others (Gray & O'Reilly, 2001).

KEY CONCEPT A **Mental Health Act** is a law that gives certain powers and sets the conditions (including time limits) for those powers, to stipulated health care professionals and designated institutions regarding the admission and treatment of individuals with a mental disorder. It also provides a framework for mental health delivery of services and establishes rules and procedures that govern the commitment of persons suffering from mental disorders (Government of Saskatchewan, 2013).

BOX 3-7 Mental Health Acts

[Note the difference in names of the Mental Health Act in Newfoundland and Labrador, Quebec, and Saskatchewan]

Province/Territory	Website Address
Alberta	Mental Health Act
	http://www.albertahealthservices.ca/mha.asp
British Columbia	Mental Health Act
	http://www.health.gov.bc.ca/mhd/mentalhealthact.html
Manitoba	Mental Health Act
	http://web2.gov.mb.ca/laws/statutes/ccsm/m110e.php
New Brunswick	Mental Health Act
	http://www.canlii.org/en/nb/laws/stat/rsnb-1973-c-m-10/latest/rsnb-1973-c-m-10.html
Newfoundland and Labrador	Mental Health Care and Treatment Act
	http://www.health.gov.nl.ca/health/mentalhealth/mentalhealthact.html
Northwest Territories	Mental Health Act
	http://www.canlii.org/en/nu/laws/stat/rsnwt-nu-1988-c-m-10/latest/rsnwt-nu-1988-c-m-10.html
Nova Scotia	http://nslegislature.ca/legc/bills/59th_1st/1st_read/b109.htm
Nunavut	Mental Health Act
	http://www.canlii.org/en/nu/laws/stat/rsnwt-nu-1988-c-m-10/latest/rsnwt-nu-1988-c-m-10.html?search UrlHash=AAAAAQASTWVudGFsIEhlYWx0aCBBY3QgAAAAAAAE
Ontario	Mental Health Act
	http://www.e-laws.gov.on.ca/html/statutes/english/elaws_statutes_90m07_e.htm
Prince Edward Island	Mental Health Act
	http://govpe.ca/law/statutes/pdf/m-06_1.pdf
Quebec	Mental Patients Protection Act
	http://www.canlii.org/en/qc/laws/stat/rsq-c-p-41/latest/rsq-c-p-41.html
Saskatchewan	Mental Health Services Act
	http://www.publications.gov.sk.ca/details.cfm?p=626
Yukon	Mental Health Act
	http://www.gov.yk.ca/legislation/acts/mehe.pdf

BOX 3-8 Involuntary Admission Criteria in Provincial and Territorial Mental Health Acts

Is not suitable as a voluntary inpatient: A person who is willing and capable of consenting to a voluntary admission cannot be admitted with an involuntary status anywhere in Canada.

Meets the definition of mental disorder: The person must have a mental disorder. In many, but not all of the jurisdictions, it is specified that the disorder must seriously impair the person's functioning.

Meets the criteria for harm: In most jurisdictions, this is not limited to serious bodily harm; nonbodily harms are acceptable. The criterion of "danger" stipulated in some acts, however, has been interpreted by the courts to mean bodily harm.

Likely to suffer substantial mental or physical deterioration: This is included in some provinces (British Columbia, Saskatchewan, Manitoba, and Ontario) as an alternative to the harm criterion.

In need of psychiatric treatment: This is a criterion in British Columbia, Saskatchewan, and Ontario. It is possible in other jurisdictions to commit a person with a mental disorder who is dangerous, but for whom there is no treatment (e.g., antisocial personality disorder) for the purpose of preventative detention.

Refusal of treatment: By the person after admission: This is allowed in some jurisdictions but not others. In some jurisdictions, a refusal can be overruled in the person's best interests.

Review and appeal procedures regarding the validity of involuntary hospitalization: These are found in all jurisdictions.

Source: Gray, J. & O'Reilly, R. (2001). Clinically significant differences among Canadian Mental Health Acts. *Canadian Journal of Psychiatry, 46*, 315–321.

Mandatory Outpatient Treatment

In some jurisdictions, an involuntary patient may return to the community on a *conditional leave* if the admission criteria are still met and if stipulations for treatment are followed. If the stipulations (e.g., taking medication and meeting with a physician) are not followed, the person can be returned to the hospital. **Mandatory outpatient treatment (MOT)** involves legal provisions requiring people with a mental illness to comply with a treatment plan while living in the community (O'Reilly et al., 2003). A **community treatment order (CTO)**, a form of MOT, is an order to provide a comprehensive plan of community-based treatment to someone with a serious mental disorder. They are only issued for persons with severe mental illness and with a history of hospitalization who have been examined by a physician and been deemed in need of continuing treatment and care while residing in the community (Canadian Mental Health Association [CMHA], 2013). (See Box 3-9 for information regarding provincial and territorial CTOs.) CTOs are less restrictive than being detained in a psychiatric facility and serve as an alternative to hospitalization (CMHA, 2013).

BOX 3-9 Community Treatment Orders

Province	Website
Alberta	health.alberta.ca/newsroom/community-treatment-orders-MHA.html
British Columbia	francais.ccamhr.ca/resources/Community_Treatment_Orders_Alternatives.pdf
Manitoba	cpa-apc.org:8080/publications/archives/cjp/2005/january/obrien.asp
New Brunswick	ncbi.nlm.nih.gov/pmc/articles/PMC2871234
Newfoundland and Labrador	health.gov.nl.ca/health/mentalhealth/mentalhealthact.html
Nova Scotia	ncbi.nlm.nih.gov/pubmed/15600067 novascotia.ca/dhw/mental-health/documents/ipta/form9_Community_Treatment_Order.pdf
Ontario	health.gov.on.ca/en/public/programs/hepatitis/docs/cto_review_report.pdf
Saskatchewan	health.gov.sk.ca/mental-health-personal-rights

The CTO plan identifies the conditions that must be met by the individual and support system (e.g., family, friends, and health care professionals) in order to stay out of the hospital. CTOs often involve intense case management support provided by nurse managers.

For the better part of a decade, doctors and psychiatrists in most provinces in Canada have been able to issue community treatment orders compelling mentally ill patients to accept treatment, medication, and supervision as a condition of living in the community (Rynor, 2010).

All Canadian jurisdictions, with the exception of New Brunswick and the three Territories, authorize the use of community treatment orders or variations such as extended leave provisions (Rynor).

Separate from mental health legislation are the legal provisions that can require people to follow treatment as a condition of probation. The law allows for persons to be found *Not Criminally Responsible due to a Mental Disorder* for an offence if they are suffering from a mental disorder that makes them incapable of appreciating the nature of the act or knowing that what they did was wrong. In these cases, the mentally ill offender needs to comply with treatment monitored by the Criminal Code Review Boards (see Chapter 38).

● **STUDY NOTE**

In Canada, the laws governing mandated commitment and treatment for major mental disorders are at the provincial level. Nurses need to understand and be able to communicate to patients and their families the core provisions of the Mental Health Act of the province/territory in which they practise (see Box 3-7).

■ RESEARCH AND THE CONTEXT OF MENTAL HEALTH CARE

Many health professionals, advocacy groups, and policy analysts believe that greater support for research on the context of mental health issues is urgently required. "There is good evidence that culture, language, ethnicity, and religion influence the causes, manifestations, and course of mental disorders, including symptomatology and illness experience, attributions and explanations for distress, help seeking and coping, treatment adherence and response" (Gone & Kirmayer, 2010, as cited in Kirmayer, 2012, p. 251). Failure to understand these issues poses a serious threat to the health of Canadian communities. Such research should include studies on methodologies to identify the determinants of mental health disorders, to explore the prevalence of preventable causative factors related to mental illness, to determine the nature and extent of barriers to access to mental health treatment and care, and to determine whether mental health legislation is effective (Arboleda-Florez, 2005).

The Need for Evidence-Based Practice

To date, mental health services have offered a great variety of treatments, "some outlandish and all making claims of efficacy that often far exceed any evidence" (Kirmayer, 2012, p. 249). Evidence-based practice (EBP) promises a better foundation for mental health delivery, services, and outcomes. According to Kirmayer, EBP involves: "(i) an epistemological commitment to science as a method of generating evidence; (ii) a professional commitment to base clinical practice on scientific research and rational decision making; and (iii) a political commitment to use science to guide health policy and services and to arbitrate and challenge the influences of marketing and other vested interests" (pp. 249–250).

The Need for Research on the Effectiveness of Cultural Competence

Within mental health care, cultural competence is viewed as a strategy to respond to the diversity of patient needs and a way of reducing mental health disparities in terms of access to patient-centred care. However, there is little evidence thus far to indicate how cultural competence affects clinical outcomes (Kirmayer, 2012). The Canadian Nurses Association welcomes further research on cultural competence and cultural safety within the Canadian health care context. A number of projects, initiatives, studies, and guidelines are being developed on local, provincial, territorial, regional and federal levels to promote cultural competence and safety in nursing (CNA, 2010).

Further Research Into the Causes of Mental Illness

The Mental Health Strategy of Canada, 2012 notes "there is no single cause of any mental health problem or illness, and no one is immune, no matter where they live, how old or young they are or their social standing" (para 11). Research to date suggests that mental health issues and illnesses are the result of a complex mix of social, economic, psychological, biologic, and genetic factors. Ongoing research continues to expand our understanding of these factors (MHCC, 2012).

SUMMARY OF KEY POINTS

■ The term *culture* is defined as a way of life that manifests the learned beliefs, values, and accepted behaviours that are transmitted socially within a specific group.

■ Cultural safety consists of cultural awareness, cultural sensitivity, and cultural competence. It is an obligation of all Canadian nurses.

■ Aboriginal mental illness and disorders encompass the recognition of the historical, socioeconomic, and political circumstances of Aboriginal people in Canada. Mental health issues as experienced by Aboriginal people may be related to one or all of the life experiences historically confronting Aboriginal people.

■ Stigmatization occurs as a result of prejudice, discrimination, and stereotyping. Cultural groups and people with mental illness are often stigmatized.

■ Religious beliefs are closely intertwined with beliefs about health and mental illness.

■ Mental health services should be integrated as completely as possible into the helping systems currently accepted by the culture.

■ Access to mental health treatment is particularly limited for those living in rural, remote, and northern areas or for those living in poverty.

■ Progressive legislation can be an effective tool to promote access to mental health care as well as to promote and protect the rights of people with mental disorders.

CRITICAL THINKING CHALLENGES

1 Discuss to what extent "culture counts" in the treatment of mental illness and Aboriginal health in Canada.
2 Compare access to mental health services in rural and urban areas in your province or territory.
3 What does poverty look like in your local community?
4 Discuss the influence of socioeconomic factors on the mental health of Canadians.

5 Compare Canada's mental health legislation to international initiatives.

6 Outline the basic tenets of the Mental Health Act of your province or territory.

7 In your opinion, what type of research would make the greatest impact on improving the context of Canadian mental health care?

REFERENCES

Aboriginal Affairs and Northern Development Canada. (2013). *A history of Indian and Northern Affairs Canada. Government of Canada*. Retrieved from http://www.aadnc-aandc.gc.ca/eng/1314977281262/1314977321448

Aboriginal Health Glossary. (2004). *Aboriginal health and cultural diversity online glossary*. Compiled by A. Kent-Wilkinson & M. Tomtene. http://www.usask.ca/nursing/aboriginalglossary

Aboriginal Nurses Association of Canada, Canadian Association of Schools of Nursing, & Canadian Nurses Association. (2009). *Cultural competence and cultural safety in nursing education*. Ottawa, ON: Aboriginal Nurses Association of Canada.

Alexander, G. R. (2008). Cultural competence models in nursing. *Critical Care Nursing Clinics of North America, 20*(4), 415–442.

American Psychiatric Association. (1994). *Diagnostic and statistical manual of mental disorders (DSM -IV)* (4th ed). Washington, DC: Author.

American Psychiatric Association. (2013a). *Cultural concepts in DSM-5*. Arlington, VA: American Psychiatric Publishing. Retrieved from http://www.psychiatry.org/File%20Library/Practice/DSM/DSM-5/Cultural-Concepts-in-DSM-5.pdf

American Psychiatric Association. (2013b). *Diagnostic and statistical manual of mental Disorders* (5th ed). Arlington, VA: American Psychiatric Publishing.

Arboleda-Florez, J. (2003). Considerations on the stigma of mental illness. *Canadian Journal of Psychiatry, 48*(10), 645–650.

Arboleda-Florez, J. (2005). The epidemiology of mental illness in Canada. *Canadian Public Policy. Analyse de Politiques, 31*, S13–S16.

Austin, W., Gallop, R., McCay, E., Peternelj-Taylor, C., & Bayer, M. (1999). Culturally competent care for psychiatric patients who have a history of sexual abuse. *Clinical Nursing Research, 8*(1), 5–25.

Beyondblue. (2012). *Stigma and discrimination associated with depression and anxiety* [Position statement]. Retrieved from http://www.beyondblue.org

Brascoupé, S., & Waters, C. (2009). Cultural safety: Exploring the applicability of the concept of cultural safety to Aboriginal health and community wellness. *Journal of Aboriginal Health, 5*(2), 6–41.

Brasfield, C. R. (2001). Residential school syndrome. *BC Medical Journal, 43*(2), 78–81.

Browne, A. J., Varcoe, C., Smye, V., Reimer-Kirkham, S., Lynam, M. J., & Wong, S. (2009). Cultural safety and the challenges of translating critically oriented knowledge in practice. *Nursing Philosophy, 10*(3), 167–179.

Campaign 2000. (2006). *Oh Canada! Too many children in poverty for too long… 2006 Report card on child and family poverty in Canada*. Retrieved from http://www.campaign2000.ca/reportcards.html

Campaign 2000. (2012). *National report cards. 2012 Report Card. End child and family poverty in Canada*. Retrieved from http://www.campaign2000.ca/reportcards.html

Campinha-Bacote J. (2011). The process of cultural competence in the delivery of health care services. In M. K. Douglas & D. F. Pacquiao (Eds.), *Core curriculum for transcultural nursing and health care*. Thousand Oaks, CA: Sage Publications.

Canadian Medical Association. (2013). *Health care in Canada: What makes us sick?* Town Hall Report. Winnipeg, MB: CMA.

Canadian Mental Health Association. (2007) *Poverty and mental illness*. Retrieved from http://ontario.cmha.ca/public_policy/poverty-and-mental-illness/

Canadian Mental Health Association. (2013). *Community treatment orders (CTO's)*. Retrieved from http://durham.cmha.ca/programs_services/community-treatment-orders/

Canadian Nurses Association. (2010). *Promoting cultural competence in nursing* [Position statement]. Retrieved from http://www.cna-aiic.ca/~/media/cna/page%20content/pdf%20en/2013/07/26/10/37/ps114_cultural_competence_2010_e.pdf

Chircop, A., Edgecombe, N., Hayward, K., Ducey-Gilbert, C., & Sheppard-LeMoine, D. (2013). Evaluating the integration of cultural competence skills into health and physical assessment tools: A survey of Canadian schools of nursing. *Journal of Transcultural Nursing, 24*(2), 195–203.

Citizenship and Immigration Canada. (2010). *Annual report on the operation of the Canadian Multiculturalism Act 2007–2008*. Retrieved from http://www.cic.gc.ca/english/pdf/pub/multi-report2008.pdf

Correctional Service Canada. (2009). *Aboriginal community development in corrections: Demographic overview of Aboriginal peoples in Canada and Aboriginal offenders in federal corrections*. Retrieved from http://www.csc-scc.gc.ca/text/prgrm/abinit/know/10-eng.shtml

Correctional Service Canada, Federal–Provincial/Territorial Partnership. (2012). *Mental health strategy for corrections in Canada*. Retrieved from http://www.csc-scc.gc.ca/health/092/MH-strategy-eng.pdf

Foucault, M. (1967). *Madness and civilization: A history of insanity in the age of reason*. (R. Howard, Trans.). London, UK: Tavistock Publications.

Geertz, C. (1973). *The interpretation of cultures: Selected essays*. New York, NY: Basic Books.

Goffman, I. (1963). *Stigma: Notes on the management of spoiled identity*. Englewood Cliffs, NJ: Prentice Hall.

Government of Canada. (2012a). *Evaluation of the multiculturalism program*. Retrieved from http://www.cic.gc.ca/english/resources/evaluation/multi/section3.asp

Government of Canada. (2012b). *Canadian multiculturalism: An inclusive citizenship*. Retrieved from http://www.cic.gc.ca/english/multiculturalism/citizenship.asp

Government of Canada. (2013). *Canada Health Act, 1984. c. 6, s. 1*. Retrieved from Justice Laws Web site: http://laws-lois.justice.gc.ca/eng/acts/C-6/FullText.html

Government of Canada, Department of Justice. (2013). *Canadian Charter of Rights and Freedoms*. Ottawa, ON: Author.

Government of Saskatchewan. (2003). *Glossary*. Government Relations and Aboriginal Affairs (GS-GRAA). Regina, SK: Author.

Government of Saskatchewan. (2013). *Mental Health Services Act of Saskatchewan M-13.1*. Regina, SK: Publications Centre. Retrieved from http://www.publications.gov.sk.ca/details.cfm?p=626

Gray, J., & O'Reilly, R. (2001). Clinically significant differences among Canadian Mental Health Acts. *Canadian Journal of Psychiatry, 46*, 315–321.

Health Canada. (2009). Commission on the future of health care in Canada: The Romanow Commission. *Romanow Report, November 28, 2002*. Retrieved from http://www.hc-sc.gc.ca/hcs-sss/hhr-rhs/strateg/romanow-eng.php

Health Canada. (2010a). *Life expectancy: Gap in life expectancy projected to decrease between Aboriginal people and the total Canadian population*. Ottawa, ON: Author.

Health Canada. (2010b). *Canada Health Act*. Ottawa, ON: Author.

Health Canada. (2013). *Indian residential schools*. Retrieved from http://www.hc-sc.gc.ca/fniah-spnia/services/indiresident/index-eng.php

International Council of Nurses. (2007). *Cultural and linguistic competence* [Position statement]. Retrieved from http://www.icn.ch/images/stories/documents/publications/position_statements/B03_Cultural_Linguistic_Competence.pdf

Johnson, D. L. & Johnson, C. A. (1965). Totally discouraged: A depressive syndrome of the Dakota Sioux. *Transcultural Psychiatry, 2*(2), 140–143.

Josewski, V. (2012). Analysing 'cultural safety' in mental health policy reform: Lessons from British Columbia, Canada. *Critical Public Health, 22*(2), 223–234.

Kent-Wilkinson, A., Sanders, S. L., Mela, M., Peternelj-Taylor, C., Adelugba, O, Luther, G., & Wormith, J. S. (2012a). *Needs assessment of forensic mental health services and programs for offenders in Saskatchewan: Executive summary*. Study conducted by Forensic Interdisciplinary Research: Saskatchewan Team (FIRST) Centre for Forensic Behavioural Sciences and Justice Studies. Saskatoon, SK: University of Saskatchewan.

Kent-Wilkinson, A., Sanders, S. L., Mela, M., Peternelj-Taylor, C., Adelugba, O., Luther, G., & Wormith, J. S. (2012b). *Needs assessment of forensic mental health services and programs for offenders in Saskatchewan: Condensed Report*. Conducted by Forensic Interdisciplinary Research: Saskatchewan Team (FIRST). Centre for Forensic Behavioural Sciences and Justice Studies. Saskatoon, SK: University of Saskatchewan.

Kersey-Matusiak, G. (2012). Culturally competent care: Are we there yet? *Nursing Management (Springhouse), 43*(4), 34–39.

Kirmayer, L. J. (2012). Cultural competence and evidence-based practice in mental health: Epistemic communities and the politics of pluralism. *Social Science and Medicine, 75*(2), 249–256.

Kirmayer, L. J., Brass, G. M., & Tait, C. L. (2000). The mental health of Aboriginal peoples: Transformations of identity and community. *Canadian Journal of Psychiatry, 45*(7), 607–616.

Mental Health Commission of Canada (MHCC). (2012). *Changing directions, changing lives: The mental health strategy for Canada*. Calgary, AB: Author.

Mental Health Commission of Canada. (MHCC). (2013a). *Stigma: What is the issue?* Calgary, AB: Author.

Mental Health Commission of Canada. (2013b). *Making the case for investing in mental health in Canada*. Calgary, AB: Author.

Mental Health Commission of Canada. (2013c). *Opening minds. Initiatives and reports*. Calgary, AB: Author. Retrieved from http://www.mental-healthcommission.ca/English/initiatives-and-projects/opening-minds?routetoken=e77f673f87ce26092879ece385b88636&terminitial=39

Mental Health Commission of Canada. (2013d). *Why investing in mental health will contribute to Canada's economic prosperity and to the sustainability of our health care system*. Calgary, AB: Author.

Mikkonen J. & Raphael, D. (2010). *Social determinants of health: The Canadian facts*. Toronto, ON: York University School of Health Policy and Management.

Office of the Auditor General of Canada. (2008). *First nations child and family services program. 2008 May: Report of the Auditor General of Canada*. Ottawa, ON: Author.

Office of the Correctional Investigator. (2006). *Report finds evidence of systemic discrimination against Aboriginal inmates in Canada's prisons*. Ottawa, ON: Author.

Office of the Correctional Investigator. (2013). *Annual report of the Office of the Correctional Investigator 2012–2013*. Ottawa, ON: Author.

O'Reilly, R., Brooks, S., Chaimowitz, G., Neilson, G., Carr, P., Zikos, E., & Beck, P. R. (2003). Mandatory outpatient treatment. *Canadian Psychiatric Association Position Paper*. Retrieved from http://ww1.cpa-apc.org:8080/publications/position_papers/mandatory.asp

Pasco, A. (2004). Cross-cultural relationships between nurses and Filipino Canadian patients. *Journal of Nursing Scholarship, 36*(3), 239–246.

PovNet. (2006). *Canadian Aboriginal children 78th on the United Nations Human Development Index*. Retrieved from http://www.povnet.org/node/116

Public Health Agency of Canada. (2006). *Appendix 1: Using the right terms. Division of Aging and Seniors*. Ottawa, ON: Author. Retrieved from http://www.phac-aspc.gc.ca/seniors-aines/pubs/communicating_aboriginal/appendix_e.htm#ab

Public Health Agency of Canada. (2010). HIV/AIDS among Aboriginal people in Canada. In *HIV/AIDS Epi Updates* (Chapter 8). Ottawa, ON: Author.

Registered Nurses' Association of Ontario (RNAO). (2007). *Embracing cultural diversity in health care: Developing cultural competence*. Toronto, ON: Author.

Richardson, D. (2008). Cultural safety: An introduction. *Paediatric Nursing, 20*(2), 39–43.

Royal Commission of Aboriginal Peoples. (1996). *Final report*. Ottawa, ON: Communication Group.

Rynor, B. (2010). Value of community treatment orders remains at issue. *Canadian Medical Association Journal, 182*(8), E337–E338.

Skip Knox, E. L. (2004). *History of western civilization*. Retrieved from http://history.boisestate.edu/westciv/plague/10.shtml

Smetanin, P., Stiff, D., Briante, C., Adair, C. E., Ahmad, S., & Khan, M. (2011). *The life and economic impact of major mental illnesses in Canada: 2011 to 2041*. RiskAnalytica, on behalf of the Mental Health Commission of Canada.

Social Progress Imperative. (2014). Social Progress Index: Canada. Retrieved from http://www.socialprogressimperative.org/data/spi/countries/CAN

Srivastava, R. (Ed.) (2007). *The healthcare professional's guide to clinical cultural competence*. Toronto, ON: Mosby Elsevier.

Standing Senate Committee on Social Affairs, Science and Technology. (2006). *Out of the shadows at last: Transforming mental health, mental illness*

and addiction services in Canada. Ottawa, ON: Author. Retrieved from http://www.parl.gc.ca/Content/SEN/Committee/391/soci/rep/pdf/rep02may06part1-e.pdf

Statistics Canada. (2013a). *Aboriginal peoples in Canada: First Nations people, Métis and Inuit*, 2011. Retrieved from http://www12.statcan.gc.ca/nhs-enm/2011/as-sa/99-011-x/99-011-x2011001-eng.cfm

Statistics Canada. (2013b). High level indicators. *Aboriginal Peoples Survey 2012*. Retrieved from http://www23.statcan.gc.ca/imdb-bmdi/document/3250_D5_T9_V1-eng.htm

Statistics Canada. (2013c). *Canadian community health survey: Mental health, 2012* Government of Canada. Ottawa, ON: Author.

Statistics Canada. (2013d). *National Household Survey, 2011*. Ottawa, ON: Author.

Thira, D. (2005). *Beyond the four waves of colonization*. Retrieved from http://www.swaraj.org/fourwaves.htm

United Nations. (1948). *Universal declaration of human rights*. Geneva, Switzerland: Author. Retrieved from http://www.un.org/Overview/rights.html

United Nations. (1991). *Principles for the protection of persons with mental illness and the improvement of mental health care*. Adopted by General Assembly resolution 46/119 of 17 December 1991, Office of the United Nations High Commissioner for Human Rights. Geneva, Switzerland: Author.

Vedantam, S. (2005). Patients' diversity is often discounted: Alternatives to mainstream medical treatment call for recognizing ethnic, social differences. Mind and culture: Psychiatry's missing diagnosis. *Washington Post, A01*. Retrieved from http://www.washingtonpost.com/wp-dyn/content/article/2005/06/25/AR2005062500982.html

Waldram, J. B. (2004). *Revenge of the Windigo: The construction of the mind and mental health of North American Aboriginal peoples*. Toronto, ON: University of Toronto Press.

Waldram, J. B., Herring, D. A., & Young, T. K. (2006). *Aboriginal health in Canada: Historical, cultural and epidemiological perspectives* (2nd ed). Toronto, ON: University of Toronto Press.

Williamson, D., & Reutter, L. (1999). Defining and measuring poverty: Implications for the health of Canadians. *Health Promotion International, 14*, 355–364.

World Health Organization. (1990). *Declaration of Caracas*. Geneva, Switzerland: Author.

World Health Organization. (2005a). *New WHO mental health atlas shows global mental health resources remain inadequate*. Geneva, Switzerland: Author.

World Health Organization. (2005b). *WHO Resource book on mental health, human rights and legislation*. Geneva, Switzerland: Author.

World Health Organization. (2013). *MiNDbank—promoting human rights in mental health reform, December 2013* 2013b. Geneva, Switzerland: Author. Retrieved from http://www.who.int/mental_health/en/

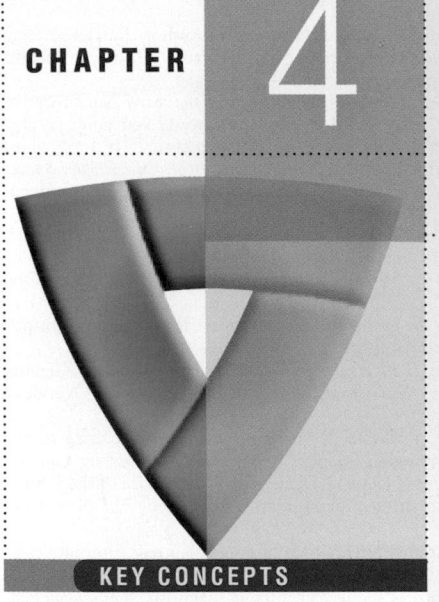
4 The Continuum of Psychiatric and Mental Health Care

Cheryl Pollard
Adapted from the chapter "The Continuum of Psychiatric and Mental Health Care" by Freida Chavez, Denise M. Gibson, and Robert B. Noud

LEARNING OBJECTIVES

After studying this chapter, you will be able to:

- Identify the different treatment settings and associated programs along the continuum of care.
- Discuss the role of the nurse along the continuum of care.
- Describe current health care trends in psychiatric services.
- Describe the importance of integrated services for people with mental illness or mental health concerns.

KEY CONCEPTS

- collaborative mental health care
- continuum of care

KEY TERMS

- case management • community-based residential services
- consultation • crisis response • empowerment • illness prevention
- integrated approach • intensive outpatient program • intensive residential services • mental health promotion • partnership • primary care
- primary health care • referral • relapse • reintegration • self-help
- stabilization • supportive employment

Health care systems need to have well-integrated psychiatric and mental health (PMH) care across the continuum, from health promotion to rehabilitation. Most mental illnesses are not caused by a single factor but are a result of a combination of factors. These causative factors relate to the complex interactions between biologic, social, psychological, and spiritual aspects of people's lives. Effective PMH care must be able to address people's needs in all of these areas. As a result, the continuum of PMH care includes a range of services.

Across all aspects of the Canadian health care system, health professionals, such as nurses, are expected to provide appropriate care to people with mental health problems and/or mental illness. Psychiatric and mental health services offer more specialized expertise in meeting the needs of people who have a mental illness. Resources that foster people's sense of self, social

inclusion and belonging, and meaning and purpose and that empower individuals to develop their capacity for well-being are important components of the PMH care continuum. Many of these resources are "outside" the formal health care system and are provided in the community by religious organizations, educational institutions, recreational associations, as well as family and peer groups.

PRIMARY HEALTH CARE APPROACH

Primary health care (not to be confused with "primary care") was adopted by the World Health Organization (WHO) in 1978 as the basis for the delivery of health services (WHO, 2008b). It is an approach that encompasses five types of care: promotive, preventive, curative, rehabilitative, and supportive/palliative. It is based on the principles of accessibility, public participation, health promotion, appropriate technology (i.e., adapted to the community's social, economic, and cultural developments), and intersectoral cooperation (necessary as health and well-being are linked to social and economic policies). Canadian nurses are expected to apply these principles in their practice across the continuum of care (Canadian Nurses Association, 2012). In 2012, the Mental Health Commission of Canada (MHCC) put forward recommendations for action that closely align with the principles of primary health care.

DEFINING THE CONTINUUM OF CARE

The **continuum of care** represents the complex, integrated system of services provided by health professionals in general and by those with specialized psychiatric and mental expertise, as well as the supports provided by informal providers and organizations within the community that help people to maintain and to restore their mental health and well-being.

The MHCC (2012) defines the concept of recovery as "living a satisfying, hopeful, and contributing life, even when there are on-going limitations caused by mental health problems and illnesses" (p. 7). Recovery also includes the concept of well-being—an individual realizing his or her potential. In order to facilitate recovery and well-being for individuals, family, groups, or communities, the approach of the services or supports provided must be founded on the principles of hope, **empowerment**, choice, and responsibility (MHCC, 2009).

The continuum begins with health promotion strategies that look for ways of keeping people from experiencing mental health problems or becoming mentally ill, as well as improving the mental health status of the whole population. In Canada, most of the services to people who experience a mental health problem or a mental illness are situated in community settings. Inpatient care (hospitalization) may be periodically necessary, but it is typically of very short duration. There are also components of the continuum that are focused on the PMH care needs of specific patient populations, such as children and families, seniors, military personnel, people with brain injuries, people who are involved with the legal system, people with addictions, and people with developmental challenges. These specialized services are typically provided by specially trained mental health professionals.

The goal of the system is to deliver the right care (appropriate medical, nursing, psychological, social, and spiritual services), by the right person, to the right person or family, at the right time and in the right place. By doing so, the continuum facilitates the stability, continuity, and comprehensiveness of service provision to an individual over the period of time. Further components

of the continuum of care range from supportive interventions by informal community support providers to professional service providers delivering clinical treatment in the community, to professional services being provided in a hospital setting. Due to the complexity of the continuum of care, individuals and families may require assistance with the coordination of their care, services, and supports.

> **KEY CONCEPT** A **continuum of care** consists of an integrated health system of supports and services designed to maximize people's health and well-being that is provided by professional health care clinicians (some who offer specialized services, such as psychiatric mental health services), as well as by nonprofessional caregivers.

Coordination of Care

Coordination of care is the integration of appropriate services so that individualized person-centred care and treatment is provided. Appropriate services are those that are tailored to promote recovery and well-being of the individual and family (when appropriate) through holistic care that supports and develops an individual's strengths, addresses vulnerabilities, promotes cultural competency and safety, inspires hope, facilitates empowerment, and offers choice and responsibility. Patients' input and opinions need to be solicited, including what they require in terms of knowledge, skills, and support to make decisions as well as their ability to participate in their own care. Patient-centred care is care that establishes a **partnership** among practitioners, patients, and their families (when appropriate) to ensure that decisions respect patients' wants, needs and preferences. The improvement of coordination care is an important factor for patient satisfaction (Health Quality Council of Alberta, 2013).

The move toward increasing professional coordination of services and social supports has occurred consistently across the Canadian health care system (Schwartz, Wright, & Lavoie-Tremblay, 2011). There are many terms that are used to describe these types of coordinating services. They include the following: **case management**, service coordination, care management, care coordination, service navigation, and transition care services. Although the terms may be different, the services provided can be described as a collaborative, client-driven process designed to support the patient's achievement of goals within a complex health, social, and fiscal environment. To meet patient goals, the coordinator of services for patients and families may need to liaise and develop collaborative and cooperative relationships among many different service partners, such as **primary care** services, public health, mental health, social services, housing, education, the workplace, and the criminal justice system, to name but a few. See Box 4-1 for guiding principles of case management and Box 4-2 for Canadian Standards of Practice for Case Management.

BOX 4-1 Guiding Principles of Case Management

- **Client-centred**
  Case management is client/caregiver centred and is sometimes driven or provided by the client. Generally, case management services benefit complex care clients the most.
- **Navigation**
  Case management provides navigation and networks through the wide spectrum of services to meet client needs. It moves beyond the boundaries of programs and service sectors.
- **Collaboration/coordination**
  Case management strategies build upon clinical expertise and the collaborative relationships/formalized partnerships amongst health care professionals, clients, and their caregivers. Health professionals work as interdisciplinary teams.
- **Health promotion/prevention**
  Case management strategies enhance health promotion, illness prevention, and risk mitigation through client education and emphasis on enhancing client self-care capacity. Case management incorporates the principles of population health and the broad determinants of health.
- **Quality of care**
  Case management incorporates evidence-based practice to promote quality of care (Health Quality Council of Alberta, 2005).
- **Resources management**
  Case management engages the family and organizes available resources.
- **Communication**
  Case management requires effective communication among health care providers, clients, and caregivers.
- **Advocating**
  Case management advocates on behalf of clients and promotes self-advocacy and independence. The challenge is that case management must balance client-focused services with effective use of resources for system sustainability.
- **Discretionary judgment**
  Professionals are empowered to use discretionary judgment, within the context of their own profession's accountability framework, in performing case management to meet a client's unique needs.
- **Flexibility**
  Degree of intensity, type of case management, and who the case manager is varies based on client characteristics, varying levels of service complexity, and the sectors/environment/programs involved in the partnerships.
- **Education**
  Case management provides clients and their families with the education and support that enables clients to understand their care needs and to be confident in providing self-care.

From Alberta Health and Wellness. (2006). *System case management for continuing care clients.* Prepared for Continuing Care Leaders Council. Edmonton, AB: Author.

BOX 4-2 Canadian Standards of Practice for Case Management

1. Clients who meet the eligibility for case management services are identified.
   This is the first step in establishing an appropriate case management service relationship.
2. In conjunction with the client, the case manager conducts and documents an individualized assessment using a structured process.
   Assessment is a dynamic and ongoing collaborative process that actively involves the client and others to secure information in a timely manner and to identify the client's values, goals, functional and cognitive capacity, strengths, abilities, preferences, resources, supports, and needs.
3. Client goals and priorities are documented and are reflected in the strategy for action agreed upon between the client and the case manager.
   The planning is designed to document the actions to achieve the client's short- and long-term goals and optimal health care outcomes. The ultimate goal is returning the client to optimal self-care and functional recovery. The plan of care explains the use of formal and informal services and resources.
4. Planned services, resources, and supports are initiated, coordinated, and adjusted as necessary.
   Implementation reflects the case manager's accountability to ensure that the client's individualized plan of care is being implemented. Implementation is the process in which all parties involved in the services/resource plan collaborate to carry out the mutually agreed-upon activities.
5. A periodic reassessment to identify the client's current needs and progress within the client's individualized plan.
   Evaluation is a part of the monitoring process and includes information from clients and others to determine the progress made by clients against the identified goals within the case management plan.
6. Transformation process that supports disengagement or shift in the mechanisms for achieving client goals.
   A redefinition of the client/case manager relationship in the evolution of the client's journey toward meeting his or her goals.

From National Case Management Network of Canada. (2009). *Canadian standards of practice for case management.* Ottawa, ON: Author.

The Nurse as Case Manager

Because of the often cyclical nature of serious mental illness, PMH nurses serve in various pivotal functions across the continuum of care. These functions can involve both direct care and coordination of the care delivered by others. The nurse when working as a case manager or care coordinator must have commanding knowledge of the patient's/family's needs, areas of strengths, and the available community resources. In order for nurses to be successful in this role, they must practice with the philosophy that recovery is defined by the patient, not the service provider, and a belief that well-being is possible for all people living with a mental illness. The nurse must also have expertise in working with the family as a unit.

The repertoire of required skills includes collaboration, teaching, management, leadership, followership, group, critical thinking, and research skills. A nurse working as a case manager arguably has one of the most diverse roles within the psychiatric services continuum.

COMPREHENSIVE MENTAL HEALTH SYSTEM: CORE PROGRAMS AND SERVICES

Each Canadian province has slightly different services to promote mental health, prevent mental illness, and provide treatment services and/or community supports to people with a mental health problem or mental illness. All, however, should be based on a commitment to patient-centred care (Canadian Nurses Association, 2012; MHCC, 2012).

Mental Health Promotion and Illness Prevention

Effective and efficient mental health service delivery systems have integrated **mental health promotion** and **illness prevention** into all aspects of the system. Mental health promotion strategies are directed toward addressing the determinants of health that can impact the population's mental health. Several mental health promotion policies and programs have been mainstreamed into Canada's government and business sectors. A few examples of these include early childhood intervention programs, such as home visiting for high-risk pregnant women; nutritional and psychosocial interventions for vulnerable populations; mental health interventions in the workplace (e.g., stress prevention programs); and community-based violence prevention that involves community policing initiatives. See Box 4-3 for a summary of best practices related to mental health promotion.

Mental illness prevention strategies are designed to keep something from happening. This something may be the illness itself, the severity or duration of the illness, or a disability associated with the illness or disease. The WHO has identified three categories of prevention strategies that will reduce the risk of experiencing an illness: (1) universal prevention: targets the general population; (2) selective prevention: targets groups or individuals at higher risk for a specific illness than the general population; and (3) indicated prevention: targets people at high risk for mental illness (WHO, 2002). An important example of illness prevention services is respite services for family caregivers of persons with a mental illness. The goals of respite programs are typically threefold:

- To validate and reinforce the necessity and value of informal caregiving within the continuum of care
- To provide support and advocacy to informal caregivers
- To prevent unnecessary long-term care placements and hospitalizations due to informal caregiver burnout. Respite services can be provided within the home, within a community living option (group home or supportive living setting), or may be provided within an inpatient setting.

Another example of a mental illness prevention strategy is the practice of providing critical incident stress debriefings. For example, if a volunteer fire crew responded to the scene of a very gruesome accident that involved one of their own members and his family, in which there was only one survivor who was severely injured and disfigured, the community mental health services may offer a critical incident stress debriefing. This intervention strategy is provided as a means to help the fire crew members avoid the potential onset of posttraumatic stress disorder.

Consumer Self-Help and Consumer/Survivor Initiatives

The knowledge and experiences of people living with mental illness are recognized and supported as part of a comprehensive mental health care system. In 2012, the MHCC identified six strategic directions to achieve its vision that "All people living in Canada have the opportunity to achieve the best possible mental health and well-being" (MHCC, 2009). Half of these strategic directions require the direct involvement of people with or who have experienced a mental illness. For example, in order to uphold patient rights and foster recovery and well-being, patients and their families need to be actively involved in decisions about services (MHCC, 2012). The importance of input from patients goes beyond decisions about their own care; it extends to the broader health care system. Expanding the "leadership role of people living with mental health problems and illnesses, and their families, in setting mental health related policy" (MHCC, 2012, p. 19) will improve knowledge and foster collaboration, which will ultimately have significant positive effects on

---

BOX 4-3   Best Practices

MENTAL HEALTH PROMOTION

1. Transform social determinants of health to affirm conditions that support mental health and reduce inequalities
2. Promote empowerment
3. Use a collaborative community process
4. Recognize that mental health is important for everyone, not just those at risk or those suffering or recovering from a mental illness

From Yearwood, E. L., & DeLeon Siantz, M. L. (2010). Global issues in mental health across the life span: Challenges and nursing opportunities. *Nursing Clinics of North America, 45*(4), 501–519.

decision making within the mental health care system. The recognition of the importance of having people with mental health problems or mental illness making decisions about their care and about the health care system is due in part to the determination and advocacy of **self-help** groups and organizations of people who have experienced mental illness (Segal, Silverman, & Temkin, 2013), many of whom refer to themselves as "consumers." Some consider themselves "survivors"—not of their illness but of their health care experience.

Two out of three Canadians with mental illness do not get the help they need (MHCC, 2009). For example, most people who receive treatment for depression in primary care receive only a single session in a year (Bilsker, Goldner, & Anderson, 2012). One strategy that is used to extend assistance to people with mental health problems or mental illness is through consumer/survivor initiatives organizations (Lurie, 2012). These are self-help organizations operated exclusively by and for people with serious mental illness. Rather than being treatment services, they are self-help groups that promote the values of member empowerment, participation, social justice, and community. The work of these organizations is helping to decrease the stigma associated with mental illness and to make care more accessible. They have also been found to be as effective as traditional services for employment, living arrangements, and reducing hospital admissions (Doughty & Tse, 2011). See Box 4-4 for best practices related to consumer self-help initiatives.

Crisis Response Systems and Psychiatric Emergency Services

Crisis intervention services are an important part of a comprehensive mental health system. An organized approach is required to treat individuals in crisis, including a mechanism for rapid access to care (24/7), telephone crisis services, mobile **crisis response**, access to crisis emergency residential services, or psychiatric emergency services in hospitals. Crisis response systems emphasize crisis supports that are flexible, portable, and person-centred (Krupa, Stuart, Mathany, Smart, & Chen, 2010). This type of short-term intervention care focuses on de-escalation, **stabilization**, symptom reduction, and prevention of **relapse** requiring inpatient services.

Crisis intervention units can be found in the emergency department of a general or psychiatric hospital or in crisis centres within a community mental health centre. Patients in crisis demonstrate severe symptoms of acute mental illness, including labile mood swings, suicidal ideation, or self-injurious behaviours. This treatment option therefore demands a high degree of nursing expertise. Patients in crisis usually require medications such as anxiolytics or benzodiazepines for symptom management. Key nursing roles include making an accurate assessment, delivering short-term therapeutic interventions, and administering medication. Nurses will also facilitate **referrals** for increased community services or support, for admission to the hospital, or for outpatient services.

Crisis Stabilization

When the immediate crisis does not resolve quickly, the next step is crisis stabilization. The primary purpose of stabilization is to control precipitating symptoms through medications, behavioural interventions, and coordination with other agencies for appropriate aftercare. The major focus of nursing care in a short-term inpatient setting is symptom

---

BOX 4-4   Best Practices

CONSUMER SELF-HELP AND CONSUMER INITIATIVES

Research Evidence
Having the support of a peer has demonstrated many positive outcomes for people living with mental health problem or illness. For example, people who have peer support have
- Reduced hospitalization
- Reduced use of other services
- Increased knowledge, information, and coping skills
- Increased employment
- Increased self-esteem, confidence, sense of well-being, and sense of being in control
- Improved social networks and support

Key Elements of Best Practice
The forms of peer support vary but typically relate to providing
- A connection to resources
- Advocacy
- Experiential sharing
- Building relationships and community
- Developing knowledge and skills training
- Providing opportunities to socialize and build self-esteem

From Jacobson, N., Trojanowski, L., & Dewa, C. (2012). What do peer support workers do? A job description. *BioMed Central Health Services Research, 12, 205.* doi:10.1186/1472-6963-12-205

BOX 4-5   Best Practices

CRISIS RESPONSE SYSTEMS AND PSYCHIATRIC EMERGENCY SERVICES

Research Evidence
There has been a shift from hospital to community-based resources. The typical location of crisis intervention services for people with mental health problems or mental illness has also shifted from hospital to community.

Key Elements of Best Practice
Key elements of community crisis services include
- 24-hour telephone crisis response
- Walk-in crisis services
- Provisional mobile response

From Krupa, T., Stuart, H., Mathany, A., Smart, J., & Chen, S. (2010). An evaluation of a community-based, integrated crisis-case management service. *Canadian Journal of Community Mental Health, 29*(5), 125–137.

management and linkage to community resources. During stabilization, the major components of nursing care are ongoing assessment; short-term, focused interventions; and medication administration while monitoring efficacy and side effects. Nurses may also provide focused group psychotherapy designed to develop and strengthen patients' personal management strategies. When treating aggressive or violent patients, the nurse monitors the appropriate use of seclusion and restraints. See Box 4-5 for a summary of best practices related to crisis response services.

Psychosocial Emergency Preparedness and Response

A national priority is to be prepared for emergencies (e.g., transportation accidents, power outages, terrorist threats) and disasters (e.g., floods, fires, tornadoes, outbreaks of disease). Most emergencies, local in nature, are handled at that level; however, partnership is a key principle of Canada's emergency management (Emergency Management Policy Directorate, 2011). The federal government, when assistance is requested or when an emergency involves more than one province or territory, mobilizes resources and coordinates federal response in the health sector through Public Safety Canada. Health Canada and the Public Health Agency of Canada play critical roles in emergency response to risks to public health. The psychosocial aspect of preparedness and response is recognized as an essential component (Health Canada, 2011).

In times of major emergencies and disasters, individuals, families, and entire communities face severe risks to psychosocial (as well as physical) well-being, and the mental health system can be overwhelmed. "The dominoes start falling backwards" was a metaphor used to describe the effects of the 2012 hurricane Sandy on New York City's mental health system ("Mental health considerations," 2013): the number of people requiring care increased dramatically while services to treat them decreased or failed due to destruction and/or lack of personnel. Canada's psychosocial preparedness and response initiative offers services to help Canadians better prepare for disasters and emergencies (e.g., resiliency building) as well as consultation during disaster response.

Primary Care

Primary care refers to the first point of access to the health care system. Provincial health care planning has typically divided the delivery of the services for physical illness and mental illness. This has resulted in a system that fragments people's needs, which is both counterproductive and harmful. An **integrated approach** is required that assists people in managing illness, regardless of its origin. The integrated approach begins with ensuring that the services and supports that are delivered are done so in a patient-centred manner. This means that people are empowered: choice is promoted, they remain in control,

and when possible remain in their community. A patient-centred approach emphasizes the partnership that the person with mental illness has with the service providers. It does not shift responsibility on people to "get themselves together," "get over it," or "deal with it." This model does not place blame on the affected individual; rather, people with mental illness are true partners in their recovery. Although the extent of a person's involvement will depend on his or her particular circumstances, it is only through involvement in their own recovery that people who experience a mental illness can expect the best possible health and well-being.

Collaborative mental health care models have been established in response to specialist mental health service-provider shortages, access issues, and the recognition that family physicians are the first point of contact for approximately 85% of people with mental illness (Kirby, 2008). These models have been described using a variety of terms: integrated care, shared care, collaborative care, and managed care, among others. In essence, collaborative care recognizes that primary care for mental health is essential, but to be fully effective it must be supported by additional levels of care as no single service setting, or provider, can meet everyone's mental health needs (WHO, 2008a). See Box 4-6 for best practices related to

---

BOX 4-6 Goals and Potential Activities of Collaborative Mental Health Care Services

Goals
- Improve access to a comprehensive range of high-quality and effective health care services.
- Improve outcomes for people who use the mental health system.
- Integrate community services across sectors.

Potential Activities
- Regular visits by a mental health care worker to a primary care setting
- Unified programs that offer mental health and physical health care through one administration and financial entity
- Regular telephone consultation between primary care and mental health providers
- Integration of specialized care providers such as psychiatrists, psychologists, nurses, social workers, pharmacists, occupational therapists, and dietitians within primary care settings
- Joint development of treatment plans by consumers and providers
- Incorporation of mental health interventions into the management of general medical conditions (e.g., diabetes)
- Meeting the primary health care needs of individuals with severe and persistent mental illness
- Strategies to improve access to community mental health services
- Development of more formal partnerships with specialized service providers

From Kates, N., et al. (2011). The evolution of collaborative mental health care in Canada: A shared vision for the future. *The Canadian Journal of Psychiatry, 56*(5), 1–10.

BOX 4-7 Benefits of Integrating Mental Health Into Primary Care

1. **The burden of mental disorders is great.** Mental disorders are prevalent in all societies. They create a substantial personal burden for affected individuals and their families, and they produce significant economic and social hardships that affect society as a whole.
2. **Mental and physical health problems are interwoven.** Many people suffer from both physical and mental health problems. Integrated primary care services help ensure that people are treated in a holistic manner, meeting the mental health needs of people with physical disorders as well as the physical health needs of people with mental disorders.
3. **The treatment gap for mental disorders is enormous.** In all countries, there is a significant gap between the prevalence of mental disorders and the number of people receiving treatment and care. Primary care for mental health helps close this gap.
4. **Primary care for mental health enhances access.** Integrating mental health into primary care is the best way of ensuring that people get the mental health care they need. When mental health is integrated into primary care, people can access mental health services closer to their homes, thus keeping their families together and maintaining their daily activities. Primary care services also facilitate community outreach and mental health promotion, as well as long-term monitoring and management of affected individuals.
5. **Primary care for mental health promotes respect of human rights.** Mental health services delivered in primary care minimize stigma and discrimination. This also removes the risk of human rights violations that occur in psychiatric hospitals.
6. **Primary care for mental health is affordable and cost-effective.** Primary mental health care services are less expensive than are psychiatric hospitals, for patients, communities, and governments alike. In addition, patients and families avoid indirect costs associated with seeking specialist care in distant locations. The treatment of common mental disorders is very cost-effective, and even small investments by governments can bring important benefits.
7. **Primary care for mental health generates good health outcomes.** The majority of people with mental health disorders treated in primary care have good outcomes, particularly when linked to a network of services at secondary level and in the community.

From World Health Organization. (2008a). *Integrating mental health into primary care: A global perspective.* Geneva, Switzerland: Author.

the goals and potential activities of collaborative mental health care services. See Box 4-7 related to the benefits of integrating mental health into primary care.

KEY CONCEPT   Collaborative mental health care refers to "care that is provided from different specialties, disciplines, or sectors that work together to offer complementary services and mutual support. As in any effective partnership, common goals, clear and equitable decision making, and open and regular communication are key" (Kates et al., 2011, p. 2).

The other levels of care required to support primary care providers include secondary service components. These components include opportunities for **consultation** and support through referrals regarding patient care needs outside the primary care provider's current competency level, as well as supervision and support to facilitate further skill development and education of the primary care provider. Collaborative mental health care also extends to include formal and informal community supports for people with mental illness, such as housing, education, and recreational organizations. It has been demonstrated that people with mental illness who receive good community care services and support have better health and mental health outcomes and better quality of life than do those people who were treated in psychiatric hospitals (WHO, 2008a). However, there is a small proportion of the population that requires very specialized services. These are people who have treatment-resistant or very complex presentations of illness, those who lack community support, and/or those requiring forensic services.

Outpatient Care

Outpatient care is a level of care that occurs outside of a hospital or institution. Outpatient services usually are less intensive and are provided to patients who do not require inpatient services. Many patients enrol in outpatient services immediately upon discharge from an inpatient setting. Others are enrolled as a means of providing treatment services when hospitalization is not required. This promotes a continued connection with their community and community **reintegration**, medication management and monitoring, and symptom management. Patients and their families have the right to choose home/community as the site for service provision. When remaining at home with their families and other supports, individuals with mental problems or mental illness are more socially integrated into society (Hair, Shortall, & Oldford, 2013). Outpatient services are provided by private practices, clinics, and community mental health centres.

Intensive Outpatient Programs

The primary focus of **intensive outpatient programs** is on stabilization and relapse prevention for highly vulnerable individuals who function autonomously on a daily basis. People who meet these criteria have returned to their previous lifestyle although their quality of life is still impacted by their mental illness (e.g., interacting with family, resuming work, or returning to school). Attendance in this type of program benefits individuals who still require frequent monitoring and support within a therapeutic milieu that enables them to remain connected to the community. The duration of treatment and level of services rendered are based on the patient's immediate needs. Treatment duration usually is time limited, with sessions offered 3 to 4 hours per day and 2 to 3 days per week for 6 to12 weeks.

BOX
4-8   Best Practices

BRIDGING THE GAPS IN INPATIENT AND OUTPATIENT CARE

Research Evidence
Well-designed follow-up studies show that
- Barriers to mental health services impede access to care
- Psychological barriers include fear of public rejection (stigmatization) and participant's judgments of the therapist
- Physical barriers include travel barriers that are caused by restricted finances, physical abilities, geographical location, or personal responsibilities (work, school, child care)
  A preliminary study results suggest that Web- and telephone-based interventions can address a number of barriers to mental health services that are traditionally delivered.

Key Elements of Best Practice
- Distance mental health delivery systems (Web- and telephone-based) can be used to overcome physical and psychological access barriers.
- Regardless of service delivery system, establishing an effective therapeutic relationship is critical to the success of therapy.
- People with mental health problems or illness continue to experience social alienation and stigma. Care providers, whether they are providing care in person or in another manner, must be aware of the potential fear of public rejection.
- The ability of the care provider to create an environment with a sense of social presence and belonging is critical to potential success of the interventions.

From Lingley-Pottie, P., McGrath, P., & Andreou, P. (2013). Barriers to mental health care: Perceived delivery system differences. *Advances in Nursing Science, 36*(1), 51–61.

See Box 4-8 for best practices related to bridging the gaps in inpatient care and outpatient care.

Housing and Community Support

With the focus on community-based care, there has been an increasing attention to housing and community support. As people have transitioned from primarily receiving services as an inpatient for serious mental illness to receiving those services within their community, it has increased the demands on families, communities, local mental health workers, and other community agencies (Sealy, 2012). Consequently, as symptoms wax and wane over the course of a chronic mental illness, families, caregivers, and workers in non–health community agencies often experience caregiving fatigue. Despite the challenges for the caregivers, one of the largest hurdles to overcome for people living with a serious and chronic mental illness is finding appropriate housing to meet their immediate social, financial, and safety needs. Most individuals with severe forms of mental illness live in some form of supervised or supported community living situation, which ranges from highly supervised congregate

settings to independent apartments. Those who lack the resources to find housing suffer higher rates of substance abuse, physical illness, incarceration, and victimization (Jakubec, Tomazewski, Powel, & Osuji, 2012). In a study that looked at 500 homeless people in three different Canadian cities, 92.8% of the participants had a mental illness (Krausz et al., 2013). A substantial illness burden resulted from illnesses related to substance dependence.

Supported Housing

There has been a paradigm shift from a reliance on the residential continuum to what is now known as supported housing. Supportive housing has site-based health and social services that are aimed at improving the health and residential stability of highly disadvantaged individuals (Hwang et al., 2011). **Community-based residential services** provide a place for people to reside during a 24-hour period or any portion of the day, on an ongoing basis. A residential facility can be publicly or privately owned. **Intensive residential services** are intensively staffed for patient treatment. These services may include medical, nursing, psychosocial, vocational, recreational, or other support services. Combining residential care and mental health services, this treatment form offers rehabilitation and therapy to people with serious and persistent mental illnesses, including chronic schizophrenia, bipolar disorder, and unrelenting depression. These services may provide short-term treatment for stays from 24 hours to 3 or 6 months, or long-term treatment for several months to years.

Nursing plays an important role in the care of people who have severe and persistent mental illnesses and who require long-term stays at residential treatment facilities. Nurses provide basic psychiatric nursing care with a focus on psychoeducation, basic social skills training, aggression management, activities of daily living training, and group living. Education on symptom management, understanding mental illnesses, and medication is essential to recovery. *Canadian Standards for Psychiatric-Mental Health Nursing* guides the nurse in delivering patient care (Canadian Federation of Mental Health Nurses, 2014) (see Chapter 5).

Supportive Employment

A key component in a comprehensive mental health system is also the provision of supports for employment. Gruhl (2012) identifies that "how people with mental serious illness spend their time has been less emphasized in care programs than whether people are compliant with medication, asymptomatic and not in hospital" (p. 379). Employment is strongly linked to a person's sense of self-worth and personal environment. **Supportive employment** services assist individuals to find work; assess individuals' skills, attitudes, behaviours, and interest relevant to work; offer vocational rehabilitation or other training; and provide work opportunities. Supportive employment programs—individual placement and support services—are highly individualized and competitive. For example, in Ontario, funding has shifted from a fee-for-service to an outcomes-based funding model (Gewurtz, Cott, Rush, & Kirsh, 2012). Service providers deliver on-site support and job-coaching services on a one-to-one basis. They occur in real work settings and are used for patients with severe mental illnesses. The primary focus is to maintain attachment between the mentally ill person and the workforce (see Chapter 16).

Acute Inpatient Care

Acute inpatient hospitalization involves the most intensive treatment and is considered the most restrictive setting in the continuum. Inpatient treatment is reserved for acutely ill patients who, because of a mental illness, meet one or more of three criteria: high risk for harming oneself, high risk for harming others, or inability to care for one's basic needs. The delivery of inpatient care can occur in a psychiatric hospital or psychiatric unit within a general hospital. Admission to inpatient environments can be voluntary or involuntary (see Chapter 3). Provincial legislation (mental health acts) describes conditions that warrant hospitalization. Length of inpatient stay is kept as short as possible without harmful effects on patient outcomes. See Box 4-9 for best practices on therapeutic relationships from psychiatric hospital to community.

BOX 4-9   Research for Best Practices

ON THE TRANSITION: FROM PSYCHIATRIC HOSPITAL TO COMMUNITY
....

Forchuk, C., et al., (2013). Preventing homelessness: After discharge from psychiatric wards: Perspectives of consumers and staff. Journal of Psychosocial Nursing and Mental Health, 51(3), 24–31.

Questions: (1) What are the effects of offering income and housing support to psychiatric clients at risk for homelessness? (2) What are the implementation issues related to the intervention? (3) What are staff perceptions of the intervention?

Method: 251 people were provided with assistance (intervention) securing housing prior to discharge. A program evaluation was conducted that included client interviews and staff focus groups to gather formative (information to improve processes within the program) and summative (information about overall program effectiveness) data.

Findings: Both recipients of the assistance and the hospital staff identified several benefits of the program. These included the recipients having an increased sense of independence and having a more efficient transition back into the community. Staff identified that they had a reduced workload as a result of the intervention.

Implications: As part of their initial assessment, mental health nurses need to assess and identify their patient's issues or concerns related to housing. These concerns can exacerbate mental health symptoms, such as depression or anxiety. Developing collaborative partnerships with income and housing support agencies can help prevent a discharge to "no fixed address."

SUMMARY OF KEY POINTS

■ The continuum of psychiatric and mental health care must be well integrated within the overall health care system and shaped by the principles of primary health care: accessibility, public participation, health promotion, appropriate technology, and intersectoral cooperation.

■ The continuum of care is a comprehensive system of services and programs spanning the range from mental health promotion and illness prevention to very specialized services designed to match the needs of the individuals and populations with the appropriate care and treatment, which vary according to levels of service, structure, and intensity of care.

■ The psychiatric and mental health nurse's specific responsibilities vary according to the setting. In most settings, nurses function as members of a multidisciplinary team. Consumers of mental health services and their families should be considered as core members of that team.

■ An integrated approach to delivering a patient-centred mental health care is required to ensure effective and efficient services.

CRITICAL THINKING CHALLENGES

1 Define the continuum of care and discuss the importance of using a patient-centred approach.
2 Differentiate the role of the nurse across the continuum of care.
3 Consider, in light of recommended best practices, the housing and community supports for people with mental disorders that are available in your community.
4 Envision an integration of services that you believe would best serve patients and their families in your community.

REFERENCES

Alberta Health and Wellness. (2006). *System case management for continuing care clients.* Prepared for Continuing Care Leaders Council. Edmonton, AB: Author.

Bilsker, D., Goldner, E., & Anderson, E. (2012). Supported self-management: A simple, effective way to improve depression care. *Canadian Journal of Psychiatry*, 57(4), 203–209. Retrieved from http://publications.cpa-apc.org

Canadian Federation of Mental Health Nurses. (2014). *Canadian standards of psychiatric and mental health nursing: Standards of practice* (4th ed.). Toronto, ON: Author.

Canadian Nurses Association. (2012). *Position statement on mental health services.* Ottawa, ON: Author.

Doughty, C., & Tse, S. (2011). Can consumer-led mental health services be equally effective? An integrative review of CLMH services in high-income countries. *Community Mental Health Journal*, 47(3), 252–266. doi: 10.1007/s10597-010-9321-5

Emergency Management Policy Directorate. (2011). *An emergency management framework for Canada* (2nd ed.). Ottawa, ON: Author.

Forchuk, C., Godin, M., Hich, J., Kingston-MacClure, S., Jeng, M., Puddy, L., … Jensen, E. (2013). Preventing homelessness: After discharge from psychiatric wards: Perspectives of consumers and staff. *Journal of Psychosocial Nursing and Mental Health*, 51(3), 24–31. doi: 10.3928/02793695-20130130-02

Gewurtz, R., Cott, C., Rush, B., & Kirsh, B. (2012). The shift to rapid job placement for people living with mental illness: An analysis of consequences. *Psychiatric Rehabilitation Journal, 35*(6), 428–434. doi: 10.1037/h0094575

Gruhl, K. (2012). Transitions to work for persons with serious mental illness in northeastern Ontario, Canada: Examining barriers to employment. *Work, 41*(4), 379–389. doi: 10.3233/WOR-2012-1315

Hair, H., Shortall, R., & Oldford J. (2013). Where's help when we need it? Developing responsive and effective brief counseling services for children, adolescents, and their families. *Social Work in Mental Health, 11*(1), 16–33. doi: 10.1080/15332985.2012.716389

Health Canada. (2011). Emergency preparedness. Retrieved from http://www.hc-sc.gc.ca/hc-ps/ed-ud/prepar/index-eng.php

Health Quality Council of Alberta. (2005). *Alberta quality matrix for health: User guide.* Calgary, AB: Author.

Health Quality Council of Alberta. (2013). *Satisfaction and experience with healthcare services: A survey of Albertans 2012.* Calgary, AB: Author.

Hwang, S., Gogosis, E., Chambers, C., Dunn, J., Hoch, J., & Aubry, T. (2011). Health status, quality of life, residential stability, substance use, and health care utilization among adults applying to a supportive housing program. *Journal of Urban Health: Bulleting of the New York Academy of Medicine, 88*(6), 1079–1090. doi: 10.1007/s11524-011-9592-3

Jacobson, N., Trojanowski, L., & Dewa, C. (2012). What do peer support workers do? A job description. *BioMed Central Health Services Research, 12,* 205. doi: 10.1186/1472-6963-12-205

Jakubec, S., Tomaszewski, A., Powell, T., & Osuji, J. (2012). "More than the house": A Canadian perspective on housing stability. *Housing, Care and Support, 15*(3), 99–108. doi: 10.1108/14608791211268518

Kates, N., Mazowita, G., Lemire, F., Jayabarathan, A., Bland, R., Selby, P., Audet, D. (2011). The evolution of collaborative mental health care in Canada: A shared vision for the future. *The Canadian Journal of Psychiatry, 56*(5-insert), 1–10.

Kirby, M. (2008). Mental health in Canada: Out of the shadows forever. *Canadian Medical Association Journal, 178*(10), 1320–1322.

Krausz, R., Clarkson, A., Strehlau, V., Torchalla, I., Li, K., & Schuetz, C. (2013). Mental disorder, service use, and barriers to care among 500 homeless people in 3 different urban settings. *Social Psychiatry and Psychiatric Epidemiology.* Advance online publication. doi: 10.1007/s00127-012-0649-8

Krupa, T., Stuart, H., Mathoany, A., Smart, J., & Chen, S. P. (2010). An evaluation of a community-based, integrated crisis-case management service. *Canadian Journal of Community Mental Health, 29*(5 Suppl), 125–137.

Lingley-Pottie, P., McGrath, P., & Andreou, P. (2013). Barriers to mental health care: Perceived delivery system differences. *Advances in Nursing Science, 36*(1) 51–61. doi: 10.1097/ANS0b013e31828077eb

Lurie, S. (2012). And now for something completely different ... Self management. *The Canadian Journal of Psychiatry, 57*(4), 201–202. Retrieved from http://publications.cpa-apc.org

Mental Health Commission of Canada. (2009). *Toward recovery and well-being: A framework for a mental health strategy for Canada.* Calgary, AB: Author.

Mental Health Commission of Canada. (2012). *Changing directions, changing lives: The mental health strategy for Canada.* Calgary, AB: Author.

Mental Health Considerations: The Unseen Effects of Disaster. (2013). *Environmental Health Perspectives, 121*(5), A159.

National Case Management Network of Canada. (2009). *Canadian standards of practice for case management.* Ottawa, ON: Author.

Schwartz, L., Wright, D., & Lavoie-Tremblay, M. (2011). New nurses' experience of their role within interpersonal health care teams in mental health. *Archives of Psychiatric Nursing, 25*(3), 153–163. doi: 10.1016/j.apnu.2010.08.001

Sealy, P. (2012). The impact of the process of deinstitutionalization of mental health services in Canada: An increase in accessing of health professionals for mental health concerns. *Social Work in Public Health, 27*(3), 229–237. doi: 10.1080/19371911003748786

Segal, S., Silverman, C., & Temkin, T. (2013). Are all consumer-operated programs empowering self-help agencies? *Social Work in Mental Health, 11*(1), 1–15. doi: 10.1080/15332985.2012.718731

World Health Organization. (2002). *Prevention and promotion in mental health.* Geneva, Switzerland: Author.

World Health Organization. (2008a). *Integrating mental health into primary care: A global perspective.* Geneva, Switzerland: Author.

World Health Organization. (2008b). *The world health report 2008: Primary health care—now more than ever.* Geneva, Switzerland: Author.

Yearwood, E. L., & DeLeon Siantz, M. L. (2010). Global issues in mental health across the life span: Challenges and opportunities. *Nursing Clinics of North America, 45*(4), 501–519. doi: 10.1016/j.cnur.2010.06.004

Foundations of Psychiatric and Mental Health Nursing Practice

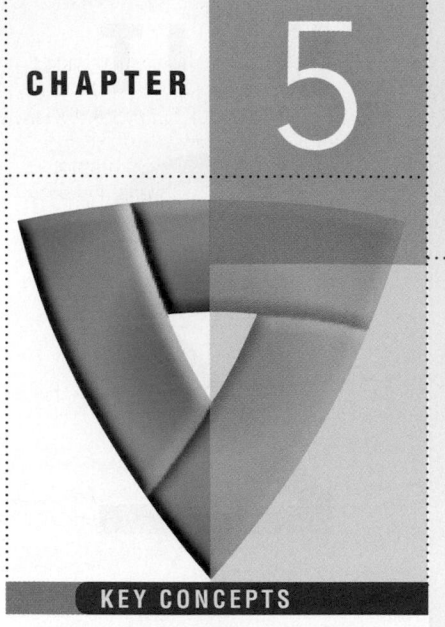

CHAPTER

5 Contemporary Psychiatric and Mental Health Nursing Practice

Wendy Austin and Margaret Osborne
Adapted from the chapters "Contemporary Psychiatric and Mental Health Nursing Practice" by Mary Ann Boyd and by Olive Yonge and Wendy Austin

LEARNING OBJECTIVES

After studying this chapter, you will be able to:

- Explain the bio/psycho/social/spiritual model as a conceptual framework for understanding and treating mental health problems and disorders.
- Explain the scope of psychiatric and mental health (PMH) nursing practice.
- Discuss the role of standards of practice for Canadian nurses.
- Provide examples of specific standards for registered nurses and for registered psychiatric nurses (RPNs).
- Specify four key components of PMH nursing.
- Discuss the current challenges of PMH nursing.
- Identify national and international organizations with relevance to PMH nursing practice.

KEY CONCEPTS

- bio/psycho/social/spiritual model
- standards of practice

KEY TERMS

- clinical decision-making • collaborative care • competencies
- critical pathways • domains of practice • interdisciplinary approach
- recovery model

This chapter introduces the bio/psycho/social/spiritual model as the approach to understanding human health that informs PMH nursing practice. The scope of PMH nursing is explained, followed by a discussion of standards of practice that explicitly describe the obligations of nurses working in Canadian PMH care settings. The discussion of the challenges of PMH nursing sets the stage for the rest of the book through an overview of the dynamic nature of this specialty.

THE BIO/PSYCHO/SOCIAL/ SPIRITUAL MODEL OF PMH NURSING

Contemporary PMH nursing uses theories from the biologic, psychological, and social sciences as a basis of practice. As well, PMH nurses are increasingly informed by knowledge from the spiritual domain of human health (Barker & Buchanan-Barker, 2004; Cobb, Rumbold, & Puchalski, 2012). This holistic approach, referred to as

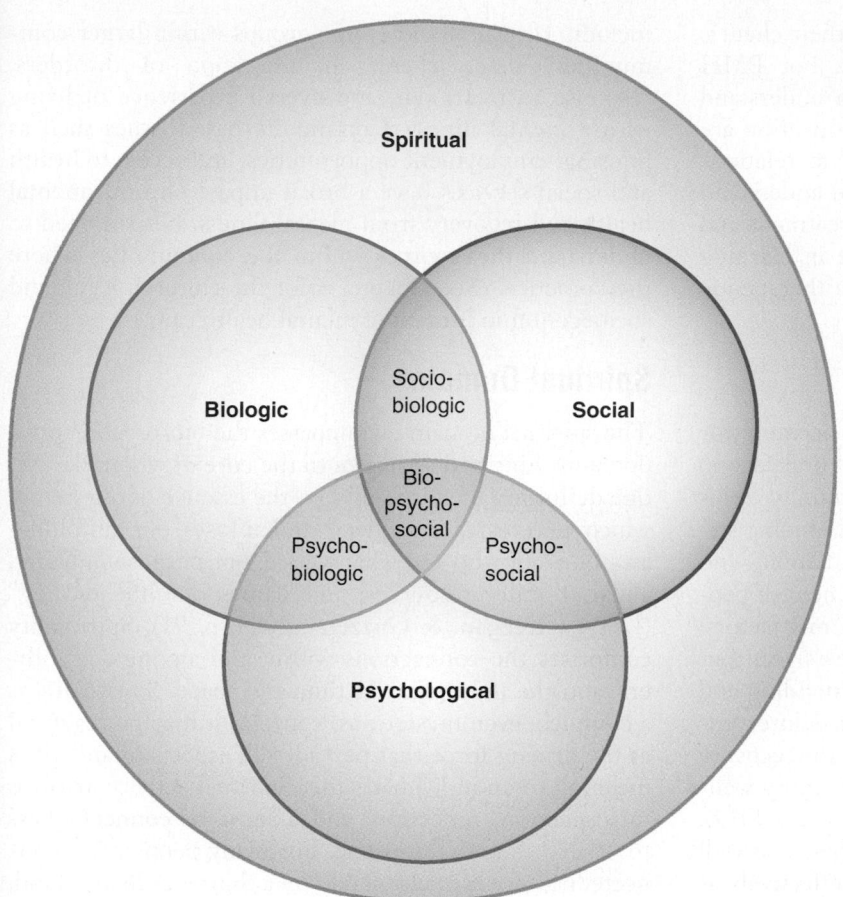

FIGURE 5-1. Bio/psycho/social/spiritual model. (Originally adapted from Abraham, I., Fox, J., & Cohen, B. (1992). Integrating the bio into the biopsychosocial: Understanding and treating biological phenomena in psychiatric–mental health nursing. *Archives of Psychiatric Nursing*, *6*(5), 296–305.)

the bio/psycho/social/spiritual model of PMH nursing, is necessary to guide understanding of the individual who is experiencing mental health problems or a mental disorder. Holism joins the biologic, psychological, social, and spiritual domains in an integrated, dynamic, evolutionary, and vital conceptualization of human health (Hood Morris, 1996). The model provides a basis for the organization of nursing care and is used throughout this text for integrating theoretic knowledge and the nursing process (Fig. 5-1).

> **KEY CONCEPT** The **bio/psycho/social/spiritual model** consists of separate but interacting domains that can be understood independently but that are mutually interdependent with the other domains.

Biologic Domain

The *biologic* domain consists of the biologic theories related to mental disorders and problems as well as all of the biologic processes related to other health problems. Today, there is evidence of neurobiologic changes in most mental disorders. Within this domain, there are also theories and concepts used as a basis of interventions focusing

on an individual's physical functioning, such as exercise, relaxation, sleep, and nutrition. In addition, the neurobiologic theories also serve as a basis for understanding such biologic treatments as pharmacologic agents and electroconvulsive therapy (see Chapter 12).

Psychological Domain

The *psychological* domain contains the theoretical basis of the psychological processes—thoughts, feelings, and behaviour (intrapersonal dynamics) that influence one's emotion, cognition, and behaviour. The psychological and nursing sciences generate theories and research that are critical to understanding an individual's symptoms and responses to mental disorders. Although mental disorders have a biologic component, they are often manifested in psychological symptoms and physical changes. The person with a thought disorder may have bizarre behaviour that needs to be interpreted within the context of the neurobiologic dysfunction of the mental disorder.

Many PMH nursing interventions are based on knowledge generated within this domain. Cognitive approaches, behaviour therapy, and client education are all based on the use of theories from the psychological domain. These interventions are explained in Unit III. PMH interventions are also based on the use of interpersonal communication techniques, which require nurses to develop awareness of their own, as well as their client's, internal thoughts, feelings, and behaviour. For PMH nurses, exploring their own and coming to understand their client's intrapersonal dynamics and motivation are critical to the development of a therapeutic relationship that motivates clients to learn about and understand their disorders and to participate in their treatment and management. Motivating clients to engage in learning activities best occurs within the context of a therapeutic relationship (see Chapter 6).

Social Domain

The *social* domain includes theories that account for the influence of social forces (including cultural forces) encompassing the client, family, and community. This knowledge base is generated from social and nursing sciences and delineates the connections within families and communities that affect the health and treatment of people with mental disorders. Understanding family factors, including origin, extended family, and other significant relationships, contributes to the total understanding and treatment of individual clients. Family-based interventions can reduce rates of relapse and improve the recovery of the client, as well as positively influence family well-being (Heru and Drury, 2006; MacCourt et al., 2013). Families need to receive information and support, as well as receive services if they are to participate effectively as part of a collaborative approach to mental health care for their relative (MacCourt et al.).

Mental disorders and their treatment can be significantly affected by the society in which the client lives. Public attitudes and beliefs about mental illness can be supportive or stigmatizing and isolating due to prejudice and discrimination (see Fig. 5-2). Community forces, including cultural and ethnic groups within larger communities, shape clients' manifestation of disorders, response to treatment, and overall experience of living with a mental illness. Community-based issues such as housing, employment opportunities, and access to health and social services have a broad impact on both mental health and recovery from mental illness. Nurses need to understand these forces within the communities where they practice. (See Chapter 3 for the cultural, legal, and socioeconomic context of mental health care.)

Spiritual Domain

The spiritual domain encompasses the bio/psycho/social domains. Spirituality relates to the core of whom we are; one definition of spirituality is "the essence of our being, which permeates our living and infuses our unfolding awareness of who and what we are, our purpose in being, and our inner resources; and shapes our life journey" (Dossey, Keegan, & Guzzetta, 2004, p. 91). Spirituality comprises the connections within and among self, others, and the universe over time and space. Spirituality is a complex, even mysterious, concept: it may be regarded as the driving force that pervades all aspects of and gives meaning to an individual's life. Spiritual activity involves introspection, reflection, and a sense of connectedness to others or to the universe. For many people, this connectedness focuses ultimately on a Supreme Being. God, Allah, Jehovah, and Creator are among the names that refer to a worshipped Supreme Being.

Although there remains a lack of agreement concerning the way spirituality should be defined, a review of the interdisciplinary literature on spirituality reveals common themes: everyone has the potential for spirituality and spiritual growth; the way one lives one's

FIGURE 5-2. Drawing by Almier, used with permission for educational purposes.

life is reflective of spirituality; spirituality is relational in nature; and there is a link among religion, spirituality, and moral norms (Catalano, 2006). Religion differs, however, from spirituality. Religion involves organized systems of rituals, patterns of beliefs, and groups of people usually congregating around the worship of a deity. A person may be spiritual but not religious, both religious and spiritual, or religious but not spiritual (Mauk & Schmidt, 2004).

Spiritual growth may be stimulated by pivotal life events, even distressing ones like being diagnosed with a mental disorder. It can be very difficult, however, to transcend one's current reality and the suffering it may entail. O'Reilly (2004) noted that individuals living with a mental illness often struggle with the loss of meaning and purpose. They may wonder "Why has this happened to me?" and be affected by religious or cultural beliefs that view mental illness as a form of punishment. The nurse can help individuals experiencing spiritual distress by supporting their efforts to find meaning in their circumstances, which may include meditation, contemplation, prayer, and other spiritual practices that may give comfort. The relationship of the body, mind, relation, and spirit in the content of human health is holistic, synergistic, and unifying.

■ STANDARDS OF PROFESSIONAL PRACTICE

As regulated health professions, nurses are given the authority to practise under provincial or territorial laws that set out governance, registration, and discipline requirements as a means of protecting the public. These laws require provincial or territorial nursing regulatory bodies to set, monitor, and enforce standards of practice that, along with a code of ethics (see Chapter 7), articulate a profession's values, knowledge, and skills. Such standards facilitate a profession's self-governance because they make explicit the profession's expectations of its members' **competencies** and performance. These standards are applicable to all nursing practice settings.

PMH nursing has been a designated Canadian Nurses Association (CNA) specialty area since 1995. The Canadian Federation of Mental Health Nurses (CFMHN) is the national association for the specialty and sets PMH nursing standards for registered nurses. National certification in this specialty can be achieved by registered nurses (RNs) who have either a minimum of 3,900 hours in the specialty area over the past 5 years or who have completed a formal post–basic nursing course/program of at least 300 hours in the past 10 years and have 2,925 hours of practice in the specialty area. As well, verification by a supervisor/consultant that the practice experience was acquired and successful completion of the CNA's PMH nursing certification examination is required. Recertification is necessary every 5 years. RNs

with certification in PMH nursing sign "CPMHN(C)," as well as "RN," after their name.

In Western Canada (Manitoba, Saskatchewan, Alberta, and British Columbia) and the Yukon, the distinct profession of RPNs is regulated by separate provincial/territorial associations. There is a national association, the Registered Psychiatric Nurses of Canada (RPNC), that publishes a code of ethics and standards of practice.

> **KEY CONCEPT Standards** are used by self-regulating professional groups to identify their expected and achievable competencies and to make explicit their obligations to the public.

CFMHN Standards of Practice

The *Canadian Standards of Psychiatric–Mental Health Nursing* were developed by expert PMH nurses in 1996 (Austin, Gallop, Harris, & Spencer, 1996), revised in 1998, 2006, and 2014 (CFMHN, 2014). The CFMHN Standards are organized by a "**domains of practice**" framework (Benner, 1984), with competencies classified within seven domains (see Boxes 5-1 to 5-7). It is acknowledged that nurses' achievement of competent practice is shaped by the nursing model they utilize as well as by the social, cultural, economic, and political factors that act on health care. Beliefs underlying the CFMHN standards include the belief that the therapeutic nurse–client relationship, based on trust and mutual respect, is at the core of PMH nursing practice and holistic, ethical, and culturally competent care. Collaborative relationships with individuals, families, communities, and different populations, as well as with interdisciplinary colleagues, are highly valued. Important to PMH nurses are the alleviation of stigma and discrimination, the protection of human rights, and the promotion of recovery and well-being for those living with mental illness. PMH nurses advocate for equitable access to health care resources, for practice environments that promote safe and positive work relationships, for research and its application to improvements in care and treatment, and for social action to promote political and social awareness that impacts health care policy. To foster action on these beliefs, PMH nurses look to fostering a legacy of moral and visionary PMH nursing leaders (CFMHN, 2014).

The RPNC Standards of Practice

Four national standards ground RPN practice: therapeutic interpersonal relationships with individuals, families, groups, and communities; application and integration of theory-based knowledge; professional responsibility for safe, competent, ethical practice; and professional ethics (RPNC, 2010). The College of the Registered Psychiatric

BOX 5-1 Canadian Standards of Psychiatric–Mental Health Nursing

STANDARD I: Provides Competent Professional Care Through the Development of a Therapeutic Relationship

A primary goal of PMH nursing is the promotion of mental health and the prevention or diminution of mental disorder. The development of a therapeutic relationship is the foundation from where the PMH nurse can "enter into partnerships with clients, and through the use of the human sciences, and the art of caring, develop helping relationships" (Registered Nurses Association of Ontario, 2002).

The nurse:

1. Assesses and clarifies the influences of personal beliefs, values, and life experience on the therapeutic relationship and distinguishes between social and therapeutic relationships
2. Works in partnership with diverse and heterogeneous populations, families, and relevant others to determine goal-directed needs and to establish an environment that is conducive to goal achievement
3. Uses a range of therapeutic verbal and nonverbal communication skills that include empathy, active listening, observing, genuineness, and curiosity
4. Recognizes the influence of age, culture, class, ethnicity, language, stigma, and social exclusion on the therapeutic process and negotiates care that is sensitive to these influences
5. Mobilizes and advocates for resources that improve community integration and increase the ability of diverse and heterogeneous populations and their families, including those isolated geographically, to access mental health services
6. Understands and responds to human reactions to distress and loss of control that may be expressed as anger, anxiety, fear, grief, helplessness, hopelessness, and humour
7. Recognizes and respects the client's expert and unique knowledge and facilitates the client's behavioural, developmental, emotional, or spiritual change while acknowledging and supporting the client's participation, responsibility, and choices in his/her care
8. Respects the client's and family's lived expertise and unique knowledge in promoting recovery
9. Fosters mutuality of the relationship by reflectively critiquing therapeutic effectiveness through client and family responses and feedback, clinical supervision, and self-evaluation
10. Understands the nature of chronic illness and applies the principles of health promotion and disease prevention when working with clients and families in the promotion of recovery

BOX 5-2 Canadian Standards of Psychiatric–Mental Health Nursing

STANDARD II: Performs/Refines Client Assessments Through the Diagnostic and Monitoring Function

Effective assessment, diagnosis, and monitoring are central to the nurse's role and depend upon theory as well as upon understanding the meaning of the health or illness experience from the perspective of the client. The nurse explains the assessment process to the client and provides feedback. Knowledge is integrated with the nurse's conceptual model of nursing practice, which provides a framework for processing client data and for developing client-focused plans of care. The nurse makes professional judgments based upon evidence and recognizes and includes the client as a valued partner.

The nurse:

1. Collaborates with clients and with other members of the health care team to gather holistic, client-centred assessments through observation, engagement, examination, interview (using respectful, recovery-focused language), and consultation, while attending to confidentiality and pertinent legal statutes
2. Assesses, documents, and analyzes data to identify health status, potential for wellness, health care deficits, potential for danger to self and others; alterations in thought content and/or process, affect behaviour, communication and decision-making abilities; substance use and dependency; and history of trauma and/or abuse (emotional, physical, neglect, sexual, or verbal)
3. Formulates and documents a plan of care in collaboration with the client and the mental health team that supports recovery and reintegration/social inclusion in the community through discharge planning and provision for ongoing support, all while recognizing variability in the client's ability to participate in the process
4. Refines and expands client assessment information by assessing and documenting significant change(s) in the client's status and by comparing new data with the baseline assessment and intermediate client goals
5. Assesses status and anticipates potential needs and risks continuously, collaborating with the client to examine his/her environment for risk factors such as self-care, housing, nutrition, economic support, psychological state, and social interactions
6. Determines the most appropriate and available therapeutic modality that meets the client's needs, and assists the client to access these resources

Nurses of Alberta (CRPNA, 2013) has provincial standards of practice that meet the conditions of Alberta's Health Professions Act, which stipulates that failure to meet the CRPNA standards constitutes unprofessional conduct.

■ KEY COMPONENTS OF PMH NURSING PRACTICE

Clinical Decision-Making

Decision-making involves critical thinking and is at the core of clinical practice. **Clinical decision-making** focuses on choices made in clinical settings. In addition to complex decisions, such as collecting, processing, and organizing information and formulating nursing approaches, many moment-to-moment decisions are made, such as deciding whether a client should receive a PRN medication. The development and implementation of efficacious interventions involve critical analysis of client, family, and community data, as well as making decisions about care. Such decision making should involve the client, family, and other significant stakeholders as much as ethically, legally, and logistically possible. Reflective thinking about the client's illness experience and personal response to the treatment and care situation is an important aspect of choosing interventions. The nurse needs to have a thorough understanding of the rationale and the theoretical underpinnings of the client's care plan.

BOX 5-3 Canadian Standards of Psychiatric–Mental Health Nursing

STANDARD III: Administers and Monitors Therapeutic Interventions

The nature of mental health problems and mental disorders raises specific practice issues for the PMH nurse in the assessment and administration of therapeutic interventions. Many clients are at risk for harm to self or others, either directly or through neglect (including self-neglect). Every effort will be made to include the client in all aspects of decision making. The PMH nurse will be alert and respond to adverse reactions.

The nurse:

1. Utilizes and evaluates evidence-based interventions to provide ethical, culturally competent, safe, effective, and efficient nursing care consistent with the mental, physical, spiritual, emotional, social, and cultural needs of the individual
2. Provides information to clients and families/significant others in accordance with relevant legislation
3. Assists, educates, and empowers clients to select choices that support informed decision making and provides information about the possible consequence(s) of the choice
4. Supports clients to draw on their own assets and resources for self-care, daily living activities, resource mobilization, and mental health promotion
5. Determines clinical intervention, using knowledge of the client's response
6. Uses technology appropriately to perform safe, effective, and efficient nursing intervention
7. Uses knowledge of age-specific implications of psychotropic medications and administers medications accurately and safely, monitoring therapeutic responses, reactions, untoward effects, toxicity, and potential incompatibilities with other medications or substances, and provides medication education with appropriate content
8. Utilizes therapeutic elements of group process
9. Incorporates knowledge of family dynamics, cultural values, and beliefs in the provision of care
10. Collaborates with the client, health care providers, and community members to access and coordinate resources, such as employment, education, and volunteering, and seeks feedback from the client and others regarding interventions
11. Encourages and assists clients to seek out mutual support groups and to strengthen social support networks as needed
12. Seeks out the client's response to, and perception of, nursing and other therapeutic interventions and incorporates it into practice
13. Ensures care for individuals of different populations (e.g., incarcerated individuals, individuals with intellectual disabilities) from therapeutic and rehabilitative perspectives

BOX 5-4 Canadian Standards of Psychiatric–Mental Health Nursing

STANDARD IV: Effectively Manages Rapidly Changing Situations

The effective management of rapidly changing situations is essential in critical circumstances that may be termed psychiatric emergencies. These situations include risk factors for self-harm, aggressive behaviours, and rapidly changing mental and physical health states (SERPN, 1996).

The nurse:

1. Utilizes the therapeutic relationship throughout the management of rapidly changing situations
2. Assesses the client using a comprehensive holistic approach for actual or potential issues, problems, risk factors, and/or crisis/emergency/catastrophic situations
3. Knows about resources required to manage actual and potential crisis/emergency/catastrophic situations and plans access to these resources
4. Monitors client safety and utilizes continual assessment to detect early changes in client status and intervenes accordingly
5. Implements timely, age-appropriate, and client-specific crisis/emergency/catastrophic interventions as necessary
6. Uses trauma-informed care when managing crisis situations with clients to minimize further trauma and interference with recovery objectives
7. Commences critical procedures when necessary, which, in an institutional setting, includes suicide precautions, emergency restraint, elopement precautions, and infectious disease management, and, in a community setting, includes community support systems, such as police, ambulance, and crisis response resources
8. Utilizes a least restraint approach to care
9. Develops and documents the management plan of care and intervention
10. Coordinates care to prevent errors and duplication of efforts where rapid intervention is imperative
11. Evaluates the effectiveness of the rapid responses with the client and modifies critical plans as necessary
12. Involves, with client collaboration, the family and significant others to identify the precipitates of the event and to plan ways to minimize risk of recurrence
13. Participates in process review with the client, family, health care team, and other service providers as needed
14. Utilizes safety measures to protect the client, self, and colleagues from potentially abusive situations in the work environment
15. Participates in and implements activities that improve client safety in the practice setting

Critical Pathways in Care Planning

Many psychiatric facilities use **critical pathways** to ensure a quality level of care in a cost-effective way. These care paths are similar to individual treatment plans in that all the disciplines' interventions are included on one plan. Critical pathways, however, are designed for a hypothetical client who has typical symptoms and who follows an expected course of treatment. Care paths are not developed for each individual client. This unification

of care can be helpful if it means that best practices shape the care received by all clients and if it facilitates the use of expert knowledge by all those providing care. It is not helpful if the unique needs and situation of each client and family are ignored, or if nurses are restrained in their provision of thoughtful, sensitive care.

● STUDY NOTE

Critical pathways, which identify key interventions and related best practices for a "typical" client with a specific mental disorder, can be helpful study tools.

BOX 5-5 Canadian Standards of Psychiatric–Mental Health Nursing

STANDARD V: Intervenes Through the Teaching-Coaching Function

All interactions are potentially teaching/learning situations. The PMH nurse attempts to understand the life experience of the client and uses this understanding to support and promote learning related to health and personal development. The nurse provides health promotion information to individuals, family, communities, and different populations.

The nurse:

1. Collaborates with clients to determine learning needs, emphasizing and supporting the client's potential for recovery
2. Plans and implements health promotion education while considering the context of the client's life experiences, readiness, culture, literacy, language, preferred learning style, and available resources
3. Explores options and resources with the client to build knowledge for making informed choices related to health needs and for accessing the system as needed
4. Incorporates knowledge of diverse learning models and principles, including the principles of recovery, when creating learning opportunities for clients
5. Provides guidance, support, and relevant information (with appropriate critiques) to clients, families, and significant others
6. Documents the teaching/learning process (assessment, implementation, client involvement, and evaluation)
7. Determines with the client the effectiveness of the educational process and collaboratively develops or adapts it to meet learning needs
8. Engages in teaching/learning opportunities as a partner with clients, families, and community agencies

---

BOX 5-6 Canadian Standards of Psychiatric–Mental Health Nursing

STANDARD VI: Monitors and Ensures the Quality of Health Care Practices

The nurse has a responsibility to advocate for clients' rights to receive the least restrictive form of care and to respect and affirm clients' right to self-determination in a safe and equitable manner. The PMH nurse must be informed about relevant legislation, its interpretation, and its implications for nursing practice.

The nurse:

1. Identifies philosophies, attitudes, values, and beliefs of the workplace that affect the nurse's performance, safety, and compassion and responds appropriately
2. Understands how the determinants of health affect community well-being and PMH nursing practice
3. Understands relevant legislation and its implications for nursing practice and utilizes it appropriately
4. Expands and incorporates knowledge of innovations and changes in mental health and psychiatric nursing practice to ensure safe, confidential, and effective care
5. Ensures and documents ongoing review and evaluation of PMH nursing care activities
6. Participates in dialogue and critical reflection about the interdependent functions of the team within the overall plan of care
7. Advocates for the client within the context of the health care environment
8. Advocates for continuous improvement to the organizational/systemic structures consistent with the principles of ethical and competent care
9. Recognizes the dynamic changes in health care locally and globally and, with stakeholders, supports strategies to manage these changes

---

Recovery as the Framework for Mental Health Care

Recovery, defined as "a process in which people with mental health problems and illnesses are empowered and supported to engage actively in their own journey of well-being," has been placed at the centre of Canada's national mental health strategy (Mental Health Commission of Canada, 2009, p. 122). The recovery process is envisioned as enabling individuals to have a meaningful, fulfilling life and is supported by the strengths of the individual, family, and community (see Chapter 8). The World Health Organization's (2013) "Mental Health Action Plan 2013–2020" acknowledges, as well, the importance of promoting and enhancing recovery, identifying the need for community-based mental health services "to encompass a recovery-based approach that puts the emphasis on supporting individuals with mental disorders and psychosocial disabilities to achieve their own aspirations and goals"(p. 14).

This vision of "recovery" that is about quality of life, rather than the more narrow notion of clinical recovery, challenges nurses and other health professionals to reassess their practice. Reorientation to a recovery-centric model is an opportunity to identify ways to improve everyday practice. It may mean that a new perspective on what constitutes "evidence" for best care will be taken or more active ways to engage family and community resources sought; or perhaps it will be greater vigilance regarding restrictive practices that evolves. Nursing associations (e.g., CFMHN, RPNC) are ensuring that a **recovery model** of practice informs practice standards. Standards are therefore excellent resources for identifying ways to enact a recovery framework in mental health care.

Collaborative Care

Although PMH care has a long tradition of using a multidisciplinary approach, with several disciplines providing services to a client, this approach can lead to fragmented care. An **interdisciplinary approach**, in which interventions from the different disciplines are integrated in the delivery of care, can be more effective. For instance, a nurse and a psychologist may simultaneously work with a client on changing a behaviour related to medication compliance. An effective interdisciplinary approach requires close collaboration with the client and family, as well as the care team to enact an integrated care plan.

BOX 5-7 Canadian Standards of Psychiatric–Mental Health Nursing

STANDARD VII: Practices Effectively Within Organizational and Work-Role Structure

Psychiatric and mental health nursing care occurs in both community and hospital settings. For the PMH nurse, care requires a therapeutic relationship involving reflective, ethical, and evidence-based practice within complex and dynamic situations. The PMH nurses must be able to plan and implement collaborative care and advocate for the mental health of their clients and others.

The nurse:
1. Collaborates with clients/families/significant others and other stakeholders to facilitate safe, supportive, and respectful environments for all persons
2. Actively participates to sustain and promote a climate that supports ethical practice and a moral community
3. Understands and utilizes quality outcome indicators and strives for continuous quality improvement
4. Seeks to utilize constructive and collaborative approaches to resolve differences among members of the health care team that may impact care
5. Participates in developing, implementing, and critiquing mental health policy, which fosters recovery and continuity of care
6. Advocates and supports a nursing leadership role
7. Supports and helps to mentor and coach new graduates
8. Utilizes knowledge of collaborative strategies for social action in working with consumer and advocacy groups
9. Pursues opportunities to reduce stigma and to promote social inclusion and community integration for clients

From Canadian Federation of Mental Health Nurses (CFMHN). (2014). *The Canadian standards of psychiatric and mental health nursing* (4th ed.). Toronto: Author.

The Canadian Collaborative Mental Health Initiative's (CCMHI's) (Gagné, 2005) vision of **collaborative care** is to have an accessible, integrated system of health care providers across various disciplines and backgrounds working together with clients and their families across the continuum of mental health care (prevention to rehabilitation). A coordinator, "case manager," or "patient/client navigator" has been found to be an important aspect of effective collaborative care (Kates et al., 2011)—a role often held by a nurse.

■ CHALLENGES OF PMH NURSING

The challenges of PMH nursing are increasing in the 21st century. New knowledge is being generated, technology is shaping health care into new dimensions, and nursing practice is becoming more specialized and autonomous. This section discusses a few of the challenges.

Knowledge Development, Dissemination, and Application

Results of new research efforts continually redefine our knowledge base relative to mental disorders and their treatment. Consider the significant advances in neurobiologic knowledge. In the 1970s, the cause of schizophrenia was hypothesized to be overactivity of dopamine. Later, it was discovered that other neurotransmitters seemed to play a role as well. Such knowledge resulted in new medications with various side effect profiles becoming available, requiring nurses to redefine their monitoring and interventions related to medication administration. Advances in our understanding of genetics and epigenetics are occurring, bringing new knowledge but also new ethical issues. The presence of comorbid medical disorders is acknowledged as significant to the treatment of mental disorders. For example, hypertension, hypothyroidism, hyperthyroidism, and diabetes mellitus can each affect the disease trajectory of mental disorders. In some settings, the nurse may be the only one who has a background in medical disorders, such as human immunodeficiency viral illness, acquired immunodeficiency syndrome, and other somatic health problems.

The challenge for nurses today is to stay abreast of the advances in holistic health care in order to provide safe, competent care to individuals with mental disorders. Nurses must strive to provide evidence-based nursing care, developing their knowledge on an ongoing basis. Accessing up-to-date information through journals, electronic databases, and continuing education programs is a recognized responsibility. Not only do nurses need to access current research studies but they also must evaluate the usefulness of the studies. For instance, one research project supporting a particular treatment approach may not be as meaningful as several statistically significant studies. The results of qualitative research studies, although not generalizable, may have important implications for practice, for instance, insights that can deepen our understanding of client experiences. Resources such as the evolving International Knowledge Exchange Network for Mental Health (IKEN-MH) will be important tools in improving care. Nurses practising in PMH settings are challenged to integrate new knowledge into a bio/psycho/social/spiritual model that includes all human responses to potential or actual health problems.

Health Care Delivery System Challenges

Continuing challenges for Canadian nurses include supporting the integration of mental health care within primary health care, articulating the influence of the determinants of health on mental health, and playing a strong, effective role in the enactment of Canada's national strategy for mental health. Nurses need to be participants in, not merely conversant with, the ongoing innovations of the Mental Health Commission of Canada (MHCC).

Consumers of mental health services and their families are gaining voice and calling for meaningful changes in the delivery of services. Inequities in health care for marginalized populations, such as those living with a chronic mental illness, are being challenged, as are paternalistic approaches to the delivery of care. One source of this challenge is the Canadian Alliance on Mental Illness and Mental Health (CAMIMH). The CAMIMH, created in 1998, consists of consumers, their families, researchers, and care providers from numerous professions. Their mission is to influence national policy, to speak in a unified voice, and to focus strategically on mental health and mental illness. CAMIMH is a member of the CCMHI. Active partnership among users of services, nurses and other health providers, and the community at large is necessary to effect the positive changes initiated by our national strategy in mental health.

Overcoming Stigma and Discrimination

Overcoming the stigma and discrimination related to mental illness, a priority of the MHCC, needs to occur within health care systems. Not only do persons with mental health disorders and their families experience stigmatization by some health care professionals' avoidance, discomfort, or even disdain, but professionals who practice in PMH settings can experience stigma by association (Halter, 2008). They may be seen as less skilled than their colleagues practising in other areas and be less respected (Halter). This can result in health science students, including those in nursing, not considering mental health care as a career choice.

e-Mental Health

The impact of communication and information technologies on mental health care and nursing is unprecedented. Nurses are challenged to gain and develop the skills to use this technology in improving care. Telehealth, for example, takes many forms, from communicating with remote sites (e.g., providing a range of services from screening to treatment) to completing educational programs. Clients and families are helped to learn about disorders, treatment, and resources. Software programs make daily functioning easier for some. E-mail and the Internet can be highly effective forms of communication. For instance, advocacy groups for consumers of mental health services use these means to organize and lobby for change locally, nationally, and internationally. Nurses can access professional development and educational resources for ongoing support in their practice.

"e-Mental Health" is the name given to these technologies that are providing cost-effective alternatives to traditional mental health care across distances and becoming important resources, given Canada's vast geography. The challenge e-Mental Health presents to nurses is to learn to use the technology effectively and ethically to connect with clients, families, and communities in a meaningful way. It is also important that nurses teach clients effective ways to critique Web sites and to question the validity of the information found (e.g., its source,

objectivity/bias, accuracy, authority, currency), as well as direct them to reliable Internet resources.

■ PMH NURSING IN A GLOBAL COMMUNITY

As members of a global community, Canadian nurses recognize their role in achieving "health for all." Mental health is a particularly disadvantaged aspect of health care around the world, so capacity building for mental health care is a pressing priority (Kakuma et al., 2011). The Faculty of Nursing at the University of Alberta is a WHO Collaborating Centre in Nursing and Mental Health, with such capacity building a prime objective of the Centre. Mental health care can be effectively delivered in primary care settings through collaboration among skilled, nonspecialist professionals, trained lay workers, consumer representatives, and caregivers when supported by mental health specialists in consultative roles for services and training (Kakuma). The International Society of Psychiatric–Mental Health Nurses (ISPN), an organization with student members, works to unite and strengthen the presence and voice of PMH nurses and to promote quality care for individuals and families with mental health problems. The World Federation for Mental Health (WFMH), an organization to which nurses belong, has as its mission, since its founding in 1948, the advancement of mental health promotion, prevention, and care among all people. It works with governments from more than 100 countries and nongovernment groups. WFMH sponsors World Mental Health Day, which occurs annually on October 10. Mental Disability Rights International (MDRI) is an advocacy group dedicated to the enforcement of rights of people with mental disabilities. Examples of their country reports on human rights, mental health, and psychiatric care include Turkey (2005), Romania (2006), Argentina (2007), and Serbia (2007). A current campaign is worldwide: to stop the institutionalization of children with disabilities. Organizations are an important pathway for nurses' contribution to the improvement of mental health and mental health care across the globe.

SUMMARY OF KEY POINTS

■ The bio/psycho/social/spiritual model focuses on separate but interdependent dimensions of biologic, psychological, social, and spiritual factors in the assessment and treatment of mental disorders. This comprehensive and holistic approach to mental disorders is the foundation for effective PMH nursing practice and is used as the basic organizational framework for this text.

■ Standards of practice set out the explicit responsibilities and competencies of a profession.

■ PMH nurses interact with other disciplines and many times act as a coordinator in the delivery of care.

■ PMH nurses need to be aware of team dynamics and their impact on care. When nurses practise in inter-disciplinary settings, there may be an overlapping of professional roles. Nurses are accountable for both discrete and shared functions that they perform in their practice.

■ Challenges facing nurses practising in PMH settings include knowledge development, dissemination, and application; e-Mental Health; addressing stigma and discrimination within health care systems; and working to make the health care system more collaborative and responsive to the mental health needs of Canadians.

■ National and international organizations are important pathways for nurses' contribution to improving mental health and mental health care worldwide.

CRITICAL THINKING CHALLENGES

1 Apply the bio/psycho/social/spiritual model to the following clinical examples:

  a A first-time father is extremely depressed after the birth of his child, who is perfectly healthy.

  b A child is unable to sleep at night because of terrifying nightmares.

  c An older woman is resentful of moving into a senior citizens' residence even though the decision was hers.

2 Visit the Web sites of the organizations (see Web Links on thePoint) and discover the role of each in promoting quality mental health care or supporting nursing practice.

3 Describe when and how nursing care plans and integrated care paths should be used.

4 What are the challenges of enacting collaborative care with other health disciplines? Is your nursing education preparing you well for collaboration with other professionals? In your opinion, what educational strategies best facilitate such preparation?

5 Reflect upon the nurse's role in a global community. Does the motto "think globally, act locally" have meaning for the improvement of mental health and mental health care?

REFERENCES

Abraham, I., Fox, J., & Cohen, B. (1992). Integrating the bio into the bio-psychosocial: Understanding and treating biological phenomena in psychiatric–mental health nursing. *Archives of Psychiatric Nursing, 6*(5), 296–305.

Austin, W., Gallop, R., Harris, D., & Spencer, E. (1996). A domain of practice approach to the standards of psychiatric and mental health nursing. *Journal of Psychiatric and Mental Health Nursing, 3,* 111–115.

Barker, P. J., & Buchanan-Barker, P. (2004). *Spirituality and mental health breakthrough.* London, UK: Whurr Publishers.

Benner, P. (1984). *From novice to expert: Excellence and power in clinical nursing practice.* Menlo Park, CA: Addison-Wesley.

Canadian Federation of Mental Health Nurses (CFMHN). (2014). *The Canadian standards of psychiatric and mental health nursing* (4th ed.). Toronto, ON: Author.

Catalano, J. T. (2006) *Nursing now: Today's issues, tomorrow's trends.* Philadelphia, PA: F. A. Davis Company.

Cobb, M., Rumbold, B., & Puchalski, C. M. (Eds.). (2012). *The Oxford textbook of spirituality in health care.* Oxford, UK: Oxford University Press.

College of Registered Psychiatric Nurses of Alberta (CRPNA). (2013). *Code of ethics and standards of psychiatric nursing practice.* Edmonton, AB: Authors.

Dossey, B. M., Keegan, L., & Guzzetta, C. E., (2004). *Holistic nursing: A handbook for practice* (4th ed.). Frederick, MD: Aspen.

Gagné, M. A. (2005). *What is collaborative mental health care? An introduction to the collaborative mental health care framework.* Mississauga, ON: Canadian Collaborative Mental Health Initiative. Available at www.ccmhi.ca

Halter, M. J. (2008). Perceived characteristics of psychiatric nurses: Stigma by association. *Archives of Psychiatric Nursing, 22*(1), 20–26.

Heru, A. & Drury, L. (2006). Overcoming barriers in working with families. *Academic Psychiatry, 30,* 379–384.

Hood Morris, L. E. (1996). A spiritual well-being model: Use with older women who experience depression. *Issues in Mental Health Nursing, 17*(5), 439–455.

Kakuma, R., Minas, H., van Ginneken, N., Dal Paz, M.R., Desiraju, K., Morris, J. E., … Scheffler, R. M. (2011). Human resources of mental health care: current situation and strategies for action. *The Lancet, 378,* 1654–1663.

Kates, N., Mazowita, G., Lemire, F., Jayabarathan, A., Bland, R., Selby, P., Isomura, T., Craven, M., Gervais, M., & Audet, D. (2011). The evolution of collaborative mental health care in Canada: A shared vision for the future: Position paper of the Canadian Psychiatric Association & the College of Family Physicians of Canada. *The Canadian Journal of Psychiatry, 56*(5), 1–10.

MacCourt, P., Family Caregivers Advisory Committee, Mental Health Commission of Canada. (2013). *National guidelines for a comprehensive service system to support family caregivers of adults with mental health problems and illnesses.* Calgary, AB: Mental Health Commission of Canada. Retrieved from http://www.mentalhealthcommission.ca

Mauk, K. & Schmidt, N. (2004). *Spiritual care in nursing practice.* New York, NY: Lippincott Williams & Wilkins.

Mental Health Commission of Canada. (2009). *Toward recovery and well-being: A framework for a mental health strategy for Canada.* Ottawa, ON: Author.

O'Reilly, M. (2004). Spirituality and mental health clients. *Journal of Psychosocial Nursing and Mental Health Service, 42*(7), 44–59.

Registered Nurses Association of Ontario. (2002). *Best practice guideline: Crisis intervention.* Toronto, ON: Author.

Registered Psychiatric Nurses of Canada (RPNC). (2010). *Code of ethics and standards of psychiatric nursing practice.* Edmonton, AB: Author.

Society for Education and Research in Psychiatric-Mental Health Nursing (SERPN) (1996). *Educational preparation for psychiatric-mental health nursing practice.* Pensacola, FL: Author.

World Health Organization. (2013). *Comprehensive mental health action plan 2013–2020.* Retrieved from http://www.who.int/mental_health/action_plan_2013/en/

6 Communication and the Therapeutic Relationship

Cheryl Forchuk

After studying this chapter, you will be able to:

- Identify the importance of self-awareness in nursing practice.
- Develop a repertoire of verbal and nonverbal communication skills.
- Develop a process for selecting effective communication techniques.
- Explain how the nurse can establish a therapeutic relationship with clients by using rapport and empathy.
- Explain the physical, emotional, social, and spiritual boundaries of the nurse–client relationship.
- Discuss the significance of defence mechanisms.
- Explain what occurs in each of the three phases of the nurse–client relationship: orientation, working, and resolution.
- Describe motivational interviewing (MI), including assumptions and techniques.
- Describe the transitional relationship model (TRM), including assumptions and components.

KEY CONCEPTS

- nurse–client relationship
- self-awareness
- therapeutic communication

KEY TERMS

- active listening • boundaries • communication blocks • content themes • countertransference • defence mechanisms • empathic linkages • empathy • nontherapeutic • nonverbal communication • orientation phase • passive listening • process recording • rapport • resolution phase • self-disclosure • symbolism • telehealth • transference • validation • verbal communication • working phase

---

Clients with mental health disorders may have special communication and relationship needs that require advanced therapeutic communication skills. In psychiatric and mental health (PMH) nursing, the nurse–client relationship is an important tool used to reach treatment goals. The purposes of this chapter are to (1) help the nurse develop self-awareness and communication techniques needed for a therapeutic nurse–client relationship, (2) examine the specific stages or steps involved in establishing the relationship, (3) explore the specific factors that make a nurse–client relationship successful and therapeutic, and (4) differentiate therapeutic from **nontherapeutic** relationships.

SELF-AWARENESS

Self-awareness is the process of understanding one's own beliefs, thoughts, motivations, biases, and limitations and recognizing how they affect others. Without self-awareness, nurses will find it impossible to establish and maintain therapeutic relationships with clients. "Know thyself" is a basic tenet of PMH nursing (see Box 6-1).

To come to self-awareness, nurses can carry out self-examination. Self-examination involves reflecting on the personal meaning of the current nursing situation. This reflection can relate to similar past situations and issues related to personal values and beliefs. Self-examination

BOX 6-1 "Know Thyself"

Do you have any physical problems or illnesses?

Have you had significant traumatic life events (e.g., divorce, death of a significant person, abuse, disaster)?

Do your family or significant others have prejudiced or embarrassing beliefs and attitudes about groups different than yours?

Would sociocultural factors in your background contribute to being rejected by members of other cultures?

Do you have strong religious beliefs that shape your daily life?

If your answer to any of these questions is yes, how would these experiences and beliefs affect your ability to care for clients with these characteristics?

can provoke anxiety and is rarely comfortable; it can occur alone or with help from others. Self-examination without the benefit of another's perspective can lead to a biased view of self. Conducting self-examination is best with a trusted individual who can give objective but realistic feedback. The development of self-awareness requires a willingness to be introspective and to examine personal beliefs, attitudes, and motivations.

KEY CONCEPT Self-awareness is the process of understanding one's own beliefs, thoughts, motivations, biases, and limitations and recognizing how they affect self and others.

THE BIO/PSYCHO/SOCIAL/ SPIRITUAL SELF

Each nurse brings a bio/psycho/social/spiritual self to nursing practice. The client perceives the biologic dimension of the nurse in terms of physical characteristics: age, gender, body weight, height, ethnic or racial background, and any other observed physical characteristics. The nurse can have a certain genetic composition, illness, or unobservable physical disability that may influence the quality or delivery of nursing care. The nurse's psychological state also influences how he or she analyzes client information and selects treatment interventions. An emotional state or behaviour can inadvertently influence the therapeutic relationship. For example, a nurse who has just learned that her child is using illegal drugs and who has a client with a history of drug use may inadvertently project a judgmental attitude toward her client, which would interfere with the formation of a therapeutic relationship. The nurse needs to examine underlying emotions, motivations, and beliefs and determine how these factors shape behaviour.

The nurse's social biases can be particularly problematic for the nurse–client relationship. Although the nurse may not verbalize these values to clients, some are readily evident in the nurse's behaviour and appearance, such as how the nurse acts or appears at work. The nurse's

spiritual beliefs or feelings can also affect interactions. For instance, beliefs about divorce, abortion, or homosexuality can affect how the nurse interacts with a client who is dealing with such issues.

UNDERSTANDING PERSONAL FEELINGS AND BELIEFS, AND CHANGING BEHAVIOUR

Nurses must understand their own personal feelings and beliefs and try to avoid projecting them onto clients. This is not an easy task. For instance, due to ethnocentrism, our own sociocultural values may not be readily apparent. It takes effort to develop self-awareness, but it will enhance the nurse's objectivity and foster a nonjudgmental attitude, which is so important in building and maintaining trust throughout the nurse–client relationship. Soliciting feedback from colleagues and supervisors about how personal beliefs or thoughts are being projected onto others is a useful self-assessment technique. One of the reasons that ongoing clinical supervision is so important is that the supervisor really knows the nurse and can continually observe for inappropriate communication and question assumptions that the nurse may hold, as well as reinforce helpful behaviour.

Once a nurse has identified and analyzed personal beliefs and attitudes, prejudicial behaviours may change. The change process requires introspective analysis that may result in viewing the world differently. Through self-awareness and conscious effort, the nurse can change learned behaviours to engage effectively in therapeutic relationships with clients. Nevertheless, a nurse may realize that some attitudes are too ingrained to support a therapeutic relationship with a client with different beliefs. In such cases, the nurse should refer the client to someone who can be therapeutically helpful.

COMMUNICATION

Effective communication skills, including verbal and nonverbal techniques, are the building blocks for all successful relationships. The nurse–client relationship is built on therapeutic communication, the ongoing process of interaction through which meaning emerges (see Box 6-2). **Verbal communication**, which is principally achieved by spoken words, includes the underlying emotion, context, and connotation of what is actually said. **Nonverbal communication** includes gestures, expressions, and body language. Both the client and the nurse use verbal and nonverbal communication. **Empathic linkages** are the direct communication of feelings. To respond therapeutically in a nurse–client relationship, the nurse is responsible for assessing and interpreting all forms of client communication.

Therapeutic and social relationships are very different. In a therapeutic relationship, the nurse focuses on the client and client-related issues, even when engaging in social activities with that client. For example, a nurse may

BOX 6-2 Principles of Therapeutic Communication

1. The client should be the primary focus of the interaction.
2. A professional attitude sets the tone of the therapeutic relationship.
3. Use self-disclosure cautiously and only when the disclosure has a therapeutic purpose.
4. Avoid social relationships with clients.
5. Maintain client confidentiality.
6. Assess the client's intellectual competence to determine the level of understanding.
7. Implement interventions from a theoretic base.
8. Maintain a nonjudgmental attitude. Avoid making judgments about the client's behaviour and giving advice. By the time the client sees the nurse, he or she has had plenty of advice.
9. Guide the client to reinterpret his or her experiences rationally.
10. Track the client's verbal interaction through the use of clarifying statements. Avoid changing the subject unless the content change is in the client's best interest.

FIGURE 6-1. The communication process. (Adapted from Boyd, M. (1995). Communication with clients, families, healthcare providers, and diverse cultures. In M. Strader & P. Decker (Eds.), *Role transition to client care management* (p. 431). Norwalk, CT: Appleton & Lange.)

take a client shopping and out for lunch. Even though the nurse is engaged in a social activity, that trip should have a definite purpose, and conversation should focus only on the client. The nurse must not attempt to meet his or her own social or other needs during the activity.

● STUDY NOTE

In analyzing nurse–client communication, nonverbal behaviours and gestures are communicated first. If a client's verbal and nonverbal communications are contradictory, priority of interpretation is given to the nonverbal behaviours and gestures since they operate on a more basic and less conscious level and are therefore harder to mask.

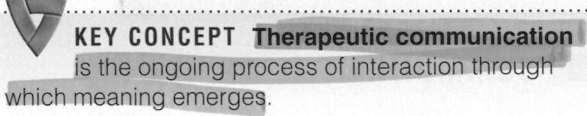

KEY CONCEPT **Therapeutic communication** is the ongoing process of interaction through which meaning emerges.

USING VERBAL COMMUNICATION

The process of verbal communication involves a sender, a message, and a receiver. The client is often the sender, and the nurse is often the receiver (Fig. 6-1), but communication always works two ways. The client formulates an idea, encodes a message (puts ideas into words), and then transmits the message with emotion. The client's words and their underlying emotional tone and connotation communicate his or her needs and emotional problems or issues. The nurse receives the message, decodes it (interprets the message, including its feelings, connotation, and context), and then responds to the client. On the surface, this interaction is deceptively simple, but unseen complexities lie beneath. Is the message that the nurse receives consistent with the client's original idea? Did the nurse

interpret the message as the client intended? Is the verbal message consistent with the nonverbal flourishes that accompany it? Validation is essential to ensure that the nurse has received the information accurately. (See section "Validation" later in this chapter for further discussion.)

Self-Disclosure

One of the most important principles of therapeutic communication for the nurse to follow is to focus the interaction on the client's concerns. **Self-disclosure**, telling the client personal information, generally is not a good idea since the conversation should focus on the client, not the nurse. If a client asks the nurse personal questions, the nurse should elicit the underlying reason for the request. The nurse can then determine how much, if any, personal information to disclose. In revealing personal information, the nurse should be purposeful and have identified therapeutic outcomes. For example, a male client struggling with the implications of marriage and fidelity asks a male nurse if he has ever had an extramarital affair. The nurse interprets the client's statement as seeking role-modelling behaviour for an adult man and judges self-disclosure in this instance to be therapeutic. He responds honestly that he does not engage in affairs and redirects the discussion back to the client's concerns.

Nurses may feel uncomfortable avoiding clients' questions for fear of seeming rude. Sometimes they disclose too much personal information because they are trying to be nice. However, being nice is not necessarily therapeutic. As appropriate, redirecting the client, giving a neutral or vague answer, or saying "Let's talk about you" may be all that is necessary to limit self-disclosure. In some instances, nurses may need to tell the client directly that they will not share personal information (Table 6-1).

Table 6-1	Self-Disclosure in Therapeutic Versus Social Relationships	

Situation	Appropriate Therapeutic Response	Inappropriate Social Response With Rationale
A client asks the nurse if she had fun over the weekend.	"The weekend was fine. How did you spend your weekend?"	"It was great. My boyfriend and I went to dinner and a movie." *(This self-disclosure has no therapeutic purpose. The response focuses the conversation on the nurse, not on the client.)*
A client asks a student nurse if she has ever been to a particular bar.	"Many people go there. I'm wondering if you have ever been there."	"Oh yes—all the time. It's a lot of fun." *(Sharing information about outside activities is inappropriate.)*
A client asks a nurse if mental illness is in his family.	"Mental illnesses do run in families. I've had a lot of experience caring for people with mental illnesses."	"My sister is being treated for depression." *(This self-disclosure has no purpose, and the nurse is missing the meaning of the question.)*
While shopping with a client, the nurse sees a friend, who approaches them.	To her friend: "I know it looks like I'm not working, but I really am. I'll see you later."	"Hi, Bob. This is Jane Doe, a client." *(Introducing the client to the friend is very inappropriate and violates client confidentiality.)*

Table 6-2	Verbal Communication Techniques		

Technique	Definition	Example	Use
Acceptance	Encouraging and receiving information in a nonjudgmental and interested manner	*Client*: I have done something terrible. *Nurse*: I would like to hear about it. It's OK to discuss it with me.	Used in establishing trust and developing empathy.
Confrontation	Presenting the client with a different reality of the situation	*Client*: My best friend never calls me. She hates me. *Nurse*: I was in the room yesterday when she called.	Used cautiously to immediately redefine the client's reality. However, it can alienate the client if used inappropriately. A nonjudgmental attitude is critical for confrontation to be effective.
Doubt	Expressing or voicing doubt when a client relates a situation	*Client*: My best friend hates me. She never calls me. *Nurse*: From what you have told me, that does not sound like her. When did she call you last?	Used carefully and only when the nurse feels confident about the details. It is used when the nurse wants to guide the client toward other explanations.
Interpretation	Putting into words what the client is implying or feeling	*Client*: I could not sleep because someone would come in my room and rape me. *Nurse*: It sounds like you were scared last night.	Used in helping the clients identify underlying thoughts or feelings.
Observation	Stating to the client what the nurse is observing	*Nurse*: You are trembling and perspiring. When did this start?	Used when a client's behaviours (verbal or nonverbal) are obvious and unusual for that client.
Open-ended statements	Introducing an idea and letting the client respond	*Nurse*: Trust means…. *Client*: That someone will keep you safe.	Used when helping the client explore feelings or gain insight.
Reflection	Redirecting the idea back to the client	*Client*: Should I go home for the weekend? *Nurse*: Should you go home for the weekend?	Used when the client is asking for the nurse's approval or judgment. Use of reflection helps the nurse maintain a nonjudgmental approach.
Restatement	Repeating the main idea expressed; lets the client know what was heard	*Client*: I hate this place. I don't belong here. *Nurse*: You don't want to be here.	Used when trying to clarify what the client has said.
Silence	Remaining quiet, but nonverbally expressing interest during an interaction	*Client*: I am angry!! *Nurse*: (Silence) *Client*: My wife had an affair.	Used when the client needs to express ideas but may not know quite how to do it. With silence, the client can focus on putting thoughts together.
Validation	Clarifying the nurse's understanding of the situation	*Nurse*: Let me see if I understand.	Used when the nurse is trying to understand a situation the client is trying to describe.

Table 6-3 Techniques That Inhibit Communication

Technique	Definition	Example	Problem
Advice	Telling a client what to do	*Client*: I can't sleep. It is too noisy. *Nurse*: Turn off the light and shut your door.	The nurse solves the client's problem, which may not be the appropriate solution and encourages dependency on the nurse.
Agreement	Agreeing with a particular viewpoint of a client	*Client*: Abortions are sinful. *Nurse*: I agree.	The client is denied an opportunity to change his or her view now that the nurse agrees.
Challenges	Disputing a client's beliefs with arguments, logical thinking, or direct order	*Client*: I'm a cowboy. *Nurse*: If you are a cowboy, what are you doing in the hospital?	The nurse belittles the client and decreases self-esteem. The client will avoid relating to the nurse who challenges.
Disapproval	Judging a client's situation and behaviour	*Client*: I'm so sorry. I did not mean to kill my mother. *Nurse*: You should be. How could anyone kill their mother?	The nurse belittles the client. The client will avoid the nurse.
Reassurance	Telling a client that everything will be OK	*Client*: Everyone thinks I'm bad. *Nurse*: You are a good person.	The nurse makes a statement that may not be true. The client is blocked from exploring feelings.

Verbal Communication Techniques

PMH nurses use many verbal techniques in establishing relationships and helping clients focus on their problems and goals. Asking a question, restating, and reflecting are examples of such techniques. These techniques may seem artificial at first, but with practice, they can be useful.

One of the most difficult but often most effective techniques is the use of silence during verbal interactions. By maintaining an open silence, the nurse allows the client to gather thoughts and to proceed at his or her own pace.

Listening is another valuable tool. Silence and listening differ in that silence consists of deliberate pauses to encourage the client to reflect and eventually respond. Listening is an ongoing activity by which the nurse attends to the client's verbal and nonverbal communication. The art of listening is developed through careful attention to the content and meaning of the client's speech. There are

BOX 6-3 Therapeutic Dialogue

GIVING ADVICE VERSUS RECOMMENDATIONS

Ms. J has just received a diagnosis of phobic disorder and been given a prescription for fluoxetine. She was referred to the home care agency because she does not want to take her medication. She is fearful of becoming suicidal. Two approaches are given below.

Ineffective Communication (Advice)
Nurse: Ms. J, the doctor has ordered the medication because it will help you.
Ms. J: I don't want to take the medication because I am afraid of becoming suicidal. I heard that some of this psychiatric medication does that. I haven't had any attacks for 2 weeks.
Nurse: This medication has rarely had that side effect. You should try it and see if you have any suicidal thoughts.
Ms. J: OK. (The nurse leaves and Ms. J does not take the medication. Within a week, Ms. J is taken to the emergency room with a panic attack.)

Effective Communication (Recommendations)
Nurse: Ms. J, how have you been doing?
Ms. J: So far, so good. I haven't had any attacks for 2 weeks.
Nurse: I understand that the doctor gave you a prescription for medication that may help with the panic attacks.
Ms. J: Yes, but I don't want to take it because I am afraid of becoming suicidal. I heard that some of this psychiatric medication does that.

Nurse: Have you ever had feelings of hurting yourself?
Ms. J: Not really.
Nurse: If you took the medication and had thoughts like that, what would you do?
Ms. J: I don't know.
Nurse: I think I see your dilemma. This medication may help your panic attacks, but the suicidal thoughts are a real fear. Is that it?
Ms. J: Yeah, that's it.
Nurse: Are there any circumstances under which you would be able to try the medication?
Ms. J: If I knew that I would not have suicidal thoughts.
Nurse: I can't guarantee that, but I could call you every few days to see if you are having any of these thoughts and help you deal with them.
Ms. J: Oh, that will be OK.
(Ms. J successfully took the medication.)

Critical Thinking Challenge
• Contrast the communication in the first scenario with that in the second.
• What therapeutic communication techniques did the second nurse employ that may have contributed to a better outcome?
• Are there any cues in the first scenario that indicate that the client will not follow the nurse's advice? Explain.

two types of listening: passive and active. **Passive listening** involves sitting quietly and letting the client talk. A passive listener allows the client to ramble and does not focus or guide the thought process. Passive listening does not foster a therapeutic relationship.

Through **active listening,** the nurse focuses on what the client is saying to interpret and respond to the message objectively. While listening, the nurse concentrates on the underlying meaning of what the client says. The nurse's verbal and nonverbal behaviours indicate active listening. The nurse usually responds indirectly, using techniques such as open-ended statements, reflection (Table 6-2), and questions that elicit additional responses from the client. In active listening, the nurse should avoid changing the subject and instead follow the client's lead although at times, it is necessary to respond directly to help a client focus on a specific topic or to clarify content, thoughts, or beliefs.

Some verbal techniques, however, block interactions and inhibit therapeutic communication (Table 6-3). One of the biggest blocks to communication is giving advice, particularly that which others likely have already given. Giving advice is different from supporting a client through decision making. The therapeutic dialogue presented in

BOX 6-4 Research for Best Practice

TELEPHONE VERSUS FACE-TO-FACE INTERVENTIONS: PERCEIVED DIFFERENCES IN THERAPEUTIC PROCESS AND TREATMENT BARRIERS

....

Lingley-Pottie, P., McGrath, P., & Andreou, P. (2013). Barriers to mental health care: Perceived delivery system differences. Advances in Nursing Science, 36(1), 51–61.

The Question: Are there differences in perceived treatment barriers between participants' experiences with distance versus face-to-face therapy?

Methods: In this "within-subject" questionnaire study, 60 participants from the *Strongest Families* telephone intervention program (Halifax, Nova Scotia) who had previous experience with face-to-face professional counselling were sampled by convenience. In the program, families who have a child with behaviour difficulties receive educational materials (handbooks, videos) and 12 weekly telephone sessions with a trained, nonprofessional coach. The questionnaire queried perceived treatment barriers using the Treatment Barrier Index (TBI) and therapeutic processes (e.g., therapeutic alliance). Questionnaires were completed by telephone, from a face-to-face perspective, and from a distance-treatment perspective.

Findings: Statistically significant differences were found between delivery system TBI scores: there were few barriers with distance treatment. Therapeutic process differences suggested enhanced therapeutic alliance and self-disclosure with distance treatment.

Implications for Practice: Increased access, convenience, and a sense of privacy (visual anonymity) are aspects of therapy using distance technologies that enhance the quality of the therapeutic experience for some individuals and families.

Box 6-3 differentiates between advice (telling the client what to do or how to act) and therapeutic communication, by which the nurse and the client explore alternative ways of viewing the client's world. The client then can reach his or her own conclusions about the best approaches to use. Refer to Box 6-4 for a summary of a research study on boundaries between clients and PMH nurses.

● **STUDY NOTE**

Self-disclosure can be used in very specific situations, but self-disclosure is not the first intervention to consider. In prioritizing interventions, active listening is one of the first methods used.

USING NONVERBAL COMMUNICATION

Gestures, facial expressions, and body language actually communicate more than do verbal messages. Under the best circumstances, body language mirrors or enhances verbal communication. However, if verbal and nonverbal messages are conflicting, the listener likely will believe the nonverbal message since it functions on a more basic level. For example, if a client says he feels fine but has a sad facial expression and is slumped in a chair away from others, a message of sadness and depression will more likely be received than the client's words. The same is true of a nurse's behaviour. If a nurse tells a client she is happy to see him, but her facial expression communicates indifference, the client will receive the message that the nurse is bored.

At times, people with mental health problems have difficulty verbally expressing themselves and interpreting the emotions of others. Nurses therefore need to assess continually the nonverbal communication needs of clients. Eye contact (or lack thereof), posture, movement (e.g., shifting in chair, pacing), facial expressions, and gestures are nonverbal behaviours that communicate thoughts and feelings. A client with low self-esteem may be unable to maintain eye contact and thus may spend a great deal of time looking toward the floor. A client who is pacing and restless may be upset or having a reaction to medication. A clenched fist usually indicates that a person feels angry or hostile.

Nonverbal behaviour is culturally specific. The nurse must therefore be careful to understand his or her own cultural context as well as that of the client. For example, in some cultures (e.g., Canadian Aboriginal nations), it is considered disrespectful to look a person straight in the eye. Other cultures see a person who makes little eye contact as "hiding something" or having low self-esteem. Other examples of nonverbal communication that may vary considerably among cultures are whether one points

FIGURE 6-2. Open and closed body language.

with the finger, nose, or eyes and how much hand gesturing one uses.

Nurses should use positive body language, such as sitting at the same eye level as the client with a relaxed posture that projects interest and attention. Leaning slightly forward helps engage the client. Generally, the nurse should not cross his or her arms or legs during therapeutic communication because such postures erect barriers to interaction. Uncrossed arms and legs project openness and a willingness to engage in conversation (Fig. 6-2). Verbal responses should be consistent with nonverbal messages.

RECOGNIZING EMPATHIC LINKAGES

Empathic linkages are the communication of feelings (Peplau, 1952). This form of communication commonly occurs with anxiety. For example, a nurse speaking with a highly anxious client may notice his own speech becoming more rapid in tandem with that of the client. The nurse may also become aware of subjective feelings of anxiety. It may be difficult for the nurse to determine whether the anxiety is communicated interpersonally or whether the nurse is personally reacting to some of the content of what the client is communicating. However, being aware of one's own feelings and analyzing them is crucial to determining the source of the feelings.

SELECTING COMMUNICATION TECHNIQUES

In therapeutic communication, the nurse chooses the best words to say and uses nonverbal behaviours that are consistent with these words. If a client is angry and upset, should the nurse invite the client to sit down and discuss the problem, walk quietly with the client, or simply observe the client from a distance and not initiate conversation? Choosing the best response begins with assessing and interpreting the meaning of the client's communication—both verbal and nonverbal.

Nurses should not necessarily take verbal messages literally, especially when a client is upset or angry. For example, a nurse enters the room of a newly admitted client who accusingly says, "You locked me up and threw away the key." The nurse could respond defensively that she had nothing to do with the client's being admitted; however, that response would end in an argument and communication would be blocked. Fortunately, the nurse recognizes that the client is communicating frustration at being in a locked psychiatric unit, and she does not take the accusation personally.

The nurse also needs to identify the desired client outcome. To do so, the nurse should engage the client with eye contact (if culturally appropriate) and quietly try to interpret the client's feelings. In the example just discussed, the desired outcome is for the client to clarify the hospitalization experience. The nurse responds by saying, "It must be frustrating to feel locked up." The nurse focuses on the client's feelings rather than the accusations, which reflects an understanding of the client's feelings. The client knows that the nurse accepts these feelings, which leads to further discussion. It may seem impossible to plan reactions for each situation, but with practice, the nurse will begin to respond consistently in a therapeutic way.

● **STUDY NOTE**

Applying communication techniques requires consideration of the ultimate goal and the client's ability to benefit from the intervention. Giving advice is rarely effective.

■ **APPLYING COMMUNICATION CONCEPTS**

When the nurse is interacting with clients, additional considerations can enhance the quality of communication. This section describes the importance of rapport, validation, empathy, and the role of boundaries and body space in nurse–client interactions.

Rapport

Rapport, interpersonal harmony characterized by understanding and respect, is important in developing a trusting, therapeutic relationship. Nurses establish rapport through interpersonal warmth, a nonjudgmental attitude, and a demonstration of understanding. A skilled nurse will establish rapport that will alleviate the client's anxiety in discussing personal problems.

People with mental health problems often feel alone and isolated. Establishing rapport helps lessen those feelings. When rapport develops, a client feels comfortable with the nurse and finds self-disclosure easier. The nurse also feels comfortable and recognizes that an interpersonal bond or alliance is developing. All these factors—comfort, sense of sharing, and decreased anxiety—are important in establishing and building the nurse–client relationship.

Validation

Validation is explicitly confirming with another person one's own thoughts or feelings with respect to a specific event or behaviour. To do so, the nurse must own his or her own thoughts or feelings by using "I" statements. Validating communication generally refers to observations, thoughts, or feelings and seeks explicit feedback. For example, a nurse who sees a client pacing the hallway before a planned family visit may conclude that the client is anxious. Validation may occur with a statement such as, "I notice you pacing the hallway. I wonder if you are feeling anxious about the family visit?" The client may agree, "Yes. I keep worrying about what is going to happen!" or

disagree, "No. I have been trying to get into the bathroom for the last 30 minutes, but my roommate is still in there!"

Empathy

The use of empathy in a therapeutic relationship is central to PMH nursing. **Empathy** is the ability to experience, in the present, a situation as another did at some time in the past. It is the ability to put oneself in another person's circumstances and feelings. The nurse does not need to have actually had the experience but has to be able to imagine the feelings associated with it. For empathy to develop, there must be a giving of self to the other individual and a reciprocal desire to know each other personally. The process involves the nurse receiving information from the client with open, nonjudgmental acceptance and communicating this understanding of the experience and feelings so that the client feels understood.

Bio/Psycho/Social/Spiritual Boundaries and Body Space Zones

Boundaries are the defining limits of individuals, objects, or relationships. Boundaries mark territory, identifying what is "mine" from what is "not mine." Human beings have many different types of boundaries. Material boundaries, such as fences around property, artificially imposed territorial lines, and bodies of water, can define territory as well as provide security and order. Within the bio/psycho/social/spiritual model, personal boundaries have physical, psychological, social, and spiritual dimensions. Physical boundaries are those established in terms of physical closeness to others—whom we allow to touch us or how close we want others to stand near us. Psychological boundaries are established in terms of emotional distance from others—how much of our innermost feelings and thoughts we want to share. Social boundaries, such as norms, customs, and roles, help us establish our closeness and place within the family, culture, and community. Spiritual boundaries, related to such things as our understanding of the meaning of life, our religious values, and/or our sense of relationship with a greater power, shape our way of being in the world. Boundaries are not fixed, but dynamic. When boundaries are involuntarily transgressed, the individual feels threatened and responds to the perceived threat. The nurse must elicit permission before implementing interventions that invade personal boundaries.

Personal Boundaries

Every individual is surrounded by four different body zones. These were identified by Hall (1990) as the intimate zone (e.g., whispering and embracing), the personal zone (e.g., for close friends), the social zone (e.g., for acquaintances), and the public zone (usually for interacting with strangers). These zones provide varying degrees of protection against unwanted physical closeness during interactions. The breadth of each zone varies according to culture. Some cultures define the intimate zone narrowly and the personal zones widely. Friends in these cultures stand and sit close while interacting. People of other cultures define the intimate zone widely and are uncomfortable when others stand close to them. The variability of intimate and personal zones has implications for nursing. For a client to be comfortable with a nurse, the nurse needs to protect the intimate zone of that individual. The client usually will allow the nurse to enter the personal zone but will express discomfort if the nurse breaches the intimate zone. For the nurse, the difficulty lies in differentiating personal and intimate zones for each client.

The nurse's awareness of his or her own need for intimate and personal space is another prerequisite for therapeutic interactions with the client. It is important that a nurse feels comfortable while interacting with clients. Establishing a comfort zone may well entail fine-tuning the size of body zones. Recognizing this will help the nurse understand occasional, inexplicable reactions to the proximity of clients.

Professional Boundaries

For nurses, professional boundaries are also essential to consider in the context of the nurse–client relationship. Clients often enter such relationships at a very vulnerable point, and nurses need to be aware of professional boundaries to avoid exploitation of the client. For example, in a friendship, there is a two-way sharing of personal information and feelings, but as mentioned previously, the focus is on the client's needs, and the nurse generally does not share personal information or attempt to meet his or her own needs through the relationship. The client may seek a friendship or sexual relationship with the nurse (or vice versa), which would be inconsistent with the professional role. Although professional boundaries are about power, influence, and control, they are not clear and precise. Professional boundaries can become blurred and ambiguous, given the familiarity, trust, and emotional intensity often involved in therapeutic relationships. It is important to be vigilant about potential abuses of power present in all such relationships (Austin, Bergum, Nuttgens, & Peternelj-Taylor, 2006). The results of a self-administered survey study of over 900 RNs and RPNs practicing in Alberta revealed that only one respondent reported having dated a current client (rarely); nine reported having dated a discharged client (rarely or sometimes), while six nurses reported having had a sexual relationship with a discharged client in the past (Campbell, Yonge, & Austin, 2005).

There are several indicators that a nurse–client relationship may be crossing professional boundaries. These include gift-giving by either party; a nurse spending inordinate time with a particular client; a nurse strenuously defending or explaining a client's behaviour in team meetings; a nurse's feeling he or she is the only one who truly understands the client; a nurse and client's keeping secrets; and a nurse's thinking frequently about a client outside of work (Forchuk et al., 2006; Gallop et al., 2002). Provincial regulatory bodies may have guidelines or firm rules, such as stipulating how long, following the termination of a therapeutic relationship,

before one may engage in a romantic or sexual relationship. Within psychiatric disciplines, a romantic or sexual relationship with a former client can be considered as always inappropriate, regardless of the length of time since the professional relationship was terminated. In nursing, the guidelines are generic and do not identify differences between specialties. Nevertheless, the professional implications of a personal relationship following a nursing relationship that involved psychotherapy are serious and must be carefully considered. Guidelines are generally vaguer about when a friendship would be appropriate, but such relationships are not appropriate when the nurse is actively providing care to the client. An exceptional case could be a relationship that preexisted that of nurse with client, for which another nurse is unavailable, such as in a nursing outpost (College of Nurses of Ontario, 2006). Similarly, relationships to meet the nurse's needs that are acquired through the nursing context, such as a relationship with a client's family member, also breach professional boundaries. It is important that the nurse be familiar with the standards of practice related to boundaries and therapeutic relationships of his or her provincial regulatory and professional associations. Table 6-4 summarizes some of these standards. When concerns arise related to therapeutic boundaries, the nurse must seek clinical supervision or transfer care of the client immediately.

Defence Mechanisms

Defence mechanisms (or coping mechanisms) are defined in the *Diagnostic and Statistical Manual of Mental Disorders-5* as "mechanisms that mediate the (client's) reaction to emotional conflicts and to external stressors. Some defense mechanisms (e.g., projection, splitting, acting out) are almost invariably maladaptive. Others (e.g., suppression, denial) may be either maladaptive or adaptive, depending on their severity, their inflexibility, and the context in which they occur" (American Psychiatric Association, 2013, p. 819). See Table 6-5 for more detailed definitions and examples of defence mechanisms. The concept of defence mechanisms originated with Freud's psychoanalytic theory and was conceived as the way the ego protected the individual from overwhelming anxiety (see Chapter 8). All healthy individuals use various defence mechanisms throughout their lives. A defence mechanism becomes pathologic when it is used so persistently that it becomes maladaptive. Suppression or denial, for instance, involves a process where anxiety-provoking information is not accepted (for suppression, this is conscious and for denial, this is unconscious). Those two defence mechanisms may be either maladaptive or adaptive depending on their severity and the context in which they occur. Other defence mechanisms such as projection (attributing one's own feelings onto another), splitting (self or others viewed as all bad or all good), and acting out (expressing unconscious feelings in actions rather than words), however, are almost invariably maladaptive.

Table 6-4	Canadian Provincial and National Standards of Practice Regarding Therapeutic Nurse–Client Relationships

Province/Territory	Standards of Practice/Best Practice Guidelines
Alberta	College and Association of Registered Nurses of Alberta: *Practice Standards for Regulated Members* (2013) with Canadian Nurses Association *Code of Ethics for Registered Nurses* (2008) *Professional Boundaries for Registered Nurses: Guidelines for the Nurse-Client Relationship* (2011) *Entry-to-Practice Competencies for the Registered Nurses Profession* (2006) College of Registered Psychiatric Nurses of Alberta: Registered Psychiatric Nurses of Canada *Code of Ethics & Standards of Psychiatric Nursing Practice* (2010)
British Columbia	College of Registered Nurses of British Columbia: *Professional Standards for Registered Nurses and Nurse Practitioners* (2012) College of Registered Psychiatric Nurses of British Columbia: Registered Psychiatric Nurses of Canada *Code of Ethics & Standards of Psychiatric Nursing Practice* (2010) *Boundaries in the Nurse–Client Relationship* (2013)
Manitoba	College of Registered Nurses of Manitoba: *Standards of Practice for Registered Nurses* (2013) *Professional Boundaries for Therapeutic Relationships* (2011) College of Registered Psychiatric Nurses of Manitoba: Registered Psychiatric Nurses of Canada *Code of Ethics & Standards of Psychiatric Nursing Practice* (2010)
New Brunswick	Nurses Association of New Brunswick: *Standards of Practice for Registered Nurses* (2012) *Practice Standard: The Therapeutic Nurse–Client Relationship* (2011)
Newfoundland and Labrador	Association of Registered Nurses of Newfoundland and Labrador: *Standards for Nursing Practice* (2013)
Northwest Territories and Nunavut	Registered Nurses Association of the Northwest Territories and Nunavut: *Standards of Nursing Practice for Registered Nurses* (2006)
Nova Scotia	College of Registered Nurses of Nova Scotia: *Standards of Practice for Registered Nurses* (2012) *Professional Boundaries and Expectations for Nurse–Client Relationships* (2002)
Ontario	College of Nurses of Ontario *Professional Standards* (2009) *Therapeutic Nurse–Client Relationships* (2006) Registered Nurses' Association of Ontario: *Establishing Therapeutic Relationships* (2002; revised 2006)
Prince Edward Island	Association of Registered Nurses of Prince Edward Island: *Standards for Nursing Practice* (2011)
Quebec	Ordre des infirmières et infirmiers du Québec: *Plan thérapeutique infirmier*
Saskatchewan	Saskatchewan Registered Nurses' Association: *Standards and Foundation Competencies for the Practice of Registered Nurses* (2007) Registered Psychiatric Nurses Association of Saskatchewan: *Standards for Psychiatric Nursing Practice* (2013)
Yukon	Yukon Registered Nurses Association: *Standards for Registered Nursing Practice in the Yukon* (2013)
National	Canadian Federation of Mental Health Nurses: *Canadian Standards of Psychiatric-Mental Health Nursing Practice* (2013)

As nurses develop therapeutic relationships, they will recognize their clients, and perhaps themselves, using defence mechanisms. (As defence mechanisms are almost always used unconsciously, it will be difficult for a nurse to readily identify his or her own without reviewing the relationship with someone else.) With experience, the nurse will evaluate the purpose of a defence mechanism and then determine whether it should be discussed with the client. For example, if a client is using humour to alleviate an emotionally intense situation, that may be very appropriate. On the other hand, if someone continually rationalizes antisocial behaviour, the use of the defence mechanism should be discussed.

● **STUDY NOTE**

When studying defence mechanisms, focus on those mechanisms and coping styles that are similar. For example, displacement, repression, and projection should be differentiated. Use these concepts in clinical assignments.

Table 6-5	Specific Defence Mechanisms and Coping Styles*	

Defence Mechanism	Definition	Example
Acting Out	Behaviours related to emotional conflicts such that the conflicts are dealt with through actions rather than reflections or feelings	A child becomes markedly more restless and disruptive in class following the loss of his father.
Denial	Refusing to acknowledge some painful aspect of external reality or subjective experience that would be apparent to others (psychotic denial is used when there is gross impairment in reality testing)	A teenager's best friend moves away, but the adolescent says she does not feel sad.
Displacement	Transferring a feeling about, or a response to, one object onto another (usually less threatening) substitute object	A child is mad at her mother for leaving for the day but says that she is really mad at the sitter for serving her food she does not like.
Dissociation	Experiencing a breakdown in the usually integrated functions of consciousness, memory, perception of self or the environment, or sensory and motor behaviour	An adult relates severe sexual abuse experienced as a child, but she does it without feeling. She says that the experience was as if she were outside her body watching the abuse.
Idealization	Attributing exaggerated positive qualities to others	An adult falls in love and fails to see the negative qualities in the other person.
Projection	Falsely attributing to another one's own unacceptable feelings, impulses, or thoughts	A child is very angry at a parent, but accuses the parent of being angry.
Rationalization	Concealing the true motivations for one's own thoughts, actions, or feelings through the elaboration of reassuring or self-serving but incorrect explanations	A man is rejected by his girlfriend, but he explains to his friends that her leaving was best because she was beneath him socially and would not be liked by his family.
Reaction formation	Substituting behaviours, thoughts, or feelings that are diametrically opposed to one's own unacceptable thoughts or feelings (this usually occurs in conjunction with their repression)	A wife finds out about her husband's extramarital affairs and tells her friends that she thinks his affairs are perfectly appropriate. She truly does not feel, on a conscious level, any anger or hurt.
Repression	Expelling disturbing wishes, thoughts, or experiences from conscious awareness (the feeling component may remain conscious, detached from its associated ideas)	A woman does not remember the experience of being raped in the basement, but she does feel anxious when going into the house.
Splitting	Compartmentalizing affect states and thus failing to integrate positive and negative aspects of the self or others	Following a messy breakup, a man refuses to acknowledge that his former partner had any redeeming qualities.
Suppression	Intentionally avoiding thoughts about disturbing problems, wishes feelings, or experiences	A woman who was abused by her husband refuses to think about the traumatic experience.
Undoing	Words or behaviours designed to negate or to make amends symbolically for unacceptable thoughts, feelings, or actions	A man has sexual fantasies about his wife's sister. He takes his wife away for a romantic weekend.

*The following defence mechanisms and coping styles are identified in the *DSM-IV-TR* as being used when the individual deals with emotional conflicts or stressors (either internal or external).

Adapted from American Psychiatric Association. (2000). *Diagnostic and statistical manual of mental disorders*. (4th ed., Text revision, pp. 811–814) Washington, DC: Author. They are not included in the *DSM-5*.

For more information on defence mechanisms see the *Handbook of psychiatric measures* (2nd ed., 2008), specifically page 727 where the use of the defence style questionnaire (DSQ) as developed by Dr. Michael Bond is discussed.

ANALYZING INTERACTIONS

Many people with mental health disorders have difficulty communicating. For example, perceptual, cognitive, and information-processing deficits, typical of people with schizophrenia, can interfere with the person's ability to express ideas, understand concepts, and accurately perceive the environment. Because of the complexity of communication, mental health professionals monitor their interactions with clients using various methods, including audio recording, video recording, and **process recording** (writing a verbatim transcript of the interaction). A video or audio recording of an interaction provides the most accurate monitoring but is cumbersome to use. Process recording, one of the easiest methods to use, is adequate in most situations. Nurses should use it when first learning therapeutic communication and during times when communication becomes a problem.

BOX 6-5 Process Recording

Setting: The living room of Mr. S's home. His parents are in the room but cannot hear the conversation. Mr. S is sitting on the couch and the nurse is sitting on a chair. This is the nurse's first visit after Mr. S's discharge from the hospital.

Client	Nurse	Comments/Interpretation
	How are you doing, Mr. S?	*Plan*: Initially develop a sense of trust and initiate a therapeutic relationship.
I'm fine. It's good to be home. I really don't like the hospital.	You didn't like the hospital?	*Interpretation*: Mr. S does not want to return to the hospital. Use reflection to begin to understand his experience.
NO. The nurses lock you up. Are you a nurse?	Yes. I'm a nurse. I'm wondering if you think that I will lock you up.	*Interpretation*: Mr. S is wondering what my role is and whether I will put him back in the hospital.
You could tell my mom to put me back in the hospital.	Any treatment I recommend I will thoroughly discuss with you first. I am here to help you stay out of the hospital. I will not discuss anything with your mother unless you give me the permission to do so.	Use interpretation to clarify Mr. S's thinking. Mr. S is wondering about my relationship with his mother. Explain my role.

In a process recording, the nurse records, from memory, the verbatim interaction immediately after the communication (Box 6-5). The nurse then analyzes the content of the interaction in terms of the words and their meaning for both the client and the nurse. The analysis is especially important because the ability to communicate verbally is often compromised in people with mental disorders. Words may not have the same meaning for the client as they do for the nurse. Clarification of meaning becomes especially important. The analysis can identify symbolic meanings, themes, and blocks in communication. **Symbolism**, the use of a word or phrase to represent an object, event, or feeling, is used universally. For example, automobiles are named for wild animals that represent speed, prowess, and beauty. In people with mental disorders, the use of words to symbolize events, objects, or feelings is often idiosyncratic, and they cannot explain their choices. For example, a person who is feeling scared and anxious may tell the nurse that bombs and guns are exploding. It is up to the nurse to make the connection between the bombs and guns and the client's feelings and then validate this with the client. Because of the client's cognitive limitations, the individual may express feelings only symbolically.

Some clients, for example, those with developmental handicaps or organic brain difficulties, may have difficulty with abstract thinking and symbolism. Conversations may be interpreted literally. For example, in response to the question "What brings you to the hospital?" a client might reply, "the ambulance." In these situations, the nurse must be cautious to avoid using symbols or metaphors. Concrete language, that is, language reflecting what can be observed through the senses, will be more easily understood.

Verbal behaviour is also interpreted by analyzing **content themes**. Clients often express concerns or feelings repeatedly in several different ways. After a few sessions, a common theme emerges. Themes may emerge symbolically, as in the case with the client who constantly talks about the "guns and bombs." Alternatively, a theme may simply be identified as a recurrent thread of a story that a client retells at each session. For example, one client always explained his early abandonment by his family. This led the nurse to hypothesize that he had an underlying fear of rejection. The nurse was then able to test whether there was an underlying fear and to develop strategies to help the client explore the fear (Box 6-6). It is important to involve clients in analyzing themes so that they may learn this skill. Within the therapeutic relationship, the person who does the work is the one who develops the competencies, so the nurse must be careful to share this opportunity with the client (Peplau, 1952/1988).

Communication blocks are identified by topic changes that either the nurse or the client makes. Topics are changed for various reasons. A client may change the topic from one that does not interest him or her to one that he or she finds more meaningful. However, an individual often changes the topic because he or she is uncomfortable with a particular subject.

BOX 6-6 Themes and Interactions

Session 1   Client discusses the death of his mother at a young age.

Session 2   Client explains that his sister is now married and never visits him.

Session 3   Client says that his best friend in the hospital was discharged and he really misses her.

Session 4   Client cries about a lost kitten.

Interpretation: Theme of loss is pervasive in several sessions.

Once a topic change is identified, the nurse or client hypothesizes the reason for it. If the nurse changes the topic, he or she needs to determine why. The nurse may find that he or she is uncomfortable with the topic or may not be listening to the client. Beginning mental health nurses who are uncomfortable with silences or trying to elicit specific information from the client often change topics.

The nurse must also record and interpret the client's nonverbal behaviour in light of the verbal behaviour. Is the client saying one thing verbally and another nonverbally? The nurse must consider the client's cultural background. Is the behaviour consistent with cultural norms? For example, if a client denies any problems but is affectionate and physically demonstrative (which is antithetical to his or her naturally stoic cultural beliefs and behaviours), the nonverbal behaviour is inconsistent with what is normal behaviour for that person. Further exploration is needed to determine the meaning of the culturally atypical behaviour.

■ THE NURSE–CLIENT RELATIONSHIP

The nurse–client relationship is a dynamic process that changes with time. It can be viewed in steps or phases with characteristic behaviours for both the client and the nurse. This text uses an adaptation of Hildegard Peplau's model that she introduced in her seminal work, *Interpersonal Relations in Nursing* (1952/1988). The nurse–client relationship is conceptualized in three overlapping phases that evolve with time: orientation phase, working phase, and resolution phase. Box 6-7 gives a recent research example testing an intervention based on this approach.

The **orientation phase** is the phase during which the nurse and client get to know each other. During this phase, which can last from a few minutes to several months, the client develops a sense of trust in the nurse. The second phase is the **working phase**, in which the client uses the relationship to examine specific problems and learn new ways of approaching them. The final stage, the **resolution phase**, is the termination stage of the relationship and lasts from the time the problems are actually resolved to the close of the relationship. The relationship does not develop in a linear manner; rather, the relationship may be predominantly in one phase but reflections of all phases can be seen in each interaction.

> ▼ **KEY CONCEPT** The **nurse–client relationship** is a dynamic process that changes with time. It can be viewed in steps or phases with characteristic behaviours for both the client and the nurse.

BOX 6-7 **Research for Best Practice**

THERAPEUTIC RELATIONSHIPS—FROM PSYCHIATRIC HOSPITAL TO COMMUNITY

Forchuk, C., Martin, M. L., Jensen, E., Ouseley, S., Sealy, P., Beal, G., ... Sharkey, S. (2012). Integrating an evidence-based intervention into clinical practice: 'Transitional relationship model'. Journal of Psychiatric and Mental Health Nursing, 20(7), 584–594.

The Question: This study identified strategies to maximize the implementation of a transitional relationship model (TRM), a model developed to sustain therapeutic relationships throughout the client's transition from the hospital to the community. While TRM had previously been shown to be an effective model of discharge (Forchuk, Jewell, Schofield, Sircelj, & Valledor, 1998), this study examined the facilitators and barriers to successful implementation.

Methods: The authors provided a history and overview of TRM. The current study included 36 tertiary care psychiatric wards that were first divided into delayed implementation and control groups. Of the implementation groups, group A included wards that had been previously implementing TRM. The remaining implementation wards were randomized into groups B and C. Group A implemented TRM first, followed by group B a year later. Lastly, group C implemented TRM in the 2nd year of the study. Group B implemented strategies suggested by group A, and group C implemented further refinements of those strategies as suggested by group B. Field notes were kept by project leaders and research assistants at each site, and focus groups were held to help streamline the suggestions made from one group to another.

Findings: A complex relationship exists between varieties of factors necessary for successful implementation of TRM. Of the implementation strategies offered to wards—educational modules, on-ward champions, and documentation systems—the effectiveness of implementation varied as a result of the staff feeling overwhelmed, poor group dynamics, and unforeseen losses of on-ward champions. This suggests the need for careful introductions of TRMs in order to continually foster ongoing support, education, and communication.

Implications for Practice: To best ensure positive outcomes for the client, work environment issues for interdisciplinary teams must be addressed.

Orientation Phase

The orientation phase begins when the nurse and client meet and ends when the client begins to identify problems to be examined within the relationship. During the orientation phase, the nurse discusses the client's expectations, explains the purpose of the relationship and its boundaries, and facilitates the development of the relationship. It is natural for the nurse and client to be more nervous during the first few sessions. The goal of the orientation phase is to develop trust and security within the nurse–client relationship. During this initial phase, the nurse listens intently to the client's history and perception of problems and begins to understand the client and identify themes. The use of empathy facilitates the development of a positive therapeutic relationship.

First Meeting

During the first meeting, it is important to outline both nursing and client responsibilities. The nurse is responsible for providing guidance throughout the therapeutic relationship, protecting confidential information, and maintaining professional boundaries. The client is responsible for attending agreed-upon sessions, interacting during the sessions, and participating in the nurse–client relationship. The nurse should also explain clearly to the client the role of the nurse as well as pragmatic issues such as meeting times, handling of missed sessions, and the estimated length of the relationship. Issues related to recording information and how the nurse will work within the interdisciplinary team should also be made explicit.

Usually, both the nurse and the client feel anxious at the first meeting. The nurse should recognize the anxieties and attempt to alleviate them before the meeting. The client's behaviour during this first meeting may indicate to the nurse some of the client's problems in interpersonal relationships. For example, a client may talk nonstop for 15 minutes or may brag of sexual conquests. What the client chooses to tell or not to tell is significant. What a client first does or says may not accurately indicate his or her true feelings or the situation. In the beginning, clients may deny problems or choose not to discuss them as defence mechanisms or to prevent the nurse from getting to know them. The client is usually nervous and insecure during the first few sessions and may exhibit behaviour reflective of these emotions, such as rambling. Often by the third session, the client can better focus on a topic.

Confidentiality in Treatment

Ideally, nurses include people who are important to the client in planning and implementing care. The nurse and client should discuss the issue of confidentiality in the first session. The nurse should be clear about any information that is to be shared with anyone else. Usually, the nurse shares significant assessment data and client progress with a supervisor and team members including a physician. Most clients expect the nurse to communicate with other mental health professionals and are comfortable with this arrangement. Boundaries around what information can be shared with whom and under what circumstances are covered under provincial/territorial legislation such as mental health acts and health information acts. It is therefore important that each nurse be aware of the legislation in the province or territory in which he or she is practising.

Testing the Relationship

This first part of the orientation phase, called the "honeymoon phase," is usually pleasant. However, the therapeutic team typically hits rough spots before completing this phase. The client begins to test the relationship to become convinced that the nurse will really accept him or her. Typical testing behaviours include forgetting a scheduled session or being late. Clients may also express anger at something a nurse says or accuse the nurse of breaking confidentiality. Another common pattern is for the client to introduce a relatively superficial issue first as if it is the major problem. The nurse must recognize that these behaviours are designed to test the relationship and establish its parameters, not to express rejection or dissatisfaction with the nurse. The student nurse often feels personally rejected during the client's testing and may even become angry with the client. If the nurse simply accepts the behaviour as testing and continues to be available to the client and consistent in responses, these behaviours usually subside. Testing needs to be understood as a normal way that human beings develop trust.

Some issues specific to mental health clients can occur. For example, a client experiencing paranoia, by definition, is going to have difficulty establishing trust and may require a longer orientation phase. A client who is depressed may have difficulty expressing needs and may require periods of silence to feel comfortable in moving forward in the relationship.

Working Phase

When the client begins identifying problems to work on, the working phase of the relationship has started. Problem identification can yield a wide range of issues, such as managing symptoms of a mental disorder, coping with chronic pain, examining issues related to sexual abuse, and dealing with problematic interpersonal relationships. Through the relationship, the client begins to explore the identified problems and develop strategies to resolve them. By the time the working phase is reached, the client has developed enough trust that he or she can examine the identified problems within the security of the therapeutic relationship. In the working phase, the nurse can use various verbal and nonverbal techniques to help the client examine problems and support the client to plan strategies to address concerns.

Transference (unconscious assignment to others of the feelings and attitudes that the client originally associated with important figures) and **countertransference** (the provider's emotional reaction to the client based on personal unconscious needs and conflicts) become important issues in the working phase. For example, a client could be hostile to a nurse because of the underlying resentment of authority figures; the nurse, in turn, could respond defensively because of earlier experiences of anger. The client uses transference to examine problems. During this phase, the client is psychologically vulnerable and emotionally dependent on the nurse. The nurse needs to recognize countertransference and prevent it from eroding professional boundaries.

Many times, nurses are eager to implement rehabilitation plans. However, this cannot be done until the client trusts the nurse and identifies what issues he or she wishes to work on in the context of the relationship.

Resolution Phase

The final stage of the nurse–client relationship is the resolution phase, which begins when the actual problems are resolved and ends with the termination of the relationship. During this phase, the client is redirected toward a life without this specific therapeutic relationship. The client connects with community resources, solidifies a newly found understanding, and practices new behaviours. The client takes responsibility for follow-up appointments and interacts with significant others in new ways. New problems are not addressed during this phase, except in terms of what was learned during the working stage. The nurse assists the client in strengthening relationships, making referrals, and recognizing and understanding signs of future relapse.

Termination begins on the 1st day of the relationship, when the nurse explains that this relationship is time-limited and was established to help handle and resolve the client's problems. Because a therapeutic relationship is dependent, the nurse must constantly evaluate the client's level of dependence and continually support the client's move toward independence. Termination is usually stressful for the client, who must sever ties with the nurse who has shared thoughts and feelings and given guidance and support over many sessions. Depending on previous experiences with terminating relationships, some clients may not handle their emotions well during termination. Some may not show up for the last session at all to avoid their feelings of sadness and separation. Many clients will also display anger about the relationship ending. Clients may express anger toward the nurse or displace it onto others. For example, a client may shout obscenities at another client after being told that his or her therapeutic relationship with the nurse will end in a few weeks. One of the best ways to handle the anger is to help the client acknowledge it, to explain that anger is a normal emotion when a relationship is ending, and to reassure the client that it is acceptable to feel angry. The nurse should also reassure the client that anger subsides once the relationship is over.

Another typical termination behaviour is raising old problems that have already been resolved. The nurse may feel frustrated if clients in the termination phase present resolved problems as if they were new. The nurse may feel that the sessions were unsuccessful. In reality, clients are unconsciously attempting to prolong the relationship and avoid its ending. Nurses should avoid addressing these problems. Instead, they should reassure clients of having already covered those issues and learned methods to control them. They should explain that the client may be feeling anxious about the relationship ending and redirect the client to newly acquired skills and abilities in forming new relationships, including support groups and social groups. The final meeting should focus on the future (see Box 6-8). The nurse can reassure the client that the nurse will remember him or her, but the nurse should not agree to see the client outside the relationship. Many clients who have difficulty establishing relationships may similarly have difficulty letting go of supportive relationships. The ending of the therapeutic relationship is a significant opportunity for client learning, including the opportunity for a healthy good-bye. The nurse needs to plan for and to support this learning.

BOX 6-8   Therapeutic Dialogue

THE LAST MEETING

Ineffective Approach

Nurse: Today is my last day.

Client: I need to talk to you about something important.

Nurse: What is it?

Client: I have been hearing voices again.

Nurse: Oh, how often?

Client: Every night. You are the only one I'm going to tell.

Nurse: I think you should tell the new nurse.

Client: She is too new. She won't understand. I feel so bad about your leaving. Is there any way you can stay?

Nurse: Well, I could check on you tomorrow.

Client: Oh, would you? I would really appreciate it if you would give me your new telephone number.

Nurse: I don't know what the number will be, but it will be listed in the telephone book.

Effective Approach

Nurse: Today is my last day.

Client: I need to talk to you about something important.

Nurse: We talked about that. Anything "important" needs to be shared with the new nurse.

Client: But, I want to tell you.

Nurse: Saying good-bye can be very hard.

Client: I will miss you.

Nurse: Your feelings are very normal when relationships are ending. I will remember you in a very special way.

Client: Can I please have your telephone number?

Nurse: No, I can't give that to you. It is important that we say good-bye today.

Client: OK. Good-bye. Good luck.

Nurse: Good-bye.

Critical Thinking Challenge

• What were some of the mistakes the nurse in the first scenario made?

• In the second scenario, how does therapeutic communication in the termination phase differ from effective communication in the working phase?

NONTHERAPEUTIC RELATIONSHIPS

Although it is hoped that all nurse–client relationships will go through the phases described in the previous section, this is not always the case. Nontherapeutic relationships also go through predictable phases (Forchuk et al., 2000). These relationships also start in the orientation phase. However, trust is not established, and the relationship moves to a *phase of grappling and struggling*. The nurse and client both feel very frustrated and keep varying their approach with each other in an attempt to establish a meaningful relationship. This is different from a prolonged orientation phase in that the efforts are not sustained; they vary constantly. The nurse may try having longer or shorter meetings, being more or less directive, and varying the therapeutic stance from warm and friendly to aloof. Clients in this phase may try to talk about the past but then change to discussions of the here and now. They may try talking about their family and in the next meeting talk about their work goals. Both the client and the nurse grapple and struggle to come to a common ground, and both become increasingly frustrated with each other. Eventually, the frustration becomes so great that the pair gives up on each other and moves to a *phase of mutual withdrawal*. The nurse may schedule seeing this client at the end of the shift and "run out of time" so that the meeting never happens. The client will leave the unit or otherwise be unavailable during scheduled meeting times. If a meeting does occur, the nurse will try to keep it short. "What's the point—we just cover the same old ground anyway." The client will attempt to keep it superficial and stay on safe topics. "You can always ask about your medications—nurses love to health teach, you know." Obviously, no therapeutic progress can be made in such a relationship. The nurse may be hesitant to ask for a therapeutic transfer, assuming that a relationship would similarly fail with another nurse. However, each relationship is unique, and difficulties in one relationship do not predict difficulties in the next. Clinical supervision early on may assist the development of the relationship, but often a therapeutic transfer to another nurse is required.

STRATEGIES WITHIN THE THERAPEUTIC RELATIONSHIP

Motivational Interviewing

One evidence-based strategy is motivational interviewing (MI). MI is a clinical method designed to facilitate change in negative client behaviour by engaging a client's own autonomous decision-making ability. Practitioners of MI seek to selectively elicit and reinforce the client's own arguments for change. Carried out in a collaborative setting, MI encourages the client to make his or her own decisions through directed counselling that addresses the source of undesirable behaviours. MI is inherently exploratory and adaptive.

Even though MI has been shown to produce statistically significant results when successfully employed, a variety of external factors may affect long-term outcomes. Often these external factors are interpersonal and social forces (Berg, Ross, & Tikkanen, 2011). The negative effect of these factors indicates that MI assumes that risky behaviours are largely under the control of individuals (Berg et al., 2011). Acknowledging this assumption helps to make clear why MI may not be effective for some clients.

As a result, MI is difficult to practice effectively, and clinicians will require frequent instruction and feedback. Topics discussed in this chapter, such as self-awareness, empathic linkages, active listening, and the avoidance of defence mechanisms, will all have to be effectively employed to achieve MI's desired results. While difficult, MI has been shown to be effective in a variety of clinical settings (Barnett, Sussman, Smith, Rohrbach, & Spruijt-Metz2012; Chen, Creedy, Lin, & Wollin, 2012; Cronk et al., 2012; Day, 2013). However, there are a broad range of techniques in which PMH nurses can be trained that significantly improve outcomes (Barwick, Bennett, Johnson, McGowan, & Moore, 2012). According to Miller and Moyers (2006), p. 3, these techniques are as follows:

- Openness to collaboration with clients' own expertise
- Proficiency in client-centered counseling, including accurate empathy
- Recognition of key aspects of client speech that guides the practice of MI
- Eliciting and strengthening client change talk
- Rolling with resistance
- Negotiating change plans
- Consolidating client commitment
- Switching flexibly between MI and other intervention styles

Transitional Relationship Model

The TRM evolved from the transitional discharge model, originally developed to help people through the discharge process. An extension of Peplau's theory, TRM is based on the assumptions that people heal in relationships and require both professional and peer therapeutic relationships. There are two essential components to this model: professional support and peer support. The professional's role is to bridge the therapeutic relationship over the discharge (or other transition) process so that the therapeutic relationship with the client is not terminated until the client enters another professional relationship with a care provider (e.g., a nurse staying involved after discharge until a community relationship is established). The peer-support component is essential during the transition from hospital to community. Peer supporters are generally trained and supported through a consumer survivor group. In other words, people need both professionals and an experienced friend. Studies have found that this approach reduces the time in hospital (Forchuk, Martin, Chan, & Jensen, 2005) and reduces readmissions (Reynolds et al., 2004.).

Technology and the Therapeutic Relationship

Traditionally, the nurse–client relationship has been face-to-face. However, changes to information and communication technologies, particularly in the past decade, have significantly changed how health professionals and their clients interact. **Telehealth is the extension of health care service delivery across distance by use of information and communication technologies such as telephone, video, and the Internet. Telehealth in Canada has been particularly effective in improving access to health professionals by clients in rural locales** (Geffen, Gordon, & Chien, 2011). In the instance of *telenursing*, telehealth can involve something as basic as a phone call between a nurse and client or something as complex as assisting with a remote surgical procedure. For the purposes of PMH nursing in particular, there are important things to consider about the communicative aspect of the therapeutic relationship in situations mediated by communication technology. Nonverbal communication, which makes up so much of an interaction between nurse and client, is lessened or largely absent; access to necessary technology may also be difficult for some clients; it can be difficult to ensure that health providers do not step outside the scope of their practice; and issues of privacy, security, and consent can be more complicated in these situations. In order to address the latter issues, many agencies presently do not allow e-mail communication. A system can be set up behind a secure hospital firewall (Forchuk et al., 2012), but access control is always a concern with sensitive information. It is important to be aware of agency policy and security before using any web-based communication. Public platforms such as Facebook do not allow privacy, sufficient security, or confidentiality for use in health care communication. The Internet can be a useful tool for health teaching or for finding resources, but its increasing use in mediating relationships, including those between health care providers and clients, raises issues of personal autonomy and consent (e.g., how a client's data are stored, exchanged, and used), persistent threats to privacy and confidentiality, and other issues of risk management.

SUMMARY OF KEY POINTS

■ To deal therapeutically with the emotions, feelings, and problems of clients, nurses must understand their own cultural values and beliefs and interpersonal strengths and limitations.

■ The nurse–client relationship is built on therapeutic communication, including verbal and nonverbal interactions between the nurse and client. Some communication skills include active listening, positive body language, appropriate verbal responses, and the ability

of the nurse to interpret appropriately and analyze the client's verbal and nonverbal behaviours.

■ Two of the most important communication concepts are empathy and rapport.

■ Defence mechanisms, used by all individuals, can be adaptive or maladaptive depending on factors like context, inflexibility, and severity.

■ In the nurse–client relationship, as in all types of relationships, certain physical, psychological, social, and spiritual boundaries and limitations need to be observed.

■ The therapeutic nurse–client relationship consists of three major and overlapping stages or phases: the orientation phase, in which the client and nurse meet and establish the parameters of the relationship; the working phase, in which the client identifies and explores problems; and the resolution phase, in which the client learns to manage the problems and the relationship is terminated.

■ The nontherapeutic relationship also consists of three major and overlapping phases: the orientation phase, the grappling and struggling phase, and the phase of mutual withdrawal.

■ Strategies that can be used within therapeutic relationships include MI and TRM.

CRITICAL THINKING CHALLENGES

1 Describe how you would communicate with a client who is concerned that a psychiatric diagnosis will negatively affect his or her social and work relationships.

2 Your client does not seem inclined to talk about his or her illness. Describe the measures you would take to initiate a therapeutic relationship with him or her. Who chooses the content to be discussed?

3 Your client does not appear for the last scheduled meeting. What will you do?

REFERENCES

American Psychiatric Association. (2000). *Diagnostic and statistical manual of mental disorders* (4th ed., Text Revision). Washington, DC: Author.

American Psychiatric Association. (2013). *Diagnostic and statistical manual of mental disorders* (5th ed.). Washington, DC: Author.

Austin, W., Bergum, V., Nuttgens, S., & Peternelj-Taylor, C. (2006). A revisioning of boundaries in professional helping relationships: Exploring other metaphors. *Ethics & Behavior, 16*(2), 77–94.

Barnett, E., Sussman, S., Smith, C., Rohrbach, L. A., & Spruijt-Metz, D. (2012). Motivational interviewing for adolescent substance use: A review of the literature. *Addictive Behaviors, 37*(12), 1325–1334.

Barwick, M. A., Bennett, L. M., Johnson, S. N., McGowan, J., & Moore, J. E. (2012). Training health and mental health professionals in motivational interviewing: A systematic review. *Children & Youth Services Review, 34*(9), 1786–1795.

Berg, R. C., Ross, M. W., & Tikkanen, R. (2011). The effectiveness of MI4MSM: How useful is motivational interviewing as an HIV risk prevention program for men who have sex with men? A systematic review. *AIDS Education & Prevention, 23*(6), 533–549.

Boyd, M. (1995). Communication with clients, families, healthcare providers, and diverse cultures. In M. Strader & P. Decker (Eds.), *Role transition to client care management* (p. 431). Norwalk, CT: Appleton & Lange.

Campbell, R. J., Yonge, O., & Austin, W. (2005). Intimacy boundaries between mental health nurses and psychiatric patients. *Journal of Psychosocial Nursing and Mental Health Services, 43*(5), 33–41.

Chen, S. M., Creedy, D., Lin, H. S., & Wollin, J. (2012). Effects of motivational interviewing intervention on self-management, psychological and glycemic outcomes in type 2 diabetes: A randomized controlled trial. *International Journal of Nursing Studies, 49*(6), 637–644.

College of Nurses of Ontario. (2006). *Practice standard: Therapeutic nurse-client relationship* (Rev. ed.). Toronto, Canada: Author.

Cronk, N. J., Russell, C. L., Knowles, N., Matteson, M., Peace, L., & Ponferrada, L. (2012). Acceptability of motivational interviewing among hemodialysis clinic staff: A pilot study. *Nephrology Nursing Journal, 39*(5), 385–391.

Day, P. (2013). Using motivational interviewing with young people: A case study. *British Journal of School Nursing, 8*(2), 97–99.

Forchuk, C., Carmichael, C., Golea, G., Johnston, N., Martin, M. L., Patterson, P., et al. (2006). *Nursing best practice guideline: Establishing therapeutic relationships* (Rev. ed.). Toronto, Canada: Registered Nurses Association of Ontario.

Forchuk, C., Jewell, J., Schofield, R., Sircelj, M., & Valledor, T. (1998). From hospital to community: Bridging therapeutic relationships. *Journal of Psychiatric and Mental Health Nursing, 5*,197–202.

Forchuk, C., Martin, M. L., Chan, Y. C., & Jensen, E. (2005). Therapeutic relationships: From psychiatric hospital to community. *Journal of Psychiatric and Mental Health Nursing, 12*, 556–564.

Forchuk, C., Martin, M. L., Jensen, E., Ouseley, S., Sealy, P., Beal, G., ... Sharkey, S. (2012). Integrating an evidence-based intervention into clinical practice: 'transitional relationship model'. *Journal of Psychiatric and Mental Health Nursing, 20*(7), 584–594.

Forchuk, C., Westwell, J., Martin, M. L., Bamber-Azzapardi, W., Kosterewa-Tolman, D., & Hux, M. (2000). The developing nurse–client relationship: Nurses perspectives. *Journal of the American Psychiatric Nurses Association, 6*(1), 3–10.

Gallop, R., Choiniere, J., Forchuk, C., Golea, G., Jonston, N., Levac, A. M., ... Wynn, F. (2002). *Nursing best practice guideline: Establishing therapeutic relationships.* Toronto, Canada: Registered Nurses Association of Ontario.

Geffen, M., Gordon, D., & Chien, E. (2011). *Telehealth benefits and adoption: Connecting people and providers across Canada.* Report commissioned by Canada Health Infoway. Retrieved from https://www.infoway-inforoute.ca/index.php/programs-services/investment-programs/telehealth

Hall, E. T. (1990). *The hidden dimension.* New York: Anchor Books.

Lingley-Pottie, P., McGrath, P., & Andreou, P. (2013). Barriers to mental health care: Perceived delivery system differences. *Advances in Nursing Science, 36*(1), 51–61.

Miller, W. R., & Moyers, T. (2006). Eight stages in learning motivational interviewing. *Journal of Teaching in the Addictions, 5*(1), 3–17.

Peplau, H. E. (1952/1988 reissued). *Interpersonal relations in nursing.* London, UK: MacMillan.

Reynolds W., Lauder W., Sharkey, S., Maciver S., Veitch T., & Cameron, D. (2004). The effect of a transitional discharge model for psychiatric patients. *Journal of Psychiatric and Mental Health Nursing, 11*(1), 82–88.

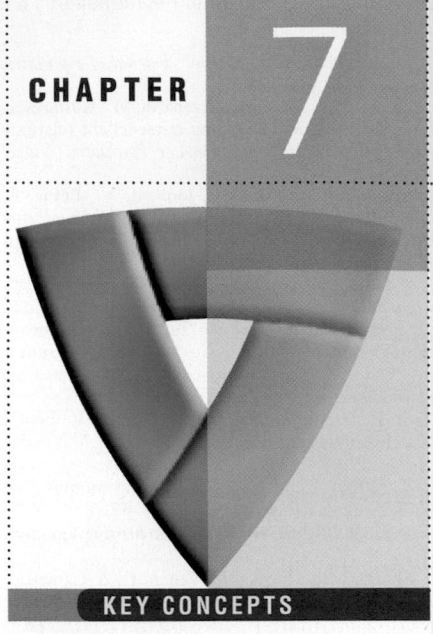

CHAPTER

7

KEY CONCEPTS

• ethics
• everyday ethics
• moral agent
• moral dilemma
• moral distress

Ethical Practice

Wendy Austin

After studying this chapter, you will be able to:

• Define ethics.
• Distinguish between the domains of ethics and law.
• Describe the nurse as a moral agent and the resources available to support this role.
• Identify the most common approaches to ethics that inform health ethics.
• Describe the components of an ethical practice environment.
• Distinguish between a moral dilemma and moral distress.
• Outline an example of an ethical decision-making framework.
• Discuss five ethical issues in psychiatric and mental health nursing.
• Identify the ethical responsibilities of nurses related to psychiatric research.

• beneficence • casuistry • confidentiality • conscientious objection • deontology • ethics of care • feminist ethics • human rights • justice • nonmaleficence • practical wisdom • principlism • relational ethics • respect for autonomy • telehealth • utilitarianism • virtue

WHAT IS ETHICS?

Ethics is about how we should live; it is *"aiming at the 'good life' with and for others in just institutions"* (Ricouer, 1992, p. 172, original italics). Ethics is about learning how to reach our potential as human beings, and so it is about values, relationships, principles, duties, rights, and responsibilities. In writing about ethics in *On Equilibrium*, Saul (2001) noted that, although we may think about ethics as something exotic or romantic, for heroes or saints, ethics is actually down to earth and practical: it needs to be an everyday part of our lives and built into our society.

Although some philosophers differentiate ethics from morality, ethics and morals can be used as interchangeable terms (*ethics* comes from *ethos*, Greek for *custom; morals* comes from *mores*, Latin for *custom*) and is so used here.

KEY CONCEPT Ethics is the consideration of the way a person should act in order to live a good life with and for others. Just institutions enable and support ethical actions.

The Legal Domain as Separate From Ethics

Law and ethics are separate domains. In a perfect world, societal laws would be totally compatible with ethical behaviours in every situation. In the real world, however, this is not always the case. Citizens may need to work to change laws that they believe to be unethical. Nurses need to be vigilant about laws and regulations that affect their practice. Psychiatric and mental health (PMH) nurses, for instance, must understand the legal context of mental health care in Canada (see Chapter 3). Nurses in forensic psychiatric settings must understand how the competing demands of the health care and justice systems affect their practice (see Chapter 38).

Health Ethics

Somerville (2000) describes Canada as a secular society, with diverse religious groups: we have no common, external, absolute moral authority. She asks, how can we know, as a society, how to respond to new approaches to science, technology, and health care? Contemporary ethics is shaped by factors such as intense individualism (the individual coming before the common good), corporatism (dominance of business interests), unprecedented advances in science and technology, the power of the media, the increased use of law as a means to resolve disputes that are inherently about values, and a loss of a sense of the sacred. She proposes that two absolute values, *profound respect for life* and *commitment to the human spirit*, will allow us to make ethical societal choices.

Somerville (2000, p. xii) uses the metaphor of a canary to signify key issues that "test the ethical air in our societal mineshaft." As canaries once served to detect toxic gas in underground mines (i.e., sick or dead canaries warned miners that the air was unsafe), these issues warn us that the ethical tone of our society is putting us at risk. The way in which Canadians address the well-being of those living with mental illness is recognizable to PMH nurses as an ethical canary.

The Ethical Nurse

Stating that "I am a nurse" is a type of moral claim. Nurses have a fiduciary relationship with the public. (*Fiducial* comes from the Latin, *fidere*, to trust.) Nurses, as professionals, profess or claim that they will use their specialized knowledge and skills for the benefit of the public in a trustworthy way. Nurses are trusted to be ethical (Austin, 2006). In polls, nurses are consistently rated the most honest and ethical professionals (Gallup, 2013). Whenever nurses enact their professional responsibilities, they are active as **moral agents**. Being ethical as a nurse requires more than having moral courage in times of crises (although it may require this); it requires the everyday expression of a commitment to the well-being of those in their care (Levine, 1977).

> **KEY CONCEPT** A **moral agent** is a person engaged in determining or expressing a moral (ethical) choice.

> **KEY CONCEPT** **Everyday ethics** involves sustained attention to ethics in daily nursing practice and to the fundamental fiduciary commitment of nurses to those in their care.

CODES OF ETHICS FOR NURSES

To guide nurses in enacting their moral agency, codes of ethics have been developed by nursing associations. These are statements of the shared values and recognized duties and commitments of the profession. They set the ethical standards for practice and inform other disciplines and the public about the ethical commitments of nurses.

The Canadian Nurses Association *Code of Ethics for Registered Nurses*

The CNA code (Canadian Nurses Association (CNA), 2008) is framed by seven values (safe, compassionate, competent, and ethical care; health and well-being; informed decision making; dignity; privacy and confidentiality; justice; and accountability) and related ethical responsibilities, grounded in nurses' professional relationships. The code document includes "ethical endeavours," an outline of ways that registered nurses (RNs) may strive, on their own and collectively, to change systems and social structures in order for greater equity for all. There is a glossary of pertinent terms and advice on responding to incompetent, noncompassionate, unsafe, or unethical care. It stipulates a provision for **conscientious objection**, defined as "a situation in which a nurse requests permission from his or her employer to refrain from providing care because a practice of procedure conflicts with the nurse's moral or religious beliefs" (College of Registered Nurses of British Columbia, 2007). Although the CNA is for RNs, it is expected by the nursing profession that students of nursing comply with the code. Those cared for by students should know the status of the student caregiver; students' caregiving should be congruent with the code. RNs are expected to share their knowledge, provide feedback, and treat students with respect (CNA, 2008). Guidelines for relationships with nursing students are provided. An *Ethics in Practice* resource is provided by CNA on such issues as whistle-blowing, ethical distress, ethical relationships and quality practice environments, social justice in practice, and use of social media (See Web Links on thePoint).

Ethics Guidelines for Registered Psychiatric Nurses

The Registered Psychiatric Nurses of Canada (RPNC)'s *Code of Ethics & Standards of Psychiatric Nursing Practice* delineates "an acceptable set of behaviours" for RPNs in British Columbia, Alberta, Saskatchewan, Manitoba, and the Yukon, as well as their legal and professional obligations (RPNC, 2010, p. 3). RPNs are expected to uphold four core values and responsibilities related to "safe, competent, and ethical practice"; "respect for the inherent worth, right of choice, and dignity of persons"; "health, mental health, and well-being"; and "quality practice" (p. 3). The document describes the profession of psychiatric nursing and its regulation and practice in Canada.

RPNs in Alberta follow a provincial code of ethics (congruent with Alberta's Health Professions Act) with the principles of beneficence, nonmaleficence, integrity, fidelity, respect for autonomy, and justice (College of RPNs of Alberta, 2013).

APPROACHES TO ETHICS

There are a number of theoretical approaches to ethical knowledge that inform ethical action in health care. Some are based on moral philosophy and others on concepts such as human rights. A brief outline of the most common approaches follows. See Table 7-1 for a summary.

Virtue Ethics

Virtue ethics, emphasizing the character of the moral agent, was the earliest approach to ethics used in nursing (Fowler, 1997). A virtuous person is one who, without strict reliance on rules, is wise enough to perceive how to act well in a particular situation. Lists of the virtues vary,

but they include compassion, courage, tolerance, prudence, honesty, humility, and trustworthiness. Aristotle (1996), the Greek philosopher whose works most inform virtue theory, believed that acquiring the virtues would assist a person to flourish as a human being. He found our moral upbringing to be important: we learn the virtues through our relationships. Observing compassion in others, for instance, can help us to develop a compassionate disposition. To acquire a virtue, it must become habitual; it is not enough, for instance, to be occasionally honest. Aristotle's concept of the virtue of *phronesis* or **practical wisdom** seems particularly relevant to nurses. It means having the sensitivity, imagination, and experience to do what is ethically fitting in difficult situations (Austin, 2007a).

In a profession with role-specific duties and responsibilities (evidenced by such things as a code of ethics), a trait that supports the good of that practice acquires the status of a moral virtue. A professional's virtues, in that sense, are necessary to his or her role (Radden & Sadler,

Table 7-1	Approaches to Ethics		
Approach	**Core Elements**	**Proponents**	**Critiques**
Virtue ethics	Character of the moral agent Some virtues: honesty, courage, compassion, practical wisdom	Aristotle Alasdair MacIntyre	Exclusive focus on the agent
Deontology	Duty based Some acts are wrong in themselves Universality Do not treat others as a means to an end (respect)	Immanuel Kant	Disregard of consequences Impartiality over relationship Emotion = irrationality
Utilitarianism	Consequence based Actions are right if they promote the best outcome (e.g., happiness, pleasure, satisfaction) for most people	Jeremy Bentham John Stuart Mill	Utility as the only principle Majority rules
Casuistry	Case based Use of paradigm cases to identify issues and courses of action for a new case	Albert Jonsen Stephen Toulmin	Keeps the status quo Can miss the broad issues
Principlism	Based on a set of principles compatible with most moral theories Nonmaleficence, beneficence, respect for autonomy, justice	Tom Beauchamp James Childress	Too abstract Which principle has a priority when different principles compete?
Ethics of care	Care based Connection/responsibility for others Emotional responsiveness	Carol Gilligan Nel Noddings	Creates a dichotomy between "care" (feminine) and "justice" (masculine) approaches to ethics Valorizes women as caregivers
Feminist ethics	Addresses power inequities, dominance, and oppression	Annette Baier Susan Sherwin	Lacks impartiality Lacks universal norms
Relational ethics	Ethical action involves relationships Context matters; emotion accepted Dialogue is supported Aims for the "fitting" response	Vangie Bergum John Dossetor	Too relativistic Lacks impartiality Lacks universality
Human rights	Rights based (negative and positive) Every person is entitled to certain basic rights	John Locke Thomas Paine United Nations	As a concept is "nonsense" Too legalistic Too individualistic

2008). In *After Virtue*, MacIntyre (1984) raises a question worthy of reflection: What would a person (nurse) lack, who lacked the virtues?

Deontology

Deontology (from the Greek *deon* or *duty*) postulates duty or obligation as the basis of doing right. This is duty not as in following external orders but as self-imposed obligation. This approach is also termed *Kantian ethics* because the work of Kant (1996), an 18th-century philosopher, laid its foundation. Kant believed that we should use reason alone to determine how to act. Reason unhampered by emotions or desires allows us to determine the types of acts that are wrong in themselves, no matter how good their consequences might be. Kant stipulated that a criterion (a *categorical imperative*) for judging the reason (or "maxim") for one's actions is universality: one should act only on a choice that one can conceive of as a universal law. Is a lie acceptable if it saves someone from danger? No, because lying cannot be willed as a universal principle. If we lie to help a person in trouble, truth will be subverted and society corrupted. In Kantian ethics, the moral worth of a person's action is determined by the intent of the person, not the effects of the action. If you act rightly, you are not responsible for bad effects.

Kant stipulated a second imperative: act so that you treat others always as an end and never as a means. Kant argued that we must treat one another with dignity and respect; it is wrong to use other people for our own purposes. Informed consent is grounded on this belief. For instance, individuals should not be used as research subjects unless they understand what will happen and agree to it. Nor should we, according to Kantian ethics, place individuals at risk in research by depriving them of the best-known treatment in order to carry out a placebo-controlled study, even though this would provide the most valid evidence.

Kant's emphasis on the individual's rational capacity as the facilitator of moral action can be seen as highly relevant to psychiatric ethics, as it is the impairment of rational capacity alone that justifies coercive or involuntary psychiatric treatment (Robertson, Morris, & Walter, 2007). Kantian ethics supports the quest for universal ethical principles, such as the efforts of the United Nations Educational, Scientific, and Cultural Organization (UNESCO) (see "Human Rights" below). It upholds that, from a moral standpoint, all persons should be treated the same. A major problem, however, is its disregard for the role of consequences in ethical action. Consequences, however, are the sole focus of the next approach.

Utilitarianism

The principle of utility is the foundation of **utilitarianism**: actions are right in proportion to their tendency to promote happiness. What is right to do is what gives the best consequences (e.g., happiness, pleasure, preference, satisfaction) for the greater number of people. Bentham (1983) and Mill (2002), philosophers of the 18th and 19th centuries, originated this theory that uses a type of cost/benefit analysis to determine the moral worth of an action.

The principle of utility can also be applied to determining which moral rules to follow. This is termed *rule utilitarianism* and holds that once we decide on the best rules, we should follow them, even if in some situations happiness is not maximized. A rule utilitarian might determine that a good rule for a PMH nurse is not to go against hospital policies except if it is necessary for the best interests of a patient. Covertly putting an antipsychotic medication in an acutely ill person's food, for instance, might be regarded as ethically acceptable in a special circumstance when such an action causes the least suffering to the ill person (Ipperciel, 2003). A Kantian would never approve of this, and, despite ethical justification from a utilitarian perspective, such an act can result in a disciplinary or legal action (Wong, Poon, & Hui, 2005).

Principlism

In the principles approach, it is believed that a few moral principles (ethical norms) can provide a basis for moral reasoning in health ethics (Beauchamp, 1994). Four *prima facie* (at first sight) principles are widely accepted: nonmaleficence, beneficence, respect for autonomy, and justice (Beauchamp & Childress, 2013). **Nonmaleficence** as a principle means that one should do no harm. **Beneficence** means that one should do, or attempt to do, good and make things better (promote benefit) for others when one can. **Respect for autonomy** (also considered as respect for persons) means an obligation to respect a person's right to be self-governing and his or her ability to make decisions. **Justice** is conceived as obligations of fairness in the distribution of benefits and risks. A criticism of **principlism** is that four principles cannot sufficiently capture moral norms (Walker, 2009). Another common criticism is that when principles compete, as they will in complex situations, there is no framework for settling the conflict.

The nature of mental illness creates situations in which respect for autonomy and beneficence conflict. How should one act when a person with a mental illness chooses to act in a way that brings harm to him or herself? For instance, what if a person with schizophrenia is living homeless on the streets? Should respect for autonomy be upheld, or should there be an intervention to bring the person to shelter? Respect for autonomy is dependent on a person's competence to make his or her own informed decisions, and evaluating such competence can be difficult.

● **STUDY NOTE**

A common ethical issue for nurses in PMH care settings is determining whether autonomy or beneficence is the most appropriate guiding principle when a patient's actions may put the patient or others at risk. The patient's capacity to make rational choices should be a predominant factor in the nurse's decision making. Admission status (i.e., voluntary or involuntary) and competency status (i.e., competent or incompetent) are important to determining such capacity (see Chapter 3).

IN A LIFE

Jan Storch (1940–)
Canadian Nurse Ethicist

Public Persona

Dr. Jan Storch's laudatory leadership in nursing ethics in Canada includes helping launch a centre of health ethics (at the University of Alberta), a provincial health ethics network (in Alberta), being the President of the Canadian Bioethics Society (CBS) and the National Council on Ethics in Human Research, doing research in ethics, publishing widely (including the ethics text, *Toward a Moral Horizon*), and speaking passionately about ethics to diverse audiences. Her guidance of the 2008 centenary revision of CNA's *Code of Ethics* was the fourth time she has contributed to CNA in this way. She serves as Chair of the Research Ethics Board for Health Canada and the Public Health Agency of Canada. Her own current research involves exploring the nature of nursing leadership and ways to create moral practice environments. She has received awards as an outstanding nurse from the nursing associations of Alberta and British Columbia, a 1:100 CNA Centennial Award, a CBS Lifetime Achievement Award, two honorary doctorates, and has been recognized as a leading public intellectual.

Personal Realities

Jan Storch is a wife, mother, grandmother, nurse, and Professor Emeritus at the University of Victoria. Her deep commitment to ethical health care and to nurses' role in it is truly inspirational.

Casuistry or Case-Based Ethics

Casuistry (pronounced kăzh' ū-ĭ;-strē), from the Latin *casus* for *case*, is the use of case comparisons to facilitate moral reasoning and decision making. It is a bottom-up approach in which one starts with the details of the present case and locates that case in a taxonomy of cases as a way to identify the pertinent ethical concerns and responses (Jonsen, 1991; Jonsen & Toulmin, 1988). The focus in casuistry is on agreement about cases, not necessarily principles or theories, and precedents are central to this approach. Past decisions about what was right or wrong in significant cases serve to inform decisions about the new case. (This is similar to what happens in legal judgments.) The nurse using this approach will need to decide how the "case" does and does not fit paradigmatic cases. There are suggested steps to use (Strong, 2000):

1. Identify the main ethical values and concerns relevant to the case.
2. Identify the main alternative courses of action that can be taken.
3. Identify the casuistic factors (i.e., the morally relevant ways the cases of this type differ).
4. Compare the case with relevant paradigm cases that have been identified.

Casuistry seems congruent with the way nurses think in practice. When a clinical situation confronts us, we often think of similar situations that we have experienced or we turn to paradigm cases to guide us. A criticism of casuistry is that there is a risk that one will miss the broad issues and that prevalent beliefs and practices will not be sufficiently questioned.

The Ethics of Care and Feminist Ethics

The **ethics of care** can be seen as a feminine approach to ethics (Sherwin, 1992). Gilligan (1982), in researching moral development, found that females seemed to differ from males in their approach to ethical decision making. Females focused on caring, connectedness, and responsibility rather than the deductive reasoning and abstract principles preferred by males. She argued that women are different from men in their approach to moral decisions, not inferior to them. (Aristotle and Kant both assumed that the moral agent was male.) The perspective of the world as a web of interdependent relationships in which our responsibility to one another is implicit is increasingly predominant in health ethics, as is the recognition that receptivity, relatedness, and responsiveness, as well as emotions, like compassion, are important components of ethical responses (Noddings, 1984; Sherwin, 1992).

Feminist ethics differs from the ethics of care in that it comes from a political perspective, offering insight into oppression (unjust, unwarranted use of power) and dominance in individual and societal-level relationships. Using understandings gained from the analysis of women's oppression, feminist ethicists illuminate negative power differentials that may be so inherent as to be invisible and remain unquestioned. Because feminist ethics combines political dimensions with the core values of care and commitment, it offers a constructive framework for challenging the oppression of people with mental illness.

Relational Ethics

Relational ethics is based on the assumption that all ethical actions are situated in relationship. Ideas of duty and utility, principles, and the character of the moral agent are accepted as important in informing action, but relationship is taken as foundational. Ethics is about how we treat one another, individually and within society, as well as how we resolve moral problems. Ethical situations are encompassed by complexity and uncertainty, and an understanding of the "messiness" of life needs to be cultivated.

Within this perspective, one strives to be responsive to the situation at hand in such a way that genuine dialogue is opened and mutual respect fostered among those involved. Feelings and emotions are viewed as a component of rational thinking and are explored, not ruled out as too subjective or confusing. Context matters. Not anything goes, but one's actions need not only to be shaped by ethical knowledge but also to be adapted to the specific circumstances of the situation. In relational ethics, one aims for the fitting response (Niebuhr, 1963). Questions can be raised within this approach (e.g., issues of power and control) that may not be raised in approaches that focus primarily on moral reasoning (Bergum & Dossetor, 2005). Refer, for example, to relational ethics perspectives

---

BOX 7-1 A Relational Ethics Decision-Making Framework

KEY QUESTIONS
1. What is happening here?
2. What are the alternatives for ethical action?
3. What is the most fitting thing to do?
4. What happened as the result of our action?

Question 1: What is happening here?
- What are the ethical questions? Their context?
- Who is involved? (Who are the moral agents?) What are their commitments to one another?
- What further information do we need?
- Are there legal, organizational, professional, cultural, religious, or any other aspects to consider? Are values in conflict?
- What resources do we have? Need?
- Patient and family resources (e.g., personal directive)?
- Health care resources (e.g., access to home care)?
- Ethics resources: principles, precedents, codes, policies, guidelines, ethicists/ethics committees, etc.?
- To what, in particular, do we need to attend?

Question 2: What are the alternatives for ethical action?
- What are the consequences for each alternative?
- What might constrain ethical action?
- What, if anything, makes me or others uncomfortable in regard to a potential action?
- Remember: refraining from making a decision is still a decision.

Question 3: What is the most fitting thing to do?
- What is the best way to carry out the decision (or plan)?
- Who is affected? Who needs to be involved?
- How may disparate views be bridged?

TAKE ACTION
Question 4: What happened as the result of our action?
- What concerns remain?
- Is anyone distressed about the result?
- Is further action desirable?
- Do we need to address systemic factors that gave rise to the situation?
- Would we act in the same way again?
- What did we learn?

Copyright: Wendy Austin, University of Alberta, Canada.

---

on responses to nurses who have an addiction (Kunyk & Austin, 2012) and on nurses' responsibilities during an epidemic (Austin, 2008). Core elements of relational ethics are mutual respect, engagement, embodied knowledge, attention to the interdependent environment, and uncertainty/vulnerability (Austin, Bergum, & Dossetor, 2003a; Bergum & Dossetor, 2005). A relational ethics decision-making framework is outlined in Box 7-1.

Human Rights

The idea of human rights dates back to 1215 and Britain's Magna Carta, to the rights language of the philosopher John Locke (Sumner, 2000) in the 17th century, and to Thomas Paine's *Rights of Man* (Paine, 1996) in the 18th century. The central assumption of **human rights** is that every person has certain claims or entitlements because he or she is a human. Rights can be conceived as negative or positive. Negative rights are usually civil or political in nature, with the state or others required to refrain from obstructing these rights (e.g., freedom of speech, freedom to worship). Positive rights are obligations of the state or others to provide a right (e.g., right to health, right to education). These rights are typically social, cultural, or economic in nature.

Rights relating to health are included in many international documents, such as the United Nations' (UN) 1948 *Universal Declaration of Human Rights* (*UDHR*) and the UN's 1991 *Principles for the Protection of Persons with Mental Illness and for the Improvement of Mental Health Care*. The Convention of the Rights of Persons with Disabilities (2006) articulates the rights of persons with disabilities to an optimal quality of life, including appropriately competent and thoughtful care from health care professionals. It is human rights law that allows for international scrutiny of a nation's health policies and practices (Gostin, 2001). In 2013, on Human Rights Day, December 10, the World Health Organization (WHO) launched MINDbank, an online platform with national and international resources related to mental health, addiction, disability, and human rights. Its purpose is to facilitate dialogue, advocacy, and research that support nations' reform of policies, laws, and service standards to be in line with international best practices and human rights (See Web Links on thePoint).

"Health" as a human right means that every person has a right to the highest attainable level of health (including a standard of living that is adequate for health) and access to health care and social services as needed. There are tangible connections between health and human rights (Mann et al., 1999). First, *health policies and practices have an impact on human rights*. For instance, mandatory outpatient treatment for persons with a mental illness is an infringement on individual rights. This infringement can only be justified if it is in the person's best interests or for the necessary protection of the public. Second, *human rights violations impact health*. Torture, for instance, may have long-lasting effects on an individual's mental health. The International Council of Nurses not only supports the United Nation's *UDHR* but also stipulates in *Torture, Death Penalty and Participation by Nurses in Executions* that nurses may not voluntarily participate in any deliberate infliction of physical or mental suffering. The World Psychiatric Association's (1996) *Madrid Declaration on Ethical Standards for Psychiatric Practice* stipulates the same for psychiatrists. Third, *health professionals have a responsibility to protect human rights by helping the public identify rights violations*. It is important to note that the (World Health Organization, 2012) claims that some of the most serious human rights violations against persons with mental illness and substance abuse problems occur in health care settings.

A rights approach is not without its critics. It has been argued that such an approach is too legalistic and the law too slow and ineffective in addressing rights violations, and that it is too individualistic, placing the individual in an antagonistic position against the community (Austin, 2001). In 2005, bioethics and human rights were brought together in the *Universal Declaration on Bioethics and Human Rights*, adopted by UNESCO. Among other things, its principles uphold respect for autonomy, the solidarity among human beings, and the need for sharing the benefits of scientific research and for protecting future generations and the planet itself.

ETHICAL PRACTICE ENVIRONMENTS

Health care environments need to be understood as moral communities where practice is grounded in compassion, empathy, and professionalism (Austin, 2012). For PMH settings to be morally habitable, a "culture of questioning" must be actively nurtured (Austin, Bergum, & Nuttgens, 2004). This means that ethical questions are to be expected as an everyday aspect of practice, not perceived as challenging or troublesome. Consultation with a clinical ethicist or ethics committee should be viewed as an acceptable option, a common use of an ethics resource.

Interprofessional communication, collaboration, and conflicts are critical factors in the ethical climate of health care areas (Austin, 2007b). Research in PMH settings has revealed for some time that the desire to get along with colleagues can trump "doing the right thing" (Carpenter, 1991; Fisher, 1995) and that staff conflict influences the way an ethical situation is resolved (Forchuk, 1991). Institutional policies, demands, and supports also play a role. Institutional constraints on a nurse's ability to advocate for patients have been identified as a common contributor to nurses' moral distress (Rittenmeyer & Huffman, 2009). In a critical incident study of nurses' perceptions of what promotes an ethical climate, it was found that being able meet the needs of patients and families "in a considerate way" and sharing responsibilities among a team were significant. These facilitated voicing care

concerns amid a collegial environment (Silén, Kjellström, Christensson, Sidenvall, & Svantesson, 2012).

MORAL DILEMMAS AND MORAL DISTRESS

A **moral dilemma** is a conflict that is morally relevant (Audi, 1995). It may be defined more narrowly as a situation in which one has an obligation to act but must choose between two incompatible alternatives. In health ethics, frameworks have been developed to facilitate the decision-making process.

The CNA Code of Ethics for RNs includes examples of ethical decision-making frameworks, such as Oberle and Raffin's (2009) framework for ethical decision making. This framework has five steps: assessing the ethics of the situation (relationships, goals, beliefs, and values), reflecting on and reviewing potential actions (recognizing available choices and how those choices are valued), selecting an ethical action (maximizing good), engaging in ethical action, and reflecting on and reviewing the ethical action (p. 62). Decision-making frameworks are tools to guide ethical deliberation, based on particular or composite approaches (see Box 7-1).

Moral distress is the anger, frustration, or anguish we feel when we are unable to fulfill our ethical obligations in the way we believe we should (Jameton, 2013). We feel a sense of responsibility and make a moral judgment about the right response, but some constraint prevents us from enacting that response (Nathaniel, 2006). A constraint may be internal (e.g., a lack of moral courage) or external (e.g., the inability to influence the actions of the care team), but when we do not act, we can feel like we participated in a moral wrongdoing. Studies of the moral distress experienced by nurses and other health care professionals in PMH settings have indicated that lack of resources, institutional demands, and unrealistic demands on the part of society that deviant behaviour be controlled are contributing factors (Austin, Bergum, & Goldberg, 2003b; Austin, Kagan, Rankel, & Bergum, 2008; Austin, Rankel, Kagan, Bergum, & Lemermeyer, 2005). Research indicates that when nurses experience moral distress, they either choose to continue giving voice to their ethical concerns or they withdraw—from ethically challenging situations, from their position, or entirely from the discipline of nursing (Pauly, Varcoe, & Storch, 2012).

When experiencing moral distress, it is helpful to identify the source of distress, to refer to one's code of ethics and other documents for guidance, and to seek support. Support may be available from peers, the health care team, or the ethics committee of one's institution or agency. It is available from one's nursing regulatory body, association, or union. For more information, refer to CNA's *Ethical Distress in Health Care Environments* that is part of its *Ethics in Practice* series (Canadian Nurses Association, 2003a).

■ SOME ETHICAL ISSUES IN PMH SETTINGS

It is not possible in this chapter to identify all the complex ethical issues of PMH settings; rather, a few significant ones are discussed. Although some issues are not unique to this specialty area (e.g., confidentiality), all are shaped by the PMH context and by the potential vulnerability of individuals living with a stigmatized illness. Such vulnerability is increased for those who have a mental disorder that can sometimes affect their competency to give informed consent to treatment and who may thus receive treatment involuntarily.

Threats to Dignity

An important aspect of ethical nursing care involves safeguarding the dignity of patients, as violated dignity can lead to suffering (Lindwall, Boussaid, Kulzer, & Wigerblad, 2012). Nurses in PMH settings, when asked about experiences that involved preserving patient dignity, described being genuinely "present" with patients (e.g., supporting a patient through emotions like anger) and being their advocate. Neglecting patients in "the space of waiting" (e.g., requests not responded to in a timely way), abusing one's power (e.g., putting own needs before the patient's), and "punishing" patients (e.g., restraining or sedating patient without first attempting other means of deescalating a situation) were cited as ways patient dignity is offended (Lindwall et al., 2012). Maureen Foy (2007), mother of a young woman with a severe and persistent mental illness, has described her experience as a family member. One example she offers occurred when her daughter was admitted to a crisis unit in a Canadian general hospital:

> Over a period of 2 to 3 hours of waiting, the staff did not speak to us or look at us once. It was as though we were not there, we were invisible. There were no words of comfort or care. There was no information given and we were left to wonder on our own what or whom we were waiting for.... Staff looked through us, around us, above us, below us, but they did not look at us. At a time of crisis and in a place where you go for help and maybe even care, this is hard to bear. This behaviour silences you (p. 1).

She notes that advancements in brain imaging, psychotropic drugs, and models of therapy are nothing if comfort and compassion are not shown to the persons needing care.

Some users of mental health care systems call themselves "survivors." They are not saying that they survived their illness, as one might say "I have survived cancer"; rather, they are saying that they survived their treatment and care (Gallop, 1993). When PMH nurses learn that care has been described in ways such as "To speak from my personal experience, being on a psychiatric ward was one of the most traumatic experiences of my life" (Kirby & Keon, 2006, p. 4) or "We need to recover from being in hospital" (Roper, 2003, p. 14), it is, and should be, very disturbing. Nurses and other health care professionals must consistently ask: What is it like to use our mental health services? What is it like to be our patient or our patient's family member? The value of respect, integral to the support of dignity, is very evident in policy documents and the literature of PMH nursing, but too frequently there is a disconnect between what is espoused and what occurs in practice; ongoing attentiveness to nursing actions that may convey disrespect is crucial to ethical practice (Cutcliffe & Travale, 2013).

Behaviour Control, Seclusion, and Restraint

The (Mental Health Commission of Canada (MHCC), 2009) points out that individuals who are at risk due to mental illness need to be protected and supported; all Canadian jurisdictions need legislation that is appropriate to ensuring this (see Chapter 3). Recovery-oriented mental health care demands, as well, that the least intrusive and restrictive interventions are used in reducing such risk. This means that individual rights, dignity, and autonomy are respected and that there is "the least possible recourse" to measures (mechanical, chemical, environmental, or physical) to limit a person's activity or to control behaviour (p. 121). Restrictive measures are to be used only when absolutely necessary and then with sensitivity and great caution. They can have serious relational consequences.

Coercion and control in psychiatric and mental health care are abiding ethical and clinical issues. A review of the empirical literature on locked doors in acute care psychiatry indicates that locked units are associated with increased patient aggression and poorer satisfaction with treatment (Van der Merwe, Bowers, Jones, Simpson, & Haglund, 2009). Studies of seclusion from the patient's perspective indicate that seclusion is often perceived as unhelpful, punitive, and as a method of control (Faschingbauer, Peden-McAlpine, & Tempel, 2013; Holmes, Kennedy, & Perron, 2004; Van der Merwe, Muir-Cochrane, Jones, Tziggili, & Bowers, 2013). Health professionals do not follow up with patients about the experience, although patients have expressed that this is essential (Larue et al., 2013). Feelings of exclusion, rejection, abandonment, and isolation can be intensified, not from seclusion per se but from the lack of contact with nurses (Holmes et al., 2004).

The concept of "protective empowering," developed by Chiovitti (2011) through research on caring in PMH settings, frames both protective and empowering dimensions of caring and facilitates nurses in "balancing patient safety with choices" (p. 88). When a patient is at high risk for self-harm or unable to accomplish activities of daily living, there may be limits to choice in PMH settings that should not exist as they recover (Chiovitti, 2011).

It is recognized that use of seclusion is shaped by a complex interaction of personal, professional, and organizational factors that include peer pressure (Holmes & Jacob, 2007). Nurses need to be very attentive to what is influencing practice decisions and ensure that ethical responsibilities are primary. Being open to questioning and addressing any use of restrictive or coercive measures is important. Trauma-informed care in inpatient PMH settings focuses on ways to eliminate seclusion and restraints (Muskett, 2014).

Other types of behavioural control in PMH care can raise ethical concerns, including electroconvulsive therapy, behaviour modification, medication, and psychosurgery. Psychotherapy can also have ramifications for one's autonomy, as when therapists expect their interpretations of clients' experiences to be accepted and acted upon (Austin et al., 2004). PMH settings should be well-designed healing places with sufficient numbers of competent, compassionate staff. When this is not so, it is an ethical issue.

Psychiatric Advance Directives

Psychiatric advance directives (PADs) are a legal resource for people to use for times when their decision-making ability is compromised by a mental illness (MHCC, 2009). Advance directives allow for designation of a surrogate decision-maker who can act on one's behalf when one is not competent to do so. It can delineate one's preferred choices to guide the surrogate and the health care team. As an individual with a bipolar disorder noted, "It will give me peace of mind to know that if I get to the point where I can't say anything, there is something in place that will represent myself" (Ambrosini, Bemme, Crocker, & Latimer, 2012, p. 4). PADs are a useful tool in communicating with physicians, avoiding side effects by identifying specific medications that an individual wishes to avoid, and preventing involuntary treatment. Autonomy is not a static value but one that can be lost and regained (Ambrosini et al., 2012). Nurses can support patients in their preparation of PADs and can actively and consistently foster autonomy through learning patient preferences and helping reduce constraints to independence (see Box 7-2).

BOX 7-2 | **Research for Best Practice**

PSYCHIATRIC ADVANCE DIRECTIVES (PADs): A COMPLEX INTERVENTION

Nicaise, P., Lorant, V., & Dubois, V. (2013). Psychiatric advance directives as a complex and multistage intervention: A realist systematic review. Health and Social Care in the Community, *21(1), 1–14.*

Question: What are the theoretical mechanisms through which a PAD is supposed to work? What are the actual conditions of its implementation?

Method: A realist systematic review, designed to assess complex interventions by identifying how they are supposed to work and examining the evidence whether expectations are/are not met, was conducted. ISI Web of Knowledge and Medline databases were searched using "advance directives" and similar terms (e.g., "joint crisis plan"); 295 papers retrieved and reviewed; 103 rejected as out of scope (e.g., about psychological aspects of end-of-life ADs). Criteria were applied to the remaining: post 1991; PAD was clinical or social intervention; had qualitative or quantitative data on health and social outcomes. Key papers were identified (most cited, conceptual papers). Thematic categories of issues related to PADs were identified. Theoretical frameworks (set of expectations) that set out how PADs are to work were synthesized and corresponding empirical data noted.

Findings: The frameworks regarding PADs were enhancement of user's autonomy, improvement of therapeutic alliance, and integration of care/partnership. There were discrepancies among stakeholders' expectations of use and utility of PADs. Users viewed the PAD as a tool to support their autonomy; clinicians, to facilitate alliance (e.g., involvement of users in treatment); family members, to improve alliance that includes carer as decision maker. Little was found related to PAD access and honouring. PADs are multistaged: defining the PAD document, its completion, the accessing and the upholding of its contents. Clarification of each stage of PADs implementation is needed, especially regarding its actual enactment and the honouring of its contents.

Relational Engagement: "Boundaries"

Engagement in therapeutic relationships is an important aspect of most, if not all, PMH care, and complex ethical issues are situated in the boundaries of these relationships (see Chapter 6). Although "boundary," the term commonly used to describe the limits of therapeutic relationships, implies clear, firm borders that should not be crossed, actual practice can be more complicated. Gift giving is an example. Although accepting a gift from a patient can be seen as an initial step down the "slippery slope" toward a boundary violation and something to be always avoided, a particular situation may be more complex (Austin, Bergum, Nuttgens, & Peternelj-Taylor, 2006). Gallop (1997) has shared her experience as a student nurse who received a gift (handmade woolen slippers) from her patient, a young woman with schizophrenia. She kept the gift a secret from her clinical teacher: "Although we were not permitted to accept gifts, I accepted the slippers, deciding the wrath of my instructor was easier to endure than the injury I would inflict by refusing her gift" (p. 28). Nurses need to be thoughtful about the meaning of a gift and seek out knowledgeable advice from members of the team and clinical supervisors.

Not unlike refusal of a gift, declining a "friend invitation" on a social networking site such as Facebook can be a complex ethical issue and require similar thoughtful deliberation (Ginory, Sabatier, & Eth, 2012). The use of email for therapeutic communication and patient-centred care raises similar issues, including that of Internet security. Interacting online with patients can be challenging and requires that professional boundaries be maintained, including the avoidance of dual relationships; nurses and health care staff need to monitor their online presence (Ginory et al., 2012).

One of the most serious types of boundary violation is the sexual harassment and abuse of patients. Despite policies of zero tolerance, abuse occurs and is known to be significantly underreported (Rodgers, 2004). Professionals who commit serious boundary violations at times argue that it was a mutual decision made with the patient. Given the power differentials in therapeutic relationships, this "defence" is unacceptable.

Transgressions of boundaries are most often discussed as "over" involvement. "Under" involvement can also be an ethical issue. Lack of time to engage with patients has been found to contribute to nurses' moral distress (Austin et al., 2003a). Countertransference experienced by the nurse may affect therapeutic availability if the nurse fails to address it appropriately (see Chapter 6). A negative response may be evoked as well, when a patient rejects care, is abusive, or is guilty of a morally reprehensible act, such as child abuse (Liaschenko, 1994). Liaschenko found that when nurses had difficulty connecting with a patient, they chose among three options: to emotionally distance themselves from the patient, to transfer the patient to another nurse, or to make a conscious effort to be respectful and provide good care. The nurses in this study recognized difficulties in "bridging the gap" to a patient as an ethical issue.

In order to engage ethically with patients, nurses must attend to their own personal and professional boundaries and must respect those of others. Education about boundaries is helpful, as are strategies such as clinical supervision and resources such as *Professional Boundaries for Registered Nurses: Guidelines for the Nurse–Client Relationship* (College and Association of Registered Nurses of Alberta, 2011).

Confidentiality and Privacy

CNA's *Code of Ethics* defines **confidentiality** as the ethical obligation to keep someone's personal and private information secret or private duty to preserve a person's privacy. (See CNA's (2003b) "Privacy and Health Information: Challenges for Nurses and for the Nursing Profession" (2003b) and "When Private Becomes Public: The Ethical Challenges and Opportunities of Social Media" (2012) in their *Ethics in Practice* series.) Privacy is a basic human right, and individuals may not wish their personal information disclosed to others or for others to intrude upon their personal space. Legislation at the federal and provincial/territorial levels protects personal health information, and there are regulations that allow individuals to access and request correction of their personal information. Privacy laws in Canada include the *Privacy Act* (Justice Canada, 2014a), which limits the collection, use, and disclosure of personal information in federal government agencies, and the *Personal Information Protection and Electronic Documents Act* (PIPEDA) (Justice Canada, 2014b) with which all provinces and territories must comply. PIPEDA regulates personal information collection, use, and disclosure that occur in commercial activities (including personal health information), requiring that organizations obtain informed consent to use individuals' personal information, secure it, and provide them with access to their own information, which they may request to have corrected.

Canada has a Privacy Commissioner who advocates for privacy rights and is able to publicly report on the handling of personal information from public and private organizations, to investigate complaints, and to promote public awareness of privacy issues (Office of the Privacy Commissioner of Canada [OPCC], 2014a). For example, when Google's online advertising service was targeting individuals with advertisements due to their online health-related searches, the OPCC investigated, as this is contrary to Canadian law. Google agreed to stop such intrusions into privacy (OPCC, 2014b).

Privacy can be particularly important in PMH settings, given the stigma and discrimination attached to mental disorders and to psychiatric care. Consent is a central factor in decisions related to privacy and confidentiality, and this factor becomes more complicated when the person involved has an illness that affects his or her ability to give consent. Overall, nurses safeguard the information learned in the context of their professional relationships, sharing it outside the health care team only with the patients' permission or as legally required.

Disclosure of information within the health care team occurs as necessary for treatment and care, but when patients confide information that is not relevant to the patient's health and well-being, this type of information is not shared. Patients and families need to be made aware that health information and care decisions are shared among the team. This is particularly important as there can be misconception that anything communicated to a health professional is protected as absolutely confidential, even within legal testimony. Such communication, however, cannot be presumed privileged in the way that attorney–client communication is held to be. As well, there are situations that legally require the reporting of information received in a patient care situation. Mandatory reporting of child abuse and abuse of adults in care are examples. (Refer to provincial and territorial legislation for reporting requirements.) Nurses are expected to intervene if others within the health care system fail to meet obligations regarding confidentiality and privacy (CNA, 2008).

Too strict observation of privacy and confidentiality rules can create problems if it means that family and other caregivers are excluded from knowledge that can help them protect and support the person with a mental disorder when he or she is at risk. A balance needs to be found between respecting the person's privacy and facilitating family assistance (MHCC, 2009). PADs are a way to address this potential problem.

Advances in Technology as a Threat to Privacy

Electronic health record systems are being adopted across Canada in an effort to improve health care services. As mental health information can be highly sensitive and potentially damaging if disclosed, due to stigma and discrimination, individuals may not seek treatment if they do not believe such systems are secure (Clemens, 2012). These information systems require nurses and others to go beyond questioning whether to share patient information. Health care staff need to question their own perusal of information: it must be on a need-to-know basis only (Griener, 2005). Other uses of technology, such as **telehealth**—"any use of technology for health purposes"—may affect privacy through security breaches and data mining, as well as involve other issues such as inaccurate data (Kaplan & Litewka, 2008, p. 401).

Neurotechnology is bringing new threats to privacy as the uses of neuroimaging that are being explored include detection of lying, prediction of criminal behaviour, and whether product preferences can be determined (Wardlaw & Schafer, 2011). The prediction of mental events has farreaching ramifications in such areas as insurance, employment, education, immigration, and counterterrorism (Kirby, 2004).

Memory manipulation is being made possible through procedures such as transcranial stimulation and deep brain stimulation and the use of pharmacologic agents (Spiers & Bendor, 2014). While understanding the way memories are formed and how memory may be enhanced or erased has clinical implications (e.g., in treatment of posttraumatic stress disorder, anxiety disorders, and drug abuse [Agren, 2014; Cestari, Rossi-Arnaud, Saraulli, & Constanzi, 2013]), there are fundamental ethical implications as well. Will using neurotechnology in such ways alter an individual's perception of "true self"? Will only pleasant memories be deemed acceptable? Will those unable to afford enhancements be at a great disadvantage in education and the workplace? In other words, what will such technology do to us?

Advances in Genetics

Advances in genetics raise other concerns, some based on past experience (Hansen, Janz & Sobsey, 2008). Eugenics (Greek for "well-born") was once a worldwide movement, beginning at the onset of the 20th century, that aimed at improving the human race. In 1939, in Nazi Germany, a program was initiated that lead to the killing of thousands of "incurable" psychiatric patients deemed to have a life "not worth living" that weakened their society. Nurses actively participated in this program (Aly & Roth, 1984; Benedict & Kuhla, 1999; McFarland-Icke, 1999). For the most part, however, eugenics involved preventing the physically and mentally disabled from reproducing; sterilization was a favoured strategy. With contemporary advances in genetic engineering, a new eugenics is evolving. Genetic testing may make possible prenatal selection and termination of a pregnancy when the foetus is at risk for a mental disorder. (It is doubtful, however, that direct linkages between a given gene and a psychiatric disorder exist; see Chapter 9.) Genetic profiles of individuals may lead to discrimination and to "genetic essentialism" (i.e., a person is defined by his or her genes) (Kirby, 2004). In considering the ethical acceptability of specific clinical genetic testing, questions should be asked, such as: What is the purpose of the test? How predictive is the test? How stigmatized is the condition being tested for? Do effective interventions exist for it? Will the testing affect third parties, such as family members? (Hoop, 2008). Increasingly, others' access to one's genetic information is a realistic concern. Private companies and researchers, hoping to develop new treatments, are seeking legal access to medical records from governments. Although data are anonymized in such cases, confidentiality remains at issue (Doward, 2013). As genetic research evolves, its risks and benefits will need to be continually assessed.

Social Justice

Conditions of fundamental equality and justice are important to optimal mental health (WHO, 2013a). Justice, a principle of fair treatment of individuals and groups within society, is a core value underpinning the CNA *Code of Ethics*. It is acknowledged that broad societal issues affect health and well-being and thus nurses need to be cognizant of these issues, including at the global level and to safeguard human rights, equity, and fairness in their practice, acting as advocates for positive change. Part II of the CNA Code describes examples of what nurses can do to address social inequities, including using the principles of primary health care for the benefit of patients and the public; advocating with others for changes to unethical social policies, legislation, and regulations; and supporting environmental preservation and restoration (CNA, 2008). The Mental Health Commission of Canada (2012) has made "Access to Services," including housing, a priority (Strategic Direction 3) of the mental health strategy for Canada.

The social injustices related to mental illness due to stigma and discrimination exist worldwide. According to the WHO, low- and middle-income countries—where 80% of the global burden of disease due to mental disorders is found—spend less than 2% of their health budget on mental health (WHO, 2011). The WHO's Mental Health Gap Action Programme (mhGAP) (WHO, 2013b) is aimed at helping nations address this mental health treatment gap and enhancing capacity for mental health promotion and care.

Research Ethics

In the history of psychiatric research in Canada, there is a strong reminder that vigilance regarding ethics is crucial. In the 1950s and early 1960s, the "depatterning" experiments of Dr. Ewen Cameron at the Allen Memorial Institute, McGill University (partially funded by the U.S. Central Intelligence Agency), attempted to erase the memories of patients and insert new "positive" ideas. Without their consent, patients were "brainwashed," with many permanently losing their memories. Although Dr. Cameron was an international leader in psychiatric medicine with the reputation of being a humanitarian, his research caused great harm (Collins, 1988). While individuals with a mental disorder may at times be more vulnerable because of their illness, they are no more vulnerable than other groups of research participants, as long as the research is conducted in an ethically sound way and without actual or perceived coercion (Miller & Rosenstein, 2009; Royal College of Psychiatrists [RCPsych], 2011).

Specific safeguards may be necessary for some groups, such as "persons with intellectual disabilities, detained patients, prisoners, children, or vulnerable groups such as refugees" (RCPsych, 2011, p. 2). For instance, research on cravings (intense desires for a drug) for the purpose of understanding their neurobiologic and cognitive bases may allow development of better treatment for addiction. However, substance-dependent research participants must be able to give genuinely informed consent and to fully understand the risks, an ability that may be diminished by potential access to their drug of addiction (Carter & Hall, 2013). Study designs in psychiatric research that raise particular ethical concerns include (1) placebo-controlled studies that deprive participants in the placebo arm of the research of existing treatment; (2) washout studies in which subjects' medications are discontinued; and (3) challenge studies, such as pharmaceutical or psychological challenges administered under controlled conditions, usually with some deception, so that the subject's response may be observed, as these can cause adverse effects (DuVal, 2004).

Research is vitally important to the improvement of the lives of persons with mental illness and their families,

as well as in the determination of ways to prevent mental illness and foster mental health and well-being. However, it is vital that risks and benefits are identified, ensuring individuals are never exploited. Canada has delineated ethics policies for federal research funding agencies in the *Tri-Council Policy Statement on the Ethical Conduct of Research Involving Humans* (Canadian Institutes of Health Research et al., 2010).

SUMMARY OF KEY POINTS

■ Ethics and law are separate domains. Nurses must be vigilant about the laws that affect their practice.

■ Key issues can warn us about the ethical tone of our society; many of these issues are situated in health care. The way in which Canadians address the well-being of persons living with mental illness is one of these issues.

■ Whenever nurses enact their professional responsibilities, they are active as moral agents. Nursing practice involves "everyday ethics," an attentiveness and responsiveness to their duties and commitments.

■ Nurses' regulatory bodies support ethical practice through codes of ethics, position statements, and resources.

■ There are theoretical approaches to ethical knowledge (based on moral philosophy and concepts such as human rights) that inform health ethics. These include virtue ethics, deontology, utilitarianism, principlism, casuistry, ethics of care, feminist ethics, relational ethics, and human rights.

■ Practice environments need to be morally habitable and support ethical questioning and dialogue.

■ Frameworks for ethical decision making are available to assist in resolving moral dilemmas. Moral distress occurs when one is unable to act on an ethical judgement and/or fulfil one's ethical obligations as one believes one should.

■ There are many complex ethical issues in PMH settings. These include issues related to threats to dignity, including behaviour control and restraint, relational engagement ("boundaries"), confidentiality and privacy, genetics, research ethics, and social justice.

■ PADs are a tool intended to support the autonomy of patients. They have been found to facilitate therapeutic alliance and promote treatment integration.

CRITICAL THINKING CHALLENGES

1 Identify a PMH nursing situation that involves an ethical dilemma. Use a decision-making framework to decide how the nurse should act in the situation.

2 Recall an experience of moral distress. What were the barriers to doing what you believed was right? Did

you discuss your concerns with others? How was the situation resolved? Was it ever resolved for you? Is there anything that you would do differently?

3 Who is your moral hero? What are his or her heroic characteristics? What, for you, constitutes moral courage?

4 In their anthology, *The Moral of the Story*, Singer and Singer (2005) have collected works that raise issues of ethics. Use this resource or select your own stories to help you explore the question: "How we should live together?"

5 In his "sci-phi" book, *The Philosopher at the End of the Universe*, Mark Rowlands (2004) addresses such issues as good and evil (*Star Wars*), the question of why one should be moral (*Hollow Man*), and the problem of free will (*Minority Report*). View two films in the science fiction genre. Identify the philosophical themes they raise.

REFERENCES

Agren, T., (2014, in press). Human reconsolidation: A reactivation and update. *Brain Research Bulletin* (online ahead of print). Available at http://www.sciencedirect.com/science/article/pii/S0361923013002062

Aly, G. & Roth, K. H. (1984). The legalization of mercy killings in medical and nursing institutions in Nazi Germany from 1938 to 1941. *International Journal of Law and Psychiatry*, 7, 145–163.

Aristotle. (1996). *Nicomachean ethics*. H. Rackham (Trans.). Ware, UK: Wordsworth Classics.

Ambrosini, D., Bemme, D., Crocker, A., & Latimer, E. (2012). Narratives of individuals concerning psychiatric advanced directives: Qualitative study. *Journal of Ethics in Mental Health*, 6, 1–9.

Audi, R. (Ed.). (1995). *The Cambridge dictionary of philosophy*. Cambridge, UK: Cambridge University Press.

Austin, W. (2001). Using the human rights paradigm in health ethics: The problems and the possibilities. *Nursing Ethics*, 8(13), 183–195.

Austin, W. (2006). Toward an understanding of trust. In J. Cutcliff & H. McKenna (Eds.), *The essential concepts of nursing* (pp. 317–330). London, UK: Churchill Livingstone.

Austin, W. (2007a). The Terminal: A tale of virtue. *Nursing Ethics*, 14(1), 54–61.

Austin, W. (2007b). The ethics of everyday practice: Healthcare environments as moral communities. *Advances in Nursing Science*, 30(1), 81–88.

Austin, W. (2008). Ethics in a time of contagion: A relational perspective. *Canadian Journal of Nursing Research*, 40(4), 10–24.

Austin, W. (2012). Moral distress and the contemporary plight of health professionals. *HEC Forum*, 24(1), 27–38.

Austin, W., Bergum, V., & Dossetor, J. (2003a). Relational ethics: An action ethic as foundation for health care. In V. Tschudin (Ed.), *Approaches to ethics* (pp. 45–52). Woburn, MA: Butterworth-Heinemann.

Austin, W., Bergum, V., & Goldberg, L. (2003b). Unable to answer the call of our patients: Mental health nurses' experiences of moral distress. *Nursing Inquiry*, 10(3), 177–183.

Austin, W., Bergum, V., & Nuttgens, S. (2004). Addressing oppression in psychiatric care: A relational ethics perspective. *Ethical Human Psychology and Psychiatry*, 6(1), 69–78.

Austin, W., Bergum, V., Nuttgens, S., & Peternelj-Taylor, C. (2006). A re-visioning of boundaries in professional helping relationships: Exploring other metaphors. *Ethics & Behaviour*, 16(2), 77–94.

Austin, W., Kagan, L., Rankel, M., & Bergum, V. (2008). The balancing act: Psychiatrists' experience of moral distress. *Medicine, Health Care and Philosophy*, 11, 89–97.

Austin, W., Rankel, M., Kagan, L., Bergum, V. & Lemermeyer, G. (2005). To stay or to go, to speak or stay silent, to act or not to act: Moral distress as experienced by psychologists. *Ethics & Behavior*, 15(3), 197–212.

Bentham, J. (1983). *Deontology together with a table on the springs of action and the article on utilitarianism*. Oxford, UK: Oxford University Press.

Beauchamp, T. (1994). The "four principles" approach. In R. Gillon (Ed.), *Principles of health care ethics* (pp. 3–12). New York, NY: John Wiley & Sons.

Beauchamp, T. & Childress, J. (2013). *Principles of biomedical ethics* (7th ed.). New York, NY: Oxford University Press.

Benedict, S. & Kuhla, J. (1999). Nurses' participation in the euthanasia programs of Nazi Germany. *Western Journal of Nursing Research*, 21(2), 246–263.

Bergum, V. & Dossetor, J. (2005). *Relational ethics: The full meaning of respect*. Hagerstown, MD: University Publishing Group.

Canadian Institutes of Health Research, Natural Sciences and Engineering Research Council of Canada, and Social Sciences and Humanities Research Council of Canada (2010). *Tri-council policy statement: ethical conduct for research involving humans*. Ottawa, ON: Authors.

Canadian Nurses Association. (2003a). Ethical distress in health care environments. *Ethics in Practice for Registered Nurses*. Retrieved from http://www.cna-aiic.ca/~/media/cna/page%20content/pdf%20en/2013/07/26/10/43/ethics_pract_ethical_distress_oct_2003_e.pdf

Canadian Nurses Association. (2003b). Privacy and health information: Challenges for nurses and for the nursing profession. *Ethics in Practice for Registered Nurses*. Retrieved from https://www.cna-aiic.ca/~/media/cna/page%20content/pdf%20en/2013/07/26/10/43/ethics_pract_privacy_health_nov_2003_e.pdf

Canadian Nurses Association (CNA). (2008). *Code of ethics for registered nurses*. Ottawa, ON: Author.

Carpenter, M. (1991). The process of ethical decision making in psychiatric nursing practice. *Issues in Mental Health Nursing*, 12, 179–191.

Carter, A. & Hall, W. (2013). Ethical implications of research on craving. *Addictive Behaviors*, 38, 1593–1599.

Cestari, V., Rossi-Arnaud, C., Saraulli, D. & Constanzi, M. (2013, in press). The MAP(K) of fear: From memory consolidation to memory extinction. *Brain Research Bulletin* [online ahead of print]. doi:10.1016/j.brainresbull.2013.09.007

Chiovitti, R. F. (2011). Theory of protective empowering for balancing patient safety and choices. *Nursing Ethics*, 18(1), 88–101.

Clemens, N. A. (2012). Privacy, consent, and the electronic mental health record: The person versus the system. *Journal of Psychiatric Practice*, 18(1), 46–50.

College and Association of Registered Nurses of Alberta. (2011). *Professional boundaries for registered nurses: Guidelines for the nurse–client relationship*. Edmonton, AB: Author.

College of Registered Psychiatric Nurses (RPNs) of Alberta. (2013). *Code of ethics and standards of psychiatric nursing practice*. Edmonton, AB: Author.

College of Registered Nurses of British Columbia. (2007). *Practice standard for Registered Nurses and Nurse Practitioners: Duty to provide care*. Vancouver, BC: Author.

Collins, A. (1988). *In the sleep room: The story of the CIA brainwashing experiments in Canada*. Toronto, ON: Lester & Orpen Dennys.

Cutcliffe, J. R. & Travale, R. (2013). Respect in mental health: Reconciling the rhetorical hyperbole with the practical reality. *Nursing Ethics*, 20(3), 273–284.

Doward, J. (2013). Sale of personal gene data condemned as 'unethical and dangerous': Critics say companies could acquire personal information that would identify NHS patients without their consent. *The Guardian*. Retrieved from http://www.theguardian.com/science/2013/feb/17/gene-genetic-database-nhs-genewatch

DuVal, G. (2004). Ethics in psychiatric research: Study design issues. *Canadian Journal of Psychiatry*, 49(1), 55–59.

Faschingbauer, K., Peden-McAlpine, C. & Tempel, W. (2013). Use of seclusion: Finding the voice of the patient to influence practice. *Journal of Psychosocial Nursing*, 51(7), 32–38.

Fisher, A. (1995). The ethical problems encountered in psychiatric nursing practice with dangerous mentally ill persons. *Scholarly Inquiry for Nursing Practice: An International Journal*, 9(2), 193–208.

Forchuk, C. (1991). Ethical problems encountered by mental health nurses. *Issues in Mental Health Nursing*, 12, 375–383.

Fowler, M. (1997). Nursing's ethics. In A. Davis, J. Liaschenko, M. Aroskar & T. Drought (Eds.), *Ethical dilemmas and nursing practice* (pp. 17–34). Stamford, CT: Appleton & Lange.

Foy, M. (2007). Thoughts on the ethics of compassion. *Journal of Ethics in Mental Health*, 2(1), 1–2.

Gallop, R. (1993). Balance of power in the provider/client relationship. *College Communiqué*, 18(3), 9–12.

Gallop, R. (1997). Caring about the client: The role of gender, empathy and power in the therapeutic process. In S. Tilley (Ed.), *The mental health nurse: Views from practice and education* (pp. 28–42). Oxford, UK: Blackwell Science.

Gallup. (2013). Honesty/ethics in professions. Retrieved from http://www.gallup.com/poll/1654/honesty-ethics-professions.aspx

Gilligan, C. (1982). *In a different voice: Psychological theory and women's development*. Cambridge, MA: Harvard University Press.

Ginory, A., Sabatier, L. M., & Eth, S. (2012). Addressing therapeutic boundaries in social networking. *Psychiatry*, 75(1), 40–48.

Gostin, L. (2001). Beyond moral claims: A human rights approach in mental health. *Cambridge Quarterly of Healthcare Ethics*, 10, 264–274.

Griener, G. (2005). Electronic health records as a threat to privacy. *Health Law Review*, 14(1), 14–17.

Hansen, N. E., Janz, H. L., & Sobsey, D. J. (2008). 21st century eugenics. *Lancet*, *372*, s104–s107.

Holmes, D. & Jacob, J. (2007). Seclusion practice: A critical examination of the nurses' decision-making process. *BMC Psychiatry*, 7(Suppl 1), S147.

Holmes, D., Kennedy, S., & Perron, A. (2004). The mentally ill and social exclusion: A critical examination of the use of seclusion from the patient's perspective. *Issues of Mental Health Nursing*, *25*(6), 559–578.

Hoop, J. (2008). Ethical considerations in psychiatric genetics. *Harvard Review of Psychiatry*, *16*(6), 322–336.

Ipperciel, D. (2003). Dialogue and discussion in a moral context. *Nursing Philosophy*, *4*, 211–224.

Jameton, A. (2013). A reflection on moral distress in nursing together with a current application of the concept. *Bioethical Inquiry*, *10*, 297–308.

Jonsen, A. (1991). Casuistry as methodology in clinical ethics. *Theoretical Medicine*, *12*, 295–307.

Jonsen, A. & Toulmin, S. (1988). *The abuse of casuistry: A history of moral reasoning*. Berkeley, CA: University of California Press.

Justice Canada. (2014a). *Privacy act, R.S.C. 1985, c. P-21*. Retrieved from http://laws-lois.justice.gc.ca/PDF/P-21.pdf

Justice Canada. (2014b). *Personal information protection and electronic documents act, S.C. 2000, c. 5*. Retrieved from http://laws.justice.gc.ca/PDF/P-8.6.pdf

Kant, I. (1996). *Practical philosophy*. M. Gregor (Trans.). Cambridge, UK: Cambridge University Press.

Kaplan, B. & Litewka, S. (2008). Ethical challenges of telemedicine and telehealth. *Cambridge Quarterly of Healthcare Ethics*, *17*, 401–416.

Kirby, M. (2004). *Interim report on mental health, mental illness and addiction of the Standing Senate Committee on Social Affairs, Science and Technology*. Retrieved from http://www.parl.gc.ca/38/1/parlbus/commbus/senate/com-e/soci-e/rep-e/repintnov04-e.htm

Kirby, M. J. L. & Keon, W. J. (2006). *Out of the shadows at last: Transforming mental health, mental illness and addiction services in Canada*. Available at Parliament of Canada website: http://www.parl.gc.ca/39/1/parlbus/commbus/senate/com-e/soci-e/rep-e/rep02may06-e.htm

Kunyk, D. & Austin, W. (2012). Nursing under the influence: a relational ethics perspective. *Nursing Ethics*, *19*(3), 380–389.

Larue, C., Dumais, A., Boyer, R., Goulet, M. H., Bonin, J. P., & Baba, N. (2013). The experience of seclusion and restraint in psychiatric settings: Perspectives of patients. *Issues in Mental Health Nursing*, *34*, 317–324.

Levine, M. (1977). Nursing ethics and the ethical nurse. *American Journal of Nursing*, *77*(5), 845–849.

Liaschenko, J. (1994). Making a bridge: The moral work with patients we do not like. *Journal of Palliative Care*, *10*(3), 83–89.

Lindwall, L., Boussaid, L., Kulzer, S., & Wigerblad, A. (2012). Patient dignity in psychiatric nursing practice. *Journal of Psychiatric and Mental Health Nursing*, *19*, 569–576.

MacIntyre, A. (1984). *After virtue* (2nd ed.). Notre Dame, IN: University of Notre Dame.

Mann, J., Gostin, L., Gruskin, S., Brennan, T., Lazzarini, Z., & Fineberg, H. (1999). Health and human rights. In J. Mann, S. Gruskin, M. Grodin, & G. Annas (Eds.). *Health and human rights: A reader* (pp. 7–20). New York, NY: Routledge.

McFarland-Icke, B. R. (1999). *Nurses in Nazi Germany: Moral choice in history*. Princeton, NJ: Princeton University Press.

Mental Health Commission of Canada (MHCC). (2009). *Toward recovery & well-being: A framework of a mental health strategy for Canada*. Calgary, AB: Authors.

Mental Health Commission of Canada (MHCC). (2012). *Changing directions, changing lives: The mental health strategy for Canada*. Calgary, AB: Author.

Mill, J. S. (2002). *The basic writings of John Stuart Mill: On liberty, the subjection of women and utilitarianism*. New York, NY: Modern Library.

Miller, F. G. & Rosenstein, D. L. (2009). Psychiatric research. In S. Bloch & S. A. Green (Eds.), *Psychiatric ethics* (4th ed., pp. 271–291). Oxford: Oxford University Press.

Muskett, C. (2014). Trauma-informed care in inpatient mental health settings: A review of the literature. *International Journal of Mental Health Nursing*, *23*, 51–59.

Nathaniel, A. (2006). Moral reckoning in nursing. *Western Journal of Nursing Research*, *28*(4), 419–438.

Nicaise, P., Lorant, V., & Dubois, V. (2013). Psychiatric advance directives as a complex and multistage intervention: A realist systematic review. *Health and Social Care in the Community*, *21*(1), 1–14.

Niebuhr, R. (1963). *The responsible self*. San Francisco, CA: Harper.

Noddings, N. (1984). *Caring: A feminine approach to ethics and moral education*. Berkeley, CA: University of California Press.

Oberle, K. & Raffin, S. R. (2009). *Ethics in Canadian nursing practice: Navigating the journey*. Toronto, ON: Pearson Education.

Office of the Privacy Commissioner of Canada (OPCC). (2014a). About the Office of the Privacy Commissioner. Retrieved from http://www.priv.gc.ca/au-ans/index_e.asp

Office of the Privacy Commissioner of Canada (OPCC). (2014b). Google ads sparked by web surfing on health sites violate privacy rights, investigation finds. Retrieved from https://www.priv.gc.ca/media/nr-c/2014/nr-c_140115_e.asp

Paine, T. (1996). *Rights of man*. Ware, UK: Wordsworth Editions.

Pauly, B. M., Varcoe, C., & Storch, J. (2012). Framing the issues: Moral distress in health care. *HEC Forum*, *24*(1), 1–11.

Radden, J. & Sadler, J. (2008). Character virtues in psychiatric practice. *Harvard Review of Psychiatry*, *16*(6), 373–380.

Registered Psychiatric Nurses of Canada (RPNC). (2010). *Code of ethics & standards of psychiatric nursing practice*. Edmonton, AB: Author.

Ricouer, P. (1992). *Oneself as another*. K. Blamey (Trans.). Chicago, IL: University of Chicago Press. (Original work published 1990).

Robertson, M., Morris, K., & Walter, G. (2007). Overview of psychiatric ethics V: Utilitarianism and the ethics of duty. *Australasian Psychiatry*, *15*(5), 402–410.

Rodgers, S. (2004). Sexual abuse by health care professionals: The failure of reform in Ontario. *Health Law Journal*, *12*, 71–102.

Roper, C. (Ed.). (2003). *Conversations between service receivers: On mental health nursing and the psychiatric service system*. Melbourne, Australia: Centre for Psychiatric Research and Practice.

Rowlands, M. (2004). *The philosopher at the end of the universe: Philosophy explained through science fiction films*. New York, NY: St. Martin's Press.

Rittenmeyer, L. & Huffman, D. (2009). How professional nurses working in hospital environments experience moral distress: A systematic review. *JBI Library of Systematic Reviews*, *7*(28), 1233–1290.

Royal College of Psychiatrists, Executive of the Faculty of Academic Psychiatry. (2011). *Ethics of psychiatric research: Position statement PS02/2011*. London, UK: Author.

Saul, J. R. (2001). *On equilibrium*. Toronto, ON: Penguin/Viking.

Sherwin, S. (1992). *No longer patient: Feminist ethics and health care*. Philadelphia, PA: Temple University Press.

Silén, M., Kjellström, S., Christensson, L., Sidenvall, B., & Svantesson, M. (2012). What actions promote a positive ethical climate? A critical incident study of nurses' perceptions. *Nursing Ethics*, *19*(4), 501–512.

Singer, P. & Singer, R. (Eds.). (2005). *The moral of the story: An anthology of ethics through literature*. Oxford, UK: Blackwell.

Somerville, M. (2000). *The ethical canary: Science, society and the human spirit*. Toronto, ON: Penguin Books.

Spiers, H. J. & Bendor, D. (2014, in press). Enhance, delete, incept: Manipulating hippocampus-dependent memories. *Brain Research Bulletin* [online ahead of print]. Available at http://www.sciencedirect.com/science/article/pii/S0361923013002074

Strong, C. (2000). Specified principlism: What is it, and does it really resolve cases better than casuistry? *Journal of Medicine and Philosophy*, *25*(3), 323–341.

Sumner, L. (2000). Rights. In H. LaFollette (Ed.), *The Blackwell guide to ethical theory* (pp. 288–305). Oxford, UK: Blackwell.

Van der Merwe, M., Bowers, L., Jones, J., Simpson, A., & Haglund, K. (2009). Locked doors in acute inpatient psychiatry: A literature review. *Journal of Psychiatric and Mental Health Nursing*, *16*(3), 293–299.

Van der Merwe, M., Muir-Cochrane, E., Jones, J., Tziggili, M., & Bowers, L. (2013). Improving seclusion practices: Implications of a review of staff and patient views. *Journal of Psychiatric and Mental Health Nursing*, *20*(3), 203–215.

Walker, T. (2009). What principlism misses. *Journal of Medical Ethics*, *35*(4), 229–231.

Wardlaw, J. M. & Schafer, B. (2011). What am I thinking and who has the right to know? Contributions from a workshop on the wider societal implications of neuroimaging [Editorial]. *Cortex*, *47*(10), 1147–1150.

Wong, J., Poon, Y., & Hui, E. (2005). I can put the medicine in his soup. *Journal of Medical Ethics*, *31*, 262–265.

World Health Organization. (2011). *Investing in mental health: Is it worth it?* Available at www.who.int/mental_health

World Health Organization (WHO). (2012). *Quality rights tool kit: Assessing and improving quality and human rights in mental health and social care facilities*. Geneva: Author.

World Health Organization (WHO). (2013a). *Investing in mental health: Evidence for action*. Geneva: Author.

World Health Organization (WHO). (2013b). WHO mental health gap action programme (mhGAP). Available at http://www.who.int/mental_health/mhgap/en/

World Psychiatric Association. (1996). Madrid declaration of ethical standards for psychiatric practice. Retrieved http://www.wpanet.org/detail.php?section_id=5&content_id=48

CHAPTER

8 Theoretic Basis of Psychiatric and Mental Health Nursing

Wendy Austin
Adapted from the chapters "Theoretic Basis of Psychiatric and Mental Health Nursing" by Ginette Pagé and by Mary Ann Boyd

KEY CONCEPT

- recovery
- theory

LEARNING OBJECTIVES

After studying this chapter, you will be able to:

- Explain the need for theory-based psychiatric and mental health (PMH) nursing practice.
- Compare the key elements of theories that provide a basis for such practice.
- Describe the common nursing theories used in PMH nursing.
- Identify theories that contribute to understanding human beings and their mental health.

KEY TERMS

- anima • animus • archetype • behaviourism • change • classical conditioning • cognition • collective unconscious • conscious • countertransference • disinhibition • ego • elicitation • empathy • extrovert • id • interpersonal relations • introvert • modelling • need • object relations • operant behaviour • preconscious • persona • reclamation • role • self-actualization • self-efficacy • self-system • shadow • superego • transaction • transference • unconditional positive regard • unconscious

---

This chapter presents an overview of some of the nursing and other theories that serve as the knowledge base for psychiatric and mental health (PMH) nursing practice. Many of the theories underlying this practice are evolving, and only some have research support to date. As acknowledged in the *Canadian Standards of Psychiatric-Mental Health Nursing*, PMH nurses use knowledge from nursing, the health sciences, and related mental health disciplines in their practice. The chapter begins, then, with selected nursing theories and moves to some of the many theories that underlie our understanding of the biologic, psychological, social, and spiritual aspects of human knowledge and experience.

NURSING THEORIES

Nursing theories are essential in conceptualizing nursing practice. Some theories described here are commonly referred to as models, not as theories, and we have followed common practice. We are not, however, differentiating between a model and a theory, as this remains an area of some debate within nursing.

A nurse may choose to base his or her practice consistently on one nursing theory or may choose to use a specific theory depending on the care situation. For example, in nursing a person with schizophrenia who has problems related to maintaining self-care, Dorothea Orem's deficit theory (1991) may be particularly useful. Peplau's model (1952) may be more helpful in addressing relationship issues. The theory or theories used by a nurse reveal the way that nurse conceives his or her practice.

▼..

> **KEY CONCEPT** A **theory** "is an imaginative grouping of knowledge, ideas, and experience that are represented symbolically and seek to illuminate a given phenomenon" (Watson, 1988, p. 1).

The Visionary: Nightingale

Florence Nightingale, the founder of modern nursing, is recognized as the first nurse researcher and the pioneer of theory development in nursing. The patterns of knowing of contemporary nursing are to be found in her work begun in the 1800s (Clements & Averill, 2006). The respect for her legacy is apparent: International Nurses Day is celebrated on her birthday, May 12, and Canada's National Nursing Week occurs that same week. Nightingale's model emerged from her clinical work in hospitals and in the Crimean War, where unhealthy physical environments for the sick prevailed (Nightingale, 1859). This is the reason that the primary focus of her model, although not neglecting psychosocial and spiritual needs, is on improving environmental conditions. Nightingale's intent was to create healthy surroundings that help alleviate suffering and promote well-being. Health, for her, included the ability to use "every power we have." For example, she considered that giving false reassurance to sick people was unacceptable behaviour. For Nightingale, the curative process was accomplished by nature alone: medicine and nursing do not cure. Nursing activities, therefore, were to "put the patient in the best condition for nature to act upon (him or her)" (p. 75).

Interpersonal Relations Models

Interpersonal Relations: Hildegard Peplau

Hildegard Peplau introduced the first systematic framework for PMH nursing in her book *Interpersonal Relations in Nursing* (1952). A major contribution was her conceptualization of the nurse-patient relationship and its phases (see Chapter 6). Although her work continues to stimulate debate, she led PMH nursing out of the confinement of custodial care into a unique model for practice.

Peplau (1992) believed in the importance of **interpersonal relations**, which included interactions between person and family, parent and child, or patient and nurse. She emphasized empathic linkage, the ability to feel in oneself the feelings experienced by another person or people. The interpersonal transmission of anxiety or panic is the most common empathic linkage, but other feelings, such as anger, disgust, and envy, can also be communicated nonverbally to others. Peplau believed that if nurses pay attention to what they feel during a relationship with a patient, they can gain invaluable observations of feelings a patient is experiencing, even those the patient has not yet recognized or spoken about.

● **STUDY NOTE**
In being empathetic as a nurse, one should know that it is not enough to attempt to understand the patient's experience. Nurses need to communicate to their patients that they are attempting to understand.

The **self-system** is an important concept in Peplau's model. Peplau defined the self as an "antianxiety system" and a product of socialization. The self proceeds through personal development that is always open to revision but tends toward stability. For example, in parent-child relationships, patterns of approval, disapproval, and indifference are used by children to define themselves. If the verbal and nonverbal messages have been derogatory, children incorporate these messages and also view themselves negatively. The concept of **need** is also important to Peplau's model. Needs are primarily of biologic origin but are met within a sociocultural environment. When a biologic need is present, it gives rise to tension that is reduced and relieved by behaviours meeting that need. According to Peplau, nurses should strive to recognize patients' patterns and style of meeting their needs in relation to their health status and help them to identify available resources, such as food and interpersonal support.

Anxiety is an important concept for Peplau, who contended that unless anxiety is understood, professional practice is unsafe. There are various levels of anxiety (mild, moderate, severe, and panic levels), each having observable behavioural cues. These cues Peplau considered "relief behaviours." For example, some people may relieve their anxiety by yelling and swearing, whereas others seek relief by withdrawing. In both instances, anxiety, according to Peplau, is generated by an unmet self-system security need.

Hildegard Peplau (1909–1999)
Psychiatric Nurse of the Century

Peplau became a nurse in 1931 in Pennsylvania. During World War II, she joined the Army Nurse Corps and worked in a neuropsychiatric clinic in London. She obtained a Master's Degree (1947) and a PhD (1953) from Columbia University. Peplau took the lead in the development of psychiatric nursing as a specialty at the Master's level and developed the theory of psychodynamic nursing. Peplau has numerous publications, with her most influential works being *Interpersonal Relations in Nursing* (1952), *Aspects of Psychiatric Nursing* (1957), and *Principles of Patient Counselling* (1964).

Her ideas regarding the centrality of relationship to nursing practice and the efficacy of the use of self as a nursing tool have had far-reaching effects. She envisioned nursing as a discipline independent from medicine and worked to ensure that this was so. Drawing on interdisciplinary knowledge from psychology, education, and pragmatic educational philosophy, she deeply influenced nursing's professional and scientific development. Her achievements occurred during a time when strong leadership from women was frowned upon, and she faced many conflicts and controversies throughout a 50-year career that included being President of the American Nurses Association and consultant to the World Health Organization in psychiatric nursing. She was named one of 50 Great Americans by Marquis' *Who's Who*. Hildegard Peplau was an honorary member of the Canadian Federation of Mental Health Nurses.

Source: Calaway, B. J. (2002). *Hildegard Peplau: Psychiatric nurse of the century.* New York: Springer.

The Dynamic Nurse–Patient Relationship: Ida Jean Orlando

In 1954, Ida Jean Orlando studied the factors that enhanced or impeded the integration of mental health principles in the basic nursing curriculum. From this study, she published *The Dynamic Nurse–Patient Relationship* (1961). A nursing situation for Orlando (1961, 1972) involves the patient's behaviour, the nurse's reaction, and anything that does not relieve the distress of the patient, which Orlando understands as related to the individual's inability to meet or communicate his or her own needs. She focuses on the whole patient, rather than on disease or institutional demands. Her ideas continue to be useful today with research supporting her model (Olson & Hanchett, 1997). For instance, in a study investigating whether Orlando's theory-based practice had a measurable impact on patients' immediate distress when compared with nonspecified nursing interventions, it was found that patients cared for in the Orlando group ($n = 19$) experienced significantly less stress than did those being cared for with traditional nursing care ($n = 11$) (Potter & Bockenhauer, 2000).

Existential and Humanistic Theoretic Perspectives

Seeking Life Meaning: Joyce Travelbee

Influenced by Peplau and Orlando, Joyce Travelbee provided an existential perspective on nursing based on the works of Viktor Frankl, an existential philosopher (see Spiritual Theories section in this chapter). Existentialists believe that humans seek meaning in their life and experiences. Travelbee believed that the nurse's spiritual values and philosophical beliefs about suffering would determine the extent to which the nurse could help ill people find meaning in their situation. She understood "suffering" as a feeling of displeasure ranging from simple and transitory mental, physical, or spiritual discomfort to extreme anguish and beyond to the malignant phase of despair (Travelbee, 1971). Travelbee expanded the area of concern of mental illness to include long-term physical illnesses. Overall, her use of the interpersonal process as a nursing intervention (Travelbee, 1969) and her focus on suffering and illness helped to define areas of concern for nursing.

Humanbecoming: Rosemarie Rizzo Parse

Quality of life as perceived by a person and his or her family is the focus of the nurse within the humanbecoming model. When Parse (2007) was asked what the practice of nurses using this model would be like in 2050, she imagined that their repertoire would remain focused on enhancing quality of life and attending to human freedom and dignity. While the quality of life will be different in 2050, it will still be unique to the individual. The individual (not to be understood as reducible to qualities or traits) is perceived as open and free to ascribe his or her own meaning to life (through values and beliefs developed) and to bear responsibility for his or her choices (Parse, 1987). Reality for an individual is cocreated with the environment. It is in the rhythm of moving closer and away from others where creativity and **change** (becoming different) occur (Leddy & Pepper, 1998). Three principles structure Parse's model:

- Meaning: "Structuring meaning is the imaging and valuing of language."
- Rhythmicity: "Configuring rhythmical patterns of relation is the revealing-concealing and enabling-limiting of connecting-separating."
- Transcendence: "Cotranscending with possible is the powering and originating of transforming." (Parse, 2007, p. 309)

Permeating these three principles are the postulates of *illimitability* (indivisible, unbounded knowing extending to infinity), *paradox* (rhythm expressed as pattern preference), *freedom* (contextually construed liberation), and *mystery* (the unexplainable). The language of human-becoming can be challenging, but the vision of person-hood that it offers can richly inform nursing practice.

Primacy of Caring: Patricia Benner

Patricia Benner has developed a particular notion of nursing as a caring relationship. As a caring profession, nursing "is guided by the moral art and ethics of care and responsibility" (Benner & Wrubel, 1989, p. xi), and nursing practice is based upon "the lived experience of health and illness" (p. 8). Based upon Heidegger's phenomenologic philosophy, Benner describes the person as "a self interpreting being … (who) gets defined in the course of a life … (and) has an effortless and nonreflective understanding of the self in the world" (p. 41). Well-being (the human experience of health or wholeness) is, as is being ill, a distinct way of being in the world. With a phenomenologic view, Benner believes the environment situates meaning. People enter situations with their own sets of meanings, habits, and perspectives, and their personal interpretations affect the way they respond in those situations. Benner and Wrubel's identification of the domains of nursing practice, as described in *The Primacy of Caring*, were used to frame the original Canadian standards of PMH nursing practice (Austin, Gallop, Harris, & Spencer, 1996).

Caring: Jean Watson

The science of caring was initiated by Jean Watson (1979) based on the belief that caring is the foundation of nursing. Watson (2005) recommends that specific theories of caring be developed in relation to specific human conditions and health and illness experiences. The science of caring is based on seven assumptions and 10 "carative" factors (Barnhart, Bennett, Porter, & Sloan, 1994). One of the assumptions is that "effective caring promotes health and individual or family growth" (p. 153); one of the carative factors is that "a trusting relationship … involves congruence, **empathy**, nonpossessive warmth, and effective communication" (p. 152). The model has evolved to address more specifically the spiritual dimension of the nurse's role, including helping the patient to grow spiritually (Watson, 1988). For Watson, spiritual well-being is the foundation of human health, and she suggests that a troubled soul can lead to illness and disease.

Watson's view is applicable to the care of those who seek help for mental illness. This model emphasizes the importance of sensitivity to self and others; the development of helping and trusting relations; the promotion of interpersonal teaching and learning; and provision for a supportive, protective, and corrective mental, physical, sociocultural, and spiritual environment. Research studies supporting the model use qualitative approaches (Baldursdottir & Jonsdottir, 2002).

The Tidal Model of Mental Health Recovery and Reclamation: Philip Barker

Philip Barker's Tidal Model (Barker & Buchanan-Barker, 2005) incorporates Barker and colleagues' Model for Empowering Interactions. It emphasizes the centrality of the lived experience of the person-in-care and is based on the assumption that people are their life stories and that they generate meaning through such stories (Barker, 2001a). It is focused on helping people to recover their lives after an arrest in development, a breakdown, or a disruption in the flow of life. This **reclamation** of one's own life story is necessary to recovery. The nurse's role is envisioned as helping the persons seeking care to discover, identify, and address the problems or challenges affecting them at this point in life. Nurses are to foster the creation of a safe haven in which the persons can

---

BOX 8-1 Ten Commitments of the Tidal Model

1. *Value the voice*: The person's own account of his or her story is the beginning and end point of the helping encounter. Records of care should represent the patient's own voice.
2. *Respect the language*: People develop their own unique way of telling their story. It is not necessary to "rewrite" the story in the language of psychiatry and psychiatric nursing.
3. *Develop genuine curiosity*: Those who seek to be of assistance to the person need to develop ways of expressing genuine interest in the story so that they might better understand the storyteller.
4. *Become the apprentice*: One is the authority on one's own life story. Professionals learn from the person what needs to be done, rather than leading.
5. *Use the available toolkit*: The person's story contains examples of "what has worked" or "what might work" for this person. These are the main tools to use in helping the person's recovery.
6. *Craft the step beyond*: The professional helper and the person work together to construct an appreciation of what needs to be done *now*. The first step is the crucial step, revealing the power of change and pointing toward the ultimate goal of recovery.
7. *Give the gift of time*: There is no value in asking "How much time do we have?" The question is "How do we use this time?"
8. *Reveal personal wisdom*: One of the key tasks for the helper is to assist in revealing the person's life wisdom that will sustain and guide his or her recovery.
9. *Know that change is constant*: The professional helper needs to become aware of how change is happening and discover the way that knowledge may steer the person out of danger and distress and help remain on the journey to recovery.
10. *Be transparent*: Both the person and the professional embody the opportunity to become a team. The professional can support this by being transparent at all times, helping the person understand *what* is being done and *why*.

Source: Buchanan-Barker, P. & Barker, P. (2008). The Tidal Commitments: Extending the value base of mental health recovery. *Journal of Psychiatric and Mental Health Nursing, 15*, 93–100.

recuperate and recover. **Recovery** is clarified by each person in a particular way but is defined in this model generally as "getting going again" (Barker & Buchanan-Barker, 2010, p. 171).

Change (i.e., becoming different) is a core element in this model (hence the metaphor of the tide), and the nurse's role will be shaped by the changing needs of patients across the continuum of care (e.g., critical, transitional, or developmental care) and the provision of interdependent services (Barker, 2001b). Box 8-1 outlines the Tidal Model's "10 commitments" of care.

The Tidal Model considers the domains of self, world, and others (see Fig. 8-1). They are metaphorical settings for the unfolding of the person's story. The process of exploring the person's experience may begin within any of the domains (Barker & Buchanan-Barker, 2010). Tidal processes, used with much flexibility, assist in exploring the person's experience within each domain. A personal security plan is considered in the self domain to help the person to feel as safe as possible. A holistic assessment is an aspect of the world domain as a means of more deeply exploring the person's lifework and problems in living. Group work in various forms is part of the process in the others domain in order to encourage individuals to share aspects of themselves as persons rather than patients (Barker & Buchanan-Barker, 2010).

The first Canadian application of this model was at the Royal Ottawa Mental Health Centre. In their evaluation of its implementation, they found that stories were captured in the holistic assessments of patients and that risk incidents (e.g., restraint use) decreased (Brookes, Murata & Tansey, 2008).

FIGURE 8-1. Tidal Model Domains. (From: Barker, P. & Buchanan-Barker, P. (2007). *The tidal model: Mental health, recovery and reclamation.* Scotland, CT: Clan Unity International.)

Systems Models

Health Promotion: The McGill Model of Nursing

This model was developed under the guidance of Dr. Moyra Allen by the students and faculty of McGill University School of Nursing. It distinguishes nursing from other health disciplines but also identifies their complementary relationships (Allen, 1977). The model's four major concepts are health, family (person), collaboration, and learning (Gottlieb & Rowat, 1987). Health is considered the focus of the practice of nursing and is seen as coexisting with illness. Coping and development are health processes that facilitate functioning and satisfaction with life; family (person) is viewed as the unit of concern. The person is perceived through his or her web of significant relationships. Family and person are considered open systems in constant interaction with their environment. The environment is viewed "as the context within which health and healthy ways of living are learned" (p. 56). Collaboration and learning are essentials for the nurse to structure a learning environment to meet "the needs, goals, and problem-solving styles of the family (person) … based upon the family (person's) strengths and resources" (p. 51). This strength-based component (rather than a deficit focus) of the McGill model makes it particularly useful in assessment, planning, and intervention with families (Feeley & Gottlieb, 2000).

Goal Attainment: Imogene M. King

The theory of goal attainment developed by Imogene M. King is based on a model that includes three interacting systems: personal, interpersonal, and social (King, 1971). King believed that human beings interact with the environment and that the individual's perceptions influence reactions and interactions. For King, nursing involves caring for the human being, with the goal of health defined as adjusting to the stressors in both internal and external environments. She defines nursing as a "process of human interactions between nurse and patient whereby each perceives the other and the situation; and through communication, they set goals, explore means, and agree on means to achieve goals" (King, 1981, p. 144). The process is initiated to help the patient cope with a health problem that compromises the ability to maintain social roles, functions, and activities of daily living (King, 1992). In this theory, the person is goal oriented and purposeful, is reacting to stressors, and is viewed as an open system interacting with the environment. It is within an interpersonal system of nurse and client that the healing process is performed. Interaction is depicted in which the outcome is a **transaction**, defined as the transfer of value between two or more people. The transaction process is what occurs in nursing situations. In the past, King's theory has been applied to group therapy for inpatient juvenile offenders, maximum security state offenders, and community parolees (Laben, Dodd, & Snead, 1991), and as a nursing framework for individual psychotherapy

(DeHowitt, 1992). It continues to be used: as example, to investigate the effectiveness of clinical pathways for a surgical procedure in terms of clinical quality, cost, and patient and staff satisfaction (Knowaja, 2006).

Systems and Stress: Betty Neuman

The purpose of Neuman's (1989) systems model is to guide the actions of the professional caregiver through the assessment and intervention processes by focusing on two major components: the nature of the relationship between the nurse and patient and the patient's response to stressors. The patient may be an individual, group (e.g., a family), or community. The nurse is an "intervener" who attempts to reduce an individual's encounter with stress and to strengthen the person's ability to deal with stressors. The patient is viewed as a collaborator in setting health care goals and determining interventions. Neuman was one of the first PMH nurses to include the concept of stressors in understanding nursing care.

The Neuman systems model has been applied in diverse settings, including community health, family therapy, renal nursing, perinatal nursing, and mental health nursing of older adults (DeWan & Ume-Nwagbo, 2006; Neuman, Newman, & Holder, 2000; Partlak Günüşen, Üstün, & Gigliotti, 2009).

Self-Care: Dorothea Orem

Self-care is the focus of the general theory of nursing initiated by Dorothea Orem in the early 1960s. The theory has three main focuses: self-care, self-care deficit, and a theory of nursing systems (Orem, 1991). Self-care is defined as those activities performed independently by an individual to promote and maintain personal well-being throughout life. Self-care deficits occur when an individual has a deficit in attitude (motivation), knowledge, or skill that impedes the meeting of self-care needs. Nurses can help individuals meet self-care requisites through five approaches: acting or doing for, guiding, teaching, supporting, and providing an environment to promote the patient's ability to meet current or future demands. The nursing systems theory refers to a series of actions a nurse takes to meet patient self-care requirements, which vary from patients totally dependent on the nurse for care to those who need only some education and support. Orem's emphasis on promoting independence of the individual and on self-care activities is of particular importance to PMH nursing (Biggs, 2008). This emphasis fits well with recovery principles and it has potential use in moving inpatient psychiatric cultures toward a recovery focus and in guiding research that explores patients' self-care agency to recovery outcomes (Seed & Torkelson, 2012).

Adaptation: Callista Roy

Callista Roy's nursing model is often selected by nurses working in inpatient psychiatric units because they find its concepts particularly relevant to their practice. Roy's adaptation model (1974), originating in 1964, describes humans as living adaptive systems with two coping mechanisms: the regulator and the cognator. The regulator copes with physiologic stimuli and the cognator with psychosociocultural stimuli. Manifestations of the coping mechanisms can be assessed by four adaptive modes: physiologic needs, self-concept, role function, and interdependence. In this model, the nursing process has six steps: "assessment of behaviour, assessment of stimuli (focal, contextual, and residual), nursing diagnosis, goal setting, intervention, and evaluation" (Lutjens, 1991a, p.10).

Unitary Human Beings: Martha Rogers

The central concept of nursing for Martha Rogers is energy fields, which are open systems (Rogers, 1970). With its principles of homeodynamics—integrality, resonancy, and helicy—her abstract system offers a perspective of **change** as continuous and evolutionary (Rogers, 1994). Health and nonhealth are considered value laden, with the purpose of nursing being the promotion of human betterment. Important concepts are accelerating change, paranormal phenomena, and rhythmic manifestation of change. Rogers' science enables us to see human phenomena differently (Lutjens, 1991b), including a psychiatric disorder (Thompson, 1990). Her influence on other nursing perspectives, such as Rosemarie Parse's health as humanbecoming, is evident. According to Lego (1973), the holistic, unitary human beings approach differentiates a nurse psychotherapist from other psychotherapists.

■ BIOLOGIC THEORIES

Biologic theories are clearly important in understanding the manifestations of mental disorders and caring for people with these illnesses. This importance is growing as we gain further knowledge of the brain. There is a separate discussion in Chapter 9 of the biologic foundations of PMH nursing. That chapter addresses many of the important neurobiologic theories and introduces other new fields of study. Further knowledge about the biologic domain can be found in Chapter 12, which focuses on psychopharmacology and other biologic treatments. In Chapter 11 can be found many of the biologically focused nursing interventions.

■ PSYCHOLOGICAL THEORIES
Psychodynamic Theories

Psychodynamic theories explain human development processes, especially in early childhood, and their effects on thought and behaviour. The study of the unconscious is a key aspect of psychodynamic theory (Ellenberger, 1970). Many important concepts in PMH

| Table 8-1 | Psychological Theories: Psychodynamic and Humanistic | | |

Theorist	Overview	Major Concepts	Applicability
Psychoanalytic			
Sigmund Freud (1856–1939)	Founder of psychoanalysis. Believed that the unconscious could be accessed through dreams and free association. Developed a personality theory and theory of infantile sexuality.	Id, ego, superego Consciousness Unconscious mental processes Libido Object relations Anxiety and defence mechanisms Free associations, transference, and countertransference	Individual therapy approach used for enhancement of personal maturity and personal growth
Anna Freud (1895–1982)	Application of ego psychology to psychoanalytic treatment and child analysis with emphasis on the adaptive function of defence mechanisms.	Refinement of concepts of anxiety, defence mechanisms	Individual therapy, childhood psychoanalysis
Neo-Freudian			
Alfred Adler (1870–1937)	First defected from Freud. Founded the school of individual psychology.	Inferiority	Added to the understanding of human motivation
Carl Gustav Jung (1875–1961)	After separating from Freud, founded the school of psychoanalytic psychology. Developed new therapeutic approaches.	Redefined libido Introversion Extroversion Persona	Personalities are often assessed on the introversion and extroversion dimensions
Karen Horney (1885–1952)	Opposed Freud's theory of castration complex in women and his emphasis on the Oedipus complex. Argued that neurosis was influenced by the society in which one lived.	Situational neurosis Character	Beginning of feminist analysis of psychoanalytic thought
Humanistic			
Abraham Maslow (1921–1970)	Concerned himself with healthy rather than sick people. Approached individuals from a holistic–dynamic viewpoint.	Needs Motivation	Used as a model to understand how people are motivated and needs that should be met
Frederick S. Perls (1893–1970)	Awareness of emotion, physical state, and repressed needs would enhance the ability to deal with emotional problems.	Reality Here-and-now	Used as a therapeutic approach to resolve current life problems that are influenced by old, unresolved emotional problems
Carl Rogers (1902–1987)	Based theory on the view of human potential for goodness. Used the term *client* rather than *patient*. Stressed the relationship between the therapist and the client.	Empathy Positive regard	Individual therapy approach that involves never giving advice and always clarifying client's feelings

nursing began with the Austrian physician Sigmund Freud (1856–1939). Psychodynamic theories initially attempted to explain the cause of mental disorders, but etiologic explanations have not been consistently supported by empiric research. These theories, however, proved to be especially important in the development of therapeutic relationships, techniques, and interventions (Table 8-1).

Psychoanalytic Theory

Study of the Unconscious

In Sigmund Freud's psychoanalytic model, the human mind was conceptualized in terms of **conscious** mental processes (an awareness of events, thoughts, and feelings with the ability to recall them) and **unconscious** mental processes (thoughts and feelings that are outside awareness and are not remembered). Freud believed that the unconscious part of the human mind is only rarely recognized by the conscious part, as in remembered dreams. The term **preconscious** was used to describe unconscious material that is capable of entering consciousness. Uncovering unconscious material to help patients gain insight into unresolved issues was basic to the psychotherapy Freud developed.

Personality and Its Development

Freud's personality structure consists of three parts: the id, ego, and superego (Freud, 1927). According to Freud, the **id** is formed by unconscious desires, primitive instincts, and unstructured drives, including sexual and aggressive tendencies that arise from the body. The **ego** consists of the sum of certain mental mechanisms, such as perception, memory, and motor control, as well as specific defence mechanisms. The ego controls movement, perception, and contact with reality. The capacity to form mutually satisfying relationships is a fundamental function of the ego, which is not present at birth but is formed throughout a child's development. The **superego** is that part of the personality structure associated with ethics, standards, and self-criticism. A child's identification with important and esteemed people in early life, particularly parents, helps form the superego.

Object Relations and Identification

Freud introduced the concept of **object relations**, the psychological attachment to another person or object. He believed that the choice of a love object in adulthood and the nature of the relationship depend on the nature and quality of the child's object relationships during the early formative years. A child's first love object is the mother, who is the source of nourishment and the provider of pleasure. Gradually, as the child separates from the mother, the nature of this initial attachment influences any future relationships. The development of the child's capacity for relationships with others progresses from a state of narcissism to social relationships, first within the family and then within the larger community. Although the concept of object relations is fairly abstract, it can be understood in terms of a child who imitates her mother and then becomes like her mother in adulthood. This child has incorporated her mother as a love object, identifies with her, and becomes like her as an adult. This process becomes especially important in understanding an abused child who, under certain circumstances, becomes the adult abuser.

Anxiety and Defense Mechanisms

For Freud, anxiety was a specific state of unpleasantness accompanied by motor discharge along definite pathways, the reaction to danger of object loss. Defence mechanisms protected a person from unwanted anxiety. Although they are defined differently than in Freud's day, defence mechanisms still play an explanatory role in contemporary PMH practice. Defence mechanisms are discussed in Chapter 6.

Sexuality

According to Freud, the energy or psychic drive associated with the sexual instinct, called the *libido*, translated from Latin as "pleasure" or "lust," resides in the id. When sexual desire is controlled and not expressed, tension results and is transformed into anxiety (Freud, 1905). Freud believed that adult sexuality is an end product of a complex process of development that begins in early childhood and involves a variety of body functions or areas (oral, anal, and genital zones) that correspond to stages of relationships, especially with parents.

Psychoanalysis

Freud (1949) developed *psychoanalysis*, a therapeutic process of accessing the unconscious and with the mature adult mind resolving the conflicts that originated in childhood. As a system of psychotherapy, psychoanalysis attempted to reconstruct the personality by examining free associations (spontaneous, uncensored verbalizations of whatever comes to mind) and the interpretation of dreams (Freud, 1955). Freud believed that therapeutic relationships had their beginnings within the psychoanalytic framework.

Transference and Countertransference

Transference is the displacement of thoughts, feelings, and behaviours originally associated with significant others from childhood onto a person in a current therapeutic relationship (Moore & Fine, 1990). For example, a woman's feelings toward her parents as a child may be transferred to the therapist: if she were unconsciously angry with her parents, she may feel inexplicable anger and hostility toward her therapist. In psychoanalysis, the therapist uses transference as a therapeutic tool to help the patient understand emotional problems and their origin. It is considered an essential aspect of therapy. **Countertransference**, on the other hand, is defined as the direction of all the therapist's feelings and attitudes toward the patient. Feelings and perceptions caused by countertransference may interfere with the therapist's ability to understand the patient.

Neo-Freudian Models

Many of Freud's followers ultimately established their own forms of psychoanalysis. The various psychoanalytic schools have adopted other names because their doctrines deviated from Freudian theory.

Adler's Foundation for Individual Psychology

Alfred Adler was a Viennese psychiatrist, founder of the school of individual psychology, and an early colleague of Freud who disagreed with Freud's focus on instinctual determination. He focused instead on the social aspects of human existence. Adler believed mental health involves love, work, and community. For Adler (1963), the motivating force in human life is a striving for superiority. Seeking perfection and security while trying to avoid feelings of inferiority can lead the individual to adopt a life goal that is unrealistic and frequently expressed as an unreasoning desire for power and dominance (i.e., *inferiority complex*). Because inferiority is intolerable, the compensatory mechanisms set up by the mind may result in self-centred attitudes, overcompensation, and a retreat from life's problems.

Adler focused on growth, lifestyle, and becoming: humans are looking to realize their potential, to flourish within their community. Adlerian theory is based on principles of mutual respect, choice, responsibility, consequences, and belonging. It informs both psychotherapy (e.g., family therapy and Ellis' (1973) Rational Emotive Therapy) and education.

Jung's Analytical Psychology

One of Freud's earliest colleagues, Carl Gustav Jung, a Swiss psychoanalyst, created a model called *analytical psychology*. For Jung, humans were influenced not only by their past but also by their hopes for the future. He not only supported the idea of a personal unconscious but also proposed a second psychic system, inherited and universal to all humans, the **collective unconscious**. Within the collective unconscious are **archetypes**, symbols common to all cultures. Images such as "mother" or "hero" or "trickster," for instance, have forms common to every society (Jung, 1959). Jung described humans as having both feminine and masculine characteristics; therapy may help an individual develop more fully as a person by embracing both aspects of himself or herself. The feminine side of men is the **anima**; the masculine side of women is the **animus**. His concept of **persona** (the mask one wears in society, one's public self) is similar to Freud's superego (Jung, 1966). The **shadow** is Jung's image for the dark side of every person, the side we do not like to recognize or show to others. To evolve as an individual, one needs to become aware of and integrate the shadow into one's personality.

Jung believed in the existence of two psychological types: the **extrovert** (who finds meaning in the world) and the **introvert** (who finds meaning within). He also described four primary modes of orientation to the world: *thinking, feeling, intuition,* and *sensation*. Although he argued that each of these functions exists in an individual, certain preferences will dominate. Our unconscious is revealed often through our least developed mode. The Myers-Briggs Type Indicator test is based on Jung's personality theory.

Horney's Feminine Psychology

Karen Horney, a German-American psychiatrist, challenged many of Freud's basic concepts and introduced principles of feminine psychology. Recognizing a male bias in psychoanalysis, Horney questioned the psychoanalytic belief that women felt disadvantaged because of their genital organs, and she rejected Freud's concept of "penis envy." She argued that there are significant cultural reasons for women to strive to obtain qualities or privileges that are defined by a society as masculine and that women truly were at a disadvantage in a paternalistic culture (Horney, 1939). She observed that men have a deep-seated dread of women that is revealed in analysis (Horney, 1932). Her primary concept was that of basic anxiety: early (childhood) feelings of helplessness and isolation which one strives to cope with and resolve. According to Horney, this anxiety underlies all of an individual's relationships and can help explain behaviour. Horney (1950) named the unrealistic expectations that one puts on oneself "tyranny of the should." With other Neo-Freudians, such as Eric Fromm, she introduced sociocultural dimensions of human behaviour into the psychoanalytical model.

Humanistic Theories

Humanistic theories were generated as a reaction against psychoanalytic premises of instinctual drives and are based on the views of human potential for goodness. Humanist therapists focus on one's ability to learn about oneself, acceptance of self, and exploration of personal capabilities. Within the therapeutic relationship, the patient begins to develop positive attitudes and views himself or herself as a person of worth. The focus is not on investigation of repressed memories but on learning to experience the world in a different way.

Rogers' Client-Centred Therapy

Carl Rogers, an American psychologist, developed new methods of client-centred therapy. Rogers (1980) defined empathy as the capacity to assume the internal reference of the client in order to perceive the world in the same way as the client. To use empathy in the therapeutic process, the counsellor must be nondirective but not passive. Thus, the counsellor's attitude and nonverbal communication are crucial. He advocated that the therapist develops **unconditional positive regard**, a nonjudgmental caring, for the client (Rogers, 1980) and believed that the therapist's emotional investment (i.e., true caring) in the client is essential to the therapeutic process. Genuineness on the part of the therapist, in contrast with the passivity of the psychoanalyst, is seen as key.

Gestalt Therapy

Another humanistic response to the psychoanalytic model was Gestalt therapy, developed by Frederick S. (Fritz) Perls. Perls believed that modern civilization inevitably produces neurotic anxiety because it forces people to repress natural desires and frustrates an inherent human tendency to adjust biologically and psychologically to the environment. For a person to be cured, unmet needs must be brought back to awareness. Perls rejected the notion that intellectual insight enabled people to change. His individual and group exercises aimed to enhance a person's awareness of emotions, physical state, and repressed needs as well as physical and psychological stimuli in the here-and-now environment (Perls, 1969).

Maslow's Hierarchy of Needs

Abraham Maslow developed a humanistic model that is used in PMH nursing today (Maslow, 1998). His major contributions were to the understanding of human needs and motivation (Maslow, 1970). He studied exemplary healthy individuals (e.g., Albert Einstein) whom he saw as self-actualizing and described their characteristics. For instance, he noted that they were creative, had a deep sense of kinship with others, and had a strong sense of ethics. People are self-actualized when they are making the most of their unique human potential. Maslow's view of human motivation was based on a hierarchy of needs, ranging from lower-level survival needs, such as air, water, basic food, and shelter, to higher-level needs, such as those for belonging and esteem and, finally, for **self-actualization**. One must meet lower-level needs before moving to the higher-level ones (see Fig. 8-2). According to Maslow's

model, values such as truth, beauty, and justice are aspects of our metaneeds, and their persistent deprivation can lead to spiritual–existential ailments often expressed as apathy, boredom, hopelessness, and powerlessness (Hoffman, 1996). Maslow's model offers a framework for assessment.

Applicability of Psychodynamic Theories to PMH Nursing

Several concepts in psychodynamic models are core elements in PMH nursing practice, such as interpersonal relationships, needs, anxiety, defence mechanisms, transference, and countertransference. Many of these concepts are further developed within nursing theories. A key psychodynamic concept, the therapeutic relationship, is recognized as a core of PMH nursing intervention.

Behavioural Theories

Behavioural theories, with roots in the discipline of psychology, offer important explanatory models for PMH nursing in terms of the way in which people act and learn (Table 8-2).

Early Stimulus–Response Theories

Pavlovian Theory

One of the earliest behavioural theorists was Ivan P. Pavlov, who was studying the gastric functioning of dogs when he noticed that stomach secretions of dogs were stimulated by triggers other than food, such as the sight and smell of food. He became interested in this anticipatory secretion. Through his experiments, he was able to stimulate secretions with a variety of other laboratory nonphysiologic stimuli. Thus, a clear connection was made between thought processes and physiologic responses.

In Pavlov's model, there is an unconditioned stimulus (not dependent on previous training) that elicits an unconditioned (i.e., specific) response. In his experiments, meat was the unconditioned stimulus, and salivation was the unconditioned response. Pavlov would then select other stimuli, such as a bell, a ticking metronome, and a triangle drawn on a large cue card, presenting this conditioned stimulus just before the meat, the unconditioned stimulus. If the conditioned stimulus was repeatedly presented before the meat, eventually salivation was elicited by the conditioned stimulus. This phenomenon was called **classical** (Pavlovian) **conditioning** (Pavlov, 1927/1960).

John B. Watson and the Behaviourist Revolution

At about the same time Pavlov was working in Russia, John B. Watson initiated the psychological revolution known as **behaviourism** in the United States. He developed two principles: frequency and recency. The principle of frequency states that the more often a given response is made to a given stimulus, the more likely the response to that stimulus will be repeated. The principle of recency states that the more recently a given response to a particular

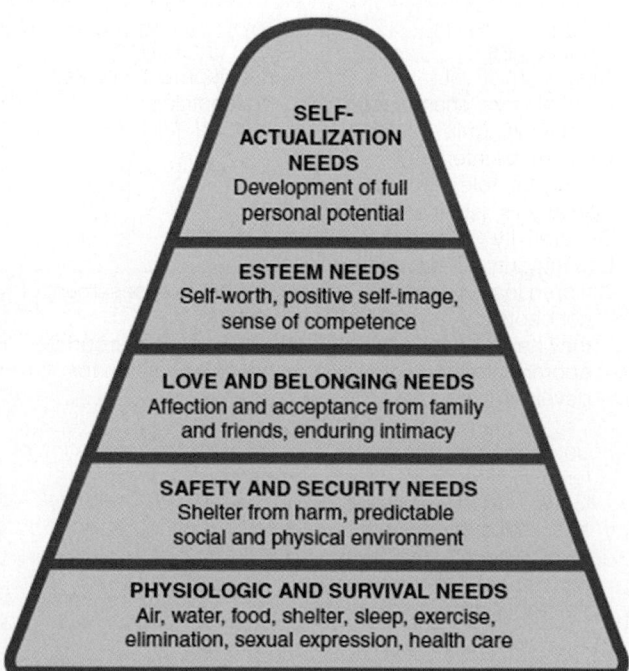

FIGURE 8-2. Maslow's Hierarchy of Needs.

SELF-
ACTUALIZATION
NEEDS
Development of full
personal potential

ESTEEM NEEDS
Self-worth, positive self-image,
sense of competence

LOVE AND BELONGING NEEDS
Affection and acceptance from family
and friends, enduring intimacy

SAFETY AND SECURITY NEEDS
Shelter from harm, predictable
social and physical environment

PHYSIOLOGIC AND SURVIVAL NEEDS
Air, water, food, shelter, sleep, exercise,
elimination, sexual expression, health care

Table 8-2	Psychological Theories: Behavioural, Cognitive, and Developmental		
Theorist	**Overview**	**Major Concepts**	**Applicability**
Stimulus–Response Theories			
Ivan P. Pavlov (1849–1936)	Classical conditioning	Unconditioned stimuli Unconditioned response Conditioned stimuli	Important in understanding learning of automatic responses such as habitual behaviours
John B. Watson (1878–1958)	Introduced behaviourism, believed that learning was classical conditioning called *reflexes*; rejected distinction between the mind and the body.	Principle of frequency Principle of recency	Focuses on the relationship between the mind and the body
Reinforcement Theories			
B. F. Skinner (1904–1990)	Developed an understanding of the importance of reinforcement and differentiated types and schedules.	Operant behaviour Respondent behaviour Continuous reinforcement Intermittent reinforcement	Important in behaviour modification
Edward L. Thorndike (1874–1949)	Believed in the importance of effects that followed behaviour.	Reinforcement	Important in behaviour modification programs
Cognitive Theories			
Albert Bandura (b. 1925)	Developed social cognitive theory, a model for understanding how behaviour is learned from others.	Modelling Disinhibition Elicitation Self-efficacy	Important in helping patients learn appropriate behaviours
Aaron Beck (b. 1921)	Conceptualized distorted cognitions as a basis for depression.	Cognitions Beliefs	Important in cognitive therapy
Kurt Lewin (1890–1947)	Developed field theory, a system for understanding learning, motivation, personality, and social behaviour.	Life space Positive valences Negative valences	Important in understanding motivation for changing behaviour
Edward Chace Tolman (1886–1959)	Introduced the concept of cognitions; believed that human beings act on beliefs and attitudes and strive toward goals.	Cognition	Important in identifying the person's beliefs
Developmental Theories			
Erik Erikson (1902–1994)	Viewed psychosocial development as influenced by environment and occurring in stages, each one having a task to resolve.	Eight stages Trust vs. mistrust Autonomy vs. shame/doubt Initiative vs. guilt Industry vs. inferiority Identity vs. role diffusion Intimacy vs. isolation Generativity vs. stagnation Ego integrity vs. despair	Allows unresolved developmental tasks to be identified
Jean Piaget (1896–1980)	Viewed intelligence as adaptation to the environment. Understood cognitive development in children to be like embryonic development: increasing differentiation in structure.	Children learn particular concepts only when they have reached the appropriate stage of development	Important in assessment of children Useful in age-appropriate health education for children
Carol Gilligan (1936–)	Gender differences in moral development.	Found a tendency for females to be more focused in relationships and issues of care in resolving moral problems, while males tend to apply abstract principles such as justice	Important in the evolution of gender studies

stimulus is made, the more likely it will be repeated. Watson's major contribution was the rejection of the distinction between body and mind and his emphasis on the study of objective behaviour (Watson & Rayner, 1917).

Reinforcement Theories

Edward L. Thorndike

A pioneer in experimental animal psychology, Edwin L. Thorndike studied the problem-solving behaviour of cats to determine whether animals solved problems by reasoning or instinct. He found that neither choice was completely correct; animals gradually learn the correct response by "stamping in" the stimulus–response connection. The major difference between Thorndike and behaviourists such as Watson was that Thorndike believed in the importance of the effects that followed the response or the reinforcement of the behaviour. He was the first reinforcement theorist, and his view of learning became the dominant view in learning theory (Thorndike, 1916, c.1906).

B. F. Skinner

One of the most influential behaviourists, B. F. Skinner recognized two different kinds of learning, each involving a separate kind of behaviour. *Respondent behaviour*, or the end result of **classical conditioning**, is elicited by specific stimuli. Given the stimulus, the response occurs automatically. The other kind of learning is referred to as **operant behaviour**. In this type of learning, the distinctive characteristic is the consequence of a particular behavioural response not a specific stimulus. The learning of operant behaviour is also known as *conditioning*, but it is different from the conditioning of reflexes. If a behaviour occurs and is followed by reinforcement, it is probable that the behaviour will recur. For example, if a child climbs on a chair, reaches the faucet, and is able to get a drink of water successfully, it is more likely that the child will repeat the behaviour (Skinner, 1935). Skinner wrote a book about a utopian community based on the principles of behaviourism that he titled *Walden II* (Skinner, 1976).

Cognitive Theories

The initial behavioural studies focused attention on human actions without attention to the internal thinking process. As complex behaviour was examined and could not be accounted for by strictly behavioural explanations, thought processes became new subjects for study. Cognitive theories, an outgrowth of different theoretic perspectives including the behavioural and the psychodynamic, attempted to link internal thought processes with human behaviour.

Albert Bandura's Social Cognitive Theory

Acquiring behaviours by learning from other people is the basis of social cognitive theory developed by the psychologist Albert Bandura, born in Mundare, Alberta. Bandura developed his ideas after being concerned about violence on television contributing to aggression in children. He believes that important behaviours are learned by internalizing behaviours of others. His initial contribution was identifying the process of **modelling**: pervasive imitation or one person trying to be like another. According to Bandura, the model may not need to be a real person but could be a character in history or generalized to an ideal person (Bandura, 1977).

The concept of **disinhibition** is important to Bandura's model and refers to the situation in which someone has learned not to make a response; then, in a given situation, when another is making the inhibited response, the individual becomes disinhibited and also makes the response. Thus, the response that was "inhibited" now becomes disinhibited through a process of imitation. For example, during severe dieting, an individual may have learned to resist eating large amounts of food. However, when at a party with a friend who eagerly fills a plate at a buffet, the person also eats large amounts of food.

In the instance of disinhibition, the desire to eat is already there, and the individual indulges that desire. However, in another instance called **elicitation**, there is no desire present, but when one person starts an activity, others want to do the same. An example of this occurs when a child is playing with a toy and the other children now want to play with the same toy even though they showed no interest in it before that time.

An important concept of Bandura's is **self-efficacy**, a person's sense of his or her ability to deal effectively with the environment (Bandura, 1997). Efficacy beliefs influence how people feel, think, motivate themselves, and behave. The stronger the self-efficacy, the higher the goals people set for themselves and the firmer their commitment to them.

Aaron T. Beck: Thinking and Feeling

American psychiatrist Aaron T. Beck of the University of Pennsylvania devoted his career to understanding the relationship between **cognition** and mental health. For Beck, cognitions are verbal or pictorial events in the stream of consciousness. He realized the importance of cognitions when treating people with depression, finding that the depression improved when patients began thinking differently. He believed that people with depression had faulty information-processing systems that led to biased cognitions. These faulty beliefs cause errors in judgment that become habitual errors in thinking. When individuals incorrectly interpret life situations, they judge themselves too harshly and jump to inaccurate conclusions. A person may, for example, truly believe that he or she has no friends and therefore no one cares. On examination, the evidence for the beliefs is based on the fact that there has been no contact with anyone because of moving from one city to another. Thus, a distorted belief is the basis of the cognition. Beck, Thase, and Wright (2003) developed cognitive therapy, a successful approach for the treatment of depression (see Chapter 22). Beck (2011) continues to develop cognitive behaviour therapy. See Chapter 13 for an overview of cognitive–behavioural techniques.

Applicability of Behavioural Theories to PMH Nursing

Interventions based on behavioural theories are important in nursing. For example, patient education interventions are usually based on learning principles derived from behavioural theories, and the teaching of new coping skills for patients in their recovery is usually based on behavioural theories. Changing an entrenched habit involves helping people to identify what motivates them, recognize cues that precede the behaviour they desire to change, and create new lifestyle habits. Examples of behavioural interventions used on inpatient hospital units include the privilege systems and token economies.

Developmental Theories

Developmental theories explain normal human growth and development and focus on **change** over time. Many are presented in terms of stages based on the assumption that normal development proceeds stage-by-stage longitudinally. Human development, however, does not necessarily unfold sequentially and in the same way for each person.

Erik Erikson: Psychosocial Development

Erik Erikson's psychosocial developmental model, an expansion of Freud's psychosexual development theory, is commonly used in nursing. Each of Erikson's eight stages is associated with a specific task that can be successfully or unsuccessfully resolved. The model is organized according to developmental conflicts by age: basic trust versus mistrust, autonomy versus shame and doubt, initiative versus guilt, industry versus inferiority, identity versus role diffusion, intimacy versus isolation, generativity versus stagnation, and ego integrity versus despair. Erikson's wife, Joan Serson Erickson, extended his theory to include old age as a ninth stage, gerotranscendence (Erikson & Erikson, 1997). Gerotranscendence theory focused on the continued growth in dimensions such as spirituality and inner strength (see Chapter 32).

Within Erickson's theory, successful resolution of a crisis leads to essential strength and virtues. For example, a positive outcome of the trust versus mistrust crisis is the development of a basic sense of trust. If the crisis is unsuccessfully resolved, the infant moves into the next stage without a sense of trust. According to this model, a child who is mistrustful will have difficulty completing the next crisis successfully and, instead of developing a sense of autonomy, will more likely be full of shame and doubt (Erikson, 1963). One of Erikson's

major contributions was the recognition of the turbulence of adolescent development. Erikson wrote extensively about adolescence, youth, and identity formation. When adolescence begins, childhood ways must be given up, and body changes must be reconciled with the individual's social position, previous history, and identifications. An identity is formed. This task of reconciling how young people see themselves and how society perceives them can become overwhelming and lead to role confusion and alienation (Erikson, 1968).

Research has explored developmental stages of this model with mixed results. For instance, in an early study, male college students who measured low on identity also scored low on intimacy ratings (Orlofsky, Marcia, & Lesser, 1973), lending support to the idea that identity precedes intimacy. Yet in another study, intimacy was found to begin developing early in adolescence, prior to the development of identity (Ochse & Plug, 1986). Studying fathers with young children, Christiansen and Palkovitz (1998) found that *generativity* (defined as the need or drive to produce, create, or effect a change) was associated with a paternal identity, psychosocial identity, and psychosocial intimacy. In a longitudinal study testing Erikson's model, 86 men were assessed at 21 years of age and then at 52 years. Fifty-six percent of the men achieved generativity, which was associated with work achievement, close friendships, successful marriage, altruistic behaviours, and mental health. Favourable predictors in young adulthood included a warm family environment and good peer relationships (Westermeyer, 2004). Research also suggests that gender influences development. One study found generativity to be associated with well-being in both males and females. In males, however, generativity seems related to the urge for self-protection, self-assertion, self-expansion, and mastery, while in women, the antecedents may be the desire for contact, connection, and union (Ackerman, Zuroff, & Moskowitz, 2000). A Canadian study that investigated grandparents' role in the socialization of children within the family queried whether midlife generativity would predict parents' descriptions of grandparenting problems. It did: generative fathers were more optimistic that problems with grandparents would be solved; both generative mothers and fathers showed higher levels of forgiveness of grandparents (Pratt, Norris, Cressman, Lawford & Hebblethwaite, 2008).

Jean Piaget: Learning in Children

One of the most influential people in child psychology was Jean Piaget, who was the first to make a systematic study of cognitive development (Piaget, 1936). Piaget viewed intelligence as an adaptation to the environment. He proposed that cognitive growth is like embryologic growth: an organized structure increasingly differentiates over time. He determined that readiness is an important consideration in children's learning. According to Piaget, a particular concept should be taught to children only when they have reached an appropriate stage of development. Piaget developed a system that explains how knowledge develops and changes. Each stage of cognitive development represents a particular structure with major characteristics (Piaget, 1957). Piaget tested his theory through observation of his own children; the theory was never subjected to formal testing.

The major strength of his model was its recognition of the central role of cognition in development and the discovery of surprising features of young children's thinking. For nursing, Piaget's model provides a framework in which to define different levels of thinking and use the data in the assessment and intervention processes.

Carol Gilligan: Gender Differentiation

Psychologist Carol Gilligan studied the ways males and females approached moral problems and identified differences (Gilligan, 1982). She wrote about these differences in moral development in her 1982 landmark work, *In a Different Voice: Psychological Theory and Women's Development*. While males tended to approach moral problems by applying abstract rules such as those related to justice, the females in her study were more likely to be concerned with preserving the relationships of those involved and with responsibilities related to care. For Gilligan, attachment within relationships is the important factor for successful female development. Thus, traditional models of development that advocate separation as a primary goal of human development, such as Erikson's, disadvantage women. They can be viewed as impaired by the importance placed on attachments. According to Gilligan, female development does not follow a progression of stages but is based on experiences within relationships. This may be the case for males, as well, in their development of a strong sense of self (Nelson, 1996).

The scientific merit of Gilligan's work has been challenged by many critics, including feminist scholars, but it has had a significant impact on the development of gender studies (Graham, 2012).

Applicability of Developmental Theories to PMH Nursing

Developmental theories are used in understanding childhood and adolescent experiences and their manifestations as adult problems. When working with children, nurses can use developmental models to help gauge development and mood. However, because most of the models are based on the assumptions of the linear progression of stages and have not been adequately tested, applicability has limitations. In addition, these models were based on a relatively small number of children who typically were raised in a Western middle-class environment. Most do not account for gender differences and diversity in lifestyles and cultures.

SOCIAL THEORIES

Numerous social theories underlie PMH nursing practice, and the nursing profession itself serves a specific societal function. This section represents a sampling of important social theories that nurses may use. This discussion is not exhaustive and should be viewed by the student as including only some of the theoretic perspectives that may be applicable.

Family Dynamics

Family dynamics are the patterned interpersonal and social interactions that occur within the family structure over the life of a family. Family dynamics models are based on systems theory describing a phenomenon in terms of a set of interrelated parts, in which the change of one part affects the total functioning of the system. A system can be "open" and interacting in the environment or "closed," completely self-contained, and not influenced by the environment. The family is viewed organizationally as an open system in which one member's actions influence the functioning of the total system. Most of the theoretic explanations have emerged from treatment case studies, rather than from systematic development of theory based on generalizable research. Consequently, the limitation of available research should be considered when these models are used to understand family interactions and plan patient care (see Chapter 15).

Applicability of Family Theories to PMH Nursing

Family theories are especially useful to nurses who are assessing family dynamics and planning interventions (Wright & Leahey, 2013). Family systems models are used to help nurses form collaborative relationships with patients and families dealing with health problems. While only nurses with specialized training in family therapy will be engaged in it, understanding family dynamics is important in every nurse's practice, and family theories must inform nurses' family interventions (see Chapter 15). The mental health problems or mental illness of a family member will have important implications for the entire family system.

Role Theories

A **role** describes an individual's social position and function within an environment. Anthropologic theories explain members' roles that relate to a specific society. For example, the universal role of healer may be assumed by a nurse in one culture and a spiritual leader in another. Societal expectations, social status, and rights are attached to these roles. Psychological theories, which are concerned about roles from a different perspective, focus on the individual and the self. The responsibilities of a parent are often in conflict with the personal needs for time alone. All of the Neo-Freudian and humanist models that have been discussed focus on reciprocal social relationships or interactions that determine how the mind develops.

Applicability of Role Theories to PMH Nursing

Role theories emphasize the importance of social inter-action in either the individual's choice of a particu-lar role or society's recognition of it. Several nursing models have role as a major concept, including King (1971), Roy (1974), and Peplau (1952). PMH nursing uses role concepts in understanding group interaction and the role of the patient in the family and community (see Chapters 14 and 15). In addition, milieu therapy approaches discussed in later chapters are based on the patient's assumption of a role within the psychiatric care environment.

Sociocultural Perspectives

Gender and culture are now recognized as significant in determining human behaviour, including the manifesta-tion of mental health problems and illness, as well as in shaping our understanding of health and disease. Critical and emancipatory scholarship is furthering our under-standing of the way power differences can stigmatize and marginalize minority groups and can take institutional-ized form. Canadian society is addressing these issues in our national mental health strategy that stresses the importance of health care services that are gender and culturally sensitive (see Chapter 3).

Gender

There is no foundational figure in the application of feminist approaches to psychotherapy, but rather many scholars who used feminist theory to inform and advance practice (Truscott, 2010).

From Horney's (1932) *Feminine Psychology* to Chesler's (1972) *Women and Madness* to Brown's (2010) *Feminist Therapy*, feminist therapists have been challeng-ing societal, political, and medical conventions that frame gender in oppressive and discriminatory ways. They have reintroduced validity to concepts such as emotions and embodied knowledge that were previously deemed irra-tional and thus dysfunctional. Throughout the develop-ment of feminist approaches to therapy, a constant has been that the constructs of gender, power, and powerless-ness inform the therapy process; feminist therapy is not just for women (Brown, 2010).

Since the 1970s, gender identity and sexual orien-tation studies have been bringing together scholarship from areas such as biology, psychology, sociology, sci-ence, philosophy, political science, and ethics to further understanding and knowledge of lesbian, gay, bisexual, transgender, and intersex identities. Such knowledge is important for health professionals.

Culture

Likewise, postcolonial theories and Marxist approaches have been introduced and call on nurses to attend to the ways that the various notions of race and class function in our understanding of psychiatric illness and mental health, respectively. "The social and moral mandate of nursing is now seen to include illumination of the experiences of those marginalized within society and within health care" (Kirkham & Anderson, 2002, p. 2).

Madeleine Leininger: Transcultural Health Care

Concern about the impact of culture on the treatment of children with psychiatric and emotional problems led Madeleine Leininger, a nurse anthropologist, to develop a new field called transcultural nursing, which is directed toward holistic, congruent, and beneficent care. She used concepts from anthropology and nurs-ing (from such theorists as Henderson (1966), Rogers (1970), and Watson (1979)) to depict universal and diverse dimensions of human caring. Because caring is an integral part of being human, as well as a learned behaviour, caring is culturally based (Leininger, 1991, 1999). Care is considered the essence of nursing, and caring manifestations include compassion, presence, and enabling (Leininger, 1993). Leininger developed a model to depict her theory symbolically. The model depicts the "world view, religion, kinship, cultural val-ues, economics, technology, language, ethnohistory, and environmental factors that are predicted to explain and influence culture care" (p. 27).

Applicability of Sociocultural Theories to PMH Nursing

Sociocultural theories are important to PMH nursing practice as the sociocultural aspect is integral to men-tal health. Adequate nursing assessments and interven-tions are not possible without consideration of the role of the individual within the family and within soci-ety and the significance of familial and cultural norms. Understanding cultural values are crucial to meaningful interactions with persons, families, and communities. Health care systems have their own cultures, as well, and it is necessary for nurses to ensure that the care environ-ment is safe and conducive to healing and recovery (see Chapter 11). Sociocultural theories inform many group interventions (see Chapter 14).

■■ SPIRITUAL THEORIES
Frankl's Logotherapy

Viktor Frankl was an Austrian psychiatrist who survived being a prisoner in Nazi concentration camps during World War II. In his book *Man's Search for Meaning*, he describes the way he discovered the importance of meaning to human existence (Frankl, 1992). Frankl wrote that each of us needs to find a reason to live. Life, otherwise, can seem empty. An existentialist therapy, logotherapy is focused on helping a person find meaning in life. Based on his experience, Frankl concluded that love was the greatest salvation. Even when one's only option is to endure suffering, contemplation of a beloved enables suffering to be endured in an honourable way (Frankl, 1992).

Yalom's Existential Psychotherapy

Influenced by Frankl's work, Irving Yalom grounds his existential psychotherapy upon what he considers central or ultimate life concerns: death, freedom, isolation, and meaninglessness. As each person attempts to confront these concerns, conflicts may arise. In his theory, Yalom (1980) describes how life concerns play a role in psychopathology and psychotherapy. For instance, "fear of death plays a major role in our internal experience; it haunts as does nothing else" (p. 27). A childhood developmental task is to deal with this fear. Often, however, we use denial to keep awareness of death at bay. Ineffective modes of facing our mortality can result in psychopathology; psychotherapy, therefore, may need to be aimed at death awareness. Yalom does not claim the existential orientation is *the* paradigm from which to understand all behaviour: the human being is too complex for this to be possible. However, existential psychotherapy is a useful, systematic approach for addressing many people's clinical situation or symptoms.

Applicability of Spiritual Theories to PMH Nursing

As well as directly influencing nurse theorists such as Travelbee, these theoretic perspectives allow nurses to explore the way the search for meaning in life and death shapes human development, experience, and understanding.

■ RECOVERY AS A FRAMEWORK FOR MENTAL HEALTH CARE

In the Canadian Senate report *Out of the Shadows at Last: Transforming Mental Health, Mental Illness and Addiction Services in Canada*, **recovery** is placed at the centre of mental health reform. It is acknowledged that recovery is an active process rather than an end point and that each individual's path to recovery is unique (Kirby & Keon, 2006, p. 5). When the framework for such a transformation of the health care system was presented (Mental Health Commission of Canada, 2009), recovery was conceived of as broader than *clinical* recovery (remission or cure). While persons with mental illness do experience clinical recovery, recovery is better understood as living a satisfying and hopeful life, even with mental health problems or illness.

Recovery

In taking a recovery orientation, many health professionals may need to significantly shift their medically centred approach to mental health care. They will need to actively engage persons with mental illness and their families in such a way that strengths, resources, and rights are acknowledged; practice in culturally safe and competent ways that respond meaningfully to diversity; address complex mental health needs in the least restrictive ways possible; and broaden the types of evidence they use to evaluate individual improvements in health and well-being. Nurses will need to assess, and perhaps adapt, their current theoretical perspectives in regard to the centrality of recovery.

> **KEY CONCEPT Recovery** is "a process in which people living with mental health problems and illnesses are empowered and supported to be actively engaged in their own journey of well-being. The recovery process builds on individual, family, cultural, and community strengths and enables people to enjoy a meaningful life in their community while striving to achieve their full potential" (Mental Health Commission of Canada, 2009; p. 122).

■ THEORIES AS MAPS

The study of theories, especially nursing theories, can be experienced as an oppressive task by students unless the meaningful link between theory and practice is made evident (Georges, 2005). If it is recognized that our theories are maps that orientate us to our care environments and guide our practice, their relevance becomes apparent. Like a map, a theory is an attempt to represent the real world and is only as useful as its correspondence to the terrain to be travelled. Just as maps need to be redrawn when the landscape changes, theories need to change with our knowledge of the human condition and the world.

SUMMARY OF KEY POINTS

■ Nursing theories form the conceptual basis for nursing practice and are useful in a variety of PMH settings.

■ The Tidal model and its focus on the person's experience and on recovery are increasingly used as an approach to care in PMH settings.

■ The traditional psychodynamic framework helped form the basis of early nursing interpersonal interventions, including the development of therapeutic relationships and the use of such concepts as transference, countertransference, empathy, and object relations.

■ The cognitive and behavioural theories are often used in strategies that help patients change behaviour and thinking.

■ Sociocultural theories remain important in understanding and interacting with patients as members of families, cultures, and society.

■ Spiritual theories offer a way to consider the human search for meaning in life and how a patient's view of life can affect his or her health and well-being.

■ The recovery orientation recommended by Canada's mental health strategy will mean significant changes in psychiatric care environments and in the practice of many health professionals.

CRITICAL THINKING CHALLENGES

1 Compare and contrast the basic ideas of the nursing theorists.

2 Discuss the similarities and differences between Freud's ideas and the Neo-Freudians, including Jung, Adler, and Horney.

3 Compare and contrast the basic ideas of psychodynamic and behavioural theories.

4 Compare and differentiate classical conditioning from operant conditioning.

5 Define the following terms and discuss their applicability to PMH nursing: *classical conditioning, operant conditioning, positive reinforcement,* and *negative reinforcement.*

6 List the major developmental theorists and their main ideas.

7 Discuss the way in which cognitive therapy approaches can be used in PMH nursing practice.

8 How might a nurse's own death awareness affect his or her ability to help patients deal with a fear of death?

9 Reflect upon your personal experience of gender. Did your family have particular expectations of you based on your gender? Do gender stereotypes influence your identity as a nurse?

REFERENCES

Ackerman, S., Zuroff, D. C., & Moskowitz, D. S. (2000). Generativity in midlife and young adults: Links to agency, communion, and subjective well-being. *International Journal of Aging and Human Development, 5*(1), 17–41.

Adler, A. (1963). *The practice and theory of individual psychotherapy.* Paterson, NJ: Littlefield, Adams.

Allen, M. (1977). Comparative theories of the expanded role in nursing and its implications for nursing practice: A working paper. *Nursing Papers/ Perspectives en Nursing, 9,* 38–45.

Austin, W., Gallop, R., Harris, D., & Spencer, E. (1996). A domains of practice approach to the standards of psychiatric and mental health nursing practice. *Journal of Psychiatric and Mental Health Nursing, 3,* 111–115.

Baldursdottir, G. & Jonsdottir, H. (2002). The importance of nurse caring behaviours as perceived by patients receiving care at an emergency department. *Heart & Lung, 31*(1), 67–75.

Bandura, A. (1977). *Social learning theory.* Englewood Cliffs, NJ: Prentice-Hall.

Bandura, A. (1997). *Self-efficacy: The exercise of control.* New York: W. H. Freeman and Company.

Barker, P. (2001a). The Tidal Model: The lived-experience in person-centred mental health nursing care. *Nursing Philosophy, 2,* 213–223.

Barker, P. (2001b). The Tidal Model: Developing a person-centred approach to psychiatric and mental health nursing. *Perspectives in Psychiatric Care, 37,* 79–87.

Barker, P. & Buchanan-Barker, P. (2005). *The Tidal Model: A guide for mental health professionals.* London, UK: Brunner-Routledge.

Barker, P. & Buchanan-Barker, P. (2010). The Tidal Model of mental health recovery and reclamation: Application in acute care settings. *Issues in Mental Health Nursing, 31,* 171–180.

Barnhart, D. A., Bennett, P. M., Porter, B. D., & Sloan, R. S. (1994). Jean Watson: Philosophy and science of caring. In A. Marriner-Tomey (Ed.), *Nursing theorists and their work* (3rd ed., pp. 148–162). St. Louis, MO: Mosby.

Beck, J. (2011). *Cognitive behavior therapy: Basics and beyond.* New York: Guilford Press.

Beck, A. T., Thase, M. D., & Wright, J. H. (2003). Cognitive therapy. In R. E. Hales & S. C. Ydofsky (Eds.), *Textbook of clinical psychiatry* (4th ed., pp. 1245–1283). Washington, DC: American Psychiatric Publishers, Inc.

Benner, P. & Wrubel, J. (1989). *The primacy of caring: Stress and coping in health and illness.* Menlo Park, CA: Addison-Wesley.

Biggs, A. (2008). Orem's self-care deficit nursing theory: Update on the state of the art and science. *Nursing Science Quarterly, 21*(3), 200–206.

Brookes, N., Murata, L., & Tansey, M. (2008). Tidal waves: Implementing a new model of mental health recovery and reclamation. *Canadian Nurse, 104*(8), 23–27.

Brown, L. (2010). *Feminist therapy.* Washington, DC: American Psychiatric Association.

Buchanan-Barker, P. & Barker, P. (2008). The Tidal Commitments: Extending the value base of mental health recovery. *Journal of Psychiatric and Mental Health Nursing, 15,* 93–100.

Calaway, B. J. (2002). *Hildegard Peplau: Psychiatric nurse of the century.* New York: Springer.

Chesler, P. (1972). *Women and madness.* Garden City, NY: Doubleday.

Christiansen, S. L. & Palkovitz, R. (1998). Exploring Erikson's psychosocial theory and development: Generativity and its relationship to paternal identity, intimacy, and involvement in childcare. *Journal of Men's Studies, 7*(1), 133–156.

Clements, P. & Averill, J. (2006). Finding patterns of knowing in the work of Florence Nightingale. *Nursing Outlook, 54,* 268–274.

DeHowitt, M. (1992). King's conceptual model and individual psychotherapy. *Perspectives in Psychiatric Care, 28*(4), 11–14.

DeWan, S. A. & Ume-Nwagbo, P. N. (2006). Using the Neuman systems model for best practices. *Nursing Science Quarterly, 19*(1), 31–35.

Ellenberger, H. (1970). *The discovery of the unconscious: The history and evolution of dynamic psychiatry.* London, UK: Lane, Penguin Press.

Ellis, A. (1973). *Humanistic psychotherapy: The rational-emotive approach.* New York: McGraw-Hill.

Erikson, E. (1963). *Childhood and society* (2nd ed.). New York: Norton.

Erikson, E. (1968). *Identity: Youth and crisis.* New York: Norton.

Erikson, E. & Erikson, J. (1997). *The lifecycle completed, extended version.* New York: Norton.

Feeley, N. & Gottlieb, L. (2000). Nursing approaches for working with family strengths and resources. *Journal of Family Nursing, 6*(1), 9–24.

Frankl, V. (1992). *Man's search for meaning: An introduction to logotherapy* (4th ed.). Boston, MA: Beacon Press.

Freud, S. (1905). Three essays on the theory of sexuality (1953). In J. Strachey, A. Strachey, & A. Tyson (Eds.). *The standard edition of the complete psychological works of Sigmund Freud* (pp. 135–248). London, UK: Hogarth Press.

Freud, S. (1927). The ego and the id (1957). In E. Jones (Ed.). *The international psycho-analytical library* (No. 12). London, UK: Hogarth Press.

Freud, S. (1949). *An outline of psychoanalysis.* New York: Norton.

Freud, S. (1955). *The interpretation of dreams.* London, UK: Hogarth Press.

Georges, J. (2005). Linking nursing theory and practice: A critical-feminist approach. *Advances in Nursing Science, 28*(1), 30–57.

Gilligan, C. (1982). *In a different voice: Psychological theory and women's development.* Cambridge, MA: Harvard University Press.

Gottlieb, L. & Rowat, K. (1987). The McGill model of nursing: A practice-derived model. *Advances in Nursing Science, 9*(4), 51–61.

Graham, R. (2012). Carol Gilligan's persistent "voice": Thirty years after the feminist classic "In a Different Voice" shook up psychology, do its claims hold up at all? In *The Boston Globe.* Retrieved from http://www.bostonglobe.com/

Henderson, V. (1966). *The nature of nursing: A definition and its implications for practice, research, and education.* New York: Macmillan.

Hoffman, E. (Ed.). (1996). *Future visions: The unpublished papers of Abraham Maslow.* Newbury Park, CA: Sage Publications, Inc.

Horney, K. (1932). *Feminine psychology.* New York: Norton.

Horney, K. (1939). *New ways in psychoanalysis.* New York: Norton.

Horney, K. (1950). *Neurosis and human growth.* New York: Norton.

Jung, C. G. (1959). *The basic writings of C. G. Jung.* New York: Modern Library.

Jung, C. G. (1966). On the psychology of the unconscious: The personal and the collective unconscious. In C. Jung (Ed.), *Collected works of C. G. Jung* (2nd ed., *Vol.* 7, pp. 64–79). Princeton, NJ: Princeton University Press.

King, I. M. (1971). *Toward a theory for nursing: General concepts of human behavior.* New York: John Wiley and Sons.

King, I. M. (1981). *A theory for nursing: Systems, concepts, process.* New York: John Wiley and Sons.

King, I. M. (1992). King's theory of goal attainment. *Nursing Science Quarterly, 5*(1), 19–26.

Kirby, M. J. L. & Keon, W. J. (2006). *Out of the shadows at last: Transforming mental health, mental illness and addiction services in Canada.* Retrieved from Parliament of Canada website: http://www.parl.gc.ca/39/1/parlbus/commbus/senate/com-e/soci-e/rep-e/rep02may06-e.htm

Kirkham, S. R. & Anderson, J. M. (2002). Postcolonial nursing scholarship: From epistemology to method. *Advances in Nursing Science, 25*(1), 1–17.

Knowaja, K. (2006). Utilization of King's interacting systems framework and theory of goal attainment with new multidisciplinary model: Clinical pathway. *Australian Journal of Advanced Nursing, 24*(2), 44–49.

Laben, J., Dodd, D., & Snead, L. (1991). King's theory of goal attainment applied in group therapy for inpatient juvenile sexual offenders, maximum security state offenders, and community parolees, using visual aids. *Issues in Mental Health Nursing, 12*(1), 51–64.

Leddy, S. & Pepper, J. M. (1998). *Conceptual basis of professional nursing* (4th ed.). Philadelphia, PA: Lippincott.

Lego, S. (1973). Nurse psychotherapists: How are we different? *Perspectives in Psychiatric Care, 11,* 144–147.

Leininger, M. (1991). *Culture care diversity and universality: A theory of nursing.* New York: National League for Nursing.

Leininger, M. (1993). Assumptive premises of the theory. In C. Reynolds & M. Leininger (Eds.), *Madeleine Leininger: Cultural care diversity and universality theory. Notes on nursing theories* (Vol. 8, pp. 15–30). Newbury Park, CA: Sage Publications, Inc.

Leininger, M. (1999). What is transcultural nursing and culturally competent care? *Journal of Transcultural Nursing, 10*(1), 9.

Lutjens, L. R. (1991a). *Callista Roy: An adaptation model.* Newbury Park, CA: Sage Publications, Inc.

Lutjens, L. R. (1991b). *Martha Rogers: The science of unitary human beings.* Newbury Park, CA: Sage Publications, Inc.

Maslow, A. (1970). *Motivation and personality* (rev. ed.). New York: Harper & Brothers.

Maslow, A. (1998). *Toward a psychology of being* (3rd ed.). New York: John Wiley & Sons.

Mental Health Commission of Canada. (2009). *Toward recovery and well-being: A framework for a mental health strategy for Canada.* Ottawa, ON: Author.

Moore, B. & Fine, B. (Eds.). (1990). *Psychoanalytic terms and concepts.* New Haven, CT: American Psychoanalytic Association and Yale University Press.

Nelson, M. (1996). Separation versus connection, the gender controversy: Implications for counseling women. *Journal of Counseling and Development, 74*(4), 339–344.

Neuman, B. (1989). *The Neuman systems model* (2nd ed.). East Norwalk, CT: Appleton & Lange.

Neuman, B., Newman, D. M. L., & Holder, P. (2000). Leadership and scholarship integration: Using the Neuman system model for 21st-century professional nursing practice. *Nursing Science Quarterly, 13*(1), 60–63.

Nightingale, F. (1859). *Notes on nursing: What it is and what it is not.* London, UK: Harrison, Bookseller to the Queen.

Ochse, R. & Plug, C. (1986). Cross-cultural investigation of the validity of Erikson's theory of personality development. *Journal of Personality and Social Psychology, 50*(6), 1240–1252.

Olson, J. & Hanchett, E. (1997). Nurse-expressed empathy, patient outcomes, and the development of a middle-range theory. *Image: The Journal of Nursing Scholarship, 29*(1), 71–76.

Orem, D. (1991). *Nursing concepts of practice* (4th ed.). St. Louis, MO: Mosby–Year Book.

Orlando, I. J. (1961). *The dynamic nurse–patient relationship.* New York: G. P. Putnam's Sons.

Orlando, I. J. (1972). *The discipline and teaching of nursing process.* New York: G. P. Putnam's Sons.

Orlofsky, J., Marcia, J., & Lesser, I. (1973). Ego identity status and the intimacy versus isolation crisis of young adulthood. *Journal of Personality and Social Psychology, 27*(2), 211–219.

Parse, R. R. (1987). *Nursing science: Major paradigms, theories, and critiques.* Philadelphia, PA: Saunders.

Parse, R. R. (2007). The humanbecoming school of thought in 2050. *Nursing Science Quarterly, 20,* 308–311.

Partlak Günüşen, N., Üstün, B., & Gigliotti, E. (2009). Conceptualization of burnout from the perspective of the Neuman systems model. *Nursing Science Quarterly, 22*(3), 200–204.

Pavlov, I. P. (1927/1960). *Conditioned reflexes.* New York: Dover Publications.

Peplau, H. (1952). *Interpersonal relations in nursing.* New York: G. P. Putnam & Sons.

Peplau, H. (1992). Interpersonal relations: A theoretical framework for application in nursing practice. *Nursing Science Quarterly, 5*(1), 13–18.

Perls, F. (1969). *In and out of the garbage pail.* Lafayette, CA: Real People Press.

Piaget, J. (1936). *Origins of intelligence in the child.* London, UK: Routledge & Kegan Paul.

Piaget, J. (1957). *Construction of reality in the child.* London, UK: Kegan Paul.

Potter, M. L. & Bockenhauer, B. J. (2000). Implementing Orlando's nursing theory. *Journal of Psychosocial Nursing and Mental Health Services, 3813,* 14–21.

Pratt, M., Norris, J., Cressman, K. Lawford, H., & Hebblethwaite, S. (2008). Parents' stories of grandparenting concerns in the three-generational family: Generativity, optimism, and forgiveness. *Journal of Personality, 76*(3), 581–604.

Rogers, M. E. (1970). *An introduction to the theoretical basis of nursing.* Philadelphia, PA: F.A. Davis.

Rogers, C. (1980). *A way of being.* Boston, MA: Houghton Mifflin.

Rogers, M. E. (1994). The science of unitary human beings: Current perspectives. *Nursing Science Quarterly, 7*(1), 33–35.

Roy, C. (1974). The Roy adaptation model. In J. P. Riehl & C. Roy, (Eds.), *Conceptual models for nursing practice* (pp. 135–144). New York: Appleton-Century-Crofts.

Seed, M. & Torkelson, D. (2012). Beginning the recovery journey in acute psychiatric care: Using concepts from Orem's self-care deficit nursing theory. *Issues in Mental Health Nursing, 33,* 394–398.

Skinner, B. F. (1935). The generic nature of the concepts of stimulus and response. *Journal of General Psychology, 12,* 40–65.

Skinner, B. F. (1976). *Walden II.* New York: Macmillan.

Thompson, J. E. (1990). Finding the borderline's border: Can Martha Rogers help? *Perspectives in Psychiatric Care, 26*(4), 7–10.

Thorndike, E. L. (1916, c.1906). *The principles of teaching, based on psychology.* New York: A. G. Seiler.

Travelbee, J. (1969). *Intervention in psychiatric nursing: Process in the one-to-one relationship.* Philadelphia, PA: F.A. Davis.

Travelbee, J. (1971). *Interpersonal aspects of nursing* (2nd ed.). Philadelphia, PA: F.A. Davis.

Truscott, D. (2010). *Becoming an effective psychotherapist: Adopting a theory of psychotherapy that is right for you and your client.* Washington, DC: American Psychological Association.

Watson, J. (1979). *Nursing: The philosophy and science of caring* (2nd ed.). Boston, MA: Little, Brown.

Watson, J. (1988). *Nursing: Human science and human care: A theory of nursing.* New York: National League for Nursing.

Watson, J. (2005). *Caring science as sacred science.* Philadelphia, PA: F.A. Davis.

Watson, J. B. & Rayner, R. (1917). Emotional reactions and psychological experimentation. *American Journal of Psychology, 28,* 163–174.

Westermeyer, J. (2004). Predictors and characteristics of Erikson's Life Cycle Model among men: A 32-year longitudinal study. *International Journal of Aging and Human Development, 58*(1), 29–48.

Wright, L. & Leahey, M. (2013). *Nurses and families: A guide to family assessment and intervention* (6th ed.). Philadelphia, PA: F.A. Davis.

Yalom, I. D. (1980). *Existential psychotherapy.* New York: Basic Books.

9

Biologic Basis of Practice

Anne Marie Creamer

Adapted from the chapter "The Biologic Foundations of Psychiatric Nursing" by Susan McCabe and Mary Ann Boyd

KEY CONCEPTS

- neurotransmitters
- plasticity

LEARNING OBJECTIVES

After studying this chapter, you will be able to:

- Describe the association between biologic functioning and symptoms of psychiatric disorders.
- Describe the approaches researchers have used to study the central nervous system and the significance of each approach.
- Locate the brain structures primarily involved in psychiatric disorders and describe the primary functions of these structures.
- Assess symptoms of common psychiatric disorders in terms of central nervous system functioning.
- Describe the mechanisms of neuronal transmission.
- Identify the location and function of neurotransmitters significant to hypotheses regarding major mental disorders.
- Discuss the basic utilization of new knowledge gained from fields of study, including psychoendocrinology, psychoimmunology, and chronobiology.
- Discuss the role of genetics in the development of psychiatric disorders.

KEY TERMS

- amino acids • animal models • autonomic nervous system • basal ganglia • biogenic amines • biologic markers • chronobiology • circadian cycle • cortex • epigenetics • frontal, parietal, temporal, and occipital lobes • genome • hippocampus • limbic system • neurohormones • neuropeptides • polymorphism • psychoendocrinology • psychoneuroimmunology • receptors • risk factors • symptom expression • synapse • zeitgebers

All behaviours recognized as human result from actions that originate in the brain and its dense interconnection of neural networks. Modern research has increased understanding of how the complex circuitry of the brain interacts with the external environment, memories, and experiences. Through the spinal column and peripheral nerves, along with other systems, such as the endocrine and immune systems, the brain constantly receives and processes information. As the brain shifts and sorts through the amazing amount of information it processes every hour, it decides on actions and initiates behaviours that allow each person to act in entirely unique and very human ways.

FOUNDATIONAL CONCEPTS

This chapter is a review of the basic information necessary for understanding neuroscience as it relates to the role of the psychiatric and mental health (PMH) nurse. The review includes basic central nervous system (CNS) structures and functions, basic mechanisms of neuro-transmission, general functions of the major neurotrans-mitters, basic structure and function of the endocrine system, genetic research, circadian rhythms, neuroim-aging techniques, and biologic tests. This chapter was written with the assumption that the reader has a basic knowledge of human biology, anatomy, and pathophysi-ology. The chapter is not intended as a full presentation of neuroanatomy and physiology but rather as an over-view of the structures and functions most critical to the role of the PMH nurse.

The Biologic Basis of Behaviour, Emotions, and Cognition

As our understanding of the brain grows, evidence accumu-lates that most human behaviours, thoughts, and emotions have a biologic basis. Whether it is responding angrily to someone, impulsively making a purchase, or struggling to make a decision, behaviours are in large part rooted in the neurocircuitry of the brain. So when common psychiatric symptoms manifest as abnormal behaviours (e.g., seeing things that are not there, attempting suicide, talking in odd or unusual ways), we look to the brain. **Symptom expres-sion** is a term referring to the behavioural symptoms seen in mental illness and the link to the neurobiologic basis of the symptom. Because symptoms of psychiatric illness are expressed mainly as behavioural disturbance and because behavioural symptoms are linked to anomalies in brain functioning, PMH nurses need to understand disease symptoms in relation to brain function.

Just as a breathing problem is often a symptom of a respiratory disorder, psychiatric symptoms are often indicators of CNS problems. Understanding this funda-mental concept makes it much easier to understand the scientific rationale for many of the nursing care and treat-ment decisions presented in this book.

As you read this chapter, think about what you know about the symptoms of mental illness. PMH nurses must be able to make the connection among (1) patients' psy-chiatric symptoms, (2) the probable alterations in brain functioning linked to those symptoms, and (3) the ratio-nale for treatment and care practices. Knowledge of the CNS is an inescapable aspect of modern PMH nursing.

Genetics

It has been noted for decades that family members of individuals who have one of the major mental disorders, such as schizophrenia, bipolar disorder, or panic disor-der, have an increased risk for the same disorder. In fact, the 1823 archives of London's Bethlehem Royal Hospital (Bedlam) noted that physicians needed to identify whether there was a hereditary component to the person's illness (McGuffin & Southwick, 2003). **Animal models** have greatly increased the ability of researchers to understand the influence of genetics on symptom expression in psy-chiatric disorders, and many of the common psychiatric

IN A LIFE
Sidney Crosby and a Life-Changing Concussion
Public Persona
Called "the best player in the world," Sidney Crosby has played in the National Hockey League since he was 18 years old. In January 2011, while playing for the Pittsburgh Penguins, he was struck on the head during a game. Later he described feeling "off, headaches, a little sick." Shortly after this, he was sidelined for the rest of the season because of a concussion. At the time of the injury, he was leading the NHL in scoring.

Realities
Concussions are common sports injuries, but they are not evident on x-rays, magnetic resonance imagings (MRIs), or computed tomography (CT) scans. They occur when the person is hit on the head or face or through a whiplash injury. When this happens, the brain strikes the inside of the skull and is bruised where it hits the skull and on the opposite side where it bounces back. As a result, the person may suffer physi-cal, cognitive, or emotional symptoms after the injury. In some cases, the symptoms can last for years. In 2010–2011, there were 2,766 hospitaliza-tions in Canada for concussion-related injuries (Morrish & Carey, 2013). June has been declared Brain Injury Awareness Month in Canada. Sidney Crosby, after missing two years of play, is back in the game.

Sources: Graves, W. (2013, January 15). "Sidney Crosby says he's free of concussion symptoms." Associated Press.

Morrish, J. & Carey, S. (2013). Concussions in Canada. *Canada Injury Compass, Spring 2013*. Toronto, Canada: Parachute.

Wyshynski, G. (2011). Sidney Crosby talks concussion, "irresponsible" blindside hits and when Penguins knew about injury. Retrieved from http://ca.sports.yahoo.com/nhl/blog/puck_daddy/post/Sidney-Crosby-talks-concussion-irresponsible-?urn=nhl-305051

disorders that nurses encounter have a known genetic component. As genetic knowledge increases, treat-ments that work at the genetic level are being developed (Pearson-Fuhrhop, Burke, & Cramer, 2012).

Genetic *processes* control how humans develop from a single-cell egg into an adult human. Genes control the regrowth of hair and skin cells, the growth and connection of nervous system cells, and our biologic reaction to stress, among other processes. Genes make humans dynamic organisms, capable of growth, change, and develop-ment. The Human Genome Project, completed in 2003, mapped the complete set of human genes, or **genome**, carried by all of us and transmitted to our offspring. There are about 30,000 genes in the human genome, with the brain accounting for only about 1% of the body's DNA. The completed human genome provided researchers with a map of the exact sequence of the 3 billion nucleotide bases that make up human organisms. If printed out, the entire human genome sequence would fill one thousand 1,000-page telephone books. Now that it is completed, the genome map is used to study the function of specific genes and their disease-inducing capacity when they mal-function. One of the things to come from the Human Genome Project is a catalogue of common human genetic variations, called the HapMap.

A gene comprises short segments of DNA and is packed with the "instructions" for making proteins that have a specific function. At a cellular level, the genes themselves do not directly control how the nerves function. Rather the genes control the proteins that regulate neural functioning. It is not an unchangeable state fixed at some point in neuronal development. Individual nerve cells may respond to neurochemical changes outside the cell, producing different proteins for adaptation to the new environment. This dynamic nature of gene function highlights the manner in which the body and the environment interact and how environmental factors influence gene expression. The diathesis–stress model holds that the diathesis (derived from a Greek word for "disposition" or "vulnerability") or biologic risk(s) interacts with environmental stressors and, depending on how successful the compensatory mechanisms work, a mental illness may or may not develop (Stahl, 2008).

When genes are absent or malfunction, protein production is altered, and bodily functions are disrupted. A gene or part of a gene can be altered, and when this change occurs commonly and has an effect on human behaviour, it is called a **polymorphism** (Pearson-Fuhrhop et al., 2012). For example, recent research has demonstrated that approximately 1% of individuals with schizophrenia have 22q11.2 deletion syndrome, a genetic subtype of schizophrenia in which there is a deletion on part of chromosome 22 (Kapadia & Bassett, 2008). This deletion has been linked with a number of abnormalities, including craniofacial and cardiovascular alterations and behavioural and learning problems.

Population Genetics

The study of molecular genetics in psychiatric disorders is quite new. Because the exact genetic bases of psychiatric disorders remain unclear and animal models are hard to produce for some disorders, much of what we know about the genetics of these disorders comes from studies that trace given disorders within groups of people. This technique, called *population genetics*, involves the analysis of genetic transmission of a trait within families and populations to determine risks and patterns of transmission. The risk of a given disorder occurring in the general population can then be compared with the risk within families and between groups of relatives. These studies rely on the initial identification of an individual who has the disorder and include the following principal methods:

- Family studies, which analyze the occurrence of a disorder in first-degree relatives (biologic parents, siblings, and children), second-degree relatives (grandparents, uncles, aunts, nieces, nephews, and grandchildren), and so on.
- Twin studies, which analyze the presence or absence of the disorder in pairs of twins. The *concordance rate* is the measure of similarity of occurrence in individuals with similar genetic makeup.

- Adoption studies, which compare the risk for the illness developing in offspring raised in different environments. The strongest inferences may be drawn from studies that involve children separated from their parents at birth.

Few traits are completely heritable. Colour blindness and blood type are examples of traits that exist because of heredity alone. Monozygotic twins have identical genetic contributions; therefore, both would have colour blindness or the same blood type if they expressed that gene. This is 100% concordance. If a disorder was completely unrelated to genetics, then monozygotic twins would have the same concordance rates as dizygotic (fraternal) twins, who share roughly the same proportion of genes that ordinary siblings do—50%. If there is a genetic contribution with environmental influence, the concordance rates would be less than 100% for monozygotic twins but significantly greater than for dizygotic twins. Such is the case with several psychiatric disorders. Although no conclusive evidence exists for a complete genetic cause of most psychiatric disorders, significant evidence suggests that strong genetic contributions exist for most (Brzustowicz & Freedman, 2011). It is likely that psychiatric disorders are *polygenic*. This means that more than one gene is involved in producing a psychiatric disorder and that the disorder develops from genes interacting, which produces a risk factor, and environmental influences that lead to the expression of the illness. The environmental factors may include stress, infections, poor nutrition, catastrophic loss, complications during pregnancy, and exposure to toxins. Thus, genetic compositions convey vulnerability, or a risk for the illness, but the right set of environmental factors must be present for the disease to develop in the at-risk individual. Additionally, specific genes may convey risk for more than one disorder (Eapen, 2012).

Using the human genome map and databases containing human samples of DNA sequences, markers for genetic variations associated with particular illnesses can be identified. Research studies using these tools are called genome-wide association studies. For example, APOE 4, a genetic polymorphism, is found in approximately 15% of the population and is linked to increased risk for atherosclerosis and Alzheimer's disease. The next step in making this research applicable is to find out whether one treatment works better in those with different genetic profiles. However, these studies remain controversial, and it is important to keep in mind that mental illnesses are not determined by one polymorphism but rather by a complex interaction between the environment and multiple genes.

When considering information regarding risks for genetic transmission of psychiatric disorders, it is important to remember several key points:

- Psychiatric disorders have been described and labelled quite differently across generations, and errors in diagnosis may occur.

- Similar psychiatric symptoms may have considerably different causes, just as symptoms such as chest pain may occur in relation to many different causes.
- Genes that are present may not always cause the appearance of the trait.
- One gene alteration may cause different symptoms in different people.
- Several genes work together in an individual to produce a given trait or disorder.
- A biologic cause is not necessarily only genetic in origin. Environmental influences alter the body's functioning and often mediate or worsen genetic **risk factors**.

As public awareness of genetic evidence grows, it is likely that a PMH nurse will be faced with patients or family members requesting genetic testing or needing information regarding their likelihood of risk for a psychiatric disorder. As a result, PMH nurses increasingly will need greater understanding of the role genetics play in mental illness.

Epigenetics

Epigenetics (*epi* meaning "above") is the study of the mechanisms by which genetic inheritance is modified without any change in an organism's genetic (DNA) sequence. It is not a new field—the term was coined in 1942 by Conrad Waddington (1957)—but 21st-century science has been making significant advances in this area, indicating that in the ancient nature-versus-nurture debate, it is not "either/or" but about interaction. Stem cell and other research are revealing that cell development is highly flexible and plastic (Shah & Allegrucci, 2013).

It has been known for some time that all cells in an individual organism have the identical genetic makeup (genotype) but can function in radically different ways (i.e., as a heart cell, a skin cell, a brain cell, etc.). As influences (environmental, lifestyle) on the genotype occur prenatally and across the life span, cell genes are distinctively expressed (phenotype) (Marques & Fleming Outeiro, 2013). An individual's *epigenome* is made up of chemicals that change or mark his or her genome (complete set of DNA) in a way that directs genetic expression (how gene information is used) (National Human Genome Research Institute, 2013). Epigenetic phenomena are related to chromatin structure and organization, chromatin being the protein–DNA complex that makes up the nucleus of a cell. The epigenome marks (turns on or off) the genome directly through DNA methylation and indirectly through histone modification; gene expression can also be silenced by RNA, a nucleic acid (Simmons, 2008).

Epigenetic changes are necessary to development and health, but some may trigger disease (National Institute on Aging, 2011). It was in 1983 that evidence of a link between epigenetic changes and disease was first noted: persons with colorectal cancer were found to have less DNA methylation in their diseased tissue than in their normal tissue (Simmons, 2008).

Epigenetics is a key research area in the quest to understand health, aging, and disease (Kundu, 2013). Scientists are, for example, using blood routinely taken from the heels of newborns and stored indefinitely by health care systems as a means to explore the way DNA methylation patterns changes in a person from birth to 3 years of age (Marx, 2012). A genome-wide association study involved researchers looking for variants in the genome among individuals with a particular health concern or trait and working to identify genes directly associated with aging (National Institute on Aging, 2011). An example of such research relevant to psychiatry and mental health is a study by Gräff et al. (2012) who found that cognitive capacities related to neurodegeneration in the brain were affected by a particular epigenetic change that may be reversible. A further example is a study by Labonté et al. (2013) in which it was discovered that there were DNA methylation changes in the hippocampal DNA of persons who had completed suicide. It is possible to imagine that some time in the future, genome sequencing might become routine in patient diagnosis, accompanied by an "epigenetic readout" (Marx, 2012, p. 147). One can imagine, as well, the ethical issues that will arise with such "routine."

Risk Factors

The concept of genetic susceptibility suggests that an individual may be at increased risk for a psychiatric disorder. Research into *risk factors* is an important avenue of study. Just as knowledge of risk factors for diabetes and heart disease led to the development of preventive interventions, learning more about risk factors for psychiatric disorders will lead to preventive care practices. Specific risk factors for psychiatric disorders are just beginning to be understood, and some of the environmental influences listed previously may be examples of risk factors. These events, circumstances, or demographic features are more likely to occur in individuals who experience a particular psychiatric disorder. In the absence of one specific gene for major psychiatric disorders, risk factor assessment may be a logical alternative for predicting who is more likely to experience psychiatric disorders or certain conditions such as aggression or suicidality. This is a growing area of PMH nursing; nurses are playing an important role in mental health promotion and illness prevention.

CURRENT RESEARCH APPROACHES AND ADVANCES

Neuroscience researchers have applied several approaches to the study of the CNS structure and function. These approaches occur with both human research and animal

Table 9-1	Approaches to the Study of Neuroanatomy	
Approach	**Purpose**	**Potential Limitations**
Comparative	Explores and compares behaviour across animal nervous systems, from a simple primitive cordlike structure in some species to the large complex structure of the human brain	Difficult to correlate animal behaviour to human, especially emotional New brain structures do not necessarily correlate to new behaviour
Developmental	Studies nervous system structure within an individual or species of animal across different stages of development	Impossible to follow one human being's neuronal development Individual variation in development complicates comparisons of individuals across a specific point of time in development
Chemoarchitectural	Identifies differences in location of neurochemicals such as neurotransmitters throughout the brain	Boundaries between regional changes are subtle and may vary across individuals
Cytoarchitectural	Identifies differences or variations in cell type, structure, and density throughout the brain, mapping these variations by location	Boundaries between regional changes are subtle and may vary across individuals
Functional	Identifies location of predominant control over various behavioural functions within the brain Studies often conducted on the basis of dysfunction from a localized injury to the brain	Several regions or structures within the brain may contribute to one behaviour, making predominant control difficult to assign Controversy exists in correlating normal brain function to damaged brain tissue

models. The approaches, highlighted in Table 9-1, include the following:

- Comparative
- Developmental
- Chemoarchitectural
- Cytoarchitectural
- Functional

These different approaches to studying the CNS have significantly increased our understanding of its normal functioning and how a disease affects behaviour and contributes to the development of psychiatric disorders. Research shows that areas of the brain, and the groups of nerve cells that constitute that area, often work together as functional units. A hierarchy of function exists in which primary sensory input is used in an increasingly more complex and integrated manner across areas of the brain. In addition, some areas of the brain, such as those that control basic levels of alertness and attention, must work correctly for information to be received, understood, and used by higher levels of the brain to organize a response. The brain's functional units work together to control or contribute to specific behaviours or emotions.

The *integrated approach* to brain development is the term used to describe the interactive working of brain areas and function. Understanding the work as an integration of parts allows us to understand that specific areas of the brain control specific functions. For example, there is a speech area in the brain, a mood area, an appetite area, and so on. Understanding the functions of areas of the brain allows nurses to assess a patient's symptoms largely as the expression of a problem in a specific brain area. Just as a person with an irregular heartbeat is experiencing disruption in normal cardiac function, a person who fails to eat because of depression is experiencing a disruption in the brain's normal appetite and mood function.

Neuroplasticity is an important concept when describing brain function. The changes in neural environment can come from internal sources such as a change in electrolytes, or from external sources such as exercise, toxins, and viruses. With neuroplasticity, nerve signals may be rerouted, cells may learn new functions, gain sensitivity, the number of cells may increase or decrease, or some nerve tissue may to some extent be regenerated. Neuroplasticity contributes to understanding how function may be restored over time after brain damage occurs or how an individual may react over time to psychotherapy or a continuous pharmacotherapy regimen.

There are several behavioural principles that impact brain plasticity (see Table 9-2). For example, brains are most plastic during infancy and early childhood, when large adaptive learning tasks should normally occur. With age, brains become less plastic, which explains why it is easier to learn a second language at the age of 5 years than at 55 years. Understanding these principles provides a framework for nurses coaching new emotional, cognitive, and behavioural skills.

KEY CONCEPT Plasticity is the ability of the brain to change its structure and function in response to internal and external pressures (Kleim & Jones, 2008).

Table 9-2	Principles of Experience-Derived Brain Plasticity	
Principle	**Example**	
1. Use it or lose it	Brain circuits not used in task performance over time can decay	
2. Use it and improve it	Through extended training, brain plasticity can be induced	
3. Learning something new	Repeating something already learned does not induce plasticity but learning something new will	
4. Repeat, repeat, repeat	Repeating a new or relearned skill may be needed to induce long-term changes	
5. Be intense but not too intense	Training too intensely can worsen things; balance is needed	
6. Brain age matters	Plasticity occurs more easily in a younger brain	
7. Timing matters	Certain types of plasticity change follow a pattern	
8. A little can go a long way	Plasticity in one set of neurons can promote ongoing development in the same or other areas of the brain	
9. Make it important	Motivation and attention are important mediators	
10. Plasticity in one form can block a different plasticity within the same circuit	Developing brain circuits to do one skill may block learning another	

Adapted from Kleim, J. & Jones, T. (2008). Principles of experience-dependent neural plasticity: Implications for rehabilitation after brain damage. *Journal of Speech, Language, and Hearing Research, 51*, S225–S239.

Neuroimaging

Since the 1980s, technologic advances in neuroimaging techniques have been a major aid to the current understanding of how the human brain functions. As knowledge grows, neuroimaging techniques are moving from research to routine clinical use, requiring PMH nurses to understand this technology. Two basic neuroimaging methods are structural and functional neuroimaging. See Table 9-3 for methods of neuroimaging.

Structural Neuroimaging

Structural neuroimaging techniques were the first form of neuroimaging that allowed visualization of brain structures. Structural images show what normal structures of the brain look like and allow clinicians to identify tissue abnormalities, changes, or damages. Commonly used structural neuroimaging techniques include computed tomography (CT) scanning and magnetic resonance imaging (MRI). Although these techniques are useful in identifying what the brain looks like, they do not reveal anything about how the brain works.

Computed Tomography (CT)

CT (also referred to as computed axial tomography or CAT) scanning first allowed scientists and clinicians to see structures inside the brain without more invasive and potentially dangerous methods. CT scans still use an X-ray beam passed through the head in serial slices. High-speed computers measure the decreased strength in the X-ray beam that results from absorption, and the computer assigns a shade of gray that reflects that change. The degree of energy absorbed by a tissue is proportionally related to its density. For example, cerebrospinal fluid (CSF) absorbs the least, so it appears the darkest, whereas bone absorbs the most and appears light. The computer then develops a 3D X-ray image. This technique is good at detecting skull fractures and injuries or abnormalities such as a subdermal hematoma requiring surgery. White matter and gray matter are more difficult to discriminate with CT technology.

CT scans can be done with or without contrast material. Contrast materials are used to increase the visibility of certain tissues or blood vessels. If a contrast agent is used, an iodinated or other material is intravenously administered to enhance the CT image. Although CT scanning is a relatively safe, noninvasive procedure, the contrast material may have some adverse effects in some patients. Some patients receiving contrast materials report a metallic taste in the mouth, and some experience mild nausea, rashes, or joint pain. In rare instances, severe allergic responses, including anaphylaxis, may develop, so nurses must closely monitor patients who have received contrast materials. In addition, because the CT equipment itself may frighten the patient, the nurse should educate the patient about the scan. Some patients may need to be accompanied by a nurse during the procedure for ongoing reassurance. Radiation exposure by a CT scan is approximately 400 times that of a standard chest X-ray (Miglioretti & Simth-Bindman, 2011).

Magnetic Resonance Imaging (MRI)

MRI is performed by placing a patient into a long tube that contains powerful magnets. The magnetic field causes hydrogen-containing molecules (primarily water) to line up and move in symmetric ways around their axes. The magnetic field is then interrupted in pulses, causing the molecules to turn 90 or 180 degrees. Electromagnetic energy is released when the molecules return to their original position. The energy released is related to the density of the tissue and is detected by the MRI device, resulting in a scan measurement of the

Table 9-3   Methods of Neuroimaging

Method	Description	Considerations
Structural Imaging		
Computed tomography (CT), also called computed axial tomography (CAT)	Uses X-ray technology to measure tissue density; is readily available; can be completed quickly, and less costly; may be used for screening, but many disease states are not clearly seen; use of contrast medium improves resolution	Contrast medium may produce allergic reactions; individuals with increased risk for contrast media complications include those with History of previous reactions Cardiac disease Hypertension Diabetes Sickle cell disease Contraindications for use of contrast: Iodine/shellfish allergies Renal disease Pregnancy
Magnetic resonance imaging (MRI)	Uses a magnetic field to magnetize hydrogen atoms in soft tissue, changing their alignment—this creates a tiny electric signal, which can be received to produce an image; produces greater resolution than a CT, diagnosing more subtle pathologic changes	Patients may experience headaches, dizziness, and nausea; symptoms of anxiety, claustrophobia, or psychosis can increase; contraindicated when patients have aneurysm clips, internal electrical, magnetic, or mechanical devices such as pacemakers, metallic surgical clips, sutures, or dental work, which distort the image; claustrophobia
Functional Neuroimaging		
Positron emission tomography (PET)	Uses positron emitting isotopes (very short-lived radioactive entities such as oxygen-15) to image brain functioning; isotopes are incorporated into specific molecules to study cerebral metabolism, cerebral blood flow, and specific neurochemicals	Images appear blurry, lacking anatomic detail, but have been extremely useful in research to study distribution of neuroreceptors and the action of pharmacologic agents; invasive procedure, use of radioactivity limits the number of scans done with a single individual
Single photon emission computed tomography (SPECT)	Like PET, SPECT uses radioisotopes that produce only one photon; data are collected as a three-dimensional volume, and two-dimensional images can be constructed on any plane; less expensive than PET technology	Less resolution and sensitivity than the PET, but inhalation methods may be used, allowing for some repeated studies; useful in drug dependency research
Functional magnetic resonance imaging (fMRI)	Combines spatial resolution of MRI with the ability to image neural activity; is able to show sequential, movie-type images of blood flow in the brain as it is happening; shows whether brain activity occurs simultaneously or sequentially in different areas of the brain while engaged in selected activities	Requires no radiation and can be completely noninvasive; individual can be imaged many times, in different clinical states, before or after treatments; removes many of the ethical constraints when studying children and adolescents with psychiatric disorders
Magnetic resonance spectroscopy (MRS)	Uses the same imaging equipment as the fMRI; by altering scanning parameters, signals represent specific chemicals in the brain	Noninvasive, repeatable, may be ideal for longitudinal studies, but has limited spatial resolution, especially with molecules that occur in low concentrations

density of the examined tissue. The MRI can produce three-dimensional images extremely clearly, allowing for gross discrimination of white and gray matters, detection of subacute haemorrhages, and rough areas of white matter damage. Sometimes contrast material is used.

MRI scans produce more information than CT images, but MRI scans also are more complicated and costly. In addition, MRI scans cannot be used for all patients. Because MRI uses magnet energy, individuals with pacemakers, metal plates, bone replacements, aneurysm clips, or other metal in their body cannot undergo the procedure;

pregnant women also cannot have MRI scans. The loud noise of the equipment and the very narrow tube in which the patient must lie still can trigger claustrophobic responses in some people. Adequate preparation of the patient by the nurse should eliminate any surprises. Assistance with shallow breathing techniques, mental distractions, or other anxiety-reducing strategies may help. Many MRI facilities are equipped with music to mask the whirring of the equipment and provide a distraction through the lengthy testing period. Some tubes are now being made of clear plastic to decrease the claustrophobic sensation.

Diffusion Tensor Magnetic Resonance Imaging (DTI)

This special type of MRI produces information on white matter not presently available through any other techniques. It cannot show what is happening to individual neurons, but it can identify what is happening at the fibre bundle level. The images are based on microscopic movement of water protons in tissues (Shenton et al., 2012). Water moves freely in CSF but is more restricted by other structures such as axons and myelin sheaths. Water can move more freely in a direction parallel to the axon but less freely perpendicular to the axon. Therefore, the directions of the axons will determine the direction of the water diffusion. If, for example, diffusion in the white matter is found to be less restricted than expected, it can mean that the myelin sheaths or axons are damaged or less dense. DTI cannot identify the cause of the diffusion changes. This technology is being used to investigate white matter changes in schizophrenia, dementia, and other psychiatric illnesses. Ongoing developments in this technique will allow scientists to visualize and measure damage in fibre tracts connecting different brain regions.

Functional Neuroimaging

Although structural imaging identifies what the brain looks like, the scans do not show how the brain is working. Functional neuroimaging techniques measure physiologic activities, providing insight into how the brain works. These methods let researchers study such activities as cerebral blood flow, neuroreceptor location and function, and distribution patterns of specific chemicals within the brain. Single photon emission computed tomography (SPECT) and positron emission tomography (PET) are the primary methods used to observe metabolic functioning. Both procedures require administering radioactive substances that emit charged particles, which are then measured by scanning equipment. SPECT and PET differ in the type of isotopes used, the method of measuring isotope uptake, and therefore the equipment used. Because these procedures measure function, the patient is usually asked to perform specific tasks during the test. The Wisconsin Card Sorting Test (WCST), which is commonly used, requires the individual to sort cards with different numbers, colours, and shapes into piles based on specified rules. This task requires the use of the brain's frontal lobe, an important area for concept formation and decision making and an area that often is disrupted in many psychiatric disorders.

Pregnant health care workers should avoid caring for patients who have had a nuclear scan for 24 hours after the scan. Caregivers need to check their institution's guide for other safety precautions when caring for patients who have been exposed to nuclear material.

Single Photon Emission Computed Tomography

SPECT is helpful in measuring regional cerebral blood flow. In one study, SPECT scans were used to study decreases in blood flow in several areas in the brains of professional football players (Amen et al., 2010). These changes in blood flow may be related to hits to the head while playing the game. SPECT scans are also used to confirm changes in cerebral blood flow caused by certain drugs. For example, caffeine and nicotine cause a generalized decrease in cerebral blood flow. At present, this technique is used more in academic settings. It is less expensive than the PET exam. New compounds have been developed recently to visualize the numbers or density of **receptors** in various areas of the brain, which may assist in understanding the effects of psychopharmacologic medications and neuroplastic changes in brain tissue over time.

Positron Emission Tomography

PET uses a radioactive particle (most commonly glucose) to measure that particle's activity in various brain regions. Because cells use glucose as fuel for cellular action, the higher the rate of glucose use detected by the PET scan, the higher the rate of metabolic activity in different areas of the brain. Abnormalities in glucose consumption, indicating more or less cellular activity, are found in Alzheimer's disease, seizures, strokes, malignancies, and a number of psychiatric disorders. Scanning may be performed while the individual is at rest or performing a cognitive task. PET scans are often used to measure regional cerebral blood flow and neurotransmitter system functions.

Bridging the Structure–Function Gap

As structural and functional neuroimaging techniques advance, attempts are being made to develop imaging procedures that detail structure and function at the same time. Magnetic resonance spectroscopy (MRS) and functional magnetic resonance imaging (fMRI) are examples. The fMRI is useful for showing structure while localizing function and providing high-resolution images. Like other forms of neuroimaging, the fMRI is noninvasive, but it requires no radioactive agent, making it economical and safer than PET and SPECT (Hennig, Speck, Koch, & Weiller, 2003).

MRS uses the same machinery as fMRI and provides precise and clear images of neuronal membranes as well as measures of metabolic cellular function (Currie et al., 2013). In addition to these procedures, magnetoencephalography (MEG) is being used. MEG testing records magnetic fields generated by neuronal activity. These results are paired with a technique that images anatomical information such as MRI, to provide both the structural and functional information. Table 9-3 summarizes these neuroimaging methods. These neuroimaging procedures are becoming useful in clinical practice.

Transcranial magnetic stimulation (TMS) is an investigational, research, and treatment tool that painlessly delivers an alternating current through a metal coil placed around the scalp. The current causes a magnetic field to be generated, and this induces an electrical current that changes firing along neurons. Depending on where and at what frequency the treatment is applied, areas of the brain may be inhibited or excited. It has been found to provide mixed results in the treatment of depression. Adverse effects can include skin burns and lesions, and in some, depression may switch to mania (Holtzheimer, 2013). TMS has been used to investigate plasticity, medication effects, and nervous propagation along nerves. Additionally, it has been used in rehabilitation and operative settings.

NEUROANATOMY OF THE CENTRAL NERVOUS SYSTEM

With advances in brain science comes greater understanding of the biologic basis of mental illnesses. Therefore, PMH nurses must increasingly be aware of the anatomic intricacy of the CNS as a foundation for modern psychiatric nursing assessments and interventions.

Although this section discusses each functioning area of the brain separately, each area is intricately connected and functions interactively with the others. The CNS contains the brain, brain stem, and spinal cord, whereas the total human nervous system includes the peripheral nervous system (PNS) as well. The PNS consists of the neurons that connect the CNS to the muscles, organs, and other systems in the periphery of the body. Whatever affects the CNS may also affect the PNS, and vice versa.

Cerebrum

The largest part of the human brain, the cerebrum, fills the entire upper portion of the cranium. The **cortex**, or outermost surface of the cerebrum, makes up about 80%

of the human brain. The cortex is several millimetres thick and is composed of cell bodies mixed with capillary blood vessels. This mixture makes the cortex grey brown, hence the term *grey matter*. The cortex contains a number of bumps and grooves in a fully developed adult brain, as shown in Figure 9-1. This "wrinkling" allows for a large amount of surface area to be confined in the limited space of the skull. The increased surface area allows for more potential connections between cells within the cortex. The grooves are called *fissures* if they extend deep into the brain and *sulci* if they are shallower. The bumps or convolutions are called *gyri*. Together, they provide many of the landmarks for the subdivisions of the cortex. The longest and deepest groove, the longitudinal fissure, separates the cerebrum into left and right hemispheres. Although these two divisions are nearly symmetric, there is some variation in the location and size of the sulci and gyri in each hemisphere. Substantial variation in these convolutions is found in the cortex of different individuals.

Left and Right Hemispheres

The cerebrum can be roughly divided into two halves, or hemispheres. Each hemisphere controls functioning mainly on the opposite side of the body. For about 95% of people, the left hemisphere is dominant, whereas about 5% of individuals have mixed dominance. The right hemisphere provides input into receptive nonverbal communication, spatial orientation, and recognition; intonation of speech and aspects of music; facial recognition and facial expression of emotion; and nonverbal learning and

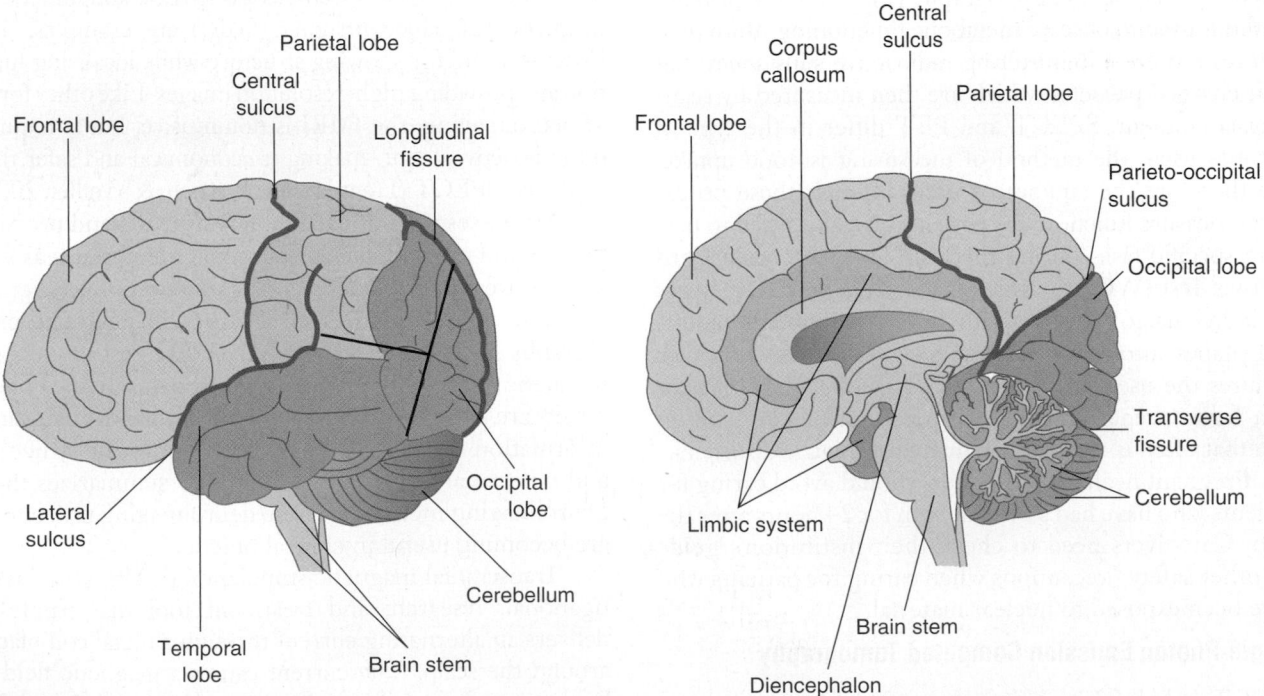

FIGURE 9-1. Lateral and medial surfaces of the brain. **Left:** the left lateral surface of the brain. **Right:** the medial surface of the right half of a sagittally hemisected brain.

memory. In general, the left hemisphere is more involved with verbal language function, including areas for both receptive and expressive speech control. In addition, the left hemisphere provides strong contributions to temporal order and sequencing, numeric symbols, and verbal learning and memory. However, the intact brain may not be neatly organized with one side being the dominant because the degree of lateralization differs across individuals. The two hemispheres are connected by the corpus callosum, a bundle of neuronal tissue that allows information to be exchanged quickly between the right and left hemispheres. An intact corpus callosum is required for the hemispheres to function in a smooth and coordinated manner.

Lobes of the Brain

The lateral surface of each hemisphere is further divided into four lobes: the **frontal, parietal, temporal, and occipital lobes** (Fig. 9-2). The lobes work in coordinated ways, but each is responsible for specific functions. Knowledge of these unique functions is helpful for understanding how damage to these areas produces the symptoms of mental illness and how medications that affect the functioning of these lobes can produce certain effects.

Frontal Lobes

The right and left frontal lobes make up about one fourth of the entire cerebral cortex and are proportionally larger in humans than in any other mammal. The precentral gyrus, the gyrus immediately anterior to the central sulcus, contains the primary motor area. Damage to this gyrus, or to the anterior neighbouring gyri, causes spastic paralysis in the opposite side of the body. The frontal lobe also contains Broca's area, which controls the motor function of speech. Damage to Broca's area produces expressive aphasia or difficulty with the motor movements of speech. The frontal lobes are also thought to contain the highest or most complex aspects of cortical functioning:

personality, working memory, executive function, intellect, and speech. Working memory is an important aspect of frontal lobe function, including the ability to plan and initiate activity with future goals in mind. Insight, judgment, reasoning, concept formation, problem-solving skills, abstraction, and self-evaluation are all abilities that are modulated and affected by the action of the frontal lobes. These skills are often referred to as *executive functions* because they modulate more primitive impulses through numerous connections to other areas of the cerebrum.

When normal frontal lobe functioning is altered, executive functioning is decreased, and modulation of impulses can be lost, leading to changes in mood and personality. The importance of the frontal lobe and its role in the development of symptoms common to psychiatric disorders are emphasized in later chapters that discuss disorders such as schizophrenia, attention-deficit hyperactivity disorder, and dementia. Box 9-1 describes how altered frontal lobe function can affect mood and personality.

Parietal Lobes

The postcentral gyrus, immediately behind the central sulcus, contains the primary somatosensory area (Fig. 9-2). The posterior areas of the parietal lobe appear to coordinate visual and somatosensory information. Damage to this area produces complex sensory deficits, including neglect of contralateral sensory stimuli and spatial relationships. The parietal lobes contribute to the ability to recognize objects by touch, calculate, write, recognize fingers of the opposite hands, draw, and organize spatial directions, such as how to travel to familiar places. They are important for speech and maintaining focused attention.

Temporal Lobes

The temporal lobes contain the primary auditory and olfactory areas. Wernicke's area, located at the posterior aspect of the superior temporal gyrus, is primarily responsible for receptive speech. The temporal lobes also integrate sensory and visual information involved in the control of written and verbal language skills, as well as visual recognition. The hippocampus, an important structure discussed in its own section later in this chapter, lies in the internal aspects of each temporal lobe and contributes to memory. Other internal structures of this lobe are involved in the modulation of mood and emotion.

Occipital Lobes

The primary visual area is located in the most posterior aspect of the occipital lobes. Damage to this area results in a condition called *cortical blindness*. In other words, the retina and optic nerve remain intact, but the individual cannot see. The occipital lobes are involved in many aspects of visual integration of information, including colour vision, object and facial recognition, and the ability to perceive objects in motion and judge distance.

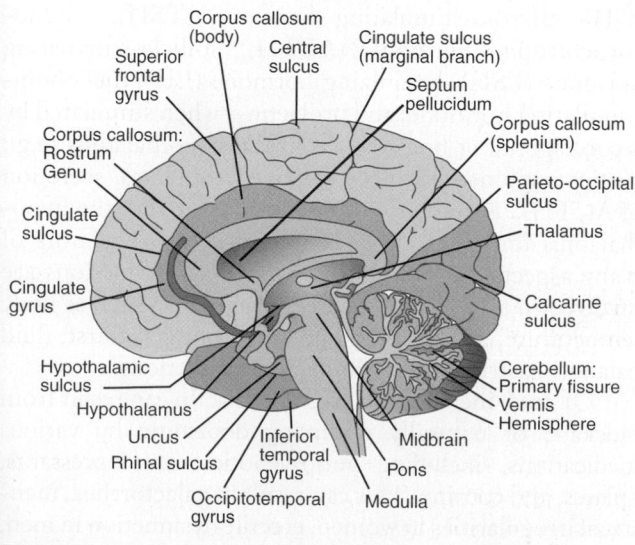

FIGURE 9-2. Gyri and sulci of the cortex.

BOX 9-1　Frontal Lobe Syndrome

In the 1860s, Phineas Gage became a famous example of frontal lobe dysfunction. Mr. Gage was a New England railroad worker who had a thick iron-tamping rod propelled through his frontal lobes by an explosion. He survived but suffered significant changes in his personality. Mr. Gage, who had previously been a capable and calm supervisor, began to show impatience, labile mood, disrespect for others, and frequent use of profanity after his injury (Harlow, 1868). Similar conditions are often called *frontal lobe syndrome*. Symptoms vary widely among individuals. In general, after damage to the dorsolateral (upper and outer) areas of the frontal lobes, the symptoms include a lack of drive and spontaneity. With damage to the most anterior aspects of the frontal lobes, the symptoms tend to involve more changes in mood and affect, such as impulsive and inappropriate behaviour.

　　The rendering shows the route the tamping rod took through Gage's skull. The angle of the rod's entry shot it behind the left eye and through the front part of the brain, sparing regions that are directly concerned with vital functions like breathing and heartbeat.

Association Cortex

Although not a lobe, the association cortex is an important area that allows the lobes to work in an integrated manner. Areas of one lobe of the cortex often share functions with an area of the adjacent lobe. When these neighbouring nerve fibres are related to the same sensory modality, they are often referred to as *association* areas. For example, an area in the inferior parietal, posterior temporal, and anterior occipital lobes integrates visual, somatosensory, and auditory information to provide the abilities required for basic academic skills. These areas, along with numerous connections beneath the cortex, are part of the mechanisms that allow the human brain to work as an integrated whole.

Subcortical Structures

Beneath the cortex are layers of tissue composed of the axons of cell bodies. The axonal tissue forms pathways that are surrounded by glia, a fatty or lipid substance, which has a white appearance and gives these layers of neuron axons their name—*white matter*. Structures inside the hemispheres, beneath the cortex, are considered subcortical. Many of these structures, essential in the regulation of emotions and behaviours, play important roles in our understanding of mental disorders. Figure 9-3 provides a coronal section view of the grey matter, white matter, and important subcortical structures.

Basal Ganglia

The **basal ganglia** are subcortical grey matter areas in both the right and left hemispheres that contain interconnected cell bodies or nuclei. These nuclei include the caudate nucleus, putamen, globus pallidus, claustrum, subthalamus, and substantia nigra. The basal ganglia are involved with motor functions and in association with both the learning and programming of behaviours or activities that are repetitive and that over time become automatic. The basal ganglia have many connections with the cerebral cortex, thalamus, midbrain structures, and spinal cord. Damage to portions of these nuclei may produce changes in posture or muscle tone. In addition, damage may produce abnormal movements, such as twitches or tremors. Parkinson's disease is the most common disorder of the basal ganglia. They can be adversely affected by some of the medications used to treat psychiatric disorders, leading to side effects and other motor-related problems.

Pituitary

The pituitary gland, often called the *master gland*, has two distinct parts, the anterior pituitary and the posterior pituitary. Located just below the hypothalamus, the anterior pituitary consists of glandular epithelial tissue and is connected to the hypothalamus by a vascular link. In contrast, the posterior pituitary is composed of neural tissue and is connected to the hypothalamus by a neural pathway. When stimulated, the posterior pituitary releases oxytocin or vasopressin (also known as antidiuretic hormone), two small peptide hormones that are produced in the hypothalamus. The anterior pituitary produces and releases seven different hormones—growth hormone (GH), thyroid-stimulating hormone (TSH), adrenocorticotropin hormone (ACTH), follicle-stimulating hormone (FSH), luteinizing hormone (LH), melatonin-stimulating hormone, and prolactin—when stimulated by a corresponding hormone from the hypothalamus (e.g., corticotrophin-releasing hormone stimulates secretion of ACTH). Together with the pituitary gland, the hypothalamus functions as one of the primary regulators of many aspects of the endocrine system. Its functions are involved in the control of visceral activities, such as body temperature, arterial blood pressure, hunger, thirst, fluid balance, gastric motility, and gastric secretions.

　　Of note, increased release of prolactin can result from blockade of naturally occurring dopamine by various medications, including antipsychotics, antidepressants, opiates, and cocaine. This can result in galactorrhea, menstrual irregularities in women, erectile dysfunction in men, and loss of libido and infertility in both men and women.

FIGURE 9-3. Three standard planes for visualizing brain structure: (**A**) sagittal, (**B**) coronal, and (**C**) horizontal cuts are made by physically slicing or rendered using imaging techniques. The transverse or cross cut (**D**) gives a view of subcortical structures. (From Bhatnagar, S. (2013). *Neuroscience for the study of communicative disorders*. Philadelphia, PA: Lippincott Williams & Wilkins.)

Limbic System

The **limbic system** is essential to understanding the many hypotheses related to psychiatric disorders and emotional behaviour in general. Basic emotions, needs, drives, and instinct begin and are modulated in the limbic system. Hate, love, anger, aggression, and caring are basic emotions that originate within the limbic system. Not only does the limbic system function as the seat of emotions but also, because emotions are often generated based on our personal experiences, the limbic system is involved with aspects of memory. Hypothesized changes in the limbic system play a significant role in many theories of major mental disorders, including schizophrenia, depression, and anxiety disorders (see Chapters 20–23). The limbic system is called a "system" because it comprises several small structures that work in a highly organized way. These structures include the hippocampus, thalamus, hypothalamus, amygdala, and limbic midbrain nuclei. See Figure 9-4 for identification and location of the structures within the limbic system and their relationship to other common CNS structures.

Hippocampus.

The **hippocampus** is involved in forming and storing memories, especially the emotions attached to a memory. Our emotional response to memories and our association with other related memories are functions of how information is stored within the hippocampus. While most neurons are formed from before birth, the neurons in the hippocampus continue to form throughout life. Although memory storage is not limited to one area of the brain, destruction of the left hippocampus impairs verbal memory, and damage to the right hippocampus results in difficulty with recognition and recall of complex visual and auditory patterns. The main body of the hippocampus extends into the temporal lobe. Deterioration of the nerves of the hippocampus and other related temporal lobe structures found in Alzheimer's disease produces the disorder's hallmark symptoms of memory dysfunction.

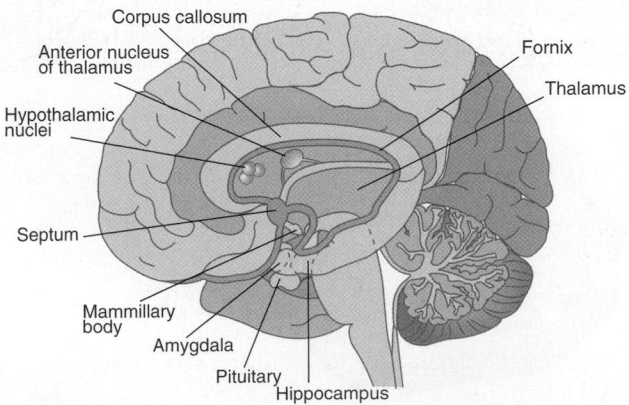

FIGURE 9-4. The structures of the limbic system are integrally involved in memory and emotional behaviour. Theories link changes in the limbic system to many major mental disorders, including schizophrenia, depression, and anxiety disorders.

Thalamus.

The thalamus is composed of several distinct subnuclei, each with its own specialized connections to many regions in the cerebral cortex. Sometimes called the "relay-switching centre of the brain," the thalamus functions as a regulatory structure to relay all sensory information, except smell, sent to the CNS from the PNS. The thalamus also relays memory, emotions, cognitions, behaviours, and motor functions. It regulates by filtering incoming information and determining what to pass on or what not to pass on to the cortex. In this fashion, the thalamus prevents the cortex from becoming overloaded with sensory stimulus. The thalamus is thought to play a part in controlling electrical activity in the cortex. Parts of the thalamus are involved in alertness, awareness, and memory. Injury to the anterior medial thalamus can cause alterations in autonomic functions, mood, and the sleep–wake cycle.

Hypothalamus.

Basic human activities, such as sleep–rest patterns, body temperature, and physical drives (e.g., hunger and sex), are regulated by the hypothalamus, which rests deep within the brain. In emotional situations, the hypothalamus perceives changes and stimulates a visceral response through the autonomic nervous system, such as an increase in heart rate when we feel angry. Dysfunction of this structure, whether from disorders or because of the adverse effects of drugs used to treat mental illness, produces common psychiatric symptoms, such as appetite and sleep problems.

Nerve cells within the hypothalamus secrete hormones such as antidiuretic hormone, which when sent to the kidneys accelerates the reabsorption of water, and oxytocin, which acts on smooth muscles to promote contractions, particularly within the walls of the uterus. Because cells within the nervous system produce these hormones, they are often referred to as **neurohormones** and form a communication mechanism through the bloodstream to control organs that are not directly connected to nervous system structures.

Deregulation of the hypothalamus can be manifested in symptoms of certain psychiatric disorders. For example, patients with schizophrenia often wear heavy coats during the hot summer months and do not appear hot. Before the role of the hypothalamus in schizophrenia was understood, psychological reasons were used to explain such symptoms. It is increasingly clear that such a symptom relates to deregulation of the hypothalamus's normal role in temperature regulation and is biologically based (Shiloh et al., 2001).

Amygdala.

The amygdala is directly connected to more primitive centres of the brain involving the sense of smell. It has numerous connections to the hypothalamus and lies adjacent to the hippocampus. The amygdala provides an emotional component to memory and is involved in modulating aggression, fear, anxiety, and sexuality. Impulsive acts of aggression and violence have been linked to deregulation of the amygdala, and erratic firing of the nerve cells in the amygdala is a focus of investigation in bipolar mood disorders (see Chapter 22). The amygdala is also the part of the brain most affected by psychoactive drugs.

Limbic Midbrain Nuclei. The limbic midbrain nuclei are a collection of neurons (including the ventral tegmental area and the locus caeruleus) that appear to play a role in the biologic basis of addiction. Sometimes referred to as the pleasure centre or reward centre of the brain, the limbic midbrain nuclei function to chemically reinforce certain behaviours, ensuring their repetition. Emotions such as feeling satisfied with good food, the pleasure of nurturing, and the enjoyment of sexual activity originate in the limbic midbrain nuclei. The reinforcement of activities such as nutrition, procreation, and nurturing young are all primitive aspects of ensuring the survival of a species. When functioning in abnormal ways, the limbic midbrain nuclei can begin to reinforce unhealthy or risky behaviours, such as drug abuse. Exploration of this area of the brain is in its infancy but offers potential insight into addictions and their treatment.

Other Central Nervous System Structures

The *extrapyramidal motor system* is a bundle of nerve fibres connecting the thalamus to the basal ganglia and cerebral cortex. Muscle tone, common reflexes, and automatic voluntary motor functioning, such as walking, are controlled by this nerve tract. Dysfunction of this motor tract can produce hypertonicity in muscle groups. In Parkinson's disease, the cells that compose the extrapyramidal motor system are severely affected, producing many involuntary motor movements. A number of medications, which are discussed in Chapter 12, also affect this system.

The *pineal body* is a pinecone-shaped organ, measuring just 5 to 8 mm in length and 3 to 5 mm in width. It is located above and medial to the thalamus. Because the pineal gland easily calcifies, it can be visualized by neuroimaging and often is a medial landmark. Its functions remain somewhat of a mystery, despite long knowledge of its existence.

It contains secretory cells that release the neurohormone melatonin and other substances. These hormones are thought to have a number of regulatory functions within the endocrine system. Darkness and hypoglycemia increase the release of melatonin. Melatonin has been associated with sleep and emotional disorders. In addition, it has been postulated that melatonin has a role in modulating immune function.

The *locus caeruleus* is a tiny cluster of norepinephrine-containing neurons that fan out and innervate almost every part of the brain, including most of the cortex, the thalamus and hypothalamus, the cerebellum, and the spinal cord. Just one neuron from the caeruleus can connect to more than 250,000 other neurons. Although it is very small, because of its wide-ranging neuronal connections, this tiny structure has influence in the regulation of attention, time perception, sleep–rest cycles, arousal, learning, pain, and mood, and it seems most involved with information processing of new, unexpected, and novel experiences. Some think its function/dysfunction may explain why individuals become addicted to substances and seek risky behaviours, despite awareness of negative consequences.

The *brain stem*, located beneath the thalamus, is composed of the midbrain, pons, and medulla and has important life-sustaining functions. Nuclei of numerous neural pathways to the cerebrum are located in the brain stem. They are significantly involved in mediating symptoms of emotional dysfunction. These nuclei are also the primary source of several neurochemicals, such as serotonin, that are commonly associated with psychiatric disorders. Table 9-4 summarizes some of the key related nuclei.

The *cerebellum* is in the posterior aspect of the skull, beneath the cerebral hemispheres. This large structure controls movements and postural adjustments. To regulate postural balance and positioning, the cerebellum receives information from all parts of the body, including muscles, joints, skin, and visceral organs, as well as from many parts of the CNS.

Table 9-4	Classic and Putative Neurotransmitters, Their Distribution and Proposed Functions		
Neurotransmitter	**Cell Bodies**	**Projections**	**Proposed Function**

Acetylcholine
Dietary precursor:
  choline
	Basal forebrain
	Pons
	Other areas
		Diffuse throughout the cortex,
		  hippocampus
		Peripheral nervous system
			Important role in learning and memory
			Some role in wakefulness and basic
			  attention
			Peripherally activates muscles and
			  is the major neurochemical in the
			  autonomic system

Monoamines
Dopamine
Dietary precursor:
  tyrosine
	Substantia nigra
	Ventral tegmental area
	Arcuate nucleus
	Retina olfactory bulb
		Striatum (basal ganglia)
		Limbic system and cerebral
		  cortex
		Pituitary
			Involved in involuntary motor
			  movements
			Some role in mood states, pleasure
			  components in reward systems,
			  and complex behaviour such as
			  judgment, reasoning, and insight

Table 9-4	Classic and Putative Neurotransmitters, Their Distribution and Proposed Functions (*Continued*)

Neurotransmitter	Cell Bodies	Projections	Proposed Function

Norepinephrine
Dietary precursor:
  tyrosine
	Locus caeruleus
	Lateral tegmental area
	  and others throughout
	  the pons and medulla
		Very widespread throughout the
		  cortex, thalamus, cerebellum,
		  brain stem, and spinal cord
		Basal forebrain, thalamus,
		  hypothalamus
			Proposed role in learning and
			  memory, attributing value in
			  reward systems; fluctuates in
			  sleep and wakefulness
			Major component of the sympathetic
			  nervous system responses,
			  including "fight-or-flight"

Serotonin
Dietary precursor:
  tryptophan
	Raphe nuclei
	Others in the pons and
	  medulla
		Widespread throughout the
		  cortex, thalamus, cerebellum,
		  brain stem, and spinal cord
			Proposed role in the control of
			  appetite, sleep, mood states,
			  hallucinations, pain perception,
			  and vomiting

Histamine
Dietary precursor:
  histidine
	Hypothalamus	Cerebral cortex
		Limbic system
		Hypothalamus
		Found in all mast cells
			Control of gastric secretions,
			  smooth muscle control, cardiac
			  stimulation, stimulation of sensory
			  nerve endings, and alertness

Amino Acids			

GABA	Derived from glutamate
	  without localized cell
	  bodies
		Found in cells and projections
		  throughout the CNS, especially
		  in intrinsic feedback loops and
		  interneurons of the cerebrum
		Also in the extrapyramidal motor
		  system and cerebellum
			Fast inhibitory response
			  postsynaptically, inhibits the
			  excitability of the neurons and
			  therefore contributes to seizure,
			  agitation, and anxiety control

Glycine	Primarily the spinal cord
	  and brain stem
		Limited projection, but especially
		  in the auditory system and
		  olfactory bulb
		Also found in the spinal cord,
		  medulla, midbrain, cerebellum,
		  and cortex
			Inhibitory
			Decreases the excitability of spinal
			  motor neurons but not cortical

Glutamate	Diffuse	Diffuse, but especially in the
		  sensory organs
			Excitatory
			Responsible for the bulk of
			  information flow

Neuropeptides			

Endogenous opioids,
  (e.g., endorphins,
  enkephalins)
	A large family of
	  neuropeptides, which
	  has three distinct
	  subgroups, all of which
	  are manufactured widely
	  throughout the CNS
		Widely distributed within and
		  outside the CNS
			Suppresses pain, modulates mood
			  and stress
			Likely involvement in reward systems
			  and addiction
			Also may regulate pituitary hormone
			  release
			Implicated in the pathophysiology of
			  diseases of the basal ganglia

Melatonin
One of its precursors:
  serotonin
	Pineal body	Widely distributed within and
		  outside the CNS
			Secreted in dark and suppressed
			  light, helps regulate the sleep–
			  wake cycle as well as other
			  biologic rhythms

Substance P	Widespread, significant in
	  the raphe system and
	  spinal cord
		Spinal cord, cortex, brain stem,
		  and especially sensory neurons
		  associated with pain perception
			Involved in pain transmission,
			  movement, and mood regulation

Cholecystokinin	Predominates in the
	  ventral tegmental area of
	  the midbrain
		Frontal cortex where it is often
		  colocalized with dopamine
		Widely distributed within and
		  outside the CNS
			Primary intestinal hormone
			  involved in satiety, also has some
			  involvement in the control of
			  anxiety and panic

Closely associated with the spinal cord, but not lying entirely within its column, is the **autonomic nervous system**, a subdivision of the PNS. It was originally given this name for being independent of conscious thought, that is, automatic. However, it does not necessarily function as autonomously as the name indicates. This system contains efferent (nerves moving away from the CNS) or motor system neurons, which affect target tissues such as cardiac muscle, smooth muscle, and the glands. It also contains afferent nerves, which are sensory and conduct information from these organs back to the CNS. The two main neurotransmitters of the ANS are acetylcholine

(Ach) and norepinephrine. It is important for nurses to recognize that any medication that impacts these neurotransmitters can have far-reaching effects in the body.

The autonomic nervous system is further divided into the sympathetic and parasympathetic nervous systems. These systems, although peripheral, are included here because they are involved in the emergency, or "fight-or-flight," response as well as the peripheral actions of many medications (see Chapter 12). Figure 9-5 illustrates the innervations of various target organs by the autonomic

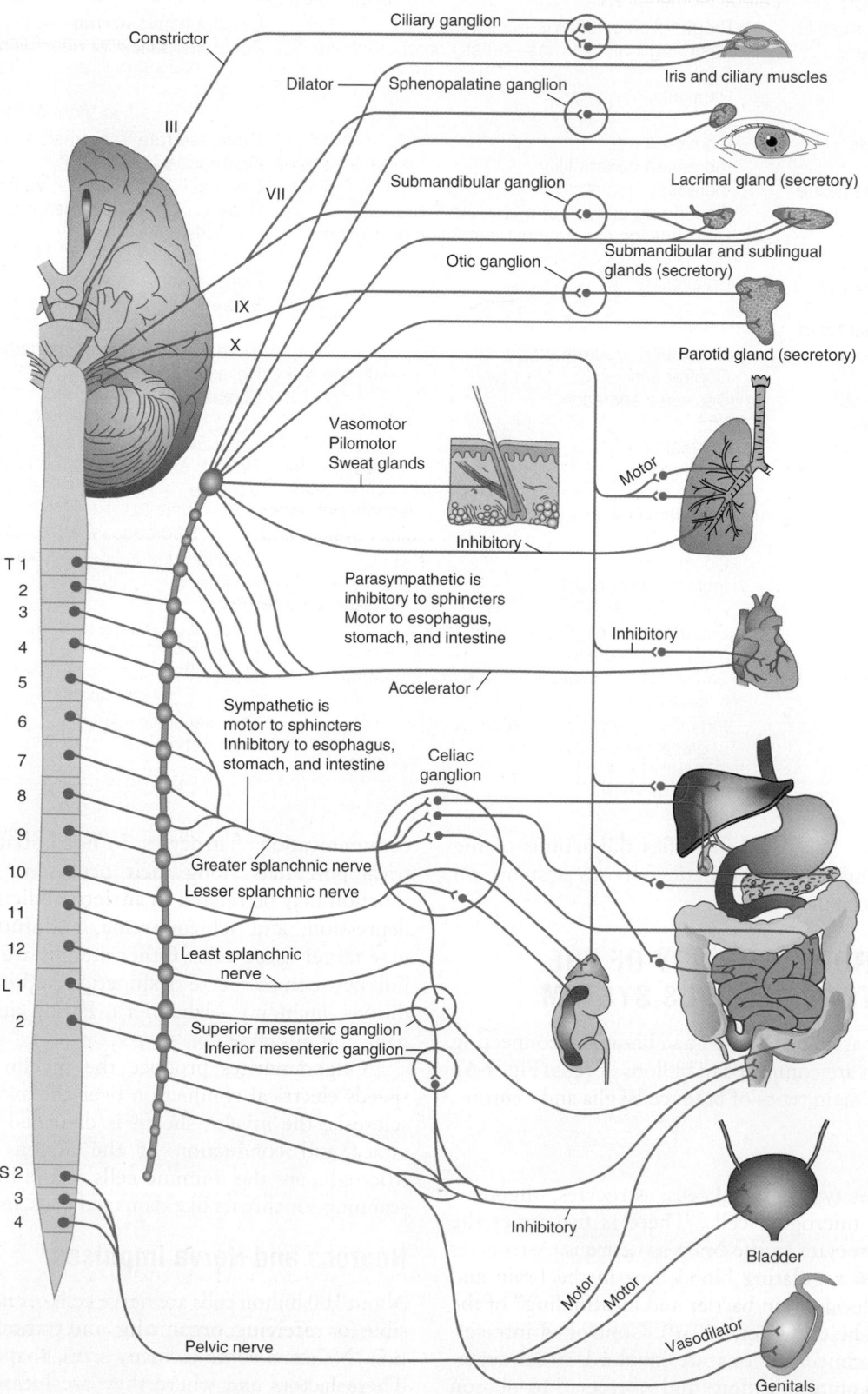

FIGURE 9-5. Diagram of the autonomic nervous system. Note that many organs are innervated by both sympathetic and parasympathetic nerves. (Adapted from Schaffe, E. E. & Lytle, I. M. (1980). *Basic physiology and anatomy.* Philadelphia, PA: J.B. Lippincott.)

Table 9-5	Peripheral Organ Response in the Autonomic Nervous System

Effector Organ	Sympathetic Response	Parasympathetic Response (Acetylcholine)
Eye		
• Iris sphincter muscle	Preganglionic neurons—acetylcholine	Constriction to normal
• Ciliary muscle	Postganglionic neurons—mostly norepinephrine	Accommodation for near vision
	Dilation	
	Relaxation	
Heart		
• Sinoatrial node	Increased rate	Decrease rate to normal
• Atria	Increased contractility	Decrease in contractility
• Atrioventricular node	Increased contractility	Decrease in conduction velocity
Blood vessels	Depending on type of sympathetic receptor, stimulation can cause constriction or dilation	Dilation of vessels supplying penis and clitoris only
Lungs		
• Bronchial muscles	Relaxation	Constriction to normal
• Bronchial glands		Secretion
Gastrointestinal Tract		
• Motility and tone	Relaxation (decreased peristalsis)	Increased (for normal peristalsis)
• Sphincters	Contraction	Relaxation
• Secretion glands	Decrease secretion	Stimulation
Urinary Bladder		
• Detrusor muscle	Relaxation	Contraction
• Trigone and sphincter	Contraction	Relaxation
Uterus	Contraction (pregnant)	Variable
	Relaxation (nonpregnant)	
Skin		
• Pilomotor muscles	Contraction	No effect
• Sweat glands	Increased secretion	No effect
Glands		
• Salivary	Stimulation of small volume of thick saliva	Stimulation of large volume of watery saliva
• Sweat	Increased secretion	None
• Adrenal medulla	Stimulation of epinephrine and norepinephrine secretion	None
• Endocrine pancreas	Inhibition of insulin secretion; stimulation of glucagon secretion	Stimulation of insulin and glucagon secretion

nervous system. Table 9-5 identifies the actions of the sympathetic and parasympathetic nervous systems on various target organs.

NEUROPHYSIOLOGY OF THE CENTRAL NERVOUS SYSTEM

At their most basic level, the human brain and connecting nervous system are composed of billions of cells (Fig. 9-6). There are two main types of brain cells: glia and neurons.

Glial Cells

There are three types of glial cells: astrocytes, oligodendrocytes, and microglial cells. There is five times the number of astrocytes in the brain as neurons. Astrocytes are involved in regulating blood flow in the brain and forming the blood–brain barrier and "scaffolding" of the CNS (Sofroniew & Vinters, 2010). Controlled intracellular calcium concentrations are involved in astrocyte-to-astrocyte communication and astrocyte-to-neuron

communication. Astrocytes do not initiate or pass electrical potentials along their processes. Astrocyte dysfunction may be related to anxiety, addiction behaviours, depression, and schizophrenia, and future treatments may target these cells. Other studies are looking at the link between astrocyte dysfunction and other CNS conditions, including Alzheimer's, Parkinson's, neuropathic pain, and migraine.

Oligodendrites produce the myelin sheath, which speeds electrical conduction over the axons. In multiple sclerosis, the myelin sheath is damaged by an immune attack and conduction of the action potential fails. Microglia are the immune cells of the brain, constantly scanning for threats like damaged cells and infection.

Neurons and Nerve Impulses

About 100 billion cells are nerve cells, or neurons, responsible for receiving, organizing, and transmitting information. Neurons come in many sizes, shapes, and lengths. These factors and where they are located in the brain

FIGURE 9-6. Cell body and organelles of an axon.

determine how they function (Fig. 9-7). Each neuron has a cell body, or soma, which holds the nucleus containing most of the cell's genetic information. The soma also includes other organelles, such as ribosomes and endoplasmic reticulum, both of which carry out protein synthesis; the Golgi apparatus, which contains enzymes to modify the proteins for specific functions; vesicles, which transport and store proteins; and lysosomes, responsible for degradation of these proteins. Located throughout the neuron, mitochondria, containing enzymes and often called the "cell's engine," are the site of many energy-producing chemical reactions. These cell structures provide the basis for secreting numerous chemicals by which neurons communicate.

It is not just the vast number of neurons that accounts for the complexities of the brain but also the enormous number of neurochemical interconnections and interactions between neurons. A single motor neuron in the spinal cord may receive signals from more than 10,000 sources of interconnection with other nerves. Although most neurons have only one axon, which varies in length and conducts impulses away from the soma, each has numerous dendrites, receiving signals from other neurons. Because

axons may branch as they terminate, they also have multiple contacts with other neurons.

Nerve signals are prompted to fire by a variety of chemical or physical stimuli. This firing produces an electrical impulse. The cell's membrane is a double layer of phospholipid molecules with embedded proteins. Some of these proteins provide water-filled channels through which inorganic ions may pass. Each of the common ions—sodium, potassium, calcium, and chloride—has its own specific molecular channel. These channels are voltage gated and thus open or close in response to changes in the electrical potential across the membrane. At rest, the cell membrane is polarized with a positive charge on the outside and about a 270-mV charge on the inside, owing to the resting distribution of sodium and potassium ions. As potassium passively diffuses across the membrane, the sodium pump uses energy to move sodium from the inside of the cell against a concentration gradient to maintain this distribution. An action potential, or nerve impulse, is generated as the membrane is depolarized and a threshold value is reached, which triggers the opening of the voltage-gated sodium channels, allowing sodium to surge into the cell. The inside of the

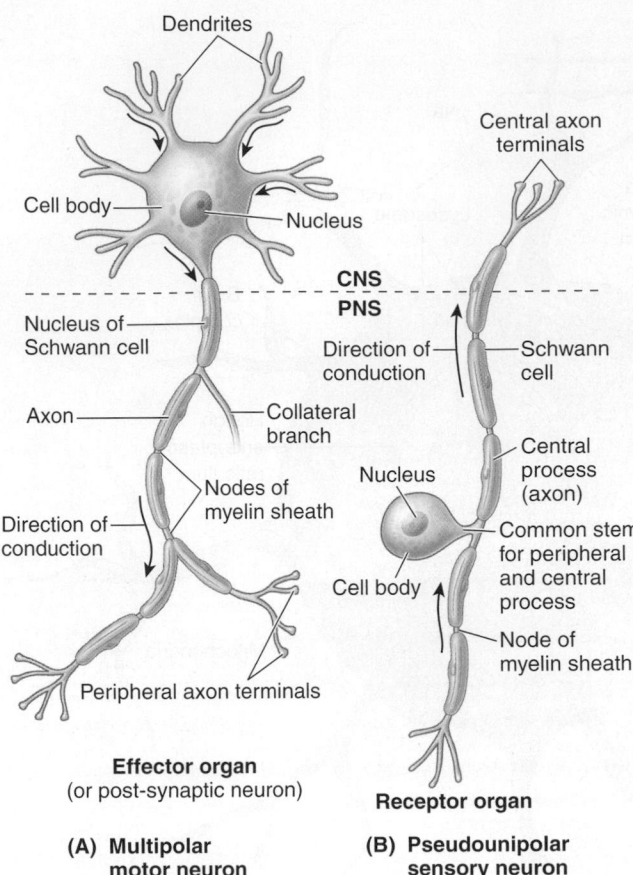

FIGURE 9-7. The two most common neurons are the (**A**) motor and (**B**) sensory neuron. (From Moore, K. L., Agur, A. M. R., & Dalley, A. F. (2014). *Clinically oriented anatomy*. Philadelphia, PA: Lippincott Williams & Wilkins.)

cell briefly becomes positively charged and the outside negatively charged. Once initiated, the action potential becomes self-propagating, opening nearby sodium channels. This electrical communication moves into the soma from the dendrites or down the axon by this mechanism.

Synaptic Transmission

For one neuron to communicate with another, the electrical process must change to a chemical communication. The synaptic cleft, a junction between one nerve and another, is the space where the electrical intracellular signal becomes a chemical extracellular signal. Various substances are recognized as the chemical messengers between neurons.

Neurotransmitters are small molecules that directly and indirectly control the opening or closing of ion channels. Neuromodulators are chemical messengers that make the target cell membrane or postsynaptic membrane more or less susceptible to the effects of the primary neurotransmitter. Some of these neurochemicals are synthesized quickly from dietary precursors, such as tyrosine or tryptophan, or enzymes inside the cytoplasm of the neuron, but most synthesis occurs in the ends of

the axons, called *terminals*, or the neuron itself. Some neurochemicals can reduce the membrane potential and enhance the transmission of the signal between neurons. These chemicals are called *excitatory neurotransmitters*. Other neurochemicals have the opposite effect, slowing down nerve impulses, and these substances are called *inhibitory neurotransmitters*.

As the electrical action potential reaches the terminals, calcium ion channels are opened, causing an influx of Ca^{++} ions into the neuron. This increase in calcium stimulates the release of neurotransmitters into the **synapse**. Rapid signaling between neurons requires a ready supply of neurotransmitters. These neurotransmitters are stored in small vesicles grouped near the cell membrane at the terminals. Because nerve terminals do not have the ability to manufacture proteins, the transmitters that fill these vesicles are small molecules, such as the bioamines (dopamine and norepinephrine) or the amino acids (glutamate or γ-aminobutyric acid [GABA]). Actions of these small molecules are discussed in the Neurotransmitters section later in this chapter. When stimulated, the vesicles containing the neurotransmitter fuse with the cell membrane, and the neurotransmitter is released into the synapse (Fig. 9-8). The neurotransmitter then crosses the synaptic cleft to a receptor site on the postsynaptic neuron and stimulates adjacent neurons. This is the process of neuronal communication.

Embedded in the postsynaptic membrane are a number of proteins that act as receptors for the released neurotransmitters. The "lock-and-key" analogy has often been used to describe the fit of a given neurotransmitter to its receptor site. Each neurotransmitter has a specific receptor, or protein, for which it and only it will fit. The target cell, when stimulated by the neurotransmitter, will respond by evoking its own action potential and either producing some action common to that cell or acting as a relay to keep the messages moving throughout the CNS. This pattern of the electrical signal from one neuron, converted to chemical signal at the synaptic cleft, picked up by an adjacent neuron, again converted to an electrical action potential and then to a chemical signal, occurs billions of times a day in billions of different brain cells. It is this electrical–chemical communication process that allows the structures of the brain to function together in a coordinated and organized manner.

When the neurotransmitter has completed its interaction with the postsynaptic receptor and stimulated that cell, its work is done and it needs to be removed. It can be removed by natural diffusion away from the area of high neurotransmitter concentration at the receptors by being broken down by enzymes in the synaptic cleft or through reuptake through highly specific mechanisms into the presynaptic terminal.

Many psychopharmacologic agents, particularly antidepressants, act by blocking the reuptake of the neurotransmitters, thereby increasing the available

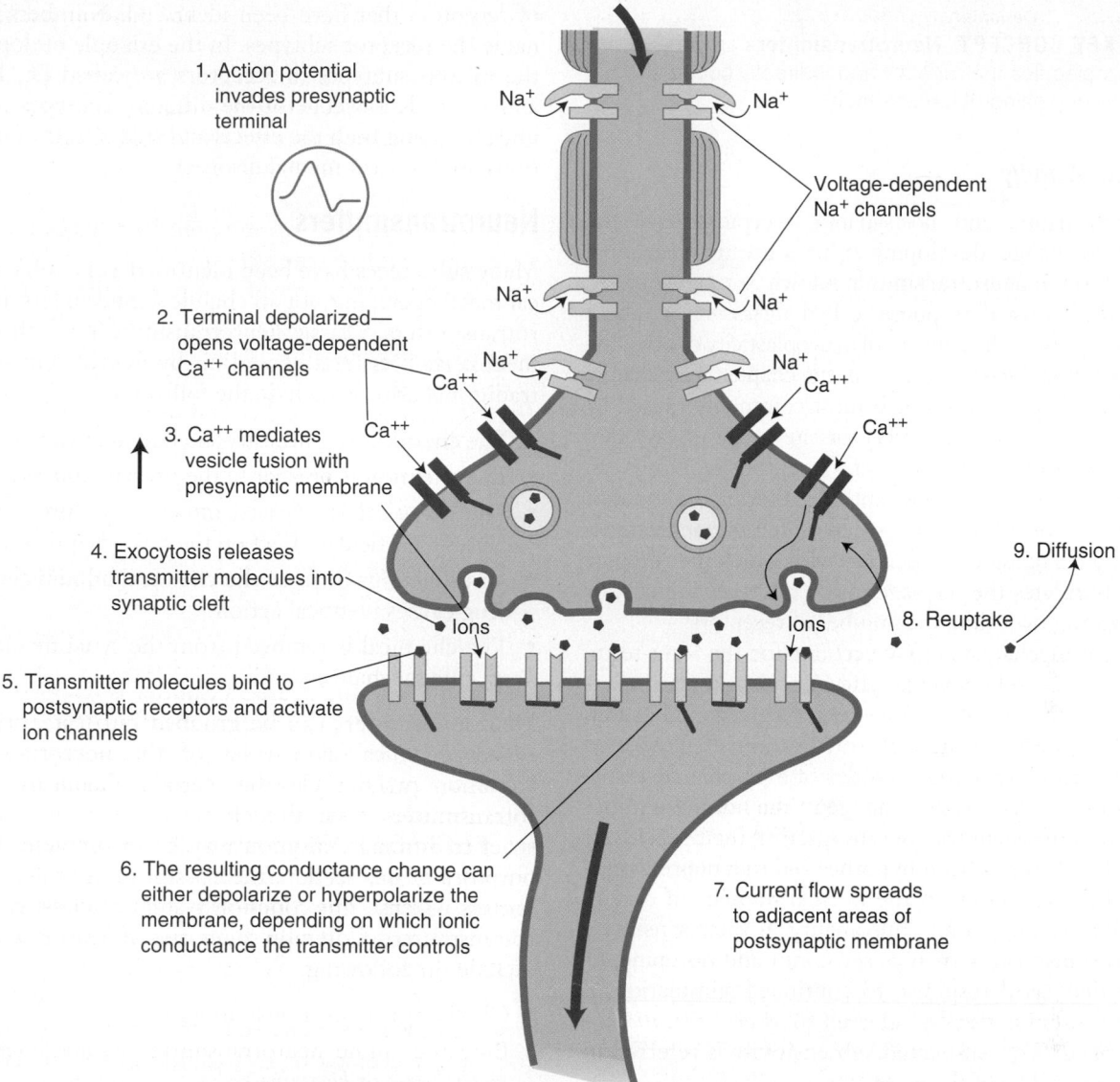

FIGURE 9-8. Synaptic transmission. The most significant events that occur during synaptic transmission: (1) the action potential reaches the presynaptic terminal; (2) membrane depolarization causes Ca++ terminals to open; (3) Ca++ mediates fusion of the vesicles with the presynaptic membrane; (4) transmitter molecules are released into the synaptic cleft, by exocytosis; (5) transmitter molecules bind to postsynaptic receptors and activate ion channels; (6) conductance changes cause an excitatory or inhibitory postsynaptic potential (excitatory and inhibitory processes are alternately referred to as depolarization and hyperpolarization), depending on the specific transmitter; (7) current flow spreads along the postsynaptic membrane; and (8) transmitter remaining in the synaptic cleft returns to the presynaptic terminal by reuptake or (9) diffuses into the extracellular fluid. (Adapted and reproduced with permission from Schauf, C., Moffett, D., & Moffett, S. (1990). *Human physiology.* St. Louis, MO: Times Mirror/Mosby.)

amount of chemical messenger. Presynaptic binding sites for neurotransmitters may serve not only as reuptake mechanisms but also as autoreceptors to perform various regulatory functions on the flow of neurotransmitters into the synapse. When these presynaptic autoreceptors are saturated, the neuron slows down or stops releasing neurotransmitters. The neurotransmitters taken back into the presynaptic neuron may be stored in vesicles for rerelease, or they may be broken down by enzymes, such as monoamine oxidase, and removed entirely.

The primary steps in synaptic transmission are summarized in Figure 9-8. The preceding discussion contains only the basic mechanisms of neuronal communication. Many other factors that modulate or contribute to the communication between neurons are only beginning to be discovered. Examples include peptides that are released into the synapse and thought to behave like neurotransmitters or that also can appear in combination with another neurotransmitter. These peptides, known as *cotransmitters*, are believed to have a modulatory effect on the primary neurotransmitter.

> **KEY CONCEPT** **Neurotransmitters** are small molecules that directly and indirectly control the opening or closing of ion channels.

Receptor Activity

Both presynaptic and postsynaptic receptors have the capacity to change, developing either a greater-than-usual response to the neurotransmitter, known as *supersensitivity*, or a less-than-usual response, called *subsensitivity*. These changes represent the concept of neuroplasticity of brain tissue, which was discussed earlier in the chapter. The change in sensitivity of the receptor is most commonly caused by the effect of a drug on a receptor site or by disease that affects the normal functioning of a receptor site. Drugs can affect the sensitivity of the receptor by altering the strength of attraction or affinity of a receptor for the neurotransmitter, by changing the efficiency with which the receptor activity translates the message inside the receiving cell, or by decreasing over time the number of receptors.

These mechanisms may account for the long-term, sometimes severely adverse, effects of psychopharmacologic drugs, the loss of effectiveness of a given medication, or the loss of effectiveness of a medication after repeated use in treating recurring episodes of a psychiatric disorder. A disease may cause a change in the normal number or function of receptors, thereby altering their sensitivity (Stahl, 2008). It has been hypothesized that depression is caused by a reduction in the normal number of certain receptors, leading to an abnormality in their sensitivity to neurotransmitters such as serotonin and norepinephrine. A decreased response to continued stimulation of these receptors is usually referred to as *desensitization* or *refractoriness*. This suspected subsensitivity is referred to as *down-regulation* of the receptors.

Receptor Subtypes

The nervous system uses many different neurochemicals for communication, and each specific chemical messenger requires a specific receptor on which the chemical can act. More than 100 different chemical messengers have been identified, with new ones being uncovered frequently as research on the functioning of the brain becomes more and more precise. In addition to the sheer number of receptors needed to accommodate these chemicals, the neurotransmitters may produce different effects at different synaptic sites. The ability of a neurotransmitter to produce different actions is, in part, because of the specialization of its receptors. The different receptors for each neurochemical messenger are referred to as *receptor subtypes* for the chemical. Each major neurotransmitter has several different subtypes of receptors, allowing the neurotransmitter to have different effects in different areas of the brain. For example, dopamine, a common neurotransmitter discussed in the next section, has five different subtypes

of receptors that have been identified. Numbers usually name the receptor subtypes. In the example of dopamine, the various subtypes of receptors are called D_1, D_2, D_3, and so on. Knowledge of the different subtypes helps in understanding both the effects and side effects of medications used to treat mental disorders.

Neurotransmitters

Many substances have been identified as possible chemical messengers, but not all chemical messengers are neurotransmitters. Classic neurotransmitters are those that meet certain criteria agreed on by neuroscientists. The traditional criteria include the following:

- The chemical is synthesized inside the neuron.
- The chemical is present in the presynaptic terminals.
- The chemical is released into the synaptic cleft and causes a particular effect on the postsynaptic receptors.
- An exogenous form of the chemical administered as a drug causes identical action.
- The chemical is removed from the synaptic cleft by a specific mechanism.

Neurotransmitters can be grouped into categories that reflect chemical similarities of the neurotransmitter. Common practice classifies certain chemicals as neurotransmitters even though their ability to meet the strict traditional definition may be incomplete. For the purposes of this section, the classification of neurotransmitters will use this common system of classifying neurotransmitters. Common categories of neurotransmitters include the following:

- Cholinergic neurotransmitters
- Biogenic amine neurotransmitters (sometimes called *monoamines* or *bioamines*)
- Amino acid neurotransmitters
- Neuropeptide neurotransmitters

Neurotransmitters are also classified by whether their action causes physiologic activity to occur or to stop occurring. All of the neurotransmitters commonly involved in the development of mental illness or affected by the drugs used to treat these illnesses are excitatory except one, GABA, which is inhibitory. The significance of this concept is discussed in the section about amino acids. Neurotransmitters are found wherever there are neurons, and neurons are contained in both the CNS and PNS. Because psychiatric mental disorders occur in the CNS, the following sections discuss neurotransmitters from the perspective of the CNS.

Cholinegeric

ACh is a primary cholinergic neurotransmitter. Found in the greatest concentration in the PNS, ACh provides the basic synaptic communication for the parasympathetic neurons and part of the sympathetic neurons, which send information to the CNS. Understanding both the action of ACh and the receptor subtypes for this neurotransmitter assists PMH nurses in understanding the complex side effects of common medications used to treat mental disorders.

Cholinergic neurons, so named because they contain ACh, follow diffuse projections throughout the cerebral cortex and limbic system, arising primarily from cell bodies in the base of the frontal lobes. Pathways from this region also project throughout the hippocampus (Fig. 9-9). These connections suggest that ACh is involved in higher intellectual functioning and memory. Individuals who have Alzheimer's disease or Down's syndrome often exhibit patterns of cholinergic neuron loss in regions innervated by these pathways (such as the hippocampus), which may contribute to their memory difficulties and other cognitive deficits. Some cholinergic neurons are afferent to these areas bringing information from the limbic system, highlighting the role that ACh plays in communicating emotional state to the cerebral cortex. ACh is an excitatory neurotransmitter, meaning that when released into a synapse, it causes the postsynaptic neuron to initiate some action.

The subtypes of ACh receptors are divided into two groups: the muscarinic receptors and the nicotinic receptors. Many psychiatric medications are anticholinergic agents, which block the effects of the muscarinic ACh receptors. This blocking effect of ACh causes common side effects, such as dry mouth, blurred vision, constipation, urinary retention, and tachycardia, which are seen in many psychotropic medications. Excessive blockade of ACh can cause confusion and delirium, especially in

older patients, as discussed in Chapter 34. Table 9-5 lists the effects of ACh on various organs in the parasympathetic system. Awareness of what organs are impacted by different medications that impact ACh and other neurotransmitters will help nurses link medications with their effects.

Biogenic Amines

The **biogenic amines** (bioamines) consist of small molecules manufactured in the neuron that contain an amine group. These include dopamine, norepinephrine, and epinephrine, which are all synthesized from the amino acid tyrosine; serotonin, which is synthesized from tryptophan; and histamine, manufactured from histidine. Of all the neurotransmitters, the biogenic amines are most central to current hypotheses of psychiatric disorders and hence are described individually in more detail.

Dopamine

Dopamine is an excitatory neurotransmitter found in distinct regions of the CNS, and it is involved in cognitive, motor, and neuroendocrine functions. Dopamine levels are decreased in Parkinson's disease, and abnormally high production of dopamine has been associated with schizophrenia (see Chapter 20). Dopamine is also the neurotransmitter that stimulates the body's natural "feel good" reward pathways, producing pleasant euphoric sensation under certain conditions. Abnormalities of dopamine use within the reward system pathways are suspected to be a critical aspect of the development of drug and other addictions. The dopamine pathways are distinct neuronal areas within the CNS in which the neurotransmitter dopamine predominates. Three major dopaminergic pathways have been identified.

The mesocortical and mesolimbic pathways originate in the ventral tegmental area and project into the medial aspects of the cortex (mesocortical) and the medial aspects of the limbic system inside the temporal lobes, including the hippocampus and amygdala (mesolimbic). Sometimes they are considered to be one pathway and at other times two separate pathways. The mesocortical pathway has major effects on cognition, including such functions as judgment, reasoning, insight, social conscience, motivation, the ability to generalize learning, and reward systems in the human brain. It contributes to some of the highest seats of cortical functioning. The mesocortical system may be linked to the positive symptoms of schizophrenia. The mesolimbic pathway also strongly influences emotions and has projections that affect memory and auditory reception. Abnormalities in the mesolimbic system may be linked with negative symptoms of schizophrenia.

Another major dopaminergic pathway begins in the substantia nigra and projects into the basal ganglia, parts

FIGURE 9-9. Cholinergic pathways. HC, hippocampal formation; PSG, parasympathetic ganglion cell; RF, reticular formation; T, thalamus. (Adapted from Nolte, J. & Angevine, J. (1995). *The human brain: In photographs and diagrams.* St. Louis, MO: Mosby.)

of which are known as the *striatum*. This pathway, called the *nigrostriatal pathway*, influences the extrapyramidal motor system, which serves the voluntary motor system and allows involuntary motor movements. Destruction of dopaminergic neurons in this pathway has been associated with Parkinson's disease.

The last dopamine pathway originates from projections of the mesolimbic pathway and continues into the hypothalamus, which then projects into the pituitary gland. Therefore, this pathway, called the *tuberoinfundibular pathway*, has an impact on endocrine function and other functions, such as metabolism, hunger, thirst, sexual function, circadian rhythms, digestion, and temperature control. Figure 9-10 illustrates the dopaminergic pathways.

As noted previously, scientists have identified at least five subtypes of dopamine receptors in the CNS. These subtypes are distributed differently throughout the brain. For example, the D_1 subtype receptor and its related receptor subtype, D_5, predominate in areas that affect memory and emotions, such as the cortex, hippocampus, and amygdala. They have not been detected in the substantia nigra. D_2 receptors are richly distributed throughout the neurons in the extrapyramidal motor system, whereas D_4 receptors are richly distributed in the frontal cortex, with few in the nigrostriatal system. Antipsychotic

medications, discussed in Chapter 12, act by blocking the effects of dopamine at the receptor sites.

Many of the medications that are most effective on the acute symptoms of psychosis have a strong attraction or affinity for D_2 receptors and a weaker but modest correlation with D_1 receptors. Because D_2 receptors predominate in the nigrostriatal pathway, medications that have a weaker blockade of D_2 will have fewer extrapyramidal motor system effects. Side effects and adverse effects from the involuntary motor system are at times extremely debilitating to individuals. Based on the assumption that these dopamine receptor subtypes have different functions in the CNS, new medications are being designed to affect more predominantly one subtype than another, presumably avoiding effects on systems containing other subtypes and thus avoiding potential side effects of the medication. Researchers are attempting to develop new antipsychotic medications that avoid or minimize the effects on D_2 and therefore diminish the occurrence of extrapyramidal effects.

Norepinephrine

Norepinephrine was first demonstrated to be the primary neurotransmitter of the PNS in 1946. Whereas it is commonly found in the PNS, norepinephrine is also critical to CNS functioning. Norepinephrine is an excitatory neurochemical that plays a major role in generating and maintaining mood states. Decreased norepinephrine has been associated with depression, and excessive norepinephrine has been associated with manic symptoms. Because norepinephrine is so heavily concentrated in the terminal sites of sympathetic nerves, it can be released quickly to ready the individual for a fight-or-flight response to threats in the environment. For this reason, norepinephrine is thought to play a role in the physical symptoms of anxiety.

Nerve tracts and pathways containing predominantly norepinephrine are called *noradrenergic* and are less clearly delineated than the dopamine pathways. In the CNS, noradrenergic neurons originate in the locus caeruleus, where more than half of the noradrenergic cell bodies are located. Because the locus caeruleus is one of the major timekeepers of the human body, norepinephrine is involved in sleep and wakefulness. From the locus caeruleus, noradrenergic pathways ascend into the neocortex, spread diffusely (Fig. 9-11), and enhance the ability of neurons to respond to whatever input they may be receiving. In addition, norepinephrine appears to be involved in the process of reinforcement, which facilitates learning. Noradrenergic pathways innervate the hypothalamus and thus are involved to some degree in endocrine function. Anxiety disorders and depression are examples of psychiatric illnesses in which dysfunction of the noradrenergic neurons may be involved.

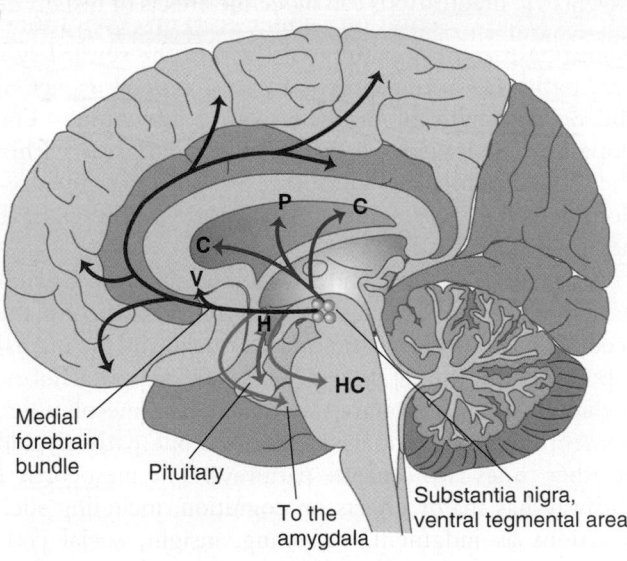

Medial forebrain bundle

Pituitary

To the amygdala

Substantia nigra, ventral tegmental area

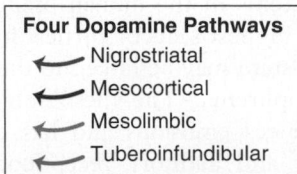

Four Dopamine Pathways
- Nigrostriatal
- Mesocortical
- Mesolimbic
- Tuberoinfundibular

FIGURE 9-10. Dopaminergic pathways. C, caudate nucleus; H, hypothalamus; HC, hippocampal formation; P, putamen; V, ventral striatum. (Adapted from Nolte, J. & Angevine, J. (1995). *The human brain: In photographs and diagrams.* St. Louis, MO: Mosby.)

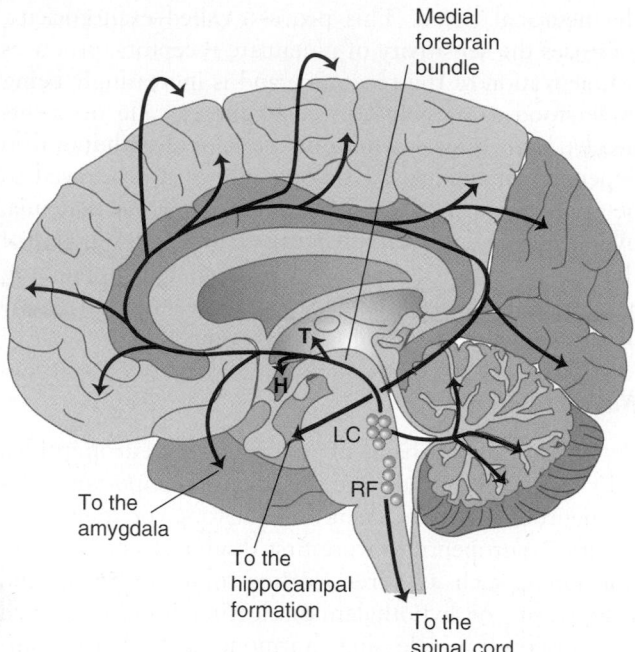

FIGURE 9-11. Noradrenergic pathways. H, hypothalamus; LC, locus caeruleus; RF, reticular formation; T, thalamus. (Adapted from Nolte, J. & Angevine, J. (1995). *The human brain: In photographs and diagrams.* St. Louis, MO: Mosby.)

Epinephrine

Epinephrine is very similar to norepinephrine chemically; however, in contrast to norepinephrine, only very small amounts of epinephrine are produced and released in the brain. Relatively few neurons in the brain use epinephrine as a neurotransmitter, and those are located in the caudal pons and the medulla. Epinephrine is found in much higher concentrations in the rest of the body, where it is secreted directly from the adrenal gland into the blood circulation.

Serotonin

Serotonin (also called 5-hydroxytryptamine or 5-HT) is primarily an excitatory neurotransmitter that is diffusely distributed within the cerebral cortex, limbic system, and basal ganglia of the CNS. Serotonergic neurons also project into the hypothalamus and cerebellum. Figure 9-12 illustrates serotonergic pathways. Serotonin plays a role in emotions, cognition, sensory perceptions, and essential biologic functions, such as sleep and appetite. During the rapid eye movement (REM) phase of sleep, or the dream state, serotonin concentrations decrease, and muscles subsequently relax. Serotonin is also involved in the control of food intake, hormone secretion, sexual behaviour, thermoregulation, and cardiovascular regulation. Some serotonergic fibres reach the cranial blood vessels within the brain and the pia mater, where they have a vasoconstrictive effect. The potency of some new medications for migraine headaches is related to their ability

to block serotonin transmission in the cranial blood vessels. Descending serotonergic pathways are important in central pain control. Depression and insomnia have been associated with decreased levels of serotonin, whereas mania has been associated with increased serotonin. Some of the most well-known antidepressant medications, such as Prozac and Zoloft, which are discussed in more depth in Chapter 12, function by raising serotonin levels within certain areas of the CNS (Stahl, 2008). Obsessive–compulsive disorder, panic disorder, and other anxiety disorders are believed to be associated with dysfunction of the serotonin pathways, explaining why antidepressant medications have several uses in treating mental disorders (Kapczinski, Lima, Souza, Cunha, & Schmitt, 2003).

Numerous subtypes of serotonin receptors also exist, and each of these appears to have a distinct function. 5-HT_{1a} is involved in the control of anxiety, aggression, and depression. Drugs such as lysergic acid diethylamide affect 5-HT_2 and produce hallucinatory effects.

Histamine

Histamine neurons originate predominantly in the hypothalamus and project to all major structures in the cerebrum, brain stem, and spinal cord. Exerting an influence in autonomic and neuroendocrine function, it is associated with many activities, including arousal, cognition, learning and memory, sleep, appetite, and seizures. Many psychiatric medications can block the effects of histamine postsynaptically and produce side effects such as sedation, weight gain, and hypotension.

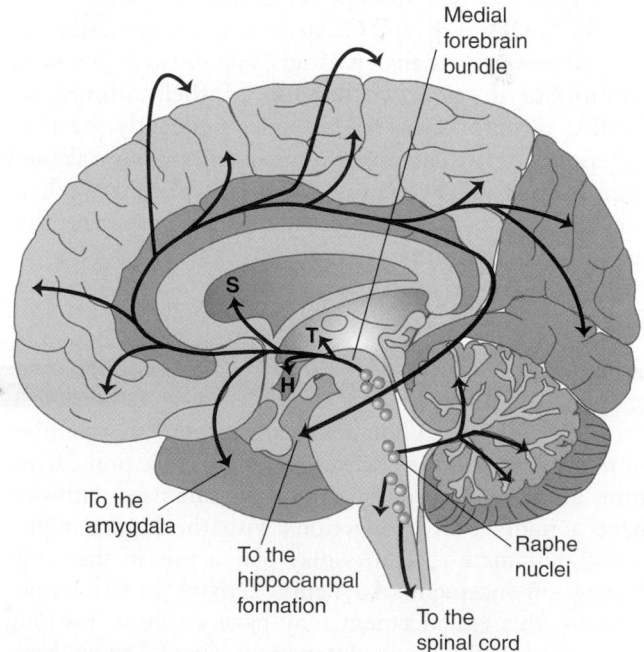

FIGURE 9-12. Serotonergic pathways. H, hypothalamus; S, septal nuclei; T, thalamus. (Adapted from Nolte, J. & Angevine, J. (1995). *The human brain: In photographs and diagrams.* St. Louis, MO: Mosby.)

Amino Acids

Amino acids are the building blocks of proteins and have many roles in intraneuronal metabolism. In addition, amino acids can function as neurotransmitters in as many as 60% to 70% of the synaptic sites in the brain. Amino acids are the most prevalent neurotransmitters. Virtually all of the neurons in the CNS are activated by excitatory amino acids, such as glutamate, and inhibited by inhibitory amino acids, such as GABA and glycine. Many of these amino acids coexist with other neurotransmitters.

γ-Aminobutyric Acid

GABA is the primary inhibitory neurotransmitter for the CNS. The pathways of GABA exist almost exclusively in the CNS, with the largest GABA concentrations in the hypothalamus, hippocampus, basal ganglia, spinal cord, and cerebellum. GABA functions in an inhibitory role in control of spinal reflexes and cerebellar reflexes. It has a major role in the control of neuronal excitability through the brain. In addition, GABA has an inhibitory influence on the activity of the dopaminergic nigrostriatal projections. GABA also has interconnections with other neurotransmitters. For example, dopamine inhibits cholinergic neurons, and GABA provides feedback and balance.

When a person feels threatened, GABA levels drop (Hasler, van der Veen, Grillon, Drevets, & Shen, 2010), and dysregulation of GABA and GABA receptors have been associated with anxiety disorders. Decreased GABA activity is involved in the development of seizure disorders. Three specific subtype receptors have been identified for GABA: A, B, and C. Alcohol, certain anaesthetics, benzodiazepine antianxiety drugs, and sedative–hypnotic barbiturate drugs work because of their affinity for GABA$_A$ receptor sites. PMH nurses frequently see alcohol used to self-treat anxiety; understanding how alcohol impacts the GABA receptors will help explain this behaviour. Interest in the beneficial effects of these drugs has led to increased interest in GABA receptor sites.

Glutamate

Glutamate, the most widely distributed excitatory neurotransmitter, is the main transmitter in the associational areas of the cortex. Glutamate can be found in a number of pathways from the cortex to the thalamus, pons, striatum, and spinal cord. In addition, glutamate pathways have a number of connections with the hippocampus. Some glutamate receptors may play a role in the long-lasting enhancement of synaptic activity. In the hippocampus, this enhancement may have a role in learning and memory. Too much glutamate is harmful to neurons, and considerable interest has emerged regarding its neurotoxic effects.

Conditions that produce an excess of endogenous glutamate can cause neurotoxicity by overexcitation of the neuronal tissue. This process, called excitotoxicity, increases the sensitivity of glutamate receptors, produces overactivation of the receptors, and is increasingly being understood as a critical piece of the cascade of events involved in physical symptoms of alcohol withdrawal in dependent individuals. Excitotoxicity is also believed to be part of the pathology of conditions such as ischemia, hypoxia, hypoglycemia, and hepatic failure. Dysfunction of the glutamate system may be involved in depression, drug addiction, psychosis, fragile X syndrome, and Parkinson's disease (Ouellet-Plamondon & George, 2012).

Neuropeptides

Peptides are short chains of amino acids. **Neuropeptides** exist in the CNS and have a number of important roles as neurotransmitters, neuromodulators, or neurohormones. Neuropeptides were first thought to be pituitary hormones, such as adrenocorticotropin, oxytocin, and vasopressin, or hypothalamic-releasing hormones, such as corticotropin-releasing hormone and thyrotropin-releasing hormone (TRH). However, when an endogenous morphine-like substance was discovered in the 1970s, the term *endorphin*, or endogenous morphine, was introduced. Although amino acids and monoamine neurotransmitters can be produced directly from dietary precursors in any part of the neuron, neuropeptides are, almost without exception, synthesized from messenger RNA in the cell body. To date, two types of neuropeptides have been identified: opioid and nonopioid. Opioid neuropeptides, such as endorphins, enkephalins, and dynorphins, act in endocrine functioning and pain suppression. Nonopioid neuropeptides, such as substance P and somatostatin, play roles in pain transmission and endocrine functioning.

There are considerable variations in the distribution of individual neuropeptides, but some areas are especially rich in cell bodies containing neuropeptides. These areas include the amygdala, striatum, hypothalamus, raphe nuclei, brain stem, and spinal cord. Many of the interneurons of the cerebral cortex contain neuropeptides, but there are considerably fewer in the thalamus and almost none in the cerebellum.

The complexities of neuronal transmission are enormous. PMH nurses have a significant role in assessing symptoms and administering and monitoring medications for patients with psychiatric disorders. Knowledge of neurotransmitters is essential because even a single dose of a drug affecting this system may cause relief of symptoms or have adverse effects. The actions of psychopharmacologic agents and related nursing responsibilities are discussed more fully in Chapter 12. In addition, many nursing interventions designed to effect changes in such functions as sleep, diet, stress management, exercise, and mood modulation affect these neurotransmitters and neuropeptides, directly or indirectly. More research is needed to understand the bio/psycho/social/spiritual aspects of nursing care.

▬▬ NEW FIELDS OF STUDY

As the complexity of the nervous system and its interrelationship with other body systems and the environment have become more fully understood, new fields of study have emerged. From the discussion of neuroanatomy and neurotransmitters, it is logical to deduce that understanding the endocrine system and its interrelationship with the nervous system is essential. Although it has long been observed that individuals under stress have compromised immune systems and are more likely to acquire common diseases, only recently have changes in the immune system been linked to some psychiatric illnesses (Capuron & Miller, 2011; Fetissov & Déchelotte, 2008). In addition, as biologic rhythms have become more fully understood and defined, new information suggests that dysfunction of these rhythms may not only result from a psychiatric illness but also contribute to its development. Therefore, the following sections provide a brief overview of psychoendocrinology, psychoneuroimmunology, and chronobiology.

Psychoendocrinology

Psychoendocrinology examines the relationships among the nervous system, endocrine system, and behaviour. Messages are conveyed within the endocrine system mainly by hormones, and neurohormones are those substances excreted by special neurons within the nervous system. Neurohormones are cellular substances and are secreted into the bloodstream and transported to a site where they exert their effect. Of the several types of hormones, peptides are the most common hormones in the CNS.

The hypothalamus sends and receives information through the pituitary, which then communicates with structures in the peripheral aspects of the body. Figure 9-13 presents an example of the communication of the anterior pituitary with a number of organs and structures. Axes, the structures within which the neurohormones are providing messages, are the most often studied aspect of the neuroendocrine system. These axes always involve a feedback mechanism. For example, the hypothalamic–pituitary–thyroid axis regulates the release of thyroid hormone by the thyroid gland using TRH hormone from the hypothalamus to the pituitary and TSH from the pituitary to the thyroid. Figure 9-14 illustrates the hypothalamic–pituitary–thyroid axis. The hypothalamic–pituitary–gonadal axis regulates estrogen and testosterone secretion through LH and FSH.

Interest in psychoendocrinology is heightened by various endocrine disorders that produce psychiatric symptoms. Addison's disease (hypoadrenalism) produces depression, apathy, fatigue, and occasionally psychosis. Hypothyroidism produces depression and some anxiety. Administration of steroids can cause depression, hypomania, irritability, and in some cases, psychosis. Some psychiatric disorders have been associated with endocrine system dysfunction. For example, some individuals with mood disorders show evidence of dysregulation in the adrenal, thyroid, and GH axes.

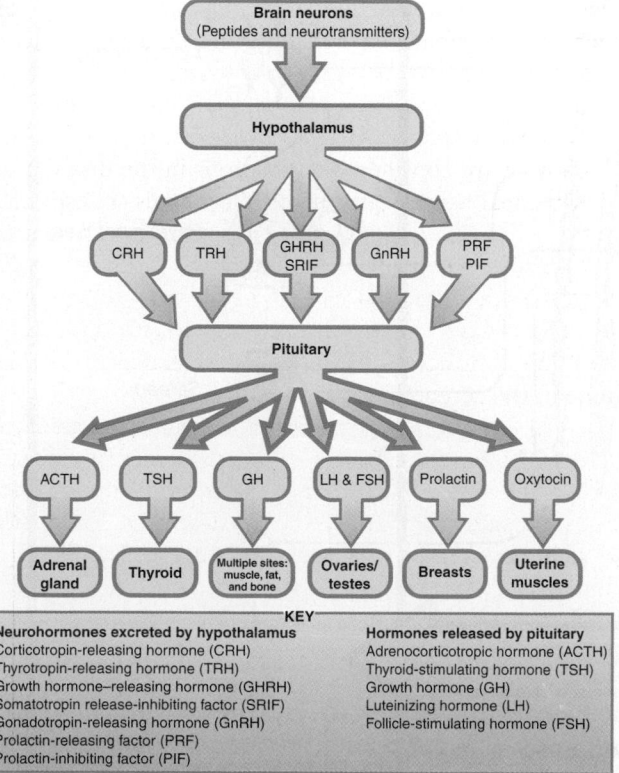

FIGURE 9-13. Hypothalamic and pituitary communication system. The neurohormonal communication system between the hypothalamus and the pituitary exerts effects on many organs and systems.

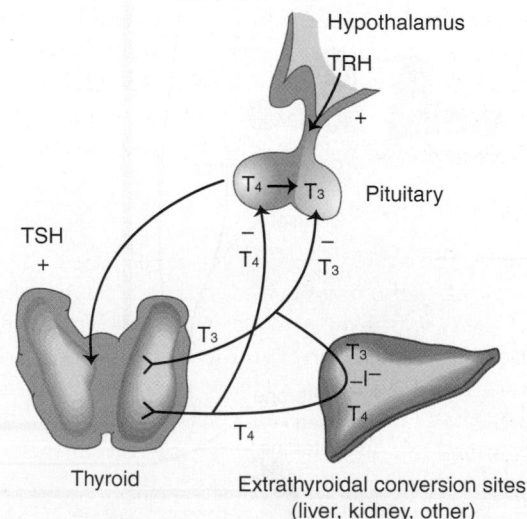

FIGURE 9-14. Hypothalamic–pituitary–thyroid axis. The regulation of thyroid-stimulating hormone (TSH or thyrotropin) secretion by the anterior pituitary. Positive effects of thyrotropin-releasing hormone (TRH) from the hypothalamus and negative effects of circulating triiodothyronine (T_3) and T_3 from intrapituitary conversion of thyroxine (T_4).

Psychoneuroimmunology

Psychoneuroimmunology is the study of immunology as it relates to emotions and behaviour. The immune system protects the body from foreign pathogens. Overactivity of the immune system can occur in autoimmune diseases such as systemic lupus erythematosus, allergies, or anaphylaxis. Too little activity may result from cancer and serious infections, as is the case with AIDS. Evidence suggests that communication between the nervous system and the immune system is bidirectional. Specific immune system dysfunctions may result

from damage to the hypothalamus, hippocampus, or pituitary and may produce symptoms of psychiatric disorders. Negative events and emotions influence catecholamines (norepinephrine and epinephrine), ACTH, cortisol, GH, and prolactin (Christensen, 2008). Each of these hormones can affect the immune function. Figure 9-15 illustrates the interaction between stress and the immune system. This figure also demonstrates the true bio/psycho/social/spiritual nature of the complex interrelationship of the nervous system, the endocrine system, the immune system, and environmental or emotional stress.

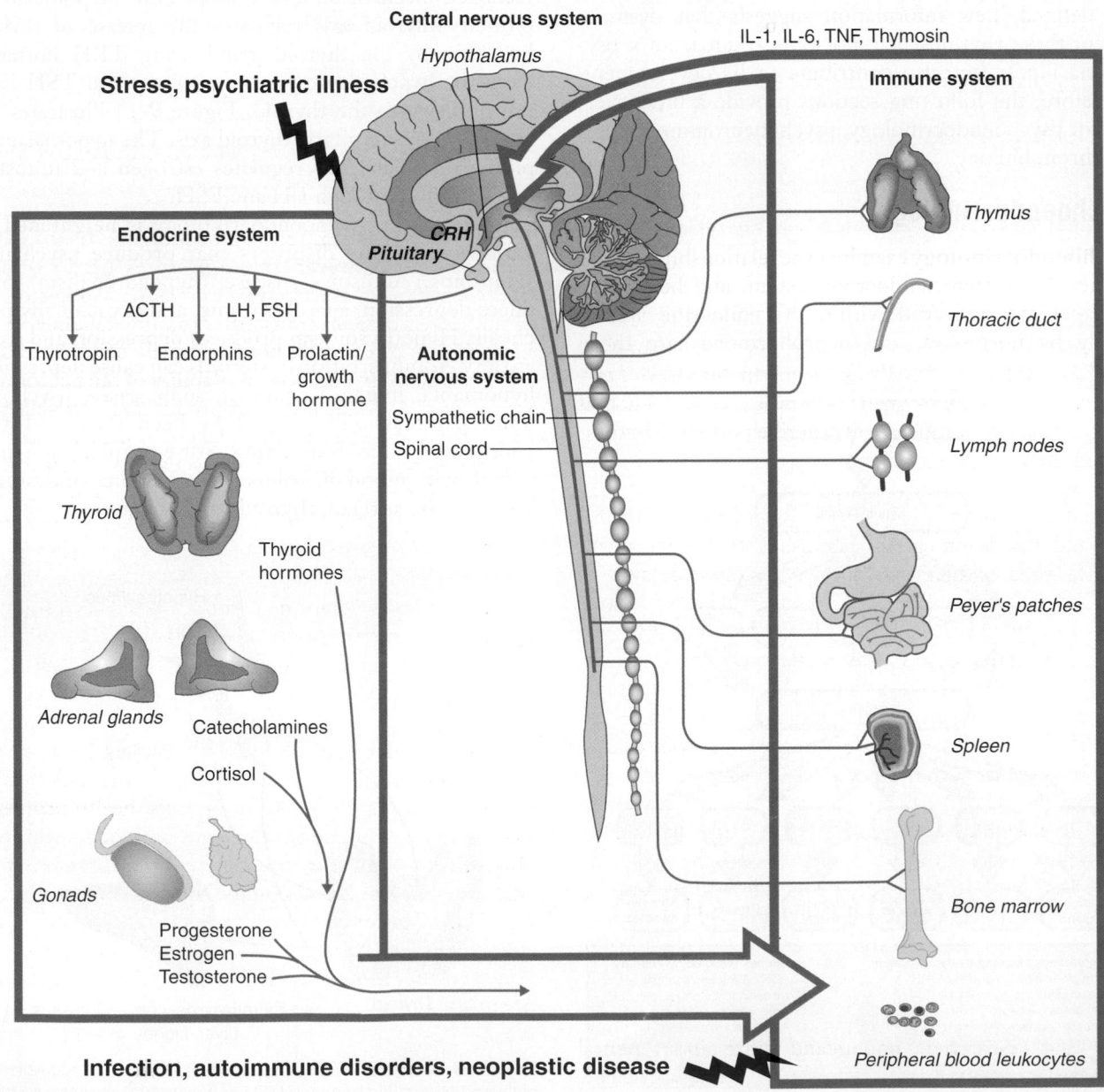

FIGURE 9-15. Examples of the interaction between stress or psychiatric illness and the immune system through the endocrine system. ACTH, adrenocorticotropic hormone; CRH, corticotropin-releasing hormone; FSH, follicle-stimulating hormone; IL, interleukin; LH, luteinizing hormone; TNF, tumour necrosis factor.

Immune dysregulation may also be involved in the development of psychiatric disorders. This can occur by allowing neurotoxins to affect the brain, damaging the neuroendocrine tissue or damaging tissues in the brain at locations such as the receptor sites. Some antidepressants have been thought to have antiviral effects. Symptoms of diseases such as depression may follow an occurrence of serious infection, and prenatal exposure to infectious organisms may be associated with the development of schizophrenia. Stress and conditioning have specific effects on the suppression of immune function.

Cytokines are hormone-like proteins that control the intensity and duration of the body's immune response. An example of a cytokine is interferon alpha, a medication used in the treatment of cancer and hepatitis. Unfortunately, up to 45% of people treated with interferon develop major depression (Capuron & Miller, 2011). Depression and anxiety are linked to cytokines that promote inflammation (Christensen, 2008). Although there is still much to learn about the relationship of psychiatric disorders and the immune system, it is clear that PMH nurses must develop and implement interventions designed to enhance immune function in psychiatric patients.

Chronobiology

Chronobiology involves the study and measure of time structures or biologic rhythms. Some rhythms have a **circadian cycle**, or 24-hour cycle, whereas others, such as the menstrual cycle, operate in different periods. Rhythms exist in the human body to control endocrine secretions, sleep–wake cycles, body temperature, neurotransmitter synthesis, and more. These cycles may become deregulated and may begin earlier than usual, known as a phase advance, or later than usual, known as a phase delay.

Zeitgebers are specific events that function as time givers or synchronizers and that set biologic rhythms. Light is the most common example of an external zeitgeber. The suprachiasmatic nucleus of the hypothalamus is an example of an internal zeitgeber. Some theorists think that psychiatric disorders may result from one or more biologic rhythm dysfunctions. For example, depression may in part be a phase advance disorder, including early-morning awakening and decreased time of onset of REM sleep. Seasonal affective disorder may be the result of shortened exposure to light during the winter months. Exposure to specific artificial light often relieves symptoms of fatigue, overeating, hypersomnia, and depression.

■ DIAGNOSTIC APPROACHES

Now that researchers understand more about neural transmission, brain functioning, and psychopharmacology, focus is shifting to applying the knowledge in order to find biologic markers for the psychiatric disorders previously thought to have only a psychological component.

Biologic markers are diagnostic test findings that occur only in the presence of the psychiatric disorder and include such findings as laboratory and other diagnostic test results and neuropathologic changes noticeable in assessment. These markers increase diagnostic certainty and reliability and may have predictive value, allowing for the possibility of preventive interventions to forestall or avoid the onset of illness.

In addition, biologic markers could assist in developing evidence-based care practices. If markers can be used reliably, they would help identify the most effective treatments and determine the expected prognosis for given conditions. The PMH nurse should be aware of the most current information on biologic markers so that information, limitations, and results can be discussed knowledgeably with the patient.

Laboratory Tests and Neurophysiologic Procedures

For many years, laboratory tests have been used in the attempt to measure levels of neurotransmitters and other CNS substances in the bloodstream. Many of the metabolites of neurotransmitters can be found in the urine and CSF as well. However, these measures have had only limited utility in elucidating what is happening in the brain. Levels of neurotransmitters and metabolites in the bloodstream or urine do not necessarily equate with levels in the CNS. In addition, availability of the neurotransmitter or metabolite does not predict the availability of the neurotransmitter in the synapse, where it must act or directly relate to the receptor sensitivity. However, in addition to neuroimaging procedures like MRIs, studies of fresh brain tissue removed in neurosurgery and postmortem studies have helped localize neurotransmitters, their function, and pharmacologic properties. These studies have provided clues but are not conclusive and therefore are not routinely used.

Although no commonly used laboratory tests exist that directly confirm a mental disorder, laboratory tests are still an active part of care and assessment of psychiatric patients. Many physical conditions mimic the symptoms of mental illness, and many of the medications used to treat psychiatric illness can produce health problems. For these reasons, the routine care of patients with psychiatric disorders includes the use of laboratory tests such as complete blood counts, thyroid studies, electrolytes, hepatic enzymes, and other evaluative tests. PMH nurses need to be familiar with these procedures and assist patients in understanding the use and implications of such tests.

Electroencephalography

Developed in the 1920s by Hans Berger, an electroencephalograph (EEG) measures electrical activity in the uppermost layers of the cortex. Electrodes are placed on

8 to 20 sites upon the patient's scalp. The EEG machine is equipped with graph paper and recording pens that trace the electrical impulses generated over each electrode. Until the use of CT scanning in the 1970s, the EEG was the only method for identifying brain abnormalities. It remains the simplest and least invasive method for identifying some disorders.

An EEG may be used in psychiatry to differentiate possible causes of a patient's symptoms. For example, some types of seizure disorders, such as temporal lobe epilepsy, head injuries, or tumours, may present with predominantly psychiatric symptoms. In addition, metabolic dysfunction, delirium, dementia, altered levels of consciousness, hallucinations, and dissociative states may require EEG evaluation.

Normal patterns seen on EEGs are called alpha, beta, theta, and delta waves; the rhythms may vary depending on the age of the person. Factors that may interfere with obtaining accurate results include being unable to remain still or cooperate during the test, being hypoglycemic or hypothermic, and hair that is dirty, oily, or treated with hair products. Spikes and wave-pattern changes are indications of brain abnormalities. Spikes may be the focal point from which a seizure occurs. However, abnormal activity often is not discovered on a routine EEG while the individual is awake. For this reason, additional methods are sometimes used. Nasopharyngeal leads may be used to get physically closer to the limbic regions. The patient may be exposed to a flashing strobe light while the examiner looks for activity that is not in phase with the flashing light, or may be asked to hyperventilate for 3 minutes to induce abnormal activity if it exists. Sleep deprivation may also be used. This involves keeping the patient awake throughout the night before the EEG evaluation. The patient may then be drowsy and fall asleep during the procedure.

Abnormalities are more likely to occur when the patient is asleep. Sleep may also be induced using medication; however, EEG wave patterns can be affected by medications such as anticonvulsants and anxiolytics, as well as by other substances that act as sedatives or stimulants. For example, the benzodiazepine class of drugs increases the rapid and fast beta activity and lithium increases theta activity. In addition to reassuring, preparing, and educating the patient for the examination, the nurse should carefully assess the history of substance use and report this information to the examiner. If a sleep deprivation EEG is to be done, caffeine or other stimulants that might help the patient stay awake should be withheld because they may change the EEG patterns.

FIGURE 9-16. Bio/psycho/social/spiritual etiologies for patients with generalized anxiety disorders. GABA, γ-aminobutyric acid; SNS, sympathetic nervous system.

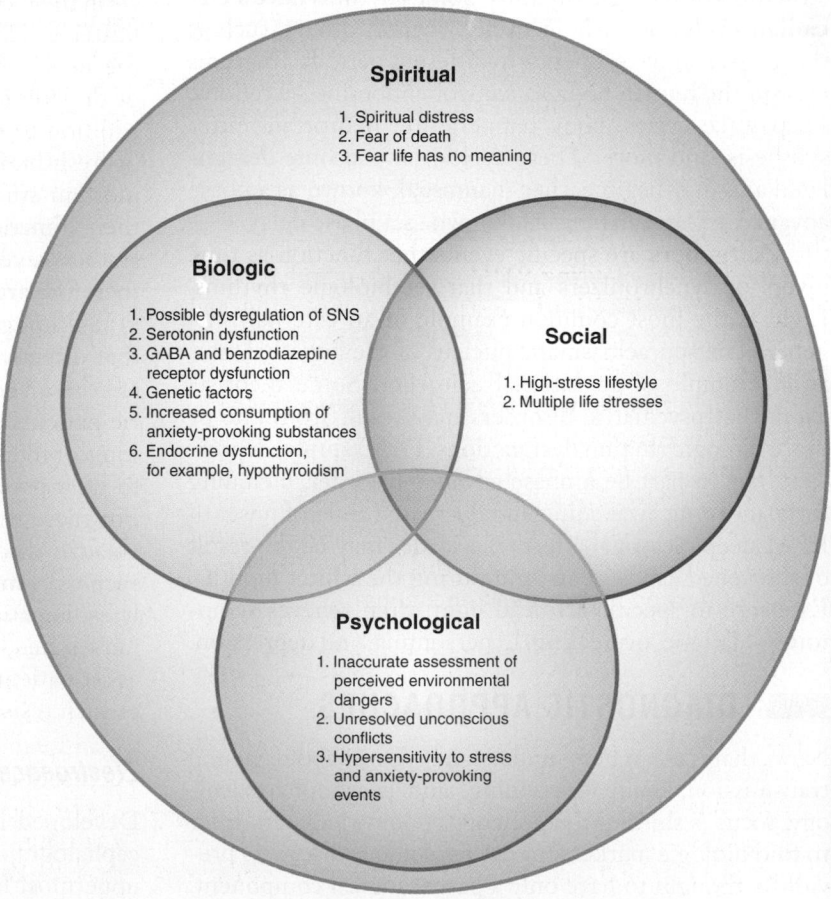

Polysomnography

Polysomnography is a special procedure that involves recording the EEG throughout a night of sleep. See Chapter 28 for a discussion of sleep studies.

Other Neurophysiologic Methods

Evoked potentials (EPs), also called event-related potentials, use the same basic principles as an EEG. They measure changes in electrical activity in the visual, somatosensory, and auditory pathways in response to a given stimulus. Electrodes placed on the scalp measure a large waveform that stands out after the administration of repetitive stimuli, such as a click or flash of light. There are several different types of EPs to be measured, depending on the sensory area affected by the stimulus, the cognitive task required, or the region monitored, any of which can change the length of time until the wave occurrence. EPs are used extensively in psychiatric research. In clinical practice, EPs are used primarily in the assessment of demyelinating disorders, such as multiple sclerosis.

● **STUDY NOTE**

A nurse who assumes that mental health problems (e.g., difficulty managing anger) are of a primarily psychosocial nature may overlook the direct influence of biologic factors.

INTEGRATION OF THE BIOLOGIC, PSYCHOLOGIC, SOCIAL, AND SPIRITUAL DOMAINS

Basic knowledge in the neurosciences has become essential content for the practising PMH nurse. In a truly holistic bio/psycho/social/spiritual model, all psychological and social influences are seen as interacting with the complex human biologic system. For example, treatment of generalized anxiety disorder would involve addressing etiologies in each of these areas (see Fig. 9-16). As research continues to increase our understanding of the biologic dimension of psychiatric disorders and mental health, nursing care will focus on human biology in increasingly sophisticated ways. PMH nurses must integrate this information into all aspects of nursing management, including

● Assessment—genetic, physical, and environmental factors that contribute to the symptoms of psychiatric disorders; biologic rhythm changes; cognitive abilities that may affect or complicate interventions; and risk factors that may predict development of psychiatric symptoms or disorders

● Diagnosis—difficulties related to diet, exercise, or sleep that may change the individual's biology; quality-of-life difficulties based on biologic changes; and knowledge deficits concerning the biologic basis of psychiatric disorders or treatment

● Interventions—designed to modify biologic changes and physical functioning; designed to enhance biologic treatments; or modified to consider cognitive dysfunction related to psychiatric disorders.

SUMMARY OF KEY POINTS

■ Neuroscientists now view behaviour and cognitive function as results of complex interactions within the CNS and its plasticity or its ability to adapt and change in both structure and function.

■ Each hemisphere of the brain is divided into four lobes. The frontal lobe controls motor speech function, personality, and working memory—often called the executive functions that govern one's ability to plan and initiate action. The parietal lobe controls sensory functions. The temporal lobe contains the primary auditory and olfactory areas. The occipital lobe controls visual integration of information.

■ The structures of the limbic system are integrally involved in memory and emotional behaviour. Dysfunction of the limbic system has been linked with major mental disorders, including schizophrenia, depression, and anxiety disorders.

■ Neurons communicate with each other through synaptic transmission. Neurotransmitters excite or inhibit a response at the receptor sites and have been linked to certain mental disorders. These neurotransmitters include Ach, dopamine, norepinephrine, serotonin, GABA, and glutamate.

■ Psychoendocrinology examines the relationship between the nervous system and endocrine system and the effects of neurohormones excreted by special neurons to communicate with the endocrine system in effecting behaviour. Psychoneuroimmunology focuses on the nervous system as regulating immune function, which may play a significant role in effecting psychological states and psychiatric disorders. Chronobiology focuses on the study and measure of time structures or biologic rhythms occurring in the body and associates dysregulation of these cycles as contributing factors to the development of psychiatric disorders.

■ Biologic markers are physical indicators of disturbances within the CNS that differentiate one disease process from another, such as biochemical changes or neuropathologic changes. These biologic markers can be measured by several methods of testing, including electroencephalography, polysomnography, EPs, CT scanning, MRI, PET, and SPECT. The PMH nurse must be familiar with each of these.

CRITICAL THINKING CHALLENGES

1 Explain the significance of mental disorders being described as *polygenetic*.

2 A patient who is scheduled for MRI asks how this test can possibly help explain why he is "all nerved up." He states that his friend had a CT scan, and he wants that instead. What would you say to assist this patient in understanding the difference between the two tests?

3 Define the five different approaches to the study of neuroanatomy and discuss their utility in understanding mental disorders.

4 A woman who has experienced a "ministroke" continues to regain lost cognitive function months after the stroke. Her husband takes this as evidence that she never had a stroke. How would you approach patient teaching and counselling for this couple to help them understand this occurrence if the stroke did damage to her brain?

5 Choose a patient for whom you are caring. Review his or her psychotropic medications and discuss their impact on the patient's CNS. Discuss what side effects might be seen and why.

6 Mr. S is unable to sleep after watching an upsetting documentary. Identify the neurotransmitter activity that may be interfering with his sleep. (Hint: fight-or-flight.)

7 Describe what behavioural symptoms or problems may be present in a patient with dysfunction of the following brain areas:
   a Basal ganglia
   b Hippocampus
   c Limbic system
   d Thalamus
   e Hypothalamus
   f Frontal lobe

8 Compare and contrast the functions of the sympathetic and parasympathetic nervous systems.

9 Discuss the steps in synaptic transmission, beginning with the action potential and ending with how the neurotransmitter no longer communicates its message to the receiving neuron.

10 Examine how a receptor's usual response to a neurotransmitter might change.

11 Compare the role of dopamine and Ach in the CNS.

12 Explain how dopamine, norepinephrine, and serotonin all contribute to endocrine system regulation. Suggest some other transmitters that may affect endocrine function.

13 Discuss how the fields of psychoendocrinology, psychoneuroimmunology, and chronobiology overlap.

14 Compare the methods used to find biologic markers of psychiatric disorders reviewed in this chapter. Consider the potential risks and benefits to the patient.

15 Determine the actions you would take in preparing a patient for an MRI scan.

16 Ask a psychiatric clinician, "What is the greatest diagnostic mystery you've encountered?"

REFERENCES

Amen, D., Newberg, A., Thatcher, R., Jin, Y., Wu, J., Keator, D., & Willeumier, K. (2010). Impact of playing American professional football on long-term brain function. *Journal of Neuropsychiatry and Clinical Neurosciences, 23*, 98–106.

Brzustowicz, L. & Freedman, R. (2011). Digging more deeply for genetic effects in psychiatric illness. *American Journal of Psychiatry, 168*, 1017–1020.

Capuron, L. & Miller, A. (2011). Immune system to brain signaling: Neuropsychopharmacological implications. *Pharmacology and Therapeutics, 130*, 226–238.

Christensen, J. (2008). Stress & disease. In M. Feldman & J. Christensen (Eds.), *Behavioral medicine: A guide for clinical practice* (3rd ed.). New York: McGraw-Hill.

Currie, S., Hadjivassiliou, M., Crave, I., Wilkinson, I., Griffiths, P., & Hoggard, N. (2013). Magnetic resonance spectroscopy of the brain. *Postgraduate Medical Journal, 89*, 94–106.

Eapen, V. (2012). Neurodevelopmental genes have not read the DSM criteria: Or have they? *Frontiers in Psychiatry, 3*, 75.

Fetissov, S. & Déchelotte, R. (2008). The putative role of neuropeptide autoantibodies in anorexia nervosa. *Current Opinion in Clinical Nutrition and Metabolic Care, 11*, 428–434.

Gräff, J., Rei, D., Guan, J. S., Wang, W. Y., Seo, I. Henning, K., … Tsai, L. H. (2012). An epigenetic blockade of cognitive functions in the neurodegenerating brain [Letter]. *Nature, 483*, 222–228.

Graves, W. (2013, January 15). "Sidney Crosby says he's free of concussion symptoms." Associated Press.

Harlow, J. M. (1868). Recovery after severe injury to the head. *Publication of the Massachusetts Medical Society, 2*, 327.

Hasler, G., van der Veen, J., Grillon, C., Drevets, W., & Shen, J. (2010). Effect of acute psychological stress on prefrontal GABA concentration determined by proton magnetic resonance spectroscopy. *American Journal of Psychiatry, 167*, 1226–1231.

Hennig, J., Speck, O., Koch, M. A., & Weiller, C. (2003). Functional magnetic resonance imaging: A review of methodological aspects and clinical applications. *Journal of Magnetic Resonance Imaging, 18*(1), 1–15.

Holtzheimer, P. E. (2013). Unipolar depression in adults: Treatment with transcranial magnetic stimulation (TMS). Retrieved from http://www.uptodate.com/index

Kapadia, R. K. & Bassett, A. S. (2008). Recognizing a common genetic syndrome: 22q11.2 deletion syndrome. *Canadian Medical Association Journal, 178*, 391–393.

Kapczinski, F., Lima, M. S., Souza, J. S., Cunha, A., & Schmitt, R. (2003). Antidepressants for generalized anxiety disorder (Cochrane Review). *Cochrane Database of Systematic Reviews, 2*, CD003592.

Kleim, J. & Jones, T. A. (2008). Principles of experience-dependent neuroplasticity: Implications for rehabilitation after brain damage. *Journal of Speech, Language, and Hearing Research, 51*, S225–S239.

Kundu, T. K. (Ed.). (2013). *Epigenetics: Development and disease*. New York: Springer.

Labonté, B., Suderman, M., Maussion, G., Lopex, J. P., Navarro-Sánchez, L., Yerko, V. G., … Turecki, G. (2013). Genome-wide methylation changes in the brains of suicide completers. *American Journal of Psychiatry, 170*(5), 511–520.

Marques, S. & Fleming Outeiro, T. (2013). Epigenetics in Parkinson's and Alzheimer's Diseases. In T. K. Kundu (Ed.), *Epigenetics: Development and disease* (pp. 507–525). New York: Springer.

Marx, V. (2012). Reading the second genomic code. *Nature, 491*, 143–147.

McGuffin, P. & Southwick, L. (2003). Fifty years of the double helix and its impact on psychiatry. *Australian and New Zealand Journal of Psychiatry, 37*, 657–661.

Miglioretti, D. & Simth-Bindman, R. (2011). Overuse of computed tomography and associated risks. *American Family Physician, 83*, 1252–1254.

Morrish, J. & Carey, S. (2013). Concussions in Canada. *Canada Injury Compass, Spring 2013*. Toronto, Canada: Parachute.

National Human Genome Research Institute. (2013). *Fact sheets: Epigenomics*. National Institutes of Health. Retrieved from http://www.genome.gov/27532724

National Institute on Aging. (2011; updated April, 2013). *Biology of aging: Research today for a better tomorrow*. US Department of Health and Human Services. Retrieved from http://www.nia.nih.gov/health/publication/biology-aging

Nolte, J. & Angevine, J. (1995). *The human brain: In photographs and diagrams*. St. Louis, MO: Mosby.

Ouellet-Plamondon, C. & George, T. (2012). Glutamate and psychiatry in 2012: Up, up and away! Retrieved from http://www.psychiatrictimes.com/bipolar-disorder/glutamate-and-psychiatry-2012%E2%80%94-and-away

Pearson-Fuhrhop, K., Burke, E., & Cramer, S. (2012). The influence of genetic factors on brain plasticity and recovery after neural injury. *Current Opinion in Neurology, 25*(6), 682–688.

Penzes, P., Cahill, M., Jones, K., VanLeeuwen, J. E., & Woolfrey, K. (2011). Dendritic spine pathology in neuropsychiatric disorders. *Nature Neuroscience, 14,* 285–293.

Schaffe, E. E. & Lytle, I. M. (1980). *Basic physiology and anatomy.* Philadelphia, PA: J.B. Lippincott.

Schauf, C., Moffett, D., & Moffett, S. (1990). *Human physiology.* St. Louis, MO: Times Mirror/Mosby.

Shah, M. & Allegrucci, C. (2013). Stem cell plasticity in development and cancer: Epigenetic origin of cancer stem cells. In T. K. Kandu (Ed.). *Epigenetics: Development and disease* (pp. 545–565). New York: Springer.

Shenton, M., Hamoda, H., Schneiderman, J., Bouiz, S., Pasternak, O., Rathi, Y., … Zafonte, R. (2012). A review of magnetic resonance imaging and diffusion tensor imaging findings in mild traumatic brain injury. *Brain Imaging and Behavior, 6,* 137–192.

Shiloh, R., Weizman, A., Epstein, Y., Rosenberg, S. L., Valevski, A., Dorfman-Etrog, P., … Hermesh, H. (2001). Abnormal thermoregulation in drug-free male schizophrenia patients. *European Neuropsychopharmacology, 11*(4), 285–288.

Simmons, D. (2008). Epigenetic influence and disease. Retrieved from http://www.nature.com/scitable/topicpage/epigenetic-influences-and-disease-895

Sofroniew, M. & Vinters, H. (2010). Astrocytes: Biology and pathology. *Acta Neuropathologica, 119,* 7–35.

Stahl, S. (2008). *Stahl's essential psychopharmacology: Neuroscientific basis and practical applications* (3rd ed.). New York: Cambridge University Press.

Waddington, C. (1957). *The strategy of the genes: A discussion of some aspects of theoretical biology.* London, UK: Allen & Unwin.

Wyshynski, G. (2011). Sidney Crosby talks concussion, "irresponsible" blindside hits and when Penguins knew about injury. Retrieved from http://ca.sports.yahoo.com/nhl/blog/puck_daddy/post/Sidney-Crosby-talks-concussion-irresponsible-?urn=nhl-305051

Interventions in Psychiatric and Mental Health Nursing Practice

UNIT
3

CHAPTER 10

The Assessment Process

Gerri Lasiuk and Kathleen Hegadoren
Adapted from the chapter "The Assessment Process" by Mary Ann Boyd

LEARNING OBJECTIVES

After studying this chapter, you will be able to:

- Identify assessment as part of the nursing process.
- Define assessment.
- Differentiate comprehensive and focused assessments.
- Explain the role of observation, interviewing, examination, and consultation in the performance of psychiatric/mental health assessment.
- Identify important areas of assessment for the biologic, psychological, and social domains of a psychiatric/mental health nursing assessment.
- Discuss the synthesis of the bio/psycho/social/spiritual assessment data.

KEY CONCEPTS

- assessment
- mental status examination

KEY TERMS

- affect • comprehensive assessment • delusion • dysphoria • euphoria • euthymic • focused assessment • hallucination • illusion • insight • judgment • level of consciousness • mental status examination • mood • nursing process • objective data • orientation • perception • promotive factors • protective factors • risk factors • subjective data • thought content • thought process

The **nursing process** is a systematic and dynamic approach to collecting and analyzing client information and is the first step in the provision of nursing care. The four essential components of the nursing process are assessment, planning, implementation, and evaluation. This chapter deals with **assessment**—activities involved with the collection, validation, analysis, synthesis, and documentation of information concerning clients' responses to health and illness.

ASSESSMENT AS A PROCESS

Standard II of the *Canadian Standards of Psychiatric and Mental Health Nursing* states:

> Effective assessment, diagnosis, and monitoring is central to the nurse's role and depends upon theory as well as upon understanding the meaning of the health or illness experience from the perspective of the client. The nurse

explains the assessment process to the client and provides feedback. Knowledge is integrated with the nurse's conceptual model of nursing practice, which provides a framework for processing client data and for developing client-focused plans of care. The nurse makes professional judgements based upon evidence, and recognizes and includes the client as a valued partner. (Canadian Federation of Mental Health Nurses, 2014, p. 7).

This statement underscores the importance of assessment as the basis for developing a plan of care.

Assessment is not a one-time activity; it is a purposeful, systematic, and dynamic process in the nurse's relationship with individuals in his or her care. Effective assessment requires that the nurse (Canadian Federation of Mental Health Nurses, 2006, p. 7)

1. Collaborates with clients and with other members of the health care team to gather holistic, client-centred assessments through observation, engagement,

examination, interview (using respectful, recovery focussed language), and consultation while attending to confidentiality and pertinent legal statutes

2. Assesses, documents, and analyzes data to identify health status, potential for wellness, health care deficits, potential for risk to self and others; alterations in thought content and/or process, affect behaviour, communication and decision-making abilities; substance use and dependency; and history of trauma and/or abuse (emotional, physical, neglect, sexual, or verbal)

3. Formulates and documents a plan of care in collaboration with the client, family, and mental health team that supports recovery and reintegration/social inclusion in the community through discharge planning and provision for ongoing support, all while recognizing variability in the client's ability to participate in the process

4. Refines and expands client assessment information by assessing and documenting significant change(s) in the client's status, and by comparing new data with the baseline assessment and client goals

5. Assesses and anticipates potential needs and risks continuously, collaborating with the client to examine his/her environment for risk factors such as self-care, housing, nutrition, economic support, psychological state, and social interactions

6. Determines the most appropriate and available therapeutic modality that meets the client's needs, and assists the client to access necessary resources

▼ **KEY CONCEPT** Assessment is a purposeful, systematic, and dynamic process in the nurse's relationship with individuals in his or her care. It involves the collection, validation, analysis, synthesis, organization, and documentation of client health–illness information.

Types of Assessment

Depending on the client's needs and the context of care, an assessment may be comprehensive or focused. A **comprehensive assessment** includes a complete health history (Table 10-1) and physical examination; considers the psychological, emotional, social, spiritual, ethnic, and cultural dimensions of health; attends to the meaning of the client's health–illness experience; and evaluates how all of this affects the individual's daily living. The purpose of a comprehensive assessment is to develop a holistic understanding of the individual's problems and needs as well as his or her strengths and resources. It is performed in collaboration with other members of the treatment team and is the basis for establishing baseline health–illness information necessary to establish a diagnosis, identify treatment goals, and develop a plan of care.

Because of its broad scope and the time it takes to develop rapport, a comprehensive assessment may take days

or even weeks to complete. Members of the health care team collect information from several sources, including the individual and his or her family, other health care providers, social service and justice personnel, educators, employers, and existing client records. All this is done while attending to issues of confidentiality and relevant legal statutes.

A **focused assessment** is the collection of specific information about a particular need, problem, or situation and may involve evaluation of such things as medication effects, risk for self-harm, knowledge deficits, or the adequacy of supports and resources. As the name suggests, focused assessments are briefer, narrower in scope, and more present oriented than are comprehensive assessments. Focused assessments may also be used to screen individuals who are at high risk for particular problems or disorders. In these instances, nurses often employ standardized assessment tools (e.g., Glasgow Coma Scale [GCS], Mini-Mental Status Examination, or Hamilton Depression Inventory).

The type of assessment required in any given situation depends on two key factors: the immediate needs of the client and the practice setting. Efforts to perform a comprehensive assessment during a psychiatric emergency (e.g., when an individual is floridly psychotic or actively suicidal) can be both dangerous and futile. The quality and trustworthiness of the information collected in these circumstances are biased by the client's symptoms and by the high emotionality of the situation. The priority in such situations is to perform a focused assessment that provides the treatment team with sufficient information to treat the client's symptoms and to ensure the safety of all involved.

The type of assessment a nurse performs is also largely determined by the setting in which he or she works. The mandate of a psychiatric and mental health (PMH) facility or program will determine the type of service it offers, which in turn dictates the nature of the assessment required. During the course of a first admission to a psychiatric unit, for example, an individual is likely to undergo a comprehensive assessment. In contrast, nurses working with a telehealth line or with a mobile mental health crisis team will collect only the information required to address the immediate problem or crisis.

● **STUDY NOTE**

STUDY NOTE Assessment is a part of all nurse–client interactions. It requires a broad theoretical knowledge of human, social, and health sciences; the ability to think critically; and psychomotor and interpersonal skills. Assessment activities include observation, examination, interview, and consultation.

Assessment Techniques

PMH assessments involve observation of the individual at different times of the day and in different circumstances, interviews with the individual and family members, analyses and synthesis of findings from physical and

Table 10-1	Health History and Significance to Psychiatric and Mental Health Problems

Data	Considerations/Significance
Source of Information	Ideally, the client is the primary source of information; consultation with secondary sources is necessary with minors or when the client is unable to provide information.
	Note the apparent reliability and consistency of the information provided.
Identification/Biographic Information	Legal name/nicknames/aliases; date and place of birth; gender; address; telephone numbers; relationship status; next of kin; ethnicity; religious/spiritual affiliation; employer; education; provincial/territorial health insurance number.
	Because this information is relatively nonthreatening, it is a safe place to begin an assessment. It also provides important clues about an individual's current living situation.
Primary Reason for Seeking Care	Record this verbatim because it speaks to the client's and family's perception of and insight into existing problems; its judgment; and goals for treatment.
Past Health	
Past illness, injury, and/or hospitalization	Note positive history of childhood diseases, especially viral infection, which have been linked to some psychiatric disorders (e.g., schizophrenia).
	Inquire about surgeries and trauma, particularly those resulting in concussion or loss of consciousness.
	Ask about parental alcohol and drug use (especially during pregnancy); birth trauma; lengthy/repeated separation from parents/caregivers because of hospitalization; a pattern of injury suggestive of childhood abuse/neglect; and surgeries.
Chronic illnesses	Chronic illnesses (e.g., diabetes and thyroid dysfunction), even when well controlled, may affect mental status.
	Highlight known allergies, type of reaction, usual treatment, and effectiveness of treatment.
Family Health History	Record the name, age, and current health status of close relatives (spouse/partner, children, parents, siblings, grandparents, and aunts/uncles). If a family member is deceased, note the date and cause of death and indications of unresolved grief/loss.
	Inquire specifically about diseases/disorders that "run in the family," particularly psychiatric disorders and addictions. A genogram is a useful tool for recording this information.
	Many psychiatric disorders are genetically linked, so a family health history provides information about the client's risk factors. It also provides clues about social roles, the availability of social support, and family resources/stressors.
	Coping strategies, both effective and ineffective, are learned early in life from our family of origin. A family health history can help to identify these.
Developmental Considerations	Note social and educational difficulties, as well as failure to achieve expected developmental milestones. These may be indicative of attentional or interpersonal deficits; behavioural problems; a chaotic family environment; acquired brain injury; or childhood mental illness.
	Ask about early parental death or separation because these may be associated with alterations in attachment and later relationship difficulties.
	The Canadian Government's practice of removing aboriginal children to residential schools traumatized children, fragmented families, decimated cultures/languages, and contributed to serious social and psychological problems that still reverberate among First Nations people.
Immunization/HIV/ Hepatitis Status	Individuals with severe and persistent mental illness often live in severe poverty and lack knowledge and resources for health promotion. In addition, many have lifestyles that put them at risk for serious communicable diseases.
Psychological Trauma	Ask: "Have you ever experienced or witnessed anything that threatened your life or safety or the life or safety of a loved one?" If yes, probe for details.
	Psychological trauma associated with natural disasters, motor vehicle crashes, combat, abuse/assault (physical or sexual), and childhood neglect is associated with a number of PMH problems (e.g., particularly posttraumatic stress disorder, other anxiety disorders, and depression).
Current Health Status	Provides information about medical conditions that affect mental status, global functioning, and quality of life.
	A systematic approach to performing a health history ensures thoroughness, helps the clinician to organize/cluster the data, and cues the informant's memory.
	Analyze significant symptoms (see Box 10-4).
Integument	Ask about problems/changes in the skin, hair, and nails. Note the presences of scars; piercings/body art; lesions/sores; rashes; discolouration; itching; or unusual sensations.
	Piercings and body art are expressions of one's personal aesthetic, which is part of self-concept. They may also indicate identification with particular social groups.
Sensory systems	Note sensory deficits and the use of eye glasses, contact lenses, hearing aids, and dentures.
	Uncorrected sensory deficits can affect an individual's day-to-day function and ability to communicate.
	Record the report of unusual perceptions or sensations because these may be related to perceptual or thought disturbances.

Table 10-1   Health History and Significance to Psychiatric and Mental Health Problems (*Continued*)

Data	Considerations/Significance
Respiratory	Note problems/disease, recurrent infections, cough, sputum, shortness of breath, noisy respirations, and smoking history.
Cardiovascular/ hematologic	Inquire about history of cardiac disease/problems; palpitations; arrhythmias; murmurs; dizzy spells; coldness/blueness/swelling of extremities; leg pain while walking.
	Individuals who experience panic episodes often present at emergency departments because their signs and symptoms mimic heart attack.
	Inquire about anemia, bleeding disorders, fatigue, blood transfusions, bruising, and cancers.
	Monitoring of some long-term neuroleptic medication use (e.g., lithium and clozapine) requires regular blood tests.
Gastrointestinal	Ask about changes in appetite, weight, and bowel patterns; nausea, vomiting, indigestion, gastroesophageal reflux disease; antacid and laxative use; history of disease (e.g., ulcers, irritable bowel syndrome, and cancer); and rectal discharge/bleeding.
	Alterations in gastrointestinal function are implicated in many psychiatric disorders. An individual may not notice hunger or have the energy to prepare food. Others may handle distressing emotions by eating more than usual.
	Anticholinergic effects of antipsychotic medication can cause constipation, whereas lithium carbonate can cause diarrhea.
Genitourinary	Note pain/burning on urination, frequency, urgency, dribbling/incontinence, hesitancy, colour of urine, history of urinary tract infection/kidney disease, and frequent nighttime urination.
	Anticholinergic effects of antipsychotic medication can cause urinary hesitancy and/or retention.
Reproductive/breasts	Ask females about menarche; usual pattern of menses (frequency, duration, colour/amount of bleeding, and recent changes); obstetrical history (pregnancies, live births, miscarriages, abortions); infertility; dysmenorrhoea (pain, excessive bleeding); past or current infection/disease (e.g., sexually transmitted infections, sores/lesions, and unusual discharge or odour); date of last Pap smear; sexual orientation; sexual activity (including level of sexual desire, change in frequency of sexual activity, satisfaction with sexual relationships, painful intercourse); and contraceptive use.
	Ask males about number of children; infertility; past or current infection/disease (e.g., sexually transmitted infections, sores/lesions, and penile/rectal discharge); date of last testicular and prostate examinations; sexual orientation; sexual activity (including level of sexual desire, change in frequency of sexual activity, satisfaction with sexual relationships, painful intercourse, erectile/ejaculatory problems); and contraceptive use.
	Ask both men and women about past disease; changes in breasts or nipples (e.g., masses/lumps, pain, and discharge); and breast self-examination. Note the date of female clients' last mammogram.
	Attitudes, beliefs, and expressions of sexuality provide important information about an individual's self-concept, gender identification, quality of relationships, and overall satisfaction with life.
	Changes in level of desire and frequency of sexual activity are common in many psychiatric disorders, including depression, anxiety, and mania.
	Side effects of selective serotonin reuptake inhibitors are decreased sexual desire and erectile/ejaculatory dysfunction.
	Suicide rates among gay and lesbian youth are higher than the national average.
Musculoskeletal	Note problems with mobility; limited range of motion; pain or weakness; joint problems; disease/injury (e.g., osteoporosis); use of prosthetics; and impairments to activities of daily living.
Endocrine	Ask about disease/illness (e.g., diabetes, hypothyroidism/hyperthyroidism, and goitre); changes in height, weight, hair and skin, appetite, and energy level; excessive thirst; frequent urination; weakness; heat/cold intolerance; and current hormone therapy.
	Diseases of the endocrine system can imitate symptoms associated with psychiatric disorders (e.g., depression, anxiety, mania, eating disorders, and dementia).
Neurologic	Ask about head trauma; alterations in consciousness; seizures; headaches; changes in cognition and memory; sensory and motor disturbances (numbness, tingling, loss of sensation, tremors, lack of coordination, balance problems, and pain). As well, inquire about alterations in personality, speech, or ability to manage activities of daily living.
	Neurologic signs and symptoms are associated with many psychiatric disorders as well as with side effects/toxicity of some neuroleptic medications (e.g., neuroleptic malignant syndrome [NMS], serotonin syndrome, and lithium toxicity).

Continued

Table 10-1	Health History and Significance to Psychiatric and Mental Health Problems (*Continued*)

Data	Considerations/Significance
Current Medications (including over-the-counter preparations and herbal remedies)	Specify the name of the medication, purpose, usual dose, frequency, effectiveness, side effects, prescriber, and the length of time the client has been taking it. This information helps to assess the client's health-promoting behaviours and potential knowledge deficits. Individuals with serious and persistent mental illness often take several different medications, which puts them at risk for drug–drug and drug–food interactions.
Health/Lifestyle Health promotion/ maintenance	Ask individuals to describe what they do on a daily, weekly, and yearly basis to promote and maintain their health. Note the dates of their last physical examination, visit to a dentist, and eye examination.
Nutritional patterns	Ask about usual eating patterns and whether there have been any recent changes. Changes in eating patterns are associated with many affective states and psychiatric disorders. Particularly note dissatisfaction with weight and shape as well as activities aimed at weight loss. Body dissatisfaction is a factor in eating disorders and contributes to self-concept. It is particularly common among girls/women, elite athletes, and those with occupations that emphasize physical appearance (e.g., modelling and dancing). Psychiatric symptoms, neuroleptic medication, and poverty can all affect nutritional status. The weight gain associated with many neuroleptic medications increases individuals' risk for type II diabetes.
Sleep/rest patterns	Changes in sleep patterns can be a response to stress or symptoms of a psychiatric disorder. Probe a positive response about alterations in usual sleep patterns. Ask about *sleep onset* (latency between going to bed and falling asleep); *sleep maintenance* (frequency of wakening during the night and ease of falling back to sleep); and *early morning wakening* (consistently waking up before one needs to be up). Also, ask about whether the individual generally feels rested/refreshed. Alterations in sleep patterns are common in many psychiatric disorders (e.g., depression, mania, and schizophrenia). For many individuals with serious and persistent mental illness, sleep disturbances are early signs of relapse.
Activity/exercise	Ask about usual activity level and type and amount of exercise. Involvement in social activities and hobbies enhances health and reduces stress. Withdrawal from these things may be early signs of illness. Two of the negative symptoms of schizophrenia are anhedonia (decreased ability to experience pleasure) and avolition (lack of motivational drive and energy). These explain why many individuals with schizophrenia sleep excessively. Alterations in usual activities are associated with many mental disorders including depression, mania, schizophrenia, and some eating disorders.
Tobacco, alcohol and nonprescription drug use, and problem gambling	*Tobacco.* Inquire about type (cigarettes, cigars, pipes, and chewing tobacco); age at first use; frequency; and efforts to stop use. *Alcohol.* Ask about age at first use; preferred type (beer, wine, or spirits); usual pattern of drinking; and any recent changes to that pattern. It is also important to explore whether the individual or those close to the individual believe that alcohol is a problem in the individual's life. If yes, probe for details. Many people use alcohol to self-medicate—that is, to cope with stress, unpleasant emotions, sleep disturbances, and so forth. *Nonprescription drugs.* Ask about the age of first use; drug(s) of choice; dose; route; and frequency of nonprescription drug use. Probe for information about the effects of drug use (physical, psychological, emotional, social, legal, and economic). *Problem gambling.* Ask at what age it began; game(s) of choice; frequency; and average amount of money lost per month. Probe for information about the consequences (physical, psychological, emotional, social, legal, and economic).

mental examinations into a care plan, and consultation with other health care providers.

Observation

Although verbal communication is vital to the assessment process, nonverbal cues also communicate important information about the client's health–illness experience (see Chapter 6). Nurses learn to engage all of their senses and to integrate assessment into all their encounters with clients. Attention to nuances of dress, behaviour, facial expression, gestures, and interactions with others (particularly when the individual is not aware of being observed) provide important information that may not otherwise be revealed through conversation. For example, as well as observing hygiene and personal grooming, the nurse considers whether the client's dress is appropriate to the season and situation. Other important observations include behavioural evidence of perceptual disturbances or disordered thoughts (e.g., listening or talking to unseen others) and apparent inconsistencies between what an individual reports and what the nurse observes.

Examination

A comprehensive health assessment includes a health history, a physical examination, and diagnostic testing. This is particularly important in the provision of holistic PMH care because, compared with the general population, individuals diagnosed with a serious mental illness are at greater risk for developing a range of chronic physical conditions, affecting almost every body system (for a full review, see Canadian Mental Health Association [CMHA], 2008). The converse is also true in that Canadians who live with chronic physical health problems are twice as likely to experience a mood or anxiety disorder compared with individuals without a chronic physical condition (Government of Canada, 2006).

Persons living with mental illness can develop physical health problems as a result of the illness itself and/or as a consequence of treatment. Mental illnesses can disrupt hormone systems and sleep–wake cycles, while psychotropic medications have side effects such as weight gain to cardiac arrhythmias (Leucht, Burkard, Henderson, Maj, & Sartorius, 2007), all of which can contribute to increased vulnerability to a range of physical conditions. Other risk factors that contribute to the development of physical illnesses include smoking, alcohol and drug use, obesity, poverty, and self-care deficits. It is also important to note that medical conditions can mask, imitate, or worsen psychiatric symptoms. The situation is further complicated because some mental illnesses cause an individual to misattribute physical sensations, making it difficult to recognize and describe his or her symptoms. For example, those who have panic attacks can attribute their symptoms to a myocardial infarction or heart attack.

The **mental status examination** (MSE) is a systematic approach to assessing an individual's psychological, emotional, social, and neurologic functioning. Although the components of the MSE are standard across clinical settings, the findings are highly subjective and rely heavily on the clinician's knowledge, communication skills, interpretation, and judgment. For this reason, it is important for clinicians to be self-reflective and to collaborate with colleagues to develop an unbiased understanding of the client's experience.

Interview

An assessment interview is a semistructured conversation aimed at building rapport, obtaining facts, clarifying perceptions and meanings, validating observations, and comparing understandings. Skillful interviewing is much more than asking an individual questions about signs and symptoms; it is both an art and a science and takes

---

BOX 10-1 Factors that Facilitate Effective Interviewing

- As much as possible, **negotiate the terms of the interview with all the participants** (e.g., choose a mutually agreeable time and place; clearly state your purpose; and continually invite the clients to express their thoughts, feelings, wants, and needs). This conveys respect, establishes a human connection, and fosters rapport.
- **The environment**. Choose a private and comfortable setting that is free from interruption.
- **Realistic time management**. Be clear at the outset how much time you have available for an interview and make a realistic plan about what you can achieve.
- **Be attentive to your nonverbal communication**. Sit at the same level as the client and maintain an open body posture. If you make notes, inform the client at the beginning of the interview; keep your notes brief so you can attend to the conversation.
- **Avoid jargon** and choose language that is clear, simple, and developmentally and culturally appropriate. Repeatedly check with the clients to ensure that they understand what you are saying.
- **Begin with a less sensitive topic and move toward sensitive issues as rapport develops**.
- Leave some time at the end of the encounter for **closure and future planning**. This involves monitoring the available time and notifying the client when the interview is coming to an end.

---

practice to develop (Box 10-1). Effective interviewers train themselves to be fully present in the situation and are genuinely warm and respectful and approach clients as collaborators working toward the same ends. Above all, competent interviewers engage in what Rogers (1975) refers to as empathic listening, which he describes as

> … being sensitive, moment by moment, to the changing felt meanings which flow in the other person and to the fear or rage or tenderness or confusion or whatever he or she is experiencing. It means temporarily living in the other's life, moving about in it delicately without making judgments (p. 4).

Because many psychiatric symptoms are beyond an individual's awareness, nurses may also interview family and friends to obtain client-related information. That being said, Canadian privacy legislation imposes obligations on government departments and public agencies, including health-serving facilities, to respect privacy rights and to limit the collection, use, and disclosure of personal information. Today, every province and territory has privacy laws, and it is the responsibility of every nurse to know the limits of information sharing under that legislation (Office of the Privacy Commission of Canada, 2012).

It is often the case that novice interviewers are so overwhelmed by their own anxieties about interviewing that they focus on their own experience and on asking questions to elicit needed information. When this happens, the client's needs and the relational nature of the interaction are forgotten. Box 10-2 identifies some interviewer behaviours that can impede effective interviewing.

BOX 10-2 Barriers to Effective Interviewing

- **Lack of clarity about the purpose and parameters of the interview** is like embarking on a journey without a clear destination. A statement such as, "Mrs. Woods, my name is Kate Donovan. I am a nurse on this unit, and I would like to spend the next hour or so getting to know more about you and completing your admission assessment. Is that okay with you?" conveys respect, informs the client of your intent, and begins the process of negotiating a contract for the encounter.
- **Asking too many closed-ended questions.** Closed-ended questions invite brief responses and are most useful for eliciting specific facts, like those needed in a focused assessment. Heavy reliance on them tends to orient the interview around the interviewer's desire for information and prevents clients from introducing or expanding on topics of importance to them.
- **Avoiding silence.** Often in response to their own discomfort or anxiety, interviewers rush to fill all silences with words. Pauses in the conversation allow both the client and the interviewer time to reflect on their experience in the moment, to formulate or elaborate on their responses, to switch speakers, or to turn the conversation to a new topic.
- **Asking complex questions.** A complex question is really several questions presented as one, as in "Why did you come to the hospital today, who brought you, and how did you get here?" These types of questions are confusing to the respondent, who often does not know which to answer first. Successful interviewers ask one question at a time, listen carefully to the answer, and probe for more detail if it is not clear.
- **Making assumptions.** Effective interviewers are those who understand that each individual experiences and understands the world in his or her own unique way. The failure to clarify and validate what the client means results in misunderstanding and inaccuracies.
- **Avoiding or ignoring expressions of emotion.** Emotions are rich communications. They provide insight into the meaning an individual assigns to an experience or event. Minimizing or ignoring an expression of emotion sends a powerful message. For example, "There are parts of you that I do not acknowledge," or "Your emotions are frightening or unimportant." Competent practitioners need to maintain a high level of self-awareness in order to remain grounded in their own experience so that they can bear witness to others.

Collaboration

Although nurses have long been vital contributors to interdisciplinary teams, a growing body of evidence stresses the importance of interprofessional collaboration. In a recent review of the evidence, the World Health Organization (2010) identified the following benefits of interprofessional practice: reduced lengths of hospital stay, improved quality of life for patients/clients and families, improved access to care, enhanced patient/client safety, and improved recruitment and retention of health care professionals. The shift toward primary health care brings with it an emphasis on teams of health professionals who are accountable for providing comprehensive services to clients. Collaborative practice among nurses, physicians, and other practitioners result in better health, improved access to services, more efficient use of resources, and higher levels of satisfaction for both consumers and health professionals.

PMH teams typically include the client and his or her family, nurses, physicians, psychologists, social workers, pharmacists, occupational therapists, and recreational therapists. Depending on the treatment setting and the client's particular needs, other professionals (e.g., teachers, clergy or spiritual leaders, other medical specialists) may be regular contributors to the team or participate on an ad hoc basis. In some settings, one member of the team may be assigned to be the client's primary therapist and takes on the role of coordinating team activities to address the client's needs. Teams meet together frequently to share information, to develop and evaluate treatment goals, and to provide ongoing support.

In most PMH treatment facilities, the interdisciplinary team works to develop a psychiatric diagnosis based on the *Diagnostic and Statistical Manual of Mental Health Disorders*, 5th edition (*DSM-5*) (American Psychiatric Association, 2013). The *DSM-5* provides a common language and standard criteria for the classification of mental disorders.

BIO/PSYCHO/SOCIAL/SPIRITUAL PSYCHIATRIC/MENTAL HEALTH NURSING ASSESSMENT

A bio/psycho/social/spiritual PMH nursing assessment rests on the assumption that humans are whole, integrated beings who live in constant and reciprocal relationship with their physical and social environments (Fig. 10-1). The bio/psycho/social/spiritual model presented in Chapter 5 provides a framework for assessing the physical, psychological, emotional, social, and spiritual dimensions of health. Whereas the goal of medical assessment is the diagnosis and treatment of disease and illness, nursing assessment aims to develop a holistic understanding of the individual's health–illness experience. In addition to identifying health problems and deficits, it attends to strengths and resources and evaluates how these affect the individual's daily living.

Types and Sources of Information

Client information or data fall into two broad categories: *objective* and *subjective*. **Objective data** (also called *signs*) are directly observable and measurable. The physical examination, vital signs, and diagnostic tests all yield objective data. In contrast, **subjective data** (*symptoms*) are neither directly observable nor measurable. Subjective data are what the client and others report about their thoughts, attitudes, beliefs, emotions, perceptions, experiences, and motivations. A health history provides this type of data. Subjective information provides a window into an individual's lifetime experiences and the meanings attached to those experiences. This experience is influenced by personal history and developmental stage; past learning; ethnicity and culture; and spirituality and offers insight into the sense an individual makes of the world.

FIGURE 10-1. Bio/psycho/social/spiritual nursing assessment.

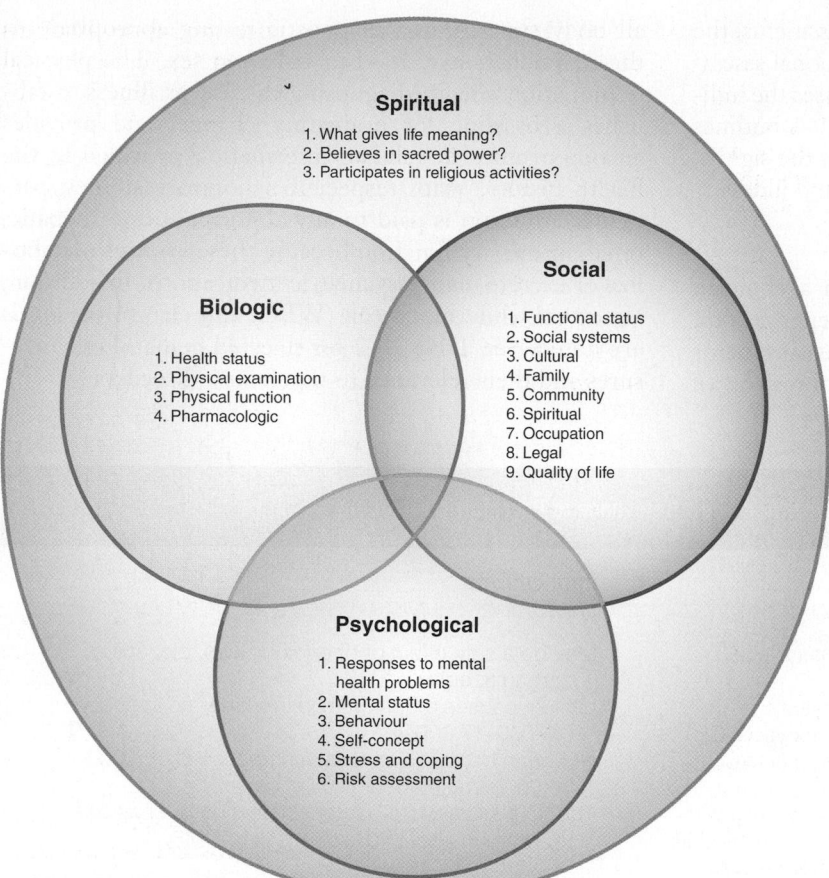

Spiritual
1. What gives life meaning?
2. Believes in sacred power?
3. Participates in religious activities?

Biologic
1. Health status
2. Physical examination
3. Physical function
4. Pharmacologic

Social
1. Functional status
2. Social systems
3. Cultural
4. Family
5. Community
6. Spiritual
7. Occupation
8. Legal
9. Quality of life

Psychological
1. Responses to mental health problems
2. Mental status
3. Behaviour
4. Self-concept
5. Stress and coping
6. Risk assessment

It is critical for nurses to remember that individuals act and react to the *meanings they assign* to events and experiences, rather than to the events or experiences themselves.

Both objective and subjective data are generated from *primary* or *secondary* sources. The individual or client is the primary source of information about himself or herself. Secondary data, on the other hand, come from all other sources, including family, other health care providers, written reports, and client records.

Documentation

Health care records are important vehicles for communication as well as being legal documents. The type of information collected and how it is documented are regulated by the program or facility in which the nurse practices. In turn, programs and facilities develop documentation policies and procedures to comply with provincial and territorial legislation.

Generally speaking, there are two common approaches to documentation: *source-oriented* and *problem-oriented* documentations. In source-oriented documentation, each discipline is assigned a section of the client record (e.g., nurse's notes or physician's notes). Although this approach clearly identifies the discipline of the person making the entry, it tends to fragment the data, which is antithetical to holistic care. In problem-oriented documentation, everyone involved with the care of an individual makes entries

in the same section of the record. This not only facilitates interdisciplinary collaboration but also keeps team members oriented toward the client's identified goals, needs, and problems.

Information may be entered in the client record in several ways, including fill-in forms, flow sheets, checklists, and narrative notes. Electronic medical records are becoming more common because they are more efficient, save time, and facilitate sharing of client information. In many settings, practitioners use the SOAP (subjective data, objective data, assessment, and plan implementation/evaluation), DAR (data, action, and plan), or PIE (problem, implementation, and evaluation) methods to organize their notes. Another approach to documentation is *charting by exception*, which involves documenting only those client health–illness responses that deviate from well-articulated standards.

Biologic Domain

Health History

The health history establishes a subjective database about the client's current and past health–illness experience, identifies strengths and resources, suggests actual and potential health problems and deficits, and is an opportunity to build rapport. Depending on the practice setting, different members of the health care team may take responsibility for sections of the health history. For example, the social worker may perform the family and social assessments, the occupational therapist undertakes the occupational assessment, and the recreational therapist often assesses the individual's exercise and leisure activities. Table 10-1 outlines the components of a health history and relates the significance of important findings to mental health and illness.

Physical Examination

Physical examination is a process by which a clinician collects objective information about the client's health. Components include anthropomorphic measurements (e.g., height and weight), vital signs, an examination of all body systems, and diagnostic testing appropriate to the individual's age, level of risk, and sex. The physical examination aids in diagnosing disease or illness, establishes a baseline for evaluating change, and provides an opportunity to validate information provided in the health history. With respect to laboratory studies, particular attention is paid to any abnormalities of hepatic, renal, or urinary function because these systems metabolize or excrete many psychiatric medications. In addition, abnormal white blood cell (WBC) and electrolyte levels are noted. See Table 10-2 for selected hematologic measures and their relevance to psychiatric disorders.

Table 10-2	**Selected Hematologic Measures and Their Relevance to Psychiatric Disorders**

Test	Result	Implications
Complete Blood Count (CBC)		
Leukocyte count (WBC)	Leukopenia ($\downarrow$ WBC)	May be a side effect of phenothiazines, clozapine, carbamazepine
	Agranulocytosis ($\downarrow$ granulocytic WCB)	Lithium causes a benign mild to moderate increase (11,000–17,000/µL).
	Leukocytosis ($\uparrow$ WCB)	NMS can be associated with increases of 15,000–30,000/mm^3 in about 40% of cases.
WBC differential	"Shift to the left"—from segmented neutrophils to band forms	This shift suggests a bacterial infection but has been reported in about 40% of cases of NMS.
Red blood cell (RBC) count	Polycythemia ($\uparrow$ RBC)	Primary form (true polycythemia) is associated with several disease states; requires further evaluation.
		Secondary form is compensation for decreased oxygenation (e.g., chronic obstructive pulmonary disease).
		Blood is more viscous, which is exacerbated by being dehydrated.
	$\downarrow$ RBCs	Associated with some types of anemia; requires further evaluation.
Hematocrit (Hct)	$\uparrow$ Hct	Associated with dehydration.
	$\downarrow$ Hct	Associated with anemia; may be related to alterations in mental status, including asthenia, depression, and psychosis.
		Twenty percent of women of childbearing age in North America have iron deficiency anemia.
Hemoglobin (Hgb)	$\downarrow$ Hgb	Indicative of anemia; evaluation of cause requires review of erythrocyte indices.
Erythrocyte indices, such as red cell distribution width (RDW)	$\uparrow$ RDW	Finding suggests a combined anemia resulting from both vitamin B$_{12}$ and folic acid deficiencies and iron deficiency, as found in chronic alcoholism.
		Oral contraceptives also decrease vitamin B$_{12}$.
Other Hematologic Measures		
Vitamin B$_{12}$	Deficiency	May be associated with neuropsychiatric symptoms such as psychosis, paranoia, fatigue, agitation, marked personality change, dementia, and delirium.
Folate	Deficiency	Associated with alcohol use and with medications such as phenytoin, oral contraceptives, and estrogens.
Platelet count	Thrombocytopenia ($\downarrow$ platelets)	Associated with use of some psychiatric medications, such as carbamazepine, phenothiazines, or clozapine and with other nonpsychiatric medications; may also cause thrombocytopenia.
		Also, associated with some disease states; requires further evaluation.

Table 10-2	Selected Hematologic Measures and Their Relevance to Psychiatric Disorders (*Continued*)	

Test	Result	Implications
Serum Electrolytes		
Sodium	Hyponatremia (serum sodium)	Associated with significant alterations in mental status. May be related to Addison's disease; the syndrome of inappropriate secretion of antidiuretic hormone; polydipsia; and carbamazepine use.
Potassium	Hypokalemia (↓ serum potassium)	Associated with weakness, fatigue, electrocardiogram changes, paralytic ileus, and muscle paresis. Common in individuals exhibiting bulimic behaviour, psychogenic vomiting, misuse of diuretics, and/or excessive laxative use. Hypokalemia may be life threatening.
Chloride	Elevation	Chloride tends to increase to compensate for lower bicarbonate.
	Decrease	Associated with binging and purging behaviour.
Bicarbonate	Elevation	Associated with binging and purging, disordered eating, excessive laxative use, and/or psychogenic vomiting.
	Decrease	May develop in individuals who hyperventilate (e.g., panic disorder).
Renal Function Tests		
Blood urea nitrogen	Elevation	Associated with alterations in mental status (e.g., lethargy and delirium), dehydration, and medications excreted by the kidney, such as lithium and amantadine.
Serum creatinine	Elevation	Indicative of decreased renal function; typically does elevate until 50% of nephrons in the kidney are damaged.
Serum Enzymes		
Amylase	Elevation	Associated with the binging and purging behaviour in eating disorders; tends to decline when these behaviours stop.
	Alanine aminotransferase (ALT)>aspartate aminotransferase (AST)	This disparity is common in acute forms of viral and drug-induced hepatic dysfunction.
ALT (formerly serum glutamic pyruvic transaminase)	Elevation	Mild elevations are common with use of sodium valproate.
AST (formerly serum glutamic oxaloacetic transaminase)	AST>ALT	Severe elevations are associated with chronic hepatic disease and myocardial infarction.
Creatine phosphokinase	Elevations of the isoenzyme related to muscle tissue	Associated with muscle tissue injury. Level is elevated in NMS and by repeated intramuscular injections (e.g., depot antipsychotics).
Thyroid Function		
Serum triiodothyronine (T_3)	Decrease	Associated with hypothyroidism and other non–thyroid-related diseases. Individuals with depression may convert less T_4 to T_3 peripherally, but not out of the normal range. Medications such as lithium and sodium valproate may suppress thyroid function, but clinical significance is unknown.
	Elevation	Indicative of hyperthyroidism; T_3 toxicosis is associated with alterations in mood, anxiety, and symptoms of mania.
Serum thyroxine (T_4)	Elevation	Indicative of hyperthyroidism.
Thyroid-stimulating hormone	Elevation	Associated with hypothyroidism, which shares features of depression with the additional physical signs of cold intolerance, dry skin, hair loss, bradycardia, and so forth. Lithium may also cause elevations.
	Decrease	Considered nondiagnostic; may be associated with hyperthyroidism, pituitary hypothyroidism, or even euthyroid status.

Psychological Domain

The psychological domain includes manifestations of PMH problems/disorders; mental status; stress and coping; and risk assessment.

Responses to Mental Health Problems

In broad terms, PMH disorders are manifest as "clinically significant patterns of behaviour or emotions that are associated with some level of distress, suffering, or impairment in one or more areas such as school, work, social and family interactions, or the ability to live independently" (Canadian Psychiatric Association, 2012). The identification and understanding of PMH conditions vary through history and across cultures. Current thinking is that mental health-illness exists on a continuum such that mental health and mental illness can coexist simultaneously within the same person. According to the WHO, more than a third of people around the globe experience problems that meet diagnostic criteria for a mental disorder. Like other illnesses, PMH disorders affect individuals and their families in many different ways. An important part of assessing the psychological domain is to explore the individual's experience of illness. Many have specific fears about losing their jobs, about their families, or about their personal safety. It is also important to identify the person's strategies for managing the illness and the effectiveness of those strategies. A simple question such as "How do you deal with your voices when you are with other people?" may initiate a discussion about a particular experience or symptom.

Mental Status Examination

The MSE (Box 10-3) is a systematic assessment of an individual's appearance, affect, behaviour, and cognitive processes. It reflects "a snapshot" of the examiner's

---

BOX 10-3 Components of the Mental Status Examination

1. Peneral observations
   a. Appearance
   b. Psychomotor behaviour
   c. Attitude toward interviewer
2. Mood
3. Affect
4. Speech characteristics
5. Perception
6. Thought
   a. Content
   b. Process/form
7. Sensorium
   a. Level of consciousness
   b. Orientation (person, place, time)
   c. Memory (immediate retention and recall; recent, short-term, and long-term)
   d. Attention and concentration
   e. Comprehension and abstract reasoning
8. Insight
9. Judgment

---

observations and impressions at the time of the interview and is performed by health practitioners across several disciplines and clinical settings to evaluate developmental, neurologic, and psychiatric disorders.

KEY CONCEPT The **mental status examination** is a systematic assessment of an individual's appearance, affect, behaviour, and cognitive processes. It reflects "a snapshot" of the examiner's observations and impressions at the time of the interview and is performed by health practitioners across several disciplines and clinical settings to evaluate developmental, neurologic, and psychiatric disorders.

General Observations

This section of the MSE provides a brief narrative summary of the examiner's observations and impressions of the individual at the time of the interview. Although an individual's health history remains relatively stable, his or her mental status is variable over time. (For a video demonstration of elements of an MSE, see http://aitlvideo.uc.edu/aitl/MSE/MSEkm.swf.)

Appearance. Describe the individual's general appearance and presentation. Note manner and appropriateness of dress, personal hygiene, odours, pupil size, and obvious identifying characteristics, such as tattoos and piercings. Physical signs such as skin tone (e.g., duskiness, pallor, or flushing), nutritional status, and energy level (e.g., catatonia, lethargy, or restlessness) provide clues to the person's general level of health–illness.

Psychomotor behaviour/activity. Observe and note the individual's behaviour during the interview, including posture, gait, motor coordination, facial expression, mannerisms, gestures, and activity. Pay particular attention to cues to the person's emotional state (e.g., muscle tension, purposeless repetitive movements, and restlessness, etc.).

Attitude toward interviewer. The individual's attitude toward the interviewer and the interview process may be described as accommodating, cooperative, open, friendly, apathetic, bored, guarded, suspicious, hostile, or evasive. The following is an example of how the interviewer may describe the individual:

> Mr. D. is a tall, thin, Caucasian man, who looks older than his stated age of 47 years. He is unshaven, his hair is uncombed, and he has a strong body odour. His clothing is stained and dishevelled but appropriate to the season. He reports feeling "jumpy," and he declined to sit during the interview, opting instead to pace around the interview room. His posture is erect and his movements are quick, purposeful, and well coordinated; he displays no unusual mannerisms. Mr. D. was cooperative with the interview process, although his verbal responses were brief and he did not maintain eye contact.

Mood and Affect

In everyday usage, the terms *emotion, feelings,* and *mood* are used interchangeably. In the context of an MSE, however, these words refer to specific phenomena. *Emotion* is the individual's experience of a feeling state, whereas **mood** is "a pervasive and sustained emotion that colours the person's perception of the world" (Saddock & Saddock, 2003). Mood is what the individual *reports* about his or her prevailing emotional state. Although mood does vary with internal and external changes, it tends to be stable over time and reflects the person's disposition or worldview. Mood can be assessed by asking a simple, open-ended question like, "How have you been feeling over the past while?" Whatever the person answers, the interviewer should probe to find whether this is typical or is a response to some recent life event. A person who is generally positive and content will remain so even when bad things happen. He or she will tend to view adversity as a temporary period of unpleasantness in a basically happy life. In contrast, an individual whose mood tends to be negative or depressed views life through dark-coloured glasses. He or she experiences life as difficult and sees happiness as fleeting.

Mood may be sustained for days or weeks, or it may fluctuate during the course of a day. For example, some depressed individuals have a diurnal variation in their mood; they experience their lowest mood in the morning, but as the day progresses, their mood lifts, and they feel somewhat better in the evening. Terms used to describe mood include **euthymic** (normal), **euphoric** (elated), and **dysphoric** (depressed, disquieted, restless).

Affect is the individual's emotional responsiveness during the interview and *is inferred by the examiner* from facial expressions, vocalizations, and behaviour. During the assessment, an individual's affect may change as he or she talks about an immediate experience or recent life events. Affect is described in terms of its *range, intensity, appropriateness,* and *stability. Affective range* can be full or constricted. Individuals who express several emotions that are consistent with their stated feelings and the content of what they are saying are described as having a full range of affect that is congruent with the situation. On the other hand, a person who speaks of the recent, tragic death of a loved one in a monotone voice with little outward expression of his or her internal feeling state is described as having constricted affect. In evaluating the *appropriateness* of a particular response, the nurse must consider both the meaning of the event to the individual and cultural norms. Descriptions of *intensity* attempt to quantify an affective response. Intensity may be characterized as heightened, blunted, or flat. An example of heightened affect is the man who reacts to deaths of the victims of the September 11, 2001 attack as if they were all his personal friends. He states that his life stopped when the World Trade Center towers came down; he cried every day and could not eat or sleep for weeks afterward.

The phrase *blunted affect* describes limited emotional expression, whereas *flat affect* is its near absence. The person whose affect is flat speaks in a monotone voice and has little or no facial expression. *Stability* of affect can be described as mobile (normal) or labile. If a person displays a wide range of strong emotions in a relatively short period of time, his or her affect is described as being labile.

Speech Characteristics

Patterns and characteristics of speech provide clues about the individual's thoughts, emotions, and cognitive processes. They also convey information about the person's understanding of the situation and ability to read and respond to social cues. Speech is described in terms of its *quantity, rate and fluency of production,* and *quality.* In assessing speech *quantity,* the individual may be described as talkative, verbose, garrulous, subdued, reticent, or taciturn. *Rate of speech production* may be slow, hesitant, fast, or pressured, whereas *fluency* refers to the apparent ease with which speech is produced. *Pressured speech* is speech that is rapid and increased in amount and difficult to understand; it is often associated with mania. Aphasic disturbances are problems of speech output and may be neurologic, cognitive, or emotional in origin. *Speech quality* refers to its characteristics, such as monotone, whispered, slurred, mumbled, staccato, or loud. During conversation, the interviewer also notes speech impediments (e.g., stuttering), response latency (the length of time it takes for the individual to respond to a question or comment), and repetition, rhyming, or unusual use of words.

Perception

Perception is the complex series of mental events involved with taking in of sensory information from the environment and the processing of that information into mental representations. Two perceptual disturbances commonly associated with mental illness are hallucinations and illusions. **Hallucinations** are false sensory perceptions not associated with external stimuli and are not shared by others. Although auditory hallucinations are the most common type, hallucinations may be experienced in any of the five major sensory modalities: auditory, visual, tactile, olfactory, or gustatory. Most people are familiar with *hypnagogic hallucinations*—false sensory perceptions that occur while falling asleep; these are not associated with mental disorder. Of more concern are *command hallucinations,* the false perception of commands or orders that an individual feels obligated to obey. For example, a person may hear voices telling him or her to harm or kill oneself or someone else. **Illusions** are the misperception or misrepresentation of real sensory stimuli (e.g., misidentifying the wind as a voice calling one's name or thinking that a label on a piece of clothing is an insect).

Thought

Because thought is not directly observable, it is assessed through language in terms of its content and process (form). **Thought content** refers to the subject matter occupying a person's thoughts; **thought process** is the manner in which thoughts are formed and expressed. Some individuals are very forthcoming about the content of their thoughts, whereas others are more reticent to talk about them. Assessing thought requires the clinician to carefully attend to and explore unusual or recurring themes in the individual's conversation. Box 10-4 lists some common disturbances of thought content.

Saddock and Saddock (2003) define thinking as "the goal-directed flow of ideas, symbols, and associations initiated by a problem or task and leading toward a reality-oriented conclusion" (p. 282). A number of mental disorders are characterized by disturbances in the form

---

BOX 10-4 Alterations in Thought Content

Delusion—a false, fixed belief, based on an incorrect inference about reality. It is not shared by others and is inconsistent with the individual's intelligence or cultural background and cannot be corrected by reasoning.

Delusions of control—the belief that one's thoughts, feelings, or will are being controlled by outside forces. The following are some specific examples of delusions of control:

- **Thought insertion**—the belief that thoughts or ideas are being inserted into one's mind by someone or something external to one's self
- **Thought broadcasting**—the belief that one's thoughts are obvious to others or are being broadcast to the world
- **Ideas of reference**—the belief that other people, objects, and events are related to or have a special significance for one's self (e.g., a person on television is talking to or about him or her)

Paranoid delusions—an irrational distrust of others and/or the belief that others are harassing, cheating, threatening, or intend one harm

Bizarre delusion—an absurd or totally implausible belief (e.g., light waves from space communicate special messages to an individual)

Somatic delusion—a false belief involving the body or bodily functions

Delusion of grandeur—an exaggerated belief of one's importance or power

Religious delusion—the belief that one is an agent of or specially favoured by a greater being

Depersonalization—the belief that one's self or one's body is strange or unreal

Magical thinking—the belief that one's thoughts, words, or actions have the power to cause or prevent things to happen; similar to Jean Piaget's notion of preoperational thinking in young children

Erotomania—the belief that someone (often a public figure) unknown to the individual is in love with them or involved in a relationship with them

Nihilism—the belief that one is dead or nonexistent

Obsession—a repetitive thought, emotion, or impulse

Phobia—a persistent, exaggerated, and irrational fear

BOX 10-5 Alterations in Thought Process

Loosening of association—the lack of a logical relationship between thoughts and ideas; conversation shifts from one topic to another in a completely unrelated manner, making it confusing and difficult to follow

Circumstantiality—the individual takes a long time to make a point because his or her conversation is indirect and contains excessive and unnecessary detail

Tangentiality—similar to circumstantiality, except that the speaker does not return to a central point or answer the question posed

Thought blocking—an abrupt pause or interruption in one's train of thoughts, after which the individual cannot recall what he or she was saying

Neologisms—the creation of new words

Flight of ideas—rapid, continuous verbalization, with frequent shifting from one topic to another

Word salad—an incoherent mixture of words and phrases

Perseveration—a persisting response to a stimulus even after a new stimulus has been presented

Clang association—the use of words or phrases that have similar sounds but are not associated in meaning; may include rhyming or puns

Echolalia—the persistent echoing or repetition of words or phrases said by others

Verbigeration—the meaningless repetition of incoherent words or sentences; typically associated with psychotic states and cognitive impairment

Pressured speech—speech that is increased in rate and volume and is often emphatic and difficult to interrupt; typically associated with mania or hypomania

---

or process of normal thinking. Box 10-5 lists some common disturbances of thought process.

Sensorium

This portion of the MSE assesses brain function and cognitive abilities. The Mini-MSE (MMSE) (Folstein, Folstein, & McHugh, 1975) is a valid and reliable instrument, widely used to screen for gross impairments in these areas. The MMSE evaluates orientation, memory, calculation, reading and writing, visuospatial ability, and language.

Level of consciousness. Evaluating level of consciousness (LOC) assesses arousal or wakefulness. An altered LOC typically indicates organic brain impairment. If the individual is not conscious, the nurse applies increasing levels of stimulation (e.g., verbal, tactile, and painful) to elicit a response. The GCS (Teasdale & Jennett, 1974) is often used to assess LOC. Terms commonly used to describe LOC include alert, awake, lethargic, somnolent, stuporous, or comatose.

Orientation. Orientation is a cognitive function involving awareness of the dimensions of time, person, and place. Alterations in orientation can be caused by a number of factors including injury, drugs, brain lesions, and dementia. The examiner determines orientation by asking questions about time, place, and person because impairments tend to exist in this order (i.e., a sense of time is impaired before a sense of place). The nurse begins with specific questions about the date, time of day, location of the interview, and name of the interviewer and moves to more general questions if necessary. For example, if the client knows the year, but not the exact date, the nurse can ask the season.

Memory. Memory function is traditionally divided into four spheres: *immediate retention and recall; recent memory; short-term memory; and remote or long-term memory.* To check immediate retention and recall, the nurse gives the person three unrelated words to remember and asks him or her to recite them immediately and at 5-and 15-minute intervals during the interview. To test recent memory, the nurse asks questions about events of the past few hours or days. Short-term memory involves things that occurred within the past few weeks or months. The nurse assesses remote or long-term memory by asking about events of years ago. If they are personal events and the answers seem incorrect, the nurse may check them with a family member.

Attention and concentration. To test attention and concentration, the nurse asks the individual to count backward, aloud, from 100 by increments of 7 (e.g., 93, 86, 79, and so on) or to start with 20 and subtract 3. The nurse must decide which is most appropriate for the patient/client considering education and understanding; subtracting 3s from 20 is the easier of the two tasks. Another way to test these areas is to ask the person to spell a simple word, such as house, backward.

Insight and Judgment

Insight and judgment are related concepts that involve the ability to examine ideas, conceptualize facts, solve problems, and think abstractly. **Insight** is understanding the reality of a set of circumstances. It reflects the person's awareness of his or her own thoughts and feelings and an ability to compare them with the thoughts and feelings of others. For example, individuals with impaired insight may not believe that they have mental illness. They may have delusions and hallucinations or be hospitalized for bizarre and sometimes dangerous behaviour but do not grasp that this is unusual or abnormal.

Judgment is the ability to reach a logical decision about a situation and to choose a course of action after examining and analyzing various possibilities. Throughout the interview, the nurse evaluates the person's problem-solving abilities and capacity to learn from past experience. For example, a nurse might conclude that an individual who repeatedly chooses partners who are abusive demonstrates poor judgment in selecting partners. Another way to assess judgment is to give a simple scenario and ask the person to identify the best response. An example of such a scenario is, "What would you do if you found a bag of money outside a bank on a busy street?" If the client responds, "run with it," his or her judgment is questionable.

Stress and Coping Patterns

Everyone lives with some degree of stress in their life (see Chapter 17 for a full discussion). For vulnerable individuals, however, stress may contribute to the development of PMH disorders. Identification of major stressors in an individual's life helps the nurse to understand and support the use of successful coping behaviours in the future. The nurse should identify the individual's current stressors and coping strategies and evaluate the effectiveness of the latter. This information is vital to the overall plan of care because it highlights both problem areas and resources.

● **STUDY NOTE**

A comprehensive assessment should always identify stressors and coping patterns. Identifying how an individual copes with stress can be used as a basis of care in all nursing situations. Review content from Chapter 17 when studying these concepts.

Assessing Risk and Protective Factors

An individual's mental health-illness is influenced by the complex interaction of individual characteristics or attributes, socioeconomic circumstances, and environmental factors (World Health Organization, 2012) (Table 10-3). Assessment takes into account both the presence and balance of risk factors, protective factors, and promotive factors. **Risk factors** are those characteristics, conditions, situations, and events that increase the individual's vulnerability to threats to safety or well-being. Throughout this text, assessment of risk factors focuses on risks to safety, risks for developing PMH disorders, and risks for increasing, or exacerbating, symptoms and impairment in individuals with an existing psychiatric disorder. **Protective factors** are attributes or conditions of an individual, family, and/or community when present reduces, mitigates, or eliminates risk. **Promotive factors** are conditions or attributes of individuals, families, and/or communities that actively enhance well-being. Taken together, protective and promotive factors increase the probability of positive, adaptive, and healthy outcomes, even in the face of risk and adversity.

Assessing safety is a priority and a part of every encounter with clients. Examples include the risk for deliberate self-harm or suicide; risk for violence toward others; and risk for adverse events, such as falls, seizures, allergic reactions, or elopement. Nurses must assess these risk factors on a priority basis. For example, they must assess the risk for violence or suicide and take measures to prevent injury, such as implementing environmental constraints, before addressing other assessment factors.

Table 10-3   Overview of Risks to Mental Health Over the Life Course

Setting	Home/Family	School	Social Media	Work	Community
Culture	Low socioeconomic status	Adverse learning environment	Discrimination/ social inequities		
Community	Poor housing/living conditions	Difficulties at school	Bullying	Unemployment	Neighbourhood violence/crime
Family	Substance use in pregnancy	Peer pressure		Job stress or insecurity	Poor civic amenities
	Trauma or maltreatment Family conflict/violence Parental mental illness				Debt/poverty
Person	Gender	Antisocial or criminal behaviour			Bereavement
	Insecure attachment Malnutrition Low self-esteem Psychoactive drug use				Elder abuse

Physical ill-health

→

| Prenatal period | Childhood | Adolescence | Adulthood | Older adulthood |

Adapted from Kieling, C., et al. (2011). Child and adolescent mental health worldwide: Evidence for action. *Lancet*, 378(9801), 1515–1525.

Suicide/Deliberate Self-Harm

A suicide risk assessment involves garnering specific details regarding

Suicidal ideation—thoughts about deliberate self-harm or of self-inflicted death

Threats of suicide—a verbal or behavioural indication (direct or indirect) that an individual is planning to end his or her life

Suicide attempt—action taken with the intent of ending one's life

To ascertain this information, the nurse asks specific questions about suicidal thoughts, previous suicide attempts (including dates and outcome), the existence and lethality of a suicide plan, access to means, and symptoms of hopelessness. See Chapter 19 for a full discussion.

- Are you currently thinking about harming or killing yourself? Have you thought of these things in the past? Do you ever wish you were dead? If the answer to any of these questions is "yes," probe for details about when these thoughts occur and their frequency and intensity.
- Have you ever tried to harm or kill yourself? If the answer is "yes," probe for details about precipitating circumstances, means, and outcome. If the individual has thought about suicide but not acted on these thoughts, determine why not.
- Do you have a plan for how you might kill yourself? If the answer is "yes," ask for details (e.g., when and by what means).

- Do you have the things you need to carry out this plan?
- Have you made preparations for your death (e.g., writing a good-bye note, putting finances in order, and/or giving away possessions)?
- What does the future hold for you? Probe for indications of hopelessness, a sense of helplessness, a loss of enjoyment in life, guilt or shame, anger, or impaired judgment.

From this assessment, the nurse and other members of the team determine the individual's level of risk for self-harm and intervene as necessary. Most PMH programs and facilities use rating scales to quantify an individual's risk for self-harm. Those deemed to be at high risk are usually hospitalized and constantly observed.

Assaultive or Homicidal Ideation

A safety assessment also includes an evaluation of the level of threat an individual poses to others. Of particular importance are delusions or hallucinations that involve harming or killing others. Questions to ask to ascertain assaultive or homicidal ideation are as follows:

- Do you intend to harm someone? If yes, whom?
- Do you have a plan for how you might do this? If yes, what are the details of the plan?
- Do you have the things that you need to carry out your plan? (If the plan requires a weapon, is it readily available?)

Social Domain

A comprehensive assessment also attends to social dimensions of an individual's life. Much of this information is elicited during the health history and the MSE, and it includes information about the individual's current living situation, the individual's family of origin, and the existence and quality of significant relationships (see Chapter 15). The treatment team also assesses work, education, and social and leisure activities. As well, the team observes the individual's interactions with those around him or her. This component of the assessment helps to identify important strengths and resources as well as problems and deficits.

Functional Status

Understanding how an individual functions in his or her day-to-day life is a vital part of assessment. The *DSM-5* recommends clinicians use the Cross-Cutting Symptom Measure at the initial interview and over time to follow changes in status and treatment response (American Psychiatric Association, 2013). Level 1 of the adult version of this tool is a self-rated survey of 13 symptom domains for adults. For children and adolescents, level 1 has 12 domains to be rated by a parent/guardian. Level 2 of the tool allows for more in-depth assessment of some domains.

The *DSM-5* also provides a Clinician-Rated Dimension of Psychosis Symptom Severity scale in which clinicians rate the severity (0–4) of eight symptom domains (e.g., hallucinations, delusions, negative symptoms, etc.) experienced by the client over the past 7 days. The use of the World Health Organization Disability Assessment Schedule 2.0 (WHODAS 2.0), a self-administered tool, is recommended for assessing the difficulties experienced over the past 30 days due to health (including mental health) conditions. It explores six domains: understanding and communicating (cognition); moving and getting around (mobility); hygiene, dressing, eating, and staying alone (self-care); interacting with other people (getting along); domestic responsibilities, leisure, work, and school (life activities); and joining in community activities (participation) (Üstün, Kostanjsek, Chatterji, & Rehm, 2010). If the individual is unable to complete the questionnaire, a knowledgeable informant is asked to complete it. (See Web Links on thePoint for the site where the WHODAS 2.0 can be found.)

Ethnic and Cultural Assessment

Ethnicity and culture profoundly affect an individual's worldview and frame the person's beliefs about life, death, health and illness, and roles and relationships. As part of a comprehensive assessment, the nurse must consider ethnic and cultural factors that influence health and illness

(see Chapter 3). To understand these, the nurse should ask the following questions:

- Do you think of yourself as belonging to a particular ethnic or cultural group? If yes, which one(s)?
- What parts of your culture are most important to you? (Probe for details about values, beliefs, personal practices, social customs, behaviours, etc.)
- What does health mean to you?
- What does illness mean to you?
- How do you define good and evil?
- What things do you do to make yourself physically and mentally healthy?
- To whom do you turn when you feel physically or mentally ill?

The *DSM-5* offers a Cultural Formulation Interview schedule for clinicians to use to obtain information about the way culture may be influencing important aspects of an individual's clinical presentation (American Psychiatric Association, 2013).

Spiritual Assessment

Nurses must be clear about their own spirituality to ensure that it does not interfere with assessment of the client's spirituality. See Chapter 5 for a definition of spirituality. Examples of questions that may foster an understanding of an individual's spirituality include

- What gives your life meaning?
- What brings joy to your life?
- Do you believe in God or a higher power?
- Do you participate in any religious activities? If yes, which ones?
- Do you feel connected with the world?

● **STUDY NOTE**

Data from spirituality assessment can serve as a basis for strengthening coping strategies.

SUMMARY OF KEY POINTS

■ **Assessment** is a purposeful, systematic, and dynamic process that is ongoing throughout the nurse's relationship with individuals in his or her care. It involves the collection, validation, analysis, synthesis, organization, and documentation of the client's health–illness information.

■ A **comprehensive assessment** includes a health history and physical examination; considers the psychological, emotional, social, spiritual, ethnic, and cultural dimensions of health; attends to the meaning of the client's health–illness experience; and evaluates how all this affects the individual's daily living.

■ A focused assessment is the collection of specific information about a particular need, problem, or situation. It is briefer, narrower in scope, and more present oriented than is a comprehensive assessment.

■ Techniques of data collection include observation, interview, physical and mental examinations, and collaboration.

■ Biologic assessment includes health history, physical examination, and diagnostic testing.

■ Assessment of the psychological domain includes understanding the individual's response to mental health problems, MSE, evaluation of stress and coping, and risk assessment.

■ The MSE is a systematic assessment of an individual's appearance, affect, behaviour, and cognitive processes. It reflects the examiner's observations and impressions at the time of the interview and is used in a variety of clinical settings to evaluate developmental, neurologic, and psychiatric disorders.

■ Risk factors are those characteristics, conditions, situations, or events that increase the individual's vulnerability to threats to safety or well-being. Examples include the risk for self-harm or suicide, violence toward others, and the risk for adverse events, such as falls, seizures, allergic reactions, or elopement.

■ Protective factors are attributes or conditions of an individual, family, and/or community that reduce, mitigate, or eliminate risk.

■ Promotive factors are conditions or attributes of individuals, families, and/or communities that actively enhance well-being.

■ The social assessment involves a family and relationship assessment, evaluation of functional status, and information about the individual's ethnicity and culture.

■ Nurses must be aware of their own spiritual beliefs and ensure that those beliefs do not affect their spiritual assessment of the client.

CRITICAL THINKING CHALLENGES

1 A 23-year-old Caucasian woman is admitted to an acute psychiatric setting because she has been depressed for most of the past month. Yesterday, she was taken to the emergency department after she cut her wrists. Her admission form states that this is her first psychiatric admission, although she reports having had bouts of depression since early adolescence. She and her fiancé have just ended their engagement and moved into separate apartments. She has not yet told anyone that she is pregnant. She reports that her mother believes that she was "living in sin" and that she would "pay for it." From this scenario, develop three assessment questions for each domain: biologic, psychological, social, and spiritual.

2 Reflect on the biologic, psychological, social, and spiritual factors that affect your own self-concept. How do your personal beliefs, values, and experiences affect your interactions with individuals with mental health/psychiatric problems? How might these things affect your practice?

REFERENCES

American Psychiatric Association. (2013). *Diagnostic and statistical manual of mental disorders* (5th ed.). Washington, DC: Author.

Canadian Federation of Mental Health Nurses. (2014). *Canadian standards of psychiatric and mental health nursing* (4th ed.). Toronto, ON: Author.

Canadian Mental Health Association [CMHA]. (2008). *The relationship between mental health, mental illness and chronic physical conditions.* Retrieved from http://ontario.cmha.ca/mental-health/connection-between-mental-and-physical-health/

Canadian Psychiatric Association. (2012). *Youth and mental illness.* Retrieved from http://publications.cpa-apc.org/browse/documents/20

Folstein, M. F, Folstein, S. E., & McHugh, P. R. (1975). Mini-mental state. A practical method for grading the cognitive state of patients for the clinician. *Journal of Psychiatric Research, 12*(3), 189–198.

Government of Canada. (2006). *The human face of mental health and mental illness in Canada.* Catalogue No. HP5-19/2006E. Ottawa, ON: Author.

Kieling, C., Baker-Henningham, H., Belfer, M., Conti, G., Ertem, I., Omigbodun, O., … Rahman, A. (2011). Child and adolescent mental health worldwide: Evidence for action. *Lancet, 378*(9801), 1515–1525.

Leucht, S., Burkard, T., Henderson, J., Maj, M., & Sartorius, N. S. (2007). Physical illness and schizophrenia: A review of the literature. *Acta Psychiatrica Scandinavica, 116*(5), 317–333.

Office of the Privacy Commission of Canada. (2012). *Privacy legislation in Canada.* Retrieved from http://www.priv.gc.ca/resource/fs-fi/02_05_d_15_e.asp

Rogers, C. R. (1975). Empathic: An unappreciated way of being. *The Counseling Psychologist, 5*(2), 2–10. Retrieved from http://tcp.sagepub.com/cgi/reprint/5/2/2-a

Saddock, J., & Saddock, V. A. (2003). *Kaplan's & Saddock's synopsis of psychiatry: Behavioral sciences and clinical psychiatry* (9th ed.). Philadelphia, PA: Lippincott Williams & Wilkins.

Teasdale, G., & Jennett, B. (1974). Assessment of coma and impaired consciousness. *Lancet, 304*(7872), 81–84.

Üstün, T. B., Kostanjsek, N., Chatterji, S., & Rehm, J. (Eds.). (2010). *Measuring health and disability: Manual for WHO Disability Assessment Schedule (WHODAS 2.0).* Geneva, IL: World Health Organization.

World Health Organization. (2010). *Framework for action on interprofessional education and collaborative practice.* Retrieved from http://www.who.int/hrh/resources/framework_action/en/

World Health Organization. (2012). *Risks to mental health: An overview of vulnerabilities and risk factors.* Retrieved from http://www.who.int/mental_health/mhgap/risks_to_mental_health_EN_27_08_12.pdf

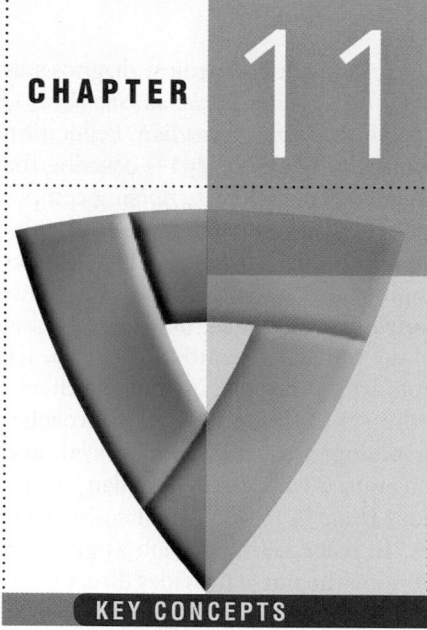

11 Diagnosis, Intervention, and Outcomes in Psychiatric and Mental Health Nursing

Nicole Snow and Christine Davis
Adapted from the chapters "Psychiatric and Mental Health Nursing Interventions" by Mary Ann Boyd and Janet Landeen, and "Diagnosis and Outcomes Development" by Doris Bell and Lorraine D. Williams

KEY CONCEPTS

- best practice guidelines
- collaboration
- client-centred care
- defining characteristics
- nursing diagnosis
- nursing interventions
- outcomes

LEARNING OBJECTIVES

After studying this chapter, you will be able to:

- Define the components of nursing diagnoses.
- Discuss the use of nursing diagnoses and outcomes in psychiatric and mental health care.
- Discuss the way clinical knowledge and judgement and a commitment to collaboration with clients and families determine the selection of nursing interventions.
- Explain the use of best practice guidelines.
- Describe the application of nursing interventions for the biologic domain.
- Describe the application of nursing interventions for the psychological domain.
- Describe the application of nursing interventions for the social domain.
- Describe the application of nursing interventions for the spiritual domain.
- Discuss the relationship between client-centred care, patient outcomes, and quality care.
- Demonstrate the process of developing individual outcome statements.

KEY TERMS

- automatic thinking • behaviour modification • behaviour therapy
- chemical restraint • cognitive interventions • conflict resolution
- counselling • cultural brokering • de-escalation • defining characteristics • diagnosis-specific outcomes • discharge outcomes
- distraction • guided imagery • home visits • illogical thinking
- indicators • initial outcomes • milieu therapy • observation
- open communication • physical restraint • psychoeducation
- recovery • reminiscence • revised outcomes • seclusion • simple relaxation techniques • spiritual care • structured interaction • token economy • validation

After completing an assessment of the individual who is to receive care, nurses generate appropriate nursing diagnoses based on the assessment data. The experienced nurse can readily cluster the assessment data to support one nursing diagnosis over another. Mutually agreed upon goals flow from nursing diagnoses and provide guidance in determining appropriate interventions. Initial outcomes are determined and then are monitored and evaluated throughout the care process. Measuring outcomes not only demonstrates clinical effectiveness but also helps to promote rational clinical decision making and is reflective of the nursing interventions.

Psychiatric and mental health (PMH) nursing interventions are nursing activities that promote mental health, prevent mental illness, assess dysfunction, assist clients to regain or improve their coping abilities, and/or prevent further disabilities. Based on clinical knowledge and judgement and a commitment to collaboration and partnership with clients and their families, nursing interventions include any treatment that a nurse performs to enhance client outcomes. These interventions are direct (performed through interaction with the client) or indirect (performed away from but on behalf of the client) (Bulechek, Butcher, Dochterman, & Wagner, 2013). Interventions can be either nurse-initiated treatment, which is an autonomous action in response to a nursing diagnosis, or physician-initiated treatment, which is a response to a medical diagnosis as a result of a physician's order. The *Canadian Standards of Psychiatric-Mental Health Nursing* (Canadian Federation of Mental Health Nurses [CFMHN], 2014) describe the scope of PMH nursing practice, delineate nursing competencies, and guide the selection of interventions for implementation in the plan of care (see Chapter 5). This chapter describes the development of nursing diagnoses, client-centred care, and individual outcomes in PMH nursing within the context of the Canadian health care system.

After many factors are considered, including a client's self-care activities, the selection of nursing approaches involves integrating biologic, psychological, social, and spiritual interventions into a comprehensive plan of care with and for the client (Fig. 11-1). PMH nurses provide care in various roles. In some settings, such as an acute care hospital or the home, the nurse provides direct nursing care. In other settings, such as the community, the nurse may assume the role of case manager, who primarily coordinates care for all disciplines, including nursing. In this instance, the nurse may be responsible for all or part of direct nursing care as well as for ensuring that agreed-on care is appropriate for the client, even if other providers deliver it. The nurse may also be the leader or manager of a nursing unit and thus responsible for delegating the care to paraprofessional and nonprofessional providers; however, he or she remains accountable for the client's care. In all of these instances, the nurse, working

FIGURE 11-1. PMH nursing interventions.

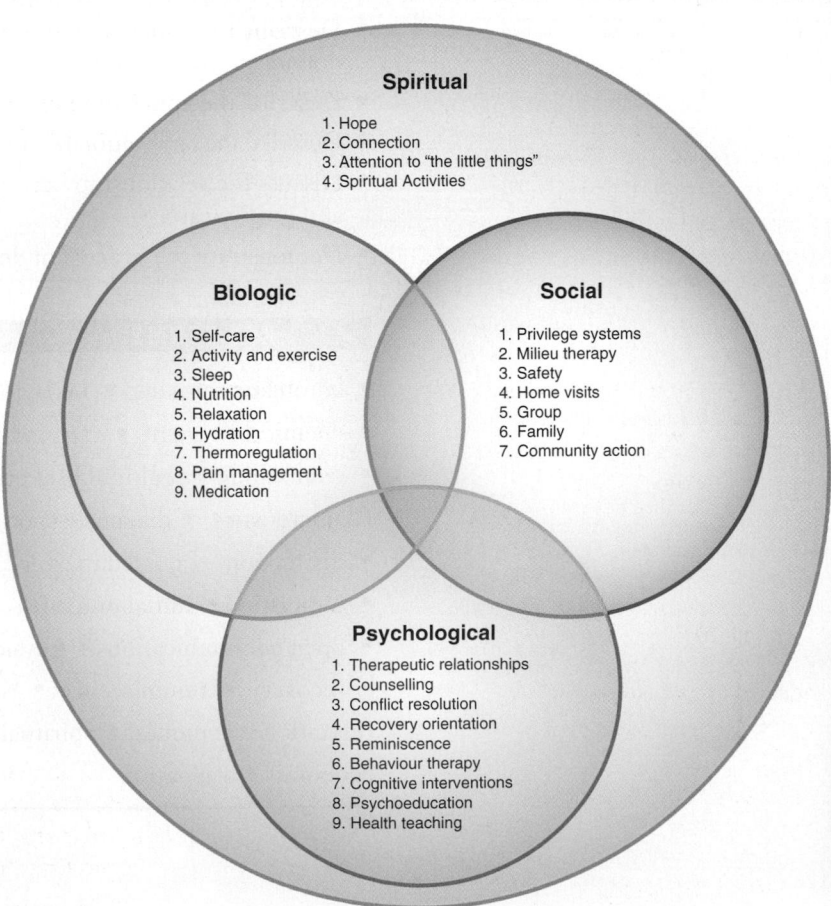

in partnership with the client and/or the client's family, plans and initiates safe and appropriate interventions.

A COMMITMENT TO COLLABORATION AND CLIENT CENTREDNESS

The current trend in nursing in Canada is away from the nurse as an expert on a client's needs and towards a client-centred approach, recognizing that individuals are unique (Registered Nurses Association of Ontario [RNAO], 2006), make meaning of their own lived experiences, and should participate as they can in all aspects of their care (Canadian Collaborative Mental Health Initiative [CCMHI], 2006). This means that plans of care are created and provided with respect for the preferences, values, and particular needs of the client and implemented as much as possible in partnership with the client and his or her family. The nurse needs to be able to discuss with them the risks and benefits of proposed interventions.

In order to enhance mental health services in primary care, the CCMHI was formed in 2004. This is a consortium of 12 national organizations representing community services, consumer, family and self-help groups, dieticians, family physicians, nurses, occupational therapists, pharmacists, psychologists, psychiatrists, and social workers. Its work centres on the needs of individual consumers of services. This consumer "centredness"—or client-centred care—involves individuals, families, and caregivers in all areas of care, from treatment choices to evaluation (Gagne, 2005).

Canadian nurses are committed to working together with clients and families. The *Canadian Collaborative Mental Health Care Charter* (CCMHI, 2006) was developed by national organizations of consumers and providers of mental health services (including the Canadian Nurses Association, the Registered Psychiatric Nurses of Canada, and the Canadian Federation of Mental Health Nurses). The charter identifies seven principles of collaborative clinical decisions and interventions: health promotion and prevention of mental health problems; holistic promotion; collaboration; partnership; respect for diversity; information exchange; and resources.

> **KEY CONCEPT** **Client-centred care** is a holistic approach and not merely about delivering services where the client is located. Client-centred care involves respecting the client's autonomous voice, self-determination, and right to participate in decision making (RNAO, 2006).

> **KEY CONCEPT** **Collaboration** is the process of working together towards common goals. Sharing knowledge and information can be an important aspect of the process.

EVOLUTION OF NURSING DIAGNOSIS AND INDIVIDUAL OUTCOMES

The concepts of nursing diagnosis and individual outcomes are not new. Florence Nightingale identified patient problems and analyzed patient outcomes during the Crimean War. Aydelotte (1962) published one of the first nursing studies involving patient outcomes. Lang and Clinton (1984) proposed nursing outcomes to include physical health status, mental health status, social and physical functioning, health attitude, knowledge and behaviour, use of professional health resources, and patient perception of the quality of nursing care. Marek (1989) identified 15 nursing outcome categories: physiologic measures; symptom control; frequency of service; home maintenance; psychosocial measures; well-being; functional status; goal attainment; patient behaviours; patient satisfaction; patient knowledge; rehospitalization; safety; cost; and resolution of nursing diagnoses. Further changes in health care provision and the nursing process in the 1990s resulted in efforts being focused on developing outcomes that could be used to evaluate nursing effectiveness. In 1998, the Nursing Outcomes Classification (NOC) taxonomy, with a structure similar to the Nursing Intervention Classification (NIC), was developed. The current fifth edition has 7 domains, 32 classes, and 490 outcomes (Moorhead, Johnson, Maas, & Swanson, 2013). Although the importance of identifying intervention outcomes has been the subject of nursing research since the 1960s, escalating health care costs have forced the demonstration of measurable outcomes. Concerns about quality, cost, and use of limited resources have contributed to the current emphasis on both evidence-based practice and individual outcomes. With the expansion of nursing knowledge gained through measuring intervention effectiveness, the nursing discipline evolves.

In Canada in the early 2000s, the RNAO was funded by the Ontario Ministry of Health and Long-Term Care to develop, implement, evaluate, and revise Best Practice Guidelines (BPGs) that would inform nursing practice in a number of areas and better ensure outcomes, thereby reducing costs (RNAO, 2012).

Box 11-1 provides examples of available RNAO guidelines. The purpose of BPGs is multifaceted: to deliver care that is effective and based on current evidence, to aid in seeking resolutions to clinical problems, to meet or exceed current quality standards in providing excellent care, to initiate use of innovations, to eliminate interventions that are not meeting best practice standards, and to foster clinical excellence through supportive work environments (RNAO, 2012).

The evidence-based practice movement, from which BPGs evolved, is not without its critics. Canadian nurse scholar and researcher David Holmes and his colleagues argue that "ready-made" guidelines can serve to impede nurses' critical thinking and thus diminish the social,

---

BOX 11-1 Examples of RNAO Practice Guidelines

Caregiving strategies for older adults with delirium, dementia, and depression
Client-centred care
Crisis intervention
Enhancing healthy adolescent development
Establishing therapeutic relationships
Postpartum depression
Suicidal ideation and behaviour
Supporting clients on methadone maintenance treatment
Supporting and strengthening families through expected and unexpected life events
Women abuse: Screening, identification, and initial response

BOX 11-2 Nursing Diagnoses Pertinent to PMH Nursing

Ineffective Coping
Disturbed Body Image
Disturbed Personal Identity
Acute Confusion
Chronic Confusion
Risk for Self-Harm
    Self-Mutilation
    Risk for Self-Mutilation
    Risk for Suicide
Ineffective Self-Health Management

From Carpenito, L. J. (2013). *Handbook of nursing diagnosis* (14th ed). Philadelphia, PA: Lippincott Williams & Wilkins.

---

political, and ethical responsibilities of the discipline. Taking the BPGs of RNAO as a case study, they suggest further that BPGs facilitate the control and regulation of nursing practice by health care organizations (Holmes, Murray, Arron, & McCabe, 2008).

KEY CONCEPT Best practice guidelines (BPGs), also termed clinical practice guidelines (CPGs), are broad or specific recommendations for health care based on the best current evidence.

DERIVING A NURSING DIAGNOSIS

Nursing diagnoses provide clearer identification of nursing knowledge and practice (Carpenito-Moyet, 2010). The basis for planning nursing interventions, they are used in diverse practice settings in multiple populations to assist individuals to achieve positive health outcomes (Delaney, Herr, Maas, & Specht, 2000). For nurses to improve their ability to make sound nursing diagnoses, they must actively apply nursing principles, concepts, and theories to the care of the individual (Kleinpell, 2003).

Clusters of data lead the nurse to choose certain diagnoses over others. For example, when assessing an individual, the nurse observes that his or her responses are often self-negating (e.g., "I always mess things up," "I never get it right"). The nurse also observes that he or she seems indecisive and lacking in problem-solving abilities (e.g., "I can never decide what the right thing to do is, and when I do finally choose, it is always wrong"). Nonverbal and verbal information are used to identify **defining characteristics**. Observations of an individual sitting with her head down, making no eye contact, and dressed in dirty clothes are important data. Such observations support the hypothesis that the individual has a disturbance in self-esteem. Further assessment will help the nurse determine whether the self-esteem disturbance is chronic or situational.

Related factors are those that influence or change the individual's health status. They are grouped into four categories: pathophysiologic, biologic, or psychological

(e.g., oxygen transport); treatment related (e.g., medications, diagnostic studies, and surgeries); situational (e.g., environmental, home, community, and person); and maturational (e.g., age-related influences on health) (Carpenito-Moyet, 2010). To continue with the assessment example, the nurse learns that the individual has lost three jobs within the past year, resulting in financial problems. These situation-related factors further support the nursing diagnosis of self-esteem disturbance. The North American Nursing Diagnosis Association (NANDA, 1990) taxonomy is not universally used in Canada. In some mental health settings, it is regarded as insufficiently client centred. See Box 11-2 for examples of nursing diagnoses pertinent to PMH nursing.

KEY CONCEPT A **nursing diagnosis** is a clinical judgement about individual, family, or community responses to actual or potential problems/life processes. Nursing diagnosis provides the basis for selection of nursing interventions to achieve outcomes for which the nurse is accountable (NANDA, 1990).

KEY CONCEPT Defining characteristics are key signs and symptoms (clues) that relate to each other and that validate a nursing diagnosis. The nurse analyzes these clues to formulate a cluster of data, which helps in making a diagnosis or diagnoses that reflects the actual or potential health status or problems of the individual.

KEY CONCEPT Outcomes are the individual's response to nursing care at a given point in time. An outcome is concise, stated in few words, and in neutral terms. Outcomes describe an individual's state, behaviour, or perception that is variable and can be measured (Table 11-1).

Table 11-1	Example of Outcomes	

Diagnosis	Outcome	Intervention
Spiritual distress Related to conflict between religious or spiritual beliefs and prescribed health regime	Will express religious or spiritual satisfaction	Provide accurate information about treatment plan. Encourage the client and the physician to consider alternative methods of therapy. Support client making informed decisions—even if decision conflicts with own values.
	Indicators a. Express decreased feelings of guilt and fear b. State that conflict has been eliminated	

From Carpenito-Moyet, L. J. (2010). *Nursing diagnosis: Application to clinical practice* (13th ed.). Philadelphia, PA: Lippincott Williams & Wilkins.

DEVELOPING INDIVIDUAL OUTCOMES

Outcomes should be individualized (Table 11-2). Individual outcomes are linked to nursing diagnoses through the nursing process. By linking outcomes to the nursing diagnosis, it is possible to monitor nursing practice and facilitate clinical decision making and knowledge development (Table 11-3).

Outcomes can be defined as an individual's response to care. Outcomes are the end result of a process, a treatment, or a nursing intervention and should be monitored and documented over time and across clinical settings. **Diagnosis-specific outcomes** show that the intervention resolved the problem or nursing diagnosis (Table 11-4). At other times, the outcome is nonspecific (i.e., not diagnosis specific, meaning it does not show resolution of the diagnosis). In that case, the outcome is abstract or general (Table 11-5). Outcomes may be used to evaluate interventions by other health care disciplines as well as nursing (Moorhead et al., 2013). For example,

occupational therapy may contribute significantly to a client's psychosocial adaptation.

Indicators answer the question, "How close is the individual moving towards the outcome?" The indicator represents the dimensions of the outcome. Outcome indicators represent or describe individual status, behaviours, or perceptions evaluated during an individual's assessment. Indicators are a measurement of individual progress in relation to the individual outcomes and can serve as intermediate outcomes in a clinical pathway or standardized care plan. See Table 11-6 for examples of NOC core outcomes for PMH nursing. In nursing care planning, outcomes can be **initial outcomes** (those written after the initial individual interview and assessment), **revised outcomes** (those written after each evaluation), or **discharge outcomes** (those outcomes to be met before discharge). Because of the decreased length of stay or days of service, discharge outcomes often are not met but are passed along to the community nurse. If these discharge outcomes continue to be relevant, they become initial outcomes in community or home care.

Table 11-2	Clinical Path: Depression			

Day	Assessment Parameters	Nursing Diagnosis	Nursing Interventions	Patient Outcomes
1	Individual admits to having a suicide plan.	Risk for self-directed violence	Institute suicide precautions.	Suicide: self-restraint
2	Maintain suicide precautions.	Suicide: self-restraint		
3	Individual is apathetic, does not wash or dress self.	Ineffective health maintenance	Help individual with personal hygiene, exhibit patience.	Self-care: dressing and bathing

From Moorhead, S., Johnson, M., & Maas, M. (2004). *Nursing outcomes classification (NOC)* (3rd ed.). St. Louis, MO: Mosby.

Table 11-3   **Results of Nursing Interventions**

Diagnosis	Patient Outcome	Nursing Intervention
Ineffective coping	The person will make decisions and follow through with appropriate actions to change provocative situations in the person environment.	Assess causative and contributing factors (Lyon, 2002). Establish rapport. Assess present coping status. Assess level of depression. Assist the client in developing appropriate problem-solving strategies. Teach problem-solving techniques. Initiate health teaching and referrals as indicated.
	Indicators a. Verbalize feelings related to emotional state. b. Focus on the present. c. Identify response patterns and the consequences of resulting behaviour. d. Identify personal strengths and accept support through the nursing relationship.	

From Carpenito, L. J. (2013). *Handbook of nursing diagnosis* (14th ed., pp. 168–175). Philadelphia, PA: Lippincott Williams & Wilkins.

Documentation of Outcomes

Nurses are accountable for documentation of individual outcomes, nursing interventions, and any changes in diagnosis, care plan, or both. Individual responses to care are documented as changes in behaviour or knowledge and can include the degree of satisfaction with the health care provided (Kleinpell, 2003). Outcomes can be expressed in terms of the individual's actual responses (e.g., no longer reports hearing voices) or the status of a nursing diagnosis at a point in time after implementation of nursing interventions, such as "caregiver role strain resolved." This documentation is important for further research and quality of care studies.

Purposes of Individual Outcomes

The primary purposes of developing individual outcomes are to ensure quality care and that the needs of the individual are being met. They provide guidelines for what is expected of the individual and direction for continuity of care that reflects current knowledge in the field of PMH nursing. The measurement of individual outcomes helps to meet the goal of continuous quality improvement.

Accountability is an important concept in health care. Nursing and other disciplines are being pressured within health service systems to justify their practice, to demonstrate to users of services that they deliver quality care, and to control health care costs. Measurement of outcomes can be used to determine quality of care during a single episode of illness and across the continuum of care and can assist in discharge planning. Outcomes also can be used to determine quality of care in different systems and between systems. Evaluation of individual outcomes can help validate nursing interventions by identifying which interventions are effective (refer to Table 11-7 for expected outcomes from nursing interventions). Outcomes can also be a

Table 11-4   **Example of Condition: Diagnosis-Specific Outcomes**

Diagnosis	Outcome
Anxiety	a. Anxiety control b. Aggression control

From Moorhead, S., Johnson, M., & Maas, M. (2004). *Nursing outcomes classification (NOC)* (3rd ed.). St. Louis, MO: Mosby.

Table 11-5   **Example of System-Specific Outcome**

Diagnosis	Outcome
Disturbed sensory perception (hallucination)	Movement disorder occurrence
	Indicators a. Initiation of antipsychotic drugs b. Demonstration of choreic movement c. Demonstration of pelvic gyrations d. Increase or decrease in dosage of antipsychotic drugs

From Moorhead, S., Johnson, M., & Maas, M. (2004). *Nursing outcomes classification (NOC)* (3rd ed.). St. Louis, MO: Mosby.

Table 11-6	Example—Linkage of Nursing Diagnosis and Outcomes	
Diagnosis	**Outcome**	
1. Disturbed Body Image	Maintenance of grooming/hygiene	
2. Chronic Confusion	Asks for validation of reality	
3. Risk for Self-Harm	Identify personal triggers for self-harm	

From Carpenito, L. J. (2013). *Handbook of nursing diagnosis* (14th ed.). Philadelphia, PA: Lippincott Williams & Wilkins.

communication tool between nurses, and with case managers, caregivers, and policy makers. They can be used to conduct program evaluations and to develop research databases.

NURSING INTERVENTIONS AND PMH NURSING

The *Nursing Interventions Classification* (NIC) (Bulechek et al., 2013) is an extensive system of specific interventions, with discrete activities for each. The NIC system is based on data collected from surveys of practising nurses, who identified the interventions that were ultimately classified. The NIC taxonomy includes classes or groups of interventions categorized according to seven domains: physiologic basic; physiologic complex; behavioural; safety; family; health system; and community. The NIC taxonomy represents both basic and specialty advanced nursing practices.

Table 11-7	Expected Outcomes from Nursing Interventions	
Nursing Intervention	**Expected Outcome**	
Provide educational information about mental illness	Knowledge: disease process	
Educational group in caregiving	Caregiver well-being	
Group therapy	Improved distorted thought control	
Weight control counselling	Knowledge: diet	
Health teaching	Knowledge: medication	
Teaching limit setting	Coping	
Reality orientation	Identity: self	
Life review	Hope	
Teaching anger management	Impulse self-control	

From Moorhead, S., Johnson, M., & Maas, M. (2004). *Nursing outcomes classification (NOC)* (3rd ed.). St. Louis, MO: Mosby.

For example, both basic and specialist nurses use interventions such as reinforcing positive behaviour; however, the advanced practice psychiatric nurse may actually develop the plan and also use it as part of psychotherapy with the client. This text uses many NIC interventions (Box 11-3) and is strongly influenced by the framework of interventions identified in the *Canadian Standards of Psychiatric-Mental Health Nursing* (CFMHN, 2014) (see Chapter 5).

Interventions for the Biologic Domain

Biologic interventions focus on physical functioning and are directed towards the client's self-care, activities and exercise, sleep, nutrition, relaxation, hydration, and thermoregulation as well as pain management and medication management. In the NIC taxonomy, these interventions are found within the physiologic basic and physiologic complex domains.

Promotion of Self-Care Activities

Self-care is the ability to perform activities of daily living (ADLs) successfully. Many clients with PMH problems can manage self-care activities such as bathing, dressing appropriately, selecting adequate nutrition, and sleeping regularly. (Although maintaining adequate nutrition and promoting normal sleep hygiene are considered self-care activities, they are discussed in separate sections because of their significance in mental health care.) Others, however, cannot manage such self-care activities, either because of their symptoms or as a result of the side effects of medications. Because nursing is concerned with maintaining the client's health and well-being, a focus on ADLs can become a nursing priority.

Orem's (1991) nursing model is based on the concept of self-care deficit (see Chapter 8). Deficits in self-care may be related to attitude (motivation), knowledge, or skill. The model identifies five nursing approaches to deficits in a client's self-care: acting or doing for; guiding; teaching; supporting; and providing an environment to promote the client's ability to meet current or future demands. The emphasis is on helping the individual develop independence. In the inpatient setting, the PMH nurse works with the client so that basic self-care activities are completed. During acute phases of psychiatric disorders, the inability to attend to basic self-care tasks (e.g., getting dressed) is very common. Therefore, the ability to complete personal hygiene activities (e.g., dental care, grooming) is monitored, and clients are assisted in completing such activities. In a psychiatric facility, clients are encouraged and expected to develop independence in completing these basic self-care activities to the best of their ability. In the community, monitoring these basic self-care activities is always a part of the nursing visit or clinic appointment.

BOX 11-3 Nursing Intervention Classification Taxonomy

1. Physiologic: Basic—Care That Supports Physical Functioning
   A. Activity and exercise management: Interventions to organize or assist with physical activity and energy conservation and expenditure
   B. Elimination management: Interventions to establish and maintain regular bowel and urinary elimination patterns and manage complications due to altered patterns
   C. Immobility management: Interventions to manage restricted body movement and the sequelae
   D. Nutrition support: Interventions to modify or maintain nutritional status
   E. Physical comfort promotion: Interventions to promote comfort using physical techniques
   F. Self-care facilitation: Interventions to provide or assist with routine ADLs
2. Physiologic: Complex—Care That Supports Homeostatic Regulation
   G. Electrolyte and acid–base management: Interventions to regulate electrolyte/acid–base balance and prevent complications
   H. Drug management: Interventions to facilitate the desired effects of pharmacologic agents
   I. Neurologic management: Interventions to optimize neurologic functions
   J. Perioperative care: Interventions to provide care before, during, and immediately after procedures (e.g., psychosurgery, electroconvulsive therapy)
   K. Respiratory management: Interventions to promote airway patency and gas exchange
   L. Skin/wound management: Interventions to maintain or restore tissue integrity
   M. Thermoregulation: Interventions to maintain body temperature within a normal range
   N. Tissue perfusion management: Interventions to optimize the circulation of blood and fluids to the tissues
3. Behavioural—Care That Supports Psychosocial Functioning and Facilitates Lifestyle Changes
   O. Behavioural therapy: Interventions to reinforce or promote desirable behaviours or alter undesirable behaviours

P. Cognitive therapy: Interventions to reinforce or promote desirable cognitive functioning or alter undesirable cognitive functioning
Q. Communication enhancement: Interventions to facilitate delivering and receiving verbal and nonverbal messages
R. Coping assistance: Interventions to assist another to build on own strengths, adapt to a change in function, or achieve a higher level of function
S. Client education: Interventions to facilitate learning
T. Psychological comfort promotion: Interventions to promote comfort using psychological techniques
4. Safety—Care That Supports Protection Against Harm
   U. Crisis management: Interventions to provide immediate, short-term help in both psychological and physiologic crises
   V. Risk management: Interventions to initiate risk reduction activities and continue monitoring risks over time
5. Family—Care That Supports the Family Unit
   W. Childbearing care: Interventions to assist in understanding and coping with the psychological and physiologic changes during the childbearing period
   X. Life span care: Interventions to facilitate family unit functioning and promote the health and welfare of family members throughout the life span
6. Health System—Care That Supports Effective Use of the Health Care Delivery System
   Y. Health system mediation: Interventions to facilitate the interface between the client/family and the health care system
   a. Health system management: Interventions to provide and enhance support services for the delivery of care
   b. Information management: Interventions to facilitate communication among health care providers
7. Community—Care That Supports the Health of the Community
   a. Community health promotion: Interventions that promote health of the community
   b. Community risk management: Interventions that assist in detecting or preventing health risk to the whole community

From Bulechek, G., Butcher, H., Dochterman, J., & Wagner, C. (eds.) (2013). *Nursing interventions classification (NIC)* (6th ed.). St. Louis, MO: Elsevier.

> **KEY CONCEPT** **Nursing interventions** are treatments or activities, based upon clinical judgement and knowledge, that are used by nurses to enhance patient or client outcomes (Bulechek et al., 2013).

Activity and Exercise Interventions

The nurse must attend to the client's level of activity. Encouraging regular activity and exercise can improve general well-being and physical health. A healthy lifestyle that includes daily exercise can help clients deal with the weight gain and type II diabetes associated with many psychotropic medications. In some psychiatric disorders (e.g., schizophrenia), people become sedentary and appear to lack the motivation to complete ADLs. This

lack of motivation is part of the disorder and requires nursing intervention. In addition, side effects of medication that include sedation and lethargy can compound the problem. It is possible for exercise behaviour to become an abnormal focus of attention, such as for some clients with anorexia nervosa.

When assuming the responsibility of a direct care provider, the nurse can help clients identify realistic activities and exercise goals. Some institutions have other professionals (e.g., recreational therapists) available for the implementation of exercise programs. As a case manager, the nurse should consider the activity needs of individuals when jointly setting goals. As a leader or manager of a psychiatric unit, the nurse can influence ward routines that promote activity and exercise.

Sleep Interventions

Many psychiatric disorders and medications are associated with sleep disturbances. Sleep is also disrupted in clients with dementia. These clients may have difficulty falling asleep or may frequently awaken during the night. In dementia of the Alzheimer type, individuals may reverse their sleeping patterns by napping during the day and staying awake at night.

Nonpharmacologic interventions are always used first for sleep disturbances because of the side-effect risks associated with the use of sedatives and hypnotics (see Chapter 12). Sleep interventions to communicate to clients include the following:

- Go to bed only when tired or sleepy.
- Establish a consistent bedtime routine.
- Avoid stimulating foods, beverages, or medications.
- Avoid naps in the late afternoon or evening.
- Eat lightly before retiring and limit fluid intake.
- Use the bed only for sleep or intimacy.
- Avoid emotional stimulation before bedtime.
- Use behavioural and relaxation techniques.
- Limit distractions.

For some clients, disrupted sleep can become chronic and quite problematic. Obtaining adequate sleep is vital for optimal daily functioning, and it is imperative that nurses assess for sleep disturbances and possible disorders and intervene appropriately. More information about sleep disorders and the nursing process involved in caring for an individual with sleep disturbances is provided in Chapter 28.

Nutrition Interventions

Psychiatric disorders and medication side effects can affect eating behaviours. For varying reasons, some clients eat too little, whereas others eat too much. For instance, homeless clients with mental illness have difficulty maintaining adequate nutrition because of their deprived lifestyle. Substance abuse also interferes with maintaining adequate nutrition, through either stimulation or suppression of appetite or through neglecting nutrition because of drug-seeking behaviour. Nutrition interventions should therefore be specific and relevant to the individual's circumstances and mental health. In addition, recommended daily allowances are important in the promotion of physical and mental health, and nurses should consider them when planning care. Resources for planning include Canada's Food Guide (Minister of Health Canada, 2011) and the Dietary Reference Intake information (Otten, Pitzi Hellwig, & Meyers, 2006).

Some psychiatric symptoms involve changes in perceptions of food, appetite, and eating habits. If a client believes that food is poisonous, he or she may eat sparingly or not at all. Interventions are then necessary to address the suspiciousness as well as to encourage adequate intake of recommended daily allowances. It may be necessary to allow clients to examine foods, participate in preparation, and test the meal's safety by eating slowly or after everyone else.

Obesity can be a problem for individuals being treated for a mental disorder. Antipsychotics, antidepressants, and mood stabilizers are associated with weight gain, which is thought to be related to changes in metabolism and appetite caused by some of these medications. Many clients stop taking medications because of the weight gain. Excessive weight gain can be especially stressful to the individual's emotional well-being, as well as detrimental to physical health. However, nurses should encourage clients to avoid quick weight loss programs because they are not effective. Furthermore, hypoglycaemia can exacerbate a depressed mood and lead to suicidal thoughts. If weight gain is a problem, the best approach is to assist the client to monitor current intake and develop realistic strategies for changing eating patterns combined with a healthy lifestyle.

Relaxation Interventions

Relaxation promotes comfort, reduces anxiety, alleviates stress, eases pain, and prevents aggression. It can diminish the effects of hallucinations and delusions. The many different relaxation techniques used as mental health interventions range from simple deep breathing to biofeedback to hypnosis. Although some techniques such as biofeedback require additional training and, in some instances, certification, nurses can easily apply simple relaxation, distraction, and imagery techniques.

Simple relaxation techniques encourage and elicit relaxation to decrease undesirable signs and symptoms. **Distraction** is the purposeful focusing of attention away from undesirable sensations. Table 11-8 provides a description of the implementation of these techniques. **Guided imagery** is the purposeful use of imagination to achieve relaxation or to direct attention away from undesirable sensations. It is especially useful in stress management. With this technique, clients imagine themselves doing something pleasurable and relaxing, such as lying on the beach or watching snow fall. They are encouraged (with permissive directions from the nurse, such as "If you wish…") to slowly experience the scene and to express how they feel and think about it. Slow, deep breathing is also encouraged (Bulechek et al., 2013). Guided imagery is an independent nursing intervention that can be used for such clients as those experiencing anxiety (Jallo, Cozens, Smith, & Simpson, 2013). However, as clients may experience unexpected, albeit therapeutic, reactions (e.g., crying) during guided imagery, students should not attempt this technique with clients unless supervised.

As a direct care provider, the nurse may teach the client relaxation exercises. As a case manager, nurses can

Table 11-8	Relaxation Techniques: Descriptions and Implementation

Simple Relaxation Techniques	Distraction
Create a quiet, nondisrupting environment with dim lights and a comfortable temperature.	Distraction techniques include music, counting, television, reading, play, and exercise, among others. Help the client choose a technique that will work for him or her. Keep in mind what may or may not be appropriate for the client based on factors such as energy level, age, literacy level, and developmental level.
Instruct the client to assume a relaxed position, wearing loose and comfortable clothing.	Advise the client to practise the distraction technique before he or she will need to use it.
Instruct the client to relax and to let the sensations happen.	Have the client develop a specific plan for how and when he or she will use distraction. Distraction can be used alone or in conjunction with other techniques.
Use a low tone of voice with a slow, rhythmic pace of words.	Teach the techniques to family members or significant others.
Instruct the client to take an initial slow, deep breath (abdominal breathing) while thinking about pleasant events.	Evaluate and document the client's response to distraction.
Use soothing music (without words) to enhance relaxation.	
Reinforce the use of relaxation by praising efforts and helping the client to schedule time regularly for it.	
Evaluate and document the client's response to relaxation.	

Adapted from Bulechek, G., Butcher, H., Dochterman, J. & Wagner, C. (eds.) (2013). *Nursing interventions classification (NIC)* (6th ed.). St. Louis, MO: Elsevier.

include relaxation exercises in the plan of care. The unit leader can be responsible for ensuring that appropriately prepared staff members implement relaxation exercises. Relaxation techniques that involve physical touch (e.g., back rubs) must be used particularly carefully, if at all, for people with mental disorders. Touching and massaging are often not appropriate for clients who have a history of physical or sexual abuse. Such clients may find touch too stimulating or misinterpret it as being sexual or aggressive. It is important for the nurse to maintain open communication with and elicit feedback from the client when providing physical interventions.

Hydration Interventions

Assessing fluid status and monitoring fluid intake and output are often important interventions. Overhydration or underhydration can be a symptom of a psychiatric disorder. For example, some clients with psychotic disorders experience chronic fluid imbalance. For these individuals, a treatment protocol that includes a target weight procedure can help prevent both overhydration and water intoxication and promote self-control (see Chapter 20). The nurse functions as the direct care provider (e.g., teaching client), unit leader (e.g., delegating weighing of the client to staff), or coordinator of the protocol.

Many psychiatric medications affect fluid and electrolyte balance (see Chapter 12). For example, when taking lithium carbonate, clients must have adequate fluid intake, with special attention paid to serum sodium levels. When sodium levels drop through perspiration, lithium is used in place of sodium, which in turn leads to lithium toxicity. Many psychiatric medications cause dry mouth, which in turn causes individuals to drink fluids excessively. Interventions that help clients understand the relationship of medications to fluid and electrolyte balance are important in their overall care.

Thermoregulation Interventions

Many psychiatric disorders can disturb the body's normal temperature regulation. Thus, clients cannot sense temperature increases or decreases and consequently cannot protect themselves from extremes of hot or cold. This problem is especially difficult for people who are homeless or live in substandard housing, such as some rooming houses. In addition, many psychiatric medications can also affect the ability to regulate body temperature.

Interventions include educating clients about the problem of thermoregulation, identifying potential extremes in temperatures, and developing strategies to protect the client from the adverse effects of temperature changes. For example, community nurses often engage in active outreach to at-risk clients during extreme weather alerts.

Pain Management

Emotional reactions are often manifested as pain. For instance, unexplained chronic pain can be a somatoform symptom (see Chapter 24). Chronic pain is particularly problematic when no cause for it is identified.

PMH nurses are more likely to provide care to clients experiencing chronic pain than acute pain. However, a single intervention is seldom successful for relieving chronic pain. In some instances, pain is managed by medication; in other instances, nonpharmacologic techniques are used, such as simple relaxation techniques, distraction, or imagery. Indeed, relaxation is one of the most widely used cognitive and behavioural approaches to pain. Psychoeducation, stress management techniques, and biofeedback are also used in pain management.

The key to managing pain is engaging the client in identifying how it is disrupting his or her personal, social, professional, and family life. Education focusing on the pain, the use of medications for treatment, and the development of cognitive skills are important pain management components. In some cases, redefining treatment success as improvement in functioning, rather than alleviation of pain, may be necessary. The interaction between stress and pain is important; that is, increased stress leads to increased pain. Clients can better manage their pain when stress is reduced (see Chapter 36).

Medication Management

The PMH nurse uses many medication management interventions to help clients maintain therapeutic regimens. Medication management involves more than the actual administration of medications. Nurses assess medication effectiveness and side effects and consider interactions with other drugs, herbal remedies, or homeopathic preparations. In addition, nurses assess any factors that may affect the client's adherence to a medication regimen, such as concerns regarding weight gain or reproductive ability, attitude towards taking medication, or cost issues. Education regarding medication must be made available to the client in appropriate ways, including information regarding the recognition and reporting of side effects. Suggesting strategies to assist the client in taking medication on time can be helpful. Treatment with psychopharmacologic agents can be lengthy because of the chronic nature of many disorders. It occurs in both acute and community care settings, as medication follow-up may include home visits as well as telephone calls. Many clients remain on medication regimens for years, never becoming medication free. Medication education is thus an ongoing intervention that requires careful documentation.

Interventions for the Psychological Domain

A major emphasis in PMH nursing is on the psychological domain: emotion, behaviour, and cognition. The nurse–client relationship serves as the basis for interventions directed towards the psychological domain. Because the therapeutic relationship is discussed extensively in Chapter 6, it is not covered in this chapter. This section covers counselling, conflict resolution, recovery orientation, reminiscence, behaviour therapy, cognitive interventions, psychoeducation, health teaching, and spiritual interventions. Chapter 8 presents the theoretic basis for many of these interventions.

Nurses in the direct care role will use all of the psychological interventions to respond to the health care problems of their clients. Nurses in case manager roles will also frequently use interventions from the psychological domain in order to promote recovery and empower the client to make changes. Case management relationships are based on trust. The nurse manager oversees the use of the psychological interventions and evaluates the staff's ability to use the interventions and assess outcomes.

Counselling Interventions

Counselling interventions are specific, time-limited interactions between a nurse and a client, family, or group experiencing immediate or ongoing difficulties related to their health or well-being. Counselling is usually short-term and focuses on improving coping abilities, reinforcing healthy behaviours, fostering positive interactions, or preventing illnesses and disabilities. Counselling strategies are discussed throughout the text. Psychotherapy is generally a long-term approach aimed at improving or helping clients regain previous health status and functional abilities. Mental health specialists, such as advanced practice nurses, use psychotherapy.

Conflict Resolution

A conflict involves an individual's perceptions, emotions, and behaviours. In a conflict, a person believes that his or her own needs, interests, wants, or values are incompatible with someone else's (Boggs, 2011). The individual experiences fear, sadness, bitterness, anger, hopelessness, or some combination of these emotions in response to the perceived threat. Misunderstandings, poor communication, value or goal differences, personality issues, and stress can interplay to contribute to this conflict and impact its resolution (Boggs, 2011).

Conflict resolution is a specific type of intervention through which the nurse helps clients resolve disagreements or disputes with family, friends, or other clients. Conflicts can be positive if individuals see the problem as solvable and providing an opportunity for growth and interpersonal understanding. The nurse may be in the position of actually resolving a family conflict or teaching family members how to resolve their own conflicts positively. In addition, because nurses are frequently in positions of leadership, they often need conflict resolution skills to settle employee conflicts.

Conflict Resolution Process

Calmness and objectivity are important in resolving any client or family conflict. The desired outcome of conflict resolution is a "win–win" situation in which each party feels positive about the outcome. The nurse will take the following steps in conflict resolution:

1. Identify conflict issues.
2. Know your own response to the conflict.
3. Separate the problem from the people involved.
4. Stay focused on the issue and the underlying motivations behind the position the other person took.
5. Identify available options.
6. Try to identify established standards to guide the decision-making process (Boggs, 2011).

It is important to be aware of what is causing the conflict. This can be difficult to discern at times, and open, honest, and respectful communication is necessary to facilitate this awareness. It is helpful when all parties involved are able to reflect on their reactions to the conflict and what triggers their emotional responses. It is best and most constructive when all involved are able to focus on the issue at hand and not be critical of the people involved. The focus needs to be on the here and now of the problem, without dwelling on issues that have occurred in the past. Once all parties understand the underlying reasons for the dispute, attention can be given to developing options on how to appropriately address it. As much as possible, this development should be a collaborative process with all parties contributing fairly to the outcome (Boggs, 2011).

Cultural Brokering in Client–System Conflicts

Clients may be marginalized within the health care system due to potentially stigmatizing factors, such as poverty, sexual orientation, lack of formal education, race, or ethnicity. Differences in cultural values and languages between clients and health care organizations can contribute to clients' feelings of powerlessness. For example, new immigrants, people who are homeless, and people who need to make informed decisions under stressful conditions may be unable to navigate the health care system. The nurse can help to resolve such conflicts through **cultural brokering**, or the use of culturally appropriate strategies that aid in bridging or mediating between the client's culture and the health care system (Bulechek et al., 2013). The health care system can be understood as a culture in and of itself, with culture shock being a potential experience for clients and families new to it.

For the "nurse-as-broker" to be effective, he or she establishes and maintains a sense of connectedness or relationship with the client. In turn, the nurse also establishes and cultivates networks with other health care facilities and resources. Cultural sensitivity enables the nurse to be aware of and sensitive to the needs of clients from a variety of cultures. Cultural competence is necessary for the brokering process to be effective (see Chapter 3).

Recovery Orientation

Recovery-focused interventions are becoming more prevalent in PMH nursing practice. The Recovery Model comes out of the mental health consumer movement and the work of Dr. William Anthony (1993). Nurses apply this orientation to their everyday interactions with their clients. For individuals struggling with addictions, self-help 12-step programs frequently refer to recovery as abstinence from the addictive behaviour. For individuals with severe persistent mental illnesses such as schizophrenia or bipolar disorder, a recovery orientation means helping the person regain functioning or "get on with life," despite having ongoing symptoms of the psychiatric illness. Recovery may refer to what the client does, how the nurse functions, or how the mental health system is organized. In taking this approach, there is recognition that a cure for the mental illness may not be possible (Mental Health Commission of Canada, 2009). According to the American Psychological Association (2012), research suggests that **recovery** involves a journey that is self-directed and person centred. The individual takes responsibility for his or her part and is empowered in a process that focuses on strengths, peer support, and respect. As a journey, the individual's path may be non-linear, with setbacks on the road to recovery. Hope for the future is a vital component. While recovery as a guiding principle in mental health care systems is increasingly accepted, there remains criticism that this model portrays recovery as a matter of will power, with an implicit message that those who are not recovering are lacking in this quality. The social implications of living with a mental illness and its effect on one's ability to cope with mental illness must be acknowledged and addressed (Canadian Mental Health Association, Ontario Division, 2003).

One approach to recovery, the Tidal Model, was created by nurses for use in mental health practice settings (Barker & Buchanan-Barker, 2010). The Tidal Model emphasizes the importance of a collaborative relationship between the nurse and the client. The client's perspectives and individual experiences are accepted and valued. Recovery is contingent on the health professional having a genuine interest in the client and his or her experiences. The process is open, transparent, and based on the mutual establishment of goals that both parties work together to achieve. It is recognized that recovery requires time and commitment from both the nurse and the client and that the process of change is enhanced through a genuine, nurturing therapeutic relationship. (See Chapter 8 for more information on this model.)

Reminiscence

Reminiscence, the thinking about or relating of past experiences, is used as a nursing intervention to enhance life review for older adults. Reminiscence encourages clients, either in individual or in group settings, to discuss their past and review their lives. Through reminiscence, individuals can identify past coping strategies that can support them in current stressful situations. Clients can also use reminiscence to maintain self-esteem, stimulate thinking, and support the natural healing process of life review. Activities that facilitate reminiscence include writing an account of past events, making a tape recording and playing it back, explaining pictures in old family albums, drawing a family tree, and writing to old friends. (See Chapter 32 for health promotion with the older person.)

Behaviour Therapy

Behaviour therapy interventions focus on reinforcing or promoting desirable behaviours or altering undesirable ones. The basic premise is that because most behaviours are learned, new functional behaviours can also be learned. Behaviours—not internal psychic processes—are the targets of the interventions. The models of behavioural theorists serve as a basis for these interventions (see Chapter 8).

Behaviour Modification

Behaviour modification is a specific, systematized behaviour therapy technique that can be applied to individuals, groups, or systems. The aim of behaviour modification is to reinforce desired behaviours and extinguish undesired ones. Desired behaviour is rewarded to increase the likelihood that clients will repeat it and, over time, replace the problematic behaviour with it. Behaviour modification is used for various problematic behaviours, such as dysfunctional eating and addictions, and often is used in the care of children and adolescents.

Token Economy

Primarily used in rehabilitative inpatient settings or schools, a **token economy** applies behaviour modification techniques to multiple behaviours. In a token economy, clients are rewarded with tokens for demonstrating selected desired behaviours. They can use these tokens to purchase meals, leave the unit, watch television, or wear street clothes, for example. In less restrictive environments, clients use tokens to purchase additional privileges, such as attending social events. Token economies can be helpful in creating a structured therapeutic environment for children with developmental delays or autism (Matson & Boisjoli, 2009), and the strategy has also been shown to work with hospitalized aggressive clients (Bisconer, Green, Mallon-Czajka, & Johnson, 2006). There has been a decline, however, in the use of token economies as a treatment approach since the 1980s. In some settings, such as forensic psychiatry, there is concern that the use of particular behaviour modification programs, such as token economies, does not respect the autonomy of the clients being served (Holmes & Murray, 2011).

Cognitive Interventions

Cognitive interventions are verbally structured interventions that reinforce and promote desirable, or alter undesirable, cognitive functioning. The belief underlying this approach is that thoughts guide emotional reactions, motivations, and behaviours. Cognitive interventions do not solve problems for clients but help clients develop new ways of viewing situations so that they can solve problems themselves. Nurses may use several models as the basis for cognitive interventions, but all models assume that by changing the cognitive appraisal of a situation (view of the world) and by examining the meaning of events, clients can reinterpret situations. In turn, emotional changes will follow the cognitive changes, and, ultimately, behaviours will change.

Because people develop their thinking patterns throughout their lifetime, many thoughts become so automatic that they are outside individuals' awareness. Thus, a person may be unaware of the automatic thoughts that influence his or her actions or other thoughts. **Automatic thinking** is often subject to errors or tangible distortions of reality that contradict objective appraisals. For example, a client with depression may be convinced that no one cares about him when, in fact, his family and friends are deeply concerned. **Illogical thinking**, another thinking error, occurs when a person draws a faulty conclusion. For example, a college student is so devastated by failing an examination that she perceives it as catastrophic and that her college career is over.

To engage in cognitive treatment, the client must be capable of introspection and reflection about thoughts and fantasies. Cognitive interventions are used in a wide range of clinical situations, from short-term crises to persistent mental disorders. Cognitive interventions also include thought stopping, contracting, and cognitive restructuring. These specific interventions are discussed in Chapter 13.

● **STUDY NOTE**
Use the principles of teaching/learning in health promotion. This applies across all areas of nursing.

Psychoeducation

Psychoeducation uses educational strategies to teach clients the skills they lack because of a psychiatric disorder. The goal of psychoeducation is a change in knowledge and behaviour. Nurses use psychoeducation to meet the educational needs of clients by adapting teaching strategies to their disorder-related issues. As clients gain skills, functioning improves. For example, some clients may need to learn how to maintain their morning hygiene.

Others may need to understand their illness and cope with hearing voices that others do not hear.

Specific psychoeducation techniques are based on adult learning principles, such as beginning at the point the learner is currently at and building on his or her current experiences. Thus, the nurse assesses the client's current skills and readiness to learn. From there, the nurse individualizes a teaching plan for each client. He or she can conduct such teaching in a one-to-one situation or in a group format.

Psychoeducation is a continuous process of assessing, setting goals, developing learning activities, and evaluating for changes in knowledge and behaviour. Nurses use it with individuals, groups, families, and communities. Psychoeducation serves as a basis for psychosocial rehabilitation, a service-delivery approach for those with severe and persistent mental illness (see Chapters 20 and 21).

● **STUDY NOTE**
Nursing competencies include intervening in mental health crises and facilitating the client's reintegration with the family and community.

Health Teaching

Teaching–coaching is one of the standards of care for the PMH nurse (CFMHN, 2014) (see Chapter 5). According to this standard, the PMH nurse "attempts to understand the life experience of the client and uses this understanding to support and promote learning related to health and personal development" (CFMHN, 2014, p. 19). Based on the principles of teaching, health teaching involves collaborating with the client to determine learning needs and transmitting new information, "while considering the context of the client's life experiences. [The nurse] considers readiness, culture, literacy, language, preferred learning style, and resources available" (CFMHN, 2014, p. 9). According to the *Canadian Standards of Psychiatric-Mental Health Nursing*, "all interactions between the nurse and patient are potentially teaching/learning situations" (CFMHN, 2014, p. 9). Thus, in health teaching, the PMH nurse attends to potential health care problems in addition to mental disorders and emotional problems. For example, if a person has diabetes mellitus and is taking insulin, the nurse provides health care teaching related to diabetes and the interaction of this problem with the mental disorder (Fig. 11-2). In addition, the nurse must also be aware of his or her own feelings when providing client education about what might be considered sensitive or culturally taboo topics. For example, some psychiatric medications have sexual side effects which significantly contribute to medication noncompliance. Nurses need

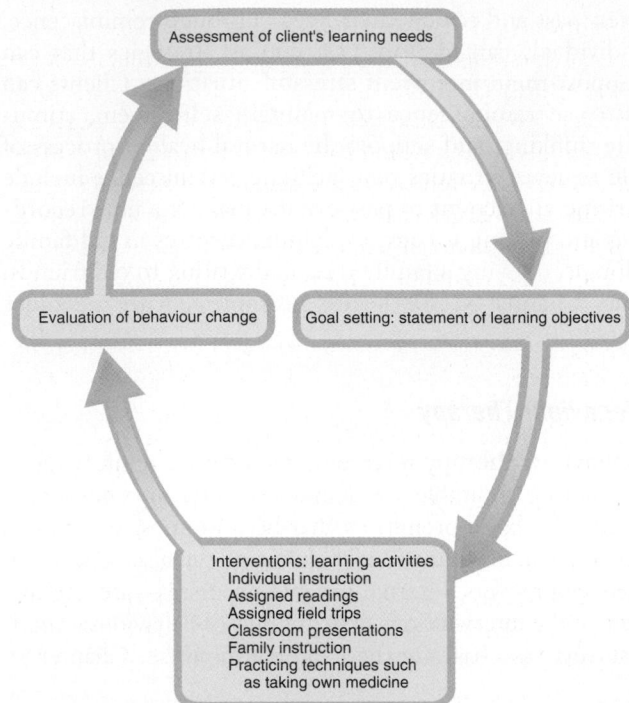

FIGURE 11-2. Teaching evaluation model. (Adapted from Rankin, S. H., Stallings, K. D., & London, F. (2005). *Patient education.* Philadelphia, PA: Lippincott Williams & Wilkins.)

to develop skills and confidence to educate clients about this important concern as many clients are embarrassed to raise it with health care professionals (Quinn, Happell, & Browne, 2012).

Interventions for the Social Domain

The social domain includes the individual's environment and its effect on his or her responses to mental disorders and distress. Interventions within the social domain are geared towards couples, families, friends, and large and small social groups, with special attention given to ethnicity and community interactions. In some instances, nurses design interventions that affect a client's environment, such as helping a family member decide to place a loved one in long-term care. In other instances, the nurse actually modifies the environment to promote positive behaviours through providing opportunities for clients to interact with others. For example, this can be accomplished through group or recreational activities for holidays or other special events, which clients can attend. Group and family interventions are discussed in Chapters 14 and 15, respectively.

Milieu Therapy

Milieu therapy provides a stable and coherent social organization to facilitate an individual's treatment. (The terms *milieu therapy* and *therapeutic environment* are often used interchangeably.) In milieu therapy, the design of the physical surroundings, structure of client activities, and promotion of a stable social structure and cultural setting enhance the setting's therapeutic potential. A therapeutic milieu facilitates client interactions and promotes personal growth. Although inpatient psychiatric units are increasingly used for intensive, short-term care of acutely and severely ill clients who are discharged as soon as possible to community care, milieu therapy remains important to these environments. In a phenomenologic study with clients hospitalized on an acute care psychiatric unit in Nova Scotia, the environment is revealed as an integral aspect of clients' illness and recovery experience. The anecdotes of the clients show that the milieu can create potential for destruction as well as healing. Clients could feel afraid and abandoned or connected and affirmed; they considered relationships as central to the milieu (Thibeault, Trudeau, d'Entremont, & Brown, 2010).

Milieu therapy is the responsibility of the nurse in collaboration with the client and other health care providers. The basic concepts of milieu therapy include safety and security, validation, open communication, and structured interaction.

Safety and Security

The milieu should be a healing place in which clients feel safe, secure, and cared for while dealing with their illness. The physical surroundings are important in this process and should be clean and comfortable, with special attention paid to promoting a noninstitutionalized environment. Pictures on walls, comfortable furniture, and soothing colours help clients relax. Most facilities encourage clients and nursing staff to wear street clothes, which helps decrease the formalized nature of hospital settings and promotes nurse–client relationships. Research suggests that the absence of a therapeutic milieu can be experienced by clients and nurses in parallel ways (Shattell, Andes, & Thomas, 2008). For instance, nurses can feel caged in by an enclosed nursing station, while clients experience similar feelings by locked unit doors.

Therapeutic milieus emphasize client involvement in treatment decisions and operation of the unit. Too often, the stigma of mental illness can exist within institutional walls, and clients can be treated in a paternalistic manner. On most inpatient psychiatric units, clients participate in maintaining the quality of the physical surroundings, such as assuming responsibility for making their own beds, attending to their own belongings, and keeping an acceptable living area. Families are viewed as a part of the client's life; family involvement is encouraged. Thus, family members should feel welcomed and safe in the milieu, as well.

Validation

In a therapeutic environment, **validation** is another process that affirms a client's individuality. Clients should feel validated as persons of worth and deserving of respect. Staff–client interactions should constantly reaffirm the client's humanity and his or her human rights. The importance of the client's personal story, history, experience, and understanding of his or her illness must be recognized in all aspects of care.

Open Communication

In **open communication**, health and treatment information is shared with clients and families. Client self-disclosure is invited within the support of a nurse–client relationship, with attention paid to the parameters of confidentiality that exist within that therapeutic relationship. These parameters may change with the care situation. For instance, if the client is undergoing a forensic assessment, information disclosed may be shared with the justice system (e.g., law courts). The client needs to understand this (see Chapter 38). Further, the environment is shaped to facilitate optimal interaction and resocialization. Support, attention, praise, and reassurance given to clients improve self-esteem and increase confidence. Client education is also a part of this support, including guidance regarding effective coping skills. Nurses and other team members should strive to role model effective communication when interacting with one another as well as with clients and families. The dynamics of team interactions can affect the milieu in both positive and negative ways.

Structured Interaction

Structured interaction is a purposeful interaction that is intended to help clients cope with particular behaviours or to learn better ways of interaction. For instance, the treatment team may assign structured interactions to specific clients as part of their treatment. Specific attitudes or approaches are assumed with individual clients or in response to particular client behaviour if beneficial to the client. These approaches include indulgence, flexibility, passive or active friendliness, matter-of-fact attitude, casualness, watchfulness, or kind firmness. For example, if and when a client becomes overexcited by daily events, the team may provide a matter-of-fact attitude when responding; or if a client's illness includes delusions that lead him or her to engage in risky behaviour, the team may intervene with an attitude of kind firmness.

Milieu treatments are based on the individual needs of the clients and include relaxation groups, discussion groups, and medication groups. Spontaneous and planned activities are possible on a short-term unit as well as in a long-term setting. In the community, it is possible to apply milieu therapy approaches in day treatment centres, group homes, and single dwellings.

Promotion of Client Safety on Psychiatric Units

A critical aspect of PMH nursing is the promotion of client safety, especially in inpatient units. It is critical because clients may be so severely ill that they engage in behaviours harmful to themselves or others. Clients experiencing delusions and hallucinations, for instance, can be responding to perceptions not based in reality. They can react with fear or in self-defence to dangers only they perceive. Sensitivity to the client's world as she or he is living it underlies nursing interventions used to keep the client safe. Interventions begin with observation and de-escalation and may evolve to the use of seclusion or restraints for clients with an involuntary status. See Chapter 7 for a discussion of ethical issues related to the use of behaviour control and restraint.

Observation

Like all hospitalized clients, individuals hospitalized on a psychiatric unit are observed by the nurses caring for them. **Observation** is the ongoing assessment of the client's status to identify and subvert any potential problem. The nature of mental disorders shapes the focus of the nurses' observations. In psychiatric settings, for instance, clients are ambulatory and thus more susceptible to environmental hazards. In addition, judgement and cognition impairment are symptoms of many psychiatric disorders. The reason for clients' admission may be, in fact, that they pose a danger to themselves or others. In PMH nursing, observation involves thoughtful, knowledgeable regard of the persons and consistent, responsible monitoring for any potential harm to themselves or others.

The intensity of the observation of the client depends on the assessed level of risk. Clients may be simply asked to "check in" at different times of the day, whereas other clients may be observed every 15 minutes by an assigned staff member. Some clients, such as those seen at a high risk for suicide, may be constantly observed by a staff member assigned to only them. Mental health facilities have policies that specify levels of observation for clients at varying degrees of risk.

De-escalation

De-escalation is an interactive process of calming and redirecting a client who has an immediate potential for violence directed towards self or others. This intervention involves assessing the situation and preventing it from escalating to one in which injury occurs to the client or others. Once the nurse has assessed the situation, he or she responds matter-of-factly to it, using various interventions that can include a request for the client and/or others to leave the situation, distraction, and conflict resolution. Psychiatric staff members are usually trained in responding to situations of aggression as a team and, thus, are often able to de-escalate such situations effectively. See Chapter 18 for information on the management of aggression and violence. Nurses can use various interventions in this situation, including distraction, conflict resolution, and cognitive interventions.

Seclusion

Seclusion is the "involuntary supervised isolation of a patient in a locked, nonstimulating room" (Van Der Merwe, Muir-Cochrane, Jones, Tziggili, & Bowers, 2013, p. 203). A client is placed in seclusion for purposes of safety or behavioural management. The nature and physical content of the seclusion room can vary. It generally has no furniture except a mattress and a blanket. The walls may be padded. The room must be environmentally safe, with no hanging devices, electrical outlets, or windows from which the client could jump. Once a client is placed in seclusion, he or she is observed at all times (i.e., continuous or constant observation).

Research regarding the experiences of using seclusion rooms has yielded conflicting data. Seclusion can be an extremely negative client experience (Van Der Merwe et al., 2013). Consequently, its use is seriously questioned, and many facilities have completely abandoned its practice. Clients have disputed the calming effects of seclusion and have perceived it as an instrument of power and control, and their outcomes may actually be worse if seclusion is used (Holmes, Kennedy, & Perron, 2004). However, clients have also reported the use of seclusion rooms in aiding them feel safe and protected (Larue et al., 2013) (see Box 11-4). Mental health staff appear to identify the potential for negative client perceptions and experiences regarding seclusion rooms but tend to feel that it can also be beneficial for clients who need that high level of restriction (Van Der Merwe et al.). If units are adequately staffed and personnel are trained in dealing with assaultive clients, seclusion is rarely needed. If seclusion is used, it must follow the same guidelines as the use of restraints.

Restraints

In Canada, the laws for restricting the freedom of clients against their will are specific to each province. Restraint is the most restrictive safety intervention and is only used in the most extreme circumstances and as a measure of last resort. Provincial mental health acts govern the situations under which restraint may be used in their jurisdiction.

Chemical restraint is the use of medication to control clients or manage their behaviour. This is distinct from medication used to treat their psychiatric illness. In several provinces, it is possible for a client to be competent to refuse medical treatment but be required to stay in the hospital for psychiatric assessment.

A **physical restraint** is any human or mechanical method that restricts the freedom of movement or normal access to one's body, material, or equipment and cannot be easily removed (National Alliance on Mental Illness, 2008). Different types of physical restraints are available. Wrist restraints restrict arm movement. Four-point restraints are applied to the wrists and ankles in

BOX 11-4   Research for Best Practice

THE EXPERIENCE OF SECLUSION AND RESTRAINT IN PSYCHIATRIC SETTINGS: PERSPECTIVES OF PATIENTS

From Larue, C., Dumais, A., Boyer, R., Goulet, M. H., Bonin, J. P., & Baba, N. (2013). The experience of seclusion and restraint in psychiatric settings: Perspectives of patients. Issues in Mental Health Nursing, 34, 317–324.

Purpose: To identify and describe clients' perceptions of the application of a seclusion and restraint protocol in a Montreal psychiatric hospital.

Method: The research was conducted using an exploratory descriptive design. Fifty clients who had experienced an episode of seclusion and restraint completed, during a face-to-face interview, a survey composed of a structured questionnaire and a series of open-ended questions. This occurred 7 to 30 days after an episode of seclusion with or without restraint.

Findings: Of the 50 clients who participated, the majority were male and were diagnosed with a psychotic disorder. Seventy-eight percent had one to five experiences with seclusion. Participants had varying perceptions about their experiences with seclusion. Some felt that it was helpful to them while others did not. The closed-ended questions were grouped into four categories: physical environment of seclusion and restraint; meeting of physical needs; support during seclusion and restraint; and postseclusion evaluation. In terms of the physical environment, clients had difficulty with their sense of time while in seclusion. Clients generally felt their physical needs were met except when it came to the need for smoking and talking. Considerable issues were identified in the support category. These included concerns with the behaviour of the health professional upon entering the seclusion room, such as demonstrating understanding, listening, and reassurance; offering help in regaining control; and explaining the situation to the client. Participants reported that there was a need for postseclusion follow-up, including debriefing about feelings and discussion about what had happened. Open-ended questions revealed the following: concerns with a lack of alternatives to seclusion being offered; seclusion as a means of addressing the need for calm, sleep, and safety; loss of freedom as difficult; and recommendations that changes to the relational interventions and physical environment are needed.

Implications for Practice: Seclusion and restraint have a negative image, and there is considerable debate regarding their use. Nurses must offer alternatives to coercive care, but when it is required as a last resort, the rationale for it must be clearly identified. The client in seclusion requires understanding, support, and reassurance. While a safe environment is necessary, nurses must also consider the client's need for comfort. Communication should be open and offer the client opportunity to discuss what happened once seclusion is discontinued.

FIGURE 11-3. Bed with five-point restraints. (Courtesy of Alberta Hospitals, photographer Pat Morrison.)

interventions before the restraint was applied. Nurses should limit the use of restraints to times when an individual is judged to be a danger to self or others. As well, they should apply restraints only until the client has gained control over his or her behaviour. When a client is in physical restraints, the nurse should closely observe the client and protect him or her from self-injury. It is the nurse's responsibility to be aware of the institutional policies that govern this.

A review of qualitative evidence on nurses' decision-making related to physical restraint suggests that nurse-based factors (e.g., perception of client's behaviour, willingness to take risks, own comfort level) and context-based factors (e.g., other team members, presence of family, the health care organization) can hinder nurses from making "an ethically balanced" decision on restraint use (Goethals, Dierckx de Casterlé, & Gastmans, 2011, p. 1207).

Given the negative consequences to the client and the impact on the nurse–client relationship, it is essential that nurses treat the client with respect and dignity at all times during a psychiatric emergency that necessitates seclusion or restraint. Every incident should be followed up by a thorough debriefing to identify how the situation might have been avoided. Education on the ethical, clinical, and legal issues related to restraint practices is very important (Kontio et al., 2009).

Home Visits

Clients usually have been hospitalized or have received treatment for acute psychiatric symptoms before being referred to a home care service. The goal of **home visits**, the delivery of nursing care in the client's living environment, is to maximize the client's functional ability within the nurse–client relationship and with the family or partner, as appropriate. The PMH nurse who makes home visits needs to be able to work independently, is skilled in teaching clients and families, can administer

bed. When five-point restraints are used, all extremities are secured, and another restraint is placed across the chest (see Fig. 11-3).

In addition to following provincial law, the nurse must also adhere to hospital policies regarding restraint. A physician's order is necessary for restraint, and nurses should document all of the previously tried de-escalation and monitor medications, and uses community resources for the client's needs. Traditional home visits are regaining popularity, particularly when the client has concomitant psychiatric and physical illnesses.

Home visits can be especially useful when helping reluctant clients to enter therapy, conducting a comprehensive assessment, strengthening a support network, and maintaining clients in the community when their condition deteriorates. Home visits are also useful in helping individuals adhere to their medication regimen. The nurse, for instance, can gain a better understanding of the barriers to taking medication as prescribed and assists the client and family to address them. One major advantage of home visits is the opportunity to provide family members with information and education and to engage them in planning and interventions.

Home visits also offer the nurse an opportunity to develop cultural sensitivity to families from a variety of backgrounds. Home-based interventions require the nurse to gain an understanding, as much as possible, of the family structure and interactions, including the roles various members play, how the family functions in terms of responsibilities, and the family life cycle (see Chapter 15). A family's cultural background influences all of these factors and is important to consider when planning interventions. The home visit also allows the nurse to identify clients who lack support from others in their daily lives.

The home visit process consists of three steps: the previsit phase, the home visit, and the postvisit phase. During previsit planning, the nurse sets goals for the home visit based on data received from other health care providers or the client. Any safety precautions that should be taken for the visit should be identified and acted upon. For instance, winter road conditions for a rural home visit or crime levels in an urban district to be visited may need to be considered. The nurse and the client agree on the time of the visit. While the nurse travels to the home, a general assessment can be made of the neighbourhood for access to services, socioeconomic factors, safety, and other factors relevant to the client's well-being within the community.

The actual visit can be divided into four parts. The first is the greeting phase, usually brief, in which the nurse begins to connect with the client and family members in their home setting. Greetings are important as they set the atmosphere for the visit and, on the part of the nurse, should be friendly but professional. In some cultures, the greeting phase may involve more formal interactions, such as taking food or tea with family members. The second phase establishes the focus of the visit. Sometimes, the purpose of the visit is medication administration, health teaching, or counselling. The client and family must be clear regarding the purpose. The implementation of the service is the next phase and should use most of the visit time. If the purpose of the visit is problem solving or decision making, the family's

cultural values may determine the types of interaction and decision-making approaches. Closure is the last phase, the end of the home visit. It is a time to summarize and clarify important points. The nurse should also schedule any additional visits and reiterate client expectations between visits. Usually, the nurse is the only provider to see the client regularly. The nurse should acknowledge family members when leaving if they were not a part of the visit.

The postvisit phase includes documentation, reporting, and follow-up planning. This time is also when the nurse meets with the supervisor and presents data from the home visit at the team meeting.

Community Action

Nurses have a unique opportunity to promote mental health awareness and support humane treatment for people with mental disorders. Activities range from being an advisor to support groups to participating in the political process through lobbying efforts and serving on community mental health boards. These unpaid activities are usually outside the realm of a particular job. However, an important role of professionals is to provide community service in addition to services through income-generating positions.

Interventions for the Spiritual Domain

Spiritual care cannot be readily separated from the bio/psycho/social components of care. It involves, rather, giving attention to all aspects of the client's life and life circumstances and takes direction from the client's reality (Sawatzky & Pesut, 2005). In doing so, the nurse identifies the spiritual needs of clients and strives to meet these needs (Pesut, 2006). The integrative nature of spirituality, and therefore of spiritual care, can make it difficult to isolate and identify spiritual needs, document spiritual interventions, and stipulate outcomes. Although spirituality always has been a core aspect of nursing care, nurses can be hesitant to address this component of their practice. However, a Canadian study of nurses' experiences of spiritual nursing care found that there was a common dimension across all the nurses' descriptions: "[S]piritual nursing care is about developing caring relationships through fostering connections to promote spiritual comfort and well-being" (Carr, 2008, p. 690). An attitude of respect and concern for the client's comfort, dignity, and well-being and recognition of the client as a person with a past, present, and future were seen as core to connection, even with individuals who appeared not to want the connection or who could not communicate. Four critical qualities for spiritual care emerged from the research data: *receptivity, humanity, competency,* and *positivity. Receptivity* involves being open to clients as a person and being genuinely present to them. It may mean simply "being with" (not just doing for) the client. *Humanity* is about being human, or put another way, being "real." It can be offering "the little things" that reveal thoughtful caring, such as knocking before entering the client's room, offering a favourite food to stimulate a client's poor appetite, or taking time to view family photos on display. *Competency* is enabling the client to know that she or he is in good hands. It reflects the integrative aspect of spiritual care that includes good bio/psycho/social care. *Positivity* describes the positive approach necessary to spiritual care. The nurse's attitude is one of hope and determination, of encouragement and good humour. Positivity is not about smiling all the time or insisting on only happy feelings being expressed. It is about fostering a positive spirit in others through one's own hopeful energy (Carr, 2008). Box 11-5 discusses a study conducted by Van Dover and Pfeiffer (2012) that described the process that clients experienced in achieving a renewed spiritual identity. These qualities of spiritual care underscore the importance of the nurse's own well-being and the therapeutic environment (see Chapter 6).

Times of illness and crisis can be opportunities for personal or spiritual growth for a person. The person may seek to connect or reconnect with others, with nature, with a power greater than him or herself (that may be named in various ways, such as God, the Creator, or Allah, or not named out of respect), or with some aspect of the sacred (Baldacchino & Draper, 2001). Nurses can support clients in their spiritual growth by listening to them as they describe their seeking; by responding to any requests for meeting with a religious leader/guide such as a minister, priest, rabbi, imam, lama, or elder; or by facilitating the use of religious ritual, such as a smudging ceremony for an Aboriginal client who requests it. Aspects of care for the spiritual domain relevant to particular disorders or age of human development may be found in the units *Care and Recovery for Persons with a Psychiatric Disorder* and *Mental Health Across the Lifespan.*

■ EVALUATION OF OUTCOMES

Evaluation of individual outcomes involves answering the following questions:

- What were the benefits for the individual?
- What was the individual's level of satisfaction?
- Was the outcome diagnosis specific or nonspecific?
- What was the cost-effectiveness of the intervention?

When measuring outcomes, nurses must consider the time frame. Identifying the intermediate outcome indicators that may be achieved in one setting versus the indicators that can be achieved in a second setting provides for a measurement of progression and enhances continuity of care. Nevertheless, not until the individual is discharged or moved to a community setting can it be known if indicators (for instance, "demonstration of confidence when alone at home," "demonstration of confidence in role skills (worker/mother)," "demonstration of self-advocacy behaviour") are achieved. Outcomes can be measured immediately after the nursing intervention or after time passes. However, outcomes based on health prevention and health promotion diagnoses can be challenging to measure and may need to occur after considerable time has passed.

BOX 11-5 Experiencing a Renewed Spiritual Identity

The provision of spiritual care in nursing is a difficult process to empirically describe. This lack of clarity is occurring at a time when clients are expecting nurses to be able to provide spiritual care. One study conducted by Van Dover and Pfeiffer (2012) used a grounded theory design to explore and portray the experience of clients of parish nurses in the context of Christian faith–based care. The parish nurses had established relationships with their clients over time. The researchers found that when clients faced a health challenge, they viewed the parish nurse as providing a "safe place." In this safe place, clients felt that they could tell their story, even if painful, and were accepted in doing so. Clients then progressed to the stage of "releasing their burdens." At this point, the client felt understood by the parish nurse and thus given permission to find a new way of living with the challenges he or she faced. This allowed clients to release their self-focus on negative experiences and to shift to a spiritual focus. Clients at this stage progressed to "changing perspectives" that aided them in the recognition of "spiritual truths" about themselves and their situation. "Adopting a revised identity" allowed clients to feel more trust and comfort in their faith. The final phase experienced was "joining or rejoining the family of faith" in which clients were able to find their place within their faith community, move on with their faith experiences, and share the process with others. While this process may not be transferrable, the provision of spiritual care in nonreligious settings may help some clients achieve a renewed spiritual identity, which could contribute to more favourable client outcomes.

From Van Dover, L. & Pfeiffer, J. (2012). Patients of parish nurses experience renewed spiritual identity: A grounded theory study. *Journal of Advanced Nursing, 68*(8), 1824–1833.

SUMMARY OF KEY POINTS

■ Nurses should work collaboratively with clients and families in determining interventions.

■ Nurses develop interventions from assessment data and may organize them around nursing diagnoses. The client's needs, values, and preferred outcomes and the *Canadian Standards of Psychiatric-Mental Health Nursing* (CFMHN, 2014) guide the selection of interventions.

■ A client's ability to manage self-care activities can fluctuate with symptom severity. The Orem (1991) self-care model can be used to conceptualize client needs (related to attitude, knowledge, and skill) and choose appropriate interventions.

■ The *Canadian Standards of Psychiatric-Mental Health Nursing* (CFMHN, 2014) supports the importance of outcome identification.

■ Outcomes must be measurable and indicative of the individual's progress.

■ More research is needed to identify individual outcomes as they relate to nursing diagnoses and interventions.

■ Nursing diagnoses, nursing interventions, and individual outcomes are initially derived from the assessment data.

■ Initial, revised, and discharge outcomes can be included in a nursing care plan.

■ Outcome statements can cover the bio/psycho/social/spiritual domains.

■ Nursing care, from assessment to outcome measurement, needs to be client centred. This means more than a recognition of the client's right to participate in health care decisions. It means genuine respect for the client's life experience and hopes for recovery.

■ Interventions focusing on the biologic domain include activity and exercise; sleep, nutrition, relaxation, hydration, and thermoregulation interventions; pain management; and medication management. Nutritional interventions are used with most clients with psychiatric disorders. Medication management is a priority because of the long-term nature of the disorders and the importance of medication compliance.

■ Interventions focusing on the psychological domain include counselling, behaviour therapy, cognitive interventions, psychoeducation, health teaching, and others. Implementation of these interventions requires a broad theoretic knowledge base.

■ Interventions focusing on the social domain include group and family approaches, milieu therapy, safety interventions, home visits, and community action. On an inpatient psychiatric unit, the nurse uses milieu therapy to maximize the treatment effects of the client's environment.

■ Interventions focusing on the spiritual domain involve a relationship and connection with the client that encompass the qualities of receptivity, humanity, competency, and positivity.

CRITICAL THINKING CHALLENGES

1   Create a nursing care plan with NANDA diagnoses for Ben, a 19-year-old man admitted to a mental health unit. Ben is an engineering student who lives at home to avoid going into debt while at university. Until recently, Ben has been a stellar student and quite an athlete, involved in hockey and lacrosse. Over the past couple of months, Ben has been struggling with exams and playoffs. He is awake all night and sleeping most of the day. At night, he has been wandering around his parents' home, rummaging in the basement. He has not eaten with the family for a while, stating that he doesn't like what his parents have made for the meal. Ben's grooming is poor; he seldom showers or changes his clothes. Ben refuses to let anyone into his bedroom, yelling at his parents to go away and leave him alone. Ben's parents can hear him inside his room talking angrily. Ben has no history of drug or alcohol use; he has never been in trouble with the law. Ben has lots of friends but now refuses to talk on the telephone with them or to go out with them. His parents are very concerned about him. What approach to this situation facing Ben and his family would be congruent with the Tidal Model?

2   What might the potential barriers be to implementing either the Tidal Model or the Recovery Model in a PMH care setting?

3   Tom, a 25-year-old man with schizophrenia, lives with his parents who want to retire to Vancouver Island. Tom goes to work each day but relies on his mother for meals, laundry, and reminders to take his medication. Tom believes that he can manage living on his own, but his mother is concerned. She asks the nurse for advice about leaving her son to manage on his own. Identify a nursing diagnosis and interventions that would meet some of Tom's potential responses to his changing lifestyle.

4   Joan, a 35-year-old married woman, is admitted to an acute psychiatric unit for stabilization of her mood disorder. She is extremely depressed but refuses to consider a recommended medication change. She asks the nurse what to do. Using a nursing intervention, explain how the nurse should approach Joan's problem.

5   A nurse reports to work for the evening shift. The unit is chaotic. The television in the day room is loud; two clients are arguing about the program. Visitors are mingling in clients' rooms. The temperature of the unit is hot. One client is running up and down the hall yelling, "Help me, help me." Using a milieu therapy approach, what might the nurse do to calm the unit?

REFERENCES

American Psychological Association. (2012). Recovery principles. *Monitor*, *43*(1), 55. Retrieved from http://www.apa.org/monitor/2012/01/recovery-principles.aspx

Anthony, W. A. (1993). Recovery from mental illness: The guiding vision of the mental health service system in the 1990's. *Psychosocial Rehabilitation Journal*, *16*, 11–23.

Aydelotte, M. K. (1962). The use of individual welfare as a criterion measure. *Nursing Research*, *11*, 10–14.

Baldacchino, D. & Draper, P. (2001). Spiritual coping strategies: A review of the nursing research literature. *Journal of Advanced Nursing*, *34*(6), 833–841.

Bisconer, S. W., Green, M., Mallon-Czajka, J., & Johnson, J. S. (2006). Managing aggression in a psychiatric hospital using a behaviour plan: A case study. *Journal of Psychiatric and Mental Health Nursing*, *13*(5), 515–521.

Boggs, K. (2011). Resolving conflict between nurse and client. In E. Arnold & K. Boggs (Eds.), *Interpersonal relationships: Professional communication skills for nurses* (6th ed., pp. 271–289). St. Louis, MO: Elsevier.

Barker, P. J. & Buchanan-Barker, P. (2010). The Tidal Model of mental health recovery and reclamation: Application in acute care settings. *Issues in Mental Health Nursing, 31,* 171–180.

Bulechek, G., Butcher, H., Dochterman, J., & Wagner, C. (Eds.) (2013). *Nursing interventions classification (NIC)* (6th ed.). St. Louis, MO: Elsevier.

Canadian Collaborative Mental Health Initiative [CCMHI]. (2006). *Canadian Collaborative Mental Health Charter.* Mississauga, ON: Author.

Canadian Federation of Mental Health Nurses (CFMHN). (2014). *Canadian standards of psychiatric-mental health nursing* (4th ed.). Toronto, ON: Author.

Canadian Mental Health Association, Ontario Division (2003). *Recovery rediscovered: Implications for the Ontario mental health system.* Available from http://www.ontario.cmha.ca/policy_positions.asp

Carpenito, L. J. (2013). *Handbook of nursing diagnosis* (14th ed.). Philadelphia, PA: Lippincott Williams & Wilkins.

Carpenito-Moyet, L. J. (2010). *Nursing diagnosis: Application to clinical practice* (13th ed.) Philadelphia, PA: Lippincott Williams & Wilkins.

Carr, T. (2008). Mapping the processes and qualities of spiritual nursing care. *Qualitative Health Research, 18*(5), 686–700.

Delaney, C., Herr, K., Maas, M., & Specht, J. (2000). Reliability of nursing diagnoses documented in a computerized nursing information system. *Nursing Diagnosis, 11*(3), 121–135.

Gagne, M. A. (2005). *What is collaborative mental health care? An introduction to the collaborative mental health care framework.* Report prepared for the Canadian Mental Health Care Initiative. Mississauga, ON: Canadian Mental Health Care Initiative.

Goethals, S., Dierckx de Casterlé, B., & Gastmans, C. (2011). Nurses' decision-making in cases of physical restraint: A synthesis of qualitative evidence. *Journal of Advanced Nursing, 68*(6), 1198–1210. doi: 10.1111/j.1365-2648.2011.05909.x

Holmes, D., Kennedy, S. L., & Perron, A. (2004). The mentally ill and social exclusion: A critical examination of the use of seclusion from the patient's perspective. *Issues in Mental Health Nursing, 25,* 559–578.

Holmes, D. & Murray, S. J. (2011). Civilizing the "barbarian": A critical analysis of behavior modification programs in forensic psychiatric settings. *Journal of Nursing Management, 19,* 293–301.

Holmes, D., Murray, S. J., Arron, A., & McCabe, J. (2008). Nursing Best Practice Guidelines: Reflecting on the obscene rise of the void. *Journal of Nursing Management, 16,* 394–403.

Jallo, N., Cozens, R., Smith, M., & Simpson, R. (2013). Effects of a guided imagery intervention on stress in hospitalized pregnant women: A pilot study. *Holistic Nursing Practice, 27*(3), 129–139.

Kleinpell, R. M. (2003). Measuring advanced practice nursing outcome, strategies and resources. *Critical Care Nurse,* (Suppl.), 6–10.

Kontio, R., Välimäki, M., Putkonen, H., Cocoman, A., Turpeinen, S., Kuosmanen, L., & Joffe, G. (2009). Nurses' and physicians' educational needs in seclusion and restraint practices. *Perspectives in Psychiatric Care, 45*(3), 198–207.

Lang, N. M. & Clinton, J. F. (1984). Assessment of quality of nursing care. *Annual Review of Nursing Research, 2,* 135–163.

Larue, C., Dumais, A., Boyer, R., Goulet, M. H., Bonin, J. P., & Baba, N. (2013). The experience of seclusion and restraint in psychiatric settings: Perspectives of patients. *Issues in Mental Health Nursing, 34,* 317–324.

Lyon, B. L. (2002). Cognitive self-care skills: A model for managing stressful lifestyles. *Nursing Clinics of North America, 37*(2), 285–294.

Marek, K. D. (1989). Outcome measurement in nursing. *Journal of Nursing Quality Assurance, 4*(1), 1–9.

Matson, J. L. & Boisjoli, J. A. (2009). The token economy for children with intellectual disability and/or autism: A review. *Research in Developmental Disabilities, 30*(2), 240–248.

Mental Health Commission of Canada (2009). *Toward recovery and wellbeing: A framework for a mental health strategy for Canada.* Ottawa, ON: Author.

Minister of Health Canada (2011). *Canada's Food Guide.* Ottawa, ON: Author.

Moorhead, S., Johnson, M., & Maas, M. (2004). *Nursing Outcomes Classification (NOC)* (3rd ed.). St. Louis, MO: Mosby.

Moorhead, S., Johnson, M., Maas, M., & Swanson, E. (2013). *Nursing Outcomes Classification (NOC): Measurement of health outcomes* (5th ed.). St. Louis, MO: Mosby.

North American Nursing Diagnosis Association (NANDA). (1990). *Proceedings of the 9th Conference on the Classification of Nursing Diagnoses.* Orlando, FL.

National Alliance on Mental Illness. (2008). *Policy topics: What are restraints and seclusion?* Retrieved from http://www.nami.org/Template. cfm?Section=Issue_Spotlights&template=/ContentManagement/ContentDisplay.cfm&ContentID=7791

Orem, D. (1991). *Nursing concepts of practice* (4th ed.). St. Louis, MO: Year Book.

Otten, J., Pitzi Hellwig, J., & Meyers, L. D. (2006). *Dietary reference intakes: The essential guide to nutrient requirements.* Washington, DC: The National Academies Press.

Pesut, B. (2006). Fundamental or foundational obligation? Problematizing the ethical call to spiritual care in nursing. *Advances in Nursing Science, 29*(2), 125–133.

Quinn, C., Happell, B., & Browne, G. (2012). Opportunity lost? Psychiatric medications and problems with sexual side function: A role for nurses in mental health. *Journal of Clinical Nursing, 21*(3/4), 415–423.

Rankin, S. H., Stallings, K. D., & London, F. (2005). *Patient education.* Philadelphia, PA: Lippincott Williams & Wilkins.

Registered Nurses Association of Ontario (RNAO). (2006). *Client-centered care—March 2006 Supplement.* Toronto, ON: Author.

Registered Nurses Association of Ontario (RNAO). (2012). *Toolkit: Implementation of best practice guidelines* (2nd ed.). Toronto, ON: Author.

Sawatzky, R. & Pesut, B. (2005). Attributes of spiritual care in nursing practice. *Journal of Holistic Nursing, 23*(1), 19–33.

Shattell, M., Andes, M., & Thomas, S. (2008). How patients and nurses experience the acute care psychiatric environment. *Nursing Inquiry, 15*(3), 242–250.

Thibeault, C., Trudeau, K., d'Entremont, M., & Brown, T. (2010). Understanding the milieu experiences of patients on an acute inpatient psychiatric unit. *Archives of Psychiatric Nursing, 24*(4), 216–226.

Van Der Merwe, M., Muir-Cochrane, E., Jones, J., Tziggili, M., & Bowers, L. (2013). Improving seclusion practice: Implications of a review of staff and patient views. *Journal of Psychiatric and Mental Health Nursing, 20,* 203–215.

Van Dover, L. & Pfeiffer, J. (2012). Patients of parish nurses experience renewed spiritual identity: A grounded theory study. *Journal of Advanced Nursing, 68*(8), 1824–1833.

12 Psychopharmacology and Other Biologic Treatments

Kathleen Hegadoren and Gerri Lasiuk
Adapted from the chapter "Psychopharmacology"
by Susan McCabe

KEY CONCEPTS

- psychopharmacology
- receptors

LEARNING OBJECTIVES

After studying this chapter, you will be able to:

- Explain the key role of neurotransmitter chemicals and their receptor sites in the action of psychopharmacologic medications.
- Explain the three major mechanisms that explain the actions of psychotropic medications in the central nervous system.
- Define the three properties that determine the strength and effectiveness of a medication.
- Describe more specific mechanisms of action for each of the major classes of psychopharmacologic medication.
- Describe the major therapeutic effects as well as prevalent side effects of various classes of psychotropic medications.
- Suggest appropriate nursing methods to administer medications that facilitate efficacy.
- Implement interventions to minimize side effects of psychopharmacologic medications.
- Differentiate acute and chronic medication-induced movement disorders.
- Identify aspects of patient teaching that nurses must implement for successful maintenance of patients using psychotropic medications.
- Analyze the potential benefits and risks associated with other forms of somatic treatments, including electroconvulsive therapy, light therapy, and nutrition therapy.
- Evaluate potential causes of nonadherence and implement interventions to improve adherence with treatment regimens.

KEY TERMS

- absorption • adherence • adverse effects • affinity • agonists
- akathisia • antagonists • bioavailability • biotransformation
- distribution • dystonia • efficacy • excretion • first-pass metabolism • half-life • intrinsic activity • kindling • metabolism
- pharmacogenomics • phototherapy • plasma protein binding
- pseudoparkinsonism • selectivity • side effects • solubility
- tardive dyskinesia • target symptoms • therapeutic index
- tolerance • toxicity • untoward effects

Throughout history, treatment choices for mental disorders have been linked to the prevailing assumptions about the aetiology of these illnesses. In the early 1900s, Emil Kraeplin classified mental disorders based on clusters of observed symptoms, providing the basic tenets of the contemporary biologic approach to understanding and treating psychiatric disorders. However, this approach fell out of favour as psychoanalytic, psychodynamic, interpersonal, and other therapies flourished, and mental disorders were increasingly assumed to have primarily a psychological aetiology. In the 1950s, when it was discovered that the phenothiazine medications, such as chlorpromazine (Thorazine), relieved many of the symptoms of psychosis and that iproniazid, a medication for treating tuberculosis, elevated mood, there was renewed interest in neurophysiology and biologic treatments for treating mental disorders.

Recent scientific and technologic developments have renewed awareness of the biologic basis of mental disorders, leading to a proliferation of new medications that act at the cellular level, producing major behavioural and psychological change. These medications provide relief from debilitating symptoms in millions of individuals with psychiatric disorders. They have become the dominant form of treatment and are the cornerstones of all psychiatric treatment.

Most psychiatric and mental health (PMH) nurses work with individuals who are receiving psychopharmacologic agents as part of their treatment. As awareness of the prevalence of mental disorders increases, these medications are increasingly prescribed in primary care settings, and even nurses working in nonpsychiatric settings now need an in-depth knowledge of these medications to care for their patients in any setting (Hegadoren, 2004).

This chapter reviews the major classes of psychopharmacologic drugs used in treating mental disorders, including antipsychotics, mood stabilizers, antidepressants, antianxiety medications, and stimulants, and provides a basis for understanding the specific biologic treatments of psychiatric disorders that are described more fully in later chapters.

The target for psychiatric medications is predominantly the central nervous system (CNS) at the cellular and synaptic levels, although the autonomic nervous system often contributes to the pharmacologic profile of psychiatric drugs. For this reason, this chapter focuses on understanding the impact of psychotropic medications on the basic unit of CNS functioning, the synapse, and on receptors embedded in neuronal cell membranes. This basic understanding allows the PMH nurse to accept the role and responsibilities of administering medications, proactively monitoring and treating side effects, and educating the patient and family, which are all crucial to successful psychopharmacologic therapy. In addition to psychopharmacologic therapy, other biologic treatments (sometimes referred to as *somatic treatments*) are used. These therapies include electroconvulsive therapy (ECT), light therapy, and nutritional therapy and are discussed later in this chapter.

> **KEY CONCEPT Psychopharmacology** is a subspecialty of pharmacology that studies medications that affect behaviour through their actions in the CNS and that are used to treat psychiatric and neurodegenerative disorders. It is important to remember, however, that many drugs used to treat other conditions, such as pain syndromes and heart disease, have powerful effects in the brain.

PHARMACODYNAMICS

A comparatively small amount of medication can have a significant and large impact on cell function and resulting behaviour. When tiny molecules of medication are compared with the vast amount of cell surface in the human body, the fraction seems disproportionate. Yet the drugs used to treat mental disorders often have profound effects on behaviour. To understand how this occurs, one needs to understand both where and how drugs work.

Targets of Drug Action: Where Drugs Act

Most drug molecules do not act on the entire cell surface, but rather at receptor sites, binding sites on enzymes, or transporters that remove neurotransmitter molecules from the synapse. Many psychopharmacologic drugs, especially older classes, act at multiple receptors. Newer agents are more specific to one type of receptor, but none are exclusive to one type of receptor. Another key to understanding drug effects is the distribution of receptors, enzymes, and transporters within the body. Different types and subtypes of receptors can be concentrated in specific brain regions. Thus, there is a close relationship between the drug effects and the functions associated with a brain region.

Receptors are proteins that are embedded within the cell membrane and have binding sites for both naturally occurring chemicals (called *endogenous substances*) and administered drugs. Endogenous brain chemicals involved in neurotransmission, such as dopamine and serotonin, bind to specific groups of receptors. Administered drugs may compete with neurotransmitters for these receptors by mimicking or blocking the action of the neurotransmitter. In this chapter, *receptor* refers only to those membrane proteins to which a neurotransmitter can specifically bind to produce a change in the cell membrane, serving a physiologic regulatory function (such as those discussed in Chapter 9). These include ligand-gated ion channels or the G-protein–coupled receptors.

KEY CONCEPT **Receptors** are associated with the work of German chemist Paul Erhlich, who in 1900 suggested that a receptive substance exists within the cell membrane. The biologic action of a drug depends on how its structure interacts with a specific receptor. Thus, a basic understanding of how receptors work is key to understanding how many drugs work in the body.

Receptors

Many drugs have been developed to act specifically at the receptor sites. When bound to the receptor, these drugs act as **agonists**—chemicals producing the same biologic action as the neurotransmitter itself—or as **antagonists**—chemicals blocking the biologic action of an agonist at a given receptor. Figure 12-1 illustrates the action of an agonist and an antagonist drug at a receptor site. A drug's ability to interact with a given receptor type may be judged by three properties: selectivity, affinity, and intrinsic activity.

Selectivity

The first property, called **selectivity**, is the ability of the drug to be specific for a particular receptor. If a drug is highly selective, it will interact only with its specific receptors in the areas of the body where these receptors occur and, therefore, not affect tissues and organs where its receptors do not occur. Using a "lock-and-key" analogy, only a specific, highly selective key will fit a given

FIGURE 12-1. Agonist and antagonist drug actions at a receptor site. This schematic drawing represents drug–receptor interactions. At **top**, drug D has the correct shape to fit receptor R, forming a drug–receptor complex, which results in a conformational change in the receptor and the opening of a pore in the adjacent membrane. Drug D is an agonist. At **bottom**, drug A also has the correct shape to fit the receptor, forming a drug–receptor complex, but in this case, there is no conformational change and, therefore, no response. Drug A is, therefore, an antagonist.

lock. The more selective or structurally specific a drug is, the more likely it will affect only the specific receptors for which it is meant. The more receptors for other neurochemicals are affected, the more unintended effects, or **side effects**, are produced. Selectivity is important to understand because it helps explain the concept of side effects caused by medications, a major cause of concern in medication treatment. The distribution of receptors in specific brain regions also plays a role in the side effect profile. For example, dopamine antagonists can produce dystonic movements because high concentrations of dopamine receptors are found in the region of the brain that controls fine motor movement.

Affinity

The second property is that of **affinity**, which is the degree of attraction or strength of the bond between the drug and its receptor. Normally, these bonds are produced by relatively weak electrochemical attractions. Basic to the action of almost all CNS drugs within the body is their ability to bind to a receptor, produce a response, and then move off the receptor. There are some exceptions to this transient bond formation, such as is seen in a class of drugs that binds to an enzyme and is discussed in that section.

Intrinsic Activity

The final property of a drug's ability to interact with a given receptor is that of **intrinsic activity**, or the ability of the drug to produce a biologic response once it becomes attached to the receptor. Some drugs have selectivity and affinity but produce no biologic response; therefore, an important measure of a drug is whether it produces a change in the cell containing the receptor. Drugs that act as agonists have all three properties: selectivity, affinity, and intrinsic activity. However, antagonists have only selectivity and affinity because they produce no biologic response by attaching to that receptor. However, in complex biologic systems, such as the brain, preventing an agonist from binding can yield multiple cellular and ultimately behavioural responses. An example of this is the antipsychotic class, all members of which are antagonists.

Some drugs act as *partial agonists*. If the endogenous molecule (like a neurotransmitter) has a greater affinity than a drug, then that drug would be called a partial agonist as it produces a weaker effect when bound than does the endogenous molecule. A drug may act as a full agonist at one receptor subtype and a partial agonist at another. For some drugs, their activity is dose dependent: at low doses, they act as agonists, but at higher doses, they act more as antagonists. Medications that have both agonist and antagonist effects are called *mixed agonist–antagonists*. Naloxone, used to treat opioid overdose, is an example of a mixed agonist–antagonist.

Ion Channels

Some drugs act directly on ion channels embedded in the nerve cell membrane. Examples include local anaesthetics that block the entry of sodium into the cell, preventing an action potential, and nicotine, which acts as an agonist at nicotinic acetylcholine receptors. Although there was some evidence that calcium channel blockers may help in the treatment of mania, a state of increased activity, euphoria, difficulty sleeping, racing thoughts, and rapid and forced speech, further research did not support its efficacy for mania or bipolar disorder (Hollister & Garza Trevino, 1999).

The benzodiazepine drugs, frequently used in psychiatry as anticonvulsants and antianxiety and hypnotic drugs to help with sleep disturbances, are an example of drugs that affect a specific ion channel of the nerve cell membrane. The benzodiazepine molecule, in such drugs as diazepam (Valium), works by binding to a region of the gamma-aminobutyric acid (GABA) receptor–chloride channel complex. The binding site for these drugs is different from where GABA itself binds. When bound, these drugs increase the frequency and duration of chloride efflux mediated by GABA. The overall effect is helping GABA to decrease the ability of that cell to conduct a nerve impulse. Thus, they are referred to as being indirect agonists or positive modulators of the $GABA_A$ channel.

Enzymes

Enzymes are complex proteins that catalyze specific biochemical reactions within cells and are the targets for some drugs used to treat mental disorders. For example, monoamine oxidase (MAO) is the enzyme required to break down most monoamine neurotransmitters, such as norepinephrine, serotonin, and dopamine, and can be inhibited by medications from a group of antidepressants called monoamine oxidase inhibitors (MAOIs). There are two types of MAO. MAO-A is more specific to norepinephrine and serotonin than it is for dopamine. This increase in available norepinephrine and serotonin is thought to initiate the cascade of cellular changes that ultimately relieve the symptoms of depression. MAO-B is more specific to dopamine and is used to treat Parkinson's disorder, a neurodegenerative disorder where dopamine neurons die off.

Instead of the on–off property in relation to drugs that bind to receptors, the older MAOIs form strong covalent bonds with the enzyme, which irreversibly inhibit the ability of the enzyme to inactivate the monoamine neurotransmitters after they have been used, resulting in increased amounts of these neurotransmitters ready for release in the nerve terminals. New enzyme molecules must be produced before any activity is restored. Although they have similar effects, some MAOIs (e.g., moclobemide) do not form covalent bonds so are called reversible.

Carrier Proteins: Uptake Receptors

Neurotransmitters are small organic molecules that are released in response to a change in the polarity of the cell membrane (called an action potential), interact with receptors, and then are transported back into the neuronal cell by carrier proteins. These transporters have binding sites specific for the type of molecule to be transported. After a neurotransmitter, such as serotonin, has activated receptors in the synapse, its actions are terminated by these transporters that take serotonin back up into the presynaptic cell. Medications specific for this site may block or inhibit this transport and, therefore, increase the amount of the neurotransmitter in the synaptic space available for action on the receptors.

A primary action of most of the antidepressants is to increase the amount of neurotransmitters in the synapse by blocking their reuptake. Older antidepressants, like the tricyclic antidepressants (TCAs), block the reuptake of more than one neurotransmitter and have affinity for other receptors, which produces increased side effects. Some antidepressants, such as fluoxetine (Prozac) and sertraline (Zoloft), are more selective for serotonin, whereas reboxetine is more selective for norepinephrine. These medications are called selective serotonin reuptake inhibitors (SSRIs) and selective norepinephrine reuptake inhibitors (NSRIs), respectively. Newer antidepressants that are selective to both serotonin and norepinephrine are called SNRIs (e.g., venlafaxine [Effexor] and duloxetine [Cymbalta]). These more selective medications have reduced the number of side effects experienced by the patients. Figure 12-2 illustrates the reuptake blockade of serotonin by an SSRI.

Efficacy and Potency: How Drugs Act

Efficacy is another characteristic of medications to be considered when selecting a drug for the treatment of a particular set of symptoms. **Efficacy** is the ability of a drug to produce a desired response. It is important to remember that the degree of receptor occupancy contributes to efficacy, yet it is not the only variable. A drug may occupy

FIGURE 12-2. Reuptake blockade of a transporter for serotonin by an SSRI.

a large number of receptors but not produce a response. In contrast, *potency* considers the amount of drug required to produce the desired biologic response. One drug may be able to achieve the same clinical effect as another drug but at a lower dose, making it more potent. Although the drug given at the lower dose is more potent, because both drugs achieve similar effects, they may be considered to have equal efficacy. However, side effects are often related to dose, so a potent drug that can produce a therapeutic response at a lower dose may be preferable.

Loss of Effect: Biologic Adaptation

In some instances, the effects of medications diminish with time, especially when they are given repeatedly, as in the treatment of chronic psychiatric disorders. This loss of effect can be a form of physiologic adaptation that may develop as the cell attempts to regain homeostatic control to counteract the effects of the drug. **Tolerance** is a gradual decrease in the action of a drug at a given dose or concentration in the blood. This decrease may take days or weeks to develop and results in the loss of therapeutic effect of a drug. This loss of effect is often called *treatment refractoriness*. There are many reasons for decreased drug effectiveness (Box 12-1). A rapid decrease can occur with some drugs because of immediate transformation of the receptor when the drug molecule binds to the receptor. Other drugs cause a decrease in the number of receptors. Some drugs may deplete cellular stores of neurotransmitters. Examples include D-amphetamine, which depletes dopamine stores, and the recreational drug "Ecstasy," which depletes serotonin stores. Drug tolerance is also caused by an increase in the *metabolism* (breakdown) of the medication, such as with barbiturates, which trigger an increase in the amount of hepatic enzymes responsible for their metabolism and results in a significant decrease in the blood level of the anticonvulsant carbamazepine (Tegretol) if used in combination with phenobarbital. Cycling female hormones can also affect response to drugs. Progesterone and its metabolites bind to the same GABA receptor as do the benzodiazepines and can affect the efficacy of benzodiazepines at certain stages of the menstrual cycle.

Other forms of physiologic adaptation result in a gradual tolerance that may be helpful in the case of unpleasant side effects, such as drowsiness or nausea. For example, the SSRIs can cause nausea and gastrointestinal upset when first started, but these side effects are

BOX 12-1 Mechanisms Causing Decrease in Medication Effects

- Change in receptor density or affinity
- Depletion of neurotransmitter stores
- Increased metabolism of the drug
- Physiologic adaptation
- Interaction with female hormones

transient. With forewarning about these temporary side effects, patients are more likely to stay on the medication and not discontinue the drug regime on their own. This information is important for the nurse to communicate to patients experiencing such side effects so that they can be reassured that the effects will subside. The PMH nurse must also know when tolerance will not occur and when a lack of tolerance to a significant side effect warrants discontinuation of the medication.

Target Symptoms and Side Effects

Psychiatric medications are indicated for specific symptoms, referred to as **target symptoms**. Target symptoms are those measurable specific symptoms expected to improve with medication use. The target symptoms for each class of medication are discussed more fully in later sections of this chapter. Because receptors for neurotransmitters such as serotonin are found in all regions of the brain and in the periphery, serotonin-related drugs produce widespread effects in many body systems. For example, these drugs interact with receptors in the gastrointestinal tract and in facial motor nerves, causing gastrointestinal upset and bruxism (clenching and grinding of teeth). These unwanted effects of medications are called **side effects** (also called **untoward effects** or **adverse effects**).

Knowledge of a medication's affinity for receptors and subtypes of receptors may give some indication of the likelihood that specific target symptoms might improve and what side effects might be predicted. Table 12-1 provides a brief summary of possible physiologic effects from drug actions on specific neurotransmitters. For example, antagonists with high affinity for acetylcholine receptors of the muscarinic subtype will be more likely to cause such side effects as dry mouth, blurred vision, constipation, urinary hesitancy or retention, and nasal congestion. This information should serve only as a guide in predicting side effects because of considerable interindividual variability in drug responses and not all underlying mechanisms have been elucidated. The PMH nurse should use this information to focus assessment on these areas. If the symptoms are mild, simple nursing interventions suggested in Table 12-2 should be implemented. If symptoms persist or are severe, the prescriber should be notified immediately. Patients need to be encouraged to report side effects and to be aware that suggestions and solutions are available to address the side effects. For example, changing from one drug to another within the same class of psychotropics can often decrease unwanted side effects.

Drug Toxicity

All drugs have the capacity to be harmful as well as helpful. **Toxicity** generally refers to the point at which concentrations of the drug in the body have gone beyond the

Table 12-1 Pharmacodynamic Properties of Antidepressants		
Neurotransmitter/Receptor Action	**Physiologic Effects**	**Examples of Drugs That Exhibit High Affinity**
Reuptake Inhibition Blockade		
Norepinephrine reuptake inhibition	Antidepressant action Potentiation of pressor effects of norepinephrine Side effects: tachycardia, tremors, insomnia, erectile and ejaculation dysfunction	desipramine reboxetine
Serotonin reuptake inhibition	Antidepressant action Antiobsessional effect Antianxiety effect Side effects: gastrointestinal distress, nausea, headache, nervousness, motor restlessness, and sexual side effects, including anorgasmia	fluoxetine paroxetine
Receptor mediated		
Histamine (H_1) receptor antagonism	Side effects: sedation, drowsiness, hypotension, and weight gain	quetiapine imipramine clozapine olanzapine
Muscarinic Acetylcholine receptor antagonism	Side effects: anticholinergic (dry mouth, blurred vision, constipation, urinary hesitancy and retention, memory dysfunction) and sinus tachycardia	imipramine amitriptyline thioridazine clozapine
Norepinephrine receptor (α_1 receptor) antagonism	Potentiation of antihypertensive effect of prazosin and terazosin Side effects: postural hypotension, dizziness, reflex tachycardia, sedation	amitriptyline clomipramine clozapine amitriptyline
Norepinephrine receptor (α_2 receptor) antagonism	Increased sexual desire (yohimbine) Interactions with antihypertensive medications, blockade of the antihypertensive effects of clonidine Side effect: priapism	clomipramine clozapine trazodone yohimbine
Norepinephrine receptor (β_1 receptor) antagonism	Antihypertensive action (propranolol) Side effects: orthostatic hypotension, sedation, depression, sexual dysfunction (including impotence and decreased ejaculation)	propranolol
Serotonin receptor (5-HT_{1a}) agonist	Antidepressant action Antianxiety effect Possible control of aggression	trazodone risperidone ziprasidone
Serotonin receptor (5-HT_2) antagonism	Antipsychotic action Some antimigraine effect Decreased rhinitis Side effects: hypotension, ejaculatory problems, weight gain, metabolic disorders	risperidone clozapine olanzapine ziprasidone haloperidol
Dopamine receptor (D_2) antagonism	Antipsychotic action Side effects: extrapyramidal symptoms, such as tremor, rigidity (especially acute dystonia and parkinsonism); endocrine changes, including elevated prolactin levels	ziprasidone

safe range and may become harmful or poisonous to the body. However, what is considered harmful? Side effects can be harmful but not toxic, and individuals vary widely in their responses to medications. Some patients experience adverse reactions more readily than others. For example, women are more likely to experience side effects than are men. **Therapeutic index**, a concept often used to discuss the toxicity of a drug, is a ratio of the maximum nontoxic dose to the minimum effective dose. A high therapeutic index means that there is a large range between the dose at which the drug begins to take effect

and a dose that would be toxic to the body. Drugs with a low therapeutic index have a narrow range and are often carefully monitored through routine assessment of blood levels. This concept has some limitations. The concept of toxicity is only vaguely defined. The range can also be affected by drug tolerance. The therapeutic index of a medication also may be greatly changed by the coadministration of other medications or drugs. For example, alcohol consumed with most CNS depressant drugs will have added depressant effects, greatly increasing the likelihood of toxicity or death.

Table 12-2	Managing Common Side Effects of Psychiatric Medications

Side Effect or Discomfort	Intervention
Blurred vision	Reassurance (generally subsides in 2–6 weeks)
Dry eyes	Warn ophthalmologist; no eye examination for new glasses for at least 3 weeks after a stable dose
	Artificial tears may be required; an increased use of wetting solutions for those wearing contact lenses
Dry mouth and lips	Frequent rinsing of the mouth, good oral hygiene, sucking sugarless candies, lozenges, lip balm, lemon juice, and glycerin mouth swabs
Constipation	High-fiber diet, encourage bran, fresh fruits, and vegetables
	Metamucil (must consume at least 16 oz of fluid with dose)
	Exercise, increase fluids
	Mild laxative
Urinary hesitancy or retention	Monitor frequently for difficulty with urination, changes in starting or stopping stream
	Notify prescriber if difficulty develops
	A cholinergic agonist, such as bethanechol, may be required
Nasal congestion	Nose drops, moisturizer, *not* nasal spray
Sinus tachycardia	Assess for infection
	Monitor pulse for rate and irregularities
	Withhold medication and notify prescriber if resting rate exceeds 120 bpm
Decreased libido and ejaculatory inhibition	Consider change to another drug in same class or change class of drug
Postural hypotension	Frequent monitoring of lying-to-standing blood pressure during dosage adjustment period, immediate changes and accommodation, measure pulse in both positions
	Advise the patient to get up slowly, sit for at least 1 minute before standing (dangling legs over side of bed), and stand for 1 minute before walking or until light-headedness subsides
	Increase hydration, avoid caffeine
	Elastic stockings if necessary
	Notify prescriber if symptoms persist or significant blood pressure changes are present
Photosensitivity	Protective clothing
	Dark glasses
Dermatitis	Use of sun block, remember to cover *all* exposed areas
	Stop medication usage
	Consider medication change, may require a systemic antihistamine
	Initiate comfort measures to decrease itching
Impaired psychomotor functions	Advise the patient to avoid dangerous tasks, such as driving
	Avoid alcohol, which increases this impairment
Drowsiness or sedation	Encourage activity during the day to increase accommodation
	Avoid tasks that require mental alertness, such as driving
	May need to adjust dosing schedule or, if possible, give single daily dose at bedtime
	May need a cholinergic medication if sedation is the problem
	Avoid driving or operating potentially dangerous equipment
	May need change to less-sedating medication
	Provide quiet and decreased stimulation when sedation is the desired effect
Weight gain	Exercise and diet teaching; regular weighing
	Caloric control and regular monitoring of blood glucose levels
Edema	Check fluid retention
	Reassurance
	May need a diuretic
Irregular menstruation	Reassurance (reversible)
Amenorrhea	May need to change class of drug
	Reassurance and counselling (does not indicate lack of ovulation)
	Instruct the patient to continue birth control measures
Vaginal dryness	Instruct in use of lubricants

Despite the limitations of the therapeutic index, it is a helpful guide for nurses, particularly when working with potentially suicidal individuals. PMH nurses must be aware of the potential for overdose and closely monitor the availability of drugs for these patients. In some cases, prescriptions may have to be dispensed every few days or each week until a suicidal crisis has passed to ensure that patients do not have a lethal dose available to them. The choice of drug can also help address toxicity. For example, the TCAs can be lethal in overdose, whereas SSRIs are not; SSRIs are thus the safer choice for higher-risk patients and adolescents.

PHARMACOKINETICS: HOW DRUGS MOVE THROUGH THE BODY

The field of pharmacokinetics describes, often in mathematical models, how a drug moves throughout the body to get to its target receptors and then is eliminated. The processes of absorption, distribution, metabolism, and excretion are of central importance. Overall, the goal in pharmacokinetics is to describe and predict the time course of drug concentrations throughout the body and factors that may interfere with these processes. Together with the principles of pharmacodynamics, this information can be helpful to the psychiatric nurse in ways such as facilitating or inhibiting drug effects and predicting behavioural response.

Absorption and Routes of Administration

The first phase of drug disposition in the human body is **absorption**, defined as the movement of the drug from the site of administration into the plasma. It is important to consider the impact of routes by which a drug is administered on the process of absorption. Not all potential routes of administration are available for medications used to treat psychiatric disorders. The primary routes available include oral (both tablet and liquid), sublingual, intramuscular (IM) (short- and long-acting agents), and intravenous (used for rapid treatment of adverse reactions and rarely for the treatment of the primary psychiatric disorder). The PMH nurse needs to know about the advantages and disadvantages of each route and the subsequent effects on absorption (Table 12-3).

Drugs taken orally are usually the most convenient for the patient; however, this route is also the most variable because absorption can be slowed or enhanced by a number of factors. Taking certain drugs orally with food or antacids may slow the rate of absorption or change the amount of the drug absorbed. For example, the β-receptor antagonist propranolol exhibits increased blood levels when taken with food. Antacids containing aluminium salts decrease the absorption of most antipsychotic drugs; thus, antacids must be given at least 1 hour before administration or 2 hours after.

Oral preparations absorbed from the gastrointestinal tract into the bloodstream first go to the liver through the portal vein. There, they may be metabolized in such a way that most of the drug is inactivated before it reaches the rest of the body. Some drugs are also subjected to metabolism in the gastrointestinal wall. These losses of orally administered drugs before entering the systemic circulation are termed **first-pass metabolism**. The consequence of first-pass metabolism is that the fraction of the drug reaching systemic circulation is reduced, sometimes substantially. First-pass metabolism explains why the dose of propranolol given intravenously is so much less than the oral dose. Oral drugs are manufactured to compensate for first-pass metabolism, such that adequate concentrations of drug will get to the site of action. Other factors affecting absorption should also be considered when administering drugs. Liver disease and dysfunction can decrease first-pass metabolism and result in increased drug levels and thus an increased risk for side effects. Gastric motility also affects how the drug is absorbed. Increasing age, many disease states, and concurrent medications can reduce motility and slow absorption. Other factors, such as blood flow in the gastrointestinal system, drug formulation, and chemical factors, may also interfere with absorption. Nurses must be aware of a patient's physical condition and use of medications or other substances that can interfere with drug absorption.

In full strength, many liquid preparations, especially antipsychotics, irritate the mucosal lining of the mouth, oesophagus, and stomach and must be adequately diluted. Nurses must be careful when diluting liquid medications because some liquid concentrate preparations are incompatible with certain juices or other liquids. If a drug is mixed with an incompatible liquid, a white or grainy precipitant usually forms, indicating that some of the drug has bound to the liquid and inactivated. Thus, the patient actually receives a lower dose of the medication than intended. Precipitants can also form from combining two liquid medications in one diluent, such as juice. Sometimes, precipitants may be difficult to see, such as in orange juice, so nurses must be aware of the compatibilities of liquid preparations. If a precipitant forms in a medication cup, it will also form in the stomach, causing additional inactivation of the drugs. Therefore, some medications should be given at least an hour apart. With new technologies come novel administration routes and drug forms, one of which is the rapid-dissolving oral pill. Manufacturers have different procedures for developing rapid-dissolving drugs, and these are patented with unique names. Common forms include the DuraSolv and Quick Tab technologies. Many drugs are currently available in rapid-dissolving form, including the atypical antipsychotic olanzapine (Zyprexa, Zydis), risperidone (Risperdal M-Tab), and mirtazapine (Remeron SolTab).

Nurses need to be aware of the special administration and patient-teaching requirements of the rapid-dissolving drug forms. To take an orally disintegrating tablet, the nurse or patient should use dry hands to peel back the foil packaging, immediately take out the tablet, and place it into the mouth. The tablet will quickly dissolve and can be swallowed with saliva. No water is needed to swallow disintegrating tablets. This is advantageous when a patient cannot swallow well or is unwilling to swallow pills, or when water is not readily available.

Table 12-3 Selected Forms and Routes of Psychiatric Medications

Preparation and Route	Examples	Advantages	Disadvantages
Oral tablet	Basic preparation for most psychopharmacologic agents, including antidepressants, antipsychotics, mood stabilizers, anxiolytics, etc.	Convenience	Variable rate and extent of absorption, depending on the drug May be affected by the contents of the intestines May show first-pass metabolism effects May not be easily swallowed by some individuals
Oral liquid	Also known as concentrates Many antipsychotics, such as haloperidol, chlorpromazine, thioridazine, risperidone The antidepressant fluoxetine Antihistamines, such as diphenhydramine Mood stabilizers, such as lithium citrate	Ease of incremental dosing Easily swallowed In some cases, more quickly absorbed	More difficult to measure accurately Depending on drug: • Possible interactions with other liquids, such as juice, forming precipitants • Possible irritation to mucosal lining of the mouth if not properly diluted
Rapid-dissolving tablet	Atypical antipsychotics, such as olanzapine and risperidone Handy for people who have trouble swallowing or for patients who let medication linger in the cheek for later expectoration Can be taken when water or other liquid is unavailable	Dissolves almost instantaneously in the mouth	The patient needs to remember to have completely dry hands and to place tablet in the mouth immediately Tablet should not linger in the hand
Sublingual	Lorazepam	Rapid action, no first-pass metabolism	Increased risk for tolerance and psychological dependence
Intramuscular	Some antipsychotics, such as haloperidol, chlorpromazine, and risperidone Anxiolytics, such as lorazepam Anticholinergics, such as diphenhydramine and benztropine mesylate No antidepressants No mood stabilizers	More rapid acting than oral preparations No first-pass metabolism	Injection-site pain and irritation Some medications may have erratic absorption if heavy muscle tissue at the site of injection is not in use High-potency antipsychotics in this form may be more prone to adverse reactions, such as NMS
IM depot (or long acting)	Haloperidol decanoate, fluphenazine decanoate, paliperidone palmitate	May be more convenient for some individuals who have difficulty following medication regimens	Significant pain at injection site
Intravenous	Anticholinergics, such as diphenhydramine, benztropine mesylate Diazepam used as an anticonvulsant	Rapid and complete availability to systemic circulation	Inflammation of tissue surrounding site Often inconvenient for the patient and uncomfortable Continuous dosage requires use of a constant-rate IV infusion

Bioavailability

Bioavailability describes the amount of the drug that actually reaches systemic circulation. The route by which a drug is administered significantly affects bioavailability. With some oral drugs, the amount of drug entering the bloodstream is decreased by first-pass metabolism and bioavailability is lower (Pandolfi et al., 2003). On the other hand, some rapid-dissolving oral medications have increased bioavailability.

Bioavailability is a concept often used to compare one drug with another, obviously implying that increased bioavailability makes one drug "better" than another. Bioavailability is used as a measure to test for equivalency of a generic drug compared with the previously patented original drug. Although a useful concept for drug development, many individual factors can affect bioavailability and thus affect the concentration of drug that gets to the site of action.

Distribution

Even after a drug enters the bloodstream, several factors affect how it is distributed in the body. **Distribution** of a drug reflects how easy it is for a drug to pass out of the systemic circulation and move into other types of tissues, such as brain, abdominal organs, skin, or bone, where target receptors are found. Factors that affect medication distribution to specific tissues in the body include the amount of blood flow or perfusion within the tissue; how lipophilic ("fat-loving") the drug is; plasma protein binding; and anatomic barriers, such as the blood–brain barrier, that the drug must cross. Highly perfused organs like the heart, liver, kidney, and brain are quickly and extensively exposed to any drug. Almost all psychotropic drugs are lipophilic, making it easier for the drug to passively cross epithelial cell membranes that line blood vessels and to cross the blood–brain barrier. Table 12-4 provides a summary of how some significant factors affect distribution. Two of these factors, ionic characteristics and protein binding, warrant additional discussion with regard to how they relate to psychiatric medications.

Ionic Characteristics of Drugs

Drugs in the bloodstream can be charged molecules (in the form of positive or negative ions) or can be uncharged. There are many charged components within cell membranes. Thus, drugs that have an electrical charge cannot passively cross through a cell membrane; instead, they must be transported by carrier proteins. Uncharged drugs (also called lipophilic or "fat-loving" drugs) can move easily across cell membranes. Most psychiatric drugs are very lipophilic and can move into major organ systems, as well as cross the blood–brain barrier. However, this characteristic means that psychopharmacologic agents can also cross the placenta. It also means that these agents can be taken into fat stores. Drugs stored in fatty tissue are only slowly released back into the systemic circulation for eventual elimination. This is why a lipophilic drug can be detected long after discontinuation in older women and overweight individuals. This effect may also account for unexpected drug–drug interactions when substitute drugs regimes are initiated quickly.

Protein Binding

Many drugs bind to large carrier proteins in the bloodstream, referred to as **plasma protein binding**. The degree to which a drug is bound to these plasma proteins affects the drug's ability to interact with receptors. Only unbound or "free" drugs can move across membranes to their target receptors. High protein binding prolongs the drug's duration of action, allowing for less frequent dosing. Many of the psychiatric drugs are more than 90% protein bound. Chronic disease and normal aging can decrease the amounts of plasma proteins, shifting the ratio of bound drug to free drug. For highly bound drugs like the classic antipsychotics, a decrease of only 10% of bound drug (e.g., from 90% to 80%) would translate into a doubling of free drug and significantly increase the risk for side effects.

Metabolism

The duration of drug action also depends on the body's ability to change or alter a drug chemically. **Metabolism**, also called **biotransformation**, is the process by which

Table 12-4 Factors Affecting Distribution of a Drug	
Factor	**Effect on Drug Distribution**
Size of the organ	Larger organs require more drug to reach a concentration level equivalent to other organs and tissues.
Blood flow to the organ	The most important contributor to distribution, the major organs have the highest blood flow (heart, lung, liver, brain, kidney) and thus have the greatest exposure.
Ionic characteristics	Drugs with no electrical charge move easily across cell membranes by passive transfer rather than needing active transport and thus will be widely distributed.
Plasma protein binding	If a drug binds well to plasma proteins, particularly to albumin, it will stay in the body longer.
Anatomic barriers	Both the gastrointestinal tract and the brain are surrounded by layers of cells that control the passage or uptake of substances. Lipid-soluble substances are usually readily absorbed and pass the blood–brain barrier.

the drug is altered, usually by adding to the drug molecule or breaking the drug molecule into smaller pieces, both processes making the molecule or the pieces more polar. Through the processes of metabolism, lipid-soluble drugs become more polar or hydrophilic so that they may be excreted more readily.

Most metabolism occurs in the liver, but it can also occur in the kidneys, lungs, and intestines. The outcome of this process is usually an inactive metabolite. However, metabolism can also produce an active metabolite with either similar or very different actions as the parent compound. For instance, the antidepressant imipramine is metabolized to a pharmacologically active substance, desipramine, which also has antidepressant effects (desipramine is also available on its own as an antidepressant). Prozac (fluoxetine), an SSRI antidepressant, is metabolized in the liver and forms an active metabolite, norfluoxetine, which has a very long half-life. This is important when changing from fluoxetine to another antidepressant to avoid potential side effects from having two antidepressants still acting in the body. Metabolism may also change an inactive drug (called a prodrug) to an active one or an active drug to a toxic metabolite. Codeine is an example of a prodrug that must be metabolized before having analgesic properties. Acetaminophen is a safe drug used in normal doses. Five to ten percent of acetaminophen is metabolized by CYP enzymes to a toxic metabolite, which is then conjugated by glutathione to a nontoxic conjugate and eliminated through bile or urine. With an overdose, stores of glutathione are depleted, the levels of the toxic metabolite rise and cause liver cell death. Death can occur from acute liver failure (Dahlin, Miwa, Lu, & Nelson, 1984).

The cytochrome P-450 superfamily of metabolic enzymes (or CYP450s) is responsible for most drug metabolism. The classification of the CYP450 superfamily uses a combination of numbers and letters to denote families, subfamilies, and individual enzymes. Specific genes encode each enzyme, but polymorphisms are common. Most psychiatric drugs are metabolized by members of the 1A, 2D, and 3A subfamilies of CYP450 enzymes. The 3A family is the most abundant, constituting more than 60% of the liver enzyme weight. The metabolizing activity of some of the CYP450 enzymes can be altered by drugs and environmental chemicals. Some drugs like phenobarbital induce CYP450 activity. This increases enzymatic action and thus decreases drug levels of any drug taken concomitantly with phenobarbital. Subthreshold drug levels may affect efficacy. Other common substances, such as tobacco smoke, alcohol, and coal tar in charcoal-broiled foods, can induce specific CYP450 enzymes. Alternately, drugs can inhibit CYP450 activity and thus increase drug levels, potentially into toxic ranges. A CYP enzyme that is responsible for a wide variety of therapeutic agents and is often inhibited is CYP2D6. Acute alcohol ingestion and the

antiulcer medication cimetidine (Tagamet), available over the counter, can inhibit CYP2D6. Some of the SSRIs are also potent inhibitors of CYP2D6. Grapefruit juice is an inhibitor of CYP3A enzymes. Not all SSRIs are equal in their potency to inhibit CYP2D6. Paroxetine (Paxil) is the most potent, producing more than 90% inhibition of this enzyme subfamily, whereas sertraline exhibits mild effects, with only 20% to 50% inhibition (Dalfen & Stewart, 2001). The newer SSRI citalopram has minimal inhibiting properties.

The metabolism of many of the older drugs has not been thoroughly investigated. Indeed, information about the specific CYP450 enzyme responsible for metabolism is available for only about 20% of commonly prescribed medications. In addition, a drug can be metabolized by more than one CYP450. A minor route of metabolism can become the major route under conditions of liver disease or dysfunction or if the individual has a genetic mutation of that enzyme, rendering it with only low intrinsic activity.

CYP450 enzymes contribute to the enormous individual differences in the overall efficacy and the side effect profiles. A Canadian study estimated that of the almost 2.5 million annual hospital admissions per year, about 185,000 were associated with an adverse event and close to 70,000 of these were potentially preventable (Baker et al., 2004). Another Canadian study of adverse events found that the elderly were most at risk and that the most common adverse events were adverse drug events (72%), therapeutic errors (16%), and nosocomial infections (11%) (Forster et al., 2004).

The differences in CYP enzyme activity often are caused by genetic variations (Dahl, 2002). DNA variants in the CYP450 system and the enzymes encoded by these genes have been investigated for several CYP enzymes in relation to specific ethnic and racial groups. For example, about 3% of Caucasians and more than 20% of Japanese are poor metabolizers of CYP2C19. About 2% of Chinese, but up to 10% of Caucasians, are poor metabolizers of CYP2D6 (Baker, Urichuk, & Coutts, 1998). The emerging science of **pharmacogenomics** blends pharmacology with genetic knowledge and is concerned with understanding and determining an individual's specific CYP450 makeup, then individualizing medications to match the person's CYP450 profile. Increasingly, psychiatric medications are prescribed after testing to determine the patient's CYP450 genotype to guide treatment with the most effective drugs for the patient and to drastically reduce potential drug–drug interactions. For example, dextromethorphan is used to assess intrinsic activity of CYP2D6 and classify the individual into low, normal, or extensive metabolizers. Within the next decade, it is expected that scientists will begin to connect DNA variants with individual responses to medical treatments, identify particular subgroups of patients, and develop drugs customized for those populations.

Nurses should remain alert to the possibilities of drug–drug interactions when patients are receiving more than one medication, especially in older adults. Pharmacology texts and dedicated Web sites are helpful reference sources. In addition, if an individual receiving a medication experiences an unusual reaction or suddenly loses effect from a medication that had previously been working, the nurse should carefully assess other substances that the person has recently consumed, including prescription medications, nonprescription remedies, dietary supplements or changes, and substances of abuse (including alcohol and tobacco). The widespread use of herbal products has introduced another potential source of drug–drug interaction. A good example of this is St. John's wort, a botanical product used extensively for mild depression. Drug–drug interactions have been reported for St. John's wort and alprazolam, amitriptyline, and cyclosporine (Izzo, 2004). There are also drug-endogenous product interactions. The most notable examples are estrogens and progesterone. Through a pharmacodynamic mechanism, progesterone can decrease the effectiveness of the benzodiazepines, but it can also affect drug concentrations as it is an inhibitor of CYP 3A enzymes. Estrogens inhibit CYP1A2. During periods of high hormone levels (ovulation, luteal phase of the menstrual cycle and pregnancy), these interactions may become clinically significant for women.

Excretion

Excretion refers to the elimination of drugs from the body either unchanged or as metabolites. *Clearance* refers to the total volume of blood, serum, or plasma from which a drug is completely removed from the bloodstream per unit of time. The driving force that determines the time required to eliminate a drug is usually the concentration of drug and the clearance rate. The elimination **half-life** ($t_{1/2}$) refers to the time required for plasma concentrations of the drug to be reduced by 50%. For example, 50% of a drug is cleared in one $t_{1/2}$. In the next $t_{1/2}$, 50% of the remaining concentration would be eliminated (leaving 25% of the original concentration), then after the third $t_{1/2}$, there would be 12.5% remaining. Thus, it usually takes four to seven half-lives for a drug to be completely eliminated from the body. Notable exceptions to this decrease by percent concentration include alcohol and acetylsalicylic acid, in which the specific enzymes responsible for metabolism limit the speed at which elimination can occur. For this reason, elimination is at a set rate irrespective of concentration, which is why in the case of alcohol, it can be calculated how many drinks it takes per hour to reach a blood alcohol level of 0.8 (a common legal level indicative of impairment) and the time required to eliminate all alcohol from the system. In the case of acetylsalicylic acid overdose, increasing the renal clearance through changes in pH or increasing fluid volume will not affect the time required for elimination because it is determined by enzyme activity, not blood flow.

As indicated previously, the goal of most metabolic processes is to decrease the lipophilic nature of drugs by increasing their ionic characteristics. Drugs that are in a more ionic form in the bloodstream can be easily removed by the kidney and excreted through urine. However, many psychiatric medications are large molecules and thus can also be removed through bile and eliminated in feces. Lithium, a mood stabilizer, is a notable exception. It is a very small cation and is dependent on renal excretion. Any impairment in renal function or renal disease, or even temporary dehydration (e.g., from flu symptoms or even strenuous exercise), may lead to severe toxic symptoms. Biliary elimination can lead to "enteroportal recirculation," a process by which active drug or metabolites that were excreted in bile into the small intestine are reabsorbed into the portal circulation, go through the liver again, and end up back into the systemic circulation. A well-known example of this is oral contraceptives. Oral antibiotics change the intestinal environment, can decrease recirculation, and thus affect the contraceptive efficacy. This same process of reabsorption may also contribute to the plasma concentration of psychiatric drugs over time.

Dosing refers to the administration of medication over time so that therapeutic levels may be achieved or maintained without reaching toxic levels. In general, it is necessary to give a drug at intervals no greater than the half-life of the medication to avoid excessive fluctuation of concentration in the plasma between doses. With repeated dosing, a certain amount of the drug is accumulated in the body. This accumulation slows as dosing continues and plateaus when absorption equals excretion. This is called *steady-state plasma concentration* or simply *steady state*. The rate of accumulation is determined by the half-life of the drug. Drugs generally reach steady state in four to five times the elimination half-life. However, because elimination or excretion rates may vary significantly, fluctuations may still occur, and dose schedules may need to be individualized.

The nurse should remember that although these principles can support best practice, they are not substitutes for ongoing individual assessment of indicators of treatment response or unwanted effects and recording individual perceptions about drug effects.

Individual Variations in Drug Effects

Many factors affect drug absorption, distribution, metabolism, and excretion. These factors may vary among individuals, depending on their age, genetics, and ethnicity. Nurses must be aware of and consider these individual variations in the effects of medications.

Age

Pharmacokinetics is influenced by life cycle stages. For example, gastric absorption changes with age. Gastric pH in a newborn is 6 to 8 and decreases to 1 to 3 over the first 24 hours (the pH remains elevated in a premature infant). This significantly affects drug absorption. Changes in drug absorption are also seen in older adults because of increased gastric pH, decreased gastric emptying, slowed gastric motility, and reduced splanchnic circulation. Normally, these changes do not significantly impair the oral absorption of a medication, but addition of common conditions, such as diarrhoea, may significantly alter and reduce absorption. The use of multiple drug therapies (termed *polypharmacy*) in older adults can also significantly alter pharmacokinetic properties of each individual drug (Hogan, Ebly, & Fung, 1995; Spina & Scordo, 2002; Turkoski, 1999).

Renal function is also altered in both very young and older adult patients. Infants who are exposed in utero to medications that are excreted through the kidneys may experience toxic reactions to these medications because renal function in the newborn is only about 20% of that of an adult. In less than a week, renal function develops to adult levels, but in premature infants, the process may take longer. Renal function also declines with age. Creatinine clearance in a young adult is normally 100 to 120 mL/min, but after the age of 40, this rate declines by about 10% per decade. Medical illnesses, such as diabetes and hypertension, may further the loss of renal function. When creatinine clearance falls below 30 mL/min, the excretion of drugs by the kidneys is significantly impaired and potentially toxic levels may accumulate.

Metabolism changes across the life span, especially in infancy and childhood. At birth, many of the liver enzymes are not fully functional, whereas in early childhood, there is evidence of increased activity compared with adulthood. For example, CYP1A2 activity is reduced in the first 4 months but increased between ages 1 and 2 years; CYP2D6 activity is reduced until ages 3 to 5 years, and CYP3A4 is reduced in the 1st month of life but increased between ages 1 and 4 (Kearns, 2000; Kearns & Winter, 2004; Leeder & Kearns, 1997). Thus, paediatric pharmacotherapeutics cannot simply be based on relative dosing by weight. With age, blood flow to the liver and the mass of liver tissue both decrease. The activities of hepatic enzymes also slow with age. As a result, the ability of the liver to metabolize medications may show as much as a fourfold decrease between the ages of 20 and 70. Again, the use of multiple drugs in older adults adds to metabolic burden, potentially increasing drug levels of each individual drug.

Most psychiatric medications are bound to proteins. Albumin is one of the primary circulating proteins to which drugs bind. The production of albumin by the liver is lower in neonates and generally declines with age. In addition, a number of medical conditions change the ability of medications to bind to albumin. Malnutrition, cancer, and liver disease decrease the production of albumin, which translates to more free drug available to interact

with target receptors and an increased risk for adverse or toxic effects.

Less information is known about age-related changes in pharmacodynamics. There is evidence of pharmacodynamic differences in cyclosporine effects in infants (Marshall & Kearns, 1999). Higher digoxin doses are required in infants because of lower affinity in target myocardial receptors (Soldin & Soldin, 2002). Changes in the parasympathetic nervous system produce a greater sensitivity in older adult patients to the anticholinergic side effects of specific psychiatric drugs.

Ethnicity and Genetic Makeup

It is clear that genetics plays a significant role in the metabolism of medications. Studies of identical and nonidentical twins show that much of the individual variability in elimination half-life of a given drug is genetically determined (Vesell, 1977). Individuals of Asian descent have decreased activities of enzymes involved in the second stage of ethanol metabolism compared with Caucasians and thus produce higher concentrations of acetaldehyde, resulting in such adverse symptoms as flushing, palpitations, and headache. Asian research subjects have been found to be more susceptible to the effects of drugs such as mephenytoin than are Caucasian individuals, whereas individuals of African descent were less sensitive (Klotz, 2007). Several case reports indicate that Asians require one half to one third the dose of antipsychotic medications required by Caucasians and that they may be more sensitive to side effects because of higher blood levels (Zhou, 2003). Lower doses of antidepressant medications are also often required for individuals of Asian descent. Although many of these variations appear to be related to the cytochrome P-450 genetic differences discussed earlier, more research is needed to understand fully the underlying mechanisms and to identify groups that may require different approaches to medication treatment.

■ PHASES OF DRUG TREATMENT

The PMH nurse is involved in all the phases of medication treatment. Considerations in terms of assessment, treatment issues such as **adherence** (keeping with the therapeutic regimen), prevalence and severity of side effects, and expected time lines for symptom relief vary across the phases of treatment, but all involve potential nursing actions. These phases include initiation, stabilization, maintenance, and discontinuation of the medication. PMH nurses must be concerned with treatment phases as a guide for what may be expected as they administer medications and monitor individuals receiving medications across each of these phases. The following subsections discuss some of the knowledge required and the assessments and interventions to be performed by the PMH nurse within each phase.

Initiation Phase

Before beginning to take medications, patients must undergo several assessments.

- A psychiatric evaluation, including past history and previous medication treatment response, will clarify diagnosis and determine target symptoms for medication use.

- An open discussion regarding adherence issues, such as attitudes toward drug treatments, patient-specific goals for the drug therapy, any lifestyle issues that affect the structuring of a drug regimen (e.g., shift work, type of occupation and current job responsibilities, reproductive issues), and any health insurance issues related to prescription benefits, will help to identify barriers to the patient's willingness and ability to manage the medication regimen.

- Physical examination and indicated laboratory tests, often including baseline determinations such as a complete blood count (CBC), liver and kidney function tests, electrolyte levels, urinalysis, and possibly thyroid function tests and electrocardiogram (ECG), will help determine whether a physical condition may be causing the symptoms and establish that it is safe to initiate use of a particular medication.

- Any other current medications, including over-the-counter medications, herbal remedies and mixtures from health food stores, or naturopathic or homeopathic visitations, and alcohol, tobacco, and other recreational drug use should be identified to prevent harmful drug interactions.

Nurses should perform their own premedication evaluations, including physical assessments that focus on preexisting symptoms, such as gastrointestinal distress, or restrictions in range of motion that may later be confused with side effects. Side effects are difficult to assess if baseline status has not been evaluated. An assessment of cognitive functioning will assist the nurse in assessing whether memory aids or other supports are necessary to assist the individual in accurately completing the medication regimen. Information from the psychosocial and lifestyle assessment should be reviewed in consultation with the prescriber and other members of the multidisciplinary team to develop a plan that is acceptable to the patient and will improve functioning, minimize side effects, and improve quality of life.

In all situations, recommendations and treatment alternatives should be developed and reviewed with input from the individual seeking treatment. Doing so will allow the patient to ask questions and receive complete information about target effects and the most common adverse effects, thus allowing for fully informed consent to the selected approach. Patients are often overwhelmed during the initial phases of treatment and may have symptoms that make it difficult for them to participate fully in treatment planning. Information is often forgotten or may need to be repeated and provided in written form for ongoing reference. Nurses must keep their detailed drug knowledge current to be able to answer questions and provide ongoing education.

When use of the medication is initiated, PMH nurses should treat the first dose as if it were a "test" dose. They should observe the patient closely for sensitivity to the medication, such as changes in blood pressure, pulse, or temperature; changes in mental status; allergic reactions; dizziness; ataxia; or gastric distress. Other common side effects that may occur with even one dose of medication should also be closely monitored. A protocol for reporting side effects and determining which ones should trigger immediate contact should be in place.

Stabilization Phase

During stabilization, the medication dosage is often adjusted to achieve the maximum amount of improvement with a minimum number of side effects. This process is sometimes referred to as *titration*. PMH nurses must continue to assess target symptoms, looking for change or improvement and side effects. If medications are being increased rapidly, such as in a hospital setting, nurses must closely monitor temperature, blood pressure, pulse, mental status, common side effects, and unusual adverse reactions.

On an outpatient basis, nurses must provide both verbal and written materials to individuals who are receiving the medication as to the expected outcome and potential side effects. This educational support should include factors that may influence the effectiveness of the medication, such as whether to take the medication with food, common interventions that may minimize side effects if they develop, and what side effects require immediate attention. Again, a plan is needed to clearly identify what to do if adverse reactions develop and what adverse reactions should prompt immediate attention. The plan should include emergency telephone numbers or available emergency treatment and should be reviewed frequently.

Therapeutic drug monitoring is important in this phase of treatment for drugs with narrow therapeutic windows, such as lithium, valproate, and carbamazepine. Nurses must be aware of when and how these levels are to be determined and assist patients in learning these procedures. Plasma levels of other psychiatric medications can be evaluated, for example, to rule them out as a potential source of treatment nonresponse related to increased metabolism.

Unfortunately, the first medication chosen often does not adequately improve the patient's target symptoms. In treatment of depression, for example, studies have shown that up to 60% of individuals fail to respond to any given antidepressant (Thase, 2002). This can be very discouraging, particularly in a population in which powerlessness and hopelessness are inherent in the disorder. This possibility must be discussed before initiating antidepressant drug therapy. Most of the time, a substitute drug from the same class or a drug from a new class will be given. Medications may also be changed when adverse reactions or seriously uncomfortable side effects occur or these effects substantially interfere with the individual's quality of life. Nurses should be familiar with the pharmacokinetics of both drugs to be able to monitor side effects and possible drug–drug interactions during this transition period.

At times, an individual may show only partial improvement from a medication, and the prescriber may try an augmentation strategy. *Augmentation* refers to the addition of another medication to enhance or potentiate the effects of the first medication. For example, a prescriber may add a mood stabilizer, such as lithium, to an antidepressant to improve the overall efficacy of the antidepressant. These strategies are often used with so-called treatment-resistant situations. *Treatment resistance* has various definitions, but most often, it means that after several medication trials, the individual has gained, at best, only partial improvement. Treatment-resistant symptoms often require multiple medications. Multiple medications may affect different physiologic processes and, in combination, provide overall synergistic or additive pharmacologic effects. Nurses must be familiar with the potential effects, side effects, drug interactions, and rationale for this type of complex treatment regimen.

Maintenance Phase

Once the individual's target symptoms have improved, medications may be continued to prevent relapse or reoccurrence. *Relapse* usually refers to reemerging symptoms in response to premature discontinuation of treatment, whereas *reoccurrence* refers to an entirely new episode that occurs over time after full remission was achieved. Higher risk for relapse in depression is associated with individuals who are older, have chronic episodes, have severe symptoms or psychotic symptoms, or have three or more previous or more frequent episodes (Viguera, Baldessarini, & Friedberg, 1988). Other reasons for reemerging symptoms, despite continued use of medication, include the loss of efficacy, metabolic induction, comorbid medical illness, psychosocial stressors, and concurrent use of prescription or nonprescription medications. Whatever the reason, patients must be educated about their target symptoms and have a plan of action if the symptoms return. The PMH nurse has a central role in assisting individuals to monitor their own symptoms, manage psychosocial stressors, and avoid other factors that may cause the exacerbation of symptoms that were previously under control.

Some side effects or adverse reactions emerge only after the individual has been receiving the medication for an extended period. Specific examples are discussed in later sections of this chapter.

Discontinuation Phase

Many psychiatric medications require a tapered discontinuation. Tapering involves slowly reducing dosage while monitoring closely for reemergence of key symptoms, such as a drop in mood, increased anxiety, sleep disturbance, thought disorder, or decreased level of self-care. Some psychiatric disorders, such as mild depression or adjustment disorder, may respond to several months of treatment and not reoccur. Other disorders, such as bipolar disorder, chronic major depressive disorder, and schizophrenia, usually require continued medication treatment for extended periods of time. A withdrawal syndrome, affecting up to 25% of individuals after abrupt cessation of the SSRIs, has been described and includes such symptoms as dizziness, restlessness, increased anxiety and mood lability, GI upset, and fatigue (Ditto, 2003). The restoration of the drug therapy relieves the symptoms within 24 hours. Untreated, the symptoms can last 1 to 3 weeks. Withdrawal effects and rebound effects (increased anxiety and/or sleep disturbance) have also been described for abrupt discontinuation of benzodiazepines.

Nurses must be aware of the potential for these symptoms, monitor them closely, and implement measures to minimize their effects. They should support individuals throughout this process, whether they can successfully stop taking the medication or must continue the treatment. Even if patients can successfully discontinue use of the medication without a return of symptoms, nurses may help implement preventive measures to avoid the reoccurrence of the psychiatric disorder. In the roles of advocate, patient educator, and provider of interpersonal support, PMH nurses often have a central role in helping patients incorporate preventive mental health strategies into their daily routine.

■ ANTIPSYCHOTIC MEDICATIONS

It is hard to image how psychiatric illnesses were treated before the development of psychopharmacologic medications. Antipsychotic medications were among the very first drugs ever used to treat psychiatric disorders. First synthesized by Paul Charpentier in 1950, chlorpromazine became the interest of Henri Lorit, a French surgeon, who was attempting to develop medications that controlled preoperative anxiety. Administered in intravenous doses of 50 to 100 mg, chlorpromazine produced drowsiness and indifference to surgical procedures. At Lorit's suggestion, a number of psychiatrists began to administer chlorpromazine to agitated psychotic patients. In 1952, Jean Delay and Pierre Deniker, two French psychiatrists, published the first report of chlorpromazine's calming effects with psychiatric patients (Granger, 1999). They soon discovered it was especially effective in relieving hallucinations and delusions associated with schizophrenia. As more psychiatrists began to prescribe the medication, the use of restraints and seclusion in psychiatric hospitals dropped sharply, ushering in a revolution in psychiatric treatment.

Since that time, numerous antipsychotic medications have been developed. Older, typical antipsychotic medications, available since 1954, are equally effective, inexpensive drugs that vary in the degree to which they cause certain groups of side effects. Table 12-5 provides a list of selected antipsychotics grouped by the nature of their chemical structure and indicating the likelihood of certain side effects. These medications treat the symptoms of psychosis, such as hallucinations, delusions, bizarre behaviour, disorganized thinking, and agitation.

Typical and Atypical Antipsychotics

Initially, the term *major tranquilizer* was applied to this group of medications. Later, major tranquilizers were known as *neuroleptics*, which more accurately describes the action of drugs such as chlorpromazine and haloperidol. Neuroleptic means "to clasp the neuron." The term reflects the common and often significant neurologic side effects produced by these types of drugs. The development of newer antipsychotic drugs that have less significant neurologic side effects has led to these older agents

being used as secondary, not first-line, drugs. The term *typical antipsychotic* now identifies the older antipsychotic drugs with greater risk for neurologic side effects, and *atypical antipsychotic* identifies the newer generation of antipsychotic drugs with fewer adverse neurologic effects within the common dosing regimes.

Indications and Mechanisms of Action

Antipsychotic medications generally are indicated for treating acute psychosis or severe agitation. Possible target symptoms for antipsychotics include hallucinations, delusions, paranoia, agitation, assaultive behaviour, bizarre ideation, disorientation, social withdrawal, catatonia, blunted affect, thought blocking, insomnia, and anorexia when these symptoms are the result of an acute exacerbation of a psychotic disorder like schizophrenia, acute hypomania associated with bipolar disorder, a psychotic response to an acute change in health status (observed with severe burns or admission to an intensive care unit), or use of specific illicit drugs.

In general, the older, typical antipsychotics, such as haloperidol (Haldol), chlorpromazine, and thioridazine (Mellaril), are equally effective in relieving hallucinations, delusions, and bizarre ideation, termed "positive" symptoms of schizophrenia. The "negative" symptoms—blunted affect, social withdrawal, lack of interest in usual activities, lack of motivation, poverty of speech, thought blocking, and inattention—do not respond as well to the typical antipsychotics and in some cases may even be

Table 12-5	Side Effect Comparison of Selected Antipsychotic Medications			
Drug Category **Drug Name**	Sedation	Extrapyramidal	Anticholinergic	Orthostatic Hypotension
Standard (Typical) Antipsychotics				
Phenothiazines				
chlorpromazine (Thorazine)	+4	+2	+3	+4
thioridazine (Mellaril)	+3	+1	+4	+4
mesoridazine (Serentil)	+3	+1	+4	+3
fluphenazine (Prolixin)	+1	+4	+1	+1
perphenazine (Trilafon)	+2	+3	+2	+2
trifluoperazine (Stelazine)	+1	+3	+1	+1
Thioxanthenes				
thiothixene (Navane)	+1	+4	+1	+1
Dibenzoxazepines				
loxapine (Loxitane)	+2	+3	+2	+3
Butyrophenones				
haloperidol (Haldol)	+1	+4	+1	+1
Dihydroindolones				
molindone (Moban)	+2	+3	+2	+1
Atypical Antipsychotics				
clozapine (Clozaril)	+4	+/0	+4	+4
risperidone (Risperdal)	+1	+/0	+/0	+2
olanzapine (Zyprexa)	+4	+/0	+2	+1
quetiapine fumarate (Seroquel)	+4	+/0	+/0	+3
ziprasidone HCl (Geodon)	+1	+/0	+1	+2
aripiprazole (Abilify)	+1	+/0	+/0	+1

worsened by such agents. Newer atypical antipsychotics, such as clozapine, risperidone (Risperdal), olanzapine (Zyprexa), quetiapine (Seroquel), and ziprasidone (Geodon), are more effective at improving negative symptoms. Although antipsychotic medications are the primary treatment for schizophrenia and related illnesses, such as schizoaffective disorder, schizophreniform disorder, and brief psychotic disorder, they are increasingly being used to treat other psychiatric and medical illnesses. Psychotic symptoms that occur during a major depressive episode, anxiety, or bipolar disorder can be treated with antipsychotics, primarily on a short-term basis. These medications reduce agitation, aggressiveness, and inappropriate behaviour in pervasive developmental disorders, such as autism or severe mental retardation. Within the typical antipsychotics, haloperidol and pimozide are approved for treating Tourette's syndrome, reducing the frequency and severity of vocal tics.

Off-label uses of the drug have also been effective. Chlorpromazine and haloperidol are both effective in treating drug-related psychosis, such as that caused by phencyclidine. Atypical antipsychotics have also been used to treat agitation and aggression seen in those acutely ill in intensive care units (often termed ICU psychosis) and with neurodegenerative disorders like Alzheimer's disease (Kirbach, Simpson, Nietert, & Mintzer, 2008; Philip, Mello, Carpenter, Tyrka, & Price, 2008; Riker & Fraser, 2005). Some evidence exists for their efficacy at very small doses in treating psychiatric sequelae of trauma, especially in the case of significant dissociation and mood reactivity arising from childhood interpersonal abuse (Grootens & Verkes, 2005). Antipsychotic medications may also be useful in treating migraine headaches, Huntington's chorea, and some other neurologic disorders.

The typical antipsychotic drugs generally are effective in decreasing the so-called positive target symptoms because they are potent postsynaptic dopamine antagonists. Chapter 20 discusses the link between dopamine and disorders such as schizophrenia, and provides additional details about how lowering dopamine levels helps reduce target symptoms. The atypical antipsychotic medications differ from the typical antipsychotics in that they block serotonin receptors that reside on dopamine neurons as well as dopamine receptors. The differences between the mechanism of action of the typical and atypical antipsychotics help to explain their differences in efficacy in relation to both positive and negative symptoms and side effect profiles.

Pharmacokinetics

Antipsychotic medications administered orally have a variable rate of absorption complicated by the presence of food, antacids, smoking, and even the coadministration of anticholinergics, which slow gastric motility. Clinical effects begin to appear in about 30 to 60 minutes.

Absorption after IM administration is less variable because this method avoids first-pass metabolism. Therefore, IM administration produces greater bioavailability but increases risk for side effects. It is important to remember that IM medications are absorbed more slowly when patients are immobile, such as when restrained for long periods of time, because erratic absorption may occur when muscles are not in use. For example, the patient's arm may be more mobile than are the buttocks. The deltoid has better blood perfusion, and thus medications are more readily absorbed. The nurse must also remember that plastic syringes may absorb some medications. This is true of the antipsychotics, and injectable medications should never be allowed to remain in the syringe longer than 15 minutes.

The metabolism of these drugs occurs almost entirely in the liver, where hepatic microsomal enzymes convert these highly lipid-soluble substances into water-soluble metabolites that can be excreted through the kidneys. Therefore, these medications are subjected to the effects of other drugs that induce or inhibit the cytochrome P-450 system described earlier. Table 12-6 summarizes many of the possible medication interactions with antipsychotics, including those resulting from changes in hepatic enzymes. Careful observance of concurrent medication use, including prescribed, over the counter, and substances of abuse, is required to avoid drug–drug interactions.

Excretion of these substances tends to be slow because the drugs can easily accumulate in fat stores. Most antipsychotics have a half-life of 24 hours or longer, but many also have active metabolites with longer half-lives. These two effects make it difficult to predict elimination time, and metabolites of some of these agents may be found in the urine months later (Altamura, Mauri, Cavallero, & Gorni, 1987). If a patient experiences side effects from a medication severe enough to discontinue the use of the drug and begin use of a new one, the adverse effects of the first drug may not necessarily immediately subside. The patient may continue to experience and sometimes need treatment for the adverse effects for several days. Similarly, patients who have discontinued the use of antipsychotic drugs may still derive therapeutic benefit for several days to weeks after drug discontinuation.

Typical antipsychotics are best administered in divided doses to minimize side effects, but the long elimination time does allow the medication to be given in once-daily dosing. This schedule increases adherence and reduces the impact of the peak occurrence of some side effects, such as sedation during the day.

High lipid **solubility**, accumulation in the body, and other factors have also made it difficult to correlate blood levels with therapeutic effects. Dose–response curves have not been established, and the dose required for an individual to experience treatment effects varies widely. Plasma levels of these medications are only partially

Table 12-6 Chemical Interactions with Antipsychotic Medications

Agent	Effect
Alcohol	Phenothiazines potentiate CNS depressant effects Extrapyramidal reactions may occur
Barbiturates	Speed action of liver microsomal enzymes so that antipsychotic is metabolized more quickly, reducing phenothiazine and haloperidol plasma levels; barbiturate levels may also be reduced by phenothiazines; potentiate CNS depressant effect
Tricyclic antidepressants	Can lead to severe anticholinergic side effects; some antipsychotics (especially phenothiazines or haloperidol) can raise the plasma level of the antidepressant, probably by inhibiting metabolism of the antidepressant
Hydrochlorothiazide and hydralazine	Can produce severe hypotension
Guanethidine	Antihypertensive effect is blocked by phenothiazines, haloperidol, and possibly thiothixene
Aluminum salts (antacids)	Impair gastrointestinal absorption of the phenothiazines, possibly reducing therapeutic effect Administer antacid at least 1 hour before or 2 hours after the phenothiazine
Tobacco	Heavy consumption requires larger doses of antipsychotic because of hepatic microsomal enzyme induction
Charcoal (and charbroiled food)	Decreases absorption of phenothiazines
Anticholinergics	May reduce the therapeutic actions of the phenothiazines, increase anticholinergic side effects, lower serum haloperidol levels, worsen symptoms of schizophrenia, increase symptoms of tardive dyskinesia
Meperidine	May result in excessive sedation and hypotension when coadministered with phenothiazines
Fluoxetine	Case report of serious extrapyramidal symptoms when used in combination with haloperidol
Lithium	May induce disorientation, unconsciousness, extrapyramidal symptoms, or possibly the risk for NMS when combined with phenothiazines or haloperidol
Carbamazepine	Decreases haloperidol serum levels, decreasing its therapeutic effects
Phenytoin	Increase or decrease in phenytoin serum levels; thioridazine and haloperidol serum levels may be decreased
Methyldopa	May potentiate the antipsychotic effects of haloperidol or may produce psychosis Serious elevations in blood pressure may occur with methyldopa and trifluoperazine
General anaesthesia (barbiturates)	Antipsychotic may potentiate effect of anesthetic; may increase the neuromuscular excitation or hypotension

Table 12-7 Antipsychotic Medications

Generic (Trade) Drug Name	Usual Dosage Range (mg/day)	Half-Life (hours)	Therapeutic Blood Level	Approximate Equivalent Dosage (mg)
Standard (Typical) Antipsychotics				
Phenothiazines				
chlorpromazine (Thorazine)	50–1,200	2–30	30–100 mg/mL	100
thioridazine (Mellaril)	50–600	10–20	1–1.5 ng/mL	100
mesoridazine (Serentil)	50–400	24–48	Not available	50
fluphenazine (Prolixin)	2–20	4.5–15.3	0.2–0.3 ng/mL	2
perphenazine (Trilafon)	12–64	Unknown	0.8–12.0 ng/mL	10
trifluoperazine (Stelazine)	5–40	47–100	1–2.3 ng/mL	5
Thioxanthenes				
thiothixene (Navane)	5–60	34	2–20 ng/mL	4
Dibenzoxazepines				
loxapine (Loxitane)	20–250	19	Not available	15
Butyrophenones				
haloperidol (Haldol)	2–60	21–24	5–15 ng/mL	2
Dihydroindolones				
molindone (Moban)	50–400	1.5	Not available	10
Atypical Antipsychotics				
clozapine (Clozaril)	300–900	4–12	141–204 ng/mL	50
risperidone (Risperdal)	2–8	20	Not available	1
olanzapine (Zyprexa)	5–10	21–54	Not available	Not available
quetiapine fumarate (Seroquel)	150–750	7	Not available	Not available
ziprasidone HCl (Geodon)	40–160	7	Not available	Not available
aripiprazole (Abilify)	10–30	75–94	Not available	Not available

helpful. Although these can be measured for a number of antipsychotics, their correlation with therapeutic response has been inconsistent. Haloperidol and clozapine correlate well and may be helpful in determining whether an adequate blood level has been reached and maintained during a trial of medication. Table 12-7 shows the therapeutic ranges available for some of the antipsychotic medications. Plasma levels may also be helpful in identifying absorption problems or metabolic differences (high or low metabolizer), determining adherence, and identifying adverse reactions from drug–drug interactions.

The potency of the antipsychotics also varies widely and is of specific concern when considering typical antipsychotic drugs. As Table 12-7 indicates, 100 mg chlorpromazine is roughly equivalent to 2 mg haloperidol and 5 mg trifluoperazine. Although drugs that are more potent are not inherently better than less potent drugs, differentiating low-potency versus high-potency antipsychotics may be somewhat helpful in predicting side effects. Roughly speaking, high-potency medications, such as haloperidol and fluphenazine, produce a greater frequency of extrapyramidal symptoms, and low-potency antipsychotics, such as chlorpromazine and thioridazine, produce more sedation and hypotension.

Ultimately, selection of medication from the group of typical antipsychotics depends predominately on predicted side effects, prior history of treatment response, whether or not a depot preparation will be needed during maintenance, concurrent medications, and other medical conditions.

Drug Formulations: Long-Acting Preparations

Currently in Canada, four antipsychotic drugs, paliperidone (the major metabolite of risperidone), haloperidol, flupentixol, and fluphenazine, are available in long-acting, depot forms (Health Canada, 2013). These antipsychotics may be administered by injection once every 2 to 4 weeks. After administration, the drug is slowly released from the injection site; therefore, these forms of the drugs are referred to as *depot preparations*. Long-acting injectable medications maintain a fairly constant blood level between injections. Because they bypass problems with gastrointestinal absorption and first-pass metabolism, this method may enhance therapeutic outcomes for the patient by decreasing individual drug concentration variability due to kinetic differences. Lower rates of relapse have been reported for patients receiving long-acting injectable medication compared with those taking oral medications (Kane et al., 1998; Bond, Pratoomsri, & Yatham, 2007). Depot preparations can be used when individuals have difficulty remembering to take their oral medications and are able to keep appointments reliably or attend a program regularly where the injection may be administered. The four agents are equally effective

in treating the symptoms of psychosis, although flupentixol is usually limited to inpatient use. Nurses should be aware that the injection site may become sore and inflamed if certain precautions are not taken. The liquids are viscous, and a large-gauge needle (at least 21-gauge) should be used to withdraw the drug from the ampoule. However, there is emerging evidence that glass particles can be drawn up with the liquid, especially if using an 18-gauge needle, and thus, a filtered needle is preferred for the long-term use of depot medications (Preston & Hegadoren, 2004). See Box 12-2 for relevant research. Because the medication is meant to remain in the injection site, the needle should be dry, and a deep IM injection should be given by the Z-track method. (Note: Do not massage the injection site. Rotate sites and document in the patient's record.) A change to depot preparation from oral antipsychotic is done on a gradual basis after the patient is fully informed and consents and has taken several oral doses to ensure that no significant immediate adverse reactions are likely to occur.

Both olanzapine and risperidone are also available in a quick-release formulation in Canada. Olanzapine is often used to treat acute agitation. In circumstances where rapid sedation is needed and the patient is able and willing to take an oral medication, this formulation maybe advantageous.

| **BOX 12-2** | **Research for Best Practice** |

GLASS CONTAMINATION IN PARENTERALLY ADMINISTERED MEDICATION

From Preston, S. T. & Hegadoren, K. (2004). Glass contamination in parenterally administered medication. Journal of Advanced Nursing, 48(3), 266–270.

The Question: Does the use of larger bore unfiltered needles increase the risk of aspirating more glass and other particles?

Method: A computer microscope was used to compare the number and size of glass particles aspirated into a syringe between two needle sizes (18 gauge [G] [130 μm lumen diameter] and 21 G [90 μm lumen diameter]) without filters and 19 G (110 μm lumen diameter) filtered needles. N = 18 in each group.

Findings: At least one glass particle was found in 22% of the 1-mL ampoules, and 56% and 39% of the 2-mL ampoules, using 18G and 21G needles, respectively, had glass contaminants. Many of the 2-mL ampoules produced multiple glass particles on opening. Use of 19G filtered needles resulted in no glass particles. There was a significant difference in mean particle size between the 18G and 21G groups of 2-mL ampoules.

Implications for Practice: The IM administration of glass particles is clinically problematic. Current nursing practice standards do not adequately address this issue in terms of aspiration or filtration techniques that can minimize risk to patients. The findings support the use of filtered needles in administering IM medications to patients who receive ongoing scheduled IM injections.

Side Effects, Adverse Reactions, and Toxicity

Various side effects and interactions can occur with antipsychotics (see Tables 12-6 and 12-7), with the typical antipsychotics producing more significant side effects than the atypical antipsychotics. The side effects vary largely based on their degree of attraction to different neurotransmitter receptors and their subtypes.

Cardiovascular Side Effects

Cardiovascular side effects, such as orthostatic hypotension, depend on the degree of blockade of α-adrenergic receptors. Low-potency typical antipsychotics, such as chlorpromazine and thioridazine, and the atypical antipsychotic clozapine have a high degree of affinity for α-adrenergic receptors and, therefore, produce considerable orthostatic hypotension. Other cardiovascular side effects from typical antipsychotics have been rare, but occasionally they cause ECG changes that have a benign or undetermined clinical effect. Thioridazine (Mellaril) and ziprasidone (Geodon) have both been associated with prolonged QT intervals and should be used cautiously in patients who have increased QT intervals or are taking other medications that may prolong the QT interval (Taylor, 2003).

Anticholinergic Side Effects

Anticholinergic side effects resulting from the blockade of muscarinic acetylcholine receptors are another common concern with the typical and some of the atypical antipsychotic drugs. Dry mouth, slowed gastric motility, constipation, urinary hesitancy or retention, vaginal dryness, blurred vision, dry eyes, nasal congestion, and confusion or decreased memory are examples of these side effects. Interventions for decreasing the impact of these side effects are outlined in Table 12-2. This group of side effects occurs with many of the medications used for psychiatric treatment. Sometimes a cholinergic medication, such as bethanechol, may reduce the peripheral effects but not the CNS effects. Using more than one medication with anticholinergic effects often increases the symptoms. Older adult patients are often more susceptible to a potential toxicity that results from high blockade of acetylcholine. This toxicity is called an *anticholinergic* crisis and is described, along with its treatment, in Chapter 20. The likelihood of anticholinergic side effects, along with sedation and extrapyramidal side effects, from antipsychotics is explored in Table 12-5.

Weight Gain

Other clinically important effects also occur with the antipsychotic medications. The exact physiologic mechanisms that contribute to weight gain are unknown, but the most promising data include investigations of the histamine H(1), 5-HT(2A), 5-HT(2C), muscarinic M(3), and adrenergic receptors (Roerig, Steffen, & Mitchell, 2011). Weight gain has been associated with antipsychotic drugs since chlorpromazine was developed but is more observed with the atypical drugs such as clozapine and olanzapine. The weight gain related to antipsychotic medications is linked to an increased risk for type II diabetes, heart disease, and hyperlipidemia. Those at higher risk for developing metabolic or cardiovascular disorders are those individuals who show more rapid weight gain in the 1st week of drug treatment. A Quebec study ($N = 19,582$) showed that the risk for initiation of a pharmacologic treatment for diabetes or dyslipidemia is significantly higher with olanzapine than with risperidone (Moisan, Gregoire, Gaudet, & Cooper, 2005). Awareness of these risks emphasizes the need for early preventive intervention with diet and exercise, as well as careful consideration in the choice of the specific atypical agent for at-risk populations (Henderson, 2008). The chronic health problems of diabetes and cardiovascular illness occur much more often in individuals with mental illness than in the general population, making it essential for nurses to assist patients in dealing effectively with issues of weight gain. Guides and food diaries have been developed to help those who are maintained on long-term atypical antipsychotic drugs.

Endocrine and Sexual Side Effects

Endocrine and sexual side effects result primarily from the blockade of dopamine in the tuberoinfundibular pathways of the hypothalamus. As a result, blood levels of prolactin may increase with almost all the typical antipsychotics but less commonly with the atypical antipsychotics. Increased prolactin causes breast enlargement and rare but potential galactorrhoea (milk production and flow), decreased sexual drive, amenorrhea, menstrual irregularities, and increased risk for growth in preexisting breast cancers. Bromocriptine, a dopamine agonist, may be helpful, but more likely, these symptoms necessitate a change in medication. Endocrine side effects can occur in males as well. Retrograde ejaculation (backward flow of semen) is rare, but it may be painful and can occur with all of the antipsychotics. A more common side effect is erectile dysfunction, including difficulty achieving and maintaining an erection. Anorgasmia, or the inability to achieve orgasm, may develop in women.

Blood Disorders

Blood dyscrasias are rare but have received renewed attention since the introduction of clozapine. Agranulocytosis is an acute reaction that causes the individual's white blood cell count to drop to very low levels, and concurrent neutropenia, a drop in neutrophils in the blood, develops. In the case of the antipsychotics, the medication suppresses the bone marrow precursors to these blood cells. The exact mechanism by which the drugs produce this effect is unknown. The most notable symptoms of this disorder include high fever, sore throat, and mouth sores. Although benign elevations in temperature have been reported in individuals taking clozapine, no fever should go uninvestigated. Untreated agranulocytosis can be life threatening. Although agranulocytosis can occur with any of the antipsychotics, the risk with clozapine is 10 to 20 times greater than with the other antipsychotics (Bilici, Tekelioglu, Efendioglu, Ovali, & Ulgen, 2003). Therefore, prescription of clozapine requires weekly blood samples for the first 6 months of treatment and then every 2 weeks after that for as long as the drug is taken. Drawing of these samples must continue for 4 weeks after clozapine use has been discontinued. If sore throat or fever develops, medications should be withheld until a leukocyte count can be obtained. Hospitalization, including reverse isolation to prevent infections, is usually required. Agranulocytosis is more likely to develop during the first 18 weeks of treatment. Some research indicates that it is more common in women (Iqbal et al., 2003). The requirement for regular blood monitoring and added cost of laboratory services with clozapine has limited its use in community psychiatry with chronically mentally ill populations.

Miscellaneous

Photosensitivity reactions to antipsychotics, including severe sunburns or rash, most commonly develop with the use of low-potency typical antipsychotics. Sun block must be worn on all areas of exposed skin when taking these drugs. In addition, sun exposure may cause pigmentary deposits to develop, resulting in the discoloration of exposed areas, especially the neck and face. This discoloration may progress from a deep orange colour to a blue grey. Skin exposure should be limited and skin tone changes reported to the prescriber. Pigmentary deposits may also develop on the retina of the eye, especially with high doses of thioridazine, even for a few days. This condition is called *retinitis pigmentosa* and can lead to significant visual impairment. Therefore, thioridazine should never be administered in doses greater than 800 mg/day.

Antipsychotics may also lower a patient's seizure threshold. Patients with an undetected seizure disorder may experience seizures early in treatment. Those who have a preexisting condition should be monitored closely.

Neuroleptic malignant syndrome (NMS) and water intoxication are two serious complications that may result from antipsychotic medications. Characterized by rigidity and high fever, NMS is a rare condition that may occur abruptly with even one dose of medication. Temperature must always be monitored when administering antipsychotics, especially high-potency medications. Water intoxication may develop gradually with long-term use. This condition is characterized by the patient's consumption of large quantities of fluid (polydipsia) and the resulting effects of sodium depletion (hyponatremia). Both of these conditions are discussed more fully in Chapter 20.

Medication-Related Movement Disorders

Medication-related movement disorders are a group of side effects or adverse reactions that are commonly caused by typical antipsychotic medications but less commonly with atypical antipsychotic drugs. These disorders of abnormal motor movements can be divided into two groups: acute extrapyramidal syndromes (EPSs), which are acute abnormal movements developing early in the course of treatment (sometimes after just one dose), and chronic syndromes, which develop from longer exposure to antipsychotic drugs. The atypical antipsychotic drugs are most likely to cause movement disorders.

Acute Extrapyramidal Syndromes

Acute EPS occurs in as many as 90% of all patients receiving typical antipsychotic medications (Chouinard & Chouinard, 2008). These syndromes include dystonia, parkinsonism, and akathisia (an involuntary movement disorder). They develop early in treatment, sometimes from as little as one dose. Although the abnormal movements are treatable, they are at times dramatic and frightening, causing physical and emotional impairments that often prompt patients to stop taking their medication. Some milder forms of EPS may occur with classes of medication other than antipsychotics, including the SSRIs. The acute EPS often are mistaken for aspects of anxiety, rather than medication side effects. Nurses play a vital role in the early recognition and treatment of these syndromes. Early recognition can save the patient considerable discomfort, fear, and impairment. All nurses must be aware of these symptoms, notifying the prescriber as soon as possible and implementing selected medication changes and other interventions. Several medications can control acute EPS (Table 12-8).

Dystonia, sometimes referred to as an *acute dystonic reaction*, is impaired muscle tone that generally is the first extrapyramidal symptom to occur, usually within a few days of initiating use of an antipsychotic. Dystonia is characterized by involuntary muscle spasms, especially of the head and neck muscles. Patients usually first complain of a thick tongue, tight jaw, or stiff neck. The syndrome can progress to a protruding tongue, oculogyric crisis (eyes rolled up in the head), torticollis (muscle stiffness in the neck, which draws the head to one side with chin pointing to the other), and laryngopharyngeal constriction. Abnormal postures of the upper limbs and torso may be held briefly or sustained. In severe cases, the spasms may progress to the intercostal muscles, producing more significant breathing difficulty for patients

Table 12-8   Drug Therapies for Acute Medication-Related Movement Disorders

Agents	Typical Dosage Ranges	Routes Available	Common Side Effects
Anticholinergics			
benztropine (Cogentin)	2–6 mg/day	PO, IM, IV	Dry mouth, blurred vision, slowed gastric motility causing constipation, urinary retention, increased intraocular pressure; overdose produces toxic psychosis
trihexyphenidyl (Artane)	4–15 mg/day	PO	Same as benztropine, plus gastrointestinal distress Older adults are most prone to mental confusion and delirium
biperiden (Akineton)	2–8 mg/day	PO	Fewer peripheral anticholinergic effects Euphoria and increased tremor may occur
Antihistamines			
diphenhydramine (Benadryl)	25–50 mg q.i.d. to 400 mg daily	PO, IM, IV	Sedation and confusion, especially in older adults
Dopamine Agonists			
amantadine (Symmetrel)	100–400 mg daily	PO	Indigestion, decreased concentration, dizziness, anxiety, ataxia, insomnia, lethargy, tremors, and slurred speech may occur on higher doses Tolerance may develop on fixed dose
β-Blockers			
propranolol (Inderal)	10 mg t.i.d. to 120 mg daily	PO	Hypotension and bradycardia Must monitor pulse and blood pressure Do not stop abruptly as this may cause rebound tachycardia
Benzodiazepines			
lorazepam (Ativan)	1–2 mg IM 0.5–2 mg PO	PO, IM	All may cause drowsiness, lethargy, and general sedation or paradoxical agitation Confusion and disorientation in older adults
diazepam (Valium)	2–5 mg t.i.d.	PO, IV	Most side effects are rare and will disappear if dose is decreased
clonazepam (Klonopin)	1–4 mg/day	PO	Tolerance and withdrawal are potential problems

who already have respiratory impairment from asthma or emphysema.

Drug-induced parkinsonism is sometimes referred to as **pseudoparkinsonism** because its presentation is identical to Parkinson's disease without the same destruction of dopaminergic cells. These symptoms include the classic triad of rigidity, slowed movements (bradykinesia), and tremor. The rigid muscle stiffness is usually seen in the arms. Bradykinesia can be observed by the loss of spontaneous movements, such as the absence of the usual relaxed swing of the arms while walking. In addition, masklike facies or loss of facial expression and a decrease in the ability to initiate movements also are present. Usually, tremor is more pronounced at rest, but it can also be observed with intentional movements, such as eating. If the tremor becomes severe, it may interfere with the patient's ability to eat or maintain adequate fluid intake. Hypersalivation is possible as well. Pseudoparkinsonism symptoms may occur on one or both sides of the body and develop abruptly or subtly, but usually within the first 30 days of treatment.

Akathisia is characterized by the inability to sit still. The person will pace, rock while sitting or standing, march in place, or cross and uncross the legs. All these repetitive motions have an intensity that is frequently beyond the explanation of the individual. In addition, akathisia may be present as a primarily subjective experience without obvious motor behaviour. This subjective experience includes feelings of anxiety, jitteriness, or the inability to relax, which the individual may or may not be able to communicate. It is extremely uncomfortable for a person experiencing akathisia to be forced to sit still or be confined. These symptoms are sometimes misdiagnosed as agitation or an increase in psychotic symptoms, but if the nurse administers an antipsychotic medication PRN (from the Latin pro re nata, which roughly translated means "as needed"), the symptoms will not abate and will often worsen. Differentiating akathisia from agitation may be aided by knowing the person's symptoms before the introduction of medication. Psychotic agitation does not usually begin abruptly after antipsychotic medication use has been started, whereas akathisia may occur after administration. In addition, the nurse may ask the patient if the experience is felt primarily in the muscles (akathisia) or in the mind or emotions (agitation).

Akathisia is the most difficult acute medication-related movement disorder to relieve. It does not usually respond well to anticholinergic medications and is uncommon in patients receiving atypical antipsychotics. It is thought that the pathology of akathisia may involve more than just the extrapyramidal motor system. It may include serotonin changes that also affect the dopamine system (Kulkarni & Naidu, 2003). A number of medications have been used to reduce symptoms, including β-adrenergic blockers, anticholinergics, antihistamines, and low-dose antianxiety agents (Pierre, 2005). The usual approach to treatment is to change to an atypical antipsychotic if possible. If not, reducing the dose of typical antipsychotic medication can be tried. During this time, PMH nurses must closely assess for worsening of symptoms. β-Adrenergic blockers, such as propranolol (Inderal), given in doses of 30 to 120 mg/day, have been most successful (Miller & Fleischhacker, 2000). Nurses must monitor the patient's pulse and blood pressure because propranolol can cause hypotension and bradycardia. If the patient's pulse falls below 60 bpm, propranolol should be withheld and the prescriber notified. Normal signs of hypoglycaemia may be blocked by propranolol; therefore, patients with diabetes must monitor their blood or urine glucose levels carefully, especially because they are under physical stress from the disorder.

A number of nursing interventions may reduce the impact of these syndromes. Individuals with acute EPS need frequent reassurance that this is not a worsening of their psychiatric condition but instead is a treatable side effect of the medication. They also need validation that what they are experiencing is real and that the nurse is concerned and will be responsive to changes in these symptoms. Physical and psychological stress appears to increase the symptoms and further frighten the patient; therefore, decreasing stressful situations becomes important. These symptoms are often physically exhausting for the patient, and nurses should ensure that the patient receives adequate rest and hydration. Because tremors, muscle rigidity, and motor restlessness may interfere with the individual's ability to eat, the nurse may need to assist the patient with eating and drinking fluids to maintain nutrition and hydration.

Risk factors for acute EPS include previous episodes of EPS and use of high-dose injected antipsychotics for acute psychotic symptoms or agitation. Listen closely when patients say they are "allergic" or have had "bad reactions" to antipsychotic medications. Often, they are describing one of the medication-related movement disorders, particularly dystonia, rather than a rash or other allergic symptoms. About 90% of the individuals who have experienced EPS in the past will again have these symptoms if the use of an antipsychotic medication is restarted (Meyer, 2007; Nasrallah, 2002). High-potency medications, such as haloperidol and fluphenazine, are more likely to cause EPS. Age and gender appear to be risk factors for specific syndromes. Acute dystonia occurs most often in young men, adolescents, and children; akathisia is more common in middle-aged women. Older adult patients are at the greatest risk for experiencing pseudoparkinsonism (Sibon, Fenelon, Quinn, & Tison, 2004). Although the occurrence of EPS is decreasing as atypical medications are more commonly used, acute EPS remains a serious clinical concern. Risperidone in high doses carries with it the same risk of EPS as does the typical antipsychotics.

Chronic Syndromes

Chronic syndromes develop from the long-term use of antipsychotics. They are serious and afflict about 20% of the patients who receive typical antipsychotics for an extended period (Pierre, 2005). These conditions can be irreversible and cause significant impairment in self-image, social interactions, and occupational functioning. Early symptoms and mild forms may go unnoticed by the person experiencing them because they frequently remain beyond the individual's awareness. Therefore, PMH nurses in contact with individuals who are taking antipsychotic medications for months or years must be vigilant for symptoms of these typical chronic conditions.

First identified in 1957, **tardive dyskinesia** is the most well known of the chronic syndromes. It involves irregular, repetitive involuntary movements of the mouth, face, and tongue, including chewing, tongue protrusion, lip smacking, puckering of the lips, and rapid eye blinking. Abnormal finger movements are common as well. In some individuals, the trunk and extremities are also involved, and in rare cases, irregular breathing and swallowing lead to belching and grunting noises. These symptoms usually begin no earlier than after 6 months of treatment or when the medication is reduced or withdrawn. Once thought to be irreversible, considerable controversy now exists as to whether or not this is true.

Part of the difficulty in determining the irreversibility of tardive dyskinesia is that any movement disorder that persists after the discontinuation of antipsychotic medication has been described as tardive dyskinesia. Atypical forms are now receiving more attention because some researchers believe that they may have different underlying mechanisms of causation. Some of these forms of the disorder appear to remit spontaneously. Symptoms of what is now called *withdrawal tardive dyskinesia* appear when use of an antipsychotic medication is reduced or discontinued and remit spontaneously in 1 to 3 months. *Tardive dystonia* and *tardive akathisia* have also been described. Both appear in a manner similar to the acute syndromes but continue after the antipsychotic medication has been withdrawn. More research is needed to determine whether these syndromes are distinctly different in origin and outcome.

The risk for experiencing tardive dyskinesia increases with age. Although the prevalence of tardive dyskinesia averages 15% to 20%, the rate rises to 50% to 70% in older adults receiving antipsychotic medications (Tariot, Salzman, Yeung, Pultz, & Rak, 2000). Cumulative incidence of tardive dyskinesia appears to increase 5% per year of continued exposure to antipsychotic medications (Levy et al., 2002). Women are at higher risk than are men. Individuals with affective disorders, particularly depression, are at higher risk than are those who have schizophrenia. Any individual receiving antipsychotic medication may experience tardive dyskinesia; therefore, nurses must be particularly alert to individuals at higher risk. Risk factors are summarized in Box 12-3. The causes of tardive dyskinesia remain unclear. Lack of a consistent theory of aetiology for the chronic medication-related movement disorder syndromes has led to inconsistent and disappointing treatment approaches. No one medication relieves the symptoms. Dopamine agonists, such as bromocriptine, and many other drugs have been tried. Even dietary precursors of acetylcholine, such as lethicin, and nutritional therapies, such as vitamin E supplements, may prove to be beneficial.

The best approach to treatment remains avoiding the development of the chronic syndromes. Preventive measures include use of atypical antipsychotics, using the lowest possible dose of typical medication, minimizing use of PRN medication, and closely monitoring individuals in high-risk groups for development of the symptoms of tardive dyskinesia. All members of the mental health treatment team who have contact with individuals taking antipsychotics for longer than 3 months must be alert to the risk factors and earliest possible signs of chronic medication-related movement disorders.

Monitoring tools, such as the Abnormal Involuntary Movement Scale (AIMS; Simpson & Angus, 1970), should be used routinely to standardize assessment and provide the earliest possible recognition of the symptoms. Standardized assessments should be performed at a minimum of 3- to 6-month intervals. The earlier the symptoms are recognized, the more likely they will resolve if

the medication can be changed or its use discontinued. Newer, atypical antipsychotic medications have a much lower risk for causing tardive dyskinesia and are increasingly being considered first-line medications for treating schizophrenia. Other medications are under development to provide alternatives that limit the risk for tardive dyskinesia.

> ● **STUDY NOTE**
> Nurses need to be particularly vigilant concerning the side effects, adverse reactions, and toxicity that may occur with antipsychotic medications when patients are unable to distinguish such reactions from their psychotic symptoms.

■ MOOD STABILIZERS (ANTIMANIA MEDICATIONS)

Mood stabilizers, or antimania medications, are psychopharmacologic agents used primarily for stabilizing mood swings, particularly those of mania in bipolar disorders. For a number of years, lithium was the only drug known to stabilize the symptoms of mania. Although it remains the gold standard of treatment for acute mania and maintenance of bipolar disorders, not all individuals experience a positive response to lithium, and increasingly other drugs are being used as first-line agents. In the 1970s, carbamazepine (Tegretol) and later valproate, both anticonvulsants approved for treating epilepsy, were found to have mood-stabilizing effects. At present, three drugs have Health Canada approval for the short-term treatment of acute mania. They include lithium, olanzapine (Zyprexa), and valproic acid (Depakote). Lithium is the only drug with approved Health Canada indication for the prevention and treatment of both manic and depressive episodes. Many other drugs, including other anticonvulsants, atypical antipsychotics, adrenergic blocking agents in conjunction with antidepressants, are used frequently to prevent episodes of hypomania or depression (Yatham et al., 2006).

Lithium

Lithium, a naturally occurring element, was first discovered in the early 1800s. It has been in medical use in a variety of forms, including tonics and elixirs, since that time. As an element that acts as a salt substitute, the unregulated use of lithium produced a number of cases of toxicity and, as a result, lost favour in the 1940s. Rediscovered in 1949 by the Australian John Cade, lithium was found to reduce agitation in some patients experiencing psychosis, and in the 1950s, Schou (1978) published reports that lithium controlled and prevented the symptoms of mania. In 1970, the FDA approved lithium for use in treating

---

BOX 12-3 Risk Factors for Tardive Dyskinesia

- Age older than 50 years
- Female
- Affective disorders, particularly depression
- Brain damage or dysfunction
- Increased duration of treatment
- Standard antipsychotic medication
- Use of acute higher doses of antipsychotic medication

manic episodes in bipolar affective disorder. Since then, it has become a mainstay in psychopharmacology. Lithium is effective in only about 40% of patients with bipolar disorder, and patients who do experience response often have limited clinical improvement. Although lithium is not a perfect drug, a great deal is known regarding its use—it is inexpensive, it has restored stability to the lives of thousands of people, and it remains the gold standard of bipolar pharmacologic treatment.

Indications and Mechanisms of Action

The target symptoms for lithium are the symptoms of mania, such as rapid speech, jumping from topic to topic (flight of ideas), irritability, grandiose thinking, impulsiveness, and agitation. Other psychiatric indications include using lithium for its mild antidepressant effects in treating depressive episodes of bipolar illness and in patients experiencing major depression that has only partially responded to antidepressants alone. Used in patients who have experienced only partial response, lithium has been used in augmentation as a potentiator (enhancing the effects) of antidepressant medications. It has also been shown to be helpful in reducing impulsivity and aggression in certain psychiatric patients.

Lithium has been effective in treating several non-psychiatric disorders, such as cluster headaches. Because lithium stimulates leukocytosis, it often improves the neutrophil counts of patients who are undergoing chemotherapy or who have other conditions that cause neutropenia. In addition, lithium has been investigated as an antiviral agent because it appears to inhibit the replication of several DNA viruses, including herpes virus. Additional research is needed to fully understand the mechanisms of these effects.

Lithium is actively transported across cell membranes, altering sodium transport in both nerve and muscle cells. It replaces sodium in the sodium–potassium pump and is retained more readily than sodium inside the cell. Conditions that alter sodium content in the body, such as vomiting, diuresis, and diaphoresis, also alter lithium retention. The results of lithium influx into the nerve cell lead to increased storage of catecholamines within the cell, reduced dopamine neurotransmission, increased norepinephrine reuptake, increased GABA activity, and increased serotonin receptor sensitivity (Bschor et al., 2003; Solomon, Keitner, & Ryan, 1998). Lithium also alters the distribution of calcium and magnesium ions and inhibits second messenger systems within the neuron. The specific mechanisms by which lithium improves the symptoms of mania are complex, most likely involving the sum of all or part of these actions and more. Genetic research in bipolar disorder considers lithium response as an important criterion for subgrouping the bipolar population (Alda, 2004).

Pharmacokinetics

Lithium carbonate is available orally in capsule, tablet, and liquid forms. Slow-release preparations are also available. Lithium is readily absorbed in the gastric system and may be taken with food, which does not impair absorption. Peak blood levels are reached in 1 to 4 hours, and the medication is usually completely absorbed in 8 hours. Slow-release preparations are absorbed at a slower, more variable rate.

Lithium is not protein bound, and its distribution into the CNS across the blood–brain barrier is slow. The onset of action is usually 5 to 7 days and may take as long as 2 weeks. The elimination half-life is 8 to 12 hours, and 18 to 36 hours in individuals whose blood levels have reached steady state and whose symptoms are stable. Lithium is almost entirely excreted by the kidneys but is present in all body fluids. Conditions of renal impairment or decreased renal function in older adults decrease lithium clearance and may lead to toxicity. Several medications affect renal function and therefore change lithium clearance. See Chapter 22 for a list of these and other medication interactions with lithium. About 80% of lithium is reabsorbed in the proximal tubule of the kidney along with water and sodium. In conditions that cause sodium depletion, such as dehydration caused by fever, strenuous exercise, hot weather, increased perspiration, and vomiting, the kidney attempts to conserve sodium. Because lithium is a salt, the kidney retains lithium as well, leading to increased blood levels and potential toxicity. Significantly increasing sodium intake causes lithium levels to fall.

Lithium is usually administered in doses of 300 mg two to three times daily. During the acute phases of mania, blood levels of 0.8 to 1.4 mEq/L are usually attained and maintained until symptoms are under control. During maintenance, the dosage is reduced, and dosages are adjusted to maintain blood levels of 0.4 to 1 mEq/L. As a drug with a narrow therapeutic range or index, blood levels are monitored frequently during acute mania, while the dosage is increased every 3 to 5 days. These increases may be slower in older adults or patients who experience uncomfortable side effects. Blood levels should be monitored 12 hours after the last dose of medication. In the hospital setting, nurses should withhold the morning dose of lithium until the serum sample is drawn to avoid falsely elevated levels. Individuals who are at home should be instructed to have their blood drawn in the morning about 12 hours after their last dose and before they take their first dose of medication.

Lithium clears the body relatively quickly after the discontinuation of its use. It is important to remember that almost half of the individuals who discontinue lithium treatment abruptly experience a relapse of symptoms within a few weeks (Goodwin & Ghaemi, 2000; Kennedy et al., 2003). Some research suggests that discontinuation of the use of lithium for individuals whose symptoms have been stable may lead to lithium losing its effectiveness when use of the medication is restarted (Kennedy et al., 2003). Patients should be warned of the risks in abruptly discontinuing their medication and should be advised to consider the options carefully in consultation with their prescriber.

Side Effects, Adverse Reactions, and Toxicity

At lower therapeutic blood levels, side effects from lithium are relatively mild. These reactions correspond with peaks in plasma concentrations of the medication after administration, and most subside during the first few weeks of therapy. Frequently, individuals taking lithium complain of excessive thirst and an unpleasant metallic-like taste. Sugarless throat lozenges may be useful in minimizing this side effect. Other common side effects include an increased frequency of urination, fine head tremor, drowsiness, and mild diarrhoea. Weight gain occurs in about 20% of the individuals taking lithium. Nausea may be minimized by taking the medication with food or by use of a slow-release preparation. However, slow-release forms of lithium increase diarrhoea. Muscle weakness, restlessness, headache, acne, rashes, and exacerbation of psoriasis have also been reported. See Chapter 22 for a summary of selected nursing interventions to minimize the impact of common side effects associated with lithium treatment. Patients most frequently discontinued their own medication use because of concerns with mental slowness, poor concentration, and memory problems.

As blood levels of lithium increase, the side effects of lithium become more numerous and severe. Early signs of lithium toxicity include severe diarrhoea, vomiting, drowsiness, muscular weakness, and lack of coordination. Lithium should be withheld and the prescriber consulted if these symptoms develop. Lithium toxicity can easily be resolved in 24 to 48 hours by discontinuing the medication, but haemodialysis may be required in severe situations. See Chapter 22 for a summary of the side effects and symptoms of toxicity associated with various blood levels of lithium.

Monitoring of creatinine concentration, thyroid hormones, and CBC every 6 months during maintenance therapy helps to assess the occurrence of other potential adverse reactions. Kidney damage is considered an uncommon but potentially serious risk for long-term lithium treatment. This damage is usually reversible after discontinuation of the lithium use. A gradual rise in serum creatinine and decline in creatinine clearance indicate the development of renal dysfunction. Individuals with preexisting kidney dysfunction are susceptible to lithium toxicity.

Lithium may alter thyroid function, usually after 6 to 18 months of treatment. About 30% of the individuals taking lithium exhibit elevations in thyroid-stimulating hormone, but most do not show the suppression of circulating thyroid hormone. Thyroid dysfunction from lithium treatment is more common in women, and some individuals require the addition of thyroxine to their care. During maintenance, thyroid-stimulating hormone levels may be monitored. Nurses should observe for dry skin, constipation, bradycardia, hair loss, cold intolerance, and other symptoms of hypothyroidism. Other endocrine system effects result from hypoparathyroidism, which increases parathyroid hormone levels and calcium. Clinically, this change is not significant, but elevated calcium levels may cause mood changes, anxiety, lethargy, and sleep disturbances. These symptoms may erroneously be attributed to depression if hypocalcaemia is not investigated.

Lithium use must be avoided during pregnancy because it has been associated with birth defects, especially when administered during the first trimester. If lithium is given during the third trimester, toxicity may develop in a newborn, producing signs of hypotonia, cyanosis, bradykinesia, cardiac changes, gastrointestinal bleeding, and shock. Diabetes insipidus may persist for months. Lithium is also present in breast milk, and women should not breast-feed while taking lithium. Women expecting to become pregnant should be advised to consult with their physician before discontinuing the use of birth control methods.

Anticonvulsants

Some anticonvulsants can be used to treat bipolar disorder: valproic acid, carbamazepine, topiramate (Topamax), lamotrigine (Lamictal), and oxcarbazepine (Trileptal). Gabapentin had been used, but controlled trials showed poor efficacy (Pande, Crockatt, Janney, Werth, & Tsaroucha, 2000). Although lithium alone has provided tremendous relief to thousands of individuals experiencing bipolar affective disorder, 20% to 40% of those affected by the disorder do not respond, most often those with rapid cycling episodes. The psychopharmacologic properties of some anticonvulsant medications have been reported since the 1960s, but it was not until the 1970s in Japan that carbamazepine was demonstrated to have mood-stabilizing effects in patients with bipolar affective disorders. Concern about blood dyscrasias delayed its release in the United States, and the increased risks for aplastic anaemia and agranulocytosis with carbamazepine use still require a close monitoring of CBCs during treatment. Valproate and its derivatives have had a similar course of development. With the exception of gabapentin (Neurontin), the benefit of anticonvulsant use in bipolar disorder has been well established (Melvin, Carey, Goodman, Oldham, & Ranney, 2008).

Indications and Mechanisms of Action

Anticonvulsant medications in general are primarily indicated for treating seizure disorders. Target symptoms for the use of anticonvulsants with bipolar disorder include all the symptoms of mania discussed earlier. However, anticonvulsants are often used for individuals who have not experienced response to lithium or who are identified as having rapid cycling. Studies have shown some common traits in these individuals. Those who do not experience response to lithium most often are those who have a dysphoric or mixed mania. These individuals experience an increase in physical activity during manic episodes without any elevation in mood. They often are referred to as *mixed states* because they have elements of both depression and mania. These individuals exhibit symptoms of high anxiety, agitation, and irritability, which are then target symptoms for the use of anticonvulsants. Empirical data show carbamazepine and valproic acid to be effective in mood stabilization.

The term *rapid cycling* is applied when individuals experience four or more episodes of either depression or mania during a 12-month period. This occurs more often in women than in men. These patients make up a group of individuals who experience poor response to lithium treatment. Mood instability is also a target symptom of anticonvulsant medications. The theory of the mechanism of action of the anticonvulsants involves the concept of kindling as it applies to mood disorders.

Kindling refers to the emergence of spontaneous firing of nerve cells in response to repeated subthreshold electrical stimulation. Once brain regions, such as the amygdala, have been "kindled," it takes considerably less stimulation to initiate a seizure. In the case of mood disorders, it is hypothesized that "kindled" brain regions include the areas associated with emotional regulation. The stimulation of these regions by increasingly minor stressors or other environmental factors produces mood swings instead of a seizure.

Anticonvulsants have "antikindling" properties and decrease the sensitization of affected cells, making them less easy to stimulate. In general, the anticonvulsant mood stabilizers have many actions, but it is their effects on ion channels, reducing repetitive firing of action potentials in the nerves, that most directly decreases manic symptoms. In addition, drugs such as carbamazepine affect the release and reuptake of several neurotransmitters, including norepinephrine, GABA, dopamine, and glutamate. They also change several second messenger systems. No single mechanism has yet accounted for the anticonvulsants' ability to stabilize mood. Divalproex sodium also has been shown to have numerous neurotransmission effects. The most widely held theory of how

it stabilizes mood swings relates to its effects on GABA. As the major inhibitory neurotransmitter in the CNS, increased levels of GABA and improved responsiveness of the neurons to GABA lead to the control of epileptic activity. Divalproex sodium increases levels of GABA in the CNS by activating its synthesis, inhibiting the catabolism (destructive metabolism) of GABA, increasing its release, and increasing receptor density (Loscher, 2002; Solomon et al., 1998). Other foci for research into the underlying mechanisms involved in mood stabilization are specific intracellular signalling pathways, in particular involving calcium signalling and inositol monophosphate (Dubovsky, Thomas, Hijazi, & Murphy, 1994; O'Donnell et al., 2000).

Pharmacokinetics

Carbamazepine is an unusual drug and is absorbed in a somewhat variable manner. The liquid suspension is absorbed more quickly than the tablet form, but food does not appear to interfere with absorption. Peak plasma levels occur in 2 to 6 hours. Because high doses influence peak plasma levels and increase the risk for side effects, carbamazepine should be given in divided doses two or three times a day. The suspension, which has higher peak plasma levels and lower trough levels, must be given more frequently than the tablet form.

Valproic acid is more rapidly absorbed, but the enteric coating of divalproex sodium adds a delay of as long as 1 hour. Peak serum levels occur in about 1 to 4 hours. The liquid form (sodium valproate) is absorbed more rapidly and peaks in 15 minutes to 2 hours (Loscher, 2002). Food appears to slow absorption but does not lower bioavailability of the drug. Valproate is a good example of the importance of considering *bioequivalence*, a term referring to the abilities of two formulations of the same drug to induce a therapeutic response of similar magnitude and duration (Zintzaras, 2005). For example, divalproex, an enteric-coated formulation, has a half-life of 12 to 16 hours; is not affected by food intake and achieves more consistent plasma levels than valproic acid, which has a shorter half-life (8 hours); should not be taken with food; and produces gastrointestinal irritation in about 40% of patients.

Carbamazepine and valproic acid are highly protein bound; therefore, patients who are older, medically ill, or malnourished may experience the effects of increased unbound levels of both drugs. When given with other drugs that are competing for the same protein-binding sites, higher levels of unbound drug may occur. In both cases, these individuals risk more side effects and fluctuations in medication plasma levels. Newer agents for the treatment of bipolar affective disorder, such as gabapentin, have little protein binding and therefore are not subject to some of these effects. Carbamazepine and valproic acid also cross easily into the CNS and move into the placenta as well. Both are associated with an increased risk for birth defects, including spina bifida, and carbamazepine accumulates in foetal tissue. Carbamazepine and valproic acid are metabolized by the cytochrome P-450 system of microsomal hepatic enzymes. However, one of the metabolites of carbamazepine is potentially toxic. When other concurrent medications inhibit the enzymes that break down this toxic metabolite, severe adverse reactions are often the result (e.g., decreased prothrombin times and hepatotoxicity; Kalapos, 2002). Medications that inhibit this breakdown include erythromycin, verapamil, and cimetidine (now available in nonprescription form).

Carbamazepine activates its own metabolism through induction of the P-450 microsomal hepatic enzymes. Patients receiving carbamazepine may experience a precipitant drop in therapeutic blood levels and a relapse in symptoms, requiring a dosage increase for as long as 2 to 3 months after steady state has been achieved. Although valproic acid is also affected by other medications that stimulate the P-450 system, it does not enhance its own metabolism. Both carbamazepine and valproic acid are available in slow-release, extended-action forms, allowing for decreased daily dosing and improved adherence.

Nurses need to educate patients about potential drug interactions, especially with nonprescription medications. Nurses can also inform other health care practitioners who may be prescribing medication that these patients are taking carbamazepine. It is important to note that oral contraceptives may become ineffective, and female patients should be advised to use other methods of birth control.

Side Effects, Adverse Reactions, and Toxicity

The most common side effects of carbamazepine are dizziness, drowsiness, tremor, visual disturbance, nausea, and vomiting. These side effects may be minimized by initiating treatment in low doses. Patients should be advised that these symptoms will diminish, but care should be taken when changing positions or performing tasks that require visual alertness. Giving the drug with food may diminish nausea. Valproic acid also causes gastrointestinal disturbances, tremor, and lethargy. In addition, it can produce weight gain and alopecia (hair loss). These symptoms are transient and should diminish with the course of treatment. Dietary supplements of zinc and selenium may be helpful to patients experiencing hair loss. Constipation and urinary retention occur in some individuals. Nurses should monitor urinary output and assist patients to increase fluid consumption to decrease constipation.

Transient elevations in liver enzymes occur with both carbamazepine and valproic acid, but rarely do symptoms of hepatic injury occur. If the patient reports abnormal pain or shows signs of jaundice, the prescriber should be notified immediately. Several blood dyscrasias are associated with carbamazepine, including aplastic anaemia, agranulocytosis, and leucopenia. Patients should be advised to report fever, sore throat, rash, petechiae, or bruising immediately. In addition, advise patients of the importance of completing routine blood tests throughout treatment.

Both valproic acid and carbamazepine may be lethal if high doses are ingested. Toxic symptoms appear in 1 to 3 hours and include neuromuscular disturbances, dizziness, stupor, agitation, disorientation, nystagmus, urinary retention, nausea and vomiting, tachycardia, hypotension or hypertension, cardiovascular shock, coma, and respiratory depression. Carbamazepine appears to be more lethal at lower doses, but valproic acid is absorbed rapidly, and gastric lavage may be ineffective, depending on time from ingestion.

Of the newer anticonvulsant drugs, lamotrigine (Lamictal) in rare cases produces severe, life-threatening rashes that usually occur within 2 to 8 weeks of treatment. This risk is highest in children. The use of lamotrigine should be immediately discontinued if a rash is noted. Topamax (Topiramate) carries an increased risk for kidney stone formation. It can also cause a decrease in serum digoxin levels and may decrease effectiveness of oral birth control agents. In addition, ongoing ophthalmologic monitoring is required because of reports of acute myopia with secondary glaucoma. In some women, these anticonvulsants may decrease the effectiveness of oral birth control agents. Because of the potentially significant adverse reactions that the anticonvulsants can produce, careful patient teaching and monitoring are required.

ANTIDEPRESSANT MEDICATIONS

Researchers in the 1950s who were investigating other drugs related to the phenothiazines for the treatment of psychosis discovered that imipramine, a related compound, relieved the symptoms of depression. Imipramine was the first of a number of medications that contained a three-ring structure in their chemical makeup and produced improvement in depression. These medications became known as TCAs. Table 12-9 lists other related TCAs still in use today.

Concurrent with the discovery of TCAs, an antibiotic, iproniazid, used in treating tuberculosis, alleviated the symptoms of depression. Iproniazid increased the bioamine neurotransmitters by inhibiting MAO, the enzyme that breaks down these neurotransmitters inside the nerve cell. Iproniazid is no longer used, but related, more effective drugs, phenelzine and tranylcypromine, make up a subgroup of antidepressants called the MAOIs. Currently, the Canadian clinical guidelines for the treatment of depressive disorders developed by the CANMAT Depression Working Group (Lam et al., 2009) as first-line treatment recommendations for a major depressive episode (based on level I evidence and little evidence of differences in efficacy or tolerability) include SSRIs, NSRIs, mirtazapine, and reboxetine. These classes and specific drugs are described below.

Table 12-9   Antidepressant Medications

Generic (Trade) Drug Name	Usual Dosage Range (mg/day)	Half-Life (hours)	Therapeutic Blood Level (ng/mL)
Tricyclic			
amitriptyline (Elavil)	50–300	31–46	110–250
clomipramine (Anafranil)	25–250	19–37	80–100
doxepin (Sinequan)	25–300	8–24	100–200
imipramine (Tofranil)	30–300	11–25	200–350
amoxapine (Asendin)	50–600	8	200–500
desipramine (Norpramin)	25–300	12–24	125–300
nortriptyline (Aventyl)	30–100	18–44	50–150
protriptyline (Vivactil)	15–60	67–89	100–200
Selective Serotonin Reuptake Inhibitors			
fluoxetine (Prozac)	20–80	2–9 days	72–300
sertraline (Zoloft)	50–200	24	Not available
paroxetine (Paxil)	10–50	10–24	Not available
fluvoxamine (Luvox)	50–300	17–22	Not available
citalopram (Celexa)	20–50	35	Not available
escitalopram (Lexapro)	10–20	27–32	Not available
Norepinephrine Selective Reuptake Inhibitors			
reboxetine	12	12	Not available
Norepinephrine and Serotonin Selective Reuptake Inhibitors			
venlafaxine	75–375	5–11	100–500
duloxetine	60–80	9–19	Not available
Other Antidepressant Medications			
trazodone (Desyrel)	150–600	4–9	650–1,600
nefazodone (Serzone)	100–600	2–4	Not available
bupropion (Wellbutrin)	200–450	8–24	10–29
mirtazapine (Remeron)	15–45	20–40	Not available
Monoamine Oxidase Inhibitors			
moclobemide (Manerix)	300–600	6–10	Not available
phenelzine (Nardil)	15–90	24 (effect lasts 3–10 days)	Not available
tranylcypromine (Parnate)	10–60	24 (effect lasts 3–10 days)	Not available

TCAS, MAOIS, and More

Throughout the 1960s and 1970s, the TCAs and MAOIs were the primary medications for treating depression. Research continued to develop new agents with increased effectiveness, while decreasing the side effects and potential lethal effects. In the 1980s, several medications that were significantly different in chemical structure were introduced. Bupropion (Wellbutrin), introduced in 1987, had actions that were significantly different from those of previous antidepressants, but concern about the risk for seizures and other side effects limited initial excitement about its use. In 1988, the release of fluoxetine (Prozac) received much public attention and resulted in an increased awareness of depression and its treatment. Fluoxetine was the first of a class of drugs that acted "selectively" on one neurotransmitter, in this case serotonin. Other similarly selective medications, sertraline (Zoloft), paroxetine (Paxil), and fluvoxamine (Luvox), soon followed and together make up the SSRIs. The newest SSRIs include citalopram (Celexa) and escitalopram oxalate (Lexapro). Reboxetine is the only norepinephrine selective reuptake inhibitor available in Canada. Two available drugs, venlafaxine (Effexor) and duloxetine (Cymbalta), are selective to both serotonin and norepinephrine. The TCAs are now considered as second-line treatments and the MAOIs as third-line treatments (Lam et al., 2009).

Citalopram is a racemate, which means it contains equal proportions of two isomers. Isomers are molecules with the same chemical formula but with a different spatial arrangement of the atoms, which may cause different effects in the human body or have different side effect profiles. The two isomers of citalopram have been separated, and escitalopram, one of the isomers, is marketed as an antidepressant in its own right.

Since the initial introduction of the SSRIs, several new chemical compounds have been introduced that have mixed or indirect actions, making them difficult to categorize. An example is mirtazapine (Remeron). Mirtazapine increases both serotonin and norepinephrine neurotransmission but not by reuptake inhibition of neurotransmitters or inhibition of catabolic enzymes; rather, it acts in part as an agonist at 5-HT$_{1A}$ receptors.

Indications and Mechanisms of Action

The TCAs have multiple effects on a variety of receptors in the CNS, including reuptake inhibition at serotonin and norepinephrine transporters; down-regulation of specific serotonin and noradrenergic receptors; and blockade of cholinergic, adrenergic, and histamine receptors. On the other hand, the MAOIs are more specific in their actions. They inhibit MAO, an enzyme that breaks down biogenic amines, such as serotonin, thereby increasing synaptic neurotransmission, resulting in clinical improvement.

The primary indication for antidepressant medications is depression, thus the name "antidepressant." Symptoms such as loss of interest in the person's usual activities (anhedonia), depressed mood, lethargy or decreased energy, insomnia, decreased concentration, loss of appetite, and suicidal ideation usually respond (see Chapter 22 for a more complete discussion of the symptoms of depression). Antidepressants are also used to treat other symptoms and disorders, and increasingly the name antidepressant is somewhat misleading.

Antidepressants are prescribed to treat the whole range of anxiety disorders (see Chapter 23). Antidepressants are also used to treat eating disorders (see Chapter 25), depression in bipolar disorders, dysthymia, chronic pain disorders, and premenstrual syndrome. More sedating antidepressants are sometimes used in small doses to address sleep disturbances. Trazodone, amitriptyline, mirtazapine, and other agents have been used alone or as adjunctive interventions for sleep disturbance. Antidepressants are also used for other sleep disorders, such as sleep apnoea. Symptoms of some psychiatric disorders of childhood (see Chapter 31), such as attention deficit hyperactivity disorder (ADHD), enuresis (bed-wetting), and school phobia, often respond to antidepressant medication.

At times, the symptoms of depression present in an "atypical" manner, which is called *atypical depression*. Individuals with atypical depression have a mixture of anxiety and depression, increased appetite and sleep rather than the typical insomnia and loss of appetite, mood reactivity rather than consistent low mood, worsening of the symptoms in the evening, and oversensitivity to such interpersonal feelings as rejection. These target symptoms of atypical depression are more often seen in women and respond better to the MAOIs, such as phenelzine (Nardil), or to the mixed action antidepressants (those that have both direct neurotransmitter receptor action and reuptake properties), such as trazodone or nefazodone (Riederer, Lachenmayer, & Laux, 2004).

Pharmacokinetics

All of the antidepressant medications are well absorbed from the gastrointestinal system; however, some individual variations exist. For example, food slightly increases the amount of trazodone absorbed but decreases its maximum blood concentrations and lengthens the time to peak effects from 1 hour on an empty stomach to 2 hours with food. Food also increases the maximum concentrations of sertraline in the bloodstream and decreases the time to peak plasma levels, whereas fluoxetine and fluvoxamine are unaffected, although food may delay the absorption of fluoxetine. Food has little effect on the TCAs.

PMH nurses should review pharmacokinetic information as it applies to each individual medication. They must consider how this information will affect the patient's use of the medication given the target symptoms for which the drug is intended. For example, if trazodone is being used on a continuous dose schedule for its antidepressant effect, the effects of food probably matter very little. However, if trazodone is being used in a small dose at bedtime to assist a patient to sleep, an empty stomach becomes important because food would lengthen the time of onset of clinical effects, in this case, sleep.

The TCAs undergo considerable first-pass metabolism but reach peak plasma concentrations in 2 to 4 hours. The TCAs are highly bound to plasma proteins, which make the association between blood levels and therapeutic clinical effects difficult. However, some plasma ranges have been established. Table 12-9 includes the available ranges for therapeutic blood levels of the TCAs. In addition, times to steady-state plasma levels have wide variations, and the effective dose of medication must be individualized. Other antidepressants are also highly protein bound, which means that drugs that compete for these binding sites may cause fluctuations in blood levels of the antidepressants. Venlafaxine has the lowest protein binding; therefore, drug interactions of this type are not expected with this medication. Blood level changes caused by the presence of other drugs competing with binding sites are not expected.

The onset of action also varies considerably, depending on specific symptoms. For example, an improvement in sleep often occurs earlier than effects on overall mood or anhedonia. Complete relief of symptoms may take several weeks (Machado-Vieira, Salvadore, Luckenbaugh, Manji, & Zarate, 2008). Full enzyme inhibition with the MAOIs may take as long as 2 weeks, but the energizing effects may be seen within a few days. Overcoming issues such as social stigma, viewing depression as a personal failing, fear about taking a medication, and the decreased energy and motivation associated with depression have made deciding to seek treatment a major hurdle. Indeed, in both US and Canadian community surveys, only about one third of individuals with depression had sought treatment for their symptoms (Patten & Beck, 2004; Rust et al., 2005). The variable onset of action may add to their sense of discouragement and powerlessness. PMH nurses and families are often involved in providing encouragement and other supportive interventions to assist the patient in "getting through" this period of time.

Although antidepressants are primarily excreted by the kidneys, their routes of metabolism vary. Most of the TCAs have active metabolites that act in much the same manner as the parent drug. Therefore, in determining the rate of elimination, one must consider the half-lives of these metabolites. Most of these antidepressants may be given in a once-daily single dose. If the medication causes sedation, this dose should be given at bedtime. Fluoxetine cause more activation of energy and must be given in the morning. Venlafaxine, nefazodone, and bupropion are examples of antidepressants whose shorter half-life periods and other factors require administration two or three times per day. Extended-release venlafaxine formulation has allowed daily dosing with this drug. Fluoxetine and its active metabolite have particularly long half-lives, remaining present for as long as 5 to 6 weeks. This may affect a number of decisions. For example, women who wish to have children and are taking fluoxetine ideally should discontinue use of the agent at least 6 weeks before attempting to conceive. They should be advised to consult their prescriber before making this decision. Fluoxetine would also not be a good choice for intermittent use for premenstrual dysphoric disorder. Table 12-9 provides information about the average elimination half-lives of most of the antidepressants.

Most of the antidepressants are metabolized by the P-450 enzyme system so that drugs that induce this system tend to decrease blood levels of the antidepressants, and inhibitors of this system increase antidepressant blood levels. This effect varies according to the subfamily that is induced. For example, fluvoxamine (Luvox) substantially inhibits CYP1A2. Thus, other drugs that are metabolized by the system experience slower metabolism. These include such medications as amitriptyline, clomipramine, imipramine, clozapine, propranolol, theophylline, and caffeine (Armstrong, Cozza, & Oesterheld, 2002). Paroxetine, fluoxetine, and duloxetine are very potent inhibitors of CYP2D6, as well as being substrates for this CYP enzyme.

Side Effects, Adverse Reactions, and Toxicity

Side effects of the antidepressant medications vary considerably. Because the TCAs act at several types of receptors, in addition to serotonin and norepinephrine receptors, these drugs have many unwanted effects. Conversely, the SSRIs are more selective for serotonin and have comparatively fewer and better tolerated side effects. Attention to a patient's ability to tolerate side effects is critical because uncomfortable side effects are the primary reason patients discontinue medication treatment. With the TCAs, sedation, orthostatic hypotension, and anticholinergic side effects are the most common sources of discomfort for patients receiving these medications. See Chapter 22 for a comparison of side effects of antidepressant medications.

Receptor affinities may be helpful in predicting which side effects are most likely to occur with a given medication. Table 12-1 provides a summary of major receptor targets for common antidepressants. Using this table in conjunction with Chapter 22, nurses may be able to predict which side effects will be most common with each medication. Interventions to assist in minimizing these side effects are listed in Table 12-2.

Tolerance develops gradually to the sedation and anticholinergic side effects caused by TCAs, but these may be minimized when the prescriber begins with a low dose and increases gradually. Other side effects of the TCAs include tremors, restlessness, insomnia, nausea and vomiting, confusion, pedal edema, headache, and seizures. Blood dyscrasias may also occur, and any fever, sore throat, malaise, or rash should be reported to the prescriber.

Sexual dysfunction is a relatively common side effect, especially with the SSRIs. Erectile and ejaculation disturbances occur in men and anorgasmia in women. This side effect is often difficult to assess if the nurse has not obtained a sexual history before the initiation of use of the medication. Anorgasmia is particularly common with the SSRIs and often goes unreported, frequently because nurses and other health care providers do not ask. Bupropion and nefazodone (Serzone) appear to be least likely to cause sexual disturbance. In addition, when sexual dysfunction is related to the medication, several treatment options are available. These include a change in dose or type of antidepressant or, less frequently, using other medications to treat this side effect. Nurses must take responsibility for discussing the potential for sexual side effects before initiation of drug treatment and for continuing to reassess during follow-up visits. The TCAs have the potential for cardiotoxicity, which limits their use in older adults. Symptoms include prolongation of cardiac conduction that may worsen preexisting cardiac conduction problems. TCAs are contraindicated with second-degree atrioventricular block and should be used cautiously in patients who have other cardiac problems. Occasionally, they may precipitate heart failure, myocardial infarction, arrhythmias, and stroke. The newer antidepressants, such as the SSRIs and bupropion, are less cardiotoxic, and nefazodone currently exhibits no evidence of cardiotoxicity.

Antidepressants that block the dopamine receptor, such as amoxapine, have the potential to produce symptoms of NMS. Mild forms of extrapyramidal symptoms and endocrine changes, including galactorrhea and amenorrhea, may develop. Amoxapine should be avoided in older adult patients because it may be associated with the development of tardive dyskinesia with this age group. Rare occurrences and only mild forms of extrapyramidal symptoms, such as tightness in the jaw and muscle spasms, may occur with any of the TCAs or SSRIs (Zullino, Delacrausaz, & Baumann, 2002).

The most common side effects of the SSRIs include headache, anxiety, insomnia, transient nausea, vomiting, and diarrhoea. Sedation may also occur, especially with fluvoxamine. Most often, these medications are given in the morning, but if daytime sedation occurs, they may be given in the evening. Venlafaxine (Effexor) has little effect on acetylcholine and histamine; thus, the risks for sedation and anticholinergic symptoms are low. However, higher doses are associated with sexual dysfunction, sedation, diastolic hypertension, increased perspiration, constipation, dry mouth, tremors, blurred vision, and asthenia or muscle weakness. Elevations in blood pressure have been described, and nurses should monitor blood pressure, especially in patients who have a preexisting history of hypertension. Nurses need to be very familiar with nefazodone (Serzone) and the clinical issues related to its side effects. Nefazodone is a phenylpiperazine antidepressant that is structurally related to trazodone. Its most common side effects include sedation, dizziness, and orthostatic hypotension; less common is increased risk for seizures. Drug–drug interactions between nefazodone and triazolam and alprazolam have been reported, with increased plasma levels of these benzodiazepines, resulting in an enhancement of the psychomotor impairment caused by these agents. Bupropion (Wellbutrin) has a chemical structure unlike any of the other antidepressants. Some of its pharmacologic profile is due to effects on dopamine systems, in addition to effects on serotonin and norepinephrine.

Bupropion's activating effects may be experienced as agitation or anxiety by some patients. Others also experience insomnia and appetite suppression. Rarely, bupropion has produced psychosis, including hallucinations and delusions. Most likely, this is secondary to the stimulation of dopamine systems. Dopamine is also associated with reward and motivated behaviour, which accounts for the increasingly common use of bupropion, under the trade name of Zyban, as a smoking cessation agent. The slightly increased risk for experiencing seizures with bupropion use has received the most attention. It has been found that if the total daily dose of bupropion is no more than 450 mg and no individual dose is greater than 150 mg, the risk for seizures with bupropion is no greater than the risk with the other TCAs (Ferry & Johnston, 2003). Most important, bupropion has not been found to cause sexual dysfunction and often is used in individuals who are experiencing these side effects.

The MAOIs can produce anticholinergic side effects (dizziness, dry mouth, blurred vision, constipation, nausea, peripheral edema, urinary hesitancy) but at a much reduced rate compared with the TCAs. Orthostatic hypotension is common; thus, frequent assessment of lying and standing blood pressures is required, especially with older adults, who may be at risk for falls and subsequent bone fractures and require assistance in changing position. Sexual dysfunction, including decreased libido, impotence, and anorgasmia, can occur with MAOIs.

The most serious side effect of the MAOIs is their interaction with food and certain medications. The food interaction occurs because MAOIs block the breakdown of tyramine, a trace amine with vasoconstrictor properties. Increased levels of tyramine can cause severe headaches and hypertension; stroke; and, in rare instances, death. Patients who are taking MAOIs are placed on a low-tyramine diet. This diet has been difficult for some individuals to follow, and concerns about the risk for severe hypertension have led many clinicians to rarely use the MAOIs (see Table 12-10).

MAOIs currently in use in Canada include phenelzine (Nardil) and tranylcypromine (Parnate). These are considered irreversible MAOIs because they form unbreakable covalent bonds with MAO. It takes at least 2 weeks to produce replacement enzyme molecules after discontinuation of use of the medication. Moclobemide is an example of a reversible MAOI that is available in Europe and Canada. Although it acts in the same way as the irreversible MAOIs, moclobemide forms weaker bonds that are short lasting. Therefore, a less restrictive diet may be used with moclobemide. In addition to food restrictions, many prescription and nonprescription medications that stimulate the sympathetic nervous system (sympathomimetics) produce the same risk for hypertensive crisis as do foods containing tyramine. The nonprescription medication interactions involve primarily diet pills and cold remedies. Patients should be advised to check the labels of any nonprescription drugs carefully for a warning against use with antidepressants, especially the MAOIs, and then consult their prescriber or pharmacist before consuming these medications. In addition, symptoms of other serious drug–drug interactions may develop, such as coma, hypertension, and fever, which may occur when patients receive meperidine (Demerol) while taking an MAOI. Patients should notify other health care providers, including dentists, that they are taking an MAOI before being prescribed or given any other medication.

Suicide is a major concern when working with individuals who are depressed. Systematic suicide risk assessment should be done routinely before initiating antidepressant therapy, in the first 2 to 4 weeks of treatment and for longer if indicated. Some of these medications are more lethal than others. For example, the TCAs pose a significant risk for overdose and are more lethal in children. Symptoms of overdose and treatment are discussed more fully in Chapter 22, but for now, it is important to remember that this potential exists. Sometimes, the prescriber will provide the patient with only small amounts of the medication, requiring more frequent visits, and will closely monitor use. In general, newer

| Table 12-10 | Example of a Tyramine-Restricted Diet |

Category of Food	Food to Avoid	Food Allowed
Cheese	All matured or aged cheeses All casseroles made with these cheeses, pizza, lasagna, etc. *Note*: All cheeses are considered matured or aged except those listed under the "Foods Allowed" column	Fresh cottage cheese, cream cheese, ricotta cheese, and processed cheese slices. All fresh milk products that have been stored properly (e.g., sour cream, yogurt, ice cream)
Meat, fish, and poultry	Fermented/dry sausage: pepperoni, salami, mortadella, summer sausage, etc. Improperly stored meat, fish, or poultry Improperly stored pickled herring	All fresh packaged or processed meat (e.g., chicken loaf, hot dogs), fish, or poultry Refrigerate immediately and eat as soon as possible
Fruits and vegetables	Fava or broad bean pods (not beans) Banana peel	Banana pulp All others except those listed in the "Food to Avoid" column
Alcoholic beverages	All tap beers	Alcohol: No more than two domestic bottled or canned beers or 4-fluid-oz glasses of red or white wine per day; this applies to nonalcoholic beer also; please note that red wine may produce a headache unrelated to a rise in blood pressure
Miscellaneous foods	Marmite concentrated yeast extract Sauerkraut Soy sauce and other soybean condiments	Other yeast extracts (e.g., brewer's yeast) Soy milk

Adapted from Gardener, D. M., Shulman, K. I., Walker, S. E., & Tailor, S. A. N. (1996). The making of a user-friendly MAOI diet. *Journal of Clinical Psychiatry, 57*, 99–104.

antidepressant medications, such as the SSRIs, are associated with less risk for toxicity and lethality in overdose. Box 12-4 highlights some of the newest antidepressants being tested in clinical trials.

ANTIANXIETY AND SEDATIVE–HYPNOTIC MEDICATIONS

Sometimes called *anxiolytics*, antianxiety medications and sedative–hypnotic medications come from various pharmacologic classifications, including benzodiazepines, nonbenzodiazepines, and nonbarbiturate sedative–hypnotics, such as chloral hydrate. These drugs represent some of the most widely prescribed medications today for the short-term relief of anxiety or anxiety associated with depression.

Benzodiazepines

Commonly prescribed benzodiazepines include chlordiazepoxide (Librium), diazepam (Valium), lorazepam (Ativan), flurazepam (Dalmane), oxazepam (Serax), and clonazepam (Rivotril).

Indications and Mechanisms of Action

Benzodiazepines act as positive modulators at $GABA_A$ ion channels, increasing the ease of GABA binding to its binding site. This enhancement of GABA binding increases both the duration and frequency of channel opening and decreases the firing rate of the nerve cell. This inhibition of nerve cell firing allows this class of drugs to act as anticonvulsants, antianxiety medications, or hypnotics, depending on dose and pharmacokinetic properties. Other neurotransmitter systems are also involved in the effects of benzodiazepines. Of the various benzodiazepines in use to relieve anxiety (and treat insomnia), oxazepam (Serax) and lorazepam (Ativan) are often preferred for patients with liver disease and for older adult patients because of their short half-lives.

Pharmacokinetics

The variable rate of absorption of the benzodiazepines determines the speed of onset. Table 12-11 provides relative indications of the speed of onset, from very fast to slow, for some of the commonly prescribed benzodiazepines.

Chlordiazepoxide (Librium) and diazepam (Valium) are slow, erratic, and sometimes incompletely absorbed when given IM, whereas lorazepam (Ativan) is rapidly and completely absorbed when given IM. Lorazepam is also well absorbed by the sublingual route.

All the benzodiazepines are highly lipid soluble and highly protein bound. They are distributed throughout the body and enter the CNS quickly. Other drugs that compete for protein-binding sites may produce drug–drug interactions. The degree to which each of these

<table>
<tr><td>

BOX 12-4 Novel Antidepressant Drug Development

Research into the neurobiology of depression has implicated other neurotransmitter and neuroendocrine systems in the aetiology of depression. This has led to the development of new antidepressants, many of which are currently in clinical trials.

For example, the hypothalamic–pituitary–adrenal (HPA) axis, a major stress hormone system, shows evidence of overactivity and blunted feedback control in depression. The principal activator of the HPA axis is a hormone called *corticotropin-releasing hormone* (CRH). This hormone is produced in the hypothalamus and stimulates the pituitary to release adrenocorticotropic hormone, which stimulates the release of cortisol from the adrenal gland. In depression, excessive CRH leads to increased levels of cortisol. Increased levels of cortisol are associated with some of the symptoms in depression, such as difficulty concentrating, sleep disturbance, and lowered energy. This led to the CRH theory of depression (Holsboer & Ising, 2008) and prompted the development of CRH antagonists and glucocorticoid receptor antagonists as potential antidepressants. Despite strong evidence that they would have antidepressant properties, no current CRH antagonists are available.

Glutamate is the major excitatory neurotransmitter and has been implicated in many psychiatric and neuropsychiatric disorders, including depression. Some evidence exists for increased glutamate in depression (Krystal et al., 2002). Thus, an open trial of a glutamate-modulating agent was completed with promise of antidepressant properties (Zarate et al., 2004). Ketamine, a specific glutamate receptor antagonist, was shown to attenuate acute suicidal ideation (DiazGranados et al., 2010).

</td></tr>
</table>

an active metabolite of diazepam, and lorazepam have no active metabolites and thus have shorter half-lives. Sustained presence of these drugs after discontinuation may be observed in older adult or obese patients.

Side Effects, Adverse Reactions, and Toxicity

The most commonly reported side effects result from the sedative and CNS depression effects of these medications. Drowsiness, intellectual impairment, anterograde memory impairment, ataxia, and reduced motor coordination are common adverse effects. If used for sleep, many of these medications, especially long-acting benzodiazepines, produce significant "hangover" effects experienced on awakening. Flunitrazepam (Rohypnol), otherwise known as the "date rape" drug because of its ability to impair anterograde memory, is illegal in Canada. Older adults receiving repeated doses of medications, such as flurazepam (Dalmane), at bedtime may experience paradoxical confusion, agitation, and delirium, sometimes after the first dose. In addition, daytime fatigue, drowsiness, and cognitive impairments may continue while the person is awake. For the older adult, drowsiness mixed with mental confusion can lead to falls and hip fractures. Current clinical guidelines for drug treatments in older adults strongly recommend avoiding benzodiazepine use in this population (Cumbler, Guerrasio, Kim, & Glasheen, 2008). For most patients, the effects subside as tolerance develops; however, alcohol increases all these symptoms and potentiates CNS depression. Indeed, benzodiazepines have a wide therapeutic index but can be lethal when used with alcohol. Individuals using these medications should be warned to be cautious when driving or performing other tasks that require mental alertness. If these tasks are part of

drugs is lipid soluble affects its duration of action. Most of these drugs have active metabolites, but the degree of activity of each metabolite affects the duration of action and elimination half-life. Most of these drugs vary markedly in the length of half-life. Oxazepam, which is itself

Table 12-11   Antianxiety and Sedative–Hypnotic Medications

Generic (Trade) Drug Name	Usual Dosage Range (mg/day)	Half-Life (hours)	Speed of Onset After Single Dose
Benzodiazepines			
diazepam (Valium)	4–40	30–100	Very fast
chlordiazepoxide (Librium)	15–100	50–100	Intermediate
clorazepate (Tranxene)	15–60	30–200	Fast
prazepam (Centrax)	20–60	30–200	Very slow
flurazepam (Dalmane)	15–30	47–100	Fast
lorazepam (Ativan)	2–8	10–20	Slow–intermediate
oxazepam (Serax)	30–120	3–21	Slow–intermediate
temazepam (Restoril)	15–30	9.5–20	Moderately fast
triazolam (Halcion)	0.25–0.5	2–4	Fast
alprazolam (Xanax)	0.5–10	12–15	Intermediate
clonazepam (Livotril)	1.5–20	18–50	Intermediate
Nonbenzodiazepines			
buspirone (BuSpar)	15–30	3–11	Very slow
zolpidem (Ambien)	5–10	2.6	Fast

the person's work requirements, another medication may be chosen. Administered intravenously, benzodiazepines often cause phlebitis and thrombosis at the intravenous sites, which should be monitored closely and changed if redness or swelling develops.

Because tolerance develops to most of the CNS depressant effects, individuals who wish to experience the feeling of "intoxication" from these medications may be tempted to increase their own dosage. Psychological dependence is more likely to occur when using these medications for a longer period, which is the reason benzodiazepines are, for the most part, to be used as short-term therapies. Abrupt discontinuation of the use of benzodiazepines may result in a recurrence of the target symptoms, such as rebound insomnia or anxiety. Other withdrawal symptoms appear rapidly, including tremors, increased perspiration, palpitations, increased sensitivity to light, abdominal discomfort or pain, and elevations in systolic blood pressure. These symptoms may be more pronounced with the short-acting benzodiazepines, such as lorazepam. Gradual tapering is recommended for discontinuing the use of benzodiazepines after long-term treatment. When tapering short-acting medications, the prescriber may switch the patient to a long-acting benzodiazepine before discontinuing the use of the short-acting drug.

Individual reactions to the benzodiazepines appear to be associated with sensitivity to their effects. Some patients feel apathy, fatigue, tearfulness, emotional lability, irritability, and nervousness. Benzodiazepines do little for depression symptoms, except for sleep disturbance, and may even exacerbate anhedonia and difficulties concentrating. As such, their use in depression, even with significant comorbid anxiety, should be closely monitored. Gastrointestinal disturbances, including nausea, vomiting, anorexia, dry mouth, and constipation, may develop. These medications may be taken with food to ease the gastrointestinal distress.

Older adults are particularly susceptible to incontinence, memory disturbances, dizziness, and increased risk for falls when using benzodiazepines. Pregnant patients should be aware that these medications cross the placenta and are associated with an increased risk for birth defects, such as cleft palate, mental retardation, and pyloric stenosis. Infants born addicted to benzodiazepines often exhibit flaccid muscle tone, lethargy, and difficulties sucking. All the benzodiazepines are excreted in breast milk, and breast-feeding women should avoid using these medications. Infants and children metabolize these medications more slowly; therefore, more drug accumulates in their bodies.

Toxicity can develop with liver dysfunction or disease. Symptoms include worsening of the CNS depression, ataxia, confusion, delirium, agitation, hypotension, diminished reflexes, and lethargy. Rarely do the benzodiazepines cause respiratory depression or death. In overdose, these medications have a high therapeutic index and rarely result in death unless combined with another CNS depressant drug, such as alcohol.

Nonbenzodiazepines: Buspirone and Zolpidem

One of the nonbenzodiazepines, buspirone (BuSpar), was first synthesized in 1968 by Michael Eison, who was searching for an improved antipsychotic medication. Later, it was found that buspirone was effective in controlling the symptoms of anxiety but had no effect on panic disorders and little effect on obsessive–compulsive disorder. Another nonbenzodiazepine, zolpidem (Ambien), is a medication for sleep that acts on the benzodiazepine–GABA receptor complex.

Indications and Mechanisms of Actions

These drugs are effective for treating anxiety disorders without the CNS depressant effects or the potential for abuse and withdrawal syndromes. Canadian treatment guidelines for generalized anxiety disorder caution against long-term use of benzodiazepines and, based on level I evidence, recommend either the SSRI, paroxetine, or the NSRI, venlafaxine (Struzik, Vermani, Coonerty-Femiano, & Katzman, 2004). Buspirone is also indicated for treating generalized anxiety disorder; therefore, its target symptoms include anxiety and related symptoms, such as difficulty in concentrating, tension, insomnia, restlessness, irritability, and fatigue. Because buspirone does not add to depression symptoms, it has been tried for treating anxiety that coexists with depression. In some instances, it is thought to potentiate the antidepressant actions of other medications.

Buspirone has no effect on the benzodiazepine–GABA complex but instead appears to control anxiety by blocking the serotonin subtype of receptor, 5-HT_{1a}, at both presynaptic reuptake and postsynaptic receptor sites. It has no sedative, muscle relaxant, or anticonvulsant effects. It also lacks potential for abuse.

Zolpidem (Ambien), which is indicated for short-term insomnia treatment, appears to increase slow-wave (deep) sleep and to modulate $GABA_A$ receptors, but with less risk for tolerance or withdrawal issues compared with benzodiazepines.

Pharmacokinetics

Buspirone is rapidly absorbed but undergoes extensive first-pass metabolism. Food slows absorption but appears to reduce first-pass metabolism, increasing the bioavailability of the medication. Buspirone is given on a continual dosing schedule of three times a day because of its short half-life of 2 to 3 hours. Clinical action depends on reaching steady-state concentrations; taking this medication with food may facilitate this process.

Buspirone is highly protein bound but does not displace most other medications. However, it does displace digoxin and may increase digoxin levels to the point of toxicity. It is metabolized in the liver and excreted predominantly by the kidneys but also through the gastrointestinal tract. Patients with liver or kidney impairment should be given this medication with caution.

Buspirone cannot be used on a PRN basis; rather, it takes 2 to 4 weeks of continual use for symptom relief to occur. It is more effective in reducing anxiety in patients who have never taken a benzodiazepine.

Buspirone does not block the withdrawal of other benzodiazepines. Therefore, a switch to buspirone must be initiated gradually to avoid withdrawal symptoms. Nurses should closely monitor patients who are undergoing this change of medication for emergence of withdrawal symptoms from the benzodiazepines and report such symptoms to the prescriber.

Zolpidem is metabolized by the liver; it crosses the placenta and enters breast milk. It has a short half-life of 3 hours, which makes it an ideal hypnotic and is excreted in the urine.

Side Effects, Adverse Reactions, and Toxicity

Common side effects from higher-dose buspirone include dizziness, drowsiness, nausea, excitement, and headache. Most other side effects occur at an incidence of less than 1%. There have been no reports of death from an overdose of buspirone alone. Older adults, pregnant women, and children have not been adequately studied. For now, buspirone can be assumed to cross the placenta and is present in breast milk; therefore, its use should be avoided in pregnant women, and women who are taking this medication should not breast-feed.

Rebound effects, such as insomnia and anxiety, from zolpidem are minimal. There are minimal effects on respiratory function and little potential for abuse. Although very rare, there have been cases of sleepwalking, sleepdriving, and other complex behaviours while asleep attributed to zolpidem use (Dolder & Nelson, 2008).

■ STIMULANTS

Amphetamines were first synthesized in the late 1800s but were not used for psychiatric disorders until the 1930s. Initially, amphetamines were prescribed for a variety of symptoms and disorders, but their high abuse potential soon became obvious.

Methylphenidate, Pemoline, and Modafinil

Among the medications known as stimulants are methylphenidate (Ritalin), used for ADHD; pemoline (Cylert), a CNS stimulant also used for hyperactivity and attention deficit disorders; and modafinil (Provigil), used for narcolepsy, a sleep disorder.

Indications and Mechanisms of Action

Medical use of these drugs is now restricted to a few disorders, including narcolepsy, ADHD—particularly in children—and obesity unresponsive to other treatments.

However, stimulants are increasingly being used as an adjunctive treatment in depression and other mood disorders to address the anhedonia and low energy common to these conditions.

Dextroamphetamine (or D-amphetamine, indicating the D-isomer; Dexedrine) indirectly stimulates the sympathetic nervous system, producing alertness, wakefulness, vasoconstriction, suppressed appetite, and hypothermia. Tolerance develops to some of these effects, such as suppression of appetite, but the CNS stimulation continues. Although the exact mechanism of action is not completely understood, stimulants cause a release of catecholamines, particularly norepinephrine and dopamine, into the synapse from the presynaptic nerve cell. They also block the reuptake of these catecholamines. Methylphenidate is structurally similar to the amphetamines but produces a milder CNS stimulation. Pemoline is structurally dissimilar from the amphetamines but produces the same pharmacologic actions. Pemoline predominantly affects the dopamine system and therefore has less effect on the sympathetic nervous system.

Although the stimulant effects of these medications may seem logically indicated for narcolepsy, a disorder in which the individual frequently and abruptly falls asleep, the indications for childhood ADHD seem less obvious. The aetiology and neurobiology of ADHD remain unclear, but psychostimulants produce a paradoxic calming of the increased motor activity characteristic of ADHD. Studies show that medication decreases disruptive activity during school hours, reduces noise and verbal activity, improves attention span and short-term memory, improves ability to follow directions, and decreases distractibility and impulsivity. Although these improvements have been well documented in the literature, the diagnosis of ADHD and subsequent use of psychostimulants with children remain a matter of controversy (see Chapter 31).

Off-Label Use

Psychostimulants have also been used for other psychiatric disorders, and nurses must be aware that these medications are outside of Health Canada–approved indications for the medications. Used alone, stimulants are not indicated for treating depression. However, research has found that these medications may be beneficial as adjunctive medications, especially in those with severe psychomotor retardation (Candy, Jones, Williams, Tookman, & King, 2008). All appetite depressants are stimulants, but most are not related to the amphetamines and have a low potential for abuse. However, psychostimulants have been used for treating obesity when other treatments have failed. In addition, these medications have relieved lethargy, boosted mood, and reduced cognitive deficits associated with chronic medically debilitating conditions, such as chronic fatigue syndrome, acquired immunodeficiency syndrome, and some types of cancer, but more research is needed. Increasingly, psychostimulants are being used to improve the residual symptoms of attention deficit disorder in adults, such as inattention, impulsivity, decreased concentration, anxiety, and irritability. This use remains a matter of controversy, and psychostimulants should be used very cautiously in individuals who have a history of substance abuse.

Modafinil (Alertec) is a new wake-promoting agent used for treating excessive daytime sleepiness (EDS) associated with narcolepsy and other health states. Patients with EDS cannot stay awake in the daytime, even after getting enough nighttime sleep. They fall asleep when they want to stay awake. Although modafinil is approved by Health Canada only for treating narcolepsy, it is being used for other mental health symptoms. For example, small studies support the use of modafinil as an augmentation to antidepressants in major depressive disorder to address fatigue (Menza, Kaufman, & Castellanos, 2000). Its use by long-distance truckers and shift workers has created controversy and significant debate (Dubljevic, 2012; Williams, Seale, Boden, Lowe, Steinburg, 2008).

Pharmacokinetics

Psychostimulants are rapidly absorbed from the gastrointestinal tract and reach peak plasma levels in 1 to 3 hours. Considerable individual variations occur between the drugs in terms of bioavailability, plasma levels, and half-life. Table 12-12 compares the primary psychostimulants used in psychiatry. Some of these differences are age dependent because children metabolize these medications more rapidly, producing shorter elimination half-lives. Methylphenidate (Ritalin) is available in a sustained release form and should not be chewed or crushed.

The psychostimulants appear to be unaffected by food in the stomach and should be given after meals to reduce the appetite-suppressant effects when indicated. However, changes in urine pH may affect the rates of excretion. Excessive sodium bicarbonate alkalizes the urine and reduces amphetamine secretion. An increased vitamin C or citric acid intake may acidify the urine and increase its excretion. Starvation from appetite suppression may have a similar effect. All these drugs are highly lipid soluble, crossing easily into the CNS and the placenta. Psychostimulants undergo metabolic changes in the liver, where they may affect, or be affected by, other drugs. They are primarily excreted through the kidneys; therefore, renal dysfunction may interfere with excretion.

The precise action of modafinil (Alertec) in promoting wakefulness is unknown. It does appear to have wake-promoting actions similar to sympathomimetic agents such as amphetamine and methylphenidate, although the pharmacologic profile is not identical. It is absorbed rapidly and reaches peak plasma concentration in 2 to 4 hours. The absorption of modafinil may be delayed by 1 to 2 hours if taken with food. Modafinil is eliminated through liver metabolism, with subsequent excretion of metabolites through renal excretion. Modafinil may interact with drugs that inhibit, induce, or are metabolized by CYP2C19 isoenzymes, including phenytoin, diazepam, and propranolol. Concurrent use of modafinil and other drugs metabolized by CYP2C19 may lead to increased circulating blood levels of the other drugs.

Psychostimulants are usually begun at a low dose and increased weekly, depending on improvement of symptoms and occurrence of side effects. Initially,

Table 12-12	Psychostimulant Medications	
Generic (Trade) Name and Half-Life	**Usual Dosage Drug Range (mg/day)**	**Side Effects**
dextroamphetamine (Dexedrine); 6–7 hours	5–40	Overstimulation
		Restlessness
		Dry mouth
		Palpitations
		Cardiomyopathy (with prolonged use or high dosage)
		Possible growth retardation (greatest risk); risk reduced with drug holidays
methylphenidate (Ritalin); 2–4 hours	10–60	Nervousness
		Insomnia
		Anorexia
		Tachycardia
		Impaired cognition (with high doses)
		Moderate risk for growth suppression
pemoline (Cylert); 12 hours (mean)	37.5–112.5	Insomnia
		Anorexia with weight loss
		Elevated liver function tests (ALT, AST, LDH)
		Jaundice
		Least risk for growth suppression

ALT, alanine aminotransferase; AST, aspartate aminotransferase; LDH, lactic dehydrogenase.

children with ADHD are given a morning dose so that their school performance may be compared from morning to afternoon. Rebound symptoms of excitability and talkativeness may occur when use of the medication is withdrawn or after dose reduction. These symptoms also begin about 5 hours after the last dose of medication, which may affect the dosing regimen for some individuals. The return of symptoms in the afternoon for children with ADHD may require that a second dose be given at school. Prescribers should work with parents to implement other interventions after school and on weekends when the psychostimulants are not used. Severity of symptoms may require that the medications be continued during these times, but this dosing schedule should be determined after careful evaluation on an individual basis. Use of these medications should not be stopped abruptly, especially with higher doses, because the rebound effects may last for several days.

Side Effects, Adverse Reactions, and Toxicity

Side effects associated with psychostimulants typically arise within 2 to 3 weeks after beginning the medication. From most to least common, these side effects include appetite suppression, insomnia, irritability, weight loss, nausea, headache, palpitations, blurred vision, dry mouth, constipation, and dizziness. Because of the effects on the sympathetic nervous system, some individuals experience blood pressure changes (both hypertension and hypotension), tachycardia, tremors, and irregular heart rates. Blood pressure and pulse should be monitored initially and after each dosage change. Pemoline is associated with elevated liver enzymes and produces hepatotoxicity in 1% to 3% of children taking the medication; therefore, liver function tests should be obtained at least every 6 months. Liver function returns to normal when use of the medication is discontinued.

Rarely, psychostimulants suppress growth and development in children. These effects are a matter of controversy, and research has produced conflicting results. Although the suppression of height seems unlikely to some researchers, others have indicated that psychostimulants may have an effect on cartilage. More reports of suppressed growth have occurred with D-amphetamine (Dexedrine) and methylphenidate (Ritalin) than pemoline (Schertz, Adesman, Alfeiri, & Bienkowski, 1996). Height and weight should be monitored several times annually for children taking these medications and compared with prior history of growth. Weight should be monitored especially closely during the initial phases of treatment. These effects also may be minimized by drug "holidays," such as during school vacations.

Rarely, individuals may experience mild dysphoria, social withdrawal, or mild to moderate depression. These symptoms are more common at higher doses and may require discontinuing the medication. Abnormal movements and motor tics may also increase in individuals who have a history of Tourette's syndrome. Psychostimulants should be avoided by patients with Tourette's symptoms or a positive family history of the disorder. In addition, dextroamphetamine has been associated with an increased risk for congenital abnormalities. Because there is no compelling reason for a pregnant woman to continue to take these medications, patients should be informed and should advise their prescriber immediately if they plan to become pregnant or if pregnancy is a possibility.

Death is rare from overdose or toxicity of the psychostimulants, but a 10-day supply may be lethal, especially in children. Symptoms of overdose include agitation, chest pain, hallucinations, paranoia, confusion, and dysphoria. Seizures may develop, along with fever, tremor, hypertension or hypotension, aggression, headache, palpitations, rashes, difficulty breathing, leg pain, and abdominal pain. Maximum dosage for children is 40 mg per day, with potential death resulting from a 400-mg dose. Parents should be warned regarding the potential lethality of these medications and take preventive measures by keeping the medication in a safe place.

Side effects associated with modafinil include nausea, nervousness, headache, dizziness, and trouble sleeping. If the effects continue or are bothersome, patients should consult the prescriber. Modafinil is generally well tolerated, with few clinically significant side effects. It is potentially habit forming and must be used with great caution in individuals with a history of substance abuse or dependence.

NEW MEDICATIONS

Each country has its own approval process for new medications. In Canada, this process is controlled by Health Canada. Through various phases of drug testing, a new drug must be determined to have therapeutic benefit based on known physiologic processes, animal testing, and laboratory models of human disease and its potential toxicity predicted at doses likely to produce clinical improvement in humans (see Box 12-5 for more information). Then, the pharmaceutical company can begin research with human volunteers after filing an *investigational new drug* (IND) application. Many new psychiatric medications, particularly the atypical antipsychotics and novel antidepressants, are in various phases of clinical testing and are expected to be released in the coming years. Keeping the phases of new drug development in mind will assist the PMH nurse in understanding what to expect from drugs newly released to the market.

OTHER BIOLOGIC TREATMENTS

Biologic treatment is the term applied to treatments that work at a somatic, physical level but are nonpharmacologic in nature. There is a long history of using somatic therapies to treat neuropsychiatric illnesses. Throughout

---

BOX 12-5 Phases of New Drug Testing

- *Phase I*: Testing defines the range of dosages tolerated in healthy individuals.
- *Phase II*: Effects of the drug are studied in a limited number of individuals with the target disorder.
- *Phase III*: Extensive clinical trials are conducted at multiple sites throughout the country with larger numbers of patients. Efforts focus on corroborating the efficacy identified in phase II. Phase III concludes with a new drug application (NDA) being submitted to Health Canada.
- *Phase IV*: Postmarketing surveillance continues to detect new or rare adverse reactions and potentially new indications. During this period, adverse reactions from the new medication are required to be reported to Health Canada.

Implications for Mental Health Nurses

Throughout the phases, side effects and adverse reactions are monitored closely. The studies are tightly controlled, and strict regulations are enforced at each step.

Clinical trials for new drugs usually involve patient populations that have no other health problems but the one under study. This is important to test the drug's effectiveness, but in clinical practice, many patients have other health problems, and postmarketing surveillance helps identify unforeseen benefits or adverse effects in most heterogeneous patient populations.

A newly approved drug is approved only for the indications for which it has been tested. However, there is often a widening of application for other health problems over time (called *off-label* uses).

In Canada, the pharmaceutical companies must follow strict guidelines in terms of product advertising and interaction with health professionals. For example, the companies are not permitted to advertise directly to the public, and there are stringent guidelines regarding any potential sales incentives offered to health professionals. This is to address potential ethical issues around influencing prescriber preferences.

---

history, numerous treatments have been developed and used to change the biologic basis of what was thought, at the time, to cause psychiatric disorders. Insulin coma, atropine coma, hemodialysis, hyperbaric oxygen therapy, continuous sleep therapy, and ether and carbon dioxide inhalation therapies are examples of some of the historical treatments that seemed to relieve some symptoms, but results could not be replicated, or potential adverse effects proved too great a risk. Although the primary biologic interventions remain pharmacologic, some somatic treatments continue to show efficacy, whereas others have gained acceptance, remain under investigation, or show promise for the future. Common somatic treatments include the following: ECT, phototherapy, nutritional therapy, and most recently, transcranial magnetic stimulation and vagus nerve stimulation (VNS).

Electroconvulsive Therapy

For hundreds of years, seizures have been known to produce improvement in some psychiatric symptoms. Camphor-induced seizures were used in the 16th century to reduce psychosis and mania. With time, other substances, such as inhalants, were tried, but most were difficult to control or produced adverse reactions, sometimes even fatalities. ECT was formally introduced in Italy in 1938. It is one of the oldest medical treatments available and remains safely in use today. Every year, over 1 million people in the world receive ECT as treatment (Payne & Prudic, 2009b). It is one of the most effective treatments for severe depression but has been used for other disorders, including mania and schizophrenia, when other treatments have failed. Although individuals with a severe form of depression, where delusions and/or paranoia are present, seem the best candidates for ECT, research has yet to determine accurate predictors of a person's response to ECT (Kellner, 2008). With ECT, a brief electrical current is passed through the brain to produce generalized seizures lasting 25 to 150 seconds. The patient does not feel the stimulus or recall the procedure. A short-acting anaesthetic and a muscle relaxant are given before induction of the current. A brief pulse stimulus, administered unilaterally on the nondominant side of the head, is associated with less confusion after ECT. However, some individuals require bilateral treatment for the effective resolution of depressive symptoms. Induction of a seizure is necessary to produce positive treatment outcomes. Because individual seizure thresholds vary and increase with age, the electrical impulse and treatment method also may vary. In general, the lowest possible electrical stimulus necessary to produce seizure activity is used. Blood pressure and the ECG are monitored during the procedure. This procedure is repeated two or three times a week, usually for a total of 6 to 12 treatments. Because there is no particular difference in treatment efficacy and a twice-weekly regimen produces less accumulative memory loss, this treatment course is often chosen. After symptoms have improved, antidepressant medications are used to prevent relapse. Some patients who cannot take or do not experience response to antidepressant treatment may go on maintenance ECT treatments. Usually, once-weekly treatments are gradually decreased in frequency to once monthly. The number and frequency of treatments vary depending on the individual's response.

Although ECT produces rapid improvement in depressive symptoms, its exact mechanism of antidepressant action remains unclear. It is known to down-regulate β-adrenergic receptors in much the same way as antidepressant medications. However, unlike antidepressant therapy, ECT produces an up-regulation in serotonin, especially 5-HT$_2$. ECT also has several other actions on neurochemistry, including increased influx of calcium and effects on second messenger systems.

Brief episodes of hypotension or hypertension, bradycardia or tachycardia, and minor arrhythmias are among the adverse effects that may occur during and immediately after the procedure but usually resolve quickly. Common aftereffects from ECT include headache, nausea, and muscle pain. Memory loss or disturbance is the most troublesome effect of ECT. Such cognitive side effects include *transient postictal* ("after seizure") *disorientation* that clears in minutes to hours and *anterograde amnesia* (amnesia for events occurring during and soon after a course of ECT) that varies in severity and for which use of a diary is helpful (Payne & Prudic, 2009a). Other possible cognitive effects are *short-term retrograde amnesia* (gaps in memory about things occurring a few weeks or months before the ECT) that usually clears within weeks and *retrograde memory loss* (persistent, severe memory deficits) that occurs rarely (Payne & Prudic, 2009a). Many patients experience no amnesia at all. Memory loss occurring as part of the symptoms of untreated depression presents a confounding factor in determining the exact nature of the memory deficits from ECT. It is important to remember that patient surveys are positive, with most individuals reporting that they were helped by ECT and would have it again (Hirose, 2002).

ECT is contraindicated in patients with an increased intracranial pressure. Risk also increases in patients with recent myocardial infarction, recent cerebrovascular accident, retinal detachment, or pheochromocytoma (a tumour on the adrenal cortex) and in patients at high risk for complications from anaesthesia.

● **STUDY NOTE**

Patients may be temporarily confused following ECT. Nurses need to monitor any confusion and reorient patients to the immediate environment as necessary.

Light Therapy (Phototherapy)

Human circadian rhythms are set by time clues (zeitgebers) inside and outside the body. One of the most powerful regulators of these body patterns is the cycle of daylight and darkness.

Research findings indicate that some individuals with depressive symptoms that worsen at specific times of the year (have a seasonal pattern) may experience disturbance in these normal body patterns or of circadian rhythms (Steinhausen, Gundelfinge, & WinklerMetzke, 2008). For example, some individuals are more depressed during the winter months, when there is less light, and they improve spontaneously in the spring. (Refer to Chapter 22 for a complete description of depression and mood disorders.) These individuals usually have symptoms that are somewhat different from classic depression, including fatigue, increased need to sleep, increased appetite and weight gain, irritability, and carbohydrate craving. Administering artificial light to these patients during winter months has reduced these depressive symptoms.

Light therapy, sometimes called **phototherapy**, involves exposing the patient to a specific type of artificial light source to relieve seasonal depression. Artificial light is believed to trigger a shift in the patient's circadian rhythm to an earlier time. Research remains ongoing. The light source must be very bright, full-spectrum light, usually 2,500 lux, which is about 200 times brighter than normal indoor lighting. Harmful ultraviolet light is filtered out. Exposure to this light source has produced improvement and relief of depressive symptoms for significant numbers of seasonally depressed individuals. It produces no change for individuals who are not seasonally depressed.

Studies have shown that morning phototherapy produces a better response than either evening or morning and evening timing of the phototherapy session (Prasko et al., 2008). Light banks with full-spectrum light may be put together by the individual or obtained from various companies now producing these light sources. Light visors, visors containing small, full-spectrum light bulbs that shine on the eyelids, have also been developed. The patient is instructed to sit in front of the lights at a distance of about 3 feet, engaging in a variety of other activities, but glancing directly into the light every few minutes. This should be done immediately on arising and is most effective before 8 AM. The duration of administration may begin with as little as 30 minutes and increase to 2 to 5 hours. One to two hours is usually sufficient, and the antidepressant response begins in 1 to 4 days, with the full effect usually complete after 2 weeks. Full antidepressant effect is usually maintained with daily sessions of 30 minutes.

Side effects of phototherapy are rare, but eye strain, headache, and insomnia are possible. An ophthalmologist should be consulted if the patient has a preexisting eye disorder. In rare instances, phototherapy has been reported to produce mania. Irritability is a more common complaint. Follow-up visits with the prescriber or therapist are needed to help manage side effects and assess positive results. Phototherapy should be implemented only by a provider knowledgeable in its use.

Nutritional Therapies

The neurotransmitters necessary for normal healthy functioning are produced from amino acids taken in with the foods we eat. Many nutritional deficiencies may produce symptoms of psychiatric disorders. Fatigue, apathy, and depression are caused by deficiencies in iron, folic acid, pantothenic acid, magnesium, vitamin C, or biotin. Logically, treating these deficiencies with nutritional supplements should improve the psychiatric symptoms. The question becomes: Can nutritional supplements actually treat psychiatric disorders?

In 1967, Linus Pauling espoused the theory that ascorbic acid deficiency produced many psychiatric disorders. He implemented a treatment for schizophrenia that included large doses of ascorbic acid and other vitamins. This treatment was referred to as *megavitamin therapy* or *orthomolecular therapy*. Many psychiatrists showed interest in Pauling's proposal, but his research and claims could never be substantiated, and most researchers and clinicians became highly sceptical of this hypothesis. Nonetheless, a small group remains committed to orthomolecular approaches.

Older theories and related diets are based on the belief that food controls behaviour. High sugar intake was once thought to produce hyperactivity in children, and Benjamin Feingold developed a diet to eliminate food additives that he believed increased hyperactivity. More recently, advances in technology have led research to new investigations regarding dietary precursors for the bioamines. For example, tryptophan, the dietary precursor of serotonin, has been most extensively investigated as it relates to low serotonin levels and increased aggression. Individuals who have low tryptophan levels are prone to have lower levels of serotonin in the brain, resulting in depressed mood and aggressive behaviour (Young & Leyton, 2002). Some individuals with mild depression do respond to large amounts of tryptophan, and tryptophan has been used as an adjunct to antidepressant drugs. Many individuals are turning to dietary herbal preparations to address psychiatric symptoms. More than 17% of the adult population has used herbal preparations to address their mood or emotions. Despite increased use of St. John's wort for depression, ginkgo for cognitive impairment, and kava for anxiety, systematic reviews provide mixed evidence for their effectiveness. Gaster and Holroyd (2000) reviewed the use of St John's wort and found evidence for its use in mild to moderate depression. Birks and Grimley Evans (2009) found no evidence for the use of ginko for dementia, and kava was removed from the market for its high risk of toxicity. Nurses need to include an assessment of these agents into their overall patient assessment to understand the needs of the patient.

Medications may also influence the development of nutritional deficiencies that may worsen psychiatric symptoms. For example, drugs with strong anticholinergic activity often produce impaired or enhanced gastric motility, which may lead to the generalized malabsorption of vitamins and minerals. In addition, many nutritional supplements have toxicities of their own when given in excess. For example, daily ingestion of more than 100 mg pyridoxine (vitamin B_6) can produce neurotoxic symptoms, photosensitivity, and ataxia. More research is needed to identify the underlying mechanisms and relationships of dietary supplements and dietary precursors of the bioamines to mood and behaviour and psychopharmacologic medications. For now, it is important for the PMH nurse to recognize that diet can have a significant impact on behaviour in sensitive individuals and that supplements can be a potential source of drug–drug interaction.

New Somatic Therapies

Repetitive transcranial magnetic stimulation (rTMS) and VNS are two emerging somatic treatments for psychiatric disorders. Both are ways to directly affect brain activity by stimulating nerve cell firing rates. Transcranial magnetic stimulation was introduced in 1985 as a noninvasive, painless method to stimulate the cerebral cortex. Underlying this procedure is the hypothesis that a time-varying magnetic field will induce an electrical field, which, in brain tissue, activates the inhibitory and excitatory neurons (Kanno, Matsumoto, Togashi, Yoshioka, & Mano, 2003), thereby modulating neuroplasticity in the brain. The low-frequency electrical stimulation from rTMS triggers lasting anticonvulsant effects in rats, and the therapeutic benefits of rTMS in humans are thought to be related to action similar to that produced by anticonvulsant medication. rTMS has been used for both clinical and research purposes. rTMS stimulation of the brain's prefrontal cortex may help some depressed patients in much the same way as ECT but without its side effects (Martin et al., 2003). Thus, it has been proposed as an alternative to ECT in managing symptoms of depression. rTMS treatment is administered daily for at least a week, much like ECT, except that subjects remain awake. Although proven effective for depression, rTMS does have some side effects, including mild headaches.

VNS is the newest of the currently available somatic treatments (Martin et al., 2003). For years, scientists have been interested in identifying how autonomic functions modulate activity in the limbic system and higher cortex. The vagus nerve has traditionally been considered a parasympathetic efferent nerve that was responsible only for regulating autonomic functions, such as heart rate and gastric tone. However, the vagus nerve (cranial X) also carries sensory information to the brain from the head, neck, thorax, and abdomen, and research has identified that the vagus nerve has extensive projections of its sensory afferent connections to many brain areas (Armitage, Husain, Hoffmann, & Rush, 2003). Although the basic mechanism of action of VNS is unknown, incoming sensory, or afferent, connections of the left vagus nerve directly project into many of the very same brain regions implicated in neuropsychiatric disorders. These connections help us to understand how VNS is helpful in treating psychiatric disorders. VNS changes levels of several neurotransmitters implicated in the development of major depression, including serotonin, norepinephrine, GABA, and glutamate (Forbes, Macdonald, Eljamel, & Roberts, 2003).

■ PSYCHOSOCIAL ISSUES IN BIOLOGIC TREATMENTS

Many factors influence successful medication and other biologic therapies. Of particular importance are issues related to adherence. Adherence refers to following the

BOX 12-6 Common Reasons for Nonadherence with Medication Regimens

- Uncomfortable side effects and those that interfere with quality of life, such as work performance or intimate relationships
- Lack of awareness of or denial of illness
- Stigma
- Feeling better
- Limited psychoeducation and follow-up
- Difficulties in access to treatment and cost of newer drug therapies
- Substance abuse

therapeutic regimen, self-administering medications as prescribed, keeping appointments, and following other treatment suggestions. Adherence exists on a continuum and can be conceived of as full, partial, or nil. Partial adherence, whereby a patient either attempts to take medications but misses doses or takes more than prescribed, is by far the most common. Recent estimates indicate that on the average, 50% or more of the individuals with schizophrenia taking antipsychotic medications stop taking the medications or do not take them as prescribed (Weiden, 2007). It should be remembered that problems with adherence are an issue with many chronic health states, including diabetes and arthritis, not just psychiatric disorders. Box 12-6 lists some of the common reasons for nonadherence. It is also important to not conclude that the patient is nonadherent until a full assessment is completed.

The most often cited reasons for nonadherence are related to side effects of the medication. Improved functioning may be observed by health care professionals but not felt by the patient. Side effects may interfere with work performance or other important aspects of the individual's life. For example, a construction worker cannot afford to be drowsy and sedated while operating a crane at a construction site or a woman in an intimate relationship may find anorgasmia intolerable. Nurses need to be sensitive to the patient's ability to tolerate side effects and to the impact that side effects have on the patient's life. Medication choice, dosing schedules, and prompt treatment of side effects may be crucial factors in helping patients to continue their treatment, even if the symptoms for which they initially sought help have improved.

Cognitive deficits associated with some psychiatric disorders may make it difficult for the individual to self-monitor, develop insight, make choices, remember to fill prescriptions, or keep appointments. Family members may have beliefs and attitudes that influence the individual not to take the medication. They may misunderstand or deny the illness; for example, "My wife's better, so she doesn't need that medicine anymore." Family members may be distressed when observable side effects occur. Akinesia, which has been linked to suicidal thoughts as a way to relieve the subjective discomfort, may be the most distressing side effect for family members of individuals who have schizophrenia (Meltzer, 2000; Niedermeyer, 2008). Patients may also be reluctant to disclose financial constraints, especially in relation to the cost of newer agents, and may try to stretch out the prescription or just not fill their prescription. Adherence concerns must not be dismissed as the patient's or family's problem. PMH nurses should actively address this issue. A positive therapeutic relationship between the nurse and the patient and family must provide a strong sense of trust that side effects and other difficulties in treatment will be addressed and minimized. When individuals report distressing side effects, the nurse should immediately respond with assessment and interventions to reduce these effects. It is important to assess adherence often, asking questions in a nonthreatening, nonjudgmental manner. It also may be helpful to seek information from others who are involved with the patient.

Adherence can be improved by psychoeducation. This approach is most helpful if it addresses the individual's specific symptoms and concerns. For example, if the patient is having difficulty with understanding the purpose of the medication, it may be helpful to link taking it to a reduction of specific unwanted symptoms or improved functioning, such as continuing to work. Family members should also be included in these discussions.

Other factors that interfere with adherence should also be assessed and plans developed to minimize their effect. For example, an individual who is being considered for clozapine therapy may have missed a number of appointments in the past. On assessment, the nurse may discover that it takes the individual 2 hours on three different busses each way to reach the clinic. The nurse can then assist with arranging for a home health nurse to visit the patient's apartment, draw blood samples for analysis, and assess side effects, thus decreasing the number of trips the patient must make to the clinic.

SUMMARY OF KEY POINTS

■ Psychopharmacology is the study of medications used to treat psychiatric disorders, including the drug categories of antipsychotics, mood stabilizers, antidepressants, antianxiety medications, and psychostimulants.

■ Pharmacodynamics refers to the actions of drugs on living tissue and the human body, with the focus primarily on drug actions at receptor sites, on transporters, and on enzyme activity.

■ The importance of receptors is recognized in current psychopharmacology. Biologic action of many drugs depends on how their structure interacts with a specific receptor, functioning either as an agonist, reproducing the same biologic action as a neurotransmitter, or as an antagonist, blocking the response.

■ A drug's ability to interact with a given receptor type may be judged on three qualities: selectivity—the ability to interact with specific types of receptors; affinity—the attraction the drug has for the binding site; and intrinsic activity—the ability to produce a certain biologic response.

■ Many characteristics of specific drugs affect how well they act and how they affect patients. PMH nurses must be familiar with characteristics, adverse reactions, and toxicity of certain drugs to administer psychotropic medications safely, educate patients regarding their safe use, and encourage therapeutic adherence.

■ Pharmacokinetics refers to how drugs move within the human body to get to their target tissues and how drugs are removed from the body. Bioavailability describes the amount of the drug that actually reaches the systemic circulation. The wide variations in pharmacokinetic properties across individuals are related to physiologic differences caused by age, genetic makeup, other disease processes, and chemical interactions.

■ Antipsychotic medications are drugs used in treating psychotic disorders, such as schizophrenia. They act primarily by blocking dopamine or serotonin postsynaptically. In addition, they have a number of actions on other neurotransmitters. Older typical antipsychotic drugs work on positive symptoms and are inexpensive, but they produce many side effects. Newer atypical antipsychotic drugs work on positive and negative symptoms; are much more expensive but have far fewer anticholinergic side effects; and are better tolerated by patients, but increase risk for metabolic disorders.

■ Medication-related movement disorders are a particularly serious group of side effects that principally occur with the typical antipsychotic medications and that may be acute syndromes, such as dystonia, pseudoparkinsonism, and akathisia, or chronic syndromes, such as tardive dyskinesia.

■ The mood stabilizers, or antimania medications, are drugs used to control wide variations in mood related to mania, but these agents may also be used to treat other disorders. Lithium and the anticonvulsants are chemically unrelated and act in different ways to stabilize mood.

■ Antidepressant medications are drugs used primarily for treating symptoms of depression but are also used extensively for anxiety disorders and eating disorders. They act by blocking the reuptake of one or more of the bioamines, especially serotonin and norepinephrine. These medications vary considerably in their structure and action. Newer antidepressants, such as the SSRIs, have fewer side effects and are less lethal in overdose than the older TCAs.

■ Antianxiety medications also include several subgroups of medications, but SSRIs, NSRIs, benzodiazepines, and nonbenzodiazepines are those principally used in psychiatry. Benzodiazepines act by enhancing the actions of GABA, whereas the nonbenzodiazepine buspirone acts on serotonin. Benzodiazepines can be used on a PRN basis, whereas buspirone must be taken regularly.

■ Psychostimulants enhance neurotransmitter activity, acting at a number of different receptor sites. These medications are most often used for treating symptoms related to ADHD and narcolepsy.

■ ECT uses the application of an electrical pulsation to induce seizures in the brain. These seizures produce a number of effects on neurotransmission that result in the fairly rapid relief of depressive symptoms.

■ rTMS and VNS are two emerging somatic treatments for psychiatric disorders. They are both means to directly affect brain function through the stimulation of the nerves that are direct extensions of the brain.

■ Phototherapy involves the application of full-spectrum light in the morning hours, which appears to reset circadian rhythm delays related to seasonal affective disorder and other forms of depression. Nutritional therapies are in various stages of investigation.

■ Adherence refers to the ability of an individual to self-administer medications as prescribed and to follow other instructions related to medication treatment. It can be full, partial, or nil. Nonadherence is related to factors such as medication side effects, cost, stigma, and family influences. Nurses play a key role in educating patients and helping them to improve adherence.

CRITICAL THINKING CHALLENGES

1 Discuss how the concepts of affinity with selectivity and intrinsic activity have meaning for nurses.

2 Discuss the usefulness of the concept of bioavailability for nurses. What does it mean to nurses, and how would nursing actions change if it were considered?

3 Delineate the ethical issues of nursing management activities associated with each phase of drug treatment: initiation, stabilization, maintenance, and discontinuation.

4 Discuss how you would go about identifying the target symptoms for a specific patient for the following medications: antipsychotic, antidepressant, and antianxiety drugs.

5 Discuss the ways in which you might explain to a patient the differences between typical and atypical antipsychotic medications.

6 Explain the health problems associated with anticholinergic side effects of the antipsychotic medications and self-care strategies that can be used to minimize these side effects.

7 Compare the type of movements that characterize tardive dyskinesia with those that characterize akathisia

and dystonia, and explore which one is easier for a patient to experience.

8 Explain how your nursing care would be different for a male patient taking lithium carbonate than for a female patient.

9 Discuss contrasting views why the antidepressant class of medications has become so commonly prescribed.

10 Discuss the efficacy of anticonvulsive therapy and its mechanism of action.

11 Compare different approaches that you might use with a patient with schizophrenia who has decided to stop taking his or her typical antipsychotic medication because of intolerance to side effects.

REFERENCES

Alda, M. (2004). The phenotype spectra of bipolar disorder. *European Neuropsychopharmacology, 14*(Suppl. 1), S94–S99.

Altamura, R., Mauri, M. C., Cavallero, R., & Gorni, A. (1987) Haloperidol metabolism and antipsychotic effect in schizophrenia. *Lancet, 4*(1), 814–815.

Armitage, R., Husain, M., Hoffmann, R., & Rush, A. J. (2003). The effects of vagus nerve stimulation on sleep EEG in depression: A preliminary report. *Journal of Psychosomatic Research, 54*(5), 475–482.

Armstrong, S. C., Cozza, K. L., & Oesterheld, J. R. (2002). Med-psych drug-drug interactions update. *Psychosomatics, 43*(1), 77–81.

Baker, G. B., Urichuk, L. J., & Coutts, R. T. (1998). Drug metabolism and metabolic drug-drug interactions in psychiatry. *Journal of Child and Adolescent Pharmacology News Supplement, 1*, 1–8.

Baker, G. R., Norton, P. G., Flintoft, V., Blais, R., Brown, A., Cox, J., ... Tamblyn, R. (2004). The Canadian Adverse Events Study: The incidence of adverse events among hospital patients in Canada. *Canadian Medical Association Journal, 170*(11), 1678–1686.

Bilici, M., Tekelioglu, Y., Efendioglu, S., Ovali, E., & Ulgen, M. (2003). The influence of olanzapine on immune cells in patients with schizophrenia. *Progress in Neuropsychopharmacology and Biological Psychiatry, 27*(3), 483–485.

Birks, J., & Grimley Evans, J. (2009) Ginkgo biloba for cognitive impairment and dementia. *Cochrane Database of Systematic Reviews*, Issue 1. Art. No.: CD003120. doi: 10.1002/14651858.CD003120.pub3.

Bond, D. J., Pratoomsri, W., & Yatham, L. N. (2007). Depot antipsychotic medications in bipolar disorder: A review of the literature. *Acta Psychiatrica Scandinavia Supplementum, 434*, 3–16.

Bschor, T., Baethge, C., Adli, M., Lewitzka, U., Eichmann, U., & Bauer, M. (2003). Hypothalamic-pituitary-thyroid system activity during lithium augmentation therapy in patients with unipolar major depression. *Journal of Psychiatry and Neuroscience, 28*(3), 210–216.

Candy, M., Jones, L., Williams, R., Tookman, A., & King, M. (2008). Psychostimulants for depression. *Cochrane Database of Systematic Reviews, 16*(2), CD006722.

Chouinard, G. & Chouinard, V. A. (2008). Atypical antipsychotics: CATIE study, drug-induced movements disorder and resulting iatrogenic psychiatric-like symptoms, supersensitivity rebound psychosis and withdrawal syndromes. *Psychotherapy and Psychosomatics, 77*(2), 69–77.

Cumbler, E., Guerrasio, J., Kim, J., & Glasheen, J. (2008). Use of medications for insomnia in the hospitalized geriatric population. *Journal of the American Geriatrics Society, 56*(3), 579–581.

Dahl, M. L. (2002). Cytochrome p450 phenotyping/genotyping in patients receiving antipsychotics: Useful aid to prescribing. *Clinical Pharmacokinetics, 41*(7), 453–470.

Dahlin, D. C., Miwa, G. T., Lu, A. Y., & Nelson, S. D. (1984). N-acetyl-p-benzoquinone imine: A cytochrome P-450-mediated oxidation product of acetaminophen. *Proceedings of the National Academy of Sciences of the United States of America, 81*(5), 1327–1331.

Dalfen, A. K. & Stewart, D. E. (2001). Who develops severe or fatal adverse drug reactions to selective serotonin reuptake inhibitors? *Canadian Journal of Psychiatry, 46*(3), 258–263.

DiazGranados, N., Ibrahim, L., Brutsche, N., Ameli, R., Henter, I. D., Luckenbaugh, D. A., ... Machado-Vieira, R. (2010). Rapid resolution of suicidal ideation after a single infusion of an NMDA antagonist in patients with treatment-resistant major depressive disorder. *Journal of Clinical Psychiatry, 71*(12), 1605–1611.

Ditto, K. E. (2003). SSRI discontinuation syndrome: Awareness as an approach to prevention. *Postgraduate Medicine, 114*, 79–84.

Dolder, C. R. & Nelson, M. H. (2008). Hypnosedative-induced complex behaviors: Incidence, mechanisms and management. *CNS Drugs, 22*(12), 1021–1036.

Dubljevic, V. (2012) Towards a legitimate public policy on cognition-enhancement drugs. *American Journal of Bioethics, 3*(3), 29–33.

Dubovsky, S. L., Thomas, M., Hijazi, A., & Murphy, J. (1994). Intracellular calcium signalling in peripheral cells of patients with bipolar affective disorder. *European Archives of Psychiatry and Clinical Neuroscience, 243*(5), 229–234.

Ferry, L. & Johnston, J. A. (2003). Efficacy and safety of bupropion SR for smoking cessation: Data from clinical trials and five years of post-marketing experience. *International Journal of Clinical Practice, 57*(3), 224–230.

Forbes, R. B., Macdonald, S., Eljamel, S., & Roberts, R. C. (2003). Cost-utility analysis of vagus nerve stimulators for adults with medically refractory epilepsy. *Seizure, 12*(5), 249–256.

Forster, A. J., Clark, H. D., Menard, A., Dupius, N., Chernish, R., Chandok, N., ... Khan, A. (2004). Adverse events among medical patients after discharge from hospital. *Canadian Medical Association Journal, 170*(3), 345–349.

Gardener, D. M., Shulman, K. I., Walker, S. E., & Tailor, S. A. N. (1996). The making of a user-friendly MAOI diet. *Journal of Clinical Psychiatry, 57*, 99–104.

Gaster, B. & Holroyd, J. (2000). St John's wort for depression: A systematic review. *Archives of Internal Medicine, 160*(2),152–156.

Goodwin, F. K. & Ghaemi, S. N. (2000). The impact of mood stabilizers on suicide in bipolar disorder: A comparative analysis. *CNS Spectrums, 5*(2), 12–19.

Granger, B. (1999). The discovery of haloperidol. *Encephale, 25*(1), 59–66.

Grootens, K. P. & Verkes, R. J. (2005). Emerging evidence for the use of atypical antipsychotics in borderline personality disorder. *Pharmacopsychiatry, 38*(1), 20–23.

Health Canada. (2013). Drug benefit list. Retrieved from http://www.hc-sc.gc.ca/fniah-spnia/alt_formats/pdf/nihb-ssna/provide-fournir/pharma-prod/med-list/list_drug_med_2013-eng.pdf

Hegadoren, K. M. (2004). Assessment and treatment of depression: A review in high risk populations. *Journal of Wound, Ostomy, and Continence Nursing, 31*, 100–112.

Henderson, D. C. (2008). Managing weight gain and metabolic issues in patients treated with atypical antipsychotics. *Journal of Clinical Psychiatry, 69*(2), e04.

Hirose, S. (2002). ECT for depression with amnesia. *Journal of ECT, 18*(1), 60.

Hogan, D., Ebly, E., & Fung, T. (1995). Regional variations in use of potentially inappropriate medications by Canadian seniors participating in the Canadian Study of Health and Aging. *Canadian Journal of Clinical Pharmacology, 2*(4), 167–174.

Hollister, L. E. & Garza Trevino, E. S. (1999). Calcium channel blockers in psychiatric disorders: A review of the literature. *Canadian Journal of Psychiatry, 44*(7), 658–664.

Holsboer, F. & Ising, M. (2008). Central CRH system in depression and anxiety—evidence from clinical studies with CRH1 receptor agonists. *European Journal of Pharmacology, 583*(2-3), 350–357.

Iqbal, M. M., Rahman, A., Husain, Z., Mahmud, S. Z., Ryan, W. G., & Feldman, J. M. (2003). Clozapine: A clinical review of adverse effects and management. *Annals of Clinical Psychiatry, 15*(1), 33–46.

Izzo, A. A. (2004). Drug interactions with St. John's Wort (Hypericum perforatum): A review of the clinical evidence. *International Journal of Pharmacology and Therapeutics, 42*(3), 139–148.

Kalapos, M. P. (2002). Carbamazepine-provoked hepatotoxicity and possible aetiological role of glutathione in the events. *Adverse Drug Reactions and Toxicological Reviews, 21*(3), 123–141.

Kane, J. M., Aguglia, E., Altamura, A. C., Ayuso Gutierrez, J. L., Brunello, N., Fleischhacker, W. W., ... Schooler, N. R. (1998) Guidelines for depot antipsychotic treatment in schizophrenia. *European Neuropsychopharmacology, 8*(1), 55–66.

Kanno, M., Matsumoto, M., Togashi, H., Yoshioka, M., & Mano, Y. (2003). Effects of repetitive transcranial magnetic stimulation on behavioural and neurochemical changes in rats during an elevated plus-maze test. *Journal of the Neurological Sciences, 211*(1–2), 5–14.

Kearns, G. L. (2000). Impact of developmental pharmacology on pediatric study design: Overcoming the challenges. *Journal of Allergy and Clinical Immunology, 106*(3), 128–138.

Kearns, G. L. & Winter, H. S. (2004). Proton pump inhibitors in pediatrics: Relevant pharmacokinetics and pharmacodynamics. *Journal of Pediatric Gastroenterology and Nutrition, 37*(Suppl. 1), S52–S59.

Kellner, C. H. (2008). ECT response prediction: From good to great. *Psychiatric Times, 25*(6), 21.

Kennedy, S. H., Segal, Z. V., Cohen, N. L., Levitan, R. D., Gemar, M., & Bagby, R. M. (2003). Lithium carbonate versus cognitive therapy as sequential combination treatment strategies in partial responders to antidepressant medication: An exploratory trial. *Journal of Clinical Psychiatry, 64*(4), 439–444.

Kirbach, S., Simpson, K., Nietert, P. J., & Mintzer, J. (2008). A Markov model of the cost effectiveness of olanzapine treatment for agitation and psychosis in Alzheimer's disease. *Clinical Drug Investigation, 28*(5), 291–303.

Krystal, J. H., Sanacora, G., Blumberg, H., Anand, A., Charney, D. S., Marek, G., ... Mason, G. F. (2002). Glutamate and GABA systems as targets for novel antidepressant and mood-stabilizing treatments. *Molecular Psychiatry, 7*(Suppl. 1), S71–S80.

Klotz, U. (2007). The role of pharmacogenetics in the metabolism of antiepileptic drugs: Pharmacokinetic and therapeutic implications. *Clinical Pharmacokinetics, 46*(4), 271–279.

Kulkarni, S. K. & Naidu, P. S. (2003). Pathophysiology and drug therapy of tardive dyskinesia: Current concepts and future perspectives. *Drugs of Today (Barcelona, Spain), 39*(1), 19–49.

Lam, R.W., Kennedy, S. H., Grigoriadis, S., McIntyre, R. S., Milev, R., Ramasubbu, R., ... Ravindran, A. V. (2009). Canadian Network for Mood and Anxiety Treatments (CANMAT) Clinical guidelines for the management of major depressive disorder in adults: III. Pharmacotherapy. *Journal of Affective Disorders, 117*, (Suppl. 1), S26–S43.

Leeder, J. S. & Kearns, G. L. (1997). Pharmacogenetics in pediatrics. *Pediatric Clinics of North America, 44*(1), 55–77.

Levy, G., Schupf, N., Tang, M. X., Cote, L. J., Louis, E. D., Mejia, H., ... Marder, K. (2002). Combined effect of age and severity on the risk of dementia in Parkinson's disease. *Annals of Neurology, 51*(6), 722–729.

Loscher, W. (2002). Basic pharmacology of valproate: A review after 35 years of clinical use for the treatment of epilepsy. *CNS Drugs, 16*(10), 669–694.

Machado-Vieira, R., Salvadore, G., Luckenbaugh, D. A., Manji, H. K., & Zarate, C. A. (2008). Rapid onset of antidepressant action: A new paradigm in the research and treatment of major depressive disorder. *Journal of Clinical Psychiatry, 22*, e1–e13.

Marshall, J. D. & Kearns, G. L. (1999). Developmental pharmacodynamics of cyclosporine. *Clinical Pharmacology and Therapeutics, 66*, 66–75.

Martin, J. L., Barbanoj, M. J., Schlaepfer, T. E., Thompson, E., Perez, V., & Kulisevsky, J. (2003). Repetitive transcranial magnetic stimulation for the treatment of depression: Systematic review and meta-analysis. *British Journal of Psychiatry, 182*, 480–491.

Meltzer, H. Y. (2000). Side effects of antipsychotic medications: Physician's choice of medication and patient compliance. *Journal of Clinical Psychiatry, 61*(Suppl. 8), 3–4.

Melvin, C. L., Carey, T. S., Goodman, F., Oldham, J. M., & Ranney, L. M. (2008). Effectiveness of antiepileptic drugs for the treatment of bipolar disorder: Findings from a systematic review. *Journal of Psychiatric Practice, 14*(Suppl. 1), 9–14.

Menza, M. A., Kaufman, K. R., & Castellanos, A. (2000). Modafinil augmentation of antidepressant treatment in depression. *Journal of Clinical Psychiatry, 61*(5), 378–381.

Meyer, J. M. (2007). Antipsychotic safety and efficacy concerns. *Journal of Clinical Psychiatry, 68*(Suppl. 14), 20–26.

Miller, C. H. & Fleischhacker, W. W. (2000). Managing antipsychotic-induced acute and chronic akathisia. *Drug Safety, 22*, 73–81.

Moisan, J., Gregoire, J., Gaudet, M., & Cooper, D. (2005). Exploring the risk of diabetes mellitus and dyslipidemia among ambulatory users of atypical antipsychotics: A population-based comparison of risperidone and olanzapine. *Pharmacoepidemiology and Drug Safety, 14*, 427–436.

Nasrallah, H. A. (2002). Pharmacoeconomic implications of adverse effects during antipsychotic drug therapy. *American Journal of Health-System Pharmacy, 59*(22 Suppl. 8), S16–S21.

Niedermeyer, E. (2008). Akinesia and the frontal lobe. *Clinical EEG and Neuroscience, 39*(1), 39–42.

O'Donnell, T., Rotzinger, S., Nakashima, T. T., Hanstock, C. C., Ulrich, M., & Silverstone, P. H. (2000). Chronic lithium and sodium valproate both decrease the concentration of myoinositol and increase the concentration of inositol monophosphates in rat brain. *Brain Research 880*(1–2), 84–91.

Pande, A. C., Crockatt, J. G., Janney, C. A., Werth, J. L., & Tsaroucha, G. (2000). Gabapentin in bipolar disorder: A placebo-controlled trial of adjunctive therapy. Gabapentin Bipolar Disorder Study Group. *Bipolar Disorders, 2*(3), 249–255.

Pandolfi, A., Grilli, A., Cilli, C., Patruno, A., Giaccari, A., DiSilvestre, S., ... Felaco, M. (2003). Phenotype modulation in cultures of vascular and smooth muscle cells from diabetic rats: Association with increased nitric oxide synthase expression and superoxide anion generation. *Journal of Cellular Physiology, 196*(2), 378–385.

Patten, S. B. & Beck, C. A. (2004). Major depression and mental health care utilization in Canada. *Canadian Journal of Psychiatry, 49*(5), 303–309.

Payne, N. & Prudic, J. (2009a). Electroconvulsive therapy Part 1. A perspective on the evolution and current practice of ECT. *Journal of Psychiatric Practice, 15*(5), 346–368.

Payne, N. & Prudic, J. (2009b). Electroconvulsive therapy Part II. A biopsychosocial perspective. *Journal of Psychiatric Practice, 15*(5), 369–390.

Philip, N. S., Mello, K., Carpenter, L. L., Tyrka, A. R., & Price, L. H. (2008). Patterns of quetiapine use in psychiatric inpatients: An examination of off-label use. *Annals of Clinical Psychiatry, 20*(1), 15–20.

Pierre, J. M. (2005). Extrapyramidal symptoms with atypical antipsychotics: Incidence, prevention and management. *Drug Safety, 28*(3), 191–208.

Prasko, J., Horacek, J., Klaschka, J., Kosova, J., Ondrackova, I., & Sipek, J. (2008). Bright light therapy and/or imipramine for inpatients with recurrent non-seasonal depression. *Neuro endocrinology Letters, 23*(2), 109–113.

Preston, S. T. & Hegadoren, K. (2004). Glass contamination in parenterally administered medication. *Journal of Advanced Nursing, 48*(3), 266–270.

Riederer, P., Lachenmayer, L., & Laux, G. (2004). Clinical applications of MAO-inhibitors. *Current Medicinal Chemistry, 11*, 2033–2043.

Riker, R. R. & Fraser, G. L. (2005). Adverse events associated with sedatives, analgesics, and other drugs that provide patient comfort in the intensive care unit. *Pharmacotherapy, 25*(5 Pt 2), 8S–18S.

Roerig, J. L., Steffen, K. J., & Mitchell, J. E. (2011). Atypical antipsychotic-induced weight gain: insights into mechanisms of action. *CNS Drugs, 25*(12), 1035–1059.

Rust, G., Daniels, E., Sacher, D., Bacon, J., Storhters, H., & Bornemann, T. (2005). Ability of community health centers to obtain health services for uninsured patients. *Journal of the American Medical Association, 293*(5), 554–556.

Schertz, M., Adesman, A. R., Alfieri, N. E., & Bienkowski, R. S. (1996). Predictors of weight loss in children with attention deficit hyperactivity disorder treated with stimulant medication. *Pediatrics, 98*(4), 763–769.

Schou, M. (1978). Lithium treatment. *Western Journal of Medicine, 128*(6), 535–536.

Sibon, I., Fenelon, G., Quinn, N. P., & Tison, F. (2004). Vascular parkinsonism. *Journal of Neurology, 252*(12), 513–524.

Simpson, G. M. & Angus, J. W. S. (1970). A rating scale for extrapyramidal side effects. *Acta Psychiatrica Scandinavica, 212*(Suppl.), 11–19.

Soldin, O. P. & Soldin, S. J. (2002). Review: Therapeutic drug monitoring in pediatrics. *Therapeutic Drug Monitoring, 24*, 1–8.

Solomon, D. A., Keitner, G. I., & Ryan, C. E. (1998). Lithium plus valproate as maintenance polypharmacy for patients with bipolar I disorder: A review. *Journal of Clinical Psychopharmacology, 5*(2), 19–28.

Spina, E. & Scordo, M. G. (2002). Clinically significant drug interactions with antidepressants in the elderly. *Drugs and Aging, 19*(4), 299–320.

Steinhausen, H. C., Gundelfinger, R., & WinklerMetz, C. (2008). Prevalence of self-reported seasonal affective disorders and the validity of the seasonal pattern assessment questionnaire in young adults: Findings from a Swiss community study. *Journal of Affective Disorders, 115*(3), 347–354.

Struzik, L., Vermani, M., Coonerty-Femiano, A., & Katzman, M. A. (2004) Treatments for generalized anxiety disorder. *Expert Review of Neurotherapeutics 4*(2), 285–294.

Tariot, P. N., Salzman, C., Yeung, P. P., Pultz, J., & Rak, I. W. (2000). Long-term use of quetiapine in elderly patients with psychotic disorders. *Clinical Therapeutics, 22*(9), 1068–1084.

Taylor, D. (2003). Ziprasidone in the management of schizophrenia: The QT interval issue in context. *CNS Drugs, 17*(6), 423–430.

Thase, M. (2002). Studying new antidepressants: If there were a light at the end of the tunnel, could we see it? *Journal of Clinical Psychiatry, 63*(Suppl. 2), 24–28.

Turkoski, B. (1999). Meeting the challenge of medications reactions in the elderly. *Orthopaedic Nursing, 7*, 85–95.

Vesell, E. S. (1977). Genetic and environmental factors affecting drug disposition in man. *Clinical Pharmacology and Therapeutics, 22*, 659–665.

Viguera, A. C., Baldessarini, R. J., & Friedberg, J. (1988). Discontinuing antidepressant treatment in major depression. *Harvard Review of Psychiatry, 5*, 293–306.

Weiden, P. J. (2007). Understanding and addressing adherence issues in schizophrenia: From theory to practice. *Journal of Clinical Psychiatry, 68*(Suppl. 14), 14–19.

Williams, J. S., Seale, C., Boden, S., Lowe, P., Steinburg, D. L. (2008). Waking up to sleepiness: Modafinil, the media and the pharmaceuticalisation of everyday/night life. *Sociology of Health and Illness, 30*(6), 839–855.

Yatham, L. N., Kennedy, S. H., O'Donovan, C., Parikh, S. V., MacQueen, G., McIntyre, R. S., ... Kapczinski, F. (2006). Canadian Network for Mood and Anxiety Treatments (CANMAT) guidelines for the management of patients with bipolar disorder: Update 2007. *Bipolar Disorders, 8*(6), 721–739.

Young, S. N. & Leyton, M. (2002). The role of serotonin in human mood and social interaction: Insight from altered tryptophan levels. *Pharmacology, Biochemistry and Behavior, 71,* 857–865.

Zarate, C. A., Payne, J. L., Quiroz, J., Sporn, J., Denicoff, K. K., Luckenbaugh, D., Charney, D. S., Manji, H. K. (2004). An open-label trial of Riluzole in patients with treatment-resistant major depression. *American Journal of Psychiatry, 161,* 171–174.

Zhou, H. (2003). Pharmacokinetic strategies in deciphering atypical drug absorption profiles. *Journal of Clinical Pharmacology, 43*(3), 211–227.

Zintzaras, E. (2005). Statistical aspects of bioequivalence testing between two medicinal products. *European Journal of Drug Metabolism and Pharmacokinetics, 30*(1–2), 41–46.

Zullino, D., Delacrausaz, P., & Baumann, P. (2002). The place of SSRIs in the treatment of schizophrenia. *Encephale, 28*(5 Pt 1), 433–438.

CHAPTER 13

Cognitive–Behavioural Techniques

Wendy Austin
Adapted from the chapter "Cognitive-Behavioural Therapy" by Tracey Tulley and Ruth Gallop

LEARNING OBJECTIVES

After studying this chapter, you will be able to:

- Explain the cognitive model.
- Describe the levels of cognition, including core beliefs, intermediate beliefs, automatic thoughts, and their interrelationship.
- Name and describe the 10 principles of cognitive–behavioural therapy.
- Identify cognitive treatment techniques.
- Identify behavioural treatment techniques.
- Define mindfulness.

KEY CONCEPTS

- cognitive–behavioural therapy
- cognitive restructuring

KEY TERMS

- automatic thoughts • behavioural experiment • cognitive schema
- core beliefs • intermediate beliefs • mindfulness

One of the more significant achievements in modern psychotherapy is the knowledge gained of the central role of thought (cognition) in the development of core beliefs about self and the world. Cognitive–behavioural therapy (CBT) is a form of psychotherapy that uses that knowledge to identify, analyze, and ultimately change the habitually inflexible and negative cognitions about oneself, others, and the world at large that contribute to distressing emotional states and problematic behaviours (Beck, 2011). When thinking is modified, emotion and behaviour also change. The cognitive interventions in CBT are used to modify maladaptive thinking or beliefs; its behavioural interventions are aimed at decreasing maladaptive responses while increasing adaptive ones and at the learning of new behavioural practices (Craske, 2010).

Although special training is required to become a cognitive–behavioural (CB) therapist, its knowledge base is highly useful to nurses. Such knowledge can be used not only to help persons change unhealthy behaviours (e.g., poor eating habits), overcome avoidance behaviours, and deal with stress and anxiety but as an important approach to health promotion. Knowledge of CBT interventions also allows nurses to support persons undergoing CBT as a means of improving their lives.

CBT is the most widely researched form of psychotherapy and, given the robust findings from numerous controlled clinical trials, is recognized as an effective treatment for many mental health problems and disorders, including general anxiety disorder (GAD), social phobia, posttraumatic stress disorder (PTSD), bulimia nervosa, panic disorder, depression, and pathological gambling. There is evidence indicating that CBT delivered via teleconferencing (Marchand et al., 2011) and via the internet (iCBT) (Carlbring, Degerman, Johnson, & Anderson, 2012; Paxling et al., 2011; Tilfors et al., 2008) is effective. As research shows that CBT for mental disorders is cost-effective, it is argued that greater access to publicly funded CBT in Canada may not only improve outcomes but result in cost savings (Myhr & Payne, 2006).

> **KEY CONCEPT Cognitive–behavioural therapy** is a psychotherapy focused on identifying, analyzing, and ultimately changing the habitually inflexible and negative cognitions about oneself, others, and the world that contribute to distress and problematic behaviours.

BOX 13-1 Preparing for the NCLEX: A Cognitive–Behavioural Approach

There is much at stake for nursing students taking credentialing examinations. Writing an examination like the NCLEX can create such anticipatory anxiety that examination performance is diminished. Distorted thinking translates into poor test-taking preparation and behaviour. Recognition of the way thinking impacts performance is an important first step to dealing with the issue. Self-assessment allows for the identification of specific knowledge deficits to be overcome, but negative thinking and problematic behaviours should also be identified. CB techniques such as cognitive restructuring, thought stopping, and visual imagery can then be used to help a student address test anxiety.

One university devised a course for senior nursing students identified by a predictor examination as at-risk for NCLEX failure. In addition to development of a study plan, identification of test-taking strategies, and test question practice, the course included CB techniques for individual students. Students often saw a significant improvement, not only on practice test scores but also in their performance in other classes. Positive feedback on the course included "I've had problems taking tests my whole life, but not anymore. I passed the NCLEX on my first try!" (Poorman, Mastorovish, Liberto, & Gerwick, 2010, p. 175).

From Poorman, P., Mastorovish, M., Liberto, T., & Gerwick, M. (2010). A Cognitive Behavioral Course for At-risk Senior Students Preparing to Take the NCLEX. *Nurse Educator, 15*(4), 172–175.

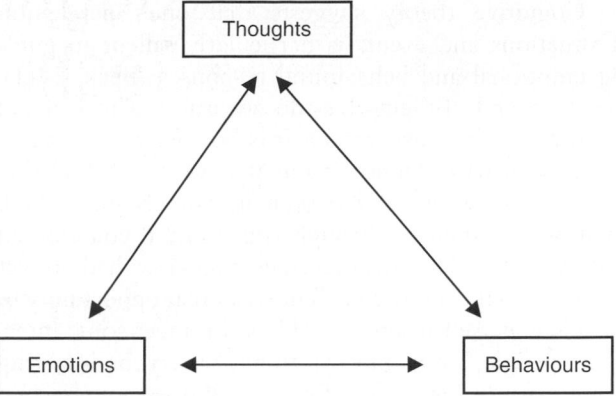

FIGURE 13-1. Interconnection between thoughts, emotions, and behaviours.

thoughts all interact in complex and interconnected ways; however, the cognitive model places particular importance on thoughts as the "director" of our experiences (Fig. 13-1).

BOX 13-2 Effect of Cognition on Feelings and Behaviour

In this example, four student nurses in the same clinical group respond to the same situation in four different ways, owing to different patterns of thinking, feeling, and acting.

The Situation: A nursing instructor informs the clinical group that by the end of their shift each student is expected to seek out an opportunity to insert his or her first intravenous line. All students received the appropriate classroom teaching and lab practice with this skill.

Susanne thinks, "I have been waiting so long to perform advanced clinical skills. I can hardly wait to give it a try." She feels excited and responds behaviourally by informing all staff in the morning report of her learning opportunity. She requests that any new intravenous starts be directed to her.

Dylan thinks, "I understand the theory behind intravenous insertion, but I did not have much success in the lab. I know I need to fulfill this requirement, but I am not sure how I am going to do it without hurting someone and embarrassing myself." He feels anxious and uncertain and responds behaviourally by reluctantly informing his buddy nurse, midway through the shift, that he is required to meet this expectation.

Jasmine thinks, "There is absolutely no way I am ready for this. I do not have the confidence or skill set to perform this task." She feels terrified and responds behaviourally by speaking to the clinical instructor privately informing her that she is feeling nauseous and must return home for the day.

Ella thinks, "Once again I'm being told what to do without any regard for my own learning needs. No one can force me to comply." She feels outraged and angry and responds behaviourally by refusing to complete the skill as required.

All the students were presented with the identical situation, and all received similar training to perform the required skill. The way in which each student *thought about* the situation, however, was very different and consequently led to emotions as varied as excitement and terror and behaviours as varied as approach and avoidance. It is not the situation itself that influenced how each of the students responded, but rather each individual's unique interpretation of the situation.

Although the assumptions underlying CBT can be traced back to ancient times and the Stoic philosopher Epictetus, psychiatrist Aaron Beck and psychologist Albert Ellis are acknowledged as having founded CBT as we know it today. From the mid-1950s to the early 1960s, when experimental and clinical psychology and psychiatry were ruled by behaviourism and psychoanalytic theory, Ellis and Beck, independently of each other, became increasingly dissatisfied with the ability of psychoanalysis to explain the struggles of their patients and its lack of scientific rigour. In treating their patients, they noted certain biases toward irrational and inflexible thought patterns that negatively influenced mood and behaviour. A radical idea at the time, they proposed that if these rigid and negative thought patterns could be changed, mood would improve and behaviour would become more functional. Although CBT is a mental health treatment, it is based on a cognitive model that is applicable to the experience of all humans in all situations. Life skills for coping with distress and problem solving can be learned using this model (see Box 13-1).

THE COGNITIVE MODEL

The cognitive model forms the foundation of CBT, the essence of which is that humans respond primarily to cognitive representations of the environment, and that cognition mediates affect and behaviour (Beck, 2011). In simpler terms, the way we *think* about situations influences our emotions and our behaviour. Our emotions, behaviours, and

Cognitive theory suggests that one's perception of situations and events is particularly salient in guiding emotional and behavioural responses (Beck, 2011). Events in and of themselves do not cause us to feel and act in particular ways; rather, it is how we *understand* or think about what happens to us that affects how we feel about it and what we do about it. For example, think about what would go through your mind if you entered a party where the only other guest you knew had not yet arrived. Would you think, "This is a great opportunity to introduce myself to others. Maybe I'll meet some interesting people," or would you think, "Everyone is staring at me because I'm alone. If my friend does not show up in the next 15 minutes, I'm leaving"? The party itself is a relatively neutral event, but how you interpret the event will affect how you feel at the party and what you do or how you act. If your thought process tends toward the former, your emotions of excitement and enjoyment will propel you to stay and mingle with the other partygoers (your behaviour). If your thought process is more consistent with the latter, your anxiety and uncertainty will compel you to flee (your behaviour).

The different ways that individuals evaluate and respond to a particular situation or event are as varied as the individuals themselves. The particular reasons why individuals are so varied in their perceptions of situations and thereby their emotional and behavioural responses are in part accounted for by their core beliefs. See Box 13-2 for an example of students responding differently to the same situation. In summary, the cognitive model posits that when an emotion is felt, a thought is behind it, and when behaviour is enacted, a thought is behind it.

■ LEVELS OF COGNITION

Cognition is given primary importance in CBT. There are three levels of cognition that are considered: core beliefs, intermediate beliefs, and automatic thoughts.

Core Beliefs

Cognitive theory posits the existence of core knowledge structures that hold, organize, and interpret all information about one's view of self, others, and the world (Beck, 2011; Craske, 2010). These structures, referred to as **core beliefs** or **cognitive schema**, comprise basic beliefs so fundamental that they are often not articulated in explicit words but rather are accepted as absolute truths (Beck, 2011). Core beliefs assist in evaluating and assigning meaning to events and influencing the subsequent range of affective and behavioural responses (Beck & Emery, 1985). The deeply rooted nature of core beliefs and their difficulty in being accessed, or explicitly identified, mean that they are difficult to change. Examples of core beliefs are "I am inadequate"; "I am unlovable"; "others are not trustworthy"; and "the world is an unsafe place."

Core beliefs hold both general and specific information about the self, others, and the world and influence the manner in which one negotiates one's way through life. If, for example, an individual holds the belief that she is a person worthy of love and that she will likely engage in mutually respectful and fulfilling relationships. Conversely, if the world is believed to be a hostile place in which people are not to be trusted, she may have an approach of hypervigilance and suspiciousness and may experience relationships as potentially dangerous. As one moves through life gathering and considering information, beliefs are processed in a way that is consistent with the view of self, others, and the world and become solidified. As such, core beliefs are self-confirming and self-perpetuating in nature, which contribute to their rigidity and global application (Beck, 2011).

Intermediate Beliefs

Existing at a more accessible level than core beliefs are cognitive products, which are often separated into two categories: **intermediate beliefs** and **automatic thoughts** (Beck, 2011). Intermediate beliefs consist of attitudes, rules or expectations, and assumptions that influence one's perceptions, affect, and behaviours. They often take the form of "if... then," "should," or "must" statements that are rigid and unrealistic. Assumptions, rules, and expectations may have arisen from the direct teaching or observation of important others early in life. One's cultural background also plays a role in one's understanding and tolerance of what is acceptable. Examples of intermediate beliefs include the following:

- If I'm not liked by everyone, it means I've failed.
- Assume the worst will happen because it usually does.
- If I show my vulnerability, I make myself open to attack.
- I must be the best in everything that I endeavour.
- Relationships make you open to rejection.

Automatic Thoughts

At an even more superficial level than intermediate beliefs are automatic thoughts. Automatic thoughts are the "knee-jerk," in-the-moment words and images generated in a particular situation (Beck, 2011). They may not be logical and are often difficult to "shut off." Automatic thoughts are the most superficial and accessible of the levels of cognition and thus are generally the first to be targeted in treatment. Although automatic thoughts are accessible, we are not always immediately conscious of their presence. Instead, we may be more aware of the accompanying emotion rather than the preceding spontaneous thought. In fact, the presence of a strong emotion is often a signal that an important thought is present. For example, when a car cuts you off on the freeway, you might be more likely to respond with anger than to be aware of the thought behind the emotion of anger ("Who do you think you are? You put the safety of my family at risk."). Part of the early therapeutic work

Situation:	I am standing in line and someone steps into the position in front of me.
↓	
Automatic thoughts:	This person must not have realized I was already in line.
	I will tell him that I was first in line so that he can take his place behind me.
↓	
Intermediate beliefs, rules, expectations:	People do not intend to be malicious, but can cause inconvenience.
	It is necessary to follow social norms.
	The ability to assert myself is important.
↓	
Core belief:	I am a valuable person worthy of respect.

FIGURE 13-2. The relationship between levels of cognition.

of CBT is to bring automatic thoughts into our awareness and help us evaluate their impact (Beck, 2011).

Relationship Between Levels of Cognition

The relationship between automatic thoughts, intermediate beliefs, and core beliefs is demonstrated in the following two examples. There is a situation in which an individual is standing in a line and someone steps into the position in front of her. In the moment, the individual tells herself, "This person must not have realized I was already in line. I will tell him that I was first in line so that he can take his place behind me." These automatic thoughts occur spontaneously and reside at the most superficial level of cognition. The deeper intermediate beliefs, rules, and expectations that support these automatic thoughts may be "People do not intend to be malicious but can cause inconvenience," "It is necessary to follow social norms," and "The ability to assert oneself is important." Underlying these automatic thoughts and intermediate rules and expectations is a core belief, the deepest level of cognition, of "I am a valuable person who is worthy of respect." This example of the relationship between the three levels of cognition is illustrated in Figure 13-2. Another individual may process this same situation very differently. The same three levels of cognition still exist, although the content of each level is different. She may tell herself, "This person saw me standing here, and he intentionally stepped in front of me. He must think I am someone who can be easily exploited." The intermediate beliefs and rules that gave rise to these automatic thoughts are "I am not capable of speaking up for myself," "I expect that people will treat me with a lack of respect," and "I can't

speak up for myself; therefore, I'll never get anywhere in life." In this example, the automatic thoughts and expectations are driven by core beliefs rooted in a sense of unworthiness, such as "I'm not deserving of respect."

Early experiences, past events, messages from others, and direct observations contribute to the formation of core beliefs and subsequent intermediate beliefs and automatic thoughts. In the individual whose early experiences were primarily nurturing, reliable, and positive, core beliefs are generally an accurate, realistic, and functional reflection of reality. However, the individual who experienced inconsistency, emotional unavailability, and cruelty may develop hypercritical beliefs about the self, others, and the world that are rigid, overgeneralized, and an inaccurate reflection of the current reality. These core beliefs contribute to emotions and behaviours that are intensely negative and harmful.

● **STUDY NOTE**

Understanding the way thinking affects emotions and behaviours can be helpful in working with patients who are having difficulty adhering to treatment regimens.

PRINCIPLES OF COGNITIVE–BEHAVIOURAL THERAPY

CBT is grounded in a set of specific principles. Treatment strategies employed in CBT are specific to the disorder being treated; however, the basic principles remain common across disorders. The 10 principles that appear in

---

BOX 13-3 Ten Principles of CBT

1. CBT is based on an evolving CB formulation of the patient.
2. CBT requires a sound therapeutic alliance.
3. CBT emphasizes collaboration and active participation.
4. CBT is goal oriented and problem focused.
5. CBT initially emphasizes the present.
6. CBT is educative and emphasizes relapse prevention.
7. CBT aims to be time-limited.
8. CBT sessions are structured.
9. CBT teaches how to identify, evaluate, and respond to dysfunctional thoughts and beliefs.
10. CBT uses a variety of techniques to change thinking, mood, and behaviour.

From Beck, J. (2011). *Cognitive therapy: Basics and beyond* (2nd ed.). New York, NY: Guilford Press.

Box 13-3 and are discussed below are based on the work of Beck (2011).

Cognitive–Behavioural Formulation

A CB formulation begins during the patient's initial assessment and is reviewed and revised over the course of therapy. It outlines the typical thoughts and problematic behaviours that contribute to the current distress. The patient who presents with social anxiety may have the thoughts, "Showing my nervousness is a sign of weakness" and "I appear incompetent when I make presentations." Problematic behaviours that flow from these negative thoughts may include avoidance of any situation in which he or she might be the centre of attention (e.g., speaking up in meetings), overpreparing (e.g., memorizing a brief statement to be made during a meeting), and use of alcohol (e.g., reliance on several glasses of beer before attending a party where socializing is an expectation). The next component of the formulation involves collecting information on the factors that precipitated the onset of the current problem. The precipitating factor for the socially anxious patient may be starting a new job where there is an expectation to chair meetings, conduct staff training, and give presentations to outside agencies. A CB formulation also outlines the developmental issues that contributed to and continue to reinforce the current problem. For example, harsh criticism by parents for being less than perfect, being ridiculed and mocked by students while speaking in front of the class, and receiving below-average grades on oral presentations may all be predisposing factors for the socially anxious patient. Over his or her life, he or she may have systematically ignored his or her multiple successes and amplified his or her perceived social failures, which served to strengthen his or her beliefs about weakness and inadequacy.

The CB formulation is shared and modified with the patient as part of the collaborative relationship (see Box 13-3, principles 2 and 3). It is a framework that can be modified as new information becomes available. In addition to providing both a framework for guiding treatment and a means to enhancing therapeutic collaboration, it also demonstrates to the patient how part of one's experience can be broken down in order to gain a better understanding of the whole, and that one's "overwhelming" problems are composed of smaller, more manageable parts.

Strong Therapeutic Alliance

Therapeutic change would not be achievable without a strong therapeutic relationship consisting of trust, mutual respect, safety, empathy, warmth, and acceptance. Most patients enter therapy afraid, uncertain, and perhaps unsure if it will be helpful. Many have struggled for years on their own, perhaps too ashamed to seek help. Further, the personal histories of some patients render them highly mistrustful of those in positions of perceived power. It is the primary task of the therapist to create an environment in which patients feel free to disclose their anxieties and take risks, in which they feel attended to, listened to, and understood. The therapeutic relationship is discussed further in Chapter 6.

Time Limited and Brief

Many forms of psychotherapy are open-ended with respect to the length of treatment. Psychodynamic therapy, for instance, may continue for years. In contrast, CBT is a short-term treatment. An assumption of CBT is that the therapist will transfer knowledge and skills to the person in therapy and then further therapy becomes unnecessary (Butler, Fennell, & Hackmann, 2008). As example, the American Psychiatric Association recommends one CBT session per week for 10 to 15 weeks for persons with panic disorder (American Psychiatric Association, 2009). Maintenance CBT sessions lessen the likelihood of relapse for such patients (White et al., 2013). Severity and duration of the presenting problem, patient motivation, and the patient's ability to form and maintain a therapeutic relationship will determine the duration of CBT for a particular individual. The *Suitability for Short-term Cognitive Therapy Rating Scale* (SRS) developed at the Centre for Addiction and Mental Health in Toronto has predictive value regarding potential for CBT to be successful with a particular patient (Myhr, Talbot, Annable, & Pinard, 2007).

Goal Oriented, Problem Focused, and Change Oriented

Patients enter CBT with a clear idea of their struggles. With the therapist, they set realistic, measurable goals to be attained within the treatment period. Using cognitive and behavioural strategies (to be discussed), the patient works toward analyzing the current accuracy and logic of negative thinking patterns. Distortions in thinking are tested and are replaced with more accurate and flexible ways of evaluating self, others, and the world. Potential barriers to goal attainment are considered, and methods to overcome these obstacles are planned.

Structured and Directive

Although the content of each therapy session changes from week to week, sessions follow a similar structure throughout treatment. The structure of CBT provides clarity, reassurance, and a sense of control to the patient; it maintains focus and maximizes the ability to use the session effectively. It prepares the patient to be his or her own therapist upon therapy termination.

The therapist begins the session with a mood check, asks for a brief summary of the patient's week, collaboratively decides which problem areas will be discussed in the session (often referred to as agenda setting), requests feedback about the previous session, reviews and discusses the self-reflective exercise, addresses the agenda items, provides new self-reflective exercises, and elicits feedback about the session. Throughout the session, the therapist offers summaries of key areas. As the therapy progresses, the patient takes on the responsibility of providing these summaries and managing the structure in general.

Educative

The initial sessions of CBT are more therapist directed than later sessions and include education about the patient's presenting problem and the cognitive model of his or her particular disorder in addition to socializing the patient to CBT. Further on in CBT, therapists teach patients how to engage in cognitive restructuring, the process whereby habitually negative thought patterns are identified, evaluated, and modified. Providing patients information on the nature and course of their disorder not only helps them to understand their current struggles but also empowers them to engage in a collaborative approach to their care. An additional benefit of the educative nature of CBT is that it assists in preparing patients for the process of self-therapy; that is, it helps ensure that patients adopt the skills necessary to continue to change and prevent relapse after the specific therapy has ended.

Therapeutic Collaboration

CBT is a collaborative effort, with patient and therapist each bringing essential but different ingredients to the relationship and vital to achieving change. The patient assumes the role of equal partner in agenda setting, problem solving, and generating self-reflective exercises (see Box 13-3, principle 3). Because the content and the process of CBT are demystified and made transparent, it is possible for patients to truly take on a collaborative role. The therapist remains an active participant in the treatment; neither a neutral nor a authoritative stance would be appropriate in CBT.

Inductive Reasoning

Patients entering therapy often view their thoughts and feelings as facts and unshakeable truths: for example, "I know I am a stupid person. When I'm depressed, it means I'm weak." Patients of CBT are encouraged to view their thoughts and feelings as hypotheses; they are not rigid facts but are plausible explanations that will be put to test and revised as needed. The goal is to assist patients in attending to all the available facts and information in their hypothesis testing, not merely the "old ruts" of thinking in which they generally find themselves stuck. Patients are encouraged to "think like a scientist and search for objective facts" or "play detective to find all the evidence" when examining the validity and accuracy of their thoughts.

Socratic Questioning

CB therapists adopt a questioning stance, referred to as Socratic questioning, as a method to help patients to evaluate their thinking (e.g., negative thought patterns) and to aid in developing balanced thoughts. When a question is posed by the therapist, possible answers are generated. The patient is encouraged to view these answers as hypotheses capable of being examined and tested in the therapy. Socratic questioning is a reasoned dialogue; the intention is not for the patient to feel interrogated; rather, it is for the patient to come to his or her own broader perspective about the validity, accuracy, and functionality of his or her thought process (Beck, 2011).

Self-Reflective Exercises

One of the most effective ways of helping patients reflect on and practice newly developed skills and monitor progress is through the use of self-reflective exercises, sometimes referred to as homework exercises. Research indicates that homework compliance is a significant predictor of positive treatment outcome (Kazantzis, Whittington, & Dattilio, 2010). Self-reflective exercises are provided at the end of each session with the expectation that the patient will work on them throughout the week and be prepared to discuss them at the beginning of the following session. Providing the patient with materials that facilitate recollection of the assignment promotes homework completion. It is essential that therapists review the assigned exercise with the patient at the following session because this reinforces the therapist's commitment and investment in the process. Patients will be less likely to complete the exercises if they have little accountability and if they do not observe the therapist valuing the assignments. Review of the exercises also provides the therapist with clinically useful information. If patients state that they do not feel like completing the exercise, are too busy, or do not see the point, this provides the therapist with clinically relevant material that should be explored further in the therapy. For example, a patient may avoid attempting the exercises because he or she does not feel as though it will be done "right" or "good enough" or that he or she will appear "stupid, just like I always do," which would lead to humiliation. The therapist would then take the opportunity to explore these thoughts, as they may represent negative patterns of thinking that are generalized to situations beyond the completion of the exercises and warrant analyzing and modification. If the patient indicates an inability to complete the exercises because time is lacking, further exploration may reveal that either the exercises as assigned were in fact too detailed and labour intensive or that the patient has difficulty committing the personal time necessary to effect therapeutic change. It is important for the therapist to know whether the patient is experiencing new insights and a sense of accomplishment through completing the exercises: this assists in gauging where to direct therapy.

▨ TREATMENT STRATEGIES

Both cognitive and behavioural techniques are used to effect change. Basic CBT strategies are outlined here. Advanced CBT strategies are beyond the scope of this text. Although treatment strategies are described here, advanced training and clinical supervision are essential to treatment delivery.

Cognitive Techniques

Cognitive techniques revolve primarily around cognitive restructuring, a process that follows a particular path of identifying, analyzing, and modifying the three levels of cognition, beginning with automatic thoughts and working through to core beliefs.

▼ **KEY CONCEPT Cognitive restructuring** is a process in which cognitions (automatic thoughts and intermediate and core beliefs) are identified, analyzed, and modified to effect positive change in mood and behaviour.

Identifying Automatic Thoughts

Awareness of one's thinking is the first step toward change. Early in treatment, patients are often unaware of their running internal negative dialogues about themselves, others, and the world. The accompanying emotion may be much more apparent to patients than the underlying negative, inflexible thoughts. When introducing patients to the skill of identifying automatic thoughts, a useful place to begin is to have them attend to shifts in or intensification of their emotions. When a strong emotion is felt or a new emotion is experienced, the

question is asked, "What was going through your mind?" (Beck, 2011). This question often helps patients to attend to the thinking that drives their emotional experience. Another technique to elicit automatic thoughts is to ask the patient to recount a very recent problematic situation. The patient is encouraged to play back the situation in his or her mind using all the senses. As the patient visualizes the details of what happened, he or she is asked, "What does this situation say about you?" "What does it mean for how others will view you?" "What about this situation is bothering you the most?" "If the worst case scenario came from this situation, what do you think would happen?" (Greenberger & Padesky, 1995). Once automatic thoughts are identified, evaluation of their accuracy and usefulness is undertaken.

Evaluating Automatic Thoughts

The goal of evaluating automatic thoughts is to examine thoughts in detail to determine their accuracy. Patients consider both supporting and unsupporting evidence in relation to their automatic thoughts. They need to focus on objective facts rather than interpretations, assumptions, or opinions when generating evidence, although initially this may be difficult (Greenberger & Padesky, 1995). Finding evidence that is unsupportive of automatic thoughts can be aided by key questions such as, "What experiences have I had that show this thought is not always completely true?" "If someone I cared deeply about had this thought, what would I tell them?" "If someone who cared deeply about me knew I was thinking this, what would they say to me?" "What evidence is there that this thought is not 100% true?" (Greenberger & Padesky, 1995). When evaluating automatic thoughts, often patients conclude that the evidence for the automatic thought is weaker than the evidence against, and therefore that the thought is no longer as accurate and valid as it was once believed to be.

The following case example illustrates the process of evaluating automatic thoughts. A patient, Elizabeth, was reprimanded by her employer for not completing her monthly report, an essential part of her job. After exploring the emotions she experienced in this situation (fear and shame), she identified several negative automatic thoughts, including "My boss hates me," "I might lose my job," "He thinks I'm incompetent," "I'm not a responsible or trustworthy employee," and "I'm nothing but a screwup." The therapist helped Elizabeth determine which automatic thought was most distressing to her ("I'm nothing but a screwup"), and it was this thought that became the one to be evaluated. Elizabeth was asked to find evidence to support the thought, "I'm nothing but a screwup." Given that she was instructed to consider only objective information, and not her opinion, the following evidence was generated: "I failed two courses in one semester during my 1st year of university because I partied more than I studied," "I am sometimes late paying my credit card bill," and "I once had a boyfriend who told me I wouldn't get anywhere in life." Elizabeth's next task was to find evidence that does not support her thought, "I'm nothing but a screwup." Reviewing key questions with her therapist, she was able to find non-supporting evidence: "I generally receive above-average yearly performance appraisals from my boss," "In addition to working this job, I volunteer in my son's classroom two times a month, and I have been called invaluable," and "My best friend tells me that I'm a very organized mother."

Evaluating one's automatic thoughts also involves identifying cognitive distortions (thinking errors or problematic thinking styles). These are the characteristic and habitual ways people err in thinking about themselves or others (Burns, 1989). Thinking errors are problematic as they keep people locked into patterns of negative thinking and behaviour. Burns initially identified 10 types of thinking errors, a list that has been adapted and added to by others over time (Box 13-4). People tend to have

---

BOX 13-4 Ten Thinking Errors

1. **All-or-nothing thinking:** The tendency to see things in black-and-white categories, with no shades of grey. Things are seen in extremes, either very good or very bad. "If I don't get a perfect evaluation, I'm a failure."
2. **Overgeneralization:** The assumption that one error/problem means a lifetime of the same error/problem. "If I lose this job, I will never succeed in making a living."
3. **Mental filter:** Filtering out the good things that happen and retaining only the negative. "When I received that award, I could see that Jane didn't think I deserved it."
4. **Magnification/minimization:** Overexaggeration of fears, imperfections, or errors. "There is absolutely no way I could have passed that exam. I've totally blown the course."
5. **Jumping to conclusions:** Concluding things that are not justified based on available evidence. "I saw Peter yawn during my presentation. Everyone was bored." It includes **mind reading:** "My coworker didn't say hello to me today because she's starting to dislike me" and **fortune telling:** "He didn't call me tonight. That's it. He'll never call again."
6. **Labelling:** Putting a negative label on yourself or others, a way to believe that no one can change. "My roommate is a slob. I have to keep everything tidy."
7. **Personalization and blame:** Making yourself feel responsible for things out of your control. "It is my fault our team lost the game. If only I hadn't dropped the ball in the first half."
8. **Should/must statements:** Thinking in terms of "should" and "must." "I must make no mistakes during the skill laboratory, no matter what."
9. **Discounting the positives:** Refusing to credit the positive aspects of situations. "John said that I looked great today. He must think that I look terrible most days."
10. **Emotional reasoning:** Believing something must be true because one "feels" it so strongly, ignoring any evidence to the contrary. "I know I've had people in my life who say I'm a good person, but it's hard to believe because I feel like I'm so bad."

From Burns, D. D. (1989). *The feeling good handbook: Using the new mood therapy in everyday life.* New York, NY: Morrow.

---

a consistent pattern of thinking errors across a variety of situations. All people engage in distorted thinking; it is not a phenomenon limited to people with mental disorders. In CBT, the therapist works with the patient to first identify which thinking errors are being used. Patients are commonly given a handout listing all the cognitive errors with relevant examples of each. Such a handout guides patients through the process of identifying and labelling thinking errors. The next step is to examine the usefulness and validity of this style of thinking so that patients can respond to their thoughts in a more realistic, balanced manner. Through the process of correcting thinking errors, patients see that the negative automatic thoughts and beliefs they held about themselves, others, and the world at large are no longer valid. It is important to catch oneself when making the errors and inject a clearer way of looking at the situation. When we give ourselves more options for how to think, we give ourselves more options for how to feel and how to respond.

Returning to the case of Elizabeth, she identified that she routinely engages in distorted thinking by jumping to conclusions ("I might lose my job." "He thinks I'm incompetent.") and overgeneralization ("I'm not a responsible or trustworthy employee. I'm nothing but a screwup"). Elizabeth worked with her therapist to increase her awareness of how frequently she engages in this style of thinking. Further, her therapist helped Elizabeth to realize the inaccuracy and destructiveness of this style of thinking.

Modifying Automatic Thoughts

Modification of automatic thoughts is an essential component of CBT. The patient uses what he or she has learned about identifying and evaluating automatic thoughts to move toward modification. Modifying thoughts involves weighing evidence for and against an automatic thought in an effort to generate a new, more balanced way of thinking. This new way of thinking does not simply involve replacing negative thoughts with positive ones. Unquestioning acceptance of a positive stance can be as destructive as negative thinking because it does not take into account all available evidence (Greenberger & Padesky, 1995). The new way of thinking considers all aspects of one's experience so that one can arrive at a more broadened way of viewing oneself, others, or the world. In Elizabeth's case, she examined all her available evidence and recognized an alternative way of understanding her situation: "I have exceedingly high expectations of myself and find it very hard to give myself a break when I've done something I perceive as less than acceptable. I have screwed up in the past, but it's been relatively infrequently, and I do learn from my mistakes." A summary statement of the evidence regarding an automatic thought can be useful in the development of balanced thinking. For example,

Elizabeth summarized her evidence by saying, "I've done things that are not responsible and have received negative messages from others of the same kind, but I also am currently successful in juggling many demanding roles and receive praise for my efforts." With this expanded view, patients generally report that they experience a positive shift in mood.

A useful, commonly used tool in CBT is the Thought Record (Greenberger & Padesky, 1995). It is a structured worksheet that records all the pertinent information about problematic and distressing situations and helps patients to make sense of why they feel and react in particular ways. Thought Records take all aspects of one's experience and organize them into information presented in seven columns: the situation, moods, automatic thoughts, evidence that supports the thoughts, evidence that does not support the thoughts, formation of balanced or alternative thoughts, and rerating of moods. At various points throughout the Thought Record, thoughts and emotions are rated and rerated on their degree of strength and believability (0% to 100%). Once the Thought Record is completed, the goal is for patients to experience a balanced or alternative thought that is rated as more believable than their original negative automatic thought accompanied by a decrease in the intensity of their originally identified emotions. Thought Records are completed during and between therapy sessions whenever problematic or distressing situations arise.

Students undergoing CB training routinely complete their own Thought Records to gain an increased awareness of their own thinking patterns and resulting emotions and behaviours, to encourage self-reflection and self-monitoring, and to become acquainted with the process of using the record. Thought Records may be shared with supervisors and discussed in supervision sessions.

Identifying and Modifying Intermediate Beliefs

The techniques of identifying and modifying automatic thoughts are used with intermediate beliefs or assumptions, as well as other techniques to get to the deeper level assumptions. Identifying assumptions can be aided by attending to the patterns of negative thoughts that emerge over the course of therapy, as these themes may suggest an underlying assumption or core belief. Identifying the rules that patients live by and expect of others may be useful. A commonly used method to uncover assumptions behind an automatic thought is the downward arrow technique (Burns, 1980), in which the therapist questions the meaning of the patient's thought until an assumption or a core belief about self, others, or the world is revealed. See Box 13-5 for an example. This technique can be used to reveal assumptions about others (What does x mean about other people?) or the

---

BOX 13-5 A Dialogue Using the Downward Arrow Technique

Patient: I didn't do the self-reflective exercise this week because it was too hard.
Therapist: What does that say about you that you found it too hard?
Patient: It says that I didn't pay enough attention in the session last week.
Therapist: And if that were true, that you didn't pay enough attention last week, what would that say about you?
Patient: It would say that I'm lazy.
Therapist: If it was true that you were lazy, what would that say about you?
Patient: It would say that I'm useless.

---

world in general (What does x say about how the world works?). Once the assumption is revealed, the process of restructuring the assumption is initiated wherein the evidence for and against the assumption and alternative responses are considered. Behavioural experiments (to be discussed) are also an effective means to modify assumptions because they allow patients to use real-life situations to test the accuracy of beliefs.

Identifying and Modifying Core Beliefs

All the techniques discussed thus far, especially the downward arrow technique, are useful for identifying core beliefs. Deeply rooted core beliefs may require additional, advanced strategies beyond the scope of this chapter. Such strategies include discussing the early life experiences of the patient, as core beliefs may be better understood when the context in which they developed is considered. In-depth exploration wherein patients relive painful early experiences, however, is not appropriate in CBT.

Beck (2011) encourages the use of Core Belief Worksheets to identify core beliefs, to strengthen the believability of new core beliefs, and to weaken the influence of old core beliefs. The patient first identifies his or her old core belief and rates it out of 100 (e.g., "I'm undesirable," 70%), followed by his or her new core belief ("Once people get to know me, they can see that I'm a likeable person," 40%). Similar to the process of evaluating automatic thoughts, the patient gathers evidence that contradicts his or her old belief and supports his or her new belief ("Last week someone in my running group gave me her number so we can arrange to go for a run together." "I have one friend who has stayed by my side despite all the things I've been through"). The final step is to gather evidence that supports the old belief with the addition of a cognitive reframe ("When my last girlfriend broke up with me, she said she could never love a person like me, but I was struggling with depression during our relationship;

therefore, I couldn't bring much to the relationship," "People don't readily seek out my friendship, but I'm now realizing that I have given off signals to people to stay away. This was my way of protecting myself from the rejection I believed was inevitable"). Thus, a broader perspective is achieved that takes into account past and current experiences.

Behavioural Techniques

Behavioural strategies are primarily utilized in CBT as a way to test and challenge both old maladaptive thinking patterns and newly acquired rational thoughts. They may be used to modify symptoms when conducted in a manner that supports a change in cognition (Butler et al., 2008). Behavioural techniques must be considered and implemented within the larger scope of CBT. They are not employed in isolation, nor are they implemented without being linked back to the cognitive model of the particular disorder being treated.

Behavioural Strategies to Test Beliefs

Creating experiences to test and challenge core beliefs is an essential CBT treatment strategy called **behavioural experiments** (Beck, 2011). The validity and accuracy of old core beliefs are tested in real-life situations, thus increasing the believability of alternative thoughts. Without this behavioural component, the process of challenging the accuracy and validity of old thoughts and generating new thoughts may be little more than an intellectual exercise and may not lead to meaningful cognitive, emotional, or behavioural change. Behavioural experiments can be challenging for patients because the prospect of putting new thoughts into action and testing old destructive ways of thinking can be anxiety producing.

Behavioural experiments can be presented to patients as an opportunity to "test-drive" their new thoughts to see what will really happen as a result. A typical behavioural experiment consists of the therapist and the patient collaboratively constructing an experiment to test a new belief. For example, the new belief, "I'm a likeable person," could be tested by constructing an experiment in which the patient plans to call an acquaintance from his running group and invite her to go for a run. The patient makes a prediction about what might happen in the course of the experiment ("She'll agree to go with me, but she'll find me a bit uninteresting"). Potential obstacles are considered ("I will become very nervous and talk very little; therefore, she'll think I'm boring"), as well as action that can be taken to manage the obstacles ("Remind myself that being nervous is okay when you are getting to know people for the first time. Remind myself that even if I don't talk much, I can't jump to the conclusion that she will think I'm boring"). The actual result of the experiment is reported ("We ran together for 1 hour and talked about our interests.

I found out that we have many things in common, including that we both like classic films and we're both shy people. She told me that *Citizen Kane* is playing in 2 weeks and suggested that we see it together"). The patient then rates how much the result of the experiment supports his or her new belief (90%) and finally reflects on what was learned in the process of the experiment ("If I take more risks and show people who I really am, they can see that I'm a nice person and worth getting to know better"). Behavioural experiments are a powerful means of altering beliefs because they compel patients to take action on a thought. When patients are able to directly see the outcome of testing their beliefs, they are more likely to actually modify their beliefs.

Behavioural Strategies to Modify Symptoms

Numerous types of behavioural strategies for symptom reduction are available, including exposure techniques, relaxation training, and activity monitoring. Exposure therapy is utilized in panic disorder, panic disorder with agoraphobia, PTSD, social phobia, and obsessive–compulsive disorder. The common thread among all types of exposure is that they put the patient in contact with feared or avoided thoughts, emotions, behaviours, or situations (Craske, 2010). Through this process, three possible outcomes may occur: the patient's anticipated catastrophic outcome may be disconfirmed; the patient may become desensitized to the feared response; and the patient's ability to cope with the feared situation may be improved. Exposure-based techniques are very specific to the disorder being treated, and the protocols are extensive and comprehensive.

Relaxation strategies, such as controlled breathing and progressive muscle relaxation, may be employed with patients who have generalized anxiety disorder, panic disorder, and PTSD. Controlled breathing is the practice of learning how to breathe at an appropriate pace and depth so that this skill can be called on when faced with feared stimuli. The person learns to breathe from the diaphragm rather than the thorax (Craske, 2010). Patients are also educated about the effects of hyperventilation and breath holding, such as increased blood pressure and disturbance of the oxygen–carbon dioxide balance, and how these can worsen anxiety symptoms. Progressive muscle relaxation, or Jacobsonian relaxation (Jacobson, 1938), involves the practice of deliberately tensing and relaxing 12 groups of muscles, beginning with the feet and moving upward to the face. The technique teaches patients how to relax muscles and induce a sense of physical and mental calmness. Other relaxation techniques include mindfulness-based CBT (see below) and guided imagery (not discussed here).

Depressed individuals often benefit from activity scheduling, wherein daily activities and accompanying moods are recorded in a diary format (Beck, 2011). Many depressed patients become immobilized and believe that they must wait to feel better before engaging in activities. Activity monitoring encourages depressed individuals

BOX 13-6 **Research for Best Practice**

THE INFLUENCE OF THERAPISTS' REACTIONS TO CLIENTS IN CBT

Westra, H., Aviram, A., Connors, L., Kertes, A., & Ahmed, M. (2012). Therapist emotional reactions and client resistance in cognitive behavioral therapy. Psychotherapy, 49(2), 163–172.

The Aim: To investigate early reactions of therapists to clients as a possible influence on client engagement in therapy (as measured by observer-rated resistance).

Methods: Video-taped CBT session data (from a larger Toronto clinical trial study of treatment efficacy) related to 30 client participants with a principal diagnosis of GAD and who received CBT were analyzed. Before CBT was initiated, the Penn State Worry Questionnaire (PSWQ) was completed by clients. After sessions 1 and 3, therapists completed Ratings of Emotional Attitudes to Clients by Treators (REACT) to measure their response to the client. The Cognitive Therapy Rating Scale (CTRS) was used by trained coders to measure therapist competence after either session 2 or 3. The Cognitive Resistance Code (CRC) was used to rate session 1 (early treatment) and session 5 (midtreatment) in their entirety for all clients. The CRC measures resistance in therapy, defined as any behaviour that opposes, blocks, diverts, or impedes direction set by the therapist. Resistance is conceived as a measure of interpersonal progress in therapy, not a characteristic of the client.

Findings: Therapists' early emotional reactions were not related to the severity of the client's worry pre-CBT. The greater the therapist's early positive reactions to clients (particularly liking, enjoyment, attachment), the significantly lower the client's resistance at midtreatment and the more client resistance was reduced from early to midtreatment. A trend was also found indicating that higher levels of negative therapist reactions (early in treatment) were associated with higher levels of client resistance. These effects were not related to therapist competence in providing CBT.

Implications: Therapists' feelings about clients may play a greater role in client engagement and the progress of therapy than commonly recognized, a role that goes beyond therapist skill in treatment techniques.

to instead engage in activity as a way to improve mood. Activity scheduling is useful for both pleasurable and avoided tasks and monitoring moods. It is beneficial for challenging beliefs ("There isn't anything that I enjoy doing," "I'm not good at doing anything") (Beck, Rush, Shaw, & Emery, 1979). See Box 13-6 for an example of CBT research.

MINDFULNESS-BASED CBT

Mindfulness is a form of trained self-observation based on meditation practices (David, 2006). It involves learning to be present to what is happening to one in the immediate moment. Mindfulness can help people to disengage their "automatic pilot" in order to look more carefully at their convictions and thought patterns. The act of pushing away negative thoughts and emotions can actually increase distress. Mindfulness reduces that struggle and

allows for calm. For those with long-standing problems, becoming mindful can be challenging. It takes time to experience mindful self-reflection with acceptance and an attitude of curiosity and compassion rather than self-judgement and distress (Butler et al., 2008). It takes practice to develop the skill of mindfulness, but being able to respond mindfully to a situation rather than with a habitually unhelpful response can make a significant positive difference (David, 2006).

CONCLUSION

The simple idea that emotion and behaviour are influenced by cognition has generated decades of empirical study, which indicates that CBT is a highly effective and cost-efficient treatment for individuals struggling with certain mental disorders. The active and collaborative nature of CBT, combined with its orientation toward change, makes it an easy fit with nursing, as is evidenced by the interest and broad appeal of CBT among nurses. Psychiatric and mental health nurses are strong advocates of self-reflection and awareness of how one's own experiences influence the therapeutic relationship. With appropriate training, nurses will find CBT to be useful to their therapeutic repertoire. CBT offers an empirically and theoretically sound means to improve the mental health of their patients.

SUMMARY OF KEY POINTS

■ The cognitive model is based on the idea that the way we think about situations influences our emotion and behaviour.

■ CBT is based on changing negative thought patterns as a means to improve mood and behaviour.

■ CBT is the most widely researched form of psychotherapy used to treat many mental disorders, including PTSD, bulimia nervosa, panic disorder, and depression.

■ There are 10 principles of CBT: CB formulation; strong therapeutic alliance; collaborative with active participation from the patient; goal oriented and problem focused; initially emphasizes the present; educative and looks to prevent relapse; time limited; structured; teaches identification, evaluation, and response to dysfunctional thoughts and beliefs; uses a variety of techniques to change thinking, mood, and behaviour.

■ Cognitive techniques involve cognitive restructuring, a process that follows the steps of identifying, analyzing, and modifying automatic thoughts through to core beliefs.

■ Behavioural techniques are used within the cognitive model and are seen as opportunities to test new beliefs.

■ Mindfulness is a form of self-awareness training based in meditation.

CRITICAL THINKING CHALLENGES

1 How would you explain the cognitive model to a fellow student with no previous knowledge of CBT? What aspects of the model do you think are most important to emphasize?
2 Think about an incident that you experienced in the past week that caused you mild upset. Using the cognitive model, how would you differentiate between various aspects of your experience?
3 Describe the differences and interplays between core beliefs and automatic thoughts. Are there automatic thoughts that you routinely experience?
4 How do thinking errors contribute to emotional distress?
5 Why are behavioural experiments an essential aspect of CBT?
6 How are the principles of CBT different from and similar to other forms of psychotherapy you have studied?

REFERENCES

American Psychiatric Association. (2009). Practice guideline for the treatment of patients with panic disorder. *American Journal of Psychiatry, 166*(Suppl), 1–68.

Beck, J. (2011). *Cognitive therapy: Basics and beyond* (2nd ed.). New York, NY: Guilford Press.

Beck, A. T., & Emery, G. (1985). *Anxiety disorders and phobias: A cognitive perspective.* New York, NY: Basic Books.

Beck, A. T., Rush, A. J., Shaw, B. F., & Emery, G. (1979). *Cognitive therapy of depression.* New York, NY: Guilford Press.

Burns, D. D. (1980). *Feeling good: The new mood therapy.* New York, NY: Morrow.

Burns, D. D. (1989). *The feeling good handbook: Using the new mood therapy in everyday life.* New York, NY: Morrow.

Butler, G., Fennell, M., & Hackmann, A. (2008). *Cognitive-behavioral therapy for anxiety disorders: Mastering clinical challenges.* New York, NY: The Guilford Press.

Carlbring, P., Degerman, N., Johnson, J., & Anderson, G. (2012). Internet-based treatment of pathological gambling with a three-year follow-up. *Cognitive Behavior Therapy, 4*(14), 321–334.

Craske, M. (2010). *Cognitive-behavioral therapy.* Washington, DC: American Psychological Association.

David, L. (2006). *Using CBT in general practice: The 10 minute consultation.* Bloxham, UK: Scion.

Greenberger, D., & Padesky, C. A. (1995). *Mind over mood.* New York, NY: Guilford Press.

Jacobson, E. (1938). *Progressive relaxation.* Chicago, IL: University of Chicago Press.

Kazantzis, N., Whittington, C., & Dattilio, F. (2010) Meta-analysis of homework effects in cognitive and behavioral therapy. *Clinical Psychology: Science & Practice, 17*(2), 144–156.

Marchand, A., Beaulieu-Prévost, D., Guay, S., Bouchard, S., Drouin, M. S., & Germain, V. (2011). Relative efficacy of cognitive-behavioral therapy administered by video conference for posttraumatic stress disorders: A six-month follow-up. *Journal of Aggression, Maltreatment & Trauma, 20,* 304–321.

Myhr, G., & Payne, K. (2006). Cost-effectiveness of cognitive-behavioural therapy for mental disorders: Implications for public health care funding policy in Canada. *Canadian Journal of Psychiatry, 51*(10), 662–669.

Myhr, G., Talbot, J., Annable, L., & Pinard, G. (2007). Suitability for short-term cognitive psychotherapy. *Journal of Cognitive Psychotherapy: An International Quarterly, 21*(4), 334–345.

Paxling, B., Almlöv, J., Dahlin, M., Carlbring, P., Breitholtz, E., Eriksson, T., & Andersson, G. (2011). Guided internet-delivered cognitive behavior therapy for generalized anxiety disorder: A randomized controlled trial. *Cognitive Behaviour Therapy, 40*(3), 159–173.

Poorman, P., Mastorovish, M., Liberto, T., & Gerwick, M. (2010). A cognitive behavioral course for at-risk senior students preparing to take the NCLEX. *Nurse Educator, 15*(4), 172–175.

Tilfors, M., Carlbring, P., Furmark, T., Lewenhaupt, S., Spak, M., Eriksson, A., et al. (2008). Treating university students with social phobia and public speaking fears: Internet delivered self-help with or without live group exposure sessions. *Depression and Anxiety, 25,* 708–717.

Westra, H., Aviram, A., Connors, L., Kertes, A., & Ahmed, M. (2012). Therapist emotional reactions and client resistance in cognitive behavioral therapy. *Psychotherapy, 49*(2), 163–172.

White, K. S., Payne, L. A., Gorman, J. M., Shear, M. K., Woods, S. W., Saksa, J. R., & Barlow, D. H. (2013). Does maintenance CBT contribute to long-term treatment response of panic disorder with or without agoraphobia? A randomized controlled clinical trial. *Journal of Consulting and Clinical Psychology, 81*(1), 47–57.

14 Interventions With Groups

Carol Ewashen
Adapted from the chapter "Interventions with Groups"
by Mary Ann Boyd

LEARNING OBJECTIVES

After studying this chapter, you will be able to:

- Discuss group concepts that are useful in understanding and leading groups.
- Compare the different roles and responsibilities of group members.
- Identify the important aspects of leading a group, such as member selection, leadership skills, seating arrangements, and ways of intervening with challenging group members.
- Differentiate types of groups: psychoeducational, cognitive–behavioural, supportive, psychotherapeutic, and self-help.
- Compare different nursing intervention groups.

KEY CONCEPTS

- group
- group process

KEY TERMS

- closed group • formal group roles • group cohesion • group dynamics • group leadership • groupthink • informal group roles • interactive groups • leadership styles • maintenance functions • open group • self-help groups • structured groups • task functions • therapeutic factors

Participation in therapeutic groups has powerful treatment effects. Group treatment is effective and efficient for participants to further understand themselves in relation to others through interaction, gain new knowledge and social skills, conquer unwanted thoughts and feelings, and change behaviours. For effective interventions, the nurse must possess leadership skills that can shape, enhance, and monitor group interactions. The decisions regarding which interventions fit best are complex and dependent upon the purpose of the group. Competent group skill development for the psychiatric and mental health (PMH) nurse requires the ability to critically select and modify techniques to best accommodate the particular practice conditions. This applies across diverse situations from providing patient and family education or conducting support groups to direct care provision, case management, and program leadership. Understanding group skills and dynamics is

also increasingly relevant to contemporary health care service delivery with emphasis on effective interprofessional practice collaboration and teamwork (Canadian Interprofessional Health Collaborative, 2010). A challenge in group intervention is the shift from a primarily individual focus to consideration of interpersonal and whole-group interactions. This chapter presents relevant group concepts for PMH nurses. **Group leadership** is explored with special emphasis on the groups relevant to PMH nursing practice.

GROUP: DEFINITIONS AND CONCEPTS

There are many different definitions of a group. Psychoanalytic tradition draws from the work of Sigmund Freud and considers group interaction as a recapitulation of the family of origin, interpreting unconscious conflicts and reexamining them. Contemporary psychodynamic theories consider groups a combination of group dynamics and interpersonal and intrapsychic transactions (Rutan & Stone, 2001). Yalom (1998) and Yalom and Leszcz (2005) suggest that a group is a social microcosm of interpersonal dynamics and advocate a here-and-now, self-reflective approach. The cognitive–behavioural approach considers a group a social arena for corrective change in maladaptive thinking and behaviour patterns; whereas, according to systems theory, a group consists of parts or components that exist to perform some activity or purpose. As group members interact, subsystems form, challenging leaders to understand boundary realignments and the effects of subcomponents on the system and to improve interpersonal communication. A more contemporary development, drawing from the rich history of group work and apparent across a wide range of settings, is the prevention group that utilizes a full range of group processes, constructive interactions, and positive group cohesion to reduce risk while promoting health and wellness (Harpine, 2013; Harpine, Nitza, & Conyne, 2010). A global, but rather simple, definition of a group is two or more people who are in an interdependent relationship with one another. The simplicity of the definition is misleading because interactions within groups, or **group dynamics**, are anything but simple. Group dynamics influence the group's development and process. In fact, it takes an astute observer to determine the real dynamics of a group and the effects. No matter the type of group, its theoretic orientation, or its purpose, group dynamics influence the effectiveness of a group intervention.

In this text, a **group** is defined as "a social system with structure, norms, and usual ways of doing things" (Dimock & Devine, 1994, p. 54). Groups can be further defined according to the number of people or the relationship of members. A *dyad* is a group of two people, such as a married couple, siblings, or parent and child. A *triad* is a group of three people. A family is a special type of group and is discussed in Chapter 15.

> **KEY CONCEPT** A **group** is "a social system with structure, norms, and usual ways of doing things" (Dimock & Devine, 1994, p. 54).

Open Versus Closed Groups

A group can be viewed as either an open or a closed system. In an **open group**, new members are welcomed and provided time to learn group norms and expectations. For example, a newly admitted patient may join an anger management group that is part of an ongoing program in an inpatient unit. With new members, it is important to help them engage with the group by inviting member-to-member interaction. The advantage of an open group is

that participants can join at any time. In addition, these groups can function on an ongoing basis and thus can be available to more people.

In a **closed group**, all members begin at the same time, and no new members are admitted. If a member of a closed group leaves, no replacement joins. Advantages of a closed group are that the participants get to know one another over time, the group becomes more cohesive, and members move concurrently through the group process. However, implementing closed-group interventions is often difficult, especially in tertiary settings where the length of stay is short and participant readiness for group work varies greatly.

Group Size

Group size is an important consideration in forming group programs. Many mental health professionals favour small groups, but large groups can also be effective. Whether to form a large or small group depends on the age of participants, the group's purpose, the leader's abilities, participant availability, and the resources available. Small groups (usually a minimum of 3 and no more than 10 members) become more cohesive, are less likely to form subgroups, and can provide a richer interpersonal experience than large groups. Small groups may function with one group leader, although many small groups are led by two people. An ideal small group is about seven to eight people in addition to the leader or leaders (Corey, 2013; Myers & Anderson, 2008).

● **STUDY NOTE**
The size of a group will depend on the overall goals and abilities of members. Those with challenging behaviours require careful screening and assignment to smaller groups.

Small groups often are used for people who are trying to deal with complex emotional issues such as depression, anxiety, eating disorders, substance use disorder, sexual abuse, or trauma. They are also ideal for individuals or families who require more specialized intervention such as families in recovery (Zimmerman & Winek, 2013). These groups work best if they are closed to new members or if new members are gradually introduced. One disadvantage of small groups relates to the loss of members. If places are unfilled, the group dynamics change, which may alter therapeutic effectiveness.

A large group (more than 10 members) can also be therapeutic as well as cost-effective. Some research suggests that large intervention and prevention groups are effective for specific problems, such as smoking, or for settings such as schools and community (Harpine, 2013; McWhirter & McWhirter, 2010). A large group can be ongoing and open-ended. In large group intervention, a challenge for the nurse leader is to include all members in discussion, preventing a sense of alienation with the potential for member dropout.

Leading a group, whether large or small, is complex because of the number of potential interactions, relationships, and conflicts that can form. The leader needs both presentation and group leadership skills. Kottler and Englar-Carlson (2010) suggest that group work requires a different sort of mindset. It is insufficient to be purely a leader—a leader must practise in a therapeutic or facilitative manner while in the midst of a complex interactive event. Practitioners who take on *leadership* of groups require education and supervised training for competent, accountable, and ethical group practices. In large groups, the leader is often both a presenter of educative information and a facilitator of experiential learning among participants. In-depth reflection on participants' feelings and thoughts may not be the focus of group work. Depending on the theoretic orientation and the purpose of the group, leadership style and interventions must change to be effective in meeting the goals of small or large groups.

Group Development

In the same way that the development of the therapeutic relationship is a process (see Chapter 6), so too is the development of a group. Many researchers view group development as a sequence of phases, particularly in small groups (Table 14-1). Although models of group development differ, most follow a pattern of a beginning, middle, and ending stage (Jacobs, Masson, & Harvill, 2009). These stages should be thought of not as a straight line with one preceding another, but as a dynamic and iterative process with continual revisiting and reexamining of group interactions, changes, and progress toward established goals.

 KEY CONCEPT Group process is the "what is happening" in the group and how members are interacting and relating as individuals and as a whole group, including nonverbal communications.

Beginning Stage

When a group begins, group members get to know one another and the group leader. The length of the beginning stage depends on, among other variables, the purpose of the group, the number of members, and the skill of the leader. It may last for only a few sessions or several. "Honeymoon" behaviours characterize the beginning of this stage, and "conflict" emerges at the end. During the initial sessions, members usually are polite and congenial, displaying behaviours typical of those in new social situations. They are "good" and often intellectualize problems; that is, by excessively using abstract thinking or generalizations, emotional conflict or stress is minimized. Members are usually anxious and sometimes act in ways that do not truly represent their feelings. In the first few sessions, members test whether they can trust one another. Some time after the initial sessions, group members experience a period of conflict, either among themselves or with the leader. This conflict is a normal part of group development, and many believe that negotiating conflict satisfactorily is necessary to move into a productive working phase. Sometimes, one or more group members become the "scapegoat." While a scapegoat often performs a central function for the group, intervening to therapeutically process scapegoating is complex but necessary (Clark, 2002). Such situations challenge the leader to guide the group during this period by avoiding taking sides and treating all members respectfully.

Table 14-1	Comparison of Models of Group Development

Tuckman (1965)	Garland, Jones, and Kolodny (1973)	Corey, Corey, and Corey (2013)
Forming: Get to know one another and form a group	*Theme in all stages: Closeness* *Pregroup Forming*: Preparing for and deciding if this is the right group	*Preaffiliation*: Approach and avoidance; ambivalence around involvement
Storming: Tension and conflict occur; subgroups form and clash with each other	*Power and control*: Testing out and vying for status, authority, autonomy, influence and connection	*Initial stage*: Orienting; forming relations; establishing group structure and climate of trust
Norming: Develop norms for how to work with each other	*Intimacy*: More intense personal involvement and recognition of others; emergent growth	*Transition*: Emerging differences and potential for conflict
Performing: Reach consensus and develop cooperative relationships	*Differentiation*: Accept uniqueness of each with interdependence; cohesion	*Working*: Involved, interactive, and committed to engaging in productive group work
Adjourning: End of relationships and orientation to the future; sadness and appreciation	*Separation*: Moving apart; review and evaluation	*Final stage*: Consolidation of learning; sadness and anxiety with leaving

Middle (Working) Stage

The middle, or working, stage of groups involves a real sharing of ideas and the development of closeness. A group-as-a-whole culture may emerge that is distinct from the individual personalities of its members. The group develops its own rules and rituals and has its own behavioural norms; for example, groups develop regular patterns of seating and interaction. Group norms are formed through the majority of members accepting or rejecting certain behaviour (Posthuma, 2001). During this stage, the group realizes its purpose. If the purpose is education, the participants engage in learning new content or skills. If the aim of the group is to share feelings and experiences, these activities consume group meetings. During this stage, the group members take responsibility for starting on time, and the leader often needs to remind members when it is time to stop.

Ending (Termination) Stage

Ending, or termination, and saying good-byes can be difficult for a group, especially a successful therapeutic one. During the final stages, members begin to separate and may grieve the loss of the group closeness while transitioning to reestablish themselves as individuals. Individuals terminate from groups as they do from other relationships (see Chapter 6). One person may not show up at the last session, another person may bring up issues that the group has already addressed, and others may demonstrate anger or hostility. Most members of successful groups are sad as the group terminates. During the last meetings, members may make arrangements for meeting after the group ends. Although these plans rarely materialize or continue, leaders should recognize these plans as part of the farewell process—saying good-bye to the group.

Roles of Group Members

There are two **formal group roles**, the leader and the members. In small groups, however, members often assume **informal group roles** or positions in the group with rights and duties that are directed toward one or more group members. Informal roles can be categorized as task, maintenance, or individual roles. One way to think of group roles is as the different hats members try on and learn from while involved in a group (Myers & Anderson, 2008; Posthuma, 2001). These roles can either facilitate or obstruct the group process and goals.

Task functions involve the business of the group or "keeping things focused." Individuals who assume this function keep the group focused on a main purpose. For any group to be successful, it must have members who assume some of these task roles, such as *information seeker* (asks for clarification), *coordinator* (spells out relationships between ideas), and *recorder* (keeper of the minutes). **Maintenance functions** facilitate the building of group-centred attitudes, behaviours, and processes. Members functioning in maintenance roles help by ensuring a consistent start time, assisting individuals to compromise, and encouraging everyone's participation. These members facilitate maintaining group cohesiveness and may have difficulty with group conflict and differentiation. The *harmonizer* (keeps the peace), *compromiser* (gives and takes), and *standard setter* (sets expectations) are examples of maintenance roles. In a successful group, members take on and learn from both group task and maintenance functions (Table 14-2). Leader and member responsibilities and functions shift depending upon the group stage and task.

Individual-centred roles are member roles that detract from group functioning (Benne & Sheats, 1948; Posthuma, 2001). These roles are considered dysfunctional to the group, often antagonistic to group building and group maintenance, and they may detract from the group purpose and cohesion; for example, someone who monopolizes the group conversation inhibits group interaction and work on task. When individual-centred roles dominate, the risk is that neither the group task nor group maintenance function is accomplished. Individual-centred role examples include the aggressor, blocker, recognition seeker, and dominator.

While acknowledged in scholarly and popular literature, member role classification and related functions in contemporary group work have become more controversial. Critiques include the dangers of decontextualizing, generalizing, and categorizing people as well as the potential "colonizing" effects when placing people in preexisting schemas that may negatively define people (Kottler & Englar-Carlson, 2010). While it is important for the leader to recognize that all groups function through a division of labour, the leader's primary responsibility is to facilitate all members in learning the functions of productive group work in relation to self, others, and group goals.

Group Communication

One of the responsibilities of *group leadership* is to facilitate both verbal and nonverbal communication to meet the treatment goals of the individual members and the entire group. Because of the number of people involved, developing trusting relationships within groups is more complicated than developing a single relationship with another person. The communication techniques used in establishing and maintaining individual relationships are similar for groups, but the leader also attends to the communication patterns among the members.

Verbal Communication

Group interaction can be viewed as a relational communication network that becomes patterned and predictable. In a group, verbal comments are linked in a chain formation.

Table 14-2   **Leader and Member Responsibilities and Functions**

Group Stage	Leader	Member
Pregroup: Formation of a group *Informed decision making:* How does this group fit with this member this purpose?	*Design and plan the group*: Purpose, structure, process, evaluation methods. Solicit group membership. Conduct pregroup screening interviews. Determine the group composition. Provide orientation to members.	To determine: Is the group right for me? Do I have enough knowledge to understand the group purpose and process? What do I want from the group experience? How do my expectations fit with the group expectations?
Initial Stage Orientation, exploration, and setting the structure of the group Creating a safe place Sharing information Engaging each other and as a whole group around purpose	Orient group members. Establish ground rules, norms, and expectations. Encourage all members to be involved and express expectations, reactions, and concerns. Clarify understandings. Be open with members' concerns and questions. Provide guidance yet encourage member interaction and initiative.	To work through: Will I be accepted? What will the leader think of me? What is expected of me? Establish trust. Form relations with others. Express thoughts, feelings, expectations, and reservations. Become involved. Set goals for self and self-in-relation to others. Be respectful of others. Learn well and share understandings.
Transition Increased anxiety and emergence of differences with potential for conflict Reluctance to voice concerns or frustrations	Teach members the value of recognizing conflict, naming the issue, and negotiating a win-win situation. Practise directness and tactfulness in naming issues in the here and now. Encourage members to share reactions while maintaining a safe environment. Intervene with sensitivity and prevent scapegoating of a particular member. Encourage participatory interaction. Reinforce learning of self in relation to others negotiating difference/conflict in group.	Recognize own defences and resistances. Recognize and express reactions to the group. Learn to constructively confront issues. Work through conflicts and differences rather than withdraw or form subgroups.
Working High trust High group cohesion High productivity Interactive with willingness to take risks Supportive hopeful climate	Exemplify caring confrontation, disclosure of issues, and support to others. Encourage member risk taking. Interpret meanings of behaviours and interpersonal patterns in group. Explore group themes. Encourage translating insight into action in daily living.	Practise openness with issues. Offer feedback to others. Practise new skills and behaviours in daily life. Initiate constructive challenge and support to others. Initiate active involvement with others.
Final Stage Saying good-byes Reflection on learning, relations, changes made, and challenges ahead	Encourage saying of good-byes to each other. Provide opportunity for members to provide feedback to each other. Reinforce changes made. Ensure members have the resources to enable further progress. Reemphasize the importance of confidentiality.	Acknowledge thoughts and feelings with leaving the group. Say good-bye to each member and to the leader. Review gains made and complete unfinished business. Evaluate the impact of the group. Plan for the future.

Adapted from Corey, M., Corey, G., & Corey, C. (2013). *Groups: Process and practice* (8th ed.). Belmont, CA: Brooks/Cole.

Communication Network

Asking a colleague to observe and record the content and interaction is a useful technique in determining the interaction patterns within a group; the leader may also use an audio or video recorder. In some groups, one person may always change the subject when another raises a sensitive topic. One person may always speak after another. People who sit next to each other tend to communicate among themselves. By analyzing the content and patterns, the leader can determine the existence of communication pathways—who is most liked in the group, who occupies a position of power, what subgroups have formed, and who is isolated from the group. Burtis and Turman's (2006) network analysis for group discussion provides a way to diagram connections among members, frequency of connections, and interactional patterns. Usually, those who are well liked or display leadership abilities tend to be chosen for interactions more often than those who are less well liked (Fig. 14-1). In one study of communication networks, members who exhibited more dominant behaviours or who the group perceived as being dominant emerged as more central to the group's communication networks and both sent and received more messages. The study also found that the task at hand affects the communication network. Groups that worked on low-complexity tasks had more centralized communication than when they worked on high-complexity tasks (Brown & Miller, 2000).

Group Themes

Group themes are the collective socioemotional and conceptual underpinnings of a group and express the members' underlying concerns or feelings, regardless of the group purpose. Themes that emerge in groups

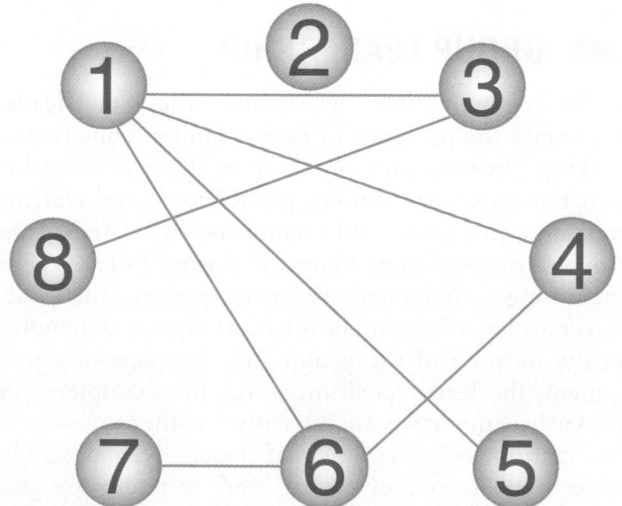

FIGURE 14-1. Network analysis of group discussion. In this analysis, response pattern was recorded during member interaction. Group members interacted with number 1 the most. Therefore, number 1 is the overchosen person. Numbers 5 and 7 are underchosen. Number 2 is never chosen and is determined to be the isolate.

help members to understand group dynamics. Different groups have different themes. For example, three themes emerged for a support group for grieving children, including vulnerability, the importance of maintaining memories, and the contribution of the group to the process of grieving (Graham & Sontag, 2001). Although some predictable themes occur in groups, the obvious or assumed themes at the beginning may actually wind up differing as the process continues. In one hospice support group, the members seemed to be focusing on the memories of their loved ones. However, upon closer examination of the thematic content of group interactions, the discussion was revolving around financial planning for the future.

Nonverbal Communication

Nonverbal communication is important to understanding group behaviour. All members, not just the group leader, observe the eye contact, posture, and body gestures of the participants. What is expressed is the result of individual and group, as well as internal and external, processes. For example, if one member is explaining a painful experience and another member looks away and tries to engage still another, the self-disclosing member may feel devalued and rejected because he or she interprets the disruptive behaviour as disinterest. However, if the leader interprets the disruptive behaviour as anxiety over the topic, he or she may try to engage the other member in discussing the source of the anxiety.

The leaders should remain attuned to the nonverbal behaviour of group members during each session and the effect on group climate and process. Often, one or two people can set the overall mood of the group. Someone who comes to a session very sad or angry can set a tone of sadness or anger for the whole group. An astute group leader recognizes the effects of an individual's mood on the total group. If the purpose of the group is to deal with emotions, the group leader may invite the member to discuss emotional issues at the beginning of the session. The leader thus acknowledges the mood of the one person experiencing it and encourages discussion regarding the effect on other group members. If the group's purpose is inconsistent with self-disclosure of personal problems, the nurse should acknowledge the individual member's distress yet set limits while maintaining the group focus. In this instance, the nurse would limit repeated episodes of self-disclosure from that member or others and redirect discussion to the group task.

Group Norms and Standards

Groups develop norms or rules and standards that establish acceptable group behaviours. Some norms are formalized, such as meeting as a group on time, but others are never really formalized. These standards encourage conformity of behaviour among group members. The group discourages deviations from these established norms. A group member has four options in relation to norms: conform, change the norm, be deviant, or leave the group (Posthuma, 2001). Open discussion that encourages healthy interaction while addressing unhelpful or problematic behaviours is one of the most successful ways of renegotiating group norms. *Leadership* is critical in establishing group norms consistent with the group goals to effect desired changes.

Group Cohesion

One of the goals of most group leaders is to foster **group cohesion**, a sense of "we-ness" as a group, with high levels of participation and involvement among members. Group cohesion is analogous to the therapeutic alliance in one-to-one relationships (MacKenzie, 1997). One of the first tasks of a good leader is to develop group cohesion through engaging all members in the group process. This involves close monitoring of the group atmosphere to develop a sense of belonging and commitment to the group goals. A particularly effective intervention for enhancing group cohesion is encouraging member-to-member interaction. In supportive and educational groups, leaders can promote social interaction with minimal supervision through organizing refreshment periods and team-building exercises. Cohesiveness is especially important in health education groups that focus on health maintenance behaviours such as exercise and weight control.

Dimock and Devine (1994) state that cohesion is like the glue that holds the group together and that if cohesion decreases, the group may begin to fall apart. Cohesion is a powerful force that motivates members and correlates with outcomes. In cohesive groups, members are committed to the existence of the group. In large heterogeneous groups, cohesiveness tends to be decreased, with subsequent decreased performance among group members in completing tasks. When members are strongly committed to completing a task and the leader encourages equal participation, cohesiveness promotes job satisfaction and higher performance (Steinhardt, Dolbier, Gottlieb, & McCalister, 2003). However, cohesiveness can be a double-edged sword. In very cohesive groups, members are more likely to transgress personal boundaries. Too much cohesiveness can exert powerful social pressure to conform to group standards with low tolerance for difference, while too little cohesiveness can result in mistrust, lack of engagement, and eventual disbanding of the group.

Groupthink and Decision Making

Groups that are strong and healthy encourage creativity, risk taking, differentiation, and change while remaining respectful of all members. Healthy groups encourage aligning with group norms and standards while remaining respectful of each member's unique contributions. However, if feelings of unity become too intense and members are overly invested in maintaining the status quo, the phenomenon of groupthink can occur. **Groupthink** is the tendency of group members to isolate as a group, avoid conflict, maintain homogeneity, and adopt a closed-mindedness that is often congruent with a lack of impartial group leadership (Janis, 1982; Myers & Anderson, 2008). With groupthink, striving for uniformity overrides realistic, fair and just appraisal of alternative courses of action. Members may not give honest feedback to each other for fear of censure. Catastrophes such as the explosion of the space shuttle *Challenger*, the Bay of Pigs invasion, and the Enron scandal have been attributed to groupthink, but the empiric evidence of the effects of groupthink in organizations is lacking. Studies have shown that a closed *leadership* style and an external threat, particularly time pressure, appear to promote symptoms of groupthink and defective decision making (Neck & Moorhead, 1995).

Nurse leaders are responsible for mobilizing **therapeutic factors** to support healthy group development and prevent a stagnating groupthink consensus. What factors to mobilize and when depend on the type, purpose, and stage of the group. Supportive factors often emerge spontaneously and include universality, altruism, hope, and acceptance (MacKenzie, 1997). Other therapeutic factors proposed by Yalom and Leszcz (2005) are imparting information, corrective recapitulation of the primary family group, development of socializing techniques, imitative behaviours, catharsis, existential factors, cohesiveness, and interpersonal learning (Box 14-1).

■ GROUP LEADERSHIP

In the beginning stage of a group, the group leader establishes the presence of each member; constructs a working environment; builds a working relationship with the group and among participants; and clarifies outcomes, processes, and commitments related to the group purpose (Corey, Corey, & Corey, 2013). While attempting to understand the group process, the leader also considers when and how to participate. Depending on the purpose of the group and the stage of development, the leader position shifts, for example, from primarily supportive to educative with provision of information to interpretive of group dynamics. The leader reflects on, evaluates, and responds to promote effective group work. Leader intervention skills include attention to process while considering timing of interventions, when to clarify and when to interpret, when to intervene with individuals, and when to intervene with the group as a whole. Various techniques

Research for Best Practice

USING THE CORE-R BATTERY TO IMPROVE GROUP PRACTICES

From Burlingame, G., Strauss, B., Joyce, A. S., MacNair-Semands, R., MacKenzie, R., Ogrodniczuk, J., et al. (2005). The American Group Psychotherapy Association's CORE Battery – Revised (CORE-R). New York: American Group Psychotherapy Association.

The Project: Collaborative project (Humboldt Foundation and the American Group Psychotherapy Association Research Special Interest Group) with the aim to revise and update the AGPA CORE battery (Clinical Outcomes Results Standardized measures), to develop clinically useful measures sensitive to patient change, to graph patient change, and to provide immediate feedback on patient status.

Questions: Does this group treatment work for this diagnostic category? What group treatment components are most important? Is this treatment working for this patient?

Method: Extensive review and metasynthesis of group literature from an empirical and a clinical perspective. The original CORE battery as well as AGPA Roy MacKenzie and Gary Burlingame course on group process and outcome instruments were reviewed. The CORE-R battery, an international tool to measure group processes and outcomes, was developed.

Findings: Meta-analysis indicates that empirically supported treatment techniques explain only 10% of patient improvement. The claim of superior outcomes on one treatment over another has little empirical support. Recommend evidence-based models coupled with patient-focused treatment that consider patient response and therapist variability. Specific areas addressed by the CORE-R battery include selection of patients for group; pregroup preparation; and an extensive, empirically validated selection of group process and outcome measures.

Implications for Practice: Clinical uses of the CORE-R *process measures* include gauging the quality of the group therapeutic environment, frequent process assessments to clarify the nature of group development over time, clarifying process dimensions that may be absent or negatively affect individual participants or the group as a whole, and increasing awareness of group dynamics. Clinical use of CORE-R *outcome measures*: It supplements clinical judgment, expands patient communication through written and verbal involvement, and provides ongoing feedback to the group leader regarding how much change as well as clinically significant changes.

and strategies enhance the leader's ability to lead the group effectively and help the group attain its goals (Table 14-3).

One of the most important group leadership skills is active listening. A leader who practises active listening provides group members with someone who is responsive to what he or she says. A group leader who listens also models listening behaviour for others, helping them improve their skills. Listening enables the leader to process events and track interactions. The leader should be able to listen to the group members and formulate responses based on an understanding of the discussion. Members may need to learn to listen to one another, track discussions without changing the subject, and learn to not speak while others are talking.

The leader tracks the verbal and nonverbal interactions throughout the group. Depending on the group purpose, the leader may keep this information private to understand the group process or may share the observations with the group. For example, if the purpose of the group is psychoeducational, the leader may use the information to facilitate the best learning environment. If the purpose of the group is to improve the self-awareness and interaction skills of members, the leader may point out patterns of interaction. The leader needs to be clear about the purpose of the group and tailor leadership strategies accordingly.

Understanding different group **leadership styles** can be useful in deciding which style fits which group situation. Leadership style is influenced by the group leader's personal characteristics and behaviours, theoretic background, and the group structure and purpose. Often leaders have a dominant style that fits more comfortably with who they are; however, developing a repertoire of different styles offers a wider range of interventions. Regardless of style, a leader remains fair and respectful, avoiding favouritism and encouraging participation and involvement of all members with each other. Other important skills include providing everyone with an opportunity to contribute and respecting everyone's ideas. A leader must also consider the degree of member disclosure warranted in each situation. In supportive and educative groups, leaders tend to be more expressive and interactive. A good rule of thumb in relation to leader self-disclosure is to consider whether the disclosure furthers the purposes of the group. A leader is responsible for understanding the intent and impact of leader self-disclosure on both individual members and the group as a whole. It is also assumed that a leader will engage in continuous learning through ongoing critical reflection with opportunity for regular supervision.

Some generally accepted guidelines in leading groups include establishing group structure and norms by setting start and stop times, arranging for the introduction of new members, and listening while other people talk. Leaders explain these group norms or rules at the first group meeting and continue structuring as an ongoing process. An important group rule is to always begin and end at the scheduled time. This sets a clear and reliable structure that helps reduce initial anxieties, educate members about group process, and encourage members to acquire skills that contribute to a successful group experience.

Typology of Leadership Styles

Whatever the leader's theoretic background, leadership styles can be viewed more traditionally as a continuum from direct to indirect, or, in keeping with contemporary

Table 14-3	Techniques in Leading Groups	

Technique	Purpose	Example
Support: giving feedback that provides a climate of emotional support	Helps a person or group continue with ongoing activities Informs group about what the leader thinks is important Creates a climate for expressing unpopular ideas Helps the more quiet and fearful members speak up	"We really appreciate your sharing that experience with us. It sounds like it was quite painful."
Confrontation: challenging a participant (needs to be done in a supportive environment)	Helps individuals learn something about themselves Helps reduce some forms of disruptive behaviour Helps members deal more openly and directly with one another	"Tom, this is the third time that you have changed the subject when we have talked about spouse abuse. Is something going on?"
Information and suggestions: sharing expertise and knowledge that the members do not have	Provides information that members can use once they have examined and evaluated it Helps focus group's task and goals	"The medication that you are taking may be causing you to be sleepy."
Summarizing: statements at the end of the session that highlight the session's discussion, any problem resolution, and unresolved problems	Provides continuity from one session to the next Brings to focus still-unresolved issues Organizes past in ways that clarify Brings to focus themes and patterns of interaction	"This session we discussed Sharon's medication problems, and she will be following up with her physicians."
Clarification: restatement of an interaction	Checks on the meanings of the interaction and communication Avoids faulty communication Facilitates focus on substantive issues rather than allowing members to be sidetracked into misunderstandings	"What I heard you say was that you are feeling very sad right now. Is that correct?"
Probing and questioning: a technique for the experienced group leader that asks for more information	Helps members expand on what they were saying (when they are ready to) Gets at more extensive and wider range of information Invites members to explore their ideas in greater detail	"Could you tell us more about your relationship with your parents?"
Repeating, paraphrasing, highlighting: a simple act of repeating what was just said	Facilitates communication among group members Corrects inaccurate communication or emphasizes accurate communication	*Member*: "I forgot about my wife's birthday." *Leader*: "You forgot your wife's birthday."
Reflecting feelings: identifying feelings that are being expressed	Orients members to the feelings that may lie behind what is being said or done Helps members deal with issues they might otherwise avoid or miss	"You sound upset."
Reflecting behaviour: identifying behaviours that are occurring	Gives members an opportunity to see how their behaviour appears to others and to evaluate its consequences Helps members to understand others' perceptions and responses to them	"I notice that when the topic of sex is brought up, you look down and shift in your chair."

Adapted from Sampson, E. & Marthas, M. (1990). *Group process for the health professions* (pp. 222–224). Albany, NY: Delmar.

literature, as transformational, authentic, and/or situational (Benson, 2010; Crowell, 2011). In the *direct leadership style*, the leader is actively authoritarian and controls the interaction by giving directions and information and allowing little discussion. The authoritarian leader literally tells the members what to do. On the other end of the continuum is *indirect leadership*, a form of laissez-faire, where the leader is primarily passive, reflects the group members' discussion, and offers little guidance or information to the group. Leadership is inadequate and lacking. Effective *group leadership* is flexible and considers the group task and when to intervene in situations that require attention. The challenge of providing leadership is to know what to do in specific situations so that the group and member goals can be met and group process furthered with enough freedom that members can make mistakes and recover in a supportive, caring learning environment. In transformational leadership, both leaders and members gain from one another, energized to perform beyond initial expectations (Grossman & Valiga, 2012), while authentic leadership promotes high ethical standards and relational transparency and instills powerful social processes that positively influence members and the group climate as a whole (Walumbwa, Luthans, Avey, & Oke, 2009). Nielsen (2013) examined the effect of leadership style on the occurrence of bullying in work groups. Laissez-faire leadership was associated with increased risk of exposure to bullying while transformational and authentic leadership was associated with less risk.

Selecting the Members

Individuals can self-refer or be referred to groups. The leader is responsible for assessing the individual's suitability to the group. In instances where a new group is forming, the leader preplans, sets criteria for group membership, and invites members with the aim that the group can be well functioning and beneficial for each member. The leader should consider the following criteria when selecting members:

- Does the purpose of the group match the treatment goals of the potential member?
- Does the potential member have the social skills to function comfortably in the group?
- Can the potential member make a commitment to attending group meetings?

Arranging Seating

Spatial seating arrangements contribute to group comfort and interactive group communication. Over time, group members tend to sit in the same places. Where a person sits may offer different insights into group interaction. For example, those who consistently sit close to the group leader may desire power more so than those who sit far away, or those sitting closer to the leader may feel safer. Arranging a group in a circle with chairs comfortably close to one another without a table focuses group work on relations with each other and on communication. In therapeutic interactive groups, no one should sit outside the group, as this often indicates exclusion and/or resistance. If a table is necessary, a round table is preferable to a rectangular one that spatially identifies two distinct positions of power for those who sit at the ends.

Ideally, the session is held in a quiet, pleasant room with no distractions, adequate space, and the assurance of privacy and confidentiality. Holding a session in too large or too small a room may inhibit engaged communication and a sense of comfort.

Intervening With Challenging Group Behaviours

Behaviours problematic to the group task can occur in all groups. They can be challenging to the most experienced group leaders and frustrating to new leaders. When intervening with any problematic behaviour or situation, the leader must remember to support the integrity of the individual members and the group as a whole. It is important for the group leader to consider what might be escalating difficult behaviours and to remember that challenging or deviant members may serve a function for the group (American Group Psychotherapy Association, 2007). This could include releasing uncomfortable tension, speaking the unspeakable, or deflecting anger. One of the simpler therapeutic interventions with difficult member behaviour is to describe what is observed and let the member know how it is affecting others (Corey, 2013).

Monopolizing Group Time

Some people tend to monopolize a group by frequent talking or interrupting others. This behaviour is common in the beginning stages of group formation and usually represents anxiety that the member displaying such behaviour is experiencing. Within a few sessions, this person usually relaxes and spends less time monopolizing the group. However, for some people, monopolizing discussions is an established interpersonal style that will continue. Other group members usually find the behaviour mildly irritating in the beginning and extremely annoying as time passes. Members may drop out of the group to avoid that person. The leader needs to decide if, how, and when to intervene. The best case scenario is when savvy group members remind the monopolizer to let others speak. The leader can then support the group in reinforcing rules that allow everyone the opportunity to participate. However, the group often waits for the leader to act. There are a couple of ways to manage the situation. The leader can interrupt the monopolizer by acknowledging the member's contribution but redirecting the discussion to others, or the leader can become more directive and limit the discussion time per member.

"Yes, But…"

Some people have a patterned response to any suggestions from others. Initially, they agree with suggestions others offer them, but then they add "yes, but…" and give several reasons why the suggestions will not work for them. Leaders and members can easily identify this patterned response. In such situations, it is best to avoid problem solving for the member and encourage the person to develop his or her own solutions. The leader can role model problem-solving behaviour for the other members and encourage them to let the member develop a solution that would work specifically for him or her.

Disliked Member

In some groups, members clearly dislike one particular member. This situation can be challenging for the leader because it can result in considerable tension and conflict. This person could become the group scapegoat, a phenomenon that requires therapeutic intervention (Clark, 2002). Depending on the group structure and purpose, one solution may be to move the person to a better-matched group. Whether the person stays or leaves, the group leader must stay neutral and avoid displaying negative verbal and nonverbal behaviours that indicate that he or she too dislikes the group member or that he or she is displeased with the other members for their behaviour. Often, the group leader intervenes by showing respect for the disliked member and acknowledging his or her contribution. In some instances, getting supervision from a more experienced group leader is useful. Defusing the situation may be possible by using conflict resolution strategies and discussing the underlying issues.

Group Conflict

Most groups experience periods of conflict. It is the avoidance of conflict that is problematic for a group. It is important that conflicts be acknowledged and the leader then decide how best to address the issues. Member-to-member conflict can be negotiated by using the conflict resolution process discussed in Chapter 11. Leader-to-member conflict is more complicated and often difficult for members to express because the leader has the hierarchical position of greater power. In this instance, the leader can use conflict resolution strategies, including encouraging members to directly express concerns, while remaining sensitive to the power differential. Group cohesion often increases as conflictual issues are effectively addressed.

■ TYPES OF GROUPS

Different types of groups are identified by the group goals and interactive processes or dynamics. The group leader assumes responsibility for ensuring group processes are in keeping with the group goals. Not every type of group is a therapy group.

Structured Groups

Structured groups have an explicit structure predetermined by the group leader. These groups are often short term, oriented to education, and focus on a specific theme such as smoking prevention, substance abuse prevention, stress management, self-esteem for children, and parenting skills. Group goals focus primarily on education, psychosocial skill development, and task completion.

Psychoeducational Groups

Psychoeducational groups are directed to specific concepts and teaching–learning aims. The process is primarily didactic with opportunity for questions, discussions, and activities related to the topic. The group leader primarily imparts information, promotes discussions, and facilitates experiential learning through structured activities. Psychoeducational groups include task groups that focus on completion of specific activities (e.g., planning a week's menu) and teaching groups that are used to enhance knowledge, improve skills, or solve problems. Other examples include medication groups, anger management groups, and stress management groups. Psychoeducational groups are formally planned, and members are purposefully selected. Members are asked to join specific groups because of the focus of the group. These groups are time limited and last for only a few sessions (Box 14-2).

BOX 14-2   **Research for Best Practice**

PSYCHOEDUCATIONAL CODEPENDENCY SUPPORT GROUPS FOR OLDER ADULTS

From McInnis-Perry, G. J., & Good, J. M. (2006). A psychoeducational codependency support group for older adults who reside in the community: Friends supporting friends. Journal of Gerontological Nursing, 32, *32–42.*

Question: What are the benefits of a psychoeducational support group for older adults with codependency issues?

Method: To promote well-being and reduce adverse effects of codependency among older adults, a pilot psychoeducational codependency support group curriculum was developed by the authors. A convenience sample of 22 older adults (age 65 years and older) who resided in an eastern Canadian community participated in six 90-minute psychoeducational group sessions held over a 2-month period. Most were females (68%). All participants had a loved one with an addiction (82% an adult child; 18% a spouse). A pretest and posttest were administered. Yalom's (1998) Therapeutic factors were used to evaluate the group process.

Findings: Results indicated that older adults do benefit from a psychoeducational support group format. Twenty-one participants demonstrated positive change post–group intervention. A majority improved on knowledge and learning of addictions, effective communication, and establishing healthy boundaries. Increased self-esteem, reduced personal isolation, and a reduction in codependency issues were seen. Some participants continued to struggle with finding ways to nurture self. Strengths of the group process included identification and support regarding the suffering of each in having an addicted family member, gain in information, the sharing of emotions, and the instillation of hope.

Implications for Practice: Using a time-limited psychoeducational group model to promote self-care for older adults who live in a codependent relationship can be effective. Providing a supportive group environment in which life experiences and coping strategies are shared allows older adults to work through sensitive and painful issues while supporting each other. Considerations for future research include using a larger sample size, a more diverse group of seniors, and standardized pretest and posttest instruments.

Cognitive–Behavioural Groups

The leader in cognitive groups identifies specific distorted thought patterns as the focus of change, whereas in behavioural groups, the leader targets specific behaviours to be modified. Cognitive and behavioural interventions may be combined to offer cognitive–behavioural group interventions. Cognitive interventions aim to modify distortions in attitudes and beliefs about self, the situation, and the future. Behavioural interventions modify behavioural excess, such as overly aggressive or sexual behaviour; behavioural deficits, such as social isolation or extreme passivity; and behaviours interfering with living, such as phobias and panic attacks (see Chapter 13). Cognitive–behavioural groups are often very structured with homework expectations for members.

Interactive Groups

Interactive groups include counselling and therapy groups. They may be focused and short-term or long-term experiential. Although some structure is predetermined by the group leader, group work primarily emphasizes dynamic, interactive group processes to allow for personal and interpersonal growth through experiential teaching and learning. The group becomes a microcosm of society. Group goals focus on addressing personal and interpersonal problems in living as well as modifying and changing more long-standing maladaptive patterns of behaviour.

Supportive Therapy Groups

Supportive therapy groups are usually less intense than psychotherapy groups and focus on helping individuals cope with their illnesses and problems as well as build interpersonal connections. Implementing supportive therapy groups is one of the basic functions of the PMH nurse. In conducting this type of group, the nurse focuses on helping members cope with situations that are common for other group members. Counselling strategies are used. For example, a group of patients with bipolar illness, whose illness is stable, may discuss at a monthly meeting how to tell other people about the illness or how to cope with a family member who seems insensitive to the illness. Family caregivers of people with mental illnesses benefit from the support of the group as well as additional information about providing care for an ill family member.

Psychotherapy Groups

Groups that rely primarily on interpretive interventions are known as group psychotherapies. Psychotherapy groups differ depending on the theoretic perspective, including psychodynamic, interpersonal, and existential. These groups focus primarily on increasing cognitive and emotional insight as well as on improving interpersonal relations to help members face their life situations. In group psychotherapy, "therapeutic change is an enormously complex process" (Yalom, 1998, p. 7). At times, these groups can be extremely intense. Psychotherapy groups provide an opportunity for members to examine and resolve psychological and interpersonal issues within a safe environment. Mental health specialists who have a minimum of a master's degree and are trained in group psychotherapy lead such groups. When providing nursing care, communication with the group therapist is important for continuity and collaboration of care.

Self-Help Groups

Self-help groups are led by lay people, often a mental health consumer who has experienced a specific problem or life crisis. These groups are generally structured, with supportive interaction among members. These groups do not explore psychodynamic issues in depth. Professionals usually do not attend these groups or serve as consultants. Alcoholics Anonymous, Overeaters Anonymous, and One Day at a Time (a grief group) are examples of self-help groups.

COMMON NURSING INTERVENTION GROUPS

Common intervention groups led by nurses include medication, symptom management, anger management, self-care, and reminiscence groups. In addition, nurses lead many other groups, including stress management, relaxation groups, and women's groups. The key, as a nurse, to being a good group leader is to critically select and modify group interventions to best accommodate the primary focus of therapeutic change in relation to the unique conditions of the setting and the group membership (Garrick & Ewashen, 2001).

Medication Groups

Nurse-led medication groups are common in psychiatric nursing. Not all medication groups are alike, so the nurse must be clear regarding the purpose of each specific medication group (Box 14-3). A medication group can be used primarily to transmit information about medications, such as action, dosage, and side effects, or it can focus on issues related to medications, such as compliance, management of side effects, and lifestyle adjustments. Many nurses incorporate both perspectives.

To determine what an individual would like to learn, it is important to assess a potential member's medication knowledge before he or she joins the group. People with mental illness may have difficulty remembering new information, so assessment of cognitive

---

BOX 14-3 Medication Group Protocol

Purpose: Develop strategies that reinforce a self-medication routine.

Description: The medication group is an open, ongoing group that meets once a week to discuss topics germane to self-administration of medication. Members will not be asked to disclose the names of their medications.

Member Selection: The group is open to any person taking medication for a mental illness or emotional problem who would like more information about the medication, side effects, and staying on a regimen. Referrals from mental health providers are encouraged. Each person will meet with the group leader before attending the group to determine if the group will meet the individual's learning needs.

Structure: Format is a small group, with no more than eight members and one PMH nurse group leader facilitating a discussion about the issues. Topics are rotated.

Time and Location: 2 to 3 PM, every Wednesday at the Mental Health Centre.

Cost: No charge for attending.

Topics:
- How Do I Know if My Medications are Working?
- Side Effect Management: Is it Worth it?
- Hints for Taking Medications Without Missing Doses!
- Health Problems That Medication Affects
- (Other topics will be developed to meet the needs of group members.)

Evaluation: Short pretest and posttest for the instructor's use only.

---

abilities is important. Assessing attention span, memory, and problem-solving skills gives valuable information that nurses can use in designing the group. The nurse should determine the members' reading and writing skills to select effective patient education materials.

An ideal group is one in which all members use the same medication. In reality, this situation is rare; typically, the group members use various medications. The nurse should know which medications each member is taking, but to avoid violating patient confidentiality, the nurse needs to be careful not to divulge that information to other patients. If group members choose, they can share the names of their medications with one another. A small-group format works best, and the more interaction, the better. Using a lecture method of teaching is less effective than involving the members in the learning process. The nurse should expose the members to various audio and visual educational materials, including workbooks, videotapes, and handouts. The nurse should ask members to write down information to help them remember and learn through various modes. Evaluation of the learning outcomes begins with the first class. Nurses can develop and give pretests and posttests, which in combination can measure learning outcomes.

Symptom Management Groups

Nurses often lead groups that focus on helping patients with severe and persistent mental illnesses. Handling hallucinations, being socially appropriate, and staying motivated to complete activities of daily living are a few common topics. In symptom management groups, prevention of relapse is often a focus. Members learn when a symptom indicates that relapse is imminent and what to do to avoid relapse.

Anger Management Groups

Anger management is another common topic for a nurse-led group, often in the inpatient setting. The purposes of an anger management group are to discuss the concept of anger, identify antecedents to aggressive behaviour, and develop new strategies to deal with anger other than verbal and physical aggression (see Chapter 19). The treatment team refers individuals with a history of being verbally and physically abusive, usually to family members, to these groups to help them better understand their emotions and behavioural responses. Impulsiveness and emotional lability are problems for many of the group members. Anger management usually includes a discussion of associated stressful situations, events that trigger anger, feelings about the situation, and unmet personal needs.

■■ SELF-CARE GROUPS

Another common nurse-led psychiatric group is a self-care group. People with psychiatric illnesses often have self-care difficulties and benefit from the structure that a group provides. These groups are challenging because members usually know how to perform these daily tasks (e.g., bathing, grooming, performing personal hygiene), but their illnesses cause a decrease in the motivation to complete them. The leader not only reinforces the basic self-care skills but also, more importantly, helps identify strategies that maintain motivation and provide structure to their daily lives.

Reminiscence Groups

Reminiscence therapy has been shown to be a valuable intervention for older adults. In this type of group, members are encouraged to remember events from past years. Such a group is easily implemented. Usually, a simple question about an important family event will spark memories. Reminiscence groups are typically associated with people who have dementia and are having difficulty with recent memory. Recalling distant memories is comforting to older people and improves well-being. Reminiscence groups can also be used in caring for people with depression (Jones & Beck-Little, 2002) and in conjunction with cognitive therapy for affective symptoms in older adults (Puentes, 2004).

SUMMARY OF KEY POINTS

■ The definition of group can vary according to theoretic orientation. A general definition of group is "a social system with structure, norms, and usual ways of doing things" (Dimock & Devine, 1994, p. 54). Group dynamics are the interactions within a group that constitute group development and process.

■ Groups can be *open*, with every session available to new membership, or *closed*, with membership determined at the first session. Leading a group, whether small or large, is complex because dynamics change depending on different sizes of groups and clinical conditions.

■ The group development process occurs in stages: beginning, middle (working), and ending (termination). These stages are not fixed but dynamic. Each stage challenges the leader to intervene in different ways. Success at the beginning stage prepares the group to take responsibility for addressing its purpose during the middle (working) stage.

■ Although there are only two formal group roles—leader and member—there are many informal group roles. These roles are usually categorized according to purpose—task functions, maintenance functions, and individual-centred roles. Members who assume task functions encourage the group members to stay focused on the group's task. Those who assume maintenance functions concern themselves more with the group working together than the task itself. Individual-centred roles can detract from the work of the group while member roles enhance group work.

■ Verbal communication includes the communication network and group themes. Nonverbal communication is more complex and involves eye contact, body posture, and mood of the group.

■ Nurse leaders are responsible for mobilizing therapeutic factors to support healthy group development and prevent a stagnating groupthink. What factors to mobilize and when depend on the type, purpose, and developmental stage of the group.

■ Seating arrangements affect group interaction. Fewer physical barriers, such as tables, improve potential for interactive communication. Everyone should be engaged as a member of the group and be invited to join in. Interactive groups should take place in a comfortable space with members facing one another in a circle arrangement.

■ Leadership skills involve active listening, tracking verbal and nonverbal behaviours, remaining fair and respectful, avoiding favouritism, and encouraging participation and involvement of all members with each other.

■ The leader should address challenges to the leadership, group process, or other members to determine whether to intervene and how. In some instances, the leader redirects a monopolizing member; at other times, the leader supports group members to provide feedback on the effects of the behaviour. Periods of group conflict occur in most groups during the transition from the beginning to the middle (working) phase.

■ There are many different types of groups. PMH nurses lead psychoeducational and supportive therapy groups. Mental health specialists trained to provide intensive therapy lead psychotherapy groups and cognitive–behavioural groups. Self-help groups are led by participants themselves, and professionals assist only as requested.

■ Medication, symptom management, anger management, self-care, and reminiscence groups are common nurse-led groups.

CRITICAL THINKING CHALLENGES

1 Group members are very polite to one another and are superficially discussing topics. You would assess the group as being in which phase? Explain your answer.

2 After three sessions of a supportive therapy group, two members begin to share their frustration with having a mental illness. The group is moving into which phase of group development? Explain your answer.

3 Define the roles of the task and maintenance functions in groups. Observe your clinical group and identify classmates who are assuming task functions and maintenance functions.

4 Observe a patient group for at least five sessions. Discuss the seating pattern that emerges. Identify the communication network and the group themes. Then identify the group norms and standards.

5 Discuss the conditions that lead to groupthink. When is groupthink positive? When is groupthink negative? Explain.

6 List at least six characteristics that are important for effective group leadership. Justify your answers.

7 During the first meeting, one member seems very anxious and tends to monopolize the conversation. Discuss how you would assess the situation and whether you would intervene.

8 At the end of the fourth meeting, one group member angrily accuses another of asking too many questions. The other members look on quietly. How would you assess the situation? Would you intervene? Explain.

REFERENCES

American Group Psychotherapy Association. (2007). *Practice guidelines for group psychotherapy*. New York: Sage.

Benne, K. & Sheats, P. (1948). Functional roles of group members. *Journal of Social Issues, 4*(2), 41–49.

Benson, J. (2010). *Working more creatively with groups* (3rd ed.). New York: Routledge.

Brown, T. & Miller, C. (2000). Communication networks in task-performing groups: Effects of task complexity, time, pressure, and interpersonal dominance. *Small Group Research, 31*(2), 131–157.

Burlingame, G., Strauss, B., Joyce, A. S., MacNair-Semands, R., MacKenzie, R., Ogrodniczuk, J., et al. (2005). *American Group Psychotherapy Association's CORE Battery—Revised (CORE-R)*. New York: American Group Psychotherapy Association.

Burtis, J. & Turman, P. (2006). *Group communication pitfalls: Overcoming barriers to an effective group experience*. Thousand Oaks, CA: Sage.

Canadian Interprofessional Health Collaborative. (2010). *A national interprofessional competency framework*. Retrieved from http://www.cihc.ca/files/CIHC_IPCompetencies_Feb1210.pdf

Clark, A. (2002). Scapegoating: Dynamics and interventions in group counseling. *Journal of Counseling & Development, 80*, 271–276.

Corey, G. (2013). *Theory and practice of group counseling* (8th ed.). Belmont, CA: Brooks/Cole.

Corey, M., Corey, G., & Corey, C. (2013). *Groups: Process and practice* (8th ed.). Belmont, CA: Brooks/Cole.

Crowell, D. (2011). *Complexity leadership: Nursing's role in health care delivery*. Philadelphia, PA: F.A. Davis.

Dimock, H. G. & Devine, I. (1994). *Making workgroups effective* (3rd ed.). North York, ON: Captus Press.

Garland, J., Jones, H., & Kolodny, R. (1973). A model of stages of development in social work groups. In S. Bernstein (Ed.), *Explorations in group work: Essays in theory and practice* (pp. 17–71). Boston, MA: Milford House.

Garrick, D. & Ewashen, C. (2001). An integrated model for adolescent inpatient group therapy. *Journal of Psychiatric and Mental Health Nursing, 8*, 165–171.

Graham, M. & Sontag, M. (2001). Art as an evaluative tool: A pilot study. *Art Therapy, 18*(1), 37–43.

Grossman, S. & Valiga, T. (2012). *The new leadership challenge: creating the future of nursing* (4th ed.). Philadelphia, PA: F.A. Davis.

Harpine, E. (2013). *Prevention groups*. Los Angeles, CA: Sage.

Harpine, E., Nitza, A., & Conyne, R. (2010). Prevention groups: Today and tomorrow. *Group Dynamics: Theory, Research, and Practice, 14*, 268–280.

Jacobs, E., Masson, R., & Harvill, R. (2009). *Group counseling strategies and skills*. Belmont, CA: Brooks/Cole.

Janis, I. (1982). *Groupthink* (2nd ed.). Boston, MA: Houghton-Mifflin.

Jones, E. D. & Beck-Little, R. (2002). The use of reminiscence therapy for the treatment of depression in rural-dwelling older adults. *Issues in Mental Health Nursing, 23*, 279–280.

Kottler, J. & Englar-Carlson, M. (2010). *Learning group leadership: An experiential approach*. Thousand Oaks, CA: Sage.

MacKenzie, R. K. (1997). *Time-managed group psychotherapy: Effective clinical applications*. Washington, DC: American Psychiatric Press.

McInnis-Perry, G. J. & Good, J. M. (2006). A psychoeducational codependency support group for older adults who reside in the community: Friends supporting friends. *Journal of Gerontological Nursing, 32*, 32–42.

McWhirter, P. & McWhirter, J. (2010). Community and school violence and risk reduction: Empirical supported prevention. *Group Dynamics: Theory, Research, and Practice, 14*, 242–256.

Myers, S. & Anderson, C. (2008). *The fundamentals of small group communication*. Thousand Oaks, CA: Sage.

Neck, C. P. & Moorhead, G. (1995). Groupthink remodeled: The importance of leadership, time pressure, and methodical decision-making procedures. *Human Relations, 48*(5), 537–557.

Nielsen, M. B. (2013). Bullying in work groups: The impact of leadership. *Scandinavian Journal of Psychology, 54*, 127–136.

Posthuma, B. (2001). *Small groups in counseling and therapy: Process and leadership* (4th ed.). Boston, MA: Pearson Education.

Puentes, W. J. (2004). Cognitive therapy integrated with life review techniques: An eclectic treatment approach for affective symptoms in older adults. *Journal of Clinical Nursing, 13*, 84–89.

Rutan, J. S. & Stone, W. N. (2001). *Psychodynamic group psychotherapy* (3rd ed.). New York: Guilford Press.

Sampson, E. & Marthas, M. (1990). *Group process for the health professions* (pp. 222–224). Albany, NY: Delmar.

Steinhardt, M. A., Dolbier, C. L., Gottlieb, N. H., & McCalister, K. T. (2003). The relationship between hardiness, supervisor support, group cohesion, and job stress as predictors of job satisfaction. *American Journal of Health Promotion, 17*(6), 382–389.

Tuckman, B. W. (1965). Development sequence in small groups. *Psychological Bulletin, 63*, 384–399.

Walumbwa, F., Luthans, F., Avey, J., & Oke, A. (2009). Authentically leading groups: the mediating role of collective psychological capital and trust. *Journal of Organizational Behavior, 32*, 4–24.

Yalom, I. D. (1998). *The Yalom reader: Selections from the work of a master therapist and storyteller*. New York: Basic Books.

Yalom, I. D. & Leszcz, M. (2005). *The theory and practice of group psychotherapy* (5th ed.). New York: Basic Books.

Zimmerman, J. & Winek, J. (2013). *Group activities for families in recovery*. Thousand Oaks, CA: Sage.

15 Family Assessment and Interventions

Peggy (Margaret) Simpson

LEARNING OBJECTIVES

After studying this chapter, you will be able to:

- Discuss the role families and caregivers provide in the support, advocacy, and recovery of people living with mental illness.
- Develop a genogram that depicts family history, relationships, and health patterns across three generations.
- Develop an ecomap to explore family networks of support that includes strengths and resources.
- Identify current family needs and concerns related to the mental illness.
- Develop a plan together with the family and health care team to address the identified family needs and concerns.

KEY CONCEPTS

- comprehensive family assessment
- family
- 15-minute family interview

KEY TERMS

- ecomap • extended family • family development • family life cycle
- family structure • genogram • nuclear family • resources
- strengths • transition times

M ental illness affects families across the life span. Currently, an estimated 1.2 million Canadian children and youth are affected by mental illness, and one in four Canadian seniors lives with a mental health problem or illness (MacCourt, 2013). The unique role of families is being recognized in promoting well-being, providing care, and facilitating recovery across the life span. Serious mental illness changes lives and relationships of families forever, and family involvement is vital to successful management of the mental illness (Marshall & Harper-Jaques, 2008; Nordby, Kjonsberg, & Hummelvoll, 2010; Ward-Griffin, Schofield, Vos, & Coatsworth-Puspoky, 2005).

Evidence suggests that family-based interventions reduce relapse rates and improve recovery of patients while increasing family well-being. Family-based interventions are shown to be effective for patients with schizophrenia, borderline personality disorder, alcoholism, bipolar disorder in adults and potentially beneficial for bipolar disorder in children. In outpatients with major depression, couples therapy is as effective as medication and often more acceptable to patients. This shows that

well-supported family caregivers play an important role in the recovery journey of their ill relative.

There are now Canadian National guidelines that provide recommendations for mental health services that recognize and address the needs of family caregivers of adults with mental health problems and illnesses (MacCourt, 2013). The purpose of this chapter is to provide an overview of key concepts from the recommendations as well as other sources to facilitate nurses in their work together with families suffering from mental illness. This chapter will include ideas on how to assess family needs and concerns and how to enhance family **strengths** and **resources** as they support the person in the recovery process.

CHARACTERISTICS OF CANADIAN FAMILIES

The portrait of Canadian families continues to change (Statistics Canada, 2011). In the last decade, while marriage and the traditional **family structure** remain important, there is more diversity in the way families are configured. Married couples continue to form the predominant family structure in Canada, accounting for two thirds of all families. Since 2006, there are more common-law couples and lone-parent families. Between 2006 and 2011, common-law couples outnumbered lone-parent families. The number of same-sex married couples nearly tripled, reflecting the first full 5-year period for which same-sex marriage has been legal across the country.

Living arrangements of children within Canadian families showed that two thirds of children aged 14 and under lived with married parents in 2011 and an increasing number lived with common-law parents. One in 10 children aged 14 and under lived in stepfamilies, while 0.5% of children in this age group were foster children in private households.

Over the past decade, more seniors aged 65 and over lived as part of a couple in a private household. During the same period, the proportion of senior women who lived alone declined, while it remained relatively stable for senior men. About 1 in every 12 seniors lived in a collective dwelling, such as a nursing home or a residence for senior citizens. These characteristics are important when we begin to conceptualize **family** in the current Canadian context.

Traditional definitions of family suggest that families are unique in that, unlike other organizations, they generally incorporate new members by birth, adoption, or marriage, and members leave only by divorce or death. Nuclear families were defined as two or more people living together and related by blood, marriage, or adoption. An **extended family** consisted of several nuclear families whose members may or may not live together but function as one group. A more inclusive definition that focuses on belonging, affection, and durability of the relationships in the context of a person's life is conceptualized by Wright and Leahey (2013) as "the family is who they say they are." Another way of conceptualizing family is a complex process where economics, emotion, context, and experiences are interwoven and multilayered (Doane & Varcoe, 2005). The last two conceptualizations seem to be an appropriate "fit" for the changing portrait of Canadian families.

Nurses interact with families in various ways. Because of the interpersonal and chronic nature of many mental illnesses, psychiatric and mental health (PMH) nurses may have frequent and long-term contact with families. Involvement may range from brief telephone contact to meeting family members face to face once or twice to treating the whole family as the unit of care. Families often share a unique history and investment in their relationships, caring for each other and promoting the welfare of family members. When one family member experiences a serious health issue, such as mental illness, the other members of the family often become caregivers. The caregiving role can

be challenging because of the unpredictable nature of many mental illnesses, the current barriers to family involvement in the mental health system, and the stigma associated with mental illness. In spite of such obstacles, family members fulfil an important role by providing support, advocating for the ill person, and contributing to the recovery process.

Nurses are obliged to provide family members with ongoing access to information, guidance, and support so that they may fulfil their caregiving responsibilities effectively and still enhance their own health and well-being. The Mental Health Commission of Canada (MHCC) (MacCourt, 2013) has national guidelines regarding support to family caregivers, recognizing that when well supported, they can enhance the recovery journey of their ill relative and improve his or her quality of life and do so with less caregiving stress than when unsupported. The unpaid care provided by family caregivers makes a major contribution to Canada's health and social service systems.

KEY CONCEPT **Family** is a group of people defined as "who they say they are" and involved relationally in a complex process where economics, emotion, context, and experiences are interwoven and multilayered (Doane & Varcoe, 2005; Wright & Leahey, 2013).

FAMILY CAREGIVERS

In 2002, a national survey was conducted of family caregivers, including those caring for people with mental illness. Characteristics of caregivers indicated that 70% are women; 60% are employed; 20% provide care not only to a person with a mental illness but also to another ill or disabled person, and 47% have been providing care for more than 5 years.

Caregiving takes time, energy, financial, emotional, and other resources. Families caring for adults living with mental illness may assist with shopping, banking, paying bills, preparing meals, housekeeping, monitoring symptoms, managing behaviours, situations and crises, and providing companionship and emotional and financial support. In addition, they may provide housing and transportation, personal safety and hygiene, guidance, encouragement, and motivation. They may provide childcare for the ill person. Caregivers often need to find services and resources for the ill member, advocate on their behalf, navigate the health and social services systems, and provide continuity of care through coordination and "case management." This often results in a high level of caregiver burden; it has been equated with burden reported by dementia caregivers (Hebert, Bravo, & Preville, 2000).

Meeting the Needs of Families

Family caregivers have not been consistently acknowledged or supported as partners in the ill person's recovery process. Rather, they often feel blamed for the problems and issues associated with the mental illness. They are confronted with issues that can arise when health care professionals must balance the family need for information and support with the rights of the individual suffering the mental illness. Family caregivers who participated in the development of national guidelines for services to support family caregivers of adults with mental illness identified several ways health care providers can address their needs (MacCourt, 2013). Families need to:

- Know their relative is receiving adequate care and services that facilitate his or her ability to achieve a reasonable quality of life.
- Have their relationships and caregiving roles recognized by mental health service providers.
- Be meaningfully involved in the assessment and treatment planning.
- Receive information, skills, support and services from knowledgeable mental health care providers, so they can effectively provide care to their relative.
- Receive family support and services to sustain their own health and emotional well-being.

Failure to address the needs of family caregivers increases their risk for developing mental health issues, compromises their physical health, and reduces the effectiveness of their support of their ill relative. Consequently, such failure increases costs to health and social service systems. On the other hand, enhancing caregiving capacity is clinically significant in terms of positive outcomes related to the relative's illness, family relationships with the ill person, improved medication adherence, fewer relapses, and fewer hospitalizations (Falloon, 2005; Miklowitz, George, Richards, Simoneau, & Suddath, 2003; Veltman, Cameron, & Stewart, 2002).

CONTEXTUAL ISSUES TO CONSIDER WHEN WORKING WITH FAMILIES

Access to Services

Families identify access to needed medical and social services as crucial to recovery. The social services include housing, income assistance, and legal and employment support. Information needs to be provided in an appropriate format and education level. It must be understandable to the family members.

Stigma

The stigma of mental illness can affect family members. They may delay seeking help, which may in turn increase their sense of isolation and decrease their ability to cope.

Diversity of Families

Canada is a multicultural and diverse society. Diversity includes ethnicity, cultural diversity, faith, gender, income, language, and sexual orientation. As these factors may influence a person's role and experience as a caregiver, nurses need to assess their effect, recognizing that social disparities and power imbalances may need to be addressed in the plan of care.

Diversity is also apparent in the characteristics of individual family members, including the individual experiencing mental illness. Life cycle stage, gender, age, type and severity of illness, and type of treatments may influence needs. Education and income will also play a role.

Based on Canadian census data (Statistics Canada, 2011), family configurations may be nuclear, blended, or extended. A family may have a single parent or be a lesbian, gay, bisexual, or transgendered (LGBT) family. If "family" is defined as "who they say they are," then those in the circle of care that protects the mentally ill individual and supports his or her independence may include unrelated individuals.

Determining the needs of families is a vital component of a comprehensive nursing assessment. When asked, families will let nurses know what has meaning, significance, and importance for them (Doane & Varcoe, 2005; Turner, Weiling, & Allen, 2004). Inquiring how the mental illness is influencing all members of the family will help the nurse understand the reciprocity between the illness and family functioning. In this way, nurses can gain understanding of the complex dynamics of familial context as it is shaped by culture. They can learn about the way a particular family thinks about and organizes themselves around their member's mental illness, including the way the illness is interpreted, symptoms are managed, and mental health care resources are accessed and used.

FAMILY ASSESSMENT

The Canadian national guidelines for services to support family caregivers of adults with mental problems and illness advocate a recovery-focused process (MacCourt, 2013). This means that caregivers as well as individuals with an illness are supported on their journey toward recovery and well-being. Principles in a recovery-focused approach include building relationships that foster hope, empowerment, self-determination, and responsibility. Five principles and values are outlined that are viewed as integral components of services. These include family engagement, respect and dignity, choice, determination

---

BOX 15-1 Family Mental Health Assessment

Family Name: _____

Family Members Present At Interview: _____

_____

_____

_____

Nurse Interviewer: _____

1. Referral route and presenting problem (include psychiatric diagnosis and current treatment) _____

_____

_____

2. Family composition (complete and attach a family genogram)
3. Family life cycle stage (include stage and any pertinent transitional issues)

_____

4. Pertinent history of the problem:
   a. Explore what the family's most urgent concerns or needs are at this point in time
   b. Explore the effects of the mental health concern on all family members
   c. Developmental history (including family of origin, health or medical events)
   d. Communication patterns (for solving day-to-day issues or problems)
   e. Previous solutions
   f. Ethnicity/culture
   g. Ecomap showing social supports (internal and external), including financial, housing, educational and legal resources
5. Strengths and problems (identify the family strengths, resources, and capabilities): _____

_____

_____

6. Summary (include urgent concerns and needs of family, strengths and resources, degree to which they wish to collaborate in care and discharge planning, any pertinent history, positive or negative relational patterns affecting illness symptoms, and preferred communication) _____

_____

7. Goals/plans (list interventions and family responses)

_____

_____

---

and independence, family caregiver needs, and family caregiver sustainability. These will be discussed in the context of a family nursing assessment model.

A comprehensive family assessment involves the collection of all relevant data related to family health, psychological and spiritual well-being, and social functioning. In this way, the nurse can identify problems, enhance family strengths, and generate solutions with the family to address their needs and concerns.

The assessment usually consists of a face-to-face interview with family members (although telephone- or videoconferencing may be an alternative) and may be conducted over several sessions. A comprehensive family assessment is appropriate when an individual is admitted to the hospital for psychiatric or mental health treatment. If the individual's admission status is voluntary and he or she is deemed competent to make treatment decisions, permission to contact the family is in order (Box 15-1). Providing support to family caregivers does not require patient consent as long as confidentiality of patient information is respected.

Engagement

In preparing for a family assessment, the nurse must take steps to promote a positive nurse–family relationship by enabling an atmosphere of trust, respect, dignity, and cooperation. This begins with the simple act of an introduction. The nurse provides an introduction by using his or her name and explaining his or her role for the meeting and the purpose of the meeting. During the meeting, the nurse calls the patient and family by name (Wright & Leahey, 2013). Many families do not know what to expect from the nurse, and this is the first step in decreasing their anxiety. Each family is unique and its needs, understanding

> **KEY CONCEPT** A **comprehensive family assessment** is the collection of all relevant data related to family health, psychological well-being, and social functioning to identify problems for which the nurse can generate solutions with the family and enhance family strengths.

of the situation, expectations for care, and previous experiences with the health care system are just some factors that should be explored at the beginning of a therapeutic relationship. More than the initial meeting may be necessary to build the relationship and complete the assessment.

The nurse must show understanding, competence, and caring. Listening to family members, valuing their contribution, acknowledging their knowledge and expertise, and addressing their immediate needs build confidence and trust with them. For example, a family that needs shelter or food is not ready to discuss a member's medication regimen until these basic needs are met. Families are encouraged to participate in the diagnosis, treatment, and recovery process of their ill family member, an approach that is balanced with the rights of that person that include privacy and confidentiality.

Genograms

Genograms are both engagement and assessment tools. The **genogram** is a structural assessment tool that may be used by the nurse to collect diverse information about the family members, their relationships, and health and illness patterns over time. The tool is simple to use, requiring only a pencil and paper, or alternatively some computer programs have this feature.

Genograms are schematic diagrams of families, listing family members and their relationships to one another. A genogram includes the age, dates of marriage/union and death, and geographic location of each member. Squares represent men and circles represent women; ages are listed inside the figures. Horizontal lines represent marriages/unions, with the date written on the line; vertical lines connect parents and children. Genograms can be particularly useful in understanding family history, composition, relationships, and illnesses (Fig. 15-1).

Genograms vary from simple to complex. The needs of the patient and family guide the level of assessment detail. In a small family with few concerns, the genogram can be simple. In a larger family with multiple concerns, the genogram can reflect these complexities. Nurses can explore important events such as marriages, divorces, deaths, and geographic movements in relation to the presenting concern. PMH nurses should always include mental health issues and other significant health problems in the genogram. Questions are more meaningful to the family if they are designed to address the family's particular area of concern rather than a general exploration. The nurse can begin the interview by explaining to family members they will be having a conversation, so the nurse can better understand their situation, their needs and concerns, and their family or support network. The genogram as a tool should be explained and the offer made to provide family members with a copy should they desire one.

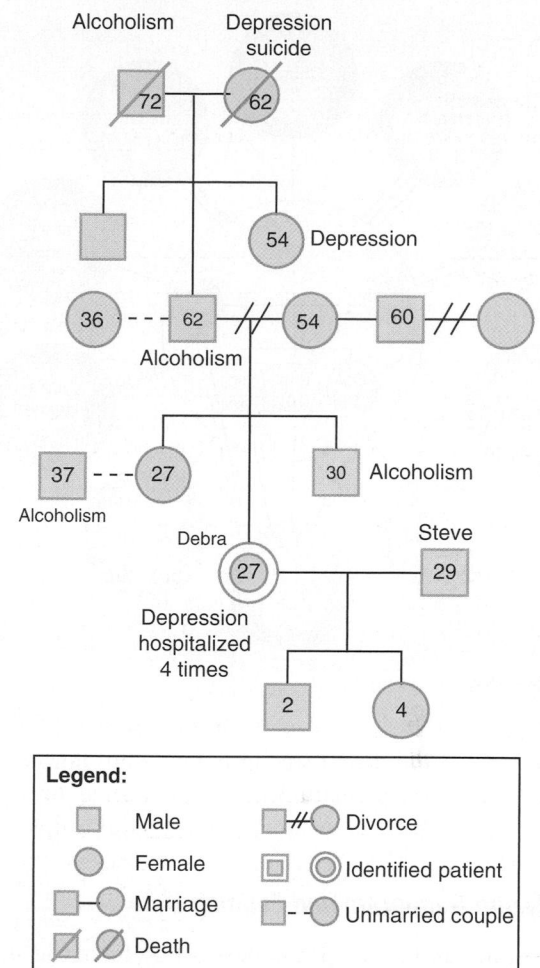

FIGURE 15-1. Analysis of genogram for Debra. Illness patterns are depression (maternal aunt and grandmother [suicide]) and alcoholism (brother, father, and grandfather). Relationship patterns show that parents are divorced and neither sibling is married.

Ecomap

The purpose of the ecomap is to explore the context for family living. The **ecomap** is a diagram of the way the family is linked to the community, culture, and resources (Fig. 15-2). This is particularly useful to determine current and past access to mental health inpatient or outpatient/community services, support networks, cultural or religious affiliations, education, employment, and housing. The ecomap can be used as a starting point to identify family needs as well as family strengths and positive connections in terms of promoting family health. It can be most informative early in the assessment process and can be used to plan for discharge. Family members can actively participate in working on the ecomap during the assessment phase.

The family genogram is placed in a centre circle and labelled family or household. Outer circles represent significant people, organizations, and service providers in the context for living. Lines are drawn from the family to the outside circle and indicate the nature of the relationship.

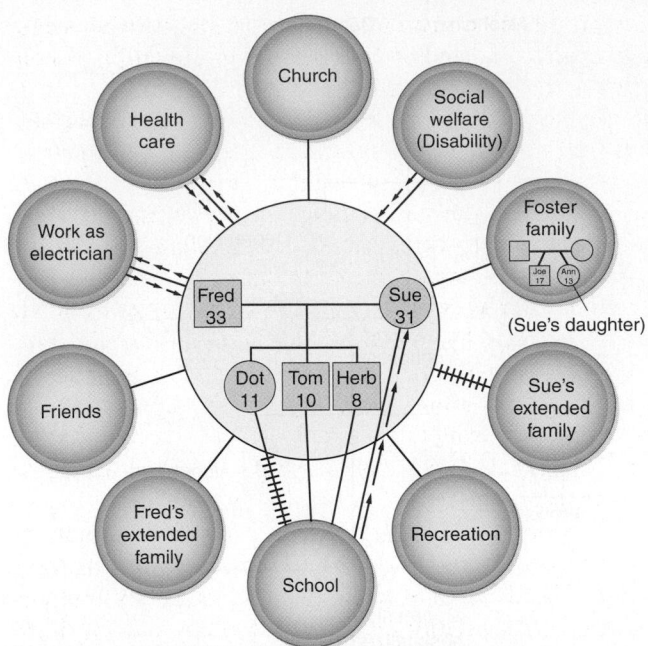

FIGURE 15-2. Ecomap.

Straight lines indicate a strong connection, dotted lines indicate a tenuous relationship, and slashed or jagged lines indicate stressful or nonexistent relationships.

Analyzing Genogram and Ecomap Data

Genograms and ecomaps can be most useful in the assessment when the nurse analyzes the data for family composition, patterns of mental health in the family, individual family needs, and relationship strengths and problems (particularly related to the mental health concern).

Nurses can begin with family composition. Who is considered to be family? How large is the family? Where do family members live? In what way do the family members show support? A large family whose members live in the same city may have more support than a family in which distance separates members. Of course, this is not always the case. The nurse could also study the genogram for relationship and illness patterns. Who in the family are closer and further apart? How might marriage and divorce influence the relationships? What illness patterns might be observed across relationships or generations? For example, depression, gambling, or alcohol addiction might be evident in past generations and may be risk factors for present and future generations. Exploring the significance and meaning of these health issues with the family is important. This can lead to conversations with the family about family strengths and solution strategies that they have tried. It can improve their understanding of health promotion and illness prevention related to family health risks.

The ecomap may be constructed to further explore family connections. The nurse may ask questions like

"What community agencies are you involved with now?" "Which are most and least helpful?" "How might you describe your work or school relationships?" "Which of your outside connections fosters your sense of well-being and gives you the most hope?" "What activities do you do, as a family, find rejuvenating?"

■ FAMILY ASSESSMENT IN THE BIO/PSYCHO/SOCIAL/SPIRITUAL DOMAINS

Biologic Domain

Family assessment includes discussion of family members' physical and mental health status and how they affect family functioning. A family with multiple health problems, both physical and mental, will be trying to manage the symptoms and treatments, as well as obtain the financial and health care resources it needs.

Directly and matter of factly, the nurse should ask the family to identify any members who have had or have a physical or mental illness. The nurse can record family health status information on the genogram. This may include current and past physical or mental illness and disabilities. Stresses currently placed on the family and its resources may be indicated in the ecomap and in narrative form. It is important for the nurse to explore how the physical and mental health problems are affecting family functioning. For example, if a member requires frequent visits to a provider or hospitalizations, the whole family may feel the effects of focusing more time and financial resources on that member.

Exploring a family's history and experience with a mental disorder must be approached with respect and sensitivity. In most cultures, mental health problems are associated with stigma and shame (Mental Health Commission of Canada, 2012). How and with whom families share information about their ill member varies greatly.

If family members do not know if there is a family history of mental illness, the nurse could ask if anyone was treated for "nerves" or had a "nervous breakdown." Overall, a comprehensive family history of mental illness across multiple generations helps the nurse understand the significance of mental illness in the current generation. If one family member has a serious mental illness, the whole family can be affected. Exploring how this is unique to each family is important to planning care.

Psychological Domain

Assessment of the family's psychological domain focuses on the family's development and life cycle, communication patterns, stress and coping abilities, and problem-solving skills. One aim of the assessment is to understand how family members communicate with each other as they negotiate developmental and life transitions, including illness. It is important in terms of the recovery process for the nurse to explore coping styles and problem-solving abilities of family members relevant to the management of both crisis and long-term issues associated with their relative's mental illness.

Family Development

Family development is a broad term that refers to all the processes connected with the growth of a family, including changes associated with its economic situation, geographic location, migration, acculturation, and serious illness. In optimal family development, family members are relatively differentiated (capable of autonomous functioning) from one another, anxiety is low, and individuals have good emotional relationships with their own families of origin.

Family Life Cycles

There is a distinction between family life cycles and family development (McGoldrick, Carter, & Garcia-Preto, 2011). Family development refers to the unique path a family makes and that is shaped by predictable and unpredictable events, such as illness or environmental disaster, and societal trends, such as an economic downturn. Family life cycle refers to a "typical" path most families go through related to the arrival and departure of family members through birth and death, couple unions and separations, and the raising and launching of children. It is important for PMH nurses to model inclusivity and respect for diversity of family forms.

As well as the traditional **nuclear family** of father, mother, and children, a family may comprise lesbian and gay couples, single parents and their children, or children raising children without a parent. The parents may be unmarried, separated, or divorced and the children, biologic, adopted, or fostered. The family may be extended, including several generations in the same home. The nurse's focus regarding family development is not on categorizing the family but rather on understanding the relational processes that occur as the family evolves and responds to its member's mental illness.

The **family life cycle** is a process of expansion, contraction, and realignment of relationship systems to support the entry, exit, and development of family members in a functional way (McGoldrick and Garcia-Preto, 2011) (Table 15-1). A family's life cycle is conceptualized in terms of stages throughout the years. To move from one stage to the next, the family system undergoes changes.

Structural and potential structural changes within stages can usually be handled by rearranging the family system (first-order changes), whereas transition from one stage to the next requires changes in the system itself (second-order changes). In first-order changes, the family system is rearranged, such as when the youngest child enters schooling and the stay-at-home parent returns to work. The system is rearranged, but the structure remains the same. In second-order changes, the family structure does change, such as when a member moves away from the family home to live independently. Families may be transitioning through more than one stage depending on the family configuration. As suggested, the nurse may use this model to explore potential areas of stress related to the family transitions. Multiple transitions can trigger or exacerbate symptoms of mental illness.

Transition times are any times of addition, subtraction, or change in status of family members. During transitions, family stresses are more likely to cause symptoms or difficulties. Significant family events, such as the death of a member or the introduction of a new member, also affect the family's ability to function. During these times, families may need help from the mental health system.

Diversity

Given Canada's multicultural climate, it is important for nurses in psychiatric settings to consciously attend to diversity. One method for increasing sensitivity to culture has been by trying to identify distinctive characteristics or responses to life cycle transitions or disruptions such as mental illness within specific ethnic communities. Becoming conscious of the characteristics of particular ethnic groups is an important step toward developing an appreciation for diversity, as long as these norms are remembered to be gross generalizations. Labelling and categorizing ethnic groups' behaviours according to general rules can help raise our awareness of difference, but it can equally obscure the uniqueness of each family that we encounter. For the nurse, appreciating and validating ethnic differences, while at the same time acknowledging similarities, can feel like a delicate balancing act. Nurses must be mindful of the personal biases they bring to their practice. In the clinical example provided in Box 15-2, a particular generalization is at play in the description of Judy's rich familial connections and her location in a particular geographic region of Canada. This is another example of a cultural assumption.

Developing sensitivity to one's own beliefs about what constitutes normalcy and functionality in a family is a challenging and important endeavour. It is only in this process of self-reflection that the nurse will develop an awareness of the cultural norms and values that are guiding and creating the template against which the nurse is judging and assessing even the family life cycle (Doane & Varcoe, 2005). It is the dominant, white, middle-class,

Table 15-1	Stages of the Family Life Cycle	
Family Life Cycle Stage	**Emotional Transition**	**Required Family Changes**
1. Leaving home: emerging young adults	Accepting emotional and financial responsibility for self	Differentiation of self in relation to family of origin Development of intimate peer relationships Establishment of self regarding work and financial independence Establishment of self in community and larger society Spirituality
2. The joining of families through marriage/union	Commitment to new system	Formation of partner systems Realignment of relationships with extended family, friends, and larger community and social system to include new partners
3. Families with young children	Accepting new members into the system	Adjusting couple system to make space for children Collaboration in child-rearing, financial, and housekeeping tasks Realignment of relationships with extended family to include parenting and grandparenting roles Realignment of relationships with community and larger social system to include new family structure and relationships
4. Families with adolescents	Increasing flexibility of family boundaries to include children's independence and grandparents' frailties	Shifting of parent–child relationships to permit the adolescent to move in and out of system Refocus on midlife couple and career issues Beginning shift toward caring for older generation Realignment with community and larger social system to include shifting family of emerging adolescent and parents to new formation of relating
5. Launching children and moving on at midlife	Accepting multitude of exits from and entries into the system	Renegotiation of couple system as a dyad Development of adult–adult relationships between grown children and parents Realignment of relationships to include in-laws and grandchildren Realignment of relationships with community and a larger social system to include new structure and constellation of family relationships Exploration of new interests/career given the freedom from childcare responsibilities Dealing with care needs, disabilities and death of parents (grandparents)
6. Families in middle age	Accepting the shifting of generational roles	Maintaining own and or couple functioning and interests in face of psychological decline, exploring new familial and social role options Support for a more central role of middle generation Realignment of the system in relation to community and a larger social system to acknowledge changed pattern of family relationships of this stage Making room in the system for the wisdom and experience of the elders Supporting the older generation without overfunctioning for them
7. Families nearing the end of life	Accepting the realities of limitations and death and the completion of one cycle of life	Dealing with loss of spouse, siblings, and other peers Making preparations for death and legacy Managing reversed roles in caregiving between middle and older generations Realignment of relationships with a larger community and social system to acknowledge changes in the life cycle relationship

BOX 15-2 John and Judy Jones

John and Judy Jones were married 3 years ago, after their graduation from a small University in Eastern Canada. Judy's career choice required that she live on the East Coast, where she would be near her large family. John willingly moved with her and quickly found a satisfying position. After about 6 months of marriage, John became extremely irritable and depressed. He kept saying that his life was not his own. Judy was very concerned but could not understand his feelings of being overwhelmed. His job was going well, and they had a very busy social life, mostly revolving around her family, whom John loved. They decided to seek counselling and completed the genogram below.

After looking at the genogram, both John and Judy began to realize that part of John's discomfort had to do with the number of family members who were involved in their lives. Judy and John began to redefine their social life, allowing more time with friends and each other.

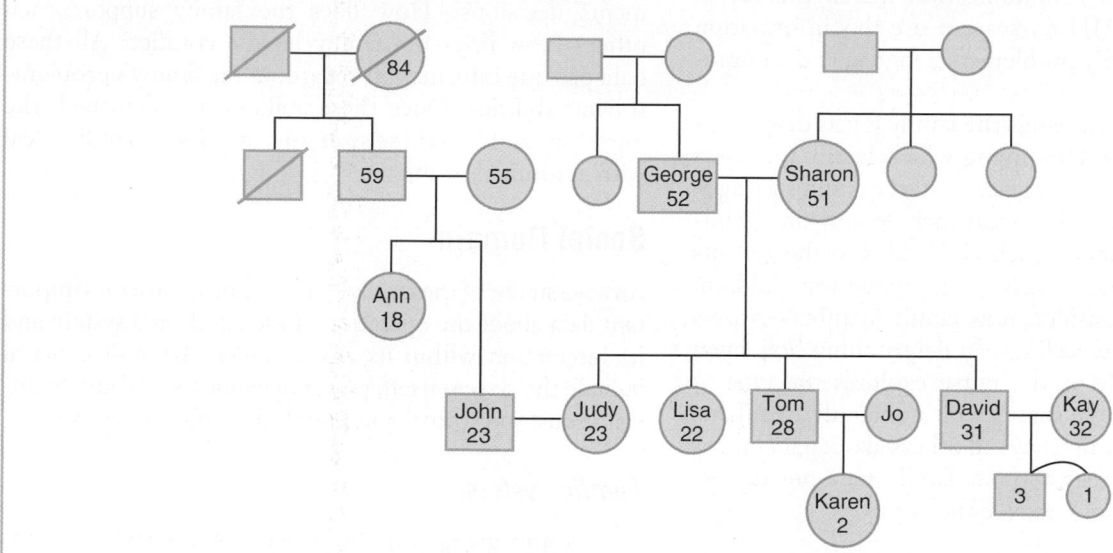

cultural rules that generally become the gold standard, the norm against which all other ethnic groups are measured and assessed. This can be problematic if the nurse is not aware of the power, and hence oppression, that might accompany these norms. Developing and maintaining sensitivity to ethnicity, culture, and power are important in helping the nurse to recognize issues of diversity (see Chapter 3).

Low-Income Families

Rates of psychological distress and mental disorders, including that of substance-related disorders and addiction, are much higher in the low-income population. These differences are statistically consistent across the Canadian sociodemographic strata: region/province, gender, age, marital status, immigration, first language, and ethnic origin (Caron & Liu, 2010). People living in poverty struggle to make ends meet, and family members may face difficulties in meeting their own or other members' basic developmental needs. They may be homeless or living in unsafe conditions. To be poor does not mean that a family is dysfunctional, but poverty is an important factor that can force even the healthiest families to crumble.

The life cycle may be condensed, such that family members leave their home, mate, have children, and become grandparents at much earlier ages than their working-class and middle-class counterparts do. Consequently, many individuals in such families assume new roles and responsibilities before they are developmentally capable. The condensed life cycle creates adolescents whose educational opportunities are compromised (no time to complete school given the family demands), limiting their employment skills. The cycle of poverty is thus reinforced.

Families living in poverty are subject to disruption via abrupt loss of members, loss of unemployment compensation, illness, death, imprisonment, or alcohol or drug addiction. Men may die relatively young compared with their middle-class counterparts. Ordinary problems, such as transportation or a sick child, can become major crises because of a lack of resources.

Reliance on institutional supports is another distinguishing characteristic of families in poverty. Poor families are often forced to seek public assistance, which ultimately can result in additional stress in having to deal with a governmental agency.

Communication Patterns

Family communication patterns develop over a lifetime. Some family members communicate more openly and freely than others. In addition, family subgroups may have unique communication patterns with one another. During the assessment, the nurse should observe the verbal and nonverbal communication of the family members. Who sits next to each other? Who talks to whom? Who answers most questions? Who volunteers information? Who changes the subject? Which subjects seem acceptable to discuss? Which topics are not discussed? How are partners intimate with each other? How are the family secrets or sensitive topics revealed? Does the nonverbal communication match the verbal communication? PMH nurses can use this information to help identify family problems, strengths, and communication issues.

Nurses should also assess the family for its daily communication patterns. Identifying which family members confide in one another is a place to start examining ongoing communication. Other areas include how often children talk with parents, which child talks to the parents most, and who is most likely to discipline the children. Another question considers how family members express positive and negative feelings. In determining how open or closed the family is, the nurse explores the type of information the family shares with nonfamily members. For example, one family may tell others about a member's mental illness, whereas another family may not discuss any illnesses with those outside the family.

Stress and Coping Abilities

One of the most important assessment tasks is to determine how family members deal with major and minor stressful events and their available coping skills. Some families seem able to cope with overwhelming stresses, such as the death of a member, major illness, or severe conflict, whereas other families seem to fall apart over relatively minor events. It is important for the nurse to listen to which situations a family appraises as stressful and help the family identify usual coping responses. The nurse can then evaluate these responses. Identifying what the family does well and acknowledging the family for these strengths are important. If the family's responses are detrimental to health (e.g., substance abuse, physical abuse), the nurse may discuss the need to develop coping skills that lead to family well-being (see Chapter 17).

● **STUDY NOTE**

Consider the following two questions.

How might a family transitioning through various life cycle stages experience the emotional process and second-order changes when one family member is experiencing an acute mental illness episode?

How might a family be affected when several life cycle stages are interrupted at the same time? For example, the death of a parent, job loss, and separation from a partner?

Problem-Solving Skills

Nurses assess family problem-solving skills by focusing on the more recent problems the family has experienced and determining the process that members used to solve them. For example, a child is sick at school and needs to go home. Does the mother, father, grandparent, or babysitter receive the call from the school? Who then cares for the child? Underlying the ability to solve problems is the decision-making process. Who makes and implements decisions? How does the family support each other? How does the family handle conflict? All these data provide information regarding the family's problem-solving abilities. Once these abilities are identified, the nurse can build on these strengths in helping families deal with additional problems.

Social Domain

An assessment of the family's social domain provides important data about the operation of the family as a system and its interaction within its environment. Areas of concern include the system itself, power dynamics, social and financial status, and formal and informal support networks.

Family Systems

Just as any group can be viewed as a system, a family can be understood as a system with interdependent members. Family system theories view the family as an open system whose members interact with their environment as well as among themselves. One family member's change in thoughts or behaviour can cause a ripple effect and change everyone else's. For example, a mother who decides to reinforce her child's positive efforts rather than focusing on negative actions may notice a change in the child's behaviour, which may in turn result in a reduction of the stress she feels when interacting with the child.

One common scenario in the mental health field is the effect of a patient's improvement on the family. With new medications and treatment, patients are more likely to be able to live independently, which subsequently changes the responsibilities and activities of family caregivers. Although family members may be relieved that their caregiving burden is lifted, they will be also adjusting to changes in the demands on their time and energies. This transition may not be easy because it is often less stressful to maintain familiar activities than to venture into uncharted territory. Families may seem as though they want to keep an ill member dependent but, in reality, they are struggling with the change in their family system.

The Calgary Family Assessment Model (CFAM) and the Calgary Family Intervention Model (CFIM) are Canadian family nursing models that have been implemented successfully in mental health care settings (Leahey & Harper-Jaques, 2010; Marshall, Bell, & Moules, 2010). They are relational practice nursing models based on postmodernism, systems, cybernetics, communication and change theories, and the biology of cognition (Wright & Leahey, 2013). These two models are multidimensional frameworks that conceptualize the family into structural, developmental, and functional categories. Each assessment category contains several subcategories. Structure is further categorized into internal (family, gender, sexual orientation, etc.), external (extended family and larger systems), and contextual (ethnicity, race, social class, religion, spirituality, environment). Family developmental assessment is organized according to stages, tasks, and attachments. Functional assessment areas include instrumental (activities of daily living) and expressive (communication, problem solving, roles, beliefs, influence, power, and alliances).

When the nurse uses CFAM/CFIM, relational practice develops and evolves during four stages: engagement, assessment, intervention, and termination. The nurse and the family are partners in care as each brings specialized expertise in managing health problems, as well as strengths and resources, to the relationship.

The *engagement* stage is the initial stage in which the family is greeted and made comfortable. In the *assessment* stage, needs are identified and relationships develop between family and health providers. During this stage, the nurse invites the family to tell its story. The nurse asks key questions and listens to the patient's and family members' expectations, hopes, questions, and ideas. The *intervention* stage is the core of the clinical work and involves providing a context in which recovery is facilitated (see Family Interventions section in this chapter). The nurse communicates regularly with the family to provide cognitive and emotional support. The *termination* phase refers to the process of evaluating the family interviews, recognizing the family efforts in their recovery journey, providing referrals if necessary, and, depending on the family's needs, extending an invitation for further interviews. The role of the family in promoting well-being and providing care to their loved one is to be recognized and their needs to be supported (Mental Health Commission of Canada, 2009).

Perspectives on Understanding Families

PMH nurses are looking to the ideas of postmodernism and social constructivism to enrich their understanding of families. These ideas support exploring how families make meaning in their lives and how they construct their reality in relation to their social environment. For instance, the constructivist influence invites PMH nurses to understand that what they are seeing is a product of their own assumptions about people, families, and problems and their interactions with families. It is recognized that people are highly influenced by their current relationships and the environments in which they perceive their realities. Persons with mental illness and their families should therefore be encouraged to express their perspectives (their own

"truth") on their situation. Nurses need to be respectful of family stories and viewpoints, within the parameters of values about human safety and rights, including self-determination and protection from interpersonal violence.

PMH nurses are also using a critical lens derived from feminist, poststructural, and postcolonial theories that support considerations of power, oppression, culture, economic conditions of life, social change, and emancipation. This critical perspective draws the nurse's attention to the sociopolitical, economic, and linguistic contexts within which families are situated and constituted. The focus can then be on exposing underlying sociopolitical structures that are advantaging some people/families and disadvantaging others. The goals are to explore social conditions and revise structures in ways that address inequities.

Social and Financial Status

Social status is often linked directly to financial status. The nurse should identify the occupations of the family members. Who works outside the home and inside the home? Who is primarily responsible for the family's financial support? Families of low social status are more likely to have limited financial resources, which can place additional stresses on the family. This information can be recorded on the ecomap and in narrative form. Nurses can use information on the family's financial status to determine whether to refer the family to social services.

Formal and Informal Support Networks

Networks both formal and informal are important in providing support to individuals and families. These networks are the links among the individual, family, and the community. Assessing the extent of formal support (e.g., hospitals, agencies) and informal support (e.g., extended family, friends, and neighbours) gives a clearer picture of the availability of support. In assessing formal support, the nurse could ask about the family's involvement with government institutions and self-help groups such as Alcoholics Anonymous. Assessing the informal network is particularly important in cultural groups with extended family networks or close friends, because these individuals can be major sources of support to patients. This is important information to include in the ecomap. If the nurse does not ask about the informal network, these important people may be missed. Nurses can inquire whether family members volunteer at schools, local hospitals, or nursing homes. They can also ask whether the family attends religious services or activities.

Spiritual Domain

Families may find that their spiritual or religious beliefs and practices help promote their recovery by helping them to understand their experiences while strengthening their sense of meaning and purpose. For many families, their religious affiliations will play a key role in their everyday lives. These affiliations can influence the family's understanding of health and illness and of healing and treatment. Religious and spiritual practices can foster family and community support and may be a major resource to families. It is increasingly recognized that, in all faith groups, the help and guidance of clergy are frequently sought by families who have a mentally ill member (Aaron, 2008). Yet, research suggests that a majority of clergy (Christian clergy were studied) feel inadequate regarding their knowledge of mental illness (Farrell & Goebert, 2008). Unfortunately, mental health professionals do not tend to view clergy collaboratively (Leavey, Lowenthal, & King, 2007). Collaboration, however, could be of significant use to both groups, especially to individuals and families requiring assistance. Clergy can provide community-based support and assist health professionals, such as nurses, to understand patients' beliefs, which is important to informing treatment planning and to improving response to crisis. Nurses and colleagues in turn can assist clergy to understand mental disorders and mental health problems and their treatment. Open communication can facilitate, for instance, appropriate use of complementary healing practices that can be a part of a group's religious beliefs. It may promote better trust in psychiatric treatment and care.

In addressing the spiritual domain of family nursing, it is important for the PMH nurse to recognize that family members may differ widely in their religious beliefs and approach to spirituality. Such variation among members' perspectives, if it exists, should inform the family assessment. It may be a source of enrichment or distress, or both, for the family.

■■ THE PYRAMID OF FAMILY CARE FRAMEWORK

The pyramid of the Family Care Framework, in the MHCC's national guidelines, identifies five levels of tasks for meeting the support needs of family caregivers (MacCourt, 2013). As one moves from the bottom to the top of the pyramid, the intensity of family intervention increases while the number of families who require the intervention decreases (Fig. 15-3). Nurses have the knowledge, skill, and competency to provide these services based on their level of education and advanced practice.

Levels 1 (*connection and assessment*) and 2 (*general education*) indicate the minimum level of service that should be available to all family caregivers. The need for level 1 and level 2 interventions should be assessed at each point of contact. One of the most important family interventions is education and health teaching related to the mental illness. As families have a central role in the treatment of mental illnesses, members need to learn about mental disorders, medications, actions, side effects, and overall

treatment approaches and outcomes. For example, families are often reluctant to have members take psychiatric medications because they believe the medications will "drug" the patient or become addictive. The family's beliefs about mental illnesses and treatment will often affect how patients manage their illness.

Level 3 (*family psychoeducation*) refers to interventions in which recommendations are made to the family caregivers regarding coping strategies or specific ways to deal with the challenges of the mental illness. Level 4 (*consultation*) may be required by family caregivers with significant challenges in supporting an individual living with mental illness. Level 5 (*family therapy*) refers to interventions that work on family relationships and is designed to facilitate change in the family interactional system. Family therapy is useful for families who are having difficulty maintaining family integrity. Various theoretical perspectives are used in family therapy: more recently, therapies influenced by postmodernism, hermeneutics, and social constructionism have developed. These focus on collaborative, conversational approaches and narrative and solution-based therapies. Family therapy can be short term or long term and is conducted by mental health specialists, including advanced practice PMH nurses. Few families require level 4 or 5.

■■ FAMILY INTERVENTIONS

Each conversation the nurse has with a family member can be meaningful and healing, and it can effect change in the patient's and the family members' bio/psycho/social/spiritual integrity and functioning. Families with loved ones suffering from mental illness have reported that even a short meaningful conversation with a health care professional is significant (Box 15-3). Therapeutic conversation in a brief family interview is purposeful and time limited. It is an opportunity to acknowledge and affirm the illness experience and patient and family expertise. Listening to the illness story is part of ethical nursing practice. Nurses have an opportunity to focus the conversations using language of recovery and strength while still addressing the needs and concerns of the family. In therapeutic conversation, information sharing, emotional support, and patient and family involvement in decision making can take place. Efforts should be made to enhance the family's choice, determination, and independence.

The "15-minute family interview" has been used effectively as a framework for family intervention. It is being evaluated in psychiatric care settings. The following are some specific ideas for conducting a healing, productive, and efficient 15-minute family interview. They are condensed ideas from the CFAM & CFIM (Wright & Leahey, 2013) and consist of five key components: manners, therapeutic conversations, genogram and ecomap, therapeutic questions, and commending individual and family strengths.

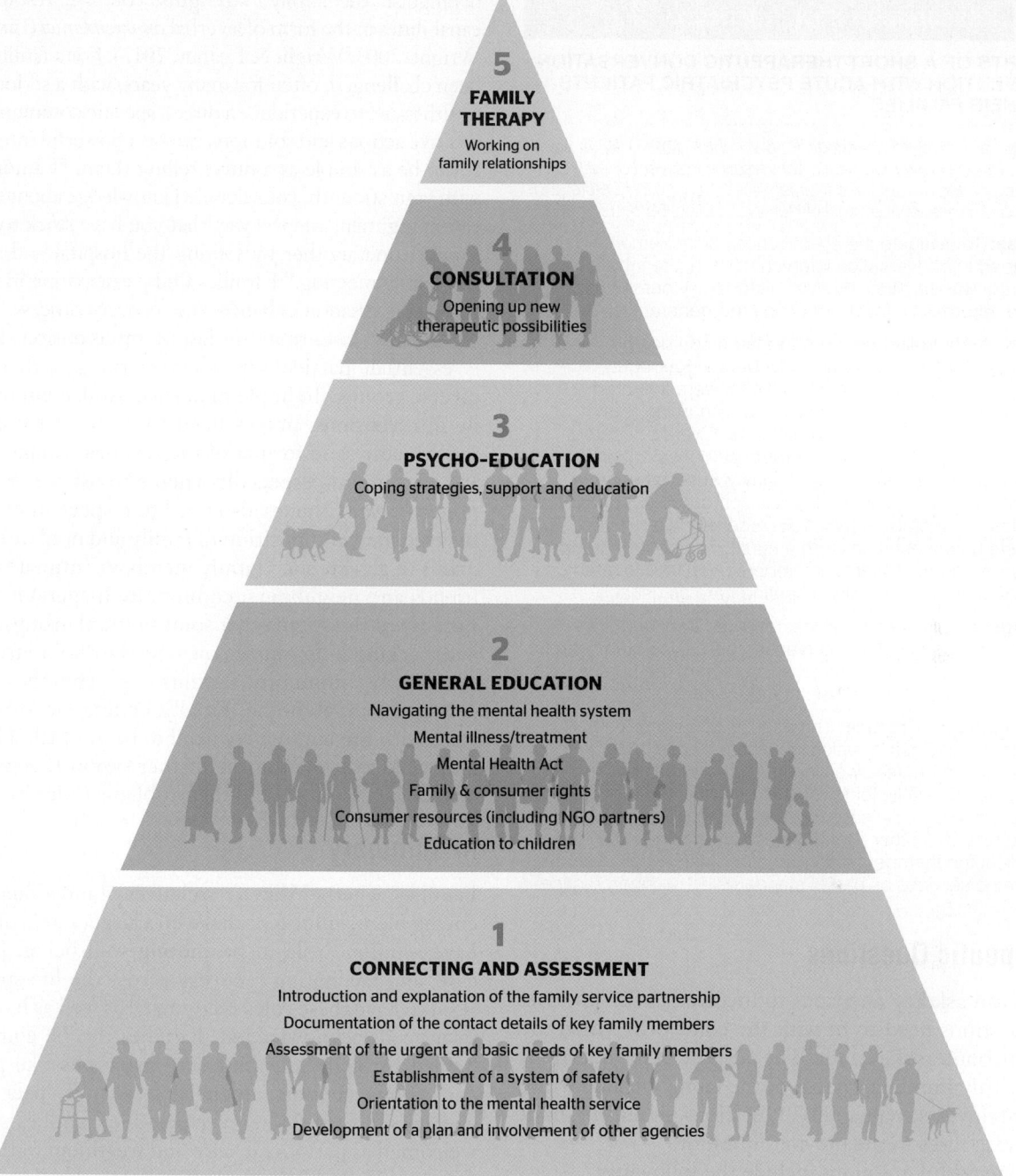

FIGURE 15-3. Pyramid of family care framework. (From: Mottaghipour, Y. & Bickerton, A. (2005). The Pyramid of family care: A framework for family involvement with adult mental health services. *Australian e-Journal for the Advancement of Mental Health*, 4(3), 210–217.)

- Begin the therapeutic conversation with a purpose in mind that can be accomplished in the period you will be together with the family.
- Use manners to engage with the family by first introducing yourself with your name and your role.
- Provide a brief overview about the purpose of the interview.
- Assess, with a genogram and ecomap, the key areas of internal/external structure, function, and relationships.
- Identify family needs or concerns by asking key therapeutic questions.

- Commend the family on one or two strengths.
- Evaluate the usefulness of the meeting, and conclude the conversation.

KEY CONCEPT The 15-minute family interview is an assessment/intervention framework that consists of five key components: manners, therapeutic conversations, genogram and ecomap therapeutic questions, and commending individual and family strengths.

BOX
15-3 **Research for Best Practice**

BENEFITS OF A SHORT THERAPEUTIC CONVERSATION INTERVENTION WITH ACUTE PSYCHIATRIC PATIENTS AND THEIR FAMILIES
....
Sveinbjarnardottir, E, Svararsdottir, E., & Wright, L. (2013). What are the benefits of a short therapeutic conversation intervention with acute psychiatric patients and their families? A controlled before and after study. International Journal of Nursing Studies, 50(5), 593–602.

Purpose: To evaluate the effectiveness of implementing a therapeutic conversation intervention in acute inpatient psychiatry with families, by evaluating family perceived support, expressive family function, and general well-being.

Method: A controlled before-and-after study design was used. Patients and family members at four acute psychiatric units at a university hospital were selected for the implementation of family systems nursing (FSN). The nurses on one acute psychiatric unit were educated, trained, and supervised in a therapeutic conversation intervention built on the Calgary Family Assessment and Interventions models. In the intervention group, 68 patients and 68 family members (N = 136) received two to five therapeutic conversations with a nurse. The control groups of 74 patients and 74 family members (N = 148) located on the three other units received nursing care as usual.

Findings: Family members who received the short therapeutic conversation intervention perceived significantly higher cognitive and emotional support from the nurses than family members who received standard care.

Implications for Practice: The benefits of a specific short-term therapeutic conversation intervention are evident and valuable for nurses working in acute psychiatry. These positive results for families of psychiatric patients should encourage clinical educators, clinical nurses, nurse researchers, and other health professionals to develop and implement the therapeutic conversation intervention in acute psychiatric services as part of standardized nursing practice.

Therapeutic Questions

Nurses can ask key questions to involve families in care. The questions need to fit with the context in which the nurse encounters the family. The purpose of the questions is to identify imminent needs of the family in supporting their caregiver sustainability. Questions should be built on the responses to the previous question.

Some useful questions include the following:

- What are your main concerns about this hospitalization or illness?
- What information would be most helpful for you at this time?
- How can we be most supportive to you now?
- Who in the family is most affected by the patient's illness?
- What is the most meaningful way to involve you in the care and treatment plan?

Commending Family and Individual Strengths

It is important to enhance the family's sense of worth. One way the nurse can accomplish this is to actively notice and distinguish the family's strengths, courage, resources, and capabilities in the form of a verbal *commendation* (Limacher & Wright, 2003; Wright & Leahey, 2013). For a family that has been challenged, often for many years, with a serious mental health issue, to experience a direct, specific comment on their positive actions and solutions can be a powerful intervention. It can be as simple as a nurse telling them, "I am impressed with your strength, your detailed knowledge about the medication regimen, and the way that you have stuck together to support one another by visiting the hospital and attending this family meeting." Families find participating in strength-based conversation enhances the recovery process.

In implementing any family intervention, flexibility is essential, particularly when working with culturally diverse groups. To implement successful, competent family interventions, nurses need to be open to modifying the structure and format of the sessions. Longer sessions are often useful, especially when a translator or an interpreter is used. Nurses also need to respect and work with the changing composition of family and nonfamily participants (e.g., extended family members, intimate partners, friends and neighbours, community helpers) in sessions. Because of the stigma that some cultural groups associate with seeking help, nurses may need to hold intervention sessions in community settings (e.g., churches, schools) or at the family's home. Finally, ending face-to-face sessions with the family may need to be gradual. The family may need information for further support, consultation, or reengagement should the problems reoccur.

In Summary

Families, whether they are relatives of individuals experiencing mental illness or make up a larger circle of support, have a unique role in promoting well-being, providing care, and facilitating recovery across the life span. They need to have these roles recognized as well as having their own needs acknowledged. Families can be engaged and helped through education and programs like parenting and sibling support, financial assistance, peer support, and respite care. Wherever possible, families should be welcomed as partners in care and treatment of their loved ones and should be included in decision making in a way that respects consent, confidentiality, and privacy (Mental Health Commission of Canada, 2009).

SUMMARY OF KEY POINTS

■ Family is a group of people defined as "who they say they are" and involved relationally in a complex process where economics, emotion, context, and experiences are interwoven and multilayered. Families come in various compositions, including nuclear, extended, multigenerational, single-parent, same-gender, and blended families. Cultural values and beliefs define family composition and roles.

■ Nurses complete a comprehensive family assessment when they care for families for extended periods or if a patient has complex mental health problems.

■ In building relationships with families, nurses must establish credibility and competence with the family. Unless the nurse listens and addresses the family's immediate needs first, the family will have difficulty engaging in the challenges of caring for someone with a mental disorder.

■ The genogram is an assessment and intervention tool that is useful in understanding health, relationships, and social functioning across several generations.

■ In assessing the family biologic domain, the nurse determines physical and mental health status and its effects on family functioning.

■ Family members are often reluctant to discuss the mental disorders of family members because of the stigma associated with mental illness. In many instances, family members do not know whether mental illnesses were present in other generations.

■ The family psychological assessment focuses on family development, the family life cycle, communication patterns, stress and coping abilities, problem-solving skills, strengths, hope, and resourcefulness. Determining how these occur in relationships is key.

■ The family life cycle is a process of expansion, contraction, and realignment of the relationship systems to support the entry, exit, and development of family members in a functional way. Families have unique patterns based on their context for living.

■ The ecomap is a tool used to assess the family social domain, which includes relationships within formal and informal support networks. The ecomap is particularly useful in care planning and discharge.

■ Clergy of all faiths may be a significant support to families with a mentally ill member in making meaning of their situation and in maintaining hope and spiritual strength.

■ Family interventions focus on supporting the family's bio/psycho/social/spiritual integrity and functioning as defined by its members. Family PMH nursing interventions include counselling, promotion of self-care activities, eliciting strengths and resources, purposefully commending the family, supportive therapy, education and health teaching, and the use of genograms and ecomaps. Mental health specialists, including advanced practice nurses, conduct family therapy.

■ Education of the family is one of the most useful interventions. Teaching the family about mental disorders, life cycles, family systems, and family interactions can help the family develop a new understanding of family functioning and the effects of mental disorders on the family.

CRITICAL THINKING CHALLENGES

1 Differentiate between a nuclear family, extended family, and "family is who they say they are." What would these three configurations have in common?

2 Interview a family with a member who has a mental illness and identify the family's most urgent concerns at this time.

3 Interview someone from a different ethnic background regarding family beliefs about mental illness. Compare them with your own.

4 Develop a genogram for your own family. Analyze the genogram in terms of its pattern of health problems, family and individual strengths and resources, and relationship patterns.

5 Develop an ecomap for your own family. Analyze the pattern of relationships around internal and external resources and other contextual issues, including social and economic functioning.

6 A female patient, divorced with two small children, reports that she is reluctant to tell anyone about her bipolar disorder. However, she worries about who will look after her children, ages 5 and 7, if she experiences another psychotic episode. Using ideas about family development and life cycle transitions, develop a plan for structuring the counselling session.

7 A family is finding it difficult to provide transportation to a support group for an adult member with mental illness. The family is committed to his treatment but is also experiencing severe financial stress because of another family illness. Using a problem-solving approach, outline a plan for helping the family explore solutions to the transportation problem.

8 Discuss with a local religious leader or clergy his or her experiences related to mentally ill members of the community and their families. What is this leader's perspective on assisting individuals and their families to make meaning of the experience and maintain hope?

REFERENCES

Aaron, M. (2008). Spirituality, the heart of caring. *A Life in the Day*, *12*(4), 23–26.

Caron, J. & Liu, A. (2010). A descriptive study of the prevalence of psychological distress and mental disorders in the Canadian population: Comparison between low-income and non-low-income populations. *Chronic Diseases in Canada*, *30*(3), 84–94.

Doane, G. & Varcoe, C. (2005). *Family nursing as relational inquiry: Developing health-promoting practice*. Philadelphia, PA: Lippincott Williams & Wilkins.

Fallon, I. (2005). Research on family interventions for mental disorders: Problems and perspectives. In N. Sartorius, J. Leff, J. J. López-Ibor, M. Maj, & A. Okasha (Eds.), *Families and mental disorders: From burden to empowerment* (pp. 235–257). Chichester, UK: Wiley.

Farrell, J. & Goebert, D. (2008). Collaboration between psychiatrists and clergy in recognizing and treating serious mental illness. *Psychiatric Services*, *59*, 437–40.

Hebert, R., Bravo, G., & Preville, M. (2000). Reliability, validity and reference values of the Zarit Burden Interview for assessing informal caregivers of community dwelling older persons with dementia. *Canadian Journal on Aging*, *19*, 494–507.

Leahey, M. & Harper-Jaques, S. (2010). Integrating family nursing into a mental health urgent care practice framework: Ladders for learning. *Journal of Family Nursing*, *16*(2) 196–212.

Leavey, G., Lowenthal, K., & King, M. (2007). Challenges to sanctuary. *Social Science and Medicine, 65*(3), 548–559.

Limacher, L. H. & Wright, L. M. (2003). Commendations: Listening to the silent side of a family intervention. *Journal of Family Nursing, 9*(2), 130–150.

MacCourt, P. (2013). Family Caregivers Advisory Committee, Mental Health Commission of Canada. *National Guidelines for a Comprehensive Service System to Support Family Caregivers of Adults with Mental Health Problems and Illnesses.* Calgary, AB: Mental Health Commission of Canada. Retrieved from http://www.mentalhealthcommission.ca

Marshall, A., Bell, J., & Moules, N. (2010). Beliefs, suffering, and healing: A clinical practice model for families experiencing mental illness. *Perspectives in Psychiatric Care, 46*(3), 182–196.

Marshall, A. & Harper-Jaques, S. (2008). Depression and family relationships. *Journal of Family Nursing, 14*(1), 56–73.

McGoldrick, M., Carter, B., & Garcia-Preto, N. (Eds.). (2011). *The expanded family life cycle: Individual, family, and social perspectives* (4th ed.). Boston, MA: Allyn & Bacon.

Mental Health Commission of Canada. (2009). *Toward recovery and well-being: A framework for a mental health strategy for Canada.* Calgary, AB: Author.

Mental Health Commission of Canada. (2012). *Opening Minds program overview.* Retrieved from http://www.mentalhealthcommission.ca/English/node/5233

Miklowitz, D., George, E., Richards, J., Simoneau, T., & Suddath R. (2003). A randomized study of family-focused psycho-education and pharmacotherapy in the outpatient management of bipolar disorder. *Archives of General Psychiatry, 60,* 904–912.

Mottaghipour, Y. & Bickerton, A. (2005). The Pyramid of family care: A framework for family involvement with adult mental health services. *Australian e-Journal for the Advancement of Mental Health, 4*(3), 210–217.

Nordby, K., Kjonsberg, K., & Hummelvoll, J. (2010). Relatives of persons with recently discovered serious mental illness: In need of support to become resource persons in treatment and recovery. *Journal of Psychiatric and Mental Health Nursing, 17*(4), 304–311.

Statistics Canada. (2011). *Fifty years of families in Canada: 1961 to 2011.* Retrieved from http://www12.statcan.gc.ca/census-recensement/2011/as-sa/98-312-x/98-312-x2011003_1-eng.cfm

Sveinbjarnardottir, E., Svararsdottir, E., & Wright, L. (2013). What are the benefits of a short therapeutic conversation intervention with acute psychiatric patients and their families? A controlled before and after study. *International Journal of Nursing Studies, 50*(5), 593–602.

Turner, W. L., Wieling, E., & Allen, W. D. (2004). Becoming culturally effective family-based research programs: Implications for family therapists. *Journal of Maritial and Family Therapy, 30*(3), 257–270.

Veltman, A., Cameron, J., & Stewart, D. E. (2002). The experience of providing care to relatives with chronic mental illness. *Journal of Nervous and Mental Disease, 190*(2), 108–114.

Ward-Griffin, C., Schofield, R., Vos, S., & Coatsworth-Puspoky, R. (2005). Canadian families caring for members with mental illness: A vicious cycle. *Journal of Family Nursing, 11*(2), 140–161.

Wright, L. M. & Leahey, M. (2013). *Nurses and families: A guide to family assessment and intervention* (6th ed.). Philadelphia, PA: F.A. Davis.

16 Psychological Health and Safety in the Workplace

Wendy Austin

Adapted from the chapter "Mental Health in the Workplace" by Wendy Austin and Marion Healey-Ogden

LEARNING OBJECTIVES

After studying this chapter, you will be able to:

- Identify the relationship between work and mental health.
- Describe a psychologically healthy and safe workplace.
- Explain work–life balance.
- Discuss gender differences in paid work.
- Outline aspects of an inclusive work culture.
- Identify threats to workplace psychological health and safety.
- Define bullying and discuss workplace violence.
- Evaluate a health care environment for healthy workplace attributes.

KEY CONCEPTS

- workplace health
- work
- workplace violence

KEY TERMS

- bullying • burnout • compassion fatigue • hazard • inclusive work culture • individual placement and support (IPS) • job attitude • job strain • risk • role overload • underemployed • unemployed • work–life balance • work–life conflict

---

The workplace has great potential as a setting in which the health of workers and their families can be protected and promoted. It offers a venue for health education, for workers to access preventive health services, and for links to primary health care (World Health Organization [WHO], 2009). This potential is being addressed globally through the WHO's Global Plan of Action on Workers' Health (2008–2017), which is aimed at strengthening the links between workplace health, public health, and health systems and at improving working conditions everywhere. These aims, however, are far from being achieved.

Psychological health issues make up the greatest number of disability claims among Canadians; in a recent survey of human resources and health benefit managers, 83% and 85% of respondents cited mental health conditions as the reason for short- and long-term disability claims, respectively (Towers Watson, 2011). Almost 25% of Canadian workers are affected by mental health problems or disorders that will lead to absence from work, a significant drop in productivity ("presenteeism"), or job turnover. The economic loss is estimated at $20 billion (Shain, Arnold, & GermAnn, 2013).

Of particular concern is the health and well-being of the health workforce: the health of everyone depends upon it (WHO, 2006). Nurses in particular are nearly twice as likely as other workers in Canada to be absent due to illness or injury (Berry & Curry, 2012). Nurses need to be able to address workplace health issues so that better health promotion, prevention, and care are available to all Canadians, and they must recognize that their own health and that of their colleagues plays a significant role in doing so. How can safe, compassionate, competent, ethical care be provided by individuals who are unhealthy, fatigued, and burned out? The rationale behind instructing airline passengers to put on their own oxygen mask before helping others can be applied here. Nurses must attend to their own well-being if they are to carry out their practice effectively.

Significant strides have been made in Canada towards improving workplace mental health. We are the first country to create national standards for psychological health and safety in the workplace (CSA Group, 2013). The standards, though voluntary, are a significant achievement, developed from legal and scientific research and through consultation with occupational health and safety experts, industry, unions, professional associations, and government agencies.

This chapter addresses psychological health and safety in the workplace. It considers the relation of work to health and well-being and the attributes of a healthy workplace. Outlined are some ways in which workplaces may support and accommodate individuals at risk for, or who have, mental health concerns. Workplace violence, including bullying, is discussed, and health care environments are considered as workplaces, particularly from the perspective of nurses.

■ WORK

Work is the term used to signify our paid employment, the job or task we perform to earn a living. In the lives of most people, however, work in its broadest sense is not restricted to places of employment. Some individuals work entirely within their homes, are not employees of any organization, and do not receive any monetary remuneration for their contribution to family, home, and community life.

Job attitudes, how people think and feel about their job, are important because one's job is important to his or her identity, health, and satisfaction with life (Judge & Kammeyer-Mueller, 2012). Facets of job satisfaction include satisfaction with work, supervision, coworkers, pay, and promotions. Of these, it is satisfaction with the work itself that is key to overall satisfaction (Herzberg, Mausner, & Bloch Snyderman, 2009; Judge & Kammeyer-Mueller, 2012). While the quality of workplace environments, particularly potential **hazards** (i.e., sources of physical and/or psychological harm), must be addressed, the quality of the work itself matters, too.

> **KEY CONCEPT Work** is "the job, occupation, or task one performs as a means of providing a livelihood" (Venes, 2009, p. 2502).

The Changing Nature of Work

Economic and technologic changes to the workplace, which are aimed at increasing short-term productivity and maximizing profits, continue to shape the nature of contemporary work. These changes include organizational restructuring and downsizing, decreased job stability, the frantic pace of work and life, and decreases in leisure time. The landscape of work continues to be transformed by factors such as the increasing turnover of work to machines and robotic devices, digital technology that allows production to occur anywhere on the globe while

managed from a central location, and a decline in the need for middle management that contributes to downsizing (Blustein, 2008). This transformation of the nature of work has direct effects on the work life of Canadians.

One in three Canadians says he or she is a "workaholic" (Statistics Canada, 2007). Comparisons of available statistics, the 1991 and 2001 National Work-Life Conflict Surveys, reveal that time in work seems to have increased across all job groups (Duxbury & Higgins, 2009). Whereas 1 in 10 respondents in the 1991 survey worked 50 or more hours per week, in 2001 the number had climbed to 1 in 4. The number of employees performing unpaid overtime has nearly doubled. It appears that employees find it increasingly difficult to complete their work during regular hours. Unsurprisingly, the survey comparisons reveal that the perceived level of stress and depression among workers has also increased (Duxbury & Higgins, 2009). Work has the potential to be a positive factor in sustaining health and well-being, but work, or the lack of it, can have a negative effect on existing health problems and can contribute to the development of new ones.

Unemployment

Most governments identify an individual as **unemployed** when the person does not have paid employment, wants to be employed, and is actively seeking work. This definition, however, does not encompass individuals who are **underemployed**—those with insufficient work relative to hours, skills, income, or status—nor does it include "discouraged workers"—those who want to work but have given up seeking it (Dooley, 2003; Dooley & Catalano, 2003). When considering a person's employment status, it may be more useful to consider employment along a continuum rather than as a dichotomous state of employed or unemployed.

Unemployment places individuals at risk for adverse health effects. A meta-analysis of the unemployment literature found that the unemployed had lower psychological and physical well-being than their employed counterparts (McKee-Ryan, Song, Wanberg, & Kinicki, 2005). When individuals have a strong attachment to the labour market or prior workplace, have high "breadwinning" responsibilities, or are disadvantaged in terms of occupational class, wage, or job quality, there is greater likelihood that unemployment will impair their mental health (Backhans & Hemmingsson, 2011). The WHO (2008) identifies the adverse effects of unemployment as including

- Elevated blood pressure
- Increased depression and anxiety
- Increased visits to general medical practitioners
- Increased symptoms of coronary disease
- Greater stress

- Increased psychological morbidity
- An increase in the number of health problems
- An increase in family problems, particularly financial hardships

Social capital (i.e., social networks and social activities) does not seem to mediate the effect of unemployment on well-being (Winkelmann, 2009). Obtaining permanent employment after being in an unstable employment situation, however, can be health promoting as the probability of psychological symptoms decreases (Reine, Novo, & Hammarström, 2008). The adverse effects of job change go beyond those who have lost jobs. Family members of those who have lost their jobs can experience hardship and stigma (Dooley & Catalano, 2003). Insecurity regarding one's job contributes to a sense of insecurity regarding the future. Sharp and/or sustained rise in unemployment negatively impacts a community's well-being as people lose jobs, acquire debt, and become unable to maintain their lifestyle. When appropriate measures are not in place, such as adequate unemployment benefits, social services, and community support, the level of stress and mental health problems in a community rises (Gunnell, Platt, & Hawton, 2009).

Work and Gender

In industrialized nations, women make up nearly half of the paid workforce but remain underrepresented in decision-making positions (the "glass ceiling" continues to exist) and on the average are paid less than men (WHO, 2011). While gender stereotypes are less influential in determining job and career choices than they once were, males and females continue to be segregated into different types of work. Registered nurses in Canada, for instance, are overwhelmingly females (about 94%), despite recent increases in males entering nursing programs ("Surge in numbers of male nursing students," 2012).

Gender segregation in types of work means that exposure to **risk**—the likelihood that harm may occur plus the severity of that harm (CSA Group, 2013)—differs between genders. For example, in a Statistics Canada survey, nearly one half of male nurses reported being physically assaulted by a patient the previous year, compared with one third of female nurses. It may be that the higher risk of abuse among male nurses involves greater exposure to violent patients and/or that male nurses tend to assume a primary role in responding to patient aggression and are protective of female staff (Shields & Wilkins, 2009).

Responses to workplace hazards may also have gender-based variation. Biologically, men and women may be affected differently by such hazards as toxins, due to hormonal differences; psychologically, women report work-related stress more frequently, perhaps due to less power and autonomy or vulnerability to harassment (WHO, 2011). Low control over work environment and conditions, however, has been found to correlate with hypertension in male workers but not in females (Smith, Mustard, Lu, & Glazier, 2013). Biology may shape response to job demands and control, as well.

Until rates of work-related injuries and disease are analyzed by gender, our understanding of its influence on workplace health will be insufficient. The dearth of research related to risks and health issues encountered in unpaid work (e.g., cooking, cleaning, care of family members, tending to the family business) contributed most often by women also leaves an important knowledge gap (WHO, 2011).

■ HEALTHY WORKPLACES

According to the WHO's framework, a healthy workplace exists when workers and managers continually collaborate to address health and safety concerns in the physical and psychosocial work environment, including the organization of work and workplace culture, and attend to health resources in the workplace and the community (Burton, 2010). The healthy workplace is an **inclusive work culture**: open, accessible, and accepting of workers with diverse backgrounds, demographics, and skills. Disparities between groups of workers or difficulties affecting specific workers (e.g., due to gender, ethnicity, or disability) are minimized or eliminated (Burton, 2010). A survey of over 4,000 Canadians found that 7 in 10 employed individuals considered their workplace to be healthy and their employer supportive of their personal needs (Ipsos Reid, 2007).

KEY CONCEPT Workplace health is the promotion and maintenance of the health and well-being of workers through policies, programs, and practises that promote safety, minimize risk, and create a positive, responsive, equitable workplace culture and a supportive workplace climate.

The Psychologically Healthy and Safe Workplace

A psychologically healthy and safe workplace is one where workers understand their roles and believe that they can contribute to decisions about how their work is carried out. There is much evidence that both worker well-being and performance are improved when organizations understand the importance of flexible work design and give their employees as much choice and control as possible (Lowe, 2010). The Mental Health Commission of Canada's recognition of the key contribution that healthy workplaces can make towards the well-being of Canadians has informed the development of several resources for employers. The psychosocial factors for a healthy and safe workplace have been identified (see Table 16-1) and free resources to help employers assess and address

Table 16-1 **Thirteen Psychosocial Factors in Workplace Health, Safety, and Well-Being**

Factor	Objective for the Workplace	Benefits to Employees
1. Psychological support	Coworkers and supervisors provide support and appropriate responses to employees' psychological and mental health concerns	Improved psychological health Increased productivity Reduced absenteeism and disability Successful and sustainable return to work
2. Organizational culture	An environment characterized by trust, honesty, and fairness	Higher job satisfaction and morale Improved teamwork and productivity Enhanced retention and recruitment Positive image in the community
3. Clear leadership and expectations	Effective leadership and support that help employees know what they need to do, how their work contributes, and whether there are impending changes	Clear expectations for job responsibilities and roles Positive morale and resiliency, particularly in times of stress and change Lessened frustration and conflict Greater trust in the employer
4. Civility and respect	An environment where employees are respectful and considerate in their interactions with one another, as well as with clients and the public	Effective teamwork and positive morale Reduced conflict Fewer grievances and lessened legal risk Improved relationships with clients
5. Psychological competencies and requirements	There is a good fit between employees' interpersonal and emotional competencies and the requirements of the position they hold	Enhanced performance and overall productivity Greater job satisfaction Increased retention of skilled staff Enhanced recruitment success
6. Growth and development	Employees receive encouragement and support in the development of their interpersonal, emotional, and job skills	Increased employee competency Retention of skilled staff Effective succession planning/internal promotion Enhanced service quality
7. Recognition and reward	Appropriate, fair, and timely acknowledgement and appreciation of employees' efforts	Greater employee satisfaction, motivation, and loyalty Improved teamwork and positive employee morale Increased retention and enhanced recruitment of skilled staff Enhanced employee/labour relations
8. Involvement and influence	Employees are included in discussion about how their work is done and how important decisions are made	Enhanced performance and productivity Greater employee motivation and job satisfaction Employees actively address challenges at work Positive employee/labour relations
9. Workload management	Tasks and responsibilities can be accomplished successfully within the time available	Enhanced performance and productivity Reduced stress and/or burnout Fewer job-related errors, incidents, accidents, and injuries Increased retention
10. Engagement	Employees feel connected to their work and motivated to do their job well	Enhanced performance and productivity High morale and motivation Enhanced recruitment and increased retention of skilled staff Improved relationships with clients
11. Balance	An environment where there is recognition of the need for balance between the demands of work, family, and personal life	Greater job satisfaction and morale Reduced stress and burnout Enhanced performance and productivity Reduced absenteeism and disability
12. Psychological protection	An environment where employees' psychological safety is ensured	Reduced absenteeism and disability Reduced conflict Fewer job-related errors, incidents, accidents, and injuries Fewer grievances and lessened legal risk
13. Protection of physical safety	Management takes appropriate action to protect the physical safety of employees	Improved physical and psychological health and safety Fewer job-related errors, incidents, accidents, and injuries Reduced absenteeism and disability Improved labour-management relations Reduced legal and regulatory costs

these factors developed (Samra, Gilbert, Shain, & Bilsker, 2012). The characteristics of psychologically *unsafe* workplaces with increased risks to mental health have similarly been identified (Shain et al., 2013) (see Box 16-1).

The National Standard of Canada for Psychological Health and Safety in the Workplace outlines a systematic framework for employers to use in creating and sustaining healthy, safe workplaces. It includes ways to identify and eliminate environmental hazards and how to assess and control risks associated with hazards that cannot be removed (e.g., inherent job demands and stressors). The standard includes several application annexes with evidence-informed resources including sample implementation models, scenarios, and audit tools (CSA Group, 2013).

Work–Life Balance

A challenge for many people is to balance the demands of their paid employment with other aspects of their lives, such as family and community. Individuals have many roles beyond that of an employee. Nonwork roles, such as educational, cultural, recreational, and volunteer activities, are important to life satisfaction and contribute to the cohesion of a society (Lero, Richardson, & Korabik, 2009). **Work–life balance** is achieved when an individual finds a satisfactory interaction among all the domains of his or her life. This balance will not be the same for everyone but will differ based on personal values, family structure, life situations and expectations, and societal norms.

Work–life conflict occurs when work–life balance is upset, when the demands of work and nonwork roles directly interfere with an individual's ability to meet one or more of the roles. At the beginning of the 21st century, Health Canada funded the National Study on Balancing Work, Family and Lifestyle from which six reports on work–life conflict in Canada were produced (see Web Links on thePoint). It was noted that many workplaces operate as if the world of work is separate from the rest of an individual's life. For instance, about 40% of employee respondents stated that it was difficult to arrange their work schedules to meet personal or family commitments; about 75% noted that it was very difficult to be home from work when their children arrived after school; and about 25% either delayed or decided not to start a family or had fewer children because they did not believe that they could balance the demands of work and family (Duxbury & Higgins, 2009).

Heavy job demands (e.g., heavy workload; multiple and/or time-pressured tasks) are a primary antecedent of work–life conflict. In an attempt to meet job demands, workers may stay on the job after regular hours, take work home, or work on days off. These strategies interfere with successful fulfillment of other roles, such as those within the family. Working long hours can keep one from attending family celebrations and children's school and sport events; preoccupation with or stress from work can strain family relationships. Family roles and responsibilities, in turn, can interfere with fulfilling one's role at work, as when caring for an ill family member means being absent from the job, or trouble at home impedes work functioning. **Role overload** occurs when an individual is unable to satisfy role demands. See Box 16-2 for categories of work–life conflict.

Both the number of demands and the control an individual feels over such demands are factors in work–life conflict (Duxbury & Higgins, 2009; Lero et al., 2009). Such work and family conflicts are associated with health issues such as stress, anxiety, depression, sleep disturbances, suppressed immune functioning, poor dietary habits, lack of exercise, hypertension, and medication use, among others (Lero et al., 2009). Many individuals suffering role overload will cut back on sleep hours to try to complete more during the day; over 50% of full-time workers and 70% of evening-shift workers cut back on sleep (Williams, 2008).

The quality and availability of community supports, such as day care or dependent care, can mitigate pressures on individuals and families, as can flexible working practices, such as varied hours of work, teleworking, opportunity for leave, and "family-friendly" workplaces (Lero et al., 2009; Lowe, 2010). In fact, flexible work design has been identified as the most effective solution for improving employee well-being, particularly when it is conceived in a holistic and systemic way (Lowe, 2010). This means that it encompasses elements related to supervisor and coworker support, job control (having some autonomy over how one's job is done and discretion to make job-related decisions), and job security, with employee assistance programs viewed as complementary (not separate) resources. More critical than formal policies of flexibility are employees' perceptions: if employees know that their supervisors will back them up when they make a decision, they will perceive they have flexibility; if they believe that taking advantage of work–family policies will have negative consequences for their career, they will not use them (Lowe, 2010). The perception of give and take in a workplace matters: workers need to feel they have some influence over their own work lives (Lowe, 2010).

■ THREATS TO WORKPLACE PSYCHOLOGICAL HEALTH AND SAFETY

Stress

Stress at work does not necessarily have a negative effect on employees; it depends upon the nature, intensity, and duration of the stress and upon the presence of protective factors (e.g., employees feel they have some control regarding their work situation) (Burton, 2010; WHO, 2005). Indications that an individual's stress is work related include awareness that he or she functions without any difficulty outside of the workplace and that stress is experienced when preparing for work or when thinking primarily about workplace issues (see Chapter 17 for a detailed discussion of stress).

When organizations commit to meeting Canada's voluntary national standard of psychological health and safety, they contribute to creating a less stressful workplace for their employees. There are many freely available resources for them to use, including the Comprehensive Workplace Health and Safety program of the Canadian Centre for Occupational Health and Safety, which addresses psychosocial work environment, workplace health promotion, and organizational community involvement (see Web Links on thePoint). Proactive initiatives are to an organization's advantage: there are huge costs related to absenteeism, presenteeism, and voluntary employee turnover (Lowe, 2010; Shain et al., 2013).

Burnout

Burnout is a term used to indicate "exhaustion due to chronic job stress" (Venes, 2009, p. 332). It has been conceived further as "a psychological syndrome in response to chronic interpersonal stressors on the job with three dimensions: exhaustion, cynicism and detachment, and lack of a sense of accomplishment" (Maslach, Schaufeli, & Leiter, 2001, p. 399). The individual may initially experience physiologic arousal (e.g., anxiety, high blood pressure, insomnia) and then enter a phase of energy conservation (e.g., tiredness, apathy) leading to exhaustion (e.g., headaches, depression) (Pompili et al., 2006). Burnout has been associated with diseases of the circulatory, musculoskeletal, and respiratory systems (Toppinen-Tanner, Ojajärvi, Väänänen, Kalimo, & Jäppinen, 2005).

Workplace Violence

Workplace violence encompasses far more than physical assault; it includes any type of intimidation, harassment, or abuse directed against a person in his or her place of employment. It is gaining attention as a serious global health, safety, and organizational problem rooted in broad cultural and socioeconomic factors (Chappell & Di Martino, 2006).

Some workers are at increased risk for violence due to factors related to their work situation. The Canadian Centre for Occupational Health and Safety (2012) has identified heightened workplace risk for employees who

- Work with the public
- Handle money, valuables, or prescription drugs (e.g., cashiers, pharmacists)
- Carry out inspection or enforcement duties (e.g., government employees)
- Provide service, care, advice, or education (e.g., health care staff, teachers)
- Work in premises where alcohol is served (e.g., food and beverage staff)
- Work in community-based settings (e.g., nurses, social workers, and other home visitors)
- Have a mobile workplace (e.g., taxicab)

KEY CONCEPT Workplace violence is the intimidation, harassment, abuse, or assault of an individual in his or her place of employment.

Table 16-2		Four Types of Bullying		

Physical	Relational	Verbal	"Cyber"
Threatening violence	Spreading gossip or rumours	Name-calling	Online verbal or relational bullying
Pushing	Withholding job information	Verbal intimidation	Sending false emails under victim's
Tripping	Overmonitoring of work	Insulting	name
Punching	Excessive or unjustified criticism	Mocking	Forwarding private emails, pictures
Kicking	Setting unrealistic goals	Attacking personal attributes	Online threats
Stalking		Attacking private life	Cyberstalking
Forcibly confining			

Adapted from Department of Criminal Justice Canada (2003), Canadian Council on Learning (2008), and Public Services Health and Safety Association (2010).

Bullying

Bullying has three defining characteristics: it occurs repeatedly; there is intent to do emotional and/or physical harm; and a power difference exists between the victim and the aggressor (Canadian Council on Learning, 2008). Recognizing these is crucial to eliminating bullying. Labelling every conflict or criticism bullying diminishes the latter's seriousness, as does dismissing bullying behaviour as "joking" or "roughhousing." Forms of bullying are found in Table 16-2.

Under Canada's Criminal Code, physical bullying, which includes threats of physical aggression, can constitute assault; physical or cyberstalking can constitute criminal harassment. The police can be called to investigate such incidents by employees as well as employers.

Persons who are targets of bullying can experience a wide range of reactions, including anxiety, fatigue, chest and back pain, high blood pressure, headaches, sleep disturbance, recurrent nightmares, concentration difficulties, irritability, depression, and posttraumatic stress (Felblinger, 2008; Public Services Health & Safety Association, 2010). A wide range of psychosocial and professional support is therefore necessary to address bullying's many potentially traumatic effects.

Emergencies and Disasters

Traumatic events that constitute an emergency or disaster can affect those involved both physically and emotionally. A traumatic event can be an emergency such as a transportation accident, large chemical spill, nuclear incident, power outage, or terrorist threat, or it can involve a natural disaster such as a disease outbreak, fire, flood, earthquake, or tornado. The workplace can be affected directly by such events, but employees can also bring to the workplace the effect of such events on their personal lives. Health Canada has established a psychosocial emergency preparedness and response team to assist federal employees exposed to traumatic events such as emergencies and natural disasters (Health Canada, 2012). This group of

professionals provides training in "resiliency building" for employees and managers, as well as consultation service to deal with the aftermath of a traumatic event.

The workplace may be a good and familiar place for employees to be following a traumatic event, as colleagues can comfort, console, and support one another. Responses to trauma can be planned and enacted together (e.g., holding memorial ceremonies, visiting the injured, attending funerals, setting up a relief fund for families). See Chapter 17 regarding response to trauma events.

■ MENTAL HEALTH PROBLEMS AND DISORDERS IN THE WORKPLACE

Awareness of the potential for mental health issues among employees is an essential component of a psychologically healthy and safe workplace. It is important to recognize, for instance, that some employees may be more vulnerable than others, in the short or long term, to stress and other work-related threats to mental health. Such vulnerability may be associated with factors such as gender, age, health status, family situation, or life history.

Workplace strategies can be put in place to assist and support specific workers or groups of workers (Burton, 2010; WHO, 2005). Examples include workshops for employees nearing retirement, counselling for those exposed to traumatic events, interventions for those with substance-related problems, and support groups for single parents. Individuals with chronic health problems may require individually negotiated support, such as an adaption of work hours to include rest periods. Strategies can also include educating managers about particular topics (e.g., cross-cultural issues to enable them to assist recently immigrated employees).

While there is rarely a direct link between an individual's work situation and the onset of a mental disorder (except for severe trauma occurring on the job), workplace factors can affect the likelihood of mental health problems and disorders, increase the severity of an existing disorder, or impede treatment and rehabilitation

Table 16-3	Work-Related Symptoms of Common Mental Disorders		
Depression	**Anxiety Disorders**	**Burnout**	
• Trouble concentrating • Trouble remembering • Trouble making decisions • Impairment of performance at work • Sleep problems • Loss of interest in work • Withdrawal: family, friends, coworkers • Feeling pessimistic, hopeless • Feeling slowed down • Fatigue	• Feeling apprehensive, tense • Difficulty managing daily tasks • Difficulty concentrating	• Becoming cynical, sarcastic, critical at work • Difficulty coming to work and getting started once at work • More irritable and less patient with coworkers, clients, customers • Lack of energy to be consistently productive at work • Tendency to self-medicate with alcohol or drugs	

From Burton, J. (2010). *WHO healthy workplace framework and model: Background and supporting literature and practices* (37). Geneva, Switzerland: World Health Organization.

(Samra et al., 2012). The workplace can also play a role in the prevention and early detection of disorders by improving knowledge of mental health problems and disorders within the organization. For instance, in regards to substance-use problems, healthier attitudes and beliefs about the use of tobacco and psychoactive substances can be promoted and assistance made available to employees needing to deal with such a problem (Shain et al., 2002). The Mental Health Commission of Canada offers Mental Health First Aid programs in which individuals learn how to recognize the signs and symptoms of a mental health problem or illness and how to find appropriate help (see Web Links on thePoint). Using such a resource is not unlike employers' and employees' accessing training in first aid for physical injuries and illness. See Table 16-3 for work-related symptoms of common mental disorders.

Addressing mental health is economically worthwhile. Mental health problems (including burnout, subclinical depression) are estimated to cost Canadian businesses $33 billion per year (Shain et al., 2002). Annual Canadian productivity losses due to depression, anxiety, and substance abuse are estimated to be over $11 billion (Burton, 2010).

Accommodation

Employers in Canada are expected to provide reasonable accommodation to special needs of current or potential employees. While an employer can show that a discriminatory policy or standard is necessary for a particular job (e.g., good vision for ambulance drivers), accommodation is otherwise a requirement under labour laws and human rights acts and prevents discriminatory employment practices. Accommodation involves primarily simple, low-cost strategies. Examples of reasonable accommodation for people with mental health problems and disorders include the following (WHO, 2005):

- Changes in communication (e.g., requests put in writing for a clerk who becomes anxious with verbal instructions; positive feedback given, not just criticisms; opportunities for self-appraisal prior to evaluation; planning sessions with a coworker as needed)
- Modifications to the physical environment (e.g., quiet work space provided)
- Job modifications (e.g., opportunities to work at home; hiring an assistant)
- Schedule modification (e.g., flexible working hours; rest periods or recuperation time; time allowed for medications or for treatment appointments; opportunity to start part-time work and move to full time)

There is strong research evidence that disability management programs are effective and that accommodating employee needs increases productivity and promotes greater trust between workers and employers (Burton, 2010).

Work and Persons Living With a Mental Disorder

Individuals living with mental disorders want, as others do, self-determination and life satisfaction through work. Work can help achieve relief from poverty, diminish reliance on social assistance, and promote social inclusion. Work can play an important role in recovery from mental illness and is a means to integrate persons with mental disorders back into their community. Nevertheless, finding appropriate employment remains difficult for persons with a mental disorder diagnosis: research has shown that a mental disorder may be a bigger barrier to employment than a physical disability (WISE Employment, 2012).

Individual placement and support (IPS) employment programs are a way to assist individuals with severe mental disorders to enter the workplace. IPS involves a rapid job search that is based on the individual's personal preferences and then continuing support to both the individual and the employer from an employment specialist working with the mental health service team. Research indicates that supported employment programs are effective (Hoffmann, Jäckel, Glauser, & Kupper, 2012). The Canadian Mental Health Association's Vancouver-Burnaby branch reported in 2012 that 70% of new clients obtained employment in the first year of their IPS program (Canadian Mental Health Association, 2012).

NURSES AND WORKPLACE PSYCHOLOGICAL HEALTH AND SAFETY

The education, recruitment, and retention of workers in the health sector are a pressing global concern (WHO, 2006). Nurses are the largest component of the health care workforce. They work across a wide range of settings, primarily on shift-work schedules, engaging with patients and families and all other members of the health care workforce (Kerr & Mustard, 2007). Nurses' health

is a barometer of workplace health in the health sector. See Table 16-4 for recommendations for the workplace health, safety, and well-being of the nurse.

Nurses, Job Strain, and Burnout

The first Canadian National Survey of the Work and Health of Nurses revealed that psychosocial and interpersonal factors (e.g., work stress, low autonomy, and lack of respect) are more closely associated with health problems among nurses who work overtime (Statistics Canada, 2006). In this survey of approximately 19,000 regulated nurses, nearly one third had high **job strain**, defined as what happens when the psychological demands of a job exceed the worker's discretion of how to enact it. Many nurses (45% of female nurses and 51% of male nurses) believed they had only low support from coworkers. This percentage compared unfavourably with employed Canadians in general, of whom approximately 33% described low support. About 20% of nurses indicated that in the previous month their mental health had made handling their workload difficult. Although burnout is usually considered as "long-term exposure

Table 16-4	Recommendations for Workplace Health, Safety, and Well-Being of the Nurse
Organization practice recommendations	Organizations/nursing employers create and design environments and systems that promote safe and healthy workplaces, including such strategies as
	Creating a culture, climate, and practices that support, promote, and maintain staff health, safety, and well-being
	Ensuring that the organization's annual budget includes adequate resources (human and fiscal) to implement and evaluate health and safety initiatives
	Establishing organizational practices that foster mutual responsibility and accountability by individual nurses and organizational leaders to ensure a safe work environment
	Being aware of the impact of organizational changes (such as restructuring and downsizing) on the health, safety, and well-being of nurses and be responsible and accountable for implementing appropriate supportive measures
	Implementing and maintaining education and training programs aimed at increasing awareness of health and safety issues for nurses (e.g., safe-lift initiative, employee rights, hazard awareness, etc.)
	Integrating health and safety best practices across all sectors of the health care system
Research recommendations	Researchers actively collaborate with health care partners to demonstrate the effectiveness of interventions aimed at improving nurse health, safety, and well-being using rigorous research and evaluation methodologies
	Researchers make full use of existing databases on nurse health, including the National Survey on the Work and Health of Nurses, in order to improve understanding of the key factors contributing to healthy work environments for nurses and to develop and test best practice indicators
Education recommendations	Nursing education institutions model the integration of health, safety, and well-being into their own workplace culture
	Nursing education institutions incorporate information about the health, safety, and well-being of the nurse into the core curriculum of nursing education programs
System recommendations	Governing/accreditation bodies incorporate the Organization Practice Recommendations from this Healthy Work Environments Best Practice Guideline in their quality health and safety standards for health care service and education organizations

From Registered Nurses' Association of Ontario. (2008). *Workplace health, safety and well-being of the nurse.* Toronto, Canada: Registered Nurses' Association of Ontario.

to a work situation that is beyond the person's capacity to cope" (WHO, 2005, p. 18), newly graduated nurses in a Quebec study reported a high level of psychological distress (43%), and a majority (62%) stated that they planned to quit their current position and seek another job in nursing; some (13%) intended to quit nursing itself (Lavoie-Tremblay et al., 2008).

Another Canadian study found that nurses' burnout and mental health problems did not arise from empathic engagement with patients but rather from the way their work was organized, so that nurses found their sense of identity, self-esteem, and worth to be compromised (Alderson, 2008). The researcher pointed to problems with an organizational paradigm in which nurses' work is framed from an industrial perspective of productivity. Nurses find meaning in their work in their relationships with patients and families; these relationships "reinforce their identity and preserve their mental health" (p. 171).

Burnout is a serious threat to the quality of health care. Its effects reach far beyond the impact on an individual, harming the entire health care system as care standards are not met. For instance, researchers found that when burnout was reduced by 30%, there were 6,239 fewer nosocomial infections, with cost savings in the millions (Cimiotti, Aiken, Sloane, & Wu, 2012).

Nurses' Fatigue

In a survey study of 6,312 Canadian nurses, fatigue was identified as a major negative influence on safe practice. Organizational factors cited as preventing nurses from responding to their fatigue included workload, professional responsibility to be there for patients, feelings of not wanting to let down their colleagues, and the culture of doing more with less. Causes of fatigue reported by the nurses were workload, shift work, patient acuity, lack of time for professional development and mentoring, a decline in organizational leadership and decision-making processes, and inadequate time for "recovery" during and following work shifts (Canadian Nurses Association and Registered Nurses' Association of Ontario, 2010). That nurses' fatigue seriously affects safe practice is further evident in the finding that medication errors were positively associated with nurses working overtime on a regular basis, role overload, perceived staffing or resource inadequacy, as well as with low coworker support, and low job security (Wilkins & Shields, 2008).

Compassion Fatigue

Compassion fatigue is the term used by caregiving professionals when they experience weariness, numbing of feelings like empathy, and relational disengagement from patients. Although it can appear as burnout, compassion fatigue seems to be rooted in prolonged exposure to others' suffering, coupled with one's own empathic responses. A review of the research literature suggests that the risk of compassion fatigue is increased by factors such as burnout and stress, heightened emotions of patients' families, the inability of the caregiver to maintain self-care, lack of social support, uncontrolled work stressors, lack of defined boundaries, degree of traumatic exposure, and lack of experience (Austin et al., 2013). In a qualitative study of registered nurses and registered psychiatric nurses with compassion fatigue, nurses described feelings of disconnection and disengagement from patients: "I couldn't give or open myself up to interact with the patients and their families… You're going through the motions but there is some disconnection … [you're] not really feeling their suffering." (Austin, Goble, Leier, & Byrne, 2009, p. 204). The nurses tried to overcome compassion fatigue by changing their practice area and schedule and by seeking out new knowledge, but they noted that changes to the health care system that improved support for compassionate caregiving were needed. The health care workplace has a role in preventing compassion fatigue.

Violence in the Health Care Workplace

Health care practitioners are at particularly high risk of workplace violence, and nurses are most at risk (Shields & Wilkins, 2009). Statistics Canada has reported that in the course of 1 year of providing direct care in hospitals or long-term care facilities, 34% of nurses were physically assaulted and 47% were emotionally abused by their patients (Shields & Wilkins, 2009). Factors identified by nurses who experienced abuse included being male, being relatively experienced, usually working noonday shifts, inadequate staffing and resources, poor nurse–physician relationships, and lack of support from coworkers and supervisors. Although many of these factors can be modified, nurses indicate that there is a culture of silence around incidents of violence, and many incidents go undocumented. The negative outcomes for nurses who experience abuse in the workplace include anger, fear, depression, anxiety, sleep disruption, increased sick leave, symptoms of posttraumatic stress disorder, and job dissatisfaction (Shields & Wilkins, 2009).

Standard IV of the Canadian Federation of Mental Health Nurses (CFMHN) practice standards—effectively manages rapidly changing situations—requires the psychiatric–mental health nurse to utilize safety measures to protect client, self, and colleagues from potentially abusive situations in the work environment (CFMHN, 2014) (see Chapter 5). The place to start is the identification of sources of violence, so discussion can begin and strategies be adopted for its prevention. Strategies may be as simple as providing timely information to patients and their friends and family, as this effectively lessens the risk of assault in health care settings, particularly in cases involving distress and long waiting periods (Chappell & Di Martino, 2006). Assigning tasks based on competencies and experience can also reduce contributing factors. Organizational pressures should be addressed. For example, appropriate staffing levels and shift lengths can reduce stress and avert aggression among staff and between workers and the public. Debriefing with those involved in the incident is helpful; counselling by qualified staff or outside specialists may be necessary in more serious cases.

Perhaps, the most essential approach to reducing violence in health care settings, however, is to ensure that everyday practice is grounded in courtesy, decency, and civility (Hesketh et al., 2003). Acceptable behaviours may require definition, systemic recognition, and support, while incivil behaviour should be confronted and addressed in a professional manner.

● **STUDY NOTE**

Nurses who are the victims of violence in the workplace may need support to deal with their reaction to the incident. A debriefing with those involved is important to the resolution of the violence and the prevention of further incidents.

SUMMARY OF KEY POINTS

■ Work influences self-identity, provides income, and plays a significant role in an individual's health and well-being. Unemployment and underemployment can cause psychological distress and negatively affect an individual's mental health. There are also adverse effects related to job change that go beyond those who have lost jobs.

■ The nature of work has been changing across the globe due to economic and technologic developments; these changes are affecting the mental health of workers.

■ Achieving work–life balance can be difficult. Work–life conflict occurs when one role interferes with meeting the demands of another.

■ Gender differences continue to influence the situation of paid workers.

■ Nurses need to understand the psychosocial factors that contribute to a healthy and inclusive workplace and the need for flexibility in sustaining a healthy workplace and for accommodating employees at risk for stress and/or mental health problems.

■ Work can help persons with mental disorders in their recovery and in the improvement of their well-being. Independent placement and support facilitates acquiring and maintaining employment for persons with severe mental disorders.

■ Bullying (physical, relational, verbal, and "cyber") involves repeated, intended harm to a person with less power than the aggressor.

■ Nurses need to overcome a culture of silence related to workplace violence in health care settings.

CRITICAL THINKING CHALLENGES

1 Listen to the TedTalk by Dan Ariely, "What makes us feel good about our work?" (ted.com/talks/dan_ariely_what_makes_us_feel_good_about_our_work.html). Are the simple experiments he describes convincing? What makes you feel good about your work?

2 Imagine your "dream" workplace as a practising nurse. What would it be like? What would be the barriers to making this dream come true?

3 Identify the strategies in place at your educational institution for the support of the mental health of students, faculty, and staff. Are there additional strategies that you believe should be in place?

4 Consider your experience as a student in a health care environment. What factors do you find cause or increase stress for you? What factors mitigate stress for you?

5 Have you been affected by an incident of workplace violence? Consider the immediate and long-term influences that may have influenced the occurrence of this incident. What was done, if anything, to prevent it from happening again?

6 Do you know the emergency response plan of your institution? Do you have a personal and family emergency plan?

REFERENCES

Alderson, M. (2008). Work structure in the chronic care setting: Possible consequences for nurses' mental health. *Canadian Journal of Nursing Research, 40*(3), 160–178.

Austin, W., Brintnell, S., Goble, E., Kagan, L., Kreitzer, L., Larsen, D., & Leier, B. (2013). *Lying down in the ever-falling snow: Canadian health professionals' experience of compassion fatigue.* Waterloo, ON: Wilfrid Laurier University Press.

Austin, W., Goble, E., Leier, B., & Byrne, P. (2009). Compassion fatigue: The experience of nurses. *Ethics and Social Welfare, 3*(2), 195–214.

Backhans, M., & Hemmingsson, T. (2011). Unemployment and mental health—who is (not) affected? *European Journal of Public Health, 22*(3), 429–433.

Berry, L., & Curry, P. (2012). *Nursing workload and patient care.* Ottawa, ON: Canadian Federation of Nurses Unions.

Blustein, D. (2008). *The psychology of working: A new perspective for career development, counseling, and public policy.* Mahwah, NJ: Lawrence Erlbaum Associates Inc.

Burton, J. (2010). *WHO healthy workplace framework and model: Background and supporting literature and practices.* Geneva, Switzerland: World Health Organization.

Canadian Centre for Occupational Health and Safety. (2012). *Workplace violence.* Retrieved from http://www.ccohs.ca/oshanswers/psychosocial/violence.html

Canadian Council on Learning. (2008). *Bullying in Canada: How intimidation affects learning.* Retrieved from http://www.ccl-cca.ca/pdfs/LessonsInLearning/Mar-20-08-Bullying-in-Canad.pdf

Canadian Federation of Mental Health Nurses (CFMHN). (2014). *Canadian standards of psychiatric-mental health nursing* (4th ed.). Toronto, ON: Author.

Canadian Mental Health Association. (2012). *Individual placement and support model of supported employment.* Retrieved from http://vancouver-burnaby.cmha.bc.ca/how-we-can-help/employment-services

Canadian Nurses Association and Registered Nurses' Association of Ontario. (2010). *Nurse fatigue and patient safety: Research report.* Retrieved from http://www2.cna-aiic.ca/cna/practice/safety/full_report_e/files/fatigue_safety_2010_report_e.pdf

Chappell, D., & Di Martino, V., (Eds.) (2006). *Violence at work* (3rd ed.). Geneva, Switzerland: International Labour Organization.

Cimiotti, J. P., Aiken, L. H., Sloane, D. M., & Wu, E. S. (2012). Nurse staffing, burnout, and health care-associated infection. *American Journal of Infection Control, 40*(6), 486–490.

CSA Group. (2013). National Standard of Canada, CAN/CSA-Z1003-13/BNQ 9700-803/2013: *Psychological health and safety in the workplace—Prevention, promotion, and guidance to staged implementation.* Retrieved from http://shop.csa.ca/en/canada/occupational-health-and-safety-management/cancsa-z1003-13bnq-9700-8032013/invt/z10032013

Department of Criminal Justice Canada. (2003). *Stalking is a crime called criminal harassment.* Retrieved from http://canada.justice.gc.ca/eng/pi/fv-vf/pub/har/har.html

Dooley, D. (2003). Unemployment, underemployment, and mental health: Conceptualizing employment status as a continuum. *American Journal of Community Psychology, 32*(1/2), 9–20.

Dooley, D., & Catalano, R. (2003). Introduction to underemployment and its social costs. *American Journal of Community Psychology, 32*(1/2), 1–7.

Duxbury, L., & Higgins, C. (2009). *Work-life conflict in Canada in the new millennium: Key findings and recommendations from the 2001 National Work-Life Conflict Study.* Ottawa, ON: Public Health Agency of Canada.

Felblinger, D. M. (2008). Incivility and bullying in the workplace and nurses' shame responses. *Journal of Obstetric, Gynecologic and Neonatal Nursing, 37*(2), 234–241.

Gunnell, D., Platt, S., & Hawton, K. (2009). Editorial: The economic crisis and suicide: Consequences may be serious and warrant early attention. *British Medical Journal, 338,* 1456–1457.

Health Canada. (2012). *Psychosocial emergency preparedness and response.* Retrieved from http://www.hc-sc.gc.ca/ewh-semt/occup-travail/empl/psychosoc-eng.php

Herzberg, F., Mausner, B., & Bloch Snyderman, B. (2009). *The motivation to work.* Piscataway, NJ: Transaction Publishers.

Hesketh, K. L., Duncan, S. M., Estabrooks, C. A., Reimer, M. A., Giovanetti, P., Hyndman, K., & Acorn, S. (2003). Workplace violence in Alberta and British Columbia hospitals. *Health Policy, 63,* 311–321.

Higgins, C., Duxbury, L., & Lyons, S. (2008). *Reducing work-life conflict: What works? What doesn't?* Retrieved from Health Canada website: http://www.hc-sc.gc.ca/ewh-semt/pubs/occup-travail/balancing-equilibre/index-eng.php

Hoffmann H., Jäckel D., Glauser S., & Kupper Z. (2012). A randomised controlled trial of the efficacy of supported employment. *Acta Psychiatrica Scandinavica, 125*(2), 157–167.

Ipsos Reid. (2007). *Mental health in the workplace: Largest study ever conducted of Canadian workplace mental health and depression.* Public release. Retrieved from http://www.mentalhealthroundtable.ca/dec_07/Ipsos%20Reid%20Nov%202007%20MentalHealthReport.pdf

Judge, T. A., & Kammeyer-Mueller, J. D. (2012). Job attitudes. *Annual Review of Psychology, 63,* 341–367.

Kerr, M., & Mustard, C. (2007). The challenge of effective workplace change in the health sector. *Healthcare Papers, 7*(Sp), 69–73.

Lavoie-Tremblay, M., Wright, D., Desforges, N., Gélinas, C., Marchionni, C., & Drevniok, U. (2008). Creating a healthy workplace for new-generation nurses. *Journal of Nursing Scholarship, 40*(3), 290–297.

Lero, D., Richardson, J., & Korabik, K. (2009). *Cost-benefit review of work-life balance practices—2009.* Gatineau, QC: Canadian Association of Administrators of Labour Legislation.

Lowe, G. (2010). *Creating sustainable organizations: How flexible work improves wellbeing and performance.* Retrieved from http://www.grahamlowe.ca/documents/258/

Maslach, C., Schaufeli, W. B., & Leiter, M. P. (2001). Job burnout. *Annual Review of Psychology, 52,* 397–422.

McKee-Ryan, F. M., Song, Z., Wanberg, C. R., & Kinicki, A. J. (2005). Psychological and physical well-being during unemployment: A meta-analytic study. *Journal of Applied Psychology, 90*(1), 53–76.

Pompili, M., Rinaldi, G., Lester, D., Girardi, P., Ruberto, A., & Tatarelli, R. (2006). Hopelessness and suicide risk emerge in psychiatric nurses suffering from burnout and using specific defence mechanisms. *Archives of Psychiatric Nursing, 20*(3), 135–143.

Public Services Health and Safety Association. (2010). *Bullying in the workplace: A handbook for the workplace.* Toronto, Canada: Author.

Registered Nurses' Association of Ontario. (2008). *Workplace health, safety and well-being of the nurse.* Toronto, Canada: Author.

Reine, I., Novo, M., & Hammarström, A. (2008). Does transition from an unstable labour market position to permanent employment protect mental health? Results from a 14-year follow-up of school-leavers. *BMC Public Health, 8.* Retrieved from http://www.biomedcentral.com/1471-2458/8/159

Samra, J., Gilbert, M., Shain, M., & Bilsker, D. (2012). *GuardingMinds@ Work.* Vancouver, Canada: Centre for Applied Research in Mental Health and Addiction (CARMHA). Retrieved from http://www.guardingmindsatwork.ca

Shain, M., Arnold, I., & GermAnn, K. (2013). *The road to psychological health and safety: Legal, scientific and social foundations for a national standard for psychological safety in the workplace.* A working paper for the Mental Health Commission of Canada. Retrieved from www.mentalhealthcommission.ca

Shain, M., Bender, A., Brenneman Gibson, J., Gnam, W., Siu, M., & Suuvali, H. (2002). *Mental health and substance use at work: Perspectives from research and implications for leaders.* A background paper prepared by the Scientific Advisory Committee to the Global Business and Economic Roundtable on Addiction and Mental Health. Retrieved from http://www.mentalhealthroundtable.ca/documents.html

Shields, M., & Wilkins, K. (2009). *Factors related to on-the-job abuse of nurses by patients.* Retrieved from Statistics Canada website: http://www.statcan.gc.ca/pub/82-003-x/2009002/article/10835-eng.htm

Smith, P., Mustard, C., Lu, H., & Glazier R. (2013). Comparing the risk associated with psychosocial work conditions and health behaviours on incident hypertension over a nine-year period in Ontario, Canada. *Canadian Journal of Public Health, 104*(1), e82–e86.

Statistics Canada. (2006). National survey of the work and health of nurses. *The Daily.* Retrieved from http://www23.statcan.gc.ca/imdb/p2SV.pl?Function=getSurvey&SDDS=5080&Item_Id=13648&lang=en

Statistics Canada. (2007). Workaholics and time perception. *The Daily.* Retrieved from http://www.statcan.gc.ca/daily-quotidien/070515/dq070515c-eng.htm

"Surge in numbers of male nursing students". (2012). *Canadian Nurse.* Retrieved from http://www.canadian-nurse.com/index.php?option=com_content&view=article&id=597%3Asurge-in-numbers-of-male-nursing-students&catid=4%3Aperspectives&Itemid=39&lang=en

Toppinen-Tanner, S., Ojajärvi, A., Väänänen, A., Kalimo, R., & Jäppinen, P. (2005). Burnout as a predictor of medically certified sick-leave absences and their diagnosed causes. *Behavioral Medicine, 31,* 18–27.

Towers Watson. (2011). *Towers Watson study: Investing in workforce health generates higher productivity.* Financial Post [Online]. Retrieved from www.financialpost.com

Venes, D. (Ed.) (2009). *Taber's cyclopedic medical dictionary* (21st ed.). Philadelphia, PA: F.A. Davis Company.

Wilkins, K., & Shields, M. (2008). Correlates of medication error in hospitals. *Health Reports, 19*(2), Statistics Canada catalogue 82–003.

Williams, C. (2008). *Work-life balance of shift workers.* Retrieved from Statistics Canada website: http://www.statcan.gc.ca/pub/75-001-x/2008108/pdf/10677-eng.pdf

Winkelmann, R. (2009). Unemployment, social capital, and subjective well-being. *Journal of Happiness Studies, 10*(4), 421–430.

WISE Employment. (2012). *SMEs attitudes to employing people who have a mental illness.* Retrieved from http://www.wiseemployment.com.au/uploads/publications/Empowermental-McNair_Research.pdf

World Health Organization (WHO). (2005). *Mental health policies and programmes in the workplace.* Geneva, Switzerland: Author.

World Health Organization (WHO). (2006). *World Health Report 2006: Working together for health.* Geneva, Switzerland: Author.

World Health Organization (WHO). (2008). *World Health Report 2008: Primary health care: now more than ever.* Geneva, Switzerland: Author.

World Health Organization (WHO). (2009). *Occupational health.* Retrieved from http://www.who.int/occupational_health/en/index.html

World Health Organization (WHO). (2011). *Gender, work and health.* Retrieved from http://whqlibdoc.who.int/publications/2011/9789241501729_eng.pdf

Challenges to Mental Health

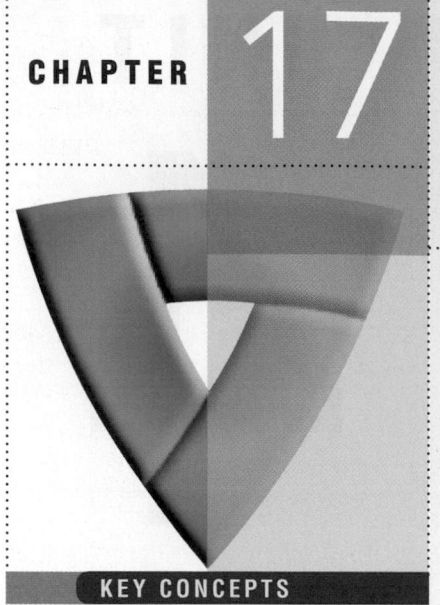

17 Trauma- and Stressor-Related Disorders, Crisis, and Response to Disaster

Gerri Lasiuk, Kathleen Hegadoren, and Wendy Austin
Adapted from the chapter "Stress, Crisis, and Disaster Management" by Lorraine D. Williams and Mary Ann Boyd

KEY CONCEPTS

- coping
- crisis
- disaster
- stress
- traumatic stressor

LEARNING OBJECTIVES

After studying this chapter, you will be able to:

- Discuss the evolution of the concept of stress.
- Use the transactional model to assess an individual's stress, adaptation, and coping abilities.
- Differentiate problem-focused and emotion-focused coping.
- Define *stress, traumatic stressor, crisis*, and *disaster* and describe human responses to them.
- Explain nursing assessment and interventions of trauma- and stressor-related disorders.
- Identify adaptive and maladaptive responses to disaster and indicators that a survivor may require psychiatric services.

KEY TERMS

- adaptation • allostatic load • allostasis • arousal • avoidance
- bereavement • cognitive appraisal • crisis intervention • dissupport
- duty to provide care • emotion-focused coping • emotions
- freeze-hide response • grief • homeostasis • mourning • negative cognitions and mood • person–environment relationship • problem-focused coping • psychological first aid • reappraisal • reexperiencing • social functioning • social support network • social support • stress–diathesis model • stressors

Although stress has been the focus of considerable scientific, clinical, and general interest over the past century, most of us would be hard-pressed to explain what it is. As Selye (1980, p. 127) quipped, "stress, like relativity, is a scientific concept which has suffered the mixed blessing of being too well known, and too little understood." In this chapter, the concepts of stress, trauma, crisis, and disaster are described and the way that nurses can identify and address the needs of individuals experiencing these events explained.

STRESS

The Evolution of the Concept of Stress

The word *stress* comes from the Latin word *stringere*, meaning to draw tight (Cooper & Dewe, 2004), and the Middle English word *stresse*, which refers to hardship or distress (Harper, 2001). Throughout the 18th and 19th centuries, the word "stress" was used to denote *force, pressure*, or *strain*, which explains why the word "stress" was used almost exclusively by engineers before the beginning of the 20th century.

The early decades of the 20th century saw the rise of *psychosomatic medicine* and a shift away from the prevailing view of the body as a machine (Cooper & Dewe, 2004). Proponents of psychosomatic medicine believed that a mechanistic model was reductionistic and could not explain the role of the mind and spirit in health and illness. It was in this context that the concept of stress as hardship was taken up by biologic and social scientists as a possible explanation of disease and illness (Bartlett, 1998). Throughout the last century, our understanding of stress evolved through three distinct periods in which it was conceptualized as a physiologic response, as a stimulus, and finally, as a transaction.

Stress As a Response

Walter Cannon and Hans Selye, two pioneers in the study of stress, both conceptualized stress as a response to changing environmental conditions. Cannon (1939), a noted Harvard physiologist, is considered by many to be the father of modern stress research. In his book *The Wisdom of the Body*, he coined the term **homeostasis** to describe the body's ability to maintain a stable internal environment despite changing environmental conditions. Cannon's thesis was that environmental changes are perceived as threats to personal integrity or safety and signal a compensatory response mediated by the sympathetic branch of the autonomic nervous system (ANS). He also believed that strong **emotions** like fear and anger are fundamental to the stress response and have evolved because of their high survival value. "Fear," he wrote, "has become associated with the instinct to run, to escape; and anger or aggressive feeling, with the instinct to attack" (p. 227). This notion, later dubbed the *fight or flight* response, remains a key concept in any discussion of stress.

Working at McGill University in Montreal, Selye (1956, 1974) developed his general adaptation syndrome. In it, Selye differentiated **stress** (a nonspecific response of the body to any demand placed on it) from **stressors** (events that initiate the response) and argued that stressors can be physical (e.g., infection, intense heat or cold, surgery, debilitating illnesses), psychological (e.g., psychological trauma, interpersonal problems), or social (e.g., lack of social support). Stressors can also be short term (acute) or long term (chronic). According to Selye, the perception of a stressor triggers an automatic, total-body response. The first stage of this response is the *alarm reaction*, during which virtually all body systems (e.g., sense organs, brain, heart and blood vessels, lungs, digestive system, immune system) respond in a coordinated effort to mediate the stressor. If this effort is successful, the body returns to its normal state. If it is not successful and the stressor remains present for hours or days, the organism moves into the *stage of resistance*, and efforts to adapt continue. In circumstances in which the stressor becomes chronic or is extreme, the body moves into the *stage of exhaustion*, during which the individual's resources deplete, and exhaustion and death ensue. Selye believed that many diseases, including hypertension, peptic ulcer, and autoimmune illnesses, are caused by prolonged adaptive reactions in which corticosteroids play a pathogenic role.

Although Selye made significant contributions to our understanding of human stress, he was criticized for his notion that stress is a nonspecific response to diverse environmental stimuli. Selye's challengers (e.g., Mason, 1971; Mikhail, 1981) pointed out that many neuroendocrine responses are not general at all but very specific. Selye's critics argued that all stressors do not necessarily produce the same response in every individual, and what is a stressor for one person may not be a stressor for another (Lazarus & Folkman, 1984). The conceptualization of stress solely as a response was also challenged for its circular reasoning (i.e., an event is stressful because it elicits a stress response).

Stress As a Stimulus

Before the 1960s, the study of stress was a physiologic concept. By the middle of the last century, the disciplines of psychology and psychiatry were on the rise, and researchers and clinicians became interested in the psychological and emotional aspects of stress. With this came the notion that life changes or events were the stimuli (i.e., stressors) that evoked the stress response (e.g., Dohrenwend & Dohrenwend, 1974; Holmes & Rahe, 1967). Within this perspective, stress, researchers explored associations between significant life events (e.g., marriage, divorce, relocation, death) and stress. One of the most widely used tools in this type of research is the *Recent Life Changes Questionnaire* (RLCQ; Holmes & Rahe, 1967; see Table 17-1). A major problem with this conceptualization of stress is that stress-provoking stimuli can be identified only in retrospect, that is, only after a response occurs. Other criticisms are that it does not take into consideration the meaning an individual assigns to an item, the individual's coping abilities, or the implications of chronic or recurrent events (see Jones & Kinman, 2001).

Stress As a Person–Environment Transaction

The mid-1970s to the early 1990s was a critical period in stress research. During this period, a debate raged in the literature between two camps of stress researchers. One group favoured the view that critical life events (i.e., the presence of an objective event) mediate the experience of stress. Supporters "urged researchers to measure pure events, uncontaminated by perceptions, appraisals, or reactions" (Dohrenwend & Shrout, 1985, p. 782). On the other side, Lazarus, DeLongis, Folkman, and Gruen (1985) maintained that it is the appraisal of an event (i.e., the subjective evaluation of an event or situation) that is critical to the stress experience. Although the debate centred on measurement and other methodologic problems, Lazarus (1999) later wrote that what was at issue

Table 17-1	Recent Life Changes Questionnaire	
Social Area	**Life Changes**	**LCU Values***
Family	Death of spouse	105
	Marital separation	65
	Death of close family member	65
	Divorce	62
	Pregnancy	60
	Change in health of family member	52
	Marriage	50
	Gain of new family member	50
	Marital reconciliation	42
	Spouse begins or stops work	37
	Son or daughter leaving home	29
	In-law trouble	29
	Change in number of family get-togethers	26
Personal	Jail term	56
	Sex difficulties	49
	Death of a close friend	46
	Personal injury or illness	42
	Change in living conditions	39
	Outstanding personal achievement	33
	Change in residence	33
	Minor violations of the law	32
	Begin or end school	32
	Change in sleeping habits	31
	Revision of personal habits	31
	Change in eating habits	29
	Change in church activities	29
	Vacation	29
	Change in school	28
	Change in recreation	28
	Christmas	26
Work	Fired at work	64
	Retirement from work	49
	Trouble with boss	39
	Business readjustment	38
	Change to different line of work	38
	Change in work responsibilities	33
	Change in work hours or conditions	30
Financial	Foreclosure of mortgage or loan	57
	Change in financial state	43
	Mortgage (home, car, etc.)	39
	Mortgage or loan less than $10,000 (stereo, etc.)	26

Directions: Total the LCUs for your life change events during the past 12 months.

250 to 400 LCUs per year: Minor life crisis

More than 400 LCUs per year: Major life crisis

*LCU, Life change unit. The number of LCUs reflects the average degree or intensity of the life change.

Source: Rahe, R. H. (2000). Recent Life Changes Questionnaire (RLCQ) (1997). In T. H. Holmes, American Psychiatric Association (Eds.). *Task Force for the Handbook of Psychiatric Measures. Handbook of psychiatric measures* (pp. 235–237). Washington, DC: American Psychiatric Association.

was the fundamental nature of stress and the **person–environment relationship**. In the end, the latter group prevailed, and the view of stress as a relationship between the person and his or her environment has become the dominant explanatory model.

In their seminal work *Appraisal and Coping*, Lazarus and Folkman (1984) conceptualized stress as resulting from a perceived imbalance between an individual's resources and the demands placed on them. Within their Transactional Model, stress depends on how a stressor is appraised in relation to the individual's resources for coping with it. The central premise is that stress is "neither an environmental stimulus, a characteristic of the person, nor a response, but a relationship between demands and the power to deal with them without unreasonable or destructive costs" (Coyne & Holroyd, 1982, p. 108).

Cognitive Appraisal

Lazarus and Folkman (1984) use the term **cognitive appraisal** to describe the process by which an individual examines the demands and constraints of a situation in relation to his or her personal and network resources. Cognitive appraisal has two levels—primary and secondary. In primary appraisal, the individual evaluates the situation and determines whether he or she is in danger or under threat. If yes, they go on to secondary appraisal, during which he or she considers the options for dealing with the situation. According to Lazarus and Folkman, stress is the perception of threat or harm (primary appraisal) for which an individual has no effective response (secondary appraisal). Figure 17-1 depicts Lazarus's (1999, p. 59) seesaw analogy illustrating stress as a balance between environmental demands and personal resources.

> **KEY CONCEPT** According to the Transactional Model (Lazarus & Folkman, 1984), **stress** is the relationship between the person and the environment that is appraised as exceeding the person's resources and endangering his or her well-being.

New Understandings of the Stress and the Stress Response

In recent years, the concept of stress has been increasingly criticized for its lack of precision and specificity. Lazarus (1999) argued that while the concept of stress is a useful one, it is not a single, unitary phenomenon. This sentiment is echoed by Woolfolk, Kehre, and Allen (2007) who contend that stress "is probably best thought of as a generic, nontechnical term, analogous to disease or to addiction" (p. 10). Until the term "stress" is replaced by a more precise label, it is a useful heuristic to aid communication among laypersons, health professionals, and researchers.

Allostasis

A recent refinement in our understanding of stress is the concept of **allostasis**. The word, which literally means *maintaining stability through change*, was coined by Sterling and Eyer (1988) to describe how the cardiovascular system adjusts to resting and active states of the body. Unlike the concept of homeostasis, which posits a single optimum state, allostasis reflects the notion that different environmental circumstances or conditions require different set points. For instance, individuals' ideal blood

---

A.   Demands   **Resources**

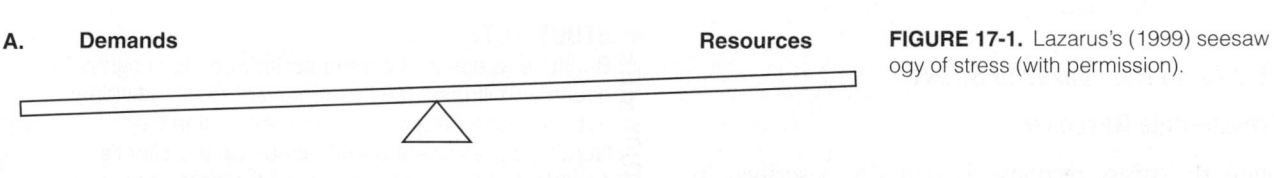

A good balance between demands and resources implies modest amounts of stress or not stress.

FIGURE 17-1. Lazarus's (1999) seesaw analogy of stress (with permission).

B.   Demands

                                                        Resources

High demands with few resources can result in a high stress balance.

                                                        Resources

C.

Demands

A low stress balance, which could imply boredom.

pressure when asleep is very different from their ideal blood pressure if they are bungee jumping (Sapolsky, 2004). Maintaining an allostatic balance in wide-ranging circumstances calls for continuous systemic adjustments throughout the whole body. For example, the hypothalamus regulates sleep and wakefulness and the production of adrenocortical hormones in response to the light–dark cycle that occurs as the earth rotates on its axis every day. When the light–dark cycle is altered (e.g., long flights across several time zones), the production of adrenocortical hormones is disrupted and alterations occur in the usual patterns of sleep, activity, appetite, and cognitive function (i.e., jet lag).

The term **allostatic load** (McEwen, 1998) refers to the cumulative negative effects on the body of continually having to adapt to changing environmental conditions and psychosocial challenges. It is mediated by the efficiency of the body's response to these changing conditions and to the number of stressors an individual experiences throughout his or her lifetime. Allostatic load is more than "chronic stress;" it is the sum total of the "wear and tear" on the body that accumulates from the constant effort required to maintain normal body rhythms in the face of changing environmental conditions, the challenges of daily life, and the adverse physiologic consequences of harmful lifestyle choices (e.g., fat-rich diet, excessive alcohol, smoking).

New Views on Responses to Stress

The Freeze–Hide Response

Although the stress response is typically described in terms of an individual organism defending itself against threat by fighting or fleeing, other responses to stress have also been observed. One of these is the **freeze–hide response**, which is the tendency to produce a passive response to stress (Korte, Koolhaas, Wingfield, & McEwen, 2005). As Korte and colleagues explain, there is an evolutionary advantage for different organisms to develop different behavioural strategies to cope with stress. Natural selection supports the development of different traits by preserving genes for high aggression (e.g., hawks) and low aggression (e.g., doves) within a population and between and across genders within the species. Although research related to the freeze–hide response has been done with animals, it suggests that the stress response may actually be more differentiated than Canon predicted.

Tend and Befriend

Another line of research into the human stress response is one proposed by Shelley Taylor and her colleagues Taylor et al. (2000, 2002) who argue that males and females respond differently to stress. They theorize that women have the same physiologic response to stress

but their resultant behaviours differ. They propose another alternative to fight-or-flight-type behavioural responses—which they call the *tend-and-befriend* behavioural responses—and explain that it is characteristic of females of various species. According to the authors, the tend-and-befriend response also has evolutionary advantages and reflects the inclination of females towards affiliation, cooperation, and caretaking.

Tending involves nurturant activities designed to protect the self and offspring that promote safety and reduce distress; befriending is the creation and maintenance of social networks that may aid in this process (Taylor et al., 2000, p. 411).

As Taylor et al. (2000, 2002) explain, the biologic mediators of the tend-and-befriend response appear to involve oxytocin and female reproductive hormones. Oxytocin, dubbed the "love hormone," appears to have a role in a range of social behaviours including social memory, attachment, and bonding; sexual and maternal behaviour; trust; and aggression (Lee, Macbeth, Pagani, & Young, 2009). It is also believed that disorders characterized by difficulties with social interactions (e.g., autism and schizophrenia) may also involve oxytocin. The possibility that the stress response may be gendered opens new horizons for exploring human stress responses.

● **STUDY NOTE**

STUDY NOTE

Because stress and coping contribute significantly to health and illness, they are relevant to all individuals, not just those diagnosed with mental illnesses. Nursing assessment should focus on the client's appraisal of the stressful event. Understanding a person's beliefs, values, commitment, and typical response patterns will help in the identification of stressors and coping resources.

Physiologic Stress Responses

The appraisal of a situation as dangerous or threatening to one's personal integrity triggers an automatic, total-body response. Structures in the brain receive and integrate simultaneous inputs from a number of sources and coordinate a series of physiologic and behavioural responses that enhance an individual's chances of survival.

The physiologic response to stress begins in the central nervous system (CNS) but quickly involves all body systems, as Table 17-2 illustrates. The hypothalamus is responsible for maintaining the body's internal environment and for initiating the body's stress response, which it orchestrates through its dense neural connections with the posterior pituitary gland, brainstem, and spinal cord and through its endocrine links with the anterior pituitary gland (Kindlen, 2003). The hypothalamus activates the sympathetic branch of the ANS, which stimulates the adrenal medulla to secrete catecholamines and mediates

Table 17-2	Physiologic Stress-Related Symptoms
System	**Symptom**
Cardiovascular	Headache
	Chest pain
	Increased pulse
	Palpitations
	Fainting (blackouts, spells)
	Increased blood pressure
Respiratory	Shortness of breath
	Smoking history
	Increased rate and depth of breathing
	Chest discomfort (pain, tightness, ache)
Gastrointestinal	Nausea
	Vomiting
	Abdominal pain (cramps, stomachache)
	Change in appetite
	Change in stool
	Obesity/frequent weight changes
Musculoskeletal	Pain
	Weakness
	Fatigue
Genitourinary	Menstrual changes
	Urinary discomforts (pain, burning, urgency, hesitancy)
	Sexual difficulty (pain, impotence, altered libido, anorgasmia)
Dermatologic	Itching
	Rash
	"Sweats"
	Eczema

Adapted from Carpenito-Moyet, L. (2009). *Nursing diagnosis: Application to clinical practice* (13th ed.). Philadelphia, PA: Lippincott Williams & Wilkins.

vigilance, arousal, activation, and mobilization (Sapolsky, 2004; see Fig. 17-2). It also secretes corticotrophin-releasing hormone (CRH) to signal the anterior pituitary gland to release adrenocorticotropic hormone into the systemic circulation, which stimulates the adrenal cortex to secrete cortisol. Also through CRH, the hypothalamus excites firing of the locus coeruleus in the brainstem to increase norepinephrine in the CNS. The hypothalamus also synthesizes arginine vasopressin or antidiuretic hormone (AVP/ADH), which is released by the posterior pituitary gland and increases blood pressure by causing vasoconstriction and water retention.

The activities of the hypothalamic–pituitary–adrenocortical (HPA) axis and the sympathetic–adrenal medullary system operate within different time frames to provide the body with a wide range of defensive responses. Because the neural response of the ANS is instantaneous, it is the body's first line of defence against stressors. The release of AVP/ADH and corticosteroids is slightly slower and augments ANS effects. In the short term, these responses mobilize energy reserves (mainly in the form of glucose to skeletal muscles) and prepare the body to deal with the stressor by running away or fighting it off. If the stressor is prolonged, the body must make longer-term metabolic adjustments that ensure a sufficient supply of energy. Cortisol is essential to the body's sustained stress response because it mobilizes lipid stores and skeletal protein for energy, which allows the conservation of glucose energy for neural tissue. It also acts on the liver to elevate and stabilize blood glucose levels through gluconeogenesis and lipolysis. As well as having these metabolic effects, cortisol is an anti-inflammatory. By reducing the dilation and permeability of blood vessels, which is part of the inflammatory response, cortisol aids in the maintenance of blood pressure and minimizes fluid loss to the tissue. At the same time, chronically elevated cortisol prolongs healing and leaves the body vulnerable to infection.

Social Support and Stress

Animal and human research consistently demonstrates that social support enhances health and well-being and, conversely, that a lack of social support increases the risk of morbidity and mortality.

Social Support

Broadly defined as resources provided to us by others (Cohen & Wills, 1985), **social support** has been shown to moderate the adverse effects of stress (Haslam, O'Brien, Jetten, Vormedal, & Penna, 2005; Park, 2007). Although it takes various forms, social support is broadly categorized as either *functional* or *structural* (Cropley & Steptoe, 2005). Functional support refers to the quality of the relationships and the degree to which an individual believes that help is available; structural support relates to the quantitative characteristics of a **social support network** (e.g., size, number of interconnections).

Much of the research on how social support mediates the effects of stress has focused on two hypotheses (Cohen & Wills, 1985). As its name suggests, the *direct effect hypothesis* proposes that social support enhances health directly by providing an individual with positive experiences and a set of stable, socially rewarding roles regardless of stress levels. The second hypothesis, the *buffering* or *moderating hypothesis*, holds that the positive effects of social support are apparent only during periods of high stress. In a study of the relationships between life stress, social support, and physical symptom reporting, Cropley and Steptoe (2005) found that social support had no general beneficial effects on the symptom reporting (i.e., health) of individuals who had not experienced recent stress. It did, however, have a moderating effect on the health of individuals reporting recent high stress, which lends credence to the stress-buffering hypothesis. The same study found that social support did not moderate the effects of chronic stress. The authors

FIGURE 17-2. Physiologic responses to stress.

concluded that chronically stressed individuals (even those who had high levels of social support) may not perceive their social support as helpful or are unable to mobilize their social support to specifically help address their circumstances.

From this, we may conclude that social support is a dynamic process that is in constant flux and varies with life events and health status (Yeager & Roberts, 2003). It is also important to keep in mind that not all interpersonal interactions within a network are supportive; an individual can have a large, complex social network but little social support. The concept of **dissupport** (Malone, 1988) derives from the observation that some relationships can be harmful, stressful, and even damaging to an individual's self-esteem. Examples of dissupport include verbal, physical, or emotional abuse; discounting

an individual's opinions, feelings, behaviours, or values; blocking access to resources; or consuming an individual's material resources. As one might expect, social dissupport can hinder growth, is emotionally destructive, and depletes resources. Even more complex are those relationships that are both supportive and dissupportive, such as those that provide tangible support (e.g., money) but are also emotionally destructive.

Social Network

We all live within networks of relationships among a defined set of people with whom we have regular face-to-face contact (Clegg, 2001). It is through these relationships that we are socialized and acquire emotional support, material aid, services, and information (Majer,

Jason, Ferrarie, Venable, & Olson, 2002). An individual's social network can be a resource, enhance the ability to cope with change, and influence the course of illness (Jones & Johnston, 2000).

Contacts within a social network are categorized into three levels:

1. *Level I*—6 to 12 people with whom the person has intimate contact (e.g., one's closest family and friends)
2. *Level II*—30 to 40 people whom the person sees regularly (e.g., more distant family and friends, neighbours, coworkers)
3. *Level III*—the several hundred people with whom an individual has direct contact, but incidental contact in the course of his or her day-to-day life (e.g., acquaintances, the grocer, mail carrier)

The various levels of an individual's social network often intersect with each other; for example, a friend may be a confidant, a neighbour, and a workout buddy. Generally speaking, the larger and more interconnected a social network is, the more support that is available to its members. An ideal network is dense and interconnected so that each individual within the network relates to the other at various levels. Dense networks are typically better able to respond in times of stress and crisis because they represent a large reservoir of social, emotional, and instrumental resources.

Intensity and reciprocity are two concepts important to understanding social networks. *Intensity* is the degree or closeness of a relationship. Some relationships are naturally more intense than others, and ideally, an individual's social network reflects a balance between intense and less intense relationships. Intense relationships can restrict a person's opportunity to interact with other network members, but without at least a few intense relationships, a person lacks intimacy. *Reciprocity* is the extent to which there is balanced give-and-take in a relationship. Network members provide and receive support, aid, services, and information from each other; sometimes members are on the giving side; at other times, they receive. Reciprocity represents a necessary equilibrium between the two states.

Emotional Responses to Stress

Although it is clear that emotion is key to the human stress response, there is still debate about the relationship between emotion and cognition. On one side is the argument that emotions are primary and influence both the form and content of our perceptions, while opponents believe that cognition is primary and gives rise to emotion. Consistent with his transactional view of stress, Lazarus (1991) takes a more integrative approach and contends that cognition and emotion are essentially simultaneous and interdependent. He and his colleagues define emotion as "complex, organized psychophysiologic reactions consisting of cognitive appraisals, action impulses, and patterned somatic reactions" (cited in Folkman & Lazarus, 1991, p. 209).

Cognitive appraisal is fundamental to the experience of emotion because it colours the meaning of a situation or an event. Based on their research, Lazarus and colleagues believe that there are 15 basic emotions, each of which is elicited in response to a particular perception of what a situation or an event means to the individual (see Table 17-3). Anxiety, for example, is typically associated

Table 17-3   Fifteen Basic Emotions

Emotion	Relational Meaning
Anger	A demeaning offense against me and mine
Anxiety	Facing an uncertain, existential threat
Fright	Facing an immediate, concrete, and overwhelming physical danger
Guilt	Having transgressed a moral imperative
Shame	Having failed to live up to an ego ideal
Sadness	Having experienced an irrevocable loss
Envy	Wanting what someone else has
Jealousy	Resenting a third party for the loss of or a threat to another's affection
Disgust	Taking in or being too close to an indigestible object or idea (metaphorically speaking)
Happiness	Making reasonable progress towards the realization of a goal
Pride	Enhancement of one's ego identity by taking credit for a valued object or achievement, either our own or that of someone or a group with whom we identify
Relief	A distressing goal-incongruent condition that has changed for the better or gone away
Hope	Fearing the worst but yearning for better
Love	Desiring or participating in affection, usually but not necessarily reciprocated
Compassion	Being moved by another's suffering and wanting to help

Source: Adapted from Lazarus, R. S. (1999). *Stress and emotion: A new synthesis.* New York, NY: Springer.

with the perception of a nonspecific threat or some uncertainty, whereas happiness reflects an appraisal of the person–environment condition that is beneficial. Patterned somatic reactions are the individual's own, unique experience of the physiologic changes associated with an emotion. For one person, a rush of energy is the salient feature of anger, whereas for another person, it is trembling and a feeling of weakness. These physical reactions motivate or inhibit action impulses. For example, the person who feels energized may attack an aggressor, whereas the person who experiences trembling and weakness is likely to withdraw.

Coping

According to Lazarus (1998), the following three principles are vital to an understanding of *coping*: (1) it continually changes over the course of an encounter, (2) it must be assessed independently of its outcomes, and (3) it consists of what an individual thinks and does in response to the perceived demands of a situation. With those principles in mind, coping is defined as "the efforts we take to manage situations we have appraised as being potentially harmful or stressful" (Kleinke, 2007, pp. 290–291). Coping reflects an individual's continual reappraisal of the person–environment relationship in light of changing conditions, as well as the success of his or her efforts to mitigate the situation. Those who evaluate their coping responses as effective are likely to feel competent and to repeat those responses in the future. Conversely, individuals who see their efforts as ineffective are likely to feel helpless and overwhelmed. Positive coping leads to **adaptation**, which is characterized by well-being and maximum social functioning. The inability to cope leads to maladaptation and contributes to ill health, a diminished self-concept, and deterioration in **social functioning**. These ideas are captured in the stress, coping, and adaptation models presented in Figures 17-3 and 17-4.

There are two general approaches to coping: problem focused and emotion focused. As Kleinke (2007) explains, **problem-focused coping** may be inner or outer directed. Outer-directed strategies attempt to eliminate or alter a situation or another's behaviour, while inner-directed strategies aim at altering one's own beliefs, attitudes, skills, responses, and so forth. In **emotion-focused coping**, the individual seeks to manage his or her emotional distress (e.g., through exercise, prayer/meditation, expressing emotions, talking to friends). Table 17-4 contrasts problem-focused and emotion-focused coping.

Coping involves the continuous reevaluation or reappraisal of the changing person–environment relationship. **Reappraisal** incorporates feedback about the effects of coping and allows for continual processing of new information. No single coping strategy is effective in all situations. Throughout life a repertoire of coping strategies is developed and adapted to suit different situations,

and these strategies become ingrained into patterned responses. Well-adapted individuals are realistic in their appraisal of the demands upon them, are flexible in their use of coping resources, and remain open to learning new coping strategies. Poor reality testing, impaired judgement, inflexibility, limited coping strategies, and an unwillingness to acquire new resources can render individuals vulnerable to stress-related problems and illness.

> **KEY CONCEPT Coping** is an individual's constantly changing cognitive and behavioural efforts to manage specific external or internal demands that are appraised as taxing or exceeding the individual's resources.

Stress and Health Illness

There is more than 50 years of accumulated research demonstrating a relationship between stress and illness. Animal experiments in the 1950s and 1960s demonstrated that a number of stressors (e.g., isolation, crowding, exposure to predators, electrical shock) increased morbidity and mortality from tumours and infections (Saddock & Saddock, 2003). In humans, acute academic exam stress is linked to a reduction in natural killer cells and increased activation of latent viruses (Glaser, Rice, Sherridan, & Fertel, 1987). Other studies demonstrate a correlation between exam stress and an increase in cytokines—proteins (produced by lymphocytes and other cells) that promote or inhibit an immune response (Lui et al., 2002). As well, Segerstrom and Miller's (2003) meta-analysis of 30 years of research on the effects of chronic stress associated with caring for a relative with dementia found a reduction in most measures of immune function.

The **stress–diathesis model** offers one explanation about the relationship between stress and mental health illness (Stanley & Burrows, 2005). This model proposes that preexisting genetic, biologic, and psychological vulnerabilities interact with negative or stressful life events to cause illness. Further, the model predicts an inverse relationship between vulnerability and stress such that the more vulnerable the individual, the smaller the stressor required to cause illness. Several lines of research conclude that the tendency to "nervousness, emotionality, 'neuroticism,' negative affect, anxiety, and being 'high strung' runs in families and has a high genetic component, with 50% of these characteristics arising from genetic or biologic vulnerability" (Stanley & Burrows, 2005, p. 90). In a large community-based study, Kendler, Neale, Kessler, Heath, and Eaves (1992) found that generalized anxiety disorder and depression share a common genetic predisposition and that episodes of illness are related to environmental stressors.

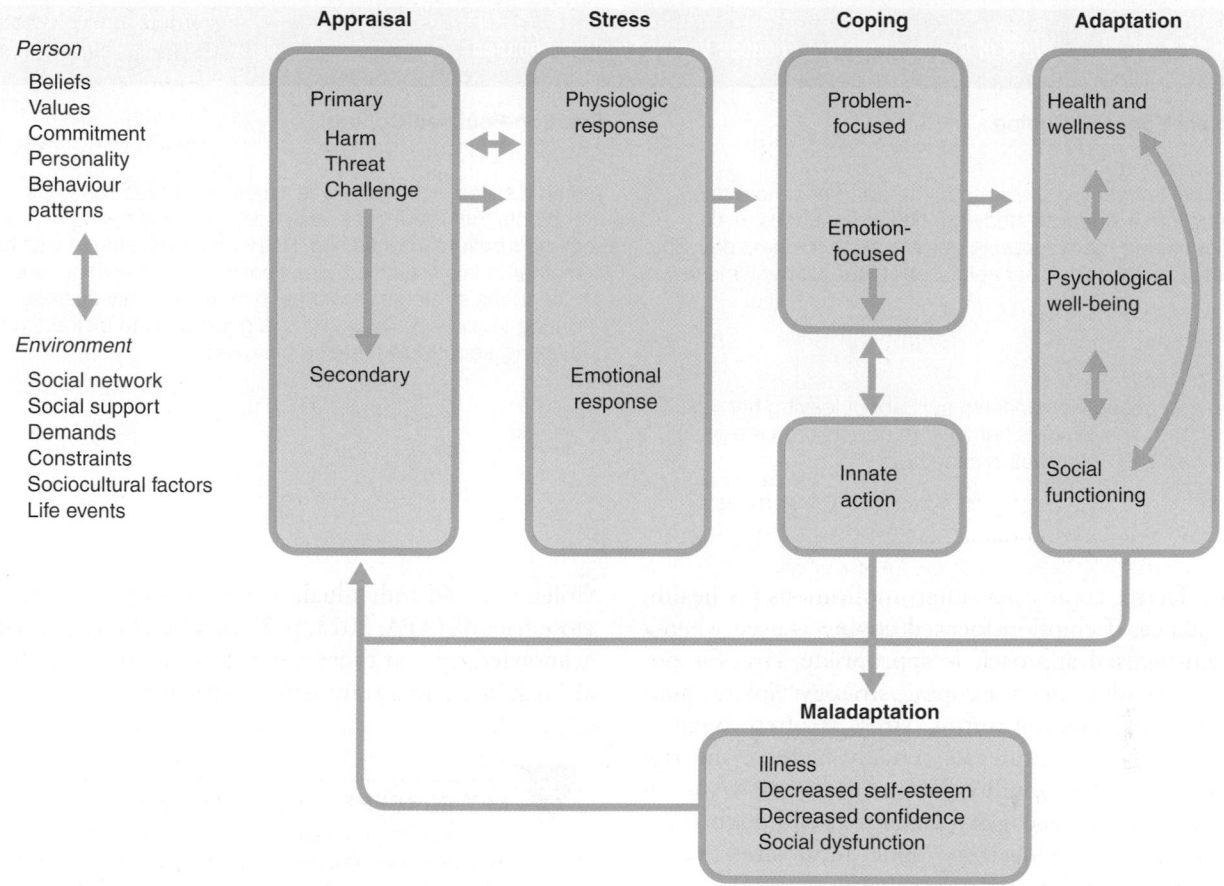

FIGURE 17-3. Stress, coping, and adaptation model.

FIGURE 17-4. Bio/psycho/social/spiritual adaptation.

Table 17-4	Ways of Coping: Problem-Focused Versus Emotion-Focused

Problem-Focused Coping	Emotion-Focused Coping
Outer directed When noise from the television in the apartment next door interrupts a student's studying, she experiences anxiety about being ready for an important exam the next day. She responds by asking her neighbour to turn the volume down. *Inner directed* When an abused woman feels guilt about leaving her husband, she reminds herself that her children are much happier and doing well in school.	A man dislikes visiting his wife's mother because she has two cats that roam her house freely, and the cat hair on all of the furniture irritates him. Rather than refusing to visit his mother-in-law, which causes conflict in his marriage, the man plans strategies that help him manage his distress during visits (e.g., long walks, a good book to distract him, thinking about how pleased his wife is).

Ineffective coping has other implications for health. For instance, if emotion-focused coping is used when a problem-focused approach is appropriate, stress is not relieved. In addition, if a coping strategy violates gender, ethnic, or cultural norms, stress is often exaggerated. Some coping strategies actually increase the risk for mortality and morbidity, such as the excessive use of alcohol, drugs, tobacco, or overeating. Although these strategies may provide some short-term stress relief, they often cause long-term secondary stress. The corollary is that healthy coping strategies such as exercising, adequate sleep, leisure activities, and good nutrition reduce the negative effects of stress and promote health and well-being.

Trauma- and Stressor-Related Disorders

Although historical and literary documents dating back to the third century BCE describe human responses to extreme stress (e.g., natural disasters, combat, physical/sexual assault; Birmes, Hatton, Brunet, & Schmitt, 2003), modern psychiatry did not officially recognize them until 1980, when posttraumatic stress disorder (PTSD) appeared in the *Diagnostic and Statistical Manual of Mental Disorders (DSM*; American Psychiatric Association [APA], 1980); 14 years later, acute stress disorder (ASD) was added as a diagnostic label (APA, 1994).

In the latest version of the *DSM* (APA, 2013), both PTSD and ASD were removed from the list of anxiety disorders and placed in a new category of disorders called *trauma- and stressor-related disorders*. All of the disorders in this category specify exposure to a traumatic or extremely stressful event as a diagnostic criterion. *Trauma* is from the Greek for *wound* and refers to an injury, physical and/or psychic (Oxford English Dictionary Online, 2013). A traumatic stressor is considered in the *DSM-5* to be "any event (or events) that may cause or threaten death, serious injury, or sexual violence to an individual, a close family member, or a close friend" (APA, 2013, p. 830). This change in criteria acknowledges that there are wide variations in individuals' responses to a traumatic experience.

> **KEY CONCEPT** A **traumatic stressor** is "any event (or events) that may cause or threaten death, serious injury, or sexual violence to an individual, a close family member, or a close friend" (APA, 2013, p. 830).

Acute Stress Disorder

The diagnostic label of ASD first appeared in the *DSM-IV* (APA, 1994) to address the lack of a diagnosis for acute pathologic reactions that occur within the 1st month of exposure to an extremely stressful or traumatic event. The authors of the *DSM-IV* conceptualized ASD as an acute and transient response that may be evident immediately after exposure and usually resolves on its own without treatment within 2 to 3 days. In the *DSM-IV*, the primary difference between ASD and PTSD was the duration of the symptoms and the emphasis on dissociative reactions to the trauma in ASD. A *DSM-IV* diagnosis of ASD required that one experience, witness, or be confronted with an event that involved actual or threatened death or serious injury to oneself or others. As well, the individual had to experience at least three dissociative symptoms: symptoms of hyperarousal, numbing, and/or avoidance and significant impairment in functioning.

In the *DSM-5*, the stressor criteria for ASD is changed from the *DSM-IV* and is explicit about whether the traumatic event was experienced directly, witnessed, or experienced indirectly. In addition, the emphasis on dissociative symptoms is reduced. According to the *DSM-5*, a diagnosis of ASD is made if an individual has experienced, witnessed, or been confronted with an event that involved actual or threatened death or serious injury, or a threat to the physical integrity of self or others. In addition, s/he must experience dissociative symptoms (numbing, depersonalization, amnesia); marked arousal; reexperiencing of traumatic event; intrusion symptoms (including flashbacks); avoidance of stimuli related to trauma; and significant impairment in function.

Posttraumatic Stress Disorder

According to the *DSM-5* (APA, 2013), a diagnosis of PTSD is made if an individual is exposed to actual or threatened death, serious injury, or sexual violation during which the individual

- directly experiences the traumatic event;
- witnesses the traumatic event in person;
- learns that the traumatic event occurred to a close family member or close friend (with the actual or threatened death being either violent or accidental); or
- experiences firsthand repeated or extreme exposure to aversive details of the traumatic event (not through media, pictures, television, or movies unless work-related).

The person must also report at least one of the following four clusters of symptoms: reexperiencing, avoidance, negative cognitions and mood, and arousal. **Reexperiencing** includes recurring and persistent thoughts and images, nightmares, or flashbacks (i.e., vivid reliving) of the stressful event. **Avoidance** is manifested as attempts to block out all reminders of the stressful event and may involve avoiding people, places, or activities associated with the event; inability to remember some or all aspects of the event; feeling detached from others; and/or a lack of interest or participation in usual activities. In an effort to numb or block out their thoughts and feelings, some individuals may turn to alcohol or drugs. **Negative cognitions and mood** reflect a range of thoughts and feelings, from persistent and distorted sense of blame of self or others, to estrangement from others, to an inability to remember key aspects of the event. Finally, **arousal** results from activation of the ANS and the HPA axis and may include startling easily, difficulty concentrating, sleep disruption, irritability, and hyperarousal.

Although more than half of individuals will experience a traumatic event at some time in their lives, most people will not develop PTSD (National Collaborating Centre for Mental Health, 2005). According to the National Comorbidity Study (Kessler, Sonnega, Bromet, Hughes, & Nelson, 1995), a large U.S. population–based study, 60.7% of men and 51.2% of women reported being exposed to at least one traumatic event during their lifetime. This estimate increases to 80% when clinical populations are surveyed. A survey study of adults in Ottawa regarding perceived personal threat in response

to the terrorist attacks of September 11, 2001 found that the higher the appraisal of personal threat and distress experienced, the more likely it was that positive life changes (e.g., closer to family, refocused priorities) were made; these changes were reported to remain stable nearly a year later (Davis & Macdonald, 2004). Adversity fosters resilience, not psychopathology for most people. Preferred coping mechanisms tend to be to (1) focus on brief time intervals (e.g., think only about the next step), (2) maintain a view of oneself as competent and a view of others as willing and able to provide support, and (3) focus on the current implications of the trauma and avoid regretting past decisions and actions.

Factors that predict the development of PTSD include female gender, type and severity of the trauma, past trauma (including childhood physical, sexual, and emotional abuse), and availability of support at the time of the stressful event (Richardson, Naifeh, & Elhai, 2007). Since women are more likely to experience more high-impact trauma, they are more likely than men to develop PTSD. It is the type of experience, such as interpersonal violence, that accounts for some of this difference (Amstadter et al., 2013; Kelly et al., 2011; Maguen et al., 2012; Rees et al., 2011). Women in the perinatal period have higher rates of PTSD compared with other times across the lifespan, likely due to exacerbation of preexisting PTSD symptoms (Seng et al., 2010). Some studies (Luxton, Skopp, & Maguen, 2010; Washington, Davis, Martirosian, & Yano, 2013) but not all (Haskell et al., 2010) of veterans of military deployment have found that women are more vulnerable to PTSD. Children (particularly those under the age of 10 years) are less likely to experience PTSD after trauma than are adults (National Collaborating Centre for Mental Health, 2005).

Treatments for PTSD include cognitive–behavioural therapy, psychotherapy, and medication. Treatment may need to be prolonged, and there are many who live with chronic persistent symptoms. Neurobiologic studies related to PTSD first began with Vietnam war veterans who still met criteria for PTSD 20 to 30 years after the war.

Nursing Care of Individuals Affected by Stress

Nursing assessment of individuals experiencing stress attends to biologic, psychological, emotional, and environmental (physical and social), as well as coping, resources. In particular, the nurse should explore recent changes (positive or negative) in the individual's life (e.g., trauma, loss, developmental milestones).

The overall goals of care for those individuals actively experiencing a stress response are to eliminate or moderate the stressor (if possible), to reduce untoward effects of the stress response, and to facilitate the maintenance or development of positive coping skills. The goals of care for individuals who are at high risk for stress (e.g., are experiencing significant life changes, have preexisting vulnerabilities, have limited coping mechanisms) are to recognize the potential for stress and to strengthen or develop positive coping skills. It is also important to educate clients about human stress responses as a way to help normalize bodily, emotional, and social responses, thereby helping the client to reappraise his or her own interpretation of these responses.

Biologic Domain

Biologic Assessment

Biologic data are essential for analyzing an individual's physical responses to stress, coping efforts, and adaptation. This information comes from the health history, physical examination, and diagnostic testing (as indicated; see Chapter 9). Nurses should pay particular attention to

- Signs and responses indicating sympathetic and parasympathetic arousal (see Chapter 9)
- Alterations in vegetative functions (e.g., appetite and eating patterns, sleep, energy level, sexual activity)

IN A LIFE

Maria Campbell (1940–)

Maria Campbell is a Métis woman and the eldest daughter of seven children. She was born in Park Valley, Saskatchewan, to parents of Scottish, Indian, and French descent. Her autobiography, *Halfbreed* (1973), recounts the first 33 years of her life and tells of how Maria lost her mother when she was only 12 years old, leaving her to care for her younger siblings. In an effort to keep her family together, young Maria married an abusive white man who reported her to child welfare authorities, and her siblings were placed in foster homes. Devastated, Maria moved to Vancouver, where her husband deserted her, and she turned to a life of drugs and prostitution. Alone and desperate, she attempted suicide twice and was hospitalized for psychiatric care. It is in the hospital that Maria joined Alcoholics Anonymous and began a journey of healing.

In the book, Maria Campbell not only tells her own story but also speaks of the discrimination and racism that affect all Métis people. In the book's introduction, she writes, "I write this for all of you, to tell you what it is like to be a half-breed woman in this country. I want to tell you about the joys and sorrows, the oppressing poverty, the frustrations and the dreams" (p. 8). Although Maria's story is one of stress and crises, it is also a story of courage and resilience. She is no longer a scared little girl but a strong, independent woman full of hope for herself and her people. She is a mother, grandmother, and great-grandmother.

Today, Maria is a Métis cultural leader and an Officer of the Order of Canada (2008). She continues to write; her translated work, *Stories of the Road Allowance People*, was republished in 2010. In 2012, she retired from the University of Saskatchewan, was awarded a Pierre Elliott Trudeau Fellowship, and joined the Métis Research Group, Institute of Canadian Studies, University of Ottawa. She is the recipient of many writing awards, including the Chalmers Award for best new play, and has four Honorary Doctorate degrees.

From Campbell, M. (1973). *Halfbreed*. Halifax, NS: Goodread Biographies.

- Chronic illness or conditions with a strong stress component (e.g., hypertension, migraine, chronic pain syndromes, irritable bowel syndrome)
- Evidence of immune system suppression (e.g., frequent infections)
- Physical appearance (e.g., deficits in grooming and hygiene; nonverbal indications of muscle tension, anxiety, or depression)
- Alterations in activity and exercise patterns

As well, the biologic assessment of stress and coping considers the use of pharmacologic agents, including prescription and nonprescription medications, over-the-counter and herbal preparations, alcohol, tobacco, and illicit drugs. As noted previously, some individuals begin or increase the frequency of using these agents as a way of coping with stress. At the same time, however, reliance on relaxants or mood-altering substances can become a secondary stressor and contribute to maladaptation. Understanding patterns of use (e.g., frequency, dose, circumstances, and effects) is important to assessing their role in stress management. The more important the substances are to a person's handling of stress, the greater the potential for abuse and addiction.

Interventions for the Biologic Domain

Individuals experiencing or at risk for untoward stress responses may benefit from a number of biologic interventions.

- The importance of (re)establishing regular routines for activities of daily living (e.g., eating, sleeping, self-care, leisure time) cannot be overstated. As well as ensuring adequate nutrition, sleep and rest, and hygiene, a routine may help to structure an individual's time and give him or her a sense of personal control or mastery.
- Exercise can reduce the emotional and behavioural responses to stress. In addition to the physical benefits of exercise, regular exercise can provide structure to a person's life, enhance self-confidence, and increase feelings of well-being. Under stress, many individuals are not receptive to the idea of exercise, particularly if it has not been a part of their life. Exploration of usual activity patterns, as well as knowledge and beliefs about the value of exercise, will help to identify where the nurse may intervene.
- Activities such as yoga, meditation, deep breathing, and progressive muscle relaxation can help individuals mediate the physical stress response, improve sleep, and reduce pain. Nurses should also consider referring clients for hypnosis or biofeedback when indicated.
- Health teaching in such areas as nutrition, sleep hygiene, and medication management may also be a part of nursing interventions in this domain.

Psychological Domain

Psychological Assessment

Information about the psychological and emotional dimensions of stress may be forthcoming throughout the assessment process. In particular, the nurse should do the following:

- Observe for behavioural and affective indicators of stress response (e.g., energy level and general presentation; appearance, grooming, and hygiene; psychomotor agitation and retardation; facial expression; speech characteristics).
- Explore reports of recent changes in mood or current emotional distress (e.g., anxiety, fear, irritability, anger, tension, pressure, depression).
- Note alterations or impairment in mental status (e.g., suicidal ideation; self-deprecatory thoughts; impulsivity; ruminations; impaired concentration, problem solving, or memory).
- Explore the individual's appraisal of significant life events (e.g., losses, physical or sexual abuse or assault, motor vehicle crashes, natural disasters, combat experience), the effect of those experiences, and the commitment to particular outcomes.
- Ask about alterations in day-to-day function or inability to fulfil responsibilities (e.g., family, work, school).
- Explore the individual's current resources and effectiveness of usual coping strategies.

Interventions for the Psychological Domain

Nursing interventions that support psychological functioning and facilitate lifestyle changes for persons coping with stress include cognitive–behavioural interventions (see Chapter 13), psychoeducational (individual or group) interventions (see Chapter 14), relaxation therapy, and assertiveness training.

Social Domain

Social Assessment

Information from a social assessment is invaluable to understanding an individual's coping resources. The ability to make healthy lifestyle changes is strongly influenced by one's social support system. Even the expression of stress is related to social factors, particularly ethnic and cultural expectations and values.

Social assessment also includes identification of the person's social network. The nurse should elicit the following information:

- Size and extent of the network, both relatives and non-relatives, and the length and quality of the relationships
- Functions the network serves (e.g., intimacy, social integration, nurturance, reassurance of worth, guidance and advice, access to new contacts)
- Degree of reciprocity between the individual and others in the network (i.e., Whom provides support to the client? Whom does the client support?)
- Degree of interconnectedness among network members

Interventions for the Social Domain

Individuals who are coping with stressful situations often benefit from interventions that facilitate social functioning and promote the health and welfare of social network members. The education of the family regarding the client's disorder and their supportive involvement can be significant. The family and individual members may also require support, including respite. Referral to family therapy may be indicated.

Spiritual Domain

The challenges faced by individuals in times of stress and crisis can lead to an acute questioning about one's life choices and situation, about one's relationships, and about the meaning of one's very existence. Making sense of what is happening to you is fundamental to being human. If we want to believe in a "just world," one response may be to search for reasons that one deserves to be "punished" (Hafer & Bàgue, 2005). In his book *When Bad Things Happen to Good People*, Kushner (1981) describes how a personal tragedy compelled him to "rethink everything" he had been taught about God and God's ways (p. 1). He could not make sense of what was happening to his family and felt "a deep aching sense of unfairness" (p. 2). Ultimately, Rabbi Kushner concluded that suffering happens in our natural world and that there are no exceptions for nice people; God gives humans strength to cope with their misfortunes and does not leave them to suffer alone. While his book reveals the search for meaning that a life crisis can inspire, his conclusions are his own. Others, even those in very similar circumstances, may choose a different resolution. For instance, lasting anger at the sacred power in which one believes may be the response if one feels totally abandoned or one may view the crisis situation as revealing direction for personal growth.

Nurses attending to the spiritual domain of their practice need to recognize the likely occurrence of such searching on the part of clients under duress or in crisis. Nurses need to refrain from providing their own answers to questions of meaning; rather, through listening, they need to provide support. Thoughtful questions may be helpful in understanding the client's perspective: Has your current stressful situation influenced the way you understand the world? Have your beliefs been affected? If so, in what way? What is sustaining you through this time? Are there spiritual acts, such as prayer or ritual, which you are finding helpful? What, if anything, can you take from this experience to help you in the future?

When a traumatic or crisis event is catastrophic in its scope, entire communities can struggle to understand the cause of what has happened and the meaning of the loss suffered. At one time in Western societies, disasters were understood as evidence of the wrath of the gods or God (Grandjean, Rendu, MacNamee, & Scherer, 2008). The Lisbon earthquake of 1755 is used to mark the beginnings of change in societal attitudes towards disaster: it is called the first modern disaster as it was attributed to "natural" rather than "supernatural" causes. The type of disaster influences this struggle, of course, and can affect the community's recovery (Furedi, 2007).

Spirituality can positively influence the response to disaster. In a study of psychiatric morbidity following a tsunami in a community with diverse religious beliefs, it was found that altruistic behaviour on the part of community leaders, religious faith, and spirituality (along with family systems and social support) were factors that positively affected the early coping of survivors (Math et al., 2008). In addition to their professional challenges, nurses responding to a disaster in their own community will have to address their personal reaction as members of the community with their own spiritual questions.

Evaluation and Treatment Outcomes

Evaluation is guided by treatment goals established in the plan of care. The goals of individual care relate to improved health, well-being, and social function. Depending on the level of intervention, there may also be goals for the family and other members of the client's social network. Family outcomes may relate to improved communication or social support (e.g., reduced caregiver stress). Social network outcomes focus on strengthening the social network and improving its function.

■ CRISIS

Our current understanding of the bio/psycho/social/spiritual implications of a crisis has its roots in Lindeman's (1944) study of **bereavement** among friends and relatives of the Coconut Grove nightclub fire in Boston in 1942. Four hundred and thirty-nine individuals died in that fire, which at the time was the worst single building fire in U.S. history. In the course of his research, Lindeman learned that family and friends of those who died experienced somatic symptoms, feelings of anger and guilt, and preoccupation with the deceased. From this work, he developed a model that describes **grief** as progressing through three stages: shock and disbelief, acute **mourning**, and resolution. Lindeman concluded that grief is both a natural response to loss and necessary to survivors' mental health. He later extended his ideas about crisis to more common, yet significant, life events (e.g., the birth of a child, marriage, death) and hypothesized that the changes associated with these events cause emotional strain and require individuals to adapt to a new reality (Lindeman, 1956). These adaptive efforts either lead to mastery (psychological growth)

or impaired functioning. Lindeman was convinced that by helping individuals through the bereavement process, mental health professionals could prevent later psychological and emotional problems. This thinking reflected two important trends that were germinating in psychiatry around the globe: the recognition of the potential for and the value of early intervention to prevent emotional and psychological problems and the movement from hospital-based to community-based psychiatric treatment.

Although Lindeman did much of the foundational work in the area of crisis, Gerald Caplan is widely acknowledged as the master architect of **crisis intervention**. A psychiatrist and close colleague of Lindeman's, Caplan (1961) equated mental health with a strong, mature ego, which he defined as: (1) the capacity to withstand stress and maintain equilibrium, (2) an accurate perception of reality, and (3) a balanced repertoire of coping strategies based on sound reality testing. Under the aegis of the Harvard School of Public Health, Caplan established the Harvard Family Guidance Centre, an interdisciplinary crisis research and consultation project that studied the impact of four stressors: premature birth, birth of children with congenital abnormalities, birth of twins, and tuberculosis. Caplan is believed to be the first to apply the term *crisis* in psychiatry, to relate the concept of homeostasis to crisis intervention, and to describe the stages of a crisis.

Caplan defined crisis as occurring "when a person faces an obstacle to important life goals, that is, for a time, insurmountable through the utilization of customary methods of problem solving" (1961, p. 18). More specifically, a crisis is a response in which psychological equilibrium is disrupted, usual coping methods are ineffective in restoring that equilibrium, and there is evidence of functional impairment (Caplan, 1961; Flannery & Everly, 2000). This disequilibrium causes a rise in inner tension and anxiety that, if it continues, engenders emotional upset and an inability to function (Caplan, 1961). Figure 17-5 summarizes the phases of crisis.

Although crises force individuals into uncharted territory, Caplan (1961) recognized that most individuals achieve resolution without professional help within 4 to 6 weeks. He viewed this time as a period of transition in which the individual, family, or group is more vulnerable to harm and at the same time more open to outside intervention. This prompted him to advocate for community-based crisis services aimed at identifying maladaptive responses and intervening early to assist those involved to transform problems into opportunities for personal growth and new learning.

KEY CONCEPT A **crisis** response occurs when an individual encounters an obstacle or problem that might affect his or her life goals and that cannot be solved by customary problem-solving methods. It is acute, time limited, and may be developmental, situational, or interpersonal in nature.

FIGURE 17-5. Phases of crisis response.

A problem arises that contributes to increase in anxiety levels. The anxiety stimulates the implementation of usual problem-solving techniques of the person.

↓

The usual problem-solving techniques are ineffective. Anxiety levels continue to rise. Trial-and-error attempts are made to restore balance.

↓

The trial-and-error attempts fail. The anxiety escalates to severe or panic levels. The person adopts automatic relief behaviours.

↓

When these measures do not reduce anxiety, anxiety can overwhelm the person and lead to serious personality disorganization, which signals the person is in crisis.

Types of Crises

Situational Crisis

A situational crisis is any event that overwhelms an individual's coping resources and upsets his or her equilibrium. The precipitating event may be positive or negative, physiologic, psychological, or social in nature. Examples of situational crises include illness, the death of a loved one, separation or divorce, job loss, school problems, physical or sexual assault, or an unplanned pregnancy. Situational crises also result from less common occurrences such as accidents, natural or human-caused disasters, and acts of terrorism. Box 17-1 discusses the death of a loved one, a situational crisis that each of us will encounter in our lifetime.

Developmental Crisis

Theorists such as Erikson (1959) propose that human development proceeds sequentially through a series of stages, each with a new set of social roles and responsibilities. Stage theorists hold that demands from the social environment exert pressure on an individual to move on to the next developmental stage and that a failure to meet these new expectations precipitates a developmental crisis. Successful resolution of this crisis is necessary for movement into the next stage. Developmental crises are an expected part of maturation and are a time during which individuals acquire new skills and resources.

The concept of developmental crisis assumes that psychosocial development progresses in an orderly, easily identifiable process. Other developmental theories, such as those of Miller (1994) and Gilligan (1994), refute the notion that human development advances in stages (see Chapter 8). That being said, the concept of developmental crisis is useful for describing unfavourable person–environment relationships that relate to maturational events, such as leaving home for the first time, completing school, or the birth of one's first child.

Crisis or Not? The Effects of Balancing Factors

Aguilera (1998) believes that a stressful event's developing into a crisis depends on three *balancing factors*: perception of the event, available situational supports, and coping mechanisms. As Figure 17-6 illustrates, the timely and successful resolution of a crisis is more likely if an individual has a realistic view of the situation, adequate supports available, and effective coping mechanisms.

Nursing Care of Individuals Experiencing Crisis

Crisis Intervention

Crisis intervention is the provision of emergency psychological care to assist victims in returning to an adaptive level of functioning and to prevent or moderate the potentially negative effects of psychological trauma (Everly & Mitchell, 1999). Although there are several models of crisis intervention, virtually all of them incorporate the following principles (Flannery & Everly, 2000):

1. **Early intervention.** By their nature, crises are acute and distressing events that overwhelm an individual's coping resources. Inability to resolve a crisis in a timely manner renders those affected at higher risk for long-term health problems. Crisis intervention services are typically community based and operate 24 hours/day. Crisis teams provide telephone triage and counselling but may also travel to the scene of the crisis, where they work closely with other emergency service personnel (e.g., police officers, firefighters, and hospital emergency staff).

BOX 17-1 Death of a Loved One: A Crisis Event

One of the most common crisis-provoking events is the loss of a loved one through death. Although death is a certainty for all of us, Western culture "denies and defies death. Death is often seen as a defeat, a failure, and an outcome to be avoided at all costs. As a result, the bereaved often feel profoundly isolated" (Roberts & Berry, 2002, p. 53).

Definition of Terms
Bereavement is typically understood to be the objective event or occurrence of having suffered a loss (Rando, 1993).

Grief is the subjective experience (e.g., thoughts, feelings, behaviours, body sensations) that accompanies the perception of a loss (Rando, 1993).

Mourning is the external manifestation of grief, which is highly influenced by gender, ethnicity, culture, religion, and the cause of death (Wolfelt, 1999).

Tasks of Mourning
Worden (2003) describes the four tasks of mourning, which are necessary to the process of adapting to loss and reestablishing equilibrium. Unlike other theorists who conceptualize mourning in terms of *stages* or *phases*, which connote linearity, Worden emphasizes the issues that bereaved individuals must face and successfully negotiate as they come to terms with their new reality:

1. *Accepting the reality of the loss.* The first task of grieving is to accept the reality and full consequence of the loss. A part of this is recognizing the permanence of death and that life as it was is over forever.
2. *Working through the pain of grief.* It is important for the bereaved individual to experience and acknowledge the pain of grief. Denial or suppression of this pain prolongs grieving.
3. *Adapting to an environment in which the deceased is absent.* This adaptation requires the bereaved individual to adjust to a new reality, which involves developing a new self-identity (e.g., as a widow or single person) and taking on new social roles and responsibilities.
4. *Developing a new relationship with the deceased and reengaging with life.* In coming to terms with the loss, the bereaved individual does not forget the deceased but

rather establishes a new relationship with the deceased. This involves healing the wound of the severed attachment so that new attachments can be formed.

Resolution of grief is manifested by the gradual return of feelings of well-being and the ability to continue with life. The bereaved person does not deny his or her former life or forget the loved one but finds a way to weave memories of the past into the current reality.

It is important to keep in mind that although the experience of loss is universal, individual responses vary widely, and there is no one clearly defined course or process of bereavement or grieving. Grief is influenced by age, development, gender, history of loss and/or trauma, history of depression, the nature and quality of the relationship with the deceased, and the type of loss (e.g., anticipated, violent, traumatic). Research underscores that the experience and expressions of grief are influenced by such factors as familial relationships and expectations, social and cultural factors, and religion (Center for the Advancement of Health, 2003).

Complicated Grief
Complicated grief is also termed abnormal, pathologic, chronic, or exaggerated grief. It refers to grief that does not seem to be advancing the bereaved individual towards acceptance and reorganization. Grief is complicated when an individual does not accomplish one or more of the tasks of mourning. Examples of this include denying the reality of one's loss; prolonged and intense emotions that do not seem to lessen over time; the apparent absence of mourning; and the inability to reinvest in life.

Role of Health Care Teams in Supporting Grief
As members of the health care team, nurses participate in supporting bereaved individuals through the process of grieving. The goals of this care are to assist bereaved individuals with the tasks of mourning and to prevent complicated grief. Activities may include sitting in silence with the bereaved, active listening, assistance with practical needs, and referral for ongoing support.

---

2. **Stabilization.** An immediate goal of all crisis intervention efforts is to prevent the situation from worsening. Stabilization involves mobilizing resources and support networks with the aim of minimizing harm and quickly restoring some semblance of order and routine.
3. **Facilitating understanding.** An important part of crisis intervention is helping individuals to develop an accurate understanding of the situation and its potential consequences. This usually involves listening to individuals' accounts of their experience and assisting them to identify and articulate their feelings about what is happening. Facilitating a clear understanding of a situation helps individuals to develop a realistic appraisal of the demands on them and aids the integration of the crisis into their cognitive schema.
4. **Focusing on problem solving.** A primary task of crisis intervention is the identification and prioritization of immediate problems. Once achieved, interventions

focus on assisting those involved to find short-term solutions.
5. **Encouraging self-reliance.** Encouraging and supporting individuals to participate in identifying and solving problems facilitate their return to independent function and the development of a sense of mastery.

The case study in Box 17-2 uses Roberts' Seven-Stage Crisis Intervention Model (Fig. 17-7; Roberts, 1991) to illustrate the application of these principles to a clinical situation.

● STUDY NOTE
The goals of crisis intervention are to assist individuals to return to an adaptive level of functioning and to prevent or moderate the potentially negative effects of extreme stress. Principles of crisis intervention include early intervention, stabilization, facilitating understanding, a focus on problem solving, and encouragement of self-reliance.

FIGURE 17-6. The effect of balancing factors in a stressful event (From Aguilera, D. C. (1998). *Crisis intervention: Theory and methodology* (8th ed). St. Louis, MO: Mosby.).

Telephone Help Lines

Many health authorities now have telephone help lines, typically staffed by mental health professionals or trained volunteers, which offer support for problems such as child abuse, suicide, and family stress. These lines permit immediate access to a spectrum of support and intervention services for individuals who are experiencing a crisis or need help to manage life stressors.

Short-Stay Hospitalization and Community-Based Emergency Housing

Some health authorities also designate a few beds on their psychiatric units for short-stay crisis stabilization. Individuals are admitted to these beds for a brief period of inpatient care (typically 72 hours) when they

have no supports in the community, need to have their medications assessed or stabilized, or require some other health service. There is also often community-based emergency housing, such as shelters for children and youth who cannot remain at home, shelters for victims of domestic violence, and short- and long-term accommodations for individuals with serious and persistent mental illness. These settings provide users with food, a place to stay, emotional support, and referrals to other community services.

Response to Disaster

Disasters are sudden, severe, and social phenomena. Defined, a disaster occurs when a hazard, originating in the geophysical or biologic environment or as the result of

---

BOX 17-2 Case Study Demonstrating Roberts' Seven-Stage Crisis Intervention Model

The mobile mental health crisis unit in a large Canadian city receives a call from Theresa, the maternal aunt of 19-year-old Billy, an Aboriginal male whose 12-year-old brother died 4 months ago from sniffing gasoline. On hearing of his brother's death, Billy quit college and went on a 5-day drinking binge. At the time of the call, he is lying on his bed in the dark. Theresa tells the crisis nurse that Billy has been eating very little for the past several weeks and has been sleeping 12 to 14 hours/day. He rarely leaves his room and speaks only when addressed directly. What little conversation he does offer is preoccupied with his brother and their parents, who died in a car crash a number of years earlier. Theresa has tried everything she can think of to convince Billy to get help; she is worried about leaving him alone for fear he will harm himself.

STAGE 1: Conduct Crisis and Bio/Psycho/Social/Spiritual Assessment (Including Lethality Assessment). Joanne, the crisis intervention nurse, performs a focused assessment and, using direct questions, ascertains important details about the situation (e.g., caller name, address, and telephone number; nature of emergency; presence of/potential for injury or loss of life; availability of weapons or other potentially dangerous items). Within 2 or 3 minutes, she determines that Billy has experienced major losses (one of them very recently); that his behaviour is suggestive of acute mourning and/or depression; that he is at high risk for self-harm; and that his aunt, who is his primary social support, has exhausted her resources for dealing with the situation. The nurse tells Theresa that she and a colleague are on their way to talk with Billy and that they will be bringing police assistance. The nurse decides to involve the police for two reasons. The first is that by their nature, crises are unpredictable situations and have some potential for violence; a police presence sometimes deters aggressive acting out, and if it does not, it ensures that there are trained personnel to effectively contain it. The second reason is that the police have authority, under provincial mental health legislation, to transport individuals for psychiatric assessment, even against their will. In order to do this, they must have evidence that the individual is in imminent danger to himself or herself or someone else.

STAGE 2: Establish Rapport and a Working Therapeutic Relationship. Joanne establishes rapport with Theresa on the telephone by listening carefully to her, validating her concerns, and offering concrete and specific assistance. When the nurse and other members of the crisis team arrive at the home, Joanne stays with Theresa while her colleague Don begins talking with Billy through his locked bedroom door. Don uses his well-developed interpersonal skills (see Chapter 6) to make a connection with the young man and to convince him to come out of his room and talk face to face. When it becomes apparent that Billy is not a danger to himself or others, the police leave.

STAGE 3: Identify Dimensions of Presenting Problem. Fortunately, when the crisis team speaks with Billy, they learn that he has not done anything to harm himself. He is experiencing a great deal of emotional pain for which he has few words, has lost his sense of meaning in life, and has only a vague plan of shooting himself. He does not have immediate access to a firearm. In his conversation with Don, Billy acknowledges that the loss of his parents was devastating, but it is his brother's death that caused his "world to crash apart."

STAGE 4: Explore Feelings and Emotions. Don encourages Billy to talk about his experience and offers him words for the things he is feeling. Eventually, Billy agrees to include his aunt and Joanne in the conversation.

STAGE 5: Generate and Explore Alternatives. Billy, Theresa, Don, and Joanne sit around the kitchen table with cups of tea discussing the supports available to the family.

STAGE 6: Develop a Plan. Theresa states that praying to the creator every day and speaking to a local elder help her to get through many difficult times. Billy says that he will pray with her every day, signs a written safety contract, and agrees to see an intake worker at the mental health centre for an assessment the next day. The safety contract specifies a number of things that Billy will do if he begins to feel overwhelmed again, including praying, talking to Theresa, and calling the crisis line.

STAGE 7: Develop a Follow-up Plan. Joanne calls Theresa the next afternoon and learns that she and Billy had spent the evening talking and praying together. He had eaten breakfast and showered this morning before attending his appointment at the mental health centre. The intake worker referred Billy to a men's grief support group and was going to speak with the student counselling service at his college to arrange one-to-one counselling.

---

unintentional or malicious human action, exceeds a community's ability to cope (Ministers Responsible for Emergency Management, 2011). The complexity of global risk for disasters appears to be increasing (Arora & Arora, 2013), along with severe financial, infrastructure, and human costs.

The suffering caused by a disaster event can last for years. Malicious acts of terrorism have the greatest impact on mental health morbidity, while disasters caused by human and technologic error have a more moderate impact, and natural disasters have the least (Math, Kumar, Christine, & Cherian, 2013). Yet even natural disasters such as floods can create extensive and sustained social and mental health problems, challenging the resilience of all those affected (Stanke, Murray, Amlôt, Nurse, & Williams, 2012).

The Canada Disaster Database (CDC) contains information on disasters that have occurred since 1900 that directly affected Canadians and tracks significant disaster events (see Web Links on thePoint; Figures 17-8 and 17-9).

Disasters are categorized in the CDC as natural, conflict, or technology (see Table 17-5 for types of disasters). Disaster management needs to be intersectoral, community based, and involve planning, mitigation, response, and recovery. Avoidance of disaster through prevention measures is critical, given the human and financial cost of these catastrophic events. The psychosocial and mental health aspects of disaster management and response must be integrated in a holistic way across the phases of disaster management, rather than as an auxiliary endeavour.

> **KEY CONCEPT** A **disaster** is a social phenomenon that occurs when a hazard, originating in the geophysical or biologic environment or as the result of unintentional or malicious human action, exceeds a community's ability to cope (Ministers Responsible for Emergency Management, 2011).

FIGURE 17-7. Roberts' (1991) Seven-Stage Crisis Intervention Model.

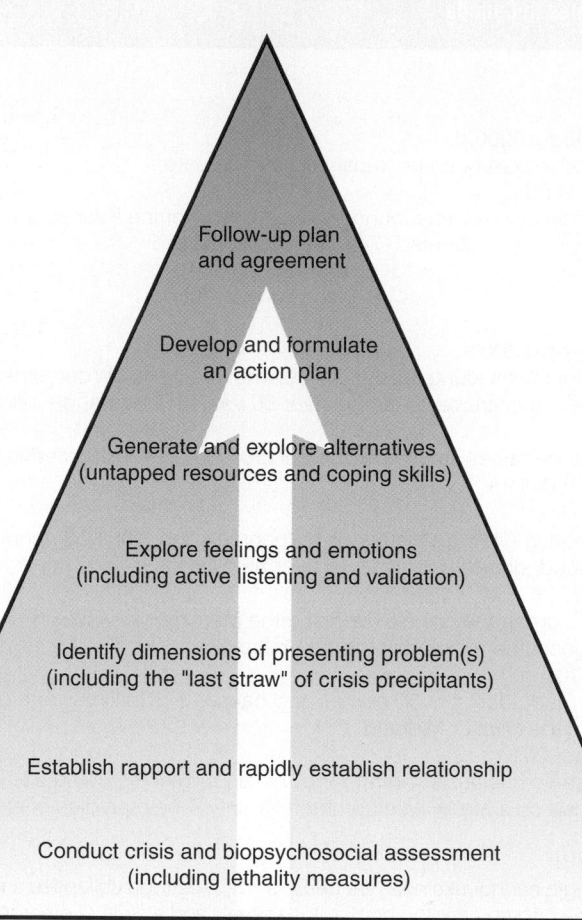

Follow-up plan and agreement

Develop and formulate an action plan

Generate and explore alternatives (untapped resources and coping skills)

Explore feelings and emotions (including active listening and validation)

Identify dimensions of presenting problem(s) (including the "last straw" of crisis precipitants)

Establish rapport and rapidly establish relationship

Conduct crisis and biopsychosocial assessment (including lethality measures)

● **STUDY NOTE**
Disasters are defined by a number of interacting factors, including natural versus human causation, proximity and degree of personal impact, magnitude and scope, visible end or low point, and probability of recurrence. Individually and collectively, these factors influence the nature, intensity, and duration of the stress associated with a disaster.

Emergency Preparedness and Response

The Role of Government

Canadians can expect their federal, provincial, and territorial governments to help them and their communities to mitigate and prepare for disaster and to assist them during

FIGURE 17-8. Kevan Yeats swims after his cat Momo to safety in High River, Alberta, on June 20, 2013. (Photo courtesy of the Canadian Press/Jordan Verlage.)

FIGURE 17-9. Smoke rises from railway cars that were carrying crude oil after derailing in downtown Lac-Mégantic, Québec, on July 6, 2013. (Photo courtesy of the Canadian Press/Paul Chiasson.)

Table 17-5 — Types of Disasters With Selected Examples in Canada

Category	Subtype	Event type	Example
Natural	Biologic	Epidemic	March–August 2003 SARS outbreak, 44 deaths, most in city of Toronto
		Infestation	October 2005 *Escherichia coli* bacteria found in water supply of the Kashechewan reserve. 1,100 people evacuated, 74 people hospitalized
		Pandemic	
	Meteorological–hydrological	Avalanche	January–April 2003 Rocky Mountains along the British Columbia–Alberta border experience deadliest avalanche season in over 30 years. Thirty people killed
		Drought	1990 Parts of the Prairies stricken by cereal crop drought, estimated losses of half a billion dollars
		Flood	June 2013 Worst flood in Alberta's history—four people killed, 100,000 people displaced, damages estimated over $5 billion
		Hurricane	August 2011 Tropical storm Irene hits Québec and the Maritime provinces. Power outages throughout the region, two people killed
		Tornado	June 2010 An F2 tornado destroys 50 homes and causes $15 million worth of damage around the town of Midland, ON
		Winter storm	December 2010 Canadian Forces assist Ontario Provincial Police in rescuing 237 motorists stranded on a highway in Lambton County. One man dies of exposure
	Geologic	Earthquake	June 2010 5.0-strength earthquake near Val-de-Bois, QC. A bridge collapses and a highway is closed. Three hundred houses lose power and a state of emergency is called
		Landslide	January 2005 Landslide of mud, debris, and snow destroys two homes in North Vancouver. One person is killed and 100 homes are evacuated
		Tsunami	
Conflict	Arson		January 1980 Arsonists set fire to a social club in Chibougamau, QC, killing 45 people and injuring 55
	Civil event		June 2011 Hockey fans take to the streets of Vancouver, rioting, burning, and looting. 140 people taken to hospital with minor injuries, four serious injuries
	Hijacking		
	Terrorist		May 1984 Shooting at the National Assembly of Québec kills three, injures 13
Technologic	Fire		July 2007 Hundreds of Edmonton residents affected by "wall of fire" that sweeps through neighbourhood, destroying 18 townhomes and damaging 76 more
	Hazardous chemicals		
	Infrastructure failure		August 2003 Fifty million people throughout Ontario and the eastern United States affected by blackout (with power outages lasting over 48 h) caused by sagging transmission lines and untrimmed trees in Ohio
	Transportation		August 2011 Flight en route from Yellowknife, NT to Resolute Bay, NU strikes a hill and crashes, killing four crewmembers and eight passengers
	Explosion		July 2013 Train carrying crude oil derails in the town of Lac-Mégantic, QC. Explosions kill 42 people, 5 missing and presumed dead. Half the town's centre is destroyed
	Space event		January 1978 Space debris falls upon the Northwest Territories

Adapted from the Canadian Disaster Database. (2013). *List of event types.* Retrieved from http://cdd.publicsafety.gc.ca/srchpg-eng.aspx

such an event. When a disaster occurs here, our federal government mobilizes resources, coordinated through Public Safety and Preparedness Canada, when assistance is requested or when more than one province or territory is involved. Public Safety Canada is responsible for national policy, standards, and response systems related to disaster. The Public Health Agency of Canada's Centre for Emergency Preparedness and Response (CEPR) has information for the public concerning response to chemical, biologic, radiologic, and nuclear threats, as well as scenarios illustrating a natural and a possible bioterrorism threat and CEPR's role (see Web Links on thePoint).

Health Canada is responsible for providing emergency health care to First Nations and Inuit communities, for working to decrease the adverse effects (health, economic) due to disaster, as well as for coordination of the response to a nuclear or radiologic emergency. Environmental and workplace health, including in emergencies and disasters, is also an area of activity (see Chapter 16 for information on emergencies in the workplace). Provincial and territorial governments' responsibilities, policies, and disaster plans can be found on their public Web sites. For example, British Columbia's disaster psychosocial response planning and delivery is addressed on their Web site (see Web Links on thePoint).

Canada assists other nations in times of disaster and shares resources and information related to disaster mitigation, responsiveness, and recovery. For instance, Canada is a member of the International Initiative for Mental Health Leadership in which countries (e.g., Australia, New Zealand, England, USA) work together to improve mental health components of disaster planning and response.

The Role of Nurses

Health care professionals play a key role across all phases of disaster: planning, mitigation, response, and recovery. Their society depends upon them to respond responsibly in times of disaster, with skill and expertise; they depend upon their society to reduce the risks they encounter in doing so (e.g., provision of antivirals, protective equipment, risk management protocols) and to plan for recovery and support in the aftermath (e.g., life and disability insurance; practical support). This reciprocal relationship must be evident in the planning phase onward, including the identification of threats to health care staff and their families and ways to mitigate them (e.g., child and elder care facilities for responders' family during a disaster).

The Canadian Nurses Association's (CNA) *Code of Ethics for Registered Nurses* (2008a) identifies, as an obligation, nurses' **duty to provide care** (with appropriate precautions) during a pandemic or other disaster. It is acknowledged that there may be circumstances when it is acceptable for a nurse to withdraw or refuse to provide care. Family responsibilities, obligations to self, and level

of risk will be factors that influence such circumstances. The Code provides examples of ethical decision-making models to assist the individual nurse and CNA's (2008b) *Nurses' Ethical Considerations in a Pandemic or other Emergency*, part of the *Ethics in Practice for Registered Nurses* series, is a further resource.

The severe acute respiratory syndrome (SARS) global outbreak in 2003 is an example of the dangers nurses can face: 43% of the 251 confirmed cases in Canada were health care workers; three died and others were left with physical and psychosocial ailments, including respiratory problems and PTSD (O'Sullivan, 2009). A study of nurses' experiences during the SARS epidemic found that nurses did not feel prepared for a large-scale disaster and that they experienced role conflict as they put their families at risk (O'Sullivan, 2009). A relational ethics approach, with its focus on relationship, environmental context, ethical decisions as embodied actions, and the importance of dialogue, may be particularly useful to nurses in preparation for and response to disaster (Austin, 2008). CNA's (2012) position statement on emergency preparation and response supports ICN's demand that nurses use strategies that respect human rights, social justice, and equity of access to health and social services for those affected by disaster.

It is of concern that many nurses do not believe that they are well prepared to respond to disaster events (see Box 17-3). A Canadian survey study of nurses ($n = 1,543$) from emergency departments and intensive care units indicated that 40% of respondents were unaware if their hospital had an emergency plan for a large-scale outbreak; nurses reported inadequate access to resources to support disaster response capacity; and expressed a low degree of confidence in the preparedness of Canadian health care institutions for disasters/attacks, particularly (O'Sullivan et al., 2008).

The Role of Individuals and Families

Public Safety Canada in collaboration with other government and nongovernment agencies has a *Get Prepared* initiative that assists Canadians and their families to prepare for the first 3 days following a disaster event. *Get Prepared* has three main components: know the risks and get prepared; make an emergency plan; and get an emergency kit. Guides to doing so, as well as a list of federal–provincial–territorial resources, are available for free (see Web Links on thePoint); there is an emergency plan guide for persons with disabilities or special needs. A mobile "get prepared" site provides key steps to follow in particular types of emergencies such as floods, wildfires, and so on, as well as how to respond to an evacuation order (see Web Links on thePoint).

As well as educating individuals and families in getting prepared for disaster, nurses have an obligation themselves to "anticipate, deliberate, and prepare" for disaster (CNA, 2008b; World Health Organization & the International Council of Nurses, 2006). They need to

BOX 17-3　Research for Best Practice

RURAL NURSES' READINESS TO MANAGE DISASTERS

Baack, S. & Alfred, D. (2013). Nurses' preparedness and perceived competence in managing disasters. Journal of Nursing Scholarship, 45(3), 281–287.

Question: Do hospital-based nurses in rural communities perceive themselves prepared and competent for disaster management? What factors among individual differences (age, years of experience, previous disaster experience), self-regulation (motivation), and health care climate influence nurses' perceptions of their competence for managing disaster events? Is there a predictive relationship between self-regulation scores and perceived competence in disaster management?

Method: The 58-item Disaster Readiness Questionnaire was used to survey hospital-based nurses (*n* = 620; 25% response rate) in rural communities in Texas, using a link through hospital intranet sites. The theoretical framework underpinning the study was aspects of Deci's self-determination theory in which the claim is that individuals seek challenges to promote their personal growth. Perceived readiness for disaster is then viewed as being influenced by individual differences, self-regulation of behaviour, perceived competence, and health care climate.

Findings: Most nurses were not confident of their ability to respond competently to a disaster event, although approximately 20% of the survey respondents worked in critical care and emergency departments. The perceived competence scores were consistently below the midpoint range. Those who were confident were more likely to have previous participation in a disaster or prior work in a postdisaster shelter. Self-regulation was significantly predictive as a factor only in relation to the willingness of the nurse to assume the risk of participation in a disaster situation.

Implication for Practice: Nurses are involved in planning, mitigation, response, and recovery to disaster. Preparation for these roles is necessary. Nurses, supported by their health care institutions and agencies, need to seek out opportunities to participate in actual disaster events, in mock drills, and in other education for disaster preparation.

ensure that they and their family are prepared to cope on their own for 72 hours in the event of a disaster situation.

Phases of Disaster

Although the experience of disaster is unique to each individual and community, various phases of disaster can be delineated. It is important to recognize such phases (e.g., preparation, response, recovery, mitigation) as multilayered, complex, and influenced by the interaction of persons–community–environment rather than as discrete and constant categories. Phases of disaster focused on possible psychological and social responses from 1 to 3 days to 1 to 3 years are shown in Figure 17-10 (DeWolfe, 2000).

There are critical factors of disaster that can potentially shape aftermath reactions and postdisaster stress. These include causation (natural or human), degree of personal impact, size and scope, visible impact/low point, and the probability of recurrence (DeWolfe, 2000). When human intent causes a disaster (e.g., bombing), the stress reaction is greater than when the cause is "natural" (an "act of God"). Causes are not always clearly defined, such as when environmental degradation contributes to flooding. If an individual has high exposure to a disaster event or intimate personal loss, the disaster impact will usually be more intense; a disaster that destroys an entire community will have more negative and lasting impact than one of lesser scope. The recovery process is impeded when disasters are neither clearly visible nor defined (i.e., there is no "it's over and the rebuilding begins" moment), as in the case of toxic spills and nuclear accidents. With such disasters, the devastating consequences continue for years, resulting in chronic stress, fear, and anxiety. When there is a high probability that a disaster will reoccur in a community, the ongoing threat will affect recovery, particularly if disaster mitigation is not occurring (DeWolfe, 2000).

An international review of the effects of disaster on over 60,000 individuals in 102 different events indicates that effects are the greatest when two of the following are present:

- Extreme and widespread property damage.
- Serious and ongoing finance problems for the community.
- Human intent was the cause.
- High prevalence of trauma: injuries, loss of life (Norris, Friedman, & Watson, 2002, p. 246).

The spiritual impact that loss of home, possessions, community, and sense of belonging can have is difficult to quantify and to address (Hagen & Hagen, 2013).

Response to Mental Health and Illness in a Disaster

Natural recovery processes and community-based sources of help are foundational to disaster response. Disaster events can result in greater social cohesion within a community (Cocking, 2013). The everyday cooperation of community members as survivors are comforted, fed, sheltered, and supported is as important as heroic acts and crucial to recovery. It is helpful to keep people in their normal groups if relocation is necessary and to facilitate their return to normal activities as soon as possible; disaster response should not undermine natural helping networks (Norris et al., 2002).

Key to community-level disaster response is the provision of accurate, timely information that allows informed action in meeting the rapidly changing circumstances inherent to disasters. In Canada, there is mandatory broadcaster participation in the public alerting system regarding disaster. Social networking (e.g., YouTube, Facebook, Twitter) has the potential to facilitate communication in times of disaster: it is broad in reach,

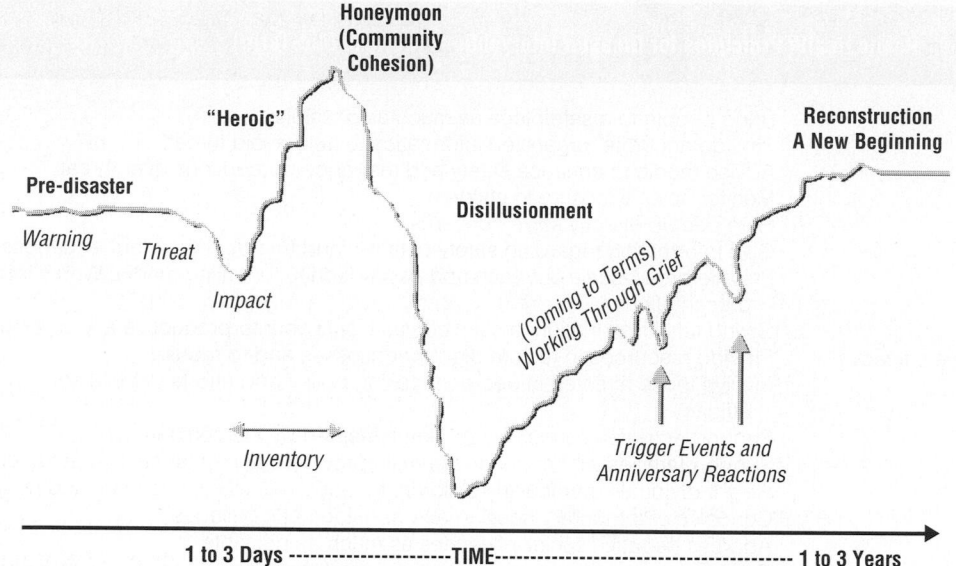

FIGURE 17-10. Sociopsychological phases of disaster. (Source: Zunin, L. M. & Meyers, D. (2000). *Phases of disaster: Training manual for human service workers in major disasters* (2nd ed, p. 5). Washington, DC: Department of Health and Human Services, Substance Abuse and Mental Health Services Administration, Center for Mental Health Services; DHHS Publication No. ADM 90-538.)

user friendly, and free. Nevertheless, there remain privacy, information accuracy, and trustworthiness concerns related to its use (Trainer & Goel, 2013). Information after disaster should be brief, basic, and focused on promoting coping among survivors. Three components to such information are recommended: reassurance and explanation about normal, to-be-expected reactions; advice to return to daily routines as soon as possible; and guidance regarding where to find help if needed (European Commission, 2008).

Psychological First Aid

The common model for mental health care delivery following a disaster is **psychological first aid (PFA)** (Rodriquez & Kohn, 2008; World Health Organization, War Trauma Foundation, & World Vision International, 2011). As with medical first aid, PFA involves intervention with the purpose of immediate relief of distress and the prevention of pathologic sequelae and can be performed by prepared nonprofessionals (Math et al., 2013). Much of the distress experienced at such times will be normative (i.e., grief, anger, and stress related to the trauma of a disaster event) and not require professional treatment (Prewitt Diaz, 2013). PFA involves promoting five key responses: sense of safety, calming, sense of self and community efficacy, connectedness, and hope (Hobfoll, Watson, & Bell, 2007; Prewitt Diaz, 2013). Hope for recovery can be supported through practical action: the provision of necessary services, housing and relocation, replacement of household goods, and employment help (Prewitt Diaz). See Table 17-6 for public health principles for disaster interventions.

The indications that an individual is not successfully coping with stress following a disaster event and may need assistance with stress management are listed in Box 17-4. Although it was once believed that PTSD, the mental disorder most often diagnosed in disaster-affected communities, could be prevented by psychological debriefing, the evidence now indicates otherwise. Single-session debriefing may even be harmful (European Commission, 2008). Professional help may be required for those experiencing persistent and complex grieving (Math et al., 2013).

Vulnerable Populations in Disaster

There are persons who are particularly "at risk" in a disaster situation. These include persons with communication difficulties (e.g., those who do not speak the area's dominant language); those who are physically impaired (e.g., blind, deaf, mobility impaired); those who are cognitively or psychologically impaired; those who are geographically or culturally isolated; and those who lack a means of transportation when evacuation becomes necessary (Hagen & Hagen, 2013, p. 582). Issues for some at-risk populations are described below.

Children and Adolescents

Children and adolescents will be strongly influenced in their response to disaster by the reactions of the adults around them. As with adults, assessment of children's and adolescents' reaction to a disaster event and their resulting mental health needs involves two components: screening and then clinical evaluation for those who are identified during screening as at risk for psychiatric disturbance and for those who (or whose family/close associates) were

Table 17-6	Public Health Principles for Disaster Interventions (Early to Mid-Term)
Safety	Bring people to a safe place as much as possible
	Provide accurate, organized information to help avoid threat
	Advise media to enhance safety and resilience perceptions over threat
	Monitor news exposure to children
Calming	Help people directly solve concerns
	Give information regarding safety of family and friends, and if further danger is expected
	Provide broad-scale outreach and psychoeducation using media, Web sites, and presentations
	Giving false information to calm community is counterproductive and undermines credibility
Self- and collective efficacy	Provide resources to restore dignity and losses and to rebuild
	Involve those affected in decision-making policy and efforts to build self- and collective efficacy
	Support activities conceived and implemented by the community
	Support families who are often the main providers of mental health care after disasters
Connectedness	Help individuals, particularly children, to reconnect with loved ones and neighbours
	Conceive of temporary housing and assistance as "villages"
	Address negative social influences as much as possible
Hope	Create advocacy programs to deal with "red tape" and the complex tasks that follow disaster
	Support rebuilding of local economies
	Involve community leaders in helping link the community with those who survived similar disasters; in memorializing and making meaning; in helping people adapt to the change in their lives and environment, to build on their strengths

Adapted from Hobfoll, S. E., Watson, P., & Bell, C. C. (2007). Five essential elements of immediate and mid-term mass trauma intervention: Empirical evidence. *Psychiatry, 70*, 283–315.; Rodriquez, J. J. & Kohn, R. (2008). Use of mental health services among disaster survivors. *Current Opinion in Psychiatry, 21*, 370–378.

directly exposed to the disaster (Pfefferbaum & North, 2013). PFA and related psychosocial interventions, such as use of play and art activities, can be effective in addressing normative psychological distress. Involving adolescents appropriately in disaster response tasks can help mitigate their distress. When clinical evaluation is required, it will involve a diagnostic assessment for psychopathology (such as PTSD) and the need for referral to professional care (Pfefferbaum & North, 2013).

BOX 17-4 Indicators of Need for Assistance With Stress Management After a Traumatic Event

The following signs occurring for more than 2 to 4 weeks indicate that assistance with stress may be necessary:

Confusion; disorientation
Problems concentrating; short attention span
Continuous crying; frequent mood swings
Feelings of hopelessness
Overwhelming self-doubt
Fear of crowds, leaving home, or being alone
Increased use of alcohol and/or other drugs, including prescription medication

Adapted from Substance Abuse and Mental Health Services Administration (SAMHSA). (2005). *Tips for survivors of a disaster or traumatic event: What to expect in your personal, family, work and financial life.* Rockville, MA: Author.

Persons With an Existing Mental Disorder

As well as those individuals who develop mental health problems or symptoms of mental disorders (e.g., PTSD) as a result of experiencing a disaster event, persons with existing psychiatric disorders are at high risk for exacerbation of their symptoms, for poor emergency coping responses, and for difficulty achieving good recovery from their experience (Hagen & Hagen, 2013). During a disaster, mental health care infrastructures may be seriously damaged, displacing the resources normally accessed for ongoing care at a time when the need for services increases. The World Health Organization (2013) projects that, during emergencies, rates of severe mental disorder among adult populations increase from pre-emergency rates of 2%–3% to 4%–5% and mild mental disorders from 10% to 15%–20%. It is important that PTSD is not exclusively the focus in disaster management so that persons with other mental disorders, including addictions, will also receive assistance.

Disabled Persons

The disruption of infrastructure and support systems during a disaster disproportionally affects persons with disabilities: they are more likely to be left behind in evacuations, and disability can be a discriminating factor in allocation of scare resources. The needs and perspectives of persons with disabilities must be included across all phases of disaster management if their vulnerability and risk are to be reduced. Article 11 in the United Nations Convention on the Rights of Persons with Disabilities (United Nations, 2006) identifies the obligation of nations to do so. Public Safety Canada's Emergency Preparedness Guide for People with Disabilities/Special Needs provides information about emergency packs, resources, tips for helping persons with disabilities/special needs, and addresses particular types of disability (e.g., mobility, hearing, vision, non-visible disabilities like mental illness, heart disease) (see Web Links on thePoint).

Aboriginal Peoples and Disaster

As Aboriginal communities in Canada are often geographically remote, as well as too often marginalized and dealing with poverty and lack of health and social services, they may be particularly vulnerable to disaster events. Problems that increase vulnerability have been lack of funding for on-reserve mitigation efforts and a complicated process for securing the necessary federal financial support after a disaster (Puxley, 2013). Getting the communities the necessary resources in a timely and culturally sensitive way seems key to good recovery, as the collective wisdom of many indigenous communities regarding survival in adverse conditions is already strong. Increasingly, experts are recognizing that lessons are to be learned from such traditional knowledge, lessons that can inform effective disaster management as a whole (Hagen & Hagen, 2013).

Ethnic Minorities

The symptoms of stress, anxiety disorders, and PTSD are identical across cultures (European Commission, 2008). Stress and distress can be reduced if disaster response information to ethnic minority communities is available in their mother tongue and if recovery efforts are culturally appropriate and involve key community figures. When possible, responders should adapt their approach to a person's culture. Things to consider include gender issues, touching, need for certain clothing items, and religious beliefs that will influence the meaning given to the disaster event (WHO et al., 2011).

Disaster Relief Workers

Volunteers are a major source of rescue and recovery assistance in times of disaster. The research on the post-disaster mental health of volunteer responders indicates that, compared with professional workers, volunteers have higher complaint levels, with the factors contributing to this being determined as "identification with victims as a friend, severity of exposure to gruesome events during disaster work, anxiety sensitivity, and lack of post-disaster social support" (Thormar et al., 2010, p. 529).

Summary

It is important that nurses understand the human experience of stress, crisis, and trauma so that they may respond appropriately to individuals, families, and communities in need. Such knowledge is important to nurses' professional self-development, as well, so that they can be confident and safe as they meet the challenges of health care practice. Being prepared to respond to disaster events is a responsibility that nurses share with other professionals; such preparation requires institutional support. Despite the adversity and challenges that disasters bring, there is also opportunity at such times to positively transform a community's approach to mental health care (WHO, 2013).

SUMMARY OF KEY POINTS

■ Many personal factors, such as personality patterns, beliefs, values, and commitment to an outcome, interact with environmental demands and constraints that produce a person–environment relationship.

■ Stress occurs when a person–environment relationship is appraised as being unfavourable. Stress responses are simultaneously emotional and physiologic, leading to an innate tendency to act.

■ Within the social network, social support can help a person cope with stress.

■ Effective coping can be either problem focused or emotion focused. The outcome of successful coping is enhanced health, psychological well-being, and social functioning.

■ A crisis is a severely stressful situation that causes exaggerated stress responses. The nursing process is similar for the person experiencing a stress response, except that increased attention is paid to safety issues.

■ Nurses have an obligation to respond competently across all phases of disasters: planning, mitigation, response, and recovery.

■ Natural recovery processes and community-based sources of help are foundational to successful disaster response and need to be supported. Timely information is key.

■ Psychological first aid (PFA) is the common model for mental health delivery following a disaster.

CRITICAL THINKING CHALLENGES

1 Compare and contrast Selye's stress response to Lazarus and Folkman's model of stress, coping, and adaptation.

2 Explain why two individuals may experience the same stressful event or situation very differently.

3 Briefly explain the physiologic stress response.

4 An 18-year-old man is admitted to a psychiatric unit for psychotic behaviour and is eventually given the diagnosis of schizophrenia. His parents refuse to accept this and take him all over the country seeking other opinions. Is this an example of problem-focused or emotion-focused coping? Explain your answer.

5 After the death of his mother, a 24-year-old single man with schizophrenia moves into an apartment. He continues to take his medication but feels sad about his mother's death. He is not adjusting well to living alone and tells his nurse that he no longer wants to go to work. In tears, he admits that he is lonely and can no longer manage the day-to-day demands of his apartment. The nurse generates the following nursing diagnosis: Ineffective coping related to inadequate support system. Develop a plan of care for this young man.

6 Define *stress*, *crisis*, and *disaster*. Compare and contrast each of these with a psychiatric emergency.

7 You are a nurse working with a mobile mental health crisis team. An elderly woman calls to say that she has just been robbed at knifepoint on her way home from shopping. What assessment questions would you ask her? Explain your answer.

8 Are you and your family/friends prepared for an emergency or disaster event? Identify the elements of such preparation. For instance, what will you do if you are not together and phones and e-mail are unavailable? Are there particular risks given your geographical location? As a student nurse, do you have a role in a health services' disaster management plan?

REFERENCES

Aguilera, D. C. (1998). *Crisis intervention: Theory and methodology* (8th ed.). St. Louis, MO: Mosby.

American Psychiatric Association [APA]. (1980). *Diagnostic and statistical manual of mental disorders* (3rd ed). Washington, DC: Author.

American Psychiatric Association [APA]. (1994). *Diagnostic and statistical manual of mental disorders* (4th ed.) Washington, DC: Author.

American Psychiatric Association [APA]. (2013). *Diagnostic and statistical manual of mental disorders* (5th ed.) Washington, DC: Author.

Amstadter, A., Aggen, S., Knudsen, G. P., Reichborn-Kjennerud, T., & Kendler, F. (2013). Potentially traumatic event exposure, posttraumatic stress disorder, and Axis I and II comorbidity in a population-based study of Norwegian young adults. *Social Psychiatry and Psychiatric Epidemiology*, *48*(2), 215–223.

Arora, R. & Arora, P. (2013). Prologue: A holistic view to managing the inevitable in high-tech and resource-poor settings. In R. Arora & P. Arora (Eds.), *Disaster management: Medical preparedness, response and homeland security* (pp. 3–25). Wallingford, Oxfordshire: CABI.

Austin, W. (2008). Relational ethics. In L. Given (Ed.), *The SAGE encyclopedia of qualitative research methods* (pp. 749–750). Thousand Oaks, CA: SAGE Publications, Inc.

Baack, S. & Alfred, D. (2013). Nurses' preparedness and perceived competence in managing disasters. *Journal of Nursing Scholarship*, *45*(3), 281–287.

Bartlett, D. (1998). *Stress: Perspectives and processes*. Philadelphia, PA: Open University Press.

Birmes, P., Hatton, L., Brunet, A., & Schmitt, L. (2003). Early historical literature for post-traumatic symptomatology. *Stress and Health*, *19*, 17–26.

Campbell, M. (1973). *Halfbreed*. Halifax, NS: Goodread Biographies.

Canadian Nurses Association. (2008a). *Code of ethics for registered nurses*. Retrieved from http://www.cna-aiic.ca/~/media/cna/files/en/codeofethics.pdf

Canadian Nurses Association. (2008b). *Nurses' ethical considerations in a pandemic or other emergency*. Retrieved from http://www.cna-aiic.ca/~/media/cna/page%20content/pdf%20en/2013/07/26/10/43/ethics_in_practice_august_2008_e.pdf

Canadian Nurses Association. (2012). *Position Statement (PS119): Emergency preparedness and response*. Toronto, ON: Authors.

Cannon, W. B. (1939). *The wisdom of the body*. New York, NY: WW Norton.

Caplan, G. (1961). *An approach to community mental health*. New York, NY: Grune & Stratton.

Carpenito-Moyet, L. (2009). *Nursing diagnosis: Application to clinical practice* (13th ed.). Philadelphia, PA: Lippincott Williams & Wilkins.

Center for the Advancement of Health. (2003). *Report on bereavement and grief research*. Retrieved from http://www.cfah.org/pdfs/griefreport.pdf

Clegg, A. (2001). Occupational stress in nursing: A review of the literature. *Journal of Nursing Management*, *9*(2), 101–106.

Cocking, C. (2013). Collective resilience versus collective vulnerability after disasters: A social psychological perspective. In R. Arora & P. Arora (Eds.) *Disaster management: medical preparedness, response and homeland security* (pp. 449–63). Wallingford, UK: CABI.

Cohen, S. & Wills, T. A. (1985). Stress, social support, and the buffering hypothesis. *Psychological Bulletin*, *98*(2), 310–357.

Cooper, G. L. & Dewe, P. (2004). *Stress: A brief history*. Malden, MA: Blackwell Publishing.

Coyne, J. C. & Holroyd, K. (1982). Stress, coping and illness: A transactional perspective. In T. Milton, C. Green, & R. Meagher (Eds.), *Handbook of clinical health psychology* (pp. 103–127). New York, NY: Plenum Press.

Cropley, M. & Steptoe, A. (2005). Social support, life events and physical symptoms: A prospective study of chronic and recent life stress in men and women. *Psychology, Health and Medicine*, *10*(4), 317–325.

Davis, C. G. & Macdonald, S. L. (2004). Threat appraisals, distress and the development of positive life changes after September 11th in a Canadian sample. *Cognitive Behaviour Therapy*, *33*(2), 68–78.

DeWolfe, D. J. (2000). *Training manual for mental health and human service workers in major disasters* (2nd ed.). Rockville, MD: Substance Abuse and Mental Health Services Administration (DHHS/PHS). Retrieved from http://www.samhsa.gov/dtac/FederalResource/Response/4-Training_Manual_MH_Workers.pdf

Dohrenwend, B. S. & Dohrenwend, B. P. (1974). *Stressful life events: Their nature and their effects*. New York, NY: Wiley & Sons.

Dohrenwend, B. P. & Shrout, P. E. (1985). "Hassles" in the conceptualization and measurement of stress variables. *American Psychologist*, *40*(7), 780–785.

Erikson, E. H. (1959). *Identity and the life cycle*. New York, NY: International Universities Press.

European Commission. (2008). *European multidisciplinary guideline: Early psychosocial interventions after disaster, terrorism and other shocking events*. Amsterdam, The Netherlands: Impact, the Dutch Knowledge & Advice Centre for Post-disaster Psychosocial Care.

Everly, G. S. & Mitchell, J. T. (1999). *Critical incident stress management: A new era and standard of care in crisis intervention* (2nd ed). Ellicott City, MD: Chevron.

Flannery, R. B. & Everly, G. S. (2000). Crisis intervention: A review. *International Journal of Emergency Mental Health*, *2*(2), 119–125.

Folkman, S. & Lazarus, R. S. (1991). The concept of coping. In A. Monatand & R. S. Lazarus (Eds.), *Stress and coping: An anthology* (3rd ed., pp. 209–227). New York, NY: Columbia University Press.

Furedi, F. (2007). The changing meaning of disaster. *Area*, *39*(4), 482–489.

Gilligan, C. (1994). Joining the resistance: Psychology, politics, girls and women. In M. Berger (Ed.), *Women beyond Freud: New concept of feminine psychology* (pp. 99–145). New York, NY: Brunner Mazel.

Glaser, R., Rice, J., Sherridan, J., & Fertel, R. (1987). Stress-related immune suppression: Health implications. *Brain, Behavior, and Immunity*, *1*(1), 7–20.

Grandjean, D., Rendu, A.-C., MacNamee, T., & Scherer, K. R. (2008). The wrath of the gods: Appraising the meaning of disaster. *Social Science Information*, *47*(2), 187–204.

Hafer, C. & Bègue, L. (2005). Experimental research on just-world theory: Problems, developments, and future challenges. *Psychological Bulletin*, *131*(1), 128–167.

Hagen, J. & Hagen, S. (2013). The immediate post-disaster reconstruction phase: Alternative care site settings and vulnerable populations. In R. Arora & P. Arora (Eds.) *Disaster management: medical preparedness, response and homeland security* (pp. 575–590). Wallingford, UK: CABI.

Harper, D. (2001). *Online etymology dictionary*. Retrieved from http://www.etymonline.com

Haskell, S., Gordon, K., Mattocks, K., Duggal, M., Erdos, J., Justice, A., & Brandt, C. (2010). Gender differences in rates of depression, PTSD, pain, obesity, and military sexual trauma among Connecticut war veterans of Iraq and Afghanistan. *Journal of Women's Health*, *19*(2), 267–271.

Haslam, S. A., O'Brien, A., Jetten, J., Vormedal, K., & Penna, S. (2005). Taking the strain: Social identity, social support, and the experience of stress. *British Journal of Social Psychology*, 44(Pt 3), 355–370.

Hobfoll, S. E., Watson, P., & Bell, C. C. (2007). Five essential elements of immediate and mid-term mass trauma intervention: Empirical evidence. *Psychiatry*, 70, 283–315,

Holmes, T. & Rahe, R. (1967). The Social Readjustment Patient Scale. *Journal of Psychosomatic Research*, 11(2), 213–218.

Jones, F. & Kinman, G. (2001). Approaches to studying stress. In F. Jones & J. Bright (Eds.), *Stress: Myth, theory & research* (pp. 17–44). London, UK: Prentice Hall.

Jones, M. C. & Johnston, D. W. (2000). Reducing distress in first level and student nurses: A review of the applied stress management literature. *Journal of Advanced Nursing*, 32(1), 66–74.

Kelly, U. A., Skelton, K., Patel, M. & Bradley, B. (2011). More than military sexual trauma: Interpersonal violence, PTSD, and mental health in women veterans. *Research in Nursing and Health*, 34(6), 457–467.

Kendler, K. S., Neale, M. C., Kessler, R. C., Heath, A. C., & Eaves, L. G. (1992). Major depression and generalized anxiety disorder. Same genes, (partly) different environments. *Archives of General Psychiatry*, 49(9), 716–722.

Kessler, R. C., Sonnega, A., Bromet, E., Hughes, M., & Nelson, C. B. (1995). Posttraumatic stress disorder in the National Comorbidity Survey. *Archives of General Psychiatry*, 52(12), 1048–1060.

Kindlen, S. (2003). Injury and illness. In S. Kindlen (Ed.), *Physiology for health care and nursing* (2nd ed.). Edinburgh, UK: Churchill Livingstone.

Kleinke, C. L. (2007). What does it mean to cope? In A. Monat, R. S. Lazarus, & G. Reevy (Eds.), *The Praeger handbook on stress and coping* (pp. 289–308). Westport, CT: Praeger.

Korte, S. M., Koolhaas, J. M., Wingfield, J. C., & McEwen, B. S. (2005). The Darwinian concept of stress: Benefits of allostasis and costs of allostatic load and the trade-offs in health and disease. *Neuroscience and Biobehavioral Reviews*, 29(1), 3–38.

Kushner, H. (1981). *When bad things happen to good people*. New York, NY: Random House Inc.

Lazarus, R. (1991). *Emotion and adaptation*. New York, NY: Oxford University Press.

Lazarus, R. S. (1998). *The life and work of an eminent psychologist: An autobiography of Richard S. Lazarus*. New York, NY: Springer.

Lazarus, R. S. (1999). *Stress and emotion: A new synthesis*. New York, NY: Springer.

Lazarus, R. S., DeLongis, A., Folkman, S., & Gruen, R. (1985). Stress and adaptation outcomes: The problem of confounded measures. *American Psychologist*, 40(7), 770–779.

Lazarus, R. S. & Folkman, S. (1984). *Stress, appraisal and coping*. New York, NY: Springer.

Lee, H. J., Macbeth, A. H., Pagani, J. H., & Young, W. S. (2009). Oxytocin: The great facilitator of life. *Progress in Neurobiology*, 88(2), 27–51.

Lindeman, E. (1944). Symptomatology and management of acute grief. *American Journal of Psychiatry*, 151(6 Suppl.), 155–160.

Lindeman, E. (1956). The meaning of crisis in individual and family. *Teachers College Record*, 57, 310.

Lui, L. Y., Coe, C. L., Swenson, C. A., Kelly, E. A., Kita, H., & Busse, W. W. (2002). School examinations enhance airway inflammation to antigen challenge. *American Journal of Respiratory and Critical Care Medicine*, 165(8), 1062–1067.

Luxton, D., Skopp, N., & Maguen, S. (2010). Gender differences in depression and PTSD symptoms following combat exposure. *Depression and Anxiety*, 27(11), 1027–1033.

Maguen, S., Luxton, D., Skopp, N., & Madden, E. (2012). Gender differences in traumatic experiences and mental health in active duty soldiers redeployed from Iraq and Afghanistan. *Journal of Psychiatric Research*, 46, 311–316.

Majer, J. M., Jason, L. A., Ferrarie, J. R., Venable, L. B., & Olson, B. D. (2002). Social support and self-efficacy for abstinence: Is peer identification an issue? *Journal of Substance Abuse Treatment*, 23(3), 209–215.

Malone, J. (1988). The social support and dissupport continuum. *Journal of Psychosocial Nursing and Mental Health Services*, 26(12), 18–22.

Mason, J. W. (1971). A re-evaluation of the concept of 'non-specificity' in stress theory. *Journal of Psychiatric Research*, 8(3), 323–333.

Math, S. B., John, J. P., Girimaji, S. C., Benegal, V., Sunny, B., Krishnakanth, K., ... Nagaraja, D. (2008). Comparative study of psychiatric morbidity among the displaced and non-displaced populations in the Andaman and Nicobar Islands following the tsunami. *Prehospital and Disaster Medicine*, 23(1), 29–34.

Math, S. B., Kumar, N. C., Christine, M. N., & Cherian, A. V. (2013). Disaster mental health: A paradigm shift from curative to preventative psychiatry. In R. Arora & P. Arora (Eds.), *Disaster management: Medical preparedness, response and homeland security* (pp. 477–494). Wallingford, UK: CABI.

McEwen, B. S. (1998). Protective and damaging effects of stress mediators. *The New England Journal of Medicine*, 338(3), 171–179.

Mikhail, A. (1981). Stress: A psychophysiological conception. *Journal of Human Stress*, 7(2), 9–15.

Miller, J. (1994). Women's psychological development: Connections, disconnections, and violations. In M. Berger (Ed.), *Women beyond Freud: New concept of feminine psychology* (pp. 79–97). New York, NY: Brunner Mazel.

Ministers Responsible for Emergency Management. (2011, January). *An emergency management framework for Canada* (2nd ed.). Ottawa, ON: Emergency Management Policy Division, Public Safety Canada. Retrieved from http://www.publicsafety.gc.ca/cnt/rsrcs/pblctns/mrgnc-mngmnt-frmwrk/index-eng.aspx

National Collaborating Centre for Mental Health. (2005). *Posttraumatic stress disorder: The management of PTSD in adults and children in primary and secondary care*. NICE Clinical Guidelines, No. 26. Gaskell. Retrieved from http://publications.nice.org.uk/posttraumatic-stress-disorder-ptsd-cg26

Norris, F. H., Friedman, M. J., & Watson, P.J. (2002). 60,000 disaster victims speak: Part II. Summary and implications of the disaster mental health research. *Psychiatry*, 65(3), 240–260.

O'Sullivan, T. (2009, April). Spotlight on research: Caring about health workers project. *Health Policy Research Bulletin*, (15), 41–42.

O'Sullivan, T. L., Dow, D., Turner, M. C., Lemyre, L., Corneil, W., Krewski, D., ... Amaratunga, C. A. (2008). Disaster and emergency management: Canadian nurses' perceptions of preparedness on hospital front lines. *Prehospital and Disaster Medicine*, 23(Supp 1), 11–18.

Oxford English Dictionary Online. (2013, December). "trauma, n." Retrieved from http://www.oed.com.login.ezproxy.library.ualberta.ca/view/Entry/205242?redirectedFrom=trauma

Park, K. O. (2007). Social support for stress prevention in hospital settings. *Journal of the Royal Society of Health*, 127(6), 260–264.

Pfefferbaum, B. & North, C. (2013). Assessing children's disaster reactions and mental health needs: Screening and clinical evaluation. *Canadian Journal of Psychiatry*, 58(3), 135–142.

Prewitt Diaz, J. O. (2013). Community-based psychosocial support: an overview. In R. Arora & P. Arora (Eds.), *Disaster management: Medical preparedness, response and homeland security* (pp. 464–476). Wallingford, UK: CABI.

Puxley, C. (2013, Nov 19). *First Nations to get disaster relief sooner, Ottawa says*. The Canadian Press. Retrieved from theglobeandmail.com

Rahe, R. H. (2000). Recent Life Changes Questionnaire [RLCQ] [1997]. In T. H. Holmes, American Psychiatric Association (Eds.). *Task Force for the Handbook of Psychiatric Measures. Handbook of psychiatric measures*. (pp. 235–237). Washington, DC: American Psychiatric Association.

Rando, T. (1993). *Treatment of complicated mourning*. Champaign, IL: Research Press.

Rees, S., Silove, D., Chey, T., Ivancic, L., Steel, Z., Creamer, M., ... Forbes, D. (2011). Lifetime prevalence of gender-based violence in women and the relationship with mental disorders and psychosocial function. *Journal of the American Medical Association*, 306(5), 513–521.

Richardson, J. D., Naifeh, J. A., & Elhai, J. D. (2007). Posttraumatic stress disorder and associated risk factors in Canadian peacekeeping veterans with health-related disabilities. *Canadian Journal of Psychiatry*, 52(8), 510–518.

Roberts, A. R. (1991). Conceptualizing crisis theory and the crisis model. In A. R. Roberts (Ed.), *Contemporary perspectives on crisis intervention and prevention* (pp. 3–17). Englewood Cliffs, NJ: Prentice-Hall.

Roberts, K. F. & Berry, P. H. (2002). Grief and bereavements. In K. K. Kuebler, P. H. Berry, & D. E. Heidrich (Eds.), *End of life care: Clinical practice guidelines* (pp. 53–63). Philadelphia, PA: WB Saunders.

Rodriquez, J. J. & Kohn, R. (2008). Use of mental health services among disaster survivors. *Current Opinion in Psychiatry*, 21, 370–378.

Saddock, B. J. & Saddock, V. A. (2003). *Kaplan and Saddock's synopsis of psychiatry* (9th ed.). Philadelphia, PA: Lippincott Williams & Wilkins.

Sapolsky, R. M. (2004). *Why zebras don't get ulcers* (3rd ed.) New York, NY: Henry Holt.

Segerstrom, S. C. & Miller, G. E. (2003). Psychological stress and the immune system in humans: A meta-analytic view of 30 years of inquiry. *Psychological Bulletin*, 130(4), 601–630.

Selye, H. (1956). *The stress of life*. New York, NY: McGraw-Hill.

Selye, H. (1974). *Stress without distress*. Philadelphia, PA: JB Lippincott.

Selye, H. (1980). The stress concept today. In I. L. Kutash, L. B. Schlesinger, and Associates (Eds.), *Handbook on stress and anxiety* (pp. 127–143). San Francisco, CA: Jossey-Bass.

Seng, J., Rauch, S., Resnick, H., Reed, C., King, A., Low, L., ... Liberzon, I. (2010). Exploring posttraumatic stress disorder symptom profile among pregnant women. *Journal of Psychosomatic Obstetrics and Gynecology*, 31(3), 176–187.

Stanke, C., Murray, V., Amlôt R., Nurse, J., & Williams, R. (2012). The effects of flooding on mental health: Outcomes and recommendations from a review of the literature. *PLOS Currents, 1*. doi: 10.1371/4f9f1fa9c3cae

Stanley, R. O. & Burrows, G. D. (2005). The role of stress in mental illness: The practice. In C. L. Cooper (Ed.), *Handbook of stress medicine and health* (2nd ed., pp. 87–100). Boca Raton, FL: CRC Press.

Sterling, P. & Eyer, J. (1988). Allostasis: A new paradigm to explain arousal pathology. In S. Fisher & J. Reason (Eds.), *Handbook of life stress, cognition and health* (pp. 629–649). New York, NY: John Wiley & Sons.

Substance Abuse and Mental Health Services Administration (SAMHSA). (2005). *Tips for survivors of a disaster or traumatic event: What to expect in your personal, family, work and financial life.* Rockville, MA: Author.

Taylor, S. E., Klein, L. C., Lewis, B. P., Gruenewald, T. L., Gurung, R. A., & Updegraff, J. A. (2000). Biobehavioral responses to stress in females: Tend-and-befriend, not fight-or-flight. *Psychological Review, 107*(3), 411–429.

Taylor, S. E., Lewis, B. P., Gruenewald, T. L., Gurung, R. A. R., Updegraff, J. A., & Klein, L. C. (2002). Sex differences in biobehavioral responses to threat: Reply to Geary and Flinn. *Psychological Review, 109*(4), 751–753.

Thormar, S. B., Gersons, B. P., Juen, B., Marschang, A., Djakababa, M. N., & Olff, M. (2010). The mental health impact of volunteering in a disaster setting: a review. *Journal of Nervous and Mental Disorders, 198*(8), 529–538.

Trainer, M. & Goel, A. (2013). The role of social networking in disaster management. In Arora, R. & Arora, P. (Eds.) *Disaster management: medical preparedness, response and homeland security* (pp. 67–94). Wallingford, UK: CABI.

United Nations. (2006). *Convention on the rights of persons with disabilities.* Retrieved from http://www.un.org/disabilities/documents/convention/convoptprot-e.pdf

Washington, D., Davis, T., Martirosian, C., & Yano, E. (2013). PTSD risk and mental health care engagement in a multi-war era community sample of women veterans. *Journal of General Internal Medicine, 28*(7), 894–900.

Wolfelt, A. D. (1999). *Dispelling 5 common myths about grief.* Retrieved from http://www.griefwords.com/index.cgi?action=page&page=articles%2Fhelping7.html&site_id=2

Woolfolk, R. L., Lehre, P. M., & Allen, L. M. (2007). Conceptual issues underlying stress management. In P. M. Lehrer, R. L. Woolfolk, & W. E. Sime (Eds.), *Principles and practice of stress management* (3rd ed., pp. 3–15). New York, NY: Guilford.

Worden, J. W. (2003). *Grief counseling and grief therapy: A handbook for the mental health practitioner.* New York: Brunner-Routledge.

World Health Organization (WHO). (2013). *Building back better: Sustainable mental health care after emergencies.* Geneva, Switzerland: Author.

World Health Organization and the International Council of Nurses. (2009). *ICN framework of disaster nursing competencies.* Available at http://www.icn.ch/images/stories/documents/networks/DisasterPreparednessNetwork/Disaster_Nursing_Competencies_lite.pdf

World Health Organization, War Trauma Foundation and World Vision International. (2011). *Psychological first aid: Guide for field workers.* Geneva, Switzerland: WHO.

Yeager, K. R. & Roberts, A. R. (2003). Differentiating among stress, acute stress disorder, crisis episodes, trauma, and PTSD: Paradigm and treatment goals. *Brief Treatment and Crisis Intervention, 3*(1), 145–167.

18 Anger, Aggression, and Violence

Yvonne Savard

Adapted from the chapter "Management of Aggression and Violence" by Sandy Harper-Jaques and Marlene Reimer

LEARNING OBJECTIVES

After studying this chapter, you will be able to:

- Explore feelings about the experience and expression of anger.
- Discuss the bio/psycho/social/spiritual factors that influence the expression of aggressive and violent behaviour.
- Discuss the theories used to explain anger, aggression, and violence.
- Identify the behaviour or actions that escalate and de-escalate violent behaviour.
- Recognize the risk for aggression towards nurses.
- Generate options for responding to the expression of anger and violent behaviour in clinical nursing practice.
- Apply the nursing process to the management of anger, aggression, and violence in clients.

KEY CONCEPTS

- aggression
- anger
- assertiveness

KEY TERMS

- catharsis • emotional circuit • mindfulness • restraint • seclusion
- violence

A nger is considered a universal human emotion, identifiable across cultures, by theorists who believe that prototypical emotions exist (DiGiuseppe & Tafrate, 2007). We get our knowledge about emotion in several ways: personal knowledge, knowledge about others' emotions, social norms, and conceptual knowledge that is evolving as we study emotion (Faucher & Tappolet, 2008). Definitions of anger, aggression, and violence vary and are influenced by experience, beliefs, culture, and gender. Individuals and groups develop their own views of acceptable and unacceptable words and actions. Theoretic distinctions can be made among anger, aggression, and violence, but clinically, their expression may be blurred. Each phenomenon may occur alone or in combination with one or both of the others.

Most societies develop norms for acceptable and unacceptable behaviour; some groups at some point in time have accepted all forms of aggression and violence. Today, images and stories about aggressive and violent acts throughout the world appear daily in the media. Incidents such as mass killings are very rare but receive enormous coverage that strongly impacts public perception of the risk for violence, especially that posed by the mentally ill (Friedman & Michels, 2013). The societal debate remains ongoing over the significance of the effect of violence in movies, television, and video games on an individual's propensity for violence.

Like other places, health care settings are not immune to expressions of anger, aggression, and violence. In any setting, aggression and violence are a reflection of the values of the individual, family, community, and society. Many people tend to minimize the frequency and severity of aggressive and violent acts; for example, couples who interact violently downplay the severity and effects of the episodes (Belknap, 2003). The expression of anger, aggression, and violence by clients and, sometimes, by their families is a tremendous challenge for nurses. This chapter discusses prominent theories about the nature of these phenomena and offers varying, sometimes controversial, models, theories, and evidence, with each discussion attempting to explain the phenomena of anger, aggression, and violence. Clinicians can choose a particular model as a basis for assessment, nursing diagnosis, planning, intervention, and evaluation. The chapter also explores how the nurse can apply the nursing process in managing angry, aggressive, or violent clients and in preventing or de-escalating situations that may lead to aggression or violence.

ANGER

Anger is "a strong, uncomfortable emotional response to a provocation that is unwanted and incongruent with one's values, beliefs, or rights" (Thomas, 1998). Anger is usually described as a temporary state of emotional arousal, in contrast to hostility, which is associated with a more enduring negative attitude (Thomas, 2001; see Chapter 37). Anger is part of the fight/flight response; although anger is portrayed as a bad emotion that always leads to aggression, this is often not the case. Thomas (2001) asserts that the expression of anger may prevent aggression and help to resolve a situation.

Language pertaining to anger is imprecise and confusing. The word *anger* is used to describe a wide range of feelings, from annoyance at having to wait at a red light when in a hurry to a severe emotional reaction to the news that a family member has been physically assaulted. Some of the words used interchangeably with anger include annoyance, frustration, temper, resentment, hostility, hatred, and rage. In addition, the word *angry* is used to describe both a transient emotional state and a personality trait (Thomas, 1993). This imprecision is related to varying beliefs and theories, including the following (Gerloff, 1997; Novaco, 2007; Shannon, 2000):

- Anger is a fixed quantity that either dams up or floods the system.
- Anger and aggression are linked. Anger is the feeling, and aggression is the behaviour; both result from an innate instinct.
- Anger is the instinctive response to a threat or to the inability to meet goals or desires.
- If outward expression of anger is blocked, then it turns inwards and develops into depression.
- Anger arises out of feelings of hurt or anxiety.

Box 18-1 invites the reader to explore variations in responses to anger through the use of an experiential exercise.

▼ **KEY CONCEPT Anger** is an affective state experienced as the motivation to act in ways that warn, intimidate, or attack those who are perceived as challenging or threatening. It occurs when there is a threat, delay, thwarting of a goal, or conflict between goals.

BOX 18-1 Self-Awareness Exercise: Personal Experience of Anger

People's reactions differ when they experience anger. Some people report a sense of power, control, and calmness different from their usual experience; others report feeling shaky, tearful, and on the verge of collapse. Still others describe physical sensations of nausea and dizziness.

Think about the last time that you felt angry. List the body sensations and other emotions that you experienced. Now ask a friend, colleague, or family member to do the same. Compare lists. What are the similarities and differences between you? How will awareness of these differences help you in your clinical practice?

Experience of Anger

The experience of anger is an internal event that involves thoughts, images, and bodily sensations (Kassinove & Tafrate, 2006). The experience of anger can serve as a warning that demands are greater than available resources (Thomas, 2001). Yet, with the exception of anger that arises from specific neurologic damage or biochemical imbalances, angry episodes can be viewed also as social events (Thomas, 1998). The meaning of angry episodes develops from the beliefs held about anger and the interpretation given to the episode (Shannon, 2000), and these are shaped by influences such as culture, language, and gender (Thomas, 2006). Anger is a normal human emotion; it is the dysfunctional expression of anger that may be threatening to the self or others.

Expression of Anger

Verbal (e.g., yelling) and motor behaviours (e.g., stomping one's foot) are involved in the expression of anger. Difficulties in expressing anger have often been associated with psychiatric health problems. Anger turned inwards has been implicated as a contributor to mood disorders, especially depression (Koh, Kim, & Park, 2002). Several medical disorders have also been positively correlated with the suppression of anger, including essential hypertension, migraine headaches, psoriasis, rheumatoid arthritis, and Raynaud's disease. Evidence from the Nova Scotia Health Survey (Davidson & Mostofsky, 2010) associated decreased constructive anger (discussing anger to resolve the situation) in men and increased destructive anger justification (blaming others for one's anger) in men and women with increased risk of coronary artery disease over a 10-year period.

Behavioural expressions of anger vary. In the 19th century, anger was viewed as sinful, dangerous, and destructive—an emotion to be contained, controlled, and denied. This negatively viewed emotion was to be dominated and conquered, and an ideal family life was free of anger. Husbands and wives were discouraged from expressing anger towards each other; parenting manuals promoted the suppression of anger in children (Thomas, 1993). This view contributed to the development of a powerful taboo against feeling and expressing anger. People who have accepted this persistent taboo may have difficulty even knowing when they are angry (Shannon, 2000).

During the early 20th century, Freud and Lorenz advocated the use of **catharsis**, the release of ideas through talking and expressing appropriate emotion, in the expression of anger. However, catharsis has been shown empirically to promote, not reduce, anger (Thomas, 1998). There is an old joke that expresses what research has shown: "How do you become a great performer?" Answer: "Practice, practice, practice." "How do you become a really angry person?" Answer: "Practice, practice, practice" (DiGiuseppe & Tafrate, 2007). In recent years, interest has grown in developing communication techniques that promote the expression of anger in nondestructive ways (Gerloff, 1997; Shannon, 2000). These varying beliefs have added to the confusion about anger. Differences in expectations about how men and women should express anger also contribute to the confusion. Varying beliefs about appropriate ways to express anger become apparent when a client and a nurse enter into a therapeutic relationship. Genetic predisposition, emotional development during infancy and childhood, and family environment influence the variations in expression for both the nurse and the client (Thomas, 2001, 2009). Previous experiences in expressing anger and reactions from others are also

influential. Frequency, duration, intensity, and mode of expression are aspects of anger that can be explored and considered (Novaco, 2007). When the expression of anger has negative outcomes for the person in terms of personal distress (e.g., shame) and consequences (e.g., lost relationships), it may be considered dysfunctional (Kassinove & Tafrate, 2006).

AGGRESSION AND VIOLENCE

While anger is an emotion, aggression and violence are actions. In this chapter, aggression is defined as "verbal statements against someone that are intended to intimidate or threaten the recipient." A study of verbal aggression on psychiatric units indicated that the types of verbal aggression by prevalence were abusive language, shouting, threats, expressions of anger, and racist comments (Stewart & Bowers, 2013). **Violence** is defined as "a physical act of force intended to cause harm to a person or an object and to convey the message that the perpetrator's point of view is correct and not the victim's" (Harper-Jaques & Reimer, 1992, p. 312). Aggression and violent behaviour reflect a continuum from suspicious behaviour to extreme actions that threaten the safety of others or result in injury or death (see Table 18-1 for examples).

Research focused on inpatient psychiatric units has found that higher levels of aggression were associated with clients detained under mental health legislation (Bowers et al., 2011), high client turnover, unit doors being locked, and higher staffing ratios (Bowers et al., 2009).

Table 18-1	Examples of Behaviours on the Continuum of Aggression and Violence	
Term	**Description**	**Clinical Example**
Suspicious behaviour	Hypervigilance to external cues Attends more to cues that fit with current thinking patterns	A female client with a long history of delusional disorder (including the belief that her family wants to "lock her away") questions the motives of a community mental health nurse when she asks the client about her medication regimen. The client misperceives the nurse's inquiry as evidence of a conspiracy against her
Verbal hostility	Verbal comments that are sarcastic or blaming and often expressed with the intent to hurt others May be used as a means of getting attention or inviting others to take action	When administration of PRN medication is delayed, a client's mother comes to the nursing station and starts to yell. She states that the nurses do not care, are lazy, and should work harder. She also demands that someone give her daughter the analgesic. (Family members have been previously reported as using demanding behaviours to have needs met.)
Physical violence	Act of striking out, throwing an object, pushing, etc., that appears to be intended to cause harm to a person or object	A young man attending a mental health clinic has missed his appointment with the psychiatrist. When he finds out he cannot be scheduled to see her for another week, he yells at the receptionist, bangs his fist on the desk, and then picks up a chair and throws it at her

FIGURE 18-1. Aetiologies for clients with aggression.

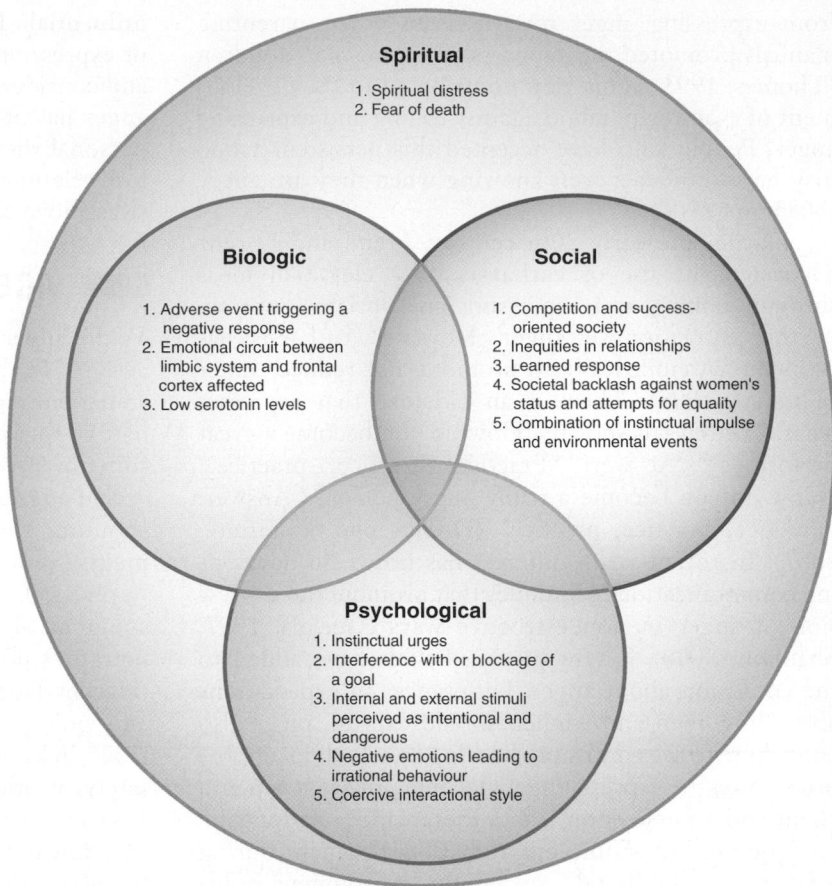

The imposition of restrictions on clients appeared to be associated with increased rather than reduced aggression. Reasons for aggression in these settings as identified by staff and patients included patient factors (e.g., psychotic symptoms), staff factors (e.g., lack of skill), and environmental factors (e.g., overcrowding, lack of access to outside space) (Bowers et al., 2011). Increasingly, the complexity of aggression and violence occurring in health care settings is being recognized. For instance, a systemic perspective of aggression and violence in mental health care has been proposed that identifies four related phenomena: environmental (e.g., layout of the unit, noise level), intrapersonal/client (e.g., age, gender, trauma, diagnosis), clinician (e.g., skills, stress level, attitude towards aggression), and mental health care system (e.g., policies, cultural factors, control orientation) (Cutcliffe & Riahi, 2013a, 2013b).

Aggression does not occur in a vacuum. Therefore, a multidimensional framework (Fig. 18-1) is essential for understanding and responding to these behaviours (Morrison & Carney Love, 2003).

> **KEY CONCEPT** **Aggression** is defined as verbal statements and/or physical actions that are intended to threaten.

MODELS OF ANGER, AGGRESSION, AND VIOLENCE

This section discusses some of the dominant theoretical explanations for anger, aggression, and violence. A single model or theory cannot yet fully explain anger, aggression, and violence; instead, the nurse must choose the most useful models for explaining a particular client's experience and for planning interventions.

Biologic Theories

From a biologic viewpoint, a tendency to have more frequent angry episodes may partially originate from developmental deficits, anoxia, malnutrition, toxins, tumours, or neurodegenerative diseases or trauma affecting the brain. Clients with a history of damage to the cerebral cortex are more likely to exhibit increased impulsivity, decreased inhibition, and decreased judgement than are those who have not experienced such damage. The interaction of neurocognitive impairment and social history of abuse or family violence increases the risk for violent behaviour (Scarpa & Raine, 1997). The odds of violent behaviour also increase when separate risk factors, such as schizophrenia, substance abuse, and not taking prescribed medications, coexist in the same person (Citrome & Volavka, 1999). Before reading

BOX 18-2 Self-Awareness Exercise: Intensity of Anger

Imagine This Scene: You are coming home late at night. You've been at the library studying for midterm examinations and are tired. As you come up the front walk, you trip over a skateboard, probably left by one of the neighbourhood children. Before you know it, you are sprawled across the front step.

What emotions threaten to overwhelm you at that moment? What contributes to the intensity of the anger that you feel?

- The pain where you scraped your leg across the cement?
- Your general state of tiredness?
- The fact that you skipped dinner?
- The five cups of coffee you had today?
- The careless children who left a toy in your way?

If the same thing had happened when you were well rested and feeling good, would the feeling and the intensity be the same?

additional research evidence, try the anger exercise in Box 18-2. What does daily experience suggest about biologically based aspects of the experience and expression of anger?

Cognitive Neuroassociation Model

The cognitive neuroassociation model is one explanation for the interplay of biologic and other internal influences (Berkowitz, 1989; Miller, Pedersen, Earleywine, & Pollock, 2003). Initially, an adverse event (e.g., pain from tripping over a skateboard) triggers a primitive negative response. Peripheral receptors communicate this response to the spinal cord through the spinothalamic tract to the hypothalamus. The hypothalamus, which synthesizes input from throughout the nervous system, is part of the limbic system. The limbic system mediates primitive emotion and basic drives to produce behaviours for survival, such as the fight-or-flight response (Harper-Jaques & Reimer, 1992).

At first, cognitive appraisal is not involved in these rudimentary feelings of fear or anger, other than identifying the stimulus as aversive; however, higher-order cognitive processing quickly begins to take over. The brain associates the current experience of physiologic sensations with memories, ideas, and previously experienced expressive motor reactions. It then interprets and differentiates the experience. Depending on prior experience and associations, the response may be intensified or suppressed. It is this latter part of the process that is most amenable to modification through psychotherapy.

● **STUDY NOTE**

In caring for a potentially aggressive client, the nurse should recognize that biochemical imbalance contributes to the person's inability to control aggression.

Neurostructural Model and the Emotional Circuit

The brain structures most frequently associated with aggressive behaviour are the limbic system and the cerebral cortex, particularly the frontal and temporal lobes. Harper-Jaques and Reimer (1992) propose the phrase **emotional circuit** to describe the interrelationship between the emotional processes of the limbic system and the neurocognitive processes of the frontal lobe and other parts of the cortex. They hypothesize that the functioning of this system determines the meaning a person gives to a particular situation. Thus, meaning is influenced by physiologic capability to perceive incoming messages, prioritize among competing stimuli, and interpret these messages in relation to stored ideas, beliefs, and memories.

Neurochemical Model and Low Serotonin Syndrome

In recent decades, knowledge has exploded about the complex role of neurotransmitters in human behaviour. Serotonin is a major neurotransmitter involved in mood, sleep, and appetite. Low serotonin levels are associated not only with depression but also with irritability, increased pain sensitivity, impulsiveness, aggression, vulnerability to alcoholism, and obsessive–compulsive behaviour (Heinz, Mann, Weinberger, & Goldman, 2001).

Serotonin is sensitive to fluctuations in dietary intake of its precursor, tryptophan, which is found in high-carbohydrate foods. Once it crosses the blood–brain barrier, tryptophan is synthesized into serotonin within the 5-hydroxytryptophan neurons by interaction with the enzyme tryptophan hydroxylase. Normally, the amount of tryptophan available in the plasma is below saturation (i.e., below the amount that could be used if available). Tryptophan intake and the availability of binding sites on the plasma proteins affect the synthesis of serotonin. Thus, assessing overall dietary intake is relevant, particularly of good tryptophan sources, such as wheat, flour, corn, milk, and eggs. Preliminary research evidence suggests that tryptophan depletion may increase anger levels in individuals already prone to aggressive behaviour (Schmeck et al., 2002).

People with a history of aggressive behaviour have been found to have a lower-than-average level of serotonin. Studies of humans with known aggressive tendencies, such as violent offenders, have repeatedly shown lower-than-average concentrations of 5-hydroxyindoleacetic acid (5-HIAA), the major metabolite for serotonin (Soloff, Lynch, & Moss, 2000) and prefrontal cortex dysfunction (Best, Williams, & Coccaro, 2002). Similarly, the plasma concentration of tryptophan is lower in people with alcoholism who have a history of aggressive behaviour than in people with alcoholism and no such history. Criminals whose acts of violence were committed impulsively have lower levels of 5-HIAA than do criminals whose acts of violence were premeditated. Impulsivity and difficulty controlling anger are characteristic of borderline personality disorder, another condition associated with lower-than-normal serotonin levels (Paris, 2005). Hyperarousal, such as may occur through being constantly vigilant against possible attack (e.g., in guerrilla warfare), also may contribute to aggressive behaviour.

This evidence for a biologic component to aggressive behaviour does not mean that only biologic means of treatment can be effective. Feedback between human behaviour and biochemistry is continuous; verbal suggestions and even early life stressors can affect biochemistry, just as biochemistry affects behaviour (Heinz et al., 2001; Pardo, Pardo, & Raichle, 1993). Environmental and learned behaviours influence the type and degree of aggression expressed, even by those for whom there is a biologic component (Soloff et al., 2000).

Psychological Theories

Several psychological explanations exist for aggressive and violent behaviours. This section discusses psychoanalytic, behavioural, and cognitive theories.

Psychoanalytic Theories

Psychoanalytic theorists view emotions as instinctual urges. They view suppression of these urges as unhealthy and as possible contributors to the development of psychosomatic or psychological disorders (Thomas, 1998). Freud struggled to understand the nature and expression of human aggressive behaviour. In his early works, he linked aggression with libidinal factors; however, this association did not explain destructive actions during wars and armed conflict. In his later writings, Freud identified aggression as a separate instinct, like the sexual instinct. He viewed aggression as an innate human quality that could be expressed when a person is provoked or abused. In doing so, he challenged the commonly held belief that human beings are essentially good.

Freud explained aggressive or violent behaviour as a combination of instinctual impulses and events in the environment that stimulated release of the instinctual urge. Freud's view fostered the use of catharsis. Therapeutic approaches, such as primal scream and nursing interventions that direct the client to "let it out" by pounding a pillow, find their origins in this theory (Tavris, 1989; Thomas, 1990). However, recent studies have not shown catharsis to be helpful in reducing anger. Venting can also have negative consequences when the action taken is hurtful to or blaming of others or damages property.

Erich Fromm (1900–1980), an American psychoanalyst best known for his application of psychoanalytic theory to social and cultural problems, believed that animals and humans share a form of aggression he called *benign*. This genetically programmed response was designed as a defence to protect oneself against a threat. The distinction between humans and animals is that human beings could reason. This capability provided them with options that are not available to animals. Thus, unlike animals, human beings are capable of behaving aggressively for reasons other than self-preservation. Fromm (1973) defined aggression in humans as any behaviour that causes or intends to cause damage to another person, animal, or object. Humans may foresee both real and perceived threats. Perceived threats that are based on distorted perceptions may lead to aggressive and violent behaviours; for example, the cognitive and information-processing deficits of clients with psychosis or schizophrenia (see Chapters 20 and 21) are frequently implicated in episodes of aggression and violence.

Behavioural Theories

The goal of behaviourists is to predict and control behaviour. Introspection has no role in these theories. One behavioural theory, drive theory, suggests that violent behaviour originates externally. A person experiences anger and acts violently in response to interference with or blocking of a goal. Laboratory experiments and the reality of everyday experience have proved the limitations of this theory (Thomas, 1990). Not all situations in which one's goal is blocked lead to anger or violence.

Another behavioural theory is social learning theory. In his research, Bandura (1973) drew attention to the role of learning and rewards in the expression of anger and violence. He studied interactions between mothers and children. The children learned that anger and aggressive behaviour helped them get what they wanted from their mothers. The children learned aggressive behaviour in a context that may have made them understand aggressive behaviour as appropriate. According to this view, people learn to be aggressive by participating in an aggressive environment. There is evidence, for instance, that playing violent video games is correlated with delinquency and violence even when other factors such as age, sex, race, and psychopathic personality traits are considered (DeLisi, Vaughn, Gentile, Anderson, & Shook, 2013).

Cognitive Theories

Cognitive theorists are interested in how people transform internal and external stimuli into useful information. They emphasize understanding how a person takes new information and fits it into an already developed schema. Beck (1976) proposed that cognitive schemas such as judgments, self-esteem, and expectations influence angry responses. In a situation perceived as intentional, dangerous, and unprovoked, the recipient's reaction will be intensified. The person's reaction will be further intensified if he or she views the offender as undesirable. In psychological disorders, cognitive processing may be compromised (Rubinsztein, Sahakian, & Dolan, 2002; Sergi & Green, 2003).

Rational–emotive theory, a type of cognitive theory, considers cognition, affect, and behaviour to be interrelated psychological processes (Ellis, 1977). This theory regards anger as an inappropriate negative emotion because it stems from irrational beliefs. Change is directed at altering irrational beliefs by identifying and working to change them and their associated psychological processes. Cognitive theories inform us about how not to get angry in the first place not about what to do when we become angry (Novaco, 2007).

Sociocultural Theories

Sociocultural theories suggest violent behaviour has multiple determinants, including social experiences in family and peer settings and the social consequences (positive and negative) of physical aggression. These determinants can be influenced by the gender of the individual and the way that gender differences are conceived and enacted within a society (Snyder, Schrepferman, Brooker, & Stoolmiller, 2007).

Western society often is characterized by a competitive, success-oriented ideology that values the individual and individual accomplishments over collaboration and a sense of community. Self-esteem, particularly for men, may be based on social and economic status and influence over others and the environment (Thomas, 2003). The pursuit of status produces inequities in relationships, whereby one person is superior and the other is subordinate. A hazard inherent in the pursuit of status is the view that a person is entitled to have influence and control, and that the "entitled person" has the right to use whatever means necessary to obtain status (Jenkins, 1990). These means may include force or disregarding the rights and needs of others. The entitled person may also begin to consider other people responsible for his or her thoughts, feelings, or actions. Such a belief in entitlement can be used to justify such actions as threatening, hurting, or murdering less powerful individuals.

Violence against women is a pressing global health issue. In 2001, the United Nations (UN) Commission on Human Rights issued a resolution towards eliminating it, asking countries to develop policies and provide funding for violence prevention and treatment programs. This resolution provides governments with a rationale to challenge men's position of entitlement and calls for societies to view women as equal partners with men. It has had an impact: women now have greater access to education, increased economic independence, and opportunities to control the frequency and number of pregnancies. Some believe, however, that these changes have led to a backlash against women's efforts to be equal, evident in continuing violence towards women (Tajaden & Thoennes, 2000).

A World Health Organization (WHO) study in 2005 revealed that the incidence of violence against women varies considerably across countries. For instance, the percentage of violence against a woman by a male partner ranged from 13% in Japan to 61% in Peru. Social factors related to violence against women included degree of economic inequality between males and females, level of women's mobility and autonomy, societal attitudes towards gender and towards violence, whether extended family or neighbours would intervene, and the level of crime and male-to-male violence (WHO, 2005).

Interactional Theory

Morrison (1998) challenges research and theories suggesting that aggression and violence are biologically or psychologically based. She asserts that these views lead to excusing the person's behaviour. She proposes that violence among people in psychiatric settings is the same as violence in other settings. Therefore, the client's behaviour should be considered a social problem and responded to on that basis. This challenge is grounded in several studies that examined the interactional style of the aggressive and violent individual. People with interactional styles that were argumentative or coercive were more likely to engage in aggressive or violent interchanges. Such people are often described as having a "chip on their shoulders." Morrison clearly states her view that the antecedent variables (e.g., history of violence, psychiatric diagnosis, length of hospitalization) and the mediating variable of interactional style are the primary reasons for the behaviour.

A life span approach to understanding aggressive behaviour can be taken, one that considers risks factors across the developmental spectrum (Liu, Lewis, & Evans, 2013). See Table 18-2 for characteristics and risk factors for aggressive behaviour across age groups.

Nursing Management: Human Response to Anger and Aggression

Aggression and violence often arise from an individual's belief that his or her view of a situation is the only correct one. The first party considers other views wrong and in need of change. A second party's refusal to give in to the view of the first may lead to violence (Capra, 2002). Box 18-3 illustrates such a scenario in the clinical setting.

Contrary to popular belief, many clients who have mental health problems do not behave aggressively or violently. To develop a means of predicting aggressive and violent behaviours, some researchers have attempted to determine the relationship between medical diagnosis and violence. Others have focused on the role of a person's history in predicting violence or examined demographics, client characteristics, and unit climate.

Table 18-2	Characteristics and Risk Factors for Aggressive Behaviour Across Age Groups	

Age Group	Characteristics	Underlying and Contextual Risk Factors
Toddlers	Crying, screaming, biting, kicking, throwing and breaking objects	Genetic and biologic factors (e.g., birth complications, nutritional deficit)
School-age children	Aggressive behaviour peaks before age 2	Imitation of others' aggression (social learning theory)
	Teasing, irritability, bullying, fighting, cruelty to animals, and fire setting	After repeated exposure to specific social stimuli (social information-processing theory)
	Nonphysical aggressive behaviour (e.g., verbal, psychological) increases	Psychosocial and environmental factors (such as poor parenting)
	Symptoms of sexual or physical abuse to the child. It is important to assess for potential abuse in these patients	
Adolescents	More serious aggressive behaviours and even violence appear	Aggressive behaviour that appears in only adolescence and disappears in later life (adolescence-limited antisocial behaviour)
	Gang activities including stealing, truancy, etc.	Learned aggressive behaviour in childhood that carried over into adolescence
	Cross-gendered aggressive behaviours, including dating violence, date rape, and sexual assault	Depression, family and other relationship difficulties, and a family history of suicide (or personal history of suicide attempts) may place an adolescent at greater risk for suicidal behaviour
	Suicide is the third leading cause of death for this group	Substance abuse
Adults	Domestic violence, sexual abuse, child abuse, and homicide	Drug use
	Highest homicide rate among age groups	Traumatic brain injury to areas responsible for managing aggression and impulse control
Elderly	Older adults in nursing homes due to daily interactions with staff and other residents	The emergence of dementias such as Alzheimer's disease may result in misunderstanding of motives. Aggression may result from this confusion
	Aggressive behaviours aimed at caregivers centre on intimate care practices or those that cause pain	The annual incidence of homicide–suicide is higher in adults 55 years and older and typically occurs more among couples
	Aggressive behaviour aimed at fellow residents in the context of excessive vocalization, territoriality, arguments with roommates, and general loneliness or frustration	Multifactorial aetiology

Adapted from Liu, J., Lewis, G., & Evans, L. (2013). Understanding aggressive behaviour across the lifespan. *Journal of Psychiatric and Mental Health Nursing, 20*(2), 156–168. Licensed © 2012 Blackwell Publishing.

Although media attention highlights violence related to mental illness, research shows that "the mentally ill as a group pose little risk of violence" (Friedman & Michels, 2013, p. 455). Persons with severe mental illness, such as schizophrenia or bipolar depression may be at a slightly higher risk for violent behaviour (Elbogen & Johnson, 2009; Swanson et al., 2006) but they are overwhelmingly more likely to be victims of violent crime (prevalence 6 to 23 times greater than others (Teplin, McClelland, Abram & Weiner, 2005). Many possible causes have been identified for aggressive behaviours in individuals experiencing a psychiatric disorder, including the presence of comorbid substance abuse, dependence, and intoxication (Citrome & Volavka, 2002; Elbogen & Johnson, 2009). As well, individuals experiencing symptom manifestation of hallucina-

tions or delusions or those with neuropsychiatric deficits are identified as posing an increased risk for violence. Individuals with underlying antisocial personality traits may use violent acts as a means to achieve specific goals. Finally, environmental factors that are associated with aggressive behaviours are identified, including a chaotic or unstable home or hospital situation, which may further encourage maladaptive aggressive behaviours (Citrome & Volavka; Elbogen & Johnson). An important consideration for the nurse is the course of violence related to changes in symptomatology (Bernstein & Saladino, 2007).

Research, nevertheless, suggests that particular characteristics are predictive of violent behaviours. Low self-esteem that may be further eroded during hospitalization or treatment may influence a client to use force to meet

BOX 18-3 Clinical Vignette

PAUL'S ANGER

Paul, a new client on the unit, appears to be experiencing auditory hallucinations. The nurse approaches Paul, careful not to invade his personal space, and begins to walk with him. In an attempt to assess his current mental status, the nurse points out that he seems restless and asks if the voices have returned. Paul responds, "They are telling me this place isn't safe. The angel in the corner is signalling to me. She wants me to leave!" Paul starts to walk towards the door. In an attempt to offer an alternative point of view and orient him to the present, the nurse understands that what the client is seeing and hearing are hallucinations. The nurse attempts to increase Paul's feeling of safety by identifying his perceptions as hallucinations and reassuring him of his safety. "No I won't stay and you can't make me." Paul pushes the nurse aside and runs to the door.

What Do You Think?

If you were the nurse in this situation, what would be your next response? How would you acknowledge Paul's concerns and encourage him to stay?

his or her needs or to experience some sense of empowerment. Many people who have chronic mental health problems "fight" the experience and have difficulty accepting medical treatment. When admitted to the hospital, they may experience turmoil from both the illness and the anger at the additional loss of control that hospitalization mandates. Clients may resort to violence to force change or to regain or maintain control. Rewards from violence include attention from nursing staff and/or status and prestige among the client group (Harris & Morrison, 1995). For example, the client who behaves violently is observed more frequently and has more opportunities to discuss concerns with nurses. Impaired communication, disorientation, and depression have been found to be consistently associated with aggressive behaviour among nursing home residents with dementia (Talerico, Evans, & Strumpf, 2002).

Nurses bring their own perceptions and reactions to clinical settings. They respond to the behaviours of the clients and families for whom they care. Clients and families, in turn, react to nurses (Leahey & Harper-Jaques, 1996). Nurses' beliefs about themselves as individuals and professionals will influence their responses to aggressive behaviours. For example, the nurse who considers any expression of anger or aggression inappropriate will approach an agitated client in a manner different from that used by the nurse who considers agitated behaviour to be meaningful. In a phenomenologic study of client experiences of violent encounters (Carlsson, Dahlberg, Ekebergh, & Dahlberg, 2006), participants described wanting caregivers who were calm and confident and who did not respond to client anger by disconnecting (e.g., becoming cool and distant). They said that such reactions on the part of caregivers increased their despair and, with it, their aggression. When a caregiver genuinely related to the client as a person and seemed to recognize the suffering

being experienced, the client's anger was diffused. The researchers found the clients to be "longing for authentic personal care" (p. 287). It is interesting to note that the Kings College London review of the literature found that reports of consequences of inpatient violence tended to focus on injuries of staff only (Bowers et al., 2011).

Duxbury and Whittington (2005) studied clients' ($N = 80$) and nurses' ($N = 82$) perspectives on inpatient aggression and violence. Clients believed poor communication on the part of staff played a significant role; nurses believed it was clients' mental illness that was most significant. Both noted that environmental conditions (e.g., restrictive and underresourced) play a role. Clients advocated for communication training for staff, while nurses looked for organizational deficits to be addressed. The nurse's ability to maintain personal control is challenged when faced with angry, provoking clients. Some clients who are experiencing emotional problems have an uncanny ability to verbally target a nurse's vulnerable characteristics. It is a usual response to become defensive when one feels vulnerable. However, when nurses lose control of their own responses, the potential for punitive interventions or the use of threats or sarcasm is greater.

Nurses in all areas of clinical practice need to understand angry emotions, know how to prevent aggression and violence, and respond assertively. To better prepare themselves to respond to different types of behaviour, many nurses take assertiveness training courses and workshops. Many nursing schools also teach assertiveness. Nurses should understand the phenomena of anger, aggression, and violence as meaningful behaviours that warrant attention rather than as disruptive behaviours to control.

KEY CONCEPT Assertiveness is a set of behaviours and a communication style that is open, honest, direct, and confident. Assertiveness enables the expression of emotions, including anger, in a manner that assumes responsibility. It allows placement of boundaries and prevents acceptance of inappropriate aggression from others.

Predictors of Violence

When assessing a client, his or her history is probably the most important predictor of potential for violence. Important markers include previous episodes of rage and violent behaviour, escalating irritability, intruding angry thoughts, and fear of losing control. Brain injury, substance use or abuse, and temporal lobe epilepsy have also been discussed as possible predictors of violence (Harper-Jaques & Reimer, 1992; Mesulam, 2000). Whether a relationship exists between temporal lobe epilepsy and aggressive behaviour remains a matter of controversy (Citrome & Volavka, 1999). Aggressive behaviour that occurs in the interictal period (i.e., between seizures)

| Table 18-3 | Physiologic and Behavioural Cues to Anger |

Internal Signs	External Signs
• Increased pulse, respirations, and blood pressure • Chills and shudders • Prickly sensations • Numbness • Choking sensations • Nausea • Vertigo	• Increased muscle tone • Changes in body posture, clenched fists, set jaw • Changes to the eyes: eyebrows lower and draw together, eyelids tense, eyes assume a "hard" appearance • Lips pressed together to form a thin line, or in a square shape • Flushing or pallor • Goose bumps • Twitching • Sweating

may also be related to the intense frustration that people who have epilepsy often experience and could lead to violent behaviour. Certain antiepileptic drugs, particularly barbiturates, may contribute to irritability and aggressive behaviour. However, mood-stabilizing medications such as carbamazepine (Tegretol) and divalproex sodium (Depakote) have reduced aggressive behaviour. The nurse should include any history of seizures, current medications, and compliance with pharmacotherapy in client assessments. Some physiologic and behavioural cues to anger are listed in Table 18-3.

Analysis and Outcome Identification

The nurse analyzes all assessment data across the biologic, psychological, and social domains to understand the dangers that the client's behaviour poses for self or others. The most common nursing diagnoses for clients experiencing intense anger and aggression are Risk for Self-Directed Violence and Risk for Other-Directed Violence (North American Nursing Diagnosis Association [NANDA], 2005). Outcomes focus on aggression control.

Planning and Implementing Interventions

This section emphasizes the development of a partnership between the nurse and client, who work together to find solutions to prevent the recurrence of explosive episodes and to de-escalate volatile situations. However, sometimes the client's condition (e.g., advanced dementia) or the situation will prevent the development of a partnership. In such instances, the nurse must take charge. The nurse who intervenes from within the context of the therapeutic relationship must be cognizant of the fit of a particular intervention. The nurse's action is based on his or her response to the client. The client's affective, behavioural, and cognitive response to the intervention provides information about its effects

and guides the nurse's next response (Wright & Leahey, 2005; Fig. 18-2).

The following assumptions are important to consider in planning interventions with this client population (Harper-Jaques & Masters, 1994):

• The nurse and client collaborate to find solutions and alternatives to aggressive and violent outbursts.

• Anger is a normal emotion. All people have the right to express their anger. All people have a responsibility to express their anger in a way that does not, emotionally or physically, threaten or harm others.

• In most instances, the person who behaves aggressively or violently can assume responsibility for the behaviour.

• The nurse views the client from the perspective of acknowledging that the client has solved problems before and is only temporarily in need of help.

• The nurse understands that norms for behaviour are created within the context of a particular environment and are influenced by the client's history and culture.

Nurses who work collaboratively with potentially violent clients must also keep in mind that they can take certain actions to minimize personal risk:

• Using nonthreatening body language

• Respecting the client's personal space and boundaries

• Positioning themselves so that they have immediate access to the door of the room in case they need to leave the room

• Choosing to leave the door open to an office while talking to a client

• Knowing where colleagues are and making sure those colleagues know where they are

• Removing or not wearing clothing or accessories that could be used to harm them, such as scarves, necklaces, or dangling earrings

When a violent outburst appears imminent or occurs, immediate intervention is required and should be directed by a designated leader. Health care facilities will have protocols that outline leader designation and the crisis response process (see Box 18-4). It is each nurse's responsibility to be knowledgeable about the process in place so that an informed, coordinated team response can occur.

The nurse who works with potentially aggressive clients does so with respect and concern. The goal is to work with clients to find solutions. The nurse approaches these clients calmly, being mindful to use nonthreatening body language and to avoid violation of boundaries. In dealing with aggression, as in other aspects of nursing practice, the nurse will find that at times the best intervention is silence. It is easy to equate intervention with activity, the sense that "I must do something." But quiet calmness on the nurse's part may be enough to help a client regain control of his or her behaviour and perspective on the situation.

FIGURE 18-2. Interventions for clients with aggression.

FIGURE 18-2. Interventions for clients with aggression.

Spiritual

1. Support consideration of spiritual issues
2. Support spiritual activities
3. Support hope for change

Biologic

1. Administer psychotropic agents
2. Monitor hepatic function
3. Encourage proper nutrition
4. Administer vitamins, such as thiamine and niacin
5. Reduce intake of caffeinated beverages
6. Modify environmental stimuli
7. Anticipate need for bladder and bowel elimination

Social

1. Develop family support groups
2. Use restraints and seclusion only as a last resort
3. Encourage use of resources for information and support

Psychological

1. Use past experiences to normalize and validate client's experiences
2. Explore beliefs about expressing aggression
3. Assist with taking charge of situation
4. Explain behavioural limits and consequences clearly
5. Develop written contracts
6. Plan to prevent escalation
7. Allow choices if possible

BOX 18-4   Emergency

GUIDELINES FOR CRISIS RESPONSE TO THREATENING OR VIOLENT CLIENT BEHAVIOUR

1. Clear the immediate area of other persons.
2. Call for staff assistance as designated in unit policy. If possible to do so, safely, remove objects that may impede movement during a team response.
3. Brief responders and designated team leader regarding the status of the client, the situation preceding the threatening or violent behaviour, and any action that has been taken.
4. With team leader, plan intervention, including specific staff roles in the intervention. Responders should remove any items from their persons that may cause injury (e.g., watches, pens, pagers, jewellery).
5. The crisis response leader speaks clearly and calmly with the client, and makes the response team's presence evident. The primary goal is to defuse the situation and prevent harm.
6. The options for intervention depend on the client's response. These include calming the patient verbally and helping him/ her to a safe area (e.g., client's room) or inviting the client to go with a staff member to "talk things over"; moving the client to a "time-out" space, sensory room, or seclusion area; using chemical (i.e., medication) or physical restraints. The client may be offered a choice of these options by the team leader.
7. The team debriefs the crisis incident. Medical and/or supervisory staff are informed, as necessary. A report of the crisis incident is recorded.
8. There is postincident debriefing for the client, as appropriate.

Trying to clarify what has upset the client is important. The nurse can use therapeutic communication techniques to prevent a crisis or defuse a critical situation (see Box 18-5). During daily interactions with clients, nurses intervene in many creative and useful ways. The intervention alone does not serve as the solution; it is the process or art of offering the intervention within the context of the nurse–client relationship that is successful. These interventions will not be successful with all clients all the time. However, it is not the nurse or client's fault when an intervention is ineffective. The intervention simply did not fit the situation at that particular time.

Biologic Domain

Biologic Assessment

The nurse may encounter clients whose aggressive tendencies have been exacerbated by a biochemical imbalance. However, nurses must recognize that biologic alterations are neither necessary nor sufficient to account for most aggressive behaviours. In taking the client's history, the nurse listens for evidence of industrial exposure to toxic chemicals, missed doses of medications, alcohol intoxication, and withdrawal or premenstrual dysphoric disorder. Similarly, a history of even minor structural

BOX 18-5 Therapeutic Dialogue

THE POTENTIALLY AGGRESSIVE CLIENT

Paul is a 23-year-old client in the high observation area of an inpatient unit. He is pacing back and forth. He is pounding one fist into his other hand. In the past 24 hours, Paul has been more cooperative and less agitated. The behaviour the nurse observes now is more like the behaviour that Paul displayed 2 days ago. Yesterday, the psychiatrist told Paul that he would be granted more freedom in the unit if his behaviour improved. The psychiatrist has just seen Paul and refused to change the restrictions on Paul's activities.

Ineffective Approach

Nurse: Paul, I can understand this is frustrating for you.

Paul: How can you understand? Have you ever been held like a prisoner?

Nurse: I do understand Paul. Now you must calm down or more privileges will be removed.

Paul: (voice gets louder) But I was told that calm behaviour would mean more privileges. Now you are telling me calm behaviour only gets me what I have got! Can't you talk to the doctor for me?

Nurse: No, Paul. I can't talk to the doctor. (Paul appears more frustrated and agitated as the conversation continues.)

Effective Approach

Nurse: Paul, you look upset (observation). What happened in your conversation with the psychiatrist? (seeking information)

Paul: Yesterday, he said calmer behaviour would mean more freedom in the unit. I have tried to be calmer and not to swear. You said you noticed the difference. But today he says "no" to more freedom.

Nurse: Some people might feel cheated if this happened to them (validation). Is that how you feel?

Paul: Yeah, I feel real cheated. Nothing I do makes a difference. That's the way it is here and that's the way it is when I am out of the hospital.

Nurse: Sounds like experiences like this leave you feeling pretty powerless (validation).

Paul: I don't have any power, anywhere. Sometimes when I have no power I get mean. At least then people pay attention to me.

Nurse: In this situation with your doctor, what would help you feel that you had some power? (Inviting client partnership).

Paul: Well if he would listen to me; if he would read my chart.

Nurse: I am a bit confused by the psychiatrist's decision. I won't make promises that your privileges will change but would it be okay with you if I talk with him?

Paul: That would make me feel like someone is on my side.

Critical Thinking Challenge

- In the first scenario, how did the nurse escalate the situation?
- Compare the first scenario with the second. How are they different?

---

changes resulting in trauma, haemorrhage, or tumour may contribute to lowering a client's anger threshold and thus requires investigation.

Aggressive episodes that are mainly biologic in origin share certain characteristics (Corrigan, Yudofsky, & Silver, 1993):

- The client has a history or evidence of central nervous system lesion or dysfunction.
- Onset of the episode is sudden and relatively unprovoked.
- The outburst is less controlled than those associated with external influences.
- The episode has a clear beginning and ending.
- The client expresses remorse after the episode.

Sensory Impairment

The most common impairments are hearing loss and reduced visual acuity. A common component of nursing assessment documents is visual and hearing impairments. If a client cannot provide information about his or her hearing and vision, the nurse should ask a family member or friend. If there are impairments, the nurse should ensure that hearing aids are working for clients who use them and assess clients for access to glasses or contact lenses.

Interventions for the Biologic Domain

Administering and Monitoring Medications

Several classes of drugs are used in the management of aggressive behaviour. Important points for the nurse to consider in making decisions about client and family teaching, medication administration, and consultation with physicians and pharmacists are as follows:

- Evidence supports the use of *atypical antipsychotics*, such as clozapine (Clozaril), risperidone (Risperdal), and olanzapine (Zyprexa), in reducing agitation (Chakos & Lieberman, 2001). As with other psychotropic medications, the action of atypical antipsychotics is not fully understood. It is thought that they block dopamine and serotonin receptors. Extrapyramidal side effects are few, which makes these drugs easier to tolerate than the typical antipsychotics (see the drug profile on risperidone [Risperdal] in Chapter 12 for more information).
- *Selective serotonin reuptake inhibitors* (e.g., fluoxetine [Prozac], paroxetine [Paxil]) are increasingly being used for their antiaggressive effects, as well as for their antidepressant effects. Their effects on aggressive behaviour usually occur before their effects on depression.
- *β-Adrenergic receptor blockers*, such as propranolol (Inderal), may be used for their effect in decreasing the peripheral manifestations of rage that are associated

with excitement of the sympathetic nervous system (Silver et al., 2000).

- *Lithium carbonate* has been effective in treating aggressive behaviour associated with brain injury (Burke, Loeber, & Birmaher, 2002).
- *Divalproex sodium* and *carbamazepine* have been shown to reduce aggressive behaviour.
- Psychotropic drugs often interact with antiepileptic and antispasmodic agents, altering pharmacokinetics. For example, chlorpromazine may increase the risk for seizures in clients taking antiepileptic drugs (Fahs, Potiron, Senon, & Perivier, 1999).
- The liver metabolizes most psychotropic drugs (except lithium). The nurse should be alert to possible hepatic dysfunction in clients with a history of alcohol or drug abuse.

Managing Nutrition

Clients with long-standing poor dietary habits (e.g., indigent clients, clients with alcoholism) often have deficiencies of thiamine, niacin, and folic acid (Young, 2002). Prolonged use of alcohol can block as much as 70% of thiamine uptake. Increased irritability, disorientation, and paranoia may result. Encouraging clients to eat more whole grains, nuts, fruits, vegetables, organ meats, and milk, instead of "junk" foods, is important. The nurse may need to help clients with obtaining the resources needed to buy and prepare healthier food choices.

Caffeine is a potent stimulant (Lorist & Tops, 2003). Some inpatient psychiatric units have reduced clients' accessibility to coffee and other caffeinated beverages as a means of trying to reduce aggressive behaviour. Results have been mixed.

Psychological Domain

Psychological Assessment

The nurse interested in working with clients to prevent and manage aggressive and violent behaviours should observe them for disturbances in thought processing. Clients may have disordered thoughts for various reasons, including associated psychiatric diagnoses. Some common diagnostic categories that the nurse needs to look for in the client's history are major depressive episode, bipolar disorder, delusional disorders, posttraumatic stress disorder, schizophrenia, and depersonalization. The nurse should also look for a current or past history of substance abuse because clients who abuse drugs, alcohol, or solvents may also exhibit disordered thought processing. Intoxication can trigger erratic thought processes and unpredicted violence. Some form of thought disorder may remain after a person is detoxified, becoming a permanent feature of the person's way of processing ideas. In addition, the nurse must look for acute and chronic medical conditions, such as brain tumour, encephalitis,

electrolyte imbalance, and hepatic failure, which may also alter thought processing (Citrome & Volavka, 1999). The thought processes of greatest interest to the nurse in assessing a client's potential for aggression and violence are perception and delusion.

Perception

Perception is awareness of events and sensations and the ability to make distinctions between them. Clients with disordered perceptions may misinterpret objects or events. Such misperception is called an *illusion*. For example, a client may assume that a person walking towards him or her is going to strike out and thus take action to defend against this illusionary foe. The nurse can explore a client's perception by asking such questions as, "I noticed you were looking very cautious as I approached you. I wonder what you are thinking."

Delusions

Clients may maintain false or unreasonable beliefs, known as delusions, despite attempts to dissuade them from their point of view. The nurse may not notice any abnormalities in the client's behaviour or appearance until the client begins to discuss delusional ideas. Discussion of the delusions may precipitate aggressive or violent behaviour. To explore these false beliefs, the nurse could, with the client's consent, ask questions respectfully. The nurse should match the pacing of such questions to the client's responses. Attempts to dissuade the client from his or her beliefs are usually ineffective.

Interventions for the Psychological Domain

Psychological interventions help clients gain control over their expression of anger and aggressive behaviour. In some instances, these interventions eliminate the need for chemical (medications) or mechanical restraints. De-escalating potential aggression is always preferable to challenging or provoking a client.

Affective Interventions

Affective interventions are designed to reduce or increase intense emotions that may hinder the client from finding alternatives to the use of aggression or violence (Wright & Leahey, 2005). They include validating, listening to the client's illness experience, and exploring beliefs.

Validating. Clients who experience intense anger and rage can feel isolated. The nurse can reduce the client's feelings of isolation by acknowledging these intense feelings. By drawing on past experience with other client's, the nurse can also reassure the client that others have felt the same way.

Listening to the Client's Illness Experience. Often, clients and their family members are invited to provide details about past medical treatments, medications, hospitalizations, and therapies. What is overlooked is

BOX 18-6   Clinical Vignette

MARY'S RAGE

Mary, a 22-year-old single woman, was a regular client at the crisis centre. During previous visits, she came alone or with her mother and demanded immediate attention. This time she comes with her mother. The receptionist groans and rolls her eyes as she describes this family to the new intake nurse. "They are obnoxious. It is best to handle them fast and get them out of here!"

Before the interview, the nurse reviews Mary's extensive file. She notes that on many occasions Mary was aggressive and violent while in the centre. The mother has complained to the local health authority about the centre on at least two occasions.

During the interview, the nurse asks the mother and daughter the following questions:

• What was the most useful thing that has happened during previous contacts at the centre?
• What was the least useful thing about previous contacts at the centre?

The family looks surprised to be asked these questions. They state that previous visits were useful only in providing them with written proof that Mary could not work. That information required by the social service agency ensured continuation of Mary's disability checks. Furthermore, Mary and her mother state that they often left the centre feeling that the nurses were not interested in their concerns and believed that if Mary tried harder, her hallucinations would decrease. They add that they often waited 1 to 2 hours to be seen, whereas other clients were seen more quickly. Mary admits that she sometimes made a lot of noise in the waiting room to be seen sooner.

The nurse then asks, "What would need to happen during your visit today to make you feel that coming here was worthwhile?" The mother expresses interest in receiving information about hallucinations and how she could help Mary when she experiences them. Mary says she wants to know how to handle angry feelings.

the experience of the health problem or the experience of interactions with professionals. Inviting clients and families to talk about their previous experience with the health care system may highlight both their concerns and resources. See Box 18-6 for an example of how a nurse uses this intervention to improve a client's care.

Exploring Beliefs. Exploring the client's beliefs about the expression of angry feelings can be useful. Discussion of beliefs that prevent the client from seeking alternate ways of handling distressing emotions and situations may help him or her to take charge of the situation.

Cognitive Interventions

Cognitive interventions are usually those that provide new ideas, opinions, information, or education about a particular problem. The nurse offers a cognitive intervention with the goal of inviting the client to consider other possibilities (Wright & Leahey, 2005). Examples include giving commendations, offering information, providing education, and using thought stopping and contracting.

● **STUDY NOTE**
The best time to teach the client techniques for managing anger and aggression is when the client is not experiencing the provoking event. Cognitive therapy approaches are useful and can be prioritized according to responses.

Giving Commendations. A commendation focuses on the client's behaviour pattern over time and highlights his or her strengths and resources (Limacher & Wright, 2003). For example, commending a client's decision to request medication or to remove herself from an overstimulating environment highlights the woman's ability to assume responsibility for thoughts and feelings that have previously invited aggressive behaviour.

Offering Information. Nurses can offer information or arrange opportunities for clients to receive information from other professionals. Clients may sometimes become agitated and threaten to harm the nurse because they do not know what is expected of them or they do not remember why they need to be in treatment. The nurse can tell them about unit expectations or the reasons for hospitalization. The nurse can also determine the client's information needs by asking questions. One option in providing information, education, and support is to develop a family support group, which can provide a forum for responding to general concerns and questions at the same time.

In the mental health setting, the nurse must make behavioural limits and consequences clear. When possible, the nurse should match consequences to the client's interests and desires. For example, Jane was slamming doors and banging down dishes in the kitchen of the group home. The nurse approached her to discuss other means of expressing her anger. During the conversation, the nurse reminded Jane that further agitated behaviour would mean that Jane would not participate in a shopping trip planned that day. The trip was important to Jane, so she chose to discuss her concern with the nurse.

Providing Education. Nurses can offer education to clients and families about various topics, including anger management and strategies to control aggressive behaviours. Greater understanding about mental health problems and altered mental status may help to prevent aggression by clarifying misunderstandings. Effective use of debriefing techniques following a crisis situation can also provide nurses and clients insights to ineffective coping and further allow for client learning in the development of strategies for future behavioural change.

Thought Stopping. In thought stopping, the nurse asks the client to identify thoughts that heighten feelings of anger and invites the client to "turn the thoughts off" by focusing on other thoughts or activities (Burns, 1999). Ideas of other activities include talking to someone, reading, baking, or thinking about a future event.

Contracting.

A contract is a written document that the nurse and client develop. The document clearly states acceptable and unacceptable behaviours, consequences and rewards, and the role of both the client and nurse in preventing and managing aggressive behaviour (Morrison, 1998).

Behavioural Interventions

Behavioural interventions are designed to assist the client to behave differently (Wright & Leahey, 2005). Examples of such interventions include assigning behavioural tasks, using bibliotherapy, interrupting patterns, and providing choices.

Assigning Behavioural Tasks.

Sometimes, the nurse may assign a behavioural task as a way to help the client maintain or regain control over aggressive behaviours. Behavioural tasks might include writing down a list of grievances that the client will discuss with the nurse or observing how other people take charge of anger and aggression. For example, the nurse may ask the client to observe clients or staff on the unit, people at a shopping mall, or particular movies or television shows to evaluate how other people in real or fictitious situations handle anger.

Using Bibliotherapy.

In bibliotherapy, the nurse may ask the client to read a particular pamphlet or article on anger management. The nurse and client then discuss what the client read to decide which, if any, of the ideas the client can use when angry.

Interrupting Patterns.

Although clients are not usually aware of it, escalation of feelings, thoughts, and behaviour from calmness to violence usually follows a particular pattern. Disruption of the pattern can sometimes be a useful means for preventing escalation and can help the client regain composure. Nurses can suggest several strategies to interrupt patterns:

- Counting to 10 or using a mantra (sacred name repetition)
- Removing oneself from interactions or stimuli that may contribute to increased distress
- Doing something different (e.g., reading, exercising, watching television)

Providing Choices.

When possible, the nurse should provide the client with choices, particularly clients who have little control over their situation because of their condition. For example, the client who is experiencing a manic episode and is confined to her room may have few options in her daily schedule. However, she may be allowed to make choices about food, personal hygiene, and which pyjamas to wear.

Social Domain

Social Assessment

The nurse should evaluate factors related to the social domain that may be contributing to aggression or violence in a client. For example, are conditions in the client's home, family, or community leading to aggression or violent episodes? Are financial or legal troubles placing stress on the client that places him or her at risk?

Interventions for the Social Domain

Reducing Stimulation

Normally, people adjust their environments to suit their needs: some people like their music loud, whereas others want it soft; some people seek out the thrill of high-risk sports, whereas others prefer to be spectators. Within the context of a brain disorder or an unusually restrictive environment, such adjustments may not be within the client's control. A client with a brain injury, progressive dementia, or distorted vision may be experiencing intense and highly confusing stimulation, even though the environment, from the nurse or family's perspective, seems calm and orderly.

For people whose perceptions or thoughts are disordered from brain damage, degeneration, or other thought-processing difficulties, modification of the environment may be one of the main interventions. Likewise, introducing more structure into a chaotic environment can help decrease the risk for aggressive behaviour (Citrome & Volavka, 1999). The nurse can make stimuli meaningful or can simplify and interpret the environment in many practical ways, such as by identifying people or equipment that may be unfamiliar, providing cues as to what is expected (e.g., posting signs with directions, putting toothbrush and toothpaste by the sink), and removing or silencing unnecessary stimuli (e.g., turning off paging systems). Considering the environment from the client's viewpoint is essential. For instance, if the surroundings are unfamiliar, the client will need to process more information. Lack of a recognizable pattern or structure further taxes the client's capacity to encode information. Appropriate interventions include clarifying the meaning and purpose of people and objects in the environment, enhancing the client's sense of control and the predictability of the environment, and reducing other stimuli as much as possible (Stolley, Gerdner, & Buckwalter, 1999).

Anticipating Needs

The nurse can anticipate many needs of clients. In assuming responsibility for clients with cognitive impairment, the nurse needs to know when the client last voided and the pattern of bowel movements. Regular toileting routines are not just interventions to prevent incontinence.

Similarly, the anticipation of basic needs such as thirst and hunger is important, especially when working with adults or children who cannot readily express their needs. Other discomforts can arise from such conditions as ingrown toenails and adverse medication reactions.

The urge to void can be a powerful stimulus to agitated behaviour. It is not uncommon in a neurologic observation unit to see a young man with a recent head injury become violent just before spontaneously voiding. From a biologic perspective, such a client is probably normally sensitive or even hypersensitive to a full bladder. He probably also has sufficient cognitive function to recognize his need to void. Even some level of social inhibition may be operational in that he recognizes that voiding while lying on his back in bed, with strangers around, is inappropriate. But if he cannot speak or ask for help, he may become increasingly panic stricken. Thrashing around in bed, unable to communicate his need, he may strike out at staff.

The following scenario is the true account of how one graduate student dealt with another common situation. A 75-year-old woman was pacing around the nursing station of a psychogeriatric unit in a nursing home, crying for her mother. Various people spoke kindly to her, trying to explain that her mother was not there. Donna, a graduate student, was studying the wandering behaviours of clients with Alzheimer's disease on the unit. Hypothesizing that there is purpose behind these actions, she walked alongside the woman. After talking a bit with her about the client's mother, Donna asked the client what she would like to do if her mother were there. Gradually, the client confided that she needed her mother to help her find the bathroom. Donna then offered to help the woman, walking her to the bathroom. After voiding copiously, the client seemed greatly relieved and settled down.

Using Seclusion and Restraint

Seclusion and **restraint** are controversial interventions to be used judiciously and only when other interventions have failed to control the client's behaviour. The availability of effective psychotropic medications since the 1950s has reduced the need for these interventions of last resort. Reasons usually cited for using them are to protect the client from injury to self or others, to help the client reestablish behavioural control, and to minimize disruption of unit treatment regimens. The controversy over these interventions and their potential to be applied punitively heightens the need for clear institutional standards for their use. The development and use of clear practice standards can reduce the likelihood that these interventions will be misused (College of Registered Psychiatric Nurses of British Columbia, 2008). Postseclusion debriefing for clients is being studied as a means of identifying and reducing traumatic effects of this intervention (Whitecross, Seeary, & Lee, 2013).

Lewis (2002) challenges the use of restraint as a primary intervention in forensic settings. Lewis presents nontouch interventions as an alternative to restraint. In contrast, Hibbs (2000) proposes the use of cognitive interventions with clients while they are restrained. These interventions are designed to challenge thought patterns that contribute to aggressive behaviours.

Evaluation is also important in tracking the use of seclusion and restraint. In a Quebec audit study of the use of a secure room/security guard in a rural hospital, it was found that only 1.1/1,000 emergency room visits occasioned such use, most commonly indicated by physicians' perception of client risk for suicide or self-harm (Brock, Gurekas, Gelinas, & Rollin, 2009). Only 10% of use of these measures was related to staff safety. Most stays in the secure room were less than two nights. On inpatient psychiatric units, the monitoring of restraints/seclusion as part of a primary prevention approach to restraint/seclusion reduction should also include such strategies as building staff skills and teamwork, promoting relationship-based care, using consultation for difficult cases, and making physical design safer (Johnson, 2010).

Spiritual Domain

In addressing the spiritual domain of care for the client who is experiencing anger and aggression issues, contemplative practices, such as **mindfulness**, may be valuable to both the client and nurse (see Chapter 13). Mindfulness is being fully attentive in the "here and now" moment (Marlatt & Kristeller, 1999). The process of paying attention (without judgment) to what is happening can promote a connection to one's inner being and spirit. Acknowledging the present moment of reality is the beginning of transforming that reality (Kabat-Zinn, 1993). Mindfulness is similar to meditation: awareness of breathing and of the body is central to it. As well, it is about acting with attentiveness and concentration as one walks, eats, looks about, and carries out daily tasks of living. It is about being consciously aware of our body and mind, rather than thinking "about" experience (Sherman & Siporin, 2008). This meditative act can bring a sense of calmness within minutes.

Mindfulness can be found within most religious and spiritual traditions (Sherman & Siporin, 2008). It is a way to recognize one's connection with something beyond oneself, to realize that one is not separate nor alone, to experience serenity (Kreitzer, Gross, Waleekhachonloet, Reilly-Spong, & Byrd, 2009), and/or to search for meaning and purpose (Reed, 1992). Shapiro (2008, p. 3), who researches mindfulness, finds that `individuals "often find their faith is deepened as a result of becoming more mindful."

Mindfulness in the health literature, however, is most often discussed as a cognitive behavioural technique. This practice tends to utilize a brief, structured format called Mindfulness Based–Stress Reduction (MBSR). MBSR programs, initially designed by Kabat-Zinn (1990, 1994), involve three basic techniques: meditation, body scan (involves directing one's attention through the entire body), and yoga. In addition to the resource of health care team members trained to teach mindfulness to clients, there are local community programs and educational tools, such as books and videos, which are available to learn about this contemplative practice.

Lown (2007) calls for mindfulness on clinicians' part when addressing anger in the clinician–client/family relationship. He notes that mindfulness in such an encounter allows one to be both a participant and an observer. In taking a moment to assess one's own response to the situation (e.g., anxiety; anger) and to focus on being present in a genuine way to the client/family member, one is better able to respond.

Interactional Processes

When the nurse develops a collaborative relationship with the client, he or she can assist the client to not exhibit aggressive behaviour. Johnson, Martin, Guha, and Montgomery (1997) explored the experience of thought-disordered individuals before an aggressive incident. Three themes emerged from interviews with 12 clients who had a diagnosis of a thought disorder and a history of aggressive incidents:

• The strong influence of the external environment
• The use of aggressive behaviours to feel empowered briefly in a situation
• The occurrence of aggressive incidents, despite knowledge of strategies to control anger

A review of the research by Hamrin, Iennaco, and Olsen (2009) regarding factors affecting violence on psychiatric units showed that violence is influenced by complex interactions among clients, staff, and unit culture. For instance, a qualitative study of experienced mental health nurses found that participants identified workplace stressors (e.g., poor staffing skill mix, inadequate workplace design, and unsupported involuntary admissions) as contributing to increased pressure, fear, and uncertainty on units (Ward, 2013). A positive culture has appropriate levels of stimulation and meaningful client activities, as well as positive staff attitudes and values towards client care. Good assessment of client factors, including violence history, plays an important role. Therapeutic relationship strategies, including being available, being a client advocate, providing client education, and collaborating with the client in treatment planning, can decrease the potential for violence. An emerging theme in the literature is client and staff power struggles as precipitants for violence.

The skills the nurse uses in interactions with the client may invite escalation or de-escalation of a tense situation (Morrison, 1998). When the nurse uses communication skills to draw out the client's experience, together the nurse and client coevolve an alternative view of the problem. Some nursing writers (Leahey & Harper-Jaques, 1996; Wright & Leahey, 2005) have highlighted the importance of attending to notions of reciprocity and circularity when providing nursing care. For example, the nurse explores the meaning of the expression of aggressive behaviours with the client and the client's beliefs about the ability to control aggressive impulses. Or, the nurse and client could discuss the effects of the nurse's behaviours on the client and the effects of the client's behaviours on the nurse. Such an approach facilitates the development of an accepting and equal nurse–client relationship. The client is a partner invited to assume responsibility for inappropriate actions. This approach is in contrast to a hierarchical nurse–client relationship that emphasizes the nurse's role in controlling the client's behaviours and defining changes the client must make. In a collaborative approach, the nurse values the client's experience and acknowledges his or her strengths. The nurse asks the client to use those strengths to either maintain or resume control of behaviour.

In Western cultures, events are typically thought of in a linear fashion (Wright & Leahey, 2005). The nurse who uses a linear causality frame of reference to think about client aggression and violence will view the problem as follows:

PACING → leads to → THREATENING
                                 BEHAVIOURS
(Event A)   (Event B)

From this linear perspective, the nurse labels the client as the problem, and other factors assume secondary importance. The nurse might decide, first, to gain control over the client's behaviour. The nurse may base this decision on his or her affective response and previous experience (e.g., that threatening behaviours frighten other clients and disrupt the unit routine). The nurse's response to a client's behaviour could be to ask the client to stop yelling, to inform the client that the behaviour is inappropriate, or to suggest the use of medication if the client does not calm down. When one thinks based on linear causality, he or she assumes that event A (pacing) causes event B (threatening behaviour).

When one thinks using circular causality, he or she attempts to understand the link between behaviours and to determine how the threatening behaviour will influence a continuation or cessation of pacing. The nurse who engages in circular thinking will also know that his or her responses to the client will influence the situation. The nurse's responses will be in the domains of cognition (ideas, concepts, and beliefs), affect (emotional state), and behaviour (Tomm, 1980). The nurse will be aware of the reciprocal influences of the nurse and client's behaviours (Wright & Leahey, 2005). In viewing the situation from a circular perspective, the nurse is interested in understanding how people are involved, rather than in discovering who is to blame. This perspective does not ignore individual responsibility for aggressive or violent actions, and it does not blame the victim. It does invite the nurse to consider the multiple influences on the expression of aggressive and violent behaviour (Robinson, Wright, & Watson, 1994).

Responding to Assault

In recent years, compelling scientific evidence that violence portrayed in the media is harmful to children has fostered debate about violence and its effects. As a result, television networks have taken both voluntary and legislated actions to limit violent programming during hours when children are generally watching programs. However, these gains in limiting access to violence have been countered by the growing availability of violent video games and websites.

Given today's societal context, it is not surprising that aggression and violence directed towards nurses are often ignored. Close proximity to clients by health care workers presents a higher risk to experience acts of violence. Approximately 40% of time loss claim–related violence is from health care workers (Rotin, 2005). Aggression and violence by clients can threaten the safety of nurses, other clients, other health care professionals, family members, and visitors. Family members may also direct aggression and violence towards nurses, especially if family members have increased stress levels and ineffective coping skills and/or experience long wait times and/or use substances (Ferns, 2007). Ineffective communication between nurses and families can contribute to increased aggression (Ferns).

In health care settings, nurses assume an active role in preventing and managing aggressive and violent behaviours. A review of the literature related to inpatient violence and aggression by the Mental Health Nursing Section of Kings College London's Institute of Psychiatry (Bowers et al., 2011) found that a majority of nurses reported experiencing violence at least once during their career, a rate much higher than that of psychiatrists. Categories of antecedents to violent and/or aggressive incidents identified across studies were staff–client interaction, client behavioural cues (e.g., agitation, attention-seeking behaviour, increased motor activity, boisterousness, and confusion), client symptoms, mood cues, external/personal issues, and no clear cause (Bowers et al., 2011). Involuntary (as opposed to voluntary) admission to a psychiatric facility or altered mental status in any setting may constrain the development of a trusting relationship between the nurse and client. Nurses are more likely than physicians to be involved with clients who are aggressive or potentially violent because of the amount of time they are in close contact with clients. Nurses also have a major role in setting limits and defining boundaries (Bostrom, Boyd, & White, 2006).

Concern and investigation of assaults on nurses have been growing. Research shows that the incidence and severity of violence directed towards nurses are on the rise with the most common form of violence being verbal abuse followed by threatening behaviours (Luck, Jackson, & Usher, 2006). The Nova Scotia Department of Health (2006) indicated that 32% of nurses reported being physically assaulted by clients within the past year. Nurses commonly report emotional abuse, with 44% experiencing emotional abuse from a client (Canadian Institute for Health Information, 2005). Reported violence is higher in long-term care, general hospitals, and psychiatric facilities, but nurses who work in ambulatory care settings or community clinics are not immune to assault (Gerberich et al., 2004). Banerjee et al. (2008) report Canadian personal support workers in long-term care facilities to be seven times more likely to experience violence directed towards them than their Nordic counterparts. The most common injury experienced by health care workers due to violence include strains to the body, such as the back (65%) and bruises/contusions (18%; WCB Statistical Services, 2005).

Variations in statistics can result from differences in definitions of violence, reporting practices, data collection and analysis, and underreporting. Rationale for underreporting is common and includes time constraints, staff attitudes, conflict between the traditional caring role and reporting the violence, belief that an individual will be blamed or perceived as inadequate, minimization of the event by the nurses involved or by their colleagues, and lack of understanding in the importance of data collection (Munro, 2002). Data, as identified by the WHO (2002), provide important information in the development of strategies to minimize violence. Lack of data limits health care facilities' ability to enact measures to protect their workers and others.

Reports of inpatient violence tend to be exclusively from the staff's perspective. Although data indicate one third of incidents are unprovoked, it may be that staff are not recognizing or not recording the antecedents of an incident. Clients' experiences need to be captured if the scope of antecedents is to be better understood (Bowers et al., 2011). Data collected should include specific information, such as gender (Ferns, 2006).

Assaults on nurses by clients can have immediate and long-term consequences (Henderson, 2003). Reported assaults range from verbal threats and minor altercations to severe injuries, rape, and murder. Any assault can produce severe consequences for the victim. Nonphysical violence towards nurses by clients or others can have long-lasting effects on nurses, such as posttraumatic stress disorder (Gerberich et al., 2005).

Lanza's research (Lanza, 1992) indicates that nurses experience a wide range of responses (Table 18-4) similar to those of victims of any other type of trauma. However, because of their role as caregivers, nurses may suppress

Table 18-4 Nurses' Responses to Assault

Response Type	Personal	Professional
Affective	• Irritability • Depression • Anger • Anxiety • Apathy	• Erosion of feelings of competence, leading to increased anxiety and fear • Feelings of guilt or self-blame • Fear of potentially violent clients
Cognitive	• Suppressed or intrusive thoughts of assault	• Reduced confidence in judgment • Consideration of job change
Behavioural	• Social withdrawal	• Possible hesitation in responding to other violent situations • Possible overcontrolling • Possible hesitation to report future assaults • Possible withdrawal from colleagues • Questioning of capabilities by coworkers
Physiologic	• Disturbed sleep • Headaches • Stomach aches • Tension	• Increased absenteeism from somatic complaints

the normal range of feelings after an assault, believing that it is wrong to experience strong feelings of anger and fear in this situation. This belief may relate to the conflict nurses experience in having to care for clients who have hurt them.

Steps can be taken at a clinical and management level to reduce the risk for assaults on nurses by clients. A nursing-based framework that identifies three staff factors that are important to reduction of conflict in inpatient psychiatric units is the City Model (Bowers, 2009; Björkdahl, Hansebo, & Palmstierna, 2013). These factors are positive appreciation of patients (i.e., psychological understanding of difficult behavior promoted; humanistic values), self-regulation of emotional responses (i.e., awareness and control of feelings), and effective structure of rules and routine (i.e., teamwork, organizational support, clarity of rules, teamwork). This model, which aims to reduce conflict and containment, may not be fully applicable to forensic services, where the highest rates of violence are to be found and which can require high levels of containment (Bowers et al., 2011).

Clinically, nurses must be provided with training programs in the prevention and management of aggressive behaviour. These programs, like courses on cardiopulmonary resuscitation (CPR), impart both knowledge and skills. Like CPR training, the courses need to be made available to nurses and students regularly so that they have opportunities to reinforce and update what they have learned. Nurses who have participated in preventive training programs as students or as professionals are more likely to effectively manage and reduce aggressive or violent situations. Additionally, training programs can raise awareness as to the nature of the problem, develop the nurses' knowledge and skills, and improve attitudes towards clients who have a propensity for violence (Deans, 2004). Less experienced staff with poor communication skills are at higher risk for assault (Wright, Dixon, & Tompkins, 2003). Training programs need to address the complex interplay of factors related to violent client behaviour. Such training would inform staff about risk assessment, staff interactions, unit milieu (primary); how to use de-escalation techniques (secondary); and how to control, manage, and perform a postassessment and documentation of an incident of violent patient behaviour (Björkdahl et al., 2013).

Evaluation and Treatment Outcomes

Treatment outcomes can be considered at both individual and aggregate levels. The desired outcome at the individual level is for the client to regain or maintain control over aggressive or potentially aggressive thoughts, feelings, and actions. *Aggression control* is the term used in the *Nursing Outcomes Classification* (Moorhead, Johnson, & Maas, 2003). The nurse may observe that the client shows decreased psychomotor activity (e.g., less pacing), has a more relaxed posture, speaks more directly about feelings of anger and personal needs, requires less sedating medication, shows increased tolerance for frustration and the ability to consider alternatives, and makes effective use of other coping strategies. Evidence of a reduction in risk factors may include decreased noise and confusion in the immediate environment, calmness on the part of nursing staff and others, and a climate of clear expectations and mutual acceptance and respect. In units, day hospitals, or group home settings, indicators of positive treatment outcomes might be a reduction in the number and severity of assaults on staff and other clients, fewer incident reports, and increased staff competency in de-escalating potentially violent situations.

Continuum of Care

Anger and aggression occur in all settings. During periods of extreme aggression, in which people are a danger to themselves or others because of a mental disorder, they are admitted to an acute psychiatric unit. Removing individuals from their environment and hospitalizing them in a locked psychiatric unit provide enough safety that the aggressive behaviour dissipates. Because uncontrolled anger and aggression interfere with their ability to function, people who have problems in these areas require

BOX 18-7   Research for Best Practice

THE LANGUAGE OF VIOLENCE IN MENTAL HEALTH CARE

Alex, M., Whitty-Rogers, J., & Panagopoulos, W. (2013). The language of violence in mental health: Shifting the paradigm to the language of peace. *Advances in Nursing Science, 36(3),* 229–242.

Proposal: The oppressive and stigmatizing language used within mental health nurse–client relationships should be changed to a language of peace.

Method: A philosophical inquiry approach is used to identify and discuss a problem that can occur in psychiatric settings: language used in regard to clients and families can be violent in its nature and create disharmony and distrust. The connections between and among the concepts of peace, health, and relational ethics in terms of nurses' responsibilities, current health care realities, and the language of nursing are made. Peace is described as involving relationships that nuture harmony, trust, and constructive solutions. Stigma and historical prejudices in the treatment of mentally distressed persons are explored with a focus on language.

It is argued that psychiatric diagnostic representations can be used to medicalize human experience and pathologize experiences of anger, despair, and distress. Victim blaming may occur, such as blaming mothers for their children's health problems without considering families' life situation. A discourse analysis of end-of-shift nursing reports is cited, revealing language that can be deemed disrespectful and stigmatizing. Clients are described with such terms as "space cadet, out to lunch, off his rocker." "Elderspeak," a way of speaking to elders hospitalized in institutional settings, is another form of language addressed. It has two forms: "singsong, overly nurturing talk" appropriate to young children and "brief, authoritarian commands" (p. 238). The authors of this inquiry make the argument that language may be used in mental health settings in ways that stop, rather than support, communication and thus create a confusing, threatening milieu.

Conclusions: "Everyday language that we use in clinical care can be part of shifting the (violent) paradigm to the language, imagery, and attitudes of peace" (p. 240–241).

Implications for Practice: Nurses need to be attentive to the language used in mental health care settings. In moving from terms that can do violence to the dignity of others to language that supports human dignity, nurses can act to promote trust and harmony.

referral to appropriate resources before these destructive behaviours erupt.

Additional understanding of the phenomena of anger, aggression, and violence as they occur in the clinical setting is needed. Research studies that have illuminated this problem from a nursing perspective need to be continued and expanded. Specific areas of study need to examine the links among biology, neurology, and psychology. In addition, further explorations of the reciprocal influence of client interactional style and treatment setting culture will assist in the development and management of humane treatment settings. See Box 18-7 for research that considers nurses' language that may be

deemed oppressive and violent. Finally, and perhaps most importantly, nurses must research the effectiveness of particular nursing interventions.

SUMMARY OF KEY POINTS

■ Theories used to explain anger, aggression, and violence include the following types:
- Neurobiologic, including the cognitive neuroassociation model, the neurostructural model (the emotional circuit), and the neurochemical model (low serotonin syndrome)
- Psychological, including psychoanalytic theories, behavioural theories (e.g., drive theory, social learning theory), and cognitive theories (e.g., rational–emotive theory)
- Sociocultural theories
- Interactional theory

■ Biologic factors to assess in clients who display aggressive and violent behaviours include exposure to toxic chemicals, use of medications, substance abuse, premenstrual dysphoric disorder, trauma, haemorrhage, and tumour.

■ Biologic intervention choices include administering medications and managing nutrition.

■ Psychological factors to assess in clients who display aggressive and violent behaviours include thought processing (e.g., perception, delusion) and sensory impairment.

■ Psychological intervention choices can be affective (e.g., validating, listening, exploring beliefs), cognitive (e.g., giving commendations, offering information, providing education, using thought stopping, contracting), or behavioural (e.g., assigning tasks, using bibliotherapy, interrupting patterns, providing choices).

■ Social intervention choices include reducing stimulation, anticipating needs, and using seclusion or restraints.

■ Mindfulness can be a component of addressing the spiritual domain of care. It is a contemplative practice that both clients and nurses may find useful in dealing with anger and situations involving aggression.

■ Client aggression and violence are serious concerns for nurses in all areas of clinical practice. Training in and policies and procedures for the prevention and management of aggressive episodes should be available in all work settings.

CRITICAL THINKING CHALLENGES

1 Mary Jane, a 24-year-old single woman, has just been admitted to an inpatient psychiatry unit. She was transferred to the unit from the emergency room, where she

was treated for a drug overdose. She is sullen when she is introduced to her roommate and refuses to answer the questions the nurse has that are part of the admission procedure. The nurse tells Mary Jane that he will come back later to see how she is. A few minutes later, Mary Jane approaches the nursing station and asks in a demanding tone to talk with someone and complains that she has been completely ignored since she came into the unit. What frameworks can the nurse use to understand Mary Jane's behaviour? At this point in time, what data does he have to develop a plan of care? What interventions might the nurse choose to use to help Mary Jane behave in a manner that is consistent with the norms of this inpatient unit?

2 Discuss the influence of gender and cultural norms on the expression of anger. When a nurse is caring for a client from a culture that the nurse is not familiar with, what could the nurse ask to ensure that his or her expectations of the client's behaviour are consistent with the gender and cultural norms of the client?

3 Under what circumstances should people who are aggressive or violent be held accountable for their behaviour? Are there any exceptions?

4 When a nurse minimizes verbally abusive behaviour by a client, family member, or health care colleague, what implicit message does he or she send?

5 In what way does our understanding of sociocultural theories influence the relationships that we, as nurses, develop with clients and families? Does this understanding also influence the relationships between nurses and other health professionals?

6 Paul is sitting quietly reading a newspaper. Jane sits down next to him and starts talking to him about the weather. Paul responds by pushing Jane off the couch. How do you understand Paul's behaviour? Could Paul's action have been prevented?

REFERENCES

Alex, M., Whitty-Rogers, J., & Panagopoulos, W. (2013). The language of violence in mental health: Shifting the paradigm to the language of peace. *Advances in Nursing Science, 36*(3), 229–242.

Bandura, A. (1973). *Aggression: A social learning analysis*. New York: Prentice-Hall.

Banerjee, A., Daly, A., Armstrong, H., Armstrong, P., Lafrance, S., & Szebehely, M. (2008). "Out of control": Violence against personal support workers in long-term care. York University/Carleton University. Retrieved from http://www.yorku.ca/mediar/special/out_of_control__english.pdf

Beck, A. T. (1976). *Cognitive therapy and emotional disorders*. New York: International Universities Press.

Belknap, R. A. (2003). Understanding abuse and violence against women: A two-day immersion course. *Nurse Educator, 28*(4), 170–174.

Berkowitz, L. (1989). Frustration-aggression hypothesis: Examination and reformulation. *Psychological Bulletin, 106*(1), 59–73.

Bernstein, K. S. & Saladino, J. P. (2007). Clinical assessment and management of psychiatric patients' violent and aggressive behaviours in general hospital. *Medsurg Nursing, 16*(5), 301–331.

Best, M., Williams, J. M., & Coccaro, E. F. (2002). Evidence for a dysfunctional prefrontal circuit in clients with an impulsive aggressive disorder. *Proceedings of the National Academy of Sciences, 99*(12), 8448–8453.

Björkdahl, A., Hansebo, G., & Palmstierna, T. (2013). The influence of staff training on the violence prevention and management climate in psychiatric inpatient units. *Journal of Psychiatric and Mental Health Nursing, 20*, 396–404.

Bostrom, A. C., Boyd, M., & White, D. (2006). Coping with aggressive behavior in patients with schizophrenia. *Psychiatric Nurse: Counseling Points, 1*(2), 4–12.

Bowers, L. (2009). Association between staff factors and levels of conflict and containment on acute psychiatric wards in England. *Psychiatric Services, 60*(2), 231–239.

Bowers, L., Allan, T., Simpson, A., Jones, J., Van Der Merwe, M., & Jeffery, D. (2009). Identifying key factors associated with aggression on acute inpatient psychiatric wards. *Issues in Mental Health Nursing, 30*, 260–271.

Bowers, L., Stewart, D., Papadopoulos, C., Dack, C., Ross, J., Khanom, H., & Jeffery, D. (2011). *Inpatient violence and aggression: A literature review. Report from the Conflict and Containment Reeducation Research Programme*. London: Institute of Psychiatry, King's College London.

Brock, G., Gurekas, V., Gelinas, A. F., & Rollin, K. (2009). Use of a "secure room" and a security guard in the management of the violent, aggressive or suicidal patient in a rural hospital: A 3-year audit. *Canadian Journal of Rural Medicine, 14*(1), 16–20.

Burke, J. D., Loeber, R., & Birmaher, B. (2002). Oppositional defiant disorder and conduct disorder: A review of the past 10 years, Part II. *Journal of the American Academy of Child and Adolescent Psychiatry, 41*(11), 1275–1293.

Burns, D. (1999). *Feeling good: The new mood therapy*. New York: Avon Books.

Canadian Institute for Health Information. (2005). *A summary of highlights from the 2005 national survey of the work and health of nurses*. Ottawa: Statistics Canada.

Capra, F. (2002). *The hidden connections: Integrating the biological, cognitive and social dimensions of life into a science of sustainability*. New York: Doubleday.

Carlsson, G., Dahlberg, K., Ekebergh, M., & Dahlberg, H. (2006). Patients longing for authentic personal care: A phenomenological study of violent encounters in psychiatric setting. *Issues in Mental Health Nursing, 27*(3), 287–305.

Chakos, M. & Lieberman, J. A. (2001). Effects of clozapine, olanzapine, risperidone, and haloperidol on hostility among clients with schizophrenia. *Psychiatric Services, 52*(11), 1510–1514.

Citrome, L. & Volavka, J. (1999). Violent clients in the emergency setting. *Psychiatric Clinics of North America, 22*(4), 789–801.

Citrome, L. & Volavka, J. (2002). Aggression. Retrieved from http://www.emedicine.com/Med/topic3005.htm

College of Registered Psychiatric Nurses of British Columbia. (2008). *The use of physical restraint & seclusion as psychiatric nursing interventions: Position statement*. Port Moody, BC: Author.

Corrigan, P. W., Yudofsky, S. C., & Silver, J. M. (1993). Pharmacological and behavioral treatment for aggressive psychiatric in-patients. *Hospital & Community Psychiatry, 44*(3), 125–133.

Cutcliffe, J. & Riahi, S. (2013a). Systematic perspective of violence and aggression in mental health care: Towards a more comprehensive understanding and conceptualization: Part 1. *International Journal of Mental Health Nursing, 22*, 558–567.

Cutcliffe, J. & Riahi, S. (2013b). Systematic perspective of violence and aggression in mental health care: Towards a more comprehensive understanding and conceptualization: Part 2. *International Journal of Mental Health Nursing, 22*, 568–578.

Davidson, K. & Mostofsky, E. (2010). Anger expression and risk of coronary heart disease: Evidence from the Nova Scotia Health Survey. *American Heart Journal, 159*(2), 199–206.

Deans, C. (2004). The effectiveness of a training program for emergency department nurses in managing violent situations. *Australian Journal of Advanced Nursing, 21*(4), 17–22.

DeLisi, M., Vaughn, M., Gentile, D., Anderson, C., & Shook, J. (2013). Violent video games, delinquency and youth violence. *Youth Violence and Juvenile Justice, 11*(2), 132–142.

DiGiuseppe, R. & Tafrate, R. (2007). *Understanding anger disorders*. Oxford, UK: Oxford University Press.

Duxbury, J. & Whittington, R. (2005). Causes and management of patient aggression and violence: Staff and patient perspectives. *Journal of Advanced Nursing, 50*(5), 469–478.

Elbogen, E. & Johnson, S. (2009). The intricate link between violence and mental disorder: Results from the national epidemiologic survey on alcohol and related conditions. *Archives of General Psychiatry, 66*(2), 152–161.

Ellis, A. (1977). *Anger: How to live with and without it*. Secaucus, NJ: Citadel Press.

Fahs, H., Potiron, G., Senon, J. L., & Perivier, E. (1999). Anticonvulsants in agitation and behavior disorders in demented subjects. *Encephale, 25*(2), 169–174.

Faucher, L. & Tappolet, C. (2008). *The modularity of emotions*. Calgary, AB: University of Calgary Press.

Ferns, T. (2006). Underreporting of violent incidents against nursing staff. *Nursing Standard, 21*(40), 41–45.

Ferns, T. (2007). Factors that influence aggressive behaviours in acute care settings. *Nursing Standard, 21*(33), 41–45.

Friedman, R. A. & Michels, R. (2013). How should the psychiatric profession respond to the recent mass killings (Editorial). *American Journal of Psychiatry, 170*(5), 455–458.

Fromm, E. (1973). *The anatomy of human destructiveness.* New York: Holt, Rinehart and Winston.

Gerberich, S. G., Church, T. R., McGovern, P. M., Hansen, H., Nachreiner, N. M., Geisser, M. S., & Jurek, A. (2005). Risk factors for work-related assaults on nurses. *Epidemiology, 16,* 704–709.

Gerberich, S. G., Church, T. R., McGovern, P. M., Hansen, H. E., Nachreiner, N. M., Geisser, M. S., & Watt, G. (2004). An epidemiological study of the magnitude and consequences of work related violence: The Minnesota nurses' study. *Occupational and Environmental Medicine, 61,* 495–503.

Gerloff, L. (1997). Anger management. *Arkansas Nursing News, 14*(1), 5–7.

Hamrin, V., Iennaco, J., & Olsen, D. (2009). A review of ecological factors affecting inpatient psychiatric unit violence: Implications for relational and unit culture improvements. *Issues in Mental Health Nursing, 30,* 214–226.

Harper-Jaques, S. & Masters, A. (1994). Powerful words: The use of letters with sexual abuse survivors. *Journal of Psychosocial Nursing and Mental Health Services, 32*(8), 11–16.

Harper-Jaques, S. & Reimer, M. (1992). Aggressive behavior and the brain: A different perspective for the mental health nurse. *Archives of Psychiatric Nursing, 6*(5), 312–320.

Harris, D. & Morrison, E. F. (1995). Managing violence without coercion. *Archives of Psychiatric Nursing, 9*(4), 203–210.

Heinz, A., Mann, K., Weinberger, D. R., & Goldman, D. (2001). Serotonergic dysfunction, negative mood states, and response to alcohol. *Alcoholism, Clinical and Experimental Research, 25*(4), 487–495.

Henderson, A. D. (2003). Nurses and workplace violence: Nurses' experiences of verbal and physical abuse at work. *Canadian Journal of Nursing Leadership, 16*(4), 82–98.

Hibbs, A. (2000). Cognitive therapy: A complementary strategy for expressed anger during the restraint of an aggressive individual. *The British Journal of Forensic Practice, 2*(2), 19–29.

Jenkins, A. (1990). *Invitations to responsibility.* Adelaide, Australia: Dulwich Centre Publications.

Johnson, M. E. (2010). Violence and restraint reduction efforts on inpatient psychiatric units. *Issues in Mental Health Nursing, 31,* 181–187.

Johnson, B., Martin, M. L., Guha, M., & Montgomery, P. (1997). The experience of thought disordered individuals preceding an aggressive incident. *Journal of Psychiatric and Mental Health Nursing, 4,* 213–220.

Kabat-Zinn, J. (1990). *Full catastrophe living: Using the wisdom of your body and mind to face stress, pain, and illness.* New York: Dell.

Kabat-Zinn, J. (1993). Mindfulness meditation: Health benefits of an ancient Buddhist practice. In D. Goleman & J. Gurin (Eds.), *Mind/body medicine* (pp. 259–276). New York: Consumer Reports Books.

Kabat-Zinn, J. (1994). *Wherever you go, there you are: Mindfulness meditation in everyday life.* New York: Hyperion.

Kassinove, H. & Tafrate, R. C. (2006). Anger-related disorders: Basic issues, models, and diagnostic considerations. In E. L. Feindler (Ed.), *Anger-related disorders: A Practitioner's guide to comparative treatments* (pp. 1–28). New York: Springer.

Koh, K. B., Kim, C. H., & Park, J. K. (2002). Predominance of anger in depressive disorders compared with anxiety disorders and somatoform disorders. *Journal of Clinical Psychiatry, 63*(6), 486–492.

Kreitzer, M. J., Gross, C. R., Waleekhachonloet, O. A., Reilly-Spong, M., & Byrd, M. (2009). The brief serenity scale: A psychometric analysis of a measure of spirituality and well-being. *Journal of Holistic Nursing, 27*(1), 7–16.

Lanza, M. L. (1992). Nurses as client assault victims: An update, synthesis, and recommendations. *Archives of Psychiatric Nursing, 6*(3), 163–171.

Leahey, M. & Harper-Jaques, S. (1996). Family–nurse relationship: Core assumptions and clinical implications. *Journal of Family Nursing, 2*(2), 133–151.

Lewis, D. M. (2002). Responding to a violent incident: Physical restraint or anger management as therapeutic interventions. *Journal of Psychiatric and Mental Health Nursing, 9*(1), 57–63.

Limacher, L. H. & Wright, L. M. (2003). Commendations: Listening to the silent side of a family intervention. *Journal of Family Nursing, 9*(2), 130–150.

Liu, J., Lewis, G., & Evans, L. (2013). Understanding aggressive behaviour across the lifespan. *Journal of Psychiatric and Mental Health Nursing, 20*(2), 156–168.

Lorist, M. M. & Tops, M. (2003). Caffeine, fatigue, and cognition. *Brain and Cognition, 53*(1), 82–94.

Lown, B. (2007). Difficult conversations: Anger in the clinician-patient/family relationship. *Southern Medical Journal, 100*(1), 34–39.

Luck, L., Jackson, D., & Usher, K. (2006). Survival of the fittest, or socially constructed phenomena? Theoretical understandings of aggression & violence towards nurses. *Contemporary Nurse, 21*(2), 251–263.

Marlatt, G. A. & Kristeller, J. L. (1999). Mindfulness and meditation. In W. R. Miller, (Ed.), *Integrating spirituality into treatment.* Washington, DC: American Psychological Association.

Mesulam, M. (2000). *Principles of behavioral and cognitive neurology* (2nd ed.). Oxford, UK: Oxford University Press.

Miller, N., Pedersen, W. C., Earleywine, M., & Pollock, V. E. (2003). Artificial theoretical model of triggered displaced aggression. *Personality and Social Psychology Review, 7*(1), 57–97.

Moorhead, S., Johnson, M., & Maas, M. (2003). *Nursing outcomes classification* (3rd ed.). Philadelphia, PA: Elsevier.

Morrison, E. F. (1998). The culture of caregiving and aggression in psychiatric settings. *Archives of Psychiatric Nursing, 12*(1), 21–31.

Morrison, E. F. & Carney Love, C. (2003). An evaluation of four programs for the management of aggression in psychiatric settings. *Archives of Psychiatric Nursing, 17*(4), 146–155.

Munro V. (2002). 'Why Do Nurses Neglect to Report Violent Incidents?' *Nursing Times, 98*(17), 38–40.

North American Nursing Diagnosis Association (NANDA). (2005). *Nursing diagnoses: Definitions and classification 2005–2006.* Philadelphia, PA: Author.

Nova Scotia Department of Health. (2006). *The National Survey of the Work and Health of Nurses, 2005.* Halifax, NS: Author.

Novaco, R. (2007). Anger dysregulation. In T. Cavell & K. Malcolm (Eds.), *Anger, aggression, and interventions for interpersonal violence* (pp. 3–54). London, UK: Lawrence Erlbaum Associates.

Pardo, J. V., Pardo, P. J., & Raichle, M. E. (1993). Neural correlates of self-induced dysphoria. *American Journal of Psychiatry, 150*(5), 713–719.

Paris, J. (2005). Borderline personality disorder. *Canadian Medical Association Journal, 172*(12), 1579–1583.

Reed, P. G. (1992). An emerging paradigm for the investigation of spirituality in nursing. *Research in Nursing & Health, 15,* 349–357.

Robinson, C., Wright, L., & Watson, W. (1994). A non-traditional approach to family violence. *Archives of Psychiatric Nursing, 8*(1), 30–37.

Rotin, J. (2005). Preventing workplace violence. *WorkSafe Magazine, 4,* 12–14.

Rubinsztein, E. R., Sahakian, B. J., & Dolan, R. J. (2002). The neural basis of mood congruent processing biases in depression. *Archives of General Psychiatry, 59*(7), 597–604.

Scarpa, A. & Raine, A. (1997). Psychophysiology of anger and violent behavior. *Psychiatric Clinics of North America, 20*(2), 375–394.

Schmeck, K., Sadigorsky, S., Englert, E., Demisch, L., Dierks, T., Barta, S., & Poustka, F. (2002). Mood changes following acute tryptophan depletion in healthy adults. *Psychopathology, 35*(4), 234–240.

Sergi, M. J. & Green, M. F. (2003). Social perception and early visual processing in schizophrenia. *Schizophrenia Research, 59*(2–3), 233–241.

Shannon, J. W. (2000). *Understanding and managing anger: Diagnosis, treatment and prevention.* Presentation by Mind Matters Seminar, April 2000, Calgary, Alberta.

Shapiro, S. L. (2008). Exploring the effects of mindfulness meditation on health, well-being, and spirituality. *Spirituality in Higher Education, 4*(2), 1–5.

Sherman, E. & Siporin, M. (2008). Contemplative theory and practice for social work. *Journal of Religion & Spirituality in Social Work, 27*(3), 259–274.

Silver, J. M., Yudofsky, S. C., Slater, J. A., Gold, R. K., Stryer, B. L., Williams, D. T., … Endicott, J. (2000). Propranolol treatment of chronically hospitalized aggressive clients. *The Journal of Neuropsychiatry and Clinical Neuroscience, 11*(3), 328–335.

Snyder, K., Schrepferman, L., Brooker, M., & Stoolmiller, M. (2007). The roles of anger, conflict with parents and peers, and social reinforcement in the early development of physical aggression. In T. Cavell & K. Malcolm (Eds.), *Anger, aggression, and interventions for interpersonal violence* (pp. 187–214). London, UK: Lawrence Erlbaum Associates.

Soloff, P. H., Lynch, K. G., & Moss, H. B. (2000). Serotonin, impulsivity, and alcohol use disorders in the older adolescent: A psychobiological study. *Alcoholism, Clinical and Experimental Research, 24*(11), 1609–1619.

WCB Statistical Services. (2005). *Fact sheet: Violence in health care and social assistance provincial overview.* Vancouver, BC: Author.

Stewart, D. & Bowers, L. (2013). Inpatient verbal aggression: Content, targets and patient characteristics. *Journal of Psychiatric and Mental Health Nursing, 20,* 236–243.

Stolley, J. M., Gerdner, L. A., & Buckwalter, K. C. (1999). Dementia management. In G. M. Bulechek & J. C. McCloskey (Eds.), *Nursing interventions: Effective nursing treatments* (3rd ed., pp. 533–548). Philadelphia, PA: WB Saunders.

Swanson, J., Schwartz, M., Van Dorn, R., Elbogen, E., Wagner, H.R., Rosenheck, R., … Lieberman, J. (2006). A national study of violent behavior of persons with schizophrenia. *Archives of General Psychiatry, 63*(5), 490–499.

Tajaden, P. & Thoennes, N. (2000). *Findings from national violence against women survey.* Washington, DC: U.S. Department of Justice.

Talerico, K. A., Evans, L. K., & Strumpf, N. E. (2002). Mental health correlates of aggression in nursing home residents with dementia. *Gerontologist, 42*(2), 169–177.

Tavris, C. (1989). *Anger: The misunderstood emotion.* New York: Simon & Schuster.

Teplin, L., McClelland, G., Abram, K., & Weiner, D. (2005). Crime victimization in adults with severe mental illness: Comparison with the National Crime Victimization Survey. *Archives of General Psychiatry, 62*(8), 911–921.

Thomas, S. P. (1990). Theoretical and empirical perspectives on anger. *Issues in Mental Health Nursing, 11,* 203–216.

Thomas, S. P. (1993). *Women and anger.* New York: Springer.

Thomas, S. P. (1998). Assessing and intervening with anger disorders. *Nursing Clinics of North America, 33*(1), 121–133.

Thomas, S. P. (2001). Teaching healthy anger management. *Perspectives in Psychiatric Care, 37*(2), 41–48.

Thomas, S. P. (2003). Men's anger: A phenomenological exploration of its meaning in a middle class sample of American men. *Psychology of Men & Masculinity, 4*(2), 163–175.

Thomas, S. P. (2006). Culture and gender considerations in the assessment and treatment of anger-related disorders. In E. L. Feindler (Ed.), *Anger-related disorders: A practitioner's guide to comparative treatments* (pp. 71–96). New York: Springer.

Thomas, S. P. (2009). *Transforming nurses' stress and anger: Steps toward healing* (3rd ed.). New York: Springer.

Tomm, K. (1980). Towards a cybernetic systems approach to family therapy at the University of Calgary. In D. Freeman (Ed.), *Diagnosis and assessment in family therapy* (pp. 101–122). London, UK: Aspen.

United Nations High Commission on Human Rights. (2001). *Human rights resolution 2001.49. Declaration on the elimination of violence against women.* Retrieved from http://www.unhchr.ch/huridocda/huridoca.nsf/(symbol)/a.res.48.104.en

Ward, L. (2013). Ready, aim fire! Mental health nurses under siege in acute inpatient facilities. *Issues in Mental Health Nursing, 34,* 281–287.

Whitecross, F., Seeary, A., & Lee, S. (2013). Measuring the impacts of seclusion on psychiatry inpatients and the effectiveness of a pilot single-session post-seclusion counselling intervention. *International Journal of Mental Health Nursing, 22,* 512–521.

World Health Organization. (2002). *World report on violence and health.* Geneva: Author.

World Health Organization. (2005). *Multi-country study on women's health and domestic violence against women.* Geneva: WHO Press.

Wright, L. M. & Leahey, M. (2005). *Nurses and families: A guide to family assessment and intervention* (3rd ed.). Philadelphia, PA: FA Davis.

Wright, N. M. J., Dixon, A. J., & Tompkins, C. N. E. (2003). Managing violence in primary care: An evidence-based approach. *British Journal of General Practice, 53,* 557–562.

Young, S. N. (2002). Clinical nutrition. 3. The fuzzy boundary between nutrition and psychopharmacology. *Canadian Medical Association Journal, 166*(2), 205–209.

Self-Harm and Suicidal Behaviour

B. Lee Murray and Wendy Austin
Adapted from the chapter "Self-harm and Suicidal Behaviour:
Children, Adolescents and Adults" by Emily J. Hauenstein

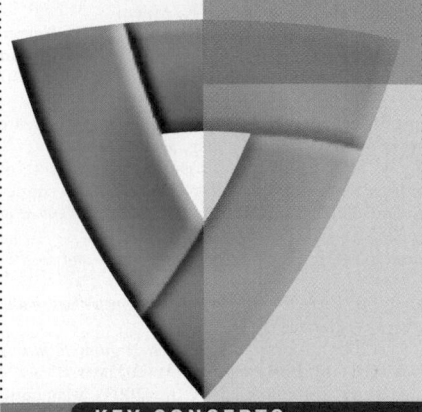

LEARNING OBJECTIVES

After studying this chapter, you will be able to:

- Define suicide, suicidal ideation, self-harm, parasuicide, and suicidal behaviour.
- Describe population groups that have high rates of suicide.
- Discuss the rights of patients and other legal issues in the care of suicidal patients.
- Determine factors that affect the nurse's responsibility in assessment and intervention with suicidal individuals, including adolescents.
- List screening measures for depression, suicide intent, and psychiatric diagnostic measures.
- Discuss the process of a comprehensive suicide risk assessment.
- Describe factors that increase the risk for suicide completion.
- Describe the no self-harm contract (contracting for safety).
- Describe the nurse's responsibilities in promoting short- and long-term recovery in suicidal adult inpatients.
- Discuss the patient's and nurse's responsibilities in discharging the patient to the community.

KEY TERMS

- beneficence • confidentiality • informed consent • involuntary hospitalization • least restrictive environment • no self-harm contract • parasuicide • self-harm • suicidal behaviour • suicidal ideation • suicide • suicide cluster • suicide contagion • voluntary hospitalization

---

The definition of **suicide** is simple: the voluntary and intentional act of killing oneself. The complexities associated with suicide, however, are grounded in an individual's perceptions and experiences of life, specifically those relating to sexuality, mental health, family factors, age, and gender. Two dimensions of suicide that need to be considered are attempt of suicide and completed suicide. An *attempt of suicide* can be characterized as living through an experience of suicide despite having expected or intended to die. Though the individual may receive support, help, and

hospitalization and be grateful for such services, the intent to end life was present. Conversely, a *completed suicide* is the engagement of suicidal behaviour that results in death. People who attempt suicide and survive tend to differ substantially in their thinking from those who complete suicide (Freedenthal, 2008). Acts of suicide, despite the actual outcome, are defined as **suicidal behaviour**. Likewise, the thought of suicide is known as *suicide ideation*. **Parasuicide** is a self-injurious behaviour or self-harm that may mimic suicidal behaviour, but the primary motivating force of action is not to kill oneself

(Kreitman, 1970; Zor et al., 2005). Death, however, may occur as a result of parasuicidal actions (Bergen et al., 2012; Welch, 2001). It is important to understand that parasuicide is *not* suicide (Kreitman, Philip, Greer, & Bagley, 1969). Understanding of parasuicide is incomplete. Furthermore, its prevalence may be seriously underestimated because being counted requires that the individual have contact with health or social services. Research is needed to more clearly define this phenomenon (Guo, Scott, & Bowker, 2003). There has been little comparison between deliberate self-harm and suicide rates (Hawton & Harriss, 2008). Self-harm exists in the suicide and parasuicide paradigms. **Self-harm** is characterized as any behaviour or act that causes harm to the body. The nature of the self-harm itself is dependent on the intent of the individual.

Many lives are deeply affected by suicide and the struggle to know what to do when a patient, colleague, friend, or loved one is suicidal. Self-harm and suicidal behaviours are very challenging for nurses and other health care professionals to address. It is important to try to understand the meaning of the self-harm and suicidal behaviours, particularly because such behaviours can be a means of communicating to others one's despair.

Suicide, like mental illness, is stigmatized in contemporary Western society. The stigma against suicide also has deep roots in some religions, including Christianity, Islam, and Hinduism. Until a few decades ago, suicide was considered a crime in Western nations and remains a crime in some places, such as India. The stigma of suicide can prevent people from voicing their suicidal thoughts or asking for help. When a suicidal act is unsuccessful, the visibility of medical intervention can trigger stigmatization by others (Cvinar, 2005). Stigma may also be experienced by the survivors of someone who completed suicide if blame for the loss is affixed to him or her. Those grieving the suicide may feel responsible for their loss and may not seek support. In this way, the stigma of suicide can significantly complicate bereavement (Cvinar, 2005).

Suicide remains a significant public health problem in Canada and places heavy demands on the health care system, despite efforts at both policy and clinical levels (e.g., to identify risk and protective factors, as well as to provide appropriate interventions). Suicide prevention is difficult because suicide is "the outcome of complex interactions among neurobiologic, genetic, psychobiologic, social, cultural, and environmental risk and protective factors" (Guo et al., 2003, p. 2). Nurses are in a unique position to contribute to preventive efforts. With knowledge of early risk assessment and interventions—understood within the context of a person's family, social world, and broader community—as well as with knowledge of how to engage with and respond to the actively suicidal person, nurses can make a difference. They can prevent the escalation or chronicity of the behaviour

(Murray, 2003). Nurses can do much to demystify suicide and prevent the stigmatization of those at risk through individual and public education. The content of this chapter provides the information needed to understand suicidal and parasuicidal behaviours, as well as the tools to respond appropriately to them.

CANADA'S SUICIDE PREVENTION STRATEGY

Canada's mental health strategy, *Changing Directions, Changing Lives*, contains a comprehensive suicide prevention strategy that cuts across the six identified strategic directions (Mental Health Commission of Canada, 2012). It includes improving front-line practitioner suicide prevention training, supporting suicide awareness and prevention programs in schools and workplaces, decreasing the stigma associated with suicide, supporting the families of persons who are suicidal, improving screening for suicidality, supporting research into suicide and its causes, and addressing social factors like poverty that increase suicide risk for specific groups. For the strategic directions of Canada's mental health strategy, see Chapter 1, Box 1-3.

EPIDEMIOLOGY OF SUICIDAL BEHAVIOUR

Suicide occurs in all age groups, social classes, and cultures. The World Health Organization (WHO, 2012) reports that nearly 1 million people kill themselves each year. Globally, suicide is a greater cause of death than war and homicide combined (Bertolote, Fleischmann, Butchart, & Besbelli, 2006). Prevalence estimates in low- and middle-income countries are similar to those in high-income countries for suicidal ideation (3.1%–12.4% versus 3.0% to 15.9%, respectively), suicide plan (0.9% to 4.1% versus 0.7% to 5.6%, respectively), and suicide attempt (0.7% to 4.7% versus 0.5% to 5.0%, respectively) (Nock et al., 2008). Although reliable data are lacking on the full impact of uncompleted suicide, it is recognized that it can result in injury, hospitalization, emotional trauma, and mental trauma.

BOX 19-1 World Suicide Prevention Day

World Suicide Prevention Day is September 10th each year. It is significant that the **World Suicide Report (WSR)** is released on this day. In 2014, the report follows the adoption of the Mental Health Action Plan 2013 to 2020 by the World Health Assembly, which commits all 194 member states to reducing their suicide rates by 10% by 2020. The WSR presents the status of suicide prevention internationally. See iasp.info/wspd and suicideprevention.ca

Canada ranks 41st in the world for reported suicides (WHO, 2012) and, within Canada, suicide is the ninth leading cause of death overall (Statistics Canada, 2012). The rate of suicide in 2011 was 10.8 per 100,000 (Statistics Canada, 2014). It is the leading cause of death for men aged 25 to 29 and 40 to 49 years and for women aged 30 to 34 years. It is also the leading cause of nonaccidental death for those aged 15 to 34 years. In the decade from 2000 to 2009, the most common means of death by suicide were by hanging, including strangulation and suffocation (44%), poisoning (25%), and firearms (16%) (Statistics Canada, 2012). It is generally accepted that prevalence rates are underestimated. Death by suicide can be difficult to identify as it may be disguised as a motor vehicle collision or homicide, especially in young people, and there is time lag between the reporting of a death and identifying it as a suicide (Statistics Canada, 2012).

Suicide is more common among groups with specific risk factors and has been associated with loss, unemployment, transience, recent life events (e.g., divorce, moving, problems with children), interpersonal distress, and earlier attempts. See Box 19-2 for a discussion of suicide and the Canadian military. Research indicates that, universally, suicide is strongly associated with chronic depression (Satyanarayana, Enns, Cox, & Sareen, 2009). The best predictor for suicide is a previous attempt. See Box 19-3 for a list of risk and protective factors.

KEY CONCEPTS Hopelessness is a perception of having no hope that one's life situation or circumstance will change or improve. It is characterized by feelings of inadequacy and an inability to act on one's own behalf.

KEY CONCEPTS Helplessness is the perception of having limited ability or ambition to change one's current life situation. It is characterized by a sense of being unable to help oneself and a sense that there is a lack of support or protection.

KEY CONCEPTS Powerlessness is the perception of having no power or control over one's life circumstance; feeling that the world will never be fair; feeling helpless and totally ineffectual; or feeling one lacks legal or other authority.

Age

Prepubertal Children

Suicide is rare among children who are younger than 10 years of age. There were two reports of self-harm resulting in completed suicide in Canadian children this age in 2011 (Statistics Canada, 2014). However, suicides by children this age may be significantly underestimated, as many question whether children can fully understand the finality of death and intentionally kill themselves.

Preadolescents and Adolescents

More teenagers die from suicide than from cancer, heart disease, birth defects, stroke, pneumonia, influenza, and chronic lung disease combined. In 2004, 156,000 adolescent deaths worldwide were the result of suicide (WHO, 2012). In 2011, 29 Canadian children aged 10 to 14 years (12.7% of all deaths within this age group) died due to intentional self-harm (Statistics Canada, 2014). Statistics Canada (2014) reports suicide to be the second leading cause of death for youth aged 15 to 24 years (499 deaths), making up 24.5% of all deaths in this age group. In 2011, 198 individuals aged 15 to 19 completed suicide. This represented one quarter (24.9%) of all deaths in this age group (Statistics Canada, 2014). Preadolescent and adolescent males are over three times more likely to complete suicide than their female peers (17.9 versus 5.3 per 100,000). Male and female Aboriginal youths in Canada, however, both die from

---

BOX 19-2 Suicide and the Canadian Military

When Canadian Forces (CF) confirmed eight suicides in the first 3 months of 2014, this sudden spike prompted public concern (Brewster, 2014). Yet, suicides in the CF are significantly lower than in the general population (Belik, Stein, Asmundson, & Sareen, 2010). Some factors related to suicide ideation and attempts appear to affect CF personnel differently than civilians. Women in CF, for instance, have a greater likelihood of suicide attempts than women in the general population; single soldiers are at less risk of suicide ideation than their civilian peers. Although research is needed to explain these differences, some possible explanations include the greater risk for female than male soldiers for negative impact to combat exposure and for sexual trauma during deployment. Single soldiers may have a stronger sense of social connection than civilian peers due to the "band of brothers" phenomenon of military life (Belik et al., 2010). A study that examined the association between suicidal ideation and self-reported symptoms of PTSD (see Chapter 17), major depressive disorder (see Chapter 22), and alcohol use disorder (see Chapter 26) in CF combat and peace-keeping veterans seeking treatment at an Ontario operational stress injury clinic found that, although PTSD alone is associated with suicidal ideation, it was self-reported depressive symptom severity that was its most significant predictor (Richardson et al., 2012). Suicide accounts for 17% of CF deaths, the fourth leading cause of death after motor vehicle crashes (22%), neoplasms (22%), and cardiovascular disease (22%). Combat deaths account for less than 5% (Tien, Acharya, & Redelmeier, 2010). Of note is that the proportion of Canadian soldiers using firearms in suicide (21%) is much lower than in the U.S. military (approximately 60%). About one quarter of Canadian military deaths are due to individual behaviours, particularly suicide, alcohol consumption, and tobacco use. The "healthy solider effect" means that other risks seen in the general population due to lack of physical activity and poor diet are uncommon. Combat soldiers, however, are more likely to smoke to deal with the stress of deployment and to abuse alcohol upon return; combat veterans are more likely to have mental health problems. Targeting these behaviours seems key to a preventive mental health strategy (Tien et al., 2010).

BOX 19-3 Risk and Protective Factors for Suicide

Risk Factors

Demographic or social factors
- Being an older adult
- Being male
- Poverty
- Being Aboriginal
- Being single (widowed > divorced > separated > single)
- Social isolation, including new or worsening estrangement, and rural location
- Economic or occupational stress, loss, or humiliation
- New incarceration
- History of gambling
- Easy access to firearms

Clinical factors
- Past and current major psychiatric illness (especially depression)
- Personality disorder (borderline, narcissistic, antisocial)
- Impulsive or violent traits by history
- Current medical illness
- Family history of suicide
- Previous suicide attempts or other self-injurious or impulsive acts
- Current anger, agitation, or constricted preoccupation
- Current abuse of alcohol or drugs
- Easy access to lethal toxins (including prescribed medication)
- Formulated plan, preparations for death, or suicide note
- Low ambivalence about dying versus living

Factors specific to youth
- All of the above
- Lack of family support
- History of abuse
- School problems
- Social ostracism, humiliation
- Conduct disorder
- Struggle with sexual orientation
- Recent marriage, unwanted pregnancy

Precipitants
- Recent stressors (especially losses of emotional, social, physical, or financial security)

Protective Factors
- Intact social supports
- Active religious affiliation or faith (may also be a risk factor if shame/guilt about behaviour is involved)
- Marriage and presence of dependent children
- Ongoing supportive relationship with a caregiver
- Absence of depression or substance abuse
- Access to medical and mental health resources
- Impulse control
- Proven problem-solving and coping skills

Presence of risk and protective factors should be noted in the patient's chart as part of the risk assessment.

Adapted from http://www.medceu.com/course-no-test.cfm?CID=308

---

suicide at rates higher than non-Aboriginal teens (Kirmayer, 2012), with Inuit males aged 15 to 19 committing suicide 40 times the rate (500 per 100,000) of non-Inuit males the same age (Eggertson, 2013). Suffocation is now the most common method used by Canadian adolescents, rather than firearms (Kirmayer, 2012).

Although the number of completed suicides is disturbingly high, the rate of attempted suicide is equally alarming. The World Health Organization (2012) reports that, worldwide, suicidal behaviours of young people ages 15 to 25 have been increasing at an alarming rate and estimates this age group to be the most at risk in one third of countries. It estimates that for every suicide, there are 20 suicide attempts. Although exact suicide attempt rates in Canada are difficult to track, Langlois and Morrison (2002) reported that, in 1999, 40.8, 152.2, and 117.9 per 100,000 Canadian youth aged 10 to 14, 15 to 19, and 20 to 29 years, respectively, attempted suicide.

Adults

Worldwide trends indicate that the suicide rate increases with age (WHO, 2012). In Canada, however, suicide rates are at their highest at midlife (age 45 to 59) (Statistics Canada, 2014). Single people in this age group have double the suicide rates of other age groups. Divorced people aged 45 to 59 have a suicide rate 1.7 times higher than divorced people of other ages, while the suicide rate in persons widowed aged 40 to 59 years is 2.1 times higher than for the widowed 60 and older (Statistics Canada,

2012). By age 55 to 60 years, however, suicide is the sixth leading cause of death and falls to 17th by age 70 to 75 (Statistics Canada, 2014). As age increases, suicide rates as a cause of death within the age group decline, indicative of an increase in pathologic deaths occurring from cancers, heart attacks, and so on.

Many adults who complete suicide have a psychiatric diagnosis, with depression being the most common condition (Mishara & Chagnon, 2011). Other factors linked to suicide include childhood physical and sexual abuse, child hunger, and other psychosocial issues (Marshall, Galea, Wood, & Kerr, 2013; McIntyre, Williams, Lavorato, & Patten, 2013). Marriage is a protective factor across all age groups, while divorce correlates to an increased risk of suicide (Statistics Canada, 2012). It is hypothesized that the social support and companionship provided by marriage help decrease the probability of suicide, while divorce increases a person's chance of developing depression (Statistics Canada, 2012).

Older Adults

Although other causes of death are more prominent, suicide risk is high among older adults (O'Connell, Chin, Cunningham, & Lawlor, 2004) and is an often-overlooked problem (Monette, 2012). Nationally, the ratio of suicide attempts to completions in older adults is 4 to 1. Older adults generally have a stronger intent to die, plan their suicide more carefully, and are more likely to use more lethal means of killing themselves than are younger people (Conwell & Duberstein, 2001). Of those aged

60 and older, 30% use hanging and 26% use a firearm as a means to complete suicide (Statistics Canada, 2012). The often frail health of older adults may contribute to the rate of completed suicides, and because many older adults live alone, the chance of a suicide's being thwarted is often less than among younger people. Of all suicides in Canada in 2001, 19% were by people older than 60 years of age. Suicide is less stigmatized for this age group and may be viewed as more acceptable.

For older adults, suicide is associated with less education, widowhood, previous attempts, depressive disorder, social isolation, financial difficulties, poor physical health and functioning, substance abuse, and loss of autonomy (Conwell, Duberstein, & Caine, 2002; Conwell, van Orden, & Caine, 2011). As in other age groups, major depressive disorder (MDD) is a significant factor in suicide. However, comorbid physical illnesses often make recognition of MDD difficult. In 2011, 71% to 95% of elderly people who completed suicide had a major psychiatric disorder at the time of death (Conwell, van Orden, & Caine, 2011).

> **KEY CONCEPTS Lethality** refers to the probability that a person will complete suicide. Lethality is determined by the seriousness of the person's intent and the likelihood that the planned method will result in death. High lethality includes firearms, hanging, carbon monoxide poisoning, drowning, suffocation, or jumping from a great height.

> **KEY CONCEPTS Risk/rescue ratio** refers to the lethality of means and the likelihood of rescue. Suicidal risk carries with it a progression of seriousness from suicidal ideation to completed suicide. Risk is lowest when intent is weak and the method used has low lethality. The likelihood of rescue is dependent on communication of intent and lower lethality of means.

Gender

Worldwide, males complete suicide at a rate three times that of females, although women are four times more likely to attempt suicide than men (Health Canada, 2003; WHO, 2012). In Canada in 2011, a total of 2,781 males committed suicide (16.3 deaths per 100,000), compared to 947 females (5.4 deaths per 100,000) (Statistics Canada, 2014). The reasons for the difference are not entirely understood. Men are seven times more likely to use firearms than women (20% versus 3% of completed suicides), whereas women are twice as likely to die by poisoning (42%). Conversely, females are three to four times more likely to attempt suicide than males, and hospitalization for attempts is 1.5 times greater in females than males (Statistics Canada, 2012).

Factors that affect suicide risk differently by gender include experiences of violence, family upbringing, and economic deprivation. Exposure to violence, sexual assault, or both also increases women's risk for suicide (Koplin & Agathen, 2002; Nelson et al., 2002), while having a small child reduces it (Qin, Agerbo, Westergård-Nielson, Erikson, & Mortenson, 2000). Having a parent with a psychotic or affective disorder increases the risk for both sexes, but especially for women (von Borczyskowski, Lindlad, Vinnerlkjung, & Hjern, 2010). Being of low socioeconomic status increases the risk of suicide for men (but not women), while living in a highly urbanized environment increases the risk for women (von Borczyskowski et al., 2010). Economic deprivation is more likely to precipitate suicide in men but not necessarily in women (Piérard & Grootendort, 2014). Although unemployment has long been associated with suicide in men, research has shown that for the long term, unemployed women also are at serious risk for suicide: unemployed women had a suicide rate three times that of employed women in a follow-up study of 9 years (Kposowa, 2001).

Aboriginal People

"I am here today because my ancestors, starving as they often were, fought to survive. Why did the old people strive to live … and the young people now want to die?" (NANYouth, 2004). In 2000, the Aboriginal suicide rate was twice the national rate (White & Jodoin, 2003). From 1999 to 2003, the Inuit suicide rate was more than 10 times the national rate (Government of Canada, 2006; Masecar, 2009), with Inuit males aged 15 to 19 years 40 times more likely to kill themselves than their non-Inuit peers (Eggertson, 2013). Unfortunately, many young Inuit see suicide as a viable option to cope with an untenable and hopeless living situation (Masecar, 2009). Among the Aboriginal people of Canada, hanging is the most common method of committing suicide (49.2% for males, 45.8% for females), followed by firearms for men and drug overdoses for women (Kirmayer et al., 2007).

Over a third of all deaths among Aboriginal youth are attributable to suicide (Health Canada, First Nations and Inuit Health Branch, 2003). Conversely, the suicide rate for Aboriginal people over the age of 70 drops below that for the general population. The risk factors for suicide among Aboriginal people are the same as for non-Aboriginals (depression, abuse, poverty, isolation, etc.) (Kirmayer et al., 2007), but are compounded by the effects of Aboriginal-specific experiences such as colonization, the residential school system, and children being taken off reserves to be fostered or adopted by non-Aboriginal families (Olson, 2013).

It is important to note that Aboriginal suicide rates may be underreported. Data collected by Statistics Canada pertain only to status Aboriginals, thus excluding nonstatus First Nations, Métis, and Inuit people from the Aboriginal suicide data. As well, the rate of accidental deaths among Aboriginal people is four to five times

BOX 19-4 Cultural Continuity and Protective Factors Against Risk for Suicide Among Aboriginal Communities

Cultural continuity is identified in terms of six protective factors that may explain the differences in suicidal rates between Aboriginal communities. Those factors listed in terms of importance are
- Self-government
- Land claims
- Education services
- Police and fire services
- Health services
- Cultural facilities

From Chandler, M. J. & Lalonde, C. (1998). Cultural continuity as a hedge against suicide in Canada's First Nations. *Transcultural Psychiatry, 35*(2), 191–219.

higher than in the general population, and up to 25% of these deaths may be from suicide (Royal Commission on Aboriginal Peoples, 1995; White & Jodoin, 2003).

Although the rate of suicide is higher for Aboriginal people as compared with other Canadians, not every Aboriginal community in Canada experiences high rates of suicide (Kirmayer et al., 2007; White & Jodoin, 2003). Marked differences can be noted between provinces and regions, and even between communities in the same geographic region. In studying suicide among British Columbia's Aboriginal communities, Chandler and Lalonde (1998) discovered that some communities had suicide rates 800 times the national average, while in other communities suicide was virtually unknown. They also identified six protective factors that may explain the differences in suicidal rates between communities (see Box 19-4). According to a Health Canada (2003) report, community wellness strategies may have the best chance of making a difference in suicide rates between Aboriginal communities. Guidelines were suggested in developing such a strategy (see Box 19-5).

BOX 19-5 Aboriginal Community Wellness Strategies

- Develop locally initiated, owned, and accountable programs.
- Suicide prevention should be the responsibility of the entire community.
- Focus on behavioural patterns of children and young people is crucial and requires the involvement of family and community.
- Suicide prevention must be addressed from the biologic, psychological, sociocultural, and spiritual perspectives.
- Long-term crisis and intervention programs must be developed.
- Suicide intervention strategies must be evaluated as needed.

From Health Canada, First Nations and Inuit Health Branch. (2003). *A statistical profile on the health of First Nations in Canada.* Ottawa, ON: Government of Canada.

Despite widespread concern about the high rates of suicide in Aboriginal populations, there are still no studies comparing rates across Aboriginal groups, nor are there data showing the origins and effective interventions concerning suicide among Aboriginal groups (Health Canada, 2003; Kirmayer et al., 2007). In Aboriginal communities where there is autonomy and a strong sense of ownership, culture, and community, however, there are much lower rates of suicide (Kirmayer et al., 2007).

Sexual Orientation

In recent years, sexual orientation has been more openly addressed as a risk factor for suicide. "Coming out" can be a risk factor because of the possible negative reactions of others, particularly peers and family; being unable to disclose sexual identity because it is unsafe to do so may contribute to a deep sense of isolation. During adolescence, when the major focus of a youth's life is on peers and sexuality, a gay, lesbian, bisexual, or transgender (GLBT) youth's search for self-identity may heighten depression and suicidal behaviour (Zhao, Montoro, Igartua, & Thombs, 2010). GLBT youth are also at a higher risk for suicide if they self-present with high levels of gender nonconformity (Liu & Mustanksi, 2012) or report being unsure as to their sexual identity (Zhao et al., 2010). As a predictor, GLBT victimization was the strongest—after suicide attempt history—for self-harm, associated with a 2.5-fold increased risk. (Liu & Mustanksi, 2012). It is important to note that the risk factors associated with GLBT individuals are in addition to those common to all ages and sexual orientations.

Regional Variations

Provincial statistics from 2009 show varied rates of suicide across Canada (see Table 19-1). Eastern and central regions of the far north have some of the highest mortality rates from suicide in Canada (Statistics Canada, 2012). As of 2009, the suicide rate per 100,000 people for Nunavut was 56.9, while for the Northwest Territories it was 21.9 and for Québec, 13.7 (see Table 19-1). These higher suicide rates may be due to a combination of factors. Most people in these regions live in rural or semirural environments where hunting (and ready access to firearms) is common; social isolation can occur due to low population per square kilometre; and the population is predominantly Aboriginal, who have rates of suicide higher than the national average. Within each province, rates of suicide are not consistent, because urban centres tend to have suicide rates lower than the national average, and demographic, social, cultural, and geographic factors affect rates of suicide.

Guns and Suicide

Almost 60% of all firearm deaths are suicides, and firearms are used in nearly 20% of all suicide fatalities (Canada Safety Council, 2014). Gagné, Robitaille, Hamel, and St-Laurent (2010) report that when firearm

Table 19-1	Canadian Suicide Statistics (2009)

Province/Territory	Suicide Rate*
Alberta	12.7
British Columbia	9.6
Manitoba	12.5
New Brunswick	13.2
Newfoundland and Labrador	8.8
Northwest Territories	21.9
Nunavut	56.9
Quebec	13.7
Saskatchewan	12.8
Yukon	5.7
National Average	10.4

*Per 100,000 people.

restrictions were introduced in Canada, male firearm suicides declined. Although the accessibility of firearms is usually associated with rural areas, urban areas show the highest rates of completed suicides by firearms.

Suicidal Ideation and Self-Harm

It is estimated that 36,560 (0.1%) people have unstated thoughts of suicide or **suicidal ideation** (Statistics Canada, 2012). Suicidal acts tend to be seen as "cries for help" rather than overt expressions of a desire to die (Health Canada, 1994). A 17-country study found that, across all countries examined, 60% of people transitioned from suicidal ideation to their first suicide attempt within the 1st year of ideation onset (Nock et al., 2008). MDD and physical, psychological, and social risk factors contribute to suicidal ideation. Physical factors include medical illness and alcohol and drug use; psychological factors include hopelessness, psychological distress, and low self-esteem; and external social risk factors include lack of social support, family problems, financial hardship, and legal problems. Childhood trauma (including physical abuse, sexual abuse, and childhood hunger) has been linked to both parasuicide and suicidal ideation in adulthood (McIntyre et al., 2013; Molnar, Berkman, & Buka, 2001).

Suicidal ideation and self-harm are more common among adolescents than other age groups. Self-harm behaviour in adolescents is often a way to communicate needs or wants, and often the need is for attention or care (Murray, 2003). As such, self-harm is an unacceptable means to acceptable ends and may communicate that the adolescent believes that something is wrong, life is tough, and things are becoming unbearable. Parasuicidal behaviour (e.g., cutting or self-mutilation) may also relieve or release certain emotions and feelings and may produce a tangible, physical pain to substitute for unfamiliar, unbearable psychological suffering. Self-punishment is often identified with self-loathing, anger, guilt, and shame (Murray, 2003). Research assessing the risk of nonsuicidal self-injury

using the Inventory of Statements about Self-Injury found, consistent with previous studies, that those who self-harm do so for a myriad of reasons, including self-punishment, sensation seeking, interpersonal influence, and marking distress (Klonsky & Glenn, 2009). Behaviour escalates if the purpose of the self-harm is not achieved, so feeling unheard or misunderstood can result in escalation of self-harm. Even if the purpose of self-harm behaviour is recognized, ignoring or minimizing the behaviour may escalate its intensity and frequency with increased attempts to get the message across (Murray, 2003).

■ AETIOLOGY OF SUICIDAL BEHAVIOUR

Suicidal behaviour occurs in the context of an individual's physiologic, psychological, and social situation and is usually triggered by stressors that are unmanageable and exceed typical coping efforts. Vulnerabilities are enhanced by engagement in risky behaviours, often used in an effort to cope with stress. Risky behaviours related to suicide include fast, dangerous driving; tempting death; promiscuity; use of alcohol or drugs; and purchase of a handgun. Appropriate interventions guided by a comprehensive assessment of risk at this point can reduce the likelihood of suicidal behaviour. Most who attempt suicide have seen a health care professional at least 1 year prior to the attempt (Morrison & Laing, 2011). Edwin Schneidman (1985), a clinical psychologist and leading authority on suicide, has described common characteristics of suicide in his book *Definition of Suicide* (see Box 19-6).

A comprehensive assessment identifies the physical, psychological, and social factors that contribute to feelings of self-harm (Fig. 19-1). These factors include changes in central nervous system neurotransmitters, engaging in negative thinking and risky behaviours, and deterioration of social relationships. The convergence of biologic, psychological, social, and spiritual factors can be directly linked to suicidal behaviour. Most will agree that suicide, like many other aspects of humanness, does not solely lie within a single sphere of the bio/psycho/social/spiritual model. However, in order to facilitate learning, suicide will be discussed in relation to each of these spheres.

Biologic Theories

Biologic theories of suicide attempt to clarify the phenomenon of suicide by recognizing and interpreting physiologic, neurophysiologic, and hormonal changes. Psychopathologic changes are evident in most suicidal people. MDD, sometimes comorbid with other psychiatric illnesses, is prevalent. Moreover, because suicide rates tend to be higher in families in which suicide has occurred, genetic and familial factors will be explored in this section. As well, a biologic explanation of increased

BOX 19-6 Schneidman's Common Characteristics of Suicide

1. **The common stimulus for suicide is unendurable psychological pain.**
   Faced with intolerable emotion and unacceptable anguish, people will sometimes opt for a cessation of consciousness. The core ambivalence in suicide reflects the conflict between survival and unbearable stress. The main clinical rule is Reduce the suffering, often just a little bit, and the individual will choose to live.

2. **The common stressor in suicide is frustrated psychological needs.**
   Suicides are born, negatively, out of needs. Most suicides represent combinations of various needs. The clinical rule is address the frustrated needs and the suicide will not occur.

3. **The common purpose of suicide is to seek a solution.**
   Suicide is not a random act. It is a way out of a problem, dilemma, or crisis. It is the answer—seemingly the only available answer—to a real puzzler: How to get out of this? It is important to view each suicidal act as an urgently felt effort to answer a question, to resolve an issue, and to solve a problem.

4. **The common goal of suicide is "cessation of consciousness."**

5. **The common emotions in suicide are hopelessness and helplessness.**
   Often people on the edge of committing suicide would be willing to live if things—life—were only a little bit better, a just noticeable difference. The common fear is that the inferno is endless and that one has to draw the line on one's suffering somewhere.

6. **The common internal attitude towards suicide is ambivalence.**
   Something can be both "A" and "not A." We can both love and hate the same person. A prototypical suicidal state is one in which the individual feels that she or he has to do it and simultaneously yearns, and even plans for rescue and intervention.

7. **The common cognitive state in suicide is "constriction" (tunnel vision).**
   Suicide cannot be understood as a psychosis, a neurosis, or a character disorder. It is a transient psychological constriction of affect and intellect. It is a narrowing of the range of options that leads to either/or thinking.

8. **The common interpersonal act in suicide is communication of intention.**
   The communication of suicidal intention is not always a cry for help. First, it is not always a cry; it can be a shout or a murmur or the nonverbal communication of something unspoken. The communication is not always for help; it can be for autonomy or any number of needs. Nonetheless, in most cases of suicide, there is some interpersonal communication related to that intended final act.

9. **The common action in suicide is regression or escape.**
   Suicide is a death in which the decedent removes him- or herself from intolerable pain and simultaneously from others in the world.

10. **Suicide is consistent with lifelong coping patterns.**
    "You can't fire me; I quit." "I'll leave her before she leaves me." Schneidman believes that suicide is not a random act and sometimes is reasonably predictable.

From Schneidman, E. (1985). *Definition of suicide.* New York, NY: John Wiley & Sons.

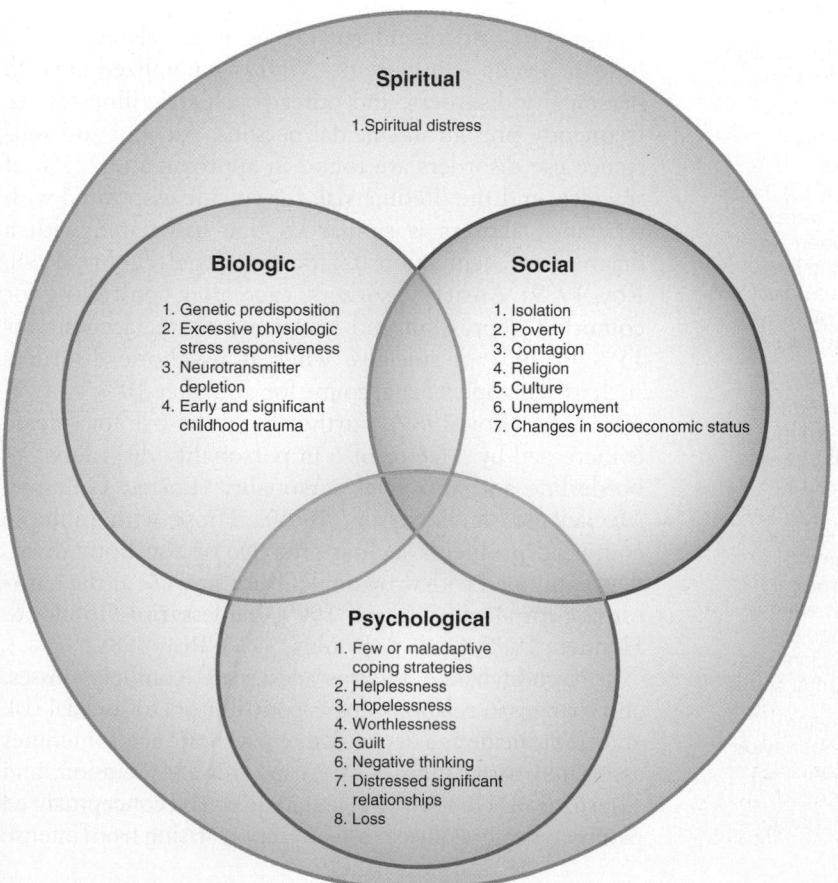

FIGURE 19-1. Bio/psycho/social/spiritual aetiologies of suicide.

suicide risk among those who experienced childhood sexual abuse and among those who have experienced a traumatic injury is considered (see Box 19-7 for the latter).

MDD tends to develop when a person who is vulnerable to it (because of genetic or other factors) is subjected to repeated or sustained stress. Stress responsiveness in them ultimately changes neurotransmitter and hormonal functioning to affect a depressed state (Hauenstein, 1996). Those who complete suicide have extremely low levels of the neurotransmitter serotonin, 5-hydroxytryptamine (5-HT; Mann, Oquendo, Underwood, & Arango, 1999), or lower levels of the neurotransmitter dopamine (Pitchot et al., 2001).

Considerable evidence exists showing a familial trend in suicide (McGuffin, Marusic, & Farmer, 2001; Qin, Agerbo, & Mortenson, 2003). First-degree relatives of individuals who have completed suicide have two to eight times the risk for suicide than do individuals in the general population (McGuffin et al., 2001). The genetic link to suicide is evident in studies of twins. Qin and colleagues showed that suicidal behaviour in one monozygotic twin increased the risk 11-fold for suicidal behaviour in the cotwin. Among

adolescent female twins, genetic factors played a part in 35% of suicide attempts (Glowinski et al., 2001). Adoption studies have shown that among adults who experience mood disorders and were adopted as children, the suicide rate among the biologic relatives of the adoptees is much higher than the rate among the adoptive relatives. Genetic abnormalities in the serotonergic neurotransmitter system may be responsible for the heightened familial risk for suicide (Mann, Brent, & Arango, 2001). Collectively, these studies demonstrate that the biologic risk for suicide appears to be independent of environmental factors.

Child abuse has been described as a specific vulnerability for psychopathology and suicide (MacMillan et al., 2001). Enhanced vulnerability to MDD and suicide associated with child abuse are attributable to changes in the hypothalamic–pituitary–adrenal axis caused by intractable stress and altered serotonin and dopamine metabolism (Skodol et al., 2002). Evidence from twin studies suggests that the link between childhood sexual abuse and biologic alterations contributing to psychopathology may be independent of other environmental influences. Several studies show that adult psychopathology is greater in abused twins when compared with nonabused cotwins (Bulik, Prescott, & Kendler, 2001; Kendler et al., 2000; Nelson et al., 2002). Additional specific features of the abuse, including severity, contributed to worse outcomes in the abused twins.

Psychological Theories

Coming to understand suicide as it is related to the human psyche is important. MDD, generalized anxiety, personality disorders, and other psychiatric illnesses are frequently present in suicidal persons. Alcohol and substance use disorders are found in approximately 25% of suicides, and the lifetime risk for suicide associated with substance abusers is similar to that associated with a diagnosis of depression (Clark & Goebel-Fabbri, 1998; Roy, 1989). Anxiety disorders, even after controlling for comorbid depression and substance abuse, account for 15% to 20% of suicides, whereas psychotic disorders such as schizophrenia account for a further 10% to 15% of suicides (Roy, 1989). Furthermore, the risk for suicide is increased by a factor of 6 in personality disorders like borderline and antisocial personality (Foster, Gillespie, McClelland, & Patterson, 1999). Those with multiple comorbid problems such as affective or psychotic disorders combined with drug or alcohol abuse are at the highest risk for suicide (Angst, 1999; Baldessarini, Tondo, & Hennen, 1999; Guze & Robins, 1970; Roy, 1989).

Psychodynamic theories designate conflicts, losses, and changes in relationships as contributors to suicidal risk and view suicide as a depressive or psychotic act, sometimes associated with fantasies of escape, reward, reunion, and resurrection (Hendin, 1991). Suicide can be conceptualized psychologically as an excessive reaction arising from intense

BOX 19-7	**Research for Best Practice**

INCREASED RISK FOR SUICIDE FOLLOWING MAJOR TRAUMA

March, J., Sareen, J., Gawazjuk, J. P., Doupe, M., Chateau, D., Hoppensack, M., ... Logsetty, S. (2014). Increased suicidal activity following major trauma: A population-based study. Journal of Trauma and Acute Care Surgery, 76(1), 180–184.

Question: What is the risk of suicidality for individuals who have experienced a major traumatic injury as compared with a matched cohort?

Method: A population-level retrospective study, this research involved adults (>18 years) who had an unintentional major injury (Injury Severity Score > 12), had no suicide attempts in the previous 5 years, and were on the registry of a trauma centre in Manitoba between April 1, 2001, and March 31, 2011; n = 2,198. Each of these individuals was matched (i.e., on age, sex, date of injury) with five control cases from the general population, using provincial administrative databases (n = 10,990). The rate of suicidality was compared between groups.

Findings: Suicidality (suicides and suicide attempts) was higher in the trauma group. This persisted even when adjusted for anxiety, mood disorders, and substance use, as well as for residence (urban/rural), income (average household income), and physical comorbidities. This study is unique in that it controlled for preexisting mental illness and excluded individuals from the data with premorbid suicide attempts. The relationship between trauma and suicide may be direct or it may be indirect and mediated through postinjury factors such as physical immobility, mental health problems or disorders, or changes in social circumstances, including social support and marital status.

Implications for Practice: As individuals with major traumatic injuries are at a higher risk for suicidal behaviour after injury as compared to the general population, it is important to identify and assess those who may need mental health interventions and follow-up on discharge.

preoccupation with humiliation and disappointment (Leenaars, 1998). It can be driven by intolerable aloneness and isolation (Adler & Buie, 1996). Cognitive approaches also attribute suicide to learned helplessness and hopelessness as an automatic and pervasive pathologic scheme for organizing and interpreting experience. The widely used cognitive theory of depression espoused by Aaron Beck and his associates (Beck, 2011; Beck, Rush, Shaw, & Emery, 1979) accounts for how negative thoughts occur, how they tend to be repetitive and intrusive, and how they can lead to suicidal behaviour (see Chapter 13).

Attachment theory explains social isolation and disrupted interpersonal relationships as being a part of the spectrum of suicide (Lopez & Brennan, 2000). In this theory, adult behaviour is shaped by early interactions with the primary caregiver during infancy. Disturbed attachment results in the individual's inability to form meaningful relationships, or in a constant concern about the viability of a lasting relationship. Suicide, then, is the result of conflicted or distant adult relationships and the social isolation that arises (Eng, Rimm, Fitzmaurice, & Kawacki, 2002). Muehlenkamp, Brausch, Quigley, & Whitlock (2013) suggest that treatments should focus on strengthening interpersonal bonds alongside emotion regulation.

Social Theories

Social factors are particularly important to the aetiology of suicide. As humans, we are inherently a part of the social fabric in which we exist. To be alive is to be in the world. Suicide, then, is the desire to estrange oneself from the world. Some suicidal people describe a desire to "feel nothing for a while," a temporary respite from life and the world.

Studying the social factors that contribute to rates of suicide, sociologist Emile Durkheim, at the end the 19th century, developed a theoretical framework outlining the social causes of suicide. Durkheim (1897, 2006) classified suicide under four headings: egoistic suicide, altruistic suicide, anomic suicide, and fatalistic suicide. These classifications of suicide are based on the degree of imbalance between social integration and moral regulation (Kendall, Lothian-Murray, & Linden, 2004).

Durkheim believed that the degree of social integration was a variable affecting rates of suicide. *Egoistic suicide* occurs among individuals who are not significantly bound to society. Some believe that the social isolation of single people is causally related to their higher rates of suicide when compared with their married counterparts. Conversely, *altruistic suicide* occurs when individuals become overly connected to society, for example, a patriotic soldier who kills him- or herself after a defeated battle because he or she is shamed.

Durkheim also acknowledged that extreme cases of social stability and social consensus contribute to rises in suicide rates. A society lacking a sense of purpose, social regulation, or community values experiences *anomic suicide*. This type of suicide occurs during times of financial depression. Contrastingly, in areas of overregulation and oppression, *fatalistic suicides* occur. Although Durkheim discussed little about fatalistic suicide, many use the suicide of slaves as an exemplar.

Contemporary sociologic investigations seek social structure models of influence on suicide. A theory explicated by Cohen and colleagues (2003) contends that socioeconomic status is a driving factor in what happens to an individual, affecting the physical and social structures available to him or her. For example, poverty represented by substandard housing affects other important neighbourhood social structures, such as schools, voluntary organizations, and jobs. People wishing to teach in these schools, help out, or conduct business in the neighbourhood are deterred by the neighbourhood deterioration. Poverty also reduces exposure to opportunities for individual advancement. Poverty affects health outcomes directly, because of environmental hazards, or indirectly, through inadequate access to health care. Substantial data exist to support this model of suicide. Cohen et al. (2003) found that the percentage of boarded-up buildings in a neighbourhood was positively associated with suicide. Socioeconomic deprivation and unemployment were found to be associated with suicide in several studies (Cubbin, LeClere, & Smith, 2000; Goodman, 1999; Hawton, Harriss, Hodder, Simkin, & Gunnell, 2001; Kposowa, 2001; Steenland, Halperin, Hu, & Walker, 2003). Unemployment may also pose an indirect risk for suicide through family tension arising from the loss of income and a normal social role. This loss may then lead to indignity, isolation, hopelessness, alcohol abuse, and violence (Platt, 1993). Wealth, too, brings with it a distinct set of worries and concerns. Importantly, suicide is at its greatest rates when a substantial change in social status occurs.

Suicide and Religion

Research regarding the impact of religion on suicide has not yielded consistent results (Rasic, Kisely, & Langille, 2011). It has been hypothesized that not only personal but also contextual differences in religious beliefs may determine an individual's willingness to consider suicide (Neeleman & Lewis, 1990). Greater moral objections to suicide in those with a religious affiliation may be protective against suicide attempts (Dervic et al., 2004). However, social scientists do not find that not believing in God or lack of religiosity is a causative factor leading to suicide. Rather, it is likely that an individual's belief that suicide is wrong is a strong deterrent to the act of suicide (Hilton, 2002).

Suicide Contagion and Suicide Clusters

A social phenomenon, seen most frequently among adolescents, is **suicide contagion**. Several studies have shown that when one teenager takes his or her life, several more may follow (Olson, 2013; Poijula, Wahlberg, & Dyregrov, 2001; Zenere, 2009). The occurrence of suicide contagion can result in the development of a **suicide cluster**, which is defined as multiple suicidal behaviours or suicides that fall within a specific time frame and often specific geographical area (Olson, 2013). A *mass cluster* is often associated with media reports related to the suicide of celebrities (e.g., Marilyn Monroe and Kurt Cobain), or other cases of completed suicide with overwhelming attention generated by media saturation (e.g., Amanda Todd). Celebrity suicide is associated with increased completed suicides; considerable care must be taken when reporting suicides, particularly high-profile ones (Niederkrotenthaler et al., 2012). There is a direct relationship between media coverage of suicide and contagion (Scherr & Reinemann, 2011). This social phenomenon was originally termed the "Werther Effect," after the young lover in Goethe (1774/1989) whose suicide inspired copycat suicides among young male readers. Some scholars, however, suggest that individuals who are influenced by such stories are already in a vulnerable state as a result of other precipitating factors and may not necessarily be influenced by media exposure of suicide (Westerlund, Schaller, & Schmidtke, 2009). Nevertheless, media guidelines have been developed to address the potential harm of suicide coverage, such as those of the Centres for Disease Control, the World Health Organization, and the Canadian Psychiatric Association. These guidelines emphasize collaboration between mental health professionals and the media to ensure that reporting is done in a way to reduce copycat suicidal behaviour. However, the realities of 21st-century technology—in which information about a person's suicide can readily be made available through YouTube, Twitter, and Facebook—can in part defeat the purpose of such guidelines.

In contrast to mass clusters, *point clusters* are suicides that occur close in time and space and often occur in settings such as hospitals, schools, prisons, and specific communities (Olson, 2013). Point clusters can be a major problem in Aboriginal communities as individuals on reserves are closely related and share the same social predicaments: a single suicide affects the entire community (Kirmayer et al., 2007). This can also manifest as *echo clusters* that occur over an extended period of time after the original cluster (Masecar, 2009).

Bullying, Cyber Bullying, and Suicide

Traditional bullying has been defined as aggressive intentional "harm doing" by one person or a group, generally carried out repeatedly over time, and which usually involves a power differential (Nansel et al., 2001). See Chapter 16, Table 16-2 for examples of the four types of bullying: physical, verbal, relational, and "cyber." Cyber bullying has been defined as "willful and repeated harm inflicted through the use of computers, cell phones, and

IN A LIFE

Rehtaeh Parsons (1995–2013)
Cyber Bullying, Suicide, and Public Response

On April 4th, 2013, 17-year-old Rehtaeh Parsons attempted suicide and died 3 days later. Her suicide was preceded by 17 months of bullying following a gang rape of Rehtaeh that had been photographed and circulated online. Although Rehtaeh's rape had been reported to authorities at the time, RCMP and the prosecutor deemed there to be insufficient evidence to charge the perpetrators (Huffington Post, 2013, April 11). According to Rehtaeh's family, her suicide was prompted by depression brought on by the rape, the ongoing distribution of the photograph, bullying by her peers, and a continuous barrage of sexually explicit texts and Facebook posts. In the year prior to her death, Rehtaeh had been voluntarily hospitalized to treat her suicidality.

Rehtaeh's suicide was widely publicized and became a flash point online and across Canada about cyber bullying and victims' rights. Following the wishes of their daughter, who wanted to contact the media before her death, Rehtaeh's parents, Leah Parsons and Glenn Canning, have openly described what happened to her (Canadian Press, 2013, October 3). Leah Parsons also created a Facebook Memorial page that went viral in popularity.

There was national outrage at what was perceived as a failure of the justice system (Huffington Post Canada, 2013, April 15). Online, the activist group Anonymous threatened to publicly identify Rehtaeh's rapists but stopped after Rehtaeh's mother requested the issue be settled in court (Huffington Post Canada, 2013; Ross, 2013, April 9). Initially, the Nova Scotia justice minister refused to open the case but, due to public pressure, it was later reopened (Huffington Post Canada, 2013).

Not all publicity, however, was in support of Rehtaeh. Locally, a poster campaign was started in support of the accused, drawing concerns about vigilanteeism. Nationally, questions were raised about whether the sex was consensual (Blatchford, 2013, April 26), which drew the ire of many, including Rehtaeh's parents, as a case of victim blaming (Cross, 2013, April 26).

In the year since Rehtaeh's death, numerous changes have resulted. In August 2013, Nova Scotia passed a new Cyber-Safety Act that would protect victims' identities during the investigative period, allow victims to sue aggressors, and, in the case of underage cyber bullies, hold their parents financially liable. Changes were also made to the province's Education Act, requiring principals to address known cases of bullying even if it happens off school property. A CyberSCAN Unit, the first in Canada, was also established in the province to investigate cases of cyber bullying (CBC News, 2013a, August 7). As well, both the school district where Rehtaeh was a student and the hospital that treated her a year earlier have investigated their handling of the situation and revised their practice. Following the renewed police investigation, two men were arrested and charged with the distribution of child pornography and one with the creation of child pornography (CBC News, 2013b, August 8). Supporters continue to hold sexual assault and cyber bullying awareness rallies (CTVNews, 2014, April 5), while Glenn Canning and Leah Parsons continue to petition the Government to improve national cyber bullying laws and mental health services for cyber bullying victims.

other electronic devices" (Hinduja & Patchin, 2010, p. 208). Across studies of the prevalence of cyber bullying, it seems that about 15% to 35% of students have been victims of cyber bullying while about 10% to 20% of students admit to cyber bullying others (Hinduja

& Patchin, 2010). A survey of nearly 2,000 randomly sampled adolescents at school revealed that those who had experienced cyber bullying, either as a victim or as an offender, were more likely to attempt suicide than those who had not experienced this form of peer aggression. Victimization had a stronger relationship to suicidal thoughts and behaviour than bullying (Hinduja & Patchin, 2010). Fisher and colleagues (2012) found that among 2,141 children aged 12 who had self-harmed, 56% were exposed to frequent bullying. This higher rate of self-harm existed even after children's premorbid emotional and behavioural problems, low IQ, and family environmental risks were taken into account. Fisher and colleagues also found that the adolescents who did engage in self-harm were more likely to experience physical maltreatment by an adult, have a family history of suicidal behaviours, and suffer from mental illness such as conduct disorder and depression. Frequently, adolescents who completed suicide after experiencing bullying or cyber bullying had emotional and psychosocial issues in their lives such as low self-esteem and depression (Zetter, 2008), struggles with social and academic life (Flowers, 2006), and stressful life circumstances (Hinduja & Patchin, 2010). Many countries including Canada have initiated antibullying legislation and school policies.

Spiritual Theories

Spirituality has reemerged as an important component of nursing care only in the last decade (Tinley & Kinney, 2007). Increasingly, it is recognized as a key component of holistic care. Spirituality, which can mean a search for meaning, connectedness (both intrapersonal and interpersonal), energy, and a person's worldview (Pesut, 2003, 2008), is being recognized as a source of resilience and coping (Martin, 2002). Studies have shown that people with spiritual involvement were at a decreased risk of substance abuse, addiction, and suicide (Benson, 1992; Koenig & Larson, 2001) and that, for some people with mental illness, spirituality was used as a coping resource and lowered the risk of substance abuse and suicide (Larson & Larson, 2003).

■ EFFECTS OF SUICIDE
Effect on Survivors

Worldwide, about 1 million people die from suicide each year (WHO, 2012). If each suicide impacts only six or seven survivors, approximately 6 to 7 million people each year will lose someone close to them as a result of suicide. Suicide has devastating effects on everyone it touches, especially family and close friends. Prolonged suffering can be caused by the sudden shock, unanswered questions of "why," and potentially the discovery of the body (Knieper, 1999). Suicide bereavement is different than that experienced by families whose loved one's death is not self-inflicted. One's reaction to suicide death is very individual and depends on personal, sociocultural, and situational factors (Grad, 2011). Furthermore, those grieving the loss of someone from suicide are at an increased risk of developing suicidal ideation (Grad) and other mental health issues (Bolton et al., 2013). The grieving over the way the death occurred, the social processes that ensue, and the effect of the suicide on the family converge to establish a grieving process that is unique (Jordan, 2001).

Family survivors of suicide report stigmatization, shame, and rejection. Insensitivity by others such as the media, police, medical examiners, and health care professionals may exacerbate grief. Nurses need to ensure that their response to survivors of suicide is compassionate and nonjudgemental. Simplistic explanations and clichés should be avoided. Survivors of suicide may need help in their search to understand of what has happened. As their personal search for meaning regarding the death transpires, their coping abilities will mediate their grief response. It is an ongoing task, but recovery can be made easier by social support that helps address related psychological trauma (Mitchell, Gale, Garand, & Wesner, 2003).

Economic Effects

Estimating the economic cost of suicide is difficult. In Canada, the average cost of hospitalization for suicide and attempted suicide was $5,500 per admission, ranging from $3,000 to $31,000 (HereToHelp, 2003). The Centre for Suicide Prevention reports that in 2004, nearly $2.5 billion was spent in Canada on direct (e.g., funeral costs, treatment, and police/coroner investigations) and indirect (e.g., lost years of life expectancy, compensation claims) costs of suicide (SmartRisk, 2009).

■ SUICIDE AND THE LAW

Revealing the evolution of social and religious attitudes, attempted suicide was removed from the provisions of the Canadian Criminal Code in 1972. Counselling or assisting suicide, however, remains a criminal act (Section 241, *Criminal Code of Canada* [Government of Canada, 1985]). Nevertheless, there is increasing debate in Canada regarding changing legislation to allow euthanasia and physician-assisted suicide. Two high-profile cases of women with amyotrophic lateral sclerosis who sought the right to physician-assisted suicide, Sue Rodriguez in 1992 and Gloria Taylor in 2012, gave sustained national attention to the issue. In January 2013, a Québec expert panel recommended health care legislation to treat euthanasia as part of end-of-life care. Such legislation was proposed, but the bill died when a provincial election was called. See Box 19-8 for the arguments for and against physician-assisted suicide, including concerns about "opening the door" to potential changes that would affect vulnerable populations such as persons with mental illness.

BOX 19-8 Arguments for and Against Physician-Assisted Suicide

Justifications for Euthanasia
- Individual autonomy and freedom of choice.
- Necessary as a right under the *Canadian Charter of Rights and Freedoms* as the able-bodied can commit suicide; those with physical limitations cannot.
- Limitations of the effectiveness of palliative care in alleviating suffering of all individuals.
- Euthanasia occurs, despite its illegality, and without adequate controls.
- Distinction between withholding/withdrawing treatment (acceptable acts) and assisted suicide does not stand up to scrutiny, as no true moral significance to distinction between acts and omissions.

Arguments Against Euthanasia
- Social value of respect for life is fundamental; killing is intrinsically wrong.
- The expectation that physicians, trained to preserve life, should be willing to "euthanize" a patient is not reasonable.
- There could be abuse of euthanasia, particularly with respect to vulnerable people.
- Euthanasia might be sought for insufficient financial and institutional resources.
- "Slippery slope" argument: euthanasia for competent people could lead to changes in law with respect to those not competent to give consent (e.g., individuals <18 years of age; those with mental illness or cognitive disabilities).
- Legal euthanasia could limit efforts to develop palliative care.
- Pain control interventions are well developed; access to them and palliative care are the real issues.

Adapted, in part, from Butler, M., Tiedemann, M., Nicol, J., & Valiquet, D. (2010/Revised, 2013). *Euthanasia and assisted suicide in Canada (Background paper). Parliamentary Information and Research Service.* Publication No. 2010-68-E. Ottawa, ON: Library of Parliament.

Involuntary Admission and the Provincial Health Acts

When a patient will not or cannot (because of noncompetent status) agree to enter the hospital voluntarily, **involuntary hospitalization** may be initiated. Considerable controversy surrounds the notion of involuntary hospitalization and treatment. See Chapter 3 for a discussion of provincial legislation that empowers physicians and peace officers to detain, without consent, a person whom they consider to be of danger to him- or herself or others (Health Canada, 1994). Changing social attitudes towards human rights, together with the influence of the 1982 Canadian Charter of Rights and Freedoms, has led to more stringent criteria for involuntary committal. For example, Ontario's Mental Health Act requires that a physician assess the situation and state, in writing, that because of a mental disorder, the individual is at risk for serious bodily harm to self or other unless admitted (Health Canada). Legislative changes in many provinces have reinforced the individual's right to refuse admission and treatment except in narrowly defined circumstances.

Health care practitioners must make every effort to obtain the patient's permission to enter the hospital voluntarily, for both legal and therapeutic reasons. Legally, **voluntary hospitalization** protects the rights of patients, permitting them some freedom in negotiating discharge from the hospital. Therapeutically, voluntary admission reinforces patients' control of the situation as partners in their own care and preserves their dignity.

Caring for Suicidal People

Canadians have legal rights that health care providers must consider during suicide prevention and treatment. They cannot deprive patients of their right to self-determination unless no other course is available to ensure a patient's safety. Patients have the right to be free from harm. Physically restraining or hospitalizing a patient against his or her will has the potential for both physical and emotional harm. Such action should be taken only when the patient is under the threat of imminent suicide or when the patient's status is "noncompetent" under the relevant mental health act and is a risk to self and/or others. Nurses must be familiar with their provincial mental health legislation (see Chapter 3) and thus be able to understand patients' legal rights and to explain them clearly.

Confidentiality

Disclosing information without a patient's permission violates his or her rights to privacy and anonymity and may damage the therapeutic relationship. Patients lose trust when the nurse shares the patients' suicidal intent with others unless the nurse has specifically explained the limits of confidentiality. When informing the patient of existing limits of confidentiality, the nurse must be very clear and specific. The Canadian Nurses Association (CNA) has articulated the concept of **confidentiality** as safeguarding information acquired within a professional relationship, except when doing so, would cause significant harm (CNA, 2002).

The CNA code of ethics is consistent with provincial legislation. Namely, the patient has a right to confidentiality unless he or she is at risk for harming self or others or discloses any form of abuse of minors, including neglect, sexual, physical, psychological, and emotional abuses. In those situations, the nurse can enlist the help of others (e.g., outside of the health care team) to protect the patient's or others' safety.

Protecting the patient's right to confidentiality is a special concern when a minor child has suicidal intent. As with adult patients, the nurse is required to describe the right to confidentiality and its limits. The nurse must always consider informing parents or legal guardians of a child who has suicidal intent. The parents of a minor child retain the privilege to determine the right care for their child, and they need sufficient information to make good decisions. Before beginning any suicide risk assessment, nurses must let a child know that disclosure of self-harm may be shared with parents. Honesty about what the nurse can and cannot keep confidential ultimately increases a child's trust and often results in a more therapeutic relationship.

Informed Consent

Obtaining fully **informed consent** from the patient protects his or her right to self-determination. However, nurses must inform suicidal patients about limits to their self-determination and make efforts to obtain their cooperation. From the time that the nurse encounters a suicidal patient until a suitable placement is made in consultation with other members of the interprofessional team, the nurse must share with the patient his or her right to be placed in the **least restrictive environment** that will ensure safety. The least restrictive environment is the setting that puts the fewest constraints on the patient's rights while still ensuring the patient's safety. By informing a patient about his or her choices, the nurse gains the patient's trust and decreases the likelihood that involuntary hospitalization will be necessary.

The ethical requirement of **beneficence**, doing no harm, is critical when restraining patients against their will. Caring for patients who are suicidal and determined to get away is difficult without touching and actively restraining them. Still, nurses must do their best to disclose to patients the specifics of planned treatments, including restraints, and attempt to obtain their consent to proceed. Respect for the patient needs to be maintained throughout the process. (For further discussion of these issues, see Chapter 11)

Documentation

The nurse must thoroughly document encounters with suicidal patients. This action is for the patient's ongoing treatment and the nurse's protection. The nursing notes must reflect that the nurse took every reasonable action to provide for the patient's safety. If a **no self-harm contract** has been instituted, the record must contain specific aspects of the contract.

■ NURSING ASSESSMENT AND INTERVENTIONS

Suicidal behaviours are seriously underreported and often not recognized by health care professionals. For example, a Statistics Canada study found that in Alberta, almost 60% of Albertans who committed suicide had recently visited an emergency room; nearly 90% had had a health visit (on average 17 visits) during the year before death (Morrison & Laing, 2011). Nurses can play important roles in suicide prevention because they practise in diverse health care settings and thus work with many different kinds of patients. Acutely suicidal behaviour is a true psychiatric emergency. Nurses must act immediately and vigorously to prevent the patient's death.

Bio/psycho/social/spiritual Domains

Nursing interventions based on a comprehensive assessment of risk provide a holistic approach to nursing care of the suicidal patient. The process of risk assessment will be discussed, followed by a discussion of nursing interventions in relation to the biologic, psychological, social, and spiritual aspects of the suicidal person.

Comprehensive Assessment of Risk

Comprehensive assessment provides a clear picture of self-harm behaviour and guides possible interventions. (See Box 19-9 for questions to guide a comprehensive assessment of risk; see Box 19-10 for suicide assessment tools.) A model developed by Murray emphasizes an approach that views patients in context of their social world, including intergenerational perspective and use of the genogram (Murray & Wright, 2006). (For family assessment, see Chapter 15.)

Assessment includes collection of adequate data to provide a clear picture of the patient's life and relevant stressors from the patient's perspective. This includes a good understanding of the patient's family, peers, and social relationships as well as workplace issues. Changes related to loss need to be explored to identify possible precipitating factors. Issues of abuse need to be discussed with thoughtfulness and sensitivity.

The broad spectrum of symptoms related to depression should be explored. (See Chapter 22 for assessment of depression.) Such symptoms include isolating or withdrawing from friends and family, sleep and eating disturbances, and not enjoying or participating in activities that were enjoyed in the past. Engaging in risky behaviours such as rebellion, noncompliance, or drug or alcohol use is commonly associated with suicide.

The patient should be assessed for other psychiatric disorders, especially those most commonly associated with suicidal behaviour (e.g., MDD, panic disorder, severe anxiety disorder, schizophrenia, substance abuse, borderline personality disorder, and antisocial personality disorder). Severity of MDD is associated with a greater likelihood of suicide completion. For adolescents, a key question is whether any family member has attempted or completed suicide. Alcoholism is another prominent factor in suicide. The 8-item Suicide Intent Scale (Beck, Brown, & Steer, 1997) is short and useful in determining whether a patient has a strong intent to die.

● **STUDY NOTE**
When completing a comprehensive suicide assessment, engaging nonjudgementally with the patient is crucial (Murray, 2003). Stressors, signs and symptoms, prior suicidal ideation and behaviour, current plan, and available resources and support should be delineated.

BOX 19-9 Questions to Guide a Comprehensive Assessment of Risk

Stressors

What is troubling you most at the moment?

Explore with curious questions in terms of all areas of the patient's life.

Explore each area, asking the patient to tell you more.

The idea is to get a clear picture of the patient's life situation and presenting stressors as the patient perceives them.

Symptoms

Can you tell me about your sleep patterns?

Explore using curious questions:

Are you having difficulty sleeping?

Do you want to stay in bed and sleep through the day?

Can you tell me about your eating habits?

Explore using curious questions:

Have you lost your appetite?

Do you eat in an attempt to cope with difficulties?

What do you do for enjoyment?

Explore with curious questions:

Do you find you no longer enjoy activities you thought were enjoyable?

How often do you use drugs or alcohol to cope?

Prior Behaviour

Have you ever thought of harming yourself?

Explore with curious questions:

Can you tell me about that? (time, place, situation, feelings, meaning)

What was the self-harm about?

What happened?

What did you expect to happen?

What did you want to happen?

Current Plan

Do you currently have a plan to harm yourself?

Explore with curious questions:

What would you do?

Do you have access to the pills? (other methods)

Have you picked a specific day or time?

Resources and Support

Do you have someone you recognize as supportive?

Explore with curious questions:

Who can you talk to about your concerns?

Who can you confide in?

Offer suggestions of a number of people the patient may not have thought of (e.g., parent's friend, colleague, clergy, coach).

Assessing Self-Harm

Assessing the context of each act of prior self-harm behaviour begins to paint a picture of motivation behind the behaviour. An exploration of prior behaviour also gives a message of interest and concern on the part of

BOX 19-10 Suicide Assessment Tools

There are tools that can assist with risk assessment, such as the *Beck Scale for Suicide Ideation*, *Nurses' Global Assessment of Suicide Risk*, and the *Suicide Intent Scale* (see Perlman, Neufeld, Martin, Goy, & Hirdes, 2012). Suicide risk assessment within the *Tidal Model* (Barker & Buchanan-Barker, 2005) includes a global assessment of risk to determine the person's need for care and ongoing monitoring and reassessment. Its dimensions include initial screening, focused assessment; integration of the risk assessment; care planning, intervention, and implementation; and monitoring and reassessment.

Alternatively, the *Inventory of Motivation for Suicide Attempts* (IMSA), developed by May and Klonsky (2013), identifies two motivations. *Intrapersonal* motivations reveal the need to escape or relieve internal emotions and thoughts and can be assessed using scales of hopelessness, psychache, escape burdensomeness, low belonging, and fearlessness. *Interpersonal* motivations reveal the desire to communicate with or influence another individual and can be assessed using scales of interpersonal influence and help seeking. To assess intent, the IMSA has 54 statements to be answered using a five-point Likert scale (e.g., "I attempted suicide because I.."; "...was so lonely I couldn't handle it"; "...hated myself so much"; "...didn't fit in anywhere").

The *Suicide Risk Assessment Model* (Murray, 2003; Murray & Wright, 2006) can be used by nurses in any care setting and includes stressors, symptoms, prior behaviour, current plan, and available resources and support. It can be integrated as part of the focused suicide risk assessment in the Tidal Model.

the health professional. A nonblaming, nonjudgemental approach allows further exploration and understanding of the patient's situation as the patient begins to trust the therapeutic relationship.

Assessment includes exploration of self-harm behaviour from the perspective of the patient. Self-harm behaviour can be imitative, especially if it is interpreted as a way of coping with frustration and anger or a way of punishing self or others (Rew, Thomas, Horner, Resnick, & Beuhring, 2001). Others' reaction to self-harm behaviour needs to be explored, whether or not the response was the expected or desired one. Understanding this can be the first step in helping the patient meet needs and wants in more healthy ways.

Having a Current Plan

Suicide requires intent, a plan, knowledge of how to carry out the act, and few obstacles to completing it. Patients who complete suicide have developed a workable method of killing themselves. They are less likely to have young children or other immediate responsibilities and may not be concerned with religious prohibitions concerning the act. The relationship between the availability of a method of suicide and the suicide completion is strong. It is important for the nurse to ask whether the patient has a current plan for suicide. Further exploration of the plan gives the nurse a more accurate assessment of risks and guides appropriate interventions.

In contrast to those who carefully prepare to take their own lives are those who decide impulsively to end their lives. The latter are usually adolescents, people who abuse alcohol or drugs, or people with personality disorders. Patients with psychoses may respond impulsively to "voices" that direct them to kill themselves. Patients with psychoses are at considerable risk because of their inability to separate psychotic thinking from reality.

Resources and Support

Lack of resources and support may put patients at the greatest risk for self-harm behaviour. Suicidal people often feel socially isolated and struggle to identify and accept support from people in their immediate environment; therefore, it is important to explore supportive people in the patient's life. Interest in the patient's life and attention received during a thorough assessment are therapeutic and can also provide connectedness and engagement with the patient and family (see Box 19-11).

Nursing Diagnoses and Outcome Identification

Several nursing diagnoses may be useful when dealing with a suicidal patient, including risk for suicide, interrupted family processes, ineffective health maintenance, risk for self-directed violence, impaired social interaction, ineffective coping, chronic low self-esteem, disturbed sleep pattern, social isolation, and spiritual distress.

Planning and Implementing Nursing Interventions

Thorough assessment becomes part of the intervention process. The health professional's genuine interest, concern, and exploration begin to establish a needed trusting relationship. Using this approach, health care professionals help patients identify what and who needs to change in their environment. This approach uncovers concrete areas of improvement or change. This empowerment addresses their feelings of hopelessness, helplessness, and powerlessness.

Understanding the purpose and meaning of the self-harm behaviour guides the intervention strategies. It also gives the patient and their family a sense of hope that things can change and that someone understands their situation and is willing to assist them in making changes. If behaviour is understood as a means of communication, then interventions need not only change behaviours but also the "cry for help" that underpins the acts. Therefore, ignoring self-harm behaviour is not helpful, although family members may not know what to do and may hope it will go away (Hall, Oliver, & Murphy, 2001). This response may actually escalate the behaviour. Punishment and overreaction are also not helpful.

If some or many of the risk factors for suicide are present in a member of a high-risk group, the nurse must determine what is necessary to ensure the patient's ongoing safety, which is the nurse's first priority. Until the nurse has identified a patient's safety needs and implemented a plan to ensure the patient's safety, the nurse must not leave the acutely suicidal person alone for any reason, not even briefly. Nursing care of acutely suicidal persons requires a team approach, including consultation.

Contracting for Safety

Contracting for safety—having the patient agree and commit, in writing, to no self-harm for an agreed upon period of time—is an intervention used extensively in

---

BOX 19-11   Research for Best Practice

SUICIDE RISK ASSESSMENT MODEL

Murray, B. L. & Wright, K. (2006). Integration of a suicide risk assessment and intervention approach: The perspective of youth. Journal of Psychiatric and Mental Health Nursing, 13(2), 157–164.

Question: What is the experience of suicide assessment and intervention for an adolescent when it is conducted by a clinical nurse specialist (CNS) using a described risk assessment model?

Method: Adolescent participants were interviewed using a phenomenologic approach to explore their lived experience of suicide risk assessment and intervention.

Findings: The major themes that emerged from the data were change, hope, and connection. Participants described the initial assessment interview as *helpful, beneficial, reducing their anxiety* and giving them a sense of *getting things under control.* They described a change in their thinking, other intrapersonal changes, and a change in interpersonal relationships over time as a result of the assessment. They spoke of their *hope* that things could or would change and how they shifted from a sense of giving up hope to hopefulness. They also spoke of recognizing their ability to deal with problems and issues and of the importance of not feeling alone. The participants spoke of feeling *connected* to the CNS and of feeling that someone cared.

Implications for Practice: Nurses' use of an assessment model that focuses on understanding the suicidal person's world and the meaning of his or her behaviour was experienced as helpful by adolescents. The first step in establishing a meaningful relationship with the adolescent is connecting with the adolescent and engaging him or her in the relationship. This requires genuine interest on the part of the nurse and an ability to set aside one's own values and beliefs while allowing adolescents to tell their story from their point of view. Active listening and open-ended questioning are necessary for a meaningful exchange of ideas and solutions. The challenging behaviour of adolescents needs to be viewed in the context of their family, social and school environment, and broader community. A focus on the adolescent's strengths and resources often promotes a shift towards cooperation and away from problematic, inappropriate, self-harm behaviours. The nurse's expectation and confidence in the adolescent's ability to act appropriately promote responsible participation, self-direction, and self-control.

some psychiatric settings (Knesper, 2011). Such contracts can only be negotiated after a thorough assessment of the patient has been completed. The nurse must consider patient competency in terms of being able to enter into a contract of this nature. The patient cannot be in a psychotic state or under the influence of alcohol or other drugs. Patients who have made a previous suicide attempt or who are extremely isolated are not good candidates for safety contracting. Legal and professional scholars disagree on the ability of children and adolescents to make decisions of this gravity on their own behalf. Involving parents in the decision about the appropriate environment for their suicidal child is important. Advantages and disadvantages of no self-harm contracts and several examples of contracts can be found in a review by Range and colleagues (2002). However, the use of safety contracts is underresearched; while their effectiveness depends upon the patient's ability to keep a commitment of this kind, the factors influencing this are not fully known or understood (Knesper, 2011).

Inpatient Care and Acute Treatment

Suicidal patients were once hospitalized for extended periods to ensure that the suicidal crisis had passed and to provide sufficient time to establish a solid base of treatment for the underlying psychiatric disorder. This is no longer the case. Hospitals are overly restrictive environments that may inhibit the patient's development of the self-reliance needed to return to the community. Objectives of hospitalization are to maintain the patient's safety, reduce or eliminate the suicidal crisis, decrease the level of suicidal ideation, initiate treatment for the underlying disorder, evaluate for substance abuse, and reduce the patient's level of social isolation.

If the patient is assessed as acutely suicidal and is at considerable risk for completing suicide, the decision must be made whether to hospitalize the patient for the patient's safety. Safety in such cases is commonly determined by whether a patient may be a threat to self or others. Provincial law requires the patient to be hospitalized only when he or she cannot make reasoned decisions to ensure his or her safety. The law also requires that the restriction of the patient occurs only when it provides a therapeutic effect. In considering the hospitalization of a patient, the nurse must consider how hospitalization will be useful in ensuring safety and relieving the patient's suicidal crisis.

Interventions for the Biologic Domain

Ensuring Safety

During the early part of the hospitalization, the most important way to reduce stress is to help the patient feel more secure and hopeful. Nurses can do so by ensuring the patient's safety with as little intrusion as possible on the person's exercise of free will. Achieving this goal can be difficult. The major deterrent to patients' completing suicide in psychiatric hospitals is their engagement in a therapeutic relationship and regular observation by nurses. Each hospital has its own specific protocol for maintaining patients' safety. In addition to nursing standards of care, hospital staffing and other policies that affect the degree to which a suicidal patient can be restrained may influence the procedures mandated for caring for patients.

Maintaining a safe environment includes observing the patient regularly for suicidal behaviour, removing dangerous objects, and providing counselling opportunities for the patient. Part of ensuring patient safety is helping patients to reestablish personal control by including them in decisions about their care and restricting their behaviour only as necessary. Ongoing and effective communication with the patient is key to allowing patients to disclose and discuss their life situation and the resulting emotions and behaviour. Patients often feel shaky in the first hours of psychiatric hospitalization, and it is comforting to know that a caring person is nearby. Observational periods can be used to help the patients express a broad range of feelings and strengthen their belief in their own abilities to keep themselves safe. The nurse can help the patient who is not skilled in self-expression or self-management skills to describe feelings more effectively and cite ways of managing safety needs. Then, at the next observation time, the nurse may have the opportunity to reinforce the patient's own safety behaviour. Thus, the observation period can be transformed from something negative (e.g., "The patient can't be trusted," "I am out of control") to something positive (e.g., "The patient is becoming safer," "Maybe I can keep myself safe after all"; Cardell & Pitula, 1999). As the patient becomes more confident in understanding and controlling self-harm behaviour, the frequency of observation periods can be reduced.

Seclusion and restraint are two modalities sometimes used in the inpatient settings to maintain patient safety. However, these restrictive interventions are extremely stressful for patients and may interfere with their recovery. Moreover, seclusion and restraint often are used to compensate for inadequate staffing numbers. Unduly restraining patients to prevent their suicide interferes with the development of trusting relationships between patients and health care providers. The stress associated with restraints contributes to the biochemical disarray of their underlying psychiatric disorders. Restraints prevent patients from managing their own dysphoric and anxiety symptoms and reinforce their sense of hopelessness and helplessness. Restraints also enhance patients' fears that they are "crazy" and incapable of controlling their impulses. These methods reinforce a patient's perception of being out of control and lessen his or her ability to form a partnership with mental health providers.

Assisting With Somatic Therapies

Suicidal patients who are seriously depressed will likely receive somatic therapies, and patients' response to them must be monitored. The major somatic therapies used in the treatment of suicidal behaviour are antidepressant medications and electroconvulsive therapy (ECT). ECT may be useful for selected patients with intractable suicidal ideation and severe depression. ECT may be used for people who do not experience response to medication or who do not tolerate antidepressant medications, such as older adults and those with comorbid medical disorders. Although the decision to use ECT must be made carefully, ECT can be a life-saving procedure for the acutely suicidal patient with depression. Nurses need to be able to support patients in accepting and understanding this treatment (see Chapter 12).

The objective of medication for suicidal behaviour is to raise serotonin rapidly to a level that reduces suicide risk. To that end, third-generation and newer antidepressant medications should be used for those who are in imminent danger of harming themselves. These include fluoxetine (Prozac), sertraline (Zoloft), paroxetine (Serzone), bupropion (Wellbutrin), venlafaxine (Effexor), and citalopram (Celexa). These drugs generally are nontoxic and cause few side effects, especially after being taken for 1 to 2 weeks. They often are faster acting than the older drugs, but their onset of action varies. Especially useful are fluoxetine and paroxetine, which may be taken once a day. Sertraline also can be taken once a day, but achieving the proper dose can sometimes be difficult. Patients who take an overdose of these medications have much better outcomes than those who abuse first- and second-generation antidepressants.

The first- and second-generation antidepressants, including tricyclics and monoamine oxidase inhibitors, are equally effective for severe depression (Sutherland, Sutherland, & Hoehns, 2003). However, for those with suicidal behaviour, they may not be the best choice because these are highly toxic medications that people with suicidal intent can use to kill themselves. The resuscitation of a patient who has taken large amounts of one of these medications can be difficult because they are cardiotoxic. Medical sequelae may be long term if the patient is saved. Also, the side effects of these early antidepressants may result in the patient stopping the use of prescribed medication while still having suicidal thoughts. The need for laboratory assessment for therapeutic drug levels is another disadvantage of these drugs. Blood monitoring requires the patient's cooperation when his or her motivation may be at its lowest.

Assisting With Treatment for Substance Use

Suicidal behaviour is often associated with substance use disorders, especially among men. When substance use is an issue for the suicidal patient, the use must be addressed, or inpatient treatment of suicidal behaviour is only palliative, and the danger of the patient repeating a suicidal attempt is high. For men, substance use disorder may be the primary psychiatric disorder, with depression a side effect of it. For women, depression commonly is the primary psychiatric disorder, and substance use disorders result from attempts to medicate the underlying depressive condition. The nurse should help the patient understand the role that alcohol and drugs play in his or her suicidal behaviour. Treatment for substance use disorders should be part of the treatment plan, as appropriate, including referral to specific inpatient or community-based programs.

Interventions for the Psychological Domain

It is important for nurses to use the hospitalization period to find out what may have precipitated or contributed to the suicidal crisis. Precipitating factors, and how the patient's coping process began to break down, often become evident. After identifying extreme stressors experienced by the patient, the nurse and patient can help determine ways for the patient to avoid those stressors in the future or, if they cannot be avoided, to manage them more effectively.

During hospitalization, the nurse should evaluate the patient's ways of thinking about problems and generating solutions. Some patients, by virtue of their depressive illness or social learning, have an unusually negative view of life. They often think such thoughts as, "I am no good," "Everything I do is useless," "I have no future," or "Nobody has ever liked me, and nobody ever will." Often patients are unable to recognize the connection between their stressors and their suicidal behaviour. Many patients have had very difficult and abusive experiences in their lives, and their ability to cope is threatened. It is important for the nurse to help the patient identify what needs to change in his or her life and how that change can come about most effectively. The prevention of further suicidal behaviour is dependent on the patient's belief that he or she can make changes with the necessary support and resources and that there is hope for the future. (See Box 19-12 for examples of effective and ineffective dialogue with a patient.)

Interventions for the Social Domain

Improving Communication

Some suicidal patients can identify family and friends who are willing to help, but in many cases, patients are concerned about burdening these people or do not feel comfortable sharing their concerns with others. Helping the suicidal patient express these concerns and arrive at ways of reducing them is important. In other cases, because of trauma and abuse, the patient may have difficulty identifying anyone in his or her life as supportive. These patients are usually at a high risk for suicide because of their perception of aloneness and lack of

BOX 19-12   Therapeutic Dialogue

SUICIDE

When Caroline sought medical care from her nurse practitioner for a cold, the nurse observed more than a cough and runny nose. Caroline appeared downcast and unusually sad. As the nurse and patient talked, the subject of family life came up, and Caroline began to cry softly. As the words tumbled out, she said that she had been unhappy for a long time. When she was very young, she recalled being happy, but things changed when her brother was born, 4 years after her. When she was 5-years-old, her father began to abuse her sexually, continuing to do so until he moved out when she was 12. Caroline suspects her mother knew of the abuse, but did nothing about it. Two years ago, Caroline's father completed suicide. She feels relieved about his death but frustrated that she never got a chance to tell him how angry she was with him. Caroline's relationship with her mother has not improved. She says that her mother favours her brother and is always telling her she won't amount to anything. Caroline begins to cry harder.

Ineffective Approach

Nurse: Clearly, many things are troubling you. Don't you think that things seem worse now because you have a cold?

Caroline: Well, that could be. What are you going to do to make me feel better?

Nurse: Give you some medicine to help you sleep and clear your nose. I think you should see a psychiatrist, too.

Caroline: I don't need a psychiatrist. I came here for my cold.

Nurse: I know you did, but you seem to be depressed.

Caroline: What are you, some kind of social worker? I am just tired.

Nurse: I am a nurse, and you seem down to me. Are you thinking about suicide?

Caroline: I don't think you know what you're talking about. I want to go now. Could you give me my medicine?

Effective Approach

Nonjudgemental, curious questions; painting a picture helps the nurse and the patient.

Nurse: It seems as though many things have been piling up on you. Does it seem that way to you, too?

Caroline: It sure does. I've just been trying to get through one day at a time, but now with this cold and no sleep, I feel like I can't go on.

Nurse: When you say you can't go on, what do you mean by that?

Caroline: Lately, I have been thinking about running away to some place where I can't be found and maybe starting over. But then I think, where would I go? Where would I stay? Who would take care of me?

Nurse: When you think that your plan for escape won't work, what happens?

Caroline: (Starting to cry again.) Then I think that maybe it would be better if I just did what my father did. I really don't think anyone would miss me.

Nurse: So you think you might take your life, like your Dad did?

Caroline: Yeah, and what really scares me is lately I have been thinking about that a lot. I keep saying to myself, "You're just tired," but I am so exhausted now that I can't chase the thoughts away.

Nurse: So, do you think about suicide every day?

Caroline: It seems like I never stop thinking about it.

Nurse: Is there anything you can do to make the thoughts go away?

Caroline: Nothing. (Silence.)

Nurse: What would you do?

Caroline: I think I would get as many pills as I could find, drink a lot of alcohol, and maybe smoke some pot and just go to sleep.

Nurse: Do you have enough pills at home to kill yourself?

Caroline (wan smile): I was hoping that sleeping medicine from you might do the job.

Nurse: It seems like you might need help getting through this time in your life. Would you like some help?

Caroline: I honestly don't know—I just want to sleep for a long time.

Critical Thinking Challenge

- In the first interaction, the nurse made two key blunders. What were they? What effect did they have on the patient? How did they interfere with the patient's care?
- What did Caroline do that might have contributed to the nurse's behaviours in the first interaction?
- In the second interaction, the nurse did several things that ensured reporting of Caroline's suicidal ideation. What were they? What differences in attitude might differentiate the nurse in the first interaction from the nurse in the second?

---

connection with any significant other. The nurse needs to assist the patient in identifying people in the patient's life who may be supportive and make appropriate referrals to professionals with expertise in the area. Within the confines of therapeutic boundaries, the nurse can also be one of the supportive people in the patient's life if the nurse is successful in establishing a professional relationship with the patient.

Networking and Discharge Planning

A final concern may be the patient's embarrassment about the hospitalization and his or her emotional state. Through education, the nurse can do much to destigmatize the situation for both the patient and significant others. Before discharge, it is ideal for the patient to be able to name people who can act as a support. When supportive people are present, with the patient's permission, the nurse can work with them to begin to develop a network for the patient to rely on to remain safe. It is important for the patient and supportive family and friends to have a plan to contact another person, either a confidante or a mental health care provider, when they have questions or distressing thoughts or feel unable to manage or control suicide thoughts and behaviours.

Educating the Patient and Family

The objectives of patient and family education are to increase the patient's understanding of the origins of his or her suicidal behaviour, establish effective treatment for depression, provide for ongoing and seamless outpatient treatment, devise a plan for managing future suicidal ideation, identify supportive others in the community, establish a plan to make contact with these people and community resources, and continue with drug and alcohol treatment. These objectives are demanding for both the nurse and patient during a brief hospitalization.

In addition to trying to reduce the stigma that the patient and family may associate with suicide, the nurse must educate them about depression, suicidal behaviour, and treatments. When possible, the nurse should schedule educational sessions to include significant others so that they will better understand the patient's illness and also learn what is necessary in providing outpatient care.

Interventions for the Spiritual Domain

There can be a gap between how a patient defines his or her spirituality and the ability of health care professionals to understand and participate in their patient's spirituality in a therapeutic way (Tacey, 2003; Webb, 2005). Nurses not only must understand the influences within the bio/psycho/social/spiritual domains on their patients' experiences but also must understand how a person's spirituality, his or her meaning and purpose of life, encompasses the other three domains. In order to understand suicide from the patient's perspective, it is important to be open to the patient's concept of spirituality, his or her thoughts and feelings around the meaning of suicide, and what it is like to contemplate killing oneself (Tacey, 2003). The lived experience of suicide contemplation needs to be heard in a caring way. Nurses, by providing a patient with the time and space to explore their meaning of life, their spirituality, and their concept of death and dying, may gain insight into the factors that precipitate the patient's suicidal thoughts and behaviours.

Evaluation and Treatment Outcomes

The most desirable treatment outcome is the patient's return to the community. Because most hospitalizations for suicidal behaviour are brief, discharge planning must begin immediately after the patient is admitted. The nurse needs to explain to the patient that hospitalization is likely to be short term and should immediately begin to form a partnership with the patient and family to ensure a smooth transition to the community. *Partnering* means empowering the patient to engage in self-care as soon as possible by helping to provide the tools he or she needs to manage.

Identifying Continuing Sources of Social Support

Appropriate referrals to professionals in the community and available resources and support are important. The community nurse or therapist requires adequate information to continue with effective interventions after discharge. In addition, engaging family and friends in the patient's ongoing care and finding sources of help in the community, such as church groups, clubhouses, drop-in centres, or other social groups, is a necessary task. A patient's inability to name any significant others or social groups often means a poor outpatient course.

Establishing an Outpatient Care Plan

At the time of discharge, the patient is still considered very ill. Most suicides occur during the first week after discharge, and many happen within the first 24 hours. Before the patient's release, a specific, concrete plan for outpatient care must be in place. The care plan includes scheduling an appointment for outpatient care, providing for continuing medication until the first outpatient treatment visit, ensuring postrelease contact between the patient and significant others, providing for access to emergency psychiatric care, and arranging the patient's environment so that it provides both structure and safety.

At discharge, the patient should have enough medication on hand to last until the first community nurse visit. At that time, the community nurse can assess the patient's level of stability and determine whether a full prescription can be given safely to the patient. At that visit, the patient and community nurse can establish a plan of care that specifies the intensity of outpatient care. Very unstable patients may need two to three outpatient visits per week in the early days after hospitalization to maintain their safety in the community.

The patient and significant others must have a plan for the patient's ongoing supervision. This plan must be established in such a way that the patient does not feel undermined in his or her ability to manage self-care but is reassured that help will be available when needed. The family members or friends involved must feel that they are resources for the patient but not responsible for the patient's life or death. In the end, it is the patient, not supporters, who must bear responsibility for his or her safety. The patient who feels connected to but not dependent on significant others will be most likely to maintain safety in the community.

The patient's outpatient environment should be made as safe as possible before discharge. The nurse must share the care plan with family members so that they can remove any objects in the patient's environment that could be of assistance in completing suicide. The nurse must explain this measure to the patient to reinforce his or her sense of self-control. It is important to be reasonable in deciding what to remove from the environment. Patients who are truly determined to kill themselves after discharge may ultimately complete suicide.

Finally, there should be some continuity between inpatient and outpatient care. The nurse must tell the patient specifically how to obtain emergency psychiatric care. He or she should place written instructions near the patient's telephone. It is helpful for the community nurse, in addition to visits, to call periodically during the few first weeks after discharge to determine whether the patient is improving. This contact will help the patient to feel valued and connected to others. Lack of continuity is thought to contribute to significant suicide mortality after hospital discharge (Hulten & Wasserman, 1998).

Short-Term Outcomes

Short-term outcomes for the suicidal patient include maintaining the patient's safety, averting suicide, and mobilizing the patient's resources. Whether the patient is hospitalized or cared for in the community, his or her emotional distress must be reduced. This often is accomplished in an environment that restricts suicidal behaviour and provides sustained emotional support. The treatment during the suicidal crisis should also set the stage for meeting long-term objectives.

Long-Term Outcomes

Long-term outcomes must focus on maintaining the patient in psychiatric treatment, enabling the patient and family to identify and manage suicidal crises effectively, and widening the patient's support network.

Avoiding Compassion Fatigue

Professional work centred on relief of emotional suffering involves empathy as a key tool. Over time, being empathetic can become exhausting, even when the caregiver is diligently maintaining self-care skills. Compassion fatigue is a genuine concern and one that may result in diminished capacity to function at work, at home, and within personal and professional relationships. The symptoms of compassion fatigue include intrusive thoughts or images of patients' situations or trauma, difficulty separating work from personal life, lower frustration tolerance, hypervigilance, decreased feelings of confidence, diminished sense of purpose or enjoyment of career, and sleep disturbances or nightmares. The nurse may begin to avoid the stress through absenteeism or presenteeism (i.e., being physically present but not truly engaged in one's role). These signal that a nurse's health is at risk. Caring for suicidal patients who are close to one's own age or who have a history of being abused or neglected in childhood enhances the risks.

To care successfully for suicidal patients or others in crisis, the nurse must attend to his or her own well-being. Self-care with attention to nutrition, rest, and exercise facilitates managing stress physiologically. Self-awareness is integral to good nursing practice, particularly in terms of one's feelings of anxiety and vulnerability. Debriefing (i.e., sharing experiences and feelings) about stressful situations and one's response to them with a colleague and developing supports within the team so that members do not feel isolated but that care burdens are shared are helpful strategies. Compassion fatigue may not be recognized as such by the fatigued health care professional; it is often caring others who realize their colleague is

in trouble (Austin et al., 2013). Many health regions in Canada are ensuring that their staff are knowledgeable regarding compassion fatigue, as well as self-care, stress management strategies, and critical stress debriefing.

SUMMARY OF KEY POINTS

■ Suicidal behaviour is a means of communicating that something is wrong in one's life—that life is difficult or intolerable.

■ Suicide is a common and major public health problem that accompanies 15% of all cases of major depression.

■ More than half of all suicides are completed on the first attempt.

■ Parasuicide is more common among women than among men.

■ Men have a higher rate of completed suicide because of the use of more lethal means (e.g., guns, hanging).

■ People who engage in parasuicide are likely to do so repeatedly.

■ Suicidal behaviour may be associated with genetic and biologic origins, as well as psychological, social, and spiritual factors.

■ People who threaten suicide have rights that must be preserved.

■ The "no self-harm" contract (i.e., contracting for safety) is a potential means of increasing the suicidal patient's safety in the community.

■ The major objectives of brief hospital care are to maintain the patient's safety, reestablish the patient's biologic equilibrium, strengthen the patient's cognitive coping skills, and develop an outpatient support system.

■ The nurse who cares for suicidal patients is vulnerable to compassion fatigue and must take steps to sustain personal mental health.

CRITICAL THINKING CHALLENGES

1 A religious woman who lives with her three children, husband, and mother in rural Québec comes to her primary care provider. She is tearful and very depressed. What factors should be investigated to determine her risk for suicide and the need for hospitalization?

2 You are the primary health care nurse on a First Nations reservation. You want to implement a youth suicide prevention program. Discuss how you would proceed and some potential challenges that you might face.

3 Analyze lyrics of popular music that have a message about suicide and consider their possible effects on listeners. For instance, REM's "Everybody Hurts" (*Automatic for the People*) and David Bowie's "Rock and Roll Suicide" (*Ziggy Stardust*).

REFERENCES

Adler, G. & Buie, D. H., Jr. (1996). Aloneness and borderline psychopathology: Possible relevance of child development issues. In J. T. Maltsberger & M. J. Goldblatt (Eds.), *Essential papers on suicide* (pp. 356–378). New York, NY: New York University Press.

Angst, J. (1999). Major depression in 1998: Are we providing optimal therapy? *Journal of Clinical Psychiatry, 60*(Suppl. 6), 5–9.

Austin, W., Brintnell, E. S., Goble, E., Kagan, L., Kreitzer, L., Larsen, D. J., & Leier, B. (2013). *Lying down in the ever-falling snow: Canadian health professionals' experience of compassion fatigue.* Ottawa, ON: Wilfrid Laurier Press.

Baldessarini, R. J., Tondo, L., & Hennen, J. (1999). Effects of lithium treatment and its discontinuation on suicidal behaviour in bipolar manic-depressive disorders. *Journal of Clinical Psychiatry, 60*(Suppl. 2), 77–84.

Barker, P. & Buchanan-Barker, P. (2005). *The Tidal Model: A guide for mental health professionals.* New York, NY: Brunner-Routledge.

Beck, A. T. (2011). *Cognitive behavior therapy: Basics and beyond* (2nd ed). New York, NY: Guilford.

Beck, A. T., Brown, G. K., & Steer, R. A. (1997). Psychometric characteristics of the scale for suicide ideation with psychiatric outpatients. *Behaviour Research and Therapy, 35,* 1039–1046.

Beck, A. T., Rush, A. J., Shaw, B. F., & Emery, G. (1979). *Cognitive therapy in depression.* New York, NY: Guilford Press.

Belik, S-L., Stein, M. B., Asmundson, G. J. G., & Sareen, J. (2010). Are Canadian soldiers more likely to have suicidal ideation and suicide attempts than Canadian civilians? *American Journal of Epidemiology, 172*(11), 1250–1258.

Benson, P. (1992). Religion and substance use. In J. E. Schumaker (Ed.), *Religion and mental health* (pp. 211–220). New York, NY: Oxford University Press.

Bergen, H., Hawton, K., Ness, J., Cooper, J., Steeg, S., & Kapur, N. (2012). Premature death after self-harm: A multicenter cohort study. *Lancet, 380,* 1568–1574.

Bertolote, M., Fleischmann, A., Butchart, A., & Besbelli, N. (2006). Suicide, suicide attempts and pesticides: A major hidden public health problem. *Bulletin of the World Health Organization, 84*(4). Retrieved from http://www.who.int/bulletin/volumes/84/4/editorial30406html/en/

Blatchford, C. (2013). Why there may never be a case against the alleged Rehtaeh Parsons rapists. *The National Post.* Retrieved from http://fullcomment.nationalpost.com/2013/04/26/christie-blatchford-why-there-will-never-be-a-case-against-the-rehtaeh-parsons/

Bolton, J. M., Au, W., Leslie, W. D., Martens, P. J., Enns, M. W., Roos, L. L. … Sareen, J. (2013). Parents bereaved by offspring suicide: A population-based control case–control study. *JAMA Psychiatry, 70*(2), 158–167.

Brewster, M. (2014). Military top doc confirms 8 suicides in 2014. Retrieved from *National Newswatch* website, http://www.nationalnewswatch.com/2014/04/08/military-top-doc-confirms-8-suicides-in-2014/#.U44XoSjyK_I.

Bulik, C. M., Prescott, C. A., & Kendler, K. S. (2001). Features of childhood sexual abuse and the development of psychiatric and substance use disorders. *British Journal of Psychiatry, 179,* 444–449.

Butler, M., Tiedemann, M., Nicol, J., & Valiquet, D. (2010/Revised, 2013). *Euthanasia and assisted suicide in Canada (Background paper).* Parliamentary Information and Research Service. Publication No. 2010-68-E. Ottawa, ON: Library of Parliament.

Canada Safety Council. (2014). *Proper handling and storage of firearms.* Retrieved from https://canadasafetycouncil.org/safety-canada-online/article/proper-handling-and-storage-firearms

Canadian Nurses Association. (2002). *Code of ethics for registered nurses.* Ottawa, ON: Author.

Canadian Press. (2013). Rehtaeh Parsons wanted to go public before her death. *CBC News.* Retrieved from http://www.cbc.ca/news/canada/nova-scotia/rehtaeh-parsons-wanted-to-go-public-before-her-death-1.1895085

CBC News, August 7. (2013). Child porn charges against 2 teens in Rehtaeh Parsons case. *CBC News.* Retrieved from http://www.cbc.ca/news/canada/nova-scotia/child-porn-charges-against-2-teens-in-rehtaeh-parsons-case-1.1320438

CBC News, August 8. (2013). N.S. cyberbullying legislation allows victims to sue. *CBC News.* Retrieved from http://www.cbc.ca/news/canada/nova-scotia/n-s-cyberbullying-legislation-allows-victims-to-sue-1.1307338

Cardell, R. & Pitula, C. R. (1999). Suicidal inpatients' perceptions of therapeutic and non-therapeutic aspects of constant observation. *Psychiatric Services, 50*(8), 1066–1070.

Chandler, M. J. & Lalonde, C. (1998). Cultural continuity as a hedge against suicide in Canada's First Nations. *Transcultural Psychiatry, 35*(2), 191–219.

Clark, D. C. & Goebel-Fabbri, A. E. (1998). Lifetime risk of suicide in major affective disorders. In D. Jacobs (Ed.), *Harvard Medical School guide to assessment and intervention in suicide* (pp. 270–286). San Francisco, CA: Jossey-Bass.

Cohen, D. A., Mason, K., Bedimo, A., Sckibner, R., Basolo, V., & Farley, T. A. (2003). Neighborhood physical conditions and health. *American Journal of Public Health, 93*(3), 467–471.

Conwell, Y. & Duberstein, P. R. (2001). Suicide in elders. *Annals of the New York Academy of Sciences, 932,* 132–150.

Conwell, Y., Duberstein, P. R., & Caine, E. D. (2002). Risk factors for suicide in later life. *Biological Psychiatry, 52,* 193–204.

Conwell, Y., van Orden, K., & Caine, E. D. (2011). Suicide in older adults. *Psychiatric Clinics of North America, 34*(2), 451–468.

Cross, A. (2013). 'It's always about the victim': Rehtaeh Parsons' parents respond to Christie Blatchford's column. *The National Post.* Retrieved from http://news.nationalpost.com/2013/04/26/its-always-about-the-victim-rehtaeh-parsons-father-responds-to-christie-blatchfords-column/

CTVNews. (2014). Rehtaeh Parsons' supporters march for awareness. *CTVNews.* Retrieved from http://www.ctvnews.ca/canada/rehtaeh-parsons-supporters-march-for-awareness-1.1762455

Cubbin, C., LeClere, F. B., & Smith, G. S. (2000). Socioeconomic status and injury mortality: Individual and neighbourhood determinants. *Journal of Epidemiology and Community Health, 54*(7), 517–524.

Cvinar, J. (2005). Do suicide survivors suffer social stigma? A review of the literature. *Perspectives in Psychiatric Care, 41*(1), 14–21.

Dervic, K., Oquendo, M. A., Grunebaum, M. F., Ellis, S., Burke, A. K., & Mann, J. J. (2004). Religious affiliation and suicide attempt. *American Journal of Psychiatry, 161,* 2303–2308.

Durkheim, E. (1897, 2006). *On suicide.* London, UK: Penguin.

Eggertson, L. (2013). Risk of suicide 40 times higher for Inuit boys. *CMAJ, 185*(15), E701–E702.

Eng, P. M., Rimm, E. B., Fitzmaurice, G., & Kawachi, I. (2002). Social ties and change in social ties in relation to subsequent total and cause-specific mortality and coronary heart disease incidence in men. *American Journal of Epidemiology, 155*(8), 700–709.

Fisher, H. L., Moffitt, T. E., Houts, R. M., Belsky, D. W., Arseneault, L., & Caspi, A. (2012). Bullying victimization and risk of self harm in early adolescence: Longitudinal cohort study. *British Medical Journal, 344,* e2683. doi: 10.1136/bmj.e2683, 2012.

Flowers, J. (2006). *Cyber-bullying hits community. Addison County Independent.* Retrieved from http://www.addisonindependent.com/node/280

Foster, T., Gillespie, K., McClelland, R., & Patterson, C. (1999). Risk factors for suicide independent of *DSM-III-R* Axis I disorder: Case–control psychological autopsy study in Northern Ireland. *British Journal of Psychiatry, 175,* 175–179.

Freedenthal, S. (2008). Assessing the wish to die: A 30-year review of the Suicide Intent Scale. *Archives of Suicide Research, 12*(4), 277–298.

Gagné, M., Robitaille, Y., Hamel, D., St-Laurent, D. (2010). Firearms regulation and declining rates of male suicide in Quebec. *Injury Prevention, 16*(4), 247–253.

Glowinski, A. L., Bucholz, K. K., Nelson, E. C., Fu, Q., Madden, P., Reich, W., & Heath, A. C. (2001). Suicide attempts in an adolescent female twin sample. *Journal of the American Academy of Child and Adolescent Psychiatry, 40*(11), 1300–1307.

Goethe, J. W. (1774/1989). *The sorrows of young Werther* (Trans. M. W. Hulse). Harmondsworth, UK: Penguin.

Goodman, E. (1999). The role of socioeconomic status gradients in explaining differences in U.S. adolescents' health. *American Journal of Public Health, 89,* 1522–1528.

Government of Canada. (1985). *Criminal code of Canada.* Ottawa, ON: Author.

Government of Canada. (2006). *The human face of mental health and mental illness in Canada 2006.* Ottawa, ON: Minister of Public Works and Government Services of Canada.

Grad, O. (2011). The sequelae of suicide: Survivors. In R. C. O'Connor, S. Platt, & J. Gordon (Eds.), *International handbook of suicide prevention: Research, policy and practice* (pp. 561–576). New York, NY: John Wiley and Sons.

Guo, B., Scott, A., & Bowker, S. (2003). *Suicide prevention strategies: Evidence from systematic reviews. HTA 28.* Edmonton, AB: Heritage Foundation for Medical Research.

Guze, S. B. & Robins, E. (1970). Suicide and primary affective disorders. *British Journal of Psychiatry, 117,* 437–438.

Hall, S., Oliver, C., & Murphy, G. (2001). Early development of self-injurious behaviour: An empirical study. *American Journal on Mental Retardation, 106,* 395–400.

Hauenstein, E. (1996). A nursing practice paradigm for depressed rural women: Theoretical basis. *Archives of Psychiatric Nursing, 10*(5), 283–292.

Hawton, K. & Harriss, L. (2008). How often does deliberate self-harm occur relative to each suicide? A study of variations by gender and age. *Suicide and Life-Threatening Behaviour, 38*(6), 650–660.

Hawton, K., Harriss, L., Hodder, K., Simkin, S., & Gunnell, D. (2001). The influence of the economic and social environment on deliberate self-harm and suicide: An ecological and person-based study. *Psychological Medicine, 31*(5), 827–836.

Health Canada. (1994). *Suicide in Canada: Update of the report of the task force on suicide in Canada.* Ottawa, ON: Government of Canada.

Health Canada. (2003). *Acting on what we know: Preventing youth suicide in First Nations.* Retrieved from http://www.hc-sc.gc.ca/fniah-spnia/pubs/promotion/_suicide/prev_youth-jeunes/index-eng.php

Health Canada, First Nations and Inuit Health Branch. (2003). *A statistical profile on the health of First Nations in Canada.* Ottawa, ON: Author.

Hendin, H. (1991). Psychodynamics of suicide, with particular reference to the young. *American Journal of Psychiatry, 148,* 1150–1158.

HereToHelp. (2003). *Economic costs of mental disorders and addictions.* Retrieved from http://www.heretohelp.bc.ca/publications/factsheets/costs

Hilton, S. C. (2002). Active Latter-day Saints seven times less likely to commit suicide. *American Journal of Epidemiology, 155,* 413–419.

Hinduja, S. & Patchin, J. W. (2010). Bullying, cyberbullying, and suicide. *Archives of Suicide Research, 14,* 206–221.

Huffington Post. (2013). Rehtaeh Parsons, Canadian girl, dies after suicide attempt; parents allege she was raped. *The Huffington Post.* Retrieved from http://www.huffingtonpost.com/2013/04/09/rehtaeh-parsons-girl-dies-suicide-rape-canada_n_3045033.html

Huffington Post Canada. (2013). Rehtaeh Parsons suicide: Web calls on Anonymous to act after Nova Scotia Teen's death (Update: Anonymous Responds). *The Huffington Post Canada.* Retrieved from http://www.huffingtonpost.ca/2013/04/10/rehtaeh-parsons-suicide-anonymous_n_3052495.html

Hulten, A. & Wasserman, D. (1998). Lack of continuity: A problem in the care of young suicides. *Acta Psychiatrica Scandinavica, 97*(5), 326–333.

Jordan, J. R. (2001). Is suicide bereavement different? A reassessment of the literature. *Suicide and Life-Threatening Behaviour, 31*(1), 91–102.

Kendall, D., Lothian-Murray, J., & Linden, R. (2004). *Sociology: In our time* (3rd ed). Scarborough, ON: Thompson Canada Inc.

Kendler, K. S., Bulik, C. M., Silberg, J., Hettema, J. M., Myers, J., & Prescott, C. A. (2000). Childhood sexual abuse and adult psychiatric and substance use disorders in women: An epidemiological and cotwin control analysis. *Archives of General Psychiatry, 57*(10), 953–959.

Kirmayer, L. (2012). Changing patterns in suicide among young people [Commentary]. *Canadian Medical Association Journal, 184*(9), 1015–1016.

Kirmayer, L. J., Brass, G. M., Holton, T., Paul, K., Simpson, C., & Tait, C. (2007). *Suicide among Aboriginal people in Canada.* Ottawa, ON: Aboriginal Healing Foundation.

Klonsky, E. D. & Glenn, C. R. (2009). Assessing the functions of non-suicidal self-injury: Psychometric properties of the Inventory of Statements about Self-injury (ISAS). *Journal of Psychopathology and Behavioral Assessment, 31,* 215–219.

Knesper, D. J. (2011). *Suicide prevention and research: Suicide attempts and suicide details subsequent to discharge from emergency rooms and psychiatric units.* American Association of Suicidology, and Suicide Prevention Research Center. Newton, MA: Education Development Centre.

Knieper, A. J. (1999). The suicide survivor's grief and recovery. *Suicide and Life-Threatening Behaviour, 29*(4), 353–364.

Koenig, H. G. & Larson, D. B. (2001). Religion and mental health: Evidence for an association. *International Review of Psychiatry, 13,* 67–78.

Koplin, B. & Agathen, J. (2002). Suicidality in children and adolescents: A review. *Current Opinion in Pediatrics, 14,* 713–717.

Kposowa, A. J. (2001). Unemployment and suicide: A cohort analysis of social factors predicting suicide in the U.S. National longitudinal mortality study. *Psychological Medicine, 31*(1), 127–138.

Kreitman, N. S. (1970). *Parasuicide.* New York, NY: John Wiley and Sons.

Kreitman, N. S., Philip, A. E., Greer, S., & Bagley C. R. (1969). Parasuicide. *British Journal of Psychiatry, 115,* 1227–1228.

Langlois, S. & Morrison, P. (2002). Suicide deaths and suicide attempts. *Health Reports, 13*(2), 9–22.

Larson, D. & Larson, S. B. (2003). Spirituality's potential relevance to physical and emotional health: A brief review of quantitative research. *Journal of Psychology and Theology, 31,* 37–51.

Leenaars, A. A. (1998). *Suicide notes: Predictive clues and patterns.* New York, NY: Human Sciences Press.

Liu, R. T. & Mustanksi, B. (2012). Suicidal ideation and self-harm in lesbian, gay, bisexual and transgender Youth. *American Journal of Preventive Medicine, 42*(3), 221–228.

Lopez, F. G. & Brennan, K. A. (2000). Dynamic processes underlying adult attachment organization: Toward an attachment theoretical perspective on the health and effective self. *Journal of Counseling Psychology, 47*(3), 283–300.

MacMillan, H. L., Fleming, J. E., Streiner, D. L., Lin, E., Boyle, M. H., Jamieson, E., ... Beardslee, W. R. (2001). Childhood abuse and lifetime psychopathology in a community sample. *American Journal of Psychiatry, 158*(11), 1878–1883.

Mann, J. J., Brent, D. A., & Arango, V. (2001). The neurobiology and genetics of suicide and attempted suicide: A focus on the serotonergic system. *Neuropsychopharmacology, 24*(5), 467–477.

Mann, J. J., Oquendo, M., Underwood, M. D., & Arango, V. (1999). The neurobiology of suicide risk: A review for the clinician. *Journal of Clinical Psychiatry, 60*(Suppl. 2), 7–11.

March, J., Sareen, J., Gawaziuk, J. P., Doupe, M., Chateau, D., Hoppensack, M., ... Logsetty, S. (2014). Increased suicidal activity following major trauma: A population-based study. *Journal of Trauma and Acute Care Surgery, 76*(1), 180–184.

Marshall, B. D. L., Galea, S., Wood, E., & Kerr, T. (2013). Longitudinal associations between types of childhood trauma and suicidal behavior among substance users: A cohort study. *American Journal of Public Health, 103*(9), e69–e75.

Martin, G. (2002). Spirituality and suicide prevention. *Auseinetter, 15*(2), 3–4.

Masecar, D. (2009). *Suicide clusters: A discussion.* Ottawa, ON: First Nations Inuit Health Branch, Health Canada.

May, A. M. & Klonsky, E. D. (2013). Assessing motivations for suicide attempts: Development and psychometric properties of the Inventory of Motivations for Suicide Attempts. *Suicide and Life-Threatening Behavior, 43*(5), 532–546.

McGuffin, P., Marusic, A., & Farmer, A. (2001). What can psychiatric genetics offer suicidology. *Journal of Crisis Intervention and Suicide, 22*(2), 62–65.

McIntyre, L., Williams, J. V. A., Lavorato, D. H., & Patten, S. (2013). Depression and suicide ideation in late adolescence and early adulthood are an outcome of child hunger. *Journal of Affective Disorders, 150,* 123–129.

Mental Health Commission of Canada. (2012). *Changing directions, changing lives: The mental health strategy for Canada.* Calgary, AB: Author.

Mishara, B. L. & Chagnon, F. (2011). Understanding the relationship between mental illness and suicide and the implications for suicide prevention. In R. C. O'Connor, S. Platt, & J. Gordon (Eds.), *International handbook of suicide prevention: research, policy and practice* (pp. 609–623). New York, NY: John Wiley & Sons.

Mitchell, A. M., Gale, D. D., Garand, L., & Wesner, S. (2003). The use of narrative data to inform the psychotherapeutic process with suicide survivors. *Issues in Mental Health Nursing, 24,* 91–106.

Molnar, B., Berkman, L. F., & Buka, S. L. (2001). Psychopathology, childhood sexual abuse and other childhood adversities: Relative links to subsequent suicidal behaviour in the U.S. *Psychological Medicine, 31*(6), 965–977.

Monette, M. (2012). Senior suicide: An overlooked problem. *CMAJ, 184*(17), E855–E856.

Morrison, K. L. & Laing, L. (2011). Adults' use of health services in the year before death by suicide. *Health Reports, 22*(3), 1–8.

Muehlenkamp, J. J., Brausch, A. M., Quigley, K., & Whitlock, J. L. (2013). Interpersonal features and functions of non-suicidal self-injury. *Suicide and Life-Threatening Behavior, 43,* 67–80.

Murray, B. L. (2003). Self-harm among adolescents with developmental disabilities: What are they trying to tell us? *Journal of Psychosocial Nursing, 41*(11), 37–45.

Murray, B. L. & Wright, K. (2006). Integration of a suicide risk assessment and intervention approach: The perspective of youth. *Journal of Psychiatric and Mental Health Nursing, 13*(2), 157–164.

Nansel, T. R., Overpeck, M., Pilla, R. S., June Ruan, W., Simons-Morton, B., & Scheidt, P. (2001). Bullying behaviors among U.S. youth: Prevalence and association with psychosocial adjustment. *Journal of the American Medical Association, 285*(16), 2094–2100.

NANYouth. (2004). Aboriginal suicide statistics. Retrieved from https://sites.google.com/site/northernontarioaboriginalyouth/

Neeleman, J., & Lewis, G. (1990). Suicide, religion, and socioeconomic conditions. An ecological study in 26 countries. *Journal of Epidemiology and Community Health, 53,* 204–210.

Nelson, E. C., Heath, A. C., Madden, P. A. F., Cooper, M. L., Dinwiddie, S. H., Bucholz, K. K., ... Martin, N. G. (2002). Association between self-reported childhood sexual abuse and adverse psychosocial outcomes: Results from a twin study. *Archives of General Psychiatry, 59,* 139–145.

Niederkrotenthaler, T., Fu, K., Yip, P. S., Fong, D. Y. T., Stack, S., Cheng, Q., & Pirkis, J. (2012). Changes in suicide rates following media reports on celebrity suicide: A meta-analysis. *Journal of Epidemiology and Community Health.* Published online April 21, 2012, doi: 10.1136/jech-2011-200707

Nock, M. K., Borges, G., Bromet, E. J., Alonso, J., Angermeyer, M., Beautrais, A., ... Williams, D. (2008). Cross-national prevalence and risk factors for suicidal ideation, plans and attempts. *The British Journal of Psychiatry, 192,* 98–105.

O'Connell, H., Chin, A., Cunningham, C., & Lawlor, B. A. (2004). Recent developments: Suicide in older people. *British Medical Journal, 329,* 895–899.

Olson, R. (2013). *InfoExchange 10: Suicide contagion and suicide clusters.* Calgary, AB: Centre for Suicide Prevention.

Perlman, C. M., Neufeld, E., Martin, L., Goy, M., & Hirdes, J. P. (2012). *Suicide risk assessment guide: A resource for health care organizations.* Toronto, ON: Ontario Hospital Association and Canadian Patient Safety Institute.

Pesut, B. (2003). Developing spirituality in the curriculum: Intrapersonal connectedness, interpersonal connectedness. *Nursing Education Perspectives, 24,* 290–294.

Pesut, B. (2008). A conversation on diverse perspectives of spirituality in nursing literature. *Nursing Philosophy, 9,* 98–109.

Piérard, E. & Grootendorst, P. (2014). Do downturns cause desperation? The effects of economic conditions on suicide rates in Canada. *Applied Economics, 46*(10), 1081–1092.

Pitchot, W., Hansenne, M., Gonzalez Moreno, A., Pinto, E., Reggers, J., Fuchs, S., … Ansseau, M. (2001). Reduced dopamine function in depressed patients is related to suicidal behaviour but not its lethality. *Psychoneuroendocrinology, 26,* 689–696.

Platt, S. (1993). The social transmission of parasuicide: Is there a modeling effect? *Crisis, 14,* 23–31.

Poijula, S., Walberg, K. E., & Dyregrov, A. (2001). Adolescent suicide and suicide contagion in three secondary schools. *International Journal of Emergency Mental Health, 3*(3), 163–168.

Qin, P., Agerbo, E., & Mortensen, P. B. (2003). Suicide risk in relationship to socioeconomic, demographic, psychiatric, and familial factors: A national register-based study of all suicides in Denmark, 1981–1997. *American Journal of Psychiatry, 160*(4), 765–772.

Qin, P., Agerbo, E., Westergård-Nielson, N., Erikson, T., & Mortenson, P. B. (2000). Gender differences in risk factors for suicide in Denmark. *British Journal of Psychiatry, 177,* 546–550.

Range, L. M., Campbell, C., Kovac, S. H., Marion-Jones, M., Aldridge, H., Kogos, S., & Crump, Y. (2002). No-suicide contracts: An overview and recommendations. *Death Studies, 26,* 51–74.

Rasic, D., Kisely, S., & Langille, D. B. (2011). Protective associations of important of religion and frequency of service attendance with depression risk, suicidal behavior, and substance use in adolescents in Nova Scotia, Canada. *Journal of Affective Disorders, 132,* 389–395.

Rew, L., Thomas, N., Horner, S. D., Resnick, M. D., & Beuhring, T. (2001). Correlates of recent suicide attempts in a triethnic group of adolescents. *Journal of Nursing Scholarship, 33*(4), 361–367.

Richardson, J. D., St Cyr, K. C. M., McIntyre-Smith, A. M., Haslam, D., Elhai, J. D., & Sareen, J. (2012). Examining the association between psychiatric illness and suicidal ideation in a sample of treatment-seeking Canadian peacekeeping and combat veterans with posttraumatic stress disorder. *Canadian Journal of Psychiatry, 57*(8), 496–504.

Ross, S. (2013). Who failed Rehtaeh Parsons?. *Herald News.* Retrieved from http://www.thechronicleherald.ca/metro/1122345-who-failed-rehtaeh-parsons

Roy, A. (1989). Suicide. In H. I. Kaplan & B. J. Sadock (Eds.), *Comprehensive textbook of psychiatry* (pp. 1414–1427). Baltimore, MD: Williams & Wilkins.

Royal Commission on Aboriginal Peoples. (1995). *Choosing life: Special report on suicide among Aboriginal people.* Ottawa, ON: Communication Group.

Satyanarayana, S., Enns, M. W., Cox, B. J., Sareen, J. (2009). Prevalence and correlates of chronic depression in the Canadian Community Health Survey: Mental health and well-being. *Canadian Journal of Psychiatry, 54,* 389–398.

Scherr, S. & Reinemann, C. (2011). Belief in a Werther effect: Third-person effects in the perceptions of suicide risk for others and the moderating role of depression. *Suicide and Life-Threatening Behavior, 41*(6), 624–634.

Schneidman, E. (1985). *Definition of suicide.* New York, NY: John Wiley & Sons.

Skodol, A. E., Gunderson, J. G., Pfohl, B., Widiger, T. A., Livesley, J. W., & Siever, L. J. (2002). The borderline diagnosis I: Psychopathology, comorbidity, and personality structure. *Biological Psychiatry, 51,* 936–995.

SmartRisk. (2009). *The economic burden of injury in Canada.* Toronto, ON: Author.

Statistics Canada. (2012). *Health at a glance: suicide rates: an overview.* Retrieved from http://www.statcan.gc.ca/pub/82-624-x/2012001/article/11696-eng.htm

Statistics Canada. (2014). *Death and mortality rate, by selected grouped causes, age group and sex, Canada.* Retrieved from http://www5.statcan.gc.ca/cansim/a26?lang=eng&retrLang=eng&id=1020551&paSer=&pattern=&stByVal=1&p1=1&p2=37&tabMode=dataTable&csid=

Steenland, K., Halperin, W., Hu, S., & Walker, J. T. (2003). Deaths due to injuries among employed adults: The effects of socioeconomic class. *Epidemiology, 14*(1), 74–79.

Sutherland, J. E., Sutherland, S. J., & Hoehns, J. D. (2003). Achieving the best outcome in treatment of depression. *Journal of Family Practice, 53*(3), 118–126.

Tacey, D. (2003). *The spirituality revolution.* Sydney, AU: Harper Collins.

Tien, H. C. N., Acharya, S., & Redelmeier, D. A. (2010). Preventing deaths in the Canadian military. *American Journal of Preventive Medicine, 38*(3), 331–339.

Tinley, S. T. & Kinney, A. Y. (2007). Three philosophical approaches to the study of spirituality. *Advances in Nursing Science, 30,* 71–80.

von Borczyskowski, A., Lindlad, F., Vinnerlkjung, B., & Hjern, A. (2010). Gender differences in risk factors for suicide: Findings from a Swedish national cohort study. *Canadian Journal of Psychiatry, 55*(2), 108–111.

Webb, D. (2005). Bridging the spirituality gap. *Australian e-Journal for the Advancement of Mental Health, 4*(1), 1–9.

Welch, S. S. (2001). A review of the literature on the epidemiology of parasuicide in the general population. *Psychiatric Services, 52*(3), 368–375.

Westerlund, M., Schaller, S., & Schmidtke, A. (2009). The role of mass-media in suicide prevention. In D. Wasserman & C. Wasserman (Eds), *Oxford textbook of suicidology and suicide prevention: A global perspective* (pp. 515–525). Oxford, UK: Oxford University Press.

White, J. & Jodoin, N. (2003). *Aboriginal youth: A manual of promising suicide prevention strategies.* Retrieved from http://www.suicideinfo.ca/csp/go.aspx?tabid=144

World Health Organization. (2012). *Suicide prevention programme.* Retrieved from http://www.who.int/mental_health/prevention/suicide/suicideprevent/en/

Zenere, F. (2009). Suicide clusters and contagion. *Principal Leadership, 10*(2), 12–16.

Zetter, K. (2008). *Dead teen's mother testifies about daughter's vulnerability in MySpace suicide case*—update. *Wired.* Retrieved from http://www.wired.com/threatlevel/2008/11/lori-drew-pla-1/

Zhao, Y., Montoro, R., Igartua, K., & Thombs, B.D. (2010). Suicidal ideation and attempt among adolescents reporting "unsure" sexual identity or heterosexual identity plus same-sex attraction or behavior: Forgotten groups? *Journal of the American Academy of Child and Adolescent Psychiatry, 49*(2), 104–113.

Zor, F., Mustafa, D., Mehmet, B., Semih, D., Duman, H., & Sengezer, M. (2005). Psychological evaluation of self-inflicted burn patients: Suicide or parasuicide? *Burns, 31,* 178–181.

Care and Recovery of Persons With a Psychiatric Disorder

20 Schizophrenia

Jane Hamilton Wilson
Adapted from the chapter "Schizophrenia" by Hélène
Provencher, Andrea C. Bostrom, and Mary Ann Boyd

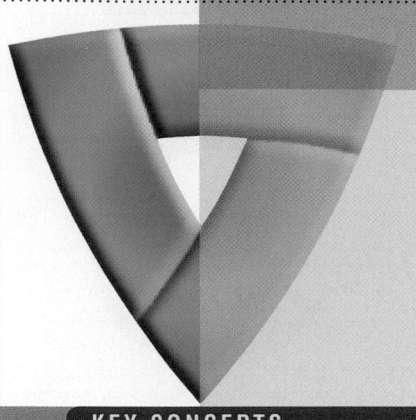

LEARNING OBJECTIVES

After studying this chapter, you will be able to:

- Distinguish key symptoms of schizophrenia.
- Analyze the prevailing biologic, psychological, and social theories that are the basis for understanding schizophrenia.
- Analyze human response to schizophrenia with emphasis on hallucinations, delusions, and social isolation.
- Formulate nursing diagnoses based on a bio/psycho/social/spiritual assessment of people with schizophrenia.
- Formulate nursing interventions that address specific diagnoses based on a continuum of care.
- Analyze special concerns within the nurse–patient relationship common to treating those with schizophrenia.
- Identify the expected outcomes and their evaluation.

KEY CONCEPTS

- disorganized symptoms
- negative symptoms
- neurocognitive impairment
- positive symptoms

KEY TERMS

- affective flattening or blunting • affective lability • aggression
- agitation • agranulocytosis • akathisia • alogia • ambivalence
- anhedonia • anosognosia • apathy • avolition • catatonic excitement • confused speech and thinking • delusions
- disorganized behaviour • echolalia • echopraxia • expressed emotion • extrapyramidal side effects • first-episode psychosis
- flight of ideas • hallucinations • hypervigilance • hypofrontality
- illusions • neuroleptic malignant syndrome • oculogyric crisis
- paranoia • polyuria • prodromal • recovery • regressed behaviour
- retrocollis • stereotypy • tangentiality • tardive dyskinesia
- torticollis • waxy flexibility • word salad

chizophrenia has fascinated and confounded healers, scientists, and philosophers for centuries. It is one of the most severe complex mental illnesses and is present in all cultures, races, and socioeconomic groups. Its symptoms have historically been attributed to possession by demons, considered punishment by gods for evils done, or accepted as evidence of the inhumanity of its sufferers. These explanations have resulted in enduring stigma for people with a diagnosis of this disorder. Today, such stigma persists despite numerous national efforts to educate the Canadian public. All nurses need to understand this disorder and advocate to correct stereotyping and misperceptions. The Mental Health Commission of Canada (MHCC) has identified combating the stigma of mental illness and preventing discrimination as important priorities in improving the mental health of Canadians (MHCC, 2007). Educating the public and the media about mental illness is a priority. In fact, in 2012, the Mental Health Commission published a strategy document entitled *Changing Directions: Changing Lives* (MHCC, 2012). This document is the first national mental health strategy, which focuses upon better mental health care for all. Canadians with serious mental illnesses such as schizophrenia are likely to be the beneficiaries of the enactment of the evidence-based approaches to enhance mental health, reduce stigmatization of those with serious mental illness, and reduce barriers to meaningful employment.

CLINICAL COURSE

In the late 1800s, Emil Kraepelin first described the course of the disorder he called *dementia praecox*. In the early 1900s, Eugene Bleuler renamed the disorder *schizophrenia*, meaning *split minds*, and began to determine that there was not just one type of schizophrenia but rather a group of schizophrenias. More recently, Kurt Schneider differentiated behaviours associated with schizophrenia as "first rank" symptoms (e.g., psychotic delusions, hallucinations) and "second rank" symptoms (all other experiences and behaviours associated with the disorder). These pioneering physicians had a great influence on the current diagnostic conceptualizations of schizophrenia that emphasize the heterogeneity of the disorder in terms of course of illness and positive and negative symptoms.

Overview of Schizophrenia

The clinical picture of schizophrenia is highly variable and complex. Individual symptoms differ from one another, and the experience for a single individual may be different from episode to episode. For some individuals, the illness onset is slow and insidious; for others, it is sudden, seemingly coming from out of the blue. Similarly, the course of schizophrenia is also unique and unpredictable. About 25% to 30% of people with schizophrenia experience a complete remission after one or several psychotic episodes (Barak & Aizenberg, 2012; Harrison et al., 2001). However, early intervention, including pharmacologic and phase-specific psychosocial interventions, shows promise for increasing the rate of recovery in people with first-onset schizophrenia (Amminger et al., 2011). Although schizophrenia is treatable, it remains a serious and potentially disabling illness. As is the case with most chronic illnesses, the emphasis must be upon maximizing wellness while minimizing the disability. It is important to note that **recovery** does not mean cure (see Box 20-1). There is not one predictable outcome for an individual with schizophrenia. There may be a variety of outcomes depending on how the illness affects the person, his or her family, and the kind and type of treatment received. Nurses in both inpatient and community settings have an

---

BOX 20-1 Recovery From Schizophrenia: The Importance of Personal Medicine

The pioneering work of individuals who have described their own "journey of recovery" from serious mental illness has significantly contributed to a better understanding of recovery from schizophrenia. Patricia Deegan (1992), a psychologist and a psychiatric consumer/advocate, in describing her own experience explains: "[R]ecovery is marked by an ever deepening acceptance of our limitations … we find our limitations are the ground from which spring our own unique possibilities. It is a way of life, an attitude of approaching the day's challenges" (p. 7). Recovery, however, does not mean cure. Rather, recovery is a highly individual process or journey that can involve the experience of growth in response to challenges and the development of a new identity that includes, but moves beyond, illness. Recovery, according to Deegan, refers to "the lived experiences of people as they accept and overcome the challenge of their disability. They experience themselves as recovering a new sense of self and of purpose within and beyond the limits of disability. Recovery is about growth. Recovery can and does happen without professional intervention. Recovery is not just specific to psychosis. Recovery is about taking back control. Recovery is about hanging in there through the long and often slow process of healing. Recovery is a process, not an end point or destination. Everyone's recovery journey is different and deeply personal. Hope is central to recovery" (p. 8).

Source: Deegan, P. (1992). The independent living movement and people with psychiatric disabilities: Taking back control over our own lives. *Psychosocial Rehabilitation Journal, 15,* 5–9.

---

opportunity to help patients live well with schizophrenia. Rates of 80% recovery following a first episode of psychosis have been reported (Picchioni & Murray, 2007).

Acute Illness Period

Initially, the illness behaviours may be both confusing and frightening to the patient and the family. At first, the changes (often called **prodromal** symptoms) may be subtle and, as they often begin in late adolescence, can even be confused with the anxiety and moodiness of teenage years. However, at some point, the changes in thought and behaviour become so disruptive or bizarre that they can no longer be overlooked. These changes herald the beginning of psychosis. Typically, family and friends become aware that something is not right. Changes might include episodes of staying up all night for several nights, withdrawal from social activities, incoherent conversations, and irritability or aggressive acts against self or others. For example, one patient's parents reported their son sneaking around their home for several days peeking out from behind the curtains and complaining that their home was under surveillance. Another father described his son's first delusional–hallucination episode as so convincing that it was frightening. His son began visiting cemeteries and making "mind contact" with the deceased. He saw his deceased grandmother walking around in the home and was certain that there were pipe bombs in objects in his home. Another patient believed

BOX 20-2 First-Episode Psychosis

First-episode psychosis simply refers to the first time someone experiences psychotic symptoms or a psychotic episode. A psychotic episode occurs in three phases. The length of each phase varies from person to person.

Phase 1. *Prodrome*: The early signs may be vague and hardly noticeable. There may be changes in the way some people describe their feelings, thoughts, and perceptions, which may become more difficult over time.

Phase 2. *Acute*: Clear psychotic symptoms are experienced, such as hallucinations, delusions, or confused thinking.

Phase 3. *Recovery*: Psychosis is treatable: Most people recover. The pattern of recovery varies from person to person. Despite common misperceptions, recovery from a first episode of psychosis is more probable than not. With help, many never have another psychotic episode.

Adapted from the Early Psychosis Prevention and Intervention Centre (http://www.eppic.org.au).

that he had been visited by space aliens who wanted to unite their world with Earth and assured him that he would become the leader of his country. These experiences are collectively referred to as indicators of **first-episode psychosis**, or the initial episode of psychosis, which most often occurs in adolescence or early adult life (see Box 20-2). This early stage of illness, defined as the first 3 to 5 years following the onset of symptoms, is considered a critical period for intervention (Melau et al., 2011). Excellent early intervention has been found to lead to more favourable recovery outcomes, leading to many early intervention programs being developed in Canada and around the world. In general, the threefold aim of these programs has been to reduce the duration of untreated psychosis (DUP), intervene appropriately at this early stage of illness, and prevent subsequent relapse and minimize the disability (Amminger et al., 2011; Malla, Norman, & Joober, 2005). These efforts have led to new hope for individuals who develop schizophrenia.

As the DUP increases, patients are less and less able to care for their basic needs, such as eating, sleeping, and bathing. Substance use is common. Functioning at school or work deteriorates. Dependence on family and friends increases, and those persons recognize the individual's need for treatment. In the acute phase, individuals with schizophrenia are at high risk for suicide and may require hospitalization to protect themselves or others.

Initial treatment for schizophrenia focuses upon thorough assessment and the alleviation of symptoms through the initiation of medications, decreasing the risk for suicide through safety measures, normalizing sleep, and reducing substance misuse. Functional deficits may persist during this period, and the patient and family must begin to learn to cope with these. Emotional blunting diminishes the ability and desire to engage in hobbies, vocational activities, and relationships. Limited

participation in social activities may spiral into numerous skill deficits, such as difficulty engaging others interpersonally. Similarly, cognitive deficits may lead to problems recognizing patterns in situations and transferring learning and behaviours from one circumstance to another similar one.

Stabilization Period

After the initial diagnosis of psychosis and the initiation of treatment, stabilization of schizophrenia symptoms becomes the focus. Symptoms become less acute but may still be present. Treatment is intense during this period as medication regimens are established and patients adapt to various medication side effects. With appropriate assistance and support, patients and their families begin to adjust to the idea of a family member having a serious mental illness. Ideally, the misuse of substances is eliminated. Socialization with others begins to increase, and rehabilitation begins.

Maintenance and Recovery Period

After the patient's condition is stabilized, his or her focus is upon recovery efforts to regain a previous level of functioning and improve quality of life. Medication treatment of schizophrenia has generally contributed to an improvement in the symptom remission of people with this disorder; however, no medication has cured it. Faithful medication management tends to make the impairments in functioning less severe when they occur and to diminish the extremes an individual might experience. As with any chronic illness, stresses of life and major crises can contribute to exacerbations of acute symptoms.

Clearly, family support and involvement are extremely important at this time. Once the initial diagnosis is made, patients and families can be educated to watch for early signs of potential relapse and know how to cope with it. This is one of the important themes throughout the nursing process for people with schizophrenia. One of the key goals in the treatment of schizophrenia is to avoid subsequent relapses after the remission of the first episode. This is a tall order indeed. The long-term prognosis with regard to relapse is most certainly influenced by a patient's willingness to remain on maintenance antipsychotic treatment and by engaging in other therapies and supports as deemed appropriate.

Relapses

Relapses can occur at any time during treatment and recovery. Relapse is not inevitable; however, it occurs with sufficient regularity to be a major concern in the treatment of schizophrenia. Relapses can occur and are detrimental to the successful management of this disorder. With each subsequent relapse, rehabilitation is prolonged, and there is a longer period of time required

Table 20-1	Fostering Recovery from Schizophrenia

Factors That Encourage Recovery	Factors That Hinder Recovery
• Early detection • Short DUP • Optimal treatment including medication, education, individual counselling, and family education and support • Supportive social network • Stable and safe living environment • Access to meaningful activity • Companionship • Attention to physical health • Quick resolution of psychotic symptoms • Hope for the future	• Late detection • Long DUP • Fragmented, inadequate, or inaccessible care • Little support from the social environment • Excess stress, tension, and conflict in the personal environment • Idleness, boredom • Isolation, loneliness • Neglect of physical health and abuse of street drugs or other substances • Persistent, unremitting psychotic symptoms • Hopelessness and despair

Adapted from Onken, S. J., Dumont, J. M., Ridgway, P., Dornan, D. H., & Ralph, R. O. (2007). Mental health recovery: What helps and what hinders? *A national research project for the development of recovery facilitating system performance indicators.* Retrieved from http://www.mhsret.org/documents/ROSIPilotMeasuresV7.pdf

to recover. Combining medications and psychosocial treatment greatly diminishes the severity and frequency of recurrent relapses (Emsley, Chiliza, Asmal, & Harvey, 2013).

One of the major reasons for relapse is nonadherence to the medication regimen. Even with newer medications, nonadherence leading to relapse continues to be a problem. Discontinuing the use of medications almost certainly leads to a relapse and may actually be a stressor that causes a severe and rapid relapse (Freudenreich & Cather, 2012). Lower relapse rates are, for the most part, among groups who were following an effective continuing treatment regimen.

Several factors contribute to relapse reduction and to optimal prognostic outcomes and recovery (see Table 20-1). Patients, their families, and members of the treatment team need to be familiar with ways to enhance recovery. It is also important to provide a realistically hopeful attitude for the future.

Many other factors can trigger a relapse: the degree of impairment in cognition and coping that leaves patients vulnerable to stressors; the accessibility of community resources, such as public transportation, housing, entry-level and low-stress employment, and social services; income supports that buffer the day-to-day stressors of living; the degree of stigmatization that the community holds for mental illness, which undermines the self-concept of patients; and the responsiveness of family members, friends, and supportive others (e.g., peers and professionals) when patients need help. ·

Diagnostic Criteria

The current definition outlined in the American Psychiatric Association's *Diagnostic and Statistical Manual of Mental Disorders*, 5th ed. (*DSM-5*; APA, 2013), states that schizophrenia is a mixture of positive and negative symptoms that present for a significant portion of a 1-month period but with continuous signs of disturbance persisting for at least 6 months.

Positive symptoms can be thought of as symptoms that exist but should not, and negative symptoms as ones that should be there but are not.

The *DSM-5* criteria for diagnosing schizophrenia include necessary symptomatology, duration of symptoms, evaluation of functional impairment, and elimination of alternate hypotheses that might account for the symptoms (APA, 2013). In the past, several schizophrenia subtypes were recognized: paranoid, disorganized, catatonic, undifferentiated, and residual. However, there was growing belief that this subtyping was not useful for predicting the course and response to treatment. The new diagnostic criteria are listed in Table 20-2.

KEY CONCEPT **Positive symptoms** reflect an excess or distortion of normal functions, including delusions and hallucinations.

KEY CONCEPT **Negative symptoms** reflect a lessening or loss of normal functions, such as restriction or flattening in the range and intensity of emotion (**affective flattening or blunting**), reduced fluency and productivity of thought and speech (**alogia**), withdrawal and inability to initiate and persist in goal-directed activity (**avolition**), and inability to experience pleasure (**anhedonia**).

Table 20-2   Key Diagnostic Characteristics of Schizophrenia

Diagnostic Criteria and Target Symptoms	Associated Findings
Diagnostic Criteria • Two or more of the following characteristic symptoms present for a significant portion of time during a 1-month period: delusions, hallucinations, disorganized speech, grossly disorganized or catatonic behaviour, and negative symptoms. (At least one of delusions, hallucination, or disorganized speech must be present.) • Disturbance in level of functioning for one or more major areas of social or occupational functioning (such as work, interpersonal relations, and self-care) markedly below the previously achieved level • Continuous signs persisting for at least 6 months • Absence or insignificant duration of major depressive, manic, or mixed episodes occurring concurrently with active symptoms • Not a direct physiologic effect of a substance or medical condition • Prominent delusions or hallucinations present when a prior history of autistic disorder or another pervasive developmental disorder exists *Target Symptoms and Associated Findings* • Inappropriate affect • Loss of interest or pleasure • Dysphoric mood (anger, anxiety, or depression) • Disturbed sleep patterns	• Lack of interest in eating or refusal of food • Difficulty concentrating • Some cognitive dysfunction, such as confusion, disorientation, and memory impairment • Lack of insight • Depersonalization, derealization, and somatic concerns • Motor abnormalities *Associated Physical Examination Findings* • Physically awkward • Poor coordination or mirroring • Motor abnormalities • Cigarette-related pathologies, such as emphysema and other pulmonary and cardiac problems *Associated Laboratory Findings* • Enlarged ventricular system and prominent sulci in the brain cortex • Decreased temporal and hippocampal size • Increased size of basal ganglia • Decreased cerebral size • Slowed reaction times • Abnormalities in eye tracking

Positive Symptoms of Schizophrenia

Delusions are erroneous fixed beliefs that usually involve a misinterpretation of experience. For example, the patient believes someone is reading his or her thoughts or plotting against him or her. Various types of delusions include the following:

• *Grandiose*: the belief that one has exceptional powers, wealth, skill, influence, or destiny
• *Nihilistic*: the belief that one is dead or a calamity is impending
• *Persecutory*: the belief that one is being watched, ridiculed, harmed, or plotted against
• *Somatic*: beliefs about abnormalities in bodily functions or structures

Hallucinations are perceptual experiences that occur without actual external sensory stimuli. They can involve any of the five senses, but they are usually *visual* or *auditory*. Auditory hallucinations are more common than are visual ones. For example, the patient hears voices carrying on a discussion about his or her own thoughts or behaviours.

Negative Symptoms of Schizophrenia

Negative symptoms are not as dramatic as positive symptoms, but they can interfere greatly with the patient's ability to function day to day. Because expressing emotion is difficult for them, people with schizophrenia laugh, cry, and get angry less often. Their affect is flat, and they show little or no emotion when personal loss occurs. They also suffer from **ambivalence**, which is the concurrent experience of equally strong opposing feelings so that it is impossible to make a decision. The avolition may be so profound that simple activities of daily living, such as dressing or combing hair, may not get done. Anhedonia prevents the person with schizophrenia from enjoying activities. People with schizophrenia may have limited speech and difficulty saying anything new or carrying on a conversation. These negative symptoms cause the person with schizophrenia to withdraw and suffer feelings of severe isolation.

Neurocognitive Impairment

Neurocognitive impairment exists in schizophrenia and may be independent of positive and negative symptoms. Neurocognition includes short- and long-term memory, vigilance or sustained attention, verbal fluency or the ability to generate new words, and executive functioning, which includes volition, planning, purposive action, and self-monitoring behaviour. Working memory is a concept that includes short-term memory and the ability to store and process information.

This impairment is independent of the positive symptoms. That is, cognitive dysfunction can exist even if the positive symptoms are in remission. Not all areas of cognitive functioning are impaired. Long-term memory and intellectual functioning are not necessarily affected. However, for many people with this disorder, symptoms may have interfered with completing educational opportunities. Neurocognitive dysfunction often is manifested in disorganized symptoms.

> **KEY CONCEPT Neurocognitive impairment** in memory, vigilance, and executive functioning is related to poor functional outcome in schizophrenia (Addington & Addington, 2006; Mesholam-Gately, Giuliano, Faraone, Goff, & Seidman, 2009).

> **KEY CONCEPT Disorganized symptoms** of schizophrenia are those things that make it difficult for the person to understand and respond to the ordinary sights and sounds of daily living. These include **disorganized speech and thinking** and **disorganized behaviour**.

Disorganized Thinking

Examples of disturbed speech and thinking patterns can be found in Chapter 10, specifically in Boxes 10-4 and 10-5.

Disorganized perceptions often create oversensitivity to colours, shapes, and background activities. **Illusions** occur when the person misperceives or exaggerates stimuli that actually exist in the external environment. This is in contrast to hallucinations, which are perceptions in the absence of environmental stimuli. Ancillary symptoms that may accompany schizophrenia include anxiety, depression, irritability, and hostility.

Disorganized Behaviour

Disorganized behaviour (which may manifest as a very slow, rhythmic, or ritualistic movement), coupled with disorganized speech, makes it difficult for someone with schizophrenia to partake in daily activities. Examples of disorganized behaviour include the following:

- **Aggression**—behaviours or attitudes that reflect rage, hostility, and the potential for physical or verbal destructiveness (usually comes about if the person believes that someone is going to do him or her harm)
- **Agitation**—inability to sit still or attend to others, accompanied by heightened emotions and tension
- **Catatonic excitement**—a hyperactivity characterized by purposeless activities and abnormal movements such as grimacing and posturing
- **Echopraxia**—involuntary imitation of another person's movements and gestures
- **Regressed behaviour**—behaving in a manner of a less mature life stage; child-like and immature

- **Stereotypy**—repetitive, purposeless movements that are idiosyncratic to the individual and to some degree outside of the individual's control
- **Hypervigilance**—sustained attention to external stimuli as if expecting something important or frightening to happen
- **Waxy flexibility**—posture held in odd or unusual fixed position for extended periods of time

Schizophrenia in Special Populations

Children

The diagnosis of schizophrenia is rare in children prior to adolescence. When it does occur in children aged 5 or 6 years, the symptoms are essentially the same as in adults. In this age group, hallucinations tend to be visual and delusions less developed. Because disorganized speech and behaviour may be explained better by other disorders that are more common in childhood, those disorders should be considered before applying the diagnosis of schizophrenia to a child (APA, 2013).

However, new studies suggest that the likelihood of children later experiencing schizophrenia can be predicted. Developmental abnormalities in childhood, including delays in the attainment of speech and motor development, problems in social adjustment, and poorer academic and cognitive performance, have been found to be present in individuals who experience schizophrenia in adulthood. Specific factors that appear to predict schizophrenia in adulthood include problems in motor and neurologic development, deficits in attention and verbal short-term memory, poor social competence, positive formal thought disorder–like symptoms, and severe instability of early rearing environment (Niemi, Suvisaari, Tuulio-Henriksson, & Lonnqvist, 2003).

Older Adults

People with schizophrenia do grow old. For older persons who have had schizophrenia since young adulthood, this may be a time in which they experience some improvement in symptoms or relapse fluctuations. For instance, admission to general hospitals for older individuals (age 65 years or older) with schizophrenia is more likely to be for an associated medical condition (Health Canada, 2002). Their lifestyle probably is dependent on the effectiveness of earlier treatment, the support systems that are in place (including relationships with family members and professionals), and the interaction between environmental stressors and the patient's functional impairments.

In late-onset schizophrenia, the diagnostic criteria are met after the age of 45 years. Women are affected more than are men. The presentation of late-onset schizophrenia is most likely to include positive symptoms, particularly paranoid or persecutory delusions. Cognitive deterioration and affective blunting occur less frequently.

Social functioning is more intact. Many individuals with diagnoses of late-onset schizophrenia have disturbances in sensory functions, primarily hearing and vision losses (APA, 2013). The cost of caring for older persons with schizophrenia remains high because many are no longer cared for in an institution, and community-based treatment has developed more slowly for this age group than for younger adults.

EPIDEMIOLOGY

Schizophrenia occurs in all cultures and countries. The incidence and prevalence rates are similar across studies, with variations explained by the definition of schizophrenia and the sampling method used. Schizophrenia occurs in about 1.3% of the population or more than 400,000 people in Canada (Goldner, Hsu, Waraich, & Somers, 2002). Its economic costs are enormous. Direct costs include treatment expenses, and indirect costs include lost wages, premature death, and incarceration. In addition, employment among people with schizophrenia is one of the lowest of any group with disabilities (Crowther, Marshall, Bond, & Huxley, 2004; MHCC, 2013a). The costs of schizophrenia in terms of individual and family suffering probably are inestimable.

People with schizophrenia tend to cluster in the lowest social classes in industrialized countries and urban communities. For some, the symptoms of the illness are so pervasive that it is difficult for these individuals to maintain any type of gainful employment. Homelessness is a problem for those with severe and persistent symptoms of mental illness (e.g., people with schizophrenia or bipolar illness). Somewhere between 30% and 40% of the homeless are estimated to be suffering from mental illness, and of those, 20% to 25% are living with concurrent disorders, that is, with addiction and other health problems (Standing Senate Committee on Social Affairs, Science and Technology, 2006). A more recent study, conducted by the MHCC (2013b) entitled *At Home/Chez Soi* reinforces the need for secure and safe housing for individuals suffering from serious mental illness.

Risk Factors

Risk factors for schizophrenia include stresses in the perinatal period (e.g., starvation, poor nutrition, infections), obstetrical complications, and genetic and family susceptibilities (Picchioni & Murray, 2007). Canadian researchers have recently discovered rare genetic changes that may be responsible for the onset of schizophrenia. This discovery gives new support to the notion that multiple rare genetic changes may contribute to schizophrenia and other brain disorders (Centre for Addiction and Mental Health, 2013). There has been evidence that parental age may also be a risk factor (Byrne, Agerbo, Ewald, Eaton, & Mortensen, 2003). Birth cohort studies suggest that the incidence of schizophrenia may be higher among individuals born in urban settings than those born in rural ones and may be somewhat lower in later-born birth cohorts (Harrison et al., 2003). Infants affected by maternal stressors may have conditions that create their own risk, such as low birth weight, short gestation, and early developmental difficulties. In childhood, stressors may include central nervous system (CNS) infections.

Age of Onset

Most people who suffer from schizophrenia have the disorder diagnosed in late adolescence or early adulthood. When schizophrenia begins prior to age 25, symptoms seem to develop more gradually, and negative symptoms predominate throughout the course of the disease. People with early-onset schizophrenia experience a greater number of neuropsychologic problems. Disruptions occur in the achievement of milestone events of early adulthood, such as achieving in education, work, and long-term relationships (Csernansky, 2003).

Gender Differences

Men are typically diagnosed with schizophrenia earlier than women are. The median age of onset for men is in the middle 20s, whereas the median age of onset for women is in the late 20s. These gender differences have received attention because of hypotheses about sex-linked genetic aetiologies. For instance, estrogen may play a protective role against the development of schizophrenia that disappears as estrogen levels drop during menopause (Kulkarni, Hayes, & Gavrilidis, 2012). This may account for the higher median age of onset and a more favourable treatment outcome in women.

Ethnic and Cultural Differences

Increasingly, efforts are being made to consider culture and ethnic origin when diagnosing the disorder and treating individuals with symptoms of schizophrenia (APA, 2013). Although symptoms of schizophrenia appear to be clearly defined, it is possible to find cultures in which what appears to be a hallucination may be considered a vision or a religious experience. In addition, behaviours such as averting eyes during a conversation or minimizing emotional expression may be culturally bound, yet easily misinterpreted by clinicians of a different cultural or ethnic background.

Individuals of various racial groups may have varying diagnosis rates of schizophrenia. However, it is important to note that these findings may reflect a misdiagnosis of the disorder based on a cultural bias of the clinician. Prevalence studies indicate a lower incidence of schizophrenia in Asian versus non-Asian countries. It is not known if this difference is due to methodologic, genetic, environmental, or sociologic variables such as stigma and underreporting (Goldner et al., 2002).

Familial Differences

First-degree biologic relatives (children, siblings, parents) of an individual with schizophrenia have a 10 times greater risk for schizophrenia than the general population (APA, 2013). Other relatives may have an increased risk for disorders within the "schizophrenia spectrum" (a group of disorders with some similarities of behaviour, such as schizoaffective disorder and schizotypal personality disorder) (APA, 2013). It is still not clear whether genetic vulnerability is present in all cases of schizophrenia. It is possible that those genetic vulnerabilities are in terms of psychosis in general and that the expression of these vulnerabilities can take various forms (Costain & Bassett, 2013; Walker, Kestler, Bollini, & Hochman, 2004).

Comorbidity

Several somatic and psychological disorders coexist with schizophrenia. It is estimated that nearly 50% of patients with schizophrenia have a comorbid medical condition, but many of these illnesses are misdiagnosed or under diagnosed (Goldman, 1999). Recently, more attention has been paid to the causes of mortality among people with schizophrenia. Several physical disorders have been identified, including vision and dental problems, heart disease, hypertension, diabetes, and sexually transmitted diseases (Hennekens, Hennekens, Hollar, & Casey, 2005; Muir-Cochrane, 2006).

Substance Abuse and Depression

Among the behavioural comorbidities, substance abuse is common (see Chapter 26). Cannabis use, in particular, has been associated with an increased risk of psychosis onset (Arseneault, Cannon, Wilton, & Murray, 2004; Carlson, 2013; Muller-Vahl & Emrich, 2008). Depression may also be observed in patients with schizophrenia. This is an important symptom for several reasons. First, depression may be the evidence that the diagnosis of a mood disorder is more appropriate (see Chapter 22). Second, depression is not unusual in all stages of schizophrenia and deserves attention. Third, the suicide rate (10%) among individuals with schizophrenia is higher than that of the general population. Risk factors for suicide are male gender, chronic illness with frequent relapses, frequent short hospitalizations, a negative attitude toward treatment, impulsive behaviour, parasuicide (nonfatal self-harm or gesture), psychosis, and depression (De Hert, McKenzie, & Peuskens, 2001). Periods of untreated psychosis exceeding 1 year and treatment with older typical antipsychotic drugs also have been associated with a higher risk for suicide attempts (Altamura, Bassetti, Bignotti, Pioli, & Mundo, 2003; Harkavy-Friedman, 2007).

Diabetes Mellitus

There is a renewed interest in the relationship of diabetes mellitus and schizophrenia. Years ago, an association was established between glucose regulation and psychiatric disorders (Franzen, 1970; Schimmelbusch, Mueller, & Sheps, 1971). In fact, insulin shock therapy was used in treating severe disorders. Research indicates that diabetes can exacerbate cognitive deficits in persons with schizophrenia, mainly in immediate memory and attention (Han et al., 2013). Also of growing concern is the possibility that people with schizophrenia may be more prone to type II diabetes, with two to three times greater prevalence than the general public (Cohn, 2012). Some suggest that this may be attributable to inherent characteristics (Leucht, Burkard, Henderson, Maj, & Sartorius, 2007; Ryan, Collins, & Thakore, 2003). Evidence that supports this view includes a higher rate of type II diabetes in first-degree relatives of people with schizophrenia and higher rates of impaired glucose tolerance and insulin resistance among people with schizophrenia. However, obesity, which is associated with type II diabetes, is a growing problem in North America, in general, and is complicated in schizophrenia treatment by the tendency of individuals to gain weight once their disease is managed with medications. Weight gain in some individuals may be attributed to a return to a healthier living situation in which regular meals are available and symptoms that interfere with obtaining food regularly (e.g., delusions) are decreased. For other individuals, weight gain may result from the antipsychotic drug (either typical or atypical) selected for the treatment. Not surprisingly, weight gain is often cited as a reason for nonadherence to antipsychotic medications.

Disordered Water Balance

Patients with schizophrenia, particularly of early onset, may experience disordered water balance. Often, this takes the form of water intoxication characterized by abnormally high water intake, followed by a rapid drop in serum sodium levels. The alteration in sodium level leads to diverse neurologic signs, ranging from ataxia to coma and possibly death. The prevalence rates of disordered water balance remain unclear.

The cause of water intoxication is also unknown. Disordered water balance generally precedes water intoxication. Patients characteristically begin compulsively drinking excessive amounts of water. Behaviourally, these patients seem to be "driven to drink" (polydipsia) and may consume between 4 and 10 L of fluid a day. They carry soda cans and water bottles with them, hoard cups or other water containers, and drink frequently from fountains and showers and sometimes from toilets. They make frequent trips to the bathroom because of the excessive need to urinate (**polyuria**). Water intoxication, a complication that is life threatening, occurs when unusually large volumes of ingested water overwhelm the kidneys' capacity to excrete water. As a result, serum sodium levels rapidly fall below the normal range of 135 to 145 mEq/L to a level of 120 mEq/L or less (acute hyponatremia).

This rapid decrease in sodium produces muscle twitching and irritability and puts the patient at risk for increased irritability, seizures, or coma (Boyd & Lapierre, 1996).

AETIOLOGY

Since the 1970s, hypothetical causes of schizophrenia have changed dramatically (Gur & Gur, 2005; Murray & Bramon, 2005; Walker et al., 2004). Purely psychological theories have been replaced by a neurobiologic model that says that patients with schizophrenia have a biologic predisposition or vulnerability that is exacerbated by environmental stressors. Individuals with schizophrenia are thought to have a genetically or biologically determined sensitivity that leaves them vulnerable to an overwhelming onslaught of stimuli from without and within. These inherent vulnerabilities include cognitive, psychophysiologic, social competence, and coping deficits that alter the individual's ability, both cognitively and emotionally, to manage life events and interpersonal situations (Box 20-3 and Fig. 20-1). This section describes the various observations and current theories about the cause of schizophrenia. However, the exact cause of schizophrenia remains elusive.

Biologic Theories

Theories and research about the biologic vulnerability for schizophrenia focus on incorporating multiple observations into a coherent explanation. These observations include the course of the illness already described,

---

BOX 20-3 Deficits That Cause Vulnerability in Schizophrenia

Cognitive Deficits
- Deficits in processing complex information
- Deficits in maintaining a steady focus of attention
- Inability to distinguish between relevant and irrelevant stimuli
- Difficulty forming consistent abstractions
- Impaired memory

Psychophysiologic Deficits
- Deficits in sensory inhibition
- Poor control of autonomic responsiveness

Social Skills Deficits
- Impairments in processing interpersonal stimuli, such as eye contact or assertiveness
- Deficits in conversational capacity
- Deficits in initiating activities
- Deficits in experiencing pleasure

Coping Skills Deficits
- Overassessment of threat
- Underassessment of personal resources
- Overuse of denial

Adapted from McGlashan, T. H. (1994). Psychosocial treatments of schizophrenia: The potential relationships. In N. C. Andreasen (Ed.), *Schizophrenia: from mind to molecule* (pp. 189–215). Washington, DC: American Psychiatric Press.

---

possible brain structure changes identified by postmortem and neuroimaging techniques, familial patterns, and pharmacologic effects on behaviour and neurotransmitter functions in the brain. One of the more recent theories about the cause of schizophrenic vulnerability focuses on neurodevelopment of the brain from the prenatal period through adolescence. Research efforts are making progress in depicting the neurobiologic substrate of schizophrenia (Kaneko & Keshavan, 2012; Keshavan, Tandon, Boutros, & Nasrallah, 2008).

Neuroanatomic Findings

Postmortem and neuroimaging brain studies of patients with schizophrenia show four consistent changes in brain anatomy:

- Decreased blood flow to the left globus pallidus early in the disease
- Absence of normal blood flow increase in frontal lobes during tests of frontal lobe functioning, such as working memory tasks
- Thinner cortex of the medial temporal lobe and a smaller anterior portion of the hippocampus
- Decreases in gray matter and enlarged lateral and third ventricles and widened sulci (Chance, Esiri, & Crow, 2003)

These findings are being used as a basis for exploring the influence of genetic loading, obstetric complications, and differences in familial and nonfamilial patients with schizophrenia (Falkai et al., 2003; McDonald et al., 2002).

Familial Patterns

Evidence supports a familial or genetic base for schizophrenia. First-degree relatives (including siblings and children) are 10 times more likely to experience schizophrenia than are individuals in the general population (APA, 2013). Concordance for schizophrenia is higher among monozygotic (identical) twins than among dizygotic (fraternal) twins, although the rate is not perfectly concordant.

Genetic researchers have sought to identify specific genes responsible for schizophrenia, but replicated results are emerging very slowly (Tsuang, Stone, & Faraone, 2001). The infrequency of reproducible results is likely attributable to the heterogeneity of the disorder, which may not be consistent with a single gene theory. A model that includes several genes is more likely to explain the development of schizophrenia. Two possible locations are on the long arm of chromosome 22 and on chromosome 6 (Kandel, Schwartz, & Jessell, 2000).

Neurodevelopment

Current theory and research attempt to explain how genes or events early in life (especially perinatal events such as infections or obstetric irregularities) would cause

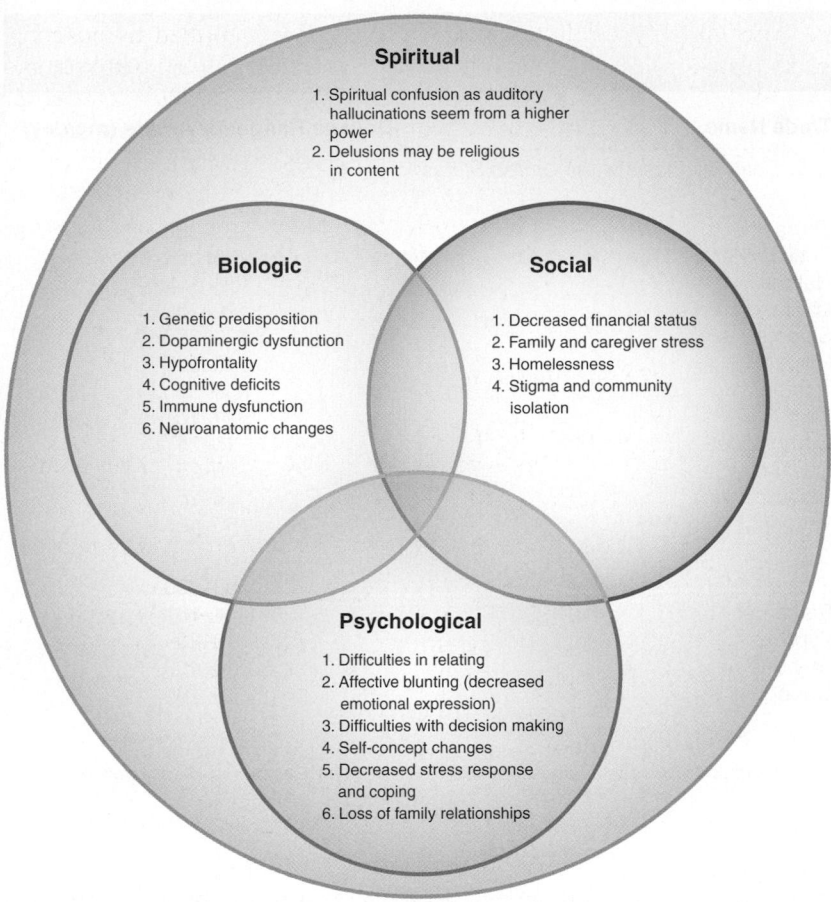

Spiritual

1. Spiritual confusion as auditory hallucinations seem from a higher power
2. Delusions may be religious in content

Biologic

1. Genetic predisposition
2. Dopaminergic dysfunction
3. Hypofrontality
4. Cognitive deficits
5. Immune dysfunction
6. Neuroanatomic changes

Social

1. Decreased financial status
2. Family and caregiver stress
3. Homelessness
4. Stigma and community isolation

Psychological

1. Difficulties in relating
2. Affective blunting (decreased emotional expression)
3. Difficulties with decision making
4. Self-concept changes
5. Decreased stress response and coping
6. Loss of family relationships

schizophrenia yet manifest symptoms only after years—in adolescence or young adulthood. The neurodevelopmental theory explains and reconciles the inconsistent neuroanatomic brain changes that have been found and links them to early development. Neurodevelopmental models of aetiology remain dominant and are fueling advances in epidemiology, imaging, and genetics. It is likely that future whole-genome association studies will further tease out the gene–gene and gene–environment interactions (Rapoport, Addington, & Frangou, 2005).

Brain development from prenatal periods through adolescence requires several coordinated molecular activities, including cell proliferation, cell migration, axonal outgrowth, pruning of neuronal connections, programmed cell death, and myelination. All these activities require coordinated development, usually through the activation and inactivation of proteins by genes. Any of these processes could be disrupted by (1) inherited genes that place the individual at risk for schizophrenia, (2) a wild-type allele of this gene that is activated in adolescence or early adulthood, or (3) genetic sensitizing that leaves the individual susceptible to environmental causes or lesioning during some adverse perinatal event. In addition, several maturational events normally occur during puberty that may affect brain development: (1) changes in dopaminergic, serotonergic, adrenergic, glutamatergic,

gamma-aminobutyric acid (GABA)-ergic, and cholinergic neurotransmitter systems and substrates; (2) a complex combination of synaptic pruning along with substantial brain growth in some areas of the cortex; and (3) changes in the steroid hormonal environment (Chou, Halldin, & Farde, 2003).

Neurotransmitters, Pathways, and Receptors

Theories about the cause and pathophysiology of schizophrenia have been generated from decades of pharmacologic research and management of the disorder. For years, the leading hypothesis about the neurobiology of schizophrenia has been based on observations of drug actions. The *dopamine hypothesis* of schizophrenia arose from observations that antipsychotic drugs (Table 20-3), which so successfully ameliorate or reduce the positive symptoms of schizophrenia, act primarily by blocking postsynaptic dopamine receptors in the brain. In addition, other drugs that enhance dopamine function, such as amphetamines or cocaine, cause behavioural symptoms similar to those of schizophrenia and paranoid subtype in humans, and bizarre stereotyped behaviour in monkeys. Antipsychotic drugs stop these drug-induced behaviours. Based on these observations, researchers concluded that schizophrenia was a syndrome of hyperdopaminergic action in the brain.

Table 20-3	Selected Antipsychotic Drugs	
Generic Name	**Trade Name**	**Dosage Range for Adults (mg/day)**
Selected Conventional Antipsychotic Drugs Used to Treat Psychosis in the United States		
First Generation		
Chlorpromazine	Thorazine	30–800
Fluphenazine	Prolixin; Permitil	0.5–20
Haloperidol	Haldol	1–15
Loxapine	Loxitane	20–250
Mesoridazine	Serentil	100–300
Molindone	Moban	15–225
Perphenazine	Trilafon	4–32
Pimozide	Orap*	1–10
Prochlorperazine	Compazine†	15–25
Thiothixene	Navane	5–25
Trifluoperazine	Stelazine	5–25
Triflupromazine	Vesprin	60–150
Second Generation		
Clozapine	Clozaril	200–600
Risperidone	Risperdal	4–16
Olanzapine	Zyprexa	10–20
Quetiapine	Seroquel	300–400
Ziprasidone	Geodon	40–160

*Approved in the United States for Tourette's syndrome.
†Adapted from Stahl, S. (2008). *Essential psychopharmacology: Neuroscientific basis and practical application* (3rd ed.). Cambridge, UK: Cambridge University Press.

This old, straightforward hypothesis of dopamine hyperactivity is clearly complicated by recent findings. Positron emission tomography (PET) scan findings suggest that in schizophrenia, there is a general reduction in brain metabolism, with a relative hypermetabolism in the left side of the brain and in the left temporal lobe. Abnormalities exist in specific areas of the brain, such as in the left globus pallidus (Sedvall, 1994). These findings support further exploration of differential brain hemisphere function in schizophrenia (Fig. 20-2).

Other PET studies show **hypofrontality** or a reduced cerebral blood flow and glucose metabolism in the prefrontal cortex of people with schizophrenia, and hyperactivity in the limbic area (Buchsbaum, 1990; Figs. 20-3 and 20-4). In addition, several types of dopamine receptors (labeled D_1, D_2, D_3, D_4, and D_5) and dopamine are found in four pathways (mesolimbic, mesocortical, nigrostriatal, and tuberoinfundibular) that innervate different parts of the brain (Kandel et al., 2000) (see Chapter 9). Based on the current understanding of schizophrenia, the following discussion relates the neurobiologic changes to the clinical symptoms.

Positive Symptoms: Hyperactivity of Mesolimbic Tract

Positive symptoms of schizophrenia (hallucinations and delusions) are thought to be caused by dopamine *hyperactivity* in the mesolimbic tract, which regulates memory and emotion. It is hypothesized that this hyperactivity

could result from an overactive modulation of neurotransmission from the nucleus accumbens (Kandel et al., 2000). Another explanation for dopaminergic hyperactivity in the mesolimbic tract is hypoactivity of the mesocortical tract, which normally inhibits dopamine activity in the mesolimbic tract by some type of feedback mechanism. In schizophrenia, the primary defect may be in the mesocortical tract, where dopaminergic function is diminished, thereby decreasing the inhibitory effects on the mesolimbic tract. This disinhibition may be responsible for the overactivity of dopamine in the mesolimbic tract, resulting in the positive symptom cluster (Kandel et al., 2000).

Support for this interconnection between the mesocortical and the mesolimbic tracts has been found in laboratory animals. Destruction of the mesocortical tract of animals resulted in increased activity in the mesolimbic tract, especially in the nucleus accumbens. A compensatory increase in mesolimbic neurons is a suggested mechanism by which this overactivity occurs.

Negative Symptoms and Cognitive Impairment: Hypoactivity of the Mesocortical Tract

Negative symptoms and cognitive impairment are thought to be related to hypoactivity of the mesocortical dopaminergic tract, which by its association with the prefrontal and neocortex contributes to motivation, planning, sequencing of behaviours in time, attention,

FIGURE 20-2. Area of abnormal functioning in a person with schizophrenia. These three views show the excessive neuronal activity in the left globus pallidus (portion of the basal ganglia next to the putamen). (Courtesy of John W. Haller, PhD, Departments of Psychiatry and Radiology, Washington University, St. Louis, MO.)

FIGURE 20-3. Metabolic activity in a control subject (**left**), a subject with obsessive–compulsive disorder (OCD) (**centre**), and a subject with schizophrenia (**right**). (Courtesy of Monte S. Buchsbaum, MD, The Mount Sinai Medical Center and School of Medicine, New York, NY.)

FIGURE 20-4. PET scan with ¹⁸F-deoxyglucose shows metabolic activity in a horizontal section of the brain in a control subject (**left**) and in an unmedicated patient with schizophrenia (**right**). Red and yellow indicate areas of high metabolic activity in the cortex; green and blue indicate lower activity in the white matter areas of the brain. The frontal lobe is magnified to show reduced frontal activity in the prefrontal cortex of the patient with schizophrenia. (Courtesy of Monte S. Buchsbaum, MD, The Mount Sinai Medical Center and School of Medicine, New York, NY.)

and social behaviour (Jibson & Tandon, 2000; Kandel et al., 2000). Negative symptoms, such as poor motivation and planning and flat affect, are remarkably similar to the symptoms of patients who underwent lobotomy procedures in the late 1940s and early 1950s to disconnect the frontal cortex from the rest of the brain. Monkeys who have had dopamine in the prefrontal cortex depleted have difficulty with cognitive tasks. Finally, PET scans of energy metabolism suggest a reduced metabolism in frontal and prefrontal areas (Davidson & Heinrichs, 2003).

Role of Other Dopamine Pathways

The tuberoinfundibular dopaminergic tract is active in prolactin regulation and may be the source of neuroendocrine changes observed in schizophrenia. The nigrostriatal dopaminergic tract modulates motor activity and is believed to be the site of the **extrapyramidal side effects** of antipsychotic drugs, such as pseudoparkinsonism and **tardive dyskinesia** (abnormal involuntary movements). This may also be the site of some motor symptoms of schizophrenia, such as stereotypic behaviour.

Role of Other Receptors

Other receptors are also involved in dopamine neurotransmission, especially serotonergic receptors. It is becoming clear that schizophrenia does not result from the dysregulation of a single neurotransmitter or biogenic amine (e.g., norepinephrine, dopamine, serotonin). Investigators are also hypothesizing a role for glutamate and GABA (Ghose et al., 2003) because of the complex interconnections of neuronal transmission and the complexity and heterogeneity of schizophrenia symptoms. The N-methyl-D-aspartate class of glutamate receptor is being studied because of the actions of phencyclidine (PCP) at these sites and the similarity of the psychotic behaviours that are produced when someone takes PCP (see Figs. 20-2–20-4).

Neural Connectivity

Manifestations of poor mental coordination include difficulty in a variety of functions, such as measuring time or space; making inferences about relationships; and coordinating the processing, priority setting, retrieval, and expression of information. It is being hypothesized that there may be a basic developmental disorder of the neural connectivity involving multiple molecular mechanisms (Benes, 2000; Penn, 2001; Sallet et al., 2003).

Psychological Theories

Several psychological frameworks have been used to explain the aetiology of schizophrenia. Before biologic and neurochemical discoveries, these psychological theories presented the primary cause of schizophrenia as dysfunctional parenting in early childhood development. Families often were blamed (e.g., the "schizophrenogenic mother" was suggested as a cause) and alienated by mental health professionals. These theories are no longer held valid, and neurochemical–biologic theories have replaced them.

Social Theories

There are no social theories believed to explain schizophrenia, but some theories focus on patterns of family interaction that seem to affect the eventual outcome and social adjustment of individuals with schizophrenia. The theory of **expressed emotion** (EE) correlates certain family communication patterns with an increase in symptoms and relapse in patients with schizophrenia. Families are classified as high-EE families when they make negative comments about family members; when there are aspects of speech that connote criticism, hostility, and negativity about the patient; and when they are emotionally "overly involved" with the patient, such as being overprotective or self-sacrificing. Low-EE families make fewer negative comments and show less overinvolvement with the patient. Families that rate high in the areas of criticism, hostility, and battles for control are hypothesized to be associated with increases in the patient's positive symptoms and relapse.

Research related to emotional expressiveness is contradictory and divisive. Although families categorized as low in EE have been shown to accept the patient as having a legitimate illness and have an understanding that interpersonal problems can exacerbate the illness (Weisman, Gomes, & Lopez, 2003), families high in EE have not been associated with either a greater family history of schizophrenia or the chronicity of the illness (Subotnik, Goldstein, Nuechterlein, Woo, & Mintz, 2002; Wuerker, Long, Haas, & Bellack, 2002).

Although this research might contribute to the understanding of how negative family interaction affects the patient, there are negative consequences to categorizing families in this dualistic manner. Professionals may tend to erroneously blame families for causing relapse or limit the patient's contact with the family, thus further alienating families who are so vital to the care and support of the patient.

There are numerous social barriers that prevent people with mental illness from getting the care they need. One of the major ones is the social stigma that surrounds mental illnesses (see Chapter 3). Box 20-4 describes the impact of living with a stigmatized illness. Another barrier is difficulty accessing recovery-oriented mental health services that provide comprehensive interventions, resources, and continuity of care. A Canadian study found that individuals experiencing symptoms of psychosis for the first time tried an average of 2.3 times to obtain help. The average length of time the psychosis remained untreated was

---

BOX 20-4

Clinical Vignette

GRADUATE STUDENT IN PERIL

BGW, born in 1985, spent most of his teenage years using drugs and alcohol, behaviour that started when he was 11. He and his small group of friends spent their teenage years outside of school running around on bicycles. He failed 8th grade, repeated it, and made it to 10th grade. He was removed permanently from school at the age of 16. His dress included a dirty denim jacket or Army fatigues, torn tee shirts with rock band logos, and tight-fitting jeans. At age 16, he was hospitalized for a psychotic episode initiated by LSD; it was the scariest moment of his life. His mind had been getting fuzzier every day; he had dabbled with black magic and Satanism. Later, he admitted that for years, he had been trapped in a fantasy land, only partially explained by his drug use.

Years of treatment followed, and even with abstinence from drugs, his mental status fluctuated. Once antipsychotic agents were prescribed, he began to feel like himself. He was motivated to complete his high school diploma and entered college. He kept his mental illness a secret. While in graduate school, his thoughts, feelings, and behaviours began to change. His thinking became delusional, his moods unpredictable, and his behaviours illogical. Finally, he was hospitalized once again, and his condition was stabilized with medications. Currently, he is reapplying to graduate school and this time vowing to keep people close to him aware of his mental status.

Adapted from Oxford University Press and the Maryland Psychiatric Research Center. (2002). Graduate student in peril: A first person account of schizophrenia. *Schizophrenia Bulletin, 28*(4), 745–755.

---

almost 2 years (Addington, van Mastrigt, Jutchinson, & Addington, 2002; Standing Senate Committee on Social Affairs, Science and Technology, 2006). Admittedly, mental health service delivery systems are often fragmented, with the quality and types of services varying between communities. Canada's remote rural regions present particular challenges to the provision of timely, comprehensive mental health care. Stigma is an ongoing issue, which prevents individuals from seeking timely mental health assistance.

■ INTERDISCIPLINARY TREATMENT

The most effective treatment approach for individuals with schizophrenia involves a variety of disciplines, including nursing, psychiatry, psychology, social work, occupational and recreational therapies, pastoral counselling, and peer support workers. Pharmacologic management is the responsibility of the physicians and nurses; all the members of the mental health team can implement various psychosocial interventions. Various professionals and paraprofessionals are necessary because of the complex nature of schizophrenia symptoms and the continuum of interventions required to enhance best outcomes. Inpatient teams are often the starting point, but the spectrum of interventions must include outpatient teams and community-based, recovery-oriented programs. Specialized assertive community teams are particularly helpful in fostering recovery from schizophrenia (see Chapter 4 for continuum of care).

A considerable amount of overlap exists among these professionals and the therapeutic interventions and services they perform. Individual, group, and family education or counselling may be performed by nurses, psychiatrists, psychologists, certified social workers, and pastoral counsellors. Nurses, along with occupational and recreational therapists, can help patients with schizophrenia cope with the disruptions in their day-to-day functioning caused by cognitive and social deficits associated with negative symptoms. Teams of professionals working in partnership with self-help and peer-support programs can shape a favourable recovery environment for stabilizing and enhancing the lives of people who have schizophrenia. However, barriers to this type of treatment abound and include inadequate funding; limitations on physician fee reimbursements; staff shortages (in particular, skilled mental health nurses); large caseloads; insufficient inpatient opportunities; and insufficient community supports, facilities, and social services. Despite these barriers, nurses can contribute significantly to interdisciplinary care given nursing's emphasis on patients' responses to their illness, their functional adaptation, holistic needs, including physical and psychosocial requirements, and their attention to family support.

PRIORITY CARE ISSUES

Several special concerns exist when working with people with schizophrenia. About 20% to 50% of people with the diagnosis of schizophrenia attempt suicide, and 10% commit suicide either as a result of psychosis in acute stages or in response to depression in the chronic phase (Canadian Psychiatric Association, 2005). A systematic review of the literature found consensus for a 5% lifetime risk for suicide for persons with schizophrenia (Hor & Taylor, 2010). Suicide assessment should always be done with a person who is experiencing a first-psychotic episode. In an inpatient unit, patient safety concerns extend to potential aggressive actions toward staff and other patients during episodes of psychoses. A priority of care during times of acute illness is treatment with antipsychotic medications.

During the recovery phase of schizophrenia, patients need help in accepting their illness and developing hopeful expectations for their future. They also need help to avoid social isolation through improved social and vocational skills and living arrangements that ensure contact with others (De Hert et al., 2001; Frese, Knight, & Saks, 2009). Interventions that focus on psychosocial goals can address the hopelessness that leads to suicide.

FAMILY RESPONSE TO DISORDER

Few families have had experience with mental illness to help them deal with the manifestations of schizophrenia.

The first episode of psychosis is often accompanied by mixed emotions of disbelief, shock, fear, and care and concern for the family member. Hope that this is an isolated or transient episode may also be present. Families initially may seek reasons for the psychotic episode, attributing it to taking illicit drugs or to extraordinary stress or fatigue. Others, particularly parents, may even blame themselves. They often do not know how to comfort their disturbed family member and may find themselves fearful of his or her behaviours. If the patient is hostile and aggressive toward family members, the family may respond with anger and hostility along with fear, confusion, and anxiety. During these episodes, some families may have to seek help from police or a crisis response team to control the situation. Coming to terms with the mental illness of a loved one is often described as an experience of catastrophic proportions (Addington, McCleery, & Addington, 2005; Hamilton Wilson, 2012).

The initial period of illness for a patient and family that receive a diagnosis of schizophrenia is extraordinarily difficult. Often, during the initial phase of treatment, families are the primary caregivers for an ill relative. This necessitates that families have opportunities for explanation, education about the illness, and access to timely support. As families acknowledge the meaning of the diagnosis and the potential long-term rehabilitation required, they often feel overwhelmed, angry, and depressed (Hamilton Wilson, 2012). We are living more than 50 years after the original theories of the schizophrenogenic family were popularized, but the notion of parents as potential causal factors in serious mental illness remains. Diagnostic labels are imbued with history and still resonate with fear and apprehension. During the early moments, when families receive the diagnostic proclamation, they generally hold the same unenlightened notions of schizophrenia as others within our culture. It is imperative then, for nurses and other health care providers to provide families with useable explanations that assist them in thinking about themselves in a way that reduces any notions of blame or self-reproach. Families are often fearful that the future they once anticipated will not be realized or will take a very different form. Nurses can help families hold the hope for their ill relative.

The issue of family caregiving for a relative with serious mental illness has recently received attention from the MHCC. A working group from the commission developed a comprehensive guide for caregivers that contains many useful recommendations. Nurses should familiarize themselves with the recommendations contained in this document entitled, *National Guidelines for a Comprehensive Service System to Support Family Caregivers of Adults with Mental Health Problems and Illnesses* (MHCC, 2013c).

Nursing Management: Human Response to Disorder

The nursing management of the patient with schizophrenia usually lasts many years. Different phases of the illness require various nursing interventions at varying intensity. During exacerbation of symptoms, many patients are hospitalized for stabilization. During periods of relative stability, the nurse helps the patient maintain a therapeutic regimen, develop positive mental health strategies, devise strategies to prepare for and cope with the stress, and reclaim his or her life as much as possible.

Because of the complexity of this major psychiatric disorder, the nursing management for each domain is discussed separately. In reality, the nursing process steps overlap in all domains. For example, medication management is a direct biologic intervention; however, the effects of medications also are seen in psychological functioning. In the clinical area, effective nursing management requires an integration of the assessment data from all domains into meaningful interventions. Nursing interventions should cover all domains, including biologic, psychological, social (including family functioning), and spiritual. See Nursing Care Plan 20-1 and Interdisciplinary Treatment Plan 20-1.

Nursing Care Plan 20-1

Patient With First-Episode Psychosis: Probable Schizophrenia

JT is a 19-year-old man who was brought to the hospital following his return from college, where he had locked himself in his room for 3 days. He was talking to nonexistent people in a strange language. His room was covered with small pieces of notepaper with single words on them. His parents were summoned and immediately made arrangements for him to be assessed and, if necessary, subsequently hospitalized.

Setting: Psychiatric Intensive Care Unit

Baseline Assessment: JT is a 6'1", 145-pound young man whose appearance is dishevelled. He has not slept for 4 days and appears frightened. He is hypervigilant, pacing, and mumbling to himself. He is vague about past drug use, but his parents do not believe that he has used drugs. He appears to be hallucinating, conversing as if someone is in the room. He is confused and unable to write, speak, or think coherently. He is disoriented to time and place. Lab values are within normal limits except Hgb, 10.2, and Hct, 32. He has not eaten for several days.

Associated Psychiatric Diagnosis	Medications
Schizophrenia	Risperidone (Risperdal), 2 mg bid, then titrate to 3 mg if needed
	Lorazepam (Ativan), 2 mg PO or IM for agitation PRN
Psychosocial and contextual issues: Educational problems (failing), social problems (withdrawn from peers)	

Nursing Diagnosis 1: Disturbed Thought Processes

Defining Characteristics	Related Factors
Inaccurate interpretation of stimuli (people thinking his thoughts)	Uncompensated alterations in brain activity
Cognitive impairment—attention, memory, and executive function impairment	
Suspiciousness	
Hallucinations	

Continued

Nursing Care Plan 20-1 *(Continued)*

Outcomes

Initial	Long Term
Decrease or eliminate hallucinations	Use coping strategies to deal with hallucinations or delusions if they reappear
Accurate interpretation of the environment (stop thinking that people are thinking his thoughts)	Communicate clearly with others
Improvement in cognitive functioning (improved attention, memory, and executive functioning)	Maintain cognitive functioning

Interventions	Rationale	Ongoing Assessment
Initiate a nurse–patient relationship by using an accepting, nonjudgemental approach. Be patient.	A therapeutic relationship will provide patient support as he begins to deal with the realization that he has experienced a first-episode psychosis and that diagnosis, although uncertain at this stage, could be the onset of schizophrenia. Be patient and offer information in small, gradual ways. Information processing is likely to be slow at this time.	Determine the extent to which JT is willing to trust and engage in a relationship.
Administer risperidone as prescribed. Observe for effects, side effects, and adverse effects. Begin teaching about the medication and its importance, once symptoms subside.	Risperidone is a D₂ and 5-HT2A antagonist and is indicated for the management of psychotic disorders.	Make sure JT swallows the pills. Monitor for relief of positive symptoms and assess side effects, especially extrapyramidal. Monitor BP for orthostatic hypotension and body temperature increase (neuroleptic malignant syndrome [NMS]).
During hallucinations and delusional thinking, assess significance (is it frightening, voices telling him to hurt himself or others?). Reassure JT that you will keep him safe. (Do not try to convince JT that his hallucinations are not real.) Redirect to the here-and-now.	It is important to understand the context of the hallucinations and delusions to be able to provide the appropriate interventions. By avoiding arguments about the content, the nurse will enhance communication.	Assess the meaning of the hallucination or delusion to the patient. Determine whether he is a danger to himself or others. Determine whether the patient can be redirected.
Assess the ability for self-care activities.	Disturbed thinking may interfere with JT's ability to carry out activities of daily living (ADLs).	Continue to assess: determine whether the patient can manage self-care.

Evaluation

Outcomes	Revised Outcomes	Interventions
Hallucinations and delusions began to decrease within 5 days.	Participate in unit activities according to Interdisciplinary Treatment Plan.	Encourage attendance at treatment activities.
He is oriented to time, place, and person. Attention and memory are improving.	Agree to continue to take antipsychotic medications as prescribed.	Teach JT about medications. Teach JT about first-episode psychosis initially and schizophrenia when diagnosis is confirmed.

Nursing Care Plan 20-1 (Continued)

Nursing Diagnosis 2: Risk for Violence

Defining Characteristics	Related Factors
Assaultive toward others, self, and environment	Frightened, secondary to auditory hallucinations and delusional thinking
Presence of pathophysiologic risk factors: delusional thinking	Poor impulse control
	Dysfunctional communication patterns

Outcomes

Initial	Long Term
Avoid hurting self or assaulting other patients or staff. Decrease agitation and aggression.	Control behaviour with assistance from staff and parents.

Interventions

Interventions	Rationale	Ongoing Assessment
Acknowledge the patient's fears, hallucinations, and delusions.	Hallucinations and delusions change an individual's perception of environmental stimuli. A patient who is frightened will respond because of his need to stay safe.	Determine whether the patient is able to hear you. Assess his response to your comments and his ability to concentrate on what is being said.
Offer the patient choices of maintaining safety: keeping distance from others, medication for relaxation, etc.	By having choices, he will begin to develop a sense of control over his behaviour.	Observe the patient's nonverbal communication for evidence of increased agitation.
Administer lorazepam, 2 mg, for agitation. Oral route is preferable over injection.	Exact mechanisms of action are not understood, but this medication is believed to potentiate the inhibitory neurotransmitter GABA, relieving anxiety and producing sedation.	Observe for a decrease in agitated behaviour.
JT gradually decreased agitated behaviour. Lorazepam was given regularly for the first 2 days.	Demonstrate control of behaviour by resisting hallucinations and delusions.	Teach JT about the effects of hallucinations and delusions. Problem-solve ways of controlling hallucinations if they occur. Emphasize the importance of taking medications.

Many nursing diagnoses apply to a person with schizophrenia. This is particularly true given that schizophrenia affects so many aspects of an individual's functioning and that symptoms can be observed in cognitive, emotional, family, social, and physical functioning. The applicable diagnoses can be categorized into the phases in which they are most likely to appear. However, it is important to note that even though they have been sorted into these categories, they may still represent recovery challenges in other phases. It is also important to note that the periods between exacerbations of symptoms are actually very important phases for pursuing recovery goals.

Biologic Domain

Biologic Assessment

The following sections highlight the important assessment areas for people with schizophrenia.

Current and Past Health Status and Physical Examination

It is important to conduct a thorough history and physical examination to rule out medical illness or substance abuse that could cause the psychiatric symptoms. It is also important to screen for comorbid medical illnesses that need to be treated, such as diabetes mellitus, hypertension,

INTERDISCIPLINARY TREATMENT PLAN 20-1

Patient With First Episode Psychosis: Probable Schizophrenia

Admission Date	Date of This Plan	Type of Plan: Check Appropriate Box
05/03/14		☐ Initial ☐ Master ☐ 30 ☐ 60 ☐ 90 ☐ Other

Treatment Team Present:
A. Barton, MD; J. Jones, RN; C. Anderson, RPN; B. Thomas, PhD; T. Toon, SW; J. Barker, Rec T; F. Huffern, OT; H. Kitchen, Peer Support Worker (PeerSW)

DIAGNOSIS (DSM-5):

Schizophreniform disorder, possible schizophrenia
Context: Educational problems (failing)
Social problems (withdrawn from peers)

ASSETS (MEDICAL, PSYCHOLOGICAL, SOCIAL, EDUCATIONAL, VOCATIONAL, RECREATIONAL):

1. First episode of psychosis. No evidence of drug use.
2. Premorbid functional level appears to be normal.
3. Maintained good grades in high school.
4. Has supportive family members.

Prob. No.	Date	Problem/Need	Code	Code	Date
1	3/5/14	Is hallucinating and had delusional thoughts. Unable to communicate with parents or staff.	T		
2	3/5/14	Is aggressive and is striking out at staff and unfamiliar people.	T		
3	3/5/14	Dropped out of college because of thoughts and behaviours.	X		
4	3/5/14	Family members are very upset about their son's psychiatric symptoms.	T		

CODE   T = Problem must be addressed in treatment.
N = Problem noted and will be monitored.
X = Problem noted, but deferred/inactive/no action necessary.
O = Problem to be addressed in aftercare/continuing care.
I = Problem incorporated into another problem.
R = Resolved.

No. 1 Problem/Need	Date Identified	Problem Resolved Discontinuation Date
Is hallucinating and has delusional thoughts. Unable to communicate with parents or staff.	3/5/14	

Objective(s)/Short-Term Goals	Target Date	Achievement Date
1. Reduce report and observations of hallucinations and delusions.	3/15/14	

Treatment Interventions	Frequency	Person Responsible
1. Antipsychotic therapy for hallucinations and delusions. Administer and monitor for adherence, effect, and side effects.	As prescribed	MD/RN
2. Monitor the frequency of hallucinations and delusions.	Close observation for 24–48 hours, then according to RN judgement	RN/RPN/LPN
3. Attend Symptom Management group as symptoms subside.	Daily	PhD, RN, RPN

INTERDISCIPLINARY TREATMENT PLAN 20.1 *(Continued)*

ASSETS (MEDICAL, PSYCHOLOGICAL, SOCIAL, EDUCATIONAL, VOCATIONAL, RECREATIONAL):

No. 2 Problem/Need	Date Identified	Problem Resolved/Discontinuation Date
Is aggressive and is striking out at staff and unfamiliar people.	3/5/14	

Objective(s)/Short-Term Goals	Target Date	Achievement Date
1. De-escalate aggressive behaviour.	3/15/14	

Treatment Interventions	Frequency	Person Responsible
1. Keep the patient in a quiet, nonstimulating environment. Assign a private room.	Ongoing	RN/RPN/LPN
2. Administer antianxiety medication as needed.	PRN	MD/RN/RPN
3. Use de-escalation techniques when approaching the patient.	Ongoing	Everyone
4. Assign to anger management group, if needed when psychotic symptoms decrease.	In 1 week	RN/RPN/LPN

No. 4 Problem/Need	Date Identified	Problem Resolved/Discontinuation Date
Family members are very upset about their son's psychiatric symptoms.	3/5/14	

Objective(s)/Short-Term Goals	Target Date	Achievement Date
Increase the family's comfort levels with mental illness.	3/15/14	

Treatment Interventions	Frequency	Person Responsible
1. Meet with the family members each time they visit. Provide support, counselling and education to the family.	Ongoing	RPN/RN/MD
2. Encourage the family to attend family support group.	Weekly	RN/SW/PeerSW
3. Provide community resources for the treatment of mental illness.	When visiting	RN/RPN/PeerSW

Responsible QMHP   **Client or Guardian**   **Staff Physician**

Signature   Date   Signature   Date   Signature   Date

---

and cardiac disease, or a family history of such disorders. People with schizophrenia have a higher mortality rate from physical illness and often have smoking-related illnesses, such as emphysema, and other pulmonary and cardiac problems. The nurse should determine whether the patient smokes tobacco, which not only affects the patient's health but also can affect the clearance of medications.

Physical Functioning

The negative symptoms of schizophrenia are often manifested in terms of impairment in physical functioning. Self-care often deteriorates, and sleep may be nonexistent during acute phases. Information regarding physical functioning may best be collected from family members.

● **STUDY NOTE**
When assessing a patient with schizophrenia, the nurse should prioritize the severity of the current responses to the disorder. If hallucinations are impairing function, then managing hallucinations is a priority, and medications are needed immediately. If hallucinations are not a problem, coping with the negative symptoms becomes a priority.

Nutritional Assessment

A nutritional history should be completed to determine baseline eating habits and preferences. Medications can alter normal nutrition, and the patient may need to limit calories or fat consumption.

Fluid Imbalance Assessment

Although quite rare, the nurse should remain alert for signs of polydipsia and polyuria to identify disordered water balance. Patients suspected of having disordered water balance should be assessed for signs and symptoms of hyponatremia, water intoxication, excessive urination, incontinence, or periodically elevated blood pressure. Signs and symptoms of hypervolemia that may be evident include puffiness of the face or eyes, abdominal distention, and hypothermia. These patients should be weighed daily, and their urine specific gravity and serum sodium levels should be monitored (Boyd & Lapierre, 1996).

Pharmacologic Assessment

Baseline information about the initial psychological and physical functioning should be obtained before the initiation of medication (or as early as possible). Side effects of medications should be assessed. Patients are often physically awkward and have poor coordination, motor abnormalities, and abnormal eye tracking. Before medication begins, standardized assessment of abnormal motor movements should be conducted using one of several assessment tools designed for that purpose, such as the Abnormal Involuntary Movement Scale (AIMS) (Guy, 1976) (see Appendix C), the Dyskinesia Identification System: Condensed User Scale (DISCUS) (Sprague & Kalachnik, 1991) (Fig. 20-5), or the Simpson-Angus Rating Scale (Simpson & Angus, 1970) (see Appendix B), which is designed for Parkinson-like symptoms.

Nursing Diagnoses for Biologic Domain

Typical nursing diagnoses focusing on the biologic domain for the person during all phases of schizophrenia include self-care deficit and disturbed sleep pattern. During a relapse, ineffective therapeutic regimen management, imbalanced nutrition, excess fluid volume, and sexual dysfunction are possible diagnoses. Constipation may occur if the patient takes anticholinergic medications.

● STUDY NOTE

Monitoring actions and side effects of medications is a priority nursing intervention. Typical and atypical antipsychotics both contribute to troublesome and uncomfortable side effects. Although most patients will be tried on atypical medications, the older typical style medications will still be used occasionally.

Interventions for Biologic Domain

Nursing interventions during the initial acute phase of schizophrenia include prompt, safe, and informed administration of antipsychotic medications. During any stage, attention to self-care needs and the patient's ability to maintain hygiene and adequate nutrition are important.

Promotion of Self-Care Activities

For many individuals with schizophrenia, the plan of care will include specific interventions to enhance self-care, nutrition, and overall health knowledge. Negative symptoms commonly leave patients unable to initiate these seemingly simple activities. Developing a daily schedule of routine activities (e.g., showering and shaving) can help the patient structure the day. Most patients actually know how to perform self-care activities (e.g., hygiene, grooming) but are not motivated (avolition) to carry them out consistently. Interventions include developing a schedule with the patient for various hygiene activities and emphasizing the importance of maintaining appropriate self-care activities.

Activity, Exercise, and Nutritional Interventions

Encouraging activity and exercise is necessary, not only to maintain a healthy lifestyle but also to counteract the side effects of psychiatric medications that cause weight gain. Because the diagnosis of schizophrenia is usually made in late adolescence or early adulthood, it is possible to establish solid exercise patterns early.

During episodes of acute psychosis, patients are unable to focus on eating. Often when patients begin atypical antipsychotic medications, normal satiety and hunger responses change, and overeating or weight gain can become a problem. Promoting healthy nutrition is a key intervention. Maintaining healthy nutrition and monitoring calorie intake also become important because of the effect many medications have on eating habits. Patients report that appetite increases and cravings for food develop when some neuroleptic medications are initiated.

Weight gain is one of the reasons some patients become resistant to taking medication. It also may be a contributing factor to the development of type II diabetes mellitus. As such, this places patients at greater risk for several health complications and early death. Monitoring for diabetes and managing weight are important activities for all care providers (Gough, 2005; Stahl, 2002). Patients should be screened for risk factors of diabetes, such as family history, obesity as indicated by a body mass index (BMI) exceeding or equal to 27, and age older than 45 years. Patients' weight should be measured at regular intervals and their BMI calculated. Blood pressure readings should be taken regularly. Laboratory findings for triglycerides, HDL cholesterol, and glucose level should be monitored and reviewed regularly as well. All providers should be alert to the development of diabetic ketoacidosis, particularly in patients known to have diabetes who begin taking new antipsychotic agents. A program to address weight gain should be initiated at the earliest sign of weight gain (probably between 5 and 10 pounds over desired body weight). Reduced caloric intake may be accomplished by increasing the patient's access to affordable, healthful, and easy-to-prepare foods. Behavioural

	NAME	I.D.

(HEALTH CARE FACILITY)
Dyskinesia Identification System:
Condensed User Scale (DISCUS)

CURRENT PSYCHOTROPICS/ANTI-
CHOLINERGIC AND TOTAL MG/DAY

_____ ____ mg
_____ ____ mg
_____ ____ mg
_____ ____ mg

See Instructions on the Other Side

EXAM TYPE (check one)
- ☐ 1. Baseline
- ☐ 2. Annual
- ☐ 3. Semi annual
- ☐ 4. D/C—1 month
- ☐ 5. D/C—2 months
- ☐ 6. D/C—3 months
- ☐ 7. Admission
- ☐ 8. Other

COOPERATION (check one)
- ☐ 1. None
- ☐ 2. Partial
- ☐ 3. Full

SCORING

0—**Not present** (movements not observed or some movements observed but not considered abnormal)

1—**Minimal** (abnormal movements are difficult to detect or movements are easy to detect but occur only once or twice in a short nonrepetitive manner)

2—**Mild** (abnormal movements occur infrequently and are easy to detect)

3—**Moderate** (abnormal movements occur frequently and are easy to detect)

4—**Severe** (abnormal movements occur almost continuously **and** are easy to detect)

NA—**Not assessed** (an assessment for an item is not able to be made)

ASSESSMENT
DISCUS Item and Score (circle one score for each item)

	Item	Score
FACE	1. Tics	0 1 2 3 4 NA
	2. Grimaces	0 1 2 3 4 NA
EYES	3. Blinking	0 1 2 3 4 NA
ORAL	4. Chewing/Lip Smacking	0 1 2 3 4 NA
	5. Puckering/Sucking/ Thrusting Lower Lip	0 1 2 3 4 NA
LINGUAL	6. Tongue Thrusting/ Tongue in Cheek	0 1 2 3 4 NA
	7. Tonic Tongue	0 1 2 3 4 NA
	8. Tongue Tremor	0 1 2 3 4 NA
	9. Athetoid/Myokymic/ Lateral Tongue	0 1 2 3 4 NA
HEAD/ NECK/ TRUNK	10. Retrocollis/Torticollis	0 1 2 3 4 NA
	11. Shoulder/Hip Torsion	0 1 2 3 4 NA
UPPER LIMB	12. Athetoid/Myokymic Finger–Wrist–Arm	0 1 2 3 4 NA
	13. Pill Rolling	0 1 2 3 4 NA
LOWER LIMB	14. Ankle Flexion/ Foot Tapping	0 1 2 3 4 NA
	15. Toe Movement	0 1 2 3 4 NA

COMMENTS/OTHER
_____
_____
_____
_____

TOTAL SCORE
(items 1–15 only)

EXAM DATE

RATER SIGNATURE AND TITLE | NEXT EXAM DATE

EVALUATION

1. Greater than 90 d neuroleptic exposure? : YES NO
2. Scoring/intensity level met? : YES NO
3. Other diagnostic conditions? : YES NO
   (if yes, specify)

   _____
   _____

4. Last exam date: _____
   Last total score: _____
   Last conclusion: _____

   Preparer signature and title for items 1–4 (if different from the physician):

5. Conclusion (circle one):

   A. No TD (if scoring prerequi- site met, list other diagnostic conditions or explain in comments)
   B. Probable TD
   C. Masked TD
   D. Withdrawal TD
   E. Persistent TD
   F. Remitted TD
   G. Other (specify in comments)

6. Comments:

   _____
   _____
   _____
   _____
   _____
   _____
   _____

CLINICIAN SIGNATURE | DATE

From Sprague, R. L., & Kalachnik, J. E. (1991). Reliability, validity, and a total score cutoff for the Dyskinesia Identification Scale System: Condensed User Scale (DISCUS) with mentally ill and mentally retarded populations. *Psychopharmacology Bulletin, 27*, 51–58.

FIGURE 20-5. The dyskinesia identification system. (From Sprague, R. L. & Kalachnik, J. E. (1991). Reliability, validity, and a total score cutoff for the Dyskinesia Identification Scale System: Condensed User Scale (DISCUS) with mentally ill and mentally retarded populations. *Psychopharmacology Bulletin, 27*, 51–58.)

management of weight gain includes keeping a food diary, diet teaching, and exercise and weight management support groups.

Thermoregulation Interventions

Patients with schizophrenia may have disturbed body temperature regulation. In winter, they may seem to be oblivious to cold weather. In the heat of summer, they may dress for winter. Observing patients' responses to temperatures helps identify problems in this area. In patients who are taking psychiatric medications, body temperature needs to be monitored, and the patient needs to be protected from extremes in temperature. Sun safety is also important, and regular use of a sunscreen product to avoid skin damage from sunburn should be recommended.

Pharmacologic Interventions

Early in the 20th century, somatic treatment of schizophrenia included hydrotherapy (baths), wet-pack sheets, insulin shock therapy, electroconvulsive therapy, psychosurgery, and occupational and physical therapies. But in the early 1950s, treatment of schizophrenia drastically changed with the accidental discovery that a drug, chlorpromazine, used to induce anesthesia also calmed patients with schizophrenia. Optimism persists as older medications continue to be used effectively while offering clues into the workings of the brain and as new discoveries about the brain lead to more precise medications for treating schizophrenia.

Antipsychotic drugs have the general effect of blocking dopamine transmission in the brain by blocking D_2 receptors to some degree (see Chapter 12). Some also block other dopamine receptors and receptors of other neurotransmitters to varying degrees. For the most part, the antidopamine effects are not specific to the mesolimbic and mesocortical tracts associated with schizophrenia, but instead travel to all the dopamine receptor sites throughout the brain. This results in desirable antipsychotic effects but also creates some unpleasant and undesirable side effects. The effects of antipsychotic drugs on other neurotransmitter systems may account for additional side effects.

The newer antipsychotic drugs risperidone (Risperdal; Box 20-5), olanzapine (Zyprexa), quetiapine (Seroquel), paliperidone (Invega), ziprasidone (Zeldox), and aripiprazole (Abilify) appear to be more efficacious and safer than conventional antipsychotics. They are available in a variety of formulations. Risperidone (Consta) and paliperidone (Invega Sustenna) are both available in a long-acting injectable form. They are effective in treating negative and positive symptoms. These newer drugs also affect several other neurotransmitter systems, including serotonin. This is believed to contribute to their overall antipsychotic effectiveness (see Chapter 9).

Monitoring and Administering Medications

Antipsychotic medications are the treatment of choice for patients with psychosis. The use of conventional or typical antipsychotics (e.g., haloperidol, Thorazine) decreased dramatically with the introduction of the second generation of antipsychotics. Generally, it takes

---

BOX 20-5 Drug Profile

RISPERIDONE (RISPERDAL; CONSTA, LONG-ACTING INJECTABLE)

Drug Class: Atypical antipsychotic.

Receptor Affinity: Antagonist with high affinity for D_2 and 5-HT_2, also histamine (H_1) and α_1- and α_2-adrenergic receptors, weak affinity for D_1 and other serotonin receptor subtypes; no affinity for acetylcholine or beta-adrenergic receptors.

Indications: Psychotic disorders such as schizophrenia, schizoaffective illness, bipolar affective disorder, and major depression with psychotic features.

Routes and Dosage: 1-, 2-, 3-, and 4-mg tablets and liquid concentrate (1 mg/mL). 25, 50, and 75 mg long-acting IM.

Adult Dosage: Initial dose typically 1 mg bid. Maximal effect at 6 mg/day. Safety not established above 16 mg/day. Use lowest possible dose to alleviate symptoms.

Geriatric: Initial dose, 0.5 mg/day, increase slowly as tolerated.

Children: Safety and efficacy with this age group have not been established.

Injection: Initiate 25 or 50 mg with oral supplementation for 2 to 3 weeks. Then, injections only, every 2 to 3 weeks. Given IM in gluteal area.

Half-Life (Peak Effect): mean, 20 hours (1 hour, peak active metabolite = 3 to 17 hours).

Select Adverse Reactions: Insomnia, agitation, anxiety, extrapyramidal symptoms, headache, rhinitis, somnolence, dizziness, headache, constipation, nausea, dyspepsia, vomiting, abdominal pain, hypersalivation, tachycardia, orthostatic hypotension, fever, chest pain, coughing, photosensitivity, and weight gain.

Warning: Rare development of NMS. Observe frequently for early signs of tardive dyskinesia. Use caution with individuals who have cardiovascular disease; risperidone can cause ECG changes. Avoid its use during pregnancy or while breast-feeding. Hepatic or renal impairments increase plasma concentration.

Specific Patient/Family Education
• Notify the prescriber if tremor, motor restlessness, abnormal movements, chest pain, or other unusual symptoms develop.
• Avoid alcohol and other CNS depressant drugs.
• Notify the prescriber if pregnancy is possible or planning to become pregnant. Do not breast-feed while taking this medication.
• Notify the prescriber before taking any other prescription or over-the-counter (OTC) medication.
• It may impair judgement, thinking, or motor skills; avoid driving or other hazardous tasks.
• During titration, the individual may experience orthostatic hypotension and should change positions slowly.
• Do not abruptly discontinue.

BOX 20-6 Drug Profile

CLOZAPINE (CLOZARIL)

Drug Class: Atypical antipsychotic

Receptor Affinity: D_1 and D_2 blockade, antagonist for 5-HT_2, H_1, α-adrenergic, and acetylcholine. These additional antagonist effects may contribute to some of its therapeutic effects. It produces fewer extrapyramidal effects than standard antipsychotics with lower risk for tardive dyskinesia.

Indications: Severely ill individuals who have schizophrenia and have not responded to standard antipsychotic treatment. Unlabelled use for other psychotic disorders, such as schizoaffective disorder and bipolar affective disorder.

Routes and Dosage: Available only in tablet form, 25- and 100-mg doses.

Adult Dosage: Initial dose of 25 mg PO bid or qid may gradually increase in 25 to 50 mg/day increments, if tolerated, to a dose of 300 to 450 mg/day by the end of the 2nd week. Additional increases should occur no more than once or twice weekly. Do not exceed 900 mg/day. For maintenance, reduce the dosage to the lowest effective level.

Children: Safety and efficacy with children younger than 16 years have not been established.

Half-Life (Peak Effect): 12 hours (1 to 6 hours).

Select Adverse Reactions: Drowsiness, dizziness, headache, hypersalivation, tachycardia, hypo/hypertension, constipation, dry mouth, heartburn, nausea/vomiting, blurred vision, diaphoresis, fever, weight gain, hematologic changes, seizures, tremor, and akathisia.

Warning: Agranulocytosis, defined as a granulocyte count of less than 500 mm^3, occurs at about a cumulative 1-year incidence of 1.3%, most often within 4 to 10 weeks of exposure, but it may occur at any time. Required registration with the clozapine. *Patient Management System*, a WBC count before initiation, and weekly WBC counts while taking the drug and for 4 weeks after its discontinuation. Rare development of NMS. No confirmed cases of tardive dyskinesia, but it remains a possibility. Increased seizure risk at higher doses. Use caution with individuals who have cardiovascular disease; clozapine can cause ECG changes. Cases of sudden, unexplained death have been reported. Avoid its use during pregnancy or while breast-feeding.

Specific Patient/Family Education
- Need informed consent regarding the risk for agranulocytosis. Weekly blood draws are required. Notify the prescriber immediately if lethargy, weakness, sore throat, malaise, or other flu-like symptoms develop.
- Notify the prescriber if pregnancy is possible or planning to become pregnant. Do not breast-feed while taking this medication.
- Notify the prescriber before taking any other prescription or OTC medication. Avoid alcohol or other CNS depressant drugs.
- It may cause drowsiness and seizures; avoid driving or other hazardous tasks.
- During titration, the individual may experience orthostatic hypotension and should change positions slowly.
- Do not abruptly discontinue.

1 to 2 weeks for antipsychotic drugs to effect a change in symptoms. During the stabilization period, the type of drug selected should be given an adequate trial, generally 6 to 12 weeks, before considering a change in the drug prescription. If treatment effects are not seen, another antipsychotic agent may be tried. Clozapine (Clozaril) use may be initiated when no other atypical antipsychotic is effective (see Box 20-6 for more information about Clozaril). Clozapine is exceptional in that it often works even when other medications have failed; however, because it requires monitoring of white blood cell counts, it is not the first choice for treatment.

Adherence to a prescribed medication regimen is the best approach to preventing relapse. Unfortunately, patient compliance with medication with atypical antipsychotic agents is not much different from that with conventional antipsychotic agents (Dolder, Lacro, Dunn, & Jeste, 2002). The use of long-acting injectable is expected to improve compliance outcomes. In these days of spending constraints and funding shortfalls, inpatient facilities are discharging patients before a judgement can be made about the efficacy of a given drug treatment. Nurses and other mental health professionals are charged to ensure the continuation of these stabilization protocols and to also ensure that outpatient caregivers assume the responsibility for maintaining this stabilization phase of treatment and

continue to monitor and manage the patient's symptoms. Outpatient systems should avoid the immediate manipulation of dosages and drugs during the stabilization phase unless a medical emergency ensues.

Given the nature of a chronic illness like schizophrenia, patients generally face a lifetime of taking antipsychotic medications. Rarely is discontinuation of medications prescribed; however, many patients stop taking medications on their own. Some situations that require the cessation of medication use are **neuroleptic malignant syndrome** (NMS) (see *Emergency!* later in this chapter) and **agranulocytosis** (dangerously low level of circulating neutrophils). Agranulocytosis is most commonly experienced with Clozaril therapy. Discontinuation is an option when tardive dyskinesia develops. Discontinuation of medications, other than in circumstances of a medical emergency, should be achieved by gradually lowering the dose over time. This diminishes the likelihood of withdrawal symptoms, which include withdrawal dyskinesia and withdrawal psychosis.

Monitoring Extrapyramidal Side Effects
Parkinsonism that is caused by antipsychotic drugs is identical in appearance to Parkinson's disease and tends to occur in older patients. The symptoms are believed to be caused by the blockade of D_2 receptors in the basal

Table 20-4	Nursing Interventions for Anticholinergic Side Effects

Effect	Intervention
Dry mouth	Sips of water; hard candies and chewing gum (preferably sugar-free)
Blurred vision	Avoid dangerous tasks; teach the patient that this side effect will diminish in a few weeks
Decreased lacrimation	Artificial tears if necessary
Mydriasis	May aggravate glaucoma; teach the patient to report eye pain
Photophobia	Sunglasses
Constipation	High-fibre diet; increased fluid intake; laxatives as prescribed
Urinary hesitancy	Privacy; run water in sink; warm water over perineum
Urinary retention	Regular voiding (at least every 2–3 h) and whenever urge is present; catheterize for residual; record intake and output; evaluate benign prostatic hypertrophy
Tachycardia	Evaluate for preexisting cardiovascular disease; sudden death has occurred with thioridazine (Mellaril)

ganglia, which throws off the normal balance between acetylcholine and dopamine in this area of the brain and effectively increases acetylcholine. The symptoms are managed by reestablishing the balance between acetylcholine and dopamine by reducing the dosage of the antipsychotic (increasing dopamine activity) or adding an anticholinergic drug (decreasing acetylcholine activity), such as benztropine (Cogentin) or trihexyphenidyl (Artane). Discontinuation of the use of anticholinergic drugs should never be abrupt, which can cause a cholinergic rebound and result in withdrawal symptoms, such as vomiting, excessive sweating, and altered dreams and nightmares. Thus, the anticholinergic drug dosage should be reduced gradually (tapered) over several days. If a patient experiences **akathisia** (physical restlessness), an anticholinergic medication may not be particularly helpful. Table 20-4 lists the anticholinergic side effects of antiparkinson drugs and several antipsychotic medications and interventions to manage them.

Dystonic reactions are also believed to result from the imbalance of dopamine and acetylcholine, with the latter being dominant. Young men seem to be more vulnerable to this particular extrapyramidal side effect. This side effect, which develops rapidly and dramatically, can be very frightening for patients as their muscles tense and their body contorts. The experience often starts with stiffness experienced in the muscles and can rapidly escalate to **oculogyric crisis**, in which the muscles that control eye movements tense and pull the eyeball so that the patient is looking toward the ceiling. This may be followed rapidly by **torticollis**, in which the neck muscles pull the head to the side, or **retrocollis**, in which the head is pulled back, or orolaryngeal–pharyngeal hypertonus, in which the patient has extreme difficulty swallowing. The patient may also experience contorted extremities. These symptoms occur early in antipsychotic drug treatment, when the patient may still be experiencing psychotic symptoms. Experiencing these side effects may compound the patient's fear and anxiety and requires a

quick response. The immediate treatment is to administer benztropine (Cogentin), 1 to 2 mg, or diphenhydramine (Benadryl), 25 to 50 mg, intramuscularly or intravenously. This is followed by daily administration of oral anticholinergic drugs and, possibly, by a decrease in antipsychotic medication (see Box 20-7 for more information about benztropine).

Akathisia appears to be caused by the same biologic mechanism as other extrapyramidal side effects. Patients are restless and report that they feel driven to keep moving. They are very uncomfortable. Frequently, this response is misinterpreted as anxiety or increased psychotic symptoms, and the patient may be inappropriately given increased dosages of the antipsychotic drug, which only perpetuates the side effect. If possible, the dose of the antipsychotic drug should be reduced. A beta-adrenergic blocker such as propranolol (Inderal), 20 to 120 mg, may be required. Failure to manage this side effect is a leading cause of patients ceasing to take antipsychotic medications.

Tardive dyskinesia (impaired voluntary movement, resulting in fragmented or incomplete movements), tardive dystonia, and tardive akathisia are less likely to appear in individuals taking atypical, rather than conventional, antipsychotics. Table 20-5 describes these and associated motor abnormalities. Tardive dyskinesia is late-appearing abnormal involuntary movements (dyskinesia). It can be viewed as the opposite of parkinsonism both in observable movements and in aetiology. Whereas muscle rigidity and the absence of movement characterize parkinsonism, constant movement characterizes tardive dyskinesia. Typical movements involve the mouth, tongue, and jaw and include lip smacking, sucking, puckering, tongue protrusion, the bon-bon sign (where the tongue rolls around in the mouth and protrudes into the cheek as if the patient were sucking on a piece of hard candy), athetoid (worm-like) movements in the tongue, and chewing. Other facial movements, such as grimacing and eye blinking, also may be present.

BOX 20-7	Drug Profile

BENZTROPINE MESYLATE (COGENTIN)

Drug Class: Antiparkinson agent

Receptor Affinity: Blocks cholinergic (acetylcholine) activity, which is believed to restore the acetylcholine/dopamine balance in the basal ganglia.

Indications: Used in psychiatry to reduce extrapyramidal symptoms (acute medication-related movement disorders), including pseudoparkinsonism, dystonia, and akathisia (not tardive syndromes), due to neuroleptic drugs such as haloperidol. Most effective with acute dystonia.

Routes and Dosage: Available in tablet form, 0.5-, 1-, and 2-mg doses, also Injectable 1 mg/mL.

Adult Dosage: For acute dystonia, 1 to 2 mg IM or IV usually provides rapid relief. No significant difference in the onset of action after IM or IV injection. Treatment of emergent symptoms may be relieved in 1 or 2 days, with 1 to 2 mg orally two to three times per day. Maximum daily dose is 6 mg/day. After 1 to 2 weeks, withdraw the drug to see if continued treatment is needed. Medication-related movement disorders that develop slowly may not respond to this treatment.

Geriatric: Older adults and very thin patients cannot tolerate large doses.

Children: Do not use in children younger than 3 years. Use with caution in older children.

Half-Life: 12 to 24 hours, very little pharmacokinetic information is available.

Select Adverse Reactions: Dry mouth, blurred vision, tachycardia, nausea, constipation, flushing or elevated temperature, decreased sweating, muscular weakness or cramping, urinary retention, urinary hesitancy, dizziness, headache, disorientation, confusion, memory loss, hallucinations, psychoses, and agitation in toxic reactions, which are more pronounced in elderly people and occur at smaller doses.

Warning: Avoid its use during pregnancy or while breast-feeding. Give with caution in hot weather due to a possible heatstroke. Contraindicated with angle-closure glaucoma, pyloric or duodenal obstruction, stenosing peptic ulcers, prostatic hypertrophy or bladder neck obstructions, myasthenia gravis, megacolon, or megaesophagus. It may aggravate the symptoms of tardive dyskinesia or other chronic forms of medication-related movement disorder. Concomitant use of other anticholinergic drugs may increase the side effects and risk for toxicity. Coadministration of haloperidol or phenothiazines may reduce serum levels of these drugs.

Specific Patient/Family Education
- Take with meals to reduce dry mouth and gastric irritation.
- Dry mouth may be alleviated by sucking sugarless candies, adequate fluid intake, or good oral hygiene; increase the intake of fiber and fluids in diet to avoid constipation; stool softeners may be required. Notify the prescriber if urinary hesitancy or constipation persists.
- Notify the prescriber if rapid or pounding heartbeat, confusion, eye pain, rash, or other adverse symptoms develop.
- It may cause drowsiness, dizziness, or blurred vision; use caution while driving or performing other hazardous tasks requiring alertness. Avoid alcohol and other CNS depressants.
- Do not abruptly stop this medication because a flu-like syndrome may develop.
- Use caution in hot weather. Ensure adequate hydration. It may increase the susceptibility to heatstroke.

Table 20-5		Extrapyramidal Side Effects of Antipsychotic Drugs

Side Effect	Period of Onset	Symptoms
Acute Motor Abnormalities		
Parkinsonism or pseudoparkinsonism	5–30 d	Resting tremor, rigidity, bradykinesia/akinesia, mask-like face, shuffling gait, and decreased arm swing
Acute dystonia	1–5 d	Intermittent or fixed abnormal postures of the eyes, face, tongue, neck, trunk, and extremities
Akathisia	1–30 d	Obvious motor restlessness evidenced by pacing, rocking, and shifting from foot to foot; subjective sense of not being able to sit or be still; these symptoms may occur together or separately
Late-Appearing Motor Abnormalities		
Tardive dyskinesia	Months to years	Abnormal dyskinetic movements of the face, mouth, and jaw; choreoathetoid movements of the legs, arms, and trunk
Tardive dystonia	Months to years	Persistent sustained abnormal postures in the face, eyes, tongue, neck, trunk, and limbs
Tardive akathisia	Months to years	Persisting, unabating sense of subjective and objective restlessness

Adapted from Casey, D. E. (1994). Schizophrenia: Psychopharmacology. In J. W. Jefferson & J. H. Greist (Eds.), *The psychiatric clinics of North America: Annual of drug therapy* (Vol. 1, pp. 81–100). Philadelphia, PA: WB Saunders.

Movements in the trunk and limbs are frequently observable. These include rocking from the hips, athetoid movements of the fingers and toes, jerking movements of the fingers and toes, guitar strumming movements of the fingers, and foot tapping. The long-term health problems for people with tardive dyskinesia are choking associated with loss of control of muscles used for swallowing and compromised respiratory function leading to infections and, possibly, respiratory alkalosis.

Because the movements resemble the dyskinetic movements of some patients who have idiopathic Parkinson's disease and who have received long-term treatment with L-dopa (a direct-acting dopamine agonist that crosses the blood–brain barrier), the suggested hypothesis for tardive dyskinesia includes the supersensitivity of the dopamine receptor in the basal ganglia.

There is no consistently effective treatment; however, antipsychotic drugs mask the movements of tardive dyskinesia and have periodically been suggested as a treatment. This is counterintuitive because these are the drugs that cause the disorder. Newer antipsychotic drugs, such as clozapine, may be less likely to cause the disorder. The best management remains prevention through prescription of the lowest possible dose of antipsychotic drug over time that minimizes the symptoms of schizophrenia, prescription of these drugs for psychotic symptoms only, and early case finding by regular systematic AIMS screening of everyone receiving these drugs (see Table 20-5).

Orthostatic hypotension is another side effect of antipsychotic drugs. The primary antiadrenergic effect is decreased blood pressure, which may be general or orthostatic. Patients may be protected from falls by teaching them to rise slowly and by monitoring blood pressure before doses of the drug. The nurse should monitor and document lying, sitting, and standing blood pressures when any antipsychotic drug therapy begins.

Hyperprolactinemia can occur and is associated with the use of haloperidol and risperidone. When dopamine is blocked in the tuberoinfundibular tract, it can no longer repress prolactin, the neurohormone that regulates lactation and mammary function. The prolactin level increases and, in some individuals, side effects appear. Gynecomastia (enlarged breasts) can occur among both sexes and is understandably distressing to individuals who may be experiencing delusional or hallucinatory body image disturbances. Galactorrhea (lactation) also may occur. Menstrual irregularities and sexual dysfunction are also possible. If these symptoms appear, the medication should be reduced or changed to another antipsychotic agent. Evidence for long-term consequences of hyperprolactinemia is still lacking.

Weight gain is related to antipsychotic agents, especially olanzapine and clozapine, which have major antihistaminic properties. Patients may gain as much as 20 or 30 pounds within 1 year. Increased appetite and weight gain are often distressing to patients. Diet teaching and monitoring may have some effect on this side effect. Another solution is to increase the accessibility of healthful, easy-to-prepare food. Although nausea and vomiting can occur with the use of these drugs, they most often mask nausea.

Sedation is another possible side effect of antipsychotic medication. Patients should be monitored for the sedating effects of antipsychotic agents that are antihistaminic. In elderly patients, sedation can be associated with falls.

Screening for new-onset diabetes in patients taking antipsychotic drugs should be conducted regularly. An association has been made between new-onset diabetes mellitus and the administration of atypical antipsychotic agents, especially olanzapine and clozapine (Gough, 2005). Patients should be assessed and monitored for clinical symptoms of diabetes. Fasting blood glucose tests are commonly ordered for these individuals.

Cardiac arrhythmias may also occur. Prolongation of the QT interval is associated with torsade de pointes (polymorphic ventricular tachycardia) or ventricular fibrillation. The potential for drug-induced prolonged QT interval is associated with many drugs. The newly approved antipsychotic agent ziprasidone (Geodon) may be more likely than other drugs to prolong the QT interval and change the heart rhythm. For these patients, baseline electrocardiograms may be ordered. Nurses should observe these patients for cardiac arrhythmias.

Agranulocytosis is a reduction in the number of circulating granulocytes and decreased production of granulocytes in the bone marrow that limits one's ability to fight infection. Agranulocytosis can develop with the use of all antipsychotic drugs, but it is most likely to develop with clozapine use. Although laboratory values below 500 cells/mm³ are indicative of agranulocytosis, often granulocyte counts drop to below 200 cells/mm³ with this syndrome.

Patients taking clozapine must have regular blood tests. White blood cell and granulocyte counts should be measured before the treatment is initiated and at least weekly or twice weekly after the treatment begins. Initial white blood cell counts should be above 3,500 cells/mm³ before treatment initiation; in patients with counts of 3,500 to 5,000 cells/mm³, cell counts should be monitored three times a week if clozapine is prescribed. Any time the white blood cell count drops below 3,500 cells/mm³ or granulocytes drop below 1,500 cells/mm³, the use of clozapine should be stopped, and the patient should be monitored for fever and infections.

A faithfully implemented program of blood monitoring, however, should not replace careful observation of the patient. It is not unusual for blood cell counts to drop precipitously in a period of 2 to 3 days. This may not be discovered when the patient is on a strict weekly blood monitoring schedule. Any reported symptoms that are reminiscent of a bacterial infection (e.g., fever, pharyngitis, weakness) should be a cause for concern, and immediate evaluation of blood count status should be undertaken. Because patients are frequently discharged before the critical period of risk for agranulocytosis, patient and family education about these symptoms is also essential so that they will report these symptoms and obtain blood monitoring if necessary. In general, granulocytes return to normal within 2 to 4 weeks after discontinuing use of the medication.

Drug–Drug Interactions

Several potential drug–drug interactions are possible when administering antipsychotic medications. One of the cytochrome P450 enzymes responsible for the metabolism of olanzapine and clozapine is 1A2. If either olanzapine or clozapine is given with another medication that inhibits this enzyme, such as fluvoxamine (Luvox), the antipsychotic blood level would increase and possibly become toxic. On the other hand, cigarette smoking can also induce 1A2 and lower concentration of drugs metabolized by this enzyme, such as olanzapine and clozapine. Smokers may require a higher dose of these medications than do nonsmokers (Levin & Rezvani, 2007).

Several atypical antipsychotic agents, including clozapine, quetiapine, and ziprasidone, are metabolized by the 3A4 enzyme. Weak inhibitors of this enzyme include the antidepressants fluvoxamine, nefazodone, and norfluoxetine (an active metabolite of fluoxetine). Potent inhibitors of 3A4 enzyme include ketoconazole (antifungal drug), protease inhibitors, and erythromycin. If these drugs are given with clozapine, quetiapine, or ziprasidone, the antipsychotic level will rise. In addition, the mood stabilizer carbamazepine (Tegretol) is a 3A4 inducer. When this drug is given with clozapine, quetiapine, or ziprasidone, the antipsychotic dose should be increased to compensate for the 3A4 induction. If the use of carbamazepine is discontinued, the dosage of the antipsychotic agent needs to be adjusted (Stahl, 2008).

Risperidone, clozapine, and olanzapine are substrates for the enzyme 2D6. Theoretically, antidepressants (fluoxetine and paroxetine) that inhibit this enzyme could increase these antipsychotics' levels. However, this is not usually clinically significant (Stahl, 2008).

 TEACHING POINTS

Nonadherence to the medication regimen is an important factor in relapse. Patients and their families must be made aware of the importance of consistently taking medications. Medication education should cover the association between medications and the amelioration of symptoms (in general as well as individualized for the patient), side effects and their management, and coaching as to when to report medication effects.

EMERGENCY !

NEUROLEPTIC MALIGNANT SYNDROME

In NMS, severe muscle rigidity develops with elevated temperature and a rapidly accelerating cascade of symptoms (occurring during the next 48 to 72 hours), which can include two or more of the following: hypertension, tachycardia, tachypnea, prominent diaphoresis, incontinence, mutism, leukocytosis, changes in the level of consciousness ranging from confusion to coma, and laboratory evidence of muscle injury (e.g., elevated creatinine phosphokinase). NMS occurs in about 1% of those who receive antipsychotic drugs, especially the conventional antipsychotics such as haloperidol and other drugs that block dopamine, such as metoclopramide (Montoya, Ocampo, & Torres-Ruiz, 2003). Up to one third of patients experiencing NMS die as a result of the syndrome. NMS is probably underreported and may account for unexplained emergency room deaths of patients taking these drugs who do not have diagnoses because their symptoms do not seem serious. The presenting symptom is a temperature greater than 37.5°C (usually between 38.3°C and 39.4°C) with no apparent cause.

The most important aspects of nursing care for patients with NMS relate to recognizing symptoms early, stopping the administration of any neuroleptic medications, and initiating supportive nursing care. In any patient with fever, fluctuating vital signs, abrupt changes in levels of consciousness, or any of the symptoms presented in Box 20-8, NMS should be suspected. The nurse should be especially alert for early signs and symptoms of NMS in high-risk patients, such as those who are agitated, physically exhausted, or

---

BOX 20-8 Diagnostic Criteria for NMS*

1. Treatment with neuroleptics within 7 days of onset (2 to 4 weeks for depot neuroleptic medications)
2. Hyperthermia
3. Muscle rigidity
4. Five of the following:
   • Change in mental status
   • Tachycardia
   • Hypertension or hypotension
   • Tachypnea or hypoxia
   • Diaphoresis or sialorrhea
   • Tremor
   • Incontinence
   • Creatinine phosphokinase elevation or myoglobinuria
   • Leukocytosis
   • Metabolic acidosis
5. Exclusion of other drug-induced, systemic, or neuropsychiatric illnesses

*All five items are required concurrently.
From Caroff, S. & Mann, S. (1993). Neuroleptic malignant syndrome. *Medical Clinics of North America, 77*, 185–202, with permission.

dehydrated, or those who have an existing medical or neurologic illness. Patients receiving parenteral or higher doses of oral neuroleptic drugs or lithium concurrently must also be carefully assessed. The nurse should carefully monitor fluid intake and fluid and electrolyte status.

● **STUDY NOTE**

Recognition of side effects, including movement disorders, tardive dyskinesia, and weight gain, should lead to interventions. NMS is a medication emergency.

To prevent NMS from developing in a patient with signs or symptoms of the disorder, the nurse should immediately discontinue the administration of any neuroleptic drugs and notify the physician. In addition, the nurse should hold any anticholinergic drugs that the patient may be taking. A common error made by nurses who fail to analyze the patient's total clinical picture (including vital signs, mental status changes, and laboratory values) is to continue the use of neuroleptic drugs. Figure 20-6 shows how to decide whether to withhold an antipsychotic medication. Medical treatment includes

administering several medications. Dopamine agonist drugs, such as bromocriptine (modest success), and muscle relaxants, such as dantrolene or benzodiazepine, have been used. Antiparkinsonism drugs are not particularly useful. Some patients experience improvement with electroconvulsive therapy.

The vital signs of the patient with symptoms of NMS must be monitored frequently. In addition, it is important to check the results of the patient's laboratory tests for increased creatine phosphokinase, elevated white blood cell count, elevated liver enzymes, or myoglobinuria. The nurse must be prepared to initiate supportive measures or anticipate emergency transfer of the patient to a medical-surgical or an intensive care unit.

Treating high temperature (which frequently exceeds 39°C) is an important priority for these patients. High body temperature may be reduced with a cooling blanket and acetaminophen. Because many of these patients experience diaphoresis, temperature elevation, or dysphagia, it is important to monitor fluid hydration. Another important aspect of care for patients with NMS is safety. Joints and extremities that are rigid or spastic must be protected from injury. The treatment of these patients depends on the facility and availability of medical support services.

FIGURE 20-6. Action tree for "holding" a neuroleptic drug because of suspected NMS.

ANTICHOLINERGIC CRISIS

There is also a potential for abuse of anticholinergic drugs. Some patients may find the anticholinergic effects of these drugs on mood, memory, and perception pleasurable. Although at toxic dosages patients may experience disorientation and hallucinations, lesser doses may cause patients to experience greater sociability and euphoria. Anticholinergic crisis is a potentially life-threatening medical emergency caused by an overdose of or sensitivity to drugs with anticholinergic properties. This syndrome (also called anticholinergic delirium) may result from an accidental or intentional overdose of antimuscarinic drugs, including atropine, scopolamine, or belladonna alkaloids, which are present in numerous prescription drugs and OTC medicines. The syndrome may also occur in psychiatric patients who are receiving therapeutic doses of anticholinergic drugs, especially when such agents are combined with other psychotropic drugs that produce anticholinergic side effects. Numerous drugs commonly prescribed in psychiatric settings produce anticholinergic side effects, including tricyclic antidepressants and some antipsychotics. As a result of either drug overdose or drug sensitivity, these anticholinergic substances may produce an acute delirium or a psychotic reaction resembling schizophrenia. More severe anticholinergic effects may occur in older patients, even at therapeutic levels (Stahl, 2008).

The signs and symptoms of anticholinergic crisis are dramatic and physically uncomfortable (Box 20-9). This disorder is characterized by elevated temperature; parched mouth; burning thirst; hot, dry skin; decreased salivation; decreased bronchial and nasal secretions; widely dilated eyes (bright light is painful); decreased ability to accommodate visually; increased heart rate; constipation; difficulty urinating; and hypertension or hypotension. The face, neck, and upper arms may become flushed because of reflex blood vessel dilation. In addition to peripheral symptoms, patients with anticholinergic psychosis may experience neuropsychiatric symptoms of anxiety, agitation, delirium, hyperactivity, confusion, hallucinations (especially visual), speech difficulties, psychotic symptoms, or seizures. The acute psychotic reaction that is produced resembles schizophrenia. The classic description of anticholinergic crisis is summarized in the following mnemonic: "Hot as a hare, blind as a bat, mad as a hatter, dry as a bone."

In general, episodes of anticholinergic crisis are self-limiting, usually subsiding in 3 days. However, if untreated, the associated fever and delirium may progress to coma or cardiac and respiratory depression. Although rare, death is generally due to hyperpyrexia and brain stem depression. Once the use of the offending drug is discontinued, improvement usually occurs within 24 to 36 hours.

SIGNS AND SYMPTOMS OF ANTICHOLINERGIC CRISIS

Neuropsychiatric Signs: confusion; recent memory loss; agitation; dysarthria; incoherent speech; pressured speech; delusions; ataxia; periods of hyperactivity alternating with somnolence, paranoia, anxiety, or coma

Hallucinations: accompanied by "picking," plucking, or grasping motions; delusions; or disorientation

Physical Signs: unreactive dilated pupils; blurred vision; hot, dry, flushed skin; facial flushing; dry mucous membranes; difficulty swallowing; fever; tachycardia; hypertension; decreased bowel sounds; urinary retention; nausea; vomiting; seizures; or coma

A specific and effective antidote, physostigmine (an inhibitor of anticholinesterase) is frequently used for treating and diagnosing anticholinergic crisis. Administration of this drug rapidly reduces both the behavioural and the physiologic symptoms. However, the usual adult dose of physostigmine is 1 to 2 mg intravenously, given slowly during a period of 5 minutes because rapid injection of physostigmine may cause seizures, profound bradycardia, or heart block. Physostigmine is relatively short acting, so it may need to be given several times during the course of treatment. This drug provides relief from symptoms for a period of 2 to 3 hours. In addition to receiving physostigmine, patients who intentionally overdose on large amounts of anticholinergic drugs are treated by gastric lavage, administration of charcoal, and catharsis. The dose may be repeated after 20 or 30 minutes.

It is important for the nurse to be alert for signs and symptoms of anticholinergic crisis, especially in elderly people and children, who are much more sensitive to the anticholinergic effects of drugs, and in patients who are receiving multiple medications with anticholinergic effects. If signs and symptoms of the syndrome occur, the nurse should discontinue the use of the offending drug and notify the physician immediately.

Other Somatic Interventions

Electroconvulsive therapy is suggested as a possible alternative when the patient's schizophrenia is not being successfully treated by medication alone. Research supports using electroconvulsive therapy as an augmentation to antipsychotic therapy (Tharyan & Adams, 2005). For the most part, this is not indicated unless the patient is experiencing catatonia or has a depression that is not treatable by other means.

Psychological Domain

Although schizophrenia is a brain disorder, the psychological manifestations are the most difficult to assess and treat. Many of these psychological manifestations improve with the use of medications, but they are not necessarily eliminated.

BOX 20-10   Rating Scales for Use With Schizophrenia

Scale for the Assessment of Negative Symptoms (SANS)
Available from Nancy C. Andreasen, MD, PhD, Department of Psychiatry, College of Medicine, The University of Iowa, Iowa City, IA 52242. Copyright 1984 (see Box 20-13).

Scale for the Assessment of Positive Symptoms (SAPS)
Available from Nancy C. Andreasen (see above) (see Box 20-12).

Abnormal Involuntary Movement Scale (AIMS)
Guy, W. (1976), *ECDEU: Assessment manual for psychopharmacology (DHEW Publication No. 76-338).* Washington, DC: Department of Health Education and Welfare, Psychopharmacology Branch.

Brief Psychiatric Rating Scale (BPRS)
Overall, J. E. & Gorham, D. R. (1988). The Brief Psychiatric Rating Scale (BPRS): Recent developments in ascertainment and scaling. *Psychopharmacology Bulletin, 24,* 97–99.

Dyskinesia Identification System: Condensed User Scale (DISCUS)
Sprague, R. L. & Kalachnik, J. E. (1991). Reliability, validity, and a total score cutoff for the Dyskinesia Identification Scale System: Condensed User Scale (DISCUS) with mentally ill and mentally retarded populations. *Psychopharmacology Bulletin, 27*(1), 51–58 (see Table 20-4).

Simpson-Angus Rating Scale
Simpson, G. M. & Angus, J. W. (1970). A rating scale for extrapyramidal side effects. *Acta Psychiatrica Scandinavica, 212*(Suppl.), 11–19. Copyright 1970, Munksgaard International Publishers, Ltd.

Psychological Assessment

Several assessment scales have been developed and received considerable reliability and validity testing to help evaluate positive and negative symptom clusters in schizophrenia. Box 20-10 lists the standardized instruments used in assessing symptoms of patients with schizophrenia. These include the Scale for the Assessment of Positive Symptoms (SAPS) (Box 20-11), the Scale for the Assessment of Negative Symptoms (SANS) (Box 20-12), and the Positive and Negative Syndrome Scale (PANSS) (Kay, Fiszbein, & Opler, 1987), which assesses both symptom clusters in the same instrument. Tools that list symptoms, such as the Brief Psychiatric Rating Scale (BPRS) (Overall & Gorham, 1988) (see Appendix A), SANS, or SAPS, can also be used to help patients self-monitor their symptoms.

Information about prediagnosis experiences usually requires retrospective reporting by the patient or the family. This reporting is generally reliable for the frankly psychotic symptoms of delusions and hallucinations; however, negative symptoms are more difficult to date. In fact, negative symptoms vary from an imperceptive deviation from normal to a clear impairment. Negative symptoms probably occur earlier than positive symptoms and are less easily noted by the patient and significant others.

Responses to Mental Health Problems

Schizophrenia robs people of mental health and imposes social stigma. People with schizophrenia struggle to maintain control of their symptoms, which affects every aspect of their life. The person with schizophrenia displays a variety of interrelated symptoms and experiences deficits in several areas. More than half of patients report the following prodromal symptoms (in order of frequency): tension and nervousness, lack of interest in eating, difficulty concentrating, disturbed sleep, decreased enjoyment and loss of interest, restlessness, forgetfulness, depression, social withdrawal from friends, feeling laughed at, more religious thinking, feeling bad for no reason, feeling too excited, and hearing voices or seeing things.

Because schizophrenia is a disorder of thoughts, perceptions, and behaviour, it is sometimes not recognized as an illness by the person experiencing the symptoms. Many people with thought disorders do not believe that they have a mental illness. Their denial of mental illness and the need for treatment poses problems for the family and clinicians. This lack of insight is also called **anosognosia**. This lack of insight or anosognosia in schizophrenia has previously been interpreted as a primary symptom of the illness, namely a defensive mechanism rather than a neurologically based condition. However, recent findings have emphasized its relationship with damage to specific brain areas. Research supports a neuropsychologic interpretation of the lack of insight in schizophrenia (Pia & Tamleto, 2006). Ideally, in lucid moments, patients recognize that their thoughts are really delusions, that their perceptions are hallucinations, and that their behaviour is disorganized. In reality, many patients do not believe that they have a mental illness but agree to treatment to please their family and clinicians.

Mental Status and Appearance

The patient with schizophrenia may look eccentric or dishevelled or have poor hygiene and bizarre dress. The patient's posture may suggest lethargy or stupor.

Mood and Affect

Patients with schizophrenia often display altered mood states. In some cases, they may show heightened emotional activity; others may display severely limited emotional responses. Affect, the outward expression of mood, is categorized on a continuum: flat (emotional expression entirely absent), blunted (expression of emotions present but greatly diminished), and full range. Inappropriate affect is marked by incongruence between the emotional expression and the thoughts expressed. Other common emotional symptoms include the following:

- **Affective lability**—abrupt, dramatic, unprovoked changes in the type of emotions expressed
- **Ambivalence**—the presence and expression of two opposing feelings, leading to inaction
- **Apathy**—reactions to stimuli are decreased; diminished interest and desire

BOX 20-11 Scale for the Assessment of Positive Symptoms

0 = None; 1 = Questionable; 2 = Mild; 3 = Moderate; 4 = Marked; 5 = Severe

Hallucinations

1. *Auditory Hallucinations* 0 1 2 3 4 5
   The patient reports voices, noises, or other sources that no one else hears.
2. *Voices Commenting* 0 1 2 3 4 5
   The patient reports a voice that makes a running commentary on his behaviour or thoughts.
3. *Voices Conversing* 0 1 2 3 4 5
   The patient reports hearing two or more voices conversing.
4. *Somatic or Tactile Hallucinations* 0 1 2 3 4 5
   The patient reports experiencing peculiar physical sensations in the body.
5. *Olfactory Hallucinations* 0 1 2 3 4 5
   The patient reports experiencing unusual smells that no one else notices.
6. *Visual Hallucinations* 0 1 2 3 4 5
   The patient sees shapes or people that are not actually present.
7. *Global Rating of Hallucinations* 0 1 2 3 4 5
   This rating should be based on the duration and severity of the hallucinations and their effect on the patient's life.

Delusions

8. *Persecutory Delusions* 0 1 2 3 4 5
   The patient believes that he or she is being conspired against or in some way persecuted.
9. *Delusions of Jealousy* 0 1 2 3 4 5
   The patient believes that his spouse is having an affair with someone.
10. *Delusions of Guilt or Sin* 0 1 2 3 4 5
    The patient believes that he has committed some terrible sin or done something unforgivable.
11. *Grandiose Delusions* 0 1 2 3 4 5
    The patient believes that he has special powers or abilities.
12. *Religious Delusions* 0 1 2 3 4 5
    The patient is preoccupied with false beliefs of a religious nature.
13. *Somatic Delusions* 0 1 2 3 4 5
    The patient believes that somehow his body is diseased, abnormal, or changed.
14. *Delusions of Reference* 0 1 2 3 4 5
    The patient believes that insignificant remarks or events refer to him or have some special meaning.
15. *Delusions of Being Controlled* 0 1 2 3 4 5
    The patient feels that his feelings or actions are controlled by some outside force.
16. *Delusions of Mind Reading* 0 1 2 3 4 5
    The patient feels that people can read his mind or know his thoughts.
17. *Thought Broadcasting* 0 1 2 3 4 5
    The patient believes that his thoughts are broadcast so that he or others can hear them.
18. *Thought Insertion* 0 1 2 3 4 5
    The patient believes that thoughts that are not his own have been inserted into his mind.
19. *Thought Withdrawal* 0 1 2 3 4 5
    The patient believes that thoughts have been taken away from his mind.
20. *Global Rating of Delusions* 0 1 2 3 4 5
    This rating should be based on the duration and persistence of the delusions and their effects on the patient's life.

Bizarre Behaviour

21. *Clothing and Appearance* 0 1 2 3 4 5
    The patient dresses in an unusual manner or does other strange things to alter his appearance.
22. *Social and Sexual Behaviours* 0 1 2 3 4 5
    The patient may do things considered inappropriate according to usual social norms (e.g., masturbating in public).
23. *Aggressive and Agitated Behaviour* 0 1 2 3 4 5
    The patient may behave in an aggressive, agitated manner, often unpredictably.
24. *Repetitive or Stereotyped Behaviour* 0 1 2 3 4 5
    The patient develops a set of repetitive actions or rituals that he must perform over and over.
25. *Global Rating of Bizarre Behaviour* 0 1 2 3 4 5
    This rating should reflect the type of behaviour and the extent to which it deviates from social norms.

Positive Formal Thought Disorder

26. *Derailment* 0 1 2 3 4 5
    A pattern of speech in which ideas slip off track onto ideas obliquely related or unrelated.
27. *Tangentiality* 0 1 2 3 4 5
    Replying to a question in an oblique or irrelevant manner.
28. *Incoherence* 0 1 2 3 4 5
    A pattern of speech that is essentially incomprehensible at times.
29. *Illogicality* 0 1 2 3 4 5
    A pattern of speech in which conclusions are reached that do not follow logically.
30. *Circumstantiality* 0 1 2 3 4 5
    A pattern of speech that is very indirect and delayed in reaching its goal idea.
31. *Pressure of Speech* 0 1 2 3 4 5
    The patient is distracted by nearby stimuli that interrupt his or her flow of speech.
32. *Distractible Speech* 0 1 2 3 4 5
    The patient's speech is rapid and difficult to interrupt; the amount of speech produced is greater than that considered normal.
33. *Clanging* 0 1 2 3 4 5
    A pattern of speech in which sounds, rather than meaningful relationships, govern word choice.
34. *Global Rating of Positive Formal Thought Disorder* 0 1 2 3 4 5
    This rating should reflect the frequency of abnormality and the degree to which it affects the patient's ability to communicate.

Inappropriate Affect

35. *Inappropriate Affect* 0 1 2 3 4 5
    The patient's affect is inappropriate or incongruous, not simply flat or blunted.

From Nancy C. Andreasen, MD, PhD, Department of Psychiatry, College of Medicine. The University of Iowa, Iowa City, IA 52242. Copyright 1984 Nancy C. Andreasen. Reprinted with permission.

BOX 20-12 Scale for the Assessment of Negative Symptoms

0 = None; 1 = Questionable; 2 = Mild; 3 = Moderate; 4 = Marked; 5 = Severe

Affective Flattening or Blunting

1. *Unchanging Facial Expression*   0 1 2 3 4 5
   The patient's face appears wooden; it changes less than expected as the emotional content of discourse changes.
2. *Decreased Spontaneous Movements*   0 1 2 3 4 5
   The patient shows few or no spontaneous movements and does not shift position, move extremities, etc.
3. *Paucity of Expressive Gestures*   0 1 2 3 4 5
   The patient does not use hand gestures, body position, etc., as an aid to expressing ideas.
4. *Poor Eye Contact*   0 1 2 3 4 5
   The patient avoids eye contact or "stares through" interviewer even when speaking.
5. *Affective Nonresponsivity*   0 1 2 3 4 5
   The patient fails to smile or laugh when prompted.
6. *Lack of Vocal Inflections*   0 1 2 3 4 5
   The patient fails to show normal vocal emphasis patterns; is often monotonic.
7. *Global Rating of Affective Flattening*   0 1 2 3 4 5
   This rating should focus on the overall severity of symptoms, especially unresponsiveness, eye contact, facial expression, and vocal inflections.

Alogia

8. *Poverty of Speech*   0 1 2 3 4 5
   The patient's replies to questions are restricted in amount and tend to be brief, concrete, and unelaborated.
9. *Poverty of Content of Speech*   0 1 2 3 4 5
   The patient's replies are adequate in amount but tend to be vague, overconcrete, or overgeneralized, and they convey little information.
10. *Blocking*   0 1 2 3 4 5
    The patient indicates, either spontaneously or with prompting, that his train of thought was interrupted.
11. *Increased Latency of Response*   0 1 2 3 4 5
    The patient takes a long time to reply to questions; prompting indicates that the patient is aware of the question.
12. *Global Rating of Alogia*   0 1 2 3 4 5
    The core features of alogia are poverty of speech and poverty of content.
13. *Grooming and Hygiene*   0 1 2 3 4 5
    The patient's clothes may be sloppy or soiled, and the patient may have greasy hair, body odor, etc.

14. *Impersistence at Work or School*   0 1 2 3 4 5
    The patient has difficulty seeking or maintaining employment, completing schoolwork, keeping house, etc. If an inpatient, he or she cannot persist at ward activities, such as OT, playing cards, etc.
15. *Physical Anergia*   0 1 2 3 4 5
    The patient tends to be physically inert. He or she may sit for hours and does not initiate spontaneous activity.
16. *Global Rating of Avolition–Apathy*   0 1 2 3 4 5
    Strong weight may be given to one or two prominent symptoms if particularly striking.

Anhedonia–Asociality

17. *Recreational Interests and Activities*   0 1 2 3 4 5
    The patient may have few or no interests. Both the quality and the quantity of interests should be taken into account.
18. *Sexual Activity*   0 1 2 3 4 5
    The patient may show a decrease in sexual interest and activity or in enjoyment when active.
19. *Ability to Feel Intimacy and Closeness*   0 1 2 3 4 5
    The patient may display an inability to form close or intimate relationships, especially with the opposite sex and family.
20. *Relationships With Friends and Peers*   0 1 2 3 4 5
    The patient may have few or no friends and may prefer to spend all of his or her time isolated.
21. *Global Rating of Anhedonia–Asociality*   0 1 2 3 4 5
    This rating should reflect the overall severity, taking into account the patient's age, family status, etc.

Attention

22. *Social Inattentiveness*   0 1 2 3 4 5
    The patient appears uninvolved or unengaged. He or she may seem "spacey."
23. *Inattentiveness During Mental Status Testing*   0 1 2 3 4 5
    Tests of "serial 7s" (at least five subtractions) and spelling "world" backward: Score: 2 = 1 error; 3 = 2 errors; 4 = 3 errors.
24. *Global Rating of Attention*   0 1 2 3 4 5
    This rating should assess the patient's overall concentration, clinically and on tests.

From Nancy C. Andreasen, MD, PhD, Department of Psychiatry, College of Medicine, The University of Iowa, Iowa City, IA 52242. Copyright 1984 Nancy C. Andreasen. Reprinted with permission.

Speech

Speech patterns may reflect obsessions, delusions, pressured thinking, loose associations, or **flight of ideas** and neologisms. Speech is an indicator of thought content and other mental processes and is usually altered. An assessment of speech should note any difficulty articulating words (dysarthria) and difficulty swallowing (dysphagia) as indicators of medication side effects. In many instances, what an individual says is as important as how it is said. Both content and speech patterns should be noted.

Thought Processes and Delusions

Delusions can be distinguished from strongly held ideas by the degree of conviction with which the belief is held despite clear contradictory evidence (APA, 2013). Culture must be considered when evaluating delusions. Delusional beliefs are those not sanctioned or held by a cultural or religious subgroup.

Bizarre delusions alone are sufficient to diagnose schizophrenia. It can often be difficult to distinguish between bizarre and nonbizarre delusions. Nonbizarre delusions generally have themes of jealousy and persecution and are derived from ordinary life experiences. For example, a woman believes that her husband, from whom she has recently separated, is trying to poison her, or a man believes that members of the Mafia are trying to kill him because, when he was in high school, he reported to the principal that several of his classmates were selling drugs at school.

Bizarre delusions are those that are implausible, not understandable, and not derived from ordinary life experiences. Bizarre delusions often include delusions of control (that some outside force controls thoughts and actions), thought broadcasting (that others can read or hear one's thoughts), thought insertion (that someone has placed thoughts into one's mind), and thought withdrawal (that someone is removing thoughts from one's mind) (APA, 2013). For example, a patient who has been with a hypnotist for 2 months reports that the hypnotist continued to read his mind and was "picking his brain away piece by piece." Another patient was convinced that a computer chip was placed in her vagina during a gynaecologic examination and that this somehow directly influenced her physical movements and her thoughts.

Assessing and judging the content of the delusion and exploring other aspects of the delusional experience are helpful in understanding the significance of these false beliefs. The underlying feeling that accompanies the delusion should be identified. Other aspects to consider include the conviction with which the delusion is held; the extent to which other aspects of the individual's life are incorporated into or affected by the delusion; the degree of internal consistency, organization, and logic evident in the delusion; and the amount of pressure (in terms of preoccupation and concern) individuals feel in their lives as a result of the delusion (see Box 20-13).

Hallucinations

Hallucinations are the most common example of disturbed sensory perception observed in patients with schizophrenia. Hallucinations can be experienced in all sensory modalities; however, auditory hallucinations are the most common in schizophrenia. Some specific hallucinations may be sufficient to diagnose schizophrenia, such as hearing voices conversing with each other or carrying on a discussion with someone who is not there. Because most individuals will not spontaneously

---

BOX 20-13 **Therapeutic Dialogue**

THE PATIENT WITH DELUSIONS

John joined the nurse in a game of pool. The following conversation occurred as they played.

Ineffective Approach

John: The RCMP put a transmitter in my molar, here (points to his right cheek).

Nurse: No one would put a transmitter in your tooth; come on, the RCMP isn't looking for you.

John: You get the striped balls. Yeah, they want to monitor me while I'm here. I know that they have the real Governor General here in the hospital. They are trying to get the Prime Minister to intervene with the Ontario Police. Mark from Ottawa told me that.

Nurse: The Governor General can't possibly be here; I saw him on television this morning.

John: Maybe—he does have lighter hair and has different-coloured contacts to disguise his eyes, but they're just trying to keep people from knowing what they're doing.

Nurse: John, he isn't in the hospital; if he were, I would know it because I work here.

John: (With anger) You don't know anything! You are probably from the RCMP also. I have nothing else to say to you.

Effective Approach

John: The RCMP put a transmitter in my molar, here (points to his right cheek).

Nurse: Oh. Which balls are mine?

John: You get the striped ones. Yeah, they want to monitor me while I'm here. I know that they have the real Governor General here in the hospital. They are trying to get the Prime Minister to intervene with the Ontario Provincial Police. Mark from Ottawa told me that.

Nurse: Do you suppose that you saw someone who looks like the Governor General?

John: Maybe—he does have lighter hair and has different-coloured contacts to disguise his eyes. But they're just trying to keep people from knowing what they're doing.

Nurse: You sound a little overwhelmed with all the information you have.

John: No, no. I can handle it. The RCMP can't do anything to me, I'll never talk. They are trying to confuse me so that I stay away from the Governor General. They all think they can keep me from my mission.

Nurse: Who is it that worries you, John?

John: Everyone in the government. The RCMP, CSIS, CRA—all those alphabets.

Nurse: It must be rather frightening to feel all these people are looking for you. You must be scared a lot of the time.

John: It's scary but I can handle it. I've handled it all my life.

Nurse: You've been in scary situations all your life?

John: Yeah. I don't know. Maybe not scary, just hard. I never seemed to be able to do as well as my parents wanted—or as I wanted.

Critical Thinking Challenge

- How did the nurse's argumentative responses cause the patient to react in the first scenario?
- What effective communication techniques did the nurse use in the second scenario?

share their hallucinatory experiences with an interviewer, the nurse may need to rely on indirect evidence in the patient's behaviour, such as (1) pauses during conversations in which the individual seems preoccupied or appears to be listening to someone other than the interviewer, (2) looking toward the perceived source of a voice, or (3) responding to the voices in some manner. Although patients may not spontaneously share their hallucinations, many validate observations of the examiner or admit to a history of hallucinations when asked (see Box 20-14).

Disorganized Communication

The other aspect of thought content and processes that may be altered in schizophrenia is the organization of expressed thoughts. Impaired verbal fluency (ability to produce spontaneous speech) is commonly present. Abrupt shifts in the focus of conversation are a typical symptom of disorganized thinking. The most severe shifts in focus may occur after only one or two words (**word salad**), after one or two phrases or sentences (flight of ideas or loose associations), or somewhat less severely as a

---

BOX 20-14 **Therapeutic Dialogue**

THE PATIENT WITH HALLUCINATIONS

The following conversation took place in a dayroom with several staff members present. The patient was potentially very violent. Although it is a good example of dealing with someone who is hallucinating, it is not a situation that should be taken lightly. Always make certain that you have a means to leave a situation (i.e., you are not in the corner of a room) and that you have sufficient staff members close by to ensure safety. Take careful note of whether the patient has a potential weapon near at hand.

Jason approached the nurse and asked to play pool. The nurse debated about playing but chose to play because Jason appeared distracted and the game might give him something to focus on.

Ineffective Approach

Nurse: Shall I break?

Jason: (Had been looking off to his right, but turns and looks directly at the nurse.) Yeah, go ahead. (Looks at the table briefly and then turns to look out the door and down the hallway.)

Nurse: (Breaking the pool balls without putting any in a pocket.) It's your turn. You can hit any ball that you'd like.

Jason: (Turning back to the table.) Huh? (Shaking his head as he stared at the table.) What?

Nurse: You know, Jason, you really should pay attention.

Jason: (Hits a ball in and moves to the other side of the table. Stops in line with the next shot but doesn't bend down to take aim. Stands very still and then shakes his head slightly and quickly. Leans down to take aim and then stands up again.)

Nurse: Jason. (Looks at the nurse.) Jason! Are you going to play or not? I don't have all day.

Jason: Oh yeah. (Leans down, takes aim, and misses.)

Nurse: (Moves to where the next shot is. Position is near where Jason is standing. The nurse watches him carefully, moving closer to him.) Please move over, Jason.

Jason: No. (Doesn't move. In peripheral vision, the nurse sees Jason's lips move and he again looks to his right and shakes his head in a staccato motion, as if trying to shake something out of his head.)

Effective Approach

Nurse: Shall I break?

Jason: (Had been looking off to his right, but turns and looks directly at the nurse.) Yeah, go ahead. (Looks at the table briefly and then turns to look out the door and down the hallway.)

Nurse: (Breaking the pool balls without putting any in a pocket.) Your turn; you can hit any ball that you'd like.

Jason: (Turning back to the table.) Huh? (Shakes his head as he stares at the table.) What?

Nurse: You can hit any ball you like. I didn't get any.

Jason: (Hits a ball in and moves to the other side of the table. Stops in line with the next shot but doesn't bend

down to take aim. Stands very still and then shakes his head slightly and quickly. Leans down to take aim and then stands up again.)

Nurse: Jason. (He looks at nurse.) Are you aiming at the 10 ball?

Jason: Oh yeah. (Leans down, takes aim, and misses.)

Nurse: (Moving to where her next shot is. The position is very close to where Jason is standing. The nurse watches him carefully while moving closer to him.) Here, let me take this shot.

Jason: Oh. (Moves back. In peripheral vision, the nurse sees Jason's lips move and again he looks to his right and shakes his head in a staccato motion, as if trying to shake something out of his head.)

Nurse: I missed again. (Moves away from the table and turns to Jason, who moves up to the table. He leans down and then stands up again. His lips move again as he turns his head to the right and then looks over his back toward the doorway.) Jason. Jason. (He looks at the nurse.) You have the striped ones.

Jason: (Nods and leans down to take a shot, which he makes. He then misses the next shot. He stands up and moves back from the table, again looking back toward the doorway. He shakes his head.)

Nurse: (Watches him closely and moves to the opposite side of the table, making the next shot. Lining up the next shot, Jason leans the pool cue against the table, looks past the nurse, and turns and walks away toward the door. Looks down the hallway, takes a few steps, stops for a minute or so, turns back into the room, and again looks past the nurse. Sits down and shakes his head again. Holds his head in his hands, with his hands covering his ears. The nurse picks up his pool cue and places both against the wall, out of the way. The nurse, recognizing that Jason is likely experiencing auditory hallucinations, remains where she can observe him, noting, as well, that another staff member is near at hand.)

Critical Thinking Challenge

- How did the nurse's impatience translate into Jason's behaviour in the first scenario?
- What effective communicating techniques did the nurse use in the second scenario?

shift that occurs when a new topic is repeatedly suggested and pursued from the current topic (**tangentiality**). In some individuals, speech may be a simple repetition of words or phrases spoken by others (**echolalia**).

Cognitive Impairments

Although cognitive impairments in schizophrenia vary widely from patient to patient, several primary problems have been identified:

- Attention may be increased and sustained on external stimuli over a period of time (hypervigilance).
- The ability to distinguish and focus on relevant stimuli may be diminished.
- Familiar cues may go unrecognized or be improperly encoded.
- Information processing may be diminished, leading to inappropriate or illogical conclusions from available observations and information (Cirillo & Seidman, 2003; Hartman, Steketee, Silva, Lanning, & Andersson, 2003; Sheffield et al., 2013).

Cognitive impairments are not easy to recognize. By relying only on clinical assessment, the nurse can miss the extent of the impairment. Using a standardized instrument such as the Mini-Mental Status Examination (MMSE), the Cognitive Assessment Screening Instrument (CASI), or the 7-Minute Screen can provide a screening measurement of cognitive function (see Chapter 10). If impairment is suspected, neuropsychologic testing by a qualified psychologist may be necessary.

Memory and Orientation

Impairments in orientation, memory, and abstract thinking may be observed. Orientation to time, place, and person may remain relatively intact unless the patient is particularly preoccupied with delusions and hallucinations. Although all aspects of memory may be affected in schizophrenia, registration or the recall within seconds of newly learned information may be particularly diminished. This affects the individual's short- and long-term memories. The ability to engage in abstract thinking may be impaired.

Insight and Judgement

Individuals display insight when they display evidence of knowing their own thoughts, the reality of external objects, and their relationship to these. Judgement is the ability to decide or act on a situation. Insight and judgement are closely related to each other and depend on cognitive functions that are frequently impaired in people with schizophrenia (Pia & Tamleto, 2006).

Behavioural Responses

During periods of psychosis, unusual or bizarre behaviour often occurs. These behaviours can usually be understood within the context of the patient's disturbed thinking. The nurse needs to understand the significance of the behaviour to the individual. One patient moved the family furniture into the yard because he thought that evil spirits were hiding in the furniture. His bizarre behaviour was an attempt to protect his family. Another patient painted a sequence of numbers on his bedroom walls. He said that the numbers were the language of the angels. His bizarre thoughts were at the basis of his behaviour.

Because of the negative symptoms, specifically avolition, patients may not seem interested or organized to complete their normal daily activities. They may stay in bed most of the day or refuse to take a shower. Many times, they will agree to get up in the morning and go to school or work, but they never get around to it. Several specific behaviours are associated with schizophrenia, including stereotypy (idiosyncratic repetitive, purposeless movements), echopraxia (involuntary imitation of others' movements), and waxy flexibility (posture held in odd or unusual fixed position for extended periods). In some cases, certain behaviours need to be evaluated carefully to distinguish them from movements that are associated with medication side effects, such as grimacing, stereotypic behaviour, or agitation.

Self-Concept

In schizophrenia, self-concept is usually poor. Patients often are aware that they are hearing voices others do not hear. They recognize that they are different from others and are often afraid of "going crazy." Many are aware of the loss of expectations for their future achievements. The pervasive stigma associated with having a mental illness contributes to the poor self-concept. Body image can be disturbed, especially during periods of hallucinations or delusions. One patient believed that her body was infected with germs and she could feel them eating away her insides.

Stress and Coping Patterns

Stressful events are often linked to psychiatric symptoms. It is important to determine stresses from the patient's perspective because a stressful event for one may not be stressful for another (see Chapter 17). It is also important to determine typical coping patterns, especially negative coping strategies, such as the use of substances or aggressive behaviour.

Risk Assessment

Because of high suicide and attempted suicide rates among patients with schizophrenia, the nurse needs to assess the patient's risk for self-injury: Does the patient speak of suicide, have delusional thinking that could lead to dangerous behaviour, and have command hallucinations telling him or her to harm self or others? Does the patient have homicidal ideations? Does the patient have access to weapons? Does the patient lack social support and the skills to be meaningfully engaged with other people or a vocation? Substance-related disorders are also common among patients with schizophrenia, and nurses should assess for substance misuse or abuse.

Nursing Diagnoses for Psychological Domain

Many nursing diagnoses can be generated from data collected assessing the psychological domain. Disturbed thought processes can be used for delusions, confusion, and disorganized thinking. Disturbed sensory perception is appropriate for hallucinations or illusions. Other examples of diagnoses include disturbed body image, low self-esteem, disturbed personal identity, risk for violence, ineffective coping, and knowledge deficit.

Interventions for Psychological Domain

All the psychological interventions, such as counselling, conflict resolution, behaviour therapy, and cognitive interventions, are appropriate for patients with schizophrenia. The following discussion focuses on applying these interventions.

Special Issues in the Nurse–Patient Relationship

The development of the nurse–patient relationship with patients with schizophrenia centres on developing trust and accepting the person as a worthy human being. People with schizophrenia are often reluctant to engage in any relationship because of previous rejection and, in some instances, an underlying suspicion that is a part of the illness. If they are having hallucinations, their images of other people may be distorted and frightening. They struggle to trust their own thoughts and perceptions, and engaging in an interaction with another human being may prove too overwhelming.

The nurse should approach the patient in a calm and caring manner. Engaging the patient in a relationship may take time. Brief interactions are best for a patient who is experiencing psychosis. Being consistent in interactions and following through on promises will help establish trust within the relationship.

Establishing a therapeutic relationship is crucial, especially with patients who deny that they are ill. Patients are more likely to agree to treatment if these recommendations are made within the context of a safe, trusting relationship. Even if some patients deny having mental illness, they may take medication and attend treatment activities because they trust the nurse.

Management of Disturbed Thoughts and Sensory Perceptions

Although antipsychotic medications may relieve positive symptoms, they do not always eliminate hallucinations and delusions. The nurse must continue helping the patient develop creative strategies for dealing with these sensory and thought disturbances. Information about the content of the hallucinations and delusions is needed, not only to determine whether the medications are effective but also to assess safety and the meaning of these thoughts and perceptions to the patient. In caring for a patient who is experiencing hallucinations or delusions, nursing actions should be guided by three general patient outcomes:

- Decrease the frequency and intensity of hallucinations and delusions.
- Recognize that hallucinations and delusions are symptoms of a brain disorder.
- Develop strategies to manage the recurrence of hallucinations or delusions.

When interacting with a patient who is experiencing hallucinations or delusions, the nurse must remember that these experiences are real to the patient. The nurse should never tell a patient that these experiences are not real. Discounting the experiences blocks communication. It also is dishonest to tell the patient that you are having the same hallucinatory experience. It is best to validate the patient's experiences and identify the meaning of these thoughts and feelings to the patient. For example, a patient who believes that he or she is under surveillance by the police probably feels frightened and suspicious of everyone. By acknowledging how frightening it must be to always feel like you are being watched, the nurse focuses on the feelings that are generated by the delusion, not the delusion itself. The nurse can then offer to help the patient feel safe within this environment. The patient, in turn, begins to feel that someone understands him or her.

 TEACHING POINTS

Teaching patients that hallucinations and delusions are part of the disorder becomes easier after the medication begins working. Once patients believe and acknowledge that they have a mental illness and that some of their thoughts are delusions and some of their perceptions are hallucinations, they can develop strategies to manage their symptoms.

Self-Monitoring and Relapse Prevention

Patients benefit greatly by learning techniques of self-regulation, symptom monitoring, and relapse prevention. By monitoring events, time, place, and stimuli surrounding the appearance of symptoms, the patient can begin to predict high-risk times for symptom recurrence. Cognitive behavioural therapy is often used in helping patients monitor and identify their emerging symptoms in order to prevent relapse (Gumley et al., 2003; Kingdon & Turkington, 2006).

Another important nursing intervention is to help the patient identify who and where to talk about delusional or hallucinatory material. Unfortunately, because self-disclosure of these symptoms immediately labels someone as having a mental illness, patients should be encouraged to evaluate the environment for negative consequences of disclosing these symptoms. It may be fine to talk about it at home but not at the grocery store.

Enhancement of Cognitive Functioning

After identifying deficits in cognitive functioning, the nurse and the patient can develop interventions that target specific deficits. The most effective interventions usually involve the whole treatment team. If the ability to focus or attend is an issue, patients can be encouraged to select activities that improve attention, such as computer games. For memory problems, patients can be encouraged to make lists and to write down important information.

Executive functioning problems are the most challenging for these patients. Patients who cannot manage daily problems may have planning and problem-solving impairments. For these patients, developing interventions that closely simulate real-world problems may help. Through coaching, the nurse can teach and support the development of problem-solving skills. For example, during hospitalizations, patients are given medications and reminded to take them on time. They are often instructed in a classroom setting but rarely have an opportunity to practise self-medication and figure out what to do if their prescription expires, the medications are lost, or they forget their medications. Yet, when discharged, patients are expected to take medication at the prescribed dose at the prescribed time. Interventions are needed that are designed to have patients actively engage in problem-solving behaviour with real problems. Cognitive remediation strategies are being developed to assist with these difficulties. Computerized remediation strategies appear promising, but more research is required (Subramaniam et al., 2012).

Another approach to helping patients solve problems and learn new strategies for dealing with problems is solution-focused therapy, which focuses on the strengths and positive attributes that exist within each person. For example, patients can be asked to identify the most important problem from their perspective. This focuses the patient on the issue that he or she deems important.

Behavioural Interventions

Behavioural interventions can be very effective in helping patients improve motivation and organize routines and daily activities, such as maintaining a regular schedule and completing activities. Reinforcement of positive behaviours (e.g., getting up on time, completing hygiene, going to treatment activities) can easily be included in a treatment plan. In the hospital, patients gain ward privileges by following an agreed-upon treatment plan.

Stress and Coping Skills

Developing skills to cope with personal, social, and environmental stresses are important to everyone, but particularly to those with a severe mental illness. Stresses

can easily trigger symptoms that patients are trying to avoid. Establishing regular counselling sessions to support the development of positive coping skills is helpful for both the hospitalized patient and those in the community. Another interesting innovation is the recent development of digital applications which are purported to assist with coping with delusions and hallucinations. One such application is *CopingTutor* (Gottlieb, 2012), which includes presentations, games, and self-help worksheets. The download is available for a small cost.

Patient Education

Cognitive deficits (difficulty in processing complex information, maintaining steady focus of attention, distinguishing between relevant and irrelevant stimuli, and forming abstractions) may challenge the nurse planning educational activities. Evidence indicates that people with schizophrenia may learn best in an errorless learning environment (O'Carroll, Russell, Lawrie, & Johnstone, 1999); that is, they are directly given correct information and then encouraged to write it down. Asking questions that encourage guessing is not as effective in helping them retain information. Trial-and-error learning is avoided. In one study, a group of people with schizophrenia who were taught using an errorless learning approach improved work skill in two entry-level job tasks (index card filing and toilet tank assembly) and performed better than the group that was instructed with conventional trial-and-error instructions (Kern, Green, Mintz, & Liberman, 2003; Kern, Liberman, Kopelowicz, Mintz, & Green, 2002).

Teaching and explaining should occur in an environment with minimal distractions. Terminology should be clear and unambiguous. Visual aids can supplement verbal information, but these materials should have simple information stated in simple language. The nurse takes care not to overcrowd the visual material or incorporate images that draw attention away from the important content. Teaching should occur in small segments with frequent reinforcement. Most important of all, teaching should occur when the patient is ready. Regular assessments of cognitive abilities with standardized instruments can help determine this readiness. These suggestions can be adapted for teaching during any phase of the illness.

Skill-training interventions should be designed to compensate for cognitive deficits. To help patients learn to process complex activities, such as catching a bus, preparing a meal, or shopping for food or clothing, nurses should break the activity into small parts or steps and list them for the patient's reference. For example:

- Make sure you have the correct bus fare in your pocket
- Leave your apartment with keys in the hand
- Close the door
- Walk to the corner
- Turn right and walk three blocks to the bus stop

BOX 20-15　Psychoeducation Checklist: Schizophrenia

When caring for the patient with schizophrenia, be sure to include the caregiver and address the following topic areas in the teaching plan:

- Psychopharmacologic agents, including drug action, dosage, frequency, and possible adverse effects. Stress the importance of adherence to the prescribed regimen
- Management of hallucinations
- Coping strategies such as self-talk, getting busy
- Management of the environment
- Use of contracts that detail the expected behaviours, with goals and consequences
- Community resources
- Community educational opportunities for families
- Family peer supports/family navigator contacts in the community

Family Education

Because having a family member with schizophrenia is a life-changing event for the family and friends who provide care and support, educating patients and their families or significant others is crucial. It is a primary concern for the mental health nurse. Family support and education are crucial to help patients maintain their treatment. Education should include information about the disease course, treatment regimens, support systems, and life management skills (see Box 20-15). The most important factor to reinforce during patient and family education ism the consistent taking of medication (Hamilton Wilson, 2012; Hamilton Wilson & Hobbs, 1999).

Social Domain

Social Assessment

Several difficulties with social functioning occur in schizophrenia. As the disorder progresses, individuals can become increasingly socially isolated. On a one-to-one basis, this occurs because the individual seems unable to connect with people in his or her environment. Several aspects of the symptoms already discussed can contribute to this, for example, emotional blunting and anhedonia (the inability to form emotional attachment and experience pleasure). Cognitive deficits that contribute to difficult social functioning include problems with the face and affect recognition, deficiencies in recall of past interactions, problems with decision making and judgement in conflictual interactions, and poverty of speech and language. Poor functioning and the inability to complete activities of daily living are manifested in poor hygiene, malnutrition, and social isolation.

Social Systems

In schizophrenia, support systems become very important in maintaining the patient in the community. The individual may become socially isolated if the treatment and management occur in long-term care facilities and group homes away from family and friends. One challenge in treating schizophrenia is to identify and maintain the patient's links with family and significant others. Assessment of the patient's formal support (e.g., family caregivers, health care providers) and informal support (e.g., neighbours, friends) should be conducted.

Quality of Life

People with schizophrenia often have a poor quality of life, especially older people who may have spent many years in a long-term hospital. The nurse should assess the patient's quality of life and how it could be improved. Simple changes, such as arranging for a different roommate or improving access to social activities by meeting transportation needs, can greatly improve a patient's quality of life. Stable housing is key to making any improvements to the patient's quality of life (MHCC, 2013b).

Family Assessment

The assessment of the family can take many forms, and the family assessment guide presented in Chapter 15 can be used. In many instances, the patient will be young and living with his or her parents. This is most often the case when a young person experiences the first episode of psychosis. Often, the nurse's first contact with the patient and family is in the initial phases of the disorder. The family is dealing with the shock and disbelief of seeing a child with a mental illness that may have lifelong consequences. Ideally, in this instance, the assessment process may be extended over several sessions to provide the family with support and education about the disorder. Certainly, the emergence of psychotic illness is a distressing and confusing time, not only for young persons experiencing these perplexing changes but also for their parents.

The family, and in particular the parents, play a critical role in early intervention for psychosis, both as a vehicle for early identification and treatment, and as a supportive context for recovery. Understanding of this caregiving experience was gleaned from a qualitative study that employed a phenomenologic approach to uncover four distinct stories: *a story of Protection, a story of Loss, a story of Stigma,* and a final story of *Enduring Love* (Hamilton Wilson, 2012). The experiences of parent caregivers suggest that health care providers, and nurses in particular, can have more discretion, insight, and discernment in clinical approaches and might also serve to shape future policies, which will recognize and affirm the strengths and resilient capacities of families. Nursing assessment and approaches, which focus upon family resilience and strengths, is most effective.

Because women with schizophrenia generally have better treatment outcomes than do men, many will marry and have children. These women experience the same life stresses as other women and may find themselves single parents, raising children in poverty-stricken conditions. Managing a psychiatric illness and trying to be an effective parent in a socially stigmatizing society are exceedingly challenging because of the lack of financial resources and social support. This family will need an extensive assessment of financial need and social support. The family life cycle model presented in Chapter 15 can also be used as a framework for the assessment.

Nursing Diagnoses for Social Domain

The nursing diagnoses generated from the assessment of the social domain are typically impaired social interaction, ineffective role performance, disabled family coping, and interrupted family processes. Outcomes will depend on the specific diagnostic area.

Interventions for Social Domain

Promoting Patient Safety

Although violence is not a consistent behaviour of people with schizophrenia, it is always a concern during the initial phase when hallucinations or delusions may put patients at risk for harming themselves or others. Nonviolent patients who are experiencing hallucinations and delusions can also be at risk for victimization by more aggressive patients. The patient who is hallucinating needs to be protected. This protection may include increased staff monitoring and, if necessary, a safer environment in a secluded area.

The nurse's best approach to avoiding violence or aggression is to demonstrate respect for the patient and the patient's personal space, assess and monitor for signs of fear and agitation, and use preventive interventions before the patient loses control. Medications should be administered as ordered. Because most antipsychotic and antidepressant medications take 1 to 2 weeks to begin moderating the patient's behaviour, the nurse must be vigilant during the acute illness.

Reducing environmental stimulation is particularly important for individuals who are experiencing hallucinations but can be helpful for all patients when signs of fear and agitation are observed. Allowing patients to use private rooms or seclusion for brief periods can be an important preventive method.

Other techniques of managing the environment (milieu management) have been found to be helpful in inpatient settings. One researcher who examined aggression and violence in psychiatric hospitals found violent behaviour to be associated with the following predictors: a history of violence, a coercive interaction style of using violence to obtain what is desired, and an environment in which violence is inadvertently rewarded, for example, by gaining staff attention (Morrison, 1992, 1993; Morrison & Carney Love, 2003). Morrison proposed the following methods to help avoid acts of violence or aggression:

- Take a thorough history that includes information about the patient's past use of violence.
- Help the patient to talk directly and constructively with those with whom he or she is angry, rather than venting anger to staff about a third person.

- Set limits with consistent and justly applied consequences.
- Involve the patient in formulating a contract that outlines patient and staff behaviours, goals, and consequences.
- Schedule brief but regular time-outs to allow the patient some privacy without the attention of staff either before or after the time-out (these time-outs may be patient activated).

Staff members need to have planned sessions after all incidents of violence or physical management in which the event is analyzed. These sessions allow staff members to learn how to better manage these situations and evaluate patients' cues. With sensitive leadership, these sessions can help staff to learn more about the interaction of patient and staff characteristics that can contribute to these incidents. (See Box 20-16 for research that shows the way conflict and containment can be reduced on inpatient units.)

Convening Support Groups

People with mental illness benefit from support groups that focus on daily problems and the stress of dealing with a mental illness. These groups are useful throughout the continuum of care and help reduce the risk for suicide. In the hospital setting, the focus of the group can be simply sharing the experience of living with a mental illness. In the community, a regular support group can provide interaction with people with similar problems and issues and the opportunity to share stories of recovery. Friendships often develop from these groups.

Implementing Milieu Therapy

Individuals with schizophrenia can be hospitalized or live in group homes for a long period of time. It is unrealistic to expect people who have an illness that interferes with their ability to live with family members to live in peace and harmony with complete strangers. Arranging the treatment environment to maximize recovery is crucial to the rehabilitation of the patient.

Developing Psychiatric Rehabilitation Strategies

Rehabilitation strategies are used to support the individual's recovery and integration into the community. Community-based psychosocial rehabilitation programs usually offer long-term intensive case management services to adults with schizophrenia. Programs provide a continuum of services to meet the changing needs of people with psychiatric disabilities. Patients set rehabilitation goals, and services are then provided to help "clients" (most programs do not use the term "patients") reach their goals. Services range from daily home visits to providing transportation, occupational training, and group support. Social skills training shows much promise for patients with schizophrenia, both individually and in groups. This is a method for teaching patients specific behaviours needed for social interactions. The skills are taught by lecture, demonstration, role-playing, and homework assignments (see Chapters 11 and 14). Nurses

BOX 20-16   **Research for Best Practice**

REDUCING CONFLICT AND CONTAINMENT ON ACUTE PSYCHIATRIC WARDS

Whitecross, F., Seeary, A., & Lee, S. (2013). Measuring the impact of seclusion on psychiatry inpatients and the effectiveness of a pilot single-session post-seclusion counseling intervention. International Journal of Mental Health Nursing, 22(6), 512–521.

Question: In order to identify the impacts that seclusion has on an individual, this intervention study used a standardized measure of trauma symptoms and measured the effectiveness of a postseclusion counselling intervention in mitigating the experience of seclusion-rated trauma and reducing time spent in seclusion.

Methods: This study evaluated a semistructured postseclusion counselling intervention, which was implemented on one inpatient ward and which compared outcomes of postseclusion trauma and time in seclusion with inpatients on another inpatient ward who received postseclusion support as usual. Outcome measures included time in seclusion and self-report of trauma symptoms related to seclusion.

Findings: Almost half (47%) of all patients who experienced seclusion met criteria for probable posttraumatic stress disorder (PTSD). Surprisingly, the semistructured counselling intervention did not reduce the trauma experience following seclusion. There was no difference in the trauma experienced between patients on the intervention ward or those secluded on the usual support wards. However, the participants who experienced the postseclusion counselling session spent significantly less time in seclusion than did those on the comparison ward with postseclusion support as usual.

Implications for Practice: The seclusion experience is considered traumatic to a large number of patients. The fact that almost half the patients who were secluded evinced a degree of trauma that met criteria for probable PTSD is in itself an important finding. It highlights the need for increasing trauma-informed care models that are sensitive and responsive to the potential for seclusion-related psychological distress. Employing less traumatic nursing interventions to avoid seclusion is worth considering. Seclusion is clearly traumatic. This finding and the implementation of a trauma-informed care model on the intervention unit resulted in a heightened awareness among nurses of the negative psychological consequences of seclusion. The nurses' heightened awareness of postseclusion trauma appeared to reduce the amount of time patents actually spent in seclusion. In order to "do no harm" to patients, we must work to minimize the use of restrictive interventions and prioritize a trauma-informed, evidence-based postseclusion response. This pilot study highlights the need for practice change.

may be team members and involved in case management or provision of services. These and other psychological treatment approaches, combined with breakthroughs in biologic therapy, continue to help improve the functioning and quality of life for patients with schizophrenia.

Family Interventions

When schizophrenia first becomes apparent, the patient and family must negotiate the mental health system for the first time (in most cases)—a challenge that almost equals that of confronting the family member's illness. In most provincial jurisdictions, the mental health system is complex and is usually ignored unless a family member becomes seriously mentally ill. The system includes inpatient and outpatient clinics supported by provincial health insurance and publicly funded community mental health clinics and hospitals.

Family members should be encouraged to participate in educational and support groups that help family members deal with the realities of living with a loved one with a mental illness. Family members should be given information about local community and provincial resources and organizations such as mental health associations and those that can help families negotiate the complex system. See Nursing Care Plan 20-2 for care of a patient with a more persistent form of schizophrenia.

Spiritual Domain

Many people living with schizophrenia find comfort in their spirituality, as well as the strength to deal with life events that interfere with their recovery journeys. Religious or spiritual beliefs can be a resource for both patients and their families. Such beliefs may help, for instance, to reappraise difficult events into a positive light (e.g., God gives us only difficulties that we are able to handle). A relationship with the sacred through ritual, prayer, worship, meditation, or other spiritual activities may offer solace, peace, and serenity. These activities may also help to structure the daily lives of individuals with schizophrenia, an important rehabilitation goal. The experience of living with a serious and chronic illness, however, can also cause a crisis of faith or lead one to question the purpose and meaning of one's life. This may be especially true if one's illness brings stigma and rejection by the members of one's community. The sense of connection and hope that supports spiritual growth may be diminished if one is labelled "crazy" by others. Spiritual nursing care actively supports patients in their efforts to sustain and enhance their spirituality. This support can take many forms, from safeguarding the dignity of the patient to understanding the potential impact of hallucinations on spiritual needs, to ensuring spiritual activities can occur. In psychiatric and mental health settings, there may be reluctance on the part of staff to consider the spirituality of a patient who is experiencing the psychotic symptoms of delusions and hallucinations, especially if there are religious overtones to the "voices" and/or fixed beliefs. Knowledge of the patient and of the disease, along with a broad, rich understanding of spirituality, should nevertheless enable the nurse and other staff to address the spiritual domain of care. Employing a relational ethics approach can move the nurse to consider the context and environment of the patient's situation to safeguard dignity (Hamilton Wilson, 2009) (see Chapter 7).

Nursing Care Plan 20-2

Patient With Schizophrenia

MP is a 53-year-old woman who was brought to the crisis support clinic by her community nurse case manager. MP had made a number of telephone calls to her case manager and to the police in rapid succession in the previous 24 hours to report that her next-door neighbour was spying on her. When the nurse case manager arrived, MP was very agitated and distrusting. The case manager also received a call from MP's landlord to report that MP has been making threatening hand gestures to neighbours from her apartment window. MP disclosed to her nurse case manager that her neighbours had tampered with her medications and that she had not been taking them for several days. MP was acutely paranoid and agreed to a hospitalization to keep her safe. She had been attending the Community Clubhouse Program but had not been there for 2 weeks. She failed to attend her follow-up appointment at the mental health clinic to pick up her biweekly dosette of pills.

Setting: Crisis Support Team: Psychosocial Rehabilitation Unit

Baseline Assessment: MP is a 5′4″, 155-pound woman whose appearance is dishevelled. She has not slept for 2 days and appears frightened. She is hypervigilant, suspicious, irritable, and wringing her hands. She is vague about when she last took her treatment medications. She is oriented to time and place and person. Lab values are within normal limits. She has a history of at least 12 former admissions to the psychiatric ward for self-discontinuation of treatment medications.

Associated Psychiatric Diagnosis	Medications
Schizophrenia Social problems/context: Landlord threatening to evict MP from her apartment. Estranged from her two adult sons. Support system limited to a few acquaintances at the clubhouse.	Olanzapine, 5 mg bid Lorazepam (Ativan), 2 mg PO or IM for agitation PRN

Nursing Diagnosis 1: Ineffective Health Maintenance

Defining Characteristics	Related Factors
MP does not remember when she last took her medications. Two weeks of pills are still in the dosette box. MP has not taken the pills for at least 2 weeks, possibly more. MP has not attended the Clubhouse program for 2 weeks. MP did not attend her appointment at the clinic to get a refill of pills in her dosette. MP has been calling the police and the case manager several times in the past 24 hours.	Paranoid delusions are contributing to her thought disturbance. Suspiciousness is contributing to her reluctance to leave her apartment. Inability to make thoughtful judgements. Ineffective individual coping.

Outcomes

Initial	Long Term
Restarts medications in the hospital. Agreement from MP to a referral to the ACT team. Increased ability to self-administer medications. Demonstrates willingness to take her medications independently while in hospital using a blister pack dosette.	MP will communicate her understanding of and demonstrate follow-through with the mutually agreed on health maintenance plan. MP will show the ability to perform health maintenance activities needed to function in her apartment independently with ACT team assistance.

Continued

Interventions

Interventions	Rationale	Ongoing Assessment
Take initial steps to help MP feel safe in the hospital setting.	When a person feels safe, trust is more likely to develop.	Determine when MP's suspiciousness is diminishing. Assess when she is ready to discuss plans for discharge.
Listen carefully, making eye contact. Make efforts to clarify what MP is thinking and feeling.	Listening attentively will help MP to feel safe and cared for.	
Contact all community care providers and convene an interdisciplinary meeting to discuss possible changes to the current community care plan.	A meeting of all care providers will provide a forum to explore alternative support/treatment solutions to improve MP's health maintenance once discharged.	Assess MP's readiness for discharge and transition to the ACT team in addition to returning to the community clubhouse.
	ACT team will be able to increase visitation to MP's home at more frequent intervals. ACT team will provide a more intense level of support.	

Evaluation

Outcomes	Revised Outcomes	Interventions
MP's delusions begin to decrease.	MP meets with the ACT team and agrees to include this team in her follow-up health maintenance plan.	Problem-solve ways for MP to respond to ongoing worries and suspicions.
MP uses some distraction techniques to draw her away from focusing upon the neighbours.		Develop a written, mutually agreed-upon relapse prevention and crisis action plan and send to all community care partners.

Nursing Diagnosis 2: Disturbed Thought Processes

Defining Characteristics	Related Factors
Inaccurate interpretation of stimuli (neighbours tampering with her medications)	Uncompensated alterations in brain activity
Cognitive impairment—attention, memory, and executive function impairment	
Suspiciousness	
Hallucinations (hears voices telling her that her sons are in danger)	

Outcomes

Initial	Long Term
Decrease or eliminate hallucinations.	Use coping strategies to deal with hallucinations or delusions if they reappear.
Have accurate interpretation of the environment.	
Exhibits some reality-based thinking.	
Demonstrates improvement in cognitive functioning (improved attention, memory, and executive functioning).	Communicate clearly with others.
Interacts appropriately with others.	Maintain cognitive functioning.

Nursing Care Plan 20-2 *(Continued)*

Interventions

Interventions	Rationale	Ongoing Assessment
Initiate a nurse–patient relationship by using an accepting, nonjudgemental approach. Be patient.	A therapeutic relationship will provide patient support as she begins to deal with the realization that she is in hospital once again. Be patient and offer reassurance as required until MP feels safe. Do not argue with the false beliefs.	Determine the extent to which MP is willing to trust and engage in a relationship. Make every effort to help MP attend to real rather than internal stimuli, orient her to the real situation, and encourage MP to focus upon distracting concrete activities. Make determined efforts to steer thinking in alternate directions.
Administer olanzapine as prescribed. Observe for effects, side effects, and adverse effects. Begin teaching about the potential switch to an injectable form of antipsychotic medication.	Olanzapine is a D_2 and $5\text{-}HT_{2A}$ antagonist and is indicated for the management of psychotic disorders.	Make sure MP swallows the pills. Monitor for relief of positive symptoms and assess side effects, especially extrapyramidal. Monitor BP for orthostatic hypotension and body temperature increase (NMS).
Assess the ability for self-care activities.	Disturbed thinking may interfere with MP's ability to carry out ADLs.	Continue to assess: determine whether the patient can manage self-care.

Evaluation

Outcomes	Revised Outcomes	Interventions
Delusions began to decrease within 6 days.	Participate in Community Clubhouse activities as soon as possible to bridge the transition from hospital back to the community.	Encourage attendance at the Clubhouse while in hospital to reconnect with the activity/recreational group which MP enjoys.

Nursing Diagnosis 3: Anxiety Related to Fears About Neighbours

Defining Characteristics	Related Factors
Constantly asking nurses for reassurance that her neighbours are not on the unit. Presence of pathophysiologic risk factors: delusional thinking.	Frightened, secondary to **paranoia** (feelings of being unsafe), and delusional thinking.

Outcomes

Initial	Long Term
MP is able to describe a reduction in anxiety. Decreased agitation, gesturing, and pacing.	MP will demonstrate decreased anxiety while at home. MP will refrain from gesturing at neighbours.

Interventions

Interventions	Rationale	Ongoing Assessment
Acknowledge MP's fear and paranoid delusions. Be genuine and empathetic.	Anxiety and delusions change an individual's perception of environmental stimuli. A patient who is frightened will respond because of her need to stay safe.	Assess her response to your comments and her ability to concentrate on what is being said.
Reassure MP verbally at frequent intervals. Make frequent brief supportive contacts. Acknowledge MP's distress.	It is helpful to validate the anxious feelings MP is experiencing.	Observe MP's nonverbal communication for evidence of increased anxiety and agitation.

Continued

Nursing Care Plan 20-2 *(Continued)*

Interventions

Administer lorazepam, 2 mg, for agitation. Oral route is preferable over injection.	Exact mechanisms of action are not understood, but this medication is believed to potentiate the inhibitory neurotransmitter GABA, relieving anxiety and producing sedation.	Observe for a decrease in anxiety.

Evaluation

Outcomes	Revised Outcomes	Interventions
MP gradually decreased anxious behaviour Lorazepam was given regularly for the first 4 days.	Demonstrate control of behaviour by resisting delusions.	Teach MP about the effects of delusions. Problem-solve ways of controlling hallucinations if they occur. Emphasize the importance of taking medications.

Evaluation and Treatment Outcomes

Outcome research related to schizophrenia has redefined previous ways of thinking about the course of the disorder. Schizophrenia was once considered to have a progressively long-term and downward course, but it is now known that schizophrenia can be successfully treated and managed. In one older but significant study, the researchers interviewed patients 20 to 25 years after diagnosis and found that 50% to 66% experienced significant improvement or recovery (Harding, Zubin, & Strauss, 1987). This study is important because it occurred before the development of atypical antipsychotic agents. Today, we can be hopeful that even more people can experience improvement or recover from schizophrenia.

Continuum of Care

Continuity of care has been identified as a major goal of community mental health systems for patients with schizophrenia, because they are at risk for becoming "lost" to services if left alone after discharge. Careful attention to discharge planning encourages follow-up care in the community. In fact, many mental health systems require an outpatient appointment before discharge to better facilitate this transition. Treatment of schizophrenia occurs across a variety of settings. Not only inpatient hospitalization but also partial hospitalization, day treatment, and crisis stabilization and continuing community care can be used effectively.

Inpatient-Focused Care

Much of the previous discussion concerns care in the inpatient setting. Today, inpatient hospitalizations are brief and focus on patient stabilization. Many times, patients are involuntarily admitted for a short period. During the stabilization period, the status is changed to voluntary admission, whereby the patient agrees to treatment.

EMERGENCY CARE !

Emergency care ideally takes place in a hospital emergency room, but the crisis often occurs in the home. Patients are usually relapsing and do not recognize their bizarre or aggressive behaviours as symptoms. In many urban communities, a specially trained crisis team is sent to assess the emergency and recommend further treatment. Patients are brought to the emergency room not only because of relapse but also because of medication side effects. Nurses should refer to the previous discussion for nursing management.

Community Care

Most of the care of patients with schizophrenia will be in the community through publicly supported mental health delivery systems. Community services include assertive community treatment, outpatient therapy, case management, and psychosocial rehabilitation, including clubhouse programs. For a very small number of patients with a community treatment order in effect that delineates the conditions required to live in the community, services must be congruent with those conditions (see Chapter 3). For all patients in the community, health care should be integrated in a holistic manner with physical

FIGURE 20-7 Bio/psycho/social/spiritual interventions for patients with schizophrenia.

Spiritual
1. Guard dignity of patient
2. Support hope
3. Support helpful sacred activities

Biologic
1. Monitor medications
2. Minimize side effects
3. Decrease impact of movement disorders
4. Address immune function
5. Address nutritional status
6. Modify cognitive deficits
7. Address sleep

Social
1. Promote economic stability
2. Decrease family/caregiver stress
3. Provide family education
4. Maintain housing
5. Increase social contact

Psychological
1. Address social skills
2. Address problem-solving skills
3. Address self-concept
4. Increase stress management skills
5. Address symptom management and relapse prevention skills
6. Address family relationships

health care. Nurses should be especially vigilant that patients with mental illnesses receive proper primary and medical health care.

● **STUDY NOTE**

Priorities in the patient with acute symptoms of schizophrenia include managing psychosis and keeping the patient safe and free from harming self or others. In the community, the priorities are preventing relapse, maintaining and improving psychosocial functioning, psychoeducation, and improving quality of life.

Mental Health Promotion

In some cases, it is less the disorder itself threatening the mental health of the person with schizophrenia than the stresses of seeking care and services. Health care systems are complex and are often at the mercy of a system rule that is outdated. Development of assertiveness and conflict resolution skills can help the person in negotiating access to systems that will provide services. Developing a positive support system for stressful periods will help promote a positive outcome (Fig. 20-7).

SUMMARY OF KEY POINTS

■ The patient with schizophrenia displays a complex myriad of symptoms typically categorized as positive symptoms (those that exist but should not), such as delusions or hallucinations and disorganized thinking and behaviour, and negative symptoms (characteristics that should be there but are lacking), such as alogia, avolition, anhedonia, and affective blunting.

■ In the past, the diagnosis and treatment of schizophrenia focused on the more observable and dramatic positive symptoms (i.e., delusions and hallucinations), but recently, scientists have shifted their focus to the disorganizing symptoms of cognition.

■ The clinical presentation of schizophrenia occurs in three phases: phase 1, first-episode psychosis, entails the initial diagnosis and first treatment; phase 2 includes periods of stabilization between episodes of overt signs and symptoms but during which the patient needs sustained treatment; and phase 3 includes periods of exacerbation or relapse that require hospitalization or more frequent contacts with mental health professionals and increased use of resources.

■ Biologic theories of what causes schizophrenia include genetic, infectious–autoimmune, neuroanatomic, and dopamine hypotheses. The last is supported by the advanced technology of PET scan findings and the understanding of the mechanisms of antipsychotic medications.

■ Biologic assessment of the patient with schizophrenia must include a thorough history and physical examination to rule out any medical illness or substance abuse problem that might be the cause of the patient's symptoms, assessment of risk for self-injury or injury to others, and documentation of baseline health information before medications are administered. Several standardized assessment tools are available to help assess characteristic abnormal motor movements.

■ Several nursing interventions address the biologic domain: promotion of self-care activities, activity, exercise, and nutritional, thermoregulation, and fluid balance interventions. In general, the antipsychotic drugs used to treat schizophrenia block dopamine transmission in the brain but also cause some troublesome and sometimes serious side effects, primarily anticholinergic side effects and extrapyramidal side effects (motor abnormalities). Newer antipsychotic agents block serotonin as well as dopamine. The nurse should be familiar with these drugs, their possible side effects, and the interventions required to manage side effects.

■ The extrapyramidal side effects of antipsychotic drugs can appear early in drug treatment and include acute parkinsonism or pseudoparkinsonism, acute dystonia, and akathisia, or they can appear late in treatment after months or years. The primary example of late-appearing extrapyramidal side effects is tardive dyskinesia, which is a severe syndrome of abnormal motor movements of the mouth, tongue, and jaw.

■ Psychological assessment must include equal attention to manifestations of both positive and negative symptoms and a concentrated focus on the cognitive impairments that make it so difficult for patients to manage their disorder. Several standardized assessment tools assess for positive and negative symptoms. Developing the nurse–patient relationship is essential in helping patients manage disturbed thoughts and sensory perceptions. Interventions should be designed to enhance cognitive functioning. Patient and family education are critical interventions for the person with schizophrenia.

■ Because schizophrenia is a lifetime disorder and patients require the continued support and care of mental health professionals and family or friends, one of the primary nursing interventions is ensuring that patients and families are properly educated about the course of the disorder, the importance of drug maintenance, and the need for consistent care and support. Research is demonstrating that interaction between patients and their families is key to the success of long-term treatments and outcomes.

CRITICAL THINKING CHALLENGES

1 Why are positive symptoms easier to track than negative symptoms?
2 Describe ways in which medical illness or substance abuse could cause a patient to show symptoms similar to schizophrenia.
3 Suggest reasons that a higher rate of schizophrenia is found in people of lower socioeconomic status from urban, industrialized communities.
4 The physical environment is important to the patient with schizophrenia. Think of the typical hospital unit. What environmental factors could be stress-producing or misleading to the person with schizophrenia?
5 Compare therapeutic and nontherapeutic communication skills when dealing with a person with schizophrenia who is actively hallucinating.
6 Explore using a simulation exercise developed by Deegan (2006), *Hearing Voices that are Distressing*, with your student group. Research suggests that students find it a valuable experience that facilitates understanding and empathy (Hamilton Wilson et al., 2009).

REFERENCES

Addington, J. & Addington, D. (2006). The impact of cognitive functioning on outcome. *Schizophrenia Research, 86*(S1), 27.
Addington, J., McCleery, A., & Addington, D. (2005). Three-year outcome of family work in an early psychosis program. *Schizophrenia Research, 79*(1), 107–116.
Addington, J., van Mastrigt, S., Jutchinson, J., & Addington, D. (2002). Pathways to care: Help seeking behaviour in first episode psychosis. *Acta Psychiatrica Scandinavica, 106*(5), 358–364.
Altamura, A. C., Bassetti, R., Bignotti, S., Pioli, R., & Mundo, E. (2003). Clinical variables related to suicide attempts in schizophrenic patients: A retrospective study. *Schizophrenia Research, 60*(1), 47–55.
American Psychiatric Association. (2013). *Diagnostic and statistical manual of mental disorders* (5th ed.). Arlington, VA: Author.
Amminger, G. P., Henry L. P., Harrigan, S. M., Harris M. G., Alvarez-Jimenez, M., Herrman, H., … McGorry, P. D. (2011). Outcome in early-onset schizophrenia revisited: Findings from the Early Psychosis Prevention and Intervention Centre long-term follow-up study. *Schizophrenia Research, 131*(1–3), 112–119.
Arseneault, L., Cannon, M., Wilton, J., & Murray, R. (2004). Causal association between cannabis and psychosis: An examination of the evidence. *British Journal of Psychiatry, 184*, 100–117.
Barak, Y. & Aizenberg, D. (2012). Clinical and psychosocial remission in schizophrenia: Correlations with antipsychotic treatment. *BioMedCentral Psychiatry, 12*(108), 1–5.
Benes, F. M. (2000). Emerging principles of altered neural circuitry in schizophrenia. *Brain Research Developmental Brain Research, 31*(2–3), 251–269.
Boyd, M. & Lapierre, E. (1996). Fluid imbalance and water intoxication: The elusive syndrome. In A. McBride & J. Austin (Eds.), *Psychiatric mental health nursing: Integration of the biological into behavioural* (pp. 396–424). Philadelphia, PA: WB Saunders.
Buchsbaum, M. (1990). The frontal lobes, basal ganglia, and temporal lobes as a site for schizophrenia. *Schizophrenia Bulletin, 16*(3), 377–387.
Byrne, M., Agerbo, E., Ewald, H., Eaton, W. W., & Mortensen, P. B. (2003). Parental age and risk of schizophrenia: A case–control study. *Archives of General Psychiatry, 60*(7), 673–678.
Canadian Psychiatric Association. (2005). Clinical practice guidelines: Treatment of schizophrenia. *Canadian Journal of Psychiatry, 50*(S1), 1–48.
Carlson, N. R. (2013). *Physiology of behavior* (11th ed.). New York, NY: Pearson.
Caroff, S. & Mann, S. (1993). Neuroleptic malignant syndrome. *Medical Clinics of North America, 77*, 185–202.
Casey, D. E. (1994). Schizophrenia: Psychopharmacology. In J. W. Jefferson & J. H. Greist (Eds.), *The psychiatric clinics of North America: Annual of drug therapy* (Vol. 1, pp. 81–100). Philadelphia, PA: WB Saunders.

Centre for Addiction and Mental Health. (2013). CAMH scientists discover genetic changes that may contribute to the onset of schizophrenia. Retrieved from http://www.camh.ca/en/hospital/about_camh/newsroom/news_releases_media_advisories_and_backgrounders/current_year/Pages/CAMH-scientists-discover-genetic-changes-that-may-contribute-to-the-onset-of-schizophrenia-.aspx

Chance, S. A., Esiri, M. M., & Crow, T. J. (2003) Ventricular enlargement in schizophrenia: A primary change in the temporal lobe? *Schizophrenia Research, 62*(1–2), 123–131.

Chou, Y. H., Halldin, C., & Farde, L. (2003). Occupancy of 5HT(1A) receptors in clozapine in the primate brain: A PET study. *Psychopharmacology, 166*(3), 234–240.

Cirillo, M. A. & Seidman, L. J. (2003). Verbal declarative memory dysfunction in schizophrenia: From clinical assessment to genetics and brain mechanisms. *Neuropsychology Review, 13*(2), 43–77.

Cohn, T. (2012). The link between schizophrenia and diabetes. *Current Psychiatry, 11*(10), 29–34, 46.

Costain, G. & Bassett, A. S. (2013). Individualizing recurrence risks for severe mental illness: Epidemiologic and molecular genetic approaches. *Schizophrenia Bulletin* [online ahead of print] doi:10.1093/schbul/sbt133

Crowther, R., Marshall, M., Bond, G., & Huxley, P. (2004). *Cochrane Database of Systematic Reviews, 1*, 1–86.

Csernansky, J. G. (2003). Treatment of schizophrenia: Preventing the progression of disease. *Psychiatric Clinics of North America, 26*(2), 367–379.

Davidson, L. L. & Heinrichs, R. W. (2003). Quantification of frontal and temporal lobe brain-imaging findings in schizophrenia: A meta-analysis. *Psychiatry Research, 122*(2), 69–87.

De Hert, M., McKenzie, K., & Peuskens, J. (2001). Risk factors for suicide in young people suffering from schizophrenia: A long-term follow-up study. *Schizophrenia Research, 47*(2–3), 127–134.

Deegan, P. (1992). The independent living movement and people with psychiatric disabilities: Taking back control over our own lives. *Psychosocial Rehabilitation Journal, 15*, 5–9.

Deegan, P. (2006). *Hearing voices curriculum: Complete training and curriculum package.* Available at http://www.power2u.org/mm5/merchant.mvc

Dolder, C. R., Lacro, J. P., Dunn, L. B., & Jeste, D. V. (2002). Antipsychotic medication adherence: Is there a difference between typical and atypical agents? *American Journal of Psychiatry, 159*(1), 103–108.

Emsley, R., Chiliza, B., Asmal, L., & Harvey, B. (2013). The nature of relapse in schizophrenia, *BMC Psychiatry, 13*, 50. Retrieved from http://www.biomedcentral.com/1471-244X/13/50

Falkai, P., Schneider-Axmann, T., Honer, W. G., Vogeley, K., Schonell, H., Pfeiffer, U., ... Tepest, R. (2003). Influence on genetic loading, obstetric complications, and premorbid adjustment on brain morphology in schizophrenia: A MRI study. *European Archives of Psychiatry and Clinical Neuroscience, 253*(2), 92–99.

Franzen, G. (1970). Plasma free fatty acids before and after an intravenous insulin injection in acute schizophrenic men. *British Journal of Psychiatry, 116*(531), 173–177.

Frese F. III, Knight, E., & Saks, E. (2009). Recovery from schizophrenia: With views of psychiatrists, psychologists, and others diagnosed with this disorder. *Schizophrenia Bulletin, 35*(2), 370–380.

Freudenreich, O. & Cather, C. (2012). Antipsychotic medication nonadherence: Risk factors and remedies. *Focus, 10*(2), 124–129.

Ghose, S., Weickert, C. S., Colvin, S. M., Coyle, J. T., Herman, M. M., Hyde, T. M., & Kleinman, J. E. (2003). Glutamate carboxypeptidase II gene expression in the human frontal and temporal lobe in schizophrenia. *Neuropsychopharmacology, 29*(1), 117–125.

Goldman, L. S. (1999). Medical illness in patients with schizophrenia. *Journal of Clinical Psychiatry, 60*(Suppl. 21), 1015.

Goldner, E. M., Hsu, L., Waraich, P., & Somers, J. M. (2002). Prevalence and incidence studies of schizophrenia disorders: A systematic review of the literature. *Canadian Journal of Psychiatry, 47*(9), 833–843.

Gottlieb, J. (2012). *CopingTutor* App, Cognitive Health Innovations Inc. Available from https://www.copingtutor.com/.

Gough, E. (2005). Diabetes and schizophrenia. *Practical Diabetes, 22*(1), 23–26.

Gumley, A., O'Grady, M., McNay, L., Reilly, J., Power, K., & Norrie, J. (2003). Early intervention for relapse in schizophrenia: Results of a 12-month randomized controlled trial of cognitive behavioural therapy. *Psychological Medicine, 33*(3), 419–431.

Gur, R. E. & Gur, R. C. (2005). Neuroimaging in schizophrenia: Linking neuropsychiatric manifestations to neurobiology. In B. J. Sadock & V. A. Sadock (Eds.), *Comprehensive textbook of psychiatry* (pp. 1396–1408). Philadelphia, PA: Lippincott Williams & Wilkins.

Guy, W. (1976). *ECDEU: Assessment manual for psychopharmacology* (DHEW Publication No. 76-338). Washington, DC: Department of Health Education and Welfare, Psychopharmacology Branch.

Hamilton Wilson, J. (2009). Moving beyond policy rhetoric: Building a moral community for early psychosis intervention. *Journal of Psychiatric and Mental Health Nursing, 16*(7), 621–628.

Hamilton Wilson, J. (2012). First episode psychosis: The experience of parent caregivers (Doctoral dissertation, University of Alberta, Edmonton, Alberta).

Hamilton Wilson, J., Azzopardi, W., Sager, S., Gould, B., Conroy, S., Deegan, P., & Archie, S. (2009). A narrative study of the experiences of student nurses who have participated in the Hearing Voices that are Distressing simulation. *International Journal of Nursing Education Scholarship, 6*(1), article 19.

Hamilton Wilson, J. & Hobbs, H. (1999). The family educator and professional resource for families. *Journal of Psychosocial Nursing and Mental Health Services, 37*(6), 22–27.

Han, M., Huang, X. F., Chen, D. C., Xiu, M., Kosten, T. R., & Zhang, X. Y. (2013). Diabetes and cognitive deficits in chronic schizophrenia: A case–control study. *PLoS ONE, 8*(6), e66299. doi:10.1371/journal.pone.0066299

Harding, C., Zubin, J., & Strauss, J. (1987). Chronicity in schizophrenia: Fact, partial fact or artifact? *Hospital and Community Psychiatry, 38*(5), 477–486.

Harkavy-Friedman, J. M. (2007). Risk factors for suicide in patients with schizophrenia. *Psychiatric Times, 25*(2). Retrieved from http://www.psychiatrictimes.com/articles/risk-factors-suicide-patients-schizophrenia

Harrison, G., Fouskakis, D., Rasmussen, F., Tynelius, P., Sipos, A., & Gunnell, D. (2003). Association between psychotic disorder and urban place of birth is not mediated by obstetric complications or childhood socioeconomic position: A cohort study. *Psychological Medicine, 33*(4), 723–731.

Harrison, G., Hopper, K., Craig, T., Laska, E., Siegel, C., Wanderling, K. ... Wiersma, D. (2001). Recovery from psychotic illness: A 15 and 25 year international follow-up study. *British Journal of Psychiatry, 178*, 506–517.

Hartman, M., Steketee, M. C., Silva, S., Lanning, K., & Andersson, C. (2003). Wisconsin Card Sorting Test performance in schizophrenia: The role of working memory. *Schizophrenia Research, 63*(3), 201–217.

Hawkes, E. (2012). *When quietness came: A neuroscientist's personal journey with schizophrenia.* Dundas, ON: Bridgecross Communication.

Health Canada. (2002). *A report on mental illnesses in Canada: Chapter 3: Schizophrenia.* Retrieved from http://www.phac-aspc.gc.ca/publicat/miic-mmac/pdf/chap_3_e.pdf

Hennekens, C., Hennekens, A., Hollar, D., & Casey, D. E. (2005). Schizophrenia and increased risks of cardiovascular disease. *American Heart Journal, 150*(6), 1115–1121.

Hor, K. & Taylor, M. (2010). Suicide and schizophrenia: A systematic review of rates and risk factors. *Journal of Psychopharmacology, 24*(Suppl. 4), 81–90.

Inman, S., (2010) *After her brain broke: Helping my daughter recover her sanity.* Dundas, ON: Bridgecross Communication.

Jibson, M. D. & Tandon, R. (2000). Treatment of schizophrenia. In D. L. Dunner, & J. E. Rosenbaum (Eds.), *The psychiatric clinics of North America annual of drug therapy* (Vol. 7, pp. 83–113). Philadelphia, PA: WB Saunders.

Kandel, E. R., Schwartz, J. H., & Jessell, T. M. (2000). *Principles of neural science* (4th ed.). New York, NY: McGraw-Hill.

Kaneko, Y. & Keshavan, M. (2012) Cognitive remediation in schizophrenia. *Clinical Psychopharmacology and Neuroscience, 10*(3), 125–135.

Kay, S. R., Fiszbein, A., & Opler, L. A. (1987). The Positive and Negative Syndrome Scale (PANSS) for schizophrenia. *Schizophrenia Bulletin, 13*, 261–276.

Kern, R. S., Green, M. V., Mintz, J., & Liberman, R. P. (2003). Does 'errorless learning' compensate for neurocognitive impairments in the work rehabilitation of persons with schizophrenia? *Psychological Medicine, 33*(3), 433–442.

Kern, R. S., Liberman, R. P., Kopelowicz, A., Mintz, J., & Green, M. F. (2002). Applications of errorless learning for improving work performance in persons with schizophrenia. *American Journal Psychiatry, 159*(11), 1921–1926.

Keshavan, M., Tandon, R., Boutros, N., & Nasrallah, H. (2008). Schizophrenia, "just the facts": What we know in 2008. Part 3: Neurobiology. *Schizophrenia Research, 106*(2–3), 89–107.

Kingdon, D. & Turkington, D. (2006). The ABCs of cognitive behavioural therapy for schizophrenia. *Psychiatric Times.* Retrieved from http://www.psychiatrictimes.com/schizophrenia/abcs-cognitive-behavioral-therapy-schizophrenia

Kulkarni, J., Hayes, E., & Gavrilidis, E. (2012). Hormones and schizophrenia. *Current Opinions in Psychiatry, 25*(2), 89–95.

Leucht, S., Burkard, T., Henderson, J., Maj, M., & Sartorius, N. (2007). Physical illness and schizophrenia: A review of the literature. *Acta Psychiatrica Scandinavica, 116*(5), 317–333.

Levin, E. & Rezvani, A. (2007). Nicotinic interactions with antipsychotic drugs, models of schizophrenia and impacts on cognitive function. *Biochemical Pharmacology, 74*(8), 1182–1191.

Malla, A., Norman, R., & Joober, R. (2005). First episode psychosis, early intervention and outcome: What have we learned? *Canadian Journal of Psychiatry, 50*(14), 881–891.

McDonald, C., Grech, A., Toulopoulou, T., Schulze, K., Chapple, B., Sham, P., ... Murray, R. (2002). Brain volumes in familial and non-familial schizophrenia probands and their unaffected relatives. *American Journal of Medical Genetics, 114*(6), 616–625.

McGlashan, T. H. (1994). Psychosocial treatments of schizophrenia: The potential relationships. In N. C. Andreasen (Ed.), *Schizophrenia: From mind to molecule* (pp. 189–215). Washington, DC: American Psychiatric Press.

Melau, M., Jeppesen, P., Thorup, A., Bertelsen, M., Peterson, L., Krarup, G., & Nordentoft, M. (2011). The effect of five years versus two years of specialised assertive intervention for first episode psychosis—OPUS II: Study protocol for a randomized controlled trial. *Trials, 12,* 72.

Mental Health Commission of Canada (MHCC). (2007). *A time for action: Tackling stigma and discrimination.* Retrieved from http://www.mentalhealthcommission.ca/English/Pages/AntiStigmaCampaign.aspx

Mental Health Commission of Canada (MHCC). (2012). *Changing directions: Changing lives. The mental health strategy for Canada.* Retrieved from http://www.mentalhealthcommission.ca/English/node/721

Mental Health Commission Canada (MHCC). (2013). *Aspiring workforce: Employment and income for people with serious mental illness.* Retrieved from http://www.mentalhealthcommission.ca/English/node/7606

Mental Health Commission of Canada (MHCC). (2013a). *At home/Chez soi.* http://www.mentalhealthcommission.ca/English/initiatives-and-projects/home?routetoken=ff8ead4644148979334f1198d0bb826f&terminitial=38

Mental Health Commission of Canada (MHCC). (2013b). *National guidelines for a comprehensive service system to support family caregivers of adults with mental health problems and illnesses.* Retrieved from http://www.mentalhealthcommission.ca/English/node/8601/#sthash.FZdfsot1.dpuf

Mesholam-Gately, R., Giuliano, A., Faraone, S., Goff, K., & Seidman, L. (2009). Neurocognition in first-episode schizophrenia: A meta-analytic review. *Neuropsychology, 23*(3), 315–336.

Montoya, A., Ocampo, M., & Torres-Ruiz, A. (2003). Neuroleptic malignant syndrome in Mexico. *Canadian Journal of Clinical Pharmacology, 10*(3), 111–113.

Morrison, E. F. (1992). A coercive interactional style as an antecedent to aggression in psychiatric patients. *Research in Nursing and Health, 15,* 421–431.

Morrison, E. F. (1993). Toward a better understanding of violence in psychiatric settings: Debunking the myths. *Archives of Psychiatric Nursing, 7,* 328–335.

Morrison, E. F. & Carney Love, C. (2003). An evaluation of four programs for the management of aggression in psychiatric settings. *Archives in Psychiatric Nursing, 17*(4), 146–155.

Muir-Cochrane, E. (2006). Medical co-morbidity factors and barriers to care for people with schizophrenia. *Journal of Psychiatric & Mental Health Nursing, 13*(4), 447–452.

Muller-Vahl, K. R. & Emrich, H. M. (2008). Cannabis and schizophrenia: Towards a cannabinoid hypothesis of schizophrenia. *Expert Review of Neurotherapeutics, 8*(7), 1037–1048.

Murray, R. M. & Bramon, E. (2005). Developmental model of schizophrenia. In B. J. Sadock & V. A. Sadock (Eds.), *Comprehensive textbook of psychiatry* (pp. 1381–1396). Philadelphia, PA: Lippincott Williams & Wilkins.

Nasar, S. (1998). *A beautiful mind: The life of mathematical genius and Nobel Laureate John Nash.* New York, NY: Touchstone.

Niemi, L. T., Suvisaari, J. M., Tuulio-Henriksson, A., & Lonnqvist, J. K. (2003). Childhood developmental abnormalities in schizophrenia: Evidence from high-risk studies. *Schizophrenia Research, 60*(2–3), 239–258.

O'Carroll, R., Russell, H., Lawrie, S., & Johnstone, E. (1999). Errorless learning and the cognitive rehabilitation of memory-impaired schizophrenic patients. *Psychological Medicine, 29,* 105–112.

Onken, S. J., Dumont, J. M., Ridgway, P., Dornan, D. H., & Ralph, R. O. (2007). Mental health recovery: What helps and what hinders? *A national research project for the development of recovery facilitating system performance indicators.* Retrieved from http://www.mhsret.org/documents/ROSIPilotMeasuresV7.pdf

Overall, J. E. & Gorham, D. R. (1988). The Brief Psychiatric Rating Scale (BPRS): Recent developments in ascertainment and scaling. *Psychopharmacology Bulletin, 24,* 97–99.

Oxford University Press and the Maryland Psychiatric Research Center. (2002). Graduate student in peril: A first person account of schizophrenia. *Schizophrenia Bulletin, 28*(4), 745–755.

Penn, A. A. (2001). Early brain wiring: Activity-dependent processes. *Schizophrenia Bulletin, 27*(3), 336–347.

Pia, L. & Tamleto, M. (2006). Unawareness in schizophrenia: Neuropsychological and neuroanatomical findings. *Psychiatry & Clinical Neurosciences, 60*(5), 531–537.

Picchioni, M. M. & Murray, R. M. (2007). Schizophrenia. *British Medical Journal, 335*(7610), 91–95.

Rapoport, J., Addington, A., & Frangou, S. (2005). The neurodevelopmental model of schizophrenia: Update 2005. *Molecular Psychiatry, 10,* 434–449.

Ryan, M. C. M., Collins, P., & Thakore, J. H. (2003). Impaired fasting glucose tolerance in first-episode, drug-naive patients with schizophrenia. *American Journal of Psychiatry, 160,* 284–289.

Sallet, P. C., Elkis, H., Alves, T. M., Oliveira, J. R., Sassi, E., Campi de Castro, C., ... Gattaz, W. F. (2003). Reduced cortical folding in schizophrenia: An MRI morphometric study. *American Journal of Psychiatry, 160*(9), 1606–1613.

Schimmelbusch, W. H., Mueller, P. S., & Sheps, J. (1971). The positive correlation between insulin resistance and duration of hospitalization in untreated schizophrenia. *British Journal of Psychiatry, 118*(545), 36–42.

Sedvall, G. (1994). Positron-emission tomography as a metabolic and neurochemical probe. In N. C. Andreasen (Ed.), *Schizophrenia: From mind to molecule* (pp. 147–155). Washington, DC: American Psychiatric Press.

Sheffield, J. M., Gold, J. M., Strauss, M. E., Carter, C. S., Macdonald, A. W. III, Ragland, J. D., ... Barch, D. M. (2014). Common and specific cognitive deficits in schizophrenia: Relationships to function. *Cognitive, Affective & Behavioral Neuroscience, 14*(1), 161–174.

Simpson, G. M. & Angus, J. W. S. L. (1970). A rating scale for extrapyramidal side effects. *Acta Psychiatrica Scandinavica, 212*(Suppl.), 11–19.

Sprague, R. L. & Kalachnik, J. E. (1991). Reliability, validity, and a total score cutoff for the Dyskinesia Identification Scale System: Condensed User Scale (DISCUS) with mentally ill and mentally retarded populations. *Psychopharmacology Bulletin, 27,* 51–58.

Stahl, S. (2002). The metabolic syndrome: Psychopharmacologists should weigh the evidence for weighing the patient. *Journal of Clinical Psychiatry, 63,* 1094–1095.

Stahl, S. (2008). *Essential psychopharmacology: Neuroscientific basis and practical application* (3rd ed.). Cambridge, UK: Cambridge University Press.

Standing Senate Committee on Social Affairs, Science and Technology. (2006). *Out of the shadows at last: Transforming mental health, mental illness and addiction services in Canada.* Retrieved from http://www.parl.gc.ca/39/1/parlbus/commbus/senate/Com-e/SOCI-E/rep-e/rep-02may06-e.htm

Subotnik, K. L., Goldstein, M. J., Nuechterlein, K. H., Woo, S. M., & Mintz, J. (2002). Are communication deviance and expressed emotion related to family history of psychiatric disorders in schizophrenia? *Schizophrenia Bulletin, 28*(4), 719–729.

Subramaniam, K., Luks, T., Fisher, M., Simpson, G., Nagarajan, S., & Vinogradov, S. (2012). Computerized cognitive training restores neural activity within the reality monitoring network in schizophrenia. *Neuron, 73*(4), 842–853.

Tharyan, P. & Adams, C. E. (2005). Electroconvulsive therapy for schizophrenia. *Cochrane Database of Systematic Reviews, 18*(2), CD000076.

Tsuang, M. T., Stone, W. S., & Faraone, S. V. (2001). Genes, environment and schizophrenia. *British Journal of Psychiatry, 178*(Suppl. 40), S18–S24.

Walker, E., Kestler, L., Bollini, A., & Hochman, K. M. (2004). Schizophrenia: Etiology and course. *Annual Review of Psychology, 55,* 401–430.

Weisman, A. G., Gomes, L. G., & Lopez, S. R. (2003). Shifting blame away from ill relatives: Latino families' reactions to schizophrenia. *Journal of Nervous and Mental Disease, 191*(9), 574–581.

Whitecross, F., Seeary, A., & Lee, S. (2013). Measuring the impact of seclusion on psychiatry inpatients and the effectiveness of a pilot single-session post-seclusion counseling intervention. *International Journal of Mental Health Nursing, 22*(6), 512–521.

Wuerker, A. K., Long, J. D., Haas, G. L., & Bellack, A. S. (2002). Interpersonal control, expressed emotion, and change in symptoms in families of persons with schizophrenia. *Schizophrenia Research, 58*(2–3), 281–292.

21 Schizoaffective, Delusional, and Other Psychotic Disorders

Diana Clarke
Adapted from the chapter "Schizoaffective, Delusional, and Other Psychotic Disorders" by Nan Roberts and Roberta Stock

LEARNING OBJECTIVES

After studying this chapter, you will be able to:

- Define schizoaffective disorder and distinguish the major differences and similarities among schizophrenia, schizoaffective, and mood disorders.
- Discuss the important epidemiologic findings related to schizoaffective disorder.
- Explain the primary elements involved in assessment, nursing diagnoses, nursing interventions, and evaluation of patients with schizoaffective disorder.
- Define delusional disorder and name the subtypes of this disorder.
- Discuss the theories related to the aetiology of delusional disorder.
- Explain the nursing care of patients with delusional disorder.
- Identify the essential features of schizophreniform disorder, brief psychotic disorder, substance/medication-induced psychotic disorder, and psychotic disorder due to another medical condition.

KEY CONCEPT

- delusions

KEY TERMS

- bipolar type • bizarre delusions • delusional disorder • depressive type
- erotomanic delusion • grandiose delusion • jealous delusion
- nonbizarre delusions • misidentification • persecutory delusion
- psychosis • schizoaffective disorder • somatic delusion

Psychiatric and mental health (PMH) nurses care for patients who have psychiatric disorders involving underlying psychoses other than schizophrenia (SCH) and mood disorders (MD). These disorders include schizoaffective, delusional, brief psychotic, and schizophreniform disorders. Psychotic disorders also may be induced by medications or other substances or be a symptom of another medical disorder. This chapter introduces these disorders and describes the associated nursing care. Their common element is the state of **psychosis** in which an individual can experience hallucinations, delusions, or disorganized thoughts, speech, or behaviour (positive symptoms) and/or diminished

emotional expression, anhedonia, and avolition (negative symptoms) (see Chapter 20 for further delineation of positive and negative symptoms).

SCHIZOAFFECTIVE DISORDER

Clinical Course

Schizoaffective disorder (SCA) is a complex and persistent psychiatric illness. This disorder was recognized in 1933 by Kasanin, who described varying degrees of symptoms of both SCH and MD, beginning in youth. All his patients were well adjusted before the sudden onset of symptoms that erupted after the occurrence of a specific

415

environmental stressor. Since Kasanin's time, debate and controversy about the status of this disorder have been extensive, resulting in many different definitions and classifications that remain under consideration (van Os, Linscott, Myin-Germeys, Delespaul, & Krabbendam, 2009). SCA was not recognized as a separate disorder in the *Diagnostic and Statistical Manual* (*DSM*) of the American Psychiatric Association (APA) until the *DSM-III-R* in 1987; its definition included symptom duration. Debate about the status of this disorder continues. A systematic review of clinical trial studies comparing SCA with SCH and MD suggests that SCA occupies an intermediate position between the latter disorders, but no clear-cut distinctions between SCA and SCH or SCA and MD could be established (Cheniaux et al., 2008). A survey of psychiatrists' attitudes towards SCA found that while almost all had used the diagnosis in clinical practice and most considered the diagnosis to be clinically useful, there was little agreement about its nature, its relationship to other mental disorders, or its aetiology (Rowe & Clark, 2008). SCA remains a separate disorder in the *DSM-5* (APA, 2013).

SCA is characterized by intervals of intense symptoms alternating with quiescent periods, during which psychosocial functioning is adequate. The episodic nature of this disorder is characteristic. It is at times marked by symptoms of SCH; at other times, it appears to be a MD. In other cases, both psychosis and pervasive mood changes occur concurrently. Patients feel that they are on a "chronic roller coaster ride" of symptoms that are often more difficult to cope with than the individual problem of either SCH or MD. The long-term outcome of SCA is generally better than that of SCH but worse than that of MD. This group of patients resembles the MD group in work function and the SCH group in social function (Bottender, Strauss, & Moller, 2010).

● **STUDY NOTE**

Patients with SCA have many similar responses to their disorder as people with SCH, with one exception. These patients have many more "mood" responses and are very susceptible to suicide.

Diagnostic Criteria

Mental health providers find SCA difficult to conceptualize, diagnose, and treat because the clinical picture is often very complex and varies from episode to episode over time. Patients often have misdiagnoses of SCH or conversely of depression with psychotic features or bipolar MD. The difficulty in conceptualizing SCA is reflected in the controversy regarding the diagnostic criteria. Although it has been argued that this disorder should be named either *schizophrenia with mood symptoms*

or *mood disorder with schizophrenia symptoms*, the fifth edition of the *DSM* (APA, 2013) has left it as a separate diagnosis midway along the SCH spectrum between SCH and schizophreniform disorder.

To receive a diagnosis of SCA, a patient must have an uninterrupted period of illness when there is a major depressive, manic, or mixed episode along with two of the following symptoms of SCH: delusions, hallucinations, disorganized speech, disorganized or catatonic behaviour, or negative symptoms (e.g., affective flattening, alogia, or avolition). In addition, although the person experiences problems with mood most of the time, the positive symptoms (delusions or hallucinations) must be present without the mood symptoms at some time during this period (for at least 2 weeks) (Table 21-1). To clarify this disorder further, two related subtypes of SCA have been identified. In the **bipolar type**, the patient exhibits manic symptoms alone or a mix of manic and depressive symptoms. Patients with the **depressive type** display only symptoms of a major depressive episode (APA, 2013). The most common disorders from which SCA must be differentiated include MD of manic, depressive, or mixed types and SCH.

Epidemiology and Risk Factors

The lifetime prevalence of SCA is estimated to be around 0.3% (APA, 2013) but is very difficult to track. This disorder occurs less commonly than does SCH. The incidence of SCA is relatively constant across populations in varied

IN A LIFE

Louis Riel (1844–1885)
Métis Leader

Public Persona

Louis Riel, leader of the Métis in Manitoba and Saskatchewan, has been remembered as the man who negotiated for the establishment of Manitoba as a province and who led the fight for the protection of Métis and Aboriginal land and rights in Western Canada. Arrested for treason in 1884, he showed symptoms of grandiosity and paranoid delusions. He was declared "sane" by the superintendent of the Asylum for the Insane in Toronto, stood trial, and was hanged in 1885.

Personal Realities

Riel had numerous episodes of profound depression, apparent psychosis, and delusional thinking throughout his life. At times, he believed he had been substituted for the real Louis Riel who had died. At other times, he talked about his "mission" to form a new religion and replace the Pope. He was hospitalized and committed to insane asylums on numerous occasions. In retrospect, he has been "diagnosed" variably in the literature with paranoid schizophrenia, SCA, and bipolar disorder.

From Perr, I. N. (1992). Religion, political leadership, charisma and mental illness: The strange story of Louis Riel. *Journal of Forensic Science, 37*(2), 574–584; Waite, P. (1987). Between three oceans: Challenges of a continental destiny. In C. Brown (Ed.), *The illustrated history of Canada* (pp. 279–373). Toronto, ON: Lester & Orpen Dennys.

Table 21-1   Key Characteristics of SCA

Diagnostic Criteria and Target Symptoms	Associated Findings
• Uninterrupted period of illness with concurrent major mood episode, (major depressive or manic) concurrent with Criterion A of SCH (see Chapter 20) • *Bipolar type*: manic episode is part of presentation; major depressive episode may also occur • *Depressive type*: only major depressive episode • Delusions or hallucinations for 2 or more weeks in the absence of a major mood episode (depressive or manic) during the lifetime duration of the illness • Symptoms of mood episode present for major portion of the active and residual periods of illness • Not a direct physiologic effect of a substance or medical condition	• Poor occupational functioning • Restricted range of social contact • Difficulties with self-care • Increased risk for suicide

Refer to APA (2013) for *DSM-5* diagnostic criteria.

geographic, climatic, industrial, and social environments. Environmental contributions are minimal.

Age of Onset

SCA can affect individuals across the life span, although in children, the disorder is rare and is often indistinguishable from early-onset SCH. In the older adult, this disorder becomes complicated because of frequent comorbid medical conditions. The typical age of onset for this disorder is early adulthood, and the most common type presented is bipolar. Cases of later onset of SCA are typically found to be of the depressive type (APA, 2013). Earlier age of onset is associated with longer illness, more severe illness, and worse outcomes (APA, 2013).

Gender

This disorder is more likely to occur in women than in men, which may be accounted for by a greater incidence of the depressive type in women (APA, 2013). It is not yet clear if this is related to biologic differences or to a diagnostic bias. Because women, on average, have more supportive social networks than men and tend to be behaviourally less violent when ill, they can more readily be cared for by family at home and may not come to the attention of mental health services in the same manner as men (MacDougall, Luckett, & Jones, 2007). While women are reported to have better outcomes than men in terms of symptom control and sometimes employment (those typically examined in research), there are other outcomes particularly relevant to women (friendships, romantic relationships, family relationships, reproductive decisions, parenting, custody loss of children, psychological and socioeconomic independence, physical attractiveness, victimization, generativity, reproductive and metabolic side effects of medications) that may contribute to mood symptoms and that have not been adequately

explored (Chernomas, Clarke, & Chisholm, 2000; Judd, Armstrong, & Kulkarni, 2009; MacDougall et al., 2007).

Ethnicity and Culture

Although some reports have indicated a connection between SCA and social class, others support no specific association with race, geographic area, or class (Siris & Lavin, 1995). Culturally sensitive assessment is crucial especially if the patient's and the clinician's cultural backgrounds differ. Some beliefs and cultural practices may appear delusional to one culture but be acceptable in another (APA, 2013).

Family

Some authorities support a familial association in SCA, but a clear familial pattern has not been established. Relatives of patients with diagnoses of SCA appear to be at increased risk for this disorder, SCH, or both (APA, 2013). Whether this familial clustering is related to genetic risk factors, nongenetic environmental and cultural factors or a combination of both is not yet clear (van Os et al., 2009).

Comorbidity

SCA may be associated with substance abuse. Men may be more likely to engage in antisocial behaviour. Twenty-five percent of patients with diagnoses of SCA experience postpsychotic depression and panic attacks. The incidence of general medical disorders for those with SCA is also found to be above the base rate for the general population (APA, 2013).

Patients with SCA are at high risk for suicide. The risk for suicide in patients with psychosis is increased by the presence of depression. Risk for suicide is increased with the use of alcohol or substances, cigarette smoking, previous attempts at suicide, and previous hospitalizations (Potkin et al., 2003; Seguin et al., 2006).

Aetiology

Biologic Theories

Although the aetiologies of SHC and MD have been investigated extensively, the aetiology of SCA remains unresolved.

Neuropathologic

Magnetic resonance imaging (MRI) and computed tomography (CT or CAT) scans have been used in the study of SCA for more than 20 years (Crow & Harrington, 1994; Lewine, Hudgins, Brown, Caudle, & Risch, 1995; Scott, Price, George, Brillman, & Rothfus, 1993). Midline brain abnormalities, especially in women, have been found. In SCA, changes in brain structure appear to be similar to those seen in bipolar disorder (Getz et al., 2002). Whether midline structural abnormality is directly causal, indirectly contributory, or an intriguing phenomenon in SCA is unclear. Research aimed at determining neuropsychological differences between SCH and SCA remains inconclusive, but it is argued that severity may be the difference between the disorders (Heinrichs, Ammari, Vaz, & Miles, 2008).

Genetic

As noted above, familial clustering may be related to genetics or environmental risk factors or both (van Os et al., 2009). Results from family, twin, and adoption studies vary but suggest that SCA may consist of phenotypic variations or expressions of a genetic interform between SCH and affective psychoses (DeLisi et al., 2002; Linney et al., 2003).

Biochemical

Before 1999, the prevailing neurochemical hypothesis, overactivity of dopamine pathways, was based on observations of the effects of psychoactive drugs on psychotic symptoms (Jacobson & Tarraza, 2013). More recently, other neurochemicals under investigation are serotonin and glutamate (Andreasen & Black, 2006; Nasrallah, 2011).

Psychological and Social Theories

No current psychodynamic, behavioural, cognitive, or developmental theories of causation explain SCA. It is clear, however, that the psychological and social sequelae of a diagnosis of SCA can be overwhelming for the patient and family. The experience of psychosis is much more than simply the symptoms and can result in issues of loss, a need to learn how to seek help, and a desire to learn how to rebuild one's life within the context of the illness (McCarthy-Jones, Marriott, Knowles, Rowse & Thompson, 2013). While historical hypotheses related to overprotective, rigid families have been disproven, family dynamics nevertheless play an important role in influencing the clinical course of the disorder (Jacobson & Tarraza, 2013).

Interdisciplinary Treatment

Because this disorder is persistent, these individuals are constantly trying to manage complex symptoms. Patients with SCA benefit from a comprehensive treatment plan and a cohesive interdisciplinary treatment team. Integral to this team is the patient (and often his or her family) who needs to be an active participant in treatment planning. Ideally, most of the treatment occurs within the patient's natural environment, and hospitalizations are limited to times of symptom exacerbation, when symptoms are so severe or persistent that extended care in a protected environment is necessary.

Pharmacologic intervention is needed to stabilize the symptoms, and it presents specific challenges. Long-term atypical antipsychotic agents are as effective as the traditional combination of a standard antipsychotic agent and an antidepressant drug. Mood stabilizers, such as lithium or valproic acid, may also be used. A combination of antipsychotic and antidepressant agents is sometimes used (see Chapter 12).

After the patient's condition has stabilized (i.e., the patient exhibits a decrease in positive and negative symptoms), the treatment that led to remission of symptoms should be continued. Titrating antipsychotic agents to the lowest dose that provides suitable protection may enable optimal psychosocial functioning, while slowing recurrence of new episodes. Patients with SCA will likely need to remain on medication for the disorder. Electroconvulsive therapy (see Chapter 12) is considered when symptoms are refractory to other interventions or when the patient's life is at risk and a rapid response is required (Swoboda, Conca, Konig, Waanders, & Hansen, 2001).

The treatment plan is revised regularly, and symptoms are monitored to guide medication management. PMH nursing interventions in hospital and in community care are guided by the nursing diagnoses. Psychotherapy may help manage interpersonal relationships and mood changes. Social services are often needed to obtain disability benefits or services. Use of advanced practice clinicians helps to provide continuity of care (Jacobson & Tarraza, 2013).

Priority Care Issues

Patients with SCA may be at least as susceptible to suicide (see Chapter 19) as those with MD (Potkin et al., 2003). Living with a persistent psychotic disorder that has a mood component makes suicide a real risk. A review of completed suicides in New Brunswick has further suggested that comorbidity with substance abuse may increase the risk (Seguin et al., 2006).

Nursing Management: Human Response to Schizoaffective Disorder

Biologic Domain

Assessment

Assessment of patients with SCA is similar to assessment of those with schizophrenia and affective disorder. A careful history from the patient and family is crucial. The history should contain a description of the full range and duration of symptoms the patient has experienced and those observed by the family; this information is important for predicting outcomes. A patient who has had symptoms for a relatively long period of time may have greater difficulty in overcoming effects of the psychosis resulting in deterioration in functioning.

A thorough system assessment is important to discover any physiologic problems the patient is experiencing, such as sleep pattern disturbances, difficulties with self-care, or poor nutritional habits.

Nursing Diagnoses for Biologic Domain

Common nursing diagnoses for the biologic domain are *disturbed thought process*, *disturbed sensory perception*, and *disturbed sleep patterns*. Because of the variety of problems in patients with SCA, almost any nursing diagnosis could be generated. The persistent nature of this disorder lends itself to numerous and varied problems that must all be addressed (see Nursing Care Plan 21-1).

Interventions for Biologic Domain

Patient Education

Interventions are based on the needs identified in the bio/psycho/social/spiritual assessment (Fig. 21-1). Helping the patient to establish a regular sleep pattern by using a routine

Nursing Care Plan 21-1

Patient With Schizoaffective Disorder

Ms. B is a 28-year-old divorced woman with a 4-year-old daughter. They reside with Ms. B's parents. Ms. B is a hairdresser and tries to work, but she becomes stressed in the workplace, which results in her being fired. She has never applied for disability. Her parents are stressed because of the exacerbations of her illness and caring for her child.

Ms. B has had numerous hospitalizations for aggressive behaviour, noncompliance with medications, and receiving medications from various physicians, which result in inappropriate psychiatric management. She is medication seeking and is often prescribed benzodiazepines and diet pills by her primary care physician.

The patient has an ingrained delusional system that makes it hard to introduce reality orientation and feedback. She believes that her ex-husband has sexually abused

their child. She has gone to numerous attorneys to try to prosecute her ex-husband to no avail because of the lack of evidence to prove any abuse.

For the last 2 years, Ms. B has believed that a bank guard is in love with her. She is adamant about him protecting her and her child. She states that he watches over them. They have no contact other than speaking to each other when she enters the bank. She has been seeing a man the past 9 months but states that she really does not care much for him and that it is hard for her to move forward in the relationship because she loves the bank guard.

Medications have included antidepressants, neuroleptics (typical and atypical), mood stabilizers, benzodiazepines, sleep medications, and anticonvulsants. She often complains of being depressed and yet does not take the antidepressant medications when they are prescribed.

Setting: Intensive Care Psychiatric Unit in a General Hospital

Baseline Assessment: Ms. B is admitted to the hospital through the ER. She was hearing voices and was delusional. She has not been taking medications for several months. She is oriented in all spheres and well nourished but unkempt. She is verbalizing delusions about a man at the bank. She cannot sleep well and reportedly goes outdoors at night and yells at a bank guard. Reality feedback increases her agitation. She denies any problems.

Associated Psychiatric Diagnosis and Other Conditions That May Be a Focus of Clinical Attention	Medications
SCA Relational problems Economic problem (no income) Occupational problem (unemployed) Nonadherence to medical treatment	None

Continued

Nursing Care Plan 21-1 *(Continued)*

Nursing Diagnosis 1: Ineffective Individual Coping

Defining Characteristics

Inability to meet role expectations
Anxiety
Delusions
Inability to problem solve

Related Factors

Chronicity of the condition
Inadequate psychological resources secondary to delusions
Inadequate coping skills
Inadequate psychological resources to adapt to residential setting

Outcomes

Initial

1. Identify coping patterns
2. Identify stressors
3. Identify personal strengths
4. Accept support through the nursing relationship

Discharge

5. Manage own behaviour
6. Adherence to medication regimen
7. Reduction of delusions

Interventions

Interventions	Rationale	Ongoing Assessment
Initiate a nurse–patient relationship to develop trust.	Through the use of the nurse–patient relationship, the patient will be able to maintain adherence to the treatment plan.	Determine whether the patient is able to relate to the nurse.
Facilitate the identification of stressors in the patient's environment.	To be able to cope with stressors, they need to be identified by the patient.	Assess whether the patient is able to identify and verbalize stressors.
Develop a wellness plan in collaboration with the patient	The patient needs to develop healthy and realistic strategies to handle environmental stressors.	Determine whether patient-identified strategies are realistic.
Help the patient to identify personal strengths.	By identifying personal strengths, the patient will increase confidence in using coping strategies.	Assess the patient's ability to incorporate coping strategies into her daily routine.
Assist the patient to understand the disorder and its management.	By understanding the disorder, the patient can develop ways to manage her disorder.	Assess the patient's level of understanding of the disease.
Facilitate emotional support for the family.	Supported family is better equipped to support the patient.	Assess the family's ability to seek emotional support from the staff.
Identify coping skills that have been effective in the past and teach new coping skills.	By developing positive coping skills, anxiety and agitation will decrease.	Assess the patient's ability to learn the skills to manage stressors.

Evaluation

Outcomes	Revised Outcomes	Interventions
Within the nursing relationship, Ms. B. was able to understand how coping skills can reduce stressors.	Support the patient's ability to recognize stressors and apply coping skills.	Discuss stressors and means of applying coping skills.
Increased insight into what behaviour is appropriate has helped the patient to decrease verbalization of delusions.	Provide ongoing support to maintain the present level of functioning.	Discuss behaviour and provide reality feedback.

Nursing Diagnosis 2: Disturbed Thought Processes

Defining Characteristics

Delusions
Impulsivity
Medication noncompliance

Related Factors

Ingrained delusions
Decreased ability to process secondary to delusions

Nursing Care Plan 21-1 *(Continued)*

Outcomes

Initial	Discharge
1. Maintain reality orientation 2. Communicate clearly with others 3. Express delusional material less frequently	4. Identify situations that contribute to delusions 5. Identify how delusions affect life situations 6. Use coping strategies to deal with delusions 7. Recognize changes in behaviour

Interventions

Interventions	Rationale	Ongoing Assessment
Promote adherence to medication regimen.	Medication will reduce delusions.	Assess for side effects: heat intolerance, neuroleptic malignant syndrome (NMS), renal failure, constipation, dry mouth, increased appetite, salivation, nausea, vomiting, tardive dyskinesia, seizures, somnolence, agitation, insomnia, dizziness, metabolic syndrome, and weight gain.
Discuss actions, effects, and side effects of planned medications and assess patient's level of tolerance for the relative side effect profiles.	The more knowledgeable patients are about medication, the more likely they will agree to take the medications.	Assess ability to understand information.
Support reality testing through helping the patient to differentiate thoughts and feelings in relation to situations.	When comparing thoughts with the situations, patients can develop skills to refute delusions.	Assess for medication compliance.
Monitor verbalization of delusional material.	To determine whether medication is reducing delusional thoughts.	Assess verbalization of delusional material.
Identify stressors that promote delusions.	If the patient is able to identify stressors that promote delusions, she can manage the stressors to effectively decrease delusions.	Assess the patient's ability to recognize stressors when they occur. Encourage use of crisis planning or wellness planning tools.
Assist the patient in developing skills to deal with delusions (recognizing delusional themes can help the patient in distinguishing between reality-based and non–reality-based patterns).	Even though medication can reduce the occurrence of delusions, they may continue in some people with decreased intensity. Cognitive–behavioural skills are important in dealing with these altered thoughts.	Monitor the patient's ability to handle delusions.

Evaluation

Outcomes	Revised Outcomes	Interventions
Delusions will be less ingrained.	Continue to practice skills in reality orientation and communication.	Support verbalization of reality-based thoughts.
The patient verbalized action, effect, dosage, and side effects of medications.	Take prescribed medication regularly.	Give positive feedback for understanding of medication.
Medication adherence		Encourage patient to be forthright about her adherence to the medication regimen.

Summary: Ms. B was discharged from the hospital. Verbalization of delusions had not decreased. She was less anxious. She is presently on Risperdal 2 mg AM and hs, Effexor XR 75 mg AM, Xanax 0.5 mg AM, and Seroquel 50 mg hs. Her mother is helping by filling a weekly medication box. At times Ms. B is questioning her delusions.

FIGURE 21-1. Bio/psycho/social/spiritual interventions for patients with SCA.

can promote or reestablish normal rest patterns. Focusing with the patient on the principles of good nutrition and identifying any barriers to healthy eating can improve nutritional status. Working with the patient can help identify self-care deficits, especially those caused by lack of motivation. For deficits created by severe mood symptoms, establishing a routine and setting goals can be useful.

Pharmacologic Interventions

An in-depth history of the patient's medication is important in evaluating response to past medications and predicting response to the present regimen. Mood and psychotic symptoms are equally important and should be evaluated throughout treatment. Atypical antipsychotic agents are generally prescribed because of their efficacy. Clozapine, reported effective for SCA by several authorities, can reduce hospitalizations and risk for suicide in treatment-refractory patients (Potkin et al., 2003; Volavka et al., 2002), although it carries with it significant side effect risk. Atypical antipsychotic agents may have thymoleptic (mood stabilizing), as well as antipsychotic, effects. Quetiapine has been found effective in this respect (Bech, 2001). Dosage is the same as that used for treating SCH, but lower dosage ranges may also be effective.

In many cases, symptoms of depression disappear when psychotic symptoms decrease. If depressive symptoms persist, adjunctive use of an antidepressant agent may be helpful. Mood stabilizers, which can decrease the frequency and intensity of episodes, may be an alternative adjunctive medication for mood states associated with the bipolar type.

● **STUDY NOTE**

The medication regimen for patients with SCA will be complex and may include antipsychotics, mood stabilizers, antidepressants, and occasional antianxiety agents.

Administering and Monitoring Medications One of the greatest challenges in pharmacologic interventions is monitoring target symptoms and identifying changes in symptom pattern. Patients can switch from being relatively calm to being very emotional. Whether the patient is overreacting to an environmental event or mood symptoms have changed and the patient requires a medication change can be determined only through careful observation and documentation.

An in-depth history of the patient's medication is important in evaluating response to past medications and predicting response to the present regimen. Investigate adherence to past treatment to determine the probability of successful intervention (see Gibson & Brand, 2013 regarding issues related to nonadherence).

Adherence to medication regimens is critical to a successful outcome. Patients need an opportunity to discuss issues with and barriers to taking the medication and subsequent adherence to the prescribed regimen. Side effects such as weight gain and sexual dysfunction can be very distressing to patients and may lead to unilateral discontinuation of the medications on the patient's part (Chernomas et al., 2000). It is crucial that prescribers engage the patient in an open and honest discussion about the patient's level of tolerance for certain side effects. Choice of medications may need to be based on side effect profiles in addition to effectiveness.

Managing Side Effects Monitoring medication side effects in patients with SCA is similar to that in patients with SCH. Patients receiving antipsychotic medications need to be aware of extrapyramidal symptoms and the possibility of developing metabolic syndrome—a triad of diabetes, dyslipidemia, and hypertension with associated obesity (DeHert, Schreurs, Vancampfort, & Winkel, 2009; Shirzadi & Ghaemi, 2006). Regular monitoring of abdominal obesity and fasting blood glucose has been shown to be a cost-effective screening test to detect patients at high risk for cardiovascular morbidity (Straker et al., 2005). Counselling regarding nutrition and healthy lifestyle choices (e.g., smoking cessation, physical exercise) is paramount with these patients.

Monitoring for Drug Interactions Avoid using lithium with antipsychotic medications. A few patients taking haloperidol and lithium have experienced an encephalopathic syndrome, followed by irreversible brain damage (Boora, Xu, & Hyatt, 2008). Lithium may interact similarly with other antipsychotic agents. It may also prolong the effects of neuromuscular blocking agents. Use of nonsteroidal anti-inflammatory drugs may increase plasma lithium levels. Diuretics and angiotensin-converting enzyme inhibitors should be prescribed cautiously with lithium, which is excreted through the kidney.

Psychological Domain

Assessment

The patient's level of insight into his or her illness may play a role in the course and treatment of SCA. Patients with SCA tend to have better insight than those with SCH (Pini, Cassano, Dell'Osso, & Amador, 2001). Stressors should be evaluated because they may trigger symptoms. Uncovering or exploratory techniques that may reveal, for example, past episodes of abuse should generally be avoided. During periods of psychosis or profound depression, mental status and reality contact may be compromised. Assessment of anxiety level or reactions to stressful situations is important because the combination of these symptoms with psychosis increases the patient's risk for suicide. Discussing the experience of the illness in the patient's life is also crucial. Understanding the symptoms and their sequelae from the

TEACHING POINTS

- Encourage the patient to discuss the side effect profiles of the medications planned. Seek patient's input on his/her level of tolerance for the side effects. If necessary, negotiate for a medication with a different side effect profile but comparable efficacy. Once a medication regimen has been decided upon, advise the patient to take medications as prescribed. Reevaluate regularly and renegotiate as needed.
- Determine whether the patient has sufficient resources to purchase and obtain medications. Explore provincial medication plans for those on social assistance.
- Have the patient write down the prescribed medication and time of administration.
- Explain the target symptom for each medication (e.g., psychosis and mood for atypical antipsychotic agents, mood for antidepressant and mood stabilizer drugs).
- Caution patients about orthostatic hypotension and instruct them to get up slowly from a lying or sitting position. Also advise them to maintain adequate fluid intake.
- Advise patients to contact their case coordinators or health care providers immediately if they experience dramatic changes in body temperature (NMS), inability to control motor movement (dystonia), or dizziness.
- Advise patients to avoid over-the-counter medications unless a prescriber is consulted.
- Advise patients taking olanzapine and clozapine to monitor body weight and report any rapid weight gain.
- Advise patients to report symptoms of diabetes mellitus (frequent urination, excessive thirst, etc.).

patient's point of view will greatly facilitate the satisfactory engagement in planning for wellness and recovery.

Nursing Diagnoses for Psychological Domain

In SCA, individuals vacillate between mood dysregulation and disturbed thinking. Typical nursing diagnoses

---

BOX 21-1 Psychoeducation Checklist: SCA

When caring for the patient with SCA, be sure to include the caregiver as appropriate and address the following topic areas in the teaching plan:
- Psychopharmacologic agents (antipsychotic or antidepressants), if used, including drug action, dosage, frequency, and possible adverse effects
- Methods to enhance adherence
- Sleep measures
- Consistent routines
- Goal setting
- Nutrition
- Support networks
- Problem solving
- Positive coping strategies
- Social and vocational skills training

21-2   **Research for Best Practice**

TESTING THE USE OF A WELLNESS PLANNER IN IMPROVING CLIENTS' PERCEPTIONS OF CONTINUITY OF CARE, EMPOWERMENT, AND QUALITY OF LIFE

From Marchinko, S. & Clarke, D. (2011). The Wellness Planner: Empowering consumers in self-care. Archives of Psychiatric Nursing, 25, 284–293.

The Question: Does using a Wellness Planner to help manage living with chronic mental illness affect personal empowerment, satisfaction with care and services, and overall quality of life?

Methods: Fifty individuals who were clients of community mental health and/or outpatient services used a Wellness Planner for 3 months. The intervention was a paper daily planner based on principles of self-management and recovery, structured in a way that allowed clients to keep track of their health care and social services providers, medications, appointments, and daily/weekly/monthly goals on physical, emotional, and spiritual issues. It also included space for a wellness/crisis plan that outlined stressors and triggers for stress with levels of possible interventions starting with strategies for self-care.

Findings: Forty-two of the fifty participants completed the study and had used the planner on a daily basis as part of their self-care. All but one said they liked the planner and would use it again. Scores on measures of empowerment (including self-efficacy and self-esteem), satisfaction with care, and quality of life significantly increased from baseline. Individuals who felt more empowered also viewed their social relationships and personal environments more favourably. Qualitative data suggested that using the planner helped structure appointments with health care providers in a positive and more collaborative way. *"I showed it to my psychiatrist and nurse; they were glad I was doing this. We filled in the planner together; we talked about symptoms/triggers, and this was very helpful in giving me more insight."*

Implications for Nursing: The positive results of this study support the use of the Wellness Planner as a means in which nurses can be instrumental in supporting mental health promotion and empowering patients in self-care and recovery.

for this domain include *hopelessness*, *powerlessness*, *ineffective coping*, and *low self-esteem*.

Interventions for Psychological Domain

Using appropriate interpersonal modalities is important to help the patient, family, and social and vocational support networks cope with the onslaught of acute episodes and recuperative periods. Patients with SCA have fewer awareness deficits than do patients with SCH. Structured, integrated, and problem-solving psychotherapeutic interventions should be used to develop or increase the patient's insight. Psychoeducational interventions can help to decrease symptoms, enhance recognition of early regression, and hone psychosocial skills (see Boxes 21-1 and 21-2.)

The collaborative development of a crisis plan or a "wellness" plan when the individual is able to do so can help the patient identify triggers and prodromal symptoms of decompensation and allow them to preplan coping mechanisms and ways to engage supports to mitigate the effects of illness (Copeland, 2005). Such plans have been well researched in the United Kingdom and have been shown to decrease the need for involuntary hospitalization (Papageorigiou, King, Jonhohamed, Davison, & Dawson, 2002; Sutherby et al., 1999). Evidence from a Manitoba study suggests that facilitating patients in planning their community care through the use of a Wellness Planner (including crisis planning and personal goal setting) can increase their sense of empowerment and improve their quality of life (Marchinko & Clarke, 2011) (see Box 21-2).

Social Domain

Assessment

Social dysfunction is common in patients with diagnosis of SCA. Premorbid adjustment, such as marital status and adolescent social adjustment, may influence both patients' level of functioning at the time of diagnosis and their prognoses. Assessment of social skill deficits and problems with interpersonal conflicts should be made. Assessment of an adult patient's childhood may provide clues to the patient's current level of social functioning. Assess the patient's use of fantasy and fighting as a means of coping. Patients who report the most severe peer rejection present with the angriest dispositions and display antisocial behaviours.

Nursing Diagnoses for Social Domain

Because of their mood and thought disturbances, these individuals will have significant problems in the social domain. Typical nursing diagnoses include *compromised family coping*, *impaired home maintenance*, and *social isolation*.

Interventions for Social Domain

Social skills training is useful for remediating social deficits and may result in positive social adjustment. Positive results include improved interpersonal competence, decreased symptom severity, and personal empowerment leading to recovery (Kurtz & Maeser, 2008). Help in identifying feelings and developing realistic goals, along with supportive therapy, can integrate insight into the disease process. Engaged and collaborative crisis planning between the patient and the mental health care provider can help the patient and family recognize oncoming decompensation and take appropriate steps to improve coping. Education focusing on conflict–resolution skills, promoting compromise, negotiation, and expression of negative feelings can help the patient achieve positive social adjustment. Social skills can be improved through role-playing and assertiveness training. Supportive, nurturing, and nonconfrontational interventions help to minimize anxiety and improve understanding (see Box 21-3).

Helping the patient to develop coping skills is essential. Teach communication skills to decrease conflicts and environmental negativity. Memory is linked with development of social skills; psychotic symptoms may interfere with retention of these skills, resulting in slower learning. These patients require long-term, intensive social training.

Families are at risk for ineffective coping. Family members face many of the same issues faced by families of patients with SCH and are often puzzled by the patient's emotional overreaction to normal daily stresses. Frequent arguments may lead to verbal and physical abuse.

BOX 21-3   Therapeutic Dialogue

MS. B'S "DELUSIONS"

Ineffective Communication

Nurse: Hello, Ms. B, what has been happening?

Patient: The guy from the bank keeps me up all night.

Nurse: That's not possible.

Patient: He's there all the time to look after me.

Nurse: No, he's not. You just think that.

Patient: No, he really is. He is helping me.

Nurse: He does not even know who you are.

Effective Communication

Nurse: Hello, Ms. B. How have you been?

Patient: That guy from the bank is really bothering me.

Nurse: What is happening?

Patient: He keeps me up all night. I go out in the street to yell at him.

Nurse: Have you actually seen him at night?

Patient: No, but I know he is there.

Nurse: Can he be there when you cannot see him?

Patient: I guess he can't.

Nurse: Does it seem that the thoughts about him come from your mind?

Patient: This might be.

Nurse: Your illness often causes thoughts that are not based in reality.

Patient: It seems real but yet so unreal. Those are sort of stupid thoughts.

Critical Thinking Challenge

- How could the nurse's approach in the first scenario have prevented development of a therapeutic relationship?
- How can the second scenario benefit the patient in developing insight into her delusions?
- Discuss the differences between the two approaches.

Spiritual Domain

As with persons living with SCH, the spiritual domain of care is very significant for persons living with SCA (see Chapter 20). Finding meaningful ways to cope with such a serious illness, one that often brings social rejection and isolation, becomes a life challenge. Religious or spiritual beliefs may be a comfort, and a relationship with the sacred through ritual, prayer, or other activities may offer daily comfort. Spiritual nursing care can support patients particularly in times of despair. With SCA, more than with SCH, the person is likely to experience emotional turmoil that is seriously disruptive to a sense of serenity the person may have achieved. Spiritual support should be understood as an ongoing need. The nurse also needs to strive to understand the potential impact of other symptoms, such as hallucinations and delusions, on spiritual needs and to assist persons with SCA to engage in spiritual activities that are satisfying to them.

Evaluation and Treatment Outcomes

Teaching skills to patients with SCA often takes longer than teaching other patients. The nurse evaluating progress related to interventions must be patient if outcomes are not completely met. Psychoeducation results in increased knowledge of the illness and treatment, increased medication compliance, fewer relapses and hospitalizations, briefer inpatient stays, increased social function, decreased family tension, and lighter family burdens (Andres, Pfammatter, Garst, Teschner, & Brenner, 2000). Maintain realistic outcomes and praise small successes to promote positive outcomes (Fig. 21-2).

Continuum of Care

Inpatient Focus Care

Hospitalization may be required during acute psychotic episodes or when suicidal ideations are present. This structured environment protects the patient from self-harm (i.e., suicidal, assaultive, financial, legal, vocational, or social). During periods of acute psychosis, offering reassurance in a soft, nonthreatening voice and avoiding confrontational stances will help the patient begin to trust the staff and nursing care (see Chapter 6). Avoid seclusion and restraint and keep environmental stimulation to a minimum. Use the patient's coping capabilities to reinforce constructive aspects of functioning and enable a return to autonomy. If the patient has advance directives, adhere to the patient's wishes as much as possible.

Family Intervention

Helping families support the patient at home or in a community placement is an integral part of nursing care. With the patient's permission, key family members can be included in home visits to learn about symptoms,

FIGURE 21-2. Bio/psycho/social/spiritual outcomes for patients with SCA.

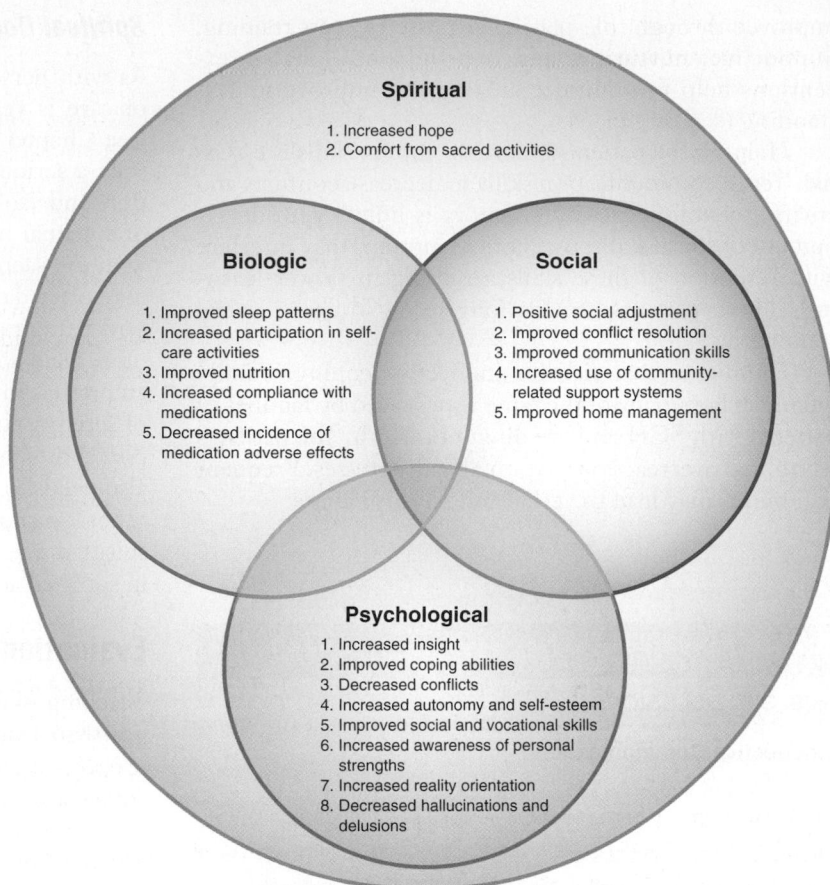

Spiritual
1. Increased hope
2. Comfort from sacred activities

Biologic
1. Improved sleep patterns
2. Increased participation in self-care activities
3. Improved nutrition
4. Increased compliance with medications
5. Decreased incidence of medication adverse effects

Social
1. Positive social adjustment
2. Improved conflict resolution
3. Improved communication skills
4. Increased use of community-related support systems
5. Improved home management

Psychological
1. Increased insight
2. Improved coping abilities
3. Decreased conflicts
4. Increased autonomy and self-esteem
5. Improved social and vocational skills
6. Increased awareness of personal strengths
7. Increased reality orientation
8. Decreased hallucinations and delusions

medications, and side effects. By collaborating with family members, the nurse can strengthen the patient's willingness to follow treatment, monitor symptoms, and continue with rehabilitation and recovery. Families should be encouraged to seek out self-help support groups in the community- and/or family-directed psychoeducation programming.

EMERGENCY CARE !

Emergency care may be needed during symptom exacerbation. Psychosis, mood disturbance, and medication-related adverse effects account for most emergency situations. During an exacerbation of psychosis, patients may become agitated or aggressive. Assaultive behaviour can be managed by using therapeutic techniques (see Chapter 18) and pharmacologic management. If medications are used, benzodiazepines such as lorazepam are usually given. Patients are then evaluated for antipsychotic therapy. Possible medication-related adverse effects include NMS as a reaction to dopamine antagonists or serotonin intoxication, especially if the patient is taking an atypical antipsychotic agent and a selective serotonin reuptake inhibitor (see Chapter 12). Suicidality (ideation and intent) must always be assessed (Clarke, Brown, & Giles-Smith, 2008) (see Chapter 19).

Community Care Within a Recovery Framework

Although this illness is episodic and chronic, within the framework of recovery, patients must be supported along their journey to becoming the best, most fulfilled persons they can be. Community supports can be on a continuum from peer support and self-help groups (such as those available through the Canadian Mental Health Association or the Schizophrenia Society of Canada) to clinics and services developed within the mental health care delivery system and delivered by mental health professionals (e.g., hospital-based outpatient clinics; assertive community treatment programs). The care and services an individual requires will depend upon the balance achieved between illness management and personal growth and will fluctuate and change along the wellness/illness trajectory. For example, an individual may be able to function in a peer support position, helping others, but then may go through a time when she/he needs the services of peer support. Programs and resources that foster building social and vocational skills should incorporate the individual's natural strengths and skills, interests, and aspirations. The Women's Group at the Manitoba Schizophrenia Society, for example, runs writing groups and annually publishes a volume of poetry, short stories, drawings, and photographs to celebrate the participants' accomplishments. Art Beat, a Winnipeg-based art studio established and run by a mental health consumer and his family, provides studio space and support for aspiring artists (from painters and potters to jewellery designers) living with mental health issues (see Web Links on thePoint). Some participants find their artistic expression allows them to cope with and find meaning in living with a mental illness, while others are enabled to make a living as artists.

DELUSIONAL DISORDER

The person with a delusional disorder is likely to be encountered in a medical–surgical rather than a psychiatric setting. As this disorder often remains undiagnosed, nurses practising in nonpsychiatric settings need to be able to recognize and understand it in order for meaningful care to be provided.

Clinical Course

Delusional disorder is a psychotic disorder characterized by nonbizarre, logical, stable, and well-systemized delusions that occur in the absence of other psychiatric disorders. **Delusions** are false, fixed beliefs unchanged by reasonable arguments. Although delusions are a symptom of many psychotic disorders, in delusional disorder, the delusions typically are **nonbizarre delusions**; that is, they are characterized by adherence to possible situations that could occur in real-life and are plausible in the context of the person's ethnic and cultural background. More rare are **bizarre delusions** that are clearly implausible and are not derived from ordinary life experiences (APA, 2013).

Examples of real-life situations include being followed, poisoned, infected, loved at a distance, or deceived by a spouse or lover. A diagnosis of delusional disorder is based on the presence of one or more nonbizarre

delusions for at least 1 month (APA, 2013). Delusions are the primary symptom of this disorder, and other psychotic features are not typically seen (APA, 2013).

The course of delusional disorder is variable. Onset can be acute, or the disorder can occur gradually and become chronic. Patients with this disorder usually live with their delusions for years, rarely receiving psychiatric treatment. They are seldom brought to the attention of health care providers unless their delusion relates to their health (somatic delusion), or they act on the basis of their delusion and violate legal or social rules. Full remissions can be followed by relapses.

Apart from the direct impact of the delusion, psychosocial functioning is not markedly impaired. The person's clarity of thinking and behaviour and emotional responses are usually consistent with the delusional focus. In general, behaviour is not odd or bizarre. In fact, behaviour is remarkably normal, except when the patient focuses on the delusion. At that time, thinking, attitudes, and mood may change abruptly. Personality does not usually change, but the patient is gradually, progressively involved with the delusional concern (APA, 2013).

 KEY CONCEPT Delusions are false, fixed beliefs unchanged by reasonable arguments.

Diagnostic Criteria

Delusional disorder is characterized by the presence of nonbizarre delusions for a duration of 1 month or longer and includes several subtypes: erotomanic, grandiose, jealous, persecutory, somatic, mixed, and unspecified (Table 21-2). These subtypes represent the prominent

Table 21-2 Key Characteristics of Delusional Disorder	
Diagnostic Criteria and Target Symptoms	**Associated Findings**

• Nonbizarre delusions of at least 1 mo. duration
• Criterion A for SCH has never been met (see Chapter 20)
• Functioning not markedly impaired; behaviour not odd or bizarre
• If concurrent with delusions, MD relatively brief in comparison with delusional periods
• Not a direct physiologic effect of substance or medical condition
   Erotomanic type: delusions that another person of usually higher status is in love with the person
   Grandiose type: delusions of inflated worth, power, knowledge, identity, or special relationship to a deity or famous person
   Jealous type: delusions that the individual's sexual partner is unfaithful
   Persecutory type: delusions that the person or someone close to the person is being malevolently treated in some way
   Somatic type: delusion that person has some physical defect or general medical condition
   Mixed type: delusions characteristic of more than one of the above types; no one theme predominates
   Unspecified type: delusion cannot be clearly identified or described
	• Social, marital, or work problems
	• Ideas of reference
	• Irritable mood
	• Marked anger and violent behaviour (especially with jealous type)

Refer to APA (2013) for *DSM-5* diagnostic criteria.

theme of the delusion. A patient who has met criterion A for SCH does not receive a diagnosis of delusional disorder (see Chapter 20 for criterion A). Although hallucinations may be present, they are not prominent and are typically related to the delusion (APA, 2013).

If mood episodes occur with this disorder, the total duration of the mood episode is relatively brief compared with the total duration of the delusional period. The delusion is not caused by the direct physiologic effects of substances (i.e., cocaine, amphetamines, marijuana) or a general medical condition (i.e., Alzheimer's disease, systemic lupus erythematosus). Because delusional disorder is uncommon and possesses features that are characteristic of other illnesses, the differential diagnosis has a clear-cut logic. It is a diagnosis of exclusion requiring careful evaluation. Distinguishing this disorder from SCH and MD with psychotic features is difficult (APA, 2013).

The prevalence of delusional disorder is estimated to be about 2 per 10,000 general population with the most common subtype being persecutory (APA, 2013). It is a rare disease even in psychiatric samples (Meloy, 1999). Research data are limited because numbers of recorded case studies and participants are small, and the studies lack systematic description, assessment, and diagnosis. Delusional disorder may be associated with dysfunction in the frontal–subcortical systems and with temporal dysfunction, particularly on the left side (Fujii, Ahmed, & Takeshita, 1999).

Subtypes

Erotomanic Delusions

The **erotomanic delusion** is characterized by the belief that the patient is loved intensely by the "loved object," who is usually married, of a higher socioeconomic status, or otherwise unattainable. The patient believes that the loved object's position in life would be in jeopardy if his or her true feelings were known. In addition, the patient is convinced that he or she is in amorous communication with the loved object. The loved object is often a public figure (e.g., movie star, politician) but may also be a common stranger. The patient may have minimal or no contact with the loved object and often keeps the delusion secret, but efforts to contact the loved object through letters, telephone calls, gifts, visits, surveillance, and stalking are also common. The patient may in many cases transfer his or her delusion to another loved object. Clinical patients are mostly women who do not usually act out their delusions. Men may more often come into contact with the law in their pursuit of the loved object or in a misguided effort to rescue the loved object from some imagined danger. This disorder is difficult to control, contain, or treat. Orders of protection are generally ineffective, and criminal charges of stalking or harassment that lead to incarceration are ineffective as a long-term solution to the problem (Petherick, 2013). The result is repeated arrests and psychiatric examinations, followed by ineffective treatment. Patients are rarely motivated to seek psychiatric treatment. Cognitive rigidity arising from frontal–subcortical dysfunction may contribute to maintaining erotic delusions and result in inability to alter a belief system (Fujii et al., 1999).

Grandiose Delusions

Patients presenting with a **grandiose delusion** are convinced they have a great, unrecognized talent or have made an important discovery. A less common presentation is the delusion of a special relationship with a prominent person (i.e., an adviser to the Prime Minister) or of actually being a prominent person (i.e., the Prime Minister). In the latter case, the person with the delusion may regard the actual prominent person as an impostor. Other grandiose delusions may be religious in nature, such as a delusional belief that he or she has a special message from a deity (APA, 2013).

Jealous Delusions

The central theme of the **jealous delusion** is the unfaithfulness or infidelity of a spouse or lover. The belief arises without cause and is based on incorrect inferences justified by "evidence" (i.e., rumpled clothing, spots on sheets) the patient has collected. The patient usually confronts the spouse or lover with a host of such evidence. An associated feature is paranoia. The patient may attempt to intervene in the imagined infidelity by secretly following the spouse or lover or by investigating the imagined lover (APA, 2013).

Delusions of jealousy are difficult to treat and may diminish only with separation, divorce, or the death of the spouse or lover. Except in the elderly, such patients generally are male. Jealousy is a powerful, potentially dangerous emotion. Aggression, even violent behaviour, may result. Litigious behaviour is common, and symptoms with forensic aspects are often seen. Care is essential in determining how to work with these patients.

Persecutory Delusions

The central theme of the **persecutory delusion** is that the individual is being conspired against, cheated, spied on, or followed, poisoned, drugged, maliciously maligned, harassed, or obstructed in his or her goals (APA, 2013). The focus of persecutory delusions is often on some injustice that must be remedied by legal action (querulous paranoia). With such delusions, patients often seek satisfaction by repeatedly appealing to courts and other government agencies (Munro, 1999). These patients are often angry and resentful and may even behave violently towards the people believed to be persecuting them (APA, 2013). The course may be chronic, although the patient's preoccupation with the delusional belief often waxes and wanes.

Somatic Delusions

The central theme of a **somatic delusion** involves bodily functions or sensations. These patients believe they have physical ailments. Delusions of this nature are fixed, inarguable, and intense, with the patient totally convinced of the physical nature of the somatic complaint. The delusion occurs in the absence of other medical or psychiatric conditions. Medication can cause tactile hallucinations that result directly from the physiologic effects of the medication; when the medication or drug is removed, the symptoms disappear. Somatic delusions are manifested in the following beliefs (Munro, 1999):

- A foul odour is coming from the skin, mouth (delusions of halitosis), rectum, or vagina
- Insects have infested the skin (delusional parasitosis)
- Internal parasites have infested the digestive system
- A certain body part is misshapen or ugly (contrary to visible evidence)
- Parts of the body are not functioning (e.g., large intestine, bowels)

The delusion of infestation by insects cannot occur without sensory perceptions, which constitute tactile hallucinations. The patient vividly describes crawling, itching, burning, swarming, and jumping on the skin surface or below the skin. The patient maintains the conviction that he or she is infested with parasites in the absence of objective evidence to the contrary.

Patients with somatic delusions present a dilemma for health care systems because of their excessive use of health care resources. They seek repeated medical consultations with dermatologists, entomologists, infectious disease specialists, and general practitioners, but they refuse psychiatric referral. If they do seek psychiatric help, these patients typically do not adhere to long-term psychiatric treatment. The somatic subtype is rare but may be underdiagnosed. Both genders are affected equally, but when onset occurs in late middle age, female patients tend to predominate. Studies of somatic delusions have been marred by methodologic uncertainties, and factors limiting investigation include rarity of the disease, lack of contact with psychiatrists, and noncompliance with the medication regimen. A differential diagnosis of delirium or a major neurocognitive disorder must be ruled out (APA, 2013). A variant of the somatic subtype is body dysmorphic disorder, which is classified under Obsessive–Compulsive and Related Disorders in the *Diagnostic and Statistical Manual of Mental Disorders*, 5th ed. (*DSM-5*).

Unspecified Delusions

In the mixed subtype, no one delusional theme predominates, and the patient presents with two or more types of delusion. In the unspecified subtype, the delusional beliefs cannot be clearly determined, or the predominant delusion is not described as a specific type. Patients are usually women who experience feelings of depersonalization and derealization and have negative-associated paranoid features. The delusions can be short-lived, recurrent, or persistent. This subtype also includes delusions of **misidentification** (i.e., illusions of doubles), wherein a familiar person is replaced by an impostor. For example, the patient may believe that close family members have assumed the persona of strangers or that people they know can change into other people at will. This type of delusion occurs rarely and is generally associated with SCH, Alzheimer's disease, or other organic conditions or dementias (APA, 2013).

Epidemiology and Risk Factors

Delusional disorder is relatively uncommon in clinical settings (APA, 2013). The best estimate of its prevalence in the population is about 0.03%, but precise information is lacking (APA, 2013). Lifetime morbidity is between 0.05% and 0.1% because of the late age of onset. Few risk factors are associated with delusional disorder. Patients can live with their delusions without psychiatric intervention because their behaviour is normal, although if delusions are somatic, patients risk unnecessary medical interventions. Acting on delusions carries a risk for intervention by law enforcement agencies or the legal system. Suicide attempts are neither more nor less common than in the general population (Grunebaum et al., 2001).

Age of Onset

Delusional disorder can begin in adolescence and occurs in middle to later adulthood. Onset occurs at a later age than among patients with SCH. A prevalence of 2% to 4% has been reported in the elderly (APA, 2013).

Gender

Gender does not appear to affect the overall frequency of most delusional disorders (APA, 2013), although men present with more severe symptoms and worse functionality (Portugal et al., 2010). Patients with erotomanic delusions are generally women; in forensic settings, most people with this disorder are men. Men also tend to experience more jealous delusions, except in the elderly population, in which women outnumber men (APA, 2013).

Ethnicity and Culture

A person's ethnic, cultural, and religious background must be considered in evaluating the presence of delusional disorder. The content of delusions varies between cultures and subcultures, as culture provides a framework for people's "bizarre and extraordinary experiences" (Jacobson & Tarraza, 2013, p. 199).

Family

No increased risk due to familial and genetic factors is known.

Comorbidity

Mood disorders are frequently found in patients with delusional disorders, who typically have mild symptoms of depression such as irritable or dysphoric mood. Delusional disorder may also be associated with obsessive–compulsive disorder and paranoid, schizoid, or avoidant personality disorder (APA, 2013).

Aetiology

The cause of delusional disorder is unknown. The only major feature of this condition is the formation and persistence of the delusions. Possible neurophysiologic and neuropsychological causes of delusional disorder have not been extensively researched, and theories of causation are contradictory. Delusional beliefs have been considered as dysfunctional extremes of cognitive and emotional mechanisms with adaptive significance but lacking in flexibility. This hypothesis places delusions on a continuum with "normalcy" and as a possible function of high vigilance towards threat and a search for safety (Abdel-Hamid & Brüne, 2008). No social theories of causation are addressed in the literature.

Possible medical reasons for delusions, especially in cases of sudden onset, need to be carefully ruled out. Disorders of the basal ganglia, toxic–metabolic conditions, dementias, and substance-related disorders can produce delusions in some persons (Sadock & Sadock, 2007).

Biologic Theories

Neuropathologic

In patients with delusional disorder, MRIs show a degree of temporal lobe asymmetry. However, these differences are subtle, so delusional disorder may involve a neurodegenerative component (Ota et al., 2003). The tactile hallucinations of somatic delusions may arise from sensory alterations in the nervous system (Abdel-Hamid & Brüne, 2008) or from sensory input that has been misinterpreted because of subtle cortical changes associated with aging.

Genetic and Biochemical

Delusional disorder is probably biologically distinct from other psychotic disorders, yet little or no attention has been paid to genetic factors. Delusions may involve faulty processing of essentially intact perceptions, whereby perceptions become linked with an interpretation that has deep emotional significance but no verifiable basis (Conway et al., 2002; McGuire, Junginger, Adams,

Burright, & Donovick, 2001). Alternately, a complex, malfunctioning dopaminergic system may lead to delusions (Morimoto et al., 2002). This explanation could lead to the argument that a particular delusion depends on the "circuit" that is malfunctioning. Denial of reality has been linked to right posterior cortical dysfunction. Some authors have proposed a combination of biologic and early life experiences as etiologic components (Bentall, Corcoran, Howard, Blackwood, & Kinderman, 2001).

Interdisciplinary Treatment

Few, if any, interdisciplinary treatments are associated with delusional disorder because patients rarely receive attention from health care providers. Pharmacologic intervention is often based on symptoms. For example, patients with somatic delusions are treated for the specific complaints with which they present. Use of benzodiazepines may be common with this disorder because complaints are vague.

Priority Care Issues

By the time a patient with a diagnosis of delusional disorder is seen in a psychiatric setting, he or she generally has had the delusion for a long time. It is deeply ingrained and many times unshakable, even with psychopharmacologic intervention. These patients rarely comply with medication regimens.

Male patients who have the erotomanic subtype are likely to require special care because they are more likely than other patients to act on their delusions (e.g., by continued attempts to contact the loved object or by stalking). This group is generally seen in forensic settings.

Nursing Management: Human Response to Delusional Disorder

Biologic Domain

Assessment

Body systems are assessed to evaluate any physical problems. In people with somatic delusional disorder, assessment may be difficult because of the number and variety of presenting symptoms. Complaints are explored to develop a complete symptom history and to determine whether symptoms have a physical basis or are delusional. Past history of each symptom should be determined because this information may affect outcome. The more recent the onset is, the more favourable the prognosis.

Most patients who receive diagnoses of delusional disorder do not experience functional difficulties or impairments. Self-care patterns may be disrupted in patients with the somatic subtype by the elaborate processes used to treat perceived illness (e.g., bathing rituals, creams). Sleep may be disrupted because of the central and overpowering nature of the delusions.

A complete medication history, past and present, is also important to determine the patient's past response and what agents the individual perceives as effective. Examining the patient's records for tests and procedures may help to substantiate the individual's symptoms.

● **STUDY NOTE**

By definition, delusions are fixed, false beliefs that cannot be changed by reasonable arguments. The nurse should assess the patient's delusion to evaluate its significance to the patient, the patient's safety, and the safety of others. The nurse should not dwell on the delusion nor try to change it.

Nursing Diagnoses for the Biologic Domain

The nursing diagnoses for the biologic domain depend on the type of delusions that are manifested and the response to these symptoms. For example, for a woman with the somatic delusion that insects are crawling on her, disturbed sensory perception (tactile) would be appropriate. For others who are fearful of poisoning, imbalanced nutrition, less than body requirements, may be a useful diagnosis. Refusal of all medication may support a nursing diagnosis of ineffective therapeutic regimen management.

Interventions for Biologic Domain

Interventions are based on the problems identified during assessment (Fig. 21-3) and addressed individually. The nurse helps the patient to establish routines that can resolve problems and promote healthy functioning. A mechanism for managing the patient's medication regimen is developed.

Somatic Interventions

Treating somatic disorder is difficult because of the patient's insistence that the problem is not psychiatrically related. Realistic and modest goals are most sensible. Establishing a therapeutic relationship is a goal for which to strive.

Pharmacologic Interventions

The literature available about using psychiatric medications in delusional disorder is sparse, and the available reports conflict. Antipsychotic agents are useful in improving acute symptoms by decreasing agitation and the intensity of the delusion. They may also be effective in the long term, but little formal information exists to support this theory.

Administering and Monitoring Medications

Patients often do not adhere to medication regimens and require monitoring of target symptoms. Look for an opportunity to discuss medications and to identify issues the patient may have with them.

FIGURE 21-3. Bio/psycho/social/spiritual interventions for patients with delusional disorder.

Managing Side Effects

Management of side effects is similar to that in other disorders that have a delusional component. The nurse assesses for NMS, extrapyramidal side effects, weight gain, and sedation.

Monitoring for Drug Interactions

Interactions are similar to those seen with medications for other disorders. A detailed list of prior and current medications must be elicited from patients, especially those with somatic delusions, because they may be receiving medications from several practitioners.

Psychological Domain

Assessment

Patients with delusional disorder show few, if any, psychological deficits, and those that do occur are generally related directly to the delusion. Use of the Minnesota Multiphasic Personality Inventory, a clinical scale that identifies paranoid symptom deviation, may be useful in substantiating the diagnosis.

Mental status is not generally affected. Thinking, orientation, affect, attention, memory, perception, and personality are generally intact. Presenting reality-based evidence in an attempt to change the person's delusion can be helpful in determining whether the belief can be altered with sufficient evidence. If mental status is altered, this fact is generally brought to the health professional's attention by a third party, such as a family member, neighbour, physician, the police, or attorney. In these cases, the person usually has acted in some manner that draws attention to him or herself. Talk with the person to grasp the nature of the delusional thinking: its theme, impact on the person's life, complexity, systematization, and related features.

Nursing Diagnosis for Psychological Domain

Numerous nursing diagnoses could be generated based on the assessment of the psychological domain. *Ineffective denial*, *impaired verbal communication*, *deficient knowledge*, and *risk for loneliness* are some examples. Nursing diagnoses of *disturbed self-concept*, *disturbed self-esteem*, *anxiety*, *fear*, and *powerlessness* may also be generated.

 TEACHING POINTS

Patients may need help and information in order to take the medication as prescribed. Determine whether the patient has sufficient resources to purchase and obtain medications and explain target symptoms for each medication. Caution patients not to take over-the-counter medications without consulting their provider.

Interventions for Psychological Domain

Patients with delusional disorder are treated most effectively in outpatient settings with supportive therapy that allays the person's anxiety. Initiating discussion of the troubling experiences and consequences of the delusion and suggesting a means for coping may be successful. Assisting the person towards a more satisfying general adjustment is desirable (see Box 21-4).

Insight-oriented therapy is not useful because there is no benefit in trying to prove the delusion is not true, arguing the person out of the delusion, or telling the individual that the delusion is imaginary. Cognitive therapy with supportive therapy that focuses on reasoning or reality testing to decrease delusional thinking, or modifying the delusion itself, may be helpful (see Chapter 13). Educational interventions can aid the patient in understanding how factors such as sensory impairment, social and physical isolation, and stress contribute to the intensity of this disorder.

In certain instances, hospitalization is needed in response to dangerous behaviour that could include aggressiveness, poor impulse control, excessive psychological tension, unremitting anger, and threats. If hospitalization is required, the person needs to be approached tactfully. Legal assistance may be necessary (Reid, 2005).

Suicide can be a concern, but most patients are not at risk. A British interview study with nurses identified as having expertise in working with acutely psychotic patients found that the nurses emphasized the importance of being respectfully attentive and supportive to these patients, including determining how their psychotic symptoms were affecting their emotions, functioning, and experiences. The nurses described the need to be empathetic, engage the patient in ordinary conversation when possible, and help them focus on the here and now. When necessary, it should be gently acknowledged that the patient's delusional ideas are not shared by the care team (Bowers, Brennan, Winship, & Theodoridou, 2009).

BOX 21-4 Psychoeducation Checklist: Delusional Disorder

When caring for the patient with delusional disorder, be sure to include the caregiver, as appropriate, and address the following topic areas in the teaching plan:
- Psychopharmacologic agents (antipsychotic or antidepressants), if used, including drug action, dosage, frequency, and possible adverse effects
- Identification of troubling experiences
- Consequences of delusions
- Realistic goal setting
- Positive coping strategies
- Safety measures
- Social training skills
- Family participation in therapy

Social Domain

Assessment

A common characteristic of individuals with delusional disorder is normal behaviour and appearance unless their delusional ideas are being discussed or acted on. The cultural background of the person with delusional disorder has to be evaluated. Ethnic and cultural systems have different beliefs that are accepted within their individual context but not outside their group. Problems can occur in social, occupational, or interpersonal areas. In general, the person's social and marital functioning is more likely to be impaired than his or her intellectual or occupational functioning. Most are employed, although generally they hold low-paying jobs. Supportive family members and friends can mean a more positive outcome for the person living with a delusional disorder.

Life difficulties are often related to the delusion; it is important to assess the person's capacity to act in response to it. What is his or her level of impulsiveness (i.e., related to behaviours of suicide, homicide, aggression, or violence)? Uncertainty in assessment can be mitigated by establishing as complete a picture of the person as possible, including his or her subjective experiences and concrete psychopathologic symptoms.

Nursing Diagnoses for the Social Domain

Several nursing diagnoses can be generated from the assessment data for the social domain. Examples are *ineffective coping*, *interrupted family processes*, and *ineffective role performance*.

Interventions for Social Domain

People with diagnoses of delusional disorder often become socially isolated. The secretiveness of their delusions and the importance the delusions have in their lives are central to this phenomenon. Social skills training tailored to the patient's specific deficits can help to improve social adaptation. Family therapy can help the person reintegrate into the family; family education and patient education will enhance understanding of the patient and the disease process. However, group therapy is usually not beneficial because the patient lacks insight into the origin of the delusion. Families face many of the same issues as families of patients with other disorders involving delusions and are at risk for ineffective coping.

Spiritual Domain

Nurses may hesitate to address the spiritual domain of a person who is experiencing delusional thinking, especially if there are religious overtones to fixed beliefs. This hesitancy may lie in an awareness that another's religious beliefs may seem so different to one's own that they may seem "fixed" and "false." Trying to understand the way a person's religious or spiritual beliefs are being shaped by his or her delusional disorder may seem a daunting task. If the nurse's response, however, is to be as sensitive and receptive as possible to the person's values (as revealed in his or her general behaviour and expression of pleasure and fears as well as by preillness choices and goals), then spiritual care may begin. Attending to the person's ultimate need to find meaning in life is what is required. This is grounded in thoughtful caring and attention to "the little things" that matter to the person, as well as through a hopeful, encouraging attitude that may foster hope in the patient (Carr, 2008).

Evaluation and Treatment Outcomes

For patients with delusional disorders, the greater the lack of insight and the poorer the adherence to treatment regimens, the more difficult it is to teach the individual. The patient rarely, if ever, develops full insight, and the symptoms related to the original diagnosis are not likely to disappear completely. In evaluating progress, the nurse must remember that outcomes are often not met completely. The nurse should maintain realistic outcomes and praise small successes to promote positive outcomes (Fig. 21-4).

Continuum of Care

Inpatient Focus Care

Hospitalization rarely occurs and is usually precipitated by legal or social violations. Insight-oriented interventions help the patient to understand his or her situation. Avoid confrontational situations; use the patient's coping abilities to reinforce constructive aspects of functioning to enable a return to autonomy.

Family Intervention

Family therapy may be helpful. By helping the family to develop mechanisms to cope with the patient's delusions, nurses help the family to be more supportive and understanding of the patient.

Community Treatment

Patients with diagnosis of delusional disorder are treated most effectively in an outpatient setting. They should be encouraged to seek psychiatric treatment. Insight-oriented therapy to develop an understanding of the

EMERGENCY CARE !

Emergency care is seldom required, unless the patient has had an incident with the law or legal system. The patient may be agitated or aggressive because the delusion, which is perceived as real, has been interrupted.

FIGURE 21-4. Bio/psycho/social/spiritual outcomes for patients with delusional disorder.

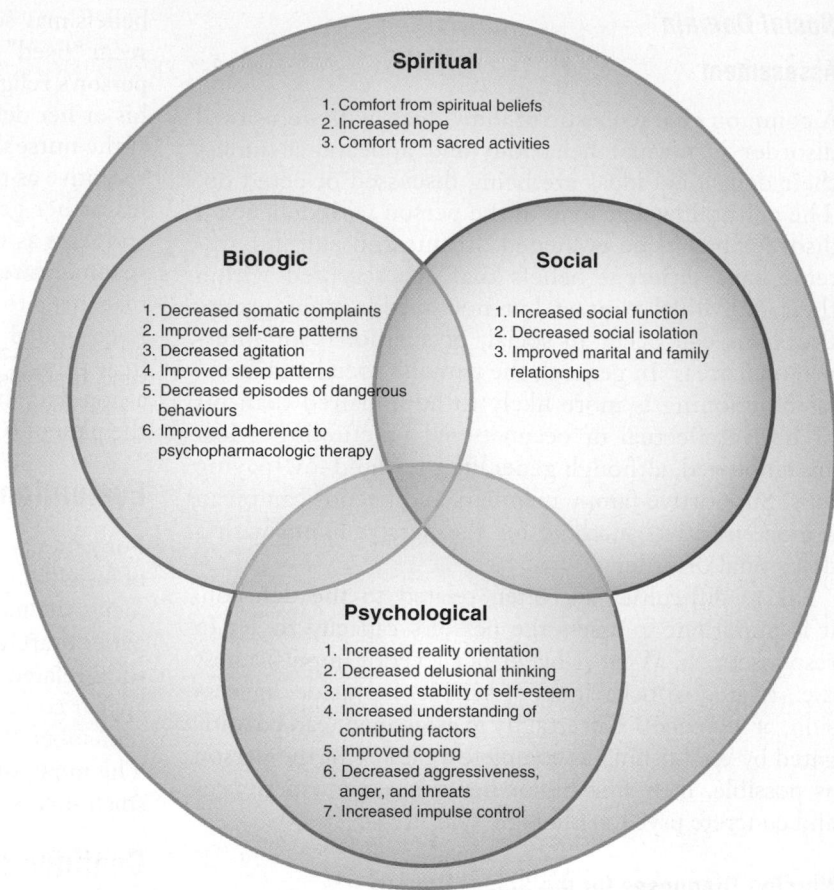

patient's delusion may be helpful. Medications are not often used with delusional disorder, but antipsychotic agents or benzodiazepines are helpful during exacerbations. Other treatments include supportive therapy, development of coping skills, cognitive therapy, and social skills training. Family therapy may be helpful.

OTHER PSYCHOTIC DISORDERS

Other disorders have psychoses as their defining features. The nursing care for patients with these disorders is not discussed specifically, but care used with other disorders can be applied to the disorders presented here (Table 21-3).

Schizophreniform Disorder

The essential features of schizophreniform disorder are identical to those of criteria A for SCH, with the exception of the duration of the illness (APA, 2013). Symptoms for schizophreniform disorder must be present for at least 1 month but less than 6 months (Table 21-4). If the symptoms persist beyond 6 months, the diagnosis should be changed to SCH. Some research has suggested that this disorder may be an early manifestation of SCH (van Os et al., 2009).

Altered social or occupational functioning may occur but is not necessary. Most patients experience interruption in one or more areas of daily functioning (APA, 2013).

Brief Psychotic Disorder

In brief psychotic disorder, the length of the episode is at least 1 day but less than 1 month. The onset is sudden and includes at least one of the positive symptoms of criteria A for SCH found in Chapter 20 (see also Table 21-4).

The person generally experiences emotional turmoil or overwhelming confusion and rapid, intense shifts of affect (APA, 2013). Although episodes are brief, impairment can be severe, and supervision may be required to protect the person. Suicide is a risk, especially in younger patients. A predisposition to develop a brief psychotic disorder may include preexisting personality disorders (APA, 2013). The person's ethnic and cultural background should also be considered in relation to the social or religious context of the symptoms presented. This disorder is uncommon but usually appears in early adulthood (APA, 2013).

Substance/Medication-Induced Psychotic Disorder

This psychotic disorder involves prominent hallucinations or delusions that are the direct physiologic effects of medication or a substance (see Table 21-4). This effect is indicated as the symptoms develop during or after intoxication or withdrawal of a substance or after exposure to medication capable of producing the symptoms. The

Table 21-3   Other Psychotic Disorders

Disorder	Definition
Schizophreniform disorder	This disorder is identical to SCH except the total duration of the illness can be <6 mo (must be at least 1 mo), and there may not be impaired social or occupational functioning
SCA	This disorder is characterized by an uninterrupted period of illness during which at some time there is a major depressive, manic, or mixed episode along with two of the following symptoms of SCH: delusions, hallucinations, disorganized speech, disorganized or catatonic behaviour, or negative symptoms (affective flattening, alogia, or avolition)
Delusional disorder	This disorder is characterized by the presence of nonbizarre delusion and includes several subtypes: erotomanic, grandiose, jealous, somatic, mixed, and unspecified
Brief psychotic disorder	In this disorder, there is a sudden onset of at least one positive psychotic symptom that lasts at least 1 d but <1 mo. Eventually, the individual has a full return to normal
Substance/medication-induced psychotic disorder	The prominent hallucinations or delusions are judged to be due to the physiologic effects or withdrawal of substances (drugs, alcohol)
Psychotic disorder due to another medical condition	Prominent hallucinations or delusions are judged to be related to the pathophysiologic consequence of another medical condition (e.g., metastatic neoplasms)

Adapted from American Psychiatric Association. (2013). *Diagnostic and statistical manual of mental disorders* (5th ed.). Washington, DC: Author.

symptoms do not occur exclusively during the course of a delirium and cause clinically significant distress or impairment of functioning (APA, 2013).

Psychotic Disorder Due to Another Medical Condition

Evidence shows that the hallucinations and/or delusions causing clinically significant distress or impairment in functioning are the direct pathophysiologic consequence

of another medical condition and are not better explained by another mental disorder or delirium (APA, 2013).

Other Specified Presentations

When symptoms characteristic of psychotic disorders cause clinically significant distress or impairment of functioning but do not meet the full criteria of a diagnostic class, they can be designated using *DSM-5* notation as "other specified" (APA, 2013). An example is *persistent*

Table 21-4   Key Characteristics for Other Psychotic Disorders

Disorder	Diagnostic Characteristics and Target Symptoms
Schizophreniform disorder	Symptoms of SCH present Delusions, hallucinations, disorganized speech, grossly disorganized or catatonic behaviour, and negative symptoms Not due to schizoaffective or MD Not due to effects of substance or general medical condition Episode lasting at least 1 mo but <6 mo
Brief psychotic disorder	Presence of delusions, hallucinations, disorganized speech, and grossly disorganized or catatonic behaviour (at least one) Duration of at least 1 d but <1 mo; returns to preillness level of functioning Not the direct physiologic effect of a substance or general medical condition; not better accounted for by other mental disorders
Substance/medication-induced psychotic disorder	Prominent hallucinations or delusions Symptoms developed during or within 1 mo of substance intoxication or withdrawal or medication use related to the disturbance Not better accounted for by other mental disorders Not occurring exclusively during delirium
Psychotic disorder due to another medical condition	Prominent hallucinations or delusions Evidence from history, physical examination, or laboratory studies that disturbance is a result of the physiologic consequences of a general medical disorder Not occurring exclusively during delirium

Refer to APA (2013) for *DSM-5* diagnostic criteria.

auditory hallucinations that occur without other features. *Shared psychotic disorder* (or *folie á deux*) was a diagnosis in the *DSM-IV*, indicating a disorder in which an individual in a close relationship with a person with a psychotic disorder comes to share some or all of that person's delusional beliefs. This diagnosis does not appear in the *DSM-5*, but rather *delusional symptoms in partner of individual with delusional disorder* is noted in the "other specified" category.

SUMMARY OF KEY POINTS

■ SCA has symptoms typical of both SCH and MD but is a separate disorder. Although these patients experience mood problems most of the time, the diagnosis of SCA depends on the presence of positive symptoms (i.e., delusions or hallucinations) without mood symptoms at some time during the uninterrupted period of illness.

■ Although controversy and discussion continue about whether SCA is truly a separate disorder, the *DSM-5* identifies it as separate.

■ Patients with SCA have fewer awareness deficits and appear to have more insight than do patients with true SCH, a fact that can be used in teaching patients to control symptoms, recognize early regression, and develop psychosocial skills.

■ Nursing care for patients with SCA is focused on minimizing psychiatric symptoms through promoting medication maintenance and on helping patients maintain optimal levels of functioning and self care. Interventions centre on developing social and coping skills through supportive, nurturing, and nonconfrontational approaches. The nurse must be constantly attuned to the mood state of the patient and help the patient learn to solve problems, resolve conflict, and cope with social situations that trigger anxiety.

■ Delusional disorder is characterized by stable, well-systematized, and logical nonbizarre delusions that could occur in reality and are plausible in the context of the patient's ethnic and cultural background. These delusions may or may not interfere with an individual's ability to function socially. Patients typically deny any psychiatric basis for their problem and refuse to seek psychiatric care. Patients whose delusions relate to somatic complaints are often seen on medical–surgical units of hospitals. Diagnosis otherwise is often made only when patients act on the basis of their delusions and violate the law or social rules.

■ Delusional disorder is further classified as a particular subtype, depending on the nature and content of the patient's delusions, including erotomanic, grandiose, jealous, somatic, mixed, and unspecified.

■ Patients with delusional disorder usually do not experience functional difficulties or mental status impairments. Their thinking, orientation, affect, attention, memory, perception, and personality generally remain intact.

■ Other psychotic disorders, distinguished particularly by duration of symptoms or specifically identified cause, include schizophreniform disorder, brief psychotic disorder, substance/medication-induced disorder, and psychotic disorder due to another medical condition.

■ The therapeutic relationship is crucial to the successful treatment of the patient with any psychotic disorder. Nurses must be aware of the patient's fragile self-esteem and unusual vulnerabilities and try to establish a trusting relationship through a flexible, nonjudgemental approach that promotes empathy, trust, and support.

CRITICAL THINKING CHALLENGES

1 Mr. J first received a diagnosis of SCH but, after experiencing extreme mood disturbances, finally receives a diagnosis of SCA. During a recent outpatient visit, he confides to a nurse that he just has stress and does not think that he really has any psychiatric problems. Identify assessment areas that should be pursued before the patient leaves his appointment. How would you confront the denial?

2 Ms. S believes she has bipolar disorder. At a recent clinic visit, she was told that she most probably has SCA. The patient asks the nurse how a bipolar disorder could turn into SCA. Identify three appropriate responses to her question.

3 A patient with SCA is prescribed an antipsychotic agent (Risperdal) and a mood stabilizer (Depakene). The patient asks you why both medications are needed. Develop the best response for this question. Be thorough.

4 At an interdisciplinary treatment team meeting, the nurse recommends that a woman with SCA attend an anger management group. The rest of the team believes that only a mood stabilizer is needed. Develop the rationale for her attending the anger management group in addition to receiving medication.

5 A patient was prescribed olanzapine (Zyprexa) and an antidepressant citalopram (Celexa) for the treatment of SCA. Since her last monthly visit, she gained 15 pounds. She is considering discontinuing her medication regimen because of the weight gain. Develop a plan that addresses her weight gain and her intention to discontinue her medication regimen.

6 J has received a diagnosis of SCA, and K has received a diagnosis of delusional disorder. How would the symptoms differ? Would there be any similarities? If so, what would they be?

7 Identify and explain each of the subtypes of delusional disorder.

8 An elderly person in a nursing home has a delusion that her husband is having an affair with her sister. Discuss nonpharmacologic nursing interventions that should be implemented with this patient. How would you explain her delusion to her husband? Choose one of the subtypes of delusion and develop a plan for clinical management, focusing on psychiatric nursing care, for a patient experiencing this condition.

9 A patient convincingly informs you that she is having an affair with a famous actor. They both attended the same college at about the same time. How would you determine whether this patient's belief is a delusion or reality? Is it important that the nurse understands whether the relationship is real? Explain the rationale for your answer.

10 A patient informs a student nurse that he is a member of the Secret Service and that he is undercover. He asks the nurse to keep the secret. The student considers several possible responses, including redirecting the patient to a different topic and confronting him with the reality of his hospitalization. Discuss the best response to this patient's comment.

REFERENCES

Abdel-Hamid, M. & Brüne, M. (2008). Neuropsychological aspects of delusional disorder. *Current Psychiatry Reports, 10,* 229–234.

American Psychiatric Association. (2013). *Diagnostic and statistical manual of mental disorders* (5th ed.). Washington, DC: Author.

Andreasen, N.C. & Black, W. (2006). *Introductory textbook of psychiatry* (4th ed.). Arlington, VA: American Psychiatric Publishing.

Andres, K., Pfammatter, M., Garst, F., Teschner, C., & Brenner, H. D. (2000). Effects of a coping-oriented group therapy for schizophrenia and schizoaffective patients: A pilot study. *Acta Psychiatrica Scandinavica, 101*(4), 318–322.

Bech, P. (2001). The significance of delusions in depressive disorders. *Current Opinions in Psychiatry, 14*(1), 47–49.

Bentall, R. P., Corcoran, R., Howard, R., Blackwood, N., & Kinderman, P. (2001). Persecutory delusions: A review and theoretical integration. *Clinical Psychology Review, 21*(8), 1143–1192.

Boora, K., Xu, J., & Hyatt, J. (2008). Encephalopathy with combined lithium-risperidone administration. *Acta Psychiatrica Scandinavia, 117,* 394–395.

Bottender, R., Strauss, A., & Moller, H. J. (2010). Social disability in schizophrenic, schizoaffective, and affective disorder 15 years post first admission. *Schizophrenia Research, 116,* 9–15.

Bowers, L., Brennan, G., Winship, G., & Theodoridou, C. (2009). *Talking with acutely psychotic people: Communication skills for nurses and others spending time with people who are very mentally ill.* London, UK: City University.

Carr, T. (2008). Mapping the processes and qualities of spiritual nursing care. *Qualitative Health Research, 18*(5), 686–700.

Cheniaux, E., Landeira-Fernandez, J., Telles, L., Lessa, J., Dias, A., Duncan, T.,& Versiani, M. (2008). Does schizoaffective disorder really exist? A systematic review of the studies that compared schizoaffective disorder with schizophrenia or mood disorders. *Journal of Affective Disorders, 106,* 209–217.

Chernomas, W., Clarke, D., & Chisholm, F. (2000). Perspectives of women living with schizophrenia. *Psychiatric Services, 51,* 1517–1521.

Clarke, D., Brown, A. M., & Giles-Smith, L. (2008). Triaging suicidal patients: Sifting through the evidence. *International Emergency Nursing, 16,* 165–174.

Conway, C. R., Bollini, A. M., Graham, B. G., Keefe, R. S., Schiffman, S. S., & McEvoy, J. P. (2002). Sensory acuity and reasoning in delusional disorder. *Comprehensive Psychiatry, 43*(3), 175–178.

Copeland, M. (2005). *Community links: Pathways to reconnection and recovery program implementation manual.* Waterbury, VT: Vermont State Department of Mental Health.

Crow, T. J. & Harrington, C. A. (1994). Etiopathogenesis and treatment of psychosis. *Annual Review of Medicine, 45,* 219–234.

DeHert, M., Schreurs, V., Vancampfort, D., & VanWinkel, R. (2009). Metabolic syndrome in people with schizophrenia: A review. *World Psychiatry, 8,* 15–22.

DeLisi, L. E., Shaw, S. H., Crow, T. J., Shields, G., Smith, A. B., Larach, V. W., et al. (2002). A genome-wide scan for linkage to chromosomal regions in 382 sibling pairs with schizophrenia or schizoaffective disorder. *American Journal of Psychiatry, 159*(5), 803–812.

Fujii, D. E., Ahmed, I., & Takeshita, J. (1999). Neuropsychologic implications in erotomania: Two case studies. *Neuropsychiatry, Neuropsychology and Behavioral Management, 12*(2), 110–116.

Getz, G. E., DelBello, M. P., Fleck, D. E., Zimmerman, M. E., Schwiers, M. L., & Strakowski, S. M. (2002). Neuroanatomic characterization of schizoaffective disorder using MRI: A pilot study. *Schizophrenia Research, 55*(1–2), 55–59.

Gibson, S. & Brand, S. (2013). Understanding treatment non-adherence in schizophrenia and bipolar mood disorder: a survey of what services users do and why. *BMC Psychiatry, 13,* 153.

Grunebaum, M. F., Oquendo, M. A., Harkavy-Friedman, J. M., Ellis, S. P., Li, S., Haas, G. L., … Mann, J. J. (2001). Delusions and suicidality. *American Journal of Psychiatry, 158*(5), 742–747.

Heinrichs, R. W., Ammari, N., Vaz, S., & Miles, A. (2008). Are schizophrenia and schizoaffective disorder neuropsychologically distinguishable? *Schizophrenia Research, 99,* 149–154.

Jacobson, L. & Tarraza, M. (2013). Integrative management of psychotic symptoms. In K.R. Tusaie & J. J. Fitzpatrick (Eds.), *Advanced practice psychiatric nursing* (pp. 182–229). New York: Springer.

Judd, F., Armstrong, S., & Kulkarni, J. (2009). Gender sensitive mental healthcare. *Australasian Psychiatry, 17,* 105–111.

Kasanin, J. (1933). The acute schizo-affective psychoses. *American Journal of Psychiatry, 13,* 97–126.

Kurtz, M. M. & Maeser, K. T. (2008). A meta-analysis of controlled research on social skills training for schizophrenia. *Journal of Consulting and Clinical Psychology, 76,* 491–504.

Lewine, R. R., Hudgins, P., Brown, F., Caudle, J., & Risch, S. C. (1995). Differences in qualitative brain morphology findings in schizophrenia, major depression, bipolar disorder, and normal volunteers. *Schizophrenia Research, 15*(3), 253–259.

Linney, Y. M., Murray, R. M., Peters, E. R., MacDonald, A. M., Rijadijk, F., & Sham, P.C. (2003). A quantitative genetic analysis of schizotypal personality traits, *Psychological Medicine, 33,* 803–816.

MacDougall, V., Luckett, K., & Jones, M. (2007). Women's experiences of psychosis: Recognition of gendered differences. In R. Velleman, E. Davis, G. Smith, & M. Drage, (Eds.), *Changing outcomes in psychosis: Collaborative cases from practitioners, users, and carers* (pp.117–34). Leicester, UK: Blackwell.

Marchinko, S. & Clarke, D. (2011). The Wellness Planner: Empowering consumers in self-care. *Archives of Psychiatric Nursing, 25,* 284–293.

McCarthy-Jones, S., Marriott, M., Knowles, R., Rowse, G., & Thompson, A. R. (2013). What is psychosis? A meta-synthesis of inductive qualitative studies exploring the experience of psychosis. *Psychosis: Psychological, Social and Integrative Approaches, 5,* 1–16.

McGuire, L., Junginger, J., Adams, S. G. Jr., Burright, R., & Donovick, P. (2001). Delusions and delusional reasoning. *Journal of Abnormal Psychology, 110*(2), 259–266.

Meloy, J. R. (1999). Erotomania, triangulation and homicide. *Journal of Forensic Science, 44*(2), 421–424.

Morimoto, K., Miyatake, R., Nakamura, M., Watanabe, T., Hirao, T., & Suwaki, H. (2002). Delusional disorder: Molecular genetic evidence for dopamine psychosis. *Neuropsychopharmacology, 26*(6), 794–801.

Munro, A. (1999). *Delusional disorder.* Cambridge, MA: Cambridge University Press.

Nasrallah, H. A. (2011). The primary and secondary symptoms of schizophrenia: Current and future management. A bridge to the future; redefining the scientific paradigm in the treatment of schizophrenia. *Current Psychiatry, 10*(Suppl, 9), S4–S9.

Ota, M., Mizukami, K., Katano, T., Sato, S., Takeda, T., & Asada, T. (2003). A case of delusional disorder, somatic type with remarkable improvement of clinical symptoms and single photon emission computed tomography findings following modified electroconvulsive therapy. *Progress in Neuro-psychopharmacology & Biological Psychiatry, 27*(5), 881–884.

Papageorgiou, A., King, M., Jonhohamed, A., Davison, D., & Dawson, J. (2002). Advanced directives for patients compulsorily admitted to hospital with serious mental illness. *British Journal of Psychiatry, 181,* 513–519.

Perr, I. N. (1992). Religion, political leadership, charisma, and mental illness: The strange story of Louis Riel. *Journal of Forensic Sciences, 37*(2), 574–884.

Petherick, W. (2013). *Profiling and serial crime* (3rd ed.). Philadelphia, PA: Elsevier Inc.

Pini, S., Cassano, G. B., Dell'Osso, L., & Amador, X. F. (2001). Insight into illness in schizophrenia, schizoaffective disorder, and mood disorders with psychotic features. *American Journal of Psychiatry, 158*(1), 122–125.

Portugal, E., Gonzalez, N., Vilaplana, M., Haro, J. M., Usall, J., & Cervilla, J. A. (2010). Gender differences in delusional disorder: Evidence from an outpatient sample. *Psychiatric Research, 177*, 235–239.

Potkin, S. G., Alphs, L., Hsu, C., Krishnan, K., Anand, R., Young, F. K., et al. (2003). Predicting suicidal risk in schizophrenic and schizoaffective patients in a prospective two-year trial. *Biological Psychiatry, 54*(4), 444–452.

Reid, W. (2005). Delusional disorder and the law. *Journal of Psychiatric Practice, 11*(2), 126–130.

Rowe, R. & Clark, T. (2008). A survey of psychiatrists' attitudes to schizoaffective disorder. *International Journal of Psychiatry in Clinical Practice, 12*(1), 25–30.

Sadock, B. J. & Sadock, V. A. (2007). *Kaplan and Sadock's synopsis of psychiatry* (10th ed.). Philadelphia, PA: Wolters Kluwer Health/Lippincott Williams & Wilkins.

Scott, T. F., Price, T. R., George, M. S., Brillman, J., & Rothfus, W. (1993). Midline cerebral malformations and schizophrenia. *Journal of Neuropsychiatry and Clinical Neurosciences, 5*(3), 287–293.

Seguin, J., Lesage, A., Chawky, N., Guy, A., Daigle, F., Girard, G., et al. (2006). Suicide cases in New Brunswick from April, 2002 to May 2003: The importance of better recognizing substance and mood disorder comorbidity. *Canadian Journal of Psychiatry, 51*, 581–586.

Shirzadi, A. A. & Ghaemi, S. N. (2006). Side effects of atypical antipsychotics: Extrapyramidal symptoms and the metabolic syndrome. *Harvard Review of Psychiatry, 14*, 152–164.

Siris, S. G. & Lavin, M. R. (1995). Other psychotic disorders. In H. Kaplan & B. Sadock (Eds.), *Comprehensive textbook of psychiatry* (6th ed.). Baltimore, MD: Williams & Wilkins.

Straker, D., Correll, L. U., Kramer-Ginsberg, E., Abdulhamid, N., Koshy, F., Rubens, E., et al. (2005). Cost-effective screening for metabolic syndrome in patients treated with second-generation antipsychotic medications. *American Journal of Psychiatry, 162*, 1217–1221.

Sutherby, K., Szmukler, G. I., Halpern, A., Alexander, M., Thornicroft, G., Johnson, C., & Wright, S. (1999). A study of 'crisis cards' in a community psychiatric service. *Acta Psychiatrica Scandinavica, 100*, 56–61.

Swoboda, E., Conca, A., Konig, P., Waanders, R., & Hansen, M. (2001). Maintenance electroconvulsive therapy in affective and schizoaffective disorder. *Neuropsychobiology, 43*(1), 23–28.

Van Os, J., Linscott, R. J., Myin-Germeys, I., Delespaul, P., & Krabbendam, L. (2009). A systematic review and meta-analysis of the psychosis continuum: Evidence for a psychosis proneness-persistence-impairment model of psychotic disorder. *Psychological Medicine, 39*, 179–195.

Volavka, J., Czobor, P., Sheitman, B., Lindenmayer, J. P., Citrome, L., McEvoy, J. P., et al. (2002). Clozapine, olanzapine, risperidone, and haloperidol in the treatment of patients with chronic schizophrenia and schizoaffective disorder. *American Journal of Psychiatry, 159*(2), 255–262.

Waite, P. (1987). Between three oceans: Challenges of a continental destiny. In C. Brown (Ed.), *The illustrated history of Canada* (pp. 279–373). Toronto, ON: Lester & Orpen Dennys.

22 Mood Disorders

Yvonne M. Hayne

Originally adapted from the chapter "Mood Disorders" by
Sandra J. Wood and Katharine P. Bailey

LEARNING OBJECTIVES

After studying this chapter, you will be able to:

- Describe the impact of underdiagnosed and untreated mood disorders as a major public health problem.
- Distinguish the clinical characteristics and the course of various mood disorders.
- Analyze human responses to mood disorders, distinguishing the experience of symptoms as distinct from the subjective experience of bearing a clinical diagnosis of such a disorder.
- Analyze prevailing biologic, psychological, and social theories, while taking into account spiritual considerations as a basis in caring for patients with mood disorders.
- Identify needs based on the holistic assessment of patients with mood disorders.
- Formulate nursing interventions on a continuum of care that address the spiritual nature of individuals experiencing specific diagnoses of mood disorder.
- Identify expected outcomes and evaluate the response to implementations of care.
- Analyze special concerns within the nurse–patient relationship common to treating people with mood disorders.

KEY CONCEPTS

- mania
- mood

KEY TERMS

- affect • bipolar • cyclothymic disorder • depressive episode • dysthymic disorder • euphoria • expansive mood • hypomanic episode • lability of mood • manic episode • mixed features • rapid cycling • unipolar

---

The World Health Organization (WHO) (2009) identifies the escalating incidence of major depression in developed and developing countries presenting as the leading cause of disease burden worldwide by the year 2030. This disorder not only directly affects a person's quality of life but impacts family and society as well (Lepine & Briley, 2011). Analysis of data from the Canadian Community Health Survey (CCHS) indicates that, from 2003 to 2009, the prevalence of mood disorders rose from 5.3% to 6.3% (CCHS, 2003). Most specifically, the prevalence was greater in the 35 to 64 age group, with women reflecting significantly higher levels than men. Indeed, studies show lifetime rate of major depression 1.7 to 2.7 times greater in women than in men, with risk increasing especially between adolescence and mid-50s, perhaps triggered by fluctuations in female hormones (Bryson, 2012). Studies also show the connection of depressive disorders with the incidence of chronic conditions such as hypertension, arthritis, back problems, and diabetes (Canadian Mental Health Association [CMHA], 2008, 2013). Further, "the risk of death by all causes is increased in depressed patients who are twice as likely to die prematurely compared with the general population" (Lepine & Briley, 2011). A significant concern is the extent that untreated mood disorders, specifically depression, are concurrent with elevated suicidality rates. The extent of these "premature and preventable" deaths prompts the WHO to declare the necessity of efforts to build awareness and improve treatments to mitigate such unfortunate consequences (WHO, 2006).

Canadian federal–provincial initiatives have developed a variety of collaborative approaches to mental health care, such as that demonstrated in the "Shared Mental Health Care" model, which aims at more effective diagnosis, assessment, and treatment of mental health patients in the context of the family physician's office (McElheran, Eaton, Rupcich, Basinger, & Johnston, 2004). Such collaborative endeavours are thought to increase efficiency in the use of health care resources by enhancing the identification of psychological and somatic complaints, accurate diagnosis, and appropriate care. In mood disorders, the potential for suicide is significant, and accurate diagnosis is vital in establishing psychological and pharmaceutical treatment. Nurses practising in any health care setting need to develop competence in assessing patients for the presence of a mood disorder and, should such a disorder be suspected, provide appropriate educational and clinical interventions or referral.

Common features of depressive disorders, and bipolar and related disorders, as described in the fifth edition of the American Psychiatric Association's *Diagnostic and Statistical Manual of Mental Disorders* (*DSM-5*) (APA, 2013), "include the presence of sad, empty, or irritable mood, accompanied by somatic and cognitive changes that significantly affect the individual's capacity to function" (p. 155). In depressive and bipolar-related disorders, the primary alteration is in mood rather than in thought or perception. Several terms describe observable expressions of mood (called **affect**) (APA, 2000), including the following:

- *Blunted*: Significantly reduced intensity of emotional expression
- *Flat*: Absent or nearly absent affective expression
- *Inappropriate*: Discordant affective expression accompanying speech content or ideation
- *Labile*: Varied, rapid, and abrupt shifts in affective expression
- *Restricted or constricted*: Mildly reduced in range and intensity of emotional expression

Primary mood disorders include both depressive (**unipolar**) and manic–depressive (**bipolar**) disorders. Although the *DSM-5* has separated its discussion of Depressive Disorders from Bipolar and Related Disorders, what endures related to both groupings are the common features noted above. Specific criteria differentiating the diagnostic classification of these disorders are detailed according to "issues of duration, timing, or presumed aetiology" (APA, 2013, p. 155). While several *mood categories*

are described in the *DSM-5*, this chapter focuses primarily on the disorders as follows:

- *Depressive disorders*: Major depressive disorder, single or recurrent; and dysthymic disorder
- *Bipolar disorders*: Bipolar I disorder, bipolar II disorder, and cyclothymic disorder
- *Mood disorder* caused by a general medical condition
- Substance-induced mood disorder

Two additional identifiers within the category of mood disorders warrant mention. First, *postpartum onset specifier* is distinguished by the onset of an episode within 3 to 4 weeks postpartum (Gavin et al., 2005; Marcus, 2009). Second, *seasonal depression* is a recognized pattern in some persons who are light-deprived (Akiskal, 2009a). This may be especially relevant to the Canadian population, for whom daylight varies widely with the seasons. This has become a recognized factor in some depressions, and phototherapy has been shown to benefit some individuals suffering depressive symptoms in such environmental situations (Akiskal, 2009a, p. 1641).

The advantage of early diagnosis of a mood disorder (e.g., early intervention, community nursing support) can be constrained by the adverse effect of a psychiatric diagnosis as a negative social label. Accessing effective care can be sabotaged by the need to keep the diagnosis hidden, even from oneself (Barney, Griffiths, Jorm, & Christensen, 2006; see Box 22-9). Increased awareness is a principal "weapon against stigma" and fundamental to combating misperceptions. Awareness would lead to clarity in detection, to acceptance by patients and their families, and ultimately to the required support and treatment (Kuhl, Kupfer, & Regier, 2011).

> **KEY CONCEPT Mood** is a pervasive and sustained emotion that colours one's perception of the world and how one functions in it. Normal variations in mood, such as sadness, euphoria, and anxiety, occur as responses to specific life experiences and are time limited, not associated with significant functional impairment.

DEPRESSIVE DISORDERS
Clinical Course

The *DSM-5* indicates that major depressive disorder can occur as a single episode, although in most cases the episode is recurrent. To constitute a **major depressive episode** (MDE), either a depressed mood or a loss of interest or pleasure in nearly all activities must be present for at least 2 weeks. Additionally, four of the following seven symptoms are usually present: disruption in sleep, appetite (or weight), concentration, or energy; psychomotor agitation or retardation; excessive guilt or feelings of worthlessness;

Table 22-1	Key Diagnostic Characteristics for Major Depressive Disorder

Diagnostic Criteria and Target Symptoms	Associated Features
• Change from previous level of functioning during a 2-week period • Depressed mood; "down in the dumps" • Markedly diminished interest or pleasure in all or almost all activities • Significant weight loss when not dieting, or weight gain or change in appetite • Insomnia or hypersomnia • Psychomotor agitation or retardation • Fatigue or loss of energy • Feelings of worthlessness or excessive or inappropriate guilt • Diminished ability to think or concentrate, or indecisiveness • Recurrent thoughts of death, recurrent suicidal ideation without a specific plan, or a suicide attempt or specific plan for committing suicide • At least one symptom is depressed mood or loss of interest or pleasure • Significant distress or impairment of social, occupational, or other important areas of functioning • Not a direct physiologic effect of substance or medical condition • Not better accounted for by bereavement, schizoaffective disorder; not superimposed on schizophrenia, schizophreniform disorder, delusional disorder, or psychotic disorder	*Associated Behavioural Findings* • Tearfulness, irritability, brooding, obsessive rumination, anxiety, phobias, excessive worry over physical health, and complaints of pain • Possible panic attacks • Difficulty with intimate relationships • Difficulties with sexual functioning • Marital problems • Occupational problems • Substance abuse, such as alcohol • High mortality rate; death by suicide • Increased pain and physical illness • Decreased physical, social, and role functioning • May be preceded by dysthymia, alternatively called persistent depressive disorder per *DSM-5* • Major depression may precede persistent depressive and MDEs and, major depression may occur during persistent depressive disorder (*DSM-5*)

American Psychiatric Association. (2013). *Diagnostic and Statistical Manual of Mental Disorders* (5th ed.). Washington, DC: Author.

and suicidal ideation (see Table 22-1). Individuals often describe themselves as depressed, hopeless, discouraged, or "down in the dumps." If individuals complain of feeling sad and empty, a depressed mood can sometimes be inferred from their facial expression and demeanour (APA, 2013). Depression may also present with behaviours such as obsessive ruminating, phobias, and panic attacks.

Major depressive disorder is commonly a progressive illness. With time, episodes tend to occur more frequently, become more severe, and last longer. Complications in the form of alcohol abuse disorders and suicidality may be the most serious of occurrences associated with major depression (Goldstein & Levitt, 2006).

Dysthymic disorder is a milder but more chronic form of major depressive disorder. The *DSM-5* criteria for dysthymic disorder are depressed mood for most days for at least 2 years, with two or more of the following symptoms present: poor appetite or overeating, insomnia or hypersomnia, low energy or fatigue, low self-esteem, poor concentration or difficulty making decisions, and feelings of hopelessness.

Depressive Disorders in Special Populations

Children and Adolescents

Depressive disorders in children have manifestations similar to those seen in adults, with a few exceptions. In major depressive disorder, children are less likely to experience psychosis, but when they do, auditory hallucinations are more common than are delusions. They are more likely to have anxiety symptoms characterized as internalizing disorders or externalizing behavioural abnormalities, such as fear of separation, and somatic symptoms, such as stomach aches and headaches. Mood may be irritable rather than sad, especially in adolescents. The risk for suicide is very real in children and adolescents and peaks during the mid-adolescent years. In Canada, the suicide rate remains alarmingly high for all age groups (Statistics Canada, 2012). Of particular concern are the rates of suicide among youth and the elderly, as well as among Aboriginal members of the population.

Older Adults

Most older patients with symptoms of depression do not meet the full criteria for major depression. However, it is estimated that 8% to 20% of older adults in the community and as many as 37% in primary care settings experience depressive symptoms. Treatment is successful in 60% to 80%, but response to treatment is slower than in younger adults. Depression in older adults often is associated with chronic illnesses, such as heart disease, stroke, and cancer; symptoms may have a more somatic focus. Suicide is a very serious risk for older adults, especially men. In Canada, significant mortality rates due to suicide are reported in people older than 80 years of age. Statistics also reflect an increase of death by suicide in this age group between the years 2005 to 2009, from 110 to 146 suicides, respectively. Rates were substantially higher among men than among women (Statistics Canada, 2012).

Epidemiology

Though individuals in the general population may occasionally describe themselves as feeling "low" or "unhappy," specific *DSM-5* criteria are used to designate major depression as a distinct disorder warranting medical treatment. The National Mental Health and Wellbeing Survey (NMHWS) (Andrews, 2008) reports on those persons who have experienced 2 weeks of depressed mood or loss of interest within a 1-year period and who fully meet the *DSM* criteria to detail three categorical descriptors. By this report, depression is said to be a *chronic disorder.* That is, only one-fifth of the individuals followed over a 15-year period were said, with treatment, to have recovered from their episode of depression and remained well. The remaining individuals, if not lost to suicide, were intermittently incapacitated through repeated episodes of depression throughout their lifetime.

IN A LIFE

James Eugene Carrey (1962–)
Canadian-born actor and comedian

Public Persona

Jim Carrey grew up in Toronto. His fame as a comedian began on *The Carol Burnett Show* at the age of 10. His stage talents ripened through the comedy routines he performed for classmates throughout his school years. Carrey, a high school dropout, began his acting career in comedy clubs and with bit-part television and movie performances. Soon his unique on-screen characteristics were recognized, and he became a box-office success. Jim Carrey is well known for his performances in such films as *The Mask, Eternal Sunshine of the Spotless Mind*, and *A Christmas Carol*. He was inducted into Canada's Walk of Fame in 2004.

Personal Reality

Carrey publicly discussed his struggle with depression on *60 Minutes* (November 2004), exposing a serious, complicated side of himself as a person who was continually questioning himself and the world. Carrey has been candid about periods of desperation in his life: the poverty, deprivation, and anger that marked some of his early childhood and adolescence; the struggles through two failed marriages; the highs and the lows bordering on despair; and the extended use of Prozac that helped him "out of a jam." Through it all, Jim, using the mask of *comedy* as a shield, maintains "life is beautiful" and that he is committed to giving full expression to the "realness" of his being.

Source: Leung, R. (2004, November). Carrey: Life is too beautiful. *60 Minutes*, CBS NEWS. Retrieved from http://www.cbsnews.com/stories/2004/11/18/60minutes/main656547.shtml

Andrews (2008), in the context of the NMHWS study, notes that *depression can occur throughout the life span*. This projection is made on the basis of three prospective cohorts: One age category from birth to 26 years, another from 24 to 50 years, and the third from the 70-to-85 age range. Beyond projections that one episode of major depression can be followed by approximately eight episodes of remission and reoccurrence in a lifetime, the report draws a disturbing conclusive summary estimate that "at least one-half of the population will experience at least one MDE during their lifetime." The magnitude of this as a major health problem to be addressed must register to all concerned. In adolescence, major depressive disorder is twice as common in female as in male populations, while prepubertal boys and girls are noted to be equally affected. Major depressive disorders are also noted to co-occur with other psychiatric and substance-related disorders, as supported by an extensive overview of the literature related to population data measures (Rush, Urbanoski, Bassani, Castel, & Wild, 2010). Further, depression is associated with a variety of comorbid medical conditions, particularly endocrine disorders, cardiovascular disease, neurologic disorders, autoimmune conditions, viral or other infectious diseases, certain cancers, and nutritional deficiencies, or as a direct physiologic effect of a substance—an example of the latter being the effects of corticosteroid treatment, which has been linked with depressive symptoms (Patten, 2010).

Ethnic and Cultural Differences

While prevalence rates in Canada are said to be unrelated to race, culture can influence the experience and communication of the symptoms of depression. Canada is a country of vast regional differences and numerous "microidentities" populated by indigenous and nonindigenous peoples. Many groups of inhabitants, such as those of Ukrainian and Asian cultures, maintain "homeland" beliefs and ideologies that may influence how individuals experience and express emotional disturbances. Depressive symptoms evidenced among Canada's Aboriginal peoples may be quite distinct coming from respective cultures, such as the Inuit, Métis, Blackfoot, Algonquian, Iroquoian, and so on (King Blood, 2005). Culture may dictate an iron resolve to keep feelings in check or unexpressed. Spiritual beliefs of First Nations peoples may complicate the detection of depression, as each group expresses and copes with feelings differently. In some cultures, somatic symptoms, rather than sadness or guilt, may predominate. Complaints of "nerves" and headaches (in Ukrainian cultures); weakness, tiredness, or "imbalance" (in Chinese and other Asian cultures); or problems of the "heart" (in Middle Eastern cultures) may be ways of expressing experience of depression. Although culturally distinctive experiences must be distinguished from symptoms, it is imperative that a symptom not be dismissed merely because it may be viewed as the norm for a culture. In this light, it is important for the nurse to be cognizant of emergent Canadian immigration trends; Latin American, south Asian, Indian, and African populations may have their own ways of characterizing a depressive disorder. The Canadian Nurses Association (CNA) recognizes that nurses must be equipped to care for an increasingly diverse population and value multiple ways of knowing, engaging, and expressing in order to make proper assessments and accurate diagnoses and to provide culturally sensitive care (Edmunds & Kinnaird-Iler, 2005).

Risk Factors

Depression is so common that it is sometimes difficult to identify risk factors. The Adverse Childhood Experiences study indicates devastating risk links between childhood emotional, physical, and sexual abuses and subsequent life experiences of depression (Felitti, 2007). Other generally acknowledged risk factors include the following:

- Prior episode of depression
- Family history of depressive disorder
- Lack of social support
- Stressful life event
- Current substance use
- Medical comorbidity
- Economic difficulties

Aetiology
Genetics

Family, twin, and adoption studies suggest a hereditary component to the aetiology of mood disorders, though strong genetic association to severe symptomatology is debated in the literature (Ebmeier, Donaghey, & Steele, 2006). Major depressive disorder, however, does demonstrate more commonly among first-degree biologic relatives of people with this disorder than among the general population, suggesting "gene–environment" interaction (Caspi et al., 2003; Uher & McGuffin, 2008). Additionally, positive correlates between "electrophysiologic deficits" and "familial risk for depression" have been reported (Zhang, Hauser, Conty, Emrich, & Dietrich, 2007). Increasingly, findings are demonstrating potential interactions between genetic, neurochemical, and cognitive influences in establishing a disposition to the experience of depression (Beck, 2008).

Neurobiologic Hypotheses

Extensive study persists as to the neurophysiologic and neurobiologic correlates to manifestations of depression. Early neurobiologic theories of the aetiology of depression emerged in the 1950s and linked with studies to advance evidence that major depression is caused by a deficiency or dysregulation in central nervous system (CNS)

concentrations of the neurotransmitters norepinephrine, dopamine, and serotonin or in their receptor functions. Research hypotheses were prompted in part from observations that some pharmacologic agents elevated mood, and subsequent studies identified their mechanisms of action (Donati & Rasenick, 2003; Thase, 2009). More recently, studies implicate a hyperactivity of the brain's amygdala as contributing to negative processing of stimuli. Ultimately, over time, it is thought that such interpretations of stimuli can result in a preponderance of negative correlates that then become associated with varied emotional stimuli and culminate in depressive episodes (Dannlowski et al., 2007). Continued study of neurophysiologic aspects will increasingly illuminate our understanding of depressive disorders.

Neuroendocrine and Neuropeptide Hypotheses

Major depressive disorder is associated with multiple endocrine alterations, specifically of the hypothalamic–pituitary–adrenal axis, the hypothalamic–pituitary–thyroid axis, the hypothalamic–growth hormone axis, and the hypothalamic–pituitary–gonadal axis. In addition, there is mounting evidence that components of neuroendocrine axes (e.g., neuromodulatory peptides such as corticotropin-releasing factor) may themselves contribute to depressive symptoms. Evidence also suggests that the secretion of these hypothalamic and growth hormones is controlled by many of the neurotransmitters implicated in the pathophysiology of depression (Beck, 2008; Hanley & Van de Kar, 2003).

Psychoneuroimmunology

Psychoneuroimmunology is a recent area of research into a diverse group of proteins known as *chemical messengers* between immune cells. These messengers, called cytokines, signal the brain and serve as mediators between immune and nerve cells. The connection between brain–immune interactions and susceptibility to major depression is a complex and ongoing study.

Psychological Theories
Psychodynamic Factors

Most psychodynamic theorists acknowledge some debt to Freud's original conceptualization of the psychodynamics of depression (Beck, 2008), which ascribes aetiology to an early lack of love, care, warmth, and protection, with resultant anger, guilt, and helplessness. Beevers (2005) proposes a more current notion of "cognitive vulnerability" to depression. This assertion theorizes that depression occurs due to patterns of uncorrected negatively biased associative processing.

Behavioural Factors

Behaviourists hold that depression occurs primarily as the result of a severe reduction in rewarding activities or an increase in unpleasant events in one's life. The resultant depression then leads to further restriction of activity, thereby decreasing the likelihood of experiencing pleasurable activities, which in turn intensifies the mood disturbance.

Developmental Factors

Developmental theorists pose that depression results from early life developmental event(s) that can become shaped and progressively evolve into dysfunctional attitudinal patterns, activated in later life by stressful events that lead to depression. The experience of parental loss in early childhood is of particular note, possibly through death, separation, or a lack of emotionally adequate parenting. This can create a "cognitive vulnerability" (Beck, 2008, p. 970) that potentially sensitizes the individual to negative experiences throughout life. Similarly viewed are the effects of varied early life adverse experiences, which can dispose to development of negative biases about oneself that then become the basis of later life depressive episodes.

Social Theories

Family Factors

Family theorists Wright and Leahey (2013) contend that the family is who they say they are (p. 55). Wright and Leahey ascribe maladaptive "circular" patterns in family interactions as contributing to the onset of depression in family members. Disruption to family dynamics deriving from multiple causes can manifest as depression experienced by a single family member. Nurses should be vigilant in identifying whether the individual's depressive experience is symptomatic of family distress. In such cases, a "family unit" assessment and assistance may be warranted and, indeed, possibly the best predictor of a positive outcome for the individual (see Chapter 15).

Social Factors

Social isolation, deprivation, and financial distress are risk factors for ensuing depression. Depression may also follow loss and adverse or traumatic life events, especially those that involve the loss of an important human relationship or role in life. Grieving after the loss of a loved one has been regarded as a normal process unless it endures for inordinate and extensive time periods and ultimately results in the symptoms equated with major depression. The dawn of the *DSM-5* has generated debate related to *grief* and whether it warrants labelling as a diagnostic mental disorder. For many, this became a contentious issue instigating debate about what "should" be considered normal, and/or normal variations of grieving, and why that should earn entry and be labelled within the rubric of mental disorder. On the one hand, grief is said to be "an inescapable part" of the human condition. Medicalizing what is regarded as normal grief would stigmatize and reduce "the normalcy and dignity of the pain" (Frances, 2010, p. 1). Others contend that both grief and depression may follow a major loss, introducing a complexity to each experience (Pies & Zisook, 2010). Thus, a case justifying the *grief diagnosis* might be thought of as a means for helping prevent complicated grief through treatment of associated depression. Akiskal (2009b) suggests that in major catastrophes a depressive episode may be more likely to occur. In such situations, bereavement reactions are characterized by primarily sympathetic arousal and restlessness, suggesting an evolutionary aspect in that the heightened physiological responses are mechanisms that occur to facilitate the "search for the lost object" (p. 1695).

Interdisciplinary Treatment

Although depressive disorders are the most commonly occurring mental disorders, they are usually treated within the primary care setting, not the psychiatric setting. Individuals with depression enter mental health settings when their symptoms become so severe that hospitalization is needed, usually for suicide attempts or if they self-refer because of incapacitation. Interdisciplinary treatment of these disorders, which are often lifelong, needs to include a wide array of health professionals in all areas. The specific goals of treatment are to

- Reduce/control symptoms and, if possible, eliminate signs and symptoms of the depressive syndrome
- Improve occupational and psychosocial function as much as possible
- Reduce the likelihood of relapse and recurrence

Priority Care Issues

The overriding concern for people with mood disorders is safety. In depressive disorders, suicide risk should always be considered, and suicide assessments should be done frequently (see Chapter 19).

Family Response to Disorder

Depression in one member affects the whole family. Spouses, children, parents, siblings, and friends experience frustration, guilt, and anger when the family member is immobilized and cannot function. It is often hard for others to understand the depth of the mood and how disabling it can be. Financial hardship can occur when the family member cannot go to work and spends days in bed. The lack of understanding and difficulty of living with a depressed person can lead to abuse. Research on families who have a member with a bipolar mood disorder reveals that families are profoundly affected by the social context of mental illness. They must manage crises, help the family member to control symptoms, and develop their own notion of "normal." Families use strategies such as being vigilant, setting limits, dealing with loss, and acknowledging the family member's strengths (Rea et al., 2003).

Nursing Management: Human Response to Depressive Disorder

The diagnosis of major depressive disorder is made when *DSM-5* criteria are met. An awareness of the risk factors for depression, a comprehensive bio/psycho/social/spiritual assessment, and a history of the patient's illness and any past treatment are key to formulating a treatment plan and to evaluating outcomes. Interviewing a family member or close friend about the patient's day-to-day functioning and specific symptoms may be helpful in determining the course of the illness, current symptoms, and level of functioning.

Depression during pregnancy and the postpartum period warrants special consideration. Symptoms of depression make it difficult for mothers to be responsive and sensitive to their infants. As a result, the maternal–infant relationship can be detrimentally affected. Infants need an environment that supports and nurtures their capabilities for emotional regulation, one that is protective and fosters a positive developmental trajectory. Depression can inhibit the mother's ability to respond in this manner. In their 1st year of life, approximately 1 in 11 infants will experience their mother's MDE (Center on the Developing Child at Harvard University, 2009). The treatment of pregnant and postpartum women with antidepressant medications presents a unique challenge due to the potential effects of these medications on the foetus and breast-feeding infants. A risk and benefit discussion about both the impact of the medications and untreated maternal depression is always necessary (American College of Obstetricians and Gynecologists, 2008; Tronick & Reck, 2009).

Biologic Domain

Assessment

Because some symptoms of depression are similar to those of some medical problems or side effects of medication therapies, biologic assessment must include a physical systems review and thorough history of medical problems, with special attention to CNS function, endocrine function, anaemia, chronic pain, autoimmune illness, diabetes, or menopause. Additional medical history includes surgeries; medical hospitalizations; head injuries; episodes of loss of consciousness; and pregnancies, childbirths, miscarriages, and abortions. A complete list of prescribed and over-the-counter (OTC) medications should be compiled, including the reason for a medication's being prescribed or its use discontinued. A physical examination is recommended with baseline vital signs and baseline laboratory tests, including a comprehensive blood chemistry panel, complete blood counts, liver function tests, thyroid function tests, urinalysis, and electrocardiograms. Biologic assessment also includes evaluating the patient for the characteristic neurovegetative symptoms listed below.

- *Appetite and weight changes* are a set criterion in major depression (APA, 2013): Changes from baseline can include decrease or increase in appetite with or without significant weight loss or gain (i.e., a change of more than 5% of body weight in 1 month). Weight loss occurs when not dieting, and weight gain presents more as an atypical feature of depression. Older adults with moderate to severe depression need to be assessed for dehydration as well as weight changes.

- *Sleep disturbance*: The most common sleep disturbance associated with major depression is insomnia. *DSM-5* (APA, 2013) addresses varied forms of insomnia, such as initial insomnia (difficulty falling asleep), middle insomnia (waking up during the night and having difficulty returning to sleep), or terminal insomnia (waking too early and being unable to return to sleep). Less frequently, the sleep disturbance is hypersomnia (prolonged sleep episodes at night or increased daytime sleep). The individual with either insomnia or hypersomnia complains of not feeling rested upon awakening (see Chapter 28).

- *Decreased energy, tiredness, and fatigue*: Fatigue associated with depression is a subjective experience of feeling tired regardless of how much sleep or physical activity a person has had. Even the smallest tasks require substantial effort (APA, 2013).

- *Loss of interest or pleasure* is to some degree always present (APA, 2013): Activities that brought pleasure in the past (e.g., hobbies, golfing, etc.) hold no interest in periods of depression.

In addition to a physical assessment, including weight and appetite, sleep habits, fatigue factors, and loss of interest, an assessment of current medications should be completed. The frequency and dosage of prescribed and OTC medications should be explored. In depression, the nurse must always assess the lethality of the medication being taken. For example, if a patient has sleep medications at home, the individual should be further queried about the number of pills in the bottle. Patients also need to be assessed for their use of alcohol, marijuana, and other mood-altering medications, as well as herbal substances because of the potential for drug–drug interactions. For example, patients taking antidepressants that affect serotonin regulation could also be taking St. John's wort (*Hypericum perforatum*) to fight depression.

● **STUDY NOTE**

In determining the severity of depressive symptoms, nursing assessment should explore changes in appetite and sleep patterns, loss of interest (anhedonia), and any decrease in energy. Considering the possibility of suicide should always be a priority, with assessment and documentation of suicide risk necessarily included in patient care.

The combined drug and herb could interact to cause serotonin syndrome (altered mental status, autonomic dysfunction, and neuromuscular abnormalities).

Nursing Diagnoses for Biologic Domain

There are several nursing diagnoses that could be formulated based on assessment data, including Disturbed Sleep Pattern, Imbalanced Nutrition, Fatigue, Ineffective Coping, and Nausea. Other diagnoses that should be considered are Ineffective Activity Planning and Sexual Dysfunction.

Interventions for Biologic Domain

Because weeks or months of disturbed sleep patterns and nutritional imbalance only make depression worse, counselling and education should aim to establish normal sleep patterns and healthy nutrition.

Teaching Physical Care

Encouraging patients to practise positive sleep hygiene and eat well-balanced meals regularly helps the patient move towards remission or recovery. Activity and exercise are also important for improving depressed mood state. Most people find that regular exercise is hard to maintain. People who are depressed may find it impossible. When teaching about exercise, it is important to start with the current level of patient activity and increase slowly. For example, if the patient is spending most of the time in bed, encouraging the patient to get dressed every day and walk for 5 or 10 minutes may be all that the patient can tolerate. Gradually, patients should be encouraged to have a regular exercise programme and to maintain a healthy diet.

Pharmacologic Interventions

An antidepressant is selected based primarily on the particular patient's target symptoms and an individual agent's side-effect profile. Other factors that may influence choice include the following:

- Prior medication response
- Drug interactions and contraindications
- Medication responses in family members
- Concurrent medical and psychiatric disorders
- Patient preference
- Age of the patient
- Cost of medication

Unlike many psychiatric disorders, depressive disorders may be time limited. As such, medication therapy should be reviewed periodically. The intensity of treatment and clinical management of psychiatric disorders is relative to the status of the presenting illness.

The primary goal of therapy for an acute illness phase is symptom reduction or remission. The objective is to choose the right match of medication and dosage for the patient. Careful monitoring and follow-up are essential during this phase to assess patient response to medications,

adjust dosage if necessary, identify and address side effects, and provide patient support and education. During the remission period, the goal is to decrease the risk for relapse. If a patient experiences a response to treatment, generally the treatment protocol will be maintained for a number of months to optimize a continued well state and minimize the prospect of residual symptoms and a risk of recurrence.

Abrupt discontinuation of medication is usually avoided as this may cause a recurrence of depressive symptoms. Sudden discontinuation of these medications can also cause physiologic symptoms, such as headaches. Medications need to be titrated down under the supervision of a physician or nurse practitioner. The decision to discontinue active treatment is generally based on factors that include the frequency and severity of past episodes, the persistence of dysthymic symptoms after recovery, the presence of comorbid disorders, and patient preference. Many patients continue taking medications for their lifetime.

● **STUDY NOTE**

Patients may be reluctant to take prescribed antidepressant medications or may self-treat depression. Continuing medication and emphasizing the potential drug–drug interactions should be included in the teaching plan.

Administering Antidepressant Medication Therapy

Antidepressant medications have proved effective in all forms of major depression. To date, controlled trials have shown no single antidepressant drug to have greater efficacy in the treatment of major depressive disorder. Antidepressant medications can be grouped as follows:

- Cyclic antidepressants, which include the tricyclic antidepressants (TCAs) and maprotiline (a tetracyclic)
- Selective serotonin reuptake inhibitors (SSRIs), which include escitalopram oxalate (Lexapro), fluoxetine (Prozac), sertraline (Zoloft), fluvoxamine (Luvox), paroxetine (Paxil), and citalopram (Celexa; see Box 22-1 for more information)
- Monoamine oxidase inhibitors (MAOIs), which include phenelzine (Nardil) and tranylcypromine (Parnate)
- "Atypical" antidepressants, which include trazodone (Desyrel), bupropion (Wellbutrin), venlafaxine (Effexor), and mirtazapine (Remeron). Table 12-9 in Chapter 12 lists antidepressant medications, usual dosage range, half-life, and therapeutic blood levels.

The first-generation drugs, the TCAs and MAOIs, are being used less often than the second-generation drugs, the SSRIs and atypical antidepressants. Second-generation drugs selectively target the neurotransmitters and receptors thought to be associated with depression in order to minimize side effects. The side-effect profiles of the two generations of drugs are significantly different as well (Table 22-2). The efficacy of the MAOIs is well established.

BOX 22-1   Drug Profile

ESCITALOPRAM OXALATE (LEXAPRO)

Drug Class: Antidepressant

Receptor Affinity: A highly selective serotonin reuptake inhibitor with low affinity for 5HT 1-7 or alpha- and beta-adrenergic, dopamine D1-5, histamine H1-3, muscarinic M1-5, and benzodiazepine receptors or for Na^+, K^+, Cl^-, and Ca^{2+} ion channels that have been associated with various anticholinergic, sedative, and cardiovascular side effects.

Indications: Treatment of depression

Routes and Dosages: Available as 5-, 10-, and 20-mg oral tablets.

Adults: Initially 10 mg once a day. May increase to 20 mg after a minimum of a week. Trials have not shown greater benefit at the 20-mg dose.

Geriatric: The 10-mg dose is recommended. Adjust dosage related to the drug's longer half-life and the slower liver metabolism of older adults.

Renal impairment: No dosage adjustment is necessary for mild to moderate renal impairment.

Children: Safety and efficacy not established in this population.

Half Life (Peak Effect): 27–32 hours (4–7 hours)

Selected Adverse Reactions: Most common adverse events include insomnia, diarrhoea, nausea, increased sweating, dry mouth, somnolence, dizziness, and constipation. Most serious adverse events include ejaculation disorder in males; serotonin syndrome if coadministered with MAOIs, St. John's wort, or SSRIs, including citalopram (Celexa), of which escitalopram (Lexapro) is the active isomer.

Specific Patient/Family Education:
- Do not take in combination with citalopram (Celexa) or other SSRIs or MAOIs. A 2-week washout period between escitalopram and SSRIs or MAOIs is recommended to avoid serotonin syndrome.
- Notify the prescriber if pregnancy is possible or being planned.
- Use caution driving or operating machinery until certain escitalopram does not alter physical abilities or mental alertness.
- Notify the prescriber of any OTC medications, herbal supplements, or home remedies being used in combination with escitalopram.

Table 22-2 **Side Effects of Antidepressant Medications**

Generic (Trade) Drug Name	Side Effects				
	Anticholinergic	Sedation	Orthostatic Hypotension	Gastrointestinal Distress	Weight Gain
Tricyclics: Tertiary Amines					
Amitriptyline (Elavil)	+4	+4	+2	0	+4
Clomipramine (Anafranil)	+3	+3	+2	+1	+4
Doxepin (Sinequan)	+2	+3	+2	0	+3
Imipramine (Tofranil)	+2	+2	+3	+1	+3
Tricyclics: Secondary Amines					
Amoxapine (Asendin)	+3	+2	+1	0	+1
Desipramine (Norpramin)	+1	+1	+1	0	+1
Nortriptyline (Aventyl, Pamelor)	+2	+2	+1	0	+1
SSRIs					
Fluoxetine (Prozac)	0/+1	0/+1	0/+1	+3	0
Sertraline (Zoloft)	0	0/+1	0	+3	0
Paroxetine (Paxil)	0	0/+1	0	+3	0
Fluvoxamine (Luvox)	0/+1	0/+1	0/+1	+3	0
Citalopram (Celexa)	0/+1	0/+1	0/+1	+3	0
Escitalopram (Lexapro)	0/+1	0/+1	0/+1	+3	0
Atypical: Antidepressants					
Venlafaxine (Effexor)	0	0	0	+3	0
Trazodone (Desyrel)	0	+1	+3	+1	+1
Bupropion (Wellbutrin)	+2	+2	+1	0	0/+1
Mirtazapine (Remeron)	+3	+4	+3	+3	+2

0, absent or rare; 0/+1, lowest likelihood; +4, highest likelihood.

Evidence suggests that their distinct advantage is treating a specific subtype of depression, so-called atypical depression (characterized in the *DSM-5* by increased appetite, mood improvement in response to actual or potential positive events, and hypersomnia). MAOIs are also used in treating depression with panic symptoms or social phobia (Schatzberg, Cole, & DeBattista, 2003). Given the complexity of their use, MAOIs usually are reserved for patients whose depression fails to respond to other antidepressants or patients who cannot tolerate typical antidepressants.

Monitoring Medications

Patients should be carefully observed when taking antidepressant medications, not only for the anticipated side effects generally associated with them but also for their less common, sometimes even lethal possibilities. Although it is essential to know the valued benefits of antidepressants, it is equally important to be cognizant of the severe adverse effects these chemical agents can provoke. For example, some studies include evidence that both SSRIs and TCAs can induce the emergence of "medication activation syndrome" (extreme anxiety, hostility, agitation) and exacerbate suicidal ideation (Lam & Kennedy, 2004), the very things they are intended to avert. When observing patients taking antidepressants, nurses must be vigilant to the range of such possibilities, knowing also that, in the depths of depression, saving medication for a later suicide attempt is possible (Box 22-2). During antidepressant treatment, there is ongoing monitoring of vital signs, plasma drug levels as appropriate, liver and thyroid function tests, complete blood counts, and blood chemistry.

BOX 22-2 Guidelines: Monitoring and Administering Antidepressant Medications

Nurses should do the following in administering/monitoring antidepressant medications:
- Observe the patient for cheeking or saving medications for a later suicide attempt.
- Monitor vital signs: obtain baseline data (e.g., orthostatic vital signs and temperature) before the initiation of medications.
- Periodically monitor liver and thyroid function, blood chemistry, and complete blood count as appropriate and compare with baseline values.
- Monitor patient symptoms for therapeutic response and report inadequate response to the prescriber.
- Monitor the patient for side effects and report to the prescriber serious side effects or those that are chronic and problematic for the patient. (Table 20-3 indicates pharmacologic and nonpharmacologic interventions for common side effects.)
- Monitor drug levels as appropriate. (Therapeutic drug levels for antidepressants are listed in Table 12-9 in Chapter 12.)
- Monitor dietary intake as appropriate, especially with regard to MAOI antidepressants.
- Inquire about patient's use of other medications, alcohol, street drugs, OTC medications, and/or herbal supplements that might alter the desired effects of prescribed antidepressants.

Responsibilities include ensuring that patients are receiving a therapeutic dosage, assessing adherence to the medication regimen, monitoring for side effects, and helping to prevent toxicity. Various pharmacologic and nonpharmacologic interventions for the side effects of antidepressant medications are listed in Table 22-3. See Chapter 12 for therapeutic blood levels for antidepressants.

Baseline vital signs should be obtained before the initiation of any medication (most particularly if administered to children, older adults, or those physiologically compromised). Thereafter, monitoring medication effects should include objective observations, vital signs, the patient's subjective reports, and the administration of rating scales over the course of treatment. Special attention should be accorded in the case of those on medications known to have an impact on vital signs (e.g., TCAs, MAOIs, or venlafaxine).

Individualizing dosages is essential for achieving optimal efficacy. When the newer antidepressants are used, this is usually done by fine-tuning the dosage based on patient feedback. The TCAs, including imipramine (Tofranil), desipramine (Norpramin), amitriptyline (Elavil), and nortriptyline (Pamelor), have standardized valid plasma levels that can be useful in determining therapeutic dosages, although therapeutic plasma levels may vary from individual to individual. Blood samples should be drawn as close as possible to 12 hours from the last dose. The newer antidepressants do not have established standardized ranges, and optimal dosing is based on efficacy and tolerability.

Monitoring and Managing Side Effects
First-Generation Antidepressants: TCAs and MAOIs The most common side effects associated with TCAs and MAOIs are the antihistaminic side effects (sedation and weight gain) and anticholinergic side effects (potentiating CNS drugs, blurred vision, dry mouth, constipation, urinary retention, sinus tachycardia, and decreased memory). TCAs are more commonly used in chronic pain patients, where depression might be a common comorbidity.

EMERGENCY !

If possible, TCAs should not be prescribed for patients at risk for suicide. Lethal doses of TCAs are only three to five times the therapeutic dose. Death may result from cardiac arrhythmia, hypotension, or uncontrollable seizures.

Serum TCA levels should be evaluated when overdose is suspected. In acute overdose, almost all symptoms develop within 12 hours. Anticholinergic effects are prominent: dry mucous membranes, warm and dry skin, blurred vision, a decreased bowel motility, and urinary retention. CNS suppression (ranging from drowsiness to coma) or an agitated delirium may occur. Basic overdose treatment includes induction of emesis, gastric lavage, and cardiorespiratory supportive care. The most common side effects of MAOIs are headache, drowsiness, dry mouth, constipation, blurred vision, and orthostatic hypotension.

Table 22-3	Interventions to Relieve Side Effects of Antidepressants

Side Effect	Pharmacologic Intervention	Nonpharmacologic Intervention
Dry mouth, caries, inflammation of the mouth	Bethanechol 10–30 mg tid Pilocarpine drops and sublingual tablets	Sugarless gum Sugarless lozenges 6–8 cups water per day Toothpaste and mouthwash for dry mouth Avoid caffeine
Nausea, vomiting	Cisapride 0.5 mg bid	Take medication with food Soda crackers, toast, tea
Weight gain	Change medication	Nutritionally balanced diet Daily exercise
Urinary hesitation Constipation	Bethanechol 10–30 mg tid Stool softener	6–8 cups water per day Laxatives as prescribed Daily exercise 6–8 cups water per day Diet rich in fresh fruits and vegetables and grains
Diarrhoea Orthostatic hypotension	OTC antidiarrheal	Maintain fluid intake Increase hydration Sit or stand up slowly
Drowsiness	Shift dosing time Lower medication dose Change medication	One caffeinated beverage at strategic time Do not drive when drowsy No alcohol or other recreational drugs Plan for rest time
Fatigue	Lower medication dose Change medication	Daily exercise
Blurred vision	Bethanechol 10–30 mg tid Pilocarpine eye drops	Temporary use of magnifying lenses until body adjusts to medication
Flushing, sweating	Terazosin 1 mg qd Lower medication dose Change medication	Frequent bathing Lightweight clothing
Tremor	β-Blockers Lower medication dose	Reassure the patient that tremor may decrease with adjustments to medication. Notify the caregiver if tremor interferes with daily functioning

EMERGENCY !

If coadministered with food or other substances containing tyramine (e.g., aged cheese, beer, red wine), MAOIs can trigger a hypertensive crisis that may be life threatening. Symptoms include sudden, severe pounding or explosive headache in the back of the head or temples, racing pulse, flushing, stiff neck, chest pain, nausea and vomiting, and profuse sweating.

MAOIs are more lethal in overdose than are the newer antidepressants and thus should be prescribed with caution if the patient's suicide potential is elevated (see Chapter 12). An MAOI generally is given in divided doses to minimize side effects. Selected adverse effects of MAOIs include headache, drowsiness, dry mouth and throat, insomnia, nausea, agitation, dizziness, constipation, asthenia, blurred vision, weight loss, and postural hypotension. Although priapism was not reported during clinical trials, the MAOIs are structurally similar to trazodone, which has been associated with priapism (prolonged painful erection).

Second-Generation Antidepressants: SSRIs and Atypical Antidepressants Serotonin syndrome is a potentially serious side effect caused by drug-induced excess of intrasynaptic serotonin (5-hydroxytryptamine [5-HT]). First reported in the 1950s, it was relatively rare until the introduction of the SSRIs. In most cases, serotonin syndrome occurs as a result of serotonin buildup when more than one drug acting on the serotonergic system (e.g., an SSRI and a TCA) is prescribed (Keogh & Doyle, 2008). Although serotonin syndrome can be life threatening, once differential diagnosis with neuroleptic malignant syndrome is made, supportive care measures generally serve in symptom recovery. Unlike neuroleptic malignant syndrome, which develops within 3 to 9 days after the introduction of neuroleptic medications, serotonin syndrome tends to develop within hours or days after initiating or increasing the dose of serotonergic medication or adding a drug with serotomimetic properties. The symptoms include altered mental status, autonomic dysfunction, and neuromuscular abnormalities. At least three of the following symptoms must be present for a diagnosis: mental status changes, agitation, myoclonus, hyperreflexia, fever, shivering, diaphoresis, ataxia, and diarrhoea. In patients who also have peripheral vascular disease or atherosclerosis, severe vasospasm and hypertension may occur in the presence of elevated serotonin levels. In addition, in a patient who is a slow metabolizer of SSRIs, higher-than-normal levels of these antidepressants may circulate in the blood. In sum, vigilance is required to detect serotonergic symptoms that can result from varied and even uncommon causes, including medications such as meperidine prescribed for pain (Koczmara, Perri, Hyland, & Rousseaux, 2005).

EMERGENCY !

The most important emergency interventions are stopping use of the offending drug, notifying the physician, and providing necessary supportive care (e.g., intravenous fluids, antipyretics, cooling blanket).

Monitoring for Drug Interactions

Although SSRIs and newer atypical antidepressants produce fewer and generally milder side effects, which improve the patient's toleration and compliance, there are some side effects to note. Among the most common are insomnia and activation, headaches, gastrointestinal symptoms, and weight gain. Sexual side effects, primarily diminished interest and performance, are also reported with some SSRIs, particularly sertraline. The most potentially harmful, but preventable, side effect/interaction of SSRIs is serotonin syndrome (Box 22-3).

BOX 22-3   Emergency

SEROTONIN SYNDROME
....

Cause: Excessive intrasynaptic serotonin

How it Happens: Combining medications that increase CNS serotonin levels, such as SSRIs + MAOIs; SSRIs + St. John's wort; or SSRIs + diet pills, dextromethorphan; or alcohol, and MAOIs, especially red wine; or SSRI + street drugs, such as LSD, MMDA, or Ecstasy.

Symptoms: Mental status changes, agitation, ataxia, myoclonus, hyperreflexia, fever, shivering, diaphoresis, diarrhoea.

Treatment: Assess all medication, supplements, foods, and recreational drugs ingested to determine the offending substances.
   Discontinue any substances that may be causative factors. If symptoms are mild, treat supportively on outpatient basis with propranolol and lorazepam and follow up with the prescriber.
   If symptoms are moderate to severe, hospitalization may be needed with monitoring of vital signs and treatment with intravenous fluids, antipyretics, and cooling blankets.

Further Use: Assess on a case-by-case basis and minimize risk factors for further medication therapy.

Trazodone administration has been associated with erectile dysfunction and priapism. Bupropion can cause seizures, particularly in patients at risk for seizures. Bupropion has also been associated with the development of psychosis because it is dopaminergic, and its use should be avoided in patients with schizophrenia. Venlafaxine can cause an increase in blood pressure, although this side effect appears to be dose related and can be controlled by lowering the dose (APA, 2002). For a listing of potential drug–drug interactions related to antidepressants, see Table 22-4.

Teaching Points

If depression goes untreated or is inadequately treated, episodes can become more frequent, more severe, and of longer duration, and they can lead to suicide. Patient education involves explaining this pattern and the importance of continuing medication use after the acute phase of treatment to decrease the risk of relapse.

The situation of patients discontinuing their prescribed medication prematurely is not uncommon. It may be natural for patients to assume that their experience of symptom relief, after short-term medication use, means their disorder has resolved. It is important for the nurse to recognize this erroneous assumption and to make clear to patients that "response" is not the same thing as "remission." Although immediate relief of symptoms may signify response, patients need to be carefully informed about the adverse possibility of depression recurring with the discontinuation of their medication. Medication should be continued for at least 6 months to 1 year after symptom relief (Markley, 2008). If the patient experiences a recurrence after tapering the first course of treatment, the regimen should be reinstituted for at least another year, and if the illness recurs, medication may be continued indefinitely (Schatzberg et al., 2003).

When on a regimen of antidepressants, patients should be cautioned about taking OTC medications such as those for hay fever and asthma or nasal decongestants. Herbal substances also pose problems. For example, the herb St. John's wort is particularly offensive in causing hypertension if taken in combination with agents containing monoamines. Consultation with a pharmacist is generally a wise course of action for patients considering impromptu combinations of medication.

Other Somatic Therapies

Electroconvulsive Therapy Although its therapeutic mechanism of action is unknown, electroconvulsive therapy (ECT) is an effective treatment for severe depression. It is generally reserved for patients whose disorder is refractory or intolerant to initial drug treatments or who are so severely ill that rapid treatment is required (e.g., patients with malnutrition, catatonia, or suicidality).

ECT is contraindicated for patients with an increased intracranial pressure. Other high-risk patients include

Table 22-4	Drug–Drug Interactions: Antidepressants	

Antidepressant	Other Drug	Effect of Interaction/Treatment
Fluvoxamine	Theophylline	Increased theophylline level: seizures. Tx: Reduce theophylline levels when administering with fluvoxamine.
Fluoxetine, paroxetine	TCAs Benzodiazepines Phenothiazines	Increased plasma levels of TCA. Tx: Reduce TCA levels when giving with fluoxetine or paroxetine.
Fluoxetine, fluvoxamine, nefazodone, triazolam	Alprazolam Benzodiazepines	Increased plasma levels of alprazolam. Tx: Reduce dose of alprazolam when administered with benzodiazepines.
Fluvoxamine	Caffeine Nicotine	Lowered levels of fluvoxamine. Tx: Increase dose of fluvoxamine in smokers or patients whose coffee, tea, or caffeinated drink intake is high.
SSRIs	Warfarin	Increased prothrombin time, bleeding. Tx: Monitor closely, decrease the dose of warfarin if giving with SSRIs.
SSRIs	Lithium TCAs Barbiturates	Increased CNS effects of SSRIs. Tx: Adjust dosage of SSRI.
SSRIs	Phenytoin	Increased serum levels of phenytoin. Tx: Adjust dosage of phenytoin.

Data from McCuistion, L. E. & Gutierrez, K. J. (2002). *Real-world nursing survival guide: Pharmacology*. Philadelphia, PA: WB Saunders; Stahl, S. (2005). *Essential psychopharmacology: A prescriber's guide*. Cambridge, MA: Cambridge University Press.

those with recent myocardial infarction, recent cerebrovascular accident, retinal detachment, or pheochromocytoma (tumour on the adrenal cortex or other tumours) and those at risk for complications of anaesthesia. Severely depressed older adults may have a more favourable response to ECT than to medication; however, the benefits of the treatment need to be considered carefully against its risks.

The CNA (2005) supports standards and best practices that uphold and effectively regulate professional nursing care for patients. For those undergoing ECT, the role of the nurse includes providing educational and emotional support for the patient and family; assessing baseline or pretreatment level of function; preparing the patient for the ECT process; and monitoring and evaluating the patient's response to the treatment, sharing it with the ECT team, and modifying treatment as needed.

Light Therapy (Phototherapy) Light therapy (described in Chapter 12) is acknowledged as an efficacious option for the treatment of seasonal affective disorder, through its effects on the circadian system. Indeed, support mounts for its value as "adjuvant" (i.e., modifies another agent with little or no direct effects by itself) to pharmacotherapy in treating nonseasonal depression as well (Even, Schroder, Friedman, & Rouillon, 2008).

Psychological Domain

Assessment

The mental status examination is an effective clinical tool to evaluate the psychological aspects of major depression because the focus is on disturbances of mood and affect, thought processes and content, cognition, memory, and attention. The comprehensive mental status examination is described in detail in Chapter 10.

Mood and Affect

The person with depression has a sustained period of feeling depressed, sad, or hopeless and may experience anhedonia (loss of interest or pleasure). The patient may report "not caring anymore" or not feeling any enjoyment in activities that were previously considered pleasurable. In some individuals, this may include a decrease in or loss of libido (sexual interest or desire) and sexual function. Depressed mood may be severe enough to provoke thoughts of suicide.

Numerous assessment scales are available for assessing depression. Easily administered self-report questionnaires can be valuable detection tools. These questionnaires cannot be the sole basis for making a diagnosis of MDE, but they are sensitive to depressive symptoms. The Beck Depression Inventory (BDI) is one such commonly used self-report scale. The Hamilton Rating Scale for Depression (HAM-D; see Appendix E) is one of several clinician-completed rating scales used and, as such, may be somewhat more precise than self-report questionnaires in detecting depression.

Thought Content

Depressed individuals often have an unrealistic, negative evaluation of their worth or have guilty preoccupations or ruminations about minor past failings. Such individuals often misinterpret neutral or trivial day-to-day events as evidence of personal defects, and they have an exaggerated sense of responsibility for untoward events. As a result, they feel helpless, hopeless, worthless, and powerless. An exploration of the individual's perspective on self, the world, and the future should be included in the overall assessment, as should the possible occurrence of disorganized thought processes (e.g., tangential or circumstantial thinking) and perceptual disturbances (e.g., hallucinations, delusions).

Suicidal Behaviour

Patients with major depression are at an increased risk for suicide. Suicide risk should be assessed initially and throughout the course of treatment. Suicidal ideation includes thoughts that range from a belief that others would be better off if the person were dead or thoughts of death (passive suicidal ideation) to actual specific plans for committing suicide (active suicidal ideation). The frequency, intensity, and lethality of these thoughts can vary and can help to determine the seriousness of intent. The more specific the plan and the more accessible the means, the more serious is the intent. Risk factors that must be carefully considered are the availability and adequacy of social supports, past history of suicidal ideation or behaviour, presence of psychosis or substance abuse, and decreased ability to control suicidal impulses.

To gain an in-depth understanding of the actual risk, questions intended to illicit behavioural indicators towards suicide are warranted. For example, the patient should be questioned whether he or she has medications to take an overdose. This differentiates whether the person has a plan and is actually acting on the plan—which indicates a more determined intent. Specific questions such as this, interfaced with a deliberate Suicide Risk Assessment (Brooks, Burata, & Tansey, 2008), would be valuable in determining the seriousness of intent.

Cognition and Memory

Many individuals with depression report an impaired ability to think, concentrate, or make decisions. They may appear easily distracted or complain of memory difficulties. In older adults with major depression, memory difficulties may be the chief complaint and may be mistaken for early signs of a dementia (pseudodementia), thus complicating the diagnostic process (Akiskal, 2009b, p. 1699; Fischer, 2002). When the depression is fully treated, the memory problem often improves or fully resolves.

Nursing Diagnoses for Psychological Domain

Nursing diagnoses focusing on the psychological domain of the patient with a depressive disorder are numerous. If patient data lead to the diagnosis of Risk for Suicide, the patient should be further assessed for plan, intent, and accessibility of means. Other nursing diagnoses include Hopelessness, Risk for Situational Low Self-Esteem, Ineffective Coping, Decisional Conflict, Spiritual Distress, and Complicated Grieving.

Interventions for Psychological Domain

Although pharmacotherapy is usually the primary treatment method for major depression, patients also can benefit from psychosocial and psychoeducational treatments. The most effective therapies for patients with severe or recurrent major depressive disorder are combinations of psychotherapy (including interpersonal therapy, cognitive–behavioural therapy [CBT], behaviour therapy) and pharmacotherapy. Adding a course of CBT may be an adjunct strategy for preventing relapse in patients who have had only a partial response to pharmacotherapy alone (see Chapter 13).

Clinical practice guidelines suggest that the combination of medication and psychotherapy may be particularly useful in more complex situations (e.g., depression in the context of concurrent, chronic general medical or other psychiatric disorders or in patients who fail to respond completely to either treatment alone). Further, depressive symptomatology can be complicated by stressful lifestyle circumstances, perhaps presenting as work-related or located in social aspects of an individual's life. CBT and other psychotherapies (individual, marital, or group) can be helpful in addressing such situational life complexities. Mindfulness-based cognitive therapy is increasingly valued as a supportive intervention modality that can be implemented in community health programmes by nurse therapists (Cowen, Harrison, & Burns, 2012, p. 250).

● **STUDY NOTE**

A cognitive therapy approach is recommended for the acute phase of depression. This approach should be included in most nursing care plans for patients with depression. Intensity of affect can result in patients' inability to attend to and follow through with cognitive interventions.

Therapeutic Relationship

One of the most effective therapeutic tools for treating any psychiatric disorder is the therapeutic alliance, a helpful and trusting relationship between clinician and patient. The alliance is built from a number of activities, including the following:

- Establishment and maintenance of a supportive relationship
- Availability in times of crisis
- Vigilance regarding dangerousness to self and/or others
- Education about the illness and treatment goals
- Encouragement and feedback concerning progress
- Guidance regarding the patient's interactions with the personal and work environment
- Realistic goal setting and monitoring

Interacting with depressed individuals is challenging because they tend to be withdrawn and have difficulty expressing feelings and engaging in interpersonal interactions. The therapeutic alliance partly depends on winning the patient's trust through a warm and empathic stance within the context of professional boundaries (see Chapter 6). Understanding the individual's personal experience of receiving a psychiatric diagnosis will enable the nurse to respond to the individual more effectively.

● **STUDY NOTE**

Establishing the patient–nurse relationship with a person who is depressed requires an empathic, quiet approach. Too much enthusiasm can block communication.

Cognitive Therapy

Cognitive therapy has been successful in reducing depressive symptoms during the acute phase of major depression (APA, 2002; see Chapter 13). This therapy uses techniques such as monitoring thoughts, emotions, and actions to identify irrational, distorted thinking and beliefs. The use of cognitive therapy in the acute phase of treatment, combined with medication, has grown in the past few years and now may be considered first-line treatment for mildly to moderately depressed outpatients. Varied modalities for implementing cognitive therapy have been made convenient through telephone and computer-assisted technology, with outcomes said to be similar to standard delivery modes (Corcoran & Walsh, 2009a).

Behaviour Therapy

Behaviour therapy for depression encompasses behavioural activation techniques, which are effective in the treatment of patients with depression and particularly when they are combined with pharmacotherapy. Therapeutic techniques include activity scheduling, self-control therapy, social skills training, and problem solving.

Interpersonal Therapy

Interpersonal therapy seeks to recognize, explore, and resolve the interpersonal losses, role confusion and transitions, social isolation, and deficits in social skills that may precipitate depressive states (APA, 2002). It maintains that losses must be mourned and related affects appreciated, that role confusion and transitions must be recognized and resolved, and that social skills deficits must be overcome to acquire social supports. Some evidence in controlled studies suggests that interpersonal therapy is more effective in reducing depressive symptoms with certain populations, such as depressed patients with human immunodeficiency virus infection, and less successful with patients who have personality disorders (APA, 2002; see Chapter 27).

Family and Marital Therapy

Patients who experience high family stress are at risk for greater future severity of illness, higher use of health services, and higher health care expenses. Marital and family problems are common among patients with mood disorders; comprehensive treatment requires that these problems be assessed. They may be an outcome of major depression but may also increase susceptibility to depression and in some instances stop recovery. Research suggests that group intervention for couples may reduce depressive symptoms and increase partners' relational satisfaction through learned abilities in regulating mood and emotions (Kirby & Baucom, 2007). Assisting the adjustment of the nondepressed partner, and of all family members, may be invaluable in averting a relapse of depression for the recovering patient. Many family nursing interventions (see Chapter 15) may be used by the generalist psychiatric nurse in providing targeted family-centred care. These include

- Monitoring patient and family for indicators of stress
- Teaching stress management techniques
- Counselling family members on coping skills for their own use
- Providing necessary knowledge of options and support services
- Facilitating family routines and rituals
- Assisting family to resolve feelings of guilt
- Assisting family with conflict resolution
- Identifying family strengths and resources with family members
- Facilitating communication among family members

Group Therapy

The role of group therapy in treating depression is based on clinical experience rather than on systematic, controlled studies. It may be particularly useful for depression associated with bereavement or chronic medical illness. Individuals may benefit from the example of others who have dealt successfully with similar losses or challenges. Survivors can gain self-esteem as successful role models for new group members. Medication support groups can provide information to the patient and to family members regarding prognosis and medication issues, thereby providing a psychoeducational forum.

Teaching Patients and Families

Patients with depression and their significant others often incorrectly believe that their illness is their own fault and that they should be able to "pull themselves up by their bootstraps" or "snap out of it." It is vital to educate patients and their families about the nature, prognosis, and treatment of depression to dispel these false beliefs and the unnecessary guilt that ensues.

BOX 22-4 Psychoeducation Checklist: Major Depressive Disorder

When caring for the patient with a major depressive disorder, be sure to include the following topic areas in the teaching plan:

- Psychoeducation about the nature of depression
- Psychopharmacologic agents, including drug action, dosing frequency, and possible adverse effects
- Risk factors for recurrence, signs of recurrence
- Adherence to therapy and treatment programme
- Nutrition
- Sleep measures
- Self-care management
- Goal setting and problem solving
- Social interaction skills
- Follow-up appointments
- Community support services

Patients need to know the full range of suitable treatment options before consenting to participate in treatment. The nurse can provide opportunities for them to question, discuss, and explore their feelings about past, current, and planned use of medications and other treatments (CNA, 2005). Developing strategies to enhance adherence and to raise awareness of early signs of relapse can be important aids to making treatment more effective. See Box 22-4 for a checklist of important topics to discuss with patients who have a major depressive disorder.

Social Domain

Assessment

Social assessment focuses on patients' developmental history, family psychiatric history, patterns of relationship, education and work history, the quality of their support system, and the impact of physical or sexual abuse on their interpersonal functioning (see Chapter 10). Including a family member or close friend in the assessment process can be helpful. Changes in patterns of relating (especially social withdrawal) and changes in level of occupational functioning are commonly reported and may represent a significant deterioration from baseline behaviour. Increased use of "sick days" may occur. The family's level of support and understanding of the disorder also need to be assessed.

Nursing Diagnoses for Social Domain

Nursing diagnoses common for the social domain include Compromised Family Coping, Ineffective Role Performance, Interrupted Family Processes, and Caregiver Role Strain (if the patient is also a caregiver).

Interventions for Social Domain

Individuals experiencing depression often withdraw from daily activities such as engaging in family routines, attending work, and participating in community events. During hospitalization, patients often withdraw to their rooms and refuse to participate in unit activities. Nurses are challenged to help the patient balance the need for privacy with the need to return to normal social functioning. Depressed patients should never be approached in an overly enthusiastic manner; this approach will irritate them and block communication. On the other hand, patients should be encouraged to set realistic goals to reconnect with family and community. Explaining to patients the importance of attending social activities, however much they may not feel like doing so, will promote the recovery process.

Milieu Therapy

While hospitalized, milieu therapy (see Chapter 11) helps depressed patients maintain socialization skills and continue to interact with others. When depressed, people are often unaware of their environment and withdraw into themselves. On a psychiatric unit, depressed patients should be encouraged to attend and participate in unit activities. These individuals have a decreased energy level and thus may be moving more slowly than others; however, their efforts should be acknowledged.

Safety

In many cases, patients are admitted to the psychiatric hospital because of a suicide attempt. Suicidality should continually be evaluated, and the patient should be protected from self-harm (see Chapter 19). During the depths of depression, patients may not have the energy to complete a suicide, but as they begin to feel better, and as their energy increases, they may be at a greater risk. If a previously depressed patient appears to have become energized overnight, he or she may have made the decision to commit suicide and thus may be relieved that the decision is finally made. The nurse may misinterpret the mood improvement as a positive move towards recovery; however, this patient may be very intent on suicide. These individuals should be carefully monitored to maintain their safety.

Other Interventions

Nurses are exceptionally well positioned to engage patients and their families in the active process of improving daily functioning, increasing knowledge and skill acquisition, and increasing independent living. Consumer-oriented support groups can help to enhance the self-esteem and the support network of participating patients and their families. Advice, encouragement, and the sense of group camaraderie may make an important contribution to recovery (CNA, 2005). Organizations providing support and information include the CMHA, the Canadian Alliance on Mental Illness and Mental Health, the Mood Disorders Society of Canada, the Native Mental Health Association of Canada, and the Organization for Bipolar Affective Disorders.

Interventions for Family Members

The family needs education and support during and after the treatment of a depressed family member. Nurses should be attentive to family distress and caregiver burden and provide appropriate support and education. Because major depressive disorder is a recurring disorder, the family needs information about specific antecedents to a family member's depression and what steps to take. For example, one patient may routinely become depressed during the fall of each year, with one of the first symptoms being excessive sleepiness. For another patient, a major loss, such as a child going to college or the death of a pet, may precipitate a depressive episode. Families of older patients need to be aware of the possibility of depression and related symptoms, which may occur after the deaths of friends and relatives. Families of children who are depressed often misinterpret depression as behaviour problems.

Spiritual Domain

Understanding the relevance of spirituality in today's varied arenas of "pluralistic" health care can be daunting and even problematic, particularly given the varied interpretations of spirituality as a concept. Koenig (2009) adds clarity to this vital area by examining spirituality in terms of religion and religious practices. Through systematic review of multiple studies in this domain, concluding statements are put forward related to the importance of religious involvement as positive correlates to better coping and less depression and suicide. This underscores the need for health care providers to take into account the religious and spiritual activities of their patients and, further, to recognize the potential of spirituality as a mental health resource (Koenig, 2009).

Assessment

Spirituality involves thoughts and feelings that contribute meaning and purpose to one's existence (Schmidt & Mauk, 2004). When a person experiences depression, he or she may have despairing thoughts and express a lack of spiritual well-being. Spiritual assessment facilitates the implementation of holistic care (Massey, Gitchett, & Roberts, 2004). The intensely personal and intimate nature of this domain justifies a cautionary and tentative approach. Patients with mood disorders may feel especially guarded in discussing their spirituality, fearing that clinicians may belittle or "pathologize" their experience. In attending to the spiritual domain, Massey and colleagues (2004) propose a mixture of subjective and objective methods, endorsing a three-phase itemized and progressive process, which entails basic spiritual screening, spiritual history taking, and, if deemed advisable, an in-depth spiritual assessment.

Spiritual Screening

An initial screening is directed to determining basic needs related to a person's religious affiliation and/or his or her desire for additional spiritual attention. The topic can be broached by questions such as: Do you wish to identify a particular religion with which you are associated? Would you like to speak with a representative of that religion (e.g., minister, priest, chaplain, elder, imam, rabbi)? Queries posed tentatively and with sensitivity are more likely to have the desired effect of eliciting concerns, should they exist. This initial assessment gives an indication of whether spirituality is an organizing principle in the patient's life and whether further assessment is appropriate (Hodge, 2006).

Spiritual History Taking

Goals of spiritual history taking include identifying themes of the patient's spiritual concerns, recognizing the impact of those concerns on the patient's condition, establishing relevant care, and identifying appropriate referrals (Massey et al., 2004). One model of spiritual history taking is based on the HOPE acronym: "H—sources of hope, meaning, comfort, strength, peace, love, and connection; O—organized religion; P—personal spirituality and practice; E—effects on medical care and end of life issues" (Anandarajah & Hight, 2001).

Spiritual Assessment

The focus is directly on patients' understanding of spirituality and its importance in their lives. The intent is an in-depth exploration of their religious history and/or spiritual practice related to whether and how they might wish to have spiritual concerns included in their work of recovery (Fallot, 2007; Wong-McDonald, 2007). Within an interdisciplinary context, this multifaceted exploration may default to (or be done in consultation with) pastoral counsellors or clinicians deemed most proficient in addressing the spiritual dimension of a patient's experience.

Nursing Diagnoses for Spiritual Domain

Nursing diagnoses pertaining to the spiritual domain focus on distress of the spirit. Very often these are specified as situational. Within the realm of mood disorders, these are often expressed as disturbances in one's belief system related to the loss of hope, the meaning of life and suffering, and discouragement and despair.

Interventions for Spiritual Domain

Spiritual interventions can have positive outcomes for individuals suffering depression and other mood disorders. Where need presents, appropriate people can intervene with patients by way of guided conversations, personal life storytelling, and ritual experiences (Massey et al., 2004). Spiritual activities can be encouraged, including prayer, the reading of religious texts, meditation, attendance at devotional services or ceremonies, and so on. Such modalities of care may serve to relieve distress, make meaning of suffering, nurture hope, and promote spiritual resolution and wellness.

Evaluation and Treatment Outcomes

The major goals of treatment are to help the patient to be as independent as possible and to achieve stability, remission, and recovery from major depression. It is often a lifelong struggle for the individual. An ongoing evaluation of the patient's symptoms, functioning, and quality of life should be carefully documented in the patient's record in order to monitor treatment outcomes.

Continuum of Care

If the prevalence of major depressive disorders in Western countries continues to escalate, it is not unrealistic to speculate that demands for services will increasingly threaten the capacity for service delivery (Carta et al., 2012). Current demands indicate that care providers can expect to encounter individuals with depressive disorders in all areas of practice. Initially, they may present in inpatient and outpatient medical and primary care settings, emergency departments, and inpatient and outpatient mental health settings (see Chapter 4). This necessitates that nurses be able to recognize depression in these patients and make appropriate interventions or referrals. The continuum, however, goes beyond these settings and may include partial hospitalization or day treatment programmes; individual, family, or group psychotherapy;

home visits; and psychopharmacotherapy. Although most patients with major depression are treated in outpatient settings, brief hospitalization may be required if the patient is suicidal or psychotic.

Nurses working on inpatient units provide a wide range of direct services, including administering and monitoring medications and monitoring target symptoms, conducting psychoeducational groups, and, more generally, structuring and maintaining a therapeutic environment. Nurses providing home care can help individuals living with a mood disorder and their families to address the everyday challenges such an illness brings. Community nurses are well situated to detect undiagnosed depressive disorders and make appropriate referrals.

Nursing practice requires a coordinated, ongoing interaction among patients, families, and providers to deliver comprehensive services. This includes using the complementary skills of other disciplines for forming overall goals, plans, and decisions and for providing continuity of care as needed (CNA, 2005). Integrated multidisciplinary care aimed at holistic interventions is key to achieving the remission of symptoms and physical well-being, restoring baseline occupational and psychosocial functioning, and reducing the likelihood of relapse or recurrence (Fig. 22-1).

FIGURE 22-1. Holistic interventions for patients with major depressive disorder.

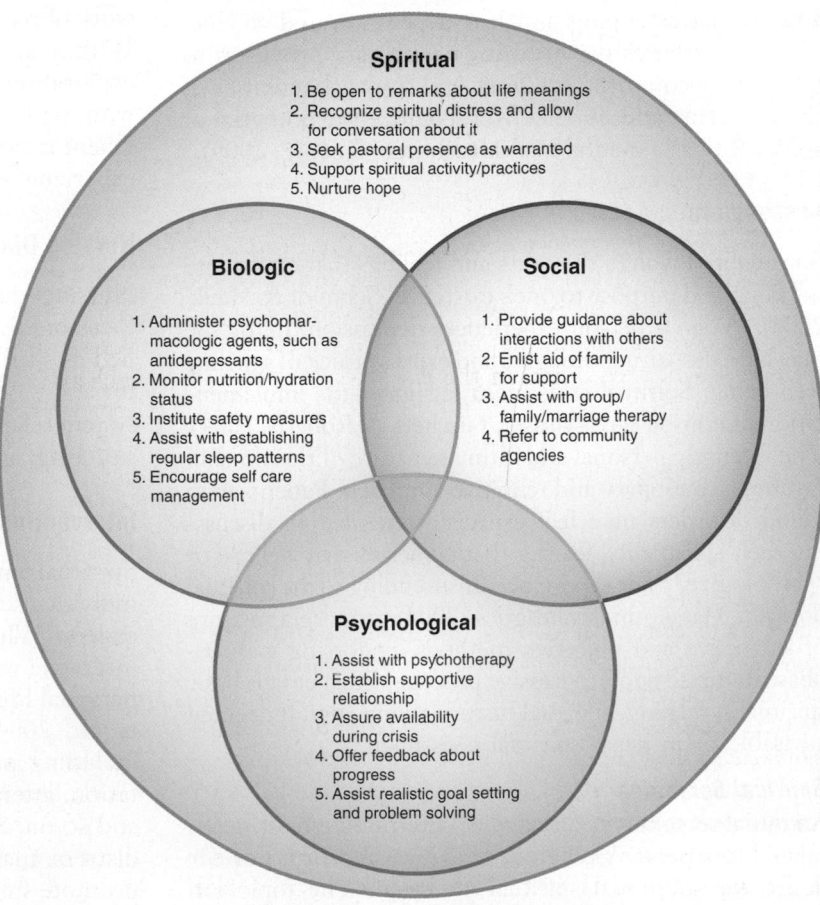

Spiritual
1. Be open to remarks about life meanings
2. Recognize spiritual distress and allow for conversation about it
3. Seek pastoral presence as warranted
4. Support spiritual activity/practices
5. Nurture hope

Biologic
1. Administer psychopharmacologic agents, such as antidepressants
2. Monitor nutrition/hydration status
3. Institute safety measures
4. Assist with establishing regular sleep patterns
5. Encourage self care management

Social
1. Provide guidance about interactions with others
2. Enlist aid of family for support
3. Assist with group/family/marriage therapy
4. Refer to community agencies

Psychological
1. Assist with psychotherapy
2. Establish supportive relationship
3. Assure availability during crisis
4. Offer feedback about progress
5. Assist realistic goal setting and problem solving

BIPOLAR DISORDERS (MANIC–DEPRESSIVE DISORDERS)

Diagnostic Criteria

Bipolar disorders are distinguished from depressive disorders by the occurrence of manic or hypomanic (i.e., mildly manic) episodes in addition to depressive episodes. The *DSM-5* divides bipolar disorders into bipolar I (characterized by one or more manic episodes generally with a major depressive occurrence), bipolar II (periods of major depression accompanied by at least one incidence of hypomania), and **cyclothymic disorder** (periods of hypomanic episodes and depressive episodes that do not meet full criteria for an MDE) (Table 22-5).

A **manic episode** is characterized by **euphoria**, a state of elation experienced as a heightened sense of well-being. During a manic episode, the individual may manifest an **expansive mood**, in which he or she shows an inappropriate lack of restraint in expressing feelings and frequently overvalues his or her own importance. Expansive qualities include an unceasing and indiscriminate enthusiasm for interpersonal, sexual, or occupational interactions. Manic episodes can also consist of irritable mood, in which the person is easily annoyed and provoked to anger, particularly when the person's wishes are challenged or thwarted. In addition, manic episodes can consist of alterations between euphoria and irritability (**lability of mood**). Other symptoms can include inflated self-esteem or grandiosity, decreased need for sleep, being more talkative or having pressured speech, flight of ideas or racing thoughts, distractibility, decrease in goal-directed activity or psychomotor agitation, and excessive involvement in pleasurable activities that have a high potential for painful consequences (Akiskal, 2009b, p. 1703). *DSM-5* criteria indicate that the disturbance must be severe enough to cause marked impairment in social activities, occupational functioning, and interpersonal relationships (APA, 2013). It is pertinent to note that decreased inhibition, impulsivity, and distractibility negatively affect cognition in the areas of *attention* and *concentration* and alter the individual's ability to learn and effectively solve problems (Osuji & Cullum 2005). Consequently, hospitalization may be required to prevent self-harm.

During a manic episode, patients experience an increase in energy that can be described as hyperactivity, and they tend to require less sleep to feel rested. The individual often remains awake for long periods at night or wakes up several times a night, full of energy. Increased motor activity and agitation, which may be purposeful at first (e.g., cleaning the house), may deteriorate into inappropriate or disorganized actions. The individual may get involved unrealistically in several new endeavours, such as a spree of overspending, or in reckless sexual encounters, drug or alcohol use, or other high-risk activities such as driving too fast or taking up dangerous sports (see Box 22-5). The individual becomes overly talkative, feels pressured to continue talking, and at times is difficult to interrupt. Thoughts become disorganized and may skip rapidly among seemingly unrelated topics. This decreased logical connection between thoughts is termed *flight of ideas*. Patients with mania have inflated self-esteem, which may range from unusual self-confidence to grandiose delusions. Other psychiatric disorders can have symptoms that resemble a manic episode. Borderline personality disorder and substance abuse involving stimulants should be ruled out when assessing for mania.

The criteria describing a **hypomanic episode** are the same as those detailed in a manic episode, excepting for a more extended duration of time noted in the expression of symptoms during the latter. As well, in hypomania, there is generally no marked impairment in social or occupational functioning. Moreover, should there be fluctuations in the way the client presents throughout the duration of an acute illness episode, for example, demonstrating high anxiety, agitation, and irritability alternating with the occurrence of depressive symptoms, the patient may be described as having **mixed features**. Such presentations can occur when the criteria for a manic or hypomanic episode are present. Mixed symptoms can also be associated with an MDE. If an individual presents with symptoms that meet full episode criteria for both mania and depression simultaneously, the diagnosis would rightfully be "manic episode, with mixed features" (*DSM-5*, APA, 2013, p. 150).

> **KEY CONCEPT** Central features of **mania** include overactivity, elevated or irritable mood, and grandiose ideas of self-importance (Cowen et al., 2012).

Secondary Mania

Mania can be caused by underlying medical disorders such as certain metabolic abnormalities, neurologic disorders, CNS tumours, and particular medications. Further, mania can be precipitated by some medical treatments, steroid therapy of particular note. As well, mania can be induced by certain substances of abuse (APA, 2013). This range of precipitants might be particularly offensive to older persons and should be suspected with those who present with no prior history of manic symptoms (Hoblyn, 2004).

Clinical Course

Bipolar disorder is a chronic, cyclic disorder (Duffy, Alda, Hajek, Sherry, & Grof, 2010).

With mixed states of mania, extreme turmoil can occur with possible suicidal ideation presenting especially high risk. Bipolar disorders can lead to severe functional

Table 22-5	Key Diagnostic Characteristics of Bipolar I Disorder

Diagnostic Criteria and Target Symptoms

- Presence of one or more manic episodes or mixed episodes, including one or more MDEs

Manic episode
- Abnormally and persistently elevated, expansive, or irritable mood for at least 1 wk
- Persistence of inflated self-esteem and grandiosity
- Decreased need for sleep
- More talkative than usual or pressure to keep talking
- Flight of ideas and subjective experience of racing thoughts
- Distractibility
- Increase in goal-directed activity or psychomotor agitation
- Excessive involvement in pleasurable activities with high potential for painful results (e.g., unrestrained buying sprees, foolish business investments)
- Sexual indiscretions
- Marked impairment in occupational functioning or in usual social activities or relationships; possible hospitalization to prevent harm; psychotic features

MDE (symptoms appear nearly every day)
- Depressed mood most of the day
- Markedly diminished interest or pleasure in all or most all activities for most of the day
- Significant weight loss when not dieting; weight gain or an increase or a decrease in appetite
- Insomnia or hypersomnia
- Psychomotor agitation or retardation
- Fatigue or loss of energy
- Feelings of worthlessness or excessive or inappropriate guilt
- Diminished ability to concentrate or indecisiveness
- Recurrent thoughts of death, suicidal ideation without a specific plan, suicide attempt or specific plan for committing suicide
- Not bereavement
- Clinically significant distress or impairment in social, occupational, or other important areas of functioning

Mixed episode
- Criteria for both manic and MDEs nearly every day for at least 1 wk
- Hospitalization to prevent harm; psychotic features
- Symptoms are observable by others

Hypomanic episode
- Distinct period of persistently elevated, expansive, or irritable mood for 4 consecutive days and present most of the day every day
- Clearly different from usual nondepressed mood
- Same symptoms as that for manic episode but does not cause impairment in social or occupational functioning or necessitate hospitalization
- Unequivocal change in function, uncharacteristic of person when asymptomatic
- Change observable by others
- Not severe enough to cause marked impairment in social or occupational functioning or to require hospitalization; no psychotic features
- Episode not better accounted for by other disorders such as schizoaffective disorder and not superimposed on schizophrenia, schizophreniform, delusional, or psychotic disorders
- Not a direct physiologic effect of substance or other medical condition

Associated Findings

Associated Behaviour Findings
Manic episode
- Resistive to efforts for treatment
- Disorganized or bizarre behaviour
- Change in dress or appearance
- Possible gambling and antisocial behaviour

MDE
- Tearfulness, irritability
- Obsessive rumination
- Anxiety
- Phobia
- Excessive worry over physical symptoms
- Complaints of pain
- Possible panic attacks
- Difficulty with intimate relationships
- Marital, occupational, or academic problems
- Substance abuse
- Increased use of medical services
- Attempted or complete suicide attempts

Mixed episode
- Similar to those for manic and depressive episodes

Hypomanic episodes
- Sudden onset with rapid escalation within 1–2 d
- Possibly precede or are followed by MDE

American Psychiatric Association. (2013). *Diagnostic and Statistical Manual of Mental Disorders* (5th ed.). Washington, DC: Author.

impairments, resulting in job losses and financial duress and culminating in alienation from family, friends, and coworkers.

Epidemiology

Distribution and Age of Onset

In Canada, the estimated 1-year prevalence for bipolar disorder (i.e., the estimated percentage of the population who have the disorder during any 1-year period) is between 0.2% and 0.6% among adults in the general population (Akiskal, 2009b; Health Canada, 2002). The estimated mean age of onset is between 21 and 30 years. The mode of onset can be variable, manifesting as a mild retarded depression or excessive sleeping for a few weeks or months that then changes abruptly to mania. Onset for others may present as an overtly psychotic episode. In this group, only when a clear manic episode is evident, does the depressive nature of the problem become apparent. Onset for another group is characterized by several depressive episodes preceding the first manic occurrence (Akiskal, 2009b).

Bipolar disorder in children is increasingly recognized as a presentation distinct from attention deficit hyperactivity disorder (ADHD). Research by Duffy and colleagues (2010) does show some intergenerational correlates between the incidence in one (or both) parents and the symptomatic manifestation of bipolar disorder in their children. Depression is more often recognized as the initial presentation in children, though the hallmark of childhood bipolar disorder not uncommonly demonstrates as intense rage. Indeed, children may display seemingly unprovoked rage episodes for as long as 2 to 3 hours. The symptoms of bipolar disorder reflect the developmental level of the child. Whereas children younger than 9 years exhibit more irritability and emotional lability, older children exhibit more classic symptoms, such as euphoria and grandiosity. The first contact with the mental health system often occurs when the behaviour becomes disruptive,

possibly 5 to 10 years after its onset. These children often have other psychiatric disorders such as ADHD and conduct disorder (Kowatch & DelBello, 2005).

Neurophysiologically, geriatric patients with mania demonstrate more abnormalities and cognitive disturbances (confusion and disorientation) than do younger patients. It generally was believed that the incidence of mania decreases with age because this population was thought to consist of only those individuals who had a diagnosis in younger years and managed to survive into old age. Recently, late-onset bipolar disorder was identified when researchers found evidence of an increased incidence of mania with age, especially in women older than 50 years and in men in their eighth and ninth decades. Late-onset bipolar disorder is more likely related to secondary mania (Hoblyn, 2004).

Gender, Ethnic, and Cultural Differences

Although no significant gender differences have been found in the lifetime prevalence of bipolar I disorder, the incidence of bipolar II disorder is reportedly 5% greater in females than males (Barnes & Mitchell, 2005). In addition, some data indicate that female patients with bipolar disorder are at greater risk for depression whereas male patients are prone to manic episodes (Corcoran & Walsh, 2009b).

While prevalence rates in Canada are said to be unrelated to race, some literature posits immigration as one risk factor for mania (Azorin et al., 2008). This invites speculation on whether adversely afflicted persons, who are subject to mood-related disorders, are those more likely to migrate from their homeland in the first place, or whether it is the process of transitioning that creates situational circumstances that dispose new migrants to affective reactivity. Is it the sense of being remote from one's homeland, feeling situationally isolated in a land where language and local customs are experienced as "strange," and where perhaps employment prospects are elusive? It does underscore the need for study to identify contextual circumstances that may dispose to possible "immigration risk." As things stand, no significant differences in prevalence have been found based on race or ethnicity (CNA, 2005).

Comorbidity

Medical comorbidity in patients with bipolar disorder is a significant issue as it complicates diagnosis and management of the illness and may have a negative impact on patient outcomes (APA, 2013, p. 145–147; Yatham et al., 2006). Two common comorbid conditions are anxiety disorders (most prevalent: panic disorder and social phobia) and substance use (most commonly alcohol and marijuana). Individuals with a comorbid anxiety disorder are more likely to experience a more severe course and characterologic aberations can intensify the challenges and course of care. A history of substance use further complicates the course of illness and results in less chance for remission and poorer treatment compliance (Goldberg, Garno, Leon, Kocsis, & Portera, 1999).

Aetiology

Current theories of the aetiology of mood disorders are associated with chronic abnormalities of neurotransmission, which are thought to result in compensatory but maladaptive changes in brain regulation. In addition, the use of controlled structural and functional imaging studies of patients with mood disorders have generated hypotheses that CNS dysfunction is associated with specific structural brain abnormalities and functional CNS alterations (Sheline, 2003; Thase, 2009).

Chronobiologic Theories

Sleep disturbance is an important aspect of depression and mania. Sleep patterns appear to be regulated by an internal biologic clock centred in the hypothalamus (see Chapter 9). Artificially induced sleep deprivation is known to precipitate mania in some patients with bipolar disorder (Grunze, Amann, Dittmann, & Walden, 2002). A number of neurotransmitter and hormone levels follow circadian patterns; therefore, sleep disruption may lead to biochemical abnormalities that affect mood. Seasonal changes in light exposure can also trigger affective episodes in some patients (Akiskal, 2009a), typically depression in winter and hypomania in the summer in the northern hemisphere (Cutler & Marcus, 1999).

Sensitization and Kindling Theory

Sensitization (increase in response to a drug with repetition of the same dosage) and the related phenomenon of kindling (subthreshold stimulation of a neuron generates an action potential; see Chapter 12) refer to animal models. Repeated chemical or electrical stimulation of certain regions of the brain produces stereotypical behavioural responses or seizures. The amount of the chemical or electricity required to evoke the response or seizure decreases with each experience. These phenomena have been used as models to explain why, over time, affective episodes, particularly those seen in patients with bipolar disorder, recur in shorter and shorter cycles and with less relation to environmental precipitants. It is hypothesized that repeated affective episodes might be accompanied by the progressive alteration of brain synapses that lower the threshold for future episodes and increase the likelihood of illness. The kindling theory also helps explain the value of using antiseizure medication, such as carbamazepine and valproic acid, for mood stabilization.

Genetic Factors

The genetic basis for the development of bipolar disorder is increasingly being explored. Results from family, adoption, and twin studies indicate that bipolar disorder

suggests a familial pattern (McCuffin et al., 2003). Such results show a 1% incidence rate in the general population, compared with a 7% incidence rate for first-degree relatives of a patient with bipolar disorder, and 60% for a monozygotic twin of a bipolar patient (Payne, Potash, & DePaulo, 2005). Modes of genetic transmission and the cumulative effects of multiple genes interacting with environmental influences have yet to be definitively identified. Compelling longitudinal study (Duffy, 2012; Duffy et al., 2010) is being done in the area of genetic associations between parents with bipolar disorder and the risks this might pose to their offspring. As evidence mounts, an increase in our understanding as to the nature of possible neurodevelopmental correlates seems probable.

Serum TCA levels should be evaluated when overdose is suspected. In acute overdose, almost all symptoms develop within 12 hours. Anticholinergic effects are prominent: dry mucous membranes, warm and dry skin, blurred vision, a decreased bowel motility, and urinary retention. CNS suppression (ranging from drowsiness to coma) or an agitated delirium may occur. Basic overdose treatment includes induction of emesis, gastric lavage, and cardiorespiratory supportive care. The most common side effects of MAOIs are headache, drowsiness, dry mouth, constipation, blurred vision, and orthostatic hypotension.

Psychological and Social Theories

Bipolar disorder encompasses two extremes of a continuum; depression locates at one end and mania at the other. In regard to depression, most psychological and social theories of mood disorders focus on loss as its cause in genetically vulnerable individuals. Mania is considered to be a biologically rooted condition, but when viewed from a psychological perspective, it is usually regarded as a condition that arises from an attempt to overcompensate for depressed feelings rather than a disorder in its own right. It is now generally accepted that environmental conditions contribute to the timing of an episode of illness rather than cause the illness (Johnson, Andersson-Lundman, Aberg-Wistedt, & Mathe, 2000).

Interdisciplinary Treatment of Disorder

Patients with bipolar disorder struggle with the complexity of their illness and must be treated by an interdisciplinary team. Nurses, physicians, social workers, psychologists, and activity therapists all have valuable expertise for bipolar patients. For children with bipolar disorder, schoolteachers and counsellors are included in the team. For older adults, the primary care physician becomes part of the team. An important treatment goal is to minimize and prevent either manic or depressive episodes, which tend to accelerate over time. The fewer the episodes, the more likely the person can live a normal, productive life. Another important goal is to provide psychoeducation and support for the client and family about the disorder so to assist them in managing it.

Priority Care Issues

During a manic episode, protection of the patient is a priority. It is during a manic episode that poor judgement and impulsivity result in risk-taking behaviours that can have dire consequences for the patient and family. For example, the person suddenly begins excessively spending money, partying, and engages in promiscuous behaviour. During either a depressive or manic phase, the patient may feel that life is not worth living. As well, during a manic episode, the patient may believe that he or she has supernatural powers, such as the ability to fly, and then may act on them. As the patient recovers from a manic episode, he or she may be so devastated by the consequences of the impulsive behaviour and poor judgement that suicide is considered as a way to deal with their shame.

Family Response to Disorder

Bipolar disorder can devastate families, who often feel that they are on an emotional roller coaster if they have difficulty understanding the mood shifts. They can be burdened by their family member's problematic behaviours (e.g., impulsive behaviour during manic episodes, such as excessive debt, assault charges, and sexual infidelities) and the disruption of household routine (Perlick et al., 2007). It is pertinent to note, however, that families do report developing coping strategies that allow them to address these issues (Goossens, van Wijngaarden, Knoppert-van der Klein, & van Achterberg, 2008).

Nursing Management: Human Response to Bipolar Disorder

The nursing care of patients with bipolar disorder can be one of the greatest challenges in psychiatric nursing. In general, the behaviour of patients with bipolar disorder is often symptom free between episodes. Nursing care of a client experiencing bipolar disorder should be approached in a multifaceted and compassionate manner during periods of acute illness and during states of remission.

Biologic Domain

Assessment

In regard to the biologic domain, the assessment emphasis is on evaluating symptoms of mania and, most particularly, changes in sleep patterns. In the manic phase of bipolar disorder, the patient may not sleep, resulting in irritability and physical exhaustion. Eating habits usually change during a manic or depressive episode, and the nurse should therefore assess changes in diet and body weight. Patients with mania may experience malnutrition

and fluid imbalance. The nurse must monitor laboratory studies, such as electrolytes and thyroid functioning. Abnormal thyroid function can be responsible for the mood and behavioural disturbances. Excessive use of alcohol and other substances may also occur, and therefore, the individual must also be assessed for these behaviours. Special attention should focus on the use of alcohol and other substances. Usually, a drug screen is ordered to determine current use of substances. A further concern during a manic phase is that patients often become hypersexual and engage in risky sexual practices. Changes in sexual practices should be explored.

Pharmacologic Assessment

When a patient is in a manic state, the previous use of antidepressants should be assessed as they can precipitate such an episode. In such cases, the use of antidepressants should be discontinued. Many times, manic or depressive episodes occur after patients 'stop taking their mood stabilizer, at which time the reason for stopping the medication should be explored. Patients may stop taking their medications because of side effects or because they no longer believe they have a mental disorder. As well, clients with known bipolar disorder who take antidepressants without attendant mood stabilizers could be at risk for a manic episode.

Nursing Diagnoses for Biologic Domain

Among nursing diagnoses in this domain are Disturbed Sleep Pattern, Sleep Deprivation, Imbalanced Nutrition, Hypothermia, Risk for Deficient Fluid Volume, and Noncompliance (related to treatment measures). If patients are in the depressive phase of illness, the previously discussed diagnoses for depression should be considered.

Interventions for Biologic Domain

Physical Care

In a state of mania, the patient's physical needs are rest, adequate hydration and nutrition, and reestablishment of physical well-being. Self-care has usually deteriorated. For a patient who is unable to sit long enough to eat, snacks and high-energy foods should be provided that can be eaten while moving. Alcohol should be avoided. Sleep hygiene is a priority but may not be realistic until medications take effect. Limiting stimuli can be helpful in decreasing agitation and promoting sleep.

> ● **STUDY NOTE**
> Ongoing assessment of patients with mania should focus on levels of irritability, fatigue, nutrition, impulsive behaviour, and the potential for impulsivity leading to harm of self or others.

Teaching Points

Once the patient's mood stabilizes, the nurse should focus on monitoring changes in physical functioning in sleep or eating behaviour and teaching patients to identify antecedents to mood episodes. A regular sleep routine should be maintained if possible. High-risk times for manic episodes, such as changes in work schedule (day to night), should be avoided if possible. Patients should be taught to monitor the amount of their sleep each night and report a pattern of decreased sleep and sleeplessness as this may indicate a shift towards a manic episode.

Intervention With Mood Stabilizers

Pharmacotherapy is essential in treating bipolar disorder to achieve two goals: the rapid control of symptoms and the prevention of future episodes—or, at least, reduction in their severity and frequency. Pharmacotherapy continues through the various phases of bipolar disorder:

- *Acute phase.* The goal of treatment in the acute phase is symptom reduction and stabilization. Therefore, for the first few weeks of treatment, mood stabilizers may need to be combined with antipsychotics or benzodiazepines, particularly if the patient has psychotic symptoms, agitation, or insomnia. If the clinical situation is not an emergency, patients usually start on a low dose and gradually increase the dose until maximum therapeutic benefits are achieved. Once stabilization is achieved, the frequency of serum level monitoring should be every 1 to 2 weeks during the first 2 months and every 3 to 6 months during long-term maintenance. Medications most commonly used for mood stabilization in bipolar disorder are listed in Table 22-6 (also see Chapter 12).

- *Continuation phase.* The treatment goal in this phase is to prevent relapse of the current episode or cycling into the opposite pole. It lasts about 2 to 9 months after acute symptoms resolve. The usual pharmacologic procedure in this phase is to continue the mood stabilizer while closely monitoring the patient for signs or symptoms of relapse.

- *Maintenance phase.* The goal of treating this phase is to sustain remission and to prevent new episodes. The great weight of evidence favours long-term prophylaxis against recurrence after the effective treatment of acute episodes. It is recommended that long-term or lifetime prophylaxis with a mood stabilizer be instituted after two manic episodes or one severe manic episode or if there is a family history of bipolar disorder.

- *Discontinuation of medication use.* Like the course of major depressive disorder, the course of bipolar disorder typically is recurrent and progressive. Therefore, the same issues and principles regarding the decision to continue or discontinue pharmacotherapy apply.

The mainstays of somatic therapy are the mood-stabilizing drugs. The agents that show significant efficacy are lithium carbonate (Lithium), divalproex sodium (Depakote), carbamazepine (Tegretol), and the atypical antipsychotic olanzapine (Zyprexa). In treating mania, Lamotrigine (Lamictal) has efficacy both as a single agent and in combination with lithium or valproate (Bowden et al., 2003). Observations suggest that it may be particularly effective for rapid cycling and in the depressed phase of bipolar illness. Anecdotal evidence suggests that gabapentin (Neurontin) may be effective for acute mania, mood stabilization, and rapid cycling. Topiramate (Topamax) has been used mostly as add-on therapy in mixed patient samples with refractory mood disorders. A characteristic of topiramate is that it is more associated with weight loss than weight gain. Controlled trials are needed to evaluate further the efficacy of these and other anticonvulsants (Schatzberg et al., 2003).

Lithium Carbonate Lithium is the most widely used mood stabilizer (see Box 22-6). Combined response rates from five studies demonstrated that 70% of patients experienced at least partial improvement with lithium therapy. However, for most patients, lithium is not a fully adequate treatment for all phases of

Table 22-6 ▼ Mood Stabilizing Medications		
Generic (Trade) Drug Name	**Usual Dosage Range (Daily)**	**Half-Life (Hours)**
Lithium (Eskalith, Lithane)	600–1,800 mg	17–36
Divalproex sodium (Depakote)	15–60 mg/kg	6–16
Carbamazepine (Tegretol)	200–1,200 mg	25–65
Olanzapine (Zyprexa)	5–20 mg	21–54
Risperidone (Risperdal)	1–6 mg	20
Lamotrigine (Lamictal/Lamictin)	Monotherapy for Bipolar disorder 100–200 mg Adjunctive treatment for bipolar disorder 100 mg/day in combination with valproate; 400 mg/day in combination with enzyme inducing antiepileptic drugs such as carbamazepine	Approximately 33 (without concomitant treatments)

BOX 22-6   Drug Profile

LITHIUM (ESKALITH)

Drug Class: Mood stabilizer

Receptor Affinity: Alters sodium transport in nerve and muscle cells, increases norepinephrine uptake and serotonin receptor sensitivity, slightly increases intraneuronal stores of catecholamines, delays some second messenger systems. Mechanism of action is unknown.

Indications: Treatment and prevention of manic episodes in bipolar affective disorder. Used successfully in a number of unlabelled uses such as prophylaxis of cluster headaches, bulimia, etc.

Routes and Dosage: 150-, 300-, and 600-mg capsules. Lithobid, 300-mg slow-release tablets; Eskalith CR, 450-mg controlled-release tablets. Lithium citrate, 300 mg/5 mL liquid form.

Adult: In acute mania, optimal response is usually 600 mg tid or 900 mg bid. Obtain serum levels twice weekly in acute phase. Maintenance: Use lowest possible dose to alleviate symptoms and maintain serum level of 0.6 to 1.2 mEq/L. In uncomplicated maintenance, obtain serum levels every 2 to 3 months. Do not rely on serum levels alone. Monitor patient side effects.

Geriatric: An increased risk for toxic effects, use lower doses, monitor frequently.

Children: Safety and efficacy in children younger than 12 years has not been established.

Half-Life (Peak Effect): Mean, 24 hours (peak serum levels in 1 to 4 hours). Steady state reached in 5 to 7 days.

Select Adverse Reactions: Weight gain. A common side effect of lithium is hand tremors and dosage needs to be monitored.

Warning: Avoid use during pregnancy or while breast-feeding. Hepatic or renal impairments increase plasma concentration.

There is a fine line between therapeutic levels and toxicity levels. Mindfulness is required in use of lithium as a treatment agent.

Specific Patient/Family Education:
- Avoid alcohol or other CNS depressant drugs.
- Notify the prescriber if pregnancy is possible or planned. Do not breast-feed while taking this medication.
- Notify the prescriber before taking any other prescription, OTC medication, or herbal supplements.
- May impair judgement, thinking, or motor skills; avoid driving or other hazardous tasks.
- Do not abruptly discontinue use.

---

the illness, and particularly during the acute phase, supplemental use of antipsychotics such as olanzapine (Zyprexa) is often beneficial. Because of its significant side-effect burden (Table 22-7), lithium is poorly tolerated in at least one-third of treated patients and has the narrowest gap between therapeutic and toxic concentrations of any routinely prescribed psychotropic agent (Belmaker & Yaroslavsky, 2000). Predictors of poor response to lithium in acute mania include a history of poor response, rapid cycling, dysphoric symptoms, mixed symptoms of depression and mania, psychiatric comorbidity, and medical comorbidity (Alda & Grof, 2000).

Lithium is a salt, and the interaction between lithium levels and sodium levels in the body and the relationship between lithium levels and fluid volume in the body remain crucial issues in its safe, effective use. The higher the sodium levels are in the body, the lower the lithium level will be and vice versa. Thus, changes in dietary sodium intake can affect lithium blood levels that, in turn, may affect therapeutic results or increase the incidence of side effects. The same applies to fluid volume. If body fluid decreases significantly because of a hot climate, strenuous exercise, vomiting, diarrhoea, or drastic reduction in fluid intake, then lithium levels can rise sharply, causing an increase in side effects, progressing to lethal lithium toxicity. See Table 22-8 for lithium interactions with medications and other substances.

● **STUDY NOTE**

STUDY NOTE

Reviewing blood levels of lithium carbonate and divalproex sodium are ongoing nursing assessments for patients receiving these medications. Side effects of mood stabilizers vary.

EMERGENCY !

If symptoms of moderate or severe toxicity (e.g., cardiac arrhythmias, blackouts, tremors, seizures) are noted, withhold additional doses of lithium, immediately obtain a blood sample to analyze the lithium level, and push fluids if the patient can take fluids. Contact the physician for further direction about relieving the symptoms. Mild side effects tend to subside or can be managed by nursing measures (see Table 22-9).

Divalproex Sodium Divalproex sodium (Depakote), an anticonvulsant, has a broader spectrum of efficacy and has about equal benefit for patients with pure mania as for those with other forms of bipolar disorder (e.g., mixed mania, rapid cycling, comorbid substance abuse, secondary mania). Moreover, in one large placebo-controlled study, patients taking divalproex sodium experienced a longer period of stable mood than did patients taking lithium or placebo (Bowden et al., 2000). Whereas divalproex is usually initiated at 250 mg twice a day or

Table 22-7	Lithium Blood Levels and Associated Side Effects

Plasma Level	Side Effects or Symptoms of Toxicity
<1.5 mEq/L Mild side effects	Metallic taste in the mouth
	Fine hand tremor (resting)
	Nausea
	Polyuria
	Polydipsia
	Diarrhoea or loose stools
	Muscular weakness or fatigue
	Weight gain
	Oedema
	Memory impairments
1.5–2.5 mEq/L Moderate toxicity	Severe diarrhoea
	Dry mouth
	Nausea and vomiting
	Mild to moderate ataxia
	Incoordination
	Dizziness, sluggishness, giddiness, vertigo
	Slurred speech
	Tinnitus
	Blurred vision
	Increasing tremor
	Muscle irritability or twitching
	Asymmetric deep tendon reflexes
	Increased muscle tone
>2.5 mEq/L Severe toxicity	Cardiac arrhythmias
	Blackouts
	Nystagmus
	Coarse tremor
	Fasciculations
	Visual or tactile hallucinations
	Oliguria, renal failure
	Peripheral vascular collapse
	Confusion
	Seizures
	Coma and death

lower, in the inpatient setting, it can be initiated in an oral loading dose using 20 to 30 mg/kg body weight (see Box 22-7). This may speed the reduction of manic symptoms and diminish the need for antipsychotics early in the course of therapy (Hirschfeld, Baker, Wozniak, Tracy, & Sommerville, 2003).

Baseline liver function tests and a complete blood count with platelets should be obtained before starting therapy, and patients with known liver disease should not be given divalproex sodium. Optimal blood levels appear to be in the range of 50 to 150 ng/mL. Levels may be obtained weekly until the patient is stable and then every 6 months. Divalproex sodium is associated with increased risk for birth defects. Cases of life-threatening pancreatitis have been reported in adults and children receiving valproate, either initially or after several years of use. Some cases were described as hemorrhagic, with a rapid progression from onset to death. If pancreatitis is diagnosed, valproate use should be discontinued.

Carbamazepine Carbamazepine, an anticonvulsant, also has mood-stabilizing effects. Data from various studies suggest that it may be effective in patients who are unresponsive to lithium. The most common side effects of carbamazepine are dizziness, drowsiness, nausea, and vomiting, which may be avoided with slow incremental dosing. Carbamazepine has both benign and severe hematologic toxicities. Frequent clinically unimportant decreases in white blood cell counts occur. Estimates of the rate of severe blood dyscrasias vary from 1 in 10,000 patients treated to a more recent estimate of 1 in 125,000 (Schatzberg et al., 2003). Mild, nonprogressive elevations of liver function test results are relatively common. Carbamazepine is associated with increased risk for birth defects.

In patients older than 12 years, carbamazepine is begun at 200 mg once or twice a day. The dosage is increased by no more than 200 mg every 2 to 4 days, to 800 to 1,000 mg a day, or until therapeutic levels or effects are achieved. It is important to monitor for blood dyscrasias and liver damage. Liver function tests and complete blood counts with differential are minimal pretreatment laboratory tests and should be repeated about 1 month after initiating treatment, and at 3 months, 6 months, and yearly. Other yearly tests should include electrolytes, blood urea nitrogen, thyroid function tests, urinalysis, and eye examinations. Carbamazepine levels are measured monthly until the patient is on a stable dosage. See Table 22-10 for carbamazepine's interactions with other drugs.

EMERGENCY !

Both valproate and carbamazepine may be lethal if high doses are ingested. Toxic symptoms appear in 1 to 3 hours and include neuromuscular disturbances, dizziness, stupor, agitation, disorientation, nystagmus, urinary retention, nausea and vomiting, tachycardia, hypotension or hypertension, cardiovascular shock, coma, and respiratory depression.

Newer Anticonvulsants In small clinical trials, case reports, and anecdotal evidence, newer anticonvulsants also show promise as mood stabilizers (Yatham et al., 2006). Oxcarbazepine is a more recent pharmacologic agent being used in treating acute mania and showing a degree of efficacy, but conclusive evidence as to its usefulness is lacking (Popova, Leighton, & Bernabarre, 2007). Likewise, agents such as levetiracetam, lamotrigine, and retigabine are recognized current medicinal treatments, but these too are said to require additional study to affirm full-scope treatment conclusions (Grunze, 2010). As large studies continue, a broadening range of atypical pharmacologic treatment agents (beyond the standard medications, e.g., lithium) are being brought to the fore of clinical practice.

Table 22-8 Lithium Interactions With Medications and Other Substances

Substance	Effect of Interaction
Angiotensin-converting enzyme inhibitors, such as: • Captopril • Lisinopril • Quinapril	Increases serum lithium; may cause toxicity and impaired kidney function
Acetazolamide	Increases the renal excretion of lithium, decreases lithium levels
Alcohol	May increase serum lithium level
Caffeine	Increases lithium excretion, increases lithium tremor
Carbamazepine	Increases neurotoxicity, despite normal serum levels and dosage
Fluoxetine	Increases serum lithium levels
Haloperidol	Increases neurotoxicity, despite normal serum levels and dosage
Loop diuretics, such as furosemide	Increases lithium serum levels but may be safer than thiazide diuretics; potassium-sparing diuretics (amiloride, spironolactone) are safest
Methyldopa	Increases neurotoxicity without increasing serum lithium levels
Nonsteroidal anti-inflammatory drugs, such as: • Diclofenac • Ibuprofen • Indomethacin • Piroxicam	Decreases renal clearance of lithium Increases serum lithium levels by 30%–60% in 3–10 d Aspirin and sulindac do not appear to have the same effect
Osmotic diuretics, such as: • Urea • Mannitol • Isosorbide	Increases renal excretion of lithium and decreases lithium levels
Sodium chloride	High sodium intake decreases lithium levels; low-sodium diets may increase lithium levels and lead to toxicity Caution warranted re salt intake
Thiazide diuretics, such as: • Chlorothiazide • Hydrochlorothiazide	Promotes sodium and potassium excretion; increases lithium serum levels; may produce cardiotoxicity and neurotoxicity
TCAs	Increases tremor; potentiates pharmacologic effects of TCAs

Table 22-9 Interventions for Lithium Side Effects

Side Effect	Intervention
Oedema of the feet or hands	Monitor intake and output, check for possible decreased urinary output Monitor sodium intake The patient should elevate the legs when sitting or lying Monitor weight
Fine hand tremor	Provide support and reassurance if it does not interfere with daily activities Tremor worsens with anxiety and intentional movements; minimize stressors Notify the prescriber if it interferes with the patient's work and compliance will be an issue More frequent smaller doses of lithium may also help
Mild diarrhoea	Take lithium with meals Provide for fluid replacement Notify the prescriber if becomes severe; may need a change in medication preparation or may be early sign of toxicity
Muscle weakness, fatigue, or memory and concentration difficulties	Provide support and reassurance; this side effect will usually pass after a few weeks of treatment Short-term memory aids such as lists or reminder calls may be helpful Notify the prescriber if becomes severe or interferes with the patient's desire to continue treatment
Metallic taste	Suggest sugarless candies or throat lozenges Encourage frequent oral hygiene
Nausea or abdominal discomfort	Consider dividing the medication into smaller doses or give it at more frequent intervals Give medication with meals
Polydipsia	Reassure the patient that this is a normal mechanism to cope with polyuria
Polyuria	Monitor intake and output Provide reassurance and explain nature of side effect Also explain that this causes no physical damage to the kidneys Withhold medication
Toxicity	Notify the prescriber Use symptomatic treatments

BOX 22-7   Drug Profile

DIVALPROEX SODIUM (DEPAKOTE)

Drug Class: Antimanic agent

Receptor Affinity: Thought to increase the level of inhibitory neurotransmitter, GABA, to brain neurons. Mechanism of action is unknown.

Indications: Treatment of bipolar disorders.

Routes and Dosage: Available in 125-mg delayed-release capsules and 125-, 250-, and 500-mg enteric-coated tablets.

Adult Dosage: Dosage depends on symptoms and clinical picture presented; initially the dosage is low and is gradually increased depending on the clinical presentation.

Half-Life (Peak Effect): 6 to 16 hours (1 to 4 hours)

Select Adverse Reactions: Sedation, tremor (may be dose related), nausea, vomiting, indigestion, abdominal cramps, anorexia with weight loss, slight elevations in liver enzymes, hepatic failure, thrombocytopaenia, transient increases in hair loss.

Warning: Contraindicated during pregnancy due to potential impact on foetus. Contraindicated in patients with hepatic disease or significant hepatic dysfunction. Administer cautiously with salicylates; may increase serum levels and result in toxicity.

Specific Patient/Family Education:
- Take with food if gastrointestinal upset occurs.
- Swallow tablets or capsules whole to prevent local irritation of the mouth and throat.
- Notify the prescriber before taking any other prescription or OTC medications or herbal supplements.
- Avoid alcohol and sleep-inducing or OTC products.
- Avoid driving or performing activities that require alertness.
- Do not abruptly discontinue use.
- Keep appointments for follow-up, including blood tests to monitor response.

Intervention With Antidepressants

Acute bipolar depression has received little scientific study in comparison with unipolar depression. Antidepressant drugs may cause either a switch to mania or a mixed state and may induce rapid cycling. Unfortunately, lithium or anticonvulsants are not as effective against depression as they are against mania. However, in a few patients, lithium or anticonvulsants can be used alone with good antidepressant effects. The most common treatment of bipolar depression is an antidepressant combined with a mood stabilizer to "protect" the patient against a manic switch. The antidepressant agents are the same as those used in unipolar illness, although they are sometimes given in lower dosages and for shorter periods of time as a precaution.

Administering and Monitoring Antipsychotic Medication

Antipsychotics are prescribed for patients who experience psychosis as a part of bipolar disorder. If patients cannot tolerate mood stabilizers, antipsychotics may be given instead of antidepressants to stabilize the moods. During acute mania, patients may not believe that they have a psychiatric disorder and refuse to take medication. Because their energy is still high, they can be very creative in avoiding medication. Once patients begin to take medications, symptom improvement should be evident. If a patient is very agitated, a benzodiazepine may be given for a short period. It is unlikely that patients will be taking only one medication; they may receive several. In some instances, one agent will be used to augment the effects of another, such as supplemental thyroid hormone to boost antidepressant response in depression (Young & Nemeroff, 2010, p. 29). Possible side effects for each medication should be listed and cross-referenced. When a side effect appears, the nurse should document the side effect and notify the prescriber so that further evaluation can be made. In some instances, medications should be changed. It is a well-established practice to combine mood stabilizers with antidepressants or antipsychotics. The previously discussed drug interactions should be considered when caring for a person with bipolar disorder. A big challenge is monitoring alcohol, drugs, OTC medications, and herbal supplements. A complete list of all medications should be maintained and evaluated for any potential interaction. (See Table 22-4 for specific drug interactions.)

Table 22-10   Selected Medication Interactions With Carbamazepine

Interaction	Drug Interacting With Carbamazepine
Increased carbamazepine levels	Erythromycin
	Cimetidine
	Propoxyphene
	Isoniazid
	Calcium channel blockers (verapamil)
	Fluoxetine
	Danazol
	Diltiazem
	Nicotinamide
Decreased carbamazepine levels	Phenobarbital
	Primidone
	Phenytoin
Drugs whose levels are decreased by carbamazepine	Oral contraceptives
	Warfarin, oral anticoagulants
	Doxycycline
	Theophylline
	Haloperidol
	Divalproex sodium
	TCAs
	Acetaminophen—increased metabolism but also increased risk for hepatotoxicity

Other Somatic Interventions: ECT

ECT may be cautiously administered to patients with severe mania who exhibit unremitting, frenzied physical activity. While ECT has the potential to intensify symptoms of mania, it has been indicated for mania that is unresponsive to antimanic agents and for patients who may be at high risk for suicide. ECT is effective treatment for patients receiving antipsychotic medications. The use of valproate or carbamazepine may require some adjustments in ECT treatment as these medications are anticonvulsant agents.

Teaching Points

For patients who are taking lithium, it is important to explain that a change in salt intake can affect the therapeutic blood level. If there is a reduction in salt intake, the body will naturally retain lithium to maintain homeostasis. This increase in lithium retention can lead to toxicity. Once stabilized on a lithium dose, salt intake should remain constant. This is fairly easy to do, except during the summer, when excessive perspiration can occur. Patients should increase salt intake during periods of perspiration, increased exercise, and dehydration. As most mood stabilizers and antidepressants can cause weight gain, patients should be alerted to this and should be instructed to monitor any changes in eating, appetite, or weight. Weight reduction techniques may need to be instituted. As always, patients should be clearly instructed to check with the nurse or physician before taking any OTC medication or herbal supplements.

Psychological Domain

Assessment

The assessment of the psychological domain should follow the process explained in Chapter 10. Individuals with bipolar disorder can usually participate in many parts of the assessment.

Mood

By definition, bipolar disorder is a disturbance of mood. If the patient is depressed, using an assessment tool for depression may help determine the severity of depression. If mania predominates, evaluating the quality of the mood (elated, grandiose, irritated, or agitated) becomes important. Usually, mania is determined by clinical observation.

Cognition

In a depressive episode, the individual may not be able to concentrate enough to complete cognitive tasks, such as those called for in the Mini-Mental State Exam. During the acute phase of a manic or depressive episode, mental status may be abnormal, and in a manic phase, judgement is impaired by extremely rapid, disjointed, and distorted thinking. Moreover, feelings such as grandiosity can interfere with normal executive functioning.

Thought Disturbances

Psychosis commonly occurs in patients with bipolar disorder, especially during acute episodes of mania. Auditory hallucinations and delusional thinking are part of the clinical picture. In children and adolescents, psychosis may not be so easily detected, due to possible differential disorders such as ADHD.

Stress and Coping Factors

Stress and coping are critical assessment areas for a person with bipolar disorder. A stressful event often triggers a manic or depressive episode. In some instances, there may be no apparent stress precipitating the episode, but it is important to discuss the possibility of a specific trigger. Determining the patient's usual coping skills for stresses lays the groundwork for developing interventional strategies. Negative coping skills, such as substance use or aggression, should be identified because these skills need to be replaced with more appropriate and functional coping.

Risk Assessment

Patients with bipolar disorder are at high risk for injury to self (Dubovsky, 2005) and others, with 10% to 15% of patients completing suicide. Child abuse, spouse abuse, or other violent behaviours may occur during severe manic episodes; thus, patients should be assessed for suicidal or homicidal risk (APA, 2000). The risk for relapse and poorer treatment outcomes are noted to have some correlation with obesity. Substantial evidence exists suggesting that bipolar disorder in and of itself is an independent risk factor for weight gain, diabetes mellitus, hypertension, dyslipidaemia, cardiovascular disease, and metabolic syndrome (Chennattucherry & Mok, 2010). How these medical problems, specifically rates of obesity, in bipolar disorder interact is difficult to determine due to confounding variables such as medication side effects and unhealthy lifestyle choices. Preventing and treating obesity in patients with bipolar disorder could decrease the morbidity and mortality related to physical illness, enhance psychological well-being, and possibly improve the course of the disorder (Chennattucherry & Mok, 2010).

Nursing Diagnoses for Psychological Domain

Nursing diagnoses associated with the psychological domain of bipolar disorder include Disturbed Sensory Perception, Disturbed Thought Processes, Defensive Coping, Risk for Suicide, Risk for Other-Directed Violence, Risk for Self-Directed Violence, and Ineffective Coping.

Interventions for Psychological Domain

Pharmacotherapy is the primary treatment for bipolar disorder, but psychotherapies and adjunctive therapy for bipolar disorder have notable benefits (Rush & Nierenberg, 2009). Family-focused therapy in particular has been shown to have primary benefit in preventing relapse. Other modalities such as interpersonal therapy and social rhythm therapy are also gaining credence as adjunct therapies in reducing relapses (Parikh & Velyvis, 2010). Integration of these therapies is fundamental to reducing depression and preventing possible relapses. Through early intervention, these therapies can be effective in promoting appropriate lifestyle management, improving medication adherence, and ultimately preempting intense symptom reoccurrence (Garland & Duffy, 2010).

In addition to obesity, the most notable of risk factors for illness reoccurrence are high rates of nonadherence to medication therapy, marital conflict, separation, divorce, unemployment, and underemployment. The goals of psychosocial interventions aim to address these risk factors and associated features, which are difficult to address with pharmacotherapy alone. Of particular importance to the intents of interventions in this domain are improving medication adherence, decreasing the number and length of hospitalizations and relapses, enhancing social and occupational functioning, improving quality of life, increasing the patient's and family's acceptance of the disorder, and reducing the suicide risk (Scott & Colom, 2005).

Psychoeducation

Psychoeducation is designed to provide information on bipolar disorder and successful treatment and recovery and usually focuses on medication adherence. Research suggests that individuals with bipolar disorder who adhere to their medication have fewer health problems and more life contentment (Darling, Olmstead, Lund, & Fairclough, 2008). The nurse can help by providing information about the illness and obstacles to recovery. Helping the patient to recognize warning signs and symptoms of relapse and to cope with residual symptoms and functional impairment are important interventions. Resistance to accepting the illness and to taking medication, the symbolic meaning of medication taking, and worries about the future can be discussed openly. In the interest of improved medication adherence, it is helpful to listen carefully to patients' concerns about the medication, its dosing schedules, any changes in dosage, and its side effects. Health teaching and weight management should be a component of any psychoeducation programme. In addition to individual variations in body weight, many of the medications (divalproex sodium, lithium, antidepressants, olanzapine) are associated with weight gain. Monitoring weight and developing individual weight management plans that include exercise can reduce the risk for relapse and increase the possibility of medication adherence. Nurses must be cognizant of the fact that poverty can negatively impact the patient's ability to maintain a healthy diet. Overall, the plan to support adherence should be made to fit the attitude, knowledge, and skills of the individual patient.

Psychotherapy

Long-term psychotherapy is an integral aspect of bipolar disorder treatment. Often treatment of the depression is overlooked due to a focus on medication adherence. In addition to addressing the depression, psychotherapy can temper the stressors that trigger episodes and increase the patient's acceptance of the need for medication. Patients should be encouraged to keep their appointments with the therapist, communicate their needs, and provide feedback on the efficacy of their treatment. Important qualitative support for the benefits of psychotherapy and medications is offered by Kay Redfield Jamison in her book *An Unquiet Mind* (1995).

Social Domain

Assessment

One of the tragedies of bipolar disorder is its effect on social and occupational functioning. Cultural views of mental illness profoundly influence the patient's acceptance of the disorder. During illness episodes, patients often behave in ways that jeopardize their social relationships. Losing a job or going through a divorce are common events. When performing an assessment of social function, the nurse should identify changes resulting from a manic or depressive episode.

Nursing Diagnoses for Social Domain

Nursing diagnoses for adults can include Ineffective Role Performance, Interrupted Family Processes, Impaired Social Interaction, Impaired Parenting, Compromised Family Coping, and Caregiver Role Strain. Another relevant diagnosis specific to children and adolescents in a family coping with a member with bipolar disorder is Delayed Growth and Development.

Interventions for Social Domain

Interventions focusing on the social domain are integral to nursing care for all ages. During mania, patients usually violate others' boundaries. Roommate selection for patients requiring hospital admittance needs to be carefully considered. If possible, a private room is ideal because patients with bipolar disorder tend to irritate others, who quickly tire of the intrusiveness. These patients may miss the cues indicating anger and aggression from others. The nurse should protect the patient with mania from self-harm, as well as harm from other patients.

Support groups are helpful for people with this disorder. Participating in groups allows the person to meet others with the disorder and learn management and preventive strategies. Support groups also are helpful in dealing with the stigma associated with mental illnesses.

BOX 22-8 Psychoeducation Checklist: Bipolar I Disorder

When caring for the family and their family member who has a bipolar I disorder, be sure to include the following topic areas in the teaching plan:
- Psychopharmacologic agents, including drug action, dosage, frequency, and possible adverse effects
- Medication regimen adherence
- Strategies to decrease agitation and restlessness
- Safety measures
- Self-care management
- Follow-up laboratory testing
- Support services

Family Interventions

Marital and family interventions are often needed at different periods in the life of a person with bipolar disorder. For the family with a child with this disorder, additional parenting skills are needed to manage the behaviours. The goals of family interventions are to help the family understand and cope with the disorder. Interventions may range from occasional counselling sessions to intensive family therapy.

Family psychoeducation strategies have been shown to be particularly useful in decreasing the risk for relapse and hospitalization. In a study of 53 patients with mania, half were assigned to a 9-month family-focused psycho-educational group and half to individually focused treatment. Those in family-focused treatment were less likely to be rehospitalized (Rea et al., 2003). For more information, see Box 22-8.

Spiritual Domain

The nursing approach to the spiritual domain in the care of the person with a bipolar disorder is the same as for the person with a major depressive disorder. See Research for Best Practice Box 22-9 for research describing the experience of receiving a psychiatric diagnosis.

Evaluation and Treatment Outcomes

Desired treatment outcomes are stabilization of mood and enhanced quality of life. Primary tools for evaluating outcomes are nursing observation and patient self-report (see Nursing Care Plan 22-1).

Continuum of Care

Inpatient Management

Inpatient admission is the treatment setting of choice for patients who are severely psychotic or who are an immediate threat to themselves or others. In acute mania, nursing interventions focus on patient safety, because such patients are prone to injury due to hyperactivity and are often unaware of injuries they sustain. Redirecting the client may also be effective when a patient is talking or acting inappropriately. Removal to a quieter environment may be necessary if other interventions have not been successful, but the patient should be carefully monitored. Because patients are often impulsive, disinhibited, and interpersonally inappropriate during acute mania, the nurse should avoid direct confrontations or challenges.

Medication management (Fig. 22-2), including control of side effects and promotion of self-care, is a major nursing responsibility during inpatient hospitalization. Nurses should be familiar with drug–drug interactions (Table 22-4) and with interventions to help control side effects.

Intensive Outpatient Programmes

When hospitalization is not necessary, or in order to prevent or shorten hospitalization, intensive outpatient programs for several weeks of acute-phase care during a manic or depressive episode are used. These programs are usually called *partial hospitalization* or *day hospitalization*. Close medication monitoring and milieu therapies that foster the restoration of a patient's previous adaptive abilities are the major nursing responsibilities in these settings.

Setting up frequent office visits and crisis telephone calls are additional nursing interventions that can help to shorten or prevent hospitalization during the acute phase of a manic episode. Psychoeducation that includes the patient and significant others are alternatives. Severely and persistently ill patients may need ongoing intensive treatment, but the frequency of visits can be decreased for patients whose conditions stabilize and who enter the continuation or the maintenance phase of treatment.

Spectrum of Care

In today's health care climate, with efforts to reduce hospitalization, most patients with bipolar disorder are treated as outpatients. Hospitalizations are usually brief, and treatment focuses on restabilization. Patients with mood disorders are likely to need long-term medication regimens and supportive psychotherapy to function in the community. Therefore, medication regimens and additional treatment planning need to be tailored to individual needs. Patients need extended and continued follow-up to monitor medication trials and side effects, reinforce self-care management, and provide continued psychosocial support (see Chapter 4).

Mental Health Promotion

Mental health promotion activities should be the focus during remissions. During this period, patients have an opportunity to learn new coping skills that promote positive mental health. Stress management and relaxation techniques can be practised for use when needed. A plan for managing emerging symptoms can also be developed during this period.

BOX 22-9

Research for Best Practice

From Hayne, Y. (2001). To be diagnosed – the experience of persons with chronic mental illness (Unpublished Dissertation). Edmonton, AB: University of Alberta.

Question: What is the lived experience of psychiatric diagnosis?

Method: Lived experience is an immediate, reflexive response to a happening in life. The experience (phenomenon) of interest in this study was the response to receiving a psychiatric diagnosis, as differentiated from experiencing the illness itself. This phenomenologic study, therefore, involved gathering concrete, detailed accounts of participants' experience of diagnosis, including self drawings (before and after diagnosis) that provided an additional means of expressing this personal experience.

Findings: Emphasized in the lived description of psychiatric diagnosis was the notion that the diagnosis places the individual in a context of reflective self-knowledge. Before and after drawings help exemplify participants' perceptions of a "legitimized/delegitimized self." Below are excerpts, including drawings, of the experiences of two participants, Matt and Jeff.

Matt desperately wanted to avoid being "abnormal." A diagnosis spelled "insanity" and he shuddered at the prospect of it. Why not "bizarre experience" or something less caustic? The diagnosis threatened to reveal "a secret he held to himself about himself," confronting him with, "I am flawed! Not, I have a flaw, but, I am flawed!" He sketches

"diagnosis" in "Before" and "After" self profiles. Prediagnosis self has a halo to arc dark (blue) hair (he interprets this as ominous). With diagnosis, there is no evading the ill-fated knowledge and Matt accommodates the diagnosis, colouring his hair bright (green) to represent hope and "self-acceptance."

Jeff views embracing the diagnosis as central in to his mental illness experience in that it supplied him "a battleground for living." Prior to diagnosis, he felt empty, forlorn, immobilized ("a scarecrow, suspended in a field"). Diagnosis resulted in "knowledge made knowledgeable" to him. With that he was able to reformulate (pictured as a snowman). Someone "cared" enough to assist this reconstituting (the therapeutic encounter). Therefore, he is not cold as a snowman (scarf); he wears a smile. Rediscovery of his personal significance (top hat) equips him to take up his future (hands outstretched).

Implications: Understanding what it is like to receive a psychiatric diagnosis is important knowledge for nurses who are caring for persons during this transformative time. With such knowledge, nurses may be better prepared to help patients sustain hope and self-acceptance. It is knowledge that may be transferred to understanding the potential life-changing ramifications of any medical diagnosis.

Diagnosis: Matt Before and After.

Diagnosis: Jeff Before and After.

Nursing Care Plan 22-1

The Patient With Bipolar Disorder

Steven was a young businessman in the oil sector. He was married with three young children and living in a large metropolitan city. When his business began to fail, he lost millions of dollars within weeks. He describes feeling desperate and going into "overdrive" trying to save the company, spare his employees from being laid off, and evade an inevitable bankruptcy. "I just wouldn't quit," he says. "Because I wouldn't quit, my mind quit. And it just literally went into la-la-land. My mind just shut down. I kind of lost contact with everything." Steven unwittingly stepped in front of a car and was hit. "I jumped up and just carried on," he says. Bystanders, however, mobilized his transport to a hospital emergency department (ED). "The doctor looked at me for eight seconds and said 'manic depressive!'"

Steven sees his condition as a gift: "I'm very likable … and creative…. With mania you think faster and when you think faster you process more. So I just process more information quicker…. "I have the energy that most people can only dream of … I mean incredible energy … I can do anything, anytime, anywhere…. And everything seems in its right space. And it can be you have no money, no house, no job, no family, no friends, no food, and you feel incredible. None of that matters! It's like the ultimate high!"

The first hospitalization established a medical regime for Steven and his health stabilized for a time. An initial manic episode very often involves treatment with lithium carbonate resulting in mood stabilization. Recurring mania with episodes of depression may benefit from treatment with TCAs and MAOIs, though this course of action was not necessary for Steven.

Steven found his psychiatric diagnosis was "a destructive (gift) of difference!" "I went from one day being gifted to the next day being mentally ill. That's a very large step." He depicts his experience in a before-diagnosis drawing, stating, "I had everything before: a wife, three children, a home! The sun shone in my world." This state is contrasted in an after-diagnosis portrayal, where "the sun is gone." "I lost it all. There is just me! No job, no friends, no home, no family! My wife thought she married a gifted person. When she realized the mental illness, she took the kids and left." Within months of his discharge from the hospital, Steven became confused and disorganized. A restaurant owner reported him for causing a disturbance. When police arrived, he was incoherent and behaving erratically. He was transported to an ED.

Setting: Acute Care Psychiatric Unit in a General Hospital

Baseline Assessment: From the ED, Steven is admitted to acute care inpatient services where he presents with symptoms of mixed bipolar mood disorder. His mood is brittle and he is easily irritated. His speech is pressured. He is unable to account for his behaviour and is exhibiting flight of ideas. Historical records indicate his prior admission and discharge on lithium, which he admits not taking. When asked why he stopped his medication he states, "I completely disagreed with it. I didn't think that my gift needed treatment."

Diagnostic Features	Medications
Bipolar I disorder	L-Thyroxine 0.1 mg q am × 1 day
Hypothyroidism	Clonazepam 0.5 mg bid for sleep and agitation
Social problems (Divorce finalized 18 months ago. Exwife has full custody of three children. Patient has supervised visitations.)	Carbamazepine added on transfer to be titrated up to 400 mg tid

Continued

Nursing Care Plan 22-1 (*Continued*)

Setting: Acute Care Psychiatric Unit in a General Hospital

Associated Features

Potential for life-threatening injury
Poor judgement and impulse control
Lack of support system

Related Factors

Elation and expansive feelings
Excitement vacillating with desolation
Loss secondary to finances/job, divorce

Goals of Care

Initial

1. Will seek out appropriate support.
2. Will comply with unit regulations.
3. Will participate in programme activities.
4. Will achieve balance in activities of daily living (e.g., rest, hydration, nutrition).

Discharge

5. Will discuss the complexity of his illness.
6. Will express antecedents of treatment related to mania and depression.
7. Will discuss need for adherence to meds.
8. Will identify antecedents and indicators of impending illness exacerbation.

Interventions	Rationale	Ongoing Assessment
Initiate a nurse–patient relationship, demonstrate acceptance of the patient as a worthwhile human being through the use of nonjudgemental statements and behaviour.	A sense of worthlessness often underlies despair. The positive therapeutic relationship can maintain the patient's dignity.	Assess the stages of the relationship and determine whether a therapeutic relationship is actually being formed. Identify indicators of trust.
Initiate suicide precautions per hospital policy. Apply vigilant observation routines.	Safety of the individual is a priority with people who have poor impulse control.	Determine risk of self-harm.
Help the client to develop a relapse prevention plan that includes seeking professional mental health support when she or he feels suicidal.	A relapse prevention plan can help the patient maintain wellness and safety by encouraging the resistance of impulses and providing a stepwise plan to address any exacerbation of symptoms. A relapse prevention plan requires an understanding of *denial* as an expected coping mechanism. This coping mechanism should be connected with the client's underlying emotional struggle with his or her illness.	Determine the patient's ability to commit to the relapse plan.

Evaluation

Outcomes	Revised Outcomes	Interventions
Has not harmed self, denies self-harm thoughts/intent.	Absence of risk or self-harm intent will continue.	Discontinue precautions incrementally; maintain ongoing assessment for safety.
Made a no self-harm contract with nurse, agrees to keep it after discharge.	Maintain a no self-harm contract with outpatient mental health provider.	Support and reinforce this contract.

Associated Impaired Sense of Self and Self-Esteem

Defining Characteristics

Expressions of grandiosity vacillating with expressions of shame and guilt.
Lack of success in business endeavours and relationships.

Related Factors

Labile mood (elation and despair noted).
Feelings of abandonment secondary to separation from significant others.
Feelings of failure secondary to bankruptcy and relationship problems.
Unrealistic expectations of self.

Nursing Care Plan 22-1 *(Continued)*

Goals of Care

Initial

1. Realistic self-appraisal.
2. Modify excessive and unrealistic self-expectations.

Discharge

3. Verbalize acceptance of personal limitations.
4. Report freedom from untoward symptoms.
5. Avoid behavioural risks.

Interventions	Rationale	Ongoing Assessment
Enhance the patient's sense of self by being attentive; validate interpretation of what is being said or experienced; help to make consistent, realistic verbalizations.	By showing respect and helping the patient frame happenings realistically, the nurse can support and help build the patient's sense of self.	Determine whether the patient confirms realistic interpretation of situations and verbalizes with moderation in rate and volume.
Assist to reframe and redefine negative statements ("not a failure, but a setback").	Reframing an event positively can help the patient view the situation in an alternative way.	Assess whether the patient can actually view the world in a different way.
Problem solve with the patient about how to approach finding satisfying employment.	Work is very important to adults. Bankruptcy can decrease self-esteem. Focusing on the possibility of a future job can provide hope.	Assess the patient's problem-solving ability. Note indicators of realistic plans.
Encourage positive physical habits (healthy eating patterns, exercise, adequate sleep).	A healthy lifestyle promotes well-being, increasing self-esteem.	Determine willingness to consider making lifestyle changes.
Teach the patient to validate consensually with others.	Low self-esteem is generated by negative interpretations of the world. Through consensual validation, the patient can determine whether others view situations in the same way.	Assess the patient's ability to participate in this process.
Teach constructive self-appraisal. Helpful exercises might include self-affirmations, imagery, use of humour, meditation/prayer, relaxation.	There are many different approaches that can be practiced to increase self-esteem.	Assess the patient's energy level and ability to focus on learning new skills.
Assist in establishing appropriate personal boundaries.	In an attempt to meet their own needs, people with a compromised sense of self often violate other people's boundaries and or allow others to take advantage of them. Helping patients establish their own boundaries will improve the likelihood of needs being met in an appropriate manner.	Assess the patient's ability to understand the concept of boundary violation and its significance.
Provide an opportunity within the therapeutic relationship to express thoughts and feelings. Use open-ended statements and questions. Encourage expression of both positive and negative statements.	The individual with compromised self-esteem may have difficulty expressing thoughts and feelings. Varied outlets for expression may help improve how thoughts and feelings are expressed.	Monitor thoughts and feelings that are expressed in order to help the patient examine them.
Explore opportunities for positive socialization.	Individuals with insecurity issues may be in social situations that reinforce artificial self-evaluation. Helping the patient identify new positive situations will present other options.	Assess whether the new situations are potentially positive or are a re-creation of other negative (self-aggrandizing) situations.
Steven began to modify excessive and unrealistic expectations of self.	Strengthen ability to affirm realistic aspects and examine expectations related to work and relationships.	Refer to mental health clinic for cognitive behavioural psychotherapy.
Verbalized defeatist thinking related to finding worthwhile employment.	Identify important aspects of tentative employment so that he can begin looking for a job that has those characteristics.	Attend a support group that focuses on job interviewing skills.
As Steven's mood stabilized, he was able to sleep through the night, and he began eating again. He also expressed positive thoughts about his future.	Maintain a stable mood to promote a positive and realistic self-concept.	Monitor mood and identify antecedents to mood escalation and/or depression.

Continued

Nursing Care Plan 22-1 *(Continued)*

Defining Characteristics

Verbalization in inability to cope or ask for help
Reported difficulty with life stressors
Compromised ability to problem solve
Alteration in social participation
Disinhibited behaviour resulting in self-risk
Distorted thought and self-control
Substance abuse

Related Factors

Altered mood (alternating mania and depression) caused by changes secondary to body chemistry (bipolar disorder)
Altered mood caused by changes secondary to intake of mood-altering substance (alcohol)
Unsatisfactory support system
Sensory overload secondary to excessive activity
Unreliable psychological resources for consistency of employment

Goals of Care

Initial

1. Accept support through the nurse–patient relationship.
2. Identify areas of ineffective coping.
3. Examine current efforts at coping.
4. Identify realistic areas of strength.
5. Learn new coping skills.

Discharge

6. Practise new coping skills.
7. Focus on realistic strengths.

Interventions	Rationale	Ongoing Assessment
Identify current stresses in Steven's life, including the acceptance of bipolar disorder.	When areas of concern are verbalized by the patient, he will be able to focus on one issue at a time. If he identifies the mental disorder as a stressor, he will more likely be able to develop strategies to deal with it.	Determine whether Steven is able to identify problem areas realistically. Continue to assess for self-risk behaviours.
Identify Steven's strengths in dealing with past stressors.	By focusing on past successes, he can identify strengths and build on them in the future.	Assess if Steven can identify any previous successes in his life.
Assist Steven in discussing, selecting, and practicing positive coping skills (jogging, yoga, volunteer work).	New coping skills take a conscious effort to learn and will at first seem strange and unnatural. Practising these skills will help build a repertoire of coping strategies.	Assess whether Steven follows through on learning new skills.
Educate the patient on the use of alcohol and its relationship to bipolar disorder.	Alcohol is an ineffective coping strategy that can exacerbate the symptoms of bipolar disorder.	Assess for the patient's willingness to control drinking.
Assist the patient in coping with bipolar disorder, beginning with education about it.	A mood disorder is a major stressor in a patient's life. To manage the stress, the patient needs a knowledge base.	Determine Steven's knowledge about bipolar disorder.
Administer lithium as ordered (give with food or milk). Reinforce the action, dosage, and side effects. Review laboratory results to determine whether lithium is within therapeutic limits. Assess for toxicity. Recommend a normal diet with normal salt intake; maintenance of adequate fluid intake.	Lithium carbonate is effective in the treatment of bipolar disorder, but it must be managed. The patient should have a thorough knowledge of the medication and side effects.	Assess for target action, side effects, and toxicity.
Administer carbamazepine as ordered, to be titrated up to 400 mg tid. Observe for presence of hypersensitivity to the drug. Teach about action, dosage, and side effects. Emphasize the possibility of drug interaction with alcohol, some antibiotics (and TCAs and MAOIs if these become a treatment option).	Carbamazepine can be effective in bipolar disorder; however, it can increase CNS toxicity when given with lithium carbonate.	Assess for target action, side effects, and toxicity.

Nursing Care Plan 22-1 *(Continued)*

Hypothyroidism Interventions	Rationale	Ongoing Assessment
Administer thyroid supplement as ordered. Review thyroid functioning laboratory results. Discuss the symptoms of hypothyroidism and how they are similar to depression. Emphasize the importance of taking lithium and L-thyroxine. Explain about the long-term effects of lithium on thyroid functioning.	Hypothyroidism can be a side effect of lithium carbonate and also mimics symptoms of depression.	Determine whether the patient understands the relationship between thyroid dysfunction and lithium carbonate.

Evaluation

Outcomes	Revised Outcomes	Interventions
Clonazepam 0.5 mg bid for sleep and agitation.		
Steven is easily engaged in a therapeutic relationship. He examined the areas in his life where he coped ineffectively.	Establish a therapeutic relationship with a therapist at the mental health clinic.	Refer to mental health clinic.
He identified his strengths and how he coped with stressors, especially his illness, in the past.	Continue to view illness as a potential stressor that can disrupt life.	Seek advice immediately if there are any problems with medications.
He learned new problem-solving skills and reported that he learned a lot about his medication. He plans to adhere to medication regimen.	Continue to practise new coping skills as stressful situations arise.	Discuss with the therapist the outcomes of using new coping skills.

FIGURE 22-2. Holistic interventions for patients with bipolar I disorder.

Spiritual
1. Openness to remarks regarding life meanings
2. Recognize spiritual distress and allow for conversation about it
3. Seek pastoral presence as warranted
4. Support spiritual activity/practices
5. Nurture hope

Biologic
1. Administer psychopharmacologic agents, such as lithium
2. Obtain serum drug levels
3. Assist with measures to enhance sleep and rest
4. Institute safety precautions
5. Plan for medication adherence

Social
1. Integrate family therapeutic interventions
2. Promote use of appropriate social skills
3. Refer to community agencies for support
4. Institute protective environmental precautions

Psychological
1. Assist with psychotherapy treatment program
2. Monitor behaviour
3. Avoid confrontation
4. Psychoeducation

SUMMARY OF KEY POINTS

■ Mood disorders are characterized by persistent or recurring disturbances in mood that cause significant psychological distress and functional impairment. Moods can be broadly categorized as manic or dysphoric (typified by exaggerated feelings of elation or irritability) or depressive or dysthymic (typified by feelings of sadness, hopelessness, loss of interest, and fatigue).

■ Primary mood disorders include both depressive disorders (unipolar depression) and manic–depressive disorders (bipolar disorders).

■ Genetics undoubtedly play a role in the aetiology of mood disorders. Risk factors include family history of mood disorders; prior mood episodes; lack of social support; stressful life events; substance abuse; and medical problems, particularly chronic or terminal illnesses.

■ The recommended depression treatment guidelines include antidepressant medication, alone or with psychotherapeutic management or psychotherapy; ECT for severe depression; or light therapy (phototherapy) for patients with seasonal depressive symptoms.

■ Nurses must be knowledgeable about antidepressant medications: their therapeutic effects and associated side effects, toxicity, dosage ranges, and contraindications. Nurses must also be familiar with ECT protocols and associated interventions. Patient education and the provision of emotional support during the course of treatment are also nursing responsibilities.

■ Many symptoms of depression, such as weight and appetite changes, sleep disturbance, decreased energy, and fatigue, are similar to those of medical illnesses. Assessment includes a thorough medical history and physical examination to detect or rule out medical or psychiatric comorbidity.

■ Bio/psycho/social/spiritual assessment includes assessing mood; speech patterns; thought content and processes; suicidal or homicidal thoughts; cognition and memory; social factors such as patterns of relationship, quality of support systems, and changes in occupational functioning; and spiritual beliefs and practices. Several self-report scales, such as the BDI, and the Hamilton Rating Scale, are helpful in evaluating depressive symptoms.

■ Establishing and maintaining a therapeutic nurse–patient relationship is key to successful outcomes. Nursing interventions that foster the therapeutic relationship include being available in times of crisis, providing understanding and education to patients and their families regarding goals of treatment, providing encouragement and feedback concerning the patient's progress, providing guidance in the patient's interpersonal interactions (within the work environment, the community), and helping to set and monitor realistic goals.

■ Psychosocial interventions for mood disorders include self-care management, cognitive therapy, behaviour therapy, interpersonal therapy, patient and family education regarding the nature of the disorder and treatment goals, marital and family therapy, and group therapy that includes medication maintenance support groups and other consumer-oriented support groups.

■ Bipolar disorders are characterized by one or more manic episodes or mixed mania (co-occurrence of manic and depressive states) that cause marked impairment in social activities, occupational functioning, and interpersonal relationships and may require hospitalization to prevent self-harm.

■ Manic episodes are periods in which the individual experiences abnormally and persistently elevated, expansive, or irritable mood characterized by inflated self-esteem, decreased need to sleep, excessive energy or hyperactivity, racing thoughts, easy distractibility, and inability to stay focused. Other symptoms can include hypersexuality and impulsivity.

■ Similar to treatment of major depressive disorder, pharmacotherapy is the cornerstone of treatment of bipolar illness, but adjunctive psychosocial interventions are also needed. Pharmacologic therapy includes treatment with mood stabilizers alone or in combination with antipsychotics or benzodiazepines if psychosis, agitation, or insomnia is present and antidepressants for unremitted depression. ECT is a valuable alternative for patients with severe mania that do not respond to other treatment.

■ Recent major advances in bipolar disorder treatment research validate the efficacy of integrated psychosocial and pharmacologic treatment involving family or couples therapies, psychoeducational programmes, and individual cognitive–behavioural or interpersonal therapies.

CRITICAL THINKING CHALLENGES

1 A patient comes into a physician's office distraught and expressing concerns about her ability to cope with her current situation. Describe how you would assess this patient for suicide risk.

2 Describe how you would approach the patient described above if you determined that she was suicidal.

3 Discuss difficulties in the differential diagnosis of bipolar disorder in the manic phase and other medical and psychiatric disorders. List the information you would use to rule out the other diagnoses when dealing with a patient who appears to have mania.

4 Describe how you would approach a patient who is expressing concern that the diagnosis of bipolar disorder will negatively affect his or her social and work relationships.

5 Your depressed patient does not seem inclined to talk about his or her depression. Describe the measures you would take to initiate a therapeutic relationship.

6 Your patient with mania is experiencing physical hyperactivity that is interfering with his or her sleep and nutrition. Describe the actions you would take to meet the patient's needs for nutrition and rest.

7 Prepare a hypothetical discussion with a patient with potential bipolar disorder concerning the advantages and disadvantages of lithium versus divalproex sodium for treatment of bipolar disorder.

8 Prepare a hypothetical discussion with a depressed patient with potential unipolar disorder concerning the advantages and disadvantages of each of the major classifications of antidepressants.

ACKNOWLEDGEMENT

The author thanks Carol Rupcich (RN, MN) for her expert analytic advice and input.

REFERENCES

Akiskal, H. S. (2009a). Mood disorders: Historical introduction and conceptual overview. In B. J. Sadock, V. A. Sadock, & P. Ruiz (Eds.), *Comprehensive textbook of psychiatry* (9th ed., vol. 1, pp. 1629–1644). Philadelphia, PA: Lippincott Williams & Wilkins

Akiskal, H. S. (2009b). Mood disorders: Clinical features. In B. J. Sadock, V. A. Sadock, & P. Ruiz (Eds.), *Comprehensive textbook of psychiatry* (9th ed., vol. 1, pp. 1693–1733). Philadelphia, PA: Lippincott Williams & Wilkins.

Alda, M. & Grof, P. (2000). Genetics and lithium response in bipolar disorders. In J. C. Soares & S. Gershon (Eds.), *Bipolar disorders: Basic mechanisms and therapeutic implications* (pp. 529–543). New York, NY: Marcel Dekker.

American College of Obstetricians and Gynecologists. (2008). *Use of psychiatric medications during pregnancy and lactation*. Washington, DC: Author.

American Psychiatric Association. (2000). *Diagnostic and statistical manual of mental disorders* (4th ed., Text revision). Washington, DC: Author.

American Psychiatric Association. (2002). *Compendium of practice guidelines for the treatment of psychiatric disorders*. Washington, DC: Author.

American Psychiatric Association. (2013). *Diagnostic and statistical manual of mental disorders* (5th ed.). Arlington, VA: Author.

Anandarajah, G. & Hight, E. (2001). Spirituality and medical practice: Using the HOPE questions as a practical tool for spiritual assessment, *American Family Physician*, 63(1), 81–89.

Andrews, G. (2008). Reducing the burden of depression. *Canadian Journal of Psychiatry*, 53(7), 420–427.

Azorin, J. M., Kaladjian, A., Adida, M., Hantouche, E., Hameg, A., Lancrenon, S., & Akiskal, A. S. (2008). Toward the delineation of mania subtypes in the French National EPIMAN-II Mille Cohort. *European Archives of Psychiatry and Clinical Neuroscience*, 258(8), 497–504.

Barnes, C. & Mitchell, P. (2005). Considerations in the management of bipolar disorder in women. *Australian and New Zealand Journal of Psychiatry*, 39(8), 662–673.

Barney, L. J., Griffiths, K. M., Jorm, A. F., & Christensen, H. (2006). Stigma about depression and its impact on help-seeking intentions. *Australian & New Zealand Journal of Psychiatry*, 40(11), 51–54.

Beck, A. T. (2008). The evolution of the cognitive model of depression and its neurobiological correlates of psychiatry. *American Journal of Psychiatry*, 165, 969–977.

Beevers, C. G. (2005). Cognitive vulnerability to depression: A dual process model. *Clinical Psychology Review*, 25, 975–1002.

Belmaker, R. H. & Yaroslavsky, Y. (2000). Perspectives for new pharmacological interventions. In J. C. Soares & S. Gershon (Eds.), *Bipolar disorders: Basic mechanisms and therapeutic implications* (pp. 507–527). New York, NY: Marcel Dekker.

Bowden, C. L., Calabrese, J. R., McElroy S. L., Gyulai, L., Wassef, A., Petty, F., … Wozniak, P. J. (2000). A randomized placebo-controlled 12-month trial of divalproex and lithium in treatment of outpatients with bipolar disorder. *Archives of General Psychiatry*, 57(5), 481–489.

Bowden, C. L., Calabrese, J. R., Sachs, G., Yatham, L. N., Asghar, S. A., Hompland, M., … Lamictal 606 Study Group. (2003). A placebo-controlled 18-month trial of lamotrigine and lithium maintenance treatment in recently manic or hypomanic patients with bipolar 1 disorder. *Archives of General Psychiatry*, 60(4), 392–400.

Brooks, N., Burata, L., & Tansey, M. (2008, October). Tidal waves: Implementing a new model of mental health recovery and reclamation. *Canadian Nurse*, 104(8), 22–27.

Bryson, C. (2012). Women's health. In *Research News. Alberta innovates—Health solutions*. Edmonton, AB: McCallum Printing Group Inc.

Canadian Community Health Survey. (2003). Mental health and well-being. Retrieved from Statistics Canada website: http://www.statcan.ca/Daily/English/030903/d030903a.htm

Canadian Mental Health Association. (2008). The relationship between mental health, mental illness and chronic physical conditions. Retrieved from http://ontario.cmha.ca/public_policy/the-relationship-between-mental-health-mental-illness-and-chronic-physical-conditions/#.UlcyghAXEno

Canadian Mental Health Association. (2013). Connection between mental and physical health. Retrieved from http://ontario.cmha.ca/mental-health/connection-between-mental-and-physical-health/.

Canadian Nurses Association. (2005). Standards and best practices. Retrieved from http://www.cna-nurses.ca/CNA/practice/standards/default_e.aspx.

Carta, M. G., Mura, G., Lecca, M. E., Moro, M. F., Bhat, K. M., Angermeyer, M. C., … Akiskal, H. S. (2012). Decreases in depression over 20 years in a mining area of Sardinia: Due to selective migration? *Journal of Affective Disorders* 141, 255–260.

Caspi, A., Sudgen, K., Moffitt, T.E., Taylor, A., Craig, I.W., Harrington, H., … Poulton, R. (2003). Influence of life stress on depression: Moderation by a polymorphism in the 5-TT gene. *Science*, 301(5631), 386–389.

Center on the Developing Child at Harvard University. (2009). Maternal depression can undermine the development of young children: Working paper no. 8. Retrieved from http://www.developingchild.harvard.edu

Chennattucherry, J. J. & Mok, Y. M. (2010). Physical health issues. In A. H. Young, I. N. Ferrier, & E. E. Michalak (Eds.), *Practical management of bipolar disorder* (pp. 106–119). New York, NY: Cambridge University Press.

Corcoran, J. & Walsh, J. (2009a). Depressive disorders. In J. Corcoran & J. Walsh (Eds.), *Mental health in social work* (pp. 189–215). Boston, MA: Pearson Education.

Corcoran, J. & Walsh, J. (2009b). Bipolar disorder. In J. Corcoran & J. Walsh (Eds.), *Mental health in social work* (pp. 216–241). Boston, MA: Pearson Education.

Cowen, P., Harrison, P., & Burns, T. (2012). Mood disorders. In P. Cowen, P. Harrison, & T. Burns (Eds.), *Shorter oxford textbook of psychiatry* (pp. 205–253). Oxford, UK: Oxford University Press.

Cutler, J. L. & Marcus, E. R. (1999). Mood disorders. In *Psychiatry*. Philadelphia, PA: W. B. Saunders.

Dannlowski, U, Ohrmann, P., Bauer, J., Kugel, H., Arolt, V., Heindel, W., … Suslow, T. (2007). Amygdala reactivity to masked negative faces is associated with automatic judgmental bias in major depression: A 3 T fMRI study. *Journal Of Psychiatry & Neuroscience*, 32(6), 423–429.

Darling, C., Olmstead, S., Lund, V., & Fairclough, J. (2008). Bipolar disorder: Medication adherence and life contentment. *Archives of Psychiatric Nursing*, 22(3), 113–126.

Donati, R. J. & Rasenick, M. M. (2003). G protein signaling and the molecular basis of antidepressant action. *Life Science*, 73(1), 1–17.

Dubovsky, S. L. (2005). Treatment of bipolar depression. *Psychiatric Clinics of North America*, 28(2), 349–370.

Duffy, A. (2012). The nature of the association between childhood ADHD and the development of bipolar disorder: A review of prospective high-risk studies. *American Journal Psychiatry*, 169(12), 1247–1255.

Duffy, A., Alda, M, Hajek, T, Sherry, S. B., & Grof, P. (2010). Early stages in the development of bipolar disorder, *Journal of Affective Disorders*, 121(1–2), 127–135.

Ebmeier, K. P., Donaghey, C., & Steele, J. D. (2006). Recent developments and current controversies in depression. *Lancet*, 367, 153–167.

Edmunds, K. & Kinnaird-Iler, E. (2005). In L. L. Stamler & L. Yiu (Eds.), *Community health nursing: A Canadian perspective* (pp. 247–264). Toronto, ON: Pearson Prentice Hall.

Even, C., Schroder, C. M., Friedman, S., & Rouillon, F. (2008). Efficacy of light therapy in nonseasonal depression: A systematic review. *Journal of Affective Disorders, 108*, 11–23.

Fallot, R. (2007). Spirituality and religion in recovery: Some current issues. *Psychiatric Rehabilitation Journal, 30*(4), 261–270.

Felitti, V. (2007). The tragic imprint of childhood adversity. In *Alberta Mental Health Board (AMHB), Mending Minds: Information Supplement.* Proceedings of the Mental Health Research Showcase, Alberta, Canada.

Fischer, C. E. (2002, June). A clinician's guide to interpreting cognitive measures in clinical trials for Alzheimer's disease. *Canadian Psychiatric Association Bulletin.* Retrieved from https://ww1.cpa-apc.org/Publications/Archives/Bulletin/2002/june/geriatricPsych.asp

Frances, A. H. (2010). Disentangling grief and depression. *DSM-5 and the medicalization of grief: Two perspectives. Psychiatric Times, 27*(5), 1–3.

Garland, E. J. & Duffy, A. (2010). Treating bipolar disorder in the early stages of illness. In A. H. Young, I. N. Ferrier, & E. E. Michalak (Eds.), *Practical management of bipolar disorder* (pp. 73–83). New York, NY: Cambridge University Press.

Gavin, N., Gaynes, B., Lohr, K., Meltzer-Brody, S., Gartlehner, G., & Swinson, T. (2005). Perinatal depression: A systematic review of prevalence and incidence. *Obstetrician Gynecology, 106,* 1071–1083.

Goldberg, J. F., Garno, J. L., Leon, A. C., Kocsis, J. H., & Portera, L. (1999). A history of substance abuse complicates remission from acute mania in bipolar disorder. *Journal of Clinical Psychiatry, 60,* 733–740.

Goldstein, B. I. & Levitt, A. (2006). Is current alcohol consumption associated with increased lifetime prevalence of major depression and suicidality? Results from a pilot community survey. *Comprehensive Psychiatry, 47*(5), 330–333.

Goossens, P., van Wijngaarden, B., Knoppert-van der Klein, E., & Van Achterberg T. (2008). Family caregiving in bipolar disorder: Caregiver consequences, caregiver coping styles, and caregiver distress. *International Journal of Social Psychiatry, 54*(4), 303–316.

Grunze, H. (2010). The treatment of mania. In A. H. Young, I. N. Ferrier, & E. E. Michalak (Eds.), *Practical management of bipolar disorder* (pp. 10–23). New York, NY: Cambridge University Press.

Grunze, H., Amann, B., Dittmann, S., & Walden, J. (2002). Clinical relevance and possibilities of bipolar rapid cycling. *Neuropsychobiology, 45*(Suppl. 1), 20–26.

Hanley, N. R. & Van de Kar, L. D. (2003). Serotonin and the neuroendocrine regulation of the hypothalamic-pituitary-adrenal axis in health and disease. *Vitamins and Hormones: Advances in Research and Applications, 66,* 189–225.

Health Canada. (2002). *A Report on mental illness in Canada.* Ottawa: Author.

Hirschfeld, R. M., Baker, J. D., Wozniak, P., Tracy, K., & Sommerville, K. W. (2003). The safety and early efficacy of oral-loaded divalproex versus standard-titration divalproex, lithium, olanzapine, and placebo in the treatment of acute mania associated with bipolar disorder. *Journal of Clinical Psychiatry, 64*(7), 841–846.

Hoblyn, J. (2004). Bipolar disorder in later life: Older adults presenting with new onset manic symptoms usually have underlying medical or neurologic disorder. *Geriatrics, 59*(6), 41–44.

Hodge, D. R. (2006). A template for spiritual assessment: A review of the JCAHO requirements and guidelines for implementation. *Social Work, 51*(4), 317–326.

Jamison, K. R. (1995). *An unquiet mind.* Toronto, ON: Random House.

Johnson, L., Andersson-Lundman, G., Aberg-Wistedt, A., & Mathe, A. A. (2000). Age of onset in affective disorder: Its correlation with hereditary and psychosocial factors. *Journal of Affective Disorders, 59*(2), 139–148.

Keogh, B. & Doyle, L. (2008). Psychopharmacological adverse effects. *Mental Health Practice, 11*(6), 28–30.

King Blood, R. J. (2005). Aboriginal Canadians. In L. L. Stamler & L. Yiu (Eds.), *Community health nursing: A Canadian perspective* (pp. 239–246). Toronto, ON: Pearson Prentice Hall.

Kirby, J. S. & Baucom, D. H. (2007). Treating emotion dysregulation in a couples context: A pilot study of a couples skills group intervention. *Journal of Marital and Family Therapy, 33*(3), 375.

Koczmara, C., Perri, D., Hyland, S., & Rousseaux, L. (2005). Meperidine (Demerol) safety issues. *Dynamics, 16*(1), 8–12.

Koenig, H. G. (2009). Research on religion, spirituality, and mental health: A review. *Canadian E- Journal of Psychiatry, 54*(5), 283–291.

Kowatch, R. A. & DelBello, M. P. (2005). Pharmacotherapy of children and adolescents with bipolar disorder. *Psychiatric Clinics of North America, 28*(2), 385–397.

Kuhl, E. A., Kupfer, D. J., & Regier, D. A. (2011). Patient-centered revisions to the *DSM-5. Virtual Mentor, 13*(12), 873–879.

Lam, R. W. & Kennedy, S. H. (2004). Prescribing antidepressants for depression in 2005: Recent concerns and recommendations. *Canadian Journal of Psychiatry, 49*(12), 1–6.

Leung, R. (2004, November). Carrey: Life is too beautiful. *60 Minutes,* CBS NEWS. Retrieved from http://www.cbsnews.com/stories/2004/11/18/60minutes/main656547.shtml

Lepine, J. P. & Briley, M. (2011). The increasing burden of depression. *Neuropsychiatric Disease and Treatment, 7*(Suppl 1), 3–7.

Marcus, S. M. (2009). Depression during pregnancy: Rates, risks and consequences–Motherisk Update 2008. *Canadian Journal Clinical Pharmacology, 16*(1), e15–e22.

Markley, V. N. (2008). Mood disorders. In P. G. O'Brien, W. Z. Kennedy, & K. A. Ballard (Eds.), *Psychiatric mental health nursing: An introduction to theory and practice* (pp. 316–334). Mississauga, ON: Jones and Bartlett Publishers.

Massey, K., Gitchett, G., & Roberts, P. A. (2004). Assessment and diagnosis in spiritual care. In N. L. Mauk & K. L. Schmidt (Eds.), *Spiritual care in nursing practice* (pp. 209–242). Philadelphia, PA: Lippincott Williams & Wilkins.

McCuffin, P., Rijsdijk, F., Andrew, J., Sham, P., Katz, R., & Cardno, A. (2003). The heritability of bipolar affective disorder and the genetic relationship to unipolar depression. *Archives of General Psychiatry, 60*(5), 497–502.

McCuistion, L. E. & Gutierrez, K. J. (2002). *Real-world nursing survival guide: Pharmacology.* Philadelphia, PA: WB Saunders.

McElheran, W., Eaton, P., Rupcich, C., Basinger, M., & Johnston, D. (2004). Shared mental health care: The Calgary model. *Families, Systems, & Health, 22*(4), 424–438.

Olympian Hughes Speaks Out On Battle With Depression. (2011). Retrieved from http://www.tsn.ca/olympics/story/?id=353141

Osuji, I. J. & Cullum, C. M. (2005). Cognition in bipolar disorder. *Psychiatric Clinics of North America, 28*(2), 427–441.

Patten, S. B. (2010). Affective disorders in Canada. In J. Cairney, & D. L. Streiner (Eds.), *Mental disorder in Canada: An epidemiological perspective* (pp. 107–125). Toronto, ON: University of Toronto Press.

Parikh, S. V. & Velyvis, V. (2010). Psychosocial interventions in bipolar disorder: Theories, mechanisms and key clinical trials. In A. H. Young, I. N. Ferrier, & E. E. Michalak (Eds.), *Practical management of bipolar disorder* (pp. 44–62). New York, NY: Cambridge University Press.

Payne, J. L., Potash, J. B., & DePaulo, J. R. (2005). Recent findings on the genetic basis of bipolar disorder. *Psychiatric Clinics of North America, 28*(2), 481–498.

Perlick, D., Rosenheck, R., Miklowitz, D., Chessick, C., Wolff, N., Kaczynski, R., ... STEP-BD Family Experience Collaborative Study Group. (2007). Prevalence and correlates of burden among caregivers of patients with bipolar disorder enrolled in the Systematic Treatment Enhancement Program for Bipolar Disorder. *Bipolar Disorders, 9*(3), 262–273.

Pies, R. & Zisook, S. (2010). Disentangling grief and depression: Rejoinder to Dr. Frances. *DSM-5 and the medicalization of grief: Two perspectives. Psychiatric Times, 27*(5), 4–5.

Popova, E., Leighton, C., & Bernabarre, A. (2007). Oxcarbazepine in the treatment of bipolar and schizoaffective disorders. *Expert Review of Neurotherapeutics, 7*(6), 617–626.

Rea, M. M., Tompson, M. C., Miklowitz, D. J., Goldstein, M. J., Hwang, S., & Mintz, J. (2003). Family-focused treatment versus individual treatment for bipolar disorder: Results of a randomized clinical trial. *Journal of Consulting Clinical Psychology, 71*(3), 482–492.

Rush, B. R., Urbanoski, K. A., Bassani, D. G., Castel, S., & Wild, T. C. (2010). The epidemiology of co-occurring substance use and other mental disorders in Canada: prevalence, service use, and unmet needs. In J. Cairney & D. L. Streiner (Eds.), *Mental disorder in Canada: an epidemiological perspective.* Toronto, ON: University of Toronto Press Incorporated.

Rush, J. A. & Nierenberg, A. A. (2009). Mood disorders: Treatment of depression. In B. J. Sadock, V. A. Sadock, & P. Ruiz (Eds.), *Comprehensive textbook of psychiatry.* (9th ed., Vol 1, pp. 1734–1813). Philadelphia, PA: Lippincott Williams & Wilkins.

Schatzberg, A. F., Cole, J. O., & DeBattista, C. (2003). *Manual of clinical psychopharmacology* (4th ed.). Washington, DC: American Psychiatric Publishing.

Schmidt, K. L. & Mauk, N. L. (2004). Spirituality as a life journey. In N. L. Mauk & K. L. Schmidt (Eds.), *Spiritual care in nursing practice* (pp. 1–19). Philadelphia, PA: Lippincott Williams & Wilkins.

Scott, J. & Colom, F. (2005). Psychosocial treatments for bipolar disorders. *Psychiatric Clinics of North America, 28*(2), 371–384.

Sheline, Y. I. (2003). Neuroimaging studies of mood disorder effects on the brain. *Biological Psychiatry, 54*(3), 338–352.

Stahl, S. (2000). *Essential psychopharmacology: A prescriber's guide.* Cambridge, MA: Cambridge University Press.

Statistics Canada (2012). *Suicides and suicide rate, by sex and by age group.* Ottawa, ON: Author. Retrieved from http://www.statcan.gc.ca/tables-tableaux/sum-som/l01/cst01/hlth66a-eng.htm

Thase, M. E. (2009). Mood disorders: Neurobiology. In B. J. Sadock, V. A. Sadock, & P. Ruiz (Eds.), *Comprehensive textbook of psychiatry* (9th ed., Vol. 1, pp. 1664–1674). Philadelphia, PA: Lippincott Williams & Wilkins.

Tronick, E. & Reck, C. (2009). Infants of depressed mothers. *Harvard Review of Psychiatry*, 17(2), 147–56.

Uher, R. & McGuffin, P. (2008). The moderation by serotonin transporter gene of environmental adversity in the aetiology of mental ill: Review and methodological analysis. *Molecular Psychiatry*, 13, 131–146.

Wong-McDonald, A. (2007). Spirituality and psychosocial rehabilitation: Empowering persons with serious psychiatric disabilities at an inner-city community program. *Psychiatric Rehabilitation Journal*, 30(4), 295–300.

World Health Organization. (2006). Building awareness—reducing risks: Suicide and mental illness. Retrieved from http://wwwo.who.int/media-centre/news/releases/2006/pr53/en/index.html

World Health Organization. (2009). *The global burden of disease: 2004 update.* Geneva, Switzerland: Author.

Wright, L. M. & Leahey, M. (2013). *Nurses and families: A guide to family assessment and intervention* (6th ed.). Philadelphia, PA: FA Davis.

Yatham, L., Kennedy, S., O'Donovan, C., Parikh, S., MacQueen, G., McIntyre, R., ... Beaulieu, S. (2006). Canadian Network for Mood and Anxiety Treatments (CANMAT) guidelines for the management of patients with bipolar disorder: Update 2007. *Bipolar Disorders*, 8, 721–739.

Young, A. H. & Nemeroff, C. B. (2010). Pharmacological treatment of bipolar depression. In A. H. Young, I. N. Ferrier, & E. E. Michalak (Eds.), *Practical management of bipolar disorder* (pp. 24–32). New York, NY: Cambridge University Press.

Zhang, Y., Hauser, U., Conty, C., Emrich, H. M., & Dietrich, D. E. (2007). Familial risk for depression and P3b component as a possible neurocognitive vulnerability marker. *Neuropsychobiology*, 55, 14–20.

23 Anxiety and Obsessive–Compulsive Disorders

Kathleen Hegadoren and Gerri Lasiuk
Adapted from the chapter "Anxiety Disorders"
by Robert B. Noud and Kathy Lee

KEY CONCEPTS

- anxiety
- compulsion
- obsession
- panic

LEARNING OBJECTIVES

After studying this chapter, you will be able to:

- Discuss anxiety as an adaptive human response to a perceived threat.
- Identify the physical, cognitive, and social manifestations of anxiety.
- Describe the neurobiologic correlates of anxiety.
- Differentiate "normal" anxiety, worry, and an anxiety disorder.
- Identify the shared and unique features of specific anxiety disorders.
- Describe the treatments available for anxiety.
- Discuss special considerations related to anxiety in children, pregnant women, and the elderly.

KEY TERMS

- allostasis • anxiolytics • cognitive–behavioural therapy
- depersonalization • derealization • distraction • exposure therapy
- existential anxiety • fear • fear conditioning • generalized anxiety disorder • obsessive–compulsive disorder • panic disorder (PD)
- paresthesia • phobias • positive self-talk • systematic desensitization
- worry

Although fear and anxiety are common human experiences, they are complex ones. Most of us would be challenged to define them precisely or explain how they are similar and different. In the literature, a few authors do argue that fear and anxiety are indistinguishable; however, most experts claim that they are distinct phenomena (Öhman, 2008) with different aetiologies, response patterns, intensity, and time courses (see Steimer, 2002 for a full discussion). In this chapter, we endorse the assumption that fear and anxiety are distinct but related emotions that function "to signal danger, threat, or motivational conflict and to trigger appropriate adaptive responses" (Steimer, p. 233). We define **fear** as an emotional response to a specific and proximal threat to an organism's life or integrity—for example, being held at gunpoint or encountering a snarling dog (Nebel-Schwalm & Davis, 2013; Pine, 2009). Anxiety, on the other hand, is an emotion characterized by the apprehension or dread of a potentially threatening or uncertain outcome (Steimer). Stated differently, fear is a "primitive alarm in response to present danger" (Barlow, 2002, p. 104), whereas anxiety is a "future-oriented" state (Barlow, p. 64) that helps one prepare for *potentially aversive* situations. Based on these definitions, the key differences between anxiety and fear relate to characteristics of the trigger (stimulus). Characteristics of the trigger include its immediacy or temporal orientation (i.e., whether it exists in the present or future) and its ambiguity or specificity (Nebel-Schwalm & Thompson). A related concept is **worry**, which Borkovec, Robinson, Pruzinsky, and DePree (1983) define as thoughts and images centring on negative outcomes that engender negative affect and are relatively uncontrollable. Fear and anxiety are emotions, and worry involves negative thoughts and images; worry is considered a symptom of fear and anxiety.

The anxiety disorders are a family of disorders that all share excessive fear or anxiety as their core symptom; specific anxiety disorders differ from one another according their key feature(s) (e.g., panic attacks, obsessions and compulsions) (American Psychiatric Association [APA], 2013). The anxiety disorders discussed in this chapter include **generalized anxiety disorder** (GAD), social anxiety disorder (social phobia), **panic disorder** (PD), and specific phobias [grouped as anxiety disorders in the *Diagnostic and Statistical Manual of Mental Disorders*, 5th edition (*DSM-5*) (APA, 2013)]. In earlier versions of the *DSM*, **obsessive–compulsive disorder** (OCD) was categorized as an anxiety disorder, but in the *DSM-5*, it is grouped under obsessive–compulsive and related disorders. Acute stress disorder (ASD) and posttraumatic stress disorder were also previously considered to be anxiety disorders but now appear in the newly created category Trauma- and Stressor-Related Disorders (discussed in Chapter 17).

Significant anxiety and anxiety disorders are not restricted to mental health practice; they are seen across all practice settings and continua of care. Indeed, inpatient psychiatric care is rare in instances where an anxiety disorder is the primary diagnosis. More common to inpatient settings are anxiety disorders that are comorbid with disorders such as severe depression or schizophrenia. Outpatient psychiatric clinics, primary care services, general practice settings, chronic disease management clinics, and private practitioners all provide various types of treatment for individuals experiencing an anxiety disorder. Anxiety disorders are often difficult to treat and symptoms often persist over many years. These disorders are thus frequently chronic in their longitudinal course, with acute episodes occurring in response to stressors or other health problems.

NORMAL VERSUS ABNORMAL ANXIETY RESPONSE

From an evolutionary perspective, an emotion is a transient response to a specific stimulus that produces an arousal reaction characterized by changes in subjective feelings and behaviour (Critchley, 2003). At low to moderate intensities, acute anxiety is an adaptive response to a perceived threat and can motivate one to act. On the other hand, when anxiety is extreme or chronic, it can produce paralysis and inaction. An anxiety disorder differs from adaptive ("normal") anxiety in that it is greater than expected in intensity and/or duration for one's age and the situation, and it interferes with one's quality of life and ability to function (APA, 2013; Peplau, 1989).

McEwen (2005) conceptualizes normal responses to stress as **allostasis**, the adaptive processes that maintain homeostasis through the production of various brain and peripheral stress-related chemicals. These mediators of the stress responses promote adaptation to perceived threat or stress. However, they also contribute to allostatic load, the cumulative wear and tear on biologic systems that over time that can increase the risk for stress-related disorders and physical health problems like cardiovascular and metabolic disorders.

The perception of a threat triggers physical and emotional changes in all individuals. A normal emotional response to anxiety consists of three parts: physiologic arousal, cognitive processes, and coping strategies. Physiologic arousal is the signal that an individual is facing a threat. This increased attention to one's environment or to the details of the situation provides more sensory inputs to the brain. Cognitive processes in the brain decipher the various inputs and yield judgements about the extent of danger and whether the perceived threat should be approached or avoided. Behaviours include "fight or flight" as described by Selye (1956) or more recently "tend and befriend" behaviours described by Taylor et al. (2000) as gender-specific responses by women. Coping strategies can be used to resolve the threat. Table 23-1 summarizes many physical, affective, cognitive, and behavioural symptoms associated with anxiety.

> **KEY CONCEPT Anxiety** is an emotion characterized by apprehension or dread of a potentially threatening or uncertain outcome. It is triggered by the perception of a threat and is manifested in physical, emotional, cognitive, and/or behavioural ways.

OVERVIEW OF ANXIETY DISORDERS

As a group, anxiety disorders represent the most common of all mental illnesses in Canada and around the globe. According to Statistics Canada's (2013) *Community Health Survey of Mental Health and Wellbeing*, approximately 2.6% of Canadians 15 years and older report symptoms that met diagnostic criteria for GAD in the previous 12 months. The same survey found that women reported higher levels of perceived stress than did men. Although anxiety disorders affect individuals of all ages, men and women aged 45 to 64 years reported the highest levels of perceived stress. Older studies conducted in Edmonton, Alberta, reported prevalence rates of anxiety disorder as 6.5% in adults 18 to 64 years of age (Bland, Newman, & Orn, 1988) and 3.1% among those 65 years and older 3.1% (Newman, Bland, & Orn, 1998).

Girls and women have higher prevalence rates for all the anxiety disorders. For example, lifetime rates of social anxiety were found to be 4.2% in men and 5.67 in women in an American community sample (Xu et al., 2012). Anxiety disorders are the psychiatric disorders most frequently treated in children and adolescents (Castellanos & Hunter, 2000; Merikangas et al., 2010).

Table 23-1	Symptoms of Anxiety

Physical

Cardiovascular	Neuromuscular	Gastrointestinal
Sympathetic	Increased reflexes	Loss of appetite
Palpitations	Startle reaction	Revulsion towards food
Heart racing	Eyelid twitching	Abdominal discomfort
Increased blood pressure	Insomnia	Diarrhoea and vomiting
	Unsteadiness	**Eyes**
Respiratory	**Skin**	Dilated pupils
Rapid breathing	Face flushed or pale	**Urinary Tract**
Difficulty getting air	Sweating	Pressure to urinate
Shortness of breath	Feeling hot or cold	
Pressure of chest		
Shallow breathing		
Lump in throat		
Choking sensations		
Gasping		

Affective	Cognitive	Behavioural
Edgy	**Sensory–Perceptual**	Inhibited
Impatient	Feeling dazed	Tonic immobility
Uneasy	Objects seem blurred/distant	Flight
Nervous	Environment seems different/unreal,	Avoidance
Wound up	feelings of depersonalization	Impaired coordination
Anxious	Self-consciousness	Restlessness
Fearful	Hypervigilance	Postural collapse
Apprehensive	**Thinking Difficulties**	Hyperventilation
Scared	Cannot recall important things	Jumpy
Frightened	Confused	Jittery
Alarmed	Difficulty focusing attention	
Terrified	Difficulty concentrating	
	Fear of losing control or not being able to cope	
	Fear of physical injury or death	
	Fear of going crazy	
	Fear of negative evaluation	
	Frightening visual images	
	Repetitive fearful ideation	

Adapted from Beck, A. T., Emery, C., & Greenberg, R. L. (1985). *Anxiety disorders and phobias: A cognitive perspective* (pp. 23–27). New York: Basic Books.

Some evidence suggests a relationship between childhood separation, anxiety disorder, and atopic disorders (asthma, hives, hay fever, and eczema) and adult-onset PD (Slattery et al., 2002). In fact, symptoms of OCD and social anxiety disorder often begin in adolescence (Regier, Rae, Narrow, Kaelber, & Schatzberg, 1998). Recent evidence points to multiple factors that contribute to the development of anxiety disorders in childhood, including genetic inheritance, as well as parental behaviours and modelling and stressful life events at key developmental stages (Murray, Creswell, & Cooper, 2009). Children and adolescents with anxiety disorders have higher rates of suicidal behaviour, early parenthood, drug and alcohol dependence, and educational underachievement later in life (Woodward, 2001). Specific anxiety disorders show more evidence of genetic vulnerability, especially PD, OCD, and phobias (Hettema, Neale, & Kendler, 2001),

compared with GAD. Of depressed elderly patients, 35% will have at least one anxiety disorder diagnosis (Lenze et al., 2000).

Anxiety may exist as a primary disorder, but as noted earlier it more often co-occurs with other psychiatric and/or physical conditions (Sareen, Cox, Clara, & Asmundson, 2005). Evidence from community-based samples tells us that persons diagnosed with an anxiety disorder will likely have at least one comorbid psychiatric disorder, either concomitantly or in their lifetime (for a full discussion, see Ries Merikangas & Alsemgeest Swanson, 2010). Individuals who live with chronic anxiety report more functional impairment; increased use of both psychiatric and nonpsychiatric health care services; and decreased productivity than those in the general population (Kessler, Chiu, Demler, Merikangas, & Walters, 2005). After adjusting for sociodemographic factors and other mental disorders, the presence of any anxiety disorder is significantly associated with suicidal ideation and suicide attempts (Sareen et al., 2005).

Generalized Anxiety Disorder

According to the *DSM-5* (APA, 2013), GAD is characterized by persistent and excessive anxiety and worry about occupational, social, and interpersonal situations or events that the individual finds difficult to control. These excessive anxiety and worry significantly impact the person's functioning and brings with it associated physical symptoms. Thus, the amount of time spent worrying; the degree of control one has over one's worrying; and the impact on personal, social, and occupational functioning are key components of the assessment of GAD. GAD can be a debilitating disorder with serious impact on quality of life (Antai-Otong, 2003; Hoffman, Dukes, & Wittchen, 2008).

GAD is a common anxiety disorder. Most community-based population studies report lifetime prevalence rates of GAD ranging between 2% and 9%, depending on the country and the definitional and measurement criteria employed (Faravelli et al., 1989; Kessler, Petukhova, Sampson, Zaslavsky, & Wittchen, 2012; Offord et al., 1996). In a Canadian sample, the rates of GAD were reported as 0.9% for men and 1.2% for women, with a total rate of 1.1% (Offord et al.). Onset of GAD is often early in life and often follows a chronic course with more severe symptoms being triggered by acute stressors. Persons living with GAD often feel powerless to change, frustrated with life, demoralized, and hopeless, and comorbid depression is very common (Ballenger et al., 2001; Mennin et al., 2008). Only one third of those with GAD have no comorbid disorder (Kessler, 2000). Rovira and colleagues (2012) reported that 7.9% of those attending a primary care setting had GAD. The elderly who have chronic cardiovascular conditions or mobility-limiting arthritic pain often become very focused on their cardiac status or their risk of falling and become highly anxious, with some developing GAD over time. Thus, assessment of persons with GAD must include the assessment of mood, somatic symptoms, specific worries, and how those worries are managed. A standardized questionnaire, such as the *Penn State Worry Questionnaire* (PSWQ) (Meyer, Miller, Metzger, & Borkovec, 1990), may help assess the severity of the symptoms and health impacts.

Obsessive–Compulsive Disorder

OCD is a psychiatric disorder characterized by severe obsessions (repetitive, intrusive thoughts), compulsions (repetitive, ritualistic behaviours), or both. A key feature of OCD is the relationship between obsessions and compulsions; the obsessions cause anxiety, and the compulsions are an attempt to reduce or eliminate it. Obsessive thinking and/or compulsive behaviours are not necessarily signs of a psychiatric disorder if they are not persistent and do not significantly interfere with the person's ability to function. However, when they are severe and persistent, obsessions can interfere with a person's reality testing and judgment to the degree that most of his or her day is spent performing actions in an attempt to minimize severe anxiety. Affected individuals feel chronically anxious and powerless to control the obsessions and compulsions.

The *DSM-5* (APA, 2013) identifies the diagnostic criteria for OCD as:

- Criterion A. The presence of obsessions or compulsions. Obsessions are (1) recurrent and persistent thoughts, images, or impulses that are intrusive and unwanted, causing marked anxiety, and (2) are not simply excessive fretting over real-life situations; and (3) the person tries to ignore or suppress the thoughts or tries to neutralize them by some other thought or action. Compulsions are (1) repetitive behaviours that the person feels driven to perform in response to the obsessions or because of rules that must be rigidly followed or (2) actions performed to prevent or reduce stress or to prevent a catastrophe from occurring. The actions and thoughts are not realistically connected and are clearly excessive to the situation.

- Criterion B. The obsessions and compulsions are time consuming and cause significant distress or impairment in social, occupational, and interpersonal functioning.

- Criterion C. The symptoms are not attributable to the physiologic effects of a substance (e.g., recreational drug) or other medical condition.

- Criterion D. The thoughts or behaviours are not better explained by another mental disorder.

Common compulsions include handwashing, checking and arranging things, and counting. Individuals who perform checking rituals repeatedly check locks, stoves, and/or switches; check for errors; or check that they have not harmed someone or their self. For example, after hitting a bump in the road, an individual may obsess hours over whether they hit someone, or parents may have recurrent intrusive thoughts that they may hurt their child. Some individuals with OCD have somatic fears and frequently seek medical treatment for physical symptoms, often just to get reassurance. Other compulsions include arranging things in perfect symmetry; counting rituals; or doing-and-undoing rituals (e.g., repeatedly turning on and off the alarm clock). Hoarding is characterized by the excessive acquisition of and inability or unwillingness to discard material possessions. Individuals who hoard may feel compelled to check their belongings repeatedly to see that all is accounted for and they may check the garbage to ensure that nothing of value was discarded.

Persons with religious obsessions ruminate over the meaning of sins and whether they have followed the letter of the law. In the case of religious obsessions and compulsions, a diagnosis of OCD is not made unless the thoughts or rituals clearly exceed cultural or religious norms, occur at inappropriate times as described by members of the same religion or culture, or interfere with social obligations.

The prevalence of OCD is similar across community samples drawn from different countries. For example, lifetime rates of OCD in a mixed Asian population were reported as 3.0% (Subramaniam, Abdin, Vaingankar, & Chong, 2012), 2.3% in an American sample (Ruscio, Stein, Chiu, & Kessler, 2010), and 3.5% in a Swiss population (Fineberg et al., 2013). All of these studies reported that men had a younger age of onset than women did. The typical age of onset of OCD is in the early 20s to mid-30s, although symptoms of OCD can begin in childhood. Despite this early onset, it is often 7 to 10 years after the onset of symptoms until individuals seek professional help (Hollander, 1997).

The most common reasons that individuals with OCD seek professional help include relationship problems, generalized anxiety, alcohol or drug problems, and major depression (Nestadt, Bienvenu, Cai, Samuels, & Eaton, 1998). Because children subscribe to myths, superstition, and magical thinking, and obsessive and ritualistic behaviours, OCD may go unnoticed in younger persons. However, it is increasing concerns about social, academic, and personal impairments that differentiate common childhood behaviours from OCD. Predictors of poorer treatment outcomes for adults include earlier age of onset; longer duration of symptoms; high symptom severity; comorbidity with other mental disorders, especially depression; a family history of OCD or other anxiety disorders; and sexual obsessions (Farrell & Boschen, 2011; Jakubovski et al., 2013). In children, the predictors of poorer outcomes also include severity and family history of OCD, but family accommodation of OCD behaviours also predicted poorer outcomes (Garcia et al., 2010).

There has been ongoing speculation about links between streptococcal infection in children and the development of tics or Tourette's syndrome and OCD. A recent attempt to examine the strength of these relationships failed to demonstrate significance, but the authors acknowledged that a link may exist in specific subpopulations of Caucasian children (Schrag et al., 2009). About two thirds of those with OCD have a comorbid disorder, such as depression (Overbeek, Schruers, Vermetten, & Greiz, 2002), social anxiety disorder, and/or PD (Rasmussen & Eisen, 1990, 1992). Substance use disorders are also common, as individuals attempt to self-medicate their anxiety symptoms.

KEY CONCEPT Obsessions are unwanted, intrusive, and persistent thoughts, impulses, or images that are incongruent with the person's usual thought patterns and cause significant anxiety and distress. The person tries to ignore, suppress or neutralize the thoughts by some other thought or action but fails in doing so.

KEY CONCEPT Compulsions are behaviours performed repeatedly, in a ritualistic fashion, with the goal of preventing or relieving anxiety and distress caused by obsessions.

Social Phobia

Social phobia (social anxiety disorder) involves a marked or intense fear of social situations in which the individual feels scrutinized and negatively evaluated by others. People with social phobia appear to be highly sensitive to disapproval or criticism; tend to evaluate themselves negatively; and have poor self-esteem and a distorted view of personal strengths and weaknesses. These individuals magnify personal flaws and underrate any talents, and the resulting fear or anxiety is out of proportion to the actual risk of being negatively evaluated. Generalized social anxiety disorder brings with it reduced quality of life (Wong, Gordon, & Heimberg, 2012) and in children brings significant decreases in school performance (Bernstein, Bernat, Davis, & Layne, 2008). Despite significant functional impairment, treatment seeking is usually related to a comorbid mental disorder (Dalrymple & Zimmerman, 2011).

The onset of social phobia is usually in early adolescence. There are two subtypes of this disorder: generalized social phobia and specific social phobia. Generalized social phobia is diagnosed when an individual experiences fears related to most social situations, including public performances and social interactions. These individuals are likely to demonstrate deficiencies in social skills, and their phobias interfere with their ability to function. Individuals with specific social phobias fear and avoid only one or two specific social situations. Classic examples of the latter are eating, writing, or speaking in public or using public bathrooms.

Social phobia has a lifetime prevalence rate of 8% to 13% (Kessler et al., 2012) in the general population. In a Canadian community sample, 12-month prevalence rates of social phobia were 2.6% for men and 3.4% for women (Xiangfei & D'Arcy, 2012). In specific populations, rates are even higher. For example, one systematic review of individuals with chronic obstructive pulmonary disorder reported rates of 5% to 11% (Willgoss & Yohannes, 2013), and in the Canadian military, the rates were 8.2% (Mather, Stein, & Sareen, 2010).

Panic Disorder

PD is characterized by repeated episodes of panic. These panic "attacks" are abrupt surges of intense fear or discomfort that peak within minutes and are associated with multiple key physical and cognitive symptoms (see Box 23-1 and Table 23-2). Panic attacks can occur in response to a serious threat but can also occur "out of the blue" with no apparent triggering environmental stimulus or stressor. PD is characterized by recurrent unexpected panic attacks and fear of prompting another attack, which limits the individual's ability to function socially, occupationally, and interpersonally.

PD is a chronic condition with exacerbations and remissions. Lifetime prevalence rates differ widely (1.4% to 20.5%), depending on the age of the sampled population and the methodologic approaches used to study it. The prevalence of PD in the United States is higher than in other countries (Lewis-Fernandez et al., 2010). Kessler and colleagues (2006) reported the lifetime prevalence rate of PD P in American adults to be 4.7%. However, the prevalence of having at least one panic attack in the same population was 28.3%. Recent longitudinal data

Table 23-2		Panic Attacks

Discrete period of intense fear or discomfort with four (or more) of the following symptoms that develop abruptly and reach a peak within 10 min:

Palpitations, pounding heart, or accelerated heart rate	Sweating
Sensations of shortness of breath or smothering	Trembling or shaking
	Nausea or vomiting
Feelings of choking	Chills or hot flushes
Chest pain or discomfort	**Derealization** (feeling of unreality)
Depersonalization (feeling detached from oneself)	Fear of dying
Paresthesias (numbness or tingling sensations)	Fear of losing control or going crazy
Feeling dizzy, unsteady, light-headed, or faint	

suggest that having panic attacks increases the risk of developing a mood and/or anxiety disorder in the future (Kinley, Walker, Enns, & Sareen, 2011). Higher rates of PD occur in women and among those 30 to 59 years, with a mean age of onset of 23 years.

Several risk factors have been implicated in the development of PD, including previous triggered panic attacks, a family history of psychological difficulties, being female, and lifetime mood disorder (King, Ollendick, & Mattis, 1994; Kinley et al., 2011). The majority of children with separation anxiety do not develop other anxiety disorders in adulthood. However, adolescents with PD may be at higher risk for suicidal thoughts or attempt suicide more often than other adolescents do (Valentiner, Gutierrez, & Blacker, 2002).

In addition to comorbid psychiatric disorders among those with PD, certain physical health problems are also common, including vertigo, cardiac disease, gastrointestinal disorders, and asthma. Persons with mitral valve prolapse, migraine headaches, and hypertension may also have an increased incidence of PD. One might ponder whether these medical conditions produce similar somatic sensations to anxiety and over time increase the risk of development of PD. The population with both physical health problems and panic symptoms reports poorer quality of life than do those without such comorbidity.

PD can occur with and without agoraphobia. Those who experience PD with agoraphobia tend to have more coexisting anxiety disorders, anxiety attacks, and anticipatory anxiety than do patients who have PD without agoraphobia. Women appear more likely to experience PD with agoraphobia and more likely than men to experience panic symptoms after remission (Sheikh, Leskin & Klein, 2002).

Panic attacks are typically accompanied by fear of death because their symptoms mimic those of a heart attack. Affected individuals often seek emergency

[handwritten margin note: crowded spaces closed ones]

BOX 23-1	Clinical Vignette

PANIC DISORDER (PD)

M, a 22-year-old man, has experienced several life changes, including a recent engagement, loss of his father to cancer and heart disease, graduation from college, and entrance to the workforce as a computer engineer in a large inner-city company. Because of his active lifestyle, his sleep habits have been poor. He frequently uses sleeping aids at night and now drinks a full pot of coffee to start each day. He has started smoking to "relieve the stress." While sitting in heavy traffic on the way to work, he suddenly experienced chest tightness, sweating, shortness of breath, feelings of being "trapped," and foreboding that he was going to die. Fearing a heart attack, he went to an emergency room, where his discomfort subsided within a half hour. After several hours of testing, the doctor informed him that his heart was healthy. During the next few weeks, he experienced several episodes of feeling trapped and slight chest discomfort on his drive to work. He fears future "attacks" while sitting in traffic and while in his crowded office cubicle.

What Do You Think?

• What risk factors does M have that might contribute to the development of panic attacks?
• What lifestyle changes do you think would help M reduce stress?

medical care because they feel as if they are dying, but most will have a negative cardiac workup. People experiencing panic attacks may also believe that the attacks stem from an underlying major medical illness (APA, 2000). Even with sound medical testing and assurance of no underlying disease, these people often remain unconvinced. However, individuals with PD continue to experience panic attacks with or without predisposing conditions (Box 23-1).

> ⬣ **KEY CONCEPT** Panic can be a normal but extreme, overwhelming form of anxiety often initiated when an individual is placed in a real or perceived life-threatening situation.

● **STUDY NOTE**
Physical symptoms of a panic attack are similar to cardiac emergencies. These symptoms are physically taxing and psychologically frightening to patients. Recognition of the seriousness of panic attacks should be communicated to the patient. Assessment of potential triggers helps to focus the patient's attention to the antecedents, which can help to develop individualized management strategies.

Agoraphobia and Other Specific Phobias

Panic attacks can lead to the development of **phobias** or persistent, unrealistic fears of situations, objects, or activities. People with phobias will go to great lengths to avoid the feared objects or situations to deter panic attacks. Box 23-2 presents examples of common phobias. *Agoraphobia*, fear of open spaces, often co-occurs

---

BOX 23-2 Common Phobias

Acrophobia (fear of heights)
Agoraphobia (fear of open spaces)
Ailurophobia (fear of cats)
Algophobia (fear of pain)
Arachnophobia (fear of spiders)
Brontophobia (fear of thunder)
Claustrophobia (fear of closed spaces)
Cynophobia (fear of dogs)
Entomophobia (fear of insects)
Haematophobia (fear of blood)
Microphobia (fear of germs)
Nyctophobia (fear of night or dark places)
Ophidiophobia (fear of snakes)
Phonophobia (fear of loud noises)
Photophobia (fear of light)
Pyrophobia (fear of fire)
Topophobia (stage fright)
Xenophobia (fear of strangers)
Zoophobia (fear of animal or animals)

---

with PD and often leads to avoidance behaviours. The process often begins with an intense, irrational fear of being in an open space, being alone, or being in a public place where escape might be difficult or embarrassing. The person fears that if a panic attack occurred, help would not be available, so he or she begins to avoid such situations. Such avoidance interferes with routine functioning and eventually renders the person afraid to leave the safety of home. Some affected individuals continue to face feared situations, but with significant trepidation (i.e., going in public only to pay bills, or to take children to school).

Specific phobia (formally simple phobia) is a disorder marked by an irrational fear of a specific object or situation that the person realizes is unreasonable. The lifetime prevalence rates differ across different subtypes, with highest rates in those with natural environment phobias (8.9% to 11.6%) and then lower rates observed with situational phobias (5.2% to 8.4%), animal phobias (3.3% to 7%), and blood injection injury phobias (3.2% to 4.5%) (LeBeau et al., 2010).

Exposure to the stimulus object or situation engenders anxiety; the intensity of anxiety is usually related to both the proximity of the object and the degree to which escape is possible. For example, anxiety heightens as a cat approaches a person who fears cats and lessens when the cat moves away. At times, the level of anxiety can escalate to a full panic attack, particularly when the person must remain in a situation from which escape is deemed impossible. Fear of specific objects is fairly common, and the diagnosis of specific phobia is not made unless the fear significantly interferes with functioning or causes marked distress.

Careful assessment differentiates simple phobia from other diagnoses with overlapping symptoms. Blood injection injury–type phobia merits special consideration here because the phobia is fairly common across all health care settings. Before beginning a procedure, nurses should routinely ask whether the person has had any prior difficulty and should continue to monitor the person closely during and afterwards. The physiologic processes exhibited during phobic exposure to a procedure or treatment (e.g., needle poke, suturing) includes a strong vasovagal response, which significantly increases blood pressure and pulse, followed by the deceleration of the pulse and lowering of blood pressure in the patient. About 40% of medical students reported fainting in relation to blood donation (Ganzeboom, Colman, Reitsma, Shen, & Wieling, 2003). Factors that predispose individuals to specific phobias include prior traumatic events; unexpected panic attacks in the presence of the phobic object or situation; observation of others experiencing a trauma; or repeated exposure to information warning of dangers, such as parents' repeatedly warning young children that dogs bite.

Charles Darwin (1809–1882)
Theory of Evolution

Public Persona

Charles Darwin, credited as the first scientist to gain wide acceptance of the theory of natural selection, might never have published his 1859 seminal work, *Origin of the Species by Means of Natural Selection,* had it not been for his psychiatric illness. Born in England, Charles Darwin, the grandson of a famous poet, inventor, and physician, was expected to accomplish great things. However, his childhood years were troublesome. When he was sent to Cambridge to study medicine, card playing and drinking became his main activities. After meeting a botanist, however, his life changed and he embarked on a 5-year expedition to the Pacific Coast of South America.

Personal Realities

Darwin described his sensation of fear, accompanied by troubled beating of the heart, sweat, and trembling of muscles. Thought to have PD, he constantly worried about what he thought he knew until he finally published his ideas on paper. He died in 1882 and was buried in Westminster Abbey.

Source: Darwin, C. (1887). *The life and letters of Charles Darwin.* New York: Appleton & Co.

AETIOLOGIC THEORIES OF ANXIETY DISORDERS

There are many similarities and overlaps among aetiologic theories of the various anxiety disorders, and the various theories are not mutually exclusive.

Genetic Theories

Genetic aetiologic theories of anxiety disorders focus on genetic vulnerabilities that increase anxiety sensitivity, childhood maltreatment, environmental stressors, and dysregulations of neurotransmitter systems or the neural circuits that underpin fear and **fear conditioning** (Cassidy, Lichtenstein-Phelps, Sibrava, Thomas, & Borkovec, 2009; Jetty, Charney, & Goddard, 2001; Scherrer et al., 2000). One meta-analysis of genetic studies of anxiety disorders found that genes account for 30% to 40% of the risk for PD and that the risk for first-degree relatives was five times that of the general population (Hettema et al., 2001). If a family member manifests PD before age 20, the risk for PD in family members jumps to 20 times that of the general population (APA, 2000). Groundbreaking findings linked a variation in the promoter region of the serotonin transporter gene to stress sensitivity (Lesch et al., 1996). This was considered a model of genetic susceptibility to mood and anxiety disorders. However, further research by others produced mixed results, more so for mood disorders than anxiety disorders, likely due to differences in how stress was measured (Caspi, Hariri, Holmes, Uher, & Moffitt, 2010). This area of research remains very active. For example, links have been shown between the serotonin transporter and specific brain enzyme polymorphisms and anxiety/rejection sensitivity in women (Enoch, Xu, Ferro, Harris, & Goldman, 2003; Melke et al., 2001). However, social conditioning may play a role in anxiety sensitivity or in overestimating the degree of threat, both of which may increase the risk to develop anxiety disorders. Mundo, Richter, Sam, Macciardi, and Kennedy (2000) discovered a link between the pathogenesis of OCD and the 5-HT$_{1D\beta}$ receptor gene. This discovery may lead to breakthroughs in pharmacologic treatments for OCD.

Neurobiology of Anxiety

The concept of learned associations provides a useful framework to understand the nature of emotional responsiveness and how anxiety can be manifested in our emotions, thoughts, and behaviour. Advances in research methods and neuroimaging techniques have also increased our understanding of the neurotransmitters and the regions of the brain involved in anxiety and specific anxiety disorders.

Fear conditioning is a type of learning during which an organism is conditioned to associate a neutral stimulus with an aversive one. Over time, the neutral stimulus elicits an automatic emotional response previously associated with the aversive one, and the individual is conditioned to respond with fear to what was once a neutral stimulus. The anxiety and fear response can further generalize to similar stimuli and become a pattern of response to stimuli that are tangentially similar to the original (e.g., a fear of dogs can generalize to all furry animals). This has led to the belief that anxiety disorders reflect an exaggeration of the normal fear response. Extinction (the gradual decrease in a conditioned fear response) can occur when repeated exposure to the conditioned stimulus does not elicit an anxiety or fear response, although the memory is still there and can be reestablished to produce the fear response in the face of a similar threat. These dynamics partially explain the chronicity of anxiety disorders and have also shaped many of the current interventions and treatments for anxiety and anxiety disorders.

The major structures of the brain involved in fear conditioning are the hippocampus and the amygdala. The hippocampus is involved with memory acquisition and storage. Short-term memory is thought to be related to enhancement of glutamate neurotransmission, while longer-term memory is considered to be the result of long-term synaptic potentiation, a process whereby synaptic activity is enhanced by increased gene expression and protein synthesis. The amygdala is a crucial area for encoding and storing fearful memories. Studies using functional magnetic resonance imaging (MRI) have shown increased amygdalar activity during associative learning (pairing stimuli with previously experienced stimuli and the prior emotional responses).

The Role of Neurotransmitters and Neuropeptides

Norepinephrine is implicated in anxiety disorders because of its effects on the systems associated with the physical sensations of anxiety—the cardiovascular, respiratory, and gastrointestinal systems via stimulation of the sympathetic arm of the autonomic nervous system. Cell bodies of norepinephrine neurons in the brain are located in the locus coeruleus, which is one of the internal regulators of sleep and alertness. Electrical stimulation of the locus coeruleus in monkeys increases fear and anxiety. Despite the relationship between this neurotransmitter and the physical symptoms of anxiety, specific norepinephrine-based drug therapies have proven to have limited efficacy for anxiety disorders. Serotonin [5-hydroxytryptamine (5-HT)] is indirectly implicated in the aetiology of anxiety disorders in that drugs that facilitate serotonergic neurotransmission are effective in treating anxiety and panic symptoms. Although various theories of how serotonin is involved in fear conditioning and anxiety disorders have been suggested but not fully elucidated (Stein & Stahl, 2000), it is clear that selective serotonin reuptake inhibitors (SSRIs) and selective serotonin and norepinephrine reuptake inhibitors are efficacious treatments.

Gamma-aminobutyric acid (GABA) is the most abundant inhibitory neurotransmitter in the brain. Very small GABA neurons (interneurons) affect the firing rates of neurons distributed throughout the brain, which explains why GABA has such pervasive effects within the brain. Although a direct role of GABA in fear conditioning or anxiety disorders has yet to be clearly demonstrated, drugs that enhance GABA neurotransmission are commonly used to treat anxiety symptoms during the day and to help with sleep disturbance that often accompanies significant anxiety.

Corticotropin-releasing hormone (CRH) is a neuropeptide and hormone found in many areas of the brain; it is the initial hormone released from the hypothalamus that activates one of the major stress response systems, the hypothalamic–pituitary–adrenal (HPA) axis. CRH receptors are widely distributed in the hypothalamus, as well as brain regions associated with fear and fear conditioning. Activation of the HPA axis results from many stimuli, including perception of threat, and increases arousal, attention to environmental cues, and glucose availability to skeletal muscles to promote survival responses like "fight or flight." Cortisol, the final output of the HPA axis in humans, is significantly elevated during panic attacks (Bandelow et al., 2000). Increasing levels of cortisol act as negative feedback to decrease further release of CRH; however, many other neurotransmitters and neuropeptides help regulate the HPA axis. CRH receptor antagonists were suggested as a mechanism to treat anxiety, but no drugs based on this mechanism are currently on the market.

Cholecystokinin (CCK) became a neuropeptide of interest when administered in challenge tests; CCK induces panic attacks in patients with PD and, to a much lesser degree, in people without PD (Bradwejn et al., 1992). High concentrations of CCK are found in the cerebral cortex, amygdala, and hippocampus—areas implicated in fear and stress responses. Although specific CCK_B receptor antagonists would be a potential treatment mechanism, these compounds did not show sufficient efficacy to be marketed. Other neurochemicals have been associated with anxiety, including growth hormone (GH), female sex hormones, arginine vasopressin (AVP), and oxytocin (OT). In healthy subjects, stimulating α-adrenergic receptors elevates GH. This process is blunted in individuals with PD (Sallee, Sethuraman, Sine, & Liu, 2000). Neuroactive steroids, including the various metabolites of progesterone, have been implicated in the development of panic attacks (Ströhle et al., 2003). AVP and OT help regulate the activity of the HPA axis in a gender-specific fashion, with AVP being able to stimulate the axis independent of CRH and OT decreasing further release of CRH, thus dampening down HPA axis activity. Indeed, OT has been central to two gender-specific theories of stress responses in women (Seng, 2010; Taylor, 2006).

Neuroimaging Data Related to Specific Anxiety Disorders

The increasing sophistication of neuroimaging techniques has enabled researchers to better understand the physiology of anxiety and the involved neural network or circuits. Most neuroimaging work related to anxiety disorders has focused on PD. No anatomical differences were found between healthy controls and those with PD (Engel, Bandelow, Gruber, & Wedekind, 2009). However, positron emission tomography (PET) studies have demonstrated consistent increases in blood supply or glucose uptake (indicators of increased neuronal activity) in the amygdala of those with PD, GAD, or social anxiety disorder (Etkin & Wager, 2007; Sakai et al., 2005; Tillfors, Furmark, Marteinsdottir, & Fredrikson, 2002). Functional MRI studies also showed abnormal activation patterns in response to provocation paradigms. Consistent findings across neuroimaging studies have led to a consensus that there is a close relationship between the prefrontal cortex and amygdala. The amygdala is activated when an individual is confronted with a novel or fearful situation. Learning from experience that a stressor can be coped with, is under control, or no longer requires attention is termed "emotional processing" and is associated with specific regions of the prefrontal cortex (Engel et al.). However, cumulative data suggest a distinction between two classes of anxiety disorders. Those disorders involving intense fear and panic (PD and specific phobias) seem to be characterized by hypoactivity of distinct prefrontal cortex areas, thus disinhibiting the amygdala.

Disorders that involve worry and rumination, such as GAD or cognitions of negative consequences in social anxiety disorder, seem to be more associated with hyperactivity of the prefrontal cortex (Engel et al.; Hermann et al., 2007; Schienle, Schäfer, Hermann, Rohrmann, & Vaitl, 2007).

Structural neuroimaging studies using computed axial tomography and MRI have revealed that a group of children with *Streptococcus*-associated OCD and/or tics have enlarged basal ganglia (caudate, putamen, and globus pallidus) compared to healthy children (Giedd, Rapaport, Garvey, Perlmutter, & Swedo, 2000). Basal ganglial structures are important in the control of fine motor movement. PET studies have also demonstrated increased activity in basal ganglion structures, the cingulate and prefrontal cortex (Baxter, 1992; Perani et al., 1995; Rauch et al., 1994).

Psychodynamic Theories

Psychodynamic theories focus on the psychological influences on human behaviour, feelings, and emotions and how these relate to early life experience. A particular contribution of psychodynamic theories to the understanding of anxiety disorders is their emphasis on the importance of the development of anxiety after separation and loss. Patients with anxiety disorders report greater numbers and severity of recent personal losses at symptom onset than do healthy controls. For example, one study of the background and personality traits of individuals with PD found the following commonalities: reports of being fearful or shy as a child; remembering their parents as angry, critical, or frightening; having feelings of discomfort with aggression; having long-term feelings of low self-esteem; and experiencing a stressful life event associated with frustration and resentment that preceded the initial onset of symptoms (Shear, Cooper, Klerman, Busch, & Shapiro, 1993). The researchers proposed that a child may possess a neurophysiologic vulnerability that predisposes him or her to fearfulness. This fearfulness is enhanced by disturbed parent–child relationships, which in turn causes the child to feel conflict about dependence and independence (separating from parents), self-doubt, and confusion regarding self-identity and personal control. These negative feelings of low self-esteem and powerlessness make the child feel extremely vulnerable to the stress of normal life events, such as going to school, getting married, or becoming a parent. The longer the child attempts to ignore these negative feelings and feels powerless to control them, the longer he or she continues to experience distress in response to stressful events. The chronic, intense fear and dread culminate in the first panic attack. However, similar dynamics can also explain the emergence of depression. Factors that determine the specific clinical presentation and health outcomes related to chronic childhood psychological problems remain elusive.

Nursing Management of Significant Anxiety Symptoms and Specific Anxiety Disorders

As indicated previously, primary anxiety disorders are usually treated in primary care settings, in outpatient clinics, or by private practitioners. Hospitalization is limited to acute exacerbation of anxiety or panic symptoms or comorbid depressive disorder not responsive to antidepressant drug therapy. That being said, significant anxiety and GAD are also very common among individuals with chronic physical health conditions such as cardiovascular problems, and assessment of anxiety should be part of the overall chronic disease management.

Assessment within a bio/psycho/social/spiritual framework is the foundation of multimodal care. Physiologic symptoms tend to be the impetus for patients to seek health care. Often, persons with PD are initially seen in emergency rooms, as they seek treatment for their panic attack. Biologic, psychological, social, and spiritual assessments unveil potential contributing factors and identify sources of strength that can guide the nurse to develop an individual action plan.

Biologic Domain

Assessment

Once it is determined that anxiety symptoms have led to significant impairment in occupational, social, and interpersonal functioning, the nurse should assess for any potential environmental triggers and obtain a detailed history of any previous similar experiences. Questions to ask the patient might include the following:

• What did you experience preceding and during times of increased anxiety or a panic attack, including physical symptoms, feelings, and thoughts?—Have you ever experienced some of these symptoms before? If so, under what circumstances?

• Has anyone in your family ever had similar experiences?

• What do you do when you have these experiences that help you to feel less anxious?

• What has helped you in the past to manage your symptoms?

Substance Use

Assessment for panicogenic substance use, such as sources of caffeine, pseudoephedrine, amphetamines, cocaine, or other stimulants, may rule out contributory issues either related or unrelated to PD. Patients with anxiety disorders may use alcohol to self-treat their symptoms. Details of typical alcohol use are an important part of the assessment.

Sleep Patterns

Sleep is often disturbed in patients with anxiety disorders. Panic attacks can occur during sleep, and the patient may fear sleep for this reason. Nurses should closely assess the impact of sleep disturbance as it can increase the risk of further panic attacks and the development of major depressive disorder.

Interventions for Biologic Domain

These interventions can assist individuals with either severe anxiety or panic symptoms.

Physical Activity

Interventions that focus on the physical aspects of anxiety and panic are particularly helpful in reducing the number and severity of the attacks, giving patients an increasing sense of accomplishment and control. Routine leisure walking can create time for reappraisal and reflection of triggering stimuli. Active participation in an exercise program may help individuals reassess automatic thinking that relates increased heart rate and shortness of breath with a physical crisis. Physical activity can also improve sleep.

Breathing Control

Hyperventilation is common. Often, people are unaware that they take rapid, shallow breaths when they become anxious. Other common sensations are choking and pressure on the chest, restricting normal breathing. Teaching breathing control is a simple intervention that has immediate results. Begin by encouraging the person to simply observe the rate, pattern, and depth of his or her breathing. Next, invite the person to perform the following abdominal or diaphragmatic breathing exercise:

- Sit in an upright position, feet flat on the floor, and arms supported on the side-arms of a chair or on your lap. (Rationale: This position increases the capacity of the lungs to fill with air and for the limbs to be comfortably supported.)
- Place your hand on your abdomen, slightly above your umbilicus (bellybutton).
- Inhale slowly through the nose to the count of four and feel your abdomen rise.
- Exhale slowly through the mouth to the count of six and feel your abdomen fall.
- As you exhale, feel all of your muscles relax and let go.
- Repeat a series of 10 slow abdominal breaths, followed by 30 seconds of normal breathing for 3 to 5 minutes.

Abdominal breathing may also be used to interrupt an episode of panic as it begins. Once individuals have learned to identify their own early signs of panic, they can use abdominal breathing to divert or decrease the severity of the attack.

Nutrition Planning

Patients need to work towards reducing and eventually eliminating stimulants such as caffeine from their diet. Many over-the-counter (OTC) remedies, especially the "energy drinks" used to boost energy or increase mental performance, have high levels of caffeine. The nurse should also assess for other potential sources of stimulants, such as some cold remedies and herbal products, and provide information about substitutes.

Relaxation Techniques

Teaching the patient relaxation techniques is another way to help with anxiety and anxiety disorders. Many individuals are unaware of the tension they carry in their bodies and first need to learn to monitor their own tension. Isometric exercises and progressive muscle relaxation are helpful methods to learn to differentiate muscle tension from muscle relaxation. This method of relaxation is also helpful when individuals have difficulty clearing the mind, focusing, or visualizing a scene, which are often required in other forms of relaxation such as meditation. Box 23-3 provides one method of progressive muscle relaxation.

BOX 23-3 Progressive Muscle Relaxation

Choose a quiet, comfortable location where you will not be disturbed for 20 to 30 minutes. Your position may be lying or sitting, but all parts of your body should be supported, including your head. Wear loose clothing and remove restrictive items such as glasses and shoes.

Begin by closing your eyes and clearing your mind. Moving from head to toe, focus on each part of your body and assess the level of tension. Visualize each group of muscles as heavy and relaxed.

Take two or three slow abdominal breaths, pausing briefly between each breath. Imagine the tension flowing from your body.

Each muscle group listed below should be tightened (or tensed isometrically) for 5 to 10 seconds and then abruptly released; visualize this group of muscles as heavy, limp, and relaxed for 15 to 20 seconds before tightening the next group of muscles. There are several methods to tighten each muscle group, and suggestions are provided below. Each muscle group may be tightened two to three times until relaxed. Do not over tighten or strain. You should not experience pain.

- Hands (tighten by making fists)
- Biceps (tighten by drawing forearms up and "making a muscle")
- Triceps (extend forearms straight, locking elbows)
- Face (grimace, tightly shutting mouth and eyes; open mouth wide and raise eyebrows)
- Neck (pull head forward to chest and tighten neck muscles)
- Shoulders (raise shoulders towards ears; push shoulders back as if touching them together)
- Chest (take a deep breath and hold for 10 seconds)
- Stomach (suck in your abdominal muscles)
- Buttocks (pull buttocks together)
- Thighs (straighten your legs and squeeze the muscles in thighs and hips)
- Leg calves (pull toes carefully towards you, avoid cramps)
- Feet (curl toes downwards and point toes away from your body)

Finally, repeat several deep abdominal breaths and mentally check your body for tension. Rest comfortably for several minutes, breathing normally, and visualize your body as warm and relaxed. Get up slowly when you are finished.

Pharmacotherapy for Anxiety and Anxiety Disorders

As mentioned previously, there are known neurotransmitter systems associated with anxiety and anxiety disorders, but not all of these associations have led to specific drug therapies. For example, drugs such as propranolol act primarily on β-adrenergic receptors and reduce the peripheral symptoms of anxiety, but they have limited effectiveness against anxiety or panic symptoms.

Serotonin-Selective and Norepinephrine- and Serotonin-Selective Reuptake Inhibitors (SSRIs and NSSRIs)

The SSRIs and NSSRIs are generally considered the first-line long-term treatment for most anxiety disorders (Bereza, Machado, Ravindran, & Einarson, 2012; Fineberg, Brown, Reghunandan, & Pampaloni, 2012; Ipser, Stein, Hawkridge, & Hoppe, 2010). Because of side effects and dietary restrictions, monoamine oxidase inhibitor antidepressants generally are only used when all other options are exhausted. Specific phobias are not generally treated with SSRIs or NSSRIs. **Anxiolytics** (antianxiety agents) may give short-term relief of phobic anxiety, but there is no evidence that they affect the course of the disorder. The treatment of choice for specific phobia is **exposure therapy** (Newman, Erickson, Przeworski, & Dzus, 2003).

The initial increase in serotonergic activity from serotonin reuptake blockade may cause temporary increases in anxiety symptoms and even panic attacks, but this is usually short-lived and can be minimized by lower starting doses (Brauer, Nowicki, Catalano, & Catalano, 2002). Full clinical response is usually seen by 4 to 6 weeks of treatment.

Administering and Monitoring Selective Reuptake inhibitors.

Overall, SSRIs produce fewer side effects than do other drugs, are safer to use, and are not lethal in the event of overdose. Details regarding these two classes of antidepressants can be found in Chapter 12.

Tricyclic Antidepressant Therapy

Like the SSRIs and the NSSRIs, the TCAs imipramine (Tofranil), nortriptyline (Pamelor), and clomipramine (Anafranil) reduce anxiety and panic symptoms, through their inhibition of serotonin and norepinephrine reuptake. However, this class of drugs also interacts with many more neurotransmitter systems, and these drugs carry with them significant side effects. Thus, they are usually only considered in the event that SSRIs or NSSRIs have failed to produce remission of symptoms. Details regarding this class of antidepressants can be found in Chapter 12.

Benzodiazepine Therapy

All benzodiazepines produce anxiolytic action, and their therapeutic onset is much faster (hours, not weeks) than that of antidepressants. Therefore, benzodiazepines are tremendously useful in treating intensely distressed patients. However, evidence to support their use in long-term treatment of anxiety disorder is limited (Ipser et al., 2010). Alprazolam (Xanax), lorazepam (Ativan), and clonazepam (Rivotril) are widely used for anxiety disorders. They are well tolerated but carry the risk for withdrawal symptoms like rebound anxiety and sleep disturbance upon discontinuation of use.

Administering and Monitoring Benzodiazepines.

Treatment may include administering benzodiazepines concurrently with antidepressants for the first 4 weeks and then tapering off the benzodiazepine. This strategy provides rapid symptom relief but avoids the complications of long-term benzodiazepine use. Details regarding this class of drugs can be found in Chapter 12. Short-acting benzodiazepines, such as alprazolam and lorazepam, are associated with rebound anxiety, or anxiety that increases after the peak effects of the medication have decreased. Medications with short half-lives should be given in three or four small doses spaced throughout the day, with a higher dose at bedtime to allay anxiety-related insomnia. Clonazepam, a longer-acting benzodiazepine, requires less frequent dosing and has a lower risk for rebound anxiety. Rebound anxiety and insomnia are also common with higher dosing regimens and the abrupt cessation of benzodiazepine treatment. Benzodiazepines should be used with extreme caution to treat anxiety in the elderly due to significantly increasing the risk of falls and anterograde memory difficulties, which can be misinterpreted as signs of dementia (Bogunovic & Greenfield, 2004).

● **STUDY NOTE**

Serotonin-selective and norepinephrine- and serotonin-selective reuptake inhibitors are the first line of treatment for anxiety disorders. Benzodiazepines are effective but should only be used for short periods of time for acute anxiety and sleep disturbance.

Psychological Domain

Assessment

A complete psychological assessment is necessary to determine patterns of anxiety, characteristic symptoms, and the person's emotional, cognitive, and behavioural responses (see Chapter 10). A comprehensive assessment includes overall mental status, suicidal tendencies and thoughts, cognitive thought patterns, avoidance behaviour patterns, and any comorbid depression symptoms. The patient's perceptions regarding his or her symptoms are discussed, as well as present and past coping strategies.

Self-Report Scales

Self-evaluation can be difficult in anxiety disorders, especially in PD. Specific triggers are often no longer

BOX 23-4 Rating Scales for Assessment of Panic Disorder and Anxiety Disorders

Panic Symptoms

Panic-Associated Symptom Scale (PASS; Argyle et al., 1991)

Acute Panic Inventory (Dillon, Gorman, Liebowitz, Fyer, & Klein, 1987)

National Institute of Mental Health Panic Questionnaire (NIMH PQ; Scupi, Maser, & Uhde, 1992)

Cognitions

Anxiety Sensitivity Index (Reiss, Peterson, & Gursky, 1986)

Agoraphobia Cognitions Questionnaire (Chambless, Caputo, Bright, & Gallagher, 1984)

Body Sensations Questionnaire (Chambless et al., 1984)

Phobias

Mobility Inventory for Agoraphobia (Chambless, Caputo, Jasin, Gracely, & Williams, 1985)

Fear Questionnaire (Marks & Matthews, 1979)

Anxiety

State-Trait Anxiety Inventory (STAI; Spielberger, Gorsuch, & Luchene, 1976)

Penn State Worry Questionnaire (PSWQ; Meyer et al., 1990)

Beck Anxiety Inventory (Beck, Epstein, Brown, & Steer, 1988)

present or have generalized so that it is difficult to be aware of subtle associations that increase symptoms. Those with PD live in fear of another panic attack with little sense of being able to control the attacks. Several tools are available to characterize and rate the patient's state of anxiety. Examples of these symptom and behavioural rating scales are provided in Box 23-4. All of these tools are self-report measures and, as such, are limited by the individual's self-awareness and openness. However, the Hamilton Rating Scale for Anxiety (HAM-A), provided in Table 23-3, is an example of a scale rated by the clinician (Hamilton, 1959). This 14-item scale reflects both psychological and somatic aspects of anxiety.

Assessment of Thought Patterns

Catastrophic misinterpretations of trivial physical symptoms can trigger intense anxiety and panic symptoms. Once identified, these thoughts should serve as a basis for individualizing patient education to counter such false beliefs. Table 23-4 presents an example of a scale to assess catastrophic misinterpretations of

Table 23-3   Hamilton Rating Scale for Anxiety

Hamilton (1959) designed this scale to help clinicians gather information about states of anxiety. The symptom inventory provides scaled information that classifies anxiety behaviour and assists the clinician in targeting behaviours and achieving outcome measures. Provide a rating for each indicator based on the following scale:

| **0** = None | **1** = Mild | **2** = Moderate |
| **3** = Severe | **4** = Severe, grossly disabling | |

Item	Symptoms	Rating
Anxious mood	Worries, anticipation of the worst, fearful anticipation, irritability	
Tension	Feelings of tension, fatigability, startle response, moved to tears easily, trembling, feelings of restlessness, inability to relax	
Fear	Fear of dark, strangers, being left alone, animals, traffic, crowds	
Insomnia	Difficulty falling asleep, broken sleep, unsatisfying sleep and fatigue on waking, dreams, nightmares, night terrors	
Intellectual (cognitive)	Difficulty concentrating, poor memory	
Depressed mood	Loss of interest, lack of pleasure in hobbies, depression, early waking, diurnal swings	
Somatic (sensory)	Tinnitus, blurred vision, hot and cold flushes, feelings of weakness, picking sensation	
Somatic (muscular)	Aches and pains, twitching, stiffness, myoclonic jerks, grinding of teeth, unsteady voice, increased muscular tone	
Cardiovascular symptoms	Tachycardia, palpitations, chest pain, throbbing of vessels, fainting feelings, heart missing beat	
Respiratory symptoms	Pressure or constriction in chest, choking feelings, sighing, dyspnea	
Gastrointestinal symptoms	Difficulty swallowing, wind, abdominal pain, burning sensation, abdominal fullness, nausea, vomiting, borborygmi (stomach rumbling), looseness of bowels, loss of weight, constipation	
Genitourinary symptoms	Frequent micturition, urgent micturition, amenorrhea, menorrhagic, development of frigidity, premature ejaculation, loss of libido, impotence	
Autonomic symptoms	Dry mouth, flushing, pallor, tendency to sweat, giddiness, tension headache, raising of hair	
Behaviour at interview	Fidgeting, restlessness or pacing, tremor of hands, furrowed brow, strained face, sighing or rapid respiration, facial pallor, swallowing, belching, brisk tendon jerks, dilated pupils, exophthalmos	

From Hamilton, M. (1959). The assessment of anxiety states by rating. *British Journal of Medical Psychology, 32,* 54.

Table 23-4	Panic Attack Cognition Questionnaire

Rate each of the following thoughts according to the degree to which you believe each thought contributes to your panic attack.

1 = Not at all   **2** = Somewhat
3 = Quite a lot   **4** = Very much

Thought	Rating
I'm going to die.	
I'm going insane.	
I'm losing control.	
This will never end.	
I'm really scared.	
I'm having a heart attack.	
I'm going to pass out.	
I don't know what people will think.	
I won't be able to get out of here.	
I don't understand what is happening to me.	
People will think I'm crazy.	
I'll always be this way.	
I am going to throw up.	
I must have a brain tumour.	
I'll choke to death.	
I'm going to act foolish.	
I'm going blind.	
I'll hurt someone.	
I'm going to have a stroke.	
I'm going to scream.	
I'm going to babble or talk funny.	
I'll be paralyzed by fear.	
Something is physically wrong with me.	
I won't be able to breathe.	
Something terrible will happen.	
I'm going to make a scene.	

Adapted from Clum, G. A. (1990). Panic attack cognitions questionnaire. In *Coping with panic: A drug-free approach to dealing with anxiety attacks.* Pacific Grove, CA: Brooks/Cole.

the symptoms of panic. Several studies have found that individuals who feel a sense of control have fewer severe panic attacks. Individuals who fear loss of control during a panic attack often make the following types of statements:

- "I feel trapped."
- "I'm afraid others will know, or I'll hurt someone."
- "I feel alone. I can't help myself."
- "I'm losing control."

Such individuals also tend to show low self-esteem, feelings of helplessness, demoralization, and overwhelming fears of experiencing panic attacks. They may have difficulty with assertiveness or expressing feelings.

Interventions and Therapies Within the Psychological Domain

Current clinical guidelines for the treatment of anxiety disorders suggest that either pharmacotherapy or specific psychotherapies can be efficacious and, in the short term, a combination of both modes of therapy can be superior to

one or the other (Baldwin & Polkinghorn, 2005). Nurses working in outpatient settings can assist individuals to identify triggers and eventually learn to manage their responses.

Peplau (1989) was one of the first to develop guidelines for nursing interventions for treating individuals experiencing problems with anxiety. These interventions help the person attend to and react to input other than the subjective experience of anxiety. Although Peplau's work is almost 25 years old, many of the interventions she described are still relevant today (see Table 23-5). Box 23-5 offers a comparison of effective and ineffective dialogue with a person with an anxiety disorder.

Distraction

Once individuals can identify the early symptoms of panic, they can learn to use **distraction** behaviours to shift their attention away from the uncomfortable physical sensations. Distraction activities include initiating a conversation with a nearby person and engaging in a physical activity (e.g., walking, gardening, house cleaning). Performing simple, repetitive activities such as snapping

Table 23-5 **Nursing Interventions Based on Degrees of Anxiety**

Degree of Anxiety	Nursing Interventions
Mild	Learning is possible. The nurse assists the patient to use the energy that anxiety provides to encourage learning.
Moderate	The nurse needs to check his or her own anxiety so that the patient does not empathize with it. Encourage the patient to talk: to focus on one experience, to describe it fully, then to formulate the patient's generalizations about that experience.
Severe	Learning is less possible. Allow relief behaviours to be used but do not ask about them. Encourage the patient to talk: ventilation of random ideas is likely to reduce anxiety to a moderate level. When this is observed by the nurse, proceed as above.
Panic	Learning is impossible. The nurse needs to stay with the patient. Allow pacing and walk with the patient. No content inputs to the patient's thinking should be made by the nurse. (They burden the patient, who will distort them.) Pick up on what the patient says, for example, Pt: "What's happening to me—how did I get here?" N: "Say what you notice." Short phrases by the nurse—direct, to the point of the patient's comment, and investigative—match the current attention span of the patient in panic and therefore are more likely to be heard, grasped, and acted on, with the patient's responses gradually reducing the anxiety in a helpful way. Do not touch the patient; patients experiencing panic are very concerned about survival, are experiencing grave threat to self, and usually distort intentions of all invasions of their personal space.

Adapted from Peplau, H. (1989). Theoretical constructs: Anxiety, self, and hallucinations. In A. O'Toole & S. Welt (Eds.), *Interpersonal theory in nursing practice: Selected works of Hildegard E. Peplau.* New York: Springer.

BOX 23-5 Therapeutic Dialogue

PANIC DISORDER WITH AGORAPHOBIA

Mark, a 55-year-old Caucasian man, was admitted 4 days ago to the psychiatric unit with exacerbation of anxiety symptoms and panic attacks during the last 3 weeks. He has a 30-year history of uncontrolled anxiety that is refractory to medications and psychotherapies. On admission, he stated that he feels suicidal at times because he thinks that his life is not within his control. He feels embarrassed, angry, and "trapped" by his disorder. During the past 24 hours, Mark is seen crying at times; he also isolates himself in his room. Michelle, Mark's nurse, enters his room to make a supportive contact and to assess his current mental status.

Ineffective Approach

Nurse: Oh…. Why are you crying?

Patient: (Looks up, gives a nervous chuckle) Obviously, because I'm upset. I am tired of living this way. I just want to be normal again. I can't even remember what that feels like.

Nurse: You look normal to me. Everyone has bad days. It'll pass.

Patient: I've felt this way longer than you've been alive. I've tried everything and nothing works.

Nurse: You're not the first depressed person that I've taken care of. You just need to go to groups and stay out of your room more. You'll start feeling better.

Patient: (Angrily) Oh, it's just that easy. You have no idea what I'm going through! You don't know me! You're just a kid.

Nurse: I can help you if you help yourself. A group starts in 5 minutes, and I'd like to see you there.

Patient: I'm not going to no damn group! I want to be alone so I can think!

Nurse: (Looks about anxiously) Maybe I should come back after you've calmed down a little.

Effective Approach

Nurse: Mark, I noticed that you are staying in your room more today. What's troubling you?

Patient: (Looks up) I feel like I've lost complete control of my life. I'm so anxious and nothing helps. I'm tired of it.

Nurse: I see. That must be difficult. Can you tell me more about what you are feeling right now?

Patient: I feel like I'm going crazy. I worry all the time about having panic attacks. They make me scared I'm going to die. Sometimes I think I'd be better off dead.

Nurse: (Remains silent, continues to give eye contact)

Patient: Do you know what it's like to be a prisoner to your emotions? I can't even go out of the house sometimes, and when I do, it's terrifying. I don't know what to think anymore.

Nurse: Mark, you have lived with this disorder for a long time. You say that the medications do not work to your liking, but what has helped you in the past?

Patient: Well, I learned in relaxation group that panic symptoms are probably caused by chemicals in my brain that are not working correctly. I learned that medications can help, but they don't work well for me. I tried an exposure plan and relaxation techniques to deal with my fears of leaving the house and my chronic anxiety. That did help some, but it's scary to do.

Nurse: It sounds like you have learned much about your illness, one that can be treated, so that you don't always have to feel this way.

Patient: This is easier to say right now when I'm here and can get help if I need it. It's hard to remember this when I'm in the middle of a panic attack and think I'm dying.

Nurse: It's harder when you're alone?

Patient: Much harder! And I'm alone so much of the time.

Nurse: Let's talk about some ways you can manage your panics when you're alone. Tell me some of the techniques you've learned.

Critical Thinking Challenge

- What tone is established by the nurse's opening question in the first scenario?
- Which therapeutic communication techniques did the nurse use in the second scenario to avoid the pitfalls encountered in the first scenario?
- What information was uncovered in the second scenario that was not touched on in the first?
- What predictions can you make about the interpersonal relationship likely to develop between the nurse and the patient in each scenario?

a rubber band against the wrist, counting backwards from 100 by threes, and counting objects along the roadway are other strategies for deterring an attack.

Positive Self-Talk

During states of increased anxiety and panic, individuals can learn to counter frightening or negative thoughts with positive coping statements, also called **positive self-talk**. Examples of positive self-talk include "This is only anxiety and it will pass"; "I can handle these symptoms"; and "I'll get through this." These positive statements are most effective when they are grounded in truth, because they offer the individual a focal point and challenge fear-provoking thoughts (e.g., "I am going to die," or "I can't handle this"). Some individuals carry positive statements written on a small card in their purse or wallet or on a handheld device. These messages can quickly be retrieved and read at the onset of panic symptoms.

Cognitive–Behavioural Therapy

Cognitive–behavioural therapy (CBT) is a model of psychotherapy developed in the late 1950s and is highly effective for treating severe anxiety, GAD, PD, and social anxiety disorder. It is also an effective treatment for depression, sleep problems, chronic pain, and eating disorders. In randomized clinical trials, CBT is as effective as an SSRI in the treatment of anxiety (Kampman, Keijsers, Hoogduin, & Hendriks, 2002). In the absence of depression, CBT is often recommended as the first line of treatment, depending on accessibility and acceptability to the patient, and appropriate when symptoms are mild to moderate in severity (Khouzam, 2009). There is evidence that individuals prefer psychological interventions such as CBT to medication, and psychosocial interventions are first-line treatment for children, adolescents, and pregnant and breast-feeding women (Khouzam, 2009). Although CBT principles are applied in many different situations, the basic principles are simple and remain constant (Burns, 1999): (1) Thoughts, feelings, behaviours (actions, choices), and body sensations affect each other. (2) Because thoughts, feelings, behaviours (actions, choices), and body sensations are connected, even small changes in one area can affect the others. (3) CBT focuses on events and situations in the "here and now" and does not try to understand how or where they began. (4) CBT encourages self-awareness. And (5) CBT emphasizes learning and practising new skills (homework).

CBT is a highly effective approach for treating severe anxiety, GAD, PD, and social anxiety disorder. The goal of CBT is to help individuals manage their anxiety by challenging anxiety-provoking thoughts. CBT strategies include psychoeducation, self-monitoring, cognitive restructuring, and somatic exercises. CBT is offered to individuals and groups and over a 12- to 20-week period, although longer treatment may be necessary to maintain an initial response. (See Chapter 13, *Cognitive–Behavioural Interventions*.)

Exposure therapy is the treatment of choice for agoraphobia, specific phobias, and OCD. The patient is repeatedly exposed increasingly complex and real or simulated anxiety-provoking situations until he or she becomes desensitized and anxiety subsides. **Systematic desensitization**, another exposure method used to desensitize patients, exposes the patient to a hierarchy of feared situations that the patient has rated from least to most feared. The patient is taught to use muscle relaxation as levels of anxiety increase through multisituational exposure. Planning and implementing exposure therapy require special training. Because of the multitude of outpatients in treatment for agoraphobia, exposure therapy would be a useful tool for home health psychiatric nurses. Outcomes of home-based exposure treatment are similar to clinic-based treatment outcomes.

Psychoeducation programs help to educate patients and families about the symptoms of anxiety and panic. Individuals with PD legitimately fear "going crazy," losing control, or dying because of their physical symptoms. Attempting to convince a patient that such fears are groundless only heightens anxiety and impedes communication. Information and physical evidence, such as electrocardiogram results and laboratory test results, should be presented in a caring and open manner that demonstrates acceptance and understanding of the patient's situation.

Box 23-6 suggests topics for individual or small-group discussion. It is especially important to cover such topics as the differences between panic attacks and heart attacks, the difference between PD and other psychiatric disorders, and the effectiveness of various treatment methods.

● STUDY NOTE

CBT is the first-line psychotherapy for anxiety disorders and has been shown to be effective within a group format or individually. Self-help manuals based on CBT principles and online structured modules have also been shown to be effective.

BOX 23-6 Psychoeducation Checklist

When caring for the patient with anxiety disorders, be sure to include the following topic areas in the teaching plan:
- Psychopharmacologic agents (anxiolytics or antidepressants) if ordered, including drug action, dosage, frequency, and possible adverse effects
- Breathing control measures
- Potential dietary triggers
- Exercise
- Progressive muscle relaxation
- Distraction behaviours
- Relevant psychotherapies and where they are available
- Time and specific stress management strategies
- Positive coping strategies

Social and Occupational Domains

Individuals with anxiety disorders often deteriorate socially as the disorder takes its toll on relationships with family and friends. Occupational success and work satisfaction are often compromised. If the disorder becomes severe enough, the person may become completely isolated. Therefore, it is an important area for assessment and active intervention if necessary.

Assessment

During the assessment, the nurse needs to assess the patient's understanding of how the anxiety or panic symptoms and associated avoidance behaviours have affected his or her social and work life along with that of the family. Pertinent questions include the following:

- How has the disorder affected your family's social life?
- How has the disorder affected your work and work–life balance?
- What limitations related to travel has the disorder placed on you or your family?
- What coping strategies have you used to manage the symptoms?
- How has the disorder affected your family members or others? (Fig. 23-1)

Cultural Factors

Cultural competence calls for the understanding of cultural knowledge, cultural awareness, cultural assessment skills, and cultural practice. Therefore, cultural differences must be considered in the assessment of anxiety disorders. Different cultures interpret anxiety-related sensations, feelings, or understandings differently. "Nervousness" may be more accepted by some cultural groups, and several cultures do not have a word to describe "anxiety" or to denote "anxiousness" but instead may use words or meanings to suggest somatic complaints. In addition, showing anxiety may be a sign of weakness in some cultures (Chen, Reich, & Chung, 2002). Many Asian OTC herbal remedies contain substances that may increase anxiety or induce panic by increasing the heart rate, basal metabolic rate, blood pressure, and sweating (Chen et al.). Diet pills and ginseng are two examples.

Interventions for Social and Occupational Domains

Individuals with anxiety disorders, especially those with significant anxiety sensitivity, may need assistance in reevaluating their lifestyle. Casual comments by friends or coworkers can be misinterpreted or overinterpreted and be triggers for intense anxiety or panic symptoms. Time management can be a useful tool. In the workplace or at home, underestimating the time needed to complete

FIGURE 23-1. Bio/psycho/social/spiritual interventions for patients with panic disorder.

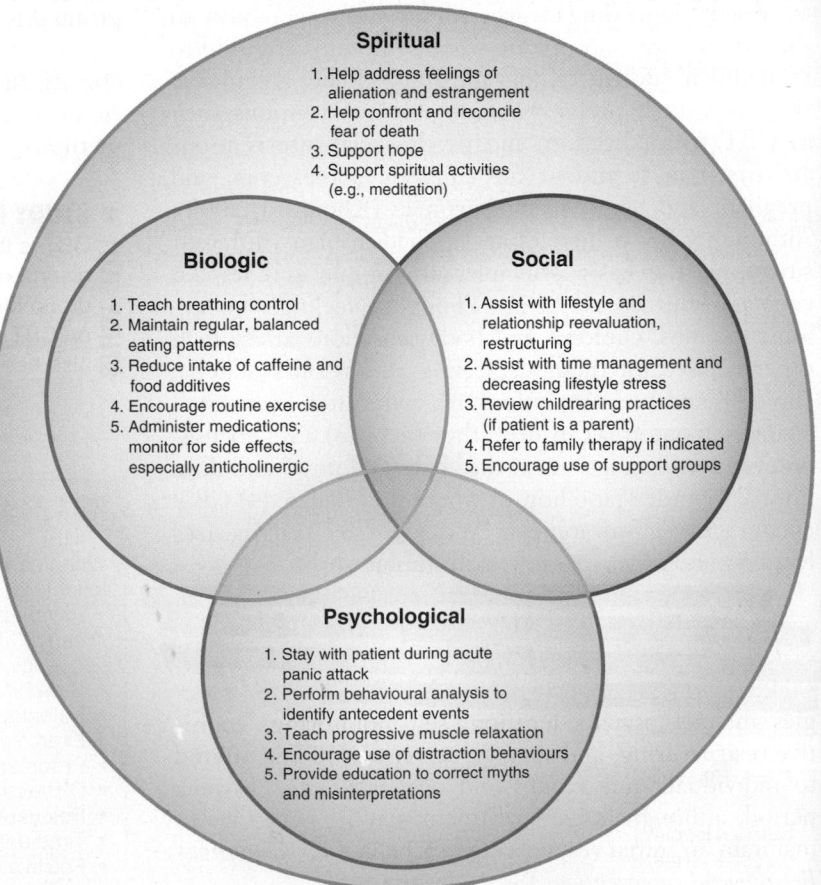

a chore or being overly involved in several activities at once increases stress and anxiety. Procrastination, lack of assertiveness, and difficulties with prioritizing or delegating tasks intensify these problems.

Writing a list of chores to be completed and estimating the time needed to complete them provide concrete feedback to the individual. Crossing-out each activity as it is completed helps the patient to regain a sense of control and accomplishment. Large tasks should be broken into a series of smaller tasks to minimize stress and maximize a sense of achievement. Rest, relaxation, and family time—frequently omitted from the daily schedule—must be included.

Family Response to Anxiety Disorders

Affected families often have difficulty with overall communication. Parents with agoraphobia may become discouraged and self-critical regarding their child-rearing abilities, which may cause their children to be overly dependent. Parents with PD may inadvertently cause excessive fears, phobias, or excessive worry in their children. Family members may get frustrated with the chronic nature of anxiety disorders and show irritation when anxiety symptoms are exacerbated by acute stressors.

Pregnancy can increase anxiety symptoms for women who have preexisting anxiety disorders. Assessment of mood and anxiety symptoms both in the antepartum and the postpartum period, as well as available resources to manage such symptoms, should be part of routine maternity care.

Spiritual Domain

Anxiety can be understood as basic to the human condition. Existentialist thinkers (see Box 23-7) argue that, because we humans are aware of our own mortality, the apprehension that death will end our existence fills us with foreboding. This **existential anxiety** must be accepted and faced, or it can subvert our everyday life. We can feel alienated and estranged (not at home) in the world. We look to find

meaning in our lives, a *raison d'etre*. Existentialists note that, as neither nature nor culture can do this for us, individual humans are, in a sense, self-making. Frankl (1992), in *Man's Search for Meaning*, wrote about how it is every human's wish to have a meaningful life (see Chapter 8 for logotherapy).

Tillich (1952), the author of *The Courage to Be* and a theistic existentialist, finds that existential anxiety involves three areas of apprehension: fate and death (the absolute threat to self), emptiness and meaninglessness (worry that there is no ultimate meaning), and guilt and condemnation (perceived threats to one's identity). Being human involves confronting and reconciling such anxiety.

Researchers are exploring the importance of understanding the relation between existential anxiety and clinical anxiety. The existential anxiety scale (EAS) has been developed, for instance, based on Tillich's theory (Weems, Costa, Dehon, & Berman, 2004). Early results suggest that existential anxiety, as measured by the EAS, is common and associated with symptoms of anxiety and depression (Weems et al.). In a critical review of the literature, Koslander, Barbosa da Silva, and Roxberg (2009) concluded that "it is evident that addressing patients' existential and spiritual needs helps them improve mentally" (p. 40). They argue that an existential perspective should be an element of mental health care.

■ EVALUATION AND TREATMENT OUTCOMES

Patients can be assisted to keep a daily log of the severity of anxiety and the frequency, duration, and severity of anxiety symptoms and panic episodes. This log will be a basic tool for monitoring progress as symptoms decrease. A number of self-help books can provide a rich source of reinforcement of simple interventions that can attenuate the intensity and frequency of panic symptoms. Rating scales may also be helpful to monitor changes in misinterpretations or other symptoms related to panic. Figure 23-2 illustrates a number of examples of bio/psycho/social/spiritual treatment outcomes for individuals with PD.

■ CONTINUUM OF CARE

As with any disorder, the continuum of patient care across multiple settings is crucial. Individuals are treated in the least restrictive environment that will meet their safety needs.

Inpatient Care

Inpatient settings provide care and treatment for individuals experiencing severe anxiety with comorbid depression, increased risk of suicide, or poor treatment response to typical treatment strategies.

BOX 23-7 Some "Existentialist" Thinkers and an Example of Their Work

Søren Kierkegaard — *Either Or: A Fragment of a Life* (1843/1944)
Friedrich Nietzsche — *Thus Spoke Zarathustra* (1883/1985)
Martin Heidegger — *Being and Time* (1927/1962)
Karl Jaspers — *On My Philosophy* (1941/1955)
Gabriel Marcel — *The Mystery of Being* (1951)
Jean-Paul Sartre — *Being and Nothingness* (1943/1956)
Simone de Beauvoir — *The Second Sex* (1949/1953)
Henrik Ibsen — *A Doll's House* (1879/1889)
Albert Camus — *The Myth of Sisyphus* (1942/1955)
Fyodor Dostoevsky — *Notes from the Underground* (1864/1918)
Samuel Beckett — *Waiting for Godot* (1953/1955)
Eugène Ionesco — *The Chairs* (1952/1958)

EMERGENCY CARE !

Because individuals with PD are likely to first present for treatment in an emergency room or primary care setting, nurses working in these settings should be involved in early recognition and referral. Consultation with a psychiatrist or mental health professional by the primary care physician can decrease both costs and overall patient symptoms (Katon, Roy-Byrne, Russo, & Cowley, 2002). Several interventions may be useful in reducing the number of emergency room visits related to panic symptoms. Psychiatric consultation and patient teaching can be provided in the emergency department, including the following:

- Stay with the person and maintain a calm demeanour. (Rationale: Anxiety often produces more anxiety, and a calm presence will help calm the patient.)

- Reassure the patient that you will not leave, that this episode will pass, and that he or she is in a safe place. (Rationale: A person experiencing a panic episode often fears dying and cannot see beyond the panic attack.)

- Give clear, concise directions, using short sentences. Do not use medical jargon. (Rationale: A person in the throes of panic is in crisis and has difficulty shifting focus away from his or her internal experience.)

- Walk or pace with the patient to an environment with minimal stimulation. (Rationale: Activity can help an individual focus excessive energy.)

- Administer PRN anxiolytic medications as ordered and appropriate. (Rationale: Benzodiazepines are effective in treating acute panic.)

After the panic attack has resolved, allow the patient to vent his or her feelings. Using a shared decision-making process, ensure a plan for follow-up is in place.

Family Interventions

The entire family will need support in adjusting to the disorder. A referral for family therapy may be indicated. Children with OCD living in families who are highly accepting of obsessive thoughts and compulsive behaviours have poorer treatment outcomes and a more chronic course (Garcia et al., 2010). Involving the entire family in the therapy process is imperative. Families experience the symptoms, treatments, clinical setbacks, and recovery from chronic anxiety and panic as a unit. Misunderstandings, misconceptions, false information, and stigma of mental illness, singly or collectively, impede recovery efforts.

FIGURE 23-2. Bio/psycho/social/spiritual outcomes for patients with PD.

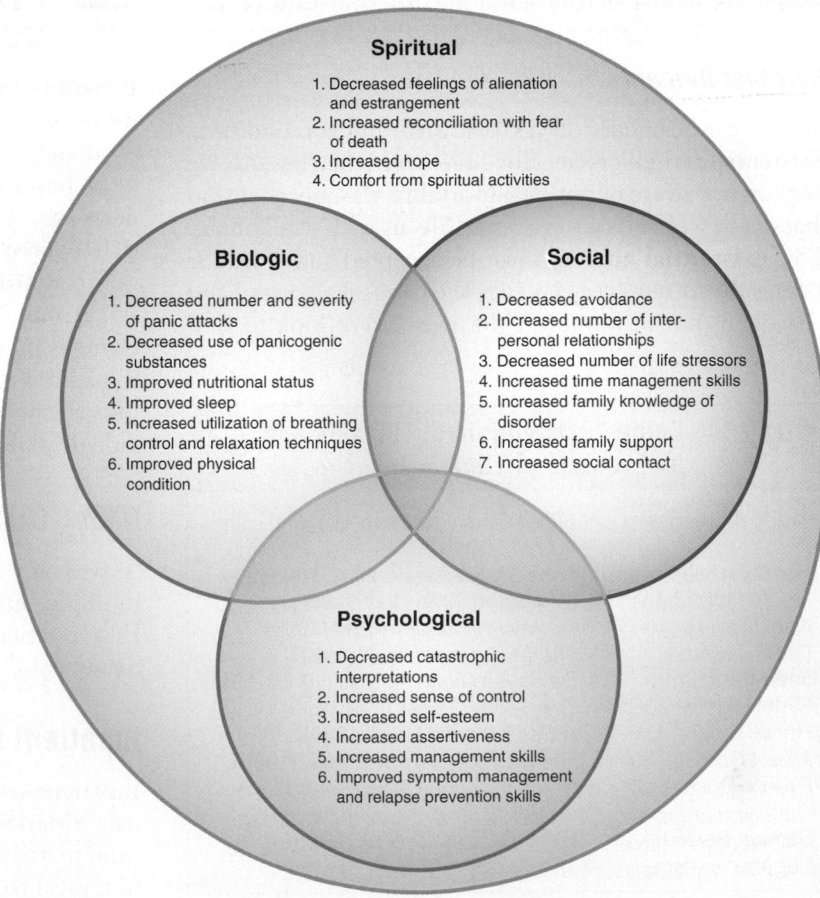

Community Treatment

Most individuals with anxiety disorders will be treated on an outpatient basis, and it is important that nurses who work in these settings have access to up-to-date lists of community resources and support groups. In outpatient or primary care settings, nurses are directly involved in treatment, conducting psychoeducation groups on relaxation and breathing techniques, and teaching symptom management. Advanced practice nurses conduct CBT and individual and family psychotherapies.

■ ASSESSMENT AND TREATMENT ISSUES SPECIFIC TO OBSESSIVE– COMPULSIVE DISORDER

Symptoms of OCD can be difficult to treat because of the pathology of the disorder, and individuals diagnosed with OCD are treated in specific outpatient programs. Short-term hospitalization may be necessary for treatment of comorbid depression and for treatment refractory symptoms. When this occurs, it is important to have a clear plan of care and to ensure that all staff members follow it consistently (Box 23-8).

Individuals with OCD do not consider their compulsions pleasurable. Often, they recognize them as odd and may initially try to resist them. Resistance eventually fails, and patients incorporate repetitive behaviours into daily routines, performing activities in a specific, ritual order. If this sequence is disturbed, the person experiences extreme anxiety until the process can be repeated in the

correct sequence. Interpersonal relationships suffer, and the patient may actively isolate himself or herself. Indeed, individuals with OCD are more likely to be young, separated or divorced, and unemployed.

Assessment

The nurse should assess the type and severity of the patient's obsessions and compulsions. Most individuals will appear neatly dressed and groomed, cooperative, and eager to answer questions. Orientation and memory are not usually impaired, but these individuals may be distracted by obsessional thoughts. Individuals with severe symptoms may be preoccupied with fears or with discussing their obsessions, but in most instances, direct questions must be asked to reveal symptoms. For example, the nurse may begin indirectly by asking how long it takes the individual to dress in the morning or leave the house, but usually follow-up questions are needed, such as "Do you find yourself frequently returning to the house to make sure that you have turned off the lights or the stove, even when you know that you have already checked this?" "Does this happen every day?" "Are you ever late for work or for important appointments?"

Although individuals with OCD do not have a higher prevalence of physical disease, some may report multiple physical symptoms. In patients with late-onset OCD (after 35 years of age) or in children who develop symptoms after a febrile illness, cerebral pathology should be excluded. Patients whose compulsions involve washing should be checked for dermatologic lesions caused by repetitive hand washing, excessive cleaning with caustic agents, or bathing. Osteoarthritic joint damage secondary to cleaning rituals may also be observed.

Identifying the degree to which the OCD symptoms interfere with the patient's daily functioning is important. Several rating scales can be used to identify symptoms and monitor improvement. Examples of these scales are provided in Box 23-9. The Yale-Brown Obsessive–Compulsive Scale (Y-BOCS) is a popular, clinician-rated 16-item scale that obtains separate subtotals for the severity of obsessions and compulsions. The Maudsley Obsessive–Compulsive Inventory is a 30-item, true–false, self-assessment tool that may help the individual to recognize individual symptoms.

BOX 23-8 Clinical Vignette

OBSESSIVE–COMPULSIVE DISORDER

Robert, a 32-year-old man, is a new patient at a local psychiatric unit. He admitted himself to have his medicines evaluated because his obsessive thoughts and depression have worsened since his recent divorce. While in the hospital, he has quickly become viewed as a "problem patient" because he hoards linens and demands a new bar of soap for each of his five daily showers. He is compelled to open and close his door five times when he leaves or enters his room but does not know why. This behaviour has led to arguments with his roommate. In an effort to "help him," the staff locked his bathroom door to prevent him from showering so frequently. He tried to enter his bathroom to shower and panicked when the staff refused to allow him to shower, telling him "You can live without it." After receiving PRN medication for extreme anxiety, Robert signed out of the hospital against medical advice because of embarrassment and anger towards the nursing staff.

What Do You Think?
- How could the staff have handled the situation differently in order not to disrupt Robert's or the unit's clinical care?
- What nursing interventions might be appropriate in providing Robert's care?

BOX 23-9 Rating Scales for Assessing Obsessive–Compulsive Symptoms

Yale-Brown Obsessive–Compulsive Scale (Y-BOCS; Goodman et al., 1989)
The Maudsley Obsessional–Compulsive Inventory (MOC; Rachman & Hodgson, 1980)
The Leyton Obsessional Inventory (Cooper, 1970)

Nurses must consider sociocultural factors when evaluating OCD. At times, cultural or religious beliefs may be misunderstood and mistaken for obsessions or compulsions. Shame and embarrassment over the irrational thoughts and behaviours often lead to social isolation and relational difficulties. The time demands related to the compulsions often lead to decreased occupational success. Assessment of current level of functioning in social, occupational, and personal spheres is therefore important.

Family Response to Disorder

Individuals whose OCD symptoms are severe are more likely to demonstrate social skill deficits and have more difficulties with intimacy; consequently, they are less likely to marry. Some studies have also shown higher divorce rates for individuals with OCD (Grabe et al., 2000). They also have higher rates of celibacy, possibly because they fear being dirty or becoming contaminated.

OCD often diminishes the quality of family relationships. Individuals with this disorder may ask family members to become involved in their rituals of checking or providing repeated reassurance (Koran, 2000). Those with OCD can become very angry and frustrated with family members for failing to comply with their requests for help with rituals. This can result in verbal and even physical altercations. Many family members find themselves modifying routines to suit a patient's symptoms and report this to be at least moderately distressing for them (Calvocoressi et al., 1999). The most troublesome symptoms of OCD for families to cope with include the patients' ruminations, long-standing unemployment, rituals, noncompliance with medication, depression, withdrawal from social and family contact, lack of motivation, and excessive arguing (Cooper, 1996). Spouses report a variety of issues such as sexual difficulties, overwhelming feelings of frustration, anger, guilt, and fatigue, and disrupted family and social life. Other relatives reported moderate to severe burden in coping with an individual with OCD. They stated that they had difficulty going on holidays, had poor social relationships, and neglected their hobbies due to their relative's illness (Magliano, Tosini, Guarneri, Marasco, & Catapano, 1996).

Treatment

Specific clinical pharmacotherapy reviews for OCD support that long-term SSRIs are the first-line treatment of choice (Eddy, Dutra, Bradley, & Westen, 2004; Fineberg et al., 2012). Although extremely rare, psychosurgery has been used to treat extremely severe OCD that has not responded to prolonged and intensive drug treatment, behavioural therapy, or a combination of the two. Modern stereotactic surgical techniques that produce lesions of the cingulum (a bundle of connective pathways between the two hemispheres) or the anterior limb of the internal capsule (a region near the thalamus and part of the circuit connecting to the cortex) may bring about substantial clinical benefit in some patients without causing significant morbidity (Kim et al., 2003). Other treatment options include radiotherapy and deep brain stimulation in which electrical current is applied through an electrode inserted into the brain (Nuttin, Cosyn, Demeulemeester, Gybels, & Meyerson, 1999).

For the patient with cleaning or handwashing compulsions, attention to skin condition is necessary. Encourage the patient to use tepid water when washing and hand cream after washing. Remove harsh, abrasive soaps and replace with moisturizing soaps. The treatment team would work with the patient to decrease the frequency of washing by structuring time schedules and time-limited washing.

Specific Psychotherapeutic Interventions for OCD

An effective behavioural intervention for patients with OCD who perform rituals is exposure with response prevention (ERP). During ERP, the person is exposed to situations or objects that are known to induce anxiety but is asked to refrain from performing the ritualistic behaviours. One goal of this procedure is to help the patient understand that resisting the rituals while exposed to the object of anxiety is less stressful and time consuming than performing the rituals. Another goal is to confound the expectation of distressing outcomes and eventually extinguish the compulsive behaviours. Cognitive restructuring is another intervention to teach the patient to restructure dysfunctional thought processes by defining and testing them (Beck, Emery, & Greenberg, 1985). Its goal is to alter the patient's immediate, dysfunctional appraisal of a situation and perception of long-term consequences. CBT has also been used extensively in the treatment of OCD. Eddy and colleagues (2004) reviewed the evidence supporting these three types of interventions in the literature. The effects sizes were similar across the three types, with about two thirds of those that completed the whole course of treatment improved. However, only one third met recovery criteria, adding support to the difficulty in obtaining full remission. In their summary, they concluded that ERP had the strongest evidence and that individual therapy is superior to group therapy.

Community Treatment

Partial hospitalization programs and day treatment programs care for most patients with OCD. They allow patients to maintain significant independence, while beginning medications and behavioural therapies. Specific day treatment psychotherapy programs for OCD are available in some larger urban centres. Specific outpatient clinics may also be available. Self-help groups and self-help books can also help patients keep their symptoms under control.

SUMMARY OF KEY POINTS

■ Anxiety-related disorders are the most common of all psychiatric disorders and significantly impair individuals' social and occupational function.

■ The anxiety disorders are a family of disorders that share excessive fear or anxiety as their core symptom; specific anxiety disorders differ from one another according their key feature(s)

■ Significant anxiety and anxiety disorders are seen across all practice settings and along the continuum of care.

■ Although anxiety can be a primary diagnosis, it is more often comorbid with other psychiatric disorders (e.g., depression, schizophrenia) and/or physical illnesses (e.g., coronary artery disease, irritable bowel disease).

■ Those experiencing anxiety disorders have high levels of physical and emotional symptoms and often experience dual diagnoses with other anxiety disorders, substance use disorder, or depression. These disorders often significantly impair individuals' ability to function socially, occupationally, and personally.

■ Treatment approaches for all anxiety-related disorders include pharmacotherapies, psychological treatments, or often a combination of both.

■ Current research points to a combination of biologic, psychological, social, and spiritual factors that cause persistent anxiety. Other research demonstrates that there are also personality traits that predispose individuals to anxiety disorders, including low self-esteem, external locus of control, some negative family influences, and some traumatic or stressful precipitating event. These components combine to yield a true bio/psycho/social/spiritual theory of causation.

■ Nurses employ interventions from each of the dimensions—biologic, psychological, social, and spiritual—in the care of persons experiencing anxiety. Approaching these individuals with knowledge of the disorders, understanding, and calm is crucial. Nurses can be instrumental in crisis intervention, medication management, and psychoeducation. Psychoeducation is crucial in the management of anxiety disorders and includes methods to help patients understand and manage anxiety symptoms (e.g., diaphragmatic breathing, stress reduction, relaxation techniques), education regarding medication side effects and management, and education of family members to understand these disorders.

CRITICAL THINKING CHALLENGES

1 How does culture affect the assessment of anxiety?
2 How might one differentiate shyness from social anxiety disorder?

3 Explain why antidepressant medications are used to treat both anxiety disorders and depression.

4 What are some of the barriers to assessing pathologic anxiety in children? Are anxiety disorders underdiagnosed or overdiagnosed in children? Explain.

5 Aside from genetics, what role might parents play in the development of anxiety disorders in their offspring?

6 What are the risks and benefits of treating anxiety disorders with benzodiazepine medications in individuals with substance abuse?

7 Pregnancy appears to protect against the development of some anxiety disorders, and postpartum onset of anxiety disorders is not uncommon. What bio/psycho/social/spiritual dynamics may be involved?

REFERENCES

American Psychiatric Association (APA). (2000). *Diagnostic and statistical manual of mental disorders* (4th ed., Text revision). Washington, DC: Author.

American Psychiatric Association (APA). (2013). *Diagnostic and statistical manual of mental disorders* (5th ed) Washington, DC: Author.

Antai-Otong, D. (2003). Current treatment of generalized anxiety disorder. *Journal of Psychosocial Nursing and Mental Health Services, 41*(12), 20–29.

Argyle, N., Deltito, J., Allerup, P., Maier, W., Albus, M., Nutzinger, D., ... Rasmussen, S. (1991). The Panic-Associated Symptom Scale: Measuring the severity of panic disorder. *Acta Psychiatrica Scandinavica, 83*, 20–26.

Baldwin, D. S. & Polkinghorn, C. (2005). Evidence-based pharmacotherapy of generalized anxiety disorder. *International Journal of Neuropsychopharmacology, 8*(2), 293–302.

Ballenger, J. C., Davidson, J. R., Lecrubier, Y., Nutt, D. J., Borkovec, T. D., Rickels K., ... Wittchen, H. U. (2001). Consensus statement on generalized anxiety disorder from the International Consensus Group on Depression and Anxiety. *Journal of Clinical Psychiatry, 62*(Suppl 11), 53–58.

Bandelow, B., Wedekind, D., Pauls, J., Brooks, A., Hajak, G., & Ruther, E. (2000). Salivary cortisol in panic attacks. *American Journal of Psychiatry, 157*, 454–456.

Barlow, D. H. (2002). *Anxiety and its disorders: The nature and treatment of anxiety and panic.* New York: Guilford Press.

Baxter, L. (1992). Neuroimaging studies of obsessive compulsive disorder. *Psychiatric Clinics of North America, 15*(4), 871–883.

Beck, A. T., Emery, C., & Greenberg, R. L. (1985). *Anxiety disorders and phobias: A cognitive perspective.* New York: Basic Books.

Beck, A. T., Epstein, N., Brown, G., & Steer, R. (1988). An inventory for measuring clinical anxiety: The Beck Anxiety Inventory. *Journal of Consulting and Clinical Psychology, 56*, 893–897.

Bereza, B. G., Machado, M., Ravindran, A. V., & Einarson, T. R. (2012). Evidence-based review of clinical outcomes of guideline-recommended pharmacotherapies for generalized anxiety disorder. *Canadian Journal of Psychiatry, 57*(8), 470–478.

Bernstein, G. A., Bernat, D. H., Davis, A. A., & Layne, A. E. (2008). Symptom presentation and classroom functioning in a nonclinical sample of children with social phobia. *Depression and Anxiety, 25*(9), 752–760.

Bland, R. C., Newman, S. C., & Orn, H. (1988). Period prevalence of psychiatric disorders in Edmonton. *Acta Psychiatrica Scandinavica, 338*(Suppl.), 33–42.

Bogunovic, O. J. & Greenfield, S. F. (2004). Practical geriatrics: Use of benzodiazepines among elderly patients. *Psychiatric Services, 55*(3), 233–235.

Borkovec, T. D., Robinson, E., Pruzinsky, T., & DePree, J. A. (1983). Preliminary exploration of worry: Some characteristics and processes. *Behaviour Research and Therapy, 21*(1), 9–16.

Bradwejn, J., Koszycki, D., du Tertre, A., Bourin, M., Palmour, R., & Ervin, F. (1992). The cholecystokinin hypothesis of panic and anxiety disorders: A review. *Journal of Psychopharmacology, 6*, 345–351.

Brauer, H., Nowicki, P., Catalano, G., & Catalano, M. (2002). Panic attacks associated with citalopram. *Southern Medical Journal, 95*(9), 1088–1089.

Burns, D. (1999). *Feeling good: The new mood therapy.* New York: Plume.

Calvocoressi, L., Mazure, C. M., Kasl, S. V., Skolnick, J., Fisk, D., Vegso, S. J., Van Noppen, B. L., & Price, L. H. (1999). Family accommodation of obsessive-compulsive symptoms: Instrument development and assessment of family behavior. *Journal of Nervous and Mental Disorders, 187*, 636–642.

Caspi, A., Hariri, A. R., Holmes, A., Uher, R., & Moffitt, T. E. (2010). Genetic sensitivity to the environment: The case of the serotonin transporter gene and its implications for studying complex diseases and traits. *American Journal of Psychiatry, 167*(5), 509–527.

Cassidy, J., Lichtenstein-Phelps, J., Sibrava, N. J., Thomas, C. L. Jr., & Borkovec, T. D. (2009). Generalized anxiety disorder: Connections with self-reported attachment. *Journal of Behavior Therapy and Experimental Psychiatry, 40*(1), 23–38.

Castellanos, D. & Hunter, T. (2000). Anxiety disorders in children and adolescents. *Southern Medical Journal, 92*(10), 946–954.

Chambless, D. L., Caputo, G. C., Bright, P., & Gallagher, R. (1984). Assessment of fear in agoraphobics: The Body Sensations Questionnaire and the Agoraphobic Cognitions Questionnaire. *Journal of Consulting and Clinical Psychology, 52*, 1090–1097.

Chambless, D. L., Caputo, G. C., Jasin, S. E., Gracely, E. J., & Williams, C. (1985). The Mobility Inventory for Agoraphobia. *Behaviour Research and Therapy, 23*, 35–44.

Chen, J-P., Reich, L., & Chung, H. (2002). Anxiety disorders. *Western Journal of Medicine, 176*(4), 249–253.

Clum, G. A. (1990). Panic attack cognitions questionnaire. In *Coping with panic: A drug-free approach to dealing with anxiety attacks.* Pacific Grove, CA: Brooks/Cole.

Cooper, J. (1970). The Leyton Obsessional Inventory. *Psychiatric Medicine, 1*, 48.

Cooper, M. (1996). Obsessive-compulsive disorder: Effects on family members. *American Journal of Orthopsychiatry, 66*, 296–304.

Critchley, H. (2003). Emotion and its disorders. *British Medical Bulletin, 65*, 35–47.

Dalrymple, K. L. & Zimmerman, M. (2011). Age of onset of comorbid social anxiety disorder in depressed outpatients. *Journal of Anxiety Disorders, 25*, 131–137.

Darwin, C. (1887). *The life and letters of Charles Darwin.* New York: Appleton & Co.

Dillon, D. J., Gorman, J. M., Liebowitz, M. R., Fyer, A. J., & Klein, D. F. (1987). Measurement of lactate-induced panic and anxiety. *Psychiatry Research, 20*, 97–105.

Eddy, K. T., Dutra, L., Bradley, R., & Westen, D. (2004). A multidimensional meta-analysis of psychotherapy and pharmacotherapy for obsessive-compulsive disorder. *Clinical Psychology Review, 24*, 1011–1030.

Engel, K., Bandelow, B., Gruber, O., & Wedekind, D. (2009). Neuroimaging in anxiety disorders. *Journal of Neural Transmission, 116*(6), 703–716.

Enoch, M. A., Xu, K., Ferro, E., Harris, C. R., & Goldman, D. (2003). Genetic origins of anxiety in women: A role for a functional catechol-O-methyltransferase polymorphism. *Psychiatric Genetics, 13*(1), 33–41.

Etkin, A. & Wager, T. D. (2007). Functional neuroimaging of anxiety: A meta-analysis of emotional processing in PTSD, social anxiety disorder, and specific phobia. *American Journal of Psychiatry, 164*(10), 1476–1488.

Faravelli, C., Guerinni Degl'Innocenti, B. G., Giardinelli, L. (1989). Epidemiology of anxiety disorders in Florence. *Acta Psychiatrica Scandinavica, 79*, 308–312.

Farrell, L. & Boschen, M. J. (2011). Treatment outcome in adult OCD: Predictors and processes of change. *Asia Pacific Journal of Counselling and Psychotherapy, 2*, 82–97.

Fineberg, N. A., Brown, A., Reghunandan, S., & Pampaloni, I. (2012). Evidence-based pharmacotherapy of obsessive-compulsive disorder. *International Journal of Neuropsychopharmacology, 9*, 1–19.

Fineberg, N. A., Hengartner, M. P., Bergbaum, C., Gale, T., Rössler, W., & Angst, J. (2013). Remission of obsessive-compulsive disorders and syndromes: Evidence from a prospective community cohort study over 30 years. *International Journal of Psychiatry in Clinical Practice, 17*(3), 179–187.

Frankl, V. (1992). *Man's search for meaning: An introduction to logotherapy* (4th ed). Boston, MA: Beacon Press.

Ganzeboom, K. S., Colman, N., Reitsma, J. B., Shen, W. K., & Wieling, W. (2003). Prevalence and triggers of syncope in medical students. *American Journal of Cardiology, 91*, 1006–1008.

Garcia, A. B., Sapyta, J. J., Freeman, J. B., Franklin, M. E., March, J. S., & Foa, E. B. (2010). Predictors and moderators of treatment outcome in pediatric obsessive compulsive treatment study (POTS I). *Journal of the American Academy of Child and Adolescent Psychiatry, 7*(10), 1024–1033.

Giedd, J., Rapaport, J., Garvey, M., Perlmutter, S., & Swedo, S. (2000). MRI assessment of children with obsessive compulsive disorder or tics associated with streptococcal infection. *American Journal of Psychiatry, 157*(2), 281–283.

Goodman, W., Price, L., Rasmussen, S., Mazure, C., Fleischmann, R. L., & Hill, C. L., (1989). The Yale-Brown Obsessive Compulsive Scale (Y-BOCS): Part 1. Development, use and reliability. *Archives of General Psychiatry, 46*, 1006–1011.

Grabe, H. J., Meyer, C., Hapke, U., Rumpf, H-J., Freyberger, H. J., Dilling, H., & John, U. (2000). Prevalence, quality of life and psychosocial function in obsessive-compulsive disorder and subclinical obsessive-compulsive disorder in northern Germany. *European Archives of Psychiatry and Clinical Neuroscience, 250*, 262–268.

Hamilton, M. (1959). The assessment of anxiety states by rating. *British Journal of Medical Psychology, 32*, 54.

Hermann, A., Schafer, A., Walter, B., Stark, R., Vaitl, D., & Schienle, A. (2007). Diminished medial prefrontal cortex activity in blood–injection–injury phobia. *Biological Psychology, 75*, 124–130.

Hettema, J. M., Neale, M. C., & Kendler, K. S. (2001). A review and meta-analysis of the genetic epidemiology of anxiety disorders. *American Journal of Psychiatry, 158*(10), 1568–1578.

Hoffman, D. L., Dukes, E. M., & Wittchen, H. U. (2008). Human and economic burden of generalized anxiety disorder. *Depression and Anxiety, 25*(1), 72–90.

Hollander, E. (1997). Obsessive-compulsive disorder: The hidden epidemic. *Journal of Clinical Psychiatry, 58*, 3–6.

Ipser, J. C., Stein, D. J., Hawkridge, S., & Hoppe, L. (2010). Cochrane review: Pharmacotherapy for anxiety disorders in children and adolescents. *Evidence-Based Child Health: A Cochrane Review Journal, 5*(2), 555–628.

Jakubovski, E., Diniz, J. B., Valerio, C., Fossaluza, V., Belotto-Silva, C., Gorenstein, C., … Miguel, E. (2013). Clinical predictors of long-term outcome in obsessive-compulsive disorder. *Depression and Anxiety, 30*(8), 763–772.

Jetty, P. V., Charney, D. S., & Goddard, A. W. (2001). Neurobiology of generalized anxiety disorder. *Psychiatric Clinics of North America, 24*(1), 75–97.

Kampman, M., Keijsers, G., Hoogduin, C., & Hendriks, G. (2002). A randomized, double-blind, placebo-controlled study of the effects of adjunctive paroxetine in panic disorder patients unsuccessfully treated with cognitive-behavioural therapy alone. *Journal of Clinical Psychiatry, 63*(9), 772–777.

Katon, W., Roy-Byrne, P., Russo, J., & Cowley, D. (2002). Cost-effectiveness and cost offset of a collaborative care intervention for primary care patients with panic disorder. *Archives of General Psychiatry, 59*(12), 1098–1104.

Kessler, R. C. (2000). The epidemiology of pure and comorbid generalized anxiety disorder: a review and evaluation of recent research. *Acta psychiatrica Scandinavica Supplementum*, (406), 7–13.

Kessler, R. C., Chiu, W. T., Demler, O., Merikangas, K. R., & Walters, E. E. (2005). Prevalence, severity, and comorbidity of 12-month DSM-IV disorders in the National Comorbidity Survey Replication. *Archives of General Psychiatry, 62*(6), 617–627.

Kessler, R. C., Chiu, W. T., Jin, R., Ruscio, A. M., Shear, K., & Walters, E. E. (2006). The epidemiology of panic attacks, panic disorder, and agoraphobia in the National Comorbidity Survey Replication. *Archives of General Psychiatry, 63*(4), 415–424.

Kessler, R. C., Petukhova, M., Sampson, N. A., Zaslavsky, A. M., & Wittchen, H. U. (2012). Twelve-month and lifetime prevalence and lifetime morbid risk of anxiety and mood disorders in the United States. *International Journal of Methods in Psychiatric Research, 21*(3), 169–184.

Khouzam, H. R. (2009). Anxiety disorders: Guidelines for effective primary care, part 2, treatment. *Consultant, 49*(4), 1–2.

Kim, C. H., Chang, J. W., Koo, M. S., Kim, J. W., Suh, H. S., Park, I. H., & Lee, H. S. (2003). Anterior cingulotomy for refractory obsessive-compulsive disorder. *Acta Psychiatrica Scandinavica, 107*(4), 241–243.

King, N. J., Ollendick, T. H., & Mattis, S. G. (1994). Panic in children and adolescents: Normative and clinical studies. *Australian Psychologist, 29*(2), 89–93.

Kinley, D. J., Walker, J. R., Enns, M. W., & Sareen, J. (2011). Panic attacks as a risk for later psychopathology: Results from a nationally representative survey. *Depression and Anxiety, 28*(5), 412–419.

Koran, L. M. (2000). Quality of life in obsessive-compulsive disorder. *Psychiatric Clinics of North America, 23*, 509–517.

Koslander, T., Barbosa da Silva, A., & Roxberg, A. (2009). Existential and spiritual needs in mental health care: An ethical and holistic perspective. *Journal of Holistic Nursing, 27*(1), 34–42.

LeBeau, R. T., Glenn, D., Liao, B., Wittchen, H. U., Beesdo-Baum, K., Ollendick, T., & Craske, M. G. (2010). Specific phobia: A review of DSM-IV specific phobia and preliminary recommendations for DSM-V. *Depression and Anxiety, 27*(2), 148–167.

Lenze, E., Mulsant, B., Shear, M., Schulberg, H., Dew, M. A., Begley, A., … Pollock, B. (2000). Comorbid anxiety disorders in depressed elderly patients. *American Journal of Psychiatry, 157*(5), 722–728.

Lesch, K. P., Bengel, D., Heils, A., Sabol, S. Z., Greenberg, B. D., Petri, S., … Murphy, D. L. (1996). Association of anxiety-related traits with a polymorphism in the serotonin transporter gene regulatory region. *Science, 274*(5292), 1527–1531.

24 Somatic Symptom and Related Disorders

D. Stewart MacLennan
Adapted from the chapters "Somatoform and Related Disorders" by Mary Ann Boyd and L. Elizabeth Hood

LEARNING OBJECTIVES

After studying this chapter, you will be able to:

• Explain the concept of somatization and its occurrence in people with mental health problems.

• Discuss epidemiologic factors related to somatic problems.

• Compare the etiologic theories of somatic symptom and related disorders from a bio/psycho/social/spiritual perspective.

• Contrast the major differences between somatic symptoms and factitious disorders.

• Discuss human responses to somatic symptom and related disorders.

• Apply the elements of nursing management to a patient with somatic symptom and related disorders.

KEY TERMS

• factitious disorder • malingering • pseudoneurologic symptoms
• psychosomatic • somatic symptom disorder

The connection between the mind and the body has been hypothesized and described for centuries. The term **psychosomatic** describes conditions in which a psychological state contributes to the development of physical illness. For example, "broken heart syndrome" or takotsubo cardiomyopathy causes the heart to enlarge and pump poorly in response to very stressful situations (such as the death of a loved one). In contrast, the term *somatization* is used when unexplained physical symptoms occur in the presence of psychological distress or psychiatric illness. This chapter explores the concept of somatization and explains the care of patients experiencing somatic symptom disorders.

Although somatization is common in many psychiatric disorders, including depression, anxiety, and psychosis, it is the *primary* symptom of somatic symptom and related disorders. Somatic symptom and related disorders occur when a person experiences physical symptoms causing psychological distress or abnormal patterns of thought. The prevalence of somatic symptom and related disorders in general practice is approximately 23%, often occurring comorbidly with anxiety or depressive disorders (Steinbrecher, Koerber, Frieser, & Hiller, 2011). A **factitious disorder** is one in which the patient simulates or inflicts injury on himself or herself or others in order to receive medical treatment. Unlike other somatic symptom disorders, the physical symptoms in a factitious disorder are deliberately produced by the patient. Due to the complexity of somatization and controversy over diagnostic validity, the American Psychiatric Association made major changes to its formulation of somatic symptom and related disorders in the fifth edition of the *Diagnostic and Statistical Manual of Mental Disorders (DSM-5)*. Somatic symptom and related disorders are now clustered into six primary clinical syndromes:

1. Somatic symptom disorder
2. Illness anxiety disorder
3. Conversion disorder
4. Psychological factors affecting other medical conditions
5. Factitious disorder
6. Other specified somatic symptom and related disorders

This chapter presents the nursing care of patients experiencing somatic symptoms and related disorders. *Somatization* is explained in detail because it is the core symptom of all somatic symptom and related disorders.

> ◢ **Key Concept Somatization** is the term used when unexplained physical symptoms are present that are related to psychological distress or psychiatric illness.

■ SOMATIZATION

Anyone who feels the pain of a sore throat or the ache of influenza has a somatic symptom (from *soma*, meaning body). Somatization, however, occurs when a person has disturbed ways of feeling, thinking, and behaving when experiencing a distressing somatic symptom. In the current way of understanding somatization, the focus is on how an individual reacts to a somatic symptom rather than the previous focus, which was on the lack of explanatory medical diagnosis. This change has the following impact: (1) fewer inappropriate mental illness diagnoses in people coping well with unexplained somatic symptoms and (2) increased diagnosis and treatment of somatic symptom and related disorders among those responding abnormally to a medically explained somatic symptom.

With somatization, individuals typically develop a preoccupation, amplify, and seek medical care for the somatic symptoms. People who somatize view their personal problems in physical rather than psychosocial terms. For example, a woman quits her job complaining of being chronically tired instead of recognizing that she is emotionally distressed from a coworker's constant harassment.

■ SOMATIC SYMPTOM DISORDER

Somatic symptom disorder is a condition characterized by emotional distress and a disruption of daily living caused by one or more physical symptoms. In 2013, the American Psychiatric Association redefined this disorder by focusing on the distress caused by somatic symptoms. The fact that an individual is experiencing physical symptoms without medical explanation is no longer sufficient to establish this diagnosis.

Clinical Course

In somatic symptom disorder, patients have one or more clinically significant somatic concerns that may involve several body systems. Physical symptoms in somatic symptom disorder occur in all body systems, such as gastrointestinal (nausea, vomiting, diarrhoea), neurologic (headache, backache), or musculoskeletal (aching legs). The physical symptom, which may be present all the time or may come and go, will typically last 6 months or longer. These individuals perceive themselves as being "sicker than sick" and report all aspects of their health as poor. They often

cannot work or take part in routine activities of daily living. Since no medical explanation of the symptom can be identified, these individuals often become frustrated with primary health care providers. Consequently, they seek opinions from many health care providers until they find one who will give them new medication, hospitalize them, or perform surgery. People with somatic symptom disorder sometimes cause frustration among health care providers. Clinicians need to recognize their feelings and deal with them in a constructive way. This may include discussing their feelings with a clinical supervisor.

Because a psychiatric diagnosis of somatic symptom disorder is made only after numerous unexplained physical problems, psychiatric and mental health (PMH) nurses do not usually care for these individuals early in the disorder; rather, these patients are more likely to have been encountered initially by nurses in primary care and medical–surgical settings.

> ● **STUDY NOTE**
> Individuals with somatic symptom disorder will seek health care from multiple providers but often avoid mental health specialists.

Diagnostic Criteria

The diagnosis is made when there is an abnormal response to a somatic symptom. Table 24-1 lists the key diagnostic criteria and target symptoms of somatic symptom disorder. A significant complaint is one that received medical treatment or for which the symptoms cause impairment in social, occupational, or other areas of functioning (APA, 2013).

Somatic Symptom Disorder in Special Populations

Evidence suggests that this disorder occurs in all populations and cultures. However, the type and frequency of somatic symptoms may differ across cultures.

Children

Although many children experience unexplained symptoms, somatic symptom disorder is not usually diagnosed until adolescence. Children often present with headaches, fatigue, and abdominal complaints for which they may miss school and/or for which their parents will seek medical opinions (APA, 2013). Greater than 50% of children with depression and 41% with anxiety are believed to experience somatic symptoms (Romero-Acosta et al., 2013).

Older Adults

While somatic symptom disorder occurs in the older adult, new onset of somatic symptoms in late life warrants a thorough investigation for hidden medical or psychiatric

Table 24-1	Diagnosis of Somatic Symptom Disorder

A. One or more somatic symptoms causing disruption in activities of daily life and significant distress
B. Excessive thoughts, feeling, or behaviours related to the somatic symptoms or associated health concerns as manifested by at least one of the following:
  a. Persistent and exaggerated thoughts about the seriousness of the symptom.
  b. High anxiety with respect to a symptom.
  c. Persistent and excessive time focusing on the symptom.
C. Although any one somatic symptom may not be continuously present, the state of being symptomatic is persistent (usually more than 6 months).
	Specify if:
	With predominant pain
	Persistent: characterized by severe symptoms, marked impairment, and long duration (more than 6 months)
	Severity:
	Mild: Only two or more of the symptoms specified in Criterion B are fulfilled.
	Moderate: Two or more of the symptoms specified in Criterion B are fulfilled.
	Severe: Two or more of the symptoms specified in Criterion B are fulfilled, plus there are multiple somatic complaints (or one very severe somatic symptom).

American Psychiatric Association. (2013). *Diagnostic and statistical manual of mental disorders* (5th ed) (p. 311). Washington, DC: Author.

disorders. Subjective lack of well-being (never feeling good), rather than objective health measures, may be an indicator of somatization (Schneider et al., 2003). In the older adult, somatic symptoms can represent many things, such as depression or bereavement.

Epidemiology

The prevalence of somatic symptom disorder, as it is currently defined, has yet to be studied. The APA (2013) estimates this disorder to occur in approximately 5% to 7% of the adult population.

Age of Onset

Although children may experience somatic symptoms, the diagnosis of somatic symptom disorder is usually delayed until adolescence (Lieb et al., 2002). Previous age restrictions pertaining to somatoform disorders, found in earlier versions of the *Diagnostic and Statistical Manual of Mental Disorders*, have been removed.

Gender, Ethnic, and Cultural Differences

Females experience somatic symptom disorder at a higher rate than do males (Bener, Ghuloum, & Burgut, 2010). The actual somatic experience appears to be different in men than in women. Researchers looking at gender differences in reporting symptoms found that women were

more likely to be diversified somatizers, who have frequent, brief sickness with a variety of complaints. Early research in this area found that men were more likely to be aesthenic somatizers, with fewer diverse complaints but who were more chronically disabled by fatigue, weakness, or common minor illnesses (Kroenke & Spitzer, 1998).

The rates and forms of somatization vary across cultural groups. Norms, values, perceptions, and expectations about illness and wellness are culturally based. In cultures where great stigma towards mental illness exists, the expression of psychological distress can occur through physical symptoms. In Iranian culture, for instance, somatization (primarily pain) is a central feature of clinical depression (Firoozabadi, Bahredar, & Seifsafari, 2013). Cultural differences also influence how nurses recognize and manage somatization.

Despite cultural and ethnic differences, the comorbidity of depression and somatic symptoms is consistent around the world (APA, 2013). In many areas, however, sets of somatic symptoms hold cultural meaning to describe feelings of distress. For instance, "burning in the head" can be an idiom for "burnout" (Kirmayer & Sartorius, 2007).

Comorbidity

Somatic symptom disorder frequently coexists with other psychiatric disorders, most commonly depression and anxiety. Somatic symptom disorder may also become more pronounced when coupled with existing impairment from other medical conditions (APA, 2013).

A disproportionately high number of people who eventually receive diagnoses of somatic symptom disorder have been treated for irritable bowel syndrome, polycystic ovary disease, and fibromyalgia and other functional somatic syndromes (Warren, Langenberg, & Clauw, 2013). Many of these patients have had prior investigations or treatments associated with a functional somatic syndrome. For instance, women with chronic pelvic pain have undergone hysterectomies while those with irritable bowel syndrome have experienced many invasive diagnostic tests such as endoscopy/colonoscopy.

Aetiology

The cause of somatic symptom disorder is unknown. The following are theories regarding the development of the disorder.

Biologic Theories

Neuropathologic Theory

The neuropathology of somatic symptom disorder is unknown. Evidence suggests decreased activity in certain brain areas, such as the caudate nuclei, left putamen, and right precentral gyrus (Garcia-Campayo, Sanz-Carrillo, Baringo, & Ceballos, 2001; Hakala et al., 2002). These findings indicate that hypometabolism may be associated with somatization.

Genetic

Although somatization disorder has been shown to run in families, the exact transmission mechanism is unclear. Because many women with somatization disorder live in chaotic families, environmental influence could explain the high prevalence in first-degree relatives.

There is research in its early stages that suggests that genetic variability within the serotoninergic and hypothalamic–pituitary–adrenal axis (HPA) may contribute to somatization (Holliday et al., 2010). This has lead to early drug trials using serotonergic agents to evaluate for clinical effect in treating somatic symptom disorders.

Biochemical Changes

Research thus far is insufficient to identify specific biochemical changes that would lead to somatization disorder. However, because these patients experience other psychiatric problems, such as depression or panic, clearly many neurobiologic changes occur. The HPA axis is currently being studied for potential links between proinflammatory cytokines and somatization (Rief, Hennings, Riemer, & Euteneuer, 2010).

Psychological Theories

Somatization has been explained as a form of social or emotional communication, meaning the bodily symptoms express an emotion that cannot be verbalized. The adolescent who experiences severe abdominal pain after her parents' argument or the wife who receives nurturing from her husband only when she has back pain are two examples of how the body expresses emotions. From this perspective, somatization may be a way of maintaining relationships. With time, physical symptoms develop automatically in response to perceived threats. Finally, somatic symptom disorder develops when somatizing begins to interfere with daily life or pervades thought. Research is indicating that lack of social support, perceived violence within the community, and external stressors can contribute to somatization (Hart, Hodgkinson, Belcher, Hyman, & Cooley-Strickland, 2013).

Social Theories

While somatic symptom disorder occurs everywhere, the symptoms may vary between cultures. The conceptualization of somatic symptom disorder is primarily a product of Western culture. In non-Western societies, where the mind–body distinction is not made and symptoms have different meanings and explanations, these physical manifestations are not labelled as a psychiatric disorder (Box 24-1). For example, within Chinese culture as well as in Latin American countries, depression is more

---

BOX 24-1 Somatization in Chinese Culture

In Chinese tradition, the health of the individual reflects a balance between positive and negative forces within the body: five elements at work in nature and in the body control conditions (fire, water, wood, earth, metal); five viscera (liver, heart, spleen, kidneys, lungs); five emotions (anger, joy, worry, sorrow, fear); and five climatic conditions (wind, heat, humidity, dryness, cold). All illness is explained by imbalances among these elements. Because emotion is related to the circulation of vital air within the body, anger is believed to result from an adverse current of vital air to the liver. Emotional outbursts are seen as results of imbalances among the natural elements, rather than results of the person's behaviour.

The stigma of mental illness in the Chinese culture is so great that it can have an adverse effect on a family for many generations. If problems can be attributed to natural causes, the individual and family are less responsible, and stigma is minimized. The Chinese have a culturally acceptable term for symptoms of mental distress—the closest translation of which would be *neuraesthenia*—which comprises somatic complaints of headaches, insomnia, dizziness, aches and pains, poor memory, anxiety, weakness, and loss of energy.

---

likely described with somatic symptoms, such as headaches, gastrointestinal disturbances, or complaints of "nerves," rather than with the sadness or guilt associated with major depression (Jorge, 2003; Yick, Shibusawa, & Agbayani-Siewert, 2003).

Risk Factors

Somatic symptom disorder tends to run in families, and children of mothers with multiple unexplained somatic complaints are themselves more likely to have somatic problems. Female gender, substance use, and anxiety disorder seem to be risk factors, and women with somatic symptom disorder appear more likely to have been sexually abused as children than do those with other psychiatric conditions, such as mood disorders (Lieb et al., 2002). Individuals with depression are especially likely to experience somatization (Silverstein et al., 2013).

Interdisciplinary Treatment

The care of patients with somatic symptom disorder involves three approaches:

- Providing long-term general management of the chronic condition
- Conservatively treating symptoms of comorbid psychiatric and physical problems
- Providing care in special settings, including group treatment

The cornerstone of management is trust. Ideally, the patient sees only one health care provider at regularly scheduled visits. During each primary care visit, the provider should conduct a partial physical examination of the organ system in which the patient has complaints. Physical symptoms are to be treated conservatively using the least intrusive approach. In the mental health setting, the use of cognitive–behaviour therapy (CBT; see Chapter 13) has produced significant clinical benefits beyond other current treatment methods (Allen, Woolfolk, Escobar, Gara, & Hamer, 2006), such as antidepressants or supportive psychotherapy (Mai, 2004). In a review of 31 clinical trials, patients treated with CBT showed more improvement than control subjects did in 71% of the studies. Benefits were observed irrespective of the amelioration of psychological distress (Kroenke & Swindle, 2000).

Nursing Management: Human Response to Disorder

Somatization is the primary response to this disorder. The defining characteristics, depicted in the bio/psycho/social/spiritual model (Fig. 24-1), are so well integrated that separating the psychological and social dimensions is difficult. The most common characteristics include the following:

- Reporting the same symptoms repeatedly
- Receiving support from the environment that otherwise might not be forthcoming (e.g., gaining a spouse's attention because of severe back pain)
- Expressing concern about the physical problems inconsistent with the severity of the illness

Biologic Domain

During the assessment interview, allow enough time for the patient to explain all medical problems; a hurried assessment interview blocks communication.

Assessment

Past medical treatment will have been ineffective because it did not address the underlying psychiatric disorder. However, PMH nurses typically see these patients for coexistent problems related to the psychiatric disorder, such as depression, rather than for the somatic symptom disorder itself. While taking the patient's history, the nurse will discover that the individual has had medical problems or multiple surgeries and realize that somatic symptom disorder is a strong possibility. If the patient has not already received a diagnosis of somatic symptom disorder, the nurse should screen for it by determining the presence of the most commonly reported problems associated with this disorder, which include dysmenorrhoea, lump in throat, vomiting, shortness of breath, burning in sex organs, painful extremities, and amnesia. If the patient has these symptoms, he or she should be seen by a mental health provider qualified to make the diagnosis.

FIGURE 24-1. Bio/psycho/social/spiritual characteristics of patients with somatic symptom disorder.

Review of Systems

Although these patients' symptoms have usually received considerable attention from the medical community, a careful review of systems is important to ensure that nothing is overlooked. Even as the nurse continues to see the patient for mental health problems, an ongoing awareness of biologic symptoms is important, particularly because these symptoms are de-emphasized in the overall management.

Pain is the most common problem in people with this disorder. Because the pain is usually related to symptoms of all the major body systems, it is unlikely that a somatic intervention such as an analgesic will be effective on a long-term basis. The nurse must remember that although there is potentially no medical explanation for the pain, the patient's pain is real and has serious psychosocial implications. A careful assessment should include the following questions:

- What is the pain like?
- What is the extent of the pain?
- When is the pain at its best? worst?
- What has worked in the past to relieve the pain?

Physical Functioning

The actual physical functioning of these individuals is often limited. They usually have problems with sleep, fatigue, activity, and sexual functioning. Assessment of these areas will generate data to be used in establishing nursing diagnoses. The amount and quality of sleep are important, as are the times when the individual sleeps. For example, an individual may sleep a total of 6 hours each diurnal cycle, but only from 2 to 6 AM, plus a 2-hour afternoon nap.

Fatigue is a constant problem, and a variety of physical problems, such as pain, interferes with normal activity. These patients report overwhelming lack of energy, which makes maintaining usual routines or accomplishing daily tasks difficult. Fatigue is accompanied by the inability to concentrate on simple functions, leading to decreased performance and disinterest in social activities. Patients tend to be apathetic and often have little energy (see Clinical Vignette, Box 24-2).

Female patients with this disorder usually have had multiple gynaecologic problems. The reason is not known, but symptoms of dysmenorrhoea, painful intercourse, and pain in the sex organs suggest involvement of the hypothalamic–pituitary–gonadal axis. Physiologic indicators, such as those produced by laboratory tests, are not available. However, a careful assessment of the patient's menstrual history, gynaecologic problems, and sexual functioning is important. The physical manifestations of somatic symptom disorder often lead to altered sexual behaviour.

BOX 24-2 Clinical Vignette

SOMATIC SYMPTOM DISORDER AND STRESS

Ms. J, age 42 years, has been coming to the mental health clinic for 2 years for her "nerves." She has seen only the physician for medication but now has been referred to the nurse's new stress management group because she is experiencing side effects of all the medications that have been tried. The psychiatrist has diagnosed somatic symptom disorder and wants her to learn to manage her "nerves" without medication.

At the first meeting with the nurse, Ms. J was preoccupied with chest pain and bloating that had been ongoing for the past 6 months. Her chest pain is constant and sharp at times. The pain does not prevent her from going to her job as a waitress but does interfere with meal preparation at night for her family and her ability to have sexual intercourse. She has numerous other physical problems, including allergies to certain perfumes, dysmenorrhoea, ovarian polycystic disease (ovarian cysts), chronic urinary tract infections, and rashes. She is constantly fatigued and has frequent leg cramps. She states that she is too tired to fix dinner for her family. On days off from work, she takes a nap in the afternoon, sleeping until evening. She is unable to fall asleep at night.

She believes that she will soon have to have her gallbladder removed because of occasional referred pain to her back and nausea that occurs a couple hours after eating. She is not enthusiastic about a stress management group and does not believe that it will help her problems; however, she has agreed to consider it, while insisting that the psychiatrist continue prescribing diazepam (Valium).

What do you think?
- How would you prioritize Ms. J's physical symptoms?
- What strategies would you use in the group to help Ms. J explore the roots of her stress and fatigue?

Pharmacologic Assessment

A psychopharmacologic assessment of these patients is challenging. Patients with somatic symptom disorder frequently see many different health care providers, perhaps seeing seven or eight different providers within a year. Because they often receive medications from each provider, they are usually taking a large number of drugs. They tend to protect their sources and may not truthfully identify the actual number of medications they are ingesting. A thorough pharmacologic best possible medication history (BPMH) and assessment of all current home medications, herbal supplements, over-the-counter vitamins, and medications is needed not only because of the number of medications but also because these individuals frequently have multiple drug–drug interactions and unusual side effects. Moreover, because of their somatic sensitivity, they often report side effects to many medications.

Patients with somatic symptom disorder spend much of their life trying to find out what is wrong with them. When one provider after another finds little or no explanation for their symptoms, they may become anxious. To alleviate their anxiety, they either self-medicate with over-the-counter medications and substances of abuse (e.g., alcohol, marijuana) or find a provider who prescribes an anxiolytic. Because the anxiety of their disorder cannot be treated within a few weeks with an anxiolytic agent, they become dependent on medication that should not have been prescribed in the first place.

Although anxiolytics have a place in therapeutics, most are addictive and therefore not recommended for long-term use. They also tend to complicate the treatment of somatic symptom disorders. Unfortunately, by the time a patient with a somatic symptom disorder sees a mental health provider, he or she has often already begun taking one or more benzodiazepine agents. Often, the reason a patient agrees to see a mental health provider is that the primary health provider has refused to continue prescribing an anxiolytic until the patient has undergone psychiatric evaluation.

Nursing Diagnoses for the Biologic Domain

Because somatic symptom disorder is a chronic illness, a patient could receive almost any one of the nursing diagnoses at some point in life. At least one nursing diagnosis likely will be related to the individual's physical state. Fatigue, pain, and disturbed sleep patterns are usually supported by the assessment data. The challenge in devising outcomes for these problems is to avoid focusing on the biologic aspects and instead help the patient overcome the fatigue, pain, or sleep problem through bio/psycho/social/spiritual approaches.

Interventions for the Biologic Domain

Nursing interventions that focus on the biologic dimension become especially important because medical treatment must be conservative, and aggressive pharmacologic treatment must be avoided. Each time a nurse sees the patient, time spent on the physical complaints should be limited. The goal is to help the person better understand the meaning behind the physical manifestations of the somatic symptom disorder. Several biologic interventions, including pain management, activity enhancement, nutrition regulation, relaxation, and pharmacologic interventions, may also be useful in caring for patients with somatic symptom disorder.

Pain Management

Pain is a primary issue, but a single approach to its management rarely works. After a careful pain assessment, the nurse should encourage nonpharmacologic management strategies (see Caudill-Slosberg, 2002). If gastrointestinal pain is frequent, for example, eating and bowel habits should be explored and modified where possible. For back pain, exercises and consultation from a physical therapist may be useful. And while headaches are particularly challenging, self-monitoring and tracking them engage the patient in the therapeutic process and help to identify psychosocial triggers.

Activity Enhancement

Helping the patient establish a daily activity routine, especially during times when the patient does not work, may alleviate some of the difficulty with sleeping. Encouraging good sleep hygiene with established patterns and times for sleeping and waking is especially helpful. Although patients typically use various reasons to avoid activity, regular exercise is important to improve the overall physical state. The nurse needs to work with the patient to foster adequate movement for healthier living.

Nutrition Regulation

Patients with somatic symptom disorder often have gastrointestinal problems including special nutritional needs. The nurse should discuss with the patient the nutritional value of foods. Because these individuals often take medications that lead to weight gain, weight control strategies may be discussed (see Chapter 11). Overweight individuals should be given suggestions for healthy, low-calorie foods. Patients should be taught about balancing dietary intake with activity levels to increase their awareness of food choices.

Relaxation

Patients taking anxiolytic medication for stress reduction can also be taught relaxation techniques. The challenge is to help a patient develop strategies for routine practice and evaluation of effect. The nurse may consider a variety of techniques, including simple relaxation techniques, distraction, and guided imagery (see Chapter 11).

Psychopharmacologic Interventions

No particular medication is recommended for somatic symptom disorder. However, psychiatric symptoms of comorbid disorders, such as depression and anxiety, may be treated pharmacologically as appropriate. Patients with this disorder often suffer from depression and anxiety. And while depressed mood itself is not an indication to initiate antidepressant treatment, if a clinical depression is present, aggressive psychopharmacologic management is indicated. A wide variety of drugs is available, including the selective serotonin reuptake inhibitors (SSRIs), tricyclic antidepressants (TCAs), and monoamine oxidase inhibitors (MAOIs; see Chapters 12 and 22). Patients with somatic symptom disorder usually take several different antidepressants throughout the course of the disorder. Evidence should be sought that the depressive symptoms are cleared before discontinuing use of the medication (see Box 24-3).

Phenelzine (Nardil) is one of the MAOIs found effective in treating not just depression (see Chapters 12 and 22) but also the chronic pain and headaches common in people with somatic symptom disorder. Food–drug interactions are the most serious side effects of MAOIs; while

BOX 24-3   Drug Profile

PHENELZINE (NARDIL)

Drug Class: Monoamine oxidase (MAO) inhibitor

Receptor Affinity: Inhibits MAO, an enzyme responsible for breaking down biogenic amines, such as dopamine, norepinephrine, and serotonin, allowing them to accumulate in neuronal storage sites throughout the central and peripheral nervous systems.

Indications: Treatment of depression characterized as "atypical, nonendogenous," or "neurotic" or of depression that is nonresponsive to other antidepressant therapy or when other antidepressant therapy is contraindicated.

Route and Dosage: Available as 15-mg tablets.

Adults: Initially, 15 mg PO tid, increasing to at least 60 mg/day at a fairly rapid pace consistent with patient tolerance. Therapy at 60 mg/day may be necessary for at least 4 weeks before response occurs. After maximum benefit is achieved, dosage is reduced gradually over several weeks. Maintenance dose may be 15 mg/day or every other day.

Geriatric: Adjust dosage accordingly because patients older than 60 years of age are more prone to develop adverse effects.

Paediatric: Not recommended for children younger than 16 years of age.

Half-Life (Peak Effects): Unknown (48 to 96 hours).

Selected Adverse Reactions: Dizziness, vertigo, headache, overactivity, hyperreflexia, tremors, muscle twitching, mania, hypomania, jitteriness, confusion, memory impairment, insomnia, weakness, fatigue, overstimulation, restlessness, increased anxiety, agitation, blurred vision, sweating, constipation, diarrhoea, nausea, abdominal pain, oedema, dry mouth, anorexia, weight changes, hypertensive crisis, orthostatic hypotension, and disturbed cardiac rate and rhythm.

Warnings: Contraindicated in patients with pheochromocytoma, congestive heart failure, hepatic dysfunction, severe renal impairment, cardiovascular disease, history of headache, and myelography within previous 24 hours or scheduled within next 48 hours. Use cautiously in patients with seizure disorders, hyperthyroidism, pregnancy, or lactation, and those scheduled for elective surgery. Possible hypertensive crisis, coma, and severe convulsions may occur if administered with TCAs; possible hypertensive crisis when taken with foods containing tyramine. Increased risk for adverse interaction is possible when given with meperidine. Additive hypoglycaemic effect can occur when taken with insulin and oral sulphonylureas.

Specific Patient/Family Education
- Take drug exactly as prescribed; do not stop taking abruptly or without consulting your health care provider.
- Avoid consuming any foods containing tyramine while taking this drug and for 2 weeks afterwards.
- Avoid alcohol, sleep-inducing drugs, over-the-counter drugs such as cold and hay fever remedies, and appetite suppressants—all of which may cause serious or life-threatening problems.
- Report any signs and symptoms of adverse reactions.
- Maintain appointments for follow-up blood tests.
- Report any complaints of unusual or severe headache or yellowing of eyes or skin.
- Avoid driving a car or performing any activities that require alertness.
- Change position slowly when going from a lying to sitting or standing position to minimize dizziness or weakness.

taking such agents, patients should avoid foods high in tyramine (see Chapter 12).

Anxiety associated with a somatic symptom disorder is more difficult than is depression to treat pharmacologically. Nonpharmacologic approaches such as biofeedback or relaxation are preferred. Benzodiazepines should be avoided because of the high potential for abuse and physiologic dependence associated with these medications. Buspirone (BuSpar), a nonbenzodiazepine, does not lead to tolerance or withdrawal and, although not as potent as benzodiazepines, may be useful for relief of anxiety. Other agents, such as the SSRIs, are effective in the management of generalized anxiety and panic disorders and may be effective in the management of anxiety associated with somatic symptom disorder.

Monitoring Medications, Interactions, and Side Effects

In somatic symptom disorder, patients are usually treated in the community, where they often use multiple over-the-counter and prescription medications. Once the nurse completes a BPMH of all current home medicinal substances, including self-prescribed and over-the-counter remedies, vitamins and herbal supplements, etc., the information should be documented and reported to the rest of the interdisciplinary team. The nurse questions and listens carefully to determine the full scope of medications, how they are used, and effects that the patient attributes to each substance. Using the BPMH, an evaluation of possible drug–drug interactions needs to be completed by the prescriber through a medication reconciliation process. The nurse needs to work with the patient, pharmacist, nurse practitioner, and physician to support the patient in maintaining a safe and effective pharmacotherapeutic regime. Individuals with somatic symptom disorder often have idiosyncratic reactions to their medications. Side effects should be assessed, but the patient should be encouraged to compare the benefits of the medication with any problems related to side effects.

In working with patients with somatization disorder, the nurse must always monitor for drug–drug interactions. Medications patients are taking for physical problems could interact with psychiatric medications. Patients may be taking alternative medicines, such as herbal supplements (i.e., Valarian for management of anxiety), and these also need to be evaluated for possible adverse interactions. The patient should be encouraged to use the same pharmacy to fill all prescriptions so that possible reactions can be checked.

Psychological Domain

The cognitive functioning of individuals with somatic symptom disorder is usually within normal limits. However, these individuals seem preoccupied with personal illnesses and often keep a record of symptoms and illnesses. They constantly focus on bodily functions, and "living with diseases" truly becomes a way of life.

Individuals with somatic symptom disorder usually have intense emotional reactions to life stressors. They often have a series of personal crises beginning at an early age. Typically, a new symptom or medical problem develops during times of emotional stress. It is critical that the physical assessment data be linked to psychological and social events. A history of major psychological events should be compared with the chronology of physical problems. Special attention should be paid to any history of sexual abuse or trauma in the patient's younger years. Early sexual abuse also may interfere with self-esteem, belonging, and sexual fulfilment in adulthood.

Response to physical symptoms is often exaggerated, such as interpreting a simple cold as pneumonia or a brief chest pain as a heart attack. Family members may not believe the physical symptoms are real, instead viewing them as attention-seeking behaviour, since the symptoms often do improve when the patient receives attention. For example, a woman who has been in bed for 3 weeks with severe back pain may suddenly feel much better once her children visit her.

● **STUDY NOTE**

Encourage patients with somatic symptom disorder to discuss and explore psychosocial and spiritual issues as well as their physical problems.

Assessment

While gathering information from the biologic domain, the nurse concurrently assesses mental status in the psychological domain. Components include appearance, psychomotor behaviour, mood, affect, perception, thought content and process, sensorium, insight, and judgement (see Chapter 10).

Nursing Diagnoses for the Psychological Domain

Nursing diagnoses related to the psychological domain and typical of people with somatic symptom disorder include anxiety, ineffective sexuality patterns, impaired social interactions, ineffective coping, and ineffective therapeutic regimen management.

Interventions for the Psychological Domain

The choice of psychological intervention depends on the specific problem the patient is experiencing. Cognitive–behavioural therapy, which helps the patient identify, connect, and change feelings, thoughts, and behaviour, is the most effective treatment for somatic symptom disorder (Mai, 2004). Supportive psychotherapy, counselling, and patient education are also useful strategies. The most important and ongoing intervention is the development and maintenance of a therapeutic relationship.

Development of a Therapeutic Relationship

The most difficult yet crucial aspect of nursing care is developing a sound, person-centred, positive, and helping nurse–patient relationship. Without it, the nurse is just one more provider who fails to meet the patient's needs and expectations. Developing this relationship requires time and patience. Therapeutic communication techniques are used to help the patient explore underlying psychosocial and spiritual problems related to the physical manifestations of the disorder (see Box 24-4).

During periods when symptoms of other psychiatric disorders surface, additional therapeutic interventions may be needed (see Chapter 6). For example, the occurrence of depression requires additional supportive or cognitive approaches.

Counselling

Counselling, with a focus on problem solving, is needed from time to time. These patients have chaotic lives and need support through a multitude of crises. Although they sometimes appear flamboyant and self-assured, their constant complaints may irritate others. The consequences of their impaired social interactions must be examined within a counselling framework. The nurse helps the patient identify stressors, explore related thoughts and feelings, and develop positive coping responses to an often chaotic lifestyle.

Patient Education: Health Teaching

Health teaching is useful throughout the nurse–patient relationship. These patients have many questions about illnesses, symptoms, and treatments. Emphasis should be upon positive health care practices rather than the effects of serious illness. Because of problems in managing medications and treatment, the therapeutic regimen needs constant monitoring; this provides ample opportunity for teaching. One area that might require special health teaching is impaired sexuality. Because of their history of physical problems related to the reproductive tract, patients may have difficulty carrying out normal sexual activity, such as masturbation, intercourse, reaching orgasm, and so forth. Basic teaching about sexual function is often needed (see Box 24-5).

BOX 24-4   Therapeutic Dialogue

ESTABLISHING A RELATIONSHIP

Ineffective Approach

Nurse: Good morning, Ms. C.

Patient: I'm in so much pain. Take that breakfast away.

Nurse: You don't want your breakfast?

Patient: Can't you see? I hurt! When I hurt, I can't eat!

Nurse: If you don't eat now, you probably won't be able to have anything until lunch.

Patient: Who cares. I have no intention of being here at lunchtime. I don't belong here.

Nurse: Ms. C, I don't think that your doctor would have admitted you unless there is a problem. I would like to talk to you about why you are here.

Patient: Nurse, I'm just here. It's none of your business.

Nurse: Oh.

Patient: Please leave me alone.

Nurse: Sure, I will see you later.

Effective Approach

Nurse: Good morning, Ms. C.

Patient: I'm in so much pain. Take that breakfast away.

Nurse: (Silently removes the tray, pulls up a chair, and sits down.)

Patient: My back hurts.

Nurse: Oh, when did the back pain start?

Patient: Last night. It's this bed. I couldn't get comfortable.

Nurse: These beds can be pretty uncomfortable.

Patient: My back pain is shooting down my leg.

Nurse: Does anything help it?

Patient: Sometimes if I straighten out my leg it helps.

Nurse: Can I help you straighten out your leg?

Patient: Oh, it's OK. The pain is going away. What did you say your name is?

Nurse: I'm Susan Miller, your nurse while you are here.

Patient: I won't be here long. I don't belong in a psychiatric unit.

Nurse: While you are here, I would like to spend time with you.

Patient: OK, but you understand I do not have any psychiatric problems.

Nurse: We can talk about whatever you want. But, since you want to get out of here, we might want to focus on what it will take to get you ready for discharge.

Critical Thinking Challenge

- What communication mistakes did the nurse in the first scenario make?
- What communication strategies helped the patient feel comfortable with the nurse in the second scenario? How is the second scenario different from the first?

Social Domain

People with somatic symptom disorder spend excessive time seeking medical care and attending to their multiple illnesses. Because they believe themselves to be very sick, they also often believe that they are disabled and cannot work; their unemployment rate is therefore high. So while these individuals are rarely satisfied with health care providers who can find no basis for a medical diagnosis, their social network may consist more of these providers than of their peers. Identifying a support network requires sorting out health care providers from their family and friends.

Assessment

It is important to identify both beneficial and harmful relationships within the patient's family. Family members

---

BOX 24-5 Psychoeducation Checklist: Somatic Symptom Disorder

When caring for the patient with somatic symptom disorder, be sure to include the following topic areas in the teaching plan:
- Psychopharmacologic agents if ordered, including drug, action, dosage, frequency, and possible adverse effects
- Nonpharmacologic approaches to pain relief
- Exercise
- Nutrition
- Social interaction
- Appropriate health maintenance practices
- Problem solving
- Relaxation and anxiety-reduction techniques
- Sexual functioning

---

may become weary of the patient's constant physical complaints. In assessing relations, however, it is important that other members with social problems and psychiatric disorders be identified, as the individual suffering from somatic symptom disorder may live in a chaotic family with multiple problems.

Symptoms of somatic symptom disorder may disrupt the family's social life. A change in routine or a major life event often precipitates a symptom's appearance. For example, a patient planning a vacation with the family may decide at the last minute that she cannot go because her back pain has returned and she will be unable to sit in the car. Such family disruptions are common.

Nursing Diagnoses for the Social Domain

Some of the nursing diagnoses related to the social domain that are typical of people with somatic symptom disorder include risk for caregiver role strain, ineffective community coping, disabled family coping, and social isolation.

Interventions for the Social Domain

Patients with somatic symptom disorders may be isolated from family and community. Strengthening relationships and encouraging social activity often become the focus of nursing care. The nurse should help the patient identify individuals with whom contact is desired, encourage him or her to reinitiate a relationship, and ask for a commitment to contact them. The nurse should counsel the patient about talking too much about his or her symptoms with these individuals and emphasize that medical information should be shared with the nurse.

Group Interventions

Although these patients may not be good candidates for insight group psychotherapy, they do benefit from cognitive–behavioural groups that focus on developing coping skills for everyday life (Lidbeck, 2003). For female patients, participation in groups that address feminist issues should be encouraged; this may help to strengthen their assertiveness skills and improve self-esteem (Fig. 24-2).

When leading a group that has members with somatic symptom disorder, redirection can keep the group from giving too much attention to a person's illness. However, these individuals need reassurance and support while in a group. The patient may report feeling as though he or she does not fit in with or belong in the group; in reality, he or she is likely feeling insecure and threatened in the situation. The group leader needs to show patience and understanding in order to engage the individual effectively in meaningful group interaction.

Family Interventions

The results of a family assessment often reveal a need for education about the disorder, helpful strategies for dealing with the patient's symptoms, and, usually, help in developing more effective communication and problem-solving strategies. Many people with somatic symptom disorder have experienced a chaotic family life and, potentially, physical and/or sexual abuse. The nurse must assess and offer interventions such as those identified through a thorough family assessment (see Chapter 15).

Spiritual Domain

The spiritual domain assesses how people with a somatic symptom disorder connect experiences, make meaning of their disorder, and find purpose in life. Somatic symptom disorder produces a continuous physical awareness of the body's pain or distress. Over time, patients may begin to resent their bodies, become bitter by living in a world of ongoing challenges, and experience conflict with their religious beliefs. A spiritual assessment provides important information needed to help patients regain spiritual health.

Assessment

To assess spiritual health, nurses enquire about topics such as meaning, ambiguity, and hope using questions such as: What is "being ill" like for you? What does "being ill" mean in your life? Personal strengths are assessed with questions such as: What brings joy and peace to you? How has your illness changed the way you understand the world? Do you have spiritual beliefs that have been affected by your illness experience? Questions to elicit information about connections

FIGURE 24-2. Bio/psycho/social/spiritual interventions for patients with somatic symptom disorder.

with self, others, and a higher power include: How are you right now? What sustains or heals your spirit? Who is significant to you? How do you feel connected to the world and events around you? Are there spiritual acts, such as prayer, that you find helpful (Burkhardt & Nagai-Jacobson, 2008)?

Nursing Diagnoses for the Spiritual Domain

Nursing diagnoses related to the spiritual domain and typical of people with somatic symptom disorder include hopelessness, spiritual distress, and potential for enhanced spiritual well-being.

Interventions for the Spiritual Domain

Individuals with somatic symptom disorders sometimes feel estranged from others. For individuals who belong to a religious group, this can include estrangement from their faith communities. Nurses intervene by creating a safe and caring environment to help the person explore deep questions related to connection, meaning, and purpose. Trust, rapport, and a mutual plan for care are developed with the use of presence, empathy, and sensitivity. Based on the person's assessed needs, nurses may also facilitate religious practices, assist with life review or reminiscence therapy, or make a referral to a spiritual care expert (Taylor, 2002).

Evaluation and Treatment Outcomes

The outcomes for patients with somatic symptom disorder must be realistic and formulated with the patient. Because this is a lifelong disorder, small successes should be expected. Specific outcomes should be identified. Over time, there should be a gradual reduction in the number of health care providers the individual contacts and gradual improvement in the ability to cope with stresses (Fig. 24-3).

Continuum of Care

For individuals experiencing somatic symptom disorder, mental health services ranging from inpatient care to health promotion may occur in various health care settings over the course of life.

Inpatient Care

Ideally, individuals with somatic symptom disorder will spend minimal time in the hospital. Inpatient stays occur when their comorbid psychiatric disorders become symptomatic. In order to provide consistency of care while in inpatient care, the patient should be the responsibility of one primary nurse who provides or oversees all the nursing care. The inpatient nurse must establish a relationship with the patient (and family) and consult other nursing staff members about this disorder.

FIGURE 24-3. Bio/psycho/social/spiritual outcomes for patients with somatic symptom disorder.

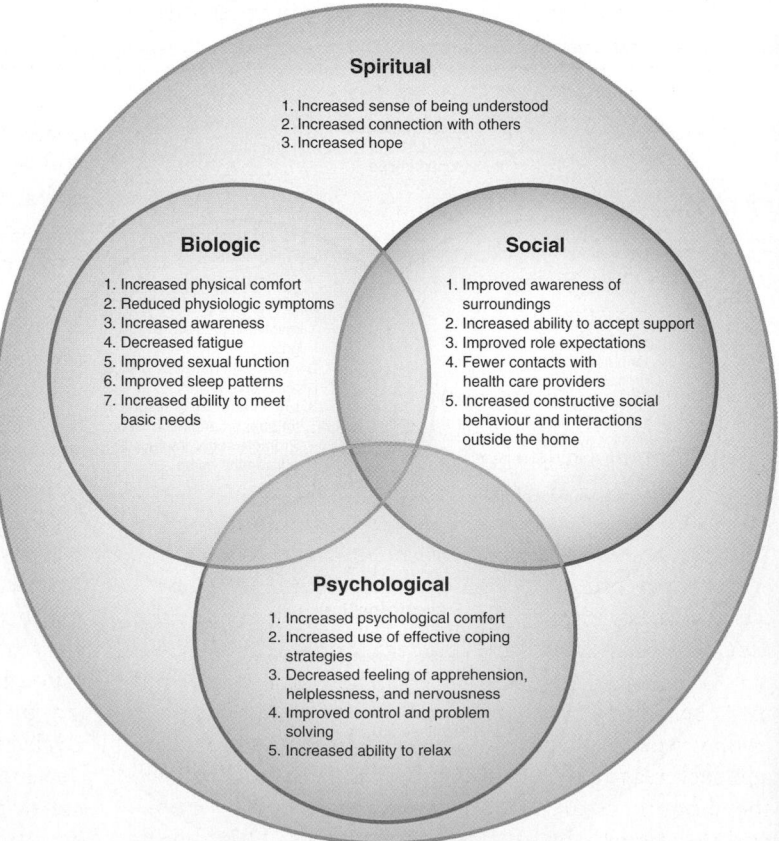

The emergencies these individuals experience may be physical (e.g., chest pain, back pain, gastrointestinal symptoms) or stress responses related to a psychosocial crisis. Careful assessment must be used so as not to overlook the symptoms of acute and/or potentially fatal illness.

Community Treatment

Individuals with somatic symptom disorder can spend a lifetime in the health care system and still have little continuity of care. Switching from provider to provider is detrimental to their long-term care. Most are outpatients. When they are hospitalized, it is usually for evaluation of physical problems. When their comorbid psychiatric disorders, such as depression, become symptomatic, these patients may also be hospitalized for a short time (see Nursing Care Plan 24-1).

Mental Health Promotion

Patients with somatic symptom disorder are encouraged to focus on staying healthy rather than on the symptoms of their illness. For these individuals, approaching the topic of health promotion usually has to be within the context of preventing further problems. Setting aside time for themselves and identifying activities that meet their psychological and spiritual needs, such as connecting with their faith group, are important in maintaining a healthy balance.

OTHER SOMATIC SYMPTOM AND RELATED DISORDERS

The following discussion summarizes other somatic symptom and related disorders and highlights the primary focus of nursing management.

Illness and Anxiety Disorder

The exclusion of hypochondriasis from the *DSM-5* has brought about the emergence of illness anxiety as a new *DSM* disorder. The condition of the majority of individuals previously diagnosed with hypochondriasis, however, fits well with the criteria for somatic symptom disorder. With *illness anxiety disorder*, patients experience excessive anxiety and preoccupation with having or acquiring a serious illness. Physical symptoms, if present, are a minor aspect of this diagnosis. Persistent worry regarding illness invades multiple aspects of an individual's life. For instance, illness becomes a frequent topic of discussion as they repeatedly discuss illness within their social circle and seek reassurance from family and friends. They will spend hours researching suspected illnesses and continuously examine their body for signs of illness. This impacts their quality of life, potentially limiting activities of daily living (looking after family, going to work) and, in extreme cases, results in the inability to go to work or school.

The prevalence rate between men and women is similar, and although the aetiology is unknown, it is proposed that a serious childhood illness or abuse may be a precursor (APA, 2013). Careful evaluation of illness anxiety disorder must be carried out and other psychiatric illnesses, such as obsessive–compulsive disorder, delusional disorder, and generalized anxiety, excluded.

Several interventions have been effective in reducing patients' fears of experiencing serious illnesses. Cognitive–behavioural therapy, stress management, and group interventions lead to a decrease in intensity and increase in control of symptoms (Fava, Grandi, Rafanelli, Fabbri, & Cazzaro, 2000). It is unknown whether the positive outcomes result from the intervention itself or from the symptom validation and increased attention given to the patient. Nursing management should include listening to the patient's report of symptoms and fears, validating it by acknowledging that the fears may be real, asking the patient to monitor symptoms in a journal, and encouraging the patient to bring the journal to clinical visits. By seeing the symptom pattern, the nurse can continue assessment and help the patient better understand the significance and implications of symptoms. The outcome of this approach should be decrease in fear and better symptom control.

Conversion Disorder

Conversion disorder, also known as functional neurologic symptom disorder, is the somatization of neurologic conditions such as paralysis. Symptoms associated with conversion disorder are called **pseudoneurologic symptoms**. Patients with conversion disorder present with symptoms of impaired coordination or balance, paralysis, aphonia (inability to produce sound), difficulty swallowing or a sensation of a lump in the throat, and urinary retention. They also may have loss of sensation, vision problems, blindness, deafness, seizures, and hallucinations (APA, 2013). Females experience conversion disorder two to three times more frequently than do males (APA, 2013). These symptoms do not follow neurologic pathways but rather the individual's conceptualization of the problem. The nurse must understand that the physical sensation is real for the patient. There is evidence of a relationship between childhood trauma (e.g., sexual abuse) or stressful life events and conversion disorder (Reuber, 2008). In approaching this patient, the nurse treats the conversion symptom as a real symptom that may have distressing psychological aspects. The nurse intervenes by acknowledging the pain and helps the patient deal with it. As trust develops within the nurse–patient relationship, the nurse can help the patient develop approaches to solving everyday problems.

Nursing Care Plan 24-1

The Patient With Somatization Disorder

SC is a 48-year-old woman who is making her weekly visit to her primary care physician for unexplained multiple somatic problems. This week, her concern is recurring abdominal pain that fits no symptom pattern. Upon physical examination, a cause of her abdominal pain could not be found. She is requesting a refill of alprazolam (Xanax), which is the only medication that relieves her pain. She is in the process of applying for disability income because of being completely disabled by neck and shoulder pain. The physician and office staff avoid her whenever possible. The physician will not refill the prescription until SC is evaluated by the consulting mental health team that provides weekly evaluations and services.

Setting: Primary Care Office

Baseline Assessment: SC is a 48-year-old obese Caucasian woman who appears very angry. She resents being forced to see a psychiatric clinician for the only medication that works to alleviate her pain. She denies any psychiatric problems or emotional distress. She is wearing a short black top and tight slacks. Her hair is in curlers; she says that it is too much trouble to comb her hair. Cognitive aspects of mental status appear normal, but she admits to being slightly depressed and takes the alprazolam for her "nerves." She says she has nothing to live for but denies any thoughts of suicide. She is dependent on her children for everything and feels very guilty about it. She spends most of her waking hours going to various doctors and taking combinations of medications to relieve her pains. She has no friends or nonfamily social contacts.

Associated Psychiatric Diagnosis and Other Conditions that May Be a Focus of Clinical Attention	Medications
R/O depression	Premarin, 1.2 mg qd
Somatic symptom disorder	Alprazolam (Xanax), 0.25 mg tid
S/P gastric bypass	Ranitidine HCL (Zantac), 150 mg bid
S/P carpel tunnel release	Simethicone, 1,235 mg qid with meals
Chronic shoulder, neck pain, vertigo	Calcium carbonate, 1,000 mg qd
	Multiple vitamin, qd
Social problems (father died 6 months ago, divorced 9 months)	Zolpidem tartrate (Ambien), 5 mg at hs PRN
Economic problems (small pension)	Ibuprofen, 600 mg q6h PRN pain
Occupational problems (potential disability)	Maalox, PRN
	Preparation H suppositories

Nursing Diagnosis 1: Chronic Low Self-Esteem

Defining Characteristics	Related Factors
Self-negating verbalizations (long standing)	Feeling unimportant to family
Hesitant to try new things	Feeling rejected by ex-husband
Expresses guilt	Constant physical problems interfering with normal social activities
Evaluates self as being unable to deal with events	

Outcomes

Initial	Long-term
Identify need to increase self-esteem	Participate in individual or group therapy for self-esteem building

Interventions

Interventions	Rationale	Ongoing Assessment
Establish rapport with the patient.	Individuals with low self-esteem feel vulnerable and may be reluctant to discuss true feelings.	Ask the patient for her perceptions of care and the helping relationship.

Interventions

Interventions	Rationale	Ongoing Assessment
Encourage the patient to spend time dressing and grooming appropriately.	Confidence and self-esteem improve when a person looks well groomed.	Monitor responses.
Encourage the patient to discuss various somatic problems, as well as psychological and interpersonal issues.	Patients with somatic symptom disorder need time to express their physical problems. It helps them feel valued. The best way to build a relationship is to acknowledge physical symptoms.	Monitor time that the patient spends explaining physical symptoms.
Explore opportunities for SC to meet other people with similar, nonmedical interests.	Focusing SC on meeting others will improve the possibilities of increasing contacts.	Observe willingness to identify other interests besides physical problems.

Evaluation

Outcomes	Revised Outcomes	Interventions
SC admitted to having low self-esteem but was very reluctant to consider meeting new people.	Focus on building self-esteem.	Identify activities that will enhance self-esteem.

Nursing Diagnosis 2: Ineffective Therapeutic Regimen Management

Defining Characteristics	Related Factors
Choices of daily living ineffective for meeting health care goal Verbalizes difficulty with prescribed regimens	Inappropriate use of benzodiazepines for nerves

Outcomes

Initial	Long term
Openly discuss the use of medications.	Use nonpharmacologic means for stress reduction.

Interventions

Interventions	Rationale	Ongoing Assessment
Clarify the frequency and purpose of taking alprazolam.	Unsupervised polypharmacy is very common with these patients. Further clarification is usually needed.	Carefully track self-report of medication use; determine whether the patient is disclosing the use of all medications.
Educate the patient about the effects of combining medications, emphasizing negative effects.	Education about combining medication is the beginning of helping the patient become effective in medication regimen.	Observe the patient's ability and willingness to consider negative effects.
Explore ways to gradually reduce the number of medications, including other means of managing physical symptoms.	Help the patient to identify appropriate ways and means to manage health care regimens.	Evaluate the patient's ability to problem solve.

Evaluation

Outcomes	Revised Outcomes	Interventions
Patient disclosed the use of medications but was unwilling to consider changing ineffective use of medication.	Identify next step if primary care physician does not refill prescription.	Discuss the possibility of not being able to obtain alprazolam. Refer the patient to mental health clinic for further evaluation.

IN A LIFE

Emily Carr (1871–1945)
Canadian Painter and Writer

Public Persona

Emily Carr was an accomplished artist and writer best known for her vivid depictions of Native culture and Canadian West Coast nature. Influenced by early educational sojourns in San Francisco, England, and France and later encouraged by the important artists known as the Group of Seven, Carr developed her unique impressionistic style in both painting and writing. Embellished with dramatizations and idealism, works like *Growing Pains* autobiographically depict the struggle of her life. Raised in a strict Victorian home, Carr has been described as rebellious, yet overweight, irritable, and socially insecure.

Personal Realities

Carr's career was interrupted many times with bouts of poor health. Just more than 100 years ago, Carr was treated in an English sanatorium. Many of the symptoms she described were representatives of what today is called illness anxiety disorder, clinical depression, and/or conversion disorder.

Table 24-2 **Diagnosis of Factitious Disorder**

Diagnostic Criteria: Imposed on Self	Diagnostic Criteria: Imposed on Others
A. Falsification of physical or psychological signs or symptoms, or induction of injury or diseases, associated with identified deception.	A. Falsification of physical or psychological signs or symptoms, or induction of injury or disease in another, associated with identified deception.
B. The individual presents himself or herself to others as ill, impaired, or injured.	B. The individual presents another individual (victim) to others as ill, impaired, or injured.
C. The deceptive behaviour is evident even in the absence of obvious external rewards.	C. The deceptive behaviour is evident even in the absence of obvious external rewards.
D. The behaviour is not better explained by another mental disorder, such as delusional disorder or another psychotic disorder.	D. The behaviour is not better explained by another mental disorder, such as delusional disorder or another psychotic disorder. The perpetrator, not the victim, receives this diagnosis.

American Psychiatric Association. (2013). *Diagnostic and statistical manual of mental disorders* (5th ed) (pp. 324–325). Washington, DC: Author.

PSYCHOLOGICAL FACTORS AFFECTING OTHER MEDICAL CONDITIONS

Within this category, patients engage in behaviours that negatively impact the outcome of an existing medical condition. In mild cases, patients may, for instance, not take their antidiabetic medication appropriately and intentionally increase their risk for diabetic complications. In more severe cases, the patient's behaviour may lead to life-threatening complications and risk of death. For example, a patient may ignore a life-threatening infection rather than seek help. This diagnosis can only be established in the absence of other diagnoses that may better characterize or explain such risky behaviour, such as major depressive disorder, delusion disorder, or posttraumatic stress disorder (APA, 2013).

FACTITIOUS DISORDERS

The other type of psychiatric disorder characterized by somatization is *factitious disorder*. Patients with this disorder intentionally cause an illness or injury to receive the attention of health care workers. These individuals are motivated solely by the desire to become a patient and develop a dependent relationship with a health care provider. There are two classes of factitious disorders: factitious disorder imposed on self and factitious disorder imposed on another. The diagnostic criteria are outlined in Table 24-2.

Factitious Disorder, Imposed on Self

Although feigned illnesses have been described for centuries, it was not until 1951 that the term *Munchausen's syndrome* was used to describe the most severe form of this disorder, which was characterized by fabricating a physical illness,

having recurrent hospitalizations, and going from one provider to another (Asher, 1951). Today, this disorder is called factitious disorder and is differentiated from **malingering**, in which the individual who intentionally produces illness symptoms is motivated by another specific self-serving goal, such as being classified as disabled or avoiding work.

Patients with factitious disorder injure themselves covertly. The illnesses are produced in such a manner that the health care provider is tricked into believing that a true physical or psychiatric disorder is present. The self-produced physical symptoms appear as medical illnesses such as seizure disorders, wound-healing disorders, the abscess processes (introduction of infectious material below the skin surface), and feigned fever (rubbing the thermometer).

Epidemiology

It is estimated that approximately 1% of psychiatric consultations completed within hospitals identify as factitious disorders (APA, 2013). The prevalence of factitious disorder is difficult to determine because its secretive nature interferes with traditional epidemiologic research methods (Krahn, Li, & O'Connor, 2003).

Nursing Management: Human Response to Disorder

The overall goal of treatment is for the patient to replace the dysfunctional, attention-seeking behaviours with positive behaviours. To begin treatment, the patient must acknowledge the deception, but confrontation does not appear to lead to acknowledgment (Krahn et al., 2003). The mental health team has to accept and value the patient as a human being who needs help. As the pattern of self-injury is well established, giving up the behaviours is difficult.

Assessment

Early childhood experiences, particularly instances of abuse, neglect, or abandonment, should be identified in order to understand the underlying psychological dynamics of the individual and the role of self-injury. Family assessment is important; relationships become strained as family members become aware of this disorder's self-inflicted nature.

Nursing Interventions

The fabrications and deceits may provoke anger and a sense of betrayal in the nurse. To be effective with these patients, the nurse must be aware of these feelings and resolve them by developing a better understanding of the underlying psychodynamic issues. Therapeutic confrontation in the context of a helping relationship can be effective if the patient feels supported and accepted and if there is clear communication between the patient, the mental health care team, and family members. All care should be centralized within one facility, and the patient should see providers regularly, even when not in active crisis. The treatment goal is recovery not confession.

Factitious Disorder, Imposed on Another

Within the category of factitious disorder, the *DSM-5* includes a rare but dramatic disorder, factitious disorder imposed on another, once called *Munchausen's by proxy*. It involves a person's inflicting injury on another—often a mother on her own child—hoping thereby to gain the attention of a health care provider. These actions include inducing seizures, poisoning, or smothering. This most severe form of child abuse is usually identified in the emergency room or by critical care nurses. The mother rarely admits to injuring the child and thus is not amenable to treatment; the child is removed from the mother's care. This form of child abuse is distinguished from other forms by the routine, unwitting involvement of health care workers, who subject the child to physical risk and emotional distress through tests, procedures, and medication trials.

SUMMARY OF KEY POINTS

■ Somatization is manifested as psychological distress and abnormal thought patterns in relation to physical symptoms, independent of whether the symptom may be medically explained or not.

■ Factitious disorders are manifested by individuals' intentionally inflicting or feigning injury or illness on themselves or others in order to gain medical attention.

■ Somatization is affected by sociocultural and gender factors. It occurs more frequently in women than in men; in those with lower levels of education or socioeconomic class; and in older adults.

■ The somatoform disorders are clustered into six different clinical syndromes: (1) somatic symptom disorder, (2) illness anxiety disorder, (3) conversion disorder, (4) psychological factors affecting other medical conditions, (5) factitious disorder, and (6) other specified somatic symptoms and related disorders.

■ Illness anxiety disorder occurs when an individual's preoccupation with having or acquiring an illness causes excessive distress.

■ Conversion disorder manifests as one or more somatic symptoms involving altered voluntary motor or sensory function. This disorder is two to three times more prevalent in females.

■ Patients with somatic symptom disorder are often seen on the medical–surgical units of hospitals and can go years without receiving a correct diagnosis. In most cases, they eventually receive mental health treatment because of comorbid conditions such as depression and panic.

■ The development of the nurse–patient relationship is crucial to assessing these patients and identifying appropriate nursing diagnoses and interventions. Because these patients deny any psychiatric basis for their problem and continue to focus on their symptoms' having a medical basis, the nurse must take a nonjudgemental, open approach that acknowledges the symptoms while helping the patient explore and understand his or her behaviour and focus on new ways of coping with stress.

■ Health teaching is important in helping the individual develop positive lifestyle changes in place of somatization responses. Identifying personal strengths and supporting the development of positive skills improve self-esteem and personal confidence. Teaching the use of biofeedback and relaxation provides the patient with positive coping skills.

CRITICAL THINKING CHALLENGES

1 A depressed young white woman is admitted to a psychiatric unit in a state of agitation. She reports extreme abdominal pain. Her admitting provider tells you that she has a classic case of somatic symptom disorder and to de-emphasize her physical symptoms. No pain medications are needed. Conceptualize how to approach, assess, and intervene with this patient.

2 Compare and contrast somatic symptom disorders with illness anxiety disorders.

3 Develop a teaching plan for an individual who has a long history of somatic symptom disorder but who

recently received a diagnosis of breast cancer. How will the patient be able to differentiate the physical symptoms of associated with somatization from those associated with the treatment of her breast cancer?

4 A woman of Chinese origin was admitted for panic attacks and numerous somatic problems, ranging from dysmenorrhoea to painful joints. Results of all medical examinations have been negative. She truly believes that her panic attacks are caused by a weak heart. What approaches should the nurse use in providing culturally sensitive nursing care?

5 A person experiencing depression with somatic features is started on a regimen of phenelzine 15 mg tid. She believes that she is allergic to most foods but insists on having wine in the evenings because it helps digest her food. Develop a teaching plan that provides the knowledge that she needs to prevent a hypertensive crisis caused by excessive tyramine but that is sensitive to the patient's food preferences.

REFERENCES

Allen, L. A., Woolfolk, R. L., Escobar, J. I., Gara, M. A., & Hamer, R. M. (2006). Cognitive-behavioral therapy for somatization disorder. *Archives of Internal Medicine, 166*, 1512–1518.

American Psychiatric Association (APA). (2013). *Diagnostic and statistical manual of mental disorders* (5th ed). Washington, DC: Author.

Asher, R. (1951). Münchausen's syndrome. *Lancet, 1*, 339–341.

Bener, A., Ghuloum, S., & Burgut, F. T. (2010). Gender differences in prevalence of somatoform disorders in patients visiting primary care centers. *Journal of Primary Care and Community Health, 37*(1), 37–42.

Burkhardt, M. A. & Nagai-Jacobson, M. G. (2008). Spirituality and health. In B. M. Dossey & L. Keegan (Eds.), *Holistic nursing: A handbook for practice* (5th ed., pp. 617–645). Toronto, ON: Jones and Bartlett Publishers.

Caudill-Slosberg, M. A. (2002). *Managing pain before it manages you* (rev. ed.). New York, NY: Guilford Press.

Fava, G., Grandi, S., Rafanelli, C., Fabbri, S., & Cazzaro, M. (2000). Explanatory therapy in hypochondriasis. *The Journal of Clinical Psychiatry, 61*(4), 317–322.

Firoozabadi, A., Bahredar, M. J., & Seifsafari, S. (2013). Somatization as central manifestation of depression in Iranian culture. *European Psychiatry, 28*(1), 1. Retrieved from http://dx.doi.org/10.1016/S0924-9338(13)75995-9

Garcia-Campayo, J., Sanz-Carrillo, C., Baringo, T., & Ceballos, C. (2001). A SPECT scan in somatization disorder patients: An exploratory study of eleven cases. *The Australian and New Zealand Journal of Psychiatry, 35*(3), 359–363.

Hakala, M., Karlsson, H., Ruotsalainen, U., Koponen, S., Bergman, J., Stenman, H., ... Niemi, P. (2002). Severe somatization in women is associated with altered cerebral glucose metabolism. *Psychological Medicine, 32*(8), 1379–1385.

Hart, S. L., Hodgkinson, S. C., Belcher, H. M. E., Hyman, C., & Cooley-Strickland, M. (2013). Somatic symptoms, peer, and school stress, and family and community violence exposure among urban elementary school children. *Journal of Behavioral Medicine, 36*, 454–465.

Holliday, K. L., MacFarlane, G. J., Nicholl, B. I., Creed, F., Thomson, W., & McBeth, J. (2010). Genetic variations in neuroendocrine gene associated with somatic symptoms in the general population: Results from the EPIFUND study. *Journal of Psychosomatic Research, 68*(5), 469–474.

Jorge, J. R. (2003). Depression in Brazil and other Latin American countries. *Seishin Shinkeigaku Zasshi, 105*(1), 9–16.

Kirmayer, L. J. & Sartorius, N. (2007). Cultural models and somatic syndromes. *Psychosomatic Medicine, 69*(9), 832–840.

Krahn, L. E., Li, H., & O'Connor, M. K. (2003). Patients who strive to be ill: Factitious disorder with physical symptoms. *The American Journal of Psychiatry, 160*(6), 1163–1168.

Kroenke, K. & Spitzer, R. (1998). Gender differences in the reporting of physical and somatoform symptoms. *Psychosomatic Medicine, 60*, 150–155.

Kroenke, K. & Swindle, R. (2000). Cognitive-behavioral therapy for somatization and symptom syndromes: A critical review of controlled clinical trials. *Psychotherapy and Psychosomatics, 69*(4), 205–215.

Lidbeck, M. (2003). Group therapy for somatization disorders in primary care: Maintenance of treatment goals of short cognitive-behavioural treatment one-and-a-half-year follow-up. *Acta Psychiatrica Scandinavica, 107*(5), 449–456.

Lieb, R., Zimmermann, P., Friis, R. H., Hofler, M., Tholen, S., & Wittchen, H. U. (2002). The natural course of *DSM-IV* somatoform disorders and syndromes among adolescents and young adults: A prospective-longitudinal community study. *European Psychiatry, 17*(6), 321–331.

Mai, F. (2004). Somatization disorder: A practical review. *Canadian Journal of Psychiatry, 49*, 652–662.

Reuber, M. (2008). Psychogenic nonepileptic seizures: Answers and questions. *Epilepsy & Behavior, 12*(4), 622–635.

Rief, W., Hennings, A., Riemer, S., & Euteneuer, F. (2010). Psychobiological differences between depression and somatization. *Journal of Psychosomatic Research, 68*(5), 495–502.

Romero-Acosta, K., Canals, J., Hernández-Martinez, C., Penelo, E., Zolog, T. C., & Domènech-Llaberia, E. (2013). Age and gender differences of somatic symptoms in children and adolescents. *Journal of Mental Health, 22*(1), 33–41.

Schneider, G., Wachter, M., Driesch, G., Kruse, A., Nehen, H. G., & Heuft, G. (2003). Subjective body complaint as an indicator of somatization in elderly patients. *Psychosomatics, 44*(2), 91–99.

Silverstein, B., Edwards, T., Gamma, A., Ajdaric-Gross, V., Rossier, W., & Angst, J. (2013). The role played by depression associated with somatic symptomatology in accounting for gender differences in the prevalence of depression. *Social Psychiatry and Psychiatric Epidemiology, 48*, 257–263.

Steinbrecher, N., Koerber, S., Frieser, D., & Hiller, W. (2011). The prevalence of medically unexplained symptoms in primary care. *Psychosomatics, 52*(3), 263–271.

Taylor, E. J. (2002). *Spiritual care: Nursing theory, research, and practice.* Upper Saddle River, NJ: Prentice Hall.

Warren, J. W., Langenberg, P., & Clauw, D. J. (2013). The number of existing functional somatic syndromes (FSSs) is an important factor for new, different FSSs. *Journal of Psychosomatic Research, 74*(1), 12–17.

Yick, A. G., Shibusawa, T., & Agbayani-Siewert, P. (2003). Partner violence, depression, and practice implications with families of Chinese descent. *Journal of Cultural Diversity, 10*(3), 96–104.

CHAPTER 25

Feeding and Eating Disorders

Kathryn Weaver
Adapted from the chapter "Eating Disorders" by Jane H. White

LEARNING OBJECTIVES

After studying this chapter, you will be able to:

- Distinguish the characteristics of feeding and eating disorders.
- Describe biologic, psychological, and social aetiologic theories of anorexia nervosa, bulimia nervosa, and binge-eating disorder within the broader spiritual dimension.
- Explain the importance of body image, body dissatisfaction, and gender identity in developmental theories that explain aetiology of anorexia nervosa, bulimia nervosa, and binge-eating disorder. Appreciate the role obesity plays in the development of anorexia nervosa and bulimia nervosa and as a consequence of binge-eating disorder.
- Describe the neurobiology, neurochemistry, and physiologic consequences associated with anorexia nervosa, bulimia nervosa, and binge-eating disorder.
- Explain the impact of sociocultural norms on the development of eating disorders.
- Describe the risk factors and protective factors associated with the development of eating disorders.
- Formulate nursing diagnoses for individuals with eating disorders.
- Identify and describe nursing interventions for individuals with anorexia nervosa, bulimia nervosa, and binge-eating disorder.
- Analyze special concerns within the nurse–client relationship for the nursing care of individuals with eating disorders.
- Identify strategies for the prevention and early detection of eating disorders.

KEY CONCEPTS

- body dissatisfaction
- body image distortion
- dietary restraint
- drive for thinness
- enmeshment
- interoceptive awareness
- maturity fears
- social comparison

KEY TERMS

- anorexia nervosa • binge eating • binge-eating disorder
- body image • body mass index • bulimia nervosa • cue elimination
- self-monitoring

Since vocalist Karen Carpenter's untimely death in 1983 raised global awareness about eating disorders, the celebrities who have disclosed eating disorders include Princess Diana, actors Dennis Quaid and Billy Bob Thornton, singer Elton John, and model Ron Saxen whose book, *The Good Eater*, describes his ordeal with binge eating. Eating disorders date to the time of ancient Greece when the rich reportedly gorged themselves and vomited, while others were reluctant to eat, believing food caused disease. In the Middle Ages, anorexia was viewed as holy and admirable (Kubersky, 1998); Saint Catherine of Siena (Cavallini, 2005) provides an example. Although in contemporary times, major religions oppose starving behaviour, restricting food can be admired as strength of character. The "starving disease" was coined in 1870 by Sir William Withey Gull (cited in Kubersky, 1998, p. 28), also using the term "nervosa." A clinical case report in the *Maritime Medical News* by New Brunswick physician Inches (1895) described a 17-year-old with low weight, loss of menses, and "almost complete refusal of food of any kind" (p. 74).

This chapter focuses on **anorexia nervosa (AN)**, **bulimia nervosa (BN)**, and **binge-eating disorder (BED)** with less common feeding and eating disorders defined. The role of obesity in the development of eating disorders and as a consequence of BED is considered. Because manifestations of eating disorders (e.g., dieting, binge eating, weight fluctuations, and preoccupation with weight and shape) overlap significantly, they may be viewed holistically within a continuum (Fig. 25-1) of eating experiences. On one end is *unrestrained eating* wherein eating and appearance are not at issue for the individual. For most, this is a time of healthy eating, exercise, weight, and body image; however, unrestrained eating can include binge eating. *Watchful eating* includes paying attention to food composition and calories, tracking calories, and physical activity for the purpose of modifying daily caloric, fat, and carbohydrate consumption. At this stage, the individual is becoming dissatisfied with body appearance and may weigh self more than usual, relating weight changes to calories ingested or expended. The individual's identity is shifting to one of a dieter and/or body sculptor. With *increasing weight and shape preoccupation*, the individual more rigidly adheres to food selection and eating patterns, insistently comparing energy expended to energy ingested and tracking weight losses and gains. A pattern of dietary restriction in response to weight gain may emerge. Chemical preparations and supplements may also be purchased and taken to target appearance ideals. Episodes of restricting or avoiding food intake, binge eating, and purging may develop. At the far end of the continuum, as the disturbed eating increases in frequency and/or duration, *clinical eating disorders* emerge as AN, BN, BED, and other disorders identified in the *Diagnostic and Statistical Manual of Mental Disorders* (5th ed.) (*DSM-5*) (American Psychiatric Association, 2013). Individuals may cycle back and forth among these disorders. Definition, clinical course, aetiologies, and interventions for the different eating disorders are considered separately in this chapter. Yet, because their risk factors and prevention strategies are similar, they are discussed under one heading.

ANOREXIA NERVOSA
Clinical Course

Although the risk of eating disorders occurs across the lifespan, the onset of AN is usually in adolescence or early adulthood. This onset is often associated with a stressful

FIGURE 25-1. Continuum of eating experiences.

transition (e.g., leaving home) and can be slow with serious dieting present long before an emaciated body is noticed. In a study of Canadian women 50 years and older, 2.6% of those 50 to 64 years and 1.8% of those over 65 years reported eating disorder symptomatology (Gadalla, 2008). Older persons who develop AN may exhibit more signs and symptoms and experience a longer duration of illness (APA, 2013).

The long-term outcome of AN has improved during the past 15 to 20 years because awareness has

IN A LIFE

Alana Ruben Free: Beginner at Life
A Canadian Success

Alana Ruben Free, a Fredericton, New Brunswick-born woman, struggled with an eating disorder as a young mother. At the age of 27, 7 months after the birth of her son, she lost her appetite and struggled for a year and a half with what she thought were digestive problems. While doing research on the Internet, she discovered she had postpartum depression and potentially anorexia nervosa. Alana contacted a well-trained nutritionist with a specialty in eating disorders who diagnosed her with atypical anorexia and put her on a treatment plan.

"Once I was diagnosed, I thought I'd be better in seven days. The nutritionist would tell me what to eat and I would eat it, and get better. But, the problem was I couldn't. I actually couldn't eat. I had no appetite. That was when the journey started." Ruben Free said it took all her strength to fight to restore what for most people is a basic human urge, the desire to eat, to put food in her mouth, chew, swallow, and sit with the sensation of satiety, fullness. "I wore yoga pants with an elastic waist for about two years so I didn't have to feel the tightness of my clothes."

Determined to live a life free of anorexia, body issues, and any eating disorder, Alana wrote and performed a stage play, *Beginner at Life*, as a means of speaking her truth, freeing herself from any lingering shame, and fully integrating and embodying her recovery. "This play is about being a human being and how difficult it is to come into our full self. I understood that anorexia was a metaphor that every human being could relate to—a condition that keeps us small and our life too small. Each of us, whether we have anorexia or not, struggles against inner forces that seem to undermine our ability to grow up into our full healthy size, as well as against voices that discourage us from asking for what we truly need and want," she said.

Beginner at Life has been translated into several languages and performed around the world. Source: Alana Ruben Free (personal email communication, August 21, 2013; CBC News: Fredericton woman's play comes to hometown stage. http://www.cbc.ca/news/canada/new-brunswick/story/2012/02/09/nb-fredericton-alana-ruben-free-play.html)

increased early detection. AN can be regarded as a chronic condition, with relapses characterized by significant weight loss; as well, conclusions from a review of 119 outcome studies revealed that 47% of individuals recovered (Steinhausen, 2002). In these and more recent studies, approximately one third of individuals go on to experience BN (Eddy et al., 2008). Furthermore, a matched control comparison of 51 persons with AN (mean age at onset = 14 years) found that 12% (n = 6) had a persisting eating disorder including three with AN, 39% met the criteria for at least one psychiatric disorder, and one in four did not have paid employment owing to psychiatric problems (Wentz, Gillberg, Anckarsäter, Gillberg, & Råstam, 2009). Poor outcome was predicted by premorbid obsessive–compulsive personality disorder, age at onset of AN, and autistic traits.

A 20-year study of the AN client population in British Columbia supports prior reports that AN has the highest mortality rate of any psychiatric disorder in young females (Birmingham, Su, Hlynsky, Goldner, & Gao, 2005). Poor outcome has been related to an initial minimum weight, less weight gain, the presence of purging (vomiting and laxative misuse), a later age of onset, substance abuse, the development of mood and anxiety disorders, and other psychological symptoms including depression (Berkman, Lohr, & Bulik, 2007; Steinhausen, Grigoriou-Serbanescu, Boyadjieva, Neumarker, & Metzke, 2008).

Diagnostic Criteria

The diagnostic criteria for AN have been refined in each edition of the *DSM*. To illustrate, the *DSM-5* does not require amenorrhoea as did previous *DSM* editions (see Table 25-1). As well, the amount of weight loss or lack of weight gain required for the diagnosis of AN has changed over time. In the *DSM-III* (APA, 1987), a weight 75% of that appropriate to age and height was required, while in the *DSM-IV-TR* (2000), a weight 85% of the appropriate weight was specified; the *DSM-5* requires "a significantly low body weight in the context of age, sex, developmental trajectory, and physical health ... defined as a weight that is less than minimally normal or, for children and adolescents, less than that minimally expected" (p. 338). The *DSM-5* use of **body mass index** (BMI) cutoffs to denote severity of AN adds consistency to the challenge of weight assessment. BMI, calculated as weight in kilograms/height in metre square, defines limits of body weight as agreed upon by the Centers for Disease Control and Prevention and the World Health Organization. For example, a BMI below 16.5 kg/m² for an adult is considered to indicate severe underweight.

AN is categorized as (1) restricting or (2) binge–purge type. The purging associated with the binge–purge type may occur through self-induced vomiting or misuse of laxatives, diuretics, or enemas even after eating a normal or small-sized meal or snack. Many of the clinical features associated with AN result from malnutrition or semistarvation. Classic research on volunteers who semistarved and observations of prisoners of war and conscientious objectors have demonstrated that these states of starvation are characterized by food preoccupation, binge eating, depression, obsession, and apathy.

Originally, the central feature of AN was thought to be a distortion in **body image**, the mental picture of one's own body (Bruch, 1973). Body image disturbance occurs when there is extreme discrepancy between how people mentally picture their bodies and how the outside world perceives them. For adolescents, body image has a complex psychological impact on overall self-concept

Table 25-1 Key Diagnostic Characteristics for Anorexia Nervosa	
Diagnostic Criteria	**Target Symptoms and Associated Findings**

A. Energy restriction leading to a significantly low body weight that is less than minimally normal or expected
B. Intense fear of gaining weight or becoming fat, or persistent behaviour interfering with weight gain, even though underweight
C. Disturbance in the way the person experiences body shape or weight, undue influence of body weight or shape on self-evaluation, or persistent lack of recognition of seriousness of current low body weight
• Restricting type: not engaged in binge-eating or purging behaviour (such as self-induced vomiting or misuse of laxatives, diuretics, or enemas) in the past 3 mo
• Binge-eating/purging type: engaging in binge eating or purging behaviour in the past 3 mo
• Current severity
  Mild: BMI > or = 17
  Moderate: BMI = 16–16.99
  Severe: BMI = 15–15.99
  Extreme: BMI < 15
• Partial remission: After all criteria for AN were previously met, either Criterion B (intense fear of gaining weight or becoming fat) or Criterion C (disturbance in self-perception of weight and shape) is still met
• Full remission: After all criteria for AN were previously met, none have been met for a sustained period
	• Depressive symptoms such as depressed mood, social withdrawal, irritability, insomnia, and diminished interest in sex
	• Obsessive–compulsive features related and unrelated to food
	• Preoccupation with thought of food
	• Concerns about eating in public
	• Feelings of ineffectiveness
	• Strong need to control one's environment
	• Inflexible thinking
	• Limited social spontaneity and overly restrained initiative and emotional expression
	
	Associated Physical Examination Findings
	• Complaints of constipation and abdominal pain
	• Cold intolerance
	• Lethargy and excess energy
	• Emaciation
	• Significant hypotension, hypothermia, and skin dryness
	• Bradycardia and possible peripheral oedema
	• Hypertrophy of salivary glands, particularly the parotid gland
	• Dental enamel erosion related to induced vomiting
	• Scars or calluses on dorsum of hand from contact with teeth for inducing vomiting
	
	Associated Laboratory Findings
	• Leucopenia and mild anaemia
	• Elevated blood urea nitrogen
	• Hypercholesterolaemia
	• Elevated liver function studies
	• Electrolyte imbalances, metabolic alkalosis, or metabolic acidosis
	• Low normal serum thyroxine levels; decreased serum triiodothyronine levels
	• Low serum oestrogen levels
	• Sinus bradycardia
	• Metabolic encephalopathy
	• Significantly reduced resting energy expenditure
	• Increased ventricular/brain ratio secondary to starvation

American Psychiatric Association. (2013). *Diagnostic and statistical manual of mental disorders* (5th ed.). Washington, DC: Author.

and is a crucial factor in determining how adolescents both interact with others and expect society to respond to them. Some individuals with AN may feel "globally overweight" while others realize they are thin but consider specific body aspects as "too fat" (APA, 2013, p. 340). Individuals with AN may cling to slenderness as "protection against a body that they loathe" (Massey-Stokes, 2001, p. 292), maintaining that the image of seeing oneself as overweight justifies subsequent restrictive behaviours.

▼ **KEY CONCEPT Body image distortion** occurs when the individual perceives his or her body disparately from how the world or society views it.

Neurobiology, Neurochemistry, and Physiologic Consequences of Anorexia Nervosa

Essential to the diagnosis of AN are semi-starvation behaviours, relentless *drive for thinness* or a morbid fear of becoming fat, and signs and symptoms resulting from the starvation. Individuals with AN ignore body signals or cues, such as hunger and weakness, and concentrate all efforts on controlling food intake. Their entire mental focus narrows to only one goal: weight loss. Typical thought patterns are "If I gain half of a kilo, I'll keep gaining. I'll never stop until I am the same size as the fat woman in the circus." Such all-or-nothing thinking keeps these individuals on rigid regimens for weight loss. Thus, the behaviour of individuals with AN becomes

BOX 25-1 Psychological Characteristics Related to Eating Disorders

Anorexia Nervosa
  Decreased interoceptive awareness
  Sexuality conflict/fears
  Maturity fears
  Ritualistic behaviours
  Perfectionism
  Dietary restraint

Bulimia Nervosa
  Impulsivity
  Boundary problems
  Limit-setting difficulties
  Dietary restraint

Binge-Eating Disorder
  Negative mood
  Self-deprecation
  Social insecurity

Anorexia, Bulimia Nervosa, and Binge-Eating Disorder
  Difficulty expressing anger
  Low self-esteem
  Body dissatisfaction
  Powerlessness
  Ineffectiveness
  Obsessiveness
  Compulsiveness
  Nonassertiveness
  Cognitive distortions

organized around food-related activities, such as preparing food, counting calories, and reading cookbooks. Much behaviour concerning what, when, and how they eat is ritualistic; for example, cutting food into tiny pieces, refusing to eat in the presence of others, or fixing elaborate meals for others which they themselves do not eat. Box 25-1 lists common psychological characteristics.

Because individuals with AN feel inadequate, many fear emotional maturation and the unknown challenges the next developmental stages would bring. For some, remaining physically small symbolizes remaining childlike; weight loss becomes a way to experience control and combat feelings of inadequacy and ineffectiveness. Every lost kilogram is viewed as a success, and weight loss often confers a feeling of virtuousness. Perfectionism is an important characteristic found in adults (Nilsson, Sundbom, & Hagglof, 2008; Pike et al., 2008) and adolescents (Bühren, 2012) with AN.

Individuals with AN may avoid conflict, have difficulty expressing negative emotions, especially anger (Miotto, Pollini, Restaneo, Favaretto, & Preti, 2008), and an overwhelming sense of guilt. In addition, they may have difficulty defining feelings because they are confused about or unsure of emotions and visceral cues, such as hunger; therefore, their responses to cues are inaccurate and inappropriate. Often they cannot name the feelings they are experiencing. This uncertainty and confusion is called a lack of *interoceptive awareness*, and it is thought to be partially responsible for developing and

maintaining this disorder (Beadle, Paradiso, Salerno, & McCormick, 2013).

Because of the ritualistic behaviours, all-encompassing focus on food and weight, and feelings of inadequacy that accompany AN, social contacts are gradually reduced and the person becomes isolated. With more severe weight loss come other symptoms, such as apathy, depression, and even mistrust of others.

The nutritional compromise associated with AN may affect most organs and can produce physiologic disturbances that include cardiac arrhythmias, loss of bone density, neuronal deficits, and hormonal changes (e.g., amenorrhoea, decreased libido). When extremely underweight, individuals with AN may exhibit major depressive disorder (APA, 2013). Table 25-2 presents the medical complications, signs, and symptoms of AN and the other eating disorders that result from starving or binge eating and purging. For instance, purging behaviours may cause electrolyte disturbances. It has been identified that individuals with AN who have diabetes mellitus may "purge" through decreasing insulin doses to subsequently decrease carbohydrate metabolism (Larrañaga, Docet, & García-Mayor, 2011).

> **KEY CONCEPT** **Drive for thinness** is an intense physical and emotional process that overrides all physiologic body cues.

> **KEY CONCEPT** **Interoceptive awareness** is a term used to describe the sensory response to emotional and visceral cues, such as hunger.

Epidemiology

The epidemiologic information for AN as per *DSM-5* criteria is unavailable; the rates given reflect the *DSM-IV-TR* (APA, 2000). The changes in *DSM-5* diagnostic criteria will likely alter the disorder frequencies (Smink, van Hoeken, & Hoek, 2012). According to the Government of Canada (Langlois, Samokhvalov, Rehm, Spence, & Connor Gorber, 2011), prevalence of AN is 0.3% to 1%, similar to that of most Western countries. AN appears to be more prevalent within ethnic minorities and in other countries than previously recognized or reported. Cultural change may be associated with increased vulnerability to eating disorders, especially when values about physical aesthetics are involved (Lam et al., 2009; Miller & Pumariega, 2001). For example, following prolonged Western satellite television exposure, key indicators of disturbed eating were significantly more prevalent among "media naive" Fiji schoolgirls who reported an interest in weight loss as a means of modelling themselves after television characters (Becker, Burwell, Gilman, Herzog, & Hamburg, 2002).

Table 25-2	Complications of Eating Disorders

Body System	Symptoms
From Starvation to Weight Loss	
Musculoskeletal	Loss of muscle mass and loss of fat (emaciation)
	Osteopaenia (*bone mineral* deficiency) and less frequently, osteoporosis
Metabolic	Hypothyroidism (symptoms include lack of energy, weakness, intolerance to cold, and bradycardia)
Cardiac	Hypoglycaemia and decreased insulin sensitivity
Gastrointestinal	Bradycardia, hypotension, loss of cardiac muscle, small heart, cardiac arrhythmias including atrial and ventricular premature contractions, prolonged QT interval, ventricular tachycardia, and sudden death
Reproductive	Delayed gastric emptying, bloating, constipation, abdominal pain, gas, and diarrhoea
	Amenorrhoea, low levels of luteinizing hormone and follicle-stimulating hormone, and irregular periods
Dermatologic	Dry, cracking skin and brittle nails due to dehydration, lanugo (fine baby-like hair over body), oedema, and acrocyanosis (bluish hands and feet); hair thinning
	Leucopenia, anaemia, thrombocytopaenia, hypercholesterolaemia, and hypercarotenaemia
Hematologic	Abnormal taste sensation (possible zinc deficiency)
Neuropsychiatric	Neurologic deficits in cognitive processing of new information; decreased total brain volume; increased brain ventricular size
	Apathetic depression, mild organic mental symptoms, sleep disturbances, and fatigue
Related to Purging (Vomiting and Laxative Abuse)	
Metabolic	Electrolyte abnormalities, particularly hypokalaemia and hypochloremic alkalosis; hypomagnesaemia; increased blood urea nitrogen
Gastrointestinal	Salivary gland and pancreatic inflammation and enlargement with increase in serum amylase; oesophageal and gastric erosion (esophagitis); dysfunctional bowel with haustral dilation; superior mesenteric artery syndrome
Dental	Erosion of dental enamel (perimyolysis), particularly frontal teeth with decreased decay
Neuropsychiatric	Seizures (related to large fluid shifts and electrolyte disturbances), mild neuropathies, fatigue, weakness, and mild organic mental symptoms
Cardiac	Ipecac cardiomyopathy arrhythmias
Binge Eating to Weight Gain	
Gastrointestinal	Heartburn; abdominal discomfort; bloating; gastric rupture; symptoms of fullness may interrupt sleep
Metabolic	Gall bladder disease; type 2 diabetes
Cardiac	Hypertension and hypercholesterolaemia
Musculoskeletal	Arthritis
Respiratory	Shortness of breath; asthma; sleep apnoea; snoring

Age of Onset

The age of onset is typically between 14 and 16 years, with the highest incidence rates for females aged 15 to 19 years. Adolescents are vulnerable because of stressors associated with their development, especially concerns about body image, autonomy, and peer pressure, and their susceptibility to such influences as the media, which extols an ideal body type and discusses dieting and exercise as ways to achieve success, popularity, and power. Unhealthy dieting behaviours are prevalent in Canadian girls as young as 10 years of age (McVey, Tweed, & Blackmore, 2004) and in boys at 13 years (Jonat & Birmingham, 2004). The incidence rate of early-onset

restrictive eating disorders diagnosed by paediatricians in Canada was 2.6 per 100,000 in children aged 5 to 12 years (Pinhas, Morris, Crosby, & Katzman, 2011).

Gender Differences

In clinical settings, females are 10 times more likely to have AN than are males (Langlois et al., 2011). This disparity may be attributed to society's influence on females to achieve an ideal body type and to men's reluctance to seek help for what is widely perceived as a female issue. Box 25-2 highlights findings about eating disorders in males, while Box 25-3 summarizes current research regarding the perspectives of male eating disorder service users.

BOX 25-2 Boys and Men With Eating Disorders

Eating disorders have been present in males for as long as in females. Morton (1694) as cited in Robinson, Mountford, and Sperlinger (2013) described the first case of loss of appetite in the absence of medical disease in a 16-year-old boy. More recently, reports in the Canadian Medical Association (Collier, 2013) and National Association of Anorexia Nervosa and Associated Disorders (Weltzin, 2010) convey a ratio of male-to-female Canadian cases of approximately 1:4. Eating disorders in men and boys are becoming more prevalent.

Woodside (2004, p. 86) questions, "Why are fewer affected men identified in formal treatment settings?" He argues that young men may tend to dismiss symptoms or attribute them to other causes (e.g., poor eating habits) because of societal expectations that persons with eating disorders are female. Feminist writer Soran (2006) further asserts that men and boys are apt to suffer in silence and isolation and be insufficiently treated because eating disorders continue to be viewed as "female" problems. However, this picture is changing as media messages increasingly target boys and men in emphasizing dieting and encouraging such surgical options as pectoral or calf implants to achieve the ideal male physique (Hatmaker, 2005).

Men are more likely to have a later onset than are women, at about the age of 20 years. Boys and men involved in an occupation or a sport in which weight control influences performance, such as wrestling (Braun, Sunday, Huang, & Halmi, 1999) and body building (Goldfield, Blouin, & Woodside, 2006), reported high rates of weight and shape preoccupation, intensive body modification practices, binge eating, and BN. In studies comparing men and women on personality characteristics, men had lower drive for thinness (Dalgliesh & Nutt, 2013; Joiner, Katz, & Heatherton, 2000) and higher attachment avoidance (Dalgliesh & Nutt, 2013), and were less at risk for perfectionism, harm avoidance, and reward dependence (Woodside et al., 2004).

Men with eating disorders report lower laxative abuse, higher vomiting episodes, and more excessive exercise than female participants do (Núñez-Navarro et al., 2012; Weltzin et al., 2012). Men and women do not differ with regard to presenting with a high percent of comorbid conditions, such as depression and substance abuse; however, 30% of men are not taking psychotropic medications when admitted (Weltzin et al., 2012). Feldman and Meyer (2007) found that a history of childhood sexual abuse related to BN but not AN and suggested that men may engage in disordered eating to cope with histories of sexual abuse. Recent research has also found premorbid overweight, particularly if bullied about the weight, to be a precipitating factor for eating disorder development in men.

Ethnic and Cultural Differences

Contextual variables that may influence eating disorders include level of acculturation, socioeconomic status, peer socialization, family structure, and immigration.

The influence of ethnic group is a significant contributing factor in eating disorder development in Canada. To illustrate, female Canadian Jewish adolescents reported more eating disordered behaviours and attitudes compared with their non-Jewish counterparts (Pinhas,

BOX 25-3 Research for Best Practice

PERSPECTIVES OF MALE EATING DISORDER SERVICE USERS

Robinson, K. J. & Sperlinger, D. J. (2013). Being men with eating disorders: Perspectives of male eating disorder service-users. Journal of Health Psychology, 18, 176–186.

The Purpose: The experiences of men with eating disorders are understudied. The study aim was to gain understanding of what men go through in seeking and receiving treatment, specifically to learn more about what men want from treatment, what they have found helpful, and the impact of the issue of gender in treatment.

Methods: A qualitative methodology was used to enable eight men from two eating disorder services in the UK to discuss the issues most important to them. Using Interpretative Phenomenological Analysis, the interviews were examined for feeling, concerns, and meanings. Emergent themes were identified from each interview, and shared themes were integrated across participants. Analysis was enhanced by independent audit of the coherence of the evidence from initial interview transcripts to the final themes, reflexive journaling, acknowledgement of researcher perspective, and provision of transcript extracts to support interpretations.

Findings: Two themes emerged: difficulty seeing self as having an eating disorder and experiences of treatment: how important is gender? The participants found it difficult to admit to themselves and others that they had an eating disorder due to lack of visibility of male eating disorders in the media, fear of negative reactions from others (e.g., others would judge or shun them; loved ones would blame themselves), and the benefits the eating disorder provided (i.e., increased sense of control; comfort for managing life stressors, feeling more accepted while also feeling self was unacceptable). Treatment was at times experienced as insufficient in duration and acceptability. The men found it helpful to feel heard about their experience. However, they often felt professionals did not understand what they needed and they were given something unwanted or nothing at all (which potentially reinforced previous trauma and life experiences). While men and women with eating disorders are more similar than different, the study participants expressed the view that each individual faces unique challenges.

Implications for Nursing: This research reinforces the importance of individual formulation of care and treatment preferences. The findings illustrate a need to raise awareness of eating disorders in men among professionals to facilitate detection, within society to assuage men's fears of a negative response, and among men themselves to assist in the process of admitting there is a problem. Nurses can direct men toward relevant literature and information.

Heinmaa, Bryden, Bradley, & Toner, 2008). Eating disorders also tend to be more common in young people who recently immigrated, even when eating disorders are not common in their country of origin (Reijonen, Prat, Patel, & Greydanus, 2003). McDonald and Kennedy (2005) found immigrants substantially less likely to be obese or overweight upon arrival to Canada and that excess weight gain with additional years in Canada is influenced by the extent to which immigrants interact with members of their ethnic group residing in the same area. Immigrants of Chinese ethnicity exhibited the lowest rates of being overweight and obese, and this did not increase over time because local Chinese-Canadian communities are sufficiently well established to reduce acculturation lifestyle choices.

Familial Predisposition

First-degree relatives of people with AN have higher rates of this disorder (Bulik, Reba, Siega-Riz, & Reichborn-Kjennerud, 2005). Female relatives also have high rates of depression, leading researchers to hypothesize that a shared genetic factor may influence the development of both disorders.

Comorbidity

Comorbid major depression and dysthymia are common in AN (Jordan et al., 2008), as are obsessive–compulsive disorder (OCD) (Reas, Rø, Karterud, Hummelen, & Pedersen, 2013) and anxiety disorders such as social phobia, posttraumatic stress, and panic disorders (Swinbourne et al., 2012; Swinbourne & Touyz, 2007). Cluster C personality disorders are also associated with AN (Kaye, Klump, Frank, & Strober, 2000). Comorbid conditions may resolve when AN has been treated successfully. At other times, symptoms of a premorbid condition, such as OCD, remain even though an individual has recovered. This finding, along with the other findings that OCD symptoms often predate the AN diagnosis, has lead many researchers to believe that (1) certain characteristics of AN, such as perfectionism and preoccupation with symmetry or specific object placement, are trait, rather than state, characteristics and may actually influence the development of the disorder, and (2) OCD may be a risk factor for AN (Anderluk, Tchanturia, Rabe-Hesketh, & Treasure, 2003; Milos, Spindler, Ruggiero, Klaghofer, & Schnyder, 2002; Swinbourne et al., 2012).

Aetiology

Some risk factors and aetiologic factors for eating disorders overlap. For example, dieting is a risk factor for the development of AN, but it is also a biologic aetiologic factor, and in its most serious form—starving—it is also a symptom. Most experts agree that eating disorders are multidimensional and multidetermined. Figure 25-2 depicts the aetiologic factors for AN within their larger spiritual dimension.

Biologic Theories

Most of what is known about the aetiology of AN is focused on psychological factors with little conclusive evidence regarding biologic theories of causation. There are many comorbid conditions, such as depression and OCD, associated with the diagnosis of AN, which may have a shared aetiology. Also, many of the biologic changes noted in AN are determined to be the result of starvation and thus state, rather than trait or causative, factors. Little evidence exists to substantiate that dysregulations in appetite–satiety systems cause AN despite significant research in the fields of endocrine function, skeletal biology, and appetite regulation (e.g., Lawson et al., 2011; Miller, 2011). Appetite dysregulation is best viewed as the end product or result of an interaction between the environment and physiology. The bio/psycho/social/spiritual model of this interaction best explains the aetiology (see Fig. 25-2).

Neuropathologic Theories

Magnetic resonance imaging and computed tomography disclose changes in the brain (e.g., cerebral ventricular enlargement, dilation of the third and lateral ventricles, and enlargement of the cortical sulci and the interhemispheric fusion) of individuals with AN who have significant weight loss. This neuropathy and the deficits in white matter reverse with weight gain. Yet, grey matter changes resulting from extreme starvation may not fully return to normal after months of weight restoration (Friederich et al., 2012; Joos et al., 2011). To date, evidence supports that brain structure changes follow rather than cause AN.

Genetic Theories

Genetic research on eating disorders is evolving. The existence of comorbid conditions makes it difficult to determine the influence of genetics on AN. Separating genetic influences from environmental influences when twins share a similar family environment is difficult, but investigators reviewing data from twin studies have demonstrated that the concordance rate for monozygotic twins is higher (44%) than for dizygotic twins (12.5%). Thus, a genetic factor may be involved in the aetiology of AN (Bulik, Sullivan, Wade, & Kendler, 2000).

Biochemical Theories

Undernutrition and weight regulatory behaviours such as vomiting and laxative abuse can lead to a range of biochemical problems in AN, most commonly, hypokalaemia and metabolic alkalosis in relation to vomiting or

FIGURE 25-2. Bio/psycho/social/spiritual aetiologies for patients with AN.

Spiritual

1. Spiritual distress

Biologic

1. Increased genetic vulnerability
2. Dieting – ➝ starving
3. Overexercising
4. Decreased awareness of hunger
5. OCD
6. Decreased serotonin activity

Social

1. Idealization of thinness – media
2. Pursuit of thinness
3. Enmeshment with family
4. Overprotective family

Psychological

1. Separation–individuation struggle
2. Sexuality conflicts
3. Decreased awareness of emotional cue
4. Feminist view – ➝ Role pressures
5. Negative body image–body dissatisfaction

diuretic use, acidosis related to laxative misuse, hyponatraemia due to excessive water ingestion and chronic energy deprivation or diuretic misuse, low urea and creatinine concentrations that may mask dehydration or renal dysfunction, hypoglycaemia, and decreased thyroid function (Winston, 2012). A review of studies of neuroendocrine, neuropeptide, vasopressin, oxytocin, and neurotransmitter functioning indicate that these systems may be related to maintaining AN (Herpertz-Dahlmann, Seitz, & Konrad, 2011). Endogenous opioids may contribute to the eventual denial of hunger in individuals with the disorder, and this is supported in studies reporting weight gain after receiving opiate antagonists (Attia & Schroeder, 2005; Brown et al., 2007). Neurotransmitter and neuroendocrine abnormalities, such as blunted serotonergic function in low-weight clients, must be viewed with caution as causative factors because these disturbances are state related and tend to normalize after symptom remission and weight gain (Bailer & Kaye, 2003). In these individuals, effects on central serotonergic function may result from starvation, rather than trigger it (Ward, Tiller, Treasure, & Russell, 2000). However, most of the investigations have been limited by small sample sizes or trial design with few controlled studies (Ramoz, Versini, & Gorwood, 2007). Based on the best evidence, these biochemical

changes may be viewed as indicating vulnerability in some individuals who under certain psychological and environmental conditions, such as cultural pressures, starve themselves (Klump, Bulik, Kaye, Treasure, & Tyson, 2009).

Psychological Theories

The most widely accepted theory of AN is psychodynamic. In this theory, key tasks of separation–individuation and autonomy are interrupted. Struggles around identity and role, body image formation, sexuality, and *maturity fears* predominate. During early adolescence, when individuals begin to establish their independence and autonomy, some girls may feel inadequate or ineffective. Dieting and weight control may be viewed as a means to defend against these feelings. In later adolescence, when separation–individuation is a developmental task, similar conflicts arise when an adolescent is ill prepared for this stage and feels inadequate and ineffective in going forward emotionally. Because AN is usually diagnosed between 14 and 18 years of age, developmental struggles of adolescence have long been an acceptable theory of causation (Bruch, 1973).

Studies have shown that girls and boys begin to differ dramatically in self-esteem just before adolescence.

At the time self-doubt increases in girls, pubertal weight gain can also occur, resulting in a more rounded, mature female shape. These normal developmental occurrences can add to confusion about identity. Such confusion and self-doubt are further promoted by conflicting messages that girls receive from society about their roles in life. Girls may interpret expectations about how they should look, what roles they should perform, and what they should achieve in society as pressures to achieve "all." They often try to please others to avoid conflicts around perceived expectations. Similarly, in a large sample of middle school boys, five types of stress (performance, relationship, education, family, and financial) were all associated with body dissatisfaction (Blodgett Salafia & Lemer, 2012). Boys who feel overwhelmed by problems may react by engaging in disordered eating behaviours such as dieting. Feminists have focused on role pressure to partly explain the increase in eating disorders and the greater prevalence in females. Box 25-4 outlines some feminist assumptions regarding role, feminism, eating disorder development, and applicability to both women and men.

BOX 25-4 Feminist Ideology and Eating Disorders

Since the 1970s, proponents of the feminist cultural model of eating disorders have advanced a position to explain the higher prevalence of these disorders in women: women today struggle in a similar way to women in the past. It is argued that during the Victorian era, "hysteria," a well-known emotional illness, developed as a result of oppression when women were "silenced" by a male-dominated society. Feminist scholars claim that women today are socialized to avoid self-expression in the face of conflict, seek attachment through putting others first, judge self by external standards, and present an outward compliant self while the inner self grows angry. Thus, eating disorders are a reaction against societal expectations and norms (Gutwill, 1994).

Feminists take issue with the biomedical explanation of eating disorders, seeing it as limiting and patriarchal. It is the recovery of society that must take place if the prevalence of eating disorders is to decrease. For this to occur, women must be emancipated, have a voice, and be socialized differently. Women need to be coresearchers, not only "subjects" so their stories and perspectives may be known.

Principles of the feminist relational model apply to males with eating disorders. Maine and Bunnell note that "pain is pain" (2008, p. 188). A feminist relational approach proposes that, in growing up, boys may long for connection but are pushed to become autonomous before they have developed the ability to identify their feelings and needs. The increase in eating disorders among males reveals a need to explore their gender roles and expectations, globalized exposure to media images of idealized male bodies, and the possibility that men express distress through their bodies. This approach focuses less on individual pathology and more on individuals' responses to pressures, expectations, roles, or environment (Malson & Ryan, 2008). Contextualizing men's body-related responses within sociopolitical realities may enable greater understanding.

> **KEY CONCEPT Maturity fears** or feeling overwhelmed by adult responsibilities are often underlying issues for individuals with AN. Starvation is viewed as a response to these fears.

Social Theories

The media, the fashion industry, and peer pressure are significant social influences in the development of eating disorders. Magazines and television shows depict young girls and adolescents with thin and often emaciated bodies as glamorous to young women (Ahzern, Bennett, & Hetherington, 2008). Women already practicing dietary restraint were found to eat less after watching slim models on television (Anschutz, Van Strien, & Engels, 2008). For younger girls, dolls such as Barbie, with her unrealistic proportions, have been found to negatively influence their views of normal body types (Dittmar, Halliwell, & Ive, 2006).

Boys also hold unfavourable perceptions of their body image. The body adolescent boys desire for themselves and believe girls are most interested in has become progressively more muscular. In contrast with the thin ideal espoused for females, adolescent males are less concerned with specific weight and more concerned with attaining an idealized masculine shape (Petrie, Greenleaf, & Martin, 2010). It is of particular concern that a significant percentage of adolescent boys were found to frequently wish they were more muscular (38.6%), to believe they would be more confident if they had a greater muscle mass (27.6%), and to sometimes think about taking anabolic steroids (41.5%) to achieve these ends (Martin & Govender, 2011).

Body dissatisfaction resulting from perceiving one's own body as falling short of an ideal may include dissatisfaction about one's weight, shape, size, or even a certain body part. In a study that compared boys and girls with AN to healthy controls, all groups overestimated parts of their bodies; however, males with AN presented a greater overestimation of shoulders, hips, and thighs, whereas adolescent females with AN demonstrated greater overestimation of thorax, waist, and hips than did controls (Darcy et al., 2012). Adolescents, including those not overweight, may act to overcome this dissatisfaction through dieting and overexercising. Moreover, the perception of oneself as overweight when at acceptable weight for height is not exclusive to adolescents. In analyzing data from the 2000/2001 Canadian Community Health Survey, Gucciardi, Wang, Badiani, and Stewart (2007) found the prevalence of distorted weight perception was 23.6% for women between the ages of 20 and 60 years and 7.8% for men with the probability of distorted perception significantly increased with age.

In addition to appearance, social competence may be compared. In a phenomenologic study, 15- to 19-year-old girls being treated for eating disorders found images from television, fashion magazines, and music videos particularly powerful because "They've got great bodies and yeah, people like them. You can see that. They jump around and are really happy. And they probably earn masses of money" (Gustafsson, Edlund, Davén, Kjellin, & Norring, 2010, p. 31). Half of the participants described feeling a pressure to be enterprising, true to themselves, and determined amid the conflicting internalized expectations to be interpersonally oriented, considerate to other people's feelings, and academically or athletically successful to ensure a good future with a glamorous or well-paid job. They recognized that their self-evaluation was negatively affected by their failure to live up to their own high expectations and the comparisons that they made of themselves with others. In other studies, too, the process of social comparison, based upon physical and/or personality features, was found to increase the likelihood of negative self-evaluation, body dissatisfaction, and disturbed eating behaviours due to feelings of insecurity (Chrisler, Fung, Lopez, & Gorman, 2013; Sharpe, Damazer, Treasure, & Schmidt, 2013; Ty & Francis, 2013).

KEY CONCEPT Body dissatisfaction is the belief that one's current body size differs from a highly valued ideal body size and that this difference deserves negative appraisal and may be expressed through comments including "I feel too fat/too gross." Body dissatisfaction has been related to low self-esteem, depression, dieting, bingeing, and purging.

KEY CONCEPT Social comparison—evaluating oneself against idealized others, such as models or attractive peers—is a major factor in body dissatisfaction, weight anxiety, and disturbed eating.

Family Responses

Early family theories and studies have classically labelled the family of the individual with AN as *enmeshed*, overprotective, rigid, and unable to resolve conflicts. In an enmeshed family, boundaries that define individual autonomy are weak: One member may relay communication from another to a third; excessive togetherness may intrude on privacy (Minuchin, Rossman, & Baker, 1978). In a study of family boundary dissolution, women with AN reported more boundary problems with mothers and fathers than did a comparison of non–eating-disordered women (Rowa, Kerig, & Geller, 2001). Specifically, higher levels of enmeshment and caregiving role reversal were reported with mothers.

Overprotectiveness is defined as acting on a high degree of concern for another. Parental overprotectiveness may hinder the child's development of autonomy and competence (Minuchin et al., 1978). Once an eating disorder has developed, the intrinsic characteristics of the disorder itself mitigate the effect of family concern (Senra, Sanchez-Cao, Seoane, & Leung, 2008). Family *rigidity* refers to maintaining the status quo and avoiding change and conflict often through being heavily committed to a strong moral code or religious orientation. Parental focus on appearance has an influence on young women who associate various types of comments about weight and size, including encouragement to control one's size, with increased body image dissatisfaction and disturbed eating symptomatology (Kluck, 2010). Some parents of daughters with eating disorders have described themselves as so attuned to their daughters that they could, as one mother did, act on gut feelings and perceptions in the absence of concrete evidence to obtain timely help when the daughter's health was in extreme danger (Weaver, 2012). Given this finding, it is reasonable to suggest that although boundary violations and overprotectiveness may be part of the pathogenesis of AN, they may also emerge as a result of living with an ill child.

KEY CONCEPT Enmeshment refers to an extreme form of intensity in family interactions.

Spiritual Theories

Core struggles in eating disorders are spiritual in nature. According to Garrett (1998), eating disorders are "an extreme form of desire; a spiritual craving expressed through the body" (p. 17). Spirituality involves developing a sense of life's meaning and purpose that includes experiences such as compassion, loving, accepting love, being able to feel hope, receiving inspiration, feeling enlightened, personal fulfillment, and being honest and congruent (Berrett, Hardman, O'Grady, & Scott Richards, 2007; Pilch, 1988). Without such spiritual development, a 23-year-old former client described feeling "unlovable. I could not give love, for I was incapable. I lost my self-respect and went against all I believed to be true. It was a downward spiral that almost led to my death" (Scott Richards, Smith, Berrett, O'Grady, & Bartz, 2007, p. 174). Indeed, individuals tend to lose the ability to affirm their self-worth and identity, defining themselves as the eating disorder and feeling distant and disconnected from family and friends (Weaver, Wuest, & Ciliska, 2005). Consideration of these spiritual constructs prevents the reduction of the eating disorder to a constellation of disease symptoms.

Historically, the example of Catherine of Sienna (1347–1380), who fasted as part of extreme asceticism, demonstrated profound preoccupation with eating not unlike modern individuals with restricting AN (Reda & Sacco, 2001). Eating practices continue to be associated with strong memories and emotions, in particular guilt, shame, well-being, and self-worth, and with religious expression (Dell & Josephson, 2007; Marsden, Karagianni, & Morgan, 2007). Garrett (1996) interpreted AN as attempting to transform self through self-control and isolation into a person more worthy to society, and recovery as reconnecting with self, others, and nature after having been strengthened through suffering and intending to never again starve, binge, and purge.

In sum, the aetiologic findings indicate no one predominant aetiologic factor for AN. Rather, biopsychosocial and spiritual factors converge to contribute to its development.

Risk Factors

Similar risk factors may put individuals at risk for AN, BN, BED. The risk factors are classified in the same way as are the aetiologic categories: biologic, psychological, social, and spiritual (Fig. 25-3).

Biologic

Biologic risk factors include dieting, altered metabolic rate, and a history of overweight or obesity. Dieting despite weight loss and an increase in basal metabolic rate are the most studied biologic risk factors. Individuals

diet because of body dissatisfaction, a need for control, an actual weight gain, and the fear of weight gain. Girls at risk for developing AN may begin to diet in response to a prepubertal weight increase. The starvation of AN may lead to binge eating followed by purging as a compensatory behaviour when restricting food intake is no longer effective or not possible to maintain (Birmingham, Touyz, & Harbottle, 2009; Zerwas et al., 2013). For individuals at risk for BN, purging ensues because of fear of becoming fat, and further dieting occurs in response to the binge eating and its associated negative effect. Those who develop obesity as a consequence of BED may have a history of "yo-yo" dieting also known as weight cycling, which has impaired their metabolic response (the amount of calories burned daily) so that over time their dieting efforts become ineffective as the cycle of gaining weight back and attempting to lose the weight recurs (Roybal, 2005).

High-level exercise and compulsive physical activity have been associated with such eating disorder symptoms as dietary restraint, weight and shape concerns, obsession with food, poor concentration, drive for thinness, body dissatisfaction, and binge eating (Meyer, Taranis, Goodwin, & Haycraft, 2011). A personal history of overweight or obesity was reported by women recovering from AN (Weaver et al., 2005) and individuals with BED

FIGURE 25-3. Bio/psycho/social/spiritual risk factors for eating disorders.

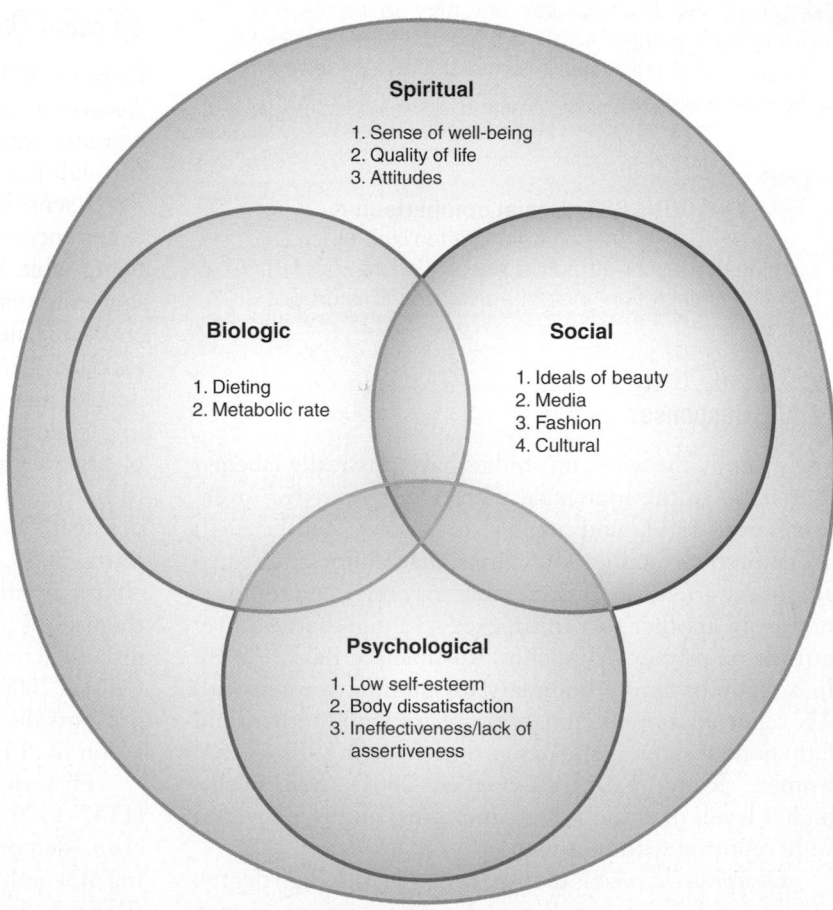

(Striegel-Moore et al., 2007). For adolescent girls, body dissatisfaction begins at the 50th BMI percentile, and body dissatisfaction is reported 1.96 times greater above the 50th BMI percentile than below the 50th percentile (Calzo et al., 2012). Higher BMI leads to dissatisfaction about the body, which can lead to dieting and increased risk for eating pathology. By contrast, boys participating in this same study reported high body dissatisfaction below the 25th BMI percentile (i.e., approaching the underweight range) as well as dramatically higher body dissatisfaction above the 75th percentile (approaching overweight and obesity).

Pubertal growth leads to a normal increase in body fat and broader hips for girls, moving them further away from society's ideal body shape for women. Thus, many girls report higher dissatisfaction and a poorer self-image that may lead them to disordered eating. In contrast, at puberty boys add muscle and their shoulder width increases, characteristics that help them fit the "ideal" cultural message for men's body shape and size. The timing of puberty rather than puberty itself may play a role in body satisfaction for boys—delayed puberty or puberty out of sync with peers may lead to feelings of alienation and depression (Petersen & Taylor, 1980). Late-maturing boys have been found to be more likely to have higher levels of body dissatisfaction, be less popular with their peers, have more conflict with parents, and show more depressive symptoms. Girls who mature early have been found to be at the greatest risk of body dissatisfaction and also tend to be less popular, have poorer self-esteem, and have higher levels of depression than do later-maturing girls.

Psychological

Results of numerous studies have shown that low self-esteem, body dissatisfaction, and feelings of ineffectiveness also put individuals at risk for an eating disorder. In general, women with AN reported lower self-esteem (Vince & Walker, 2008) and significantly higher rates of negative affectivity, perfectionism, and family discord and higher parental demands than did women with other psychiatric disorders (Pike et al., 2008). Specifically, those with the restricting subtype of AN reported higher scores on perceived physical appearance and global self-worth than did those with the binge-eating/purging subtype or BN (Obeid, Buchholz, Boerner, Henderson, & Norris, 2013). This may be because those with restrictive behaviours achieved the "thin ideal" and the goals that they set out to accomplish. Social anxiety and perceived global self-worth are negatively correlated, suggesting that if individuals have low personal feelings of acceptance and overall self-worth, then they are likely to assume that others will evaluate them in the same way (Kocovski & Endler, 2000; Obeid et al., 2013). Recent research has demonstrated that resilience or protective factors, such as academic achievement and positive self-esteem, can mediate psychological risk factors of low self-esteem, body dissatisfaction, and perceived ineffectiveness and thus prevent eating disorder development (Croll, Neumark-Sztainer, Story, & Ireland, 2002).

Childhood sexual abuse has been suggested as a risk factor for eating disorders. Gay and bisexual men with a history of childhood sexual abuse were found more likely to experience eating disorders compared with men who do not have a history of sexual abuse (Feldman & Meyer, 2007). Increasingly, researchers report childhood sexual abuse as a risk factor for the development of BN not necessarily mediated by dietary restriction (Leonard, Steiger, & Kao, 2003; Sanci et al., 2008). Also, middle school girls who were teased about their appearance or overweight by older siblings demonstrated significantly higher levels of body dissatisfaction, thin idealization, dietary restriction, bulimic behaviours, and depression, and lower levels of self-esteem than did girls who were not teased (Keery, Boutelle, van den Berg, & Thompson, 2005). In comparing the rates and parameters of abuse in women with AN and borderline personality disorder (BPD), Laporte and Guttman (2001) found that women with AN experienced less multiple abuse at an older age than did those with personality disorder. Nonetheless, sexual or physical abuse occurred in one fifth and verbal abuse in one third of the women with AN of the latter study and sexual abuse alone in 6% of the former study. Researchers have found a relationship between stress and binge eating (Harrington, Crowther, Henrickson, & Mickelson, 2006; Johnson & Wardle, 2005). Women with BN report a higher incidence of stressful life events than do women with other eating disorders (Vince & Walker, 2008), and the recent findings of Striegel-Moore and colleagues (2007) suggest that elevated levels of perceived stress prior to the age of 14 may precede the onset of BEDs. In a study with older men, Rosenberger and Dorflinger (2013) found that depressive symptoms, lower self-efficacy in sticking with healthier eating habits (e.g., eating smaller portions and sticking with healthy eating habits), higher self-classified weight, and perceived barriers to physical activity (e.g., lack of time, social support, energy level, and willpower) significantly predicted binge eating.

Sociocultural

The media, the fashion industry, and the society's focus on the ideal body type are social risk factors for eating disorders. In addition, peer pressure and attitudes influence eating behaviours by reinforcing societal messages regarding the importance of thinness or popularity. Some adolescents have reported that dieting, binge eating, and purging were learned behaviours, resulting from peer pressure and a need to conform. As demonstrated by their scores on eating behaviour scales, young women who experienced weight-related teasing by peers during childhood and adolescence were more likely to develop disturbed eating behaviours and eating disorders than were their non–weight-teased peers. Those who recalled their weight at ages 6, 12, or 16 years as being heavier than average reported having endured weight teasing more frequently and greater distress than their lighter counterparts (Quick, McWilliams, & Byrd-Bredbenner, 2013).

Although peers increase in importance throughout adolescence and romantic partners become primary sources of personal feedback and satisfaction during young adulthood, research has linked an appearance-focused family culture (including hearing weight-related comments from family members and about the hurtful importance of being thin) with increased disordered eating and body image dissatisfaction (Eisenberg, Berge, Fulkerson, & Neumark-Sztainer, 2012; Kluck, 2010; Linville, Stice, Gau, & O'Neil, 2011). In a sample of college women, those with eating issues were clustered into three groups (dysregulated, rigid, and adaptive) associated with social adjustment difficulties and specific family disturbances (Perkins, Slane, & Klump, 2013). Women in the dysregulated group reported the least parental empathy, warmth, and affection, and the most parental hostility, intrusion, and maternal overprotection. In other studies, low levels of paternal affection, communication, and time spent with daughters and sons during their childhood were associated with high rates of eating and weight problems and eating disorders during their adolescence or early adulthood (Dallos & Denford, 2008; Johnson, Cohen, Kasen, & Brook, 2002). A childhood history of family discord and high parental demands are considered risk factors for BED (Striegel-Moore et al., 2007).

Athletes are at greater risk for developing eating disorders because lower body weights give a competitive advantage. The actual performance demands of a sport and the sports environment itself can intensify body- and weight-related concerns because of such factors as pressure from coaches and parents, social comparisons with teammates, team weigh-ins, physique-revealing uniforms, and judging criteria (Greenleaf, Petrie, Carter, & Reel, 2009). Elite athletes are particularly at risk (Martinsen & Sundgot-Borgen, 2013). Ballet dancers are at high risk because of the need to maintain a particular appearance and performance; both male and female athletes are at risk for developing eating disorders. In particular, boys and men involved in weight-classed sports that necessitate weight restrictions, such as wrestling, bodybuilding, rowing, ski jumping, and swimming, are more likely to engage in pathogenic eating and weight control behaviours than are endurance athletes (Chatterton & Petrie, 2013).

Spiritual

Eating in response to emotional cues such as boredom, loneliness, and anxiety—rather than hunger—may arise from unmet basic needs, including the need for belongingness and self-esteem. Such emotional eating is

considered a risk factor in eating disorders. Women who typically evaluated their worth based on their weight or shape and held unrealistic beliefs such as "I must be perfect in every way" or "I can stop feeling guilty by not eating" may fear rejection or judgement and strive to earn external approval through physical perfection or dieting (Homan & Boyatzis, 2010). These women were found to be more vulnerable to sociocultural messages regarding weight and shape than were women who felt loved and secure in their relationship with their higher power, indicating that women who feel loved and accepted by God are protected *over time* from the harmful effects of sociocultural pressures on body image and eating.

Interdisciplinary Treatment

Treatment of the patient with AN focuses on initiating nutritional rehabilitation, resolving conflicts around body image disturbance, increasing effective coping, addressing the underlying conflicts related to maturity fears and role conflict, and assisting the family with healthy functioning and communication. The preferred method of treatment is outpatient care that includes family-based interventions if the client is a child or adolescent (Findlay, Pinzon, Taddeo, Katzman, & Canadian Paediatric Society Adolescent Health Committee, 2010/reaffirmed 2013). However, the acuity of the eating disorder is carefully monitored. Inpatient hospital admission is warranted if health deteriorates and the client meets the criteria outlined in Table 25-3. Typically, the medical complications presented in Table 25-2 and suicidality influence the decision to hospitalize an individual with an eating disorder.

Treatment goals are developed around nutritional rehabilitation, weight restoration, medical stabilization, prevention of serious medical complications and death, cessation of binge-eating and/or purging behaviours if present, reduction of eating disordered ideation including body image disturbance and dissatisfaction, and restoration of meal patterns that promote health and social connections. An end goal is the reestablishment of social engagement (Academy of Eating Disorders, 2011). Treatment requires an interdisciplinary approach. The primary care provider (usually a physician) is supported by other professionals who together strive to meet the multidisciplinary needs of the client (Central West Eating Disorders Program, 2010). Dieticians plan a weight-increasing program; physicians, nurses, psychologists, and social workers monitor the refeeding process and its effects and establish the intensive therapies that must be instituted after the refeeding phase. Team members may include a consulting psychiatrist, occupational therapist, and dentist.

Individuals with AN are often intelligent, engaging, and (with the exception of their emaciated state) appear nonimpaired. Because of this, they may be erroneously perceived as less sick (Wolfe & Gimby, 2003). It is therefore important to remember the high rates of mortality

Table 25-3 Criteria for Hospitalization of Children, Adolescents, and Adults With Eating Disorders	
Medical	**Psychiatric**

• Weight loss that is:
  <75% below ideal for age, sex, and height
  rapid, e.g., >15% in 1 mo
  associated with physiologic instability unexplained by
    another medical condition
  rapidly approaching weight at which physiologic instability
    occurred in the past
• BMI < 16 for adults
• Heart rate for children, adolescents, and adults (resting
  daytime) <40 bpm
• Cardiac dysrhythmia
• Cardiac oedema
• Blood pressure adults <90/60 mm Hg; children <80/50
  mm Hg. Orthostatic hypotension (with an increase in pulse
  of >20 bpm or drop in BP of >10–20 mm Hg/min from
  supine to standing
• Hypoglycaemia with glucose, 3.0 mmol/L for children; <60
  mg/dL for adults
• Electrolyte imbalance (serum potassium, <2.5
  mmol/L; serum Cl, <88 mmol/L, hyponatraemia,
  hypophosphataemia)
• Severe dehydration
• Hypothermic (body temperature <36°C)
• Oesophageal tears
• Intractable vomiting ± hematemesis
• Physiologic instability
• Acute medical complications due to starvation (e.g.,
  syncope, seizures, cardiac failure, pancreatitis). Also
  poorly controlled diabetes or pregnancy with adults
• Arrested growth and development as per growth chart for
  children and adolescents
	• Acute psychiatric emergencies (e.g., suicidal, psychotic)
	• Comorbid diagnosis that interferes with the treatment of
	  an eating disorder (e.g., severe depression, obsessive–
	  compulsive disorder, severe family dysfunction)
	• Failure to comply with treatment (e.g., acute refusal to eat)
	• Lack of improvement or worsening despite outpatient
	  treatment

Source: Central West Eating Disorders Program. (2010). *Putting eating disorders on the radar of primary care providers.* Available at www.shared-care.ca/files/Eating_Disorders_Toolkit.pdf

and medical complications among individuals with eating disorders. If they are severely malnourished and their somatic systems are seriously compromised, a medical unit might be the choice for the initial intensive refeeding phase that requires close monitoring (see Table 25-2).

The intensive therapies needed to help clients with their underlying issues (e.g., body dissatisfaction and low self-esteem) and families with communication usually begin after refeeding because concentration is usually impaired in the severely undernourished individual with anorexia. During this phase of treatment, a privilege-earning program is often implemented in which positive reinforcers, such as having visitors and receiving passes to go outside the hospital, are earned based on weight gain. After an acceptable weight (at least 85% of ideal) is established, the client may be discharged to a partial hospitalization program or an intensive outpatient program. Art therapy and psychodrama may be more effective than traditional group therapy for adolescents with eating disorders during the acute phases, when the concentration required for verbal therapy may

be impaired (Diamond-Raab & Orrell-Valente, 2002). Family therapy typically begins while the individual is still hospitalized.

Pharmacologic Interventions

Many experts claim that the symptoms of AN, such as body distortion and hyperactivity, are primarily the result of starvation, which causes changes in brain chemistry. Therefore, restoring weight influences symptom remission more than psychopharmacology. It is generally held that the core symptoms of AN are unresponsive to psychotropic medications; however, these medications are useful in treating comorbid psychiatric conditions and preventing relapses (Rossi et al., 2007). The use of tricyclic antidepressants is discouraged, as they generally failed to accelerate weight regain in clinical trials (Mitchell, Roerig, & Steffen, 2013) and may increase susceptibility to hypotension and cardiac arrhythmias (Kaplan & Noble, 2007). Research has demonstrated that selective serotonin reuptake inhibitors (SSRIs) are not efficacious for the early treatment of AN (Mitchell et al., 2013; Strober, Pataki, Freeman, & DeAntonio, 1999), possibly because low body weights cause low protein stores, and protein is needed for SSRI metabolism. However, some clinical experts have found that the SSRIs can be effective later, during outpatient treatment and after weight restoration to address symptoms such as obsessiveness, ritualistic behaviours, and perfectionism. SSRIs must be used with caution, and the client's weight must be constantly monitored because, during the initiation phase, some of the SSRIs may cause weight loss. Buproprion is contraindicated because of increased risk of seizures (Kaplan & Noble, 2007). Recently, the efficacy of antipsychotics in the treatment for AN was determined to not improve weight significantly (McKnight & Park, 2010), despite prior findings that the use of olanzapine for severe AN resulted in weight gain, less resistance to treatment, and reduced agitation (Jensen & Mejlhede, 2000; LaVia, Grey, & Kaye, 2000).

There is no evidence to support the efficacy of mood stabilizers (e.g., lithium) for treating AN, and these medications must be used only with extreme caution in clients with dehydration and compromised renal function (Kaplan & Noble, 2007). Investigation of prokinetic agents to alleviate gastrointestinal (GI) complaints associated with refeeding (e.g., bloating, early satiety) resulted in removal of Prepulside (cisapride) from the market because of potentially fatal cardiac effects (Quigley, 2011). Oestrogen replacement therapy in the form of oral contraceptive pills has not been found effective in preventing osteopaenia/osteoporosis in AN (Lim et al., 2010; Mehler, Cleary, & Gaudiani, 2011). A practical reason to refrain from using hormonal therapy is that it may cause resumption of menses, which in turn may give a false sense of being cured and reinforce denial in women who are still at a low weight. The use of bisphosphonates to improve bone density has generated interest, in light of a study (Miller et al., 2004) finding that bone mineral density increased substantially in the spines of clients with AN who received 5 mg of risedronate, in contrast with bone loss in the controls, despite weight gain and concerns about the safety of these agents in women of reproductive age. Bisphosphonates can persist in the body for many years after the discontinuation of treatment and possibly affect foetal bone development (Mehler et al., 2011). Research is needed to define their long-term efficacy and safety in treatment of bone density loss associated with AN.

Body weight is the most important determinant of bone density; the optimal intervention is one that promotes weight restoration early in the course of the illness. Given the concerns with pharmacologic interventions, the careful assessment of medical complications of starvation that may impede catabolism and excretion is necessary; the use of such agents is recommended only within the context of client support based on nutritional and psychotherapeutic approaches (Mehler et al., 2011; Rossi et al., 2007).

Priority Care Issues

In a 20-year study of 246 treatment-seeking female clients with AN or BN, risk of premature death among those with lifetime AN peaked within the first 10 years, resulting in a standardized mortality ratio of 7.7% (Franko et al., 2013). Predictors of mortality in AN included long duration of illness, alcohol abuse, low BMI, and poor social adjustment. Some studies report mortality rates for women with AN aged 15 to 24 years as 12 times higher than the mortality rates from all other causes for age-matched community comparison groups of women and as two times higher than for other female psychiatric populations (Eckert, Halmi, Marchi, Grove, & Crosby, 1995; Sullivan, 1995).

Stigma is an issue that may impede seeking treatment. Many girls with AN are avoided, especially in their emaciated state. Peers do not know how to approach those with AN who appear both frightening and fragile (Gowers & Shore, 1999). A university setting study found prejudice and discrimination, as evidenced by greater reported discomfort interacting with persons with AN compared with those with depression (Roehrig & McLean, 2010) and mononucleosis (Stewart, Schiavo, Herzog, & Franko, 2008). However, lower levels of blame-based stigma among university students were reported when the aetiology of AN was conceptualized as biologic rather than sociocultural (Crisafulli, Thompson-Brenner, Franko, Eddy, & Herzog, 2010).

Nursing Management: Human Response to Anorexia Nervosa Disorder

Establishing therapeutic alliance with individuals with AN may be difficult initially because they may be suspicious and mistrustful. They often express fear of adults, especially health care professionals, whom they believe want to "make them fat." Because of their low body weight and starvation, they are often impatient and irritable. A matter-of-fact, accepting approach is important. Providing a rationale for all interventions helps build trust. Power struggles over eating are common; remaining nonreactive is a challenge. In avoiding such power struggles, the nurse monitors and reduces personal feelings of frustration and need for control (see Box 25-5).

Nursing management involves bio/psycho/social/spiritual assessment and interventions (see Nursing Care Plan 25-1).

Biologic Domain

Assessment

A thorough evaluation of the client's body systems is important because many systems can be compromised by starvation. A detailed history from both the individual with AN and the family, including the length and duration of symptoms, such as avoiding meals and overexercising,

BOX 25-5   Therapeutic Dialogue

THE CLIENT WITH AN EATING DISORDER

Ineffective Approach

Nurse: You haven't eaten your lunch yet.

Client: I can't. I'm already fat.

Nurse: Look at you, you're skin and bones.

Client: I'll eat when I go out this afternoon on pass.

Nurse: You can't go on pass. You have to start realizing that you are sick. Because you can't take care of yourself, we are in charge.

Client: You're trying to control me.

Nurse: We are trying to be responsible.

Client: I won't eat!

Nurse: Then you will also lose the next pass.

Client: Well I won't go out! At least I won't get fatter.

Effective Approach

Nurse: You haven't eaten your lunch.

Client: I can't. I'm already fat.

Nurse: You're uncomfortable with how you see yourself and with eating?

Client: I'll eat when I go out on pass.

Nurse: You and I, and the other members of your treatment team wrote your behavioural plan together. You know then that you will not be able to go out because your pass is dependent on you eating both breakfast and lunch.

Client: You're trying to control me.

Nurse: The plan is to help you learn to take control over the eating disorder. It sure does mean a lot of hard work for you. How can I help you right now with this meal?

Client: What if I eat half?

Nurse: You are to eat all of it. Why don't I sit here while you eat? Eating is scary for you. We can talk about other choices you have on the unit; tonight, you can choose the movie or board games.

Client: Okay, at least I have some choices.

Critical Thinking Challenge
- What effect did the first interaction have on the client's behaviour? Why?
- In the second interaction, what theories and interventions regarding eating disorders did the nurse use in her approach to the client?

---

is necessary to assess altered nutrition. The longer the duration of these behaviours typically means more difficult and prolonged recovery.

● STUDY NOTE

Eating disorders are serious psychiatric disorders that threaten life. Careful assessment of physiologic and psychological concerns and referral for treatment are important nursing interventions.

Nursing Diagnoses for Biologic Domain

A primary nursing diagnosis is Imbalanced Nutrition: Less Than Body Requirements.

Interventions for Biologic Domain

Weight restoration is the chief intervention during the hospital or initial stage of treatment for AN (Fig. 25-4). The nurse will encounter resistance to eating and weight gain and carefully monitors and records all intake as part of the weight gain protocol. Typically starting with 1,500 cal per day, intake is increased slowly until about 3,500 cal per day is consumed in several meals and snacks. The usual plan for individuals with very low weights is a gain of between 0.5 and 1.0 kg (1 and 2 pounds) a week.

Weight-increasing protocols usually take the form of a behavioural plan, using positive reinforcements (e.g., outings or passes) and negative reinforcements (e.g., returning to bed rest) to facilitate weight gain.

The reinforcements are incremental, informed by client preferences, and based on progress. For example, phone calls, walks around the unit, and walks outside the hospital occur before the day passes and then weekend passes. These protocols provide consistent responses to food-avoidance behaviours and are carried out in a caring and supportive context. When all team members agree on a clear protocol for behaviours related to eating and weight gain, negative reactivity to the individual with AN is greatly reduced. During the implementation of negative reinforcements, the client is helped to see that these actions are not punitive. On rare occasions when the client is unable to recognize or accept the eating disorder as harmful, nasogastric tube feedings may be necessary to enable weight restoration.

Menses history also is assessed. Most young women with AN have reached menarche but may have experienced amenorrhoea for some months because of starvation. A return to regular menses signifies substantial body fat restoration. Sleep disturbance is also common, and these individuals are viewed as overly active. They may sleep little but usually awaken in an energized state. A structured, healthy sleep routine is established immediately to conserve energy and calorie expenditure. To further conserve energy, individuals are often relegated to bed rest until a certain amount of weight is regained. Exercise is generally not permitted during refeeding and only with caution after this phase. Inpatients must be closely supervised because they are often found exercising in their rooms, running in place, and doing calisthenics.

Nursing Care Plan 25-1

Nursing Care Plan for a Patient With AN

Jan is 16 years old, 165 cm (5′4″) tall and weighs 42 kg (92 pounds). She has been treated unsuccessfully in an outpatient clinic and now is being hospitalized to stabilize her weight.

She does not believe that she is too thin and resents being admitted. Her hospitalization was precipitated by being asked to leave the gymnastics team because of her low body weight.

Setting: Inpatient Psychiatric Unit

Baseline Assessment: Jan appears frail, pale, and dressed in oversized, layered clothing. She tearfully states she is depressed and angry and that she has no friends, adding "Why would anyone want to hang out with me? I'm gross! I'm a total disaster!" History and physical findings include bradycardia with pulse = 38, hypotension (80/50), constipation, amenorrhoea for 9 months, dry skin patches, cold intolerance, BMI = 15.8, dehydration, and temperature of 36°C (96.8°F). Laboratory results include hypokalaemia (K^+ = 2.5), leucopenia (WBCs < 5,000), elevated BUN, abnormal thyroid functioning, and bone density via DEXA scan of one standard deviation below mean age-adjusted scores.

Associated Psychiatric Diagnosis	Medications
Anorexia nervosa Binge-eating/purging type	Fluoxetine (Prozac), 20 mg in AM

Nursing Diagnosis 1: Imbalanced Nutrition: Less Than Body Requirements

Defining Characteristics	Related Factors
Unable to gain required weight Weight more than 20% below ideal weight	Believes she cannot eat as she feels full Purges by vomiting "because I feel so full and fat" Exercises 3–4 hours daily (usually in her room late at night) Sleep pattern disturbed by exercise

Outcomes

Initial	Long Term
Maintains daily intake of 1,500 cal Eliminates exercising while in hospital Ceases purging for 1 week	Gains 0.5–1.5 kg (1–3 pounds) per week until weight is approximately 85% of ideal weight or attains a BMI of approximately 17 Develops strategies to maintain weight

Interventions

Interventions	Rationale	Ongoing Assessment
Encourage Jan to verbalize feelings such as anxiety related to food and weight gain—develop a therapeutic relationship. Monitor meals and snacks, record the amount eaten. Provide any required supplemental intake. Do not substitute other foods for food on meal trays. Limit caffeine intake to one cup of coffee or soda daily.	Through relationship with the nurse and examining her feelings, she may be more likely to cooperate with the nutritional regimen. Severe AN is life threatening. Aggressive interventions are needed to ensure adequate intake. People with AN often "play games" with food. Prohibiting substitution encourages a more positive approach. Caffeine has appetite suppressant and diuretic effects.	Determine anxiety level when discussing food, body image, and weight gain. Assess Jan's ability to complete meals on time and without supplements. Support Jan in following her nutritional regimen.

Nursing Care Plan 25-1 *(Continued)*

Interventions	Rationale	Ongoing Assessment
Monitor Jan's behaviour after meals and snacks for purging and exercising. Weigh her daily each morning in hospital gown after she has voided. Monitor vital signs daily, electrolytes.	Physical signs of impending complications include evidence of purging, decreasing body weight, hypotension, hyperthermia, and hypokalaemia.	Monitor vital signs, weight, and electrolytes, especially potassium.
Assist Jan to identify activities to try if she feels compelled to purge or exercise.	Positive coping skills will enable her to build capacity to hold and mitigate distress.	Monitor restless behaviour.
Provide psychoeducational intervention. Teach risks of osteopaenia and role of fat-soluble vitamins.	Increase awareness of health needs and risks.	Observe comprehension of material. Repeat teaching after weight restoration if mental concentration was initially impaired.

Evaluation

Outcomes	Revised Outcomes	Interventions
Jan gains 2 kg (5 pounds) at the end of 2 weeks. Jan cooperates with meal regimen.	Ceases purging episodes for 1 week. Continues to increase her weight 0.5–1.5 kg/week (1–3 pounds/week).	Daily weights while on unsupervised meals. Praise her for her successes. Arrange for discharge to outpatient clinic or day hospital program.
She has begun to acknowledge the seriousness of her illness and the life-threatening aspects of severe dieting and purging.	Establish and maintain regular, adequate nutritional eating habits.	Participation in relapse-prevention classes.

Nursing Diagnosis 2: Disturbed Body Image/Body Experience

Defining Characteristics	Related Factors
Verbalizes that she is too fat	Inaccurate perceptions of physical appearance secondary to anorexia nervosa
Perceives herself as "gross" and unattractive	Believes that she is failing to measure up to an internalized desired ideal of beauty
Hides body in layers of baggy clothing	Equates physical fitness and attractiveness with thinness

Outcomes

Initial	Long term
Verbalizes feelings related to changing body shape and weight	Acknowledges negative consequences of too little fat on body
Identifies beliefs about controlling body size	Identifies positive aspects of her body and its ability to function

Interventions

Interventions	Rationale	Ongoing Assessment
Explore Jan's beliefs and feelings about body. Maintain a nonjudgemental approach.	To help Jan gain a more positive body image, an understanding of her own views is important.	Monitor for statements that identify perceptions of her body. Is her view *distorted* or *dissatisfied*?

Continued

Interventions

Interventions	Rationale	Ongoing Assessment
Assist Jan in identifying positive and realistic physical characteristics.	In AN, the body is viewed negatively. By focusing on parts of the body that are positive, such as the eyes or hands, or that enhance function, such as strong legs for running, Jan can begin to experience a positive image of her body.	Observe for her reaction to her body. Which areas are viewed positively? Observe for negative statements related to body size and self-esteem.
Clarify Jan's views about an ideal body.	Many societal cues idealize an unrealistically thin female body.	Monitor for statements indicating external pressures to lose weight, experiences of teasing about body changes, or evidence of sexual abuse from others.
Provide education related to normal growth of women's bodies and the protective role of fat.	Providing education will help in reinforcing a broader view of the importance of a healthy body.	Assess willingness to learn information.

Evaluation

Outcomes	Revised Outcomes	Interventions
Jan revealed her belief that she is too fat but does have positive physical traits—her eyes. She believes that those who are overweight have lost control of their lives. She knows some models who are 6′ and weigh barely 45 kg (100 pounds).	Jan accepts alternative beliefs related to her own body.	Gradually, focus on other positive physical aspects of Jan's body. Discuss grooming that encourages a more attractive look. Challenge her beliefs about body weights of models.
Willing to read information about normal body functioning.	Jan accepts a new view of body functioning as a complex phenomenon.	Discuss the biologic aspect of the development of body weight. Emphasize multiple factors that determine body weight.

Nursing Diagnosis 3: Spiritual Distress Related to Loss of Relationship With Self and Others

Defining Characteristics	Related Factors
Questions or expresses inner conflict about her self, the meaning or purpose of her life	"Why would anyone want to hang out with me?"
Evinces guilt, hopelessness, despair, and/or abandonment	Tearful, depressed, and angry
Withdrawal from, or absence of, relationships	Says she has no friends
Refers to self in a totally negative way	"I'm gross. I'm a total disaster!"

Outcomes

Initial	Long term
Begins to expresses inner distress in acceptable ways (e.g., talking, journaling, art work)	Spiritual health as evidenced by: Using a type of spiritual experience/expression that provides her comfort Connecting with others to share thoughts, feelings, and beliefs

Interventions

Interventions	Rationale	Ongoing Assessment
Model self-awareness and acceptance without harsh self-judgement.	Jan will not trust a nurse who does not demonstrate self-comfort.	Ask: How do you feel about the changes in your life that have come about because of the eating disorder?

Nursing Care Plan 25-1 (*Continued*)

Interventions	Rationale	Ongoing Assessment
Create an accepting, nonjudgemental atmosphere.	Providing ongoing, unconditional support establishes rapport and therapeutic relationship, which promotes communication, open expression, and opportunity to explore inner world of meaning and experience	Assess her ability to see and affirm her self-worth and identity. What does she sees as her strengths? Does she define herself as *the eating disorder?*
Spend nontask time with Jan.	Being with the person who is suffering gives meaning to his or her experience. It confirms to the client that he or she is important and of value. The nurse's presence helps alleviate the client's sense of isolation, anxiety, and abandonment.	Is she feeling distant and disconnected from family and friends? Does she know what she does and does not have control over? Does she accept her human limitations within the context of any traumatic experiences?
Encourage Jan to experience and verbalize feelings, perceptions, and fears	Helps her access potential healing resources to well-being. Releasing emotions can provide energy and freedom.	Assess her ability to name and identify her feelings.
Encourage her to identify values that guide her everyday behaviour and her actions in times of crisis, loss, and tragedy.	Helps her clarify values and beliefs by reflecting on past behaviours. Experience is a major source for values development.	Assess her ability to challenge counterproductive beliefs.
Observe and listen empathetically to her communication, offering patience, repetition, and reassurance over an extended period of time.	Listening to the "unacceptable" helps the process of finding meaning, healing, growth, and reentering life with a renewed sense of purpose and connection to others and self.	Assess her growth beyond any prior limiting or traumatic experiences. Does she accept herself and her past? What, if anything, would she change?
Help Jan tell her story about the eating disorder and any painful traumatic experiences in descriptive rather than evaluative terms.	Storytelling minimizes self-judgement and allows emergence of patterns that aid understanding.	Monitor her capacity for informed understanding.
Help Jan develop a healthy, positive outlook through such things as letter writing, meditation, and/or imagery.	Helps her access potential healing resources to enhance well-being and reduce negative affectivity.	Assess her ability to care for self.

Outcomes	Revised Outcomes	Interventions
She has begun to acknowledge the meaning of the eating disorder in her life and the life-threatening aspects of severe dieting and purging.	Establish and maintain appropriate self-care strategies that include adequate nutrition and eating practices and self-development.	Participation in comprehensive and individualized treatment program.

Psychological Domain

Assessment

The psychological symptoms that individuals with AN experience are listed in Box 25-1. The classic symptoms—low weight, unrealistic expectations and thinking, and ritualistic behaviours—may be noted during a clinical interview. Conflicts that underlie this disorder, such as maturity or independence fears and feelings of ineffectiveness, may not be apparent during the interview.

Assessing individuals with low self-esteem and high social anxiety may be particularly difficult, as clients may believe that the clinician is negatively evaluating them, whereas their low self-worth may make them feel that they are not worth the effort of referral or therapy.

A variety of instruments is available to clinicians and researchers for determining the presence and severity of symptoms. Box 25-6 lists well-known instruments used to assess psychological symptoms associated with eating disorders. The Eating Attitude Test is frequently

FIGURE 25-4. Bio/psycho/social/spiritual interventions for individuals with AN.

Spiritual
1. Model self awareness and acceptance
2. Suspend negative judgement
3. Encourage description of eating disorder experiences
4. Encourage expression of life history
5. Activities to promote reflection and awareness
6. Peer debriefing of countertransference experiences

Biologic
1. Assess and monitor somatic symptoms
2. Weigh daily
3. Record all intake
4. Supervise bathroom if purging
5. Establish normal sleep routine
6. Administer medication for depression
7. Monitor exercise

Social
1. Be supportive but firm with family
2. Include family in therapies and teaching
3. Suggest resources for information and support
4. Assist teachers with discharge plans and re-entry into classroom

Psychological
1. Establish trust
2. Use diary self-monitoring to help identify emotions
3. Correct cognitive distortions
4. Encourage movement–dance therapies
5. Assist with realistic goal setting
6. Provide education to clarify misconceptions

used with community and clinical populations. There is an abbreviated 26-item version of this test, EAT26 for adolescents and adults, and also a child version, the CHEAT. The test is readily available online (http://www.eat-26.com/) and is particularly useful in screening for eating disorder risk in high school, university, and in other groups such as athletes. The results can help identify the most significant symptoms and indicate if an individual should be referred for evaluation of an eating disorder.

Nursing Diagnosis for Psychological Domain

Two common nursing diagnoses in AN are Anxiety and Disturbed Body Image.

Interventions for Psychological Domain

Most individuals with AN experience interoceptive awareness problems (inability to experience visceral cues and emotions) and use a somatic complaint such as "I feel bloated" or "I'm fat" to replace a negative emotion such as guilt or anger. Although these complaints may be related to refeeding, they often are part of body dissatisfaction. Research into the experiences of women with eating disorders has demonstrated shame about one's body to be a major theme (Rørtveit, Åström, & Severinsson, 2009) influencing self-criticism (Kelly & Carter, 2012) and nondisclosure (Swan & Andrews, 2003). To make

it possible for women to speak about such feelings, the nurse can normalize the shame experience in conversation with the client and can encourage clients in keeping a journal, helping them to identify feelings by having them write a description of the "fat feeling" and list possible underlying emotions and troublesome situations next to this description.

In preparing to interact with an individual struggling with AN, the clinician must first make meaning of personal experiences with eating issues and self-preservation strategies. Self-awareness and acceptance cannot be effectively modelled without having engaged in this critical self-development. In Box 25-7, an upper-level student nurse reflected on her past experiences that influenced the development of an eating disorder. Through identifying the various perceptions, values, and pressures that guided her own actions and responses, the student was receptive to exploring underlying factors and points of interest with her clients.

Understanding Feelings

Identifying feelings, such as anxiety and fear, and especially negative emotions, such as anger, helps individuals decrease conflict avoidance and develop effective strategies for managing these feelings. It is unhelpful to attempt to change distorted body image by pointing out that the individual is actually too thin. This characteristic is often the last to resolve itself, and it may take years

BOX 25-6 Assessment Tools for Eating Disorder Symptoms

1. Screening Tools
SCOFF
Perry, L., Morgan, J., Reid, F., Brunton, J., O'Brien, A., Luck, A., & Lacey, H. (2002). Screening for symptoms of eating disorders: Reliability of the SCOFF screening tool with written compared to oral delivery. *International Journal of Eating Disorders, 32*(4), 466–472.

Eating Attitude Test (EAT)
Garner, D. M. & Garfinkel, P. E. (1979). The Eating Attitude Test: An index of the symptoms of anorexia nervosa. *Psychosomatic Medicine, 10,* 647–656.
Garner, D. M., Olmsted, M. P., Bohr, Y., & Garfinkel, P. E. (1982). The Eating Attitude Test: Psychometric features and clinical correlates. *Psychological Medicine, 12,* 871–878.

Children's Eating Attitude Test (CHEAT)
Maloney, M., McGuire, J., & Daniels, S. R. (1988). Reliability testing of a children's version of the Eating Attitude Test. *Journal of the American Academy of Child and Adolescent Psychiatry, 27,* 541–543.
Smolak, L. & Levine, M. P. (1994). Psychometric properties of the Children's Eating Attitudes Test. *International Journal of Eating Disorders, 16*(3), 275–282.

2. Assessment/Diagnostic Measures
Eating Disorder Examination
Cooper, P., Taylor, M., Cooper, Z., & Fairburn, C. (1987). The development and validation of the BSQ. *International Journal of Eating Disorders, 6,* 485–494.
Fairburn C. G. & Cooper, Z. (1993). The Eating Disorder Examination. In C. G. Fairburn & G. T. Wilson (Eds.). *Binge eating: Nature, assessment and treatment* (12th ed., pp. 317–360). New York: Guilford Press.

Eating Disorder Examination -Questionnaire (EDE-Q)
Carter, J. C., Stewart, D. A., & Fairburn, C. G. (2001). Eating Disorder Examination Questionnaire: Norms for adolescent girls. *Behaviour Research and Therapy, 39,* 625–632.
Fairburn, C. G. & Beglin, S. J. (1994). Assessment of eating disorder psychopathology: Interview or self-report questionnaire? *International Journal of Eating Disorders, 16,* 363–370.
Mond, J. M., Hay, P. J., Rodgers, B., & Owen, C. (2006). Eating Disorder Examination Questionnaire (EDE-Q): Norms for young adult women. *Behaviour Research and Therapy, 44,* 53–62.

Eating Disorder Inventory-3 (EDI-3) and EDI-3 Symptom Checklist (EDI-3-SC)
Garner, D. M. (2011). *Eating Disorder Inventory-3: Professional manual.* Odessa, FL: Psychological Assessment Resources.

Yale-Brown-Cornell Eating Disorder Scale (YBC-EDS)
Mazure, C. M., Halmi, K. A., Sunday, S. R., Romano, S. J., & Einhorn, A. M. (1994). Yale-Brown-Cornell Eating Disorder Scale: Development, use, reliability, and validity. *Journal of Psychiatric Research, 28,* 425–445.
Sunday, S. R., Halmi, K. A., & Einhorn, A. (1995). The Yale-Brown-Cornell eating disorder scale: A new scale to assess eating disorder symptomatology. *International Journal of Eating Disorders, 18*(3), 237–245.

Three-factor Eating Questionnaire-R18
de Lauzon, B., Romon, M., Deschamps, V., Lafay, L., Borys, J-M., Karlsson, J., ... Fleurbaix Laventie Ville Sante Study Group. (2004). The Three-Factor Eating Questionnaire-R18 is able to distinguish among different eating patterns in a general population. *Journal of Nutrition, 134*(9), 2372–2380.

3. Tests of Body Dissatisfaction/Body Image
Body Shape Questionnaire (BSQ)
Cooper, P., Taylor, M., Cooper, Z., & Fairburn, C. (1987). The development and validation of the BSQ. *International Journal of Eating Disorders, 6,* 485–494.
Colour-a-Person Test
Wooley, S. C., & Kearney-Cooke, A. (1986). Intensive treatment of bulimia and body image disturbance. In K. D. Brownell & J. P. Foreyt (Eds.), *Handbook of eating disorders: Physiology, psychology and treatment of obesity, anorexia, and bulimia* (pp. 476–502). New York: Basic Books.

4. Tests of Emotional and Cognitive Components
Cognitive Behavioural Dieting Scale
Martz, D. M., Sturgis, E. T., & Gustafson, S. B. (1996). Development and preliminary validation of the Cognitive Behavioral Dieting Scale. *International Journal of Eating Disorders, 19,* 297–309.
Emotional Eating Scale
Arrow, B., Kenardy, J., & Agras, W. S. (1995). The Emotional Eating Scale: The development of a measure to assess coping with negative affect by eating. *International Journal of Eating Disorders, 18,* 79–90.

Compulsive Eating Scale
Ondercin, P. A. (1979). Compulsive eating in college women. *Journal of College Student Personnel, 20,* 153–157.
Dunn, P. K. & Ondercin, P. (1981). Personality variables related to compulsive eating in college women. *Journal of Clinical Psychology, 31,* 43–49.
Golden, B. R., Buzcek, T., & Robbins, S. B. (1986). Parameters of bulimia: Examining the Compulsive Eating Scale. *Measurement and Evaluation in Counselling and Development, 19(2),* 84–92.

The Restraint Scale (RS)
Herman, C. P. & Polivy, J. (1975). Anxiety, restraint, and eating behavior. *Journal of Abnormal Psychology, 84,* 66–72.
Herman, C. P. & Polivy, J. (1980). Restrained eating. In A. J. Stunkard (Ed.), *Obesity* (pp. 208–225). Philadelphia: Saunders.

Three Factor Eating Questionnaire Cognitive Restraint Scale (TFEQ-R)
Stunkard, A. J. & Messick, S. (1985). The Three-Factor Eating Questionnaire to measure dietary restraint, disinhibition, and hunger. *Journal of Psychosomatic Research, 29,* 71–83.

5. Behavioural Tests
Test meals
Andersen, A. E. (1995). A standard test meal to assess treatment response in anorexia nervosa patients. *Eating Disorders, 3,* 47–55.
Anderson, D. A. & Maloney, K. C. (2001). The efficacy of cognitive-behavioral therapy on the core symptoms of bulimia nervosa. *Clinical Psychology Review, 21,* 971–988.
Anderson, D. A., Williamson, D. A., Johnson, W. G., & Grieve, C. O. (2001). Validity of test meals for determining binge eating. *Eating Behaviors, 2,* 105–112.

6. Risk Factors Identification
The McKnight Risk Factor Survey
Shisslak, C. M., Renger, R., Sharpe, T., Crago, M., McKnight, K. M., Gray, N., ... Taylor, C. B. (1999). Development and evaluation of the McKnight Risk Factor Survey for assessing potential risk and protective factors for disordered eating in preadolescent and adolescent girls. *International Journal of Eating Disorders, 25*(2), 195–214. (Versions available for younger and older children).

BOX 25-7 Spirituality of the Nurse: Beginning the Journey

Self-Esteem and Eating Disorders

Born into a dark world of neglect,
There wasn't a person whose expectations I met.
Always told I was "not good enough,"
These words embedded in my brain, making life tough.
Constantly teased for being overweight
And without a friend who could truly relate.
I believed I knew what I had to do,
I needed to eliminate the enemy: food!
But, I just did not realize how hard it would be
To go without something my body would need.
Results showed quickly and I was no longer ignored,
Why had I not thought to starve myself before?
Yet, I needed to be skinnier so I could meet society's needs,
After all, others are the ones I needed to please.
My bones were now visible, giving me the motivation I would need,
To work out even harder to ensure I would succeed.
My hair was dead and finger nails brittle,
But society loved me because I was little.

By Samantha Braman
University of New Brunswick

In my 3rd year of nursing, I had the privilege of working in "It's Not About Food" (INAF), a group for women around campus who were experiencing eating issues. This community clinical experience allowed me to self-reflect on my own personal struggle with anorexia nervosa that I had battled as a young teen. Writing this poem was one way that allowed me to express the many thoughts and feelings that I had experienced when working through my issue. I learned the major role that self-esteem plays in the development of an eating issue—something that I myself lacked. As well, there were several other factors contributing to my eating disorder such as family, friends, and society. I spent many years silently recovering from my eating issue until my encounter with INAF. That was when I began to take a stand for my right to be ME (and other people's rights to be themselves). Most people are too embarrassed to admit they have an issue and therefore, never seek the help they may need. It is my hope that readers will realize that eating issues often remain undisclosed and that in order to help eradicate this issue, we must raise awareness and eliminate the stigma. It is a complex issue that is well beyond the "desire" for one to starve oneself, and it typically coincides with other issues including low self-esteem, perfectionism, and obsessive–compulsive disorder. These are all issues that society influences and all issues that require immediate attention. When overcoming AN, I realized that it did not matter what my peers, family, or friends thought of me: It mattered what I thought of myself. I do not have to look, dress, or act a certain way; the only thing I have to do in this life is to be both happy and proud of myself. Overcoming the eating issue was the single hardest challenge of my life, and also my biggest accomplishment! I want to help inspire others to also embark upon what will be their most memorable journey yet.

for individuals to see their bodies realistically. Individuals may continue to fear becoming fat but no longer be driven to act on the distortion by starving. The fear of becoming fat eventually lessens with time.

The nurse can help individuals restructure the way they view the world, especially relative to food, eating, weight, and shape. Faulty ways of viewing these situations result in ineffective coping. Table 25-4 lists some cognitive distortions commonly experienced by individuals with eating disorders and some typical restructuring responses that challenge the distortion, which the nurse can present as more realistic ways of perceiving situations. Other therapies, such as movement and dance therapy, can help individuals experience pleasure from their bodies, although dance should be used cautiously during refeeding because of energy-expenditure concerns. Imagery and relaxation are often used to overcome distortions and decrease anxiety.

Psychotherapy

Interpersonal therapy (IPT) is a type of treatment that focuses on uncovering and resolving developmental and psychological issues underlying the disorder. Role transitions, conflicts, and interpersonal deficits leading to social isolation or chronically unsatisfactory relationships typically are the focus (Hilbert & Brähler, 2012; McIntosh et al., 2006). Cognitive therapy may also be incorporated to continue to address faulty beliefs about food and social interactions (Murphy, Cooper, Hollon, & Fairburn, 2009). A third treatment option, nonspecific supportive clinical management, includes education, care, support, and therapeutic alliance that promotes adherence to treatment through use of praise, reassurance, and advice. Nonspecific supportive clinical management emphasizes the resumption of normal eating and the restoration of weight; verbal and written information are provided on weight maintenance strategies, energy requirements, and relearning to eat normally (McIntosh et al., 2006).

Patient Education

As weight is restored and concentration improved, individuals with AN can maximally benefit from psychoeducation. Although these individuals have much knowledge about food and calories, they also have misinformation that needs clarifying. For example, they are often unclear about the role of "fats" in a healthy diet and try to be as "fat free" as possible. A thorough assessment of their knowledge is important because they may need information on the importance of including all nutrients in a healthy diet.

● STUDY NOTE

Because individuals with AN are often perfectionistic, they may set unrealistic goals. Teaching them to set smaller, progressive, attainable eating goals is one of the most helpful interventions for those with eating disorders.

Table 25-4	Cognitive Distortions Typical of Patients With Eating Disorders, With Restructuring Statements

Distortion	Clarification or Restructuring
Dichotomous or all-or-nothing thinking "I've gained 1 kilo (2 pounds), so I'll be up by 50 kilos (100 pounds) soon."	"You have not ever gained 50 kilos (100 pounds), but I understand that gaining 1 kilo (2 pounds) is scary."
Magnification "I binged last night, so I can't go out with anyone."	"Feeling bad and guilty about a binge are difficult feelings, but you are in treatment and you have been monitoring and changing your eating."
Selective abstraction "I can only be happy 5 kilos (10 pounds) lighter." or "People will only love me if I am thin."	"When you were 5 kilos (10 pounds) lighter, you were hospitalized. You can choose to be happy about many things in your life." "People love you for being you—your kindness, sense of humour, and so on. Let's talk about qualities that make you a good friend/sister"
Overgeneralization "I didn't eat anything yesterday and did okay, so I don't think *not* eating for a week or two will harm me."	"Any starvation harms the body, whether or not outward signs were apparent to you. The more you starve, the more problems your body will encounter."
Catastrophizing "I purged last night for the first time in 4 mo—I'll never recover." or "I am so evil—if I have whipped cream on my latte, my stomach will be over my jeans like a muffin in the tin."	"Recovery includes ups and downs, and it is expected you will still have some mild but infrequent symptoms." "No, that's not true. You are working hard to ensure you take in enough to meet your body's needs, such as the extra energy it takes you to walk all the way to the coffee shop."

 TEACHING POINTS

Individuals with AN often set unrealistic goals and end up frustrated. To help these clients learn to develop appropriate goals around food and other activities, the nurse can help them consider essential topic areas pertinent to their recovery (see Box 25-8) and patiently support them to gain skill in formulating realistic, attainable goals.

BOX 25-8 Psychoeducation Checklist: Anorexia Nervosa

When caring for the patient with AN, be sure to include the following topic areas in the teaching plan:
- Psychopharmacologic agents, if used, including drug, action, dosage, frequency, and possible adverse effects
- Nutrition and eating patterns
- Effect of restrictive eating or dieting
- Weight monitoring
- Safety and comfort measures
- Avoidance of triggers
- Self-monitoring techniques
- Trust
- Realistic goal setting
- Resources

Social Domain

Nursing Diagnosis for Social Domain

Ineffective Coping is a predominant nursing diagnosis with regard to the social domain.

Interventions for Social Domain

Younger individuals with AN who may have lost some school time because of hospitalization may find integrating back into a school and classroom setting difficult. Shame and guilt about having an eating disorder and being hospitalized needs to be addressed. Because these clients typically have isolated themselves before hospitalization and treatment, renewing friendships and relationships with peers may provoke anxiety. Involving school nurses and teachers in the reentry process may help.

When a family is informed that a member has been diagnosed with a dangerous illness such as an eating disorder, the response is often to temporarily feel out of control or afraid (Weaver, 2012; Wright & Leahey 2009). Burden, conflict regarding the seriousness of the AN and caregiving role, attitudes and actions of others, stigma directed toward the family, and social support all influence family functioning (Dimitropoulos, Carter, Schachter, & Woodside, 2008). Family members want to help the affected member but may need help themselves.

Their own emotional reactions (e.g., anger, distress, anxiety, guilt, and fear) may prevent them from expressing themselves as intended, and they may need initial direction, support, and follow-up (Gísladóttir & Svavarsdóttir, 2011). Friends as well as family may say things that are not helpful (Brown & Geller, 2006), and Box 25-9 provides a list of general strategies that may assist families and friends.

Nurses are able to help family members manage feelings, increase effective communication and capacity to provide helpful nonintrusive support, decrease protectiveness, and resolve guilt (Gísladóttir & Svavarsdóttir, 2011). In therapy with the whole family and the person with AN, an advanced practice nurse, therapist, psychologist, or social worker meet regularly with them, at least once a week. This method has been demonstrated to be more effective than family therapy that does not include the individual with AN (Eisler et al., 2000) or individual therapy on its own (Robin et al., 1999). The family are helped to focus on such issues as separation–individuation, autonomy, ineffective communication, symptom interruption, and practical issues, such as how to effectively monitor food intake. A major focus is to help family members see each other's strengths and begin to work together to address the eating issue. See Box 25-10. Many family theorists believe that eating disorders develop because of family dysfunction and as such have some unrealized meaning for each family. For example, an individual may be attempting to keep a separating, divorcing, or estranged family together with the eating disorder. In other instances, parents may be trying to prevent a daughter from separating and individuating because they are emotionally unprepared for this process. The development of an eating disorder may be a reaction to these situations. Therapy helps to uncover these meanings and to improve effective, supportive parenting. Behaviourally based family therapy (FBT or "Maudsley Family Therapy") for adolescents with eating disorders is superior to individual therapy (Couturier, Kimber, & Szatmari, 2013).

Often siblings become resentful of the attention the individual with an eating disorder gets from the parents. It is helpful to have siblings attend family sessions to discuss these feelings and the effect the illness has had on them. Further research is needed to explore social support to individuals with eating disorders and to identify best approaches that would enable nurses, and other care providers reduce the occurrence of unhelpful interactions.

Spiritual Domain

Overcoming eating disorders requires attention to the individual in his/her physical, psychological, social, and spiritual fullness. Core components of recovery can be

---

BOX 25-9 What Family and Friends Can Do to Help Those With Eating Disorders

- Tell the person you are concerned, you care, and you would like to help. Suggest that the person seek professional help from a physician or therapist.
- If the person refuses to seek professional help, encourage reaching out to an adult, such as a teacher, school nurse, or counsellor.
- Do not discuss weight, the number of calories being consumed, or particular eating habits. Do try to talk about things other than food, weight, counting calories, and exercise.
- Avoid making comments about a person's appearance. Concern about weight loss may be interpreted as a compliment; comments regarding weight gain may be felt as criticism.
- It will not help to become involved in a power struggle. You cannot force the person to eat.
- You can offer support. Ultimately, however, the responsibility and the decision to accept help and to change rest with the person.
- Read and educate yourself regarding these disorders.

BOX 25-10 Research for Best Practice

RECOVERY PERSPECTIVES OF CHILD, PARENT, AND THERAPIST

Weaver, K., Martin-McDonald, K., & Spiers, J. (2012). Mirroring voices of mother, daughter and therapist in anorexia nervosa. Forum: Qualitative Social Research, 13(3), 1–21.

Background: The experiences of children with eating disorders and the meanings drawn from these experiences are poorly represented in clinical and academic discourse.

Purpose: To examine interpersonal relationships in the context of anorexia nervosa between an adolescent, her mother, and therapist revealed in their private and intimate diaries, letters, and reflections.

Method: A narrative approach enabled access to individual meanings and to a rationalized representation of complex, dynamic processes in everyday situations of the mother and the clinical setting of eating disorder treatment. Themes identified in the analysis reflected their written dialogue, represented their stories, and were validated by participants.

Findings: The core story, mirroring voices, documents the reciprocal processing of experiences and perceptions between the daughter and mother that facilitated the daughter's recovery. Six themes of mirroring voices include "being implicitly there for each other," "writing gives us voice," "centering on ourselves," "measuring up," "anorexic bitch," and "pain has a name." The findings suggest the use of similar strategies by the daughter and mother to manage the anorexia nervosa by recasting it as an intrusion (i.e., the "anorexic bitch").

Implications for Nursing: In the core story of mirroring voices, the eating disorder served a protective function and was eventually resisted by a mother–daughter unified team effort. The mother–daughter interaction thus provided a critical piece of the puzzle of AN recovery. The major implications are that health care professionals consider the mother–daughter interaction as a resource, and that they might better support individuals and families affected by eating disorders by eliciting their stories.

sociopolitical activism and spiritual commitment (Garrett, 1998; Matusek & Knudson, 2009; Scott Richards, Hardman, & Berrett, 2007). Sociopolitical activism enables uniting voices with others to identify and begin to redress limitations to change. Spiritual interventions entail establishing trust, rapport, consistency, and support while enabling clients to voice and make meaning of their eating disorder experience. The nurse helps clients recognize patterns, identify, and clarify values. Encouraging activities that promote reflection and self-awareness helps clients access potential solutions to well-being and reduce depression, anxiety, relationship distress, social role conflict, and eating disorder symptoms (Scott Richards, Berrett, Hardman, & Eggett, 2006).

The need for ongoing self-awareness on the part of the nurse is critical when interacting with an individual whose body has served as a container for pain, suffering, and disgust and has subsequently been starved, stuffed, or purged. The nurse may encounter body countertransference or the phenomenon of experiencing a similar type of discomfort in the nurse's own body (Costin, 2009; Orbach, 2004). The nurse must be attuned to these body sensations and anticipate this phenomenon. It is necessary to understand and process countertransference issues concerning the nurse's relationship with her/his own weight, eating patterns, and body image; the client's tendency to scrutinize and comment about the nurse's body; and the degree of self-disclosure in the therapeutic relationship (Costin, 2009). Without such awareness and self-monitoring, the nurse may communicate any personal body discomfort to the client. Individual or group peer debriefing sessions are helpful to manage such countertransference.

Evaluation and Treatment Outcomes

Among the varied factors influencing the outcome of treatment for AN, discharge BMI was found the singularly best predictor of full recovery from AN; this finding emphasizes the crucial need for full weight restoration during treatment (Brewerton & Costin, 2011). Intensive ongoing outpatient treatment, including nutritional counselling and support, can prevent relapse and facilitate full recovery. Many of the instruments used to assess eating disorder symptoms (see Box 25-6) can be used throughout the individual's treatment to evaluate attitudes and thinking processes. Nurses are ideally positioned within hospital and community health treatment settings to help individuals with AN recover.

Continuum of Care
Hospitalization

AN in its acute stage requires hospitalization.

EMERGENCY CARE !

Death may result from cardiac problems associated with starvation and suicide. However, emergency care is not usually needed for individuals with AN. Family members and peers usually notice the weight loss and emaciation before the individual's systems are compromised to the degree that they require emergency treatment. The individual is usually admitted immediately for inpatient care if systems are compromised or if the individual is suicidal. In hospital, individuals are evaluated for discharge to day hospitalization or outpatient therapy, depending on the resources available, the extent of family support, and comorbidity. In both instances, the individual and family participate in a combination of individual and family therapy. Family therapy, initiated in the hospital, is continued more intensively after discharge (see Chapter 15).

Outpatient Treatment

After weight restoration, treatment of AN may take place on an outpatient basis and involve continued individual and family therapy, nutrition counselling to reinforce healthy eating patterns and attitudes, and physician visits to monitor weight and evaluate somatic recovery. Support groups, often suggested, are not substituted for therapy. This is because some self-directed support groups that lack professional leadership can actually delay or prevent needed professional treatment. The role of support groups to maintain recovery requires further study.

BULIMIA NERVOSA

Until about 35 years ago, BN was thought to be a subtype of AN. However, findings from extensive investigations identified BN as a separate entity. Individuals with BN are usually older at onset than are those with AN. The usual treatment is outpatient therapy. Outcomes are better for BN than for AN, and mortality rates are lower.

Clinical Course

There are few outward signs associated with BN. Individuals binge and purge in secret and are typically of normal weight; therefore, BN does not come to the attention of parents and peers as quickly as AN. Consequently, treatment can be delayed for years as individuals attempt on their own to get their eating under control. Once treatment is undertaken and completed, they are capable of full recovery, except when personality disorders and comorbid serious depression are also present.

Individuals with BN may present as overwhelmed and overly committed and have difficulty with setting limits and establishing appropriate boundaries. They have many rules regarding food and food restriction, and they feel ashamed, guilty, and disgusted about binge eating and purging. They may also be impulsive in other areas of their lives, such as spending.

Diagnostic Criteria

The key characteristics for the diagnosis of BN appear in Table 25-5 (also see Box 25-1). BN involves engaging in recurrent episodes of binge eating and compensatory purging in the form of vomiting; using laxatives, diuretics, or emetics; or nonpurging compensatory behaviours such as fasting or overexercising in order to avoid weight gain. These episodes must occur at least once a week for a period of at least 3 months in order to meet the *DSM-5* criteria (APA, 2013).

Binge eating is defined as rapid, episodic, impulsive, and uncontrollable ingestion of a large amount of food during a short period of time, usually 1 to 2 hours. Eating is followed by feelings of guilt, remorse, and often self-contempt, leading to purging. To assuage the out-of-control feeling, severe dieting referred to as *dietary restraint* is instituted. Restrictions are viewed as "rules," such as no sweets or no fats. Each binge seems to influence stricter rules about what cannot be consumed, leading to more frequent binge eating, subsequent guilt, and self-loathing. Purging or dietary restraint may follow (Fig. 25-5). This cycle has prompted clinicians to focus the treatment on interventions related to dietary restraint or purging behaviours. Bohon, Stice, and Burton (2009)

found dietary restraint and compensatory symptoms negatively correlated with the length of time to remission, suggesting that when dietary restraint is resolved, or purging is prevented, binge eating is decreased.

As shown in Figure 25-5, dietary restriction serves as a means to regulate painful feelings. It may also alter one's perceptual reactivation to attractive food cues, making them more irresistible. Restriction may make dieters more prone to feel distress over their dietary "failures," especially if dieting has become a way to overcome body dissatisfaction and to compensate for distress through binge eating. Whether the eating is influenced by hunger, the attraction of forbidden foods, or internal needs to assuage failure, there is evidence that restraining one's intake may instigate a drive toward repletion (Haedt-Matt & Keel, 2011) and subsequent overeating for individuals at genetic risk for binge eating (Johnson, Pratt, & Wardle, 2012; Racine, Burt, Iacono, McGue, & Klump, 2011).

KEY CONCEPT **Dietary restraint** was originally described to explain the differences between the eating patterns of obese individuals and those of normal-weight people (Herman & Mack, 1975). Restraint is often initiated as a response to weight gain, and the sustained effort to monitor and control food intake characterizes successful long-term weight maintenance.

Table 25-5 Key Diagnostic Characteristics for Bulimia Nervosa

Diagnostic Criteria	Target Symptoms and Associated Findings

A. Recurrent episodes of binge eating
Characterized by both of the following:
• eating in a discrete period of time an amount larger than most people would eat during a similar period of time and under similar circumstances;
• sense of lack of control over eating during the episode
B. Recurrent inappropriate compensatory behaviour to prevent weight gain, such as self-induced vomiting, misuse of laxatives, diuretics, enemas, or other medications; fasting; or excessive exercise
C. Binge eating and inappropriate compensatory behaviours occurring on average once a week for 3 mo
D. Self-evaluation unduly influenced by body shape and weight
E. Not occurring exclusively during episodes of anorexia nervosa
• Severity:
  Mild: (average of 1–3 episodes of compensatory behaviours/week)
  Moderate: (average of 4–7 episodes/week)
  Severe: (average of 8–13 episodes/week)
  Extreme: (average of 14 or more episodes/week)
• Partial remission: After full criteria were previously met, some but not all criteria have been met for a sustained period of time
• Full remission: If full criteria were previously met but no criteria have been met for a sustained period of time.
	• Usually within normal weight range, possible overweight or underweight
	• Restriction of total calorie consumption between binges, selecting low-calorie foods while avoiding foods perceived to be fattening or likely to trigger a binge
	• Increased frequency of depressive symptoms and anxiety symptoms
	• Possible substance abuse or dependence involving alcohol or stimulants
	Associate physical examination
	• Loss of dental enamel
	• Chipped, ragged, or moth-eaten teeth appearance
	• Increased incidence of dental caries
	• Scars on the dorsum of hand from manually inducing vomiting
	• Cardiac and skeletal myopathies from use of syrup of ipecac for vomiting
	• Menstrual irregularities
	• Dependence on laxatives
	• Oesophageal tears
	Associate laboratory findings
	• Fluid and electrolyte abnormalities
	• Metabolic alkalosis (from vomiting) or metabolic acidosis (from diarrhoea)
	• Mildly elevated serum amylase levels

American Psychiatric Association. (2013). *Diagnostic and statistical manual of mental disorders* (5th ed.). Washington, DC: Author.

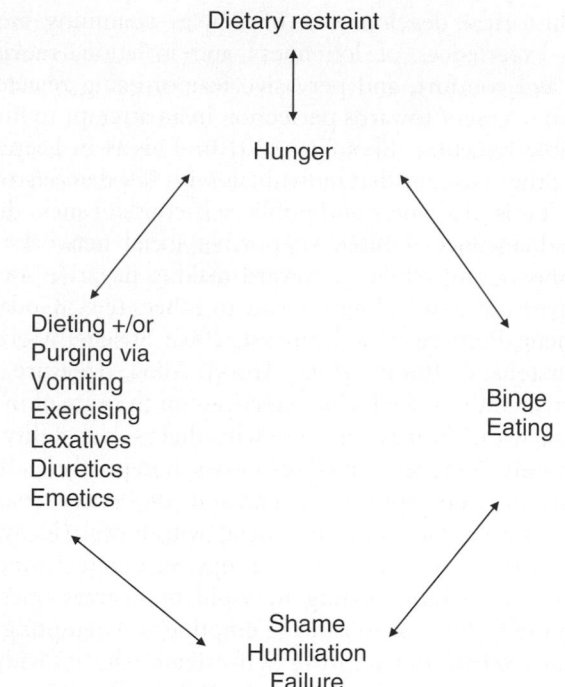

FIGURE 25-5. Binge–purge cycle.

Epidemiology

Approximately 1% to 3% of young women develop BN in their lifetime (Statistics Canada, 2012). Using symptom frequency of once a week, in concordance with the *DSM-5* criteria, the lifetime prevalence of BN is reported as 2.3% in women (Smink et al., 2012), making BN more common than AN (Gauvin, Steiger, & Brodeur, 2009).

Age of Onset

Typically, the onset of BN begins in adolescence or early adulthood (Statistics Canada, 2012) and may coincide with a developmental transition (e.g., leaving home to attend university, or psychosocial stress (Yager & Powers, 2007).

Gender Differences

In the community setting, one case in four of BN is a male (Dr. Blake Woodside, Director of the Program for Eating Disorders at Toronto General Hospital, as cited by Kirkey, 2013) (see Box 25-2).

Ethnic and Cultural Differences

BN is related to culture in the same way as AN. In Western cultures and those becoming westernized in their norms, the focus on achieving an idealized thin body underlies the dieting and dietary restraint that set up the trajectory toward a diagnosable eating disorder. Hispanic and white women have higher reported rates than do Asian and African Americans. There is a paucity of research exploring ethnic and culture differences among Canadian women.

Familial Differences

First-degree relatives of women with BN are more likely to have eating disorders than control subjects and women with other psychiatric disorders (Yager & Powers, 2007). Families of clients with BN also have higher rates of substance abuse, particularly alcoholism, affective disorders, and obesity. Traits such as impulsivity, negative affect, perfectionism, and low self-esteem are risk factors that may largely be genetically determined (Monteleone & Maj, 2008).

Comorbidity

The most common comorbid conditions are substance misuse (Carbaugh & Sias, 2010; Yilmaz, Kaplan, & Zawertailo, 2012), depression (Keski-Rahkonen et al., 2013), and anxiety disorders including OCD (Godart et al., 2006; Sallet et al., 2010). Women were found to continue having OCD after remission of their bulimic symptoms, suggesting that some comorbid conditions are trait related and may actually have a role in precipitating the disorder (Morgan, Wolfe, Metzger, & Jimerson, 2007). Cluster B, Axis II disorders, such as BPD, are also identified frequently with BN (Selby et al., 2012). Bulimic clients with BPD have reported stronger feelings of ineffectiveness and more problems with interoceptive awareness than bulimic clients without BPD (Zeeck et al., 2007).

Aetiology

Some of the predisposing or risk factors for BN overlap with theories of causality (see Fig. 25-2). For example, dieting may put an individual at risk for developing BN. The dieting can turn into dietary restraint, which can lead to binge eating and purging in vulnerable individuals. The interplay of other risk factors (e.g., body dissatisfaction and separation–individuation issues) also helps explain the development of this disorder.

Biologic Theories

Dieting may occur in girls as young as 9 years of age. Girls' weight status at 5 years was found to predict the emergence of dieting at age 9, with higher weight status conferring an elevated risk for dieting. Other predictors of early dieting included higher levels of depression, lower general self-competence, and maternal restriction of child's intake (Sinton & Birch, 2005). Canadian children in grades three and four have said they would rather lose a parent, get cancer, or live through nuclear war than be fat (National Eating Disorder Information Centre, 1998/2003). Dieting is believed to affect the neurotransmitters, including serotonin, which are involved in the appetite, satiety, and eating patterns of BN. Levels of cholecystokinin, a hormone associated with satiation, were found to be low in some individuals with BN (Fujimoto et al., 1997; Hannon-Engel, 2012). As in AN, overexercising has also contributed to some of the symptoms of BN.

Neuropathologic

The changes in the brain are the result rather than the cause of eating dysregulation. As with AN, these changes resolve when symptoms such as dietary restraint, binge eating, and purging remit.

Genetic

A specific gene responsible for BN has not been identified. However, research suggests that genes acting within the dopamine system influence both eating- and personality-related psychopathology either directly or indirectly (i.e., in interaction with traumatic childhood experiences), with the result that lower levels of dopamine neurotransmission contribute to variations in the presentation of comorbid traits and to increased psychopathology and body mass in women with bulimia disorders (Groleau et al., 2012; Thaler et al., 2012). A review of twin studies recognized the role of genetic influences as outweighing environmental influences (Bulik et al., 2007). Findings are to be treated with caution because sorting out environmental and genetic influences is difficult when twins live in the same environment.

Biochemical

The most frequently studied biochemical theory in BN relates to lowered brain serotonin neurotransmission. People with BN are believed to have altered modulation of central serotonin neuronal systems (Bailer et al., 2011; Pichika et al., 2012). Even following recovery from BN, findings of altered serotonin levels persist that potentially contribute to BN symptomatology and responses to medication.

Psychological and Social Theories

Psychological factors in the aetiology of BN have been studied extensively, and most experts believe that these factors converge with environmental or sociocultural factors within individuals with a biologic predisposition, causing symptoms to develop. As with AN, psychoanalytic developmental theories that explain separation–individuation are important in causality. Because the age of onset for BN is late adolescence/early adulthood, leaving home (e.g., for employment or college opportunities) may represent the first physical separation for some adolescents who are unprepared for the emotional separation. Analysis of interviews conducted with female and male undergraduate students revealed the life–historical development of BN as stemming from deep experiences of loneliness and isolation, seeking love and comfort, and pervasive fear of being rejected, with movement towards perfection in an attempt to limit possible rejection (Skoufalos, 2010). This is in keeping with other findings that individuals with BN demonstrate high levels of shyness and public self-consciousness during adolescence, limited supportive social networks in adulthood, and tendency toward making negative social comparisons and feeling inferior to others (e.g., Godart, Flament, Perdereau, & Jeammet, 2002; Striegel-Moore, Silberstein, & Rodin, 1993; Troop, Allan, Treasure, & Katzman, 2003). Such characteristics on the part of individuals with BN may interfere with their social ability to accurately interpret others' responses, potentially leading toward their perception of negative mental states, resulting in low self-esteem and social withdrawal (Kenyon et al., 2012). Overwhelming feelings such as resentment often lead to binge eating to avoid or distract oneself from the feelings or to assuage emptiness. Attempting to regain control and improve self-esteem, the individual may resume the cycle of dieting. Both binge eating and purging may serve as regulation strategies for coping with negative affect (Polivy & Herman, 1993).

Cognitive Theory

Cognitive theory helps explain the distorted thinking present in people with BN. This explanation is similar for depression, in which a particular thought pattern is learned (see Chapter 13 for an explanation of cognitive theory). Experts such as Cooper, Wells, and Todd (2004) and Cooper, Todd, Turner, and Wells (2007) view BN as a disorder of thinking, in that distortions are the basis of behaviours such as binge eating and purging. Psychological triggering mechanism models explain that cues such as stress related to interpersonal difficulties (e.g., an argument with a loved one), negative emotions, physiologic state (e.g., hunger, fullness), and environment (e.g., the presence of attractive food, a remark about the person's weight or how much one is eating, catching sight of self in a mirror) play a role in aetiology. The cues may activate personal negative self-beliefs (e.g., "I'm unlikeable," or "I'm a failure"), and this activation typically generates considerable emotional distress. Eating provides a distraction from negative thoughts and emotions and is commonly associated with a decrease in intensity of emotional states. Thus, eating is initially interpreted positively and linked to positive beliefs (e.g., "Eating will take away my painful feelings"). However, eating can also be closely linked with negative beliefs about the potential consequences (e.g., "I'll gain weight"). The person with BN is caught in a state of conflict in which both positive and negative beliefs about eating coexist. The binge provides only temporary relief from the original distress and is subject to negative interpretation (e.g., as a sign of failure) that, in turn, reinforces the negative self-beliefs in the first place. In contrast, purging may result when negative beliefs about eating become dominant over positive beliefs and the person switches from eating to vomiting or other compensatory behaviour. Once the compensatory behaviour has ceased, any initial sense of relief at having gotten rid of the food starts to dissipate and the negative consequences of yet another episode of binge eating and purging, negative mood, and arousal start to increase again. These cognitive and triggering theories are viewed as an explanation for maintaining the binge eating once it has been established, rather than an explanation of causality (Bergin & Wade, 2012).

The same sociocultural factors regarding societal focus on the ideal body type that underlie AN play a significant role in the development of BN.

Family

A review of studies by Vince and Walker (2008) found that families of individuals with BN were reported to be chaotic, with few rules and unclear boundaries. However, as with AN, theories of causation do not individually explain the development of BN. Rather, the convergence of many factors at a vulnerable stage of individual development contribute to causality. Originating with work at the Maudsley Hospital in London in the late 1970s, a paradigm shift directed attention away from presuming an aetiologic role for family dynamics and toward regarding the family as a resource in therapy, easing parents' guilt, and promoting an attitude of inclusion (le Grange, Lock, Loeb, & Nicholls, 2010).

Risk Factors

The risk or predisposing factors for BN are included in Figure 25-3.

Interdisciplinary Treatment

Individuals with BN benefit from a comprehensive multifaceted treatment approach that usually takes place in an outpatient setting, except when the client is suicidal or when past outpatient treatment has failed (Table 25-3). Therapy for BN focuses on psychological issues, including boundary setting and separation–individuation conflicts and on changing problematic behaviours and dysfunctional thought patterns and attitudes, especially about eating, weight, and shape. Intensive psychotherapy and pharmacologic interventions are necessary. Nutrition counselling helps stabilize and normalize eating, which means stopping the binge–purge cycle. Support groups may also be involved. Family therapy is not usually a part of the treatment, because many people with BN live on college campuses away from home or are older and on their own. Usually, the treatment becomes less intensive as symptoms remit.

Priority Care Issues

Given the comorbid conditions of depression, anxiety, substance misuse, and BPD, some individuals with BN may become suicidal. They are also often at risk for self-mutilation. Because they display high levels of impulsivity (e.g., shoplifting, overspending), financial and legal difficulties have been associated with BN.

Nursing Management: Human Response to Bulimia Nervosa Disorder

The primary nursing diagnoses for patients with BN are Imbalanced Nutrition: Less Than or More Than Body Requirements, Powerlessness, Anxiety, and Ineffective Coping.

Therapeutic Relationship

Individuals with BN experience shame and guilt and have an intense need to please and be liked. They are too ashamed to discuss their symptoms but do not want to disappoint others, so they may discuss more superficial social or unrelated issues in an attempt to engage the nurse. A nonjudgemental approach stressing the importance of the relationship and outlining its purpose is important from the outset. Explaining the nature of the relationship and the goals of therapy will help clarify the boundaries (see Chapter 6). Box 25-11 describes issues experienced by mental health trainees with personal histories of eating issues. It is important to anticipate and normalize issues of shame in eating disorder educational programs with health professional trainees and in working with clients.

Biologic Domain

Most individuals with BN maintain normal weights. Those who purge risk fluid and electrolyte abnormalities, particularly hypokalaemia that contributes to muscle weakness and fatigability, cardiac arrhythmias, palpitations, and cardiac conduction defects. Neuropsychiatric disturbances, such as poor concentration and attention, and sleep disturbances are common.

Assessment

The nurse assesses current eating patterns, determines the number of times a day the individual binges and purges, and notes dietary restraint practices. Sleep patterns and exercise habits are also important.

HUMAN RESPONSE TO EATING ISSUES

Dayal, H. (2013). From shame to shame resilience: Narratives of counsellor trainees with eating issues. Unpublished Master's of Education Thesis. Fredericton, NB: University of New Brunswick.

Mental health practitioners are expected to be free from mental health issues. However, research has identified that approximately one in every three to four eating disorder practitioners has an eating disorder history. Failure to work through such personal issues can induce feelings of shame that have been linked to concealment, secrecy, withdrawal, isolation, and reluctance to seek help.

Research Questions: To more fully understand the shame experiences of counselling students as well as the ways they develop resilience and thus stand to improve both client and practitioner wellness, these questions were asked: How do mental health counsellor trainees with present or previous eating issues overcome shame and develop resilience? How does shame influence support seeking for eating issues? What stories of shame are recounted by counsellor trainees with eating issues?

Method: Narrative inquiry was used to elicit and analyze stories of shame and resilience from seven Master's level trainees in various Canadian Counselling and Counselling Psychology programs. Individual stories were examined for common and unique features and were woven together into a single collective story that accounted for temporal, social, and situational influences. The trainees had the opportunity to refine the individual and collective stories.

Findings: A dialectical conflict between protecting shame versus prioritizing recovery emerged from the stories of shame and resilience. Five layers of shame were identified: secrecy, discounting, disconnection from others, striving for perfection, and disconnection from self. These shame layers built on one another, preventing help seeking. Threads of resilience emerged as factors that helped in overcoming shame. Resilience threads included connecting with others (finding belonging and a culture of safety) and connecting with self (invalidating perfection and redefining ideals). Various points of connection played a central role in helping or hindering the process of overcoming shame. Contact with others who also had eating issues provided unconditional acceptance and fostered recognition of the universality of shaming experiences that helped normalize the shame and decrease the isolation felt by the trainees. Lack of safety and community within trainee education programs and contact with others who discounted their experiences resulted in further shame and nondisclosure of eating issues.

Implications for Counselling and Nursing: The findings highlight the importance of mutually empathic relationships to overcome shame. This research supports the use of psychoeducational and peer support groups and the need to anticipate and address shame in the treatment of eating issues.

Nursing Diagnoses for Biologic Domain

Imbalanced Nutrition: Less Than/More Than Body Requirements and Disturbed Sleep Pattern are typical nursing diagnoses for the biologic domain.

Interventions for Biologic Domain

If the client is admitted to the hospital, all food intake is strictly monitored to normalize eating. Bathroom visits are also supervised to prevent purging. Outpatients are asked to record their intake, binges, and purges to establish a foundation for changing behaviours with psychotherapy. Because individuals with BN have chaotic lifestyles and are often overcommitted, sleep may be a low priority. Sleep-deprived individuals may assume that food would be helpful, and they begin to eat, triggering a binge. To encourage regular sleep patterns, individuals are encouraged to go to bed and rise at about the same time every day.

Pharmacologic Interventions

Pharmacotherapy is effective for symptom remission in BN. Although cognitive–behavioural therapy (CBT) is the treatment of choice for BN (Hay, 2013; Mitchell et al., 2013), CBT is not always available in all treatment settings. Therefore, pharmacotherapy may be appropriate. Antidepressant treatment may additionally benefit comorbid affective symptoms (Mitchell et al., 2013). Fluoxetine (Prozac) has been the most studied medication for BN in clinical trials (see Box 25-12). Effective doses are usually 60 mg/day, a higher dosage than that used to treat depression. Sertraline (Zoloft) and citalopram (celexa) have also been used effectively. These medications, prescribed for binge eating and purging, are effective even when depression is not present (Trunko & Kaye, 2008). Weight is monitored as decreased appetite and weight loss are common during the first few weeks of administration. It is also important to monitor the intake of medication for possible purging after administration. The effect of the medication depends on the time taken for its absorption. Bupropion (Wellbutrin) is contraindicated for the treatment of BN and AN due to its seizure risk (Mitchell et al., 2013).

 TEACHING POINTS

Individuals should be instructed to take medication as prescribed. SSRIs should be taken in the morning because they can cause insomnia. Individuals should be informed that any weight loss they initially experience is temporary and is usually regained after a few weeks, when the medication dosage has stabilized. Treatment dropout is high (Romano, Halmi, Sarkar, Koke, & Lee, 2002); monitoring adverse effects and eliciting the client's understanding of the reasons why the clinician recommended the pharmacotherapy may help direct interventions.

BOX
25-12

Drug Profile

FLUOXETINE HYDROCHLORIDE (PROZAC)

Drug Class: Selective serotonin reuptake inhibitor

Receptor Affinity: Inhibits central nervous system neuronal uptake of serotonin with little effect on norepinephrine; thought to antagonize muscarinic, histaminergic, and α-adrenergic receptors.

Indications: Treatment of depressive disorders, most effective in major depression, obesity, bulimia, and OCD

Routes and Dosage: Available in 10- and 20-mg pulvules and 20 mg/5 mL oral solution

Adults: 20 mg/day in the morning, not to exceed 80 mg/day. Full antidepressant effect may not be seen for up to 4 weeks. If no improvement, dosage is increased after several weeks. Dosages above 20 mg/day may be administered on a once-a-day (morning) or BID schedule (i.e., morning and noon). For eating disorders: typically 60 mg/day, administered in the morning, is recommended for reducing the frequency of binge eating and vomiting.

Geriatric: Administer at lower or less frequent doses; monitor responses to guide dosage.

Children: Safety and efficacy have not been established.

Half-Life (Peak Effect): 2–3 days (6–8 hours)

Selected Adverse Reactions: Headache, nervousness, insomnia, drowsiness, anxiety, tremors, dizziness, light headedness, nausea, vomiting, diarrhoea, dry mouth, anorexia, dyspepsia, constipation, taste changes, upper respiratory infections, pharyngitis, painful menstruation, sexual dysfunction, urinary frequency, sweating, rash, pruritus, weight loss, asthenia, and fever.

Warnings: Avoid use in pregnancy and while breast-feeding. Use with caution in patients with impaired hepatic or renal function and diabetes mellitus. Possible risk for toxicity if taken with tricyclic antidepressants.

Special Patient and Family Education:

- Be aware that the drug may take up to 4 weeks to get full antidepressant effect.
- Take the drug in the morning or in divided doses, if necessary.
- Report any adverse reactions.
- Avoid driving a car or performing hazardous activities because the drug may cause drowsiness or dizziness.
- Eat small, frequent meals to help with complaints of nausea and vomiting.

Psychosocial Domain

Assessment

Psychological assessment focuses on cognitive distortions—cues or stimuli that lead to dysfunctional behaviour affecting symptom development—and knowledge deficits. The psychological characteristics typical of individuals with BN are presented in Box 25-1. Examples of cognitive distortions present in BN are given in Table 23-4. These thought patterns form the basis for "rules" and lead the way to destructive eating patterns. During routine history taking, individuals may relate many of these distortions. Situations that produce feelings of being overwhelmed and powerless need to be explored, as does the individual's ability to set boundaries, control impulsivity, and maintain quality relationships. These underlying issues may precipitate binge eating. Several assessment tools are available to gauge such characteristics as body dissatisfaction and impulsivity (see Box 25-6). Body dissatisfaction should be openly explored. Mood is evaluated because many people with BN also have depression.

Nursing Diagnoses for Psychosocial Domain

Deficient Knowledge and Disturbed Thought Processes are among the common diagnoses for the psychosocial domain.

Interventions for Psychosocial Domain

Studies comparing various psychotherapy methods have demonstrated the superiority of CBT for BN (Brown & Keel, 2012; Murphy, Straebler, Cooper, & Fairburn, 2010). CBT is usually conducted in a group, with one or two sessions a week. CBT has also been effectively delivered in guided self-help format (Bailer et al., 2004; Schmidt et al., 2007). IPT has had positive outcomes but may take longer to change binge-eating and purging symptoms. Behavioural therapy alone has not been as effective as CBT. While binge eating may persist, little work can be done on underlying interpersonal issues, such as boundary setting, because the client feels out of control with eating. Therefore, cognitive therapy is begun first, to address the distorted thinking processes influencing dietary restraint, binge eating, and purging. Decreasing these symptoms will help eliminate the out-of-control feelings.

Behavioural Techniques

The behavioural techniques, such as **cue elimination** and response prevention, require self-monitoring to individualize the therapy. **Self-monitoring** is accomplished using a diary, in which the individual records binges, purges, precipitating emotions, and environmental cues including physiologic/nutritional and psychological pressures to eat, as well as individuals and situations that may be associated with negative feelings such as depression, anger, or anxiety. Self-monitoring enables further understanding of the eating problem, identifies progress, and helps clients develop awareness of what is happening *in the moment* so that they can begin to change behaviours that may have seemed automatic or beyond their control (Murphy et al., 2010). The client's records are jointly reviewed at each session, and any difficulties are addressed in the session. Emotional and environmental cues are identified, and alternative responses are formulated, tried, and reinforced. When a cue or stimulus leads to a dysfunctional or unhealthy response, the response can be eliminated, or an alternate, healthier response to the cue can be substituted,

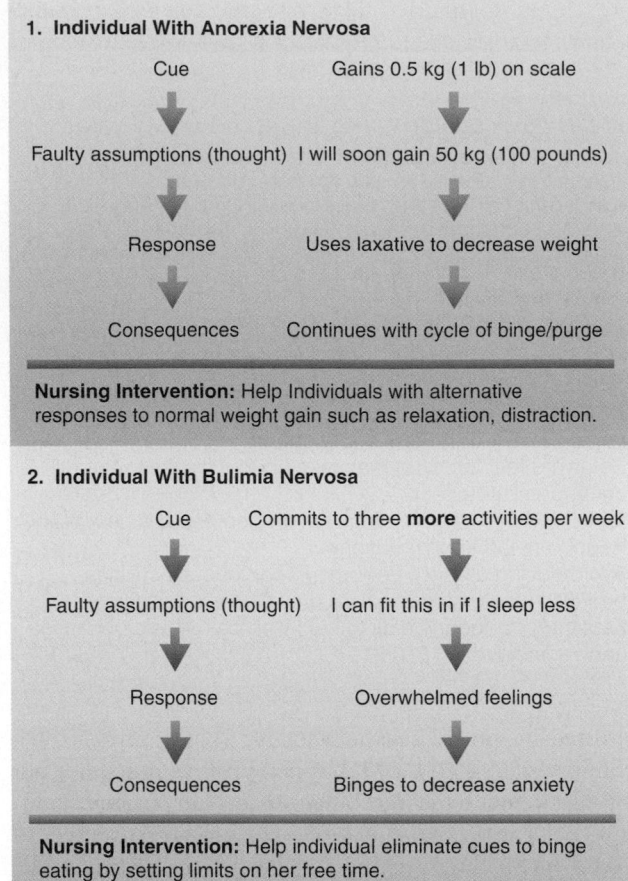

1. **Individual With Anorexia Nervosa**

Cue — Gains 0.5 kg (1 lb) on scale

↓

Faulty assumptions (thought) — I will soon gain 50 kg (100 pounds)

↓

Response — Uses laxative to decrease weight

↓

Consequences — Continues with cycle of binge/purge

Nursing Intervention: Help Individuals with alternative responses to normal weight gain such as relaxation, distraction.

2. **Individual With Bulimia Nervosa**

Cue — Commits to three **more** activities per week

↓

Faulty assumptions (thought) — I can fit this in if I sleep less

↓

Response — Overwhelmed feelings

↓

Consequences — Binges to decrease anxiety

Nursing Intervention: Help individual eliminate cues to binge eating by setting limits on her free time.

FIGURE 25-6. Examples of the relationship of cues, thoughts, and responses: behavioural interventions.

tried, and then reinforced. The client is encouraged to focus on longer-term consequences (e.g., social isolation) rather than shorter-term relief of uncomfortable feelings. Figure 25-6 gives two examples of behavioural interventions. In example 1, for the individual with AN, the response is modified or altered to a healthier one; in example 2, for the individual with BN, the cue is changed to produce a different, healthier response. Other techniques, such as postponing binges and purges through distraction, a technique to interrupt the cycle, are also effective.

Psychoeducation

The nurse can assist clients to understand the binge–purge cycle and the role of rigid rules in contributing to this cycle. The value of eating meals regularly to ward off hunger and reduce the possibility of a binge is important. Individuals who misuse laxatives are taught that although these drugs produce water-weight loss, they are ineffective for true, lasting weight loss. Moreover, individuals also need information about potassium depletion, electrolyte imbalances, dehydration, and the medical consequences of binge eating and purging. For example, laxative-dependent bowel may result from laxative misuse (Spear & Stellefson Myers, 2001). Other topics for psychoeducation are included in Box 25-13.

BOX 25-13 Psychoeducation Checklist: Bulimia Nervosa

When caring for the individual with BN, be sure to include the following topic areas in the teaching plan:
- Psychopharmacologic agents, if used, including drug, action, dosage, frequency, and possible adverse effects
- Binge–purge cycle and effects on body
- Nutrition and eating patterns
- Hydration
- Avoidance of cues
- Cognitive distortions
- Limit-setting
- Appropriate boundary setting
- Assertiveness
- Resources
- Self-monitoring and behavioural interventions
- Realistic goal setting

TEACHING POINTS

Psychoeducation for individuals with BN focuses on setting boundaries and healthy limits, developing assertiveness, learning nutritional concepts related to healthy eating, discussing societal definitions of beauty, and clarifying misconceptions about food (Hendricks & Thompson, 2005; White, 1999). Research findings related to semistarvation, weight regulation, dieting, obesity, and the sociocultural milieu that influences the development and perpetuation of eating disorders are discussed. Cognitive distortions are addressed because of their role in dietary restraint and resulting binge eating. Garner's abbreviated Eating Attitudes Test (EAT 26, 1997) can be used to assess clients' eating concerns before, during, and after psychoeducation.

Family Assessment and Intervention

Families caring for members with BN report intense emotions, including guilt, feelings of helplessness, anger, fear, and self-blame (Perkins, Winn, Murray, Murphy, & Schmidt, 2004). Winn and colleagues (2007) found that family caregivers of adolescents with BN may describe negative caregiving experiences including stigma and problems with services. The nurse explores with families the negative impact of giving care to assess its physical and psychosocial toll and to evaluate coping capacity. Strategies that families use to manage the difficulties associated with the eating disorder are thinking positively, using humour, maintaining their own interests, and actively obtaining information (Perkins et al., 2004). National eating disorder associations recommend that families engage in self-care activities such as speaking about their experiences to help lessen the shame and obtaining support (NEDA, 2013; NEDIC, 1998/2003).

Group Therapy

Group therapy is cost-effective and effectively increases learning because individuals learn from each other as well as from the nurse or other therapist. Some experts have recommended 12-step programs for treating BN. However, many clinicians who work in this specialty have noted that these programs, with their strict rules, can be counterproductive for individuals with BN, who already have stringent rules (e.g., dietary restraint) and are "abstinent" in many ways that lead to binge eating. Broad parameters regarding food choices (e.g., allowing all foods in moderation), together with knowledge about healthy eating, are encouraged instead. As symptoms subside, individuals can concentrate on underlying interpersonal issues in therapy, such as feelings of inadequacy and low self-esteem, and can work with other group members to develop assertiveness.

Spiritual Domain

Assessment

The role of spirituality in the lives of individuals with BN can be assessed through their expressions of loss and powerlessness, self-care capacity, quality of relationships, history of conflicts and painful traumatic experiences, attitudes about food and overeating, harm avoidance strategies, self-directedness, and self-judgements. Adolescents with diagnoses related to BN have been found to score higher on measures of boredom and fatigue; to be passive, socially inhibited, disorderly, and pessimistic; and to blame others; yet, they were also determined to be spiritual and unpretentious (Sancho, Arija, & Canals, 2008). The nurse must strive to see the person beyond the dieting behaviour.

Nursing Diagnoses for Spiritual Domain

Loss and Powerlessness are among the common diagnoses for the spiritual domain.

Interventions for Spiritual Domain

The nurse encourages clients to express feelings of loss and powerlessness without negative self-judgement (Berrett et al., 2007). Clients will benefit from exploring what they do and do not have control over and to accept their human limitations. Those who binge eat and purge can learn to delay these behaviours through engaging in activities such as journal writing, affirming positive self-worth, meditation, and imagery. These strategies may help clients with BN to build support from self and to help deal with comorbid depression and anxiety. Nurses can further help create the context for clients with BN to enlist support from others.

Evaluation and Treatment Outcomes

Individuals with BN may have better recovery outcomes than do those with AN. Outcomes have improved since the early 1990s, partially because of earlier detection,

research on treatments that are most effective, and neuropharmacologic research and advances. In one study, 22.7% of 88 former clients were indistinguishable from the 67 healthy controls on eating-related measures when recovery was comprehensively defined as (a) no longer meeting diagnostic criteria for an eating disorder, (b) no binge eating or compensatory behaviours for a period of 3 months, (c) maintaining a BMI of at least 18.5 kg/m², and (d) scoring within one standard deviation (SD) of normal on all subscales of the Eating Disorders Examination Questionnaire (EDE-Q) (Bardone-Cone et al., 2010). In other research that similarly defined recovery as abstinence from binge eating and purging and BMI greater than 18.5, recovery rates of 15.6% at the end of treatment and 19.8% at 62-week follow-up were reported for a sample of 96 adults with BN (Yu, Agras, & Bryson, 2013). Relapse was reported as 60% when recovery was defined as abstinence from binge eating and purging. According to the researchers, it may be more fitting to use the term "remission" for individuals who no longer binge and purge at the end of treatment and "recovered" for those maintaining abstinence for a prolonged period of follow-up (Yu et al., 2013). In a 10-year follow-up study of clients receiving residential treatment, it was found that the best predictor of a recovery outcome for BN was low vomiting and binge-eating frequency at discharge (Brewerton & Costin, 2011). This finding supports the importance of attaining complete abstinence during treatment.

Continuum of Care

Individuals with BN are less likely than those with AN to require hospitalization. However, those with extreme dehydration and electrolyte imbalance, depression and suicidality, or symptoms that have not remitted with outpatient treatment, need hospitalization. After treatment, referrals to recovery groups and support groups are important to prevent relapse.

BINGE-EATING DISORDER

BED was introduced into the *DSM-IV* as a provisional diagnosis in 2004 and included in the *DSM-5* (APA, 2013) as its own category of eating disorders. BED is more prevalent than either AN or BN and is not uncommon in men. It is associated with high comorbidity comparable to that of BN, overweight, and obesity. When diagnosed, the usual treatment is outpatient therapy.

Clinical Course

The criteria for BED consist of binge eating, which includes both the ingestion of a large amount of food in a short period of time and a sense of loss of control during the binge, distress regarding the binge, eating until uncomfortably full, and feelings of guilt or depression following the binge. Purging does not occur with BED, and this helps differentiate BED from BN. In addition, investigators have shown that individuals with BED, when compared with those with BN, have lower dietary restraint and are higher in weight, even though many are not obese. It has been estimated that 10% to 30% of obese individuals have BED. In the first moderately sized community study that completed annual diagnostic interviews (using *DSM-5* eating disorder criteria) during the entire adolescent period, the peak age for onset of BED was between 18 and 20 years and the lifetime prevalence for BED was 3.0% (Stice, Marti, & Rohde, 2013). The findings revealed the following associations between BN and BED: approximately 23% of the women in the sample with initial BN of low frequency/duration reported the later development of BED; 22% reported moving from initial BED of low frequency/duration into BN (Stice et al., 2013). In other studies, persons with BED reported significantly less nocturnal eating than those with BN but more than controls (Masheb, Grilo, & White, 2011). Those with BED have described feeling "emptiness from a terrible feeling of loneliness" (Hertz, Addad, & Ronel, 2012, p. 115) and "very depressed about just life in general" (Woolhouse, Knowles, & Crafti, 2012, p. 332), perceiving their relationship with food as an "intense … antidote to … pain; well, in the short term, at least" (McIver, McGartland, & O'Halloran, 2009, p. 1241).

Outward signs associated with BED may include overweight, obesity, and associated consequences such as gallbladder disease and arthritis. Through these manifestations, BED may come to the attention of family and peers. Treatment can be delayed for years as individuals attempt on their own or with commercial weight loss programs to control their eating. Outcomes have not been extensively studied; poor prognosis is expected given the difficulty of attempting to achieve and maintain weight loss and in cases in which mood and anxiety disorders are also present.

Individuals with BED may miss work, school, or social activities to binge eat. Those who become obese often are extremely distressed by their binge eating, feel bad about themselves, and are preoccupied with their appearance. Most feel ashamed, may avoid social gatherings, and try to hide their problem. Often they are so successful that close family members and friends do not know that they binge eat.

Diagnostic Criteria

The key criterion for the diagnosis of BED is recurrent episodes of binge eating that occur on average at least once a week for a period of 3 months (APA, 2013). Other criteria appear in Table 25-6. Binge eating is influenced by such cues as dietary restraint, hunger, and negative affective states. Persons with BED are typically ashamed of their eating and try to conceal symptoms from others. Although obesity affects approximately 65% of clients with BED and increases progressively over time (Yager, 2008), overweight

and obesity are not diagnostic criteria. According to the *DSM-5* (APA, 2013), dieting typically follows the development of binge eating in BED, whereas dieting usually precedes the development of binge eating in BN.

Binge-Eating Disorder in Special Populations

BED is more prevalent among those seeking weight loss treatment (APA, 2013). BED is more prevalent in certain clinical populations, including persons with diabetes (Yager & Powers, 2007) and obese older men (Udo Tomoko et al., 2013).

Epidemiology

BED in individuals with type 2 diabetes is more common than AN or BN. Twelve-month prevalence among American adult females and males is 1.6% and 0.8%, respectively (APA, 2013), while higher lifetime prevalences were found among adults (women 3.5%; men 2.0%) and among 13- to 18-year-old adolescents (girls 2.3%; boys 0.8%) (Smink et al., 2012). A community survey conducted by the World Health Organization in 12 nations (including the United States, New Zealand, and countries in Latin America and Europe) reported country-specific lifetime prevalence estimates for BED as consistently higher than for BN (Kessler et al., 2013).

Age of Onset

Binge eating as a disordered eating behaviour or symptom is quite common among adolescents. In a longitudinal study of 14- to 18-year-old American adolescents, the incidence rate for binge eating was 10.1 per 1,000 persons among females and 6.6 per 1,000 persons among males (Field et al., 2008). Data from the 2002 Canadian Community Health Survey identified that women aged 15 years or older who were concerned about their weight were younger and more likely overweight or obese than women unconcerned with their weight (Park & Beaudet, 2007).

Gender Differences

A ratio of 1.5 to 2 adult females to 1 male experience BED.

Ethnic and Cultural Differences

There does not appear to be a significant difference in the prevalence of BED by ethnicity. BED is considered as common among American women from racial minority groups as it is among white women (APA, 2013).

Familial Differences

BED may run in families, reflecting a genetic influence. First-degree relatives report significantly higher lifetime rates of anxiety disorders, mood disorders (in particular, bipolar I or II disorder, and any depressive disorder), and eating disorders than the first-degree relatives of those

Table 25-6 Key Diagnostic Characteristics for Binge-Eating Disorder	
Diagnostic Criteria	**Target Symptoms and Associated Findings**

A. Recurrent episodes of binge eating (eating significantly more food in a short period of time than most people would eat under similar circumstances, with episodes marked by feelings of lack of control).
B. The binge-eating episodes are associated with at least three of the following:
1. eating much more rapidly than normal
2. eating until feeling uncomfortably full
3. eating large amounts of food when not feeling physically hungry
4. eating alone because of being embarrassed by how much one is eating
5. feeling disgusted with oneself, depressed, or very guilty after overeating
C. Marked distress regarding binge eating
D. The binge eating occurs, on average, at least once a week for 3 mo.
E. The binge eating is not associated with the regular use of inappropriate compensatory behaviours (e.g., purging, fasting, excessive exercise) and does not occur exclusively during the course of anorexia nervosa or bulimia nervosa.
• Severity:
  • Mild; 1–3 episodes of binge eating per week
  • Moderate; 4–7 episodes of binge eating per week
  • Severe; 8–13 episodes of binge eating per week
  • Extreme; 14 or more episodes of binge eating per week
• Partial remission: After full criteria were previously met, binge eating occurs less than one episode per week for a sustained period of time
• Full remission: If full criteria were previously met, no criteria have been met for a sustained period of time.
	• Usually leads to overweight and less often to obesity
	• Individuals tend to binge on foods that are chocolate, high fat, sweet, or salty.
	• Depression and anxiety contribute to body dissatisfaction.
	• Those who binge eat frequently use dieting and join fitness programs to control resultant weight gain (Lyons, 1998; Williamson, 1990) These behaviours are not excessive as they are with BN–purging type.

American Psychiatric Association. (2013). *Diagnostic and statistical manual of mental disorders* (5th ed.). Washington, DC: Author.

without BED (Hudson et al., 2006; Lilenfeld, Ringham, Kalarchian, & Marcus, 2008).

Comorbidity

Hypertension is the most common organic comorbidity, as well as diabetes mellitus type 2, hypertriglyceridaemia, and low high-density lipoprotein cholesterol (Castellini et al., 2008). The most common psychiatric comorbid conditions are mood, anxiety, and substance use disorders (APA, 2013). Grilo, White, Barnes, and Masheb (2013) found that 67% of persons seeking treatment for obesity and binge eating in primary care had at least one additional lifetime psychiatric disorder and 37% had at least one current psychiatric disorder. Psychiatric comorbidity was associated with the severity of the binge eating, not the degree of obesity.

Complications

Medical complications of BED include obesity, diabetes, hypertension, high cholesterol, gallbladder disease, kidney disease and/or failure, heart disease, arthritis, certain types of cancer, bone deterioration, menstrual

irregularities, ovarian abnormalities, complications of pregnancy, depression, anxiety, and suicidal thoughts. BED is also associated with impaired quality of life and increased health care utilization. Obese individuals with BED may also experience the consequences of stigma such as increased risk of depression, economic hardship, isolation, and social withdrawal. These stigmatized individuals have negative body image, poorer psychosocial functioning, and higher incidence of binge eating. They have reported feelings of discouragement and social inadequacy, which in turn have generated insecurity, social escape, and relationship difficulties (de Lima Santos, Pasquali, & Marcon, 2012). Using national survey data with 10-year longitudinal follow-up Schafer and Ferraro (2011) found that perceived weight discrimination increased the health risks of obesity. Such findings suggest that the sense of being marginalized because of one's weight can actually contribute to health decline.

Moreover, as a stigmatized condition, obesity negatively affects the relationship between clients and health care providers. Obese clients reported feeling that health care professionals' ambivalence towards their health needs amplified the extent to which the obese persons felt personally responsible for their condition, contributing to their personal ambivalence in relation to accessing and using services (Mold & Forbes, 2011). For example, they were less probable to undergo clinical breast examination, gynaecologic examination, and Papanicolaou smear testing; they cancelled medical appointments if they believed they would be weighed.

Aetiology

It is postulated that binge-eating functions to modulate negative emotional states. Positive mood, negative mood, and tension have all been found to strongly deteriorate immediately before the first daily binge (Munsch, Meyer, Quartier, & Wilhelm, 2012), as has been also observed in BN (Engelberg, Steiger, Gauvin, & Wonderlich, 2007; Smyth et al., 2007). However, unlike in the case of BN, researchers observed a slight improvement of mood up to 30 minutes before binge eating followed by an abrupt and significant deterioration immediately after the binge (Munsch et al., 2012). These results indicate that binge eating in BED might be the result of an immediate breakdown of emotion and impulse regulation caused by sudden increases of negative affect and tension and a rapid decrease of positive affect. Regarding the long-term course of binge eating, researchers found that a lasting improvement in mood emerged several hours following the binge (Munsch et al., 2012).

Biologic Theories

While AN and BN tend to be characterized by high levels of most forms of dietary restraint, including extreme restrictive behaviours, BED tends to be associated with low levels of dietary restraint (Blomquist & Grilo, 2011).

Genetic

BED was found to be 45% heritable and 55% environmental, with 13% due to common environmental and 42% due to unique environmental factors (Mitchell et al., 2010). Higher lifetime rates of mental disorders have been shown in female relatives of women with BED when compared with female relatives of control women without BED (Lilenfeld et al., 2008).

Psychological and Social Theories

Individuals with BED show higher harm-avoidance scores than obese individuals who do not binge eat. Elevated harm avoidance may be related to attempting to avoid painful situations (Peterson et al., 2010). Among participants in a large community sample, those with binge-eating symptoms were younger and more likely to report childhood physical abuse and childhood sexual abuse than those who never binged (Sachs-Ericsson et al., 2012). Some individuals describe experiences of

dissociation and "numbing out" while binge eating (Yager & Powers, 2007, p. 23). One woman who experienced BED reported that she was "constantly feeling afraid and panicky" and that she "just want[ed] to plug that feeling up" (McIver et al., 2009, p. 1239). Obese individuals with BED are more likely to request professional psychological help than obese non–binge-eating individuals. Their greater sense of social insecurity and the impairment in interpersonal relationships associated with being overweight may contribute to this issue, and the intrinsic feeling of ineffectiveness and self-deprecation maintained by social stigmatization promotes the vicious circle leading to binge eating through negative feedback on self-esteem.

Cognitive Theory

Increasing evidence indicates that dysfunctional attitudes toward eating, weight, and shape are as central to BED as they are to AN and BN (Ramacciotti et al., 2008). Cognitive characteristics postulated to be present in individuals who engage in binge eating include high standards and expectations, aversive self-awareness, removal of inhibitions, and irrational beliefs (Heatherton & Baumeister, 1991). High standards for body shape and thinness influence individuals in becoming highly aware of self, feeling inadequate in comparison with others, and consequently in their developing low self-esteem and high self-aversion. This may lead some people to adopt, or think they should adopt, rigid dietary rules and restrict eating in unrealistic ways. Eating behaviour can be disrupted by such propensity for setting unrealistic aims for body appearance and food intake, unsuccessful striving to meet them, and equating lack of complete achievement with abject failure.

Disinhibition occurs once the "diet" is broken: The individual will no longer maintain control and will compensate through overeating (Dolan & Ford, 1991). Because of the inflexibility of these eating schemes, any minor transgression can lead to an all-or-nothing reaction whereby attempts to control eating are abandoned and result in a binge. The tendency to evaluate self-worth in terms of weight and shape, and a dichotomous (black-and-white) thinking style, together with having unrealistic weight goals, low self-efficacy, poor coping or problem-solving skills, have been identified as significant psychological predictors of weight regain in obesity (Ramacciotti et al., 2008) and higher frequency of binge eating at 12-month follow-up after completing treatments for BED (Grilo, White, Gucorguieva, Wilson, & Masheb, 2013).

Spiritual Underpinnings

Underlying reasons for eating without being hungry include subjective experiences of distress and disconnection that do not encourage trust in others, and prior relationships characterized by insecurity. One participant in an Overeaters Anonymous project explained her distress in terms of frightening emotions: "In the past I had outbursts of anger that could not be contained. Nobody could control me, and there was a great deal [of anger] within me. The message … was: cry, shout until you burst, without any empathy" (Hertz et al., 2012, p. 114). Individuals who come to regard food as a kind of substitute attachment object may use it to fill the emptiness, often hiding their food and eating from others, and thus increasing their sense of disconnection from self and others.

Risk Factors

The risk or predisposing factors for BED are included in Figure 25-3.

Interdisciplinary Treatment

The treatment methods for BED in current use include CBT, interpersonal psychotherapy, medications, self-help support groups, and commercial weight loss and exercise programs. Surgical interventions are recommended for morbidly obese (BMI > 40) adult clients for whom other weight loss attempts have failed (Neff, Olbers, & Le Roux, 2013). Individual CBT was found to reduce binge eating with abstinence for 12 months following treatment but did not result in weight loss (Grilo, Wilson, Crosby, & Masheb, 2012). Both clients and treatment providers have identified that improving self-esteem, improving body experience, and learning problem-solving skills are necessary to recovery (Vanderlinden, Buis, Pieters, & Probst, 2007).

As with the treatment of AN and BN, a comprehensive interdisciplinary approach is needed. The treatment goals focus on reducing binge eating, effecting and maintaining weight loss if overweight or obese, restructuring dysfunctional thinking about food and appearance, alleviating comorbid depression and anxiety, and addressing harassment. Treatment occurs in an outpatient setting, except for the rare time the client is hospitalized for bariatric surgery.

Nutrition counselling is an important treatment component focusing on portion size and control, the role of emotions on eating behaviours, healthy food and nutrient choices, self-monitoring, and strategies to delay binge eating. A pilot trial with chromium supplementation resulted in greater reductions in binge frequency, weight, fasting glucose, and symptoms of depression for those treated with chromium versus placebo (Brownley, Von Holle, Hamer, La Via, & Bulik, 2013). Clients may also access commercial weight loss and fitness programs. Alternative therapies monitored by holistic health professionals may also be helpful, such as relaxation and yoga.

Priority Care Issues

Comorbid obesity, overweight, depression, and anxiety can contribute to cardiac and other health crises. The risk of type 2 diabetes is significant in the presence of obesity.

Nursing Management: Human Response to Binge-Eating Disorder

The primary nursing diagnoses for patients with BED may include Imbalanced Nutrition: More Than Body Requirements, Impaired Physical Mobility, Activity Intolerance, Anxiety, Ineffective Coping, and Ineffective Health Maintenance. The nurse establishes a therapeutic relationship and through this connection helps monitor the client's self-care abilities including dietary intake and activity, teaches and models effective problem solving, and makes nutritional recommendations, taking into account the client's individual needs.

Therapeutic Relationship

Individuals with BED may experience a great deal of shame and guilt in response to negative judgements of their eating behaviours, overweight, and obesity. They often are reluctant to participate in formal fitness programs for fear of being ridiculed. They may opt out of such programs when they believe they have nothing in common with other group members. Often those who have BED suffer with the disorder for years, feeling very lonely. The nurse builds a relationship of trust through modelling self-acceptance, nonjudgemental approach, and discussing the role of the nurse–client relationship with respect to the goals of therapy (see Chapter 6).

Biologic Domain

Most individuals with BED become overweight or obese. The medical consequences of cardiovascular disease, diabetes, and arthritis as well as other health threats are considered in all aspects of the nursing process.

Assessment

The nurse assesses current binge-eating patterns and associated symptoms. In a population-based survey of 4,096 community residents, where 6.1% reported BED symptoms, BED was independently associated with acid regurgitation, heartburn, dysphagia, bloating, upper abdominal pain, diarrhoea, urgency, constipation, and feeling of anal blockage (Cremonini et al., 2009). These symptoms may interfere with sleep (Trace et al., 2012). Two implications from this work are that clients presenting with GI symptoms be questioned regarding BED, and clients presenting with BED be screened for GI symptoms. Psychosocial–spiritual assessment is also warranted given the likelihood of comorbid depression, anxiety, and stigmatization.

Nursing Diagnoses for Biologic Domain

Imbalanced Nutrition: More Than Body Requirements, Impaired Physical Mobility, and Activity Intolerance are examples of nursing diagnoses for the biologic domain.

Interventions for Biologic Domain

Clients are asked to record their intake, binges, and feelings associated with food and eating to form a foundation for changing behaviours. As noted above, symptoms of gastric distress should be assessed. Clients should be monitored for associated complications such as diabetes, cardiovascular disease, and arthritis. Physical mobility, activity, and sleep patterns are evaluated.

Pharmacologic Interventions

Topiramate and orlistat are currently used in the long-term treatment of obesity. Investigations have shown that topiramate (an antiepileptic agent) has been effective in decreasing binge eating and appetite. Topiramate has demonstrated efficacy in the treatment of BED-related obesity (Mitchell et al., 2013). Orlistat inhibits GI lipase, an enzyme that breaks down triglycerides in the intestine so that triglycerides from the diet are prevented from being hydrolyzed into absorbable free fatty acids and are excreted undigested, thus preventing approximately 30% of dietary fat from being absorbed (Grilo & Masheb, 2007). Other medications, usually SSRIs, may treat anxiety and depression symptomatology. Prozac (fluoxetine) is often used to reduce binge eating (see Box 25-12).

 TEACHING POINTS

Individuals taking the above weight loss agents should be informed that weight will be regained if the medication is stopped unless lifestyle interventions that include physical activity and stress management are incorporated. Those taking orlistat should be instructed to expect looser greasy stools. The instructions for SSRI use are contained in Chapter 12.

Psychosocial Domain

Assessment

Psychological assessment for the individual with BED is similar to that for the individual with BN, requiring identification of cognitive distortions and knowledge deficits. Dissociation is evaluated given that binge eating may be a means to escape negative emotion (La Mela, Maglietta, Castellini, Amoroso, & Lucarelli, 2010; Zeeck, Stelzer, Linster, Joos, & Hartmann, 2011). Symptoms of mood and anxiety disorders are explored in-depth in Chapters 22 and 23, respectively.

Nursing Diagnoses for Psychosocial Domain

Common diagnoses for the psychosocial domain include Anxiety, Ineffective Coping, Deficient Knowledge, and Social Isolation.

Interventions for Psychosocial Domain

Psychotherapy and structured self-help, both based on cognitive–behavioural interventions, are recommended as the first-line treatments for BED (Vocks et al., 2010). A longer course of treatment (i.e., 20 sessions or more) is associated with better BED remission than is a briefer course (Thompson-Brenner et al., 2013). Clients are taught the techniques to monitor and change their eating habits, as well as to change the way they respond to difficult and stressful situations. CBT was found superior to fluoxetine for BED in terms of decreasing the number of binge days, the number of binge episodes, and psychological features of BED such as hunger and disinhibition (Grilo et al., 2012). Therapist-led individual treatment has been associated with better outcomes of remission and treatment completion than self-help individual treatment. Compared with therapist-led group therapy, self-help group participants who received self-help in a group format were three times more likely to drop out and 3.58 times more likely to continue binge eating at termination (Thompson-Brenner et al., 2013).

Family

There is little research into family needs; families of individuals with binge eating may need support themselves.

Psychoeducation

The nurse can assist the individual with BED to eat appropriately portioned meals at regular intervals to reduce hunger and binge eating. Individuals also need information about the medical consequences of binge eating. Other topics for psychoeducation are included in Box 25-14.

Spiritual Domain

Assessment

The nurse assesses the client's reported satisfaction with relationships and lifestyle choices, watchful of expressions of self-judgement and self-acceptance, enabling the

---

> **BOX 25-14 Psychoeducation Checklist: Binge-Eating Disorder**
>
> When caring for the individual with BED, consider the following topics:
> - Health and lifestyle
> - How weight reduction can be attained
> - Applied knowledge about food and healthy eating
> - Principles of dieting
> - The importance of being present of one's body and choices
> - Relaxation techniques
> - Stress management
> - The importance of physical activity
> - Strength training; instruction and practical exercises
> - Accessing resources; computers as an aid in eating well and achieving nutritional goals
> - Planning for holidays

client to describe any painful traumatic experiences with harassment and discrimination. The nurse listens to client stories of social exclusion, developmental interruption, and denied extracurricular opportunities such as shopping for clothing, attending parties, and participating in recreational/sporting events.

Nursing Diagnoses for Spiritual Domain

Potential diagnoses for the spiritual domain include Ineffective Protection: Reduced Quality of Life and Impaired Self-Identity. Individuals with BED who binge eat in response to various biopsychosocial experiences, environmental cues, trauma, and nonevents may struggle to protect themselves from such underlying issues as isolation and discrimination, filling themselves with food without awareness of deeper unmet needs.

Interventions for Spiritual Domain

Provide BED clients opportunities to discuss any experiences of stress, relationship conflict, and trauma. Support them to narrate themes of disappointment and pain in response to stigma. Through the safety of the nurse–client relationship, they can develop their capacity to reconnect with self, others, and, when appropriate, the larger universal life force. The nurse may offer anticipatory guidance to individuals who need to catch up with missed developmental milestones such as dating and intimacy (Ciliska, 1990). Helping them attend to their growth and well-being during the course of treatment may reduce depression, anxiety, relationship distress, social role conflict, and eating disorder symptoms (Scott Richards et al., 2006).

Evaluation and Treatment Outcomes

In a random trial to test brief and long-term clinical efficacy of enhanced and standard CBT in obese patients with BED, control participants regained on average most of the weight they had lost during the inpatient treatment program, while participants receiving enhanced CBT had improved weight loss at 1-year follow-up (Cesa et al.,

 TEACHING POINTS

Keeping in mind that many BED clients are overweight or obese and may have experienced harassment, psychoeducation focuses on principles of dieting, lifestyle changes to maintain weight loss, the importance of being self-aware, relaxation techniques, strength training, and how to deal with stress. Studies report a high attrition rate for psychoeducational programs (e.g., Stahre, Tärnell, Håkanson, & Hällström, 2007). Therefore, attending to client emotional comfort, briefing, and debriefing must be considered.

2013). Munsch, Meyer, and Biedert (2012) found a strong improvement (i.e., remission of binge eating, BED diagnosis, the number of self-reported weekly binge-eating episodes, and all BED symptoms except restraint eating) at the end of treatment. Furthermore, overall improvement relative to pretreatment values was found at 6-year follow-up. BMI values at 6-year follow-up were improved relative to pretreatment though the effect size was small: Less than half of all participants still revealed comorbid mental disorders at 6-year follow-up. Rapid response during the early treatment phase was the only characteristic predictive of favourable long-term treatment outcome (Munsch et al., 2012).

Other studies of the natural course of BED reveal that at 12- to 13-year follow-up, approximately 8% to 10% were still affected by BED, while 67% to 69% no longer met criteria for an eating disorder (Fichter, Quadflieg, & Hedlund, 2008; Wade, Bergin, Tiggemann, Bulik, & Fairburn, 2006). Studies comparing methods found medication and behavioural interventions moderately effective, while self-help and other interventions were not (Brownley, Berkman, Sedway, Lohr, & Bulik, 2007).

Continuum of Care

Although individuals do not require hospitalization for BED, the consequence of obesity may involve hospitalization for surgical intervention such as gastric bypass or gastric banding surgery (Neff et al., 2013).

■■ PREVENTION OF EATING DISORDERS

Eating disorders are among the most preventable mental disorders. National eating disorder awareness and advocacy groups work toward educating the general public, those at risk, and those who work with groups at risk, such as teachers, coaches, and college student health centre staff. They promote greater awareness of early signs of eating disorders and available resources to those at risk for developing eating disorders (Tillman, Arbaugh, & Balaban, 2012). They also monitor the media, striving to remove unhealthy advertisements and articles in magazines appealing to vulnerable individuals. A list of online resources is found in the Web Links on the thePoint.

Prevention and early detection strategies for parents and schoolteachers are often the focus of school nurses and community mental health nurses. Specific strategies to promote positive body image in children have included a web-based prevention program designed for elementary school teachers (McVey, Gusella, Tweed, & Ferrari, 2009), a children's picture book called *Shapesville* that increased the appearance satisfaction and awareness of healthy eating in 5- to 9-year-old girls (Dohnt & Tiggemann, 2008), and a peer program whereby older

Table 25-7 ◢ Prevention Strategies for Parents and Children	
Parents Education	**Children Education**
Real versus ideal weight	Peer pressure regarding eating and weight
Influence of attitudes, behaviours, and teasing	Menses, puberty, and normal weight gain
Ways to increase self-esteem	Strategies for obesity
Role of media: TV and magazines	Ways to develop or improve self-esteem
Signs and symptoms	Body image traps: media and retail clothing
Interventions for obesity	Adapting and coping with problems
Boys at risk also	Reporting friends with signs of eating disorders
Observe for rituals	**Screening:** for risk factors
Supervision of eating and exercise	**Assessment:** for treatment
	Follow-up: monitor for relapse

students (fourth to seventh grades) were taught to teach younger (Kindergarten–third grade) buddies about nutrition, physical activity, and healthy body image (Stock et al., 2007). Successful overweight and obesity prevention programs are delivered in school settings with program leaders having access to specialist support (Kirk, Bornstein, Navarro, & Swanson, 2009). For example, a school intervention program targeting children in grades 4 to 6 over a 2-year period and including components of nutrition

education, nutrition policy, social marketing, and parent outreach resulted in a 50% reduction in the incidence of overweight (Foster et al., 2008). The researchers recommended further research focus (a) on school environment (e.g., physical education classes) and environment beyond schools (e.g., corner stores, fast-food outlets, homes) and (b) with younger ages given the high prevalence of children expressing body dissatisfaction in grades 4 to 6 and the rising Canadian obesity epidemic.

Other strategies for parents and children appear in Table 25-7 and are based on research of risk factors and protective factors. These protective factors, such as confidence and healthy competition in athletics (Taylor et al., 1998), paternal involvement and support (McVey, Pepler, Davis, Flett, & Abdolel, 2002), positive atmosphere at family meals, and frequent lunch intake (Neumark-Sztainer et al., 2007) have been shown to prevent the development of an eating disorder for individuals at risk. Dieting, low self-esteem, and body dissatisfaction are examples of risk factors underlying the development of eating disorders that can be reversed with early identification and intervention.

■■■ FUTURE DIRECTIONS IN EATING DISORDER KNOWLEDGE

The classification of eating disorders underwent significant revision in 2013 with the *DSM-5*. While AN, BN, and BED have been extensively discussed, other feeding and eating disorders, listed in Table 25-8, require ongoing research and development.

Table 25-8 ◢ Brief Overview of Other Feeding and Eating Disorders Presented in the *DSM-5* (APA, 2013)			
Pica	Persistently eating nonfood substances	Period of at least 1 mo	More prevalent among children with developmental delays (e.g., autism spectrum disorders or intellectual disability) (Barrett, 2008; Casey, Cook-Cottone, & Beck-Joslyn, 2012).
Rumination disorder	Repeated regurgitation of food during or after eating	Period of at least 1 mo	May be associated with malnutrition. Adolescents and adults may try to disguise by placing hand over mouth or coughing
Avoidant/restrictive food intake disorder	Persistent inability to meet appropriate nutrition or energy needs	Not specified	Previously named "feeding disorder of infancy or early childhood" (APA, 2000)
Other specified feeding or eating disorders:			
1. Atypical AN	Meet all criteria for AN except weight remains within or above normal range		
2. BN (of low frequency ± limited duration)	Meet all criteria for BN except binge eating and inappropriate compensatory behaviours occur less than once a week ± less than 3 mo		
3. BED (of low frequency ± limited duration)	Meet all criteria for BED except binge eating occurs less than once a week ± less than 3 mo		
4. Purging disorder	Recurrent purging behaviour to influence weight/shape in the absence of binge eating		
5. Night eating syndrome	Recurrent episodes of eating at night (i.e., eating after awakening from sleep, excessive food consumption after the evening meal)		
Unspecified feeding or eating disorder	Do not meet full criteria for any of the feeding and eating disorders diagnostic class		

Society has begun to engage in an effort to help young individuals resist developing eating disorders. Many of the Web links on the thePoint have online help and resources for young individuals, families, teachers, and health care professionals.

SUMMARY OF KEY POINTS

■ AN, BN, and BED have some common symptoms but are classified as discrete disorders in the *DSM 5*.

■ Eating disorders are best viewed along a continuum that includes normal unrestricted eating, mild disturbed eating, increasing weight and shape preoccupation, and clinical eating disorders. Because these symptomologic patterns occur more frequently than full eating disorders, they are often overlooked; however, once identified, they can be prevented from worsening.

■ Similar factors predispose individuals to the development of AN, BN, and BED, and these factors represent a bio/psycho/social/spiritual model of risk that threatens health and well-being. Identifying risk factors assists with prevention strategies.

■ Aetiologic factors contribute in combination to the development of eating disorders; no one factor provides a complete explanation.

■ Mood and anxiety disorders are significantly more frequent in individuals with eating disorders than the general community.

■ All of the eating disorders have physical, emotional, social, and spiritual consequences that influence health, well-being, and even life.

■ Treatment of AN almost always includes hospitalization for refeeding; BN and BED are treated primarily on an outpatient basis.

■ For individuals with BN, CBT improves symptoms sooner than does IPT. For individuals with AN, family therapy plus individual IPT are the most effective. Research on best practice for BED is in its infancy; CBT and weight reduction behavioural therapy may foster remission.

■ Pharmacotherapy can be effective for BN and BED but less so for AN, especially during acute malnourishment.

■ Individuals with eating disorders require responsive treatment addressing both specific (e.g., eating behaviour) and nonspecific (e.g., underlying) vulnerabilities.

■ The outcomes for BN are better than those for AN and BED. The type and severity of comorbid conditions and the length of the illness influence outcomes.

CRITICAL THINKING CHALLENGES

1 Discuss the potential difficulties and risks in attempting to treat a client with AN in an outpatient setting.

2 A client in the clinic is examined for BN and is prescribed fluoxetine. She reports great success immediately and attributes this to the side effect of weight lost. What are your concerns and interventions?

3 The nurse caring for an overweight BED client is obese himself. How can nurses be supported to examine personal attitudes, biases, and experiences with weight gain and loss? What are the dangers of not engaging in this type of self-development?

4 Parents are often in need of support and suggestions for how to help prevent eating disorders. Develop a teaching program and include the topics and rationale for the suggestions chosen.

5 Identify the important nursing management components of a refeeding program for a hospitalized individual with AN.

6 BN is often described as a closet disorder with secretive binge eating and purging. Identify the signs and symptoms of each body system involved for someone with this disorder.

7 Amid extensive health policy and programming to address global obesity, how do nurses best advocate for the needs of individuals and families affected by AN and BN?

8 Positive outcomes for the recovery of BED, BN, and AN are dependent on many factors. Identify the factors that promote positive outcomes and those related to poorer outcomes and prognosis.

REFERENCES

Academy of Eating Disorders. (2011). *Critical points for early recognition and medical risk management in the care of individuals with eating disorders* (2nd ed.). Retrieved from http://www.aedweb.org/AM/Template.cfm?Section=Resources_for_Professionals&Template=/CM/ContentDisplay.cfm&ContentID=2593

Ahzern, A. L., Bennett, K. M., & Hetherington, M. M. (2008). Internalization of the ultra-thin ideal: Positive implicit associations with underweight fashion models are associated with drive for thinness in young women. *Eating Disorders, 16,* 294–307.

American Psychiatric Association. (1987). *Diagnostic and statistical manual of mental disorders (DSM-III)* (3rd ed.). Washington, DC: Author.

American Psychiatric Association. (2000). *Diagnostic and statistical manual of mental disorders* (4th ed., Text revision). Washington, DC: Author.

American Psychiatric Association. (2013). *Diagnostic and statistical manual of mental disorders* (5th ed.). Washington, DC: Author.

Anderluk, M. B., Tchanturia, K., Rabe-Hesketh, S., & Treasure, J. (2003). Childhood obsessive-compulsive personality traits in adult women with eating disorders: Defining a broader eating disorder phenotype. *American Journal of Psychiatry, 160*(2), 242–247.

Andersen, A. E. (1995). A standard test meal to assess treatment response in anorexia nervosa patients. Eating Disorders. *Journal of Treatment and Prevention, 3,* 47–55.

Anderson, D. A. & Maloney, K. C. (2001). The efficacy of cognitive-behavioral therapy on the core symptoms of bulimia nervosa. *Clinical Psychology Review, 21,* 971–988.

Anderson, D. A., Williamson, D. A., Johnson, W. G., & Grieve, C. O. (2001). Validity of test meals for determining binge eating. *Eating Behaviors, 2,* 105–112.

Anschutz, D. J., Van Strien, T., & Engels, R. C. (2008). Exposure to slim images in mass media: Television commercials as reminders of restriction in restrained eaters. *Health Psychology, 27,* 401–408.

Arrow, B., Kenardy, J., & Agras, W. S. (1995). The Emotional Eating Scale: The development of a measure to assess coping with negative affect by eating. *International Journal of Eating Disorders, 18*, 79–90.

Attia, E. & Schroeder, L. (2005). Pharmacologic treatment of anorexia nervosa: Where do we go from here? *International Journal of Eating Disorders, 37*, S60–S63.

Bailer, U. F., Bloss, C. S., Frank, G. K., Price, J. C., Meltzer, C. C., Mathis, C. A., ... Kaye, W. H. (2011). 5-HT receptor binding is increased after recovery from bulimia nervosa compared to control women and is associated with behavioral inhibition in both groups. *International Journal of Eating Disorders, 44*(6), 477–487.

Bailer, U., de Zwaan, M., Leisch, F., Strnad, A., Lennkh-Wolfsberg, C., El-Giamal, N., ... Kasper, S. (2004). Guided self-help versus cognitive-behavioral group therapy in the treatment of bulimia nervosa. *International Journal of Eating Disorders, 35*, 522–537.

Bailer, U. F. & Kaye, W. H. (2003). A review of neuropeptide and neuroendocrine dysregulation in anorexia and bulimia nervosa. *Current Drug Targets. CNS and Neurological Disorders, 2*(1), 53–59.

Bardone-Cone, A. M., Harney, M. B., Maldonado, C. R., Lawson, M. A., Robinson, D. P., Smith, R., & Tosh, A. (2010). Defining recovery from an eating disorder: Conceptualization, validation, and examination of psychosocial functioning and psychiatric comorbidity. *Behaviour Research and Therapy, 48*, 194–202.

Barrett, R. P. (2008). Pica. *Brown University Child and Adolescent Behavior Letter, 22*, 1–3.

Beadle, J. N., Paradiso, S., Salerno, A., & McCormick, L. M. (2013). Alexithymia, emotional empathy, and self-regulation in anorexia nervosa. *Annals of Clinical Psychiatry, 25*(2), 107–120.

Becker, A. E., Burwell, R. A., Gilman, S. E., Herzog, D. B., & Hamburg, P. (2002). Eating behaviours and attitudes following exposure to television among ethnic Fijian adolescent girls. *British Journal of Psychiatry, 180*, 509–514.

Bergin, J. L. & Wade, T. D. (2012). A cross-sectional analysis of the cognitive model of bulimia nervosa. *International Journal of Eating Disorders, 45*(6), 776–786.

Berkman, N. D., Lohr, K. N., & Bulik, C. M. (2007). Outcomes of eating disorders: A systematic review of the literature. *International Journal of Eating Disorders, 40*, 293–309.

Berrett, M. E., Hardman, R. K., O'Grady, K., & Scott Richards, P. (2007). The role of spirituality in the treatment of trauma and eating disorders: Recommendations for clinical practice. *Eating Disorders, 15*, 373–389.

Birmingham, C. L., Su, J., Hlynsky, J. A., Goldner, E. M., & Gao, M. (2005). The mortality rate from anorexia nervosa. *International Journal of Eating Disorders, 38*, 143–146.

Birmingham, C. L., Touyz, S., & Harbottle, J. (2009). Are anorexia nervosa and bulimia nervosa separate disorders? Challenging the 'transdiagnostic' theory of eating disorders. *European Eating Disorders Review, 17*(1), 2–13.

Blodgett Salafia, E. & Lemer, J. (2012). Associations between multiple types of stress and disordered eating among girls and boys in middle school. *Journal of Child and Family Studies, 21*(1), 148–157.

Blomquist, K. K. & Grilo, C. M. (2011). Predictive significance of changes in dietary restraint in obese patients with binge eating disorder during treatment. *International Journal of Eating Disorders, 44*, 515–523.

Bohon, C., Stice, E., & Burton, E. (2009). Maintenance factors for persistence of bulimic pathology: A prospective natural history study. *International Journal of Eating Disorders, 42*, 173–178.

Braun, D. L., Sunday, S. R., Huang, A., & Halmi, K. A. (1999). More males seek treatment for eating disorders. *International Journal of Eating Disorders, 25*(4), 415–424.

Brewerton, T. D. & Costin, C. (2011). Long-term outcome of residential treatment for anorexia nervosa and bulimia nervosa. *Eating Disorders, 19*(2), 132–144.

Brown, K. E. & Geller, J. (2006). Supporting friends and family members with eating disorders: Discrepancies between intentions and reality. *Eating Disorders, 14*, 1–14.

Brown, K. M., Bujac, S. R., Mann, E. T., Campbellm, D. A., Stubbins, M. J., & Blundell, J. E. (2007). Further evidence of association of OPRD1 & HTR1D polymorphisms with susceptibility to anorexia nervosa. *Biological Psychiatry, 61*(3), 367–373.

Brown, T. A. & Keel, P. K. (2012). Current and emerging directions in the treatment of eating disorders. *Substance Abuse, 6*, 33–61.

Brownley, K. A., Berkman, N. D., Sedway, J. A., Lohr, K. N., & Bulik, C. M. (2007). Binge eating disorder treatment: A systematic review of randomized controlled trials. *International Journal of Eating Disorders, 40*, 337–348.

Brownley, K. A., Von Holle, A., Hamer, R. M., La Via, M., & Bulik, C. M. (2013). A double-blind, randomized pilot trial of chromium picolinate for binge eating disorder: Results of the Binge Eating and Chromium (BEACh) Study. *Journal of Psychosomatic Research, 75*(1), 36–42.

Bruch, H. (1973). *Eating disorders: Obesity, anorexia nervosa and the person within*. New York: Basic Books.

Bühren, K. K. (2012). Cognitive flexibility in juvenile anorexia nervosa patients before and after weight recovery. *Journal of Neural Transmission, 119*(9), 1047–1057.

Bulik, C. M., Hebebrand, J., Keski-Rahkonen, A., Klump, K. L., Reichborn-Kjennerud, T., Mazzeo, S. E., & Wade, T. D. (2007). Genetic epidemiology, endophenotypes, and eating disorder classification. *International Journal of Eating Disorders, 40*, S52–S60.

Bulik, C. M., Reba, L., Siega-Riz, A-M., & Reichborn-Kjennerud, T. (2005). Anorexia nervosa: Definition, epidemiology, and cycle of risk. *International Journal of Eating Disorders, 37*, 52–59.

Bulik, C. M., Sullivan, P., Wade, T., & Kendler, K. (2000). Twin studies of eating disorders: A review. *International Journal of Eating Disorders, 27*, 1–20.

Calzo, J. P., Sonneville, K. R., Haines, J., Blood, E. A., Field, A. E., & Austin, S. B. (2012). The development of associations among body mass index, body dissatisfaction, and weight and shape concern in adolescent boys and girls. *Journal of Adolescent Health, 51*(5), 517–523.

Carbaugh, R. J. & Sias, S. M. (2010). Comorbidity of bulimia nervosa and substance abuse: Etiologies, treatment issues, and treatment approaches. *Journal of Mental Health Counseling, 32*(2), 125–138.

Carter, J. C., Stewart, D. A., & Fairburn, C. G. (2001). Eating Disorder Examination Questionnaire: Norms for adolescent girls. *Behaviour Research and Therapy, 39*, 625–632.

Casey, C., Cook-Cottone, C., & Beck-Joslyn, M. (2012). An overview of problematic eating and food-related behavior among foster children: Definitions, etiology, and intervention. *Journal of Child and Adolescent Social Work, 29*(4), 307–322.

Castellini, G., Lapi, F., Ravaldi, C., Vannacci, A., Rotella, C. M., Faravelli, C., & Ricca, V. (2008). Eating disorder psychopathology does not predict the overweight severity in subjects seeking weight loss treatment. *Comprehensive Psychiatry, 49*(4), 359–363. Retrieved from http://dx.doi.org.proxy.hil.unb.ca/10.1016/j.comppsych.2008.01.005

Cavallini, G. (2005). *Catherine of Siena*. London, UK: Continuum.

Central West Eating Disorders Program. (2010). *Putting eating disorders on the radar of primary care providers*. Available at www.shared-care.ca/files/Eating_Disorders_Toolkit.pdf

Cesa, G. L., Manzoni, G. M., Bacchetta, M., Castelnuovo, G., Conti, S., Gaggioli, A., ..., Riva, G. (2013). Virtual reality for enhancing the cognitive behavioral treatment of obesity with binge eating disorder: Randomized controlled study with one-year follow-up. *Journal of Medical Internet Research, 15*(6), e113.

Chatterton, J. M. & Petrie, T. A. (2013). Prevalence of disordered eating and pathogenic weight control behaviors among male collegiate athletes. *Eating Disorders, 21*(4), 328–341.

Chrisler, J. C., Fung, K. T., Lopez, A. M., & Gorman, J. A. (2013). Suffering by comparison: Twitter users' reactions to the Victoria's Secret fashion show. *Body Image, 10*(4), 648–652.

Ciliska, D. (1990). *Beyond dieting: Psychoeducational interventions for chronically obese women. Brunner/Mazzel Eating Disorders Monograph Series, 5*. New York: Taylor & Francis.

Collier, R. (2013). Treatment challenges for men with eating disorders. *Canadian Medical Association Journal, 185*(3), E137–E138.

Cooper, M. J., Todd, G., Turner, H., & Wells, A. (2007). Cognitive therapy for bulimia nervosa: An A-B replication series. *Clinical Psychology and Psychotherapy, 14*, 402–411.

Cooper, M. J., Wells, A., & Todd, G. (2004). A cognitive model of bulimia nervosa. *British Journal of Clinical Psychology, 43*, 1–16.

Cooper, P., Taylor, M., Cooper, Z., & Fairburn, C. (1987). The development and validation of the BSQ. *International Journal of Eating Disorders, 6*, 485–494.

Costin, C. (2009). The embodied therapist: Perspectives on treatment, personal growth, and supervision related to body image. In M. Maine, W. Davis, & J. Shure (Eds.), *Effective clinical practice in the treatment of eating disorders: the heart of the matter* (pp. 179–192). New York: Routledge.

Cremonini, F. F., Camilleri, M. M., Clark, M. M., Beebe, T. J., Locke, G. R., Zinsmeister, A. R., ... Talley, N. J. (2009). Associations among binge eating behavior patterns and gastrointestinal symptoms: A population-based study. *International Journal of Obesity, 33*(3), 342–353.

Crisafulli, M. A., Thompson-Brenner, H., Franko, D. L., Eddy, K. T., & Herzog, D. B. (2010). Stigmatization of anorexia nervosa: Characteristics and response to intervention. *Journal of Social and Clinical Psychology, 29*(7), 756–770.

Croll, J., Neumark-Sztainer, D., Story, M., & Ireland, M. (2002). Prevalence and risk and protective factors related to disordered eating behaviors among adolescents: Relationship to gender and ethnicity. *Journal of Adolescent Health, 13*(2), 166–175.

Couturier, J., Kimber, M., & Szatmari, P. (2013). Efficacy of family-based treatment for adolescents with eating disorders: A systematic review and meta-analysis. *International Journal of Eating Disorders, 46*(1), 3–11.

Dalgliesh, J. & Nutt, K. (2013). Treating men with eating disorders in the NHS. *Nursing Standard*, 27(35), 42–46.

Dallos, R. & Denford, S. (2008). A qualitative exploration of relationship and attachment themes in families with an eating disorder. *Clinical Child Psychology and Psychiatry*, 13, 305–322.

Darcy, A. M., Doyle, A. C., Lock, J., Peebles, R., Doyle, P., & Le Grange, D. (2012). The eating disorders examination in adolescent males with anorexia nervosa: How does it compare to adolescent females? *International Journal of Eating Disorders*, 45(1), 110–114.

Dayal, H. (2013). *From shame to shame resilience: Narratives of counsellor trainees with eating issues*. Unpublished Master's of Education Thesis. Fredericton, NB: University of New Brunswick.

de Lauzon, B., Romon, M., Deschamps, V., Lafay, L., Borys, J-M., Karlsson, J., ... Fleurbaix Laventie Ville Sante Study Group. (2004). The Three-Factor Eating Questionnaire-R18 is able to distinguish among different eating patterns in a general population. *Journal of Nutrition*, 134(9), 2372–2380.

de Lima Santos, A., Pasquali, R., & Marcon, S. S. (2012). Feelings and living experiences of individuals taking part in a support group for control of obesity: An exploratory study. *Online Brazilian Journal of Nursing*, 11(1), 3–13.

Dell, M. L. & Josephson, A. M. (2007). Religious and spiritual factors in childhood and adolescent eating disorders and obesity. *Southern Medical Journal*, 100, 628–632.

Diamond-Raab, L. & Orrell-Valente, J. K. (2002). Art therapy, psychodrama, and verbal therapy: An integrative model of group therapy in the treatment of adolescents with anorexia nervosa and bulimia nervosa. *Child & Adolescent Psychiatric Clinics of North America*, 11(2), 343–364.

Dimitropoulos, G., Carter, J., Schachter, R., & Woodside, D. B. (2008). Predictors of family functioning in carers of individuals with anorexia nervosa. *International Journal of Eating Disorders*, 41, 739–747.

Dittmar, H., Halliwell, E., & Ive, S. (2006). Does Barbie make girls want to be thin? The effect of experimental exposure to images of dolls on the body image of 5- to 8-year-old girls. *Developmental Psychology*, 42, 283–292.

Dohnt, H. K. & Tiggemann, M. (2008). Promoting positive body image in young girls: An evaluation of 'Shapesville.' *European Eating Disorders Review*, 16(3), 222–233.

Dolan, B. & Ford, K. (1991). Binge eating and dietary restraint: A cross-cultural analysis. *International Journal of Eating Disorders*, 10, 345–353.

Dunn, P. K. & Ondercin, P. (1981). Personality variables related to compulsive eating in college women. *Journal of Clinical Psychology*, 31, 43–49.

Eckert, E. D., Halmi, K. A., Marchi, P., Grove, W., & Crosby, R. (1995). Ten-year follow-up of anorexia nervosa: Clinical course and outcome. *Psychological Medicine*, 25, 143–156.

Eddy, K. T., Dorer, D. J., Franko, D. L., Tahilani, K., Thompson-Brenner, H., & Herzog, D. B. (2008). Diagnostic crossover in anorexia nervosa and bulimia nervosa: Implications for *DSM-5*. *American Journal of Psychiatry*, 165, 245–250.

Eisenberg, M., Berge, J., Fulkerson, J., & Neumark-Sztainer, D. (2012). Associations between hurtful weight-related comments by family and significant other and the development of disordered eating behaviors in young adults. *Journal of Behavioral Medicine*, 35(5), 500–508.

Eisler, I., Dare, C., Hodes, M., Russell, G., Dodge, E., & LeGrange, D. (2000). Family therapy for adolescent anorexia nervosa: The results of a controlled comparison of two family interventions. *Journal of Child Psychology and Psychiatry*, 41, 727–736.

Engelberg, M., Steiger, H., Gauvin, L., & Wonderlich, S. (2007). Binge antecedents in bulimic syndromes: an examination of dissociation and negative affect. *International Journal of Eating Disorders*, 40(6), 531–536.

Fairburn, C. G. & Beglin, S. J. (1994). Assessment of eating disorder psychopathology: Interview or self-report questionnaire? *International Journal of Eating Disorders*, 16, 363–370.

Fairburn, C. G. & Cooper, Z. (1993). The Eating Disorder Examination. In C. G. Fairburn & G. T. Wilson (Eds.), *Binge eating: Nature, assessment and treatment* (12th ed., pp. 317–360). New York: Guilford Press.

Feldman, M. B. & Meyer, I. H. (2007). Childhood abuse and eating disorders in gay and bisexual men. *International Journal of Eating Disorders*, 40, 418–423.

Fichter, M. M., Quadflieg, N., & Hedlund, S. (2008). Long-term course of binge eating disorder and bulimia nervosa: Relevance for nosology and diagnostic criteria. *International Journal of Eating Disorders*, 41, 577–586.

Field, A. E., Javaras, K. M., Aneja, P., Kitos, N., Camargo, C. A. Jr, Taylor, C. B., & Laird, N. M. (2008). Family, peer, and media predictors of becoming eating disordered. *Archives of Pediatrics and Adolescent Medicine*, 162(6), 574–579.

Findlay, S., Pinzon, J., Taddeo, D., Katzman, D. K., & Canadian Paediatric Society, Adolescent Health Committee. (2013). Family-based treatment of children and adolescents with anorexia nervosa: Guidelines for the community physician. *Paediatrics and Child Health*, 15(1), 31–35.

Foster, G. D., Sherman, S., Borradaile, K. E., Grundy, K. M., Vander Veur, S. S., Nachmani, J., ... Shults, J. (2008). A policy-based school intervention to prevent overweight and obesity. *Pediatrics*, 121, 794–802.

Franko, D. L., Keshaviah, A., Eddy, K. T., Krishna, M., Davis, M. C., Keel, P. K., & Herzog, D. B. (2013). A longitudinal investigation of mortality in anorexia nervosa and bulimia nervosa. *American Journal of Psychiatry*, 170, 917–925.

Friederich, H-C., Walther, S., Bendszus, M., Biller, A., Thomann, P., Zeigermann, S., ... Herzog, W. (2012). Grey matter abnormalities within cortico-limbic-striatal circuits in acute and weight-restored anorexia nervosa patients. *Neuroimage*, 59(16), 1106–1113.

Fujimoto, S., Inui, A., Kiyota, N., Seki, W., Koide, K., Takamiya, S., ... Kasuga, M. (1997). Increased cholecystokinin and pancreatic polypeptide responses to a fat-rich meal in patients with restrictive but not bulimic anorexia nervosa. *Biological Psychiatry*, 41(10), 1068–1070.

Gadalla, T. M. (2008). Eating disorders and associated psychiatric comorbidity in elderly Canadian women. *Archives of Women's Mental Health*, 11, 357–362.

Garner, D. (1997). Psychoeducational principles in treatment. In D. M. Garner & P. E. Garfinkel (Eds.), *Handbook of treatment for eating disorders* (2nd ed., pp. 145–177). New York: Guilford Press.

Garner, D. M. (2011). *Eating Disorder Inventory-3: Professional manual*. Odessa, FL: Psychological Assessment Resources.

Garner, D. M. & Garfinkel, P. E. (1979). The Eating Attitude Test: An index of the symptoms of anorexia nervosa. *Psychosomatic Medicine*, 10, 647–656.

Garner, D. M., Olmsted, M. P., Bohr, Y., & Garfinkel, P. E. (1982). The Eating Attitude Test: Psychometric features and clinical correlates. *Psychological Medicine*, 12, 871–878.

Garrett, C. (1998). *Beyond anorexia: Narrative, spirituality, and recovery*. New York: Cambridge University Press.

Garrett, C. J. (1996). Recovery from anorexia nervosa: A Durkheimian interpretation. *Social Science and Medicine*, 10, 1489–1506.

Gauvin, L., Steiger, H., & Brodeur, J-M. (2009). Eating-disorder symptoms and syndromes in a sample of urban-dwelling Canadian women: Contributions toward a population health perspective. *International Journal of Eating Disorders*, 42, 158–165.

Gísladóttir, M. M. & Svavarsdóttir, E. K. (2011). Educational and support intervention to help families assist in the recovery of relatives with eating disorders. *Journal of Psychiatric and Mental Health Nursing*, 18(2), 122–130.

Godart, N., Berthoz, S., Rein, Z., Perdereau, F., Lang, F., Venisse, J., & Curt, F. (2006). Does the frequency of anxiety and depressive disorders differ between diagnostic subtypes of anorexia nervosa and bulimia? *International Journal of Eating Disorders*, 39(8), 772–778.

Godart, N., Flament, M., Perderau, F., & Jeammet, P. (2002). Comorbidity between eating disorders and anxiety disorders: a review. *International Journal of Eating Disorders*, 32(3), 253–270.

Golden, B. R., Buzcek, T., & Robbins, S. B. (1986). Parameters of bulimia: Examining the Compulsive Eating Scale. *Measurement and Evaluation in Counseling and Development*, 19(2), 84–92.

Goldfield, G. S., Blouin, A. G., & Woodside, D. B. (2006). Body image, binge eating, and bulimia nervosa in male bodybuilders. *Canadian Journal of Psychiatry*, 51, 160–168.

Gowers, S. G. & Shore, A. (1999). The stigma of eating disorders. *International Journal of Clinical Practice*, 53(5), 386–388.

Greenleaf, C., Petrie, T. A., Carter, J., & Reel, J. J. (2009). Female collegiate athletes: Prevalence of eating disorders and disordered eating behaviors. *Journal of American College Health*, 57, 489–495.

Grilo, C. M., & Masheb, R. M. (2007). Rapid response predicts binge eating and weight loss in binge eating disorder: Findings from a controlled trial of orlistat with guided self-help cognitive behavioral therapy. *Behaviour Research and Therapy*, 45(11), 2537–2550.

Grilo, C. M., White, M. A., Barnes, R. D., & Masheb, R. M. (2013). Psychiatric disorder comorbidity and correlates in an ethnically diverse sample of obese patients with binge eating disorder in primary care settings. *Comprehensive Psychiatry*, 54(3), 209–216.

Grilo, C. M., White, M. A., Gueorguieva, R., Wilson, G. T., & Masheb, R. M. (2013). Predictive significance of the overvaluation of shape/weight in obese patients with binge eating disorder: Findings from a randomized controlled trial with 12-month follow-up. *Psychological Medicine*, 43(6), 1335–1344.

Grilo, C. M., Wilson, G., Crosby, R. D., & Masheb, R. M. (2012). 12-month follow-up of fluoxetine and cognitive behavioral therapy for binge eating disorder. *Journal of Consulting and Clinical Psychology*, 80(6), 1108–1113.

Groleau, P., Steiger, H., Joober, R., Bruce, K. R., Israel, M., Badawi, G., ... Sycz, L. (2012). Dopamine-system genes, childhood abuse, and clinical manifestations in women with Bulimia-spectrum Disorders. *Journal of Psychiatric Research*, 46(9), 1139–1145.

Gucciardi, E., Wang, S. C., Badiani, T., & Stewart, D. E. (2007). Beyond adolescence: Exploring Canadian women and men's perception of overweight. *Women's Health Issues*, 17, 374–382.

Gustafsson, S., Edlund, B., Davén, J., Kjellin, L., & Norring, C. (2010). Perceived expectations in daily life among adolescent girls suffering from an eating disorder: A phenomenographic study. *Eating Disorders, 18*(1), 25–42.

Gutwill, S. (1994). Women's eating problems: Social context and the internalization of culture. In C. Bloom, L. Zaphiropdous, A. Gitter, S. Gutwill, & L. Kogel (Eds.), *Eating problems: A feminist psychoanalytic treatment model* (pp. 1–27). New York: Basic Books.

Haedt-Matt, A. A. & Keel, P. K. (2011). Hunger and binge eating: A meta-analysis of studies using ecological momentary assessment. *International Journal of Eating Disorders, 44*(7), 573–578.

Hannon-Engel, S. (2012). Regulating satiety in bulimia nervosa: The role of cholecystokinin. *Perspectives in Psychiatric Care, 48*(1), 34–40.

Harrington, E. F., Crowther, J. H., Payne Henrickson, H. C., & Mickelson, K. D. (2006). The relationships among trauma, stress, relationships, and binge eating. *Cultural Diversity and Ethnic Minority Psychology, 12,* 212–229.

Hatmaker, G. (2005). Boys with eating disorders. *Journal of School Nursing, 21,* 329–332.

Hay, P. (2013). A systematic review of evidence for psychological treatments in eating disorders: 2005–2012. *International Journal of Eating Disorders, 46*(5), 462–469.

Heatherton, T. F. & Baumeister, R. F. (1991). Binge eating as an escape from self-awareness. *Psychological Bulletin, 110,* 86–108.

Hendricks, P. S. & Thompson, J. K. (2005). An integration of cognitive-behavioral therapy and interpersonal psychotherapy for bulimia nervosa: A case study using the case formulation method. *International Journal of Eating Disorders, 37,* 171–174.

Herman, C. P. & Mack, D. (1975). Restrained and unrestrained eating. *Journal of Personality, 43,* 647–660.

Herman, C. P. & Polivy, J. (1975). Anxiety, restraint, and eating behavior. *Journal of Abnormal Psychology, 84,* 66–72.

Herman, C. P. & Polivy, J. (1980). Restrained eating. In A. J. Stunkard (Ed.), *Obesity* (pp. 208–225). Philadelphia: Saunders.

Herpertz-Dahlmann, B., Seitz, J., & Konrad, K. (2011). Aetiology of anorexia nervosa: From a "psychosomatic family model" to a neuropsychiatric disorder? *European Archives of Psychiatry and Clinical Neuroscience, 261*(Suppl 2), S177–S181.

Hertz, P., Addad, M., & Ronel, N. (2012). Attachment styles and changes among women members of Overeaters Anonymous who have recovered from binge-eating disorder. *Health and Social Work, 37*(2), 110–122.

Hilbert, A. & Brähler, E. (2012). Interpersonal psychotherapy for eating disorders: A systematic and practical review. *Verhaltenstherapie, 22,* 149–157.

Homan, K. & Boyatzis, C. (2010). The protective role of attachment to God against eating disorder risk factors: Concurrent and prospective evidence. *Eating Disorders, 18*(3), 239–258.

Hudson, J. I., Lalonde, J. K., Berry, J. M., Pindyck, L. J., Bulik, C. M., Crow, S. J., … Pope, H. G. Jr. (2006). Binge-eating disorder as a distinct familial phenotype in obese individuals. *Archives of General Psychiatry, 63*(3), 313–319.

Inches, P. R. (1895). Anorexia nervosa. *Maritime Medical News, 7,* 73–75.

Jensen, V. S. & Mejlhede, A. (2000). Anorexia nervosa treatment with olanzapine. *British Journal of Psychiatry, 177*(2), 87.

Johnson, F., Pratt, M., & Wardle, J. (2012). Dietary restraint and self-regulation in eating behavior. *International Journal of Obesity, 36*(5), 665–674.

Johnson, F. & Wardle, J. (2005). Dietary restraint, body dissatisfaction, and psychological distress: A prospective study. *Journal of Abnormal Psychology, 114,* 119–125.

Johnson, J. G., Cohen, P., Kasen, S., & Brook, J. S. (2002). Childhood adversities associated with risk for eating disorders or weight problems during adolescence or early adulthood. *American Journal of Psychiatry, 159,* 394–400.

Joiner, T. E., Katz, J., & Heatherton, T. F. (2000). Personality factors differentiate late adolescent females and males with chronic bulimic symptoms. *International Journal of Eating Disorders, 27,* 191–197.

Jonat, L. M. & Birmingham, C. L. (2004). Disordered eating attitudes and behaviours in the high-school students of a rural Canadian community. *Eating and Weight Disorders, 9*(4), 306–308.

Joos, A., Hartmann, A., Glauche, V., Perlov, E., Unterbrink, T., Saum, B., … Zeeck, A. (2011). Grey matter deficit in long-term recovered anorexia nervosa patients. *European Eating Disorders Review, 19*(1), 59–63.

Jordan, J., Joyce, P. R., Carter, F. A., Horn, J., McIntosh, V. V., Luty, S. E., … Bulik, C. M. (2008). Specific and nonspecific comorbidity in anorexia nervosa. *International Journal of Eating Disorders, 41,* 47–56.

Kaplan, A. S. & Noble, S. (2007). Pharmacological approaches to the outpatient treatment of anorexia nervosa. In J. Yager & P. S. Powers (Eds.), *Clinical manual of eating disorders* (pp. 138–142). Washington, DC: American Psychiatric Association.

Kaye, W. H., Klump, K. L., Frank, G. K., & Strober, M. (2000). Anorexia and bulimia. *Annual Review of Medicine, 51,* 299–313.

Kelly, A. C. & Carter, J. C. (2012). Why self-critical patients present with more severe eating disorder pathology: The mediating role of shame. *British Journal of Clinical Psychology, 52*(2), 148–161.

Keery, H., Boutelle, K., van den Berg, P., & Thompson, K. (2005). The impact of appearance-related teasing by family members. *Journal of Adolescent Health, 37,* 120–127.

Kenyon, M., Samarawickrema, N., DeJong, H., Van den Eynde, F., Startup, H., Lavender, A., … Schmidt, U. (2012). Theory of mind in bulimia nervosa. *International Journal of Eating Disorders, 45*(3), 377–384.

Keski-Rahkonen, A., Raevuori, A., Bulik, C. M., Hoek, H. W., Sihvola, E., Kaprio, J., … Rissanen, A. (2013). Depression and drive for thinness are associated with persistent bulimia nervosa in the community. *European Eating Disorders Review, 21*(2), 121–129.

Kessler, R. C., Berglund, P. A., Chiu, W. T., Deitz, A. C., Hudson, J. I., Shahly, V., … Xavier, M. (2013). The prevalence and correlates of binge eating disorder in the World Health Organization World Mental Health Surveys. *Biological Psychiatry, 73*(9), 904–914.

Kirk, S., Bornstein, P., Navarro, E., & Swanson, E. (2009). *Effective non-clinical interventions to prevent and treat childhood overweight and obesity in Newfoundland and Labrador.* St. John's, NL: Newfoundland and Labrador Centre for Applied Health Research, Memorial University.

Kirkey, S. (2013). *Anorexia hitting men increasingly hard: One in three cases in new study is male.* National Post. Retrieved from http://life.nationalpost.com/2013/01/21/anorexia-hitting-men-increasingly-hard-one-in-three-cases-in-new-study-is-male/

Kluck, A. S. (2010). Family influence on disordered eating: The role of body image dissatisfaction. *Body Image, 7*(1), 8–14.

Klump, K. L. Bulik, C. M., Kaye, W. H., Treasure, J., & Tyson, E. (2009). Academy for eating disorders position paper: Eating disorders are serious mental illnesses. *International Journal of Eating Disorders, 42,* 97–103.

Kocovski, N. L. & Endler, N. S. (2000). Social anxiety, self-regulation, and fear of negative evaluation. *European Journal of Personality, 14,* 347–358.

Kubersky, R. (1998). *Everything you need to know about eating disorders anorexia and bulimia.* New York: Rosen.

Lam, T. H., Lee, S. W., Fung, S., Ho, S. Y., Lee, P. W. H., & Stewart, S. M. (2009). Sociocultural influences on body dissatisfaction and dieting in Hong Kong girls. *European Eating Disorders Review, 17,* 152–160.

La Mela, C., Maglietta, M., Castellini, G., Amoroso, L., & Lucarelli, S. (2010). Dissociation in eating disorders: Relationship between dissociative experiences and binge-eating episodes. *Comprehensive Psychiatry, 51*(4), 393–400.

Langlois, K. A., Samokhvalov, A. V., Rehm, J., Spence, S. T., & Connor Gorber, S. K. (2011). *Health state descriptions for Canadians: Mental illnesses.* Statistics Canada, catalogue no. 82-619-MIE2005002. Ottawa, Canada: Statistics Canada.

Laporte, L. & Guttman, H. (2001). Abusive relationships in families of women with borderline personality disorder, anorexia nervosa and a control group. *Journal of Nervous and Mental Disease, 180,* 522–531.

Larrañaga, A., Docet, M. F., & García-Mayor, R. V. (2011). Disordered eating behaviors in type 1 diabetic patients. *World Journal of Diabetes, 2*(11), 189–195.

LaVia, M. C., Grey, M., & Kaye, W. H. (2000). Case reports of olanzapine treatment of anorexia nervosa. *International Journal of Eating Disorders, 27,* 363–366.

Lawson, E. A., Eddy, K. T., Donoho, D., Misra, M., Miller, K. K., Meenaghan, E., … Klibanski, A. (2011). Appetite-regulating hormones cortisol and peptide YY are associated with disordered eating psychopathology, independent of body mass index. *European Journal of Endocrinology, 164*(2), 253–261.

le Grange, D., Lock, J., Loeb, K., & Nicholls, D. (2010). Academy for eating disorders position paper: The role of the family in eating disorders. *International Journal of Eating Disorders, 43*(1), 1–5.

Leonard, S., Steiger, H., & Kao, A. (2003). Childhood and adulthood abuse in bulimic and nonbulimic women: Prevalences and psychological correlates. *International Journal of Eating Disorders, 33,* 397–405.

Lilenfeld, L. R., Ringham, R., Kalarchian, M. A., & Marcus, M. (2008). A family history study of binge-eating disorder. *Comprehensive Psychiatry, 49,* 247–254.

Lim, L. A., McGovern, L., Elamin, M. B., Swiglo, B. A., Erwin, P. J., & Montori, V. M. (2010). Effect on bone health of estrogen preparations in premenopausal women with anorexia nervosa: A systematic review and meta-analyses. *International Journal of Eating Disorders, 43,* 218–225.

Linville, D., Stice, E., Gau, J., & O'Neil, M. (2011). Predictive effects of mother and peer influences on increases in adolescent eating disorder risk factors and symptoms: A 3-year longitudinal study. *International Journal of Eating Disorders, 44*(8), 745–751.

Lyons, M. A. (1998). The phenomenon of compulsive overeating in a selected group of professional women. *Journal of Advanced Nursing, 27*(6), 1158–1164.

Maine, M. & Bunnell, D. (2008). Questions and answers. How do the principles of the feminist, relational model apply to treatment of men with eating disorders and related issues? *Eating Disorders, 16*(2), 187–192.

Maloney, M., McGuire, J., & Daniels, S. R. (1988). Reliability testing of a children's version of the Eating Attitude Test. *Journal of the American Academy of Child and Adolescent Psychiatry, 27*, 541–543.

Malson, H. & Ryan, V. (2008). Tracing a matrix of gender: An analysis of the feminine in hospital-based treatment for eating disorders. *Feminism and Psychology, 18*(1), 112–132.

Marsden, P., Karagianni, E., & Morgan, J. F. (2007). Spirituality and clinical care in eating disorders: A qualitative study. *International Journal of Eating Disorders, 40*, 7–12.

Martin, J. & Govender, K. (2011). "Making muscle junkies": Investigating traditional masculine ideology, body image discrepancy, and the pursuit of muscularity in adolescent males. *International Journal of Men's Health, 10*(3), 220–239.

Martinsen, M. & Sundgot-Borgen, J. (2013). Higher prevalence of rating disorders among adolescent elite athletes than controls. *Medicine and Science in Sports and Exercise, 45*(6), 1188–1197.

Martz, D. M., Sturgis, E. T., & Gustafson, S. B. (1996). Development and preliminary validation of the Cognitive Behavioral Dieting Scale. *International Journal of Eating Disorders, 19*, 297–309.

Masheb, R. M., Grilo, C. M., & White, M. A. (2011). An examination of eating patterns in community women with bulimia nervosa and binge eating disorder. *International Journal of Eating Disorders, 44*(7), 618–624.

Massey-Stokes, M. (2001). Communication, expressing feelings, and creative problem solving. In J. J. Robert-McComb (Ed.), *Eating disorders in women and children: Prevention, stress management, and treatment* (pp. 291–307). Boca Raton, FL: CRC Press.

Matusek, J. A. & Knudson, R. M. (2009). Rethinking recovery from eating disorders: Spiritual and political dimensions. *Qualitative Health Research, 19*, 697–707.

Mazure, C. M., Halmi, K. A., Sunday, S. R., Romano, S. J., & Einhorn, A. M. (1994). Yale-Brown-Cornell Eating Disorder Scale: Development, use, reliability, and validity. *Journal of Psychiatric Research, 28*, 425–445.

McDonald, J. T. & Kennedy, S. (2005). Is immigration to Canada associated with unhealthy weight gain? Overweight and obesity among Canada's immigrants. *Social Science and Medicine, 61*, 2469–2481.

McIntosh, V. V., Jordan, J., Luty, S. E., Carter, F. A., McKenzie, J. M., Bulik, C. M., & Joyce, P. J. (2006). Specialist supportive clinical management for anorexia nervosa. *International Journal of Eating Disorders, 39*(8), 625–632.

McIver, S., McGartland, M., & O'Halloran, P. (2009). "Overeating is not about the food": women describe their experience of a yoga treatment program for binge eating. *Qualitative Health Research, 19*(9), 234–245.

McKnight R. F. & Park, R. J. (2010). Atypical antipsychotics and anorexia nervosa: A review. *European Eating Disorders Review, 18*, 10–21.

McVey, G., Gusella, J., Tweed, S., & Ferrari, M. (2009). A controlled evaluation of web-based training for teachers and public health practitioners on the prevention of eating disorders. *Eating Disorders, 17*(1), 1–26.

McVey, G., Tweed, S., & Blackmore, E. (2004). Dieting among preadolescent and young adolescent females. *Canadian Medical Association Journal, 170*, 1559–1561.

McVey, G. L., Pepler, D., Davis, R., Flett, G. L., & Abdolel, M. (2002). Risk and protective factors associated with disordered eating during early adolescence. *Journal of Early Adolescence, 22*(1), 75–95.

Mehler, P. S., Cleary, B. S., & Gaudiani, J. L. (2011). Osteoporosis in anorexia nervosa. *Eating Disorders, 19*(2), 194–202.

Meyer, C., Taranis, L., Goodwin, H., & Haycraft, E. (2011). Compulsive exercise and eating disorders. *European Eating Disorders Review, 19*(3), 174–189.

Miller, K. K. (2011). Endocrine dysregulation in anorexia nervosa update. *Journal of Clinical Endocrinology and Metabolism, 96*(10), 2939–2949.

Miller, K. K., Grieco, K. A., Mulder, J., Grinspoon, S., Mickley, D., Yhezkel, R., ... Klibanksi, A. (2004). Effects of risedronate on bone density in anorexia nervosa. *Journal of Clinical Endocrinology and Metabolism, 89*, 3903–3906.

Miller, M. N. & Pumariega, A. J. (2001). Culture and eating disorders: A historical and cross-cultural review. *Psychiatry, 64*(2), 93–110.

Milos, G., Spindler, A., Ruggiero, G., Klaghofer, R., & Schnyder, V. (2002). Comorbidity of obsessive-compulsive disorders and duration of eating disorders. *International Journal of Eating Disorders, 36*(3), 284–289.

Minuchin, S., Rossman, B. L., & Baker, L. (1978). *Psychosomatic families.* Cambridge, MA: Harvard University Press.

Miotto, P., Pollini, B., Restaneo, A., Favaretto, G., & Preti, A. (2008). Aggressiveness, anger, and hostility in eating disorders. *Comprehensive Psychiatry, 49*, 364–373.

Mitchell, J. E., Roerig, J., & Steffen, K. (2013). Biological therapies for eating disorders. *International Journal of Eating Disorders, 46*(5), 470–477.

Mitchell, K. S., Neale, M. C., Bulik, C. M., Aggen, S. H., Kendler, K. S., & Mazzeo, S. E. (2010). Binge eating disorder: A symptom-level investigation of genetic and environmental influences on liability. *Psychological Medicine, 40*, 1899–1906.

Mold, F. & Forbes, A. (2011). Patients' and professionals' experiences and perspectives of obesity in health-care settings: A synthesis of current research. *Health Expectations, 16*(2), 119–142.

Mond, J. M., Hay, P. J., Rodgers, B., & Owen, C. (2006). Eating Disorder Examination Questionnaire (EDE-Q): Norms for young adult women. *Behaviour Research and Therapy, 44*, 53–62.

Monteleone, P. & Maj, M. (2008). Genetic susceptibility to eating disorders: Associated polymorphisms and pharmacogenetic suggestions. *Pharmacogenomics, 9*, 1487–1520.

Morgan, J. C., Wolfe, B. E., Metzger, E. D., & Jimerson, D. C. (2007). Obsessive-compulsive characteristics in women who have recovered from bulimia nervosa. *International Journal of Eating Disorders, 40*, 381–385.

Munsch, S., Meyer, A. H., & Biedert, E. (2012). Efficacy and predictors of long-term treatment success for Cognitive-Behavioral Treatment and Behavioral Weight-Loss-Treatment in overweight individuals with binge eating disorder. *Behaviour Research and Therapy, 50*(12), 775–785.

Munsch, S., Meyer, A. H., Quartier, V., & Wilhelm, F. H. (2012). Binge eating in binge eating disorder: A breakdown of emotion regulatory process? *Psychiatry Research, 195*(3), 118–124.

Murphy R., Cooper Z., Hollon, S. D., & Fairburn, C. G. (2009). How do psychological treatments work? Investigating mediators to change. *Behavior Research and Therapy, 47*, 1–5.

Murphy, R., Straebler, S., Cooper, Z., & Fairburn, C. G. (2010). Cognitive behavioral therapy for eating disorders. *Psychiatric Clinics of North America, 33*(3), 611–627.

National Eating Disorder Association (NEDA). (2013). *Eating disorders affect families for the bad and the good.* Retrieved from www.nationaleatingdisorders.org/eating-disorders-affect-families-bad-and-good

National Eating Disorder Information Centre (NEDIC). (1998/2003). *Families and eating disorders.* Retrieved from http://www.nedic.ca/knowthefacts/documents/Familiesandeatingdisorders.pdf

Neff, K. J., Olbers, T. T., & Le Roux, C. W. (2013). Bariatric surgery: The challenges with candidate selection, individualizing treatment and clinical outcomes. *BMC Medicine, 11*(1), 1–17.

Neumark-Sztainer, D. R., Wall, M. M., Haines, J. I., Story, M. T., Sherwood, N. E., & van den Berg, P. A. (2007). Shared risk and protective factors for overweight and disordered eating in adolescents. *American Journal of Preventive Medicine, 33*(5), 359–369.

Nilsson, K., Sundbom, E., & Hagglof, B. (2008). A longitudinal study of perfectionism in adolescent onset anorexia nervosa-restricting type. *European Eating Disorders Review, 16*, 386–394.

Núñez-Navarro, A., Agüera, Z., Krug, I., Jiménez-Murcia, S., Sánchez, I., Araguz, N., ... Fernández-Aranda, F. (2012). Do men with eating disorders differ from women in clinics, psychopathology and personality? *European Eating Disorders Review, 20*, 23–31.

Obeid, N., Buchholz, A., Boerner, K. E., Henderson, K. A., & Norris, M. (2013). Self-esteem and social anxiety in an adolescent female eating disorder population: Age and diagnostic effects. *Eating Disorders, 21*(2), 140–153.

Ondercin, P. A. (1979). Compulsive eating in college women. *Journal of College Student Personnel, 20*, 153–157.

Orbach, S. (2004). What can we learn from the therapist's body? *Attachment & Human Development, 6*(2), 141–150.

Park, J. & Beaudet, M. P. (2007). Eating attitudes and their correlates among Canadian women concerned about their weight. *European Eating Disorders Review, 15*, 311–320.

Perkins, P. S., Slane, J. D., & Klump, K. L. (2013). Personality clusters and family relationships in women with disordered eating symptoms. *Eating Behaviors, 14*(3), 299–308.

Perkins, S., Winn, S., Murray, J., Murphy, R., & Schmidt, U. (2004). A qualitative study of the experiences of caring for a person with bulimia nervosa. Part 1: The emotional impact of caring. *International Journal of Eating Disorders, 36*(3), 256–268.

Perry, L., Morgan, J., Reid, F., Brunton, J., O'Brien, A., Luck, A., & Lacey, H. (2002). Screening for symptoms of eating disorders: Reliability of the SCOFF screening tool with written compared to oral delivery. *International Journal of Eating Disorders, 32*(4), 466–472.

Petersen, A. C. & Taylor, B. (1980). The biological approach to adolescence. In J. Adelson (Ed.), *Handbook of adolescent psychology* (pp. 115–155). New York: Wiley.

Peterson, C. B., Thuras, P., Ackard, D. M., Mitchell, J. E., Berg, K., Sandager, N., ... Crow, S. J. (2010). Personality dimensions in bulimia nervosa, binge eating disorder, and obesity. *Comprehensive Psychiatry, 51*(1), 31–36.

Petrie, T., Greenleaf, C., & Martin, S. (2010). Biopsychosocial and physical correlates of middle school boys' and girls' body satisfaction. *Sex Roles, 63*(9/10), 631–644.

Pichika, R., Buchsbaum, M. S., Bailer, U., Hoh, C., DeCastro, A., Buchsbaum, B. R., & Kaye, W. (2012). Serotonin transporter binding after recovery from bulimia nervosa. *International Journal of Eating Disorders, 45*(3), 345–352.

Pike, K. M., Hilbert, A., Wilfley, D. E., Fairburn, C. G., Dohm, F.-A., Walsh, B. T., & Striegel-Moore, R. (2008). Toward an understanding of risk factors for anorexia nervosa: A case–control study. *Psychological Medicine, 38*, 1443–1453.

Pilch, J. L. (1988). Wellness spirituality. *Health Values, 12*(3), 28–31.

Pinhas, L., Heinmaa, M., Bryden, P., Bradley, S., & Toner, B. (2008). Disordered eating in Jewish adolescent girls. *Canadian Journal of Psychiatry, 53*, 601–608.

Pinhas, L., Morris, A., Crosby, R. D., & Katzman, D. K. (2011). Incidence and age-specific presentation of restrictive eating disorders in children: A Canadian Paediatric Surveillance Program study. *Archives of Pediatrics and Adolescent Medicine, 165*(10), 895–899.

Polivy, J. & Herman, C. P. (1993). Etiology of binge eating: Psychological mechanisms. In C. G. Fairburn & G. T. Wilson (Eds.), *Binge eating: Nature, assessment and treatment* (pp. 173–205). New York: Guilford.

Quick, V. M., McWilliams, R., & Byrd-Bredbenner, C. (2013). Fatty, fatty, two-by-four: Weight-teasing history and disturbed eating in young adult women. *American Journal of Public Health, 103*(3), 508–515.

Quigley, E. M. (2011). Cisapride: What can we learn from the rise and fall of a prokinetic? *Journal of Digestive Diseases, 12*(3), 147–156.

Racine, S. E., Burt, S. A., Iacono, W. G., McGue, M., & Klump, K. L. (2011). Dietary restraint moderates genetic risk for binge eating. *Journal of Abnormal Psychology, 120*(1), 119–128.

Ramacciotti, C. D., Coli, E., Bondi, E., Burgalassi, A., Massimetti, G., & Dell'Osso, L. (2008). Shared psychopathology in obese subjects with and without binge-eating disorder. *International Journal of Eating Disorders, 41*, 643–649.

Ramoz, N., Versini, A., & Gorwood, P. (2007). Eating disorders: An overview of treatment responses and the potential impact of vulnerability genes and endophenotypes. *Expert Opinion on Pharmacotherapy, 8*(13), 2029–2044.

Reas, D. L., Rø, O., Karterud, S., Hummelen, B., & Pedersen, G. (2013). Eating disorders in a large clinical sample of men and women with personality disorders. *International Journal of Eating Disorders, 46*, 801–809.

Reda, M. & Sacco, G. (2001). Anorexia and the holiness of Saint Catherine of Siena. *Journal of Criminal Justice and Popular Culture* (G. Newman, Trans.), *8*(1), 37–47.

Reijonen, J. H., Prat, H. D., Patel, D. R., & Greydanus, D. E. (2003). Eating disorders in the adolescent population: An overview. *Journal of Adolescent Research, 18*, 209–222.

Robin, A. L., Siegel, P. T., Moye, A. W., Gilroy, M., Dennis, A. B., & Sikand, A. (1999). A controlled comparison of family versus individual therapy for adolescents with anorexia nervosa. *Journal of the American Academy of Child and Adolescent Psychiatry, 38*(12), 1482–1489.

Robinson, K. J., Mountford, V. A., & Sperlinger, D. J. (2013). Being men with eating disorders: Perspectives of male eating disorder service users. *Journal of Health Psychology, 18*, 176–186.

Robinson, K. J. & Sperlinger, D. J. (2013). Being men with eating disorders: Perspectives of male eating disorder service-users. *Journal of Health Psychology, 18*, 176–186.

Roehrig, J. P. & McLean, C. P. (2010). A comparison of stigma toward eating disorders versus depression. *International Journal of Eating Disorders, 43*(7), 671–674.

Romano, S. J., Halmi, K. A., Sarkar, N. P., Koke, S. C., Lee, J. S. (2002). A placebo-controlled study of fluoxetine in continued treatment of bulimia nervosa after successful acute fluoxetine treatment. *American Journal of Psychiatry, 159*(1), 96–102.

Rørtveit, K., Åström, S., & Severinsson, E. (2009). The feeling of being trapped in and ashamed of one's own body. *International Journal of Mental Health Nursing, 18*, 91–99.

Rosenberger, P. H. & Dorflinger, L. (2013). Psychosocial factors associated with binge eating among overweight and obese male veterans. *Eating Behaviors, 14*(3), 401–404.

Rossi, G., Balottin, U., Rossi, M., Chiappedi, M., Fazzi, E., & Lanzi, G. (2007). Pharmacological treatment of anorexia nervosa: A retrospective study in preadolescents and adolescents. *Clinical Pediatrics, 46*(9), 806–811.

Rowa, K., Kerig, P. K., & Geller, J. (2001). The family and anorexia nervosa: Examining parent–child boundary problems. *European Eating Disorders Review, 9*(2), 97–114.

Roybal, D. (2005). Is "yo-yo" dieting or weight cycling harmful to one's health? *Nutrition Noteworthy, 7*(1). Retrieved from http://escholarship.org/uc/item/1zz4r4qk

Sachs-Ericsson, N., Keel, P. K., Holland, L., Selby, E. A., Verona, E., Cougle, J. R., & Palmer, E. (2012). Parental disorders, childhood abuse, and binge eating in a large community sample. *International Journal of Eating Disorders, 45*(3), 316–325.

Sallet, P. C., de Alvarenga, P., Ferrão, Y., de Mathis, M., Torres, A. R., Marques, A., … Fleitlich-Bilyk, B. (2010). Eating disorders in patients with obsessive–compulsive disorder: Prevalence and clinical correlates. *International Journal of Eating Disorders, 43*(4), 315–325.

Sancho, C., Arija, M. V., & Canals, J. (2008). Personality in non-clinical adolescents with eating disorders. *European Eating Disorders Review, 16*(2), 133–138.

Sanci, L., Coffey, C., Olsson, C., Reid, S., Carlin, J. B., & Patton, G. (2008). Childhood sexual abuse and eating disorders in females: Findings from the Victoria adolescent health cohort study. *Archives of Pediatrics and Adolescent Medicine, 162*, 261–267.

Schafer, M. H. & Ferraro, K. F. (2011). The stigma of obesity: Does perceived weight discrimination affect identity and physical health? *Social Psychology Quarterly, 74*(1), 76–97.

Schmidt, U., Lee, S., Beecham, J, Perkins, S., Treasure, J., Yi, I., … Eisler I. (2007). A randomized controlled trial of family therapy and cognitive behavior therapy guided self-care for adolescents with bulimia nervosa and related disorders. *American Journal of Psychiatry, 164*(4), 591–598.

Scott Richards, P., Berrett, M. E., & Hardman, R. K., & Eggett, D. L. (2006). Comparative efficacy of spirituality, cognitive, and emotional support groups for treating eating disorder inpatients. *Eating Disorders, 14*, 401–415.

Scott Richards, P., Hardman, R. K., & Berrett, M. E. (2007). *Spiritual approaches in the treatment of women with eating disorders*, Washington, DC: American Psychological Association.

Scott Richards, P., Smith, M. H., Berrett, M. E., O'Grady, K., & Bartz, J. D. (2007). A theist spiritual treatment for women with eating disorders. *Journal of Clinical Psychology, 65*, 172–184.

Selby, E. A., Doyle, P., Crosby, R. D., Wonderlich, S. A., Engel, S. G., Mitchell, J. D., & Le Grange, D. (2012). Momentary emotion surrounding bulimic behaviors in women with bulimia nervosa and borderline personality. *Journal of Psychiatric Research, 46*(11), 1492–1500.

Senra, C., Sanchez-Cao, E., Seoane, G., & Leung, Y. K. (2008). Evolution of self-concept deficits in patients with eating disorders: The role of family concern about weight and appearance. *European Eating Disorders Review, 15*, 131–138.

Sinton, M. M. & Birch, L. L. (2005). Weight status and psychosocial factors predict the emergence of dieting in preadolescent girls. *International Journal of Eating Disorders, 38*(4), 346–354.

Sharpe, H., Damazer, K., Treasure, J., & Schmidt, U. (2013). What are adolescents' experiences of body dissatisfaction and dieting, and what do they recommend for prevention? A qualitative study. *Eating and Weight Disorders, 18*(2), 133–141.

Shisslak, C. M., Renger, R., Sharpe, T., Crago, M., McKnight, K. M., Gray, N., … Taylor, C. B. (1999). Development and evaluation of the McKnight Risk Factor Survey for assessing potential risk and protective factors for disordered eating in preadolescent and adolescent girls. *International Journal of Eating Disorders, 25*(2), 195–214.

Smink, F. R. E., van Hoeken, D., & Hoek, H. W. (2012). Epidemiology of eating disorders: Incidence, prevalence and mortality rates. *Current Psychiatry Reports, 14*(4), 406–414.

Skoufalos, C. (2010). *The development of bulimia nervosa: A psychological phenomenological analysis* (Doctoral thesis). ETD Collection for Fordham University (paper AAI3438468). Available from http://fordham.bepress.com/dissertations/AAI3438468

Smolak, L. & Levine, M. P. (1994). Psychometric properties of the Children's Eating Attitudes Test. *International Journal of Eating Disorders, 16*(3), 275–282.

Smyth, J. M., Wonderlich, S. A., Heron, K. E., Sliwinski, M. J., Crosby, R. D., Mitchell, J. E., & Engel, S. G. (2007). Daily and momentary mood and stress are associated with binge eating and vomiting in bulimia nervosa patients in the the natural environment. *Journal of Consulting and Clinical Psychiatry, 75*(4), 629–638.

Soran, C. (2006). What about the boys? Addressing issues of masculinity within male anorexia nervosa in a feminist therapeutic environment. *International Journal of Men's Health, 5*, 251–267.

Spear, B. A. & Stellefson Myers, E. (2001). Nutrition intervention in the treatment of anorexia nervosa, bulimia nervosa, and eating disorder not otherwise specified (EDNOS). *Journal of the American Dietetic Association, 101*(7), 810–819.

Stahre, L., Tärnell, B., Håkanson, C., & Hällström, T. (2007). A randomized controlled trial of two weight-reducing short-term group treatment programs for obesity with an 18-month follow-up. *International Journal of Behavioral Medicine, 14*, 48–55.

Statistics Canada. (2012). *Mental illnesses Section D—Eating disorders.* Retrieved from http://www.statcan.gc.ca/pub/82-619-m/2012004/sections/sectiond-eng.htm

Steinhausen, H-C. (2002). The outcome of anorexia nervosa in the 20th century. *American Journal of Psychiatry, 159*, 1284–1293.

Steinhausen, H-C., Grigoriou-Serbanescu, M., Boyadjieva, S., Neumarker, K-J., & Metzke, C. W. (2008). Course and predictors of rehospitalization in adolescent anorexia nervosa in a multisite study. *International Journal of Eating Disorders, 41*, 29–36.

Stewart, M-C., Schiavo, R. S., Herzog, D. B., & Franko, D. L. (2008). Stereotypes, prejudice and discrimination of women with anorexia nervosa. *European Eating Disorders Review, 16*, 311–318.

Stice, E., Marti, C., & Rohde, P. (2013). Prevalence, incidence, impairment, and course of the proposed *DSM-5* eating disorder diagnoses in an 8-year prospective community study of young women. *Journal of Abnormal Psychology, 122*(2), 445–457.

Stock, S., Miranda, C., Evans, S., Plessis, S., Ridley, J., & Yeh, S. (2007). Healthy buddies: A novel, peer-led health promotion program for the prevention of obesity and eating disorders in children in elementary school. *Pediatrics, 120*, 1059–1068.

Striegel-Moore, R. H., Dohm, F-A., Kraemer, H. C., Schreiber, G. B., Taylor, C. B., & Daniels, S. R. (2007). Risk factors for binge-eating disorders: An exploratory study. *International Journal of Eating Disorders, 40*, 481–487.

Striegel-Moore, R. H., Silberstein, L. R., & Rodin, J. (1993). The social self in bulimia nervosa: Public self-consciousness, social anxiety, and perceived fraudulence. *Journal of Abnormal Psychology, 102*, 297–303.

Strober, M., Pataki, C., Freeman, R., & DeAntonio, M. (1999). No effect of adjunctive fluoxetine on eating behavior or weight phobia during the inpatient treatment of anorexia nervosa: An historical case controlled study. *Journal of Child and Adolescent Psychopharmacology, 9*(3), 195–201.

Stunkard, A. J. & Messick, S. (1985). The Three-Factor Eating Questionnaire to measure dietary restraint and hunger. *Journal of Psychosomatic Research, 29*, 71–83.

Sullivan, P. (1995). Mortality in anorexia nervosa. *American Journal of Psychiatry, 152*, 1073–1074.

Sunday, S. R., Halmi, K. A., & Einhorn, A. (1995). The Yale-Brown-Cornell eating disorder scale: A new scale to assess eating disorder symptomatology. *International Journal of Eating Disorders, 18*(3), 237–245.

Swan, S. & Andrews, B. (2003). The relationship between shame, eating disorders and disclosure in treatment. *British Journal of Clinical Psychology, 42*(4), 367–378.

Swinbourne, J., Hunt, C., Abbott, M., Russell, J., St. Clare, T., & Touyz, S. (2012). The comorbidity between eating disorders and anxiety disorders: Prevalence in an eating disorder sample and anxiety disorder sample. *Australian and New Zealand Journal of Psychiatry, 46*(2), 118–131.

Swinbourne, J. N., & Touyz, S. W. (2007). The comorbidity of eating disorders and anxiety disorders: A review. *European Eating Disorders Review, 15*, 253–274.

Taylor, C. B., Sharpe, T., Shisslak, C., Bryson, S., Estes, L. S., Gray, N., ... Killen, J. D. (1998). Factors associated with weight concerns in adolescent girls. *International Journal of Eating Disorders, 24*, 31–42.

Thaler, L., Groleau, P., Badawi, G., Sycz, L., Zeramdini, N., Too, A., ... Steiger, H. (2012). Epistatic interactions implicating dopaminergic genes in bulimia nervosa: Relationships to eating- and personality-related psychopathology. *Progress in Neuro-Psychopharmacology and Biological Psychiatry, 39*(1), 120–128.

Thompson-Brenner, H., Thompson, D. R., Boisseau, C. L., Richards, L. K., Bulik, C. M., Devlin, M. J., ... Wilson, G. (2013). Race/ethnicity, education, and treatment parameters as moderators and predictors of outcome in binge eating disorder. *Journal of Consulting and Clinical Psychology, 81*(4), 710–721.

Tillman, K. S., Arbaugh, T., & Balaban, M. S. (2012). Campus programming for National Eating Disorders Awareness Week: An investigation of stigma, help-seeking, and resource knowledge. *Eating Behaviors, 13*(3), 281–284.

Trace, S. E., Thornton, L. M., Runfola, C. D., Lichtenstein, P., Pedersen, N. L., & Bulik, C. M. (2012). Sleep problems are associated with binge eating in women. *International Journal of Eating Disorders, 45*(5), 695–703.

Troop, N. A., Allan, S., Treasure, J. L., & Katzman, M. (2003). Social comparison and submissive behaviour in eating disorder patients. *Psychology and Psychotherapy, 76*, 237–249.

Trunko, M. E. & Kaye, W. H. (2008). Pharmacological treatment of bulimia nervosa. *Psychiatric Times, 25*(6), 52, 56–58.

Ty, M. & Francis, A. J. P. (2013). Insecure attachment and disordered eating in women: The mediating processes of social comparison and emotion dysregulation. *Eating Disorders, 21*(2), 154–174.

Udo Tomoko, T., McKee, S. A., White, M. A., Masheb, R. M., Barnes, R. D., & Grilo, C. M. (2013). Sex differences in biopsychosocial correlates of binge eating disorder: A study of treatment-seeking obese adults in primary care setting. *General Hospital Psychiatry, 35*, 578–591.

Vanderlinden, J., Buis, H., Pieters, G., & Probst, M. (2007). Which elements in the treatment of eating disorders are necessary 'ingredients' in the recovery process?—A comparison between the patient's and therapist's view. *European Eating Disorders Review, 15*, 357–365.

Vince, E. & Walker, I. (2008). A set of meta-analytic studies on the factors associated with disordered eating. *Internet Journal of Mental Health, 5*(1), 2.

Vocks, S., Tuschen-Caffier, B., Pietrowsky, R., Rustenbach, S., Kersting, A., & Herpertz, S. (2010). Meta-analysis of the effectiveness of psychological and pharmacological treatments for binge eating disorder. *International Journal of Eating Disorders, 43*(3), 205–217.

Wade, T. D., Bergin, J. L., Tiggemann, M., Bulik, C. M., & Fairburn, C. G. (2006). Prevalence and long-term course of lifetime eating disorders in an adult Australian twin cohort. *Australian and New Zealand Journal of Psychiatry, 40*(2), 121–128.

Ward, A., Tiller, J., Treasure, J., & Russell, G. (2000). Eating disorders: Psyche or soma. *International Journal of Eating Disorders, 27*, 279–287.

Weaver, K. (2012). Loving her into well-being one day at a time: Narratives of caring for daughters with eating disorders. *Open Journal of Nursing, 2*, 406–419.

Weaver, K., Martin-McDonald, K., & Spiers, J. (2012). Mirroring voices of mother, daughter and therapist in anorexia nervosa. *Forum: Qualitative Social Research, 13*(3), 1–21.

Weaver, K. D., Wuest, J., & Ciliska, D. (2005). Understanding women's journey of recovering from anorexia nervosa. *Qualitative Health Research, 15*(2), 188–206.

Weltzin, T. E. (2010). Males and eating disorders. *ANAD*. Retrieved from http://www.anad.org.

Weltzin, T. E., Cornella-Carlson, T., Fitzpatrick, M. E., Kennington, B., Bean, P., & Jefferies, C. (2012). Treatment issues and outcomes for males with eating disorders. *Eating Disorders, 20*(5), 444–459.

Wentz, E., Gillberg, C. Anckarsäter, H., Gillberg, C., & Råstam, M. (2009). *The British Journal of Psychiatry, 194*, 168–174.

White, J. H. (1999). The development and clinical testing of an outpatient program for women with bulimia nervosa. *Archives of Psychiatric Nursing, 13*(4), 179–191.

Williamson, D. A. (1990). *Assessment of eating disorders: Obesity, anorexia, and bulimia nervosa*. New York: Penguin.

Winn, S., Perkins, S., Walwyn, R., Schmidt, U., Eisler, I., Treasure, J., ... Yi, I. (2007). Predictors of mental health problems and negative caregiving experiences in carers of adolescents with bulimia. *International Journal of Eating Disorders, 40*, 171–178.

Winston, A. P. (2012). The clinical biochemistry of anorexia nervosa [Review]. *Annals of Clinical Biochemistry, 49*(Pt 2), 132–143.

Wolfe, B. E. & Gimby, L. B. (2003). Caring for the hospitalized patient with an eating disorder. *Nursing Clinics of North America, 38*, 75–99.

Woodside, D. B. (2004). *Assessing and treating men with eating disorders*. Retrieved from *Psychiatric Times* website, http://www.psychiatrictimes.com/articles/assessing-and-treating-men-eating-disorders/page/0/2

Woodside, D. B., Bulik, C. M., Thornton, L., Klump, K. L., Tozzi, F., Fichter, M. M., ... Kaye, W. H. (2004). Personality in men with eating disorders. *Journal of Psychosomatic Research, 57*(3), 273–278.

Wooley, S. C. & Kearney-Cooke, A. (1986). Intensive treatment of bulimia and body image disturbance. In K. D. Brownell & J. P. Foreyt (Eds.), *Handbook of eating disorders: Physiology, psychology and treatment of obesity, anorexia, and bulimia* (pp. 476–502). New York: Basic Books.

Woolhouse, H., Knowles, A., & Crafti, N. (2012). Adding mindfulness to CBT programs for binge eating: A mixed-methods evaluation. *Eating Disorders, 20*(4), 321–339.

Wright, L. & Leahey, M. (2009). *Nurses and families: A guide to family assessment and intervention* (5th ed.). Philadelphia: F. A. Davis.

Yager, J. (2008). Binge eating disorder: The search for better treatments. *American Journal of Psychiatry, 165*, 4–6.

Yager, J. & Powers, P. S. (2007). *Clinical manual of eating disorders*. Arlington, VA: American Psychiatric Association.

Yilmaz, Z., Kaplan, A. S., & Zawertailo, L. A. (2012). Bulimia nervosa and alcohol use disorder: Evidence for shared etiology and neurobiology. *Current Psychiatry Reviews, 8*(1), 69–81.

Yu, J., Agras, W. S., & Bryson, S. (2013). Defining recovery in adult bulimia nervosa. *Eating Disorders, 21*(5), 379–394.

Zeeck, A., Birindelli, E., Sandholz, A., Joos, A., Herzog, T., & Hartmann, A. (2007). Symptom severity and treatment course of bulimic patients with and without a borderline personality disorder. *European Eating Disorders Review, 15*, 430–438.

Zeeck, A., Stelzer, N., Linster, H., Joos, A., & Hartmann, A. (2011). Emotion and eating in binge eating disorder and obesity. *European Eating Disorders Review, 19*(5), 426–437.

Zerwas, S., Lund, B. C., Von Holle, A., Thornton, L. M., Berrettini, W. H., Brandt, H., ... Bulik, C. M. (2013). Factors associated with recovery from anorexia nervosa. *Journal of Psychiatric Research, 47*(7), 972–979.

CHAPTER 26

Substance-Related and Addictive Disorders

Diane Kunyk and Charl Els

LEARNING OBJECTIVES

After studying this chapter, you will be able to:

- Conceptualize "addiction" as a prevalent, chronic, relapsing, and treatable medical disorder.
- Describe the features of the bio/psycho/social/spiritual and public health theories for understanding addiction in Canadian settings.
- Describe the principles of safe and effective treatment of substance-related and addictive disorders.
- Outline the essential components of screening, comprehensive assessment, matching patients with appropriate multimodal treatment interventions, as well as monitoring progress and effectiveness of treatment.
- Formulate an individualized nursing care plan.

KEY CONCEPTS

- addiction

KEY TERMS

- addiction • alcohol • ambivalence • brief intervention • caffeine
- cannabis • concurrent mental disorders • contemporaneous
- craving • delirium tremens • denial • detoxification • gambling disorder • hallucinogens • harm reduction • inhalants • intoxication
- motivational interviewing • multimodal • opioids • relapse
- remission • screening • sedatives, hypnotics, and anxiolytics
- stimulants • substance-related and addictive disorders • substance use disorders • substance-induced disorders • substance withdrawal
- therapeutic alliance • tobacco • tolerance • twelve-step programs

Addiction is recognized by both the major disease classification systems as a bona fide, chronic, and relapsing medical condition (American Psychiatric Association [APA], 2013; World Health Organization [WHO], 2007). Advances in brain imaging and other research have demonstrated that repeated exposure to alcohol, tobacco, and/or other psychoactive substances over time may alter brain structure, chemistry, and function in susceptible individuals, leading to a potential loss of control over their use of one or more substances and continued use despite harm or the knowledge of risk of harm. This conceptualization, along with emerging theories and understandings, has made advances in safe and effective treatment possible and provided increasingly optimistic outcomes for those affected with addiction.

Addiction may be expressed in individuals regardless of their age, gender, sexual orientation, socioeconomic status, education, culture, or occupation. Addiction is the most prevalent of all mental conditions, the leading preventable cause of death and disease globally, and the single greatest contributor to excess health care spending. For these reasons, it has been argued that addiction is the most important illness of our time (Els, 2007).

Yet addiction is often neglected and undertreated in Canadian society. There are significant barriers (e.g., stigma and resources) for persons with addiction to overcome in order to access the treatment they need, and these systemic barriers may be as intractable as the disease of addiction itself. Individuals affected with addiction are often alienated and isolated from

572

both their family and communities. Nurses encounter patients and their families who are struggling with addiction in their everyday practices and are favourably situated to help. With the necessary knowledge, skills, and attitudes conducive to health promotion and disease intervention, nurses are able to safely and effectively work with individuals and families experiencing this disorder and thereby effectively reduce this care deficit.

This chapter reviews the categories of **substance-related and addictive disorders**, current theories regarding the aetiology of substance use disorders (SUDs), and evidence-based treatment interventions. The role of the nurse is discussed in terms of early identification, assessment, and intervention planning with the purpose of helping to meet the needs of individuals and their family and to satisfy the ethical duty of patient advocacy. Also explored are selected topics of interest such as tobacco dependence in the mentally ill population and nurses with SUDs.

> **KEY CONCEPT** Addiction, a chronic, relapsing, and treatable medical condition, is a leading preventable cause of death, disability, and disease globally.

NEUROBIOLOGY

Addictive substances (licit and illicit) are used and misused for many reasons such as for their pleasurable effects, to alter mental status, to improve performance, to relieve boredom, or to self-medicate a mental disorder. These substances, when taken in excess, have in common the direct activation of the brain reward system. Stimulation of the reward pathway occurs in part through increasing extracellular dopamine concentrations in limbic regions of the brain. Dopamine is involved in many aspects of reward and pleasure and is involved in the production of memories and behavioural reinforcement. Chronic exposure to these substances may lead to pervasive changes in brain function at structural (molecular and cellular) and neurophysiologic levels, undermining the individual's voluntary control over its use (Leshner, 1997). These underlying changes in brain circuits may persist beyond withdrawal, and the behavioural effects of these changes may be exhibited in the repeated experiences of craving and relapse of individuals exposed to drug-related stimuli (APA, 2013). From a neurobiologic perspective, therefore, addiction can be considered a chronic, relapsing disease of the brain, and the associated abnormal behaviour is the result of dysfunction of brain tissue (Volkow & Li, 2011).

Given equal exposure to psychoactive substances, however, not all individuals who are exposed to addictive substances will develop addiction. Addiction comes to expression in individuals who may be considered potentially susceptible on any one or more of the following levels: biologic, psychological, social, or spiritual. For example, individuals who start using substances in adolescence are at higher risk of developing addiction than those who start later in life (Pitkanen, Lyyra, & Pulkkinen, 2005). It has also been estimated that 40% to 60% of the vulnerability to addiction is attributable to genetic factors (Volkow & Li, 2011). Gender differences have also been established, with the prevalence among males consistently demonstrating higher rates and women who regularly use or abuse substances considered more vulnerable for developing addiction (Swendsen & Le Moal, 2011). Regardless of putative vulnerabilities, the manifestation of addiction has been described as "a cluster of cognitive, behavioural, and physiologic symptoms indicating that the individual continues using the substance despite significant substance-related problems" (APA, 2013, p. 483).

DIAGNOSTIC CRITERIA

The APA's (2013) *Diagnostic and Statistical Manual of Mental Disorders*, 5th ed. (*DSM-5*) classification of substance-related and addictive disorders refers to disorders related to taking of substances of abuse and includes two categories: **substance use disorders** and **substance-induced disorders** (substance intoxication, substance withdrawal, and other substance/medication-induced mental disorders).

The diagnosis of a SUD is substance specific (e.g., alcohol, or cocaine, or tobacco use disorder). It is based on a pathologic pattern of 11 behaviours (Criteria) grouped into (1) impaired control, (2) social impairment, (3) risky use, and (4) pharmacologic categories. SUDs occur in a range of severity from mild to severe. A *mild* SUD is suggested by the presence of two or three symptoms, *moderate* by four or five, and *severe* by six or more. Changes in severity may also be observed across time. The following are the SUD Criteria (APA, 2013):

1. **Impaired control over substance use:**
   - The individual may take the substance in larger amounts or over a longer period than was originally intended (Criterion A1).
   - The individual may express a persistent desire to cut down or regulate substance use and may report multiple unsuccessful efforts to decrease or discontinue use (Criterion A2).
   - The individual may spend a great deal of time obtaining the substance, using the substance, or recovering from its effects (Criterion A3).
   - Cravings: The individual may experience a time when he or she experiences strong desire or urges to take the substance (Criterion A4).

2. **Social impairment due to substance use:**
   - Recurrent substance use resulting in failures to fulfill major role obligations at work, school, or home (Criterion A5).
   - Continued use of the substance despite having persistent or recurrent social or interpersonal problems caused or exacerbated by its effects (Criterion A6).
   - Important social, occupational, or recreational activities may be given up or reduced because of substance use (Criterion A7).

3. **Risky use of the substance:**
   - The recurrent use of the substance in situations where it is physically hazardous (Criterion A8).
   - The individual may continue substance use despite knowledge of having a persistent or recurrent physical or psychological problem that is likely to have been caused or exacerbated by the substance (Criterion A9).

4. **Pharmacologic criterion:**
   - Tolerance, characterized by requiring a markedly increased dose of the substance to achieve the desired effect or a markedly reduced effect when the usual dose is consumed (Criterion A10).
   - Withdrawal occurs when blood or tissue concentrations of a substance decline in an individual who had maintained prolonged heavy use of the substance (Criterion A11).

The substance-induced disorder of **intoxication** is described as the development of a reversible substance-specific syndrome due to the recent ingestion of (or exposure to) a substance. The maladaptive behaviours associated with intoxication (e.g., belligerence, mood lability, cognitive impairment, impaired judgement, impaired social or occupational functioning) are due to the direct physiologic effects of the substance on the central nervous system (APA, 2013). These behaviours place the individual at significant risk for adverse effects (e.g., accidents, general medical complications, disruption in social and family relationships, vocational or financial difficulties, and legal problems).

Substance withdrawal is the development of a substance-specific maladaptive behavioural change that is due to the cessation, or reduction, of heavy and prolonged substance use. This may cause clinically significant distress or impairment in social, occupational, or other important areas of functioning and, as a result, most individuals will experience craving to readminister the substance to reduce the discomforting symptoms. Some withdrawal syndromes are life threatening, others are uncomfortable, and some are even less pronounced.

Classes of Substances

Although not fully distinct, there are 10 described classes of heterogenous substances referred to in the *DSM-5*. The classification system includes **alcohol; caffeine; cannabis** (marijuana); **hallucinogens** (with separate categories for phencyclidine [PCP] [or similarly acting arylcyclohexylamines] and other hallucinogens); **inhalants; opioids; sedatives, hypnotics,** and **anxiolytics; stimulants; tobacco** (nicotine); and **other** (or unknown) **substances.** The diagnosis of a SUD can be applied to all 10 classes of substances except for caffeine. The pharmacologic mechanisms by which each of these drugs produces reward to the brain are different, but what is common to these classes of drugs is that, when they are taken in excess, the brain reward system is intensely activated (APA, 2013).

Clinical Course

Addiction is described as a *chronic disease, specifically a chronic mental disorder*—one that potentially threatens the health and well-being of individuals with the disorder as well as their family, their colleagues, and the broader community, as well as the economy. There is considerable heterogeneity among people with SUD, but it is often observed that there are periods of sustained substance use that are interrupted by periods of partial or complete **remission** (a period when symptoms have abated). In some individuals, addiction to a single substance may lead to the **contemporaneous** use of (and possible addiction to) another substance (Sridharan, Kawata, Campbell, & Tseng, 2005). Of particular note in this regard is the use of tobacco and caffeine, as these are often contemporaneously encountered with other SUD but may be uncertainly addressed in many hospitals and addiction treatment facilities. What is well acknowledged, however, is that when addiction is neglected and untreated, the course of the disease often typically progresses in severity and may even result in premature death (Kleber et al., 2006).

Substance-related and addictive disorders are widely considered to be amenable to treatment. The outcomes to evidence-based interventions are similar to those for other chronic disease conditions, including hypertension, asthma, and type 2 diabetes (McLellan, Lewis, O'Brien, & Kleber, 2000). Most persons with substance-related disorder (SRD) will have one or more **relapses** (a return to substance use after a drug-free period) during their process of recovery. Some of the most commonly cited precursors to relapse include substance-related reminder cues (e.g., sights, sounds, smells, or thoughts), negative mood states, positive mood states, and sampling the drug itself, even in small doses. Current **craving** (the experience of a strong desire or urge to take the substance) is often used as an outcome measure because it may be a signal of impending relapse (APA, 2013).

Non–Substance-Related Disorders

Ranges of other repetitive behaviours have been postulated to form part of the addiction-related disorder spectrum. These include such behaviours as "Internet gaming addiction," "sex addiction," "exercise addiction," "shopping addiction," and others. More research is needed for the non–SRDs and related conditions to reach the necessary internal consistency of criteria or the diagnostic stability for inclusion in the *DSM-5* classification system.

The *DSM-5* (APA, 2013) includes **gambling disorder** in its classification system due to the body of evidence indicating that gambling behaviours activate reward systems similar to those activated by drugs of abuse and appear to produce some behavioural symptoms comparable to those of SUD. The diagnostic criteria for persistent and recurrent maladaptive gambling behaviour leading to clinically significant impairment of distress as indicated by the individual exhibiting four (or more) of the following in a 12-month period (APA, 2013):

- Needs to gamble with increasing amounts of money in order to achieve the desired excitement (Criterion A1).
- Restlessness or irritability is experienced when attempting to cut down or stop gambling (Criterion A2).
- Repeated unsuccessful efforts to control, cut back, or stop gambling (Criterion A3).
- Often preoccupied with gambling (i.e., having persistent thoughts of reliving past gambling experiences, handicapping or planning the next venture, or thinking of ways to get money with which to gamble) (Criterion A4).
- Gambling often occurs when feeling distressed (helpless, guilty, anxious, depressed) (Criterion A5).
- After losing money gambling, the individual often returns another day to get even (Criterion A6).
- Lying to others occurs to conceal the extent of involvement with gambling (Criterion A7).
- A significant relationship, job, or educational or career opportunity has been jeopardized or lost because of gambling (Criterion A8).
- Others are relied upon to provide money to relieve a desperate financial situation caused by gambling (Criterion A9).

A disqualifier for the diagnosis of gambling disorder is added to rule out whether the gambling behaviour cannot be better accounted for by a manic episode (Criterion B).

EPIDEMIOLOGY

Nurses should be open to the possibility that patients are unlikely ever too young or old, too healthy or infirm, or too educated or wealthy to have problems with substance use. In their practices, nurses are well positioned to detect areas of potential or actual need for patients and their families in all of the settings in which nursing is practised (i.e., home, community, ambulatory, inpatient, and long-term settings). The following section addresses the most commonly used substances in Canadian society.

Tobacco

The use of tobacco products remains the most important preventable cause of death and disease globally, and it is projected to cause 1 billion deaths internationally during the 21st century (WHO, 2010). Tobacco is a risk factor for six of the eight leading causes of mortality and is responsible for 1 out of every 10 deaths of adults, and 45% of smokers will die of a tobacco-induced disorder (Lerman, Patterson, & Berrettini, 2005). In Canada, tobacco use is responsible for approximately 37,000 deaths annually from direct causes and a further 1,100 to 7,800 deaths related to second-hand smoke (Makomoaski Illing & Kaiserman, 2004). With 18% of the population currently smoking, tobacco continues to be the most commonly abused substance in Canada (Health Canada, 2011). Most Canadians initiate their use of tobacco between the ages of 11 and 15; for this reason, tobacco addiction is described as a paediatric disease that in most cases continues into adulthood unless successfully managed in childhood and adolescence. Another consideration for nurses is the effect of second-hand smoke in vehicles and third-hand smoke (referring to particulate matter from smoke that has been deposited on surfaces in homes) experienced by children and others in the family of those who smoke (U.S. Department of Health and Human Services, 2010).

Alcohol

Alcohol is consumed by over 80% of Canadians adults, and Canadians consume alcohol at a rate more than 50% above the global average (Ialomiteanu, Adlaf, Mann, & Rehm, 2009; Shield, Rylett, Gmel, Kehoe-Chan, & Rehm, 2013). In most instances, alcohol is used in moderation but, in general, for both men and women, the frequency of drinking alcohol increases with age, income, and education just as smoking and illicit drug use decrease across these variables. Alcohol is second only to tobacco in its prevalence of addiction in Canada. The prevalence rate of lifetime and 12-month alcohol abuse is 17.8% and 4.7%, respectively, while the prevalence of lifetime and 12-month alcohol dependence is 12.5% and 3.8%, respectively (Hasin, Stinson, Ogburn, & Grant, 2007).

Other Substances

Although several surveys estimate the prevalence in Canada of *substance use*, there are fewer population-level studies that have examined the prevalence of *SUDs* (excluding alcohol and tobacco). Findings from American studies based on the *DSM-IV* criteria suggest that the lifetime and 12-month prevalence for substance abuse is 7.7% and 1.4%, respectively, and the lifetime and

12-month prevalence for substance dependence is 2.6% and 0.6%, respectively (Compton, Thomas, Stinson, & Grant, 2007).

Societal Costs

Alcohol, tobacco, and other substance use exacts a heavy toll on the health of individuals, their families, and communities. Taken together, substances are implicated in over 12% of mortality worldwide, and their use constitutes the leading cause of preventable death (WHO, 2009). In 2002, the costs incurred to Canadian society were estimated at nearly $40 billion when health care (e.g., hospitalization, treatment services), the workplace (e.g., employee assistance programs, toxicologic drug testing), transfer payments (e.g., social welfare, workers' compensation), crime and law enforcement (e.g., police, courts), and lost productivity (e.g., reduced output, sick time) were considered (Rehm et al., 2006).

■■■■ AETIOLOGIC THEORIES

Addiction (used synonymously with substance dependence or the *DSM-5* designation of a SUD) can be conceptualized as a disorder with a multifactorial pathogenesis and predisposing, precipitating, and modulating factors that encompass the body, the mind (psyche), and the spirit. It is further shaped and impacted by social, environmental, cultural, economic, and political influences in the development and expression of the disease, which may impact on conceptualizing and formulating safe and effective treatment. Addiction is not all-or-none but rather a matter of degree (West, 2006, p. 3). This disease typically develops, and comes to expression, in behavioural ways with varying degrees of embedded biologic, psychological, social, and spiritual aspects that cannot be explained in isolation or with one reductive theory. Environmental or conditioned cues—of which there may be tens of thousands that individuals associate with their substance use—also become a part of the addiction, and these are experienced within a complex environment where a range of dynamic factors likely influence the course of the disease.

Biologic Theories

There is large body of evidence examining the influence of addictive substances on the brain, including sophisticated brain-imaging techniques that demonstrate structural and functional changes in the addicted brain. The addicted brain has been demonstrated to be fundamentally different from the nonaddicted brain, and this is manifested by changes in gene expression, receptor availability, metabolic activity, and responsiveness to environmental cues (Leshner, 1997). These pervasive changes in brain function may persist on molecular, cellular, structural, and functional levels long after the individual stops consuming the substance. These demonstrated changes to brain structure and function form the foundation and evidence for addiction to be classified as a "disease of the brain" and a mental disorder.

The use of addictive substances has been found to increase extracellular levels of dopamine. This dopamine-related "high" (euphoria) becomes a reinforcement mechanism in the brain. The brain, in essence, remembers this pleasure and wants it repeated, but the neurochemical status in the brain readjusts to these increased levels of dopamine as being the "normal" neurochemical state; the user then requires increased amounts of substances to produce the same dopamine-related effects (Goldstein & Volkow, 2011). This need for increased amounts of a substance to achieve (or obtain) the same results (effects) is termed **tolerance** and is considered one of the hallmark features of addiction. Cravings to use substances often dominate the thoughts and affect mood and behaviour of the addicted individual. Just as food is linked to daily survival, once the brain has become addicted to a substance, it attaches the same level of salience or significance to consuming the substance as it does to the level of life-sustaining functions or behaviour. The substance is no longer sought only for pleasure but for the need to relieve distress or withdrawal; on a subconscious level, it may be enjoyed at the same level of salience as life-sustaining elements of behaviour. Eventually, the drive to obtain and use the substance becomes one of the most important priorities despite adverse (and at times devastating) consequences.

Psychological Theories

The psychological theories refer to the relative contribution of psychological and psychiatric factors that reflect the individual's preferences, experiences, or problems. It is postulated that these factors influence the likelihood that addictive substances will be used initially or that the individual will go on to develop an addiction. These theories suggest that some individuals are born with certain temperaments and subsequently develop particular personality traits, vulnerabilities, or even personality disorders that may make them more susceptible to addiction. From this theoretical perspective, addiction is considered a behavioural disorder occurring in a vulnerable phenotype, in which an intrinsic predisposed state determines the neuroplasticity that is induced (Swendsen & Le Moal, 2011).

Research increasingly focuses on the possibility that vulnerabilities acquired early in life may predispose individuals to psychiatric conditions (including addiction). Children of mothers who experience stress during pregnancy or children who have experienced disrupted maternal care during infancy and other early adverse experiences are considered important factors associated with substance initiation and addiction (Gordon, 2002). It is postulated that the disrupted development and stress from such adverse childhood events (often defined by social and economic disadvantages) contribute to subsequent vulnerability to addiction (Swendsen & Le Moal, 2011).

There is a large body of literature demonstrating that SUDs are strongly associated with other mental disorders. Individuals with SUD often have mood, anxiety, or other psychiatric conditions. Self-medication, whereby substances are used (at least in part) as a means for reducing anxiety, depression, or other symptoms, is one explanation for this finding. The reverse causal association has also been proposed, whereby the use of substances may induce anxiety or other psychiatric conditions. By contrast, shared aetiologic models suggest that there may be specific factors that increase the risk of individuals developing more than one condition (Swendsen & Le Moal, 2011).

Social Theories

The World Health Organization has determined that there are significant differences between some countries in their prevalence of alcohol, tobacco and other substance addictions (WHO, 2009). These differences exist even between countries of similar income and geographic region. These findings may be attributable, in part, to differences in substance availability, legislation, and other health policies.

Culture is considered to be another factor influencing addiction prevalence rates. Migration studies have compared rates of addiction for homogeneous ethnic groups in the country of origin with those of the host country possessing a different culture. For example, studies of Mexican families migrating to the United States generally indicate lower rates of addiction in their country of origin than among corresponding groups in the United States (Grant et al., 2004). It has been hypothesized that the protective aspects of the country of origin may diminish over time and over generations, as a function of acculturation (Merikangas et al., 2009).

Spiritual Theories

Spirituality (which is not to be confused with *religion*) has a close relationship with the field of addiction treatment; individuals who have recovered from addiction often mention spiritual experiences or motivation as a major contributory factor in their recovery. Spirituality can be defined as the relationship between an individual and the sacred (numinous), perhaps represented by a transcendent higher being (or higher power) or force (or mind of the universe). This relationship is personal to the individual and does not require affiliation with any organized religion; religion is *not* necessary

---

BOX 26-1 The Twelve Steps of Alcoholics Anonymous

1. We admitted we were powerless over alcohol—that our lives had become unmanageable
2. Came to believe that a Power greater than ourselves could restore us to sanity
3. Made a decision to turn our will and our lives over to the care of God *as we understood Him*
4. Made a searching and fearless moral inventory of ourselves
5. Admitted to God, to ourselves, and to another human being the exact nature of our wrongs
6. Were entirely ready to have God remove all these defects of character
7. Humbly asked Him to remove our shortcomings
8. Made a list of all persons we had harmed and became willing to make amends to them all
9. Made direct amends to such people wherever possible, except when to do so would injure them or others
10. Continued to take personal inventory and, when we were wrong, promptly admitted it
11. Sought through prayer and meditation to improve our conscious contact with God as we understood Him, praying only for knowledge of His will for us and the power to carry that out
12. Having had a spiritual awakening as a result of these steps, we tried to carry this message to alcoholics and to practise these principles in all our affairs

Source: The Twelve Steps are reprinted with permission of Alcoholics Anonymous World Services, Inc. (AAWS). Permission to reprint the Twelve Steps does not mean that the AAWS has reviewed or approved the contents of this publication or that the AAWS necessarily agrees with the views expressed herein. A.A. is a program of recovery from alcoholism *only*—use of the Twelve Steps in connection with programs and activities which are patterned after A.A., but which address other problems, or in any other non-A.A. context, does not imply otherwise.

---

for an individual to develop his or her spirituality or, for that matter, to recover from addiction. Spirituality is an integral dimension of the Twelve Step tradition of Alcoholics Anonymous (AA). The 12 steps, formulated by William Wilson or "Bill W.," were empirically derived from his experiences of living with alcohol addiction. They reference "a power greater than us," "God," "Higher Power," and "a spiritual experience" (refer to Box 26-1). The spirituality of this program includes the themes of release, gratitude, humility, and tolerance and is considered to be distinct from religious dogma (Nace, 2005).

Public Health Theories

The *public health model* (also called epidemiologic homeostasis) considers the interaction between the host, agent, vector, and environment. This framework incorporates the biologic, psychological, social, and spiritual theories as they pertain to addiction in a manner that can demonstrate their interdependent relationships. It is within these relationships that interventions/policies may be designed to reduce the impact and the spread of the disease of addiction. This understanding of addiction is based on examining the interaction between individuals (*the host*) and the substance of abuse (*the agent*). These domains include the psychopharmacology of the substance of abuse and the biologic, psychological, and spiritual components of the individual. Here is where phenomena such as experimentation and family history may be examined.

Many approaches to controlling substance-related and addictive disorders at the public health level depend on broader understandings of this disease and incorporate some of the social theoretical components. One of these includes consideration of the *vector*. In addiction, these would be considered the suppliers, "mules," and "pushers" involved in the manufacture and/or distribution of addictive substances. The tobacco industry, for example, is the vector of the disease of tobacco addiction and profits massively through the making and selling of cigarettes from tobacco, by marketing its product through advertising and promotions, and by lobbying government for favoured treatment. The tobacco industry has an unparalleled history of success in its role as a vector. Secondary vectors, such as convenience stores or publications that feature advertisements of addictive substances, may also promote the disease of addiction. Nurses (e.g., in psychiatric settings) facilitating access to tobacco and its use (e.g., by dispensing tobacco to patients) may also be considered secondary vectors in spreading the disease. Examining the concept of the vector opens possibilities of controlling the spread of addiction to include interventions such as restrictions on advertising, denormalization, and advocating for corporate responsibility and liability for the damages sustained as a result of promoting dangerous products.

The other major core elements in the public health model are the cultural, political, economic, legal, and historical settings in which the agent, the host, and the vector interact. These unique and varied settings comprise the broader *environment*. Understanding the large and small environments in which the vector–agent–host interactions occur and tailoring approaches appropriate for them is as essential for effective treatment and prevention of addiction as is tailoring nursing care to the patient (host). Taxation on alcohol and tobacco are examples of interventions that change the environment to negatively impact rates of addiction. An advantage to the public health model is its ability to consider intervention at both the individual (e.g., clinical) and environmental (e.g., legislation and social marketing) levels. By placing treatment and prevention strategies into this model, it allows the nurses to better understand how their work fits into the larger picture and how they can best contribute during and beyond their day-to-day practice. An application of the public health model to the situation of tobacco in health care settings may be found in Box 26-2.

BOX 26-2 Application of the Public Health Model to Tobacco and Health Care Settings

The Situation: For decades, the use of tobacco products has been tolerated, sometimes even in health care settings. This *environment* has been culpable to the spread of the disease of tobacco addiction through measures including allowing smoking in designated areas or rooms, selling tobacco products on-site, and allowing smoking in visible outdoor areas. In these settings, the *hosts* (tobacco consumers) have been accommodated for their addiction. Furthermore, some patients, employees, physicians, and volunteers have become *incidental hosts* through their exposure to second-hand smoke during the course of care delivery. The vector of the disease in this situation is the tobacco industry that, in efforts to increase sales, has heavily marketed its product and sometimes funded health professionals and health facilities as a measure to gain credibility. Nurses (along with other health care professionals) have, at times, been a *secondary vector* in the hospital situation by storing, dispensing, lighting, and even rolling cigarettes, selling and gifting tobacco, supervising smoking, scheduling activities around "smoke breaks," and there are even reports of nurses smoking with patients as a measure to establish therapeutic relationships. There is anecdotal evidence of patients who are former smokers who relapse as a response to the smell of tobacco on nurses' clothing or breath.

Intervention: The placement of this situation into the Public Health Model allows for the development of a comprehensive tobacco control policy to limit the spread of the disease. Elements include the following:

- The closure of all designated smoking rooms and areas indoors
- Prevent nicotine withdrawal in patients through appropriate pharmacotherapy
- Eliminating tobacco sales on-site
- Reject funding and any other form of relationship with the tobacco industry
- Designating all outdoor areas as smoke free including parking areas
- Supporting nurses and other health employees to quit smoking with comprehensive and ongoing workplace wellness programs

Source: Kunyk, D., Els, C., Predy, G., & Haase, M. (2007). Development and introduction of a comprehensive tobacco control policy in a Canadian regional health authority. *Preventing Chronic Disease: Public Health Research, Practice, and Policy*, 4(2), 1–8.

■ INTERDISCIPLINARY TREATMENT

The adaptation in the brain that results from chronic substance exposure is long lasting. Therefore, addiction interventions must also reflect its chronic (and relapsing) nature. This is a similar model as for other chronic conditions (such as asthma, diabetes, hypertension, and others). Not surprisingly, the rates of recovery for addiction are comparable to those of other chronic conditions, and discontinuation of treatment is likely to result in similar rates of relapse (McLellan et al., 2000). As with other chronic diseases, effective addiction interventions require the involvement of multiple brain circuits (reward, motivation, learning, inhibitory control, and executive function), and their associated disruption of behaviour indicates the need for a multimodal approach in its treatment (Volkow & Li, 2011). Within this paradigm, relapse is not interpreted as failure but rather as a temporary setback, and recovery is conceptualized as a "process" and not as an event.

To reflect the most up-to-date treatment concepts and recommendations, the National Institute on Drug Abuse (NIDA, 2012a) updated their seminal document *Principles of Drug Addiction Treatment* in 2012. These principles are intended to address addiction to alcohol, tobacco, and other drugs and are based on the existing body of scientific evidence. They provide a critical starting point for any discussion about the treatment of addiction (Box 26-3).

Goals of Addiction Treatment

Addiction treatment programs have as their goal not simply stabilizing the patient's condition but altering the course of the substance-related disorder as well as the patient's overall functioning (Mee-Lee & Shulman, 2009). Safe and effective treatment for individuals with SRD requires the completion of screening, a comprehensive assessment, matching treatment to include the evidence-based modalities available for the particular disorder and comorbidities, monitoring of outcome,

as well as follow-up on a longitudinal basis. Treatment ought to be culturally sensitive and appropriate, taking into account the specific needs and preferences of the patient. Issues related to gay, queer, bisexual, lesbian, two-spirited, and transgender individuals, pregnant women, ethnic minorities, gender-related variables, age, and medical needs are to be considered as well in the treatment provision. Box 26-4 outlines specific goals of addiction treatment.

The **multimodal** treatment of addiction typically involves a combination of psychosocial interventions as well as pharmacotherapy where (and if) available for a particular condition. A longitudinal approach for management of this chronic disease is ideal and, in general, the iterative approach to treatment is first to screen, engage, assess, motivate, and help to retain the patient in a safe and effective evidence-based treatment setting. Treatment retention and adherence to mutually agreed-upon goals generally maximize the potential benefits of treatment and improve outcomes.

Treatment further seeks to help educate patients, their family members, caregivers, and significant others about addiction as a bona fide disease, including its causes, consequences, longitudinal approaches to, and the options for interdisciplinary treatment. In some cases and situations, **harm reduction** may be an interim step towards abstinence, and these philosophies are not considered to be mutually exclusive or incompatible. Understanding the complementary nature of these approaches is vital, and this may mean initially using a harm reduction approach under certain circumstances and thereby initially working towards reducing harm as a first step towards abstinence.

The **therapeutic alliance** (or the "helping alliance") between the nurse and the patient is a *key ingredient* for treatment success. This therapeutic alliance ideally builds a foundation of empathy, mutual trust, and nonjudgement; provides hope for recovery; and begins at the very first meeting with the patient. Nurses should aim to establish rapport and create a positive alliance with the patient, which is the trusting relationship within which change can be negotiated. A healthy treatment relationship generally facilitates treatment, improves adherence with treatment, and ultimately improves outcomes.

In order to establish a therapeutic alliance, the nurse should aim to minimize or avoid premature and inappropriate confrontations, judgement, negative interactions, advice without permission, and other approaches not congruent with motivation-based techniques. Some health professionals may experience an element of negative bias and stereotyping of people, perhaps stemming from their own particular background, psychodynamics, or their own losses or experiences with addiction. For the ethical professional, it is important to make the

BOX 26-3 Principles of Addiction Treatment

1. Addiction is a complex but treatable disease that affects brain function and behaviour. Drugs of abuse alter the brain's structure and function, resulting in changes that persist long after drug use has ceased. This may explain why drug abusers are at risk for relapse even after long periods of abstinence and despite the potentially devastating consequences.
2. No single treatment is appropriate for everyone. Treatment varies depending on the type of drug and the characteristics of the patients. Matching treatment settings, interventions, and services to an individual's particular problems and needs is critical to his or her ultimate success in returning to productive functioning in the family, workplace, and society.
3. Treatment needs to be readily available. Because drug-addicted individuals may be uncertain about entering treatment, taking advantage of available services the moment people are ready for treatment is critical. Potential patients can be lost if treatment is not immediately available or readily accessible. As with other chronic diseases, the earlier treatment is offered in the disease process, the greater the likelihood of positive outcomes.
4. Effective treatment attends to multiple needs of the individual, not just his or her drug abuse. To be effective, treatment must address the individual's drug abuse and any associated medical, psychological, social, vocational, and legal problems. It is also important that treatment be appropriate to the individual's age, gender, ethnicity, and culture.
5. Remaining in treatment for an adequate period of time is critical. The appropriate duration for an individual depends on the type and degree of his or her problems and needs. Research indicates that most addicted individuals need at least 3 months in treatment to significantly reduce or stop their drug use and that the best outcomes occur with longer durations of treatment. Recovery from drug addiction is a long-term process and frequently requires multiple episodes of treatment. As with other chronic illnesses, relapses to drug abuse can occur and should signal a need for treatment to be reinstated or adjusted. Because individuals often leave treatment prematurely, programs should include strategies to engage and keep patients in treatment.
6. Behavioural therapies—including individual, family, or group counselling—are the most commonly used forms of drug abuse treatment. Behavioural therapies vary in their focus and may involve addressing a patient's motivation to change, providing incentives for abstinence, building skills to resist drug use, replacing drug-using activities with constructive and rewarding activities, improving problem-solving skills, and facilitating better interpersonal relationships. Also, participation in group therapy and other peer support programs during and following treatment can help maintain abstinence.
7. Medications are an important element of treatment for many patients, especially when combined with counselling and other behavioural therapies. For example, methadone, buprenorphine, and naltrexone (including a new long-acting formulation) are effective in helping individuals addicted to heroin or other opioids stabilize their lives and reduce their illicit drug use. Acamprosate, disulfiram, and naltrexone are medications approved for treating alcohol dependence. For persons addicted to nicotine, a nicotine replacement product (available as patches, gum, lozenges, or nasal spray) or an oral medication (such as bupropion or varenicline) can be an effective component of treatment when part of a comprehensive behavioural treatment program.
8. An individual's treatment and services plan must be assessed continually and modified as necessary, to ensure that it meets his or her changing needs. A patient may require varying combinations of services and treatment components during the course of treatment and recovery. In addition to counselling or psychotherapy, a patient may require medication, medical services, family therapy, parenting instruction, vocational rehabilitation, and/or social and legal services. For many patients, a continuing care approach provides the best results, with the treatment intensity varying according to a person's changing needs.
9. Many drug-addicted individuals also have other mental disorders. Because drug abuse and addiction—both of which are mental disorders—often co-occur with other mental illnesses, patients presenting with one condition should be assessed for the other(s), and when these problems co-occur, treatment should address both (or all), including the use of medications as appropriate.
10. Medically assisted detoxification is only the first stage of addiction treatment and by itself does little to change long-term drug abuse. Although medically assisted detoxification can safely manage the acute physical symptoms of withdrawal and, for some, can pave the way for effective long-term addiction treatment, detoxification alone is rarely sufficient to help addicted individuals achieve long-term abstinence. Thus, patients should be encouraged to continue drug treatment following detoxification. Motivational enhancement and incentive strategies, begun at initial patient intake, can improve treatment engagement.
11. Treatment does not need to be voluntary to be effective. Sanctions or enticements from family, employment settings, and/or the criminal justice system can significantly increase treatment entry, retention rates, and the ultimate success of drug treatment interventions.
12. Drug use during treatment must be monitored continuously, as lapses during treatment do occur. Knowing their drug use is being monitored can be a powerful incentive for patients and can help them withstand urges to use drugs. Monitoring also provides an early indication of a return to drug use, signalling a possible need to adjust an individual's treatment plan to better meet his or her needs.
13. Treatment programs should assess patients for the presence of HIV/AIDS, hepatitis B and C, tuberculosis, and other infectious diseases as well as provide targeted risk reduction counselling, linking patients to treatment if necessary. Typically, drug abuse treatment addresses some of the drug-related behaviours that put people at risk of infectious diseases. Targeted counselling specifically focused on reducing infectious disease risk can help patients further reduce or avoid substance-related and other high-risk behaviours. Counselling can also help those who are already infected to manage their illness. Moreover, engaging in substance abuse treatment can facilitate adherence to other medical treatments. Substance abuse treatment facilities should provide on-site, rapid HIV testing rather than referrals to off-site testing as research shows that doing so increases the likelihood that patients will be tested and receive their test results. Those providing treatment should also inform patients that highly active antiretroviral therapy (HAART) has proven effective in combating HIV, including among drug-abusing populations and link them to HIV treatment if they test positive.

From the U.S. Government's National Institute on Drug Abuse. (Revised December 2012). Available at http://www.drugabuse.gov/sites/default/files/podat_1.pdf

BOX 26-4 Goals of Addiction Treatment

The *goals* of addiction treatment include the following:
- Treatment retention
- Reduction in severity and frequency of substance use episodes
- Reducing harm caused by substances, with the ultimate goal of total abstinence
- Management of comorbid psychiatric and medical conditions
- Improving the patient's quality of life
- Improving all areas of life affected by addiction (e.g., employment, interpersonal relationships, interface with the law/criminal justice system, physical health)
- Improving all levels of adaptive functioning
- Preventing relapse to substance use

BOX 26-5 Levels of Care for Substance-Related Disorders

LEVEL 0.5 Early intervention
Assessment and education for at-risk individuals.

LEVEL I: Outpatient treatment
This represents an organized nonresidential treatment service, or office-based outpatient practice, with provision of professionally directed substance-related and addictive disorders treatment. This treatment typically includes scheduled sessions (fewer than 9 hours per week) and may include individual therapy and/or group therapy, with or without participation in self-help groups such as Alcoholics Anonymous.

LEVEL II: Intensive outpatient treatment (including partial hospitalization)
On this level, there is provision of a structured program of substance-related and addictive disorders treatment service components to patients, with a minimum of 9 treatment hours per week. This includes full-spectrum day or evening treatment programs, but participants continue to live at home or in special residences.

LEVEL III: Medically monitored intensive inpatient treatment (residential)
This is a residential setting and represents organized addiction services including a formal regimen of around-the-clock professionally directed evaluation, care, and treatment in an inpatient (or residential) setting. This includes 24-hour observation, monitoring, and treatment where needed, and direct nursing supervision of care is available.

LEVEL IV: Medically managed intensive inpatient treatment
This is the most intensive level of care and represents 24-hour medically directed evaluation, care, and treatment in an acute care inpatient (e.g., psychiatric) setting. Patients suffering from severe withdrawal syndromes (e.g., withdrawal delirium or delirium tremens), or those with significant medical, emotional, or behavioural problems (e.g., associated with severe and persistent mental illness such as bipolar disorder, schizophrenia, borderline personality, or severe depression, or those with psychosis or suicidality), who require the level of intensity of medical and nursing services offered on this level, are also considered eligible for this inpatient level of care. Persons who have a substance overdose and who cannot be safely managed in the emergency department may also be best matched to this level of care. Individuals who have failed on a less restrictive level of care, and whose ongoing substance use poses a risk of harm to their physical or mental health, may also be offered more intensive levels of care.

effort of processing any unresolved conflicts and losses in her/his own life and to successfully work through any related issues.

The evidence clearly suggests that a confrontational interpersonal style is generally not helpful for achieving goals in addiction treatment and can lead to the patient being more defensive, displaying increased levels of **denial**, decreased levels of treatment acceptance, and even disengagement in treatment. Among the most important and valuable skills and attitudes translating into treatment success for the patient are the nurse's appropriate empathy, boundary setting, confidence, instillation of hope, and the provision of support and encouragement.

Principles of Matching Treatment

As an overarching principle, treatment should be offered on the least restrictive level of care that is proven to be safe and likely to be effective. Patients are matched to the most appropriate level of care, based on availability, along with the assessment of their condition and comorbidities, and with respect to the individuals' preference. Refer to Box 26-5 for a description of the levels of care that have been described by the American Society of Addiction Medicine (ASAM).

Screening, Brief Intervention, and Referral

It has been estimated that about one in five adults accessing primary care services reports problems related to substance use. Screening (*Ask*), brief intervention (*Advice and Assess*) and, when appropriate, referral (*Assist*), and follow-up (*Arrange*) are considered mainstays of early identification and intervention for substance-related and addictive disorders. However, the identification of SUD is often missed because of a lack of **screening**. A number of valid and reliable screening tools exist and are readily accessible. In a review of the literature, it was concluded that screening for alcohol and drug use disorders, brief intervention, and referral for treatment are feasible and effective strategies in primary care settings provided

that brief interventions and treatment facilities to which patients can be referred and treated promptly are available (Pilowsky & Wu, 2012).

Screening is used to identify patients who are likely to have an SUD as determined to their responses to certain key questions. An example of a preliminary question about alcohol use is, "Do you sometimes drink beer, wine, or other alcoholic beverages?" If a positive response, screening would occur with options such as the CAGE (Box 26-6) and MAST questionnaires. If the screen is negative, this should be followed with individually tailored advice to maintain consumption below the "at-risk"

BOX 26-6 The CAGE Questionnaire

1. Have you ever felt you should **C**ut down on your drinking?
2. Have people **A**nnoyed you by criticizing your drinking?
3. Have you ever felt bad or **G**uilty about your drinking?
4. Have you ever had a drink first thing in the morning to steady your nerves or to get rid of a hangover (**E**ye opener)?

Scoring: Item responses on the CAGE are scored 0 or 1 with a higher score an indication of alcohol problems. A total score of 2 or greater is considered clinically significant.

Source: Ewing, J. A. (1984). Detecting alcoholism: The CAGE Questionnaire. *Journal of the American Medical Association, 252,* 1905–1907.

BOX 26-7 Conversion into a Standard Drink

Alcohol consumption is measured in terms of the numbers of "standard drink," each of which contains 13.6 g of alcohol. Different beverages contain different concentrations, and conversion into a "standard drink" is described as the following:

- 43 mL (1.5 oz) spirit (40% alcohol)
- 142 mL (5 oz) table wine (12% alcohol)
- 341 mL (12 oz) regular beer (5% alcohol)
- 85 mL (3 oz) fortified wine (18% alcohol)

---

drinking limits (up to nine standard drinks per week for [nonpregnant] females and up to 14 drinks per week for males (Brands, Kahan, Selby, & Wilson, 2000). If the screen is positive, the patient may be advised to undergo more detailed diagnostic testing to confirm or rule out the disorder and/or to arrange for clinical follow-up.

Brief interventions can be defined as time-limited (i.e., 5 to 20 minutes), patient-centred counselling (talk therapy) designed to reduce substance use (Zgierska & Fleming, 2011). There is good evidence that even patients who do not meet the diagnostic criteria for alcohol addiction but are exceeding safe drinking limits (i.e., consuming alcohol at levels that may place them at risk for increased problems) can be supported and helped through screening and brief intervention. Somewhat similarly, the *Canadian Best Practice Guidelines for Smoking Cessation* recommend that the assessment of tobacco use status should be updated for all patients by health providers on a regular basis (CAN-ADAPTT, 2011). The Canadian Nurses Association (2011) agrees that all health professionals ought to be involved in tobacco cessation through assessing and documenting all forms of tobacco use, willingness to quit, and risk of exposure to second-hand smoke.

The goal of screening must also include identifying women who are pregnant or considering pregnancy and to provide advice on abstention from substance use. Alcohol, tobacco, and other substances can have harmful effects on the foetus and can be responsible for lifelong consequences such as foetal alcohol spectrum disorder (FASD). Substances are transmitted into breast milk, and the nursing mother can expose the breast-fed baby to harmful chemicals, with a range of adverse outcomes and risks. It is important for nurses to note that, due to stigma and fear, many women may underreport their consumption of alcohol (Zgierska & Fleming, 2011).

Screening and brief interventions are promising interventions, but further evidence is required regarding their use. Only one single item has been validated in primary care settings to screen for drug use: "How many times in the past year have you used an illegal drug or used a prescription medication for nonmedical reasons?"

Answering "one or more" represents a positive screen (Zgierska & Fleming, 2011). Box 26-7 provides conversion of alcohol into a standard drink.

Multidimensional Assessment

Assessment serves as an early mechanism to engage, motivate, and retain the patient in treatment and to assess for any imminent risk of harm. It further aims to guide ongoing management and allows for the measurement of progress and outcomes. The assessment process aims to gather information from many different sources that are relevant to the life of the patient affected by SUD. Assessment involves an evaluation of the following domains:

A comprehensive *substance use* assessment, including

- Onset of use or change of pattern of use
- Quantity per day or per week
- Frequency of use and periods of abstinence
- Route of use (e.g., injection, smoke, snort, oral ingestion)
- Prior treatment received (e.g., 12 steps, residential care)
- Sources of substances (e.g., black market, double doctoring, borrowing others' medication)

A comprehensive *psychiatric assessment*, including

- Obtaining a family and social history
- Details of any emotional and behavioural condition, or complications (psychiatric, emotional, behavioural status, including any potential for imminent and substantial risk of harm to self or to others; e.g., risk of suicide or risk of aggression, including homicide)

A comprehensive *physical assessment*, including

- Screening for infectious diseases (e.g., HIV, STDs, TB, hepatitis)
- The assessment of biomedical conditions and complications associated with substance use
- Focus on the risk for acute intoxication and/or withdrawal potential in the patient
- Laboratory testing (e.g., liver function testing)

Collateral information from others (with necessary consent):

- Assessment of the patient's level of *treatment acceptance* and elements of resistance, including

- Assessment of risk for relapse (relapse potential) and recovery environment

- The use of structured rating scales to help quantify clinical features and provide baseline for serial monitoring of progress

Management of Intoxication and Withdrawal

Intoxication is the result of being under the influence of, and responding to, the acute effects of alcohol or other substances of abuse. In the clinical setting, it is important to determine the substances involved, the quantity of the ingested substance, and the patient's level of consciousness. Life-threatening intoxication is of immediate concern, and the first priority is for supportive care (Wright, Cluver, & Myrick, 2011). Symptoms of intoxication and withdrawal specific to each class of substances are identified in the *DSM-5*. In general, the signs and symptoms of withdrawal are the opposite of a substance's direct pharmacologic effects. **Detoxification** is a process by which, under the care of a physician, individuals are systematically withdrawn from addictive substances in an either inpatient or outpatient setting. The American Society of Addiction Medicine (2009) offers three immediate goals for detoxification: to provide a safe withdrawal from the drug(s) of dependence and enable the patient to become substance free; to provide withdrawal from substance use that is humane and protects the patient's dignity; and to prepare the patient for ongoing treatment of his or her dependence on alcohol or other substances. It is important to recognize that detoxification is not the treatment of the SUD. Rather, it is only the management of withdrawal symptoms.

Harm Reduction

Countless examples of harm reduction exist, with varying levels of evidence to support its benefit and the most appropriate application in the context of SRD. Harm reduction, a community health intervention designed to reduce the consequences of substance use to the individual, the family, and society, has replaced a moral or criminal approach to substance abuse and addiction (Canadian Centre on Substance Abuse [CCSA], 2005). The purpose of this approach is to *reduce the risk* for adverse consequences arising from substance use, while recognizing that abstinence is ideal, and this approach works with the individual regardless of his or her commitment to reduce use. Harm reduction forms a part of the continuum of care and should not be viewed as exclusive of the overarching goal of abstinence. Fischer

---

BOX 26-8 Drinking and Driving

Driving impaired by alcohol remains the single largest cause of criminal death and one of the leading criminal causes of injury in Canada. The level of impairment resulting from the use of alcohol is determined by measuring breath or blood alcohol levels (BALs), and the level at which a person is considered to be legally impaired varies with jurisdiction and country. Under the Criminal Code of Canada, the operator of a vehicle could be charged for driving with a BAL over 0.08%. Some provinces have passed legislation allowing for progressive administrative penalties for drivers with lower BALs (i.e., between 0.03% and 0.08%). These penalties do not include criminal charges; rather, they may include vehicle seizure, licence suspension, and fines.

(2005, p. 13) suggests five general principles of harm reduction:

- Harm reduction focuses on the consequences of substance use, not on the use itself, requiring decisions about which harms to be targeted and in what order based on what is known about patient's welfare, public health, and the severity of the problem.

- Harm reduction focuses on the pragmatic and effective minimization of use-related harms.

- Meaningful and realistic efforts must be made to actively understand and consider the social and environmental context in which substance use occurs.

- Education, knowledge, and informed decision making by substance users and potential users are key pillars of harm reduction.

- Misinformed or ineffective interventions or policy can be considered sources of substance-related harms and must also be targeted for harm reduction interventions.

As an example, interventions for alcohol-related harm reduction include education about the safe use of alcohol, provision of food at bars to reduce the incidence of rapid intoxication, and encouragement of the use of a "designated driver." (Box 26-8 addresses drinking and driving).

Psychosocial Interventions

Effective psychosocial treatment exists for the addictive disorders and includes motivational interviewing (MI); cognitive–behavioural therapy (CBT); other behavioural therapies (contingency management, community reinforcement, cue exposure and relaxation training, and aversion therapy); self-help groups and 12-step facilitation; relapse prevention; psychodynamic and interpersonal therapy; group therapy and family therapy; brief therapies; self-guided therapies; and hypnotherapy.

Motivational Interviewing

Motivational interviewing is a directive, patient-centred style of counselling that helps patients to explore and resolve their **ambivalence** (the presence of both positive and negative feelings) about changing (Miller & Rollnick, 2002). It has wide application in practice for behavioural change, not only for the field of addiction. It is based, in part, on stages of change as delineated in Box 26-9. Some of the techniques in MI involve listening reflectively, eliciting motivational statements, and examining ambivalence. Those using this form of counselling avoid nontherapeutic responses such as directing and giving advice without patient permission, threatening with consequences, being coercive, and inappropriately raising concern without permission because these place the patient in an unhelpful, passive role. This model allows for the process of change to be viewed along a continuum and where concrete steps can be taken to help individuals increase readiness for changing behaviour.

MI involves at least two processes: increasing preferred behaviours and decreasing nonpreferred behaviours. Ambivalence is an expected part of the process of change, and resistance to change is to be expected. In the efforts to help patients move through the stages of change, from precontemplation through to contemplation, preparation, action, and maintenance, two critical components emerge that are iteratively assessed for their influence.

These are *conviction* (importance) and *confidence*. Strategies for increasing the patient's conviction include asking questions regarding the relative importance of changing behaviour; examining the risks and benefits of the particular behaviour and of changing; exploring concerns about behaviour; having the "hypothetical look over the fence," and exploring possible next steps. Enhancing confidence also includes brainstorming solutions, focusing on successful past efforts, and serial reassessment and repetition of the process. Asking the patient asking open-ended questions, listening reflectively, issuing affirming and summarizing statements, and also eliciting self-motivational statements from the patient conduct building motivation for change. These include problem recognition, expression of concern, the intention to change, and a sense of optimism. Refer to Box 26-10 for the principles of MI.

BOX 26-9 Stages of Change

This model provides a framework for a "staged" approach to interventions for substance use. It recognizes that quitting is not typically a singular event but rather a dynamic process. Five stages have been identified and guide the appropriate intervention for the individual at that time. These stages include the following:

1. **Precontemplation:** In this first stage, the user has no intention to quit in the next 6 months. An appropriate intervention for the nurse is to encourage consideration of the benefits and risks of continued use.
2. **Contemplation:** An individual in the contemplation stage is aware that a problem exists and is seriously thinking about quitting at some point but has not yet made a plan to do so. At this stage, the nurse, for example, may assist by reinforcing reasons for change, and exploring new ones.
3. **Preparation:** At this stage, the individual has made a decision to quit within the next 30 days and prepares to do so. An example of appropriate nursing intervention is to identify barriers to stopping and elicit solutions.
4. **Action:** The individual has quit within the past 6 months and is actively applying cessation skills. An appropriate nursing intervention is to ask how the individual is doing and advise regarding relapse prevention.
5. **Maintenance:** The individual has quit for more than 6 months. The nurse may ask how the patient is doing regarding risk situations and relapses and offer encouragement.

Many individuals will cycle through the Stages of Changes a number of times. Each attempt to quit provides new opportunities to learn new skills and techniques that will help in the next attempt.

Source: Prochaska, J., Diclemente, C., & Norcross, J. (1992). In search of how people change: Applications to addictive behaviors. *American Psychologist, 47*(9), 1102–1114.

BOX 26-10 The Principles of Motivational Enhancement

1. **Avoid arguing:** Generally, the more the therapist tells a patient "You can't do this," the more likely he or she will respond, if unconsciously, with "I will." Resistance to change is influenced by how the therapist responds to the patient's ambivalence.
2. **Express empathy:** The attitude underlying empathy might also be called acceptance, and it is not the same as approval of harmful behaviour, but rather an unconditional acceptance of where the patient is at in terms of the behaviour. Through skilful reflective listening, the therapist can seek to understand the patient's feelings and perspectives without judging, criticizing, or blaming. Paradoxically, this kind of acceptance of people as they are appears to free them to change, whereas insistence on change and nonacceptance of "where they are at" in the process of change can have the effect of keeping people as they are. It is not helpful to view the patient as "problematic," "pathologic," "unwilling to change," or "incapable of change," rather, the patient's situation is understood as one of being "stuck."
3. **Develop discrepancy:** Motivation for change is created when people perceive a discrepancy between their present behaviour and important personal goals. Thus, MI aims at developing discrepancy until it overrides attachment to the present behaviour. This is accomplished without coercion. It is the patient who gives voice to concerns and intentions to change.
4. **Roll with resistance:** When encountering resistance, the therapist acknowledges ambivalence as natural. The patient is invited to consider new information and perspectives. The responsibility for change is repeatedly handed back to the patient, but with the offer of help and support. It is not the therapist's role to generate all the solutions or to tell the patient what to do. Directive approaches may elicit "Yes, but..." responses from the patient, with little or no change following and often a disengagement and dropping out of treatment.
5. **Support self-efficacy:** This refers to the reinforcement of the patient's belief in his or her ability to carry out and succeed. Change is a stepwise approach, and each small step along the journey should be reinforced and supported. The therapist's expectations about a patient's chances for recovery can have a powerful impact on outcome.

BOX 26-11 FRAMES: Effective Elements of Brief Intervention

Feedback
Provide patients with personal feedback regarding their individual status, such as personal alcohol and other substance consumption relative to norms, information about elevated liver enzyme values, and so forth.

Responsibility
Emphasize the individual's freedom of choice and personal responsibility for change. General themes are as follows:
1. It's up to you; you're free to decide to change or not.
2. No one else can decide for you or force you to change.
3. You're the one who has to do it if it's going to happen.

Advice
Include a clear recommendation or advice on the need for change, typically in a supportive and concerned, rather than in a judgemental, manner.

Menu
Provide a menu of treatment options, from which patients may pick those that seem more suitable or appealing.

Empathic Counselling
Show warmth, support, respect, and understanding in communication with patients.

Self-Efficacy
Reinforce self-efficacy or an optimistic feeling that he or she can change.

Some of the signals of successful MI are the following: the nurse is speaking slowly; the patient is doing much more of the talking than the nurse; the patient is actively talking about behaviour change; and finally, the nurse is listening very carefully and gently directing the interview at appropriate moments. The acronym FRAMES (*feed-back*, *responsibility*, *advice*, *menu*, *empathy*, *self-efficacy*) was coined by Miller and Sanchez (1994) to summarize elements of brief interventions with patients using MI (refer to Box 26-11; see Chapter 6 for further discussion of MI).

Cognitive–Behavioural Therapy

Cognitive approaches to addiction hypothesize that if an individual can change the way he or she thinks about a situation, both the emotional reaction to it and the behavioural response will change. Psychoeducational materials, groups, and one-on-one interactions with nurses also impart information to reduce knowledge deficits related to alcohol, tobacco, and other substance dependence. For additional discussion on CBT, refer to Chapter 13.

Twelve-Step Recovery Programs

Twelve-step programs emphasize the conceptualization of addiction as an incurable, progressive disease that has spiritual, cognitive, and behavioural components. Alcoholics Anonymous (AA) was the first 12-step self-help group and started in the mid-1930s by William Wilson ("Bill W.") and a physician. The AA movement has become a worldwide fellowship of people with problems (current or past) related to alcohol, which provides support, individually and at meetings, to others who seek help. The only criterion for entry into AA is the "desire to quit drinking." Many treatment programs discuss concepts from AA, hold meetings at treatment facilities, and encourage patients to attend community meetings when appropriate. They also encourage continuing use of AA and other self-help groups as part of an ongoing plan for continued abstinence.

Twelve-step methods firmly endorse the need for abstinence and are considered by followers as lifelong programs of recovery with success attained 1 day at a time. The importance of recognizing and relying on a "higher power," or a power greater than the individual, is a central element of these programs. Members of 12-step groups can attend meetings on a self-determined or prescribed schedule that, if necessary, may be every day or even twice a day. Periods associated with high risk of relapse (e.g., holidays, weekends, family functions) are particularly appropriate times for attending meetings. A sponsor who is compatible with the patient can be particularly supportive and offer guidance through the recovery process, particularly during periods of high stress or increased craving.

The benefits from 12-step groups occur through the interplay of social interactions, prescribed behaviours, and mobilized psychological process. There is strong evidence that social support for abstinence is an important element to its success. Consistent support is also found for the benefit of two specific prescribed behaviours: meeting attendance and engagement in the program and being a sponsor. The evidence is mixed about the relative importance of spiritual/religious changes for explaining increased abstinence (Cavacuiti, Vasic, McCrady, & Tonigan, 2011). Inclusion in 12-step groups is considered a routine part of addiction treatment in most settings. However, an individual's refusal to participate in a self-help group is nonsynonymous with his or her resistance to treatment in general. Self-help groups are not beneficial for all people, and some persons may not embrace the spiritual dimension of the program. Alternative programs for sobriety, although not as widely available, have been developed to address this problem, such as Women for Sobriety and Secular Organizations for Sobriety.

There are now more than 60 different 12-step fellowships available worldwide, including Alcoholic Anonymous, Cocaine Anonymous, Narcotics Anonymous, Dual Recovery Anonymous, Sex Addicts Anonymous, among others. They do not solicit members, engage in political or religious activities, make medical or psychiatric diagnoses, engage in education about addiction to the general population, or provide mental health, vocational, or legal counselling.

Group Therapy

An integral and valuable component of the treatment regimen for many with a SUD is group therapy, and advantages of this approach include the following:

- The presence of others with an addiction may provide comfort.
- Other group members who are further along in their recovery may act as role models.
- Group members may offer a wide menu of coping strategies.
- Some members may act as "buddies" outside of the group setting.
- The public nature of group settings can act as a deterrent for relapse. It has been noted that individuals recovering from SUDs may be highly skilled at detecting each other's concealed substance use or early relapse.

The efficacy of group therapy is similar to individual therapy, and it can be a successful component of a combined treatment program. For more detailed information about group therapy, refer to Chapter 14.

Family Therapy

Long-term family therapy is often beneficial following the initial stages of detoxification and stabilization. Families can often unwittingly support addiction by, for instance, continuing to supply money to the individual, allowing adult children to live at home while continuing their substance use, and "bailing out" (rescuing) individuals from legal and other difficulties that result from substance use. Family therapy can bring these behaviours to light and assist family members to set limits on their further support. More detailed information is available in Chapter 15.

Pharmacotherapy

Pharmacotherapy, when available and appropriate, is routinely combined with psychosocial treatment and is not recommended for use in isolation from psychosocial interventions. Medications for SRD are generally utilized to treat intoxication and withdrawal, to reduce the reinforcing effects of drugs, to prevent relapse, and to treat comorbid medical or psychiatric conditions. For most of the SRD, there is not sufficient evidence for the use of pharmacotherapy. However, for the disorders related to tobacco, alcohol, and opioids, the empirical evidence supports the use of pharmacotherapy.

Relapse Prevention

Recovery from addiction can, for some, be defined as a long-term and ongoing process rather than merely an end point. Ten interventions have been identified for the

purposes of reducing relapse risk (Douaihy, Daley, Marlatt, & Spotts, 2011). These include helping patients to

- Understand relapse as a possible part of the recovery process and to learn how to identify warning signs
- Identify their own high-risk situations for relapse and develop effective cognitive and behavioural coping
- Enhance their communication skills and interpersonal relationships and to develop a recovery social network
- Reduce, identify, and manage negative emotional states (i.e., the acronym HALT warns not to become too Hungry, too Angry, too Lonely, or too Tired)
- Identify and manage cravings and any cues that may precede cravings
- Identify and challenge cognitive distortions
- Work towards a more balanced lifestyle
- Consider the use of medications in combination with psychosocial treatments
- Facilitate the transition between the levels of care between residential or hospital-based treatment programs and structured partial hospital or intensive outpatients programs
- Incorporate strategies to improve adherence to treatment and medications

Toxicology Testing/Drug Screening

Toxicology testing/drug screening can be a critical tool in the multimodal approach to addiction treatment. These tests can detect the presence of a substance (or its metabolite) in the body for a specified window period. These may be done to contribute to the confirmation of a diagnosis of SUD and to support recovery through frequent, random testing and (more increasingly) are used for workplace (i.e., preemployment, periodic, or postaccident) testing (Swotinsky & Smith, 2006). The most commonly used matrices for drug testing are urine and serum, but other body fluids may be utilized under certain circumstances. Specific protocols (e.g., chain of custody) are followed to ensure integrity of the specimens, and a medical review officer typically interprets results. With the exception of alcohol, the level of the substance detectable does not provide any reliable indication of the amount used or the level of impairment at the time of use or the time of testing. Drug testing does not have the technologic sophistication to distinguish between recreational use, drug abuse, drug misuse, accidental exposure, or addiction.

■ NURSING INTERVENTIONS FOR SPECIFIC SUBSTANCE-RELATED DISORDERS

There is no standardized intervention that will work for every individual with a substance-related disorder, because they may differ greatly with respect to severity,

BOX 26-12 Synthetic Cathinones ("Bath Salts")

The term "bath salts" refers to an emerging family of drugs containing one or more synthetic chemicals related to cathinone, an amphetamine-like stimulant found naturally in the Khat plant. Their use can produce euphoria, increased sociability, and increased sex drive. Paranoia, agitation, hallucinations, psychotic and violent behaviour, and death have also been reported with its use. Bath salts take the form of a white or brown crystalline powder and can be taken orally, inhaled, or injected. Early indications are that synthetic cathinones have high abuse and addictive potential. Another danger is that these products may contain other unknown ingredients that may have their own harmful effects.

Source: National Institute on Drug Abuse (NIDA). (2012b). DrugFacts: Synthetic cathinones ("bath salts"). Retrieved from www.drugabuse. ov/publications/drugfacts/synthetic-cathinones-bath-salts

substance of abuse, and their own unique biologic, psychological, social, and spiritual considerations. Often several approaches can work together; others may be deemed inappropriate. Treatment programs usually combine psychosocial interventions with other approaches to provide a comprehensive plan based on the individual's needs. Nursing interventions vary depending on the nature of the current problems, the status and severity of the illness, and the individual's situation. For an individual who is being detoxified, physical interventions (e.g., monitoring vital signs and neurologic functioning) are necessary. When the SUD is secondary to other physical or psychiatric problems, it may be a priority to address these concurrently.

The following section is organized by the classes of substances and addresses some of their unique features. Greater level of detail has been provided to the substances most frequently abused in Canadian society: alcohol, cannabis, caffeine, opioids, and tobacco. These are the ones nurses are more likely to encounter in everyday practice, including mental health and psychiatric settings but also other settings (i.e., community health, hospital, and primary care). Further details on addictive substances are readily available on the National Institute on Drug Abuse (NIDA) Web site. It is not uncommon for new addictive drugs and drug use trends to emerge, and one of these ("bath salts") is addressed in Box 26-12.

Alcohol-Related Disorders

The physiologic effects of alcohol are dependent on a multitude of physiologic factors that include, among many others, dose, genetic factors, the level of tolerance, gender, body mass, body fat, liver mass, and metabolic rate. The acute effects of alcohol are usually characterized by feelings of warmth, relaxation, mild sedation, and a sense of social disinhibition. In alcohol-naïve individuals, a blood alcohol concentration of 160 mg% is associated with obvious intoxication symptoms and signs, which may not be evident in persons who have developed tolerance on physiologic or behavioural levels. In progressively higher concentrations, there is a greater depressant effect on inhibition and behavioural control, producing heightened emotions, emotional lability (or mood swings), impulsivity, impaired motor and cognitive functioning (including impairment in memory, concentration, attention span, and judgement). In increasingly higher concentrations, it also leads to more severe impairment of motor functions and speech, blackouts, confusion, delirium, respiratory failure, stupor, coma (at about 400 to 560 mg%), and death. Although sedating, alcohol impairs the quality of sleep by disturbing the normal sleep architecture.

Alcohol use is also associated with worsening of certain psychiatric conditions and symptoms and may increase the risk of depression, suicide, and homicide and the risk of harm to self or others. Alcohol also induces the liver enzyme system that leads to more rapid metabolism of therapeutic (and other) compounds, with an anticipated potential for lower therapeutic effects. Excessive or long-term use of alcohol can adversely affect any or all body systems, some of which could be serious, disabling, and irreversible even if alcohol use is discontinued. These include varying degrees of cognitive impairment, amnestic disorder, dementia, and other neurologic complications, for example, neuropathies, cerebellar degeneration, and brain atrophy. In the category of alcohol-induced cognitive disorders, there are the conditions of Wernicke's syndrome and Korsakoff's syndrome. The former develops as a result of thiamine deficiency and manifests with oculomotor dysfunction, ataxia, and confusion, while the latter is characterized by retrograde and anterograde amnesia with confabulation as a key feature.

Alcohol Withdrawal

Reduction of consumption, or abstinence, in some individuals may lead to withdrawal symptoms from alcohol that may even progress into life-threatening complications. Symptoms of withdrawal typically start hours after the last consumption of alcohol and may include nausea and vomiting, tactile disturbances, tremor, auditory disturbances, paroxysmal sweats, visual disturbances, anxiety, headaches (or sensations of fullness in the head), agitation, and disturbances in orientation and clouding of the sensorium. It may also include autonomic disturbances, for example, blood pressure increases, tachycardia, and diaphoresis, and in severe cases, withdrawal may progress to seizures (tonic–clonic), delirium (**delirium tremens**), or death.

Alcohol detoxification treatment consists of achieving safe withdrawal from alcohol followed by psychosocial interventions and the option of pharmacotherapy. Management of intoxication and withdrawal (Box 26-13

BOX 26-13 Clinical Features of Alcohol Withdrawal

Minor Withdrawal: Patients are anxious and may experience nausea and vomiting, coarse tremor, sweating, tachycardia, and hypertension. Symptoms typically appear 6 to 12 hours after the last drink, or shortly after the BAL reaches 0, and are usually resolved within 48 to 72 hours.

Intermediate Withdrawal: Patients experience the symptoms of minor withdrawal in addition to seizures, dysrhythmias, and/or hallucinosis. Within 12 to 72 hours after cessation of drinking, grand mal and nonfocal seizures typically occur. Dysrhythmias range in severity from occasional ectopic beats to atrial fibrillation and supraventricular or ventricular tachycardia. Patients are aware of the unreal nature of their auditory or visual hallucinations and remain oriented and alert.

Major Withdrawal (Delirium Tremens): Patients experience severe agitation, gross tremulousness, marked psychomotor and autonomic hyperactivity, global confusion, disorientation, and auditory, visual, or tactile hallucinations. They tend to occur 5 or 6 days after severe, untreated withdrawal. Symptoms fluctuate and are often more severe at night. These may include severe diaphoresis and vomiting, tachycardia, hypertension, and fever. Sudden death can occur.

Source: Brands, B., Kahan, M., Selby, P., & Wilson, L. (2000). *Medical management of alcohol and drug-related problems: A physician's manual* (2nd ed.). Toronto, ON: Centre for Addiction and Mental Health.

discusses the clinical features of withdrawal) requires a safe environment, and hospitalization may be indicated if there is a history of seizures, delirium, or comorbid medical or psychiatric conditions. The level of withdrawal is used to determine the most appropriate dose of pharmacotherapy-assisted symptom-triggered detoxification management and is measured by conducting a brief rating scale, the Clinical Institute Withdrawal Assessment for Alcohol (CIWA-R; Revised, Clinical Institute of Alcohol Withdrawal for Alcohol, Addiction Research Foundation, or Centre for Addiction and Mental Health [CAMH] found in Appendix F). Medication administered early in the course of withdrawal (and in sufficient dosages) can prevent the development of delirium tremens.

Poor nutrition and vitamin deficiencies are often symptoms of alcohol addiction. Thiamine (vitamin B_1) may be needed when a patient is in withdrawal to decrease ataxia and other symptoms of deficiency. It is usually given orally, 100 mg four times daily, but can be given intramuscularly or by intravenous infusion with glucose. Folic acid deficiency is corrected with administration of 1 mg orally, four times daily. Magnesium deficiency has also been found in some individuals with long-term alcohol consumption. Traditionally, patients have been given magnesium to treat or prevent alcohol withdrawal syndrome (AWS). Evidence to support this practice is limited and is often based on the controversial

link between hypomagnesaemia and AWS. Magnesium sulphate, which enhances the body's response to thiamine and reduces seizures, was typically given as a prophylactic for patients with histories of withdrawal seizures. There is, however, insufficient evidence to determine whether magnesium sulphate is beneficial or harmful for the treatment or prevention of AWS. The use of benzodiazepines, multivitamins, and thiamine, as well as fluid balance should be monitored, and supportive treatment provided.

Alcohol Use Disorder

The goal of treatment depends on the nature, extent, and severity of the alcohol use disorder. Coexisting conditions are also important determinants of the therapeutic approach and methods used. The best way to match the type and intensity of treatment to the individual needs of the patient remains unclear as no superior systematic outcomes have been demonstrated for residential or intensive day program treatment compared with once- or twice-weekly outpatient treatment (Willembring, 2011). Psychosocial interventions, as described earlier, should be offered at all stages of treatment in combination with pharmacotherapy and at the appropriate level of care. The suggestion to include attendance at AA is routinely offered. The outcome monitoring for alcohol use disorder treatment includes reporting on sobriety and abstinence. Serial monitoring of liver function tests, ethyl glucoronide (ethyl glucuronide/EtG, is a metabolite of ethyl alcohol that is formed in the body by glucuronidation following exposure to ethanol), carbohydrate-deficient transferrin, and Early Detection of Alcohol Consumption (EDAC) testing can provide valuable information on the course of the condition and success of treatment and supplement the self-reported abstinence and sobriety.

Following detoxification (when necessary), there are several medication options that exist to support the treatment of alcohol addiction. These include the following:

- *Disulfiram* is a medication that blocks the effects of aldehyde dehydrogenase and leads to a severely unpleasant reaction (including flushing, nausea, vomiting, and diarrhoea) when the person consumes alcohol. It is suitable only for reliable and motivated patients. This is an adjunct therapy that deters drinking while the individual learns new coping skills and alters abuse behaviours through other treatment approaches. Disulfiram's potential adverse effects include hepatotoxicity and neuropathy, which, along with potentially severe interactions with alcohol, limit its widespread use.

- *Naltrexone*, originally used as a treatment for opioid-related disorders, targets alcohol's effects on the brain and requires relatively normal liver functions. The use of this opioid antagonist medication cannot be in conjunction with any opioid medication as it will trigger an opioid withdrawal syndrome. It is further contraindicated in pregnancy and suicidal patients. Naltrexone may be particularly useful in patients who continue to drink heavily. Targeted use of naltrexone also may be effective for decreasing alcohol consumption levels among problem drinkers who do not suffer from addiction.

- *Acamprosate* has the ability to curb cravings for alcohol and may be an effective adjunct treatment in motivated persons who are also receiving psychosocial interventions.

● **STUDY NOTE**

STUDY NOTE Alcohol use disorder requires nursing assessment and interventions in all settings (home, community, ambulatory, inpatient, and long-term settings). Nurses who are open to the possibility that no individual is too young or too old, too healthy or too infirm, or too poor or too wealthy to have substance use problems (to alcohol, tobacco, and other drugs) are well positioned to detect areas of potential or actual need. Patients who abuse alcohol for long periods of time, and especially those who are deemed physiologically addicted, are at high risk for developing medical complications during withdrawal, for example, delirium tremens. Observing for risk/signs of seizure activity is a priority of nursing intervention.

Caffeine-Related Disorders

Caffeine is the world's most popular psychoactive substance and most widely used drug. It is a mild CNS stimulant that is found in many drinks (e.g., coffee, tea, cocoa, soft drinks, and energy drinks), chocolate, and in many over-the-counter medications (e.g., analgesics, stimulants, appetite suppressants, and cold relief preparations). A typical cup of brewed coffee contains 100 mg caffeine, but the content may vary greatly depending on the type of product or beverage.

Caffeine curbs fatigue and increases mental acuity, exerts stimulating effects on both mental and motor performance, and is subjectively viewed as beneficial by some in alleviating mood. It may, however, cause or exacerbate tremors; impair motor performance; and lead to anxiety, dysphoria, and insomnia. Higher doses increase the heart rate; stimulate respiratory, vasomotor, and vagal centres and cardiac muscles, resulting in increased heart contractibility; dilate pulmonary and coronary blood vessels; and constrict blood flow to the cerebral vascular system.

Caffeine Intoxication

Symptoms of caffeine intoxication include restlessness, nervousness, excitement, insomnia, flushed face, diuresis, and gastrointestinal (GI) complaints. Symptoms that generally appear at levels of more than 1 g/day include

muscle twitching, rambling flow of thought and speech, tachycardia or cardiac arrhythmia, periods of inexhaustibility, and psychomotor agitation (APA, 2013). The symptoms usually remit within the 1st day or so and do not have any known long-lasting consequences. Caffeine intoxication has been observed among young individuals after consumption of highly caffeinated products, including energy drinks. Individuals who have consumed very high doses of caffeine may require immediate medical attention as such doses may be lethal (APA, 2013).

Caffeine Withdrawal

When used in high doses over the course of time, caffeine can be associated with unpleasant withdrawal symptoms when abruptly tapered or discontinued. Withdrawal symptoms may include headache, insomnia, abnormal dreams, drowsiness, fatigue, impaired psychomotor performance, difficulty concentrating, craving, yawning, and nausea. Heavy consumers of caffeine who drastically and rapidly reduce or discontinue consumption may be at risk for withdrawal. Preferentially, caffeine should be reduced gradually in those considered to be consuming in excess, and this may occur over the course of days or weeks. Those deemed physiologically dependent may benefit from additional support. Psychoeducation can help individuals learn about the caffeine contents of beverages and medication, providing the ability to gradually switch to decaffeinated beverages.

Cannabis-Related Disorders

Cannabis is the most widely used illicit drug in Canada, and although occasionally classified as a hallucinogenic drug, its effects are less intense than that of other hallucinogens. Depending on the dose and route of administration, its effects begin shortly after administration (when smoked) and typically last from 1 to 3 hours (or longer when swallowed). Cannabis' effects include relaxation, euphoria, at times dyscoria (abnormal pupillary reaction or shape), distortion of senses, conjunctival injection, spatial misperception, time distortion (time standing still), tachycardia, hypotension, and increased appetite/food cravings ("the munchies"). Cannabinoids are also synthetically produced and commercially available for the treatment of selected medical conditions/symptoms (e.g., appetite stimulation related to medical illness in HIV/AIDS, remedy pain, multiple sclerosis, and for the treatment of nausea) (Box 26-14 explores this topic further).

In the short term, cannabis can result in motor impairment, loss of coordination and balance, and slowing of reaction time. This translates into the potential for significant impairment in the ability to safely operate machinery or a vehicle, and studies show that approximately 4% to 14% of drivers who sustained injury or died in traffic accidents tested positive for THC (Ramaekers, Berghaus, van Laar, & Drummer, 2004). When smoked,

---

BOX 26-14 Synthetic Cannabinoids and Medical Marijuana

Cannabinoids are also synthetically produced and commercially available for the treatment of selected medical conditions/symptoms (e.g., appetite stimulation related to medical illness in HIV/AIDS, remedy pain, and multiple sclerosis and for the treatment of nausea). Only under very specific and regulated circumstances, individuals who qualify may access the drug through the federal Marihuana Medical Access Regulations. Unless the particular individual has a legal exemption, it is illegal to possess, cultivate, or sell marijuana in Canada.

Cannabinoids have a largely unproven history of medicinal use for ailments such as pain management, psychiatric illnesses (while it can make conditions like schizophrenia worse), headaches, and obstetric and gynaecologic conditions. Cannabis preparations have the disadvantages of instability, varying strength, and insolubility in water, making it difficult for the drug to enter the bloodstream from the digestive track.

---

cannabis delivers to the body similar toxic chemicals to tobacco, and exposure during pregnancy may result in cognitive problems in offspring. Long-term use may impair consolidation of memory, recall ability, and impair cognition, hence interfering with academic functioning. Weight gain can also occur as a result of chronic appetite stimulation. Persons consuming high-potency cannabis, or heavy doses, may develop psychotic symptoms, and the use of cannabis is recognized as an independent risk factor in the development of schizophrenia and psychosis.

The mainstay for the treatment of cannabis use disorders is psychosocial treatment. This includes motivational enhancement, psychodynamic and interpersonal therapy, and relapse prevention. There is no medication proven to be superior to placebo in the treatment of this condition.

Hallucinogen-Related Disorders

The hallucinogens (the psychedelics) refer to a class of drugs that are sometimes used in religious/spiritual settings, and some of the drugs in this class may also be termed "entheogens." This broad classification encompasses agents with varied chemical structures that can elicit varied pharmacologic effects but produce similar alterations of perception, mood, and cognition in users. There are more than 100 different hallucinogens with substantially different molecular structures and unique features and include the "designer drugs." They fall into two different chemical groups: serotonin or tryptamine related, and phenylethylamine or amphetamine related. In addition, miscellaneous ethnobotanical compounds are within this classification (e.g., *salvia divinorum*), but cannabis is not. Some of these substances (i.e., LSD) have a long half-life and extended duration to the extent that the user may spend a day using and/or recovering from their effects, and others are short acting (APA, 2013).

These drugs have salient effects in changing the senses (e.g., visual, auditory, gustatory, tactile, and olfactory) and may induce euphoria or dysphoria, altered body image, distorted sensory perceptions, confusion, incoordination, and impaired judgement and memory. Hallucinogens typically affect the autonomic and regulatory nervous systems first, increasing heart rate and body temperature, and slightly elevating blood pressure. The individual may experience dry mouth, dizziness, and subjective feelings of being hot or cold. Intense mood and sexual behaviour changes may occur, and the subject may feel unusually close to others or distant and isolated. In severe cases, individuals have reported paranoia, depersonalization, illusions, delusions, and hallucinations.

Phencyclidine (PCP or angel dust), not a true hallucinogen, can affect many neurotransmitter systems; it interferes with the functioning of the glutamate but also enhances dopamine release. At low to moderate doses, PCP causes altered perception of body image but rarely produces visual hallucinations. PCP can also cause effects that mimic the primary symptoms of schizophrenia, such as delusions and mental turmoil. People who use PCP for long periods of time have memory loss and speech difficulties.

Ketamine ("Special-K") is an anaesthetic drug and follows the characteristics of PCP, albeit less potent on an equivalent mass basis. Ketamine has legitimate medical utility in both human and veterinary medicine, with specific value in emergency medicine. In illicit settings it is often injected, insufflated (i.e., blown into a body cavity), smoked, or taken orally, and it has a similar physical appearance to cocaine (pure). Ketamine has been reported as a drug frequently used in "date rape" cases.

The mechanism of action on the brain is similar for both PCP and ketamine, namely to block a specific subset of protein molecules, called NMDA (*N*-methyl-D-aspartic acid) receptors, involved in memory functions of the brain. Upon administration, a state of acute mental decompensation can occur, characterized by diminished ability to think and carry on daily activities, and typically includes loss of memory (both long term and short term). A sense of detachment from the external world, or from their own body, occurs, and in these dissociative states, certain thoughts, emotions, sensations, and/or memories may not be integrated in the usual fashion when compared to a drug-free state. In sufficient doses, the appearance of disorganization can occur, possibly followed by the appearance of stupor.

Inhalant-Related Disorders

Inhalants refer to a group of chemical vapours or gasses, including organic solvents, or *volatile substances*, that are inhaled (breathed in), causing a high. These substances are not intended for human consumption, and although the effects may vary, several are considered CNS depressants. Inhalants typically are used by younger individuals in lower socioeconomic settings where they are often available, accessible, and generally affordable. Inhalants, particularly solvents, are a particular challenge in some Aboriginal communities of Canada. The inhalants are divided into four classes, but there are hundreds of different chemicals belonging to each class:

1. Volatile solvents (benzene, toluene, xylene, acetone, hexane, felt-tip markers, hobby glue, airplane glue, polyvinyl chloride cement, rubber cement, dry cleaning fluid, spot removers, degreasers, computer cleaners, paint and nail polish removers, paint thinners, correction fluids, lighter fluid)
2. Aerosols or spray cans (whipped cream and cooking oil sprays, hair spray, fluorocarbon, butane [pressurized liquids or gases], asthma sprays, deodorants, air fresheners)
3. Gases (oxide [laughing gas], chloroform, halothane, ether, butane, propane, enflurane, isoflurane, ethyl chloride)
4. Nitrates (amyl, butyl, isopropyl nitrate)

As a class, the inhalants are known to cause euphoria, sedation, emotional lability, and/or impaired judgement. In some cases, intoxication can result in respiratory depression, stupor, and coma. The chemical structure of the various types of inhalants is diverse, making it difficult to generalize about their effects. However, serious health consequences may ensue, including hearing loss, damage to the liver, kidney, lungs, and heart, as well as bone marrow suppression. Magnetic resonance imaging scans of users demonstrate severe changes in cerebral white matter, including atrophy, and a foetal solvent syndrome has been described (National Institute on Drug Abuse [NIDA], 2005a). Fatalities may occur even on the first exposure and are not thought to be dose related.

Opioid-Related Disorders

The opioids represent a broad category of psychoactive substances, consisting of both licit and illicit substances that act by attaching to the endogenous opioid receptors in the brain. The opioid family of substances include

1. Pure opioid agonists:
   a. Naturally occurring alkaloids: (opium), morphine, codeine
   b. Semisynthetic substances (e.g., heroin [diacetylmorphine])
   c. Synthetic substances (e.g., oxycodone, methadone, fentanyl, meperidine, hydrocodone, propoxyphene, tramadol)
2. Mixed agonist–antagonists (e.g., pentazocine, butorphanol)
3. Partial agonists: buprenorphine (combined with naloxone)

Opioids cause CNS depression, sleep or stupor, and analgesia, and possess strong reinforcing properties that

can quickly trigger addiction when used improperly. Opiates elicit their effects by binding to opioid receptors that are widely distributed throughout the brain and body. Two important effects produced by opioids are pleasure (or reward) and pain relief (analgesia). The brain itself also produces substances known as endorphins that activate the opiate receptors. Research indicates that endorphins are involved in many functions, including respiration, nausea, vomiting, pain modulation, and hormonal regulation (NIDA, 2005b).

Opioids may cause tolerance and physical dependence (sometimes rapidly) that appear to be specific for each receptor subtype. In the early stages, the use of opioids may be associated with euphoria in some cases. Tolerance develops particularly to the analgesic, respiratory depression, and sedative actions of the opioids. The common physical effects associated with the use of the opioids include sweating, nausea, constipation (which can progress to narcotic bowel syndrome), and dose-dependent sedation, fatigue, confusion, cognitive impairment, respiratory depression, as well as reproductive and endocrine effects (e.g., suppression of testosterone in men and menstrual irregularities in women). In some cases, the opioids are used concurrently with other sedative substances (e.g., benzodiazepines, alcohol, barbiturates, or sedating antidepressants). In these cases, the risk of CNS and respiratory depression may be especially salient, thus warranting an even higher level of vigilance in their assessment and management. There is further a phenomenon called medication-induced headaches, for example, with the chronic use of analgesics, where the analgesic drug is causally linked to the exacerbation of the headache, and improvement is noticed when the analgesic is discontinued.

Even when following a regimen as prescribed by a physician, individuals may become addicted to opioids, especially when injudiciously prescribed. Inquiry into the patterns of abuse of opioids should occur if persons report or are found to be "double-doctoring," "borrowing pain medications from others," and "buying black market medications," when individuals run out of their medication early, or if triplicate prescriptions are reported to be lost or stolen. Canada ranks as the world's second largest per-capita consumer of prescription opioids, and its rate of use increased by 203% between 2000 and 2010 (International Narcotics Control Board, 2013). In Canada, the (past-year) prevalence of nonmedical prescription opioid use was 15.5% for students and 5.9% for adults (Fischer et al., 2013).

Many Canadians initiate their use through a prescription for therapeutic purposes. In a study of opioid-dependent patients, 37% reported receiving opioids from physician prescriptions, 26% from both a prescription and "the street," and 21% from the street (Sproule, Brands, Li, & Catz-Biro, 2009). Although there is no current Canadian information, it has been estimated in the United States that the annual cost of the nonmedical use of prescription opioids is more than $50 billion, with lost productivity and crime accounting for 94% of this amount (Hansen, Oster, Edelsberg, Woody, & Sullivan, 2011).

Opioid Intoxication

Opioid intoxication typically does not require treatment except in cases where CNS or respiratory depression is a risk or where it is combined with other depressants (e.g., alcohol, barbiturates, or benzodiazepines). The use of an opioid receptor blocker, for example, naloxone or naltrexone, may be indicated in such cases, along with supportive treatment and monitoring of vital signs.

Opioid Withdrawal

When its use is discontinued or rapidly tapered after a period of continuous use, a rebound hyperexcitability withdrawal syndrome may occur. Withdrawal may be associated with severe cravings and mimics a "bad case of the flu," involving both the respiratory and GI systems. It may include symptoms of anxiety, dysphoria, nausea, vomiting, muscle aches, lacrimation or rhinorrhea, papillary dilatation, piloerection, sweating, diarrhea, yawning, fever, and insomnia. These withdrawal symptoms are not typically life threatening but can be particularly uncomfortable and may lead to significant distress. Medically ill, pregnant, very young, and very old individuals at risk of opioid withdrawal may be more prone to developing medical complications during withdrawal from opioids or combination substances.

Detoxification management is usually not associated with medical complications and serves only as the first stage of ongoing treatment for addiction to opioids. Detoxification is conducted with the use of medication options, for example, methadone, buprenorphine (combined with naloxone in Canada, suboxone), or by using a tapering regimen of the existing opioid. Clonidine is also useful in curbing withdrawal symptoms during abrupt discontinuation of opioids and can be combined with naltrexone. Care must be taken to avoid the development of orthostatic hypotension during detoxification using clonidine.

Opioid Use Disorder

For the treatment of opioid use disorders in individuals who have not achieved abstinence through psychosocial interventions, there are three pharmacologic options available in Canada: methadone, buprenorphine (Suboxone, i.e., with naloxone), and naltrexone. For the first two options, the prescribing physician is required to have completed special training and to have been granted exemption and be registered at the provincial professional regulatory body.

Sedative, Hypnotic, and Anxiolytic-Related Disorders

Sedative, hypnotic, and anxiolytic-related (antianxiety) agents are synthetic medications that are sedating, induce sleep, and reduce anxiety. Barbiturates were the first class of drugs used to treat sleep disturbances and anxiety and have largely been replaced by benzodiazepines because of their comparative safety with regard to potential toxicity and addictive qualities. Benzodiazepines are often used to sedate individuals preoperatively, to treat seizures and alcohol withdrawal, and as muscle relaxants. The effects of benzodiazepines and other sedative–hypnotics include decreased anxiety, increased sedation, muscle relaxation, and increase seizure threshold.

The abuse of sedative, hypnotic, and anxiolytic-related agents is common and complex, especially among people who abuse other drugs to enhance their effects (e.g., opioids and alcohol) or to ease the agitation of drugs that have stimulant effects, such as ecstasy or cocaine. This is extremely dangerous and can put individuals at risk for overdose, causing coma or death. The combination of benzodiazepines and alcohol also complicates withdrawal treatment because the individual may seem to improve after the AWS subsides, only to have similar symptoms emerge as the benzodiazepine withdrawal syndrome appears. The severity of symptoms during benzodiazepine withdrawal depends on the duration and dosage of regular use; symptoms include the following:

- Anxiety rebound—tension, agitation, tremulousness, insomnia, anorexia
- Autonomic rebound—hypertension, tachycardia, sweating, hyperpyrexia
- Sensory excitement—paresthesias, photophobia, hyperacusis (sensitivity to sound), illusions
- Motor excitation—hyperreflexia, tremors, myoclonus, fasciculation (visible muscle contraction), myalgia, muscle weakness, tonic–clonic convulsions
- Cognitive excitement—nightmares, delirium, depersonalization, hallucinations

Stimulant-Related Disorders

This category of substances includes amphetamine and amphetamine-type stimulants, substances that are structurally different but have similar effects, such as methylphenidate, and cocaine as they have similar effects. Amphetamines and other stimulants may be obtained by prescription for the treatment of obesity, attention deficit/hyperactivity disorder, and narcolepsy. These prescribed stimulants may be diverted to the black market.

Cocaine is a powerful and highly addictive stimulant that is snorted (powder), smoked (crack), or injected. Cocaine is highly addictive and is often coadministered with other addictive substances like alcohol or tobacco. When snorted, injected, or smoked, cocaine rapidly crosses the blood–brain barrier and peak intoxication occurs within seconds after intravenous injection or crack smoking. Injecting releases the substance directly into the bloodstream and heightens the intensity of its effects. Smoking entails the inhalation of cocaine vapour or smoke into the lungs, where absorption into the bloodstream is as rapid as by injection (NIDA, 2009). Cocaine use causes tachycardia, hypertension, dilated pupils, and rises in body temperature. It may contribute to seizures, myocardial infarcts, cerebrovascular accidents, and crosses the placenta.

When cocaine is used concomitantly with alcohol, a potentially dangerous interaction may develop. Taken in combination, the two drugs are converted by the body to cocaethylene, which has a longer duration of action in the brain and is more cardiotoxic than either drug alone. Notably, this mixture of cocaine and alcohol is the most common two-drug combination that results in drug-related death (NIDA, 2009).

Shortly after cocaine is snorted, smoked, or injected, the individual experiences a sudden burst of alertness and energy ("cocaine rush"), euphoria, increased feelings of self-confidence, being in control, and sociability. There is an increase in sense awareness (e.g., sexuality is heightened, and sound, touch, and sight are more acute). There is also a decreased need for sleep and a lowering of appetite. Along with this, anxiety and restlessness as well as agitation may occur. With the use of higher doses, there may also occur panic, mania, psychosis (hallucinations, disorganization, and delusions), and erratic and bizarre behaviours, potentially leading up to violence and potential risk of harm. The use of cocaine in an individual with a vulnerability to depression, mania, or psychosis may experience exacerbation of symptoms of related psychiatric conditions.

The high is followed by a significant and intense depressive phase (let-down effect or "cocaine crash") in which the subject feels irritable, depressed, and tired and displays increased appetite and powerful cravings for the drug. The individual may desperately seek cocaine or even other drugs, to self-medicate some of the unpleasant side effects of the crash phase. Similar to the severe anxiety, restlessness, and agitation of intoxication, these symptoms may also appear during withdrawal. These, along with drug-seeking behaviour, may last for weeks, contributing to the extremely high relapse rates observed in these persons.

Long-term cocaine use depletes norepinephrine and, when the drug is discontinued, results in a "crash" causing the user to sleep 12 to 18 hours. Upon awakening, withdrawal symptoms may occur that are characterized by sleep disturbances with rebound rapid eye movement (REM) sleep, anergia (lack of energy), decreased libido, depression with possible suicidality, anhedonia, poor concentration, and cocaine craving. Depression typically resolves, and unless an underlying major depressive disorder is demonstrated, the use of antidepressants is not indicated.

Stimulant Withdrawal

Withdrawal from cocaine is usually relatively uncomplicated. There is a high risk of relapse, and the challenge is often to establish a recovery environment in which this risk minimized. Cocaine detoxification is not typically associated with medical complications and usually requires only supportive care. However, if a patient develops psychotic symptoms (e.g., hallucinations, delusions, or paranoia) during intoxication phases, specific treatments to remedy them may be required, such as the use of atypical antipsychotics. Amphetamine withdrawal symptoms are not as pronounced as those of cocaine withdrawal and are treated similarly. Evidence in support of treatment for addiction using pharmacologic agents is limited and is similar to that used for cocaine.

Stimulant Use Disorder

Treatment is complex and involves assessing the psychobiologic, social, and pharmacologic aspects of abuse. Psychosocial interventions form the mainstay of treatment for cocaine addiction treatment, and residential care may be required in cases where relapse risk cannot be adequately managed on an outpatient basis. Stabilization of the patient's recovery environment is pivotal in achieving lasting abstinence from cocaine, and inclusion in a 12-step program is recommended (e.g., Narcotics Anonymous). Patients using cocaine should be advised to abstain from alcohol as well, and if applicable, offered opportunities to quit smoking. To date, there is no medication proven to be superior to placebo in regards to cocaine addiction treatment. However, there are promising options, for example, topiramate, disulfiram, or modafinil, which may be considered in cases where psychosocial treatment alone has failed to yield optimal results (DeLima, de Olivera Soceres, Reisser, & Farrell, 2002).

Tobacco-Related Disorders

If tobacco were introduced to the market today, it could not become a legal product because of its high lethality index. Tobacco smoke contains over 6,000 chemicals, of which there are at least 172 toxic substances, 33 hazardous air pollutants, 47 chemicals restricted as hazardous waste, and 67 known human or animal carcinogens (U.S. Department of Health and Human Services, 2004). These exist whether tobacco smoke is inhaled in the act of smoking or by non-smokers out of the air indoors or outdoors. Nicotine is an addictive substance found within the tobacco plant, has both stimulant and depressant effects, and is considered as the fundamental chemical "driver" of the process of addiction in the brain. The use of tobacco products without nicotine would not be addictive but, paradoxically, nicotine is not the harmful chemical found within tobacco products, and pharmaceutical-grade (and dosage) nicotine is generally considered to be safe. It is the tar and other substances and additives in tobacco products that threaten health.

A cigarette provides approximately 10 puffs, and a person who smokes 20 cigarettes per day (one pack) is taking 200 doses of nicotine daily. No other drug—not even cocaine—is dosed that frequently and conditioned cues to smoke become established. As a result, desiring a cigarette becomes associated with everyday events such as getting up in the morning, drinking coffee or alcohol, taking a break, and having a conversation. The quantity and power of this conditioning are unique to cigarette smoking, and it is one of the reasons that smoking is so difficult to quit. Signs of tobacco use disorder include the urge to smoke within minutes of waking, smoking at regular intervals throughout the day, and continuing to smoke despite wanting to quit. People who are addicted may become tolerant to the desired effects and may no longer experience pleasure from smoking but continue to smoke in order to avoid nicotine withdrawal.

Tobacco Withdrawal

Symptoms of tobacco withdrawal vary but may include cravings, irritability, restlessness, difficulty concentrating, depression, frustration, anxiety, insomnia, fatigue, and increased appetite. Most symptoms reach maximum intensity at 24 to 48 hours and are relieved within a few weeks, but some individuals may be unable to concentrate and have strong cravings to smoke for weeks or months after quitting smoking. In recognition of the harmful effects of second-hand smoke for the patients, staff, visitors, and others, most hospitals and health care facilities are smoke free. Some patients are often placed into involuntary tobacco withdrawal as a result of protections from second-hand smoke policies.

Detoxification interventions are safe and reliable and minimize the suffering from tobacco withdrawal. Detoxification is not considered cessation intervention and, by itself, does not contribute to long-term abstinence. Detoxification is achieved through identifying patients who smoke, offering nicotine replacement therapy (NRT) at sufficient doses and not expecting a commitment to quit smoking. Effective detoxification requires repeated opportunities to receive NRT and provision of a supportive environment that includes omission of cues to smoke. Systematic measures that are required to ensure rapid treatment delivery include standing orders for NRT, ward stock for quick access, and supplies of a broad spectrum of NRT on hospital formulary (Els, Kunyk, Barak, Thomas, & Scharf, 2012).

Tobacco Use Disorder

There are individuals who are able to stop using tobacco independently without treatment, but others require formal assistance to achieve long-term abstinence. For some, quitting can be a complex process spanning months and/or years that requires support, medication, and multiple attempts. The optimal treatment design for tobacco use disorder treatment requires a comprehensive and multimodal approach that may include psychosocial and pharmacologic

interventions. Clinical practice guidelines that can serve as a suitable template for the delivery of smoking cessation treatments by nurses can be found in Box 26-15.

There are many opportunities for nurses to positively intervene with patients who smoke, as over 70% want to quit, almost half have tried to quit at least once in the past year, and fully one-third report that they want to quit in the next month (Leatherdale & Shields, 2009). In a Cochrane review of nursing interventions, Rice and Stead (2004) concluded that smoking cessation and/or counselling given by nurses can be effective. They identified that a nursing challenge is the incorporation of smoking behavioural monitoring and smoking cessation interventions as part of their daily practice. All patients can be asked about their tobacco use and given advice and/or counselling to quit along with reinforcement and follow-up. To dramatically enhance the likelihood of a successful quit attempt, clinical findings support the offer, and provision, of simple and strategic behavioural counselling and pharmacotherapy to every person interested in quitting. Those who are not ready to make an attempt at cessation should be offered empathetic counselling designed to permit a reassessment of their reasons for continued smoking and an invitation to seek assistance with at any time. Several levels of evidence support the use of the following modalities.

Psychosocial Interventions

Psychosocial interventions, such as group, individual, telephone, office, or Web-based counselling, should be routinely offered in combination with medication for increased successful cessation rates (Cohen, Dragonetti, Herie, & Barker, 2012). The provision of simple advice regarding the avoidance of high-risk relapse situations, recognition of

---

BOX 26-15 The 5 A Approach to Tobacco Addiction Treatment

A1 = Ask—Systematically identify all tobacco users at every visit.

A2 = Advise—In a clear, strong, and personalized fashion all tobacco users should be strongly advised to quit.

A3 = Assess—Every tobacco user's willingness to make a quit attempt should be assessed.

A4 = Assist—Help the patient set a quit date, advise the patient to tell family and friends about quitting and to remove tobacco products from the home/work environment, and anticipate challenges in the weeks to come. Also offer the combination of pharmacotherapy and psychosocial interventions.

A5 = Arrange follow-up—Ensure follow-up contact and approach the treatment in a longitudinal fashion.

Source: Fiore, M., et al. (2008). A clinical practice guideline for treating tobacco use and dependence: 2008 update. A U.S. Public Health Service report. *American Journal of Preventive Medicine*, *35*(2), 158–176.

settings or circumstances where smoking has been particularly common, management of acute cravings, and development of smoke-free guidelines for home and vehicles are all important in accentuating the likelihood of cessation success. Although the evidence suggests that interventions are effective across a broad range of populations, tailored interventions may be advised for selected subpopulations (e.g., individuals with mental illness, women who are pregnant, and smokeless tobacco users).

Pharmacologic Interventions

Nicotine replacement therapy (NRT) is available in five forms: transdermal patch, chewing "gum," inhaler/vapourizer, lozenge, and spray. Individuals who smoke seek to maintain a certain individualized level of nicotine and when their nicotine levels fall, distinct and significant discomfort usually occurs (withdrawal symptoms). NRT stimulates nicotine receptors and relieves withdrawal symptoms, and its appropriate use roughly doubles success rates of quit attempts. Combinations of NRT (e.g., patch and a short-acting version concurrently) have the advantage of allowing the patient to titrate his or her nicotine intake to meet his or her unique needs and are associated with increased levels of success.

Bupropion is an antidepressant that was serendipitously found to be effective in tobacco cessation. Bupropion inhibits the reuptake of dopamine in the reward centres of the brain, as well as norepinephrine, a chemical associated with withdrawal symptoms. Its use has been shown to double success rates in those attempting to quit smoking.

Varenicline, a third-generation smoking cessation pharmacotherapy, directly and distinctly binds to $\alpha_4\beta_2$ nicotinic receptors. These receptor sites are completely blocked but only partially stimulated reducing the transmission of neurologic impulses and causing a reduced amount of dopamine to be released in the reward centres of the brain. Consequently, the patient experiences little to no withdrawal symptoms and no pleasurable sensation if a cigarette is smoked. Varenicline has been shown to be a superior pharmacotherapy for cessation when compared with NRT and bupropion, with an odds ratio of quitting of approximately 3:1.

The Canadian labelling of NRT, bupropion, and varenicline is required to have a warning to heighten the level of awareness of adverse events and mitigate potential risks in patients taking cessation medications. These warnings note the potential risk of serious mental health events including changes in behaviour, depressed mood, hostility, and suicidal thoughts when quitting smoking. It is not conclusive whether these risks are due to the medications or to the effects of quitting smoking. The tobacco plant contains a class of chemicals, the β-carbolines, which are monoamine oxidase inhibitors (like certain antidepressants). Quitting smoking stops the ingestion of these naturally found antidepressants and, for this reason, depressive symptoms may be triggered in some individuals who are quitting smoking. Risks while taking tobacco cessation medications must always be weighed against the significant health benefits of quitting smoking, and the awareness that this symptomatology may also be expressed in response to tobacco cessation. Despite the absence of evidence for a causal link between cessation medications and neuropsychiatric adverse effects, prudence suggests screening for mood issues in patients who consume tobacco products as well as those going through the quitting process (Els, 2012). Current labelling also suggests that patients should be offered NRT prior to considering the use of varenicline.

The scientific evidence does not support the use of alternative tobacco-based nicotine delivery systems (e.g., smokeless tobacco) as a smoking cessation aid. Despite claims by the tobacco industry to the contrary, these are not considered a "harm reduction" measure and may in actuality discourage or postpone cessation efforts in patients who would otherwise have quit, or may induce another form of tobacco addiction, and have associated health consequences such as pancreatic cancer. There is emerging evidence in support of the electronic cigarette (containing nicotine) as a promising intervention to assist cessation. More research is required to further explore this nicotine delivery device.

Gambling Disorder

Gambling is the activity of risk taking for the purposes of gaining an advantage or benefit, and it is a massive business in Canada, producing vast revenue for investors as well as for government. Gambling disorder typically develops over the course of years, and most individuals with the disorder gradually increase their frequency of gambling and amount of wagering. The past-year prevalence of gambling disorder is 0.2% to 0.3% in the general population. Males are more likely to have a gambling disorder (although this gap appears to be narrowing); the lifetime prevalence for males is about 0.6% (APA, 2013). More recently, the Internet has expanded the range and accessibility of gambling to younger people (Tupperman & Wanner, 2012).

The mainstay of treatment for gambling disorder is psychotherapy, specifically cognitive and behavioural modalities. Brief interventions and motivational enhancement have also shown to have benefit in improving outcomes. There are no registered pharmacotherapeutic options, although some benefits have been demonstrated with the use of opioid antagonists (e.g., naltrexone), bupropion, lithium, and selective serotonin reuptake inhibitors (e.g., paroxetine and fluvoxamine).

None of these studies have, however, examined treatment effects for longer than 6 months. Individuals report benefit from attendance at Gamblers' Anonymous (12-step–based) and in some situations voluntary self-exclusion programs may offer some degree of protection. Due to the high rates of co-occurrence of other psychiatric conditions, assessment and treatment of comorbid symptoms and syndromes are deemed prudent. The high rates of suicide in gambling addiction warrant special attention to prevention.

Nursing Care Plan 26-1

Patient With Alcohol Use Disorder

Kenneth W. is a 55-year-old lawyer with a 25-year history of alcohol use disorder. He is the youngest of three children born and raised on a farm. His mother is still living with his older sister, but his father died of cirrhosis, a complication of years of alcohol use. Kenneth is married and has two children who he rarely sees. Kenneth starting binge drinking on weekends when he was in university, and this developed into a regular pattern once he started his law practice. His drinking has escalated after he started having difficulties with his partners at work, and he reports consuming up to 2 L of vodka a day. He began smoking in his early teens and continues to smoke a pack a day of cigarettes.

Recently, Kenneth was involved in a car accident and has been charged with operating a vehicle with a BAC over 0.08%. He was admitted to the hospital through the emergency department following the collision, with a gash above his right eye. Kenneth began to have symptoms of alcohol withdrawal and became anxious shortly after admission. He requested hospital admission for alcohol detoxification and was transferred to a detoxification and brief treatment unit.

Setting: Inpatient Detoxification Unit, Psychiatric Hospital

Baseline Assessment: First admission, last drink and cigarette at 7 PM. Admission vital signs: T 99.2°F, HR 98, R 20, and BP 140/88 on admission to the ER. He has a history of withdrawal seizures and hallucinations (likely delirium tremens during past withdrawal). He had a BAL of 0.15 mg%, becoming increasingly anxious and restless over the next hour. His CIWA score was 17, and he was given diazepam, 20 mg PO, as ordered, at that time. Decision to conduct CIWA 4-hourly.

Five hours after admission, vital signs were T 99.8°F, HR 110, R 22, and BP 152/100. He continued to be anxious and was tremulous, diaphoretic, and nauseous. CIWA Score had increased to 22, and diazepam 20 mg PO stat was given. The decision was made to conduct CIWA scores hourly. The next CIWA score was 15, and 4 hours later it was 10.

Associated Psychiatric Diagnosis	Medications
Alcohol use disorder (severe)	Deferred until detoxification is complete, after which consideration will be given to acamprosate, naltrexone, or disulfiram.
Alcohol withdrawal	Thiamine Folic acid Multivitamins Diazepam, 20 mg stat, followed by CIWA score, based on elevated BP, HR, and tremors Haloperidol, 5.0 mg IM PRN, for hallucinations or agitation
Tobacco withdrawal	Transdermal nicotine patch 21 mg QD PRN Nicotine inhaler 10 mg, puff on cartridge for 45 minutes, as directed PRN
Tobacco use disorder	Deferred, but continuation of nicotine replacement is offered postdetoxification

Nursing Diagnosis 1: Risk Related to Alcohol Withdrawal

Defining Characteristics	Related Factors
Altered vital signs Altered cerebral function secondary to alcohol withdrawal Altered mood states	Withdrawal is common among patients consuming more than 40 drinks per week or in those with other risk factors. Symptoms of detoxification include fever, high blood pressure, tachycardia, tremor or sweating, confusion, and dehydration. Level of consciousness, orientation, perceptual disturbances (hallucinations or illusions), mood, and thought processes including suicide ideation and cognitive deficits

Nursing Care Plan 26-1

Outcomes

Initial	Discharge
1. Detoxification from alcohol will be monitored, based on CIWA Score, and management implemented to treat symptoms and to prevent complications	2. Bridging from inpatient from level IV care for detoxification to a regimen that is acceptable to KW and keeps him engaged in ongoing treatment

Interventions

Interventions	Rationale	Ongoing Assessment
Welcome to treatment and assure Kenneth that he is in a safe place. Inform of what he may expect during withdrawal. Start with engagement for treatment.	Begin to establish relationship, a therapeutic alliance, with the patient.	See Box 26-11.
Monitor vital signs, orientation, and identify stage of alcohol withdrawal and severity of symptoms.	The more severe the reactions, the more likely that anxiety, disorientation, confusion, and restlessness increase.	Administer (symptom triggered, CIWA) diazepam (for elevated BP, HR, and tremors) and haloperidol (for hallucinations or tremors) prn and report symptoms.
Institute seizure precautions (bed in low position, padded side rails).	Withdrawal seizures usually occur within 48 hours after last drink.	Monitor for seizure activity.
Orient the patient to surroundings and call light, and maintain consistent physical environment.	Disorientation often occurs as BAL drops. These symptoms can last several days.	Determine Kenneth's level of orientation to surroundings, and whether he can use call light.
Avoid sudden moves, loud noises, discussion of the patient at bedside, and lighting that casts shadows downwards.	Decreased environmental stimulation helps calm the patient, which in turn promotes optimal CNS responses.	Observe reactions to loud noises and monitor room environment.

Evaluation

Outcomes (at 3 days)	Revised Outcomes	Interventions
Orientated, hydrated, and no seizure activity.	Engage in the development of a recovery plan.	Continue to monitor for any signs of disorientation.

Nursing Diagnosis 2: Discomfort Related to Tobacco Withdrawal

Defining Characteristics	Related Factors
Symptoms of tobacco withdrawal include irritability, restlessness, anxiety, insomnia, and fatigue.	Discomfort related to tobacco withdrawal may be difficult to distinguish from alcohol withdrawal.

Outcomes

Initial	Discharge
1. Will be comfortable without smoking during hospitalization period	2. Will be provided additional resources and supports to extend tobacco abstinence into a cessation attempt, if desired

Continued

Nursing Care Plan 26-1 (*continued*)

Interventions

Intervention	Rationale	Ongoing Assessment
Explain that the hospital has a non-smoking policy. This is to protect patients, visitors, and staff from the harmful effects of second-hand smoke. The purpose of the policy is not to "force" Kenneth to quit smoking, or to "make his life difficult."	There are direct causes and linkages between exposure to second-hand smoke and serious health effects among nonsmokers.	Monitor Kenneth's level of comfort and assess for breakthrough cravings. Assess for sleep disruption; if present, may remove patch at bedtime.
Discuss prevention of discomfort related to tobacco withdrawal. Assess whether Kenneth's wife is a current smoker and the influence this may have on his ability to abstain. Offer a 21-mg transdermal nicotine patch qd to prevent tobacco withdrawal. This can be combined with other forms of NRT.	The blood level of nicotine begins to drop immediately following smoking a cigarette. Smell off of clothing, and cigarette products, may provide potent cues to smoke. The higher dose 21-mg nicotine patch recommended for pack-per-day smoker; may not be of sufficient dosage to prevent breakthrough cravings. Side effects may include sleep disruption.	

Evaluation

Outcomes (Day 2)	Revised Outcomes	Interventions
Refused nicotine patch, and becomes increasingly anxious to leave the unit to smoke.	Remain abstinent and engaged in the treatment regimen on the unit.	Offer prn nicotine inhaler to provide some immediate relief, and reoffer nicotine patch for longer-term effects.

■ SPECIAL POPULATIONS AND SITUATIONS

Youth

Adolescence constitutes the life stage with the greatest vulnerability to developing SUDs. It is a time of life when self-regulatory executive functions are still maturing, and this period is characterized by pronounced changes in behaviour, with increased risk taking, novelty and sensation seeking, social interactions, and high activity. At the same time, there may be low levels of anxiety regarding the risk of harm, strong emotional states, and mood instability. During this age, the prefrontal cortex and limbic systems are undergoing prominent reorganization in myelination, neuronal plasticities, and structural rearrangements, and drug exposure might result in different neuroadaptations than those that occur during adulthood. Substance use during this critical period of cortical development may lead to increased vulnerability to addiction and to lifelong changes of executive function. In general, the younger a person starts using substances, the more likely he or she is to progress and exceed occasional experimentation and to move into frequent abuse,

with a higher chance of developing addiction (Swendsen & Le Moal, 2011).

Not all young people who experiment with substances proceed to levels that bring health problems. The serious risks of substances to youth are physical (e.g., liver and heart damage, impaired brain function, impaired reproductive organ development), psychological (e.g., depression, sleep disorders, conduct disorders) and social (e.g., academic performance, relationships with family/friends, and increased exposure to risk situations). It is important to address a developing substance problem in young people as early as possible, with a recognition that they are different from adults in many ways: their unique developmental (e.g., difficulty comprehending future consequences) and psychiatric issues, differences in values and belief systems, and environmental considerations (such as strong peer influence). Family involvement plays a critical role in an adolescent's treatment and recovery.

College Students

Peak lifetime alcohol use generally occurs in an individual's late teens and early 20s. The prevalence of heavy episodic (or binge) drinking (defined as reaching a BAL of

0.08 or higher, usually by consuming five or more drinks for men, four or more for women, in a 24-hour period) and the detrimental consequences resulting from this type of drinking have led to the classification of college binge drinking as a major public heath problem (Larimer, Kilmer, & Whiteside, 2011).

Advances are being made in identifying effective strategies to reduce alcohol (and other substance) consumption and its consequences among this population. These interventions include developing CBT skills (such as identifying and planning for or avoiding risky situations using protective strategies such as drink spacing, counting drinks, and limit setting), norm clarification (correcting misperceptions about drinking norms), using MI to reduce resistance and promote change, and challenging expectations. Environmental interventions are emerging as important components of an overall prevention strategy. These include strategies such as promoting alcohol-free options, creating an environment that supports health-promoting norms, limiting alcohol availability, restricting alcohol promotion, and developing policies/laws about consumption (Larimer et al., 2011).

Pregnancy and Lactation

Alcohol, tobacco, and other drug use during pregnancy can have serious detrimental effects on the course of pregnancy, as well as on the physiologic status of the foetus and newborn. Some women are able to stop using substances when they learn they are pregnant, but others may have difficulty stopping due to the severity of the addiction or withdrawal. Nurses should be aware that the use of substances is more stigmatized in pregnancy, so that women may minimize or deny their use, its harmful effects, and the need to seek care. The nurse should be aware of special social, emotional, and legal issues involving the treatment of pregnant women and be sensitive to their special needs. For example, women may fear that, by seeking prenatal care, their drug use will be detected by urine toxicology tests and cause them to lose custody of their children. Screening for domestic violence should be routine in this population as 34% of substance-abusing pregnant women report physical abuse (Wunsch & Weaver, 2011).

In most cases, offering advice alone is insufficient to achieve sobriety/abstinence. A comprehensive approach to treatment in the perinatal period, including prenatal and perinatal care; pharmacologic interventions such as methadone maintenance programs; life skills training, such as relapse prevention and social skills training; mother–infant development assessment; and early childhood development programs and social work services, as required, is recommended. The newborn will require evaluation for neonatal intoxication and abstinence syndromes, as well as for foetal effects of psychoactive substance use. Substances are transmitted into breast milk, and the nursing mother can expose the breast-fed baby to harmful chemicals, with a range of adverse outcomes and risks. However, women actively engaged in addiction treatment should be encouraged to breast-feed as long as drug screens are clear (Wunsch & Weaver, 2011).

Aboriginal Populations

Although accurate and complete data are limited regarding the prevalence of alcohol, tobacco, and other drug use among Aboriginal communities, there is a consensus that they suffer significantly higher rates of addiction when compared to the general Canadian population (Kirby, 2006). Further, the rates of foetal alcohol spectrum disorder (FASD) and its effects are higher among the Aboriginal communities. Although the causes of the addiction problems in Aboriginal and non-Aboriginal communities may be similar, Aboriginal communities have added cultural factors that affect individuals. Addiction has been implicated as both the cause and effect of the relatively disadvantaged health of Canada's Aboriginal people. As their once-powerful role in the economic exchange systems of early Canada was displaced through economic developments, the Aboriginal people lost their traditional economies and became particularly vulnerable to the health and social problems characteristic of economically marginalized members of all industrialized societies, including crippling alcohol, tobacco, and other drug use patterns (National Native Addictions Partnership Foundation, 2000).

HIV/AIDS

Some individuals who abuse drugs and alcohol may be at high risk for sexual transmission of HIV/AIDS because they may be unable to take adequate precautions and use preventive methods while intoxicated or may engage in risky sexual encounters to obtain money or drugs. Intravenous drug users may be considered particularly at risk for HIV/AIDS infection, because some may be placed in situations where hypodermic needles, syringes, and other supplies used to inject drugs are shared.

The concurrence of a SUD and HIV/AIDS infection requires exceedingly careful assessment and intervention planning. Continued alcohol and substance use can interfere with the medical treatment of HIV/AIDS; for example, alcohol, marijuana, cocaine, and amphetamines are immunosuppressants that further impair the seriously compromised immune system of individuals with HIV/AIDS. Addicted persons infected with HIV/AIDS may have difficulty adhering to medication schedules, and some would not benefit fully from antiviral medications because of this. Other complicating factors include the financial, social, and emotional stressors (including stigma) experienced by individuals with SUDs who must also cope with the devastating diagnosis of HIV/AIDS disease.

Addiction treatment programs have an important role for individuals with HIV/AIDS disease, SUDs, and concurrent mental health problems. Because the issues facing these individuals are so complex, planning treatment and priority setting are essential. Addiction treatment is nearly always necessary for the individual to follow with other HIV/AIDS-related health and mental health interventions. At the initial diagnosis of HIV/AIDS infection, SUD issues therefore need to be evaluated and addressed.

Concurrent Substance Use and Other Mental Disorders

The risk for addiction in individuals with mental illness is significantly higher than for the general population, and many individuals with addiction also have **concurrent mental disorders** (Volkow & Li, 2011). Also known as dual disorders, dual diagnosis, and comorbid substance abuse disorders and mental disorders (Centre for Addiction and Mental Health, 2008), concurrent mental disorders can be defined as the coexistence of at least one mental disorder and at least one other SUD as defined by the *DSM-5*. Some mental disorders are in part a byproduct of long-term SUDs; some mental disorders predispose the individual to alcohol, tobacco, or other drug use. For example, alcohol addiction is 21 times more likely to occur among people with antisocial personality disorders and 4 times more likely among people with schizophrenia; among those treated for alcohol-related disorders, up to 70% to 80% may have a mental disorder (Health Canada, 2002). Nurses should be aware that individuals with SUDs often have anxiety disorders, phobias, or obsessive–compulsive and affective disorders, such as major depression and dysthymia (Fu et al., 2002). Other coexisting mental disorders include personality disorders and attention deficit hyperactivity disorder (Rosenthal & Westreich, 1999). Concurrent disorders are discussed in detail in Chapter 35. Nurses need to remember that individuals do not compartmentalize their problems, so health professionals should not either.

The Special Case of Tobacco and Mental Illnesses

There is a long-standing and robust historical relationship between people with mental illness and the use of tobacco products. When compared with the general population, individuals with mental illness are two to three times more likely to smoke and are less likely to quit (Lasser et al., 2000). Up to 90% of persons with schizophrenia also smoke (Ziedonis et al., 2008), and those with mental illness smoke almost half of all cigarettes smoked in North America (Lasser et al., 2000). Financially deprived and socially disenfranchised persons may "pick butts" because they cannot afford cigarettes, which exposes them to communicable diseases and to the higher tar content found in tobacco closer to the cigarette butt. When compared with the general population, persons living with mental illness are more likely to die of tobacco-related illness than from any other cause and have higher rates of cardiovascular and respiratory morbidity and type 2 diabetes (tobacco is a major contributor towards these conditions). The health benefits of smoking cessation are undisputed, but some persons may be discouraged from quitting out of fear of a relapse of their mental illness. There is no evidence to suggest that standard tobacco cessation interventions cannot be effective for persons with mental illness or addiction (Filimon & George, 2012).

Nurses With Substance Use Disorders

Nurses, as with other groups of health professionals, may also develop SUDs. Rather than being protected by the special knowledge, skills, or insights they may have due to education or professional experiences, there is research indicating that nurses may be at particular risk for SUD because of high job strain, disruption, and fatigue related to shift work, ease of access to medications in the workplace, and their knowledge of the benefits of medications (Lillibridge, Cox, & Cross, 2002; Trinkoff, Zhou, Storr, & Soeken, 2000). The evidence suggests that the prevalence of SRD among nurses may be similar to, or greater than, the general population (Kunyk, 2013).

When nurses abuse or become addicted to substances, more than their own health and welfare are placed at risk. There are also patient safety concerns because of the risk associated with impaired nursing practice and, when drugs are accessed from the workplace, patients may be undermedicated and suffer as a consequence. It may even place the safety of other health professionals at risk. To reduce this risk and improve the recovery of the impaired nurse, the focus of the profession must be on prevention, early identification, multimodal treatment, and return to practice with long-term supports.

Unfortunately, the issue of SUDs among nurses is extremely sensitive and appears challenging for the profession to address. Historically, nurses have concealed their addiction because of their fear of professional, employer, peer, and legal reprisals (Heise, 2003). Reducing the stigma associated with substance use by nurses is critical; nurses can help one another recognize the problem and seek treatment for it. Furthermore, the impaired nurse may not be able to recognize his or her illness and seek help, and this inability places some responsibility on others to intervene. Perhaps, one of the more difficult challenges nurses may have involves addressing a nurse colleague whom they suspect has an addiction and is practising while impaired. Nurses have a responsibility in this situation to ensure patient safety and to assist their nurse colleague in accessing appropriate care and supports (e.g., confidential employee assistance programs are available in many workplaces throughout Canada), with the goal of successful return to practice.

Evidence does not support the use of discipline as an effective remedy in reducing the risks of nurses practising while impaired by the use of substances (Kunyk, 2013) (see Box 26-16). Aftercare programs for physicians have been established as an effective mechanism for early intervention, supporting long-term recovery and detecting a

BOX 26-16 Research for Best Practice

SUBSTANCE USE AND IMPAIRED PRACTICE AMONG REGISTERED NURSES

From Kunyk, D. (2013). Substance use disorders among registered nurses: Prevalence, risks and perceptions in a disciplinary jurisdiction. Journal of Nursing Management. Advance online publication. doi: 10.111/john.12081

Purpose: To investigate substance use disorders, impaired practice, and health risks among nurses in a disciplinary environment.

Method: A convenience sample of 4,064 registered nurses responded to an Internet survey that asked questions about their health, substance use, and organizational support. Questions were also asked about their perceptions of the treatment and disposition of impaired nurses.

Findings: The prevalence of self-reported substance use disorders among nurses was similar to the general population. Most nurses who coded high risk for impaired practices were working, unknown to their regulators and employers, and not receiving treatment. When compared with their peers, nurses with substance use disorders were compromised on measures of their health and organizational support. Nurse peers viewed impaired nurses as having a treatable illness that their regulator and employer should assist and afford confidentiality.

Implications: Nursing has an important role in addressing substance use disorders among its members. In this study, discipline was not rated as effective for mitigating the risks associated with substance use, supportive of nurses with substance use disorders, or in alignment with nurse perceptions. Alternative approaches that are more in alignment with nursing values hold promise as more fitting responses for dealing well with this complex situation.

relapse upon return to work. These programs monitor for continued engagement in evidence-based treatment programs that include random drug testing. A number of studies have followed physicians in these programs and demonstrated outcomes of approximately 80% practising after 5 years (Brewster, Kaufman, Hutchinson, & MacWilliam, 2008; DuPont, McLellan, White, Merlo, & Gold, 2009; McLellann, Skipper, Campbell, & DuPont, 2008). The recognition of addiction as a treatable medical illness (as opposed to a moral weakness or lifestyle choice) places a "duty to accommodate" on the employer, and this is increasingly being reflected in employee wellness programs. For further information, see Chapter 16.

■ THE NURSE AS HEALTH ADVOCATE

The Code of Ethics for Registered Nurses (Canadian Nurses Association [CNA], 2008) serves as a foundation for nurses' ethical practice, and this includes endeavours that nurses may undertake to address social inequities. Nurses are expected to uphold principles of justice by safeguarding human rights, equity, and fairness and by promoting the public good. Individuals with addiction are among the more marginalized and impoverished

members of Canadian society. The challenges associated with their illness are often exacerbated by the experience of stigma, placing an additional burden for overcoming barriers to accessing care. Stigma includes having fixed ideas and judgements—such as thinking that people with substance use and mental health problems are not normal; that they caused their own problems; or that they can simply get over their problems if they want to do so. In its eighth *Annual National Report Card on Health Care*, the Canadian Medical Association (2008) reported on the perception of mental illness and addiction among Canadians. Their survey findings indicated that only about half of Canadians say drug addiction (51%) and alcoholism (49%) are either serious illnesses or mental illnesses. Only 21% of Canadians would socialize with a coworker who has either an alcohol or a drug addiction. The stigma and shame associated with substance dependence can, in effect, isolate those with addiction from the rest of society.

The use of substances threatens to affect the overall welfare of our nation and our health care system and poses a massive economic burden. Nurses are well positioned on the frontlines of the health care system to be provided opportunities to understand the needs and vulnerabilities of those with SUDs, to be aware of available services and resources, and to note the existing deficits. It is well within the role of the nurse to seek opportunities to reduce the stigma and misunderstanding associated with addiction, as well as to collaborate and advocate for broader societal changes through policy, legislation, and other mechanisms to improve conditions for preventing and treating addiction at a population level. In these times of health care reform, nurses may have to proactively advocate for health care systems that ensure accessibility, universality, and comprehensiveness of services in order to meet the needs of individuals with addictions and their families.

SUMMARY OF KEY POINTS

■ Addiction is recognized by the major global disease classification systems as a chronic medical disorder characterized by periods of remission and relapse. Substances of abuse alter the brain's structure and function, resulting in changes that persist long after their use has discontinued. Addiction is amenable to evidence-based treatment, yet it remains largely untreated.

■ The *DSM-5* classification of substance-related and addictive disorders includes SUDs (ranging in severity from mild to severe) and substance-induced disorders (including substance intoxication and substance withdrawal). These are classified according to the class of substance: alcohol; caffeine; cannabis (marijuana); hallucinogens; inhalants; opioids; sedatives, hypnotics, and anxiolytics; stimulants; tobacco (nicotine); and other (or unknown) substances.

■ The bio/psycho/social/spiritual model conceptualizes addiction as a disorder with multifactorial pathogenesis, including predisposing, precipitating, and modulating factors, that encompasses the body, the mind (psyche), the spirit, as well as social and environmental influences.

■ Accurate and comprehensive assessment is crucial in planning addiction treatment interventions. Assessment should consider all substances for pattern of use, including factors of tolerance; withdrawal symptoms; consequences of use; loss of control over amount, frequency, or duration of use; desire or efforts to cease or control use; social, vocational, and recreational activities affected by use; and history of previous addiction treatment. It also includes investigating family and social support systems. Treatment plans must be assessed continually and modified as necessary to ensure that they meet the changing needs of the patient.

■ In some individuals, reducing consumption or abstaining from alcohol and some other substances may lead to withdrawal symptoms that may progress into life-threatening complications. Symptoms of alcohol withdrawal may include nausea and vomiting, tactile disturbances, tremor, auditory disturbances, paroxysmal sweats, visual disturbances, anxiety, headaches (or sensations of fullness in the head), agitation, and disturbances in orientation and clouding of the sensorium. It may also include autonomic disturbances; for example, blood pressure increases, tachycardia, diaphoresis, and in the most severe cases withdrawal may progress to seizures (tonic–clonic), delirium (delirium tremens), or death.

■ Substance withdrawal can be assisted through symptom-triggered detoxification. Detoxification by itself does little to change long-term drug SUDs; it could be better described as the first stage of treatment.

■ The use of tobacco products remains the leading preventable cause of death and disease globally. Tobacco addiction is vastly undertreated; most individuals who smoke want to quit, but few are helped in doing so. Nurses can effectively intervene and, as a minimum, should incorporate the 5As (Ask, Advise, Assess, Assist, and Arrange follow-up) into their daily practice. Uptake of smokeless tobacco is not considered a treatment for smoking cessation.

■ The purpose of harm reduction is to reduce the risk for adverse consequences arising from substance use and works with the individual to achieve this goal regardless of his or her commitment to reduce use. Harm reduction forms only one part of a continuum of care and is not viewed as exclusive of the overarching goal of abstinence.

■ MI helps to explore and resolve ambivalence by examining the conviction (importance) and the confidence in the process to change. Therapeutic approaches include avoiding arguing, expressing empathy, developing discrepancy, rolling with resistance, and supporting self-efficacy, and the purpose of using these are to motivate patients, to resolve ambivalence, and to help patients change health-related behaviours.

■ Many individuals with SUDs also have other mental disorders, and patients presenting with one condition should be assessed for others. When these conditions co-occur, treatment should address both (or all) at the same time (integrated or parallel treatment).

■ Stigma can be a massive barrier for individuals with SUDs, and the nurse is well placed to reduce this stigma and misunderstanding. It is within the nursing role to collaborate and advocate for broader societal changes through policy, legislation, and other mechanisms to improve conditions for preventing and treating addiction.

CRITICAL THINKING CHALLENGES

1 What is your understanding of the aetiology of addiction? Based on this understanding, what would be your priorities for patient education?

2 Jeff H., a 35-year-old cocaine-dependent patient, has recently entered a rehabilitation program. What goals do you believe would be realistic to achieve by the end of his projected 30-day inpatient stay?

3 You are working in an orthopaedic unit, and Mary L. has been admitted for treatment for a fractured femur. She has been drinking recently and has a BAL of 0.08%. What further information in the following areas would you need to plan her care?
   a Medical
   b Alcohol, tobacco, and other substance related
   c Other psychosocial issues

4 The medical use of marijuana has been approved in Canada. How would you explain its availability and use to a patient inquiry? What do you think are the advantages and disadvantages of this public policy?

5 Hannah K. presented with suicide ideation at the emergency department. When you see her, she appears agitated and restless and expresses a desire to leave the emergency department despite the fact she has not yet received examination and attention. You note that she smokes and has been waiting at the hospital to be assessed for almost 7 hours. What steps can you take to alleviate her possible nicotine withdrawal symptoms?

6 John M. has sought treatment for depression and job stress. He came to your psychiatric assessment unit smelling of alcohol. He believes that he does not have

a drinking problem but a job problem. What interventions would you use for possible alcohol abuse or dependence?

7 Sylvia G. has been using heroin intravenously heavily for 2 years. She has come into the hospital with an abscess on her leg. What symptoms would you expect to observe as she experiences withdrawal from opiates? What medications would likely be used to ease these symptoms?

8 After Sylvia G. is free of withdrawal symptoms, she expresses interest in obtaining drug treatment. What are her options? How would you describe them to her?

9 Raymond L. has been treated for hypertension at your clinic. You notice that he complains of peripheral neuropathy and has an unsteady gait. What other medical signs would corroborate alcoholism?

10 Andre P. is being treated for cocaine dependence in a residential treatment facility. He asks you whether he should try to quit smoking at the same time. How do you respond?

REFERENCES

American Psychiatric Association. (2013). *Diagnostic and statistical manual of mental disorders* (5th ed.). Arlington, VA: American Psychiatric Association.

American Society of Addiction Medicine. (2009). *Principles of addiction medicine* (4th ed.). Philadelphia, PA: Lippincott Williams & Wilkins.

Brands, B., Kahan, M., Selby, P., & Wilson, L. (2000). *Medical management of alcohol and drug-related problems: A physician's manual* (2nd ed.). Toronto, ON: Centre for Addiction and Mental Health.

Brewster, J., Kaufmann, M., Hutchinson, S., & MacWilliam, C. (2008). Characteristics and outcomes of a dependence monitoring programme in Canada: Prospective descriptive study. *BMJ, 337,* a2098.

CAN-ADAPTT. (2011). *Canadian smoking cessation clinical practice guideline.* Toronto, ON: Canadian Action Network for the Advancement, Dissemination and Adoption of Practice-informed Tobacco Treatment, Centre for Addiction and Mental Health.

Canadian Centre on Substance Abuse. (2005). *Substance abuse in Canada: Current challenges and choices 2005.* Ottawa, ON: Author.

Canadian Medical Association. (2008). *8th Annual National Report Card on Health Care.* Retrieved from http://www.cma.ca/multimedia/CMA/Content_Images/Inside_cma/Annual_Meeting/2008/GC_Bulletin/National_Report_Card_EN.pdf

Canadian Nurses Association. (2008). *Code of Ethics for registered nurses.* Retrieved from http://www.cna-aiic.ca/CNA/practice/ethics/code/default_e.aspx

Canadian Nurses Association. (2011). *Joint position statement: The role of health professionals in tobacco cessation.* Retrieved from http://www2.cna-aiic.ca/CNA/documents/pdf/publications/JPS_Tobacco_Cessation_2011_e.pdf

Cavacuiti, C. A., Vasic, A., McCrady, B. S., & Tonigan, J. S. (2011). Recent research into twelve-step programs. In C. Cavacuiti (Ed.), *Principles of addiction medicine: The essentials* (pp. 355–361). Philadelphia, PA: Lippincott Williams & Wilkins.

Centre for Addiction and Mental Health. (2008). *Concurrent substance use & mental health disorders: Selected bibliography.* Retrieved from http://www.camh.ca/en/education/about/services/camh_library/Documents/RLGConcurrentDisorders2008.pdf

Cohen, S., Dragonetti, R., Herie, M., & Barker, M. (2012). Psychosocial interventions. In C. Els, D. Kunyk, & P. Selby (Eds.), *Disease interrupted: Tobacco reduction and cessation* (pp. 103–130). North Carolina, NC: Createspace.

Compton, W., Thomas, Y., Stinson, F., & Grant, B. F. (2007). Prevalence, correlates, disability, and comorbidity of *DSM-IV* drug abuse and dependence in the United States: Results from the National Epidemiologic Survey on Alcohol and Related conditions. *Archives of General Psychiatry, 64*(5), 566–576.

DeLima, M. S., de Olivera Soceres, B. G., Reisser, A. A., & Farrell, M. (2002). Pharmacological treatment of cocaine dependence: A systematic review. *Addiction, 97*(8), 931–949.

Douaihy, A., Daley, D. C., Marlatt, G. A., & Spotts, C. E. (2011). Relapse prevention: Clinical models and intervention strategies. In C. Cavacuiti (Ed.), *Principles of addiction medicine: The essentials* (pp. 340–344). Philadelphia, PA: Lippincott Williams & Wilkins.

DuPont, R. L., McLellan, A. T., White, W. L., Merklo, L. J., & Gold, M. S. (2009). Setting the standard for recovery: Physicians' health programs. *Journal of Substance Abuse Treatment, 36,* 159–171.

Els, C. (2007). Addiction is a mental disorder, best managed in a (public) mental health setting—but our system is failing us. *Canadian Journal of Psychiatry, 52*(3), 167–169.

Els, C. (2012). Neuropsychiatric considerations. In C. Els, D. Kunyk, & P. Selby (Eds.), *Disease interrupted: Tobacco reduction and cessation* (pp. 183–194). North Carolina, NC: Createspace.

Els, C., Kunyk, D., Barak, Y., Scharf, D., & Thomas, E. (2012). Detoxification: Treatment of the 'other' tobacco use disorder. In C. Els, D. Kunyk, & P. Selby (Eds.), *Disease interrupted: Tobacco reduction and cessation* (pp. 195–206). North Carolina, NC: Createspace.

Ewing, J. A. (1984). Detecting alcoholism: The CAGE Questionnaire. *Journal of the American Medical Association, 252,* 1905–1907.

Filimon, M. & George, T. (2012). Treatment of tobacco dependence in mental health and addictive disorders. In C. Els, D. Kunyk, & P. Selby (Eds.), *Disease interrupted: Tobacco reduction and cessation* (pp. 257–274). North Carolina, NC: Createspace.

Fiore, M., Jaén, C., Baker, T., Bailey, W. C., Benowitz, N., Curry, S. J., ... Williams, C. (2008). A clinical practice guideline for treating tobacco use and dependence: 2008 update. A U.S. Public Health Service report. *American Journal of Preventive Medicine, 35*(2), 158–176.

Fischer, B. (2005). Harm reduction. In: *Substance abuse in Canada: Current challenges and choices* (pp. 11–15). Ottawa, ON: Canadian Centre on Substance Abuse.

Fischer, B., Ialomiteanu, A., Boak, A., Adlaf, E., Rehm, J., & Mann, R. E. (2013). Prevalence and key covariates of non-medical prescription opioid use among the general secondary student and adults populations in Ontario, Canada. *Drug and Alcohol Review, 32,* 266–887.

Fu, Q., Heath, A., Bucholz, K. K., Nelson, E., Goldberg, J., Lyons, M. J., ... Eisen, S. A. (2002). Shared genetic risk of major depression, alcohol dependence, and marijuana dependence: Contribution of antisocial personality disorder in men. *Archives of General Psychiatry, 59*(12), 1125–1132.

Goldstein, R. Z. & Volkow, N. D. (2011). Dysfunction of the prefrontal cortex in addiction; neuroimaging findings and clinical implications. *Nature Reviews. Neuroscience, 12*(11), 652–669.

Gordon, H. W. (2002). Early environmental stress and biological vulnerability to drug abuse. *Psychoneuroendocrinology, 27,* 115–126.

Grant, B. F., Stinson, F. S., Hasin, D. S., Dawson, D. A., Chow, S. P., & Anderson, K. (2004). Immigration and lifetime prevalences of *DSM-IV* psychiatric disorders among Mexican Americans and non-Hispanic whites in the United States: Results from the National Epidemiologic Survey on Alcohol and Related Conditions. *Archives of General Psychiatry, 61*(12), 1226–1233.

Hansen, R. N., Oster, G., Edelsberg, J., Woody, G. E., & Sullivan, S. D. (2011). Economic costs of nonmedical use of prescription opioids. *Clinical Journal of Pain, 27,* 194–202.

Hasin, D., Stinson, F., Ogburn, E., & Grant, B. (2007). Prevalence, correlates, disability, and comorbidity of *DSM-IV* alcohol abuse and dependence in the United States: Results from the National Epidemiologic Survey on Alcohol and Related Conditions. *Archives of General Psychiatry, 64*(7), 830–842.

Health Canada. (2002). *A report on mental illness in Canada.* Ottawa, ON: Author.

Health Canada. (2011). *Canadian tobacco use monitoring survey, 2010.* Ottawa, ON: Author. Retrieved from http://www.hc-sc.gc.ca

Heise, B. (2003). The historical contact of addiction in the nursing profession: 1850–1982. *Journal of Addictions Nursing, 14,* 117–124.

Ialomiteanu, A. R., Adlaf, E. M., Mann, R. E., & Rehm, J. (2009). *CAMH Monitor eReport: Addiction & mental health indicators among Ontario adults, 1977–2007.* CAMH Research Document Series No. 25. Toronto, ON: Centre for Addiction & Mental Health.

International Narcotics Control Board. (2013). *Narcotic drugs: Estimated world requirements for 2012—Statistics for 2011.* New York, NY: United Nations.

Kirby, M. (2006). *Out of the shadows at last: Transforming mental health, mental illness and addiction services in Canada.* Ottawa, ON: Standing Senate Committee on Social Affairs, Science and Technology.

Kleber, H., Weiss, R., Anton, R., George, T., Greenfield, S., Kosten, T., ... Connery, H. S. (2006). *Practice guidelines for the treatment of patients with Substance Use Disorders* (2nd ed.). Arlington, VA: American Psychiatric Association.

Kunyk, D. (2013). Substance use disorders among registered nurses: Prevalence, risks and perceptions in a disciplinary jurisdiction. *Journal of Nursing Management.* doi: 10.1111/jonm.12081

Kunyk, D., Els, C., Predy, G., & Haase, M. (2007). Development and introduction of a comprehensive tobacco control policy in a Canadian regional health authority. *Preventing Chronic Disease: Public Health Research, Practice, and Policy,* 4(2), 1–8.

Larimer, M. E., Kilmer, J. R., & Whiteside, U. (2011). College student drinking. In C. Cavacuiti (Ed.), *Principles of addiction medicine: The essentials* (pp. 177–180). Philadelphia, PA: Lippincott Williams & Wilkins.

Lasser, K., Boyd, J., Woolhandler, S., Himmelstein, D., McCormick, D., & Bor, D. (2000). Smoking and mental illness—a population-based prevalence study. *Journal of the American Medical Association,* 284(20), 2606–2610.

Leatherdale, S. & Shields, M. (2009). Smoking cessation: Intentions, attempts and techniques. *Statistics Canada Health Reports,* 20(3), 31–39. Retrieved from http://www.statcan.gc.ca/pub/82–003-x/2009003/article/10904-eng.htm

Lerman, D., Patterson, F., & Berrettini, W. (2005). Treating tobacco dependence: State of the science and new direction. *Journal of Clinical Oncology,* 23, 311–323.

Leshner, A. (1997). Addiction is a brain disease, and it matters. *Science,* 278(3), 45–47.

Lillibridge, J., Cox, M., & Cross, W. (2002). Uncovering the secret: Giving voice to the experiences of nurses who misuse substances. *Journal of Advanced Nursing,* 39(3), 219–229.

Makomoaski Illing, E. M. & Kaiserman, M. G. (2004). Mortality attributable to tobacco use in Canada and its regions. *Canadian Journal of Public Health,* 95(1), 38–44.

McLellan, A. T., Lewis, D., O'Brien, C., & Kleber, H. (2000). Drug dependence, a chronic medical illness: Implications for treatment, insurance, and outcomes evaluation. *Journal of the American Medical Association,* 284(13), 1689–1695.

McLellann, A. T., Skipper, G. S., Campbell, M., & DuPont, R. L. (2008). Five year outcomes in a cohort study of physicians treated for substance use disorders in the United States. *BMJ,* 337, a2038.

Mee-Lee, D. & Shulman, G. D. (2009). The ASAM placement criteria and matching patients to treatment. In R. K. Reis, D. A. Fiellin, S. C. Miller, & R. Saitz (Eds.), *Principles of addiction medicine* (4th ed.). Philadelphia, PA: Lippincott Williams & Wilkins.

Merikangas, K. R., Conway, K. P., Swendsen, J., Febo, J., Dierker, L., Brunetto, W., … Canino, G. (2009). Substance use and behaviour disorders in Puerto Rican youth: A migrant family study. *Journal of Epidemiology and Community Health,* 63(4), 310–316.

Miller, W. R. & Rollnick, S. (2002). *Motivational interviewing: Preparing people for change.* New York, NY: Guilford Press.

Miller, W. R. & Sanchez, V. C. (1994). Motivating young adults for treatment and lifestyle change. In G. S. Howard & P. E. Nathan (Eds.), *Alcohol use and misuse by young adults.* Notre Dame, IN: University of Notre Dame Press.

Nace, E. P. (2005). Alcoholics anonymous. In J. H. Lowinson, P. Ruiz, R. B. Millman, & J. G. Langrod (Eds.), *Substance abuse: A comprehensive textbook* (4th ed., pp. 587–598). Baltimore, MD: Lippincott Williams & Wilkins.

National Institute on Drug Abuse (NIDA). (2005a). *Research report series: Inhalant abuse.* Publication Number 05-3818. Bethesda, MD: Author.

National Institute on Drug Abuse (NIDA). (2005b). *Research report: Heroin: Abuse and addiction.* NIH Publication Number 05-4165. Bethesda, MD: Author.

National Institute on Drug Abuse (NIDA). (2009). *Research report: Cocaine: Abuse and addiction.* NIH Publication Number 09-4166. Bethesda, MD: Author.

National Institute on Drug Abuse (NIDA). (2012a). *Principles of drug addiction treatment: A research-based guide* (3rd ed.). Rockville, MD: Author.

National Institute on Drug Abuse (NIDA). (2012b). DrugFacts: Synthetic cathinones ("bath salts"). Retrieved from www.drugabuse.ov/publications/drugfacts/synthetic-cathinones-bath-salts

National Native Addictions Partnership Foundation (NNADAP). (2000). *NNADAP renewal framework: For implementing the strategic recommendations of the 1998, General review of the National Native Alcohol and Drug Abuse Program.* Draft working paper, prepared for the Framework Subcommittee of the NNADAP, December 2000.

Pilowsky, D. J. & Wu, L. (2012). Screening for alcohol and drug use disorders among adults in primary care: A review. *Substance Abuse & Rehabilitation,* 3(1), 25–34.

Pitkanen, T., Lyyra, A. L., & Pulkkinen, L. (2005). Age of onset of drinking and the use of alcohol in adulthood: A follow-up study from age 8–42 for females and males. *Addiction,* 100, 652–661.

Prochaska, J., Diclemente, C., & Norcross, J. (1992). In search of how people change: Applications to addictive behaviors. *American Psychologist,* 47(9), 1102–1114.

Ramaekers, J. G., Berghaus, G., van Laar, M., & Drummer, O. H. (2004). Dose related risk of motor vehicle crashes after cannabis use. *Drug and Alcohol Dependence,* 23(3), 319–344.

Rehm, J., Ballunas, D., Brochu, S., Fischer, B., Gnam, W., Patra, J., … Taylor, B. (2006). *The costs of substance abuse in Canada 2002.* Ottawa, ON: Canadian Centre on Substance Abuse.

Rice, V. & Stead, L. (2004). Nursing interventions for smoking cessation (Cochrane Review). *Cochrane Library,* Issue 1. Retrieved from http://www.ncsct.co.uk/usr/pub/nursing-interventions.pdf

Rosenthal, R. N. & Westreich, L. (1999). Treatment of persons with dual diagnoses of substance use disorder and other psychological problems. In B. S. McCrady & E. E. Epstein (Eds.), *Addictions: A comprehensive guidebook* (pp. 439–476). New York, NY: Oxford University Press.

Shield, K. D., Rylett, M., Gmel, G., Keho-Chan, G., & Rehm, J. (2013). Global alcohol exposure estimates by country, territory and region for 2005—a contribution to the Comparative Risk Assessment for the 2010 Global Burden of Disease study. *Addiction,* 108, 912–922.

Sproule, B., Brands, B., Li, S., & Catz-Biro, L. (2009). Changing patterns in opioid addiction. *Canadian Family Physician,* 55(1), 68–69.

Sridharan, S., Kawata, J. H., Campbell, B., & Tseng C.W. (2005). Contemporaneous relationship between substance abuse treatment and poly-substance use: Evidence from the Persistent Effect of Treatment Studies. *Journal of Substance Abuse Treatment,* 28(Suppl 1), S83–S90.

Swendsen, J. & Le Moal, M. (2011). Individual vulnerability to addiction. *Annals of the New York Academy of Sciences,* 1216, 73–85.

Swotinsky, R. B. & Smith, D. (2006). *The medical review officer's manual* (3rd ed.). Beverly Farms, MA: OEM Press.

Trinkoff, A. M., Zhou, Q., Storr, C. L., & Soeken, K. L. (2000). Workplace access, negative proscriptions, job strain, and substance use in registered nurses. *Nursing Research,* 49(2), 83–90.

Tupperman, L. & Wanner, K. (2012). *Problem gambling in Canada.* Don Mills, ON: Oxford University Press.

U.S. Department of Health and Human Services. (2004). *The health consequences of smoking: A report of the Surgeon General.* Atlanta, GA: US Department of Health and Human Services, Centers for Disease Control and Prevention, National Center for Chronic Disease Prevention and Health Promotions, Office on Smoking and Health.

U.S. Department of Health and Human Services. (2010). *How tobacco smoke causes disease: The biology and behavioral basis for smoking-attributable disease: A report of the Surgeon General.* Atlanta, GA: U.S. Department of Health and Human Services, Centers for Disease Control and Prevention, National Center for Chronic Disease Prevention and Health Promotions, Office on Smoking and Health.

Volkow, N. D. & Li, T. (2011). Drug addiction: The neurobiology of behavior gone awry. In C. Cavacuiti (Ed.), *Principles of addiction medicine: The essentials* (pp. 1–5). Philadelphia, PA: Lippincott Williams & Wilkins.

West, R. (2006). *Theory of addiction.* Oxford, UK: Blackwell Publishing/Addiction Press.

Willembring, M. J. (2011). Treatment of heavy drinking and alcohol use disorders. In C. Cavacuiti (Ed.), *Principles of addiction medicine: The essentials* (pp. 105–109). Philadelphia, PA: Lippincott Williams & Wilkins.

World Health Organization. (2007). *International statistical classification of disease and related health problems* (10th ed.). Geneva, IL: WHO Press.

World Health Organization. (2009). *Global health risks. Morality and burden of diseases attributable to selected major risks.* Geneva, IL: WHO Press.

World Health Organization. (2010). *WHO report on the global tobacco epidemic.* Geneva, IL: WHO Press.

Wright, T. M., Cluver, J. S., & Myrick, H. (2011). Management of intoxication and withdrawal: General principles. In C. Cavacuiti (Ed.), *Principles of addiction medicine: The essentials* (pp. 199–203). Philadelphia, PA: Lippincott Williams & Wilkins.

Wunsch, M. J., & Weaver, M. F. (2011). Alcohol and other drug use during pregnancy: Management of mother and child. In C. Cavacuiti (Ed.), *Principles of addiction medicine: The essentials* (pp. 448–453). Philadelphia, PA: Lippincott Williams & Wilkins.

Zgierska, A. & Fleming, M. F. (2011). Screening and brief intervention. In C. Cavacuiti (Ed.), *Principles of addiction medicine: The essentials* (pp. 81–86). Philadelphia, PA: Lippincott Williams & Wilkins.

Ziedonis, D., Hitsman, B., Beckham, J. C., Zvolensky, M., Adler, L. E., Audrain-McGovern, J., … Riley, W. T. (2008). *Tobacco use and cessation in psychiatric disorders: National Institute of Mental Health report. Nicotine & Tobacco Research,* 10(12), 1691–1715.

27 Personality and Disruptive, Impulse-Control, and Conduct Disorders

Wendy Austin

Adapted from the chapters "Personality and Impulse-Control Disorders" by Stephen VanSlyke (2009) and by Mary Ann Boyd and Barbara J. Limandri (2005)

KEY CONCEPTS

- personality
- personality disorder
- personality traits

LEARNING OBJECTIVES

After studying this chapter, you will be able to:

- Discuss the concepts of *personality* and *personality trait*.
- Describe what is known about the aetiology of personality disorders.
- Identify the common features of personality disorders.
- Name components of (mal)adaptive personality functioning that can be used to describe the severity of a personality disorder.
- Distinguish among the three clusters of personality disorders.
- Formulate nursing assessment and interventions for clients with specific personality disorders.
- Apply the nursing process to clients with borderline personality disorder.
- Identify concerns within the nurse–client relationship common to caring for clients with personality disorders.
- Name the disruptive, impulse-control, and conduct disorders and describe these: intermittent explosive disorder, pyromania, and kleptomania.

KEY TERMS

- affective instability • attachment • cognitive schema
- communication triad • dialectical behaviour therapy (DBT)
- dichotomous thinking • dissociation • emotional dysregulation
- emotional vulnerability • emotions • identity diffusion • impulsivity
- invalidating environment • kleptomania • parasuicidal behaviour
- projective identification • pyromania • reframing • self-identity
- separation–individuation • skills groups • temperament • thought stopping • trait • trichotillomania

---

he concept of personality appears simple but is very complex. Historically, the term *personality* was derived from the Greek *persona*, the theatrical mask used by dramatic players. Originally, the term had the connotation of a projected pretence or illusion. With time, the connotation changed from being an external surface representation to the internal traits of an individual.

BOX 27-1 Shoes and Personality

Impressions about others are formed quickly from such cues as appearance. Investigating how accurately such cues might be in revealing an unknown individual's personality, researchers used shoes as the cue of interest. Photos of participants' (208 undergraduate psychology students) shoes were coded on several dimensions and found to correlate with self-reported descriptions of the shoe owners' personality, including assessment of "The Big Five" personality traits using the Ten-Item Personality Inventory (TIPI). Overall, observers were accurately able to judge age, gender, income, and attachment anxiety of shoe owners, based solely on shoe photos; for personality traits, however, only agreeableness was judged with any accuracy.

Source: Gillath, O., Bahns, A. J., Ge, F., & Crandall, C. S. (2012). Shoes as a source of first impressions. *Journal of Research in Personality, 4*, 423–430.

Today, personality is conceptualized as a complex pattern of psychological characteristics that are not easily altered and that are largely outside the person's awareness. Such characteristics or traits include the individual's specific style of perceiving, thinking, and feeling about self, others, and the environment. These styles, known as traits, are similar and coherent across many different social or personal situations and are expressed in almost every facet of functioning. Intrinsic and pervasive, they emerge from a complicated interaction of genetics, neurobiologic dispositions, psychosocial experiences, and environmental situations that ultimately make up the individual's distinctive personality (Widiger, 2012).

Psychologists are exploring personality from biologic, cognitive, and social perspectives (Maruszewski, Fajkowska, & Eysenck, 2010). While various theories about personality have evolved, the approach to understanding human personality through analyzing **traits** (i.e., core attributes of individuals that consistently shape their ideas and actions) has been taken since Hippocrates' description of temperament as being influenced by the dominance of one of four bodily humours: sanguine [blood], melancholic [black bile], choleric [yellow bile], and phlegmatic [phlegm] (Friedman & Schustack, 2012). In contemporary times, the empirically developed Big Five or five-factor model identifies key traits as **O**penness (to experience), **C**onscientiousness, **E**xtraversion, **A**greeableness, and **N**euroticism (emotional instability) (Friedman & Schustack, 2012). (Hint: Use the mnemonic **OCEAN** to remember them.) See Box 27-1.

KEY CONCEPT Personality is a complex pattern of characteristics, largely outside the person's awareness, that compose the individual's distinctive and enduring pattern of perceiving, feeling, thinking, coping, and behaving. The personality emerges from a complicated interaction of biologic dispositions, psychological experiences, and environmental situations.

KEY CONCEPT A personality trait is "a tendency to behave, feel, perceive, and think in consistent ways across time and across situations in which the trait may be manifest" (American Psychiatric Association [APA], 2013, p. 826).

PERSONALITY DISORDERS (PD)

No sharp division exists between normal and abnormal personality functioning. Instead, personalities are viewed on a continuum from normal at one end to abnormal at the other. Many of the same processes involved in the development of a "normal" personality are responsible for the development of a personality disorder (PD). Individuals do not seek treatment for a "personality disorder"; nurses will encounter these clients when they require treatment for other health problems or want help for symptoms such as hopelessness, anxiety, or relationship problems (Leahy & McGinn, 2012).

Personality disorders are delineated in the *Diagnostic and Statistical Manual of Mental Disorders*. The criteria for personality disorders remain the same in the *DSM-5* as appeared in the *DSM-IV*. Ten personality disorders are recognized as psychiatric diagnoses and are organized into three clusters (see Box 27-2). These clusters were previously based on dimensions of *odd–eccentric* (cluster A), *dramatic–emotional* (cluster B), and *anxious–fearful* (cluster C) behaviours or symptoms, but these dimensions are not stipulated in the *DSM-5*.

An alternative approach to the diagnosis of personality disorders was developed during the work for the *DSM-5*. This alternative dimensional approach characterizes PDs by impairments in personality functioning (self, i.e., identity, self-direction, and interpersonal, i.e., empathy and intimacy) and by pathologic traits (negative affectivity, detachment, antagonism, disinhibition, psychoticism). It is available in Section III of the *DSM-5* and awaits further study.

Borderline personality disorder (BPD) is highlighted in this chapter because it is severely incapacitating, its treatment is challenging, and its symptoms may provoke in the clinician negative reactions that interfere with the clinician's ability to provide effective care. Disruptive, impulse-control, and conduct disorders are summarized at the end of the chapter. These disorders commonly coexist with other mental disorders.

BOX 27-2 Personality Disorders (PDs)

Cluster A	Cluster B	Cluster C
Paranoid PD	Antisocial PD	Avoidant PD
Schizoid PD	Borderline PD	Dependent PD
Schizotypal PD	Histrionic PD	Obsessive–
	Narcissistic PD	Compulsive PD

> **KEY CONCEPT** A **personality disorder (PD)** is an enduring pattern of inner experience and behaviour that deviates markedly from the expectations of the individual's culture, is pervasive and inflexible, has an onset in adolescence or early adulthood, is stable with time, and leads to distress or impairment (APA, 2013, p. 645).

IN A LIFE

Ferdinand Waldo Demara (1921–1982)
The Great Impostor

Public Persona

Ferdinand Waldo Demara spent much of his adult life using forged, stolen, or nonexistent credentials to gain employment in numerous and varied vocations. He became most famous for his masquerade as a commissioned Surgeon-Lieutenant in the Royal Canadian Navy in 1951, having stolen the identity of the Canadian physician Dr. Joseph Cyr. Demara was apparently competent in his role as a physician, relying on medical texts and a medical assistant. Demara had similar success in other branches of the military, as a psychologist in a college, as a prison warden, and as a well-respected schoolteacher.

Personal Realities

Demara's life was patterned by the establishment of personal connections with individuals (often in the context of a religious order), theft of this person's identity, and subsequent employment using these false credentials. Once caught, he would disappear, only to reappear claiming a new identity. It was a sense of emptiness and boredom that would kindle Demara's dreams and his need to act as an impostor to fulfil his seemingly well-intentioned passions.

Source: Crichton, R. (1959). *The great impostor.* New York, NY: Random House.

Personality Disorder Versus Personality Traits

To receive a diagnosis of a personality disorder, an individual must demonstrate the criteria behaviours persistently and to such an extent that they impair the ability to function socially and occupationally. In some people, the underlying feelings and behaviours may be intermittent and interfere interpersonally without obvious impairment. Instead of having a personality disorder, the individual is said to have **traits** of the disorder. Other people, including health care professionals, can become impatient with persons who have a PD or traits of a PD, expecting them to change a way of being in the world that is less than optimal. Changing lifelong personality patterns is difficult, however, and requires much understanding and support.

Common Features and Diagnostic Criteria

The personality disorder diagnosis is based on the manifestation of abnormal, inflexible behaviour patterns of long duration, traced to adolescence or early adulthood. These behaviours are pervasive across a broad range of personal and social situations and cause significant distress or impairment to social or occupational functioning. These abnormal behaviour patterns deviate markedly from the expectations of the individual's culture and manifest in two or more of the following areas: cognition, or ways of perceiving and interpreting self, other people, and events; affectivity, or the range, intensity, lability, and appropriateness of emotional responses; interpersonal functioning; and impulse control. For immigrants who may be having difficulty learning new acceptable social and cultural behaviour patterns and adjusting to a new culture, the diagnosis of a personality disorder is often delayed to beyond this difficult adjustment period. It is highly unusual for children or adolescents to be diagnosed with a PD.

Maladaptive Cognitive Schema

Cognitive schemas are patterns of thoughts that determine how a person interprets events. Each person's cognitive schemas screen, code, and evaluate incoming stimuli. In personality disorders, maladaptive cognitive schemas cause the misinterpretation of other people's actions or reactions and of events that result in dysfunctional ways of responding. For example, if a person thinks that no one can be trusted, an innocent, friendly gesture can be interpreted as a suspicious behaviour, provoking a hostile response instead of a reciprocal friendly greeting.

Affectivity and Emotional Instability

Emotions are psychophysiologic reactions that define a person's mood and can be categorized as negative (e.g., anger, fright, anxiety, guilt, shame, sadness, envy, jealousy, disgust), positive (e.g., happiness, pride, relief, love), and neutral (e.g., hope, compassion, empathy, sympathy, contentment). Emotions can affect one's ability to learn and function by affecting one's memory and how one accesses and stores information. Emotional arousal, particularly increased negative emotional arousal characteristic of people with personality disorders, can decrease one's ability to remember new information and accurately perceive the environment (Herpertz, Kunnert, Schwenger, & Sass, 1999; Hurlemann, Hawellek, Maier, & Dolan, 2007).

Impaired Self-Identity and Interpersonal Functioning

Self-identity is central to the normal development of one's personality. Self-identity includes an integration of social and occupational roles and affiliations, self-attributed personality traits, attitudes about gender roles, beliefs about sexuality and intimacy, long-term goals, political ideologies, and religious beliefs. Without an adequately formed identity, an individual's goal-directed behaviour is impaired, and interpersonal relationships are disrupted. Each individual's abilities, limitations, and goals are shaped by one's identity. In personality disorders, self-identity is often impaired or incomplete.

Impulsivity and Destructive Behaviour

Individuals with personality disorders frequently come to the attention of mental health clinicians because their impulsive behaviour results in negative consequences to others or themselves. They seem unable to consider the consequences of their actions before acting on their impulses. Nurses working in psychiatric inpatient settings associate impulsivity with unpredictability, "identifiable precipitants, rejection/abandonment, build up/breakthrough, and intolerance for delay" (Gallop, McCay, & Esplen, 1992, p. 369). For example, an individual may feel rage towards another and lack skills to resist the impulse to attack that person physically, even though this action may be punished.

Severity of Disorder

Five reliable, clinically relevant, core components of (mal)adaptive personality functioning have been identified in a series of research studies (Verheul et al., 2008). These components and their facets are

- self-control (stable self-image, self-reflective, emotional and aggressive regulation)
- identity integration (enjoyment, purposefulness, self-respect, frustration tolerance)
- relational capacities (intimacy, enduring relationships, feeling recognized)
- responsibility (trustworthiness, responsible industry)
- social concordance (respect, cooperation)

The components are associated with the severity of the personality pathology and, using the measure that evolved from the research, the Severity Indices of Personality Problems (SIPP-118), long-term changes can be determined (Verheul et al., 2008).

Epidemiology

While Canadian prevalence data are lacking for personality disorders, the reported prevalence of PDs is very similar across studies (Torgersen, 2012). In Statistics Canada's *Health State Descriptions for Canadians* (2012, modified 2013), it is estimated that 6% to 15% of the population are affected by PDs. Among the most common PDs are obsessive–compulsive (7.7%), avoidant (6.6%), paranoid (5.6%), borderline (5.4%), and schizotypal (5.2%). Comorbidity between PDs is common. There is some consensus across studies of clinical populations that borderline personality disorder is among the most frequent PD seen. The tendency to seek and attend psychiatric care affects these rates; such a tendency is high among persons with the PDs of borderline (BPD), dependent (DPD), and narcissistic (NPD) and low among those with antisocial (ASPD), avoidant (APD), and schizoid (SPD) personality disorders (Torgersen, 2012). Among persons in substance abuse clinics, prisons, or other forensic settings, up to 70% are reported to have ASPD (APA, 2013).

Gender does not appear to affect the prevalence of PD as a whole. Men, however, are much more likely to be diagnosed with ASPD than are women (Oltmanns & Powers, 2012). Is this a genuine difference or a specious one? (See Box 27-3.) It may be that ASPD is underdiagnosed in women for such reasons as the

---

BOX 27-3　Clinical Vignette

ANTISOCIAL PERSONALITY DISORDER: MALE VERSUS FEMALE

Jackson (male) and Stasia (female) are fraternal twins, 22 years old, who received diagnoses of ASPD. The following are their clinical profiles.

Jackson

Jackson's juvenile probation officer explained that Jackson came from a very violent family and neighbourhood and described the situation by saying, "If gangs hadn't gotten him, his father would have." His lawyer described him as "a likeable guy, but I wouldn't turn my back on him."

Jackson is currently in prison for the third time. Although his juvenile records begin at age 9 and include minor assault and property damage charges, his burglary conviction is his first adult crime. His schoolteachers thought that Jackson was very bright but that he had significant difficulty with peers and authority figures. He fought regularly, was described as a bully, and seemed always to be scamming. At age 16, Jackson dropped out of school and joined a gang.

Stasia

Stasia was recently hospitalized for the sixth time when one of her male friends beat her. She has been working as a prostitute for 5 years. Her physical examination noted not only multiple bruises but also tattoos that cover 50% of her body. In addition, she has piercings of her tongue, ears, brow, lips, and nipples. She is emotionally volatile, manipulative, and angry. Stasia has many acquaintances and sexual partners, but none are truly intimate. She has periods when she uses drugs regularly.

Stasia and Jackson's mother was jailed when the twins were 18 months old and did not return until they were 6 years old. They were raised mostly by their paternal grandmother, who hated their mother and reminded Stasia frequently of how much she looked like her mother. Their father, when present, was violent towards Jackson and sexually abused Stasia.

What Do You Think?

- How might gender influence the development of symptoms?
- How might culture influence early recognition of problems and provision of early intervention to prevent future serious mental disorders?
- What are some possible outcomes in this situation?
- How does this case demonstrate the interaction between socialization, biology, and culture?

emphasis on aggression for conduct disorder or that ASPD is manifested differently in women, who are more likely to receive diagnoses of somatization (see Chapter 24) or histrionic disorders (discussed later in this chapter). It has been commonly assumed that BPD is more common in women, but this is not so. Higher prevalence rates among women seem to be an artefact of sampling in clinical settings; women are more likely to seek treatment (Hooley, Cole, & Gironde, 2012). The prevalence of disorders for which the affected individual rarely seeks help, such as pyromania, is particularly difficult to estimate.

Aetiology

For the most part, the aetiology of PDs and of the disruptive, impulse-control, and conduct disorders remains speculative and undetermined. A basic assumption underlying the category of PDs is that they evolve within the development of an individual's personality. What changes a normal personality to a disordered one might be genetic, neurobiologic, trauma- and stress-induced, environmental, or an interaction of such factors.

Temperament, a recognizable and distinctive pattern of behaviour that is evident during the first few months of life, is believed to be neurobiologically determined and may be central to understanding personality disorders. Temperament consists of the interaction of two behavioural dimensions—activity and adaptability. Activity patterns in individuals vary along a spectrum, from active or intense children, whose actions display decisiveness and vigour as they continuously relate to their environment, to passive children, who are more cautious and slow to relate to their environment (a wait-and-see pattern of behaviour). Adaptability includes a spectrum, with the extreme at one end being the child who is regular in biologic functions such as eating or sleeping, has a positive approach to new stimuli, and maintains a high degree of flexibility in response to changing conditions. At the other end of the adaptability dimension are children who display irregularity in biologic functions, withdrawal reactions to new stimuli, and minimal flexibility in response to change.

Research is exploring the influence of temperament and environment on the development of PDs. As example, a prospective, longitudinal study with adolescents explored temperament and maltreatment in predicting the emergence of BPD and ASPD. Measures of temperament, maltreatment, BPD, and ASPD symptoms were completed by 11- to 13-year-old participants ($n = 245$), most of whom ($n = 206$) were assessed again in 2 years. Childhood neglect was found to be a significant predictor of an increase in BPD symptoms, while childhood abuse predicted an increase in ASPD symptoms (Jovev et al., 2013). As well, findings suggested that high capacity for interpersonal affiliation and self-regulation may

protect children from developing such psychopathology in the presence of an adverse environment (Jovev et al., 2013).

It may be that PDs are on a continuum with more severe mental disorders. For example, there is evidence of a genetic link between STPD and schizophrenia (Matta et al., 2000). More research, however, is required before it can be determined if this disorder is actually a milder form of schizophrenia. Conversely, it is speculated in a neurodevelopmental explanation of STPD that schizotypy is due to insults to the nervous system (e.g., oxygen deprivation) at critical developmental periods. Supporting this perspective is that persons with STPD have cognitive deficits, involving the left hemisphere more than the right, and short-term memory and verbal learning difficulties (Cadenhead, Perry, Shafer, & Braff, 1999; Voglmaier et al., 2000).

A challenge of determining the aetiology of PDs can be their potential overlap with other mental disorders. For example, AVPD can overlap with social anxiety disorder (social phobia), and research indicates that frequently clients with diagnoses of social phobia also met the criteria for AVPD (Moutier & Stein, 1999). Social phobia is more pervasive and characterized by a higher level of interpersonal sensitivity (Perugi et al., 1999), however, and AVPD involves greater overall psychopathology (Boone et al., 1999). Persons with AVPD may experience aversive stimuli more intensely and more frequently than do others because they may possess an overabundance of neurons in the aversive centre of the limbic system (Millon, Millon, Meagher, Grossman, & Ramnath, 2004). A general biologic vulnerability may be inherited and interact with environmental factors. The evidence for this biologic influence is the impact of pharmacotherapies on these individuals. When taking medications (e.g., benzodiazepines, β-blockers, monoamine oxidase inhibitors), symptoms are reduced, but they resume once medication is stopped (Mattick & Newman, 1991). For BPD, genetic factors (e.g., abnormalities in serotonin neurotransmission system) and adverse life events may interact in its development, with neurobiologic evidence pointing to abnormalities in the brain's frontolimbic networks (Leichsenring, Leibing, Kruse, New, & Leweke, 2011). This is discussed further in the section on BPD.

Emotional and behavioural self-control problems characterize the disruptive, impulse-control, and conduct disorders, but the underlying causes of these problems vary greatly, even among individuals with the same diagnosis (APA, 2013). The risk factors for them may be temperamental, genetic, physiologic, environmental, or an interaction among such factors. Further research is necessary if the significant lack of clarity regarding the aetiologies of these and the personality disorders are to be resolved.

■■■ CLUSTER A DISORDERS
Paranoid Personality Disorder

The most prominent features of paranoid personality disorder (PPD) are mistrust of others and the desire to avoid relationships in which one is not in control. Individuals with PPD are suspicious, guarded, and hostile. They are consistently mistrustful of others' motives, even those of relatives and close friends. Actions of others are often misinterpreted as deception, deprecation, and betrayal, especially regarding fidelity or trustworthiness of a spouse or friend (Millon et al., 2004). Minor innocuous incidents are often misinterpreted as having sinister or hidden meaning, and suspicions are magnified into major distortions of reality. People with paranoid personalities distance themselves from others and can be outwardly argumentative and abrasive; internally, they may hold private hopes of being understood and feel powerless, fearful, and vulnerable (Hayward, 2007). Imagine living with the belief that you can trust no one and that there are some persons or organizations actively "out to get you."

Other hallmark features of PPD are persistent ideas of self-importance and the tendency to be rigid and controlled. The individual wants to appear controlled and objective, yet often reacts emotionally, displaying signs of nervousness, anger, envy, and jealousy. Fearful, the person will be hypervigilant to any environmental changes. Essentially, PPD is "a stable pattern of nonpsychotic paranoid behaviour" (Hopwood & Thomas, 2012, p. 582). If help is sought, however, it is unlikely that it will be from mental health professionals but rather from a resource, such as the police, that the person with PPD believes could stop the harm others are doing.

Narcissistic, avoidant, and obsessive–compulsive PDs can coexist with PPD, as can generalized anxiety disorder, mood disorders, and schizophrenia (Millon et al., 2004). There is some controversy regarding PPD as a unique diagnostic construct. It is questioned whether or not paranoid symptoms are unique; they may be fully explained by normal personality traits or psychotic disorders (Hopwood & Thomas, 2012).

Nursing Management

Nurses are most likely to see these clients for other health problems but will need to formulate nursing diagnoses based on the client's underlying suspiciousness (Ward, 2004). An assessment of individuals with PPD reveals disturbed or illogical thoughts that demonstrate the misinterpretation of environmental stimuli. For example, a man was convinced that his wife was having an affair with the neighbour because his wife and the neighbour left their homes for work at the same time each morning. Although the man's beliefs were illogical, he never once considered that he was wrong. He frequently followed them but never caught them together. He continued to believe that they were having an affair. When making a nursing diagnosis of disturbed thought processes, it needs to be supported by assessment data.

Because of their difficulty with developing relationships, individuals with PPD are often socially isolated and lack social support systems. Yet, the nursing diagnosis of social isolation is not appropriate for the person with PPD because the defining characteristics of feelings of aloneness, rejection, desire for contact with people, and insecurity in social situations are not met.

Nursing interventions based on the establishment of a nurse–client relationship are difficult to implement because of the person's mistrust. A professional, matter-of-fact approach and the creation of a nonthreatening environment in which the client can feel as secure as possible are helpful. Nurses must ensure that their own response to a client who does not readily accept them as trustworthy does not further impede relationship building. If a trusting relationship is established, the nurse helps the individual identify specific problematic areas, such as getting along with particular others or keeping a job. Through therapeutic techniques such as acceptance and reflection, as well as recognition by the nurse of the ramifications for client of his/her view of the world (e.g., what it feels like to believe one's spouse is having an affair), the nurse and the client can examine a problematic area to gain another view of the situation. Changing thought patterns takes time. Client outcomes are evaluated in terms of small changes in thinking and behaviour. Although antipsychotics might be considered in its treatment, no medications have been found to be specifically effective in treating PPD (Silk & Feurino, 2012).

Schizoid Personality Disorder

Individuals with schizoid personality disorder (SPD) are expressively impassive and interpersonally unengaged (Millon et al., 2004). They tend to be unable to experience the joyful and pleasurable aspects of life. They are introverted and reclusive, and clinically they appear distant, aloof, apathetic, and emotionally detached. They have difficulties making friends, seem uninterested in social activities, and appear to gain little satisfaction in personal relationships. In fact, they appear to be incapable of forming social relationships. Interests are directed at objects, things, and abstractions. As children, they engage primarily in solitary activities, such as stamp collecting, computer games, electronic equipment, or academic pursuits such as mathematics or engineering. In addition, there seems to be a cognitive deficit characterized by obscure thought processes, particularly about social matters. Communication with others is confused and lacks focus. These individuals reveal minimum introspection and self-awareness, and interpersonal experiences are described in a very mechanical way.

Nursing Management

Impaired social interactions and chronic low self-esteem are typical diagnoses of individuals with SPD. Major treatment goals are to enhance the experience of pleasure, prevent social isolation, and increase emotional responsiveness to others. Because these individuals often lack customary social skills, social skills training is useful in enhancing their ability to relate in interpersonal situations. The primary focus is to increase the person's ability to experience enjoyment. The nurse balances interventions between encouraging enough social activity that prevents the individual from retreating to a fantasy world and too much social activity that becomes intolerable.

Because persons with SPD typically shy away from interactions, establishing a therapeutic relationship can be challenging. The evaluation of outcomes should be in terms of increasing the client's feelings of satisfaction with solitary activities.

Schizotypal Personality Disorder

People with the schizotypal personality disorder (STPD) are characterized by a pattern of social and interpersonal deficits. They do not form friendships easily and may be close only to first-degree relatives. Their beliefs about their world are often are inconsistent with their cultural norms and appear odd to others. Ideas of reference (i.e., incorrect interpretations of events as having special, personal meaning) are often present, as are unusual perceptual delusions and odd, circumstantial, and metaphorical thinking and speech. Mood is constricted or inappropriate, and there are excessive social anxieties of a paranoid character that do not diminish with familiarity. Appearance and behaviour can be characterized as eccentric, or peculiar. An avoidant behaviour pattern is usually exhibited. The requirement that five of nine *DSM* criteria need to be met for a STPD diagnosis means that two individuals with STPD may share only one diagnostic feature (Kwapil & Barrantes-Vidal, 2012).

If an individual with STPD becomes psychotic, they will seem highly disoriented and confused and may exhibit posturing, grimacing, inappropriate giggling, rambling speech, and peculiar mannerisms. Fantasy, hallucinations, and bizarre, fragmented delusions may be present. Regressive acts such as enuresis and encopresis may occur. These individuals may consume food in an infantile or ravenous manner. Symptoms mirror but fall short of features that would justify the diagnosis of schizophrenia. Individuals with STPD may be unable to engage in social interaction that can keep them functional.

Nursing Management

Depending on the amount of decompensation (i.e., deterioration of functioning and exacerbation of symptoms), the assessment of a client with a STPD can generate a range of nursing diagnoses. If a person has severe symptoms, such as delusional thinking or perceptual disturbances, the nursing diagnoses are similar to those for a person with schizophrenia (see Chapter 20). If symptoms are mild, the typical nursing diagnoses include social isolation, ineffective coping, low self-esteem, and impaired social interactions.

People with STPD need help in increasing their sense of self-worth and recognizing their positive attributes. Limiting dependency and supporting self-directed activities appropriately is a focus of care. Individuals with this PD can benefit from interventions (e.g., social skills training; environmental management) that increase psychosocial functioning. As eccentric thoughts and behaviours alienate others, reinforcing and modelling socially appropriate dress and behaviour for a person with STPD can help to improve overall appearance and ability to relate (Hayward, 2007). A challenge for the person with STPD will be to generalize from one situation to another, so attention to cognitive skills is important (Waldeck & Miller, 2000).

Continuum of Care

Persons with cluster A personality disorders are rarely seen in mental health treatment unless their daily activities are seriously affected or symptoms of depression or anxiety appear. Improvement in quality of life for persons with these PDs is possible through psychotherapy, although symptoms such as suspiciousness, lack of trust, and impaired social interactions can make it difficult to establish a therapeutic relationship (Hayward, 2007). Engaging therapeutically with individuals with cluster A disorders can be at variance with the standard approach used with other clients, given the difficulty these clients have in forming emotional connections. In order to reduce the extreme anxiety that interpersonal engagement can cause, nurses will need to carefully judge appropriate therapeutic distance (Hayward, 2007). Brief interventions, including self-care assistance, reality orientation, and role enhancement, can be helpful (Bulechek, Butcher, & McCloskey Dochterman, 2008). Nurses encountering clients with cluster A PDs in non–mental health settings may need to consult with a PMH nursing specialist.

● **STUDY NOTE**

Nurses will care for individuals who have a PD in contexts other than mental health settings and in situations in which the PD is not the focus of care. When the disorder is not identified, the client may be unhelpfully labelled as "difficult."

CLUSTER B DISORDERS

Borderline Personality Disorder

Clinical Course of Disorder

In 1938, the term *border line* was first used to refer to a group of disorders that did not quite fit the definition of either neurosis or psychosis (Stern, 1938). The term evolved from the psychoanalytic conceptualization of the disorder as a dysfunctional personality structure. In 1980, Borderline Personality Disorder (BPD) was formally recognized as a distinct disorder in the *DSM-III*. Today, in the *DSM-5*, the essential feature of BPD is "a pervasive pattern of instability of interpersonal relationships, self-image, and affects, and marked impulsivity that begins by early adulthood and is present in a variety of contexts" (APA, 2013, p. 663). Instability is a core component of this disorder. Table 27-1 outlines the diagnostic characteristics of BPD. (Note: In the WHO's International Classification of Disease [ICD-10], the term "emotionally unstable disorder, borderline type" is used.)

Individuals with BPD have difficulty with interpersonal relationships in that they experience them as intensive, alternately idealize and devalue others, and become frantic if they feel that they may be abandoned. They have problems with unstable, highly reactive moods, with developing a sense of self, with feelings of emptiness, and with maintaining reality-based cognitive processes. Intense, inappropriate anger and its control can be a problem for them. Impulsive or destructive behaviour, such as suicidal or self-mutilating acts, is an ongoing possibility. Persons with BPD may appear more competent than they actually are and often set unrealistically high expectations for themselves. When these expectations are not met, they experience intense shame, self-hate, and self-directed anger. They seem to live from one crisis to another. Some of the crises are caused by the individual's dysfunctional lifestyle or inadequate social milieu, but many are simply challenging human experiences, like the death of a spouse or diagnosis of an illness, to which they react emotionally with minimal coping skills. The intensity of their dysregulation often frightens themselves and others. Friends, family members, and coworkers may come to limit their contact with them, which furthers their sense of aloneness, abandonment, and self-hatred. It also diminishes opportunities for learning self-corrective measures.

Affective Instability

Affective instability (i.e., rapid and extreme shift in mood) is a core characteristic of BPD and is evidenced by erratic emotional responses to situations and intense sensitivity to criticism or perceived slights. For example, a person may greet a casual acquaintance with intense affection, yet later be aloof with the same acquaintance. Friends describe individuals with BPD as moody, irresponsible, or intense. These individuals fail to recognize their own emotional responses, thoughts, beliefs, and behaviours.

Table 27-1 **A Summary of Diagnostic Characteristics of Borderline Personality Disorder**

Diagnostic Criteria and Target Symptoms	Associated Behavioural Findings
• Pervasive pattern of unstable interpersonal relationships, self-image, and affects • Frantic efforts to avoid real or imagined abandonment • Pattern of unstable and intense interpersonal relationships (alternating between the extremes of idealization and devaluation) • Identity disturbance (markedly and persistently unstable self-image or sense of self) • Impulsivity in at least two areas that are potentially self-damaging (spending, sex, substance abuse, reckless driving, or binge eating) • Recurrent suicidal behaviour, gestures, or threats; or self-mutilating behaviour • Affective instability due to a marked reactivity of mood (intense episodes lasting a few hours and only rarely more than a few days) • Chronic feelings of emptiness • Inappropriate, intense anger or difficulty controlling anger • Transient, stress-related paranoid ideation or severe dissociative symptoms • Beginning by early adulthood and presenting in a variety of contexts	• Pattern of undermining self at the moment a goal is to be realized • Possible psychotic-like symptoms during times of stress • Recurrent job losses, interrupted education, and broken marriages • History of physical and sexual abuse, neglect, hostile conflict, and early parental loss or separation

American Psychiatric Association. (2013). *Diagnostic and Statistical Manual of Mental Disorders* (5th ed.). Washington, DC: Author.

Clinically, when a stressful situation is encountered, the person with BPD reacts with shifts in emotions, appearing to have limited ability to develop emotional buffers to stressful situations. Regulating anger, anxiety, and sadness is particularly problematic. Difficulty with the intensity and regulation of emotion negatively affects social behaviours and relationships, including relations with health professionals (Holm & Severinsson, 2008). These affective symptoms have been shown to be long-lasting components of the disorder (Zanarini et al., 2007). Research does suggest that emotional dysregulation may play a central role in the development and maintenance of BPD (Stepp et al., 2014). When individuals with innate biologic propensity for intense emotional reactivity develop in an environment that is unsupportive of learning ways to regulate one's emotions, such a deficit will contribute to increased affective instability and dysregulated cognitions, behaviours, and interpersonal relationships. If this is so, helping the individual with BPD to develop emotional awareness and clarity and to improve their ability to cope with negative emotions may be effective in improving other BPD symptoms, as well (Stepp et al., 2014).

Identity Disturbances

Identity diffusion occurs when a person lacks aspects of personal identity or when personal identity is poorly developed (Erikson, 1968). Four factors of identity are most commonly disturbed: role absorption (i.e., narrowly defining self within a single role), painful incoherence (i.e., distressed sense of internal disharmony), inconsistency (i.e., lack of coherence in thoughts, feelings, and actions), and lack of normative commitment (Weston, Beton, & Defife, 2011). Other factors of personality identity (e.g., religious ideologies, moral value systems, and sexual attitudes) appear to be less important in identity diffusion. Clinically, these clients appear to have little sense of their own identity and direction; this becomes a source of great distress to them and is often manifested by chronic feelings of emptiness and boredom. It is not unusual for persons with BPD to direct their actions in accord with the wishes of other people. For example, as one woman with BPD described herself:

> I am a singer because my mother wanted me to be. I live in the city because my manager thought that I should. I become whatever anyone tells me to be. Whenever someone recommends a song, I wonder why I didn't think of that. My boyfriend tells me what to wear.

Unstable Interpersonal Relationships

Individuals with BPD have an extreme fear of abandonment as well as a history of unstable, insecure attachments (Meyer & Pilkonis, 2005). This abandonment likely stems from ambivalent early childhood attachment and invalidations within the early parent–child bond (Yen et al., 2002). Most have never experienced a consistently secure, nurturing relationship and thus are constantly seeking reassurance and validation. In an attempt to meet their interpersonal needs, they idealize others and establish intense relationships that violate others' interpersonal boundaries, which ultimately leads to rejection (Bartholomew & Horowitz, 1991). When these relationships do not live up to their expectations, the person with BPD devalues the other person. Continually disappointed in relationships, this individual feels estranged from others and inadequate in the face of perceived social standards. Intense shame and self-hate follow. These feelings often result in self-injurious behaviours, such as cutting the wrist, self-inflicted burns, or head banging.

In social situations, persons with BPD use elaborate strategies to structure interactions. That is, they restrict their relationships to ones in which they feel in control. They distance themselves from groups when feeling anxious (which is most of the time) and rarely use their social support system. Even if they are married or have a supportive extended family, they are reluctant to share their feelings (Krause, Mendelson, & Lynch, 2003). They do not want to burden anyone, fear rejection, and assume that others are tired of hearing them repeat the same issues (Miller, 1994).

A controversial area of BPD is separating early childhood abuse and trauma from pathologic development. In fact, persons with confirmed childhood abuse and neglect histories show a fourfold likelihood of having a personality disorder (Johnson, Cohen, Brown, Smailes, & Bernstein, 1999). Although trauma and abuse do not seem to cause BPD, they may sufficiently disturb identity and affect regulation to contribute to disordered personality development (Grover et al., 2007; Zanarini et al., 1997).

Cognitive Dysfunctions

An aspect of BPD is dichotomous thinking. Individuals with BPD will evaluate experiences, people, and objects in terms of mutually exclusive categories (e.g., good or bad, success or failure, trustworthy or deceitful); this informs extreme interpretations of events that would normally be viewed as including both positive and negative aspects. There are also times when thinking becomes disorganized. Irrelevant, bizarre notions and vague or scattered thought connections can be present, as well as delusions and hallucinations.

Another cognitive dysfunction common in BPD is **dissociation**, in which thoughts and ideas can be split off from consciousness (Martin, 2007). Dissociation can be conceptualized as lying on a continuum from minor dissociations of daily life, such as daydreaming, to a breakdown in the usually integrated functions of consciousness, memory, perception of self or the environment, and sensorimotor behaviours. For example, in driving familiar roads, people often get lost in their thoughts or dissociate and suddenly do not remember what happened during that part of the trip. Environmental stimuli are ignored, and there are changes in the perception of reality.

The individual is physically present but mentally in another place. Dissociation can be a coping strategy for avoiding disturbing events. In dissociating, the person does not have to be aware of or remember traumatic events. There is a strong correlation between dissociation and self-injurious behaviour (Zanarini, Ruser, Frankenburg, & Hennen, 2000).

Dysfunctional Behaviours

Impaired Problem Solving

In BPD, there is often a failure to engage in active problem solving. Instead, problem solving is attempted by soliciting help from others in a helpless, hopeless manner (Linehan, 1993a). Suggestions are rarely taken.

Impulsivity

Impulsivity is also characteristic of the individual living with BPD. When impulse driven, individuals will have difficulty delaying gratification or thinking through the consequences before acting on their feelings; their actions are often unpredictable. Essentially, they act in the moment and then must face the consequences afterwards. Gambling, spending money irresponsibly, binge eating, engaging in unsafe sex, and abusing substances are examples of such impulse acts. Job losses, interrupted education, and unsuccessful relationships are common to the history of persons with BPD.

Self-Injurious Behaviours

Unsuccessful interpersonal relationships and turmoil in social experiences may lead the person with BPD to undermine himself or herself when a goal is about to be reached. The most serious consequences are suicide attempts or **parasuicidal behaviours** (i.e., deliberate self-injury with intent to harm oneself). The prevalence of self-injurious behaviour is estimated to be 43% to 67% of people with BPD (Soloff, Lis, Kelly, Cornelius, & Ulrich, 2004). Self-injurious behaviour can be compulsive, episodic, or repetitive, and is more likely to occur when the individual with BPD is depressed; has highly unstable interpersonal relationships, especially problems with intimacy and sociability; and is hypervigilant (i.e., alert, watchful), and resentful (Paris, 2007; Yeomans, Hull, & Clarkin, 1994). Self-injurious behaviours associated with BPD are listed below.

- *Compulsive self-injurious behaviours* that may occur many times daily and are repetitive and ritualistic. For example, hair pulling, which can be a separate disorder (**trichotillomania**) or behaviour associated with other personality disorders, involves pulling out hair, especially from the scalp, eyebrows, and eyelashes. Hair is plucked, examined, and sometimes eaten. Hair-pulling sessions may take several hours (Boughn, 2005). Most of those afflicted do not seek help unless the symptoms are severe and then they usually consult dermatologists or family practitioners.

- *Episodic self-injurious behaviours* occur every so often. These are especially common in people with BPD and develop into habitual coping behavioural patterns during periods when stress (i.e., progressive tension manifested by feelings of anger, depression, or anxiety) rises to an intolerable level. The individual reports being numb or empty and ends this dissociated state with a self-injurious behaviour that elicits feeling. One-half to two-thirds of people with BPD with self-injurious behaviours experience little or no associated pain (Links, Heslegrave, & van Reekum, 1998); rather, endogenous endorphins (opioids) are released, which dampen pain perception and activate the brain's pleasure centre. In addition, tension is relieved and a sense of calmness or even pleasure may follow. These feelings are believed to be reinforcing, and the person learns to relieve stress and anxiety by self-mutilation. The individuals harm themselves to feel better, get rapid relief from distressing thoughts and emotions, and gain a sense of control.

- *Repetitive self-mutilation* occurs when occasional self-injury turns into an overwhelming preoccupation. The person can be labelled as a "cutter" or "burner," for example, and describes him or herself as being addicted to self-harm. In an interpretive phenomenologic study of people with BPD, Nehls (1999) described the emotional conflict when efforts to comfort oneself are interpreted by others as manipulation, resulting in care being denied. Sometimes clients and nurses determine the risk for suicide by whether the intended outcome of an episode is death or injury. The underlying assumption is that those who attempt to kill themselves are at higher risk than those who self-injure. In reality, all self-injurious behaviours should be considered potentially life threatening and taken seriously.

Aetiology

The answer to what causes BPD remains undetermined. Most likely, it will be found that BPD is caused by the interaction of genetic and biologic vulnerabilities, and environmental factors. This is a "highly individualized disorder" so the diagnosis of BPD likely reflects many "unique influences and developmental trajectories" (Hooley et al., 2012, p. 415). A brief overview of the existing knowledge related to the aetiology of BPD follows.

Neurobiologic and Genetic Factors

There is evidence that genetic factors are involved in the development of BPD: it is five times more common among "first-degree biologic relatives" of individuals with BPD than among the general population (APA, 2013, p. 665). Persons with BPD appear to have abnormal serotonergic function, associated with impulsive aggressive symptoms, and such a defect might be related to genetic factors (Leichsenring et al., 2011). BPD may be related to "stress-induced compromises" in the neural circuits underlying regulatory processes (Hooley et al., 2012, p. 428). PET studies support the hypothesis that persons with BPD have abnormalities in the prefrontal brain regions (associated with emotion control); functional MRI studies add support to the hypothesis that persons with BPD have a dysfunctional frontolimbic network. There has been speculation that individuals with BPD have reduced volume in the amygdala, but the evidence for this remains inconsistent (Leichsenring et al., 2011).

Psychosocial Risk Factors

Various studies show that maltreatment appears to be a significant risk factor for BPD: 55% to 80% of individuals with BPD have reported a history of childhood sexual abuse and/or physical abuse (Jordan, 2004). Childhood neglect has been correlated with increase in BPD symptoms (Jovev et al., 2013). Other earlier studies cite parental loss and separation (Zweig-Frank, Paris, & Guzder, 1994a, 1994b). Clearly, more studies are needed to identify risk factors for the development of BPD.

Psychological Theories

Psychoanalytic Theories

The psychoanalytic views of BPD focus on two important psychoanalytic concepts: separation–individuation and projective identification. According to this theory, a person with BPD has not achieved the normal and healthy developmental stage of **separation–individuation**, during which a child develops a sense of self, a permanent sense of significant others (object constancy), and integration of seeing both bad and good components of self (Mahler, Pine, & Bergman, 1975). Object Relations Theory explains how the objects (i.e., real and internalized relationships with significant people) contribute to personality and are expressed through defences and interpersonal interactions (Clarkin, Yeomans, & Kernberg, 2006; Magnavita, 2004). Within this theory, individuals with BPD are viewed as lacking the ability to separate from the primary caregiver and develop a separate and distinct personality or self-identity. Psychoanalytic theory suggests that these separation difficulties occur because the primary caregivers' behaviours have been inconsistent or insensitive to the needs of the child. The child develops ambivalent feelings regarding interpersonal relationships and therefore has no basis for establishing trusting and secure relationships in the future. Children experience feelings of intense fear and anger in separating themselves from others. This problem continues into adulthood, and they continue to experience difficulties in maintaining personal boundaries and in interpersonal interactions and relationships. These individuals may falsely attribute to others their own unacceptable feelings, impulses, or thoughts, termed **projective identification**. Projective

identification is believed to play an important role in the development of BPD and is a defence mechanism by which people with BPD protect their fragile self-image. For example, when overwhelmed by anxiety or anger at being disregarded by another, they defend against the intensity of these feelings by unconsciously blaming others for what happens to them. They project their feelings onto a significant other with the unconscious hope that the other knows how to deal with it. Projective identification becomes a defensive way of interacting with the world, which leads to more rejection.

Maladaptive Cognitive Processes

Cognitive schemas are important in understanding BPD. Individuals with personality disorders develop maladaptive schemas leading them to misinterpret environmental stimuli continuously, which in turn leads to rigid and inflexible behaviour patterns in response to new situations and people. Because those with BPD have been conditioned to anticipate rejection and disappointment in the past, they become entrenched in a pattern of fear and anxiety regarding encountering new people or situations. They have fears that a disaster is going to strike any minute. Early in life, individuals with BPD and other personality disorders develop maladaptive schemas or dysfunctional ways of interpreting people and events. Table 27-2 explains 18 major maladaptive schemas at work in those with personality disorders. The work of cognitive therapists is to challenge these distortions in thinking patterns and replace them with realistic ones. Therapists, too, have personal schemas regarding themselves and others; they need to identify their own schemas and ensure that therapeutic progress is not impeded by an unrecognized conflict with the schema of their clients' (Leahy & McGinn, 2012).

Biosocial Theories

The biosocial learning theory was developed by Theodore Millon, who viewed BPD as a distinct disorder that develops as a result of both biologic and psychological factors (Millon & Davis, 1999). While he supported the biologic determination of personality, he believed that a child's interaction with the environment and learning and experience could greatly affect his or her biologic predisposition. He argued that each individual possesses a biologically based pattern of sensitivities and behavioural dispositions that shapes his or her experiences, including active–passive behaviour or a tendency to take initiative versus reacting to events, sensitivity to pleasure or pain, and sensitivity behaviour to self and others. Millon believed that BPD is a particular cycloid personality pattern representing a moderately dysfunctional dependent or ambivalent orientation, often expressed in intense endogenous moods, described as patterns of recurring dejection and apathy interspersed with spells of anger, anxiety, or euphoria.

Table 27-2	Maladaptive Schemas

Domain	Schemas With Definitions
I. Disconnection and rejection	1. *Abandonment/instability* Important people will not be there 2. *Mistrust/abuse* Other people will use the client for own selfish ends 3. *Emotional deprivation* Emotional connection will not be fulfilled 4. *Defectiveness/scheme* One is flawed, bad, or worthless 5. *Social isolation/alienation* Being different from or not fitting in
II. Impaired autonomy and performance	1. *Dependence/incompetence* Belief that one is unable to function on one's own 2. *Vulnerability to harm and illness* Fear that disaster is about to strike 3. *Enmeshment/undeveloped self* Excessive emotional involvement at the expense of normal social development 4. *Failure* Belief that one has failed
III. Impaired limits	1. *Entitlement/grandiosity* Belief that one is superior to other; entitled to special rights 2. *Insufficient self-control/self-discipline* Difficulty or refusal to exercise sufficient self-control
IV. Other directedness	1. *Subjugation* Excessive surrendering of control to others because of feeling coerced 2. *Self-sacrifice* Excessive focus on voluntarily meeting the needs of others at the expense of one's own gratification 3. *Approval seeking/recognition seeking* Excessive emphasis on gaining approval, recognition, or attention
V. Overvigilance and inhibition	1. *Negativity/pessimism* Lifelong focus on the negative aspects of life 2. *Emotional inhibition* Excessive inhibition of spontaneous action, feeling, or communication 3. *Unrelenting standard/hypercriticalness* Belief that one must meet very high standards; perfectionistic, rigid 4. *Punitiveness* Belief that people should be harshly punished

Young, J. E. (1999). *Cognitive therapy for personality disorders: A schema-focused approach.* Sarasota, FL: Professional Resource Press.

A further elaboration of Millon's multidimensional model incorporates biologic explanations into the behaviour. Cloninger, Bayon, and Svrakic (1998) described personality disorder behaviours based on temperament and character dimensions derived from a factor analysis design. Cluster A disorders are associated with low-reward dependence and social attachment mediated by norepinephrine and serotonin. Cluster B disorders are associated with high novelty-seeking mediated by dopamine. Novelty-seeking behaviour includes exhilaration, exploration, impulsivity, extravagance, and irritability. Cluster C disorders are associated with high harm-avoidance mediated by γ-aminobutyric acid (GABA) and serotonin.

A current biosocial theory of BPD proposed by Marsha Linehan and colleagues is similar to Millon's theory, with a focus on the interaction of both biologic and social learning influences. Their primary focus is on the particular behavioural patterns observed in BPD, including emotional vulnerability, self-invalidation, unrelenting crises, inhibited grieving, active passivity, and apparent competence (Linehan, 1993a; Box 27-4).

This biosocial viewpoint presents BPD as a multifaceted problem, a combination of a person's innate **emotional vulnerability** and his or her inability to control that emotion in social interactions (**emotional dysregulation**) and the environment (Linehan, 1993a). The emotional dysregulation and aggressive impulsivity entail both social learning and biologic regulation. Much of the neurobiologic research is directed at neurotransmitter functions (Silk, 2000) and neural firing between the limbic system and the frontal and prefrontal cortex. When these pathways are functional, the person has a greater

---

BOX 27-4 Behavioural Patterns in BPD

1. *Emotional vulnerability.* Person experiences a pattern of pervasive difficulties in regulating negative emotions, including a high sensitivity to negative emotional stimuli, high emotional intensity, and slow return to emotional baseline.
2. *Self-invalidation.* Person fails to recognize one's own emotional responses, thoughts, beliefs, and behaviours and sets unrealistically high standards and expectations for self. May include intense shame, self-hate, and self-directed anger. Person has no personal awareness and tends to blame social environment for unrealistic expectations and demands.
3. *Unrelenting crises.* Person experiences a pattern of frequent, stressful, negative environmental events, disruptions, and roadblocks—some caused by the individual's dysfunctional

lifestyle, others by an inadequate social milieu, and many by fate or chance.
4. *Inhibited grieving.* Person tries to inhibit and overcontrol negative emotional responses, especially those associated with grief and loss, including sadness, anger, guilt, shame, anxiety, and panic.
5. *Active passivity.* Person fails to engage actively in solving own life problems but will actively seek problem solving from others in the environment; learned helplessness, hopelessness.
6. *Apparent competence.* Tendency for the individual to appear deceptively more competent than he or she actually is; usually due to failure of competencies to generalize across expected moods, situations, and time and failure to display adequate nonverbal cues of emotional distress.

From Linehan, M. (1993a). *Cognitive-behavioral treatment of borderline personality disorder* (p. 10). New York, NY: Guilford Press.

---

capacity to think about his or her emotions and modulate behaviours more responsibly.

The biosocial viewpoint supports the notion that the ability to control one's emotion is in part a learning process, learned from one's private experiences and encounters with the social environment. A risk factor associated with BPD is believed to develop when emotionally vulnerable individuals interact with an **invalidating environment**, a social situation that negates the individual's private emotional responses and communication. That is, when others whom the person respects or values are continuously insensitive to the person's core emotional responses, respond irrationally and inappropriately, or trivialize his or her painful experiences, the person receives confused messages about expressing feelings. Further, the message from significant others may be that negative emotions, in particular, are not to be expressed. Invalidation occurs as the individual's emotions are continuously dismissed, trivialized, devalued, punished, and discredited.

A minor example of invalidating environment or response follows. The parents of Emily, a 4-year-old girl, tell her that the family is going to grandmother's house for a family meal. The child responds, "I am not going to Grandma's. I hate Stevie (cousin)." The parents reply, "You don't hate Stevie. He is a wonderful child. He is your cousin, and only a spoiled, selfish little girl would say such a thing." The parents have devalued Emily's feelings and discredited her comments, thereby invalidating her feelings and sense of personal worth.

The most severe form of invalidation occurs in situations of child sexual abuse. Often, the abusing adult has told the child that this is a "special secret" between them, that the child should feel guilty if he or she tells anyone, and that telling someone would end their trust and special relationship. The child experiences feelings of fear, pain, and sadness, yet this trusted adult continuously dismisses the child's true feelings and tells the child what he or she should feel. Children often learn to endure sexual

abuse for years, suppressing their true feelings. In disclosing the secret to a nonoffending adult, the child risks not being believed or attended to, and possible punishment.

In reality, all children, not just those who are emotionally vulnerable, must learn to trust their own feelings and learn when and how to express them by interacting with their environments, including parents, families, friends, and social situations. If they constantly meet with an invalidating environment, they cannot learn to trust their own feelings—when to be angry, sad, or happy—they become emotionally dysregulated. This emotional dysregulation leads to further difficulties in identity disturbances, interpersonal relationships, and the development of impulsive, parasuicidal behaviours.

Interdisciplinary Treatment

BPD is a very complex disorder that requires the involvement of the entire mental health care team in its treatment. Although psychotherapy has not been shown to lead to remission of BPD (i.e., the diagnostic criteria are no longer met), it can help the individual better manage symptoms of the disorder (Leichsenring et al., 2011), such as dysfunctional moods, impulsive behaviours, and self-injurious behaviours. Specially trained therapists, representing a variety of mental health disciplines, including psychology, social work, and advanced practice nursing are often involved. The factors important to a psychotherapeutic approach to BPD include a strong working alliance, empathy, and a practical problem-solving approach (Paris, 2010). This can be a lifelong disorder requiring ongoing treatment as the individual copes with multiple interpersonal crises.

Dialectical Behaviour Therapy

Dialectical behaviour therapy (DBT), developed by Marsha Linehan (1993a), uses cognitive–behavioural therapy strategies but also draws on Zen principles, dialectical philosophy, and behavioural science. DBT consists of four treatment components: individual therapy, group skills training, telephone coaching, and therapist consultation team (i.e., therapy for the therapist) (Leahy & McGinn, 2012). Behaviour patterns of BPD are perceived in this treatment approach as based in a dysfunctional emotional regulation system that evolved from biologic vulnerabilities and an invalidating environment. There are three facets: sensitivity to both positive and negative emotional stimuli, emotional intensity, and slow return to emotion baseline (Lynch & Cuper, 2012, p. 786). As noted, persons with BPD have difficulty moderating their emotions; they react based on their current emotions and come to mistrust their thoughts and emotional responses (Lynch & Cuper, 2012).

For DBT to be effective, the therapists and coaches must work with clients as partners and be willing to focus on interconnected behaviours (e.g., parasuicidal and substance abuse) and not a single diagnosis. Clients actively participate in treatment by collecting information about their own behaviours, identifying behaviours to change, and working with the therapists to change them. Problem solving, exposure techniques (i.e., gradual exposure to cues that set off aversive emotions), skill training, contingency management (i.e., reinforcement of positive behaviour), and cognitive modification are core procedures used.

Skills groups are an integral part of DBT in which members practise emotional regulation, interpersonal effectiveness, core mindfulness skills, and distress tolerance. Skills taught to manage intense, labile moods involve helping the client to label and analyze the context of the emotion and to use strategies to reduce emotional vulnerability. Learning to observe and describe emotions without judging or blocking them allows the individual to experience emotions without stimulating secondary feelings that cause more distress. For example, describing the emotion of anger without judging it as being "bad" can eliminate feelings of guilt that lead to self-injury.

Interpersonal effectiveness skills include the development of assertiveness and problem-solving skills within an interpersonal context. Clients are given strategies to meet their goals in a particular situation, while at the same time maintaining relationships with others and their self-respect.

Mindfulness skills are the psychological and behavioural versions of meditation skills usually taught in Eastern spiritual practice and are used to help the person improve observation, description, and participation skills by learning to focus the mind and awareness on the current moment's activity in a nonjudgemental and effective manner (see Chapter 13).

Distress tolerance skills involve helping the individual tolerate and accept distress as a part of normal life. Self-management skills focus on helping clients learn how to control, manage, or change behaviours, thoughts, or emotional responses to events (Linehan, 1993a; van den Bosch, Verheul, Schippers, & van den Brink, 2002).

Although there is no evidence as yet to support one form of psychotherapy over another for the treatment of BPD (Leichsenring et al., 2011), there is evidence to support DBT's clinical effectiveness. When used on an inpatient basis, it requires staff commitment and reinforcement; significant improvement in depression, anxiety, and dissociation symptoms and a highly significant decrease in parasuicidal behaviour have been shown (Bohus et al., 2000). DBT is more often incorporated into a long-term outpatient treatment approach because the greatest effectiveness occurs when skills are learned over time and practised in a variety of daily living settings (Feigenbaum, 2007). Members of the treatment team maintain a positive skills-coaching role with clients. Pessimistic and oppositional attitudes towards recovery from BPD on the part of health care professionals have been a significant impediment in the treatment of persons with BPD (Horsfall, 1999; Nehls, 1998, Nehls, 1999).

Psychopharmacotherapy

Although individuals with BPD are treated with medication, the efficacy of such treatments appears to be symptomatic at best. A Cochrane collaborative systematic review of randomized controlled trials of drug treatment for BPD found that mood stabilizers (e.g., topiramate) and second-generation antipsychotics (e.g., olanzapine) can be effective for symptoms, but evidence does not support medication as treatment for overall reduction of severity of the disorder (Lieb, Völlm, Rücker, Timmer, & Stoffers, 2010). Some medications used to treat BPD symptoms have side effects that are potentially harmful (e.g., valproate semisodium for women of childbearing age) or are neurologic or metabolic in nature (e.g., antipsychotics) (Leichsenring et al., 2011). Risks/benefits must be carefully considered in the symptomatic treatment of BPD.

Family Response to Disorder

The family of clients with BPD may feel captive to the symptoms of the disorder. Family members can be afraid to disagree with them or refuse to meet their multiple needs, fearing that self-destructive behaviours will follow. During the course of the disorder, family members can get "burned out" and withdraw from the individual, only adding to the person's fear of abandonment (Hoffman, Fruzzetti, & Buteau, 2007). DBT treatment that includes the involvement of family and others has been developed (Black, Blum, Pfohl, & John, 2004; Van Wel et al., 2006).

Nursing Management

It is important to recognize that BPD is a devastating disorder that involves much emotional pain and distress and, too often, it is stigmatized (Hooley et al., 2012). Individuals living with BPD experience instability in a

BOX 27-5 Response Patterns of Individuals With BPD

Affective (mood) dysregulation
Mood lability
Problems with anger
Interpersonal dysregulation
Chaotic relationships
Fears of abandonment
Self-dysregulation
Identity disturbance or difficulties with sense of self
Sense of emptiness
Behavioural dysregulation
Parasuicidal behaviour or threats
Impulsive behaviour
Cognitive dysregulation
Dissociative responses
Paranoid ideation

Courtesy of M. Linehan, Department of Psychology, Box 351525, University of Washington, Seattle, WA 98195–1525.

variety of areas, including mood, interpersonal relationships, self-esteem, and self-identity, and they can exhibit behavioural and cognitive dysregulations. These manifest in a number of ways, the most prominent of which are listed in Box 27-5. Due to their patterns of response, clients may have problems in daily living: maintaining intimate relationships, keeping a job, and living within the law (Box 27-6).

Individuals with BPD may enter the mental health system early (young adulthood or before), but because of their chaotic lifestyle, they typically do not receive consistent treatment. They drop in and out of treatment and usually do not remain with one clinician for long-term treatment. Persons with BPD usually seek help from health care workers because of consequences of life crises, medical conditions, or other psychiatric disorders (e.g., depression) or for physical treatment of self-injury. Thus, other problems may need attention before the client's underlying personality disorder can be addressed; at times, the nurse will not know that the person has BPD. During an assessment, however, it usually becomes clear that the client is affected by things more intensely than the average person or has an inflexible view of the world. The great difficulty the client has in changing behaviour, no matter the consequences, will also become apparent. He or she faces difficulty in successfully relating to other people and struggles to live a satisfying life.

Biologic Domain

Biologic Assessment

The client with BPD is usually able to maintain personal hygiene and physical functioning. Because of the comorbidity of BPD and eating disorders and substance abuse, a nutritional assessment may be needed. The assessment should also include the use of caffeinated beverages (e.g., coffee, tea, soft drinks) and alcohol. With individuals who engage in binging or purging, an assessment should include examining the teeth for pitting and discolouration, as well as the hands and fingers for redness and calluses caused by inducing vomiting. The client should be

BOX 27-6 Clinical Vignette

BORDERLINE PERSONALITY DISORDER

JS is a 22-year-old single woman who was recently fired from her job as a data entry clerk. She is living with her mother and stepfather, who brought her to the emergency room after finding her crouched in a foetal position in the bathroom, her wrists bleeding. She seemed to be in a daze. This is her first psychiatric admission, although her mother and stepfather have suspected that she has "needed help" for a long time. In high school, she received brief treatment for a potential eating disorder. She remains very thin but is able to eat at least one meal per day. During periods of stress, however, she will go for days without eating.

JS is the second of three children. Her parents divorced when she was 3 years old. She has not seen her father since he left. Although she has pleasant memories of her father, her mother has told her that he beat JS and her sisters when he was drinking. When JS was 6 years old, her older sister died following an automobile accident. JS was in the car but was uninjured. As a child, JS was seen as a potential singing star. Her natural musical talent attracted her teachers' support, which encouraged her to develop her talent. She received singing lessons and entered provincial competitions in high school. Although she enjoyed the attention, she was never really comfortable in the limelight and felt "guilty" about having a talent that she sometimes resented. She was able to make friends but found that she was unable to keep them.

They described her as "too intense" and emotional. She had one boyfriend in high school, but she was very uncomfortable with any physical closeness. After ending the relationship with the boyfriend, she concentrated on dieting to have a "perfect body." When her dieting attracted her parents' attention, she vowed to eat just enough to keep them "off her back about it." She spent much of her leisure time with her grandmother. She attended university briefly but was unable to concentrate. It was during her time at university and after her grandmother's death that JS began cutting her wrists during periods of stress. It seemed to calm her.

After leaving university, JS returned home. She had several jobs and short-lived friendships. She was usually fired from her job because of "moodiness," and it would take her several months before she would again find another. She would spend days in her room listening to music. Her recent episode followed being fired from work and spending 3 days in her bedroom.

What Do You Think?
- How would you describe JS's mood?
- Are JS's losses (father, sister) really severe enough to affect her ability to relate to others now? Do the losses seem to relate to the self-injury?
- What behaviours indicate that there are problems with self-esteem and self-identity?

queried about physiologic responses of emotion. Sleep patterns also should be assessed because sleep alterations may suggest coexisting depression or mania.

Physical Indicators of Self-Injurious Behaviours

Clients with BPD should be assessed for self-injurious behaviours or suicide attempts. It is important to ask the individual about specific self-abusive behaviours, such as cutting, scratching, or overdosing. She or he may wear long sleeves to hide an injury on the arms. Specifically asking about thoughts of hurting oneself when experiencing a major upset provides an opportunity for prevention and for coaching the client towards alternative self-soothing measures.

Pharmacologic Assessment

The medications that clients with BPD are taking need to be identified and assessed. Initially, individuals may be reluctant to disclose all their medications as they may be concerned that some or all of their medication may be stopped. The development of rapport with special attention to a nonjudgemental approach is especially important when eliciting current medication practices. The client will play an important role in determining the efficacy of a medication in relieving targeted symptoms. The use of alcohol and street drugs should also be carefully assessed to determine drug interactions.

Nursing Diagnoses for the Biologic Domain

Nursing diagnoses focusing on the biologic domain include disturbed sleep pattern, imbalanced nutrition, self-mutilation or risk for self-mutilation, and ineffective therapeutic regimen management.

Interventions for the Biologic Domain

The interventions for the biologic domain may address a whole spectrum of problems. Usually, the individuals are managing hydration, self-care, and pain well. This section focuses on those areas most likely to be problematic.

Sleep Enhancement

The facilitation of regular sleep–wake cycles may be needed because of disturbed sleep patterns. Conservative approaches should be exhausted before recommending medication (see Chapter 28). Establishing a regular bedtime routine, monitoring bedtime snacks and drinks, and avoiding foods and drinks that interfere with sleep should be tried. If relaxation exercises are used, they should be adapted to the tolerance of the individual. Moderate exercises (e.g., brisk walking) 3 to 4 hours before bedtime activate both serotonin and endorphins, thereby enhancing calmness and a sense of well-being before bedtime. For individuals who have difficulty falling asleep and experience interrupted sleep, it helps to establish some basic sleeping routines. The bedroom should be reserved for only two activities: sleeping and sex. Therefore, the client should remove the television, computer, and exercise equipment from the bedroom. If the individual is not asleep within 15 minutes, he or she should get out of bed and go to another room to read, watch television, or listen to soft music. The client should return to bed when sleepy. If the person is not asleep in 15 minutes, the same process should be repeated.

Special consideration must be made for individuals who have been physically and sexually abused and who may be unable to put themselves in a vulnerable position (e.g., lying down in a room with other people or closing their eyes). These clients may need additional safeguards to help them sleep, such as a night light or repositioning of furniture to afford easy exit.

Nutritional Balance

The nutritional status of the person with BPD can quickly become a priority, particularly if the individual has coexisting eating disorders or substance abuse. Eating is often a response to stress, and clients can quickly become overweight. This is especially a problem when the individual has also been taking medications that can promote weight gain, such as antipsychotics, antidepressants, or mood stabilizers. Helping the client to learn the basics of nutrition, make reasonable choices, and develop other coping strategies is a useful intervention. If individuals are engaging in purging or severe dieting practices, teaching them about the dangers of both of these practices is important (see Chapter 25). Referral to an eating disorders specialist may be needed.

Prevention and Treatment of Self-Injury

Clients with BPD are usually admitted to the inpatient setting because of actual or potential self-injury. Observing for antecedents of self-injurious behaviour and intervening before an episode is an important safety intervention. Clients can learn to identify situations leading to self-destructive behaviour and develop preventive strategies. Because individuals with BPD are impulsive and may respond to stress by harming themselves, observation of the person's interactions and assessment of mood, level of distress, and agitation are important in determining the threat of self-injury.

Remembering that self-injury is an effort to self-soothe by activating endogenous endorphins, the nurse can assist the individual to find more productive and enduring ways to find comfort. Linehan (1993b) suggests using a self-soothing exercise and focusing on each of the five senses:

- Vision (e.g., go outside and look at the stars or flowers or autumn leaves)
- Hearing (e.g., listen to beautiful or invigorating music or the sounds of nature)
- Smell (e.g., light a scented candle, boil a cinnamon stick in water)
- Taste (e.g., drink a soothing, warm, nonalcoholic beverage)
- Touch (e.g., take a hot bubble bath, pet your dog or cat, get a massage)

Pharmacologic Interventions

As noted, there is no specific drug available for the treatment of BPD, but medications for target symptoms are sometimes used. These should be on a short-term basis (e.g., an antidepressant for a bout with depression). Clients with BPD may be taking medications for a comorbid disorder, such as a mood disorder or substance abuse.

 TEACHING POINTS

Clients should be educated about any medications and their interactions with other drugs and substances. Interventions include teaching individuals about the medication and how and where it acts in the brain and body, helping establish a routine for taking prescribed medication, reporting side effects, and facilitating the development of positive coping strategies to deal with daily stresses, rather than relying on medications. Eliciting the client's partnership in care improves adherence and, thereby, outcomes.

Psychological Domain

Psychological Assessment

People with BPD have usually experienced significant losses in their lives that shape their view of the world. They experience **inhibited grieving**, "a pattern of repetitive, significant trauma and loss, together with an inability to fully experience and personally integrate or resolve these events" (Linehan, 1993a, p. 89). They have unresolved grief that can last for years and avoid situations that evoke those feelings of separation and loss. During the assessment, the nurse can identify the losses (real or perceived) and explore the client's experience during these losses, paying particular attention to whether the individual has reached resolution. A history of physical or sexual abuse and an early separation from significant caregivers may provide important clues to the severity of the disturbances.

Mood fluctuations are common and can be assessed by any number of the depression and anxiety screening scales, or by asking the following questions:

- What things or events bother you and make you feel happy, sad, and angry?
- Do these things or events trouble you more than they trouble other people?
- Do friends and family tell you that you are moody?
- Do you get angry easily?
- Do you have trouble with your temper?
- Do you think you were born with these feelings, or did something happen to make you feel this way?

Appearance and activity level generally reflect the person's mood and psychomotor activity. Many of those with BPD have been physically or sexually abused and thus should be assessed for depression. A dishevelled appearance can reflect depression or an agitated state. When feeling good, these individuals can be very engaging; they tend to be dramatic in their style of dress and attract attention, such as by wearing an unusual hairstyle or heavy makeup. Because physical appearance reflects identity, clients may experiment with their appearance and seek affirmation and acceptance from others. Body piercing, tattoos, and other adornments provide a mechanism to define self.

Impulsivity

Impulsivity can be identified by asking the client if he or she does things impulsively or on the spur of the moment (e.g., "Have there been times when you were hurt by your actions or were sorry later that you acted in the way you did?"). Direct questions about gambling, choices in sexual partners, sexual activities, fights, arguments, arrests, and alcohol drinking habits can also help in identifying areas of impulsive behaviour.

From a neurophysiologic perspective, impulsively acting before thinking seems to be mediated by rapid nerve firing in the mesolimbic area. This activates psychomotor responses before pathways reach the prefrontal cortex (Best, Williams, & Coccaro, 2002). Teaching the client strategies to slow down automatic responses (e.g., deep breathing, counting to 10) allows time to think before acting.

Cognitive Disturbances

The mental status examination of those with BPD usually reveals normal thought processes that are not disorganized or confused, except during periods of stress. Those with BPD usually exhibit **dichotomous thinking**, or a tendency to view things as absolute—either black or white, good or bad—with no perception of compromise. Dichotomous thinking can be assessed by asking clients how they view other people. Evidence of dichotomous thinking is indicated with responses of "good" or "bad," "wonderful" or "terrible."

Dissociation and Transient Psychotic Episodes

The individual with BPD may experience periods of dissociation and of transient psychotic episodes. Dissociation can be assessed by asking if there are times when the person does not remember events or has the feeling of being separate from his or her body. Some individuals refer to this as "spacing out." By asking specific information about how often, how long, and when dissociation first was used, the nurse can get an idea of how important dissociation is as a coping skill. It is important to ask the person what is happening in the environment when dissociation occurs. Frequent dissociation indicates a highly habitual coping mechanism that will be difficult to change.

Because transient psychotic states occur, it is also important to elicit data regarding the presence of hallucinations or delusions along with their frequency and circumstances. Terms such as "pseudo-" or "quasi-psychotic" are misleading and should not be used (Schroeder, Fisher, & Schäfer, 2013).

Risk Assessment: Suicide or Self-Injury

It is critical that individuals with BPD be assessed for suicidal and self-damaging behaviours, including alcohol and drug abuse. (Suicide assessment is discussed in Chapter 19; substance use in Chapter 26). Suicide is a real risk; it is estimated that about 10% of clients with BPD will die of suicide, many before the age of 40 years (Hooley et al., 2012). An assessment should include direct questions, asking if the person thinks about or engages in self-injurious behaviours. If so, the nurse should continue to explore the behaviours: what is done, how it is done, its frequency, and the circumstances surrounding the self-injurious behaviour. It is helpful to explain briefly to the client that sometimes people cut, scratch, or pick at themselves as a way of bringing some relief and comfort. Although the behaviour brings temporary relief, it also places the person at risk for infection.

Approaching the assessment in this way conveys a sense of understanding and is more likely to invite the individual to disclose honestly. This is important as revealed when men (n = 15) with a recent history of suicidal behaviour as well as substance use and antisocial or borderline behaviour described their experiences with treatment services while living in Toronto. In this qualitative study, these participants noted that they were unable to express their emotions and to navigate the health care system (Strike, Rhodes, Bergmans, & Links, 2006). They felt mislabelled, as complete assessments (including contextual factors) were not carried out; that they were treated disrespectfully; and that they felt compelled to lie or to attempt suicide to have their needs met. They desired connection with the staff but perceived them as disinterested or hostile (Strike et al., 2006).

The common risk factors for suicide attempts remain true for clients with BPD: history of recent attempts and hospitalizations and a history of childhood sexual abuse (Links, Kolia, Guimond, & McMain, 2013).

● **STUDY NOTE**

Monitoring changes in the stress levels of a client with BPD is important, as increased stress (or distress) can be a trigger for self-harming behaviours, including a suicide attempt.

Nursing Diagnoses for the Psychological Domain

One of the first diagnoses to consider is the risk for self-mutilation because protection of the individual from self-injury is always a priority. If cognitive changes are present (dissociation and transient psychosis), two other diagnoses may be appropriate: disturbed thought process and ineffective coping. The disturbed thought process diagnosis is used if dissociative and psychotic episodes actually interfere with daily living. For example, a secretary could not complete processing letters because she was unable to differentiate whether the voices on the dictating machine were being transmitted by the machine or by her hallucinations. The nurse helped her learn to differentiate the hallucinations from dictation. The client learned to take her headset off, take a deep breath, and listen to her external environment. When she recognized "the voice" as her partner criticizing her, she was able to use her cognitive reframing strategies to refocus on reality.

If the individual copes with stressful situations by dissociating or hallucinating, the diagnosis of ineffective coping is used. The outcome in this instance would be the substitution of positive coping skills for the dissociations or hallucinations.

Other nursing diagnoses that are typically supported by assessment data include personal identity disturbance, anxiety, grieving, low self-esteem, powerlessness, posttrauma response, defensive coping, and spiritual distress. The identification of outcomes depends on the nursing diagnoses (Fig. 27-1).

Interventions for the Psychological Domain

The greatest challenge of working with clients with BPD is engaging the individual in a therapeutic relationship that will survive its emotional ups and downs. The client needs to understand that the nurse is there to coach her or him to develop self-modulation skills. A relationship based on mutual respect and consistency is crucial for helping the person with those skills. Self-awareness skills, along with access to supervision and collaboration, are needed by the nurse. Because individuals with BPD are frequently hospitalized, even nurses in acute care settings have an opportunity to develop a long-term relationship (Fig. 27-2). A recovery-focused approach to change can be successful, including for persons with BPD who exhibit suicidal behaviours, if clients feel supported and that their experience of what it means to live with BPD is understood (Holm & Severinsson, 2011).

A further challenge that may face nurses within this nurse–client relationship is maladaptive coping behaviour that persons with BPD may use that involves regarding a particular person as being all good or all bad, rather than seeing him or her as a complex human being. This seeing others in terms of black and white, rather than in shades of grey, can create problems for individuals with BPD in maintaining their relationships. If this happens

FIGURE 27-1. Bio/psycho/social/spiritual outcomes for individuals with BPD.

within the nurse–client relationship and/or affects the team approach to the client, it is important to respond professionally and appropriately, with understanding of the relationship dynamics.

Generalist nurses, including psychiatric and mental health nurses, do not function as the client's primary therapists, but they do need to establish a therapeutic relationship that strengthens the client's coping skills and self-esteem and supports individual psychotherapy. The therapeutic relationship helps the client to experience a model of healthy interaction with consistency, limit setting, caring, and respect for others (both self-respect and respect for the person). Clients who have low self-esteem need help in recognizing genuine respect from others and reciprocating with respect for others. In the therapeutic relationship, the nurse models self-respect by observing personal limits, being assertive, and clearly communicating expectations. Consistency is critical in building self-esteem (see Box 27-7).

Responding to Abandonment and Intimacy Fears

A key to helping individuals with BPD is recognizing their fears of both abandonment and intimacy. Informing the client of the length of the relationship as much as possible allows the individual to engage in and prepare for termination with the least pain of abandonment. If the client's hospitalization is time-limited, the nurse overtly acknowledges the limit and reminds the person with each contact how many sessions remain.

In day treatment and outpatient settings, the duration of treatment may be indeterminate, but the nurse may not be available that entire time. The termination process cannot be casual; this would stimulate abandonment fears. However, some clients end prematurely when the nurse informs them of the impending end as a way to leave before being rejected. Anticipating premature closure, the nurse explores with the individual anticipated feelings, including the wish to run away. After careful planning, the nurse anticipates, in advance, the client's feelings, discusses how to cope with them, reviews the progress the individual has made, and summarizes what the person has learned from the relationship that can be generalized to future encounters.

Establishing Personal Boundaries and Limitations

Personal boundaries are highly context-specific; for example, stroking the hair of a stranger on the bus would be inappropriate, but stroking the hair and face of one's intimate partner while sitting together would be appropriate. Our personal physical space needs (boundaries) are distinct from behavioural and emotional limits we have. These concepts apply both to the client and the nurse. Furthermore, limits may be temporary (e.g., "I can't talk with you right now, but after the change of shift, I can be available for 30 minutes.") (see Chapter 6).

Testing limits is a natural way of identifying where the boundaries are and how strong they are. Therefore, it is necessary to state clearly the enduring limits

FIGURE 27-2. Bio/psycho/social/spiritual interventions for individuals with BPD.

Spiritual
1. Teach mindfulness or other distress-reducing skills
2. Maintain compassionate attitude
3. Support hope
4. Support spiritual activities

Biologic
1. Manage medications
2. Prevent harm to self and others
3. Establish regular sleep routines
4. Encourage adequate nutrition
5. Observe for eating disorders

Social
1. Milieu management
2. Help establish new relationships for support
3. Group skills
4. Assertiveness classes

Psychological
1. Recognize abandonment and intimacy fears
2. Identify triggers for self-injury
3. Track emotion regulation
4. Teach and reinforce desired behaviours and communication skills

(e.g., the written rules or contract) and the consequences of violating them. The limits must then be consistently maintained. Clarifying limits requires making explicit what is usually implicit. Despite the clinical setting (e.g., hospital, day treatment setting, outpatient clinic), the nurse must clearly state the day, time, and duration of each contact with the client and remain consistent in those expectations. This may mean having a standing appointment in day treatment or a mental health clinic or noting the time during each shift that the nurse will talk individually with the hospitalized client. The nurse should refrain from offering personal information, which is frequently confusing to the person with BPD. At times, the person may present in a somewhat arrogant and entitled way. It is important for the nurse to recognize such a presentation as reflective of internal confusion and dissonance. Responding in a very neutral manner avoids confrontation and a power struggle, which might also unwittingly reinforce the client's internal sense of inferiority.

Some additional strategies for establishing the boundaries of the relationship include the following:

- Documenting in the client chart the agreed-on appointment expectations
- Sharing the treatment plan with the client
- Confronting violations of the agreement in a nonpunitive way
- Discussing the purpose of limits in the therapeutic relationship and applicability to other relationships

When individuals violate boundaries, it is important to respond right away but without taking the behaviour personally. For example, if a client is flirtatious, simply say something like, "I feel uncomfortable with your overly friendly behaviour. It is out of place within our professional relationship. It is important that we maintain a professional relationship so that I may help you. We cannot and will not have a different kind of relationship."

Management of Dissociative States

The desired outcome for someone who dissociates is to reduce or eliminate the dissociative experiences. The natural tendency is to want to "fix it." Unfortunately, there are limited medications for dissociation, but because the selective serotonin reuptake inhibitors (SSRIs), dopamine antagonists, and serotonin–dopamine antagonists affect other target symptoms, the dissociative experiences decrease. Because dissociation occurs during periods of stress, the best approach is to help the individual develop other strategies to deal with stress.

The nurse can teach the client how to identify when he or she is dissociating and then to use some grounding strategies in the moment. Basic to grounding is planting both feet firmly on the floor or ground, then taking a deep abdominal breath to the count of four, holding it to the count of 4, exhaling to the count of 4, and then holding it to the count of 4. This is called the four-square method of breathing. The benefit of this approach is to bring about a deep, slow breath that activates the calming mechanisms of the parasympathetic system.

BOX 27-7 Therapeutic Dialogue

BORDERLINE PERSONALITY DISORDER

Ineffective Approach

Client: Hey, you know what? You are my favourite nurse. That night nurse sure doesn't understand me the way you do.

Nurse: Oh, I'm glad you are comfortable with me. Which night nurse?

Client: You know, Sue.

Nurse: Did you have problems with her?

Client: She is terrible. She sleeps all night or she is on the telephone.

Nurse: Oh, that doesn't sound very professional to me. Anything else?

Client: Yeah, she said that you didn't know what you were doing. She said that you couldn't nurse your way out of a paper bag (smiling).

Nurse: She did, did she. (Getting angry.) She should talk.

Client: Well, I gotta go to group. Where will you be? I feel so much better if I know where you are. I don't know how I can possibly be discharged tomorrow.

Effective Approach

Client: Hey, you know what? You are my favourite nurse. That night nurse sure doesn't understand me the way you do.

Nurse: I like you, Sara. Tomorrow you will be discharged, and I'm glad that you will be able to return

home. (The nurse avoided responding to "favourite nurse" statement. Redirected the interaction to impending discharge.)

Client: That night nurse slept all night.

Nurse: What was your night like? (Redirecting the interaction to Sara's experience.)

Client: It was terrible. Couldn't sleep all night. I'm not sure that I'm ready to go home.

Nurse: Oh, so you are not quite sure about discharge? (Reflection.)

Client: I get so, so lonely. Then, I want to hurt myself.

Nurse: Lonely feelings have started that chain of events that led to cutting, haven't they? (Validation.)

Client: Yes, I'm very scared. I haven't cut myself for 1 week now.

Nurse: Do you have a plan for dealing with your lonely feelings when they occur?

Client: I'm supposed to start thinking about something that is pleasant—like spring flowers in the meadow.

Nurse: Does that work for you?

Client: Yes, sometimes.

Critical Thinking Questions

- How did the nurse in the first scenario get sidetracked?
- How was the nurse in the second scenario able to keep the client focused on herself and her impending discharge?

After the grounding exercise, the client uses one or more senses to make contact with the environment, such as touching the fabric of a nearby chair or listening to the traffic noise. As the client improves in self-esteem and the ability to relate to others, the frequency of dissociation should decrease.

The Use of Behavioural Interventions

The goal of behavioural interventions is to replace dysfunctional behaviours with positive ones. The nurse has an important role in helping individuals control emotions and behaviours by acknowledging and validating desired behaviours and by ignoring or confronting undesired behaviours. Clients often test the nurse for a response, and nurses must decide how to respond to particular behaviours. This can be tricky because even negative responses can be viewed as positive reinforcement for the client. In some instances, if the behaviour is irritating but not harmful or demeaning, it is best to ignore rather than focus on it. However, grossly inappropriate and disrespectful behaviours require confrontation. If a client throws a glass of water on an assistant because the client is angry at the treatment team for refusing to increase her hospital privileges, an appropriate intervention would include confronting the individual with her behaviour and issuing the consequences, such as losing her privileges and apologizing to the assistant.

However, this incident can be used to help the individual understand why such behaviour is inappropriate

and how it can be changed. The nurse should explore with the client what happened, what events led up to the behaviour, what were the consequences, and what feelings were aroused. Advanced practice nurses or other therapists will explore the origins of the client's behaviours and responses, but the generalist nurse needs to help the person explore ways to change behaviours involved in the current situation. The laboriousness of this analytical process may be a sufficient incentive for the client to abandon the dysfunctional behaviour.

Addressing Emotional Regulation

A major goal of cognitive therapeutic interventions is emotional regulation—recognizing and controlling the expression of feelings. Clients often fail even to recognize their feelings; instead, they respond quickly without thinking about the consequences. Remember, the time needed for taking action is shorter than the time needed for thinking before acting. Pausing makes up for the momentary lag between the limbic and autonomic response and the prefrontal response.

The nurse can help the client identify feelings and gain control over expressions such as anger, disappointment, or frustration. The goal is for individuals to tolerate their feelings without feeling compelled to act out those feelings on another person or on themselves.

A helpful technique for managing feelings is known as the **communication triad**. The triad provides a specific syntax and order for clients to identify and express their feelings and seek relief. The "sentence" consists of three parts:

- An "I" statement to identify the prevailing feeling
- A nonjudgemental statement of the emotional trigger
- What the individual would like differently or what would restore comfort to the situation

The nurse must emphasize with clients that they begin with the "I" statement and the identification of feelings, although many want to begin with the condition. If the person begins with the condition, the statement becomes accusatory and likely to evoke defensiveness (e.g., "When you interrupt me, I get mad."). Beginning with "I" allows the client to identify and express the feeling first and take full ownership. For example, the individual who is angry with another client in the group might say, "Joe, I feel angry ('I' statement with ownership of feeling) when you interrupt me (the trigger or conditions of the emotion), and I would like you to apologize and try not to do that with me (what the individual wants and the remedy)." This simple skill is easy to teach, is easy to reinforce and to encourage others to reinforce, and is a surprisingly effective way of moderating the emotional tone.

Another element of emotional regulation is learning to delay gratification. When clients want something that is not immediately available, the nurse can teach individuals to distract themselves, find alternate ways of meeting the need, and think about what would happen if they have to wait to meet the need.

The practice of **thought stopping** might also help the person to control the inappropriate expression of feelings. In thought stopping, the client identifies what feelings and thoughts exist together. For example, when the person is ruminating about a perceived hurt, the individual might say "Stop that" (referring to the ruminative thought) and engage in a distracting activity. Three activities associated with thought stopping are effective:

- Taking a quick deep breath when the behaviour is noted (this also stimulates relaxation)
- Visualizing a stop sign or saying "stop" when possible (this allows the person to hear externally and internally)
- Deliberately replacing the undesired behaviour with a positive alternative (e.g., instead of ruminating about an angry situation, thinking about a neutral or positive self-affirmation)

The sequencing and combining of the steps puts the person back in control.

Addressing Dysfunctional Thinking

The nurse can help the individual address his or her problematic, dysfunctional ways of thinking by encouraging the person to think about the event in a different way. This is termed **reframing**. The client learns to take a more positive, yet realistic, perspective on a situation or issue. When a client engages in catastrophic thinking, the

---

BOX 27-8 Challenging Dysfunctional Thinking

Ms. S had worked for the same company for 20 years with a good job record. Following an accident, she made some minor mistakes in her work that she quickly corrected. She informed her company's nurse that her work was "really slipping" and that she was fearful of her coworkers' disapproval and getting fired from her job. The nurse asked her to keep a journal of coworkers' comments for the next week. At the next visit, the following dialogue occurred:

Nurse: I noticed that you received several compliments on your work. Even a close friend of your boss expressed appreciation for your work.

Ms. S: It was a light week at work. I really don't believe they meant what they said.

Nurse: I can see how you can believe that one or two comments are not genuine, but how do you account for four and five good reports on your work?

Ms. S: Well, I don't know.

Nurse: It looks like your beliefs are not supported by your journal entries. Now, what makes you think that your boss wants to fire you after 20 years of service?

---

nurse can address such thinking by asking, "What is the worst that could happen?" and "How likely would that be to occur?" For dichotomous thinking, as when the client fixates on one extreme perception or alternates between the extremes only, the nurse can ask the person to think about any examples of exceptions to the extreme. The point of the challenge is not to debate or argue with the individual but to provide different perspectives to consider. Encouraging clients to keep journals of real interactions to process with the nurse or therapist is another effective way of testing the reality of their thinking and anticipations, affording more choices and flexibility (Box 27-8).

In problem solving, the nurse might encourage the individual to debate both sides of the problem and then search for common ground. Practising communication and negotiation skills through role playing helps the client make mistakes and correct them without harm to her or his self-esteem. The nurse also encourages clients to use these skills in their everyday lives and report back on the results, asking individuals how they feel applying the skills and how doing so affects their self-perceptions. Success, even partial success, builds a sense of competence and self-esteem (Box 27-9).

Management of Transient Psychotic Episodes

During psychotic episodes with auditory hallucinations, the client should be protected from harming self or others. In an inpatient setting, the client should be monitored closely and a determination made as to whether the voices are telling the person to engage in self-harm (command hallucinations). The client may be observed more closely and begin taking antipsychotic medications. In the community setting, the nurse should help the client develop a plan for managing the voices. For example, if the voices return, the individual contacts the clinic and

BOX 27-9 Thought Distortions and Corrective Statements

Thought Distortion	Corrective Statement
Catastrophizing	
"This is the most awful thing that has ever happened to me."	"This is a sad thing, but not the most awful."
"If I fail this course, my life is over."	"If you fail the course, you can take the course again. You can change your major."
Dichotomizing	
"No one ever listens to me."	"Your husband listened to you last night when you told him…"
"I never get what I want."	"You didn't get the promotion this year, but you did get a merit raise."
"I can't understand why everyone is so kind at first, and then always dumps me when I need them the most."	"It is hard to remember those kind things and times when your friends have stayed with you when you needed them."
Self-Attribution Errors	
"If I had just found the right thing to say, she wouldn't have left me."	"There is not a single right thing to say; and she left you because she chose to."
"If I had not made him mad, he wouldn't have hit me."	"He has a lot of choices in how to respond, and he chose hitting. You are responsible for your feelings and actions."

returns for evaluation. There may be a friend or relative who should be contacted or a case manager who can help the person get the necessary protection if it is needed. In some instances, hearing the voices is a prelude to self-injury. Another person can help the individual resist the voices. Once other aspects of the disorder are managed, the episodes of psychosis decrease or disappear.

Teaching and practising distress tolerance skills help the individual have power over the voices and control intense emotions. When not experiencing hallucinations, the client can practise deep abdominal breathing, which calms the autonomic nervous system. Using brainstorming techniques, the individual identifies early internal cues of rising distress while the nurse writes them on an index card for the client to refer to later. Next, the nurse teaches some skills for tolerating painful feelings or events. To help the client remember, suggest the mnemonic "Wise Mind ACCEPTS" with the following actions:

- **A**ctivities to distract from stress
- **C**ontributing to others, such as volunteering or visiting a sick neighbour
- **C**omparing yourself to people less fortunate than you
- **E**motions that are opposite to what you are experiencing
- **P**ushing away from the situation for awhile
- **T**houghts other than those you are currently experiencing
- **S**ensations that are intense, such as holding ice in your hand (Linehan, 1993b, pp. 165–166)

Client Education

Client education within the context of a therapeutic relationship is one of the most important, empowering interventions for the nurse to use. Teaching individuals skills to resist parasuicidal urges, improve emotional regulation, enhance interpersonal relationships, tolerate stress, and

enhance overall quality of life provides the foundation for long-term behavioural changes. These skills can be taught in any treatment setting as a part of the overall facility program (see Box 27-10). If nurses are practising in a facility where DBT is the treatment model, they can be trained in DBT and can serve as group skills leaders.

Social Domain

Social Assessment

Some individuals with BPD can function very well except during periods when symptoms erupt. They hold jobs, are active in communities, and can perform well. During periods of stress, symptoms often appear. On the other hand, some individuals with severe BPD function poorly; they are always in a crisis, which they have often created.

Social Support Systems

The identification of social supports, such as family, friends, and religious organizations, is the purpose in assessing resources. Knowing how the person obtains social support is important in understanding the quality

BOX 27-10 Psychoeducation Checklist: Borderline Personality Disorder

When caring for the client with BPD, be sure to include the following topic areas in the teaching plan:
- Management of medication, if used, including drug action, dosage, frequency, and possible adverse effects
- Regular sleep routines
- Nutrition
- Safety measures
- Functional versus dysfunctional behaviours
- Cognitive strategies (distraction, communication skills, thought stopping)
- Structure and limit setting
- Social relationships
- Community resources

of interpersonal relationships. For example, some individuals consider their "best friends" to be their nurses, physicians, and other health care personnel. Because this is a false friendship (i.e., not reciprocal), it inevitably leads to frustration and disappointment. Helping the individual find ways to meet other people and encouraging the client's efforts are more realistic.

Interpersonal Skills

An assessment of the person's ability to relate to others is important because interpersonal problems are linked to dissociation and self-injurious behaviour. Information about friendships, frequency of contact, and intimate relationships will provide data about the person's ability to relate to others. Clients with BPD often are sexually active and may have numerous sexual partners. Their need for closeness clouds their judgement about sexual partners, and it is not unusual to find these individuals in abusive, destructive relationships with people with ASPD. During assessment, nurses should use their own self-awareness skills to examine their personal response to the client. How the nurse responds to the individual can often be a clue to how others perceive and respond to this person. For example, if the nurse feels irritated or impatient during the interview, that is a sign that others respond to this person in the same way; on the other hand, if the nurse feels empathy or closeness, chances are this individual can evoke these same feelings in others.

Self-Esteem and Coping Skills

Coping with stressful situations is one of the major problems for people with BPD. An assessment of their coping skills and their ability to deal with stressful situations is important. Because the individual's self-esteem is usually very low, an assessment of self-esteem can be done with a self-esteem assessment or by interviewing the client and analyzing the assessment data for evidence of personal self-worth and confidence. Self-esteem is highly related to identifying with health care workers. Clients with BPD perceive their families and friends as being weary of their numerous crises and their seeming unwillingness to break the cycle of self-destructiveness. Feeling rejected by their natural support system, these individuals attempt to create one within the health system. During periods of crisis or affective instability, especially during the late evening, early morning, or on weekends, they call or visit various psychiatric units, asking to speak to specific personnel who formerly cared for them. They may know different nurses' scheduled days off and make the rounds to several hospitals and clinics. Sometimes they bring gifts to nurses or call them at home. Because this attempt at a new social support system must fail as it cannot provide the desired support, the person continues to feel rejected. One of the goals of the treatment is to help the individual establish a natural support network.

Family Assessment

Family members may or may not be involved with the client. Individuals with BPD are often estranged from their families. In other instances, they are dependent on them, which is also a source of stress. Childhood abuse is common in these families, and the perpetrator may be a family member. Ideally, family members are interviewed for their perspectives on the client's problem. An assessment of any mental disorder in the client's family and of the current level of functioning is useful in understanding the client and identifying potential resources for support.

Nursing Diagnoses for the Social Domain

Defensive coping, chronic low self-esteem, and impaired social interaction are nursing diagnoses that address the social problems faced by clients with BPD.

Interventions for the Social Domain: Modifying Coping Behaviours

Environmental management becomes critical in caring for a person with BPD. Because the unit can be structured to represent a microcosm of the individual's community, clients have an opportunity to identify relationship problems, boundary violations, and stressful situations. When these situations occur, the nurse can help the individual cope by finding alternative explanations for the situation and practising new skills. Individual sessions help the client try out some skills, such as putting feelings into words without actions. Role playing may help individuals experience different degrees of effectively relating feelings without the burden of hurting someone they care about. Day treatment and group settings are excellent places for clients to learn more effective feeling management and to practise these techniques with each other. The group helps members develop empathy and diffuses attachment to any one person or therapist.

Building Social Skills and Self-Esteem

In the hospital, the nurse can use groups to discuss feelings and ways to cope with them. Women with BPD often benefit from assertiveness classes and women's health issues classes. Many of the women are involved in abusive relationships and lack the ability to resolve these relationships because of their extreme anxiety regarding separating from those they love and their extreme need to feel connected. These women verbalize desires to leave, but they do not have the strength and self-confidence needed to leave. Exposing them to a different style of interaction as well as validation from other people increases their self-esteem and ability to separate from negative influences.

Exploring Social Supports

Dependency on family members is a problem for many people with BPD. In some families, a client's positive progress may be met with negative responses, and individuals in these situations need help in maintaining a separate identity while staying connected to family members for social support. Family support groups sometimes help. Usually, the nurse helps the person explore new relationships that can provide additional social contacts.

Teaching Effective Ways to Communicate

An important area of client education is teaching communication skills. Clients lack interpersonal skills in relating because they often had inadequate modelling and few opportunities to practise. The goals of relationship skill development are to identify problematic behaviour that interferes with relationships and to use appropriate behaviours in improving relationships. The starting point is with communication. The nurse teaches the individual basic communication approaches, such as making "I" statements, paraphrasing what the other party says before responding, checking the accuracy of perceptions with others, compromising and seeking common ground, listening actively, and offering and accepting reactions. Besides modelling the behaviours, the nurse guides clients in practising a variety of communication approaches for common situations. When role playing, the nurse needs to discuss not only what the skills are and how to perform them but also the feelings clients have before, during, and after the role play.

In day treatment and outpatient settings, the nurse can give the client homework, such as keeping a journal, applying role-playing skills to actual situations, and observing behaviours in others. In the hospital, the individual can experience the same process, and the nurse is available to offer immediate feedback. Whatever the setting, or even the specific problems addressed, the nurse must keep in mind and remind the client that change occurs slowly. Thus, working on the problems occurs gradually, with severity of symptoms as the guide to deciding how fast and how much change to expect.

Spiritual Domain

In addressing the spiritual domain, the qualities of the nurse that have been identified as important include receptivity (e.g., being genuinely available to the client as a person), humanity (e.g., taking time for the "little things" when giving care), competency (e.g., demonstrating safe practice), and positivity (e.g., having a hopeful attitude and fostering a positive spirit; Carr, 2008; see Chapter 11). In nursing clients with BPD, enacting these qualities may be challenging, as characteristics of BPD involving self-dysregulation and interpersonal dysregulation can sometimes promote a negative response to the person in the nurse. If the nurse does not grasp that the client's personality patterns do comprise a mental disorder, she or he may become frustrated with the lack of client behaviour change and progress. As well, trying to understand the worldview of the client with BPD can be difficult. Spiritual care is particularly important for such clients as they struggle with issues of self and connection,

purpose and meaning. A review of the research on spirituality and persons with PDs, in fact, indicates that spiritual well-being may remain high for persons with borderline personality traits, even though general well-being is low (Bennett, Shepherd, & Janca, 2013). Nurses can play an important role in helping clients sustain such well-being through respectful, knowledgeable, and supportive connection within a therapeutic relationship.

Evaluation and Outcomes

Evaluation and outcomes vary depending on the severity of the disorder, the presence of comorbid disorders, and the availability of resources. For a client with severe symptoms or continual self-injury, keeping the individual safe and alive may be a realistic outcome. Helping the person resist parasuicidal urges may take years. In contrast, individuals who rarely need hospitalization and have adequate resources can expect to recover from the self-destructive impulses and learn positive interaction skills that promote a fulfilling lifestyle. Most clients fall somewhere in between, with periods of symptom exacerbation and remission. In these individuals, increasing the symptom-free time may be the best indicator of outcomes.

Continuum of Care

Treatment of BPD involves long-term therapies. Hospitalization is sometimes necessary during acute episodes involving parasuicidal behaviour (see Box 27-11 best practices research), but once this behaviour is controlled, clients are discharged. It is important for these individuals to continue with treatment in the outpatient or day treatment setting. They often appear more competent and in control than they are, and nurses must not be deceived by these outward appearances. They need continued follow-up and long-term therapies, including individual therapy, psychoeducation, and positive role models (see Nursing Care Plan 27-1).

Antisocial Personality Disorder

Clinical Course of Disorder

In the *DSM-5*, the essential feature of ASPD is "a pervasive pattern of disregard for, and violation of, the rights of others that begins in childhood or early adolescence and continues into adulthood" (APA, 2013, p. 659). ASPD is related to, but not synonymous with the older, broader term "psychopath" (Horley, 2013). In WHO's ICD-10, the term "dissocial disorder" is used rather than ASPD. People with this disorder are behaviourally impulsive and interpersonally irresponsible, failing to conform to the ethical and social standards of their community. They display deceitfulness (e.g., repeated lying, use of aliases, "conning" others), act hastily and impulsively, and fail to plan ahead. They lack a sense of personal responsibility

BOX 27-11 | Research for Best Practice

BRIEF ADMISSION AS AN INTERVENTION FOR PERSONS WITH BPD

Helleman, M., Goossens, P. J. J., Kaasenbrood, Ad., & van Achterberg, T. (2014). Evidence base and components of brief admission as an intervention for patients with borderline personality disorder: A review of the literature. Perspectives in Psychiatric Care, 50, 65–75.

Question: What is the evidence re: the components of brief inpatient psychiatric hospital admission as an intervention for clients with BPD?

Method: A systematic literature search (time frame = January 1985 to December 2011) was conducted using MEDLINE, CINAHL, PsycINFO, and Cochrane Database of Systematic Reviews. Abstracts of retrieved articles (*n* = 1030) were screened for relevance, leaving *n* = 88; full texts of 24 articles were examined for eligibility with *n* = 10 articles meeting relevance criteria. Content analysis of components of interventions described in the studies was carried out.

Findings: Research re: intervention effectiveness for treating persons with BPD is sparse. There were methodologic shortcomings in some of the analyzed studies. Five identified components of the intervention of Brief Admission (BA) were

distinguished: "discussion of goals; organization of BA; clear admission procedure; specification of any other interventions during BA; and stipulation of conditions for premature (i.e., forced) discharge" (p. 65). Goals were to prevent self-harm and suicidal crises, as well as to avoid prolonged psychiatric hospitalization (as it tends to be counter-therapeutic) and facilitating quick return to the community. The goals and conditions of BA were discussed and agreed upon between client and clinician in advance of times of crisis. Interventions during BA varied across studies from none except contact with a nurse to active, rapid response to psychiatric, psychological, interpersonal, financial, and/or housing factors prompting admission. There were conditions for forced discharge noted in five studies (e.g., aggressive behaviour; alcohol/drug use).

Implications for Practice: As an intervention, BA can be effective in preventing self-harm and suicide in clients with BPD. It is an opportunity for nurses to support the individual with BPD to actively cope with their symptoms. The researchers recommend that qualitative studies of clients' and clinicians' experiences with BA be conducted.

Nursing Care Plan 27-1

Client With BPD

YJ, a 28-year-old single woman, was brought to the emergency department of a hospital by police officers after finding her in a fast food restaurant with superficial self-inflicted lacerations on both forearms. She pleaded with the police not to take her to the hospital. The police report noted that she fluctuated between intense crying and pleading to fighting physically and using foul language. By the time she arrived in the emergency department, however, she was calm, cooperative, pleasant, and charming. When asked why she cut herself, YJ reported that she was not sure but added that her therapist was leaving today for a 4-week trip to Europe. YJ specifically asked the staff not to call her therapist because "she will be angry with me."

After the emergency physician examined YJ, the advanced practice mental health nurse assessed her developmental and psychiatric histories and a summary of recent events, before she reached a provisional diagnosis of BPD with a primary nursing diagnosis of risk for self-mutilation related to abandonment anticipation. YJ had several previous self-destructive episodes with minor injuries, only one requiring sutures, and two hospitalizations. She lives with her boyfriend, who is currently on a business trip, and she works

part time at a bookstore. Her invalid mother lives with her younger sister. There are no other relatives. YJ's father died traumatically in an automobile accident when she was 3 years old. YJ was in the car when it crashed; she received minor injuries.

Because YJ refused to agree not to harm herself, the nurse admitted YJ to the psychiatric unit with suicide precautions. Once on the unit, YJ was assessed by a staff nurse as having a basically normal mental status examination except that her mood was very tearful at times but charming and joking at other times. She said, "Don't mind me, I cry at the drop of a hat sometimes." Towards the middle of the interview she said, "I feel safer here than I ever felt before. It must be you. Are you sure you're just a staff nurse?" YJ agreed to contract for safety just for today, but added, "Are you going to be my nurse tomorrow? I feel safest with you." When the nurse had completed her assessment, she showed YJ around the unit. As the nurse left her in the day room, YJ said, "My therapist doesn't understand me very well. I don't care if she is going out of town. After 4 years, she hasn't helped. If I had you as a therapist, I wouldn't be here now."

Setting: Inpatient Psychiatric Unit in a General Hospital

Baseline Assessment: YJ, a 28-year-old woman, came into the emergency department with superficial self-inflicted wounds on both forearms. There was a marked discrepancy in her behaviour at the scene of the incident reported by emergency medical technicians from her presentation in the emergency department and now on the inpatient unit. She was admitted this time because she refused to agree not to harm herself further if released. She is angry and sad that her therapist is leaving for 4 weeks for a vacation and does not know how she will cope while the therapist is gone. She fears that the therapist will not return.

Psychiatric Diagnosis	Medications
Borderline Personality Disorder	Sertraline (Zoloft) 150 mg qd for anxiety and depression

Nursing Care Plan 27-1 *(Continued)*

Nursing Diagnosis 1: Self-Mutilation

Defining Characteristics	Related Factors
Cuts and scratches on body Self-inflicted wounds	Fears of abandonment secondary to therapist's vacation Inability to handle stress

Outcomes

Initial	Discharge
1. Remain safe and not harm herself. 2. Identify feelings before and after cutting herself. 3. Agree not to harm herself over the next 24 hours.	4. Identify ways of dealing with self-harming impulses if they return. 5. Verbalize alternate thinking with more realistic base. 6. Identify community resources to provide structure and support while her therapist is gone.

Interventions

Interventions	Rationale	Ongoing Assessment
Monitor the client for changes in mood or behaviour that might lead to self-injurious behaviour. Discuss with the client the need for close observation and rationale to keep her safe.	Close observation establishes safety and protection of the client from self-harm and impulsive behaviours. Explanation to the client for the purpose of nursing interventions helps her cooperate with the nursing activity.	Document according to the facility policy. Continue to observe for mood and behaviour changes. Assess her response to the increasing level of observation.
Administer medications as prescribed and evaluate medication effectiveness in reducing depression, anxiety, and cognitive disorganization. After 6–8 hours, present written agreement to not harm herself.	Allows for adjustment of medication dosage based on target behaviours and outcomes. Permits the client time to return to more thoughtful ways of responding rather than her previous reactive response. Also permits her to save face and avoid embarrassment of a losing power struggle if presented much earlier.	Observe for side effects. Observe for her willingness to agree to not harm herself.
Communicate information about the client's risk to other nursing staff.	The close observation should be continued throughout all shifts until the client agrees to resist self-harm urges.	Review the documentation of close observation for all shifts.

Evaluation

Outcomes	Revised Outcomes	Interventions
Remained safe without further harming self. Identified fears of abandonment before cutting herself and relief of anxiety afterwards. She identified friends to call when fears return and hotlines to use if necessary.	Use hotlines or call friends if fears to harm self return.	Give the client hotline number and ask her to record her friends' numbers in an accessible place.
Agreed to not harm herself over the next 3 days. Enrolled in a day hospital program for 4 weeks.	Does not harm self for 3 days. Attend the day hospital program.	Remind her to call someone if urges return. Follow-up on enrolment.

Continued

Nursing Care Plan 27-1(*Continued*)

Nursing Diagnosis 2: Risk for Loneliness

Defining Characteristics	Related Factors
Social isolation	Fear of abandonment secondary to the therapist's impending vacation

Outcomes

Initial	Discharge
1. Discuss being lonely. 2. Identify previous ways of coping with loneliness.	3. Identify strategies to deal with loneliness while the therapist is away.

Interventions

Interventions	Rationale	Ongoing Assessment
Develop a therapeutic relationship.	Individuals with BPD are able to examine loneliness within the structure of a therapeutic relationship.	Assess her ability to relate and the nurse's response to the relationship.
Discuss her past experience with the therapist being gone with an emphasis on how she was able to survive it.	She has previously survived the therapist's absences. By identifying the strategies she used, she can build on those strengths.	Assess her ability to assume any responsibility for "living through it." This will become a strength.
Acknowledge that it is normal to feel angry and frightened when her therapist is gone, but there are other strategies that may help her deal with the loneliness that do no involve self-harm.	Acknowledging feelings is important. Helping the client focus on the possibility of other strategies for dealing with the anger helps her regain a sense of control over her behaviour.	Assess whether she is willing to acknowledge that there are other behavioural strategies of handling anger.
Begin immediate disposition planning with a focus on day hospitalization or day treatment for skills training and management of loneliness.	While the client is in hospital, she is out of stressful environment in which she can learn more effective behaviours and use the therapy. Moving out of the hospital and back into the outpatient therapy decreases the possibility of regression and lost learning (Linehan, 1993a, 1993b).	Assess her willingness to learn new skills within a day treatment setting.
Teach her stress management techniques. Assign her to an anger management group while she is in the hospital.	Learning about ways of dealing with feelings and stressful situations helps the client with BPD choose positive strategies rather than self-destructive ones.	Monitor attendance and response to the group. Encourage to attend and to try out what she is learning there.

Evaluation

Outcomes	Revised Outcomes	Interventions
YJ was able to verbalize her anger about her therapist leaving and fears of abandonment. The most recent times (two) that her therapist went on vacation, the client became self-injurious and was hospitalized for 2 weeks.	None.	
YJ was willing to be discharged the next day if she could attend day treatment while her therapist was gone.	Identify other strategies of dealing with the therapist vacations besides cutting.	Attend stress management, communication, and self-comforting classes.

Bulechek, G., Butcher, H., & McCloskey Dochterman, J. (Eds.). (2008). *Nursing interventions classification (NIC)* (5th ed.). St. Louis, MO: Mosby.

(e.g., fail to fulfil social and financial obligations, work responsibilities). They can be superficially charming and facile communicators. In reality, they lack empathy; are unable to express human compassion; and tend to be insensitive, callous, and contemptuous of others. Easily irritated, they often become aggressive, disregarding the safety of themselves or others. They are exploitive and lack remorse (e.g., indifferent to hurting or mistreating others) (APA, 2013). They may present with depressive mood or complaints of tension (APA, 2013). Because of its association with conduct disorders, APD is listed there as well as with PDs in the *DSM-5*. A diagnosis of ASPD cannot be given until an individual is 18 years of age. To be diagnosed with ASPD, the individual must have a history of symptoms of conduct disorder (e.g., "aggression to people and animals, destruction of property, deceitfulness or theft, or serious violation of rules") before the age of 15 years (APA, 2013, p. 659). ASPD has a chronic course, but the antisocial behaviours tend to diminish later in life (APA, 2013).

Some individuals with ASPD openly violate laws, ending up in jail. Criminal behaviour for gain without the personality features of ASPD, however, does not meet ASPD diagnostic criteria. Most individuals with ASPD will not come in conflict with the law; some find a niche in society, such as in business, the military, or politics, which rewards their competitive, tough behaviour (Millon et al., 2004). Given that ASPD is associated with low economic status in urban settings, the diagnosis may be misapplied when antisocial behaviour is an aspect of survival and protective strategies (APA, 2013, p. 662).

Comorbidity

ASPD is strongly associated with alcohol and drug abuse; substance-related disorders are common (Waldman & Slutske, 2000). Individuals with ASPD appear to be more prone to alcohol-related aggression than persons without this PD diagnosis, according to rates of alcohol dependence and alcohol-related problems and in laboratory studies. Those with ASPD who had exhibited the most aggression in the past were the most likely to be aggressive with alcohol use (Moeller & Dougherty, 2001).

Aetiology

There is no comprehensive, generally accepted explanation of the aetiology of ASPD. A genetic or innate component appears to exist. For example, pooled twin study data from North America, Japan, Norway, Germany, and Denmark showed a concordance rate for ASPD between identical twins as 51.5%, but only 23.1% between fraternal twins (Gottesman & Goldsmith, 1994). There is research evidence of neurobiologic dysregulation such as dysregulation in catecholamines with changed activity of the dopaminergic pathways in the frontal cortex (Soderstrom, Blennow, Sjodin, &

Forsman, 2003) and limbic abnormalities in affective processing (Kiehl et al., 2001).

Some studies indicate that a temperament characterized by withdrawal from novel stimuli, low adaptability, and intense emotional reactions can make one vulnerable to antisocial behaviour patterns. Four key behaviours are present in this "difficult" temperament: aggression, inattention, hyperactivity, and impulsivity. There appears to be a strong relationship between difficult temperament and problem behaviours such as those of ADHD, oppositional behaviour, and conduct disorder (Dowson, Sussams, Grounds, & Taylor, 2001; Herpertz et al., 2001; Hill, 2002, 2003; Langbehn & Cadoret, 2001).

Nursing Management

Persons with ASPD rarely seek mental health care for their disorder itself; they may, rather, seek treatment for depression, substance abuse, or uncontrolled anger, or be hospitalized in forensic psychiatric settings for evaluation (Black, Baumgard, & Bell, 1995). Nurses will most likely encounter them in medical–surgical settings. Key areas of assessment are determining the quality of relationships, impulsivity, and the extent of aggression. These individuals do not assume responsibility for their own actions and often blame others for their misfortune. Their disregard for others is manifested in their interactions. For example, one individual with human immunodeficiency virus was engaging in unprotected sex with several different women because he wanted to "have fun as long as I can." He was completely unconcerned about the possibility of transmitting the virus. These individuals often make good first impressions. Self-awareness is especially important for the nurse because of the initial charming quality of many of these individuals. Once these clients realize that the nurse cannot be used or manipulated, they lose interest in the nurse and revert to their normal, egocentric behaviours. Protection of other clients and staff from manipulative and sometimes abusive behaviour is a priority.

Nursing diagnoses for clients with ASPD are related to their interpersonal detachment, lack of awareness of others, avoidance of feelings, impulsiveness, and discrepancy between their perception of themselves and others' perception of them. Typical diagnoses are ineffective role performance (unemployment), ineffective individual coping, impaired communication, impaired social interactions, low self-esteem, and risk for violence. Outcomes should be short term and relevant to a specific problem. For example, if a person has been chronically unemployed, a reasonable short-term outcome would be to set up job interviews, rather than obtain a job.

Therapeutic relationships are difficult to establish because an individual with ASPD is often unable to use the relationship to change behaviour. A superficial alliance with health care professionals is usually formed. Even though the professional may initially believe that the foundation for a therapeutic relationship is evolving, further sessions often reveal a lack of client commitment. Individuals with ASPD tend to lose interest in trying to work on problems. The goal of the therapeutic relationship is to assist the client in identifying dysfunctional thinking patterns and developing new problem-solving behaviours.

Self-responsibility facilitation (encouraging a person to assume more responsibility for personal behaviour) is useful with clients with ASPD (Bulechek et al., 2008). The nursing activities that are particularly helpful include holding the client responsible for his or her behaviour, monitoring the extent to which self-responsibility is assumed, and discussing the consequences of not dealing with responsibilities. The nurse needs to refrain from arguing or bargaining about the unit rules, such as time for meals, use of the television room, and smoking. Instead, positive feedback is given to the individual for accepting additional responsibility or changing behaviour.

Self-awareness enhancement (exploring and understanding personal thoughts, feelings, motivation, and behaviours) is another nursing intervention that is important in helping these individuals develop a sense of understanding about relating peacefully to the rest of the world (Bulechek et al., 2008). Encouraging clients to recognize and discuss thoughts and feelings helps the nurse understand how the person views the world. The nurse can then use many of the same communication techniques discussed in the section on BPD. In teaching the client about positive health care practices, impulse control, and anger management, the best approach is to engage the individual in a discussion about the issue and then direct the topic to the major teaching points and avoid being sidetracked (Box 27-12).

These clients have a long-standing history of difficulty in interpersonal relationships. In an inpatient unit, interventions can be more intense and focus on helping the individual develop positive interaction skills and experience a consistent environment. For example, the focus of nursing interventions may be the client's continual disregard of the rights of others. On one unit, a client continually placed orders for pizzas in the name of another person on the unit. This individual had limited intelligence and was genuinely afraid of the person with ASPD. The victimized person always paid for the pizza and gave it to the other client. When the nursing staff realized what was happening, they confronted the client with ASPD about the behaviour and revoked his unit privileges.

Group interventions typically are more effective than individual modalities, with problem-solving groups that focus on identifying a problem and developing a variety of alternative solutions being particularly helpful. Within group therapy, clients are able to confront each other with dysfunctional schemas or thinking patterns. Teaching individuals with ASPD the same communication techniques as those with BPD will also encourage self-responsibility. These clients often attend groups that focus on the development of empathy.

Milieu interventions, such as providing a structured environment with rules that are consistently applied to clients who are responsible for their own behaviour, are important. While living in close proximity to others, the individual with ASPD will demonstrate dysfunctional social patterns that can be identified and targeted for correction. For example, these clients often violate ward rules, such as no smoking or limitations on the number of visitors, and may bring contraband, such as illegal drugs, to the unit.

Aggressive behaviour is often a problem for these individuals and their family members. Anger control assistance (helping to express anger in an adaptive, nonviolent manner) becomes a priority intervention; anger management techniques can be beneficial.

Social support for individuals with ASPD is often minimal as they have often taken advantage of friends and relatives who no longer trust them. Helping the client build a new support system once new skills are learned is often the only option. For new friendships to be developed and sustained and for reengagement with family members to occur, new ways of interaction must be learned by the person with ASPD. As these ways of interaction need to include empathy and attachment, such goals may never become reality.

The outcomes of interventions for individuals with ASPD need to be evaluated in terms of management of specific problems, such as maintaining employment or developing a meaningful interpersonal relationship, as well as adherence to treatment recommendations and the development of health care practices for other health care issues (e.g., reduce smoking and alcohol consumption).

BOX 27-12 Psychoeducation Checklist: Antisocial Personality Disorder

When caring for the client with ASPD, be sure to include the following topic areas in the teaching plan:
- Positive health care practices, including substance abuse control
- Effective communication and interaction skills
- Impulse control
- Anger management
- Group experience to help develop self-awareness and impact of behaviour on others
- Analyzing an issue from the other person's viewpoint
- Maintenance of employment
- Interpersonal relationships and social interactions

● **STUDY NOTE**

Within inpatient settings, the nurse may need to help clients with a Cluster B disorder set limits on their behaviour. Limit setting should be accomplished in such a way that the client recognizes that it is the behaviour that is unacceptable, not him or herself.

Histrionic Personality Disorder

"Hysteria" (a term derived from the Greek for "uterus") is one of the oldest mental disorders. It was described by early Egyptian physicians as a female illness in which the womb "wandered," producing symptoms wherever it was in the body (Blashfield, Reynolds, & Stennett, 2012). Histrionic personality disorder (HPD), however, is not a female disorder: although more females may be diagnosed with HPD in clinical settings, its prevalence is similar across genders (APA, 2013). "Attention-seeking" and "emotional" describe people with HPD, who are lively and dramatic and draw attention to themselves by their enthusiasm, dress, and apparent openness. Often the "life of the party," they appear superficially interested in others. Persistent need for attention and approval is an aspect of this PD. The person with HPD may be moody and experience a sense of helplessness when others are disinterested in them. The speech of individuals with this PD is dramatic; strong opinions without supporting facts are often expressed and readily changed. Loyalty and fidelity are lacking (APA, 2013).

Gender influences the manifestations of this disorder. Women dress seductively, may express dependency on selected men, and may play a submissive role. Men may dress in a very masculine manner and seek attention by bragging about athletic skills or successes in the job. Although they may be hypersensitive to the moods and thoughts of those they hope to please, individuals with HPD have difficulty achieving true intimacy in interpersonal relationships. Their need for constant attention can quickly alienate others; without such attention they may become depressed. As culture affects the norms for physical appearance, interpersonal behaviour, and emotional expressiveness, the traits expressed by an individual must be evaluated in context as to whether clinically significant impairment or distress exists before a diagnosis of HPD is made (APA, 2013).

This disorder may co-occur with BPD, DPD, and ASPD, as well as anxiety disorders, substance abuse, and mood disorders (Millon et al., 2004).

Nursing Management

The ultimate treatment goal for individuals with HPD is to help them change the tendency to fulfil all their needs by focusing on others to the exclusion of themselves. In the nursing assessment, the nurse focuses on the quality of the individual's interpersonal relationships. It is common that the person is dissatisfied with his or her partner, and sexual relations may be nonexistent. During the assessment, the client may make statements that indicate low self-esteem. Because these individuals assume that they are incapable of handling life's demands and that they need a truly competent person to take care of them, they have not developed a positive self-concept or adequate problem-solving abilities.

Nursing diagnoses that are usually generated include chronic low self-esteem, ineffective individual coping, and ineffective sexual patterns. Outcomes focus on helping the individual develop autonomy, a positive self-concept, and mature problem-solving skills.

A variety of interventions support the outcomes. A nurse–client relationship that allows the client to explore positive personality characteristics and develop independent decision-making skills forms the basis of the interventions. Reinforcing personal strengths, conveying confidence in the person's ability to handle situations, and examining negative perceptions of self can be done within the therapeutic relationship. Encouraging the client to act autonomously can also improve the individual's sense of self-worth (Bulechek et al., 2008). Attending assertiveness groups can help increase the individual's self-confidence and improve self-esteem.

Narcissistic Personality Disorder

The use of the term "narcissism" for excessive self-love came from an ancient Greek myth. A young man, Narcissus, upon seeing his own reflection in a forest pool, fell in love and died pining for his own image: "Unwitting youth, himself/He wants;—at once beloving, and belov'd" (Ovid, 1807/2009, p. 949). Individuals with NPD seem to possess a form of self-love that causes problems for themselves and affects their relationships with others. They present as having an inexhaustible need for admiration, a grandiose sense of their own importance, and a lack of empathy. Their sense of being very special leads them to be preoccupied with fantasies of unlimited success, power, beauty, or ideal love. Their benign arrogance is associated with a strong sense of entitlement. There are behavioural features associated with NPD that are noted in the *DSM-5* that include: "vulnerable self-esteem, feelings of shame, sensitivity, and intense reactions of humiliation, emptiness or disdain to criticism or defeat, and vocational irregularities due to difficulties tolerating criticism or competition" (Ronningstam, 2012, p. 536). Clients with these associated characteristics may present somewhat differently than those captured in the *DSM-5* criteria itself. Others' perceptions of a person with NPD may be very different from that individual's self-perception. Behind grandiose notions of self-importance, for example, there may be a sense of insecurity (Ronningstam, 2012).

Nursing Management

The nurse usually encounters persons with narcissistic personality disorder in medical settings and in psychiatric settings with a coexisting psychiatric disorder. It is important to listen carefully and attempt to understand the person's own perceptions of experiences, bearing in mind that the person may not readily self-disclose. Understanding their sense of self-agency is helpful as it reflects self-awareness, self-esteem, and self-regulation; it allows for some differentiation regarding real competence and accomplishments from grandiose or self-devaluated ones (Ronningstam, 2012). Nurses must pay close attention to their own reaction to the client: it will give clues as to the way others may respond to the client, as well as indicate any therapeutic use of self issues that need to be addressed. The client may oppose a diagnosis of NPD and consider it prejudicial (Ronningstam, 2012). Treatment for NPD, usually some form of psychotherapy, if accepted, will be community based.

■■■ CLUSTER C DISORDERS

Avoidant Personality Disorder

Avoidant personality disorder (AVPD) is characterized by a desire for affiliation that is affected by a sense of personal inadequacy and intense fear of social rejection (Sanislow, da Cruz, Gianol, & Reagan, 2012). The person with AVPD thus avoids social situations, including occupational activities, in which there is interpersonal contact with others. They engage in interpersonal relationships only when they are certain that they will receive approval and be liked. They appear timid, shy, and hesitant. They perceive themselves as socially inept, inadequate, and inferior (justifying their sense of rejection by others) and avoid new activities as they may be a new source of embarrassment. Fantasy may become a means to gratify needs and to feel confident; withdrawing into fantasies can be a means of dealing with frustration and anger. Persons with AVPD experience feelings of tension, sadness, and anger that vacillate between desire for affection, fear of rebuff, embarrassment, and numbness of feeling (APA, 2013; Millon et al., 2004). AVPD co-occurs frequently with anxiety and depressive disorders.

Nursing Management

An assessment of these individuals reveals a lack of social contacts, a fear of being criticized, and evidence of chronic low self-esteem. The nursing diagnoses of chronic low self-esteem, social isolation, and ineffective coping can be used. The establishment of a therapeutic relationship is necessary to be able to help the client meet treatment outcomes. The nurse should expect the nurse–client relationship to take time to develop, as the individual is usually inexperienced in positive interpersonal relationships and will need time to trust that the nurse will not be critical and demeaning. Interventions should focus on assisting the client to identify positive responses from others, exploring previous achievements of success, and exploring reasons for self-criticism. The person's social dimension should be examined for activities that increase self-esteem and interventions focused on multiplying such activities. Social skills training may help reduce symptoms.

Dependent Personality Disorder

Individuals with dependent personality disorder (DPD) are desperate to keep others close and will be overwilling to do anything to maintain closeness, including being submissive and without regard for self. Decision-making is difficult for persons with DPD, who adapt their behaviour to please those to whom they lean upon for guidance. Ingratiating to others but self-denigrating, the person with DPD's self-esteem is other-determined. Behaviourally, they withdraw from adult responsibilities by acting helpless and seeking nurturance from others. In interpersonal relationships, they need excessive advice and reassurance. They are compliant, conciliatory, and placating. They rarely disagree with others and are easily persuaded. Friends describe them as gullible. They are warm, tender, and noncompetitive. They timidly avoid social tension and interpersonal conflicts (APA, 2013). DPD bears resemblance to HPD; individuals with DPD demonstrate high levels of self-attributed dependency needs, while those with HPD have a greater implicit dependency and will even argue against needing others (Bornstein, 1998).

Nursing Management

Nurses can determine the extent of dependency by an assessment of self-worth, interpersonal relationships, and social behaviours. They should determine whether there is currently someone on whom the person relies (e.g., parent, spouse) or if there has been a separation from a significant relationship by death or divorce.

Nursing diagnoses that are usually generated from the assessment data are ineffective individual coping, low self-esteem, impaired social interaction, and impaired home maintenance management. Home management may be a problem if the client does not have the necessary skills and now has to make decisions related to finances, shopping, cooking, and cleaning. The challenge of caring for these individuals is to help them recognize their dependent patterns, motivate them to want to change, and teach them adult skills that have not been developed, such as balancing a cheque book, planning a weekly menu, and paying bills. Occasionally, if a client is extremely fatigued, lethargic, or anxious and the disorder interferes with efforts at developing more independence, antidepressants or antianxiety agents may be used.

These individuals readily engage in a nurse–client relationship and initially will look to the nurse to make all decisions. The nurse can support these individuals to make their own decisions by resisting the urge to tell them what to do. Ideally, these clients are in individual psychotherapy and working towards long-term personality changes. The nurse can encourage clients to stay in therapy and to practise the new skills that are being learned. Assertiveness training is helpful.

Obsessive–Compulsive Personality Disorder

OCD bears a close resemblance to obsessive–compulsive anxiety disorder. A distinguishing difference is that those with the anxiety disorder tend to use obsessive thoughts and compulsions when anxious but less so when anxiety decreases. With OCD, the person does not demonstrate obsessions and compulsions as much as an overall inflexibility, perfectionism, and need to be in mental and interpersonal control. In an attempt to maintain control, the individual is preoccupied with orderliness, details, rules, organization, schedules, and lists; they have difficulty delegating tasks and working with others who may not do things exactly as they do (APA, 2013). Their perfectionism can interfere with completion of tasks. Persons with OCD tend to be excessively devoted to work and uncomfortable with unstructured leisure time, especially vacations. They strive to maintain a highly structured, strictly organized life. Overly conscientious about morality and ethics and values, they have difficulty accepting new ideas and customs and act with rigidity and stubbornness. Some individuals with OCD have difficulty discarding useless objects, even those without sentimental value (APA, 2013).

Nursing Management

These individuals seek mental health care when they have attacks of anxiety, spells of immobilization, sexual impotence, and excessive fatigue. To change the compulsive pattern, psychotherapy is needed. There may be a short-term adjunct pharmacologic intervention with an antidepressant or anxiolytic.

The nursing assessment focuses on the client's physical symptoms (sleep, eating, sexual), interpersonal relationships, and social problems. Typical nursing diagnoses include anxiety, risk for loneliness, decisional conflict, sexual dysfunction, disturbed sleep pattern, and impaired social interactions. People with OCD realize that they can improve their quality of life, but they will find it extremely anxiety provoking to make the necessary changes. A supportive nurse–client relationship based on acceptance of the individual's need for order and rigidity will help the person have enough confidence to try new behaviours. Examining the person's belief that underlies the dysfunctional behaviours can set the stage for challenging childhood thinking. Because the compulsive pattern was established in childhood, it will take a long time to modify the behaviour.

Continuum of Care

Persons with AVPD will need long-term therapy to allow for time to make changes; they will need encouragement and support to contact the therapist when necessary and to continue with treatment. As they avoid seeking help, they may need assistance to deal with other health problems.

Persons with Cluster C PDs are typically treated in the community, unless a coexisting disorder, such as depression, requires short-term hospitalization.

> ● **STUDY NOTE**
>
> For clients with PDs, a key aspect of nursing care is working with the client to identify and address specific dysfunctional or distressing behaviours. The nurse needs to recognize that the symptoms of the PD will shape the approach to the behaviour change, including the number of incremental changes and time involved.

OTHER PERSONALITY DISORDERS

Other PD identified in the *DSM-5* are as follows:

- **General Personality Disorder**: "enduring pattern of inner experience and behaviour" that do not meet the expectations of the individual's culture, manifesting in at least two areas ("cognition, affectivity, interpersonal functioning, and impulse control"), and that cause significant distress or impairment of functioning (APA, 2013, p. 646).
- **Personality Change Due to Another Medical Condition**: "persistent personality disturbance," causing "clinically significant distress or impairment," that can be identified as the result of "direct pathophysiologic consequence of another medical condition" (APA, 2013, p. 682).
- **Other Specified Personality Disorder**: presentations for which symptoms are characteristic of a PD and cause significant distress or impairment but do not meet full criteria for a PD
- **Unspecified Personality Disorder**: presentations similar to Other Specified PD except that a specific PD disorder for which full criteria are not met is not identified due to insufficient information or clinician's choice.

DISRUPTIVE, IMPULSE-CONTROL, AND CONDUCT DISORDERS

Disruptive, impulse-control, and conduct disorders are newly combined in the *DSM-5*. They are characterized by emotional and behavioural self-control problems that lead to violation of the rights of others or bring the person into conflict with societal norms or the authority figures (APA, 2013). These disorders, which often coexist with other disorders, are identified as follows:

- Oppositional defiant disorder
- Intermittent explosive disorder
- Conduct disorder
- Kleptomania
- Pyromania

Of these disorders, intermittent explosive disorder, pyromania, and kleptomania are considered in this chapter. Oppositional defiant disorder and conduct disorder are discussed in Chapter 31, "Psychiatric Disorders Diagnosed in Children and Adolescents." Pathologic gambling, now classified as "Gambling Disorder" in the *DSM-5*, is addressed with substance-related disorders in Chapter 26. Trichotillomania (i.e., chronic, self-destructive hair pulling that results in noticeable hair loss and is associated with increasing tension immediately prior to the hair pulling and release of tension afterwards) is classified in the *DSM-5* with the obsessive–compulsive and related disorders. It is not discussed further in this text. As previously noted, ASPD is listed in the *DSM-5* with the disruptive, impulse-control, and conduct disorders as well as with the PDs.

Intermittent Explosive Disorder

Episodes of aggressiveness that result in an assault or destruction of property characterize people with intermittent explosive disorder. The severity of aggressiveness is out of proportion to the provocation. The episodes can have serious psychosocial consequences, including job loss, interpersonal relationship problems, school expulsion, divorce, automobile crashes, or imprisonment. This diagnosis is given only after all other disorders with aggressive components (e.g., delirium, dementia, head injury, BPD, ASPD, substance abuse) have been excluded. Little is known about this rare disorder.

The treatment of this disorder is multifaceted. Psychopharmacologic agents are sometimes used as an adjunct to psychotherapeutic, behavioural, and social interventions. GABAergic mood stabilizers have been used. Anxiolytics are used for obsessive clients who experience tension states and explosive outbursts. Medication alone, however, is insufficient.

Kleptomania

In **kleptomania**, individuals cannot resist the urge to steal, and they independently steal items that they could easily afford and/or that are not particularly useful or wanted. The underlying issue is the act of stealing. The term *kleptomania* was first used in 1838 to describe the behaviour of several kings who stole worthless objects (Goldman, 1992). Individuals with this disorder experience an increase in tension and then gain pleasure and relief with the theft; they usually experience much guilt and shame afterwards. It is a rare condition (0.3% to 0.6% of general population) and occurs in about 4% to 24% of arrested shoplifters (APA, 2013). In clinical settings, approximately two thirds of clients with kleptomania are female; it is concurrent with a range of other mental disorders, including a 24% concurrency rate with bulimia (Grant & Potenza, 2008). The rate of suicide attempts found in a study of persons with kleptomania was high (24.3%), with the majority attributing their suicidality specifically to their kleptomania (Odlaug, Grant, & Kim, 2012).

Kleptomania, which seems to have an early onset and a chronic trajectory, is difficult to detect (individuals with this disorder actively hide it from family and friends) and to treat. There is inconsistent success with various individual, group, and behavioural therapies; cognitive-behavioural therapy is recommended but this approach, too, awaits further research (Aboujaoude, Gamel, & Koran, 2004).

Pyromania

Pyromania is "deliberate and purposeful fire setting on more than one occasion" (APA, 2013, p. 476). Individuals with this disorder are fascinated with fire and its contexts (e.g., fire alarms, fire stations and personnel) and experience arousal, pleasure, or relief when setting or watching a fire. When they intentionally set fires or make an effort at fire setting, they are not motivated by impaired judgement (e.g., neurocognitive disorder), monetary gain, aggression, anger, vengeance, suicidal ideation, or political ideology. They may make advanced preparation for the fire (APA, 2013). This disorder occurs infrequently and mostly in males (APA, 2013). No controlled clinical trials for psychopharmacologic treatment of pyromania have been reported to date; cognitive-behavioural therapy is said to "show promise" (Burton, McNiel, & Binder, 2012, p. 358).

Continuum of Care

Hospitalization for disruptive, impulse-control, and conduct disorders is rare, except when there are comorbid psychiatric or medical disorders.

SUMMARY OF KEY POINTS

■ Personality is a complex pattern of characteristics, largely outside of the person's awareness, that compose the individual's distinctive pattern of perceiving, feeling, thinking, coping, and behaving. The personality emerges from a complicated interaction of biologic dispositions, psychological experiences, and environmental situations.

■ Personality disorder is an enduring pattern of inner experience and behaviour that deviates markedly from the expectations of the individual's culture, is pervasive and inflexible, has an onset in adolescence or early adulthood, is stable over time, and leads to distress or impairment.

■ In the *DSM*, personality disorders are organized around three clusters: A, B, and C. Prior to the *DSM-5*, cluster A disorders were termed "odd-eccentric";

B disorders, "dramatic-emotional"; and C disorders, "anxious-fearful."

■ People with cluster A personality disorders, whose odd, eccentric behaviours often alienate them from others, can benefit from interventions such as social skills training, environmental management, and cognitive skill building. Changing the patterns of thinking and behaving is difficult and takes time; client outcomes must therefore be evaluated in terms of small changes in thinking and behaviour.

■ In cluster A, paranoid personality disorder is characterized by a suspicious pattern, schizoid personality disorder by an asocial pattern, and schizotypal personality disorder by an eccentric pattern.

■ People with BPD (cluster B) have difficulties regulating emotion and have extreme fears of abandonment, leading to dysfunctional relationships; they often engage in self-injury.

■ ASPD (cluster B) includes people who have no regard for and refuse to conform to social rules, including the law.

■ Individuals with cluster B personality disorders often have difficulties with emotional regulation or being able to recognize and control the expression of feelings such as anger, disappointment, and frustration. The nurse can help these clients identify feelings and gain control over their feelings and actions by teaching communication skills and techniques, thought-stopping techniques, distraction, or problem-solving techniques.

■ Cluster C personality disorders are characterized by anxieties and fears and include avoidant, dependent, and obsessive–compulsive disorders. The obsessive–compulsive personality disorder differs from the obsessive–compulsive anxiety disorder because the individual demonstrates an overall rigidity, perfectionism, and a need for control.

■ For many persons with personality disorders, maintaining a therapeutic nurse–client relationship can be one of the most helpful interventions. Through this therapeutic relationship, the individual experiences a model of healthy interaction, establishing trust, consistency, caring, boundaries, and limitations that help to build the client's self-esteem and respect for self and others. In some personality disorders, nurses will find it more difficult to engage the individual in a true therapeutic relationship because of the person's avoidance of interpersonal and emotional attachment (e.g., ASPD or paranoid personality disorder).

■ Individuals with personality disorders rarely receive inpatient treatment, except during periods of destructive behaviour or self-injury. Treatment is delivered in the community and over time. Continuity of care

is important in helping the individual change lifelong personality patterns.

■ Although not classified as personality disorders, the impulse-control disorders share one of the primary characteristics of impulsivity, which leads to inappropriate social behaviours that are considered harmful to self or others and that give the individual excitement or gratification at the time the act is committed.

CRITICAL THINKING CHALLENGES

1 Describe your own personality. Is this difficult to do? If so, what makes it difficult? Does the Big Five model of personality traits help you to understand your personality?

2 Define the concept of *personality disorder*. What distinguishes a personality disorder from a normal personality?

3 Name the five core components of (mal)adaptive personality functioning that can be used to describe the severity of a PD.

4 Define, compare, and contrast the three PDs of cluster A.

5 Define, compare, and contrast the four PDs of cluster B.

6 Define, compare, and contrast the three PDs of cluster C.

7 Define and describe intermittent explosive disorder, pyromania, and kleptomania.

8 Read the Roman poet Ovid's version of the Narcissus myth in *The Metamorphoses*.

9 Karen, a 36-year-old woman receiving inpatient care, was admitted for depression; she also has a diagnosis of BPD. After a telephone argument with her husband, she approaches the nurse's station with her wrist dripping with blood from cutting. What nursing diagnosis best fits this behaviour? What interventions should the nurse use with the client once the self-injury is treated?

10 A 22-year-old man with BPD is being discharged from the mental health unit after a severe suicide attempt. As his primary nurse, you have been able to establish a therapeutic relationship with him but are now terminating the relationship. He asks you to meet with him "for just a few sessions" after his discharge because his therapist will be on vacation. What are the issues underlying this request? What should you do? Explain and justify.

11 The stigma attached to a personality disorder diagnosis can be evident within health care services itself. What strategies can be used to ensure that such stigma is eradicated and that the client with a PD is not labelled as "difficult"?

REFERENCES

Aboujaoude, E., Gamel, N., & Koran, L. M. (2004). Overview of klepto-mania and phenomenological description of 40 patients. *Primary Care Companion to the Journal of Clinical Psychiatry*, 6(6), 244–247.

American Psychiatric Association (APA). (2013). *Diagnostic and statistical manual of mental disorders* (5th ed.). Washington, DC: Author.

Bartholomew, K. & Horowitz, L. (1991). Attachment styles among young adults: A test of a four-category model. *Journal of Personality and Social Psychology*, 61, 226–244.

Bennett, K., Shepherd, J., & Janca, A. (2013). Personality disorders and spirituality. *Current Opinion in Psychiatry*, 26, 79–83.

Best, M., Williams, J. M., & Coccaro, E. F. (2002). Evidence for a dysfunctional prefrontal circuit in patients with an impulsive aggressive disorder. *Proceedings of the National Academy of Sciences of the Unites States of America*, 11(12), 8448–8853.

Black, D., Baumgard, C., & Bell, S. (1995). The long-term outcome of anti-social personality disorder compared with depression, schizophrenia, and surgical conditions. *The Bulletin of the American Academy of Psychiatry and the Law*, 23(1), 43–52.

Black, D., Blum, N., Pfohl, B., & John, D. (2004). The STEPPS group treatment program for outpatients with borderline personality disorder. *Journal of Contemporary Psychotherapy*, 34, 193–210.

Blashfield, R. K., Reynolds, S. M., & Stennett, B. (2012). The death of histrionic personality disorder. In T. A. Widiger (Ed.). *The Oxford handbook of personality disorders* (pp. 603–627). Oxford, UK: Oxford University Press.

Bohus, M., Haaf, B., Stiglmayr, C., Pohl, U., Böhme, R., & Linehan, M. (2000). Evaluation of inpatient dialectical-behavioral therapy for borderline personality disorder—a prospective study. *Behaviour Research and Therapy*, 38(9), 875–887.

Boone, M. L., McNeil, D. W., Masia, C. L., Turk, C. L., Carter, L. E., Ries, B. J., & Lewin, M. R. (1999). Multimodal comparisons of social phobia subtypes and avoidant personality disorder. *Journal of Anxiety Disorders*, 13(3), 271–292.

Bornstein, R. F. (1998). Implicit and self-attributed dependency needs in dependent and histrionic personality disorders. *Journal of Personality Assessment*, 71(1), 1–14.

Boughn, S. (2005). Evidence-based nursing care of patients suffering from trichotillomania. *New Jersey Nurse*, 35(3), 13.

Bulechek, G., Butcher, H., & McCloskey Dochterman, J. (Eds.). (2008). *Nursing interventions classification (NIC)* (5th ed.). St. Louis, MO: Mosby.

Burton, P. R. S., McNiel, D. E., & Binder, R. L. (2012). Firesetting, arson, pyromania, and the forensic mental health expert. *The Journal of the American Academy of Psychiatry and the Law*, 40, 355–365.

Cadenhead, K. S., Perry, W., Shafer, K., & Braff, D. L. (1999). Cognitive functions in schizotypal personality disorder. *Schizophrenia Research*, 37(2), 123–132.

Carr, T. (2008). Mapping the processes and qualities of spiritual nursing care. *Qualitative Health Research*, 18(5), 686–700.

Clarkin, J. F., Yeomans, F. E., & Kernberg, O. F. (2006). *Psychotherapy for borderline personality: Focusing on object relations*. Washington, DC: American Psychiatric Press.

Cloninger, C., Bayon, C., & Svrakic, D. (1998). Measurement of temperament and character in mood disorders: A model of fundamental states as personality types. *Journal of Affective Disorders*, 51(1), 21–32.

Crichton, R. (1959). *The great impostor*. New York, NY: Random House.

Dowson, J. H., Sussams, P., Grounds, A. T., & Taylor, J. C. (2001). Associations of past conduct disorder with personality disorders in "non-psychotic" psychiatric inpatients. *European Psychiatry: The Journal of the Association of European Psychiatrists*, 16(1), 49–56.

Erikson, E. (1968). *Identity: Youth and crisis*. New York, NY: Norton.

Feigenbaum, J. (2007). Dialectical behaviour therapy: An increasing evidence base. *Journal of Mental Health*, 16(1), 51–68.

Friedman, H. S. & Schustack, M. W. (2012). *Personality: classic theories and modern research*. Boston, MA: Allyn & Bacon.

Gallop, R., McCay, E., & Esplen, J. (1992). The conceptualization of impulsivity for psychiatric nursing practice. *Archives of Psychiatric Nursing*, 6(6), 366–373.

Gillath, O., Bahns, A. J., Ge, F., & Crandall, C. S. (2012). Shoes as a source of first impressions. *Journal of Research in Personality*, 4, 423–430.

Goldman, M. (1992). Kleptomania: An overview. *Psychiatric Annals*, 22(2), 68–71.

Gottesman, I. & Goldsmith, H. (1994). Developmental psychopathology of antisocial behavior: Inserting genes into its ontogenesis and epigenesis. In C. Nelson (Ed.), *Threats to optimal development: Integrating biological, social, and psychological risk factors* (Vol. 27, pp. 69–104). Hillsdale, NJ: Erlbaum.

Grant, J. E. & Potenza, M. N. (2008). Gender-related differences in individuals seeking treatment for kleptomania. *CNS Spectrums*, 13(3), 235–245.

Grover, K. E., Carpenter, L. L., Price, L. H., Gagne, G. G., Mello, M. F., & Tyrka, A. R. (2007). The relationship between childhood abuse and adult personality disorder symptoms. *Journal of Personality Disorders*, 21(4), 442–447.

Hayward, B. A. (2007). Cluster A personality disorders: Considering the "odd-eccentric" in psychiatric nursing. *International Journal of Mental Health Nursing*, 16(1), 15–21.

Helleman, M., Goossens, P. J. J., Kaasenbrood, Ad., & van Achterberg, T. (2014). Evidence base and components of brief admission as an intervention for patients with borderline personality disorder: A review of the literature. *Perspectives in Psychiatric Care*, 50, 65–75.

Herpertz, S. C., Kunnert, H. J., Schwenger, U. B., & Sass, H. (1999). Affective responsiveness in borderline personality disorder: A psychophysiological approach. *American Journal of Psychiatry*, 156(10), 1550–1556.

Herpertz, S. C., Wenning, B., Mueller, B., Qunaibi, M., Sass, H., & Herpertz-Dahlmann, B. (2001). Psychophysiological responses in ADHD boys with and without conduct disorder: Implications for adult antisocial behavior. *Journal of the American Academy of Child and Adolescent Psychiatry*, 40(10), 1222–1230.

Hill, J. (2002). Biological, psychological and social processes in the conduct disorders. *Journal of Child Psychology and Psychiatry and Allied Disciplines*, 43(1), 133–164.

Hill, J. (2003). Early identification of individuals at risk for antisocial personality disorder. *British Journal of Psychiatry-Supplementum*, 44, S11–S14.

Hoffman, P. D., Fruzzetti, A. E., & Buteau, E. (2007). Understanding and engaging families: An education, skills and support program for relatives impacted by borderline personality disorder. *Journal of Mental Health*, 16(1), 69–82.

Holm, A. L. & Severinsson, E. (2008). The emotional pain and distress of borderline personality disorder: A review of the literature. *International Journal of Mental Health Nursing*, 17(1), 27–35.

Holm, A. L. & Severinsson, E. (2011). Struggling to recover by changing suicidal behaviour: Narratives from women with borderline personality disorder. *International Journal of Mental Health Nursing*, 20(3), 165–173.

Hooley, J. M., Cole, S. H., & Gironde, S. (2012). Borderline personality disorder. In Widiger, T. A. (Ed.), *The Oxford handbook of personality disorders* (pp. 409–436). Oxford, UK: Oxford University Press.

Hopwood, C. J. & Thomas, K. M. (2012). Paranoid and schizoid personality disorders. In T. Widiger (Ed.), *The Oxford handbook of personality disorders* (pp. 582–602). Oxford, UK: Oxford University Press.

Horley, J. (2013). Introduction: An overview of some issues in the study of psychopathy. In J. Horley (Ed.) *Born bad? Critiques of psychopathy*. Hauppauge, NY: Nova Science Publishers, Inc.

Horsfall, J. (1999). Towards understanding some complex borderline behaviours. *Journal of Psychiatric Mental Health Nursing*, 6(6), 425–432.

Hurlemann, R., Hawellek, B., Maier, W., & Dolan, R. (2007). Enhanced emotion-induced amnesia in borderline personality disorder. *Psychological Medicine*, 37(7), 971–981.

Johnson, J. G., Cohen, P., Brown, J., Smailes, E. M., & Bernstein, D. P. (1999). Childhood maltreatment increases risk for personality disorders during early adulthood. *Archives of General Psychiatry*, 56(7), 607–608.

Jordan, J. V. (2004). Personality disorder or relational disconnection. In J. J. Magnavita (Ed.), *Handbook of personality disorders* (pp. 120–134). Hoboken, NJ: John Wiley.

Jovev, M., McKenzie, T., Whittle, S., Simmons, J. G., Allen, N. B., & Chanen, A. M. (2013). Temperament and maltreatment in the emergence of borderline and antisocial personality pathology during early adolescence. *Journal of the Canadian Academy of Child and Adolescent Psychiatry*, 22(3), 220–229.

Kiehl, K. A., Smith, A. M., Hare, R. D., Mendrek, A., Forster, B. B., Brink, J., & Liddle, P. F. (2001). Limbic abnormalities in affective processing by criminal psychopaths as revealed by functional magnetic resonance imaging. *Biological Psychiatry*, 50(9), 677–684.

Krause, E. D., Mendelson, T., & Lynch, T. R. (2003). Childhood emotional invalidation and adult psychological distress: The mediating role of emotional inhibition. *Child Abuse and Neglect*, 27, 199–213.

Kwapil, T. R. & Barrantes-Vidal, N. (2012). Schizotypal personality disorder: An integrative review. In T. A. Widiger (Ed.), *The Oxford handbook of personality disorders* (pp. 437–477). Oxford, UK: Oxford University Press.

Langbehn, D. R. & Cadoret, R. J. (2001). The adult antisocial syndrome with and without antecedent conduct disorder: Comparisons from an adoption study. *Comprehensive Psychiatry*, 42(4), 272–282.

Leahy, R. L. & McGinn, L. K. (2012). Cognitive therapy for personality disorders. In T. A. Widiger (Ed.), *The Oxford handbook of personality disorders* (pp. 727–750). Oxford, UK: Oxford University Press.

Leichsenring, F., Leibing, E., Kruse, J., New, A. S., & Leweke, F., (2011). Borderline personality disorder. *Lancet*, 377(1), 74–84.

Lieb, K., Völlm, B. Rücker, G., Timmer, A. & Stoffers, J. M. (2010). Pharmacotherapy for borderline personality disorder: Cochrane systematic review of randomized trials. *British Journal of Psychiatry*, *196*(1), 4–12.

Linehan, M. (1993a). *Cognitive-behavioral treatment of borderline personality disorder*. New York, NY: Guilford.

Linehan, M. (1993b). *Skills training manual for treating borderline personality disorder*. New York, NY: Guilford.

Links, P. S., Heslegrave, R., & van Reekum R. (1998). Prospective follow-up study of borderline personality disorder: Prognosis, prediction of outcome, and Axis II comorbidity. *Canadian Journal of Psychiatry*, *43*(3), 265–270.

Links, P. S., Kolia, N. J., Guimond, T., & McMain, S. (2013). Prospective risk factors for suicide attempts in a treated sample of patients with borderline personality disorder. *Canadian Journal of Psychiatry*, *58*(2), 99–106.

Lynch, T. R. & Cuper, P. F. (2012). Dialectical behavior therapy of borderline and other personality disorders. In T. A. Widiger (Ed.), *The Oxford handbook of personality disorders* (pp. 785–793). Oxford, UK: Oxford University Press.

Magnavita, J. J. (Ed.). (2004). The relevance of theory in treating personality dysfunction. In *Handbook of personality disorders: Theory and practice* (pp. 56–77). Hoboken, NJ: John Wiley & Sons.

Mahler, M., Pine, F., & Bergman, A. (1975). *The psychological birth of human infant: Symbiosis and individuation*. New York, NY: Basic Books.

Martin, E. A. (Ed.). (2007). *Concise medical dictionary* (7th ed.). London, UK: Oxford.

Matta, I., Sham, P. C., Gilvarry, C. M., Jones, P. B., Lewis, S. W., & Murray, R. M. (2000). Childhood schizotypy and positive symptoms in schizophrenic patients predict schizotypy in relatives. *Schizophrenia Research*, *44*(2), 129–136.

Mattick, R. & Newman, C. (1991). Social phobia and avoidant personality disorder. *International Review of Psychiatry*, *3*(2), 163–173.

Meyer, B. & Pilkonis, P. A. (2005). An attachment model of personality disorders. In M. F. Lenzenweger & J. F. Clarkin (Eds.), *Major theories of personality disorders* (pp. 231–281). New York, NY: Guilford.

Miller, S. (1994). Borderline personality disorder from a patient's perspective. *Hospital and Community Psychiatry*, *45*(12), 1215–1219.

Millon, T. & Davis, R. (1999). *Personality disorders in modern life*. New York, NY: John Wiley.

Millon, T., Millon, C., Meagher, S., Grossman, S., & Ramnath, R. (2004). *Personality disorders in modern life* (2nd ed.). New York, NY: John Wiley.

Moeller, F. G. & Dougherty, D. M. (2001). Antisocial personality disorder, alcohol, and aggression. *Alcohol Research and Health*, *25*(1), 5–11.

Moutier, C. Y. & Stein, M. B. (1999). The history, epidemiology, and differential diagnosis of social anxiety disorder. *Journal of Clinical Psychiatry*, *60*(Suppl. 9), 4–8.

Maruszewski, T., Fajkowska, M., & Eysenck, M. W. (2010). An integrative view of personality. In Maruszewski, T., Fajkowska, M., & Eysenck, M. W. (Ed.), *Warsaw lectures in personality and social psychology, Vol. 1: Personality from biological, cognitive, and social perspectives* (pp. 1–9). Clinton Corners, NY: Eliot Werner Publications, Inc.

Nehls, N. (1998). Borderline personality disorder: Gender stereotypes, stigma and limited system of care. *Issues in Mental Health Nursing*, *19*(2), 97–112.

Nehls, N. (1999). Borderline personality disorder: The voice of patients. *Research in Nursing and Health*, *22*(4), 285–293.

Odlaug, B. L., Grant, J. E., & Kim, S. W. (2012). Suicide attempts in 107 adolescents and adults with kleptomania. *Archives of Suicide Research*, *16*, 348–359.

Oltmanns, T. F. & Powers, A. D. (2012). Gender and personality disorders. In Widiger, T. A. (Ed.). *The Oxford handbook of personality disorders* (pp. 206–218). Oxford, UK: Oxford University Press.

Ovid. (1807/2009). The metamorphoses of Publius Ovidus Naso in English blank verse, Vols. I & II. J. J. Howard (Trans.). Project Gutenberg EBook. Retrieved from http://www.gutenberg.org/files/28621/28621-h/28621-h.htm

Paris, J. (2007). *Half in love with death: Managing the chronically suicidal patient*. Mahwah, NJ: Lawrence Erlbaum.

Paris, J. (2010). Effectiveness of different psychotherapy approaches in the treatment of borderline personality disorder. *Current Psychiatry Reports*, *12*(1), 56–60.

Perugi, G., Nassini, S., Socci, C., Lenzi, M., Toni, C., Simonini, E., & Akiskal, H. S. (1999). Avoidant personality in social phobia and panic-agoraphobia disorder: A comparison. *Journal of Affective Disorders*, *54*(3), 277–282.

Ronningstam, E. (2012). Narcissistic personality disorder: The diagnostic process. In T. A. Widiger (Ed.), *The Oxford handbook of personality disorders* (pp. 527–549). Oxford, UK: Oxford University Press.

Sanislow, C. A., da Cruz, K. L., Gianol, M. O., & Reagan, E. M. (2012). Avoidant personality disorder, traits, and types. In T. A. Widiger (Ed.), *The Oxford handbook of personality disorders* (pp. 549–565). Oxford, UK: Oxford University Press.

Schroeder, K., Fisher, H. L., & Schäfer, I. (2013). Psychotic symptoms in patients with borderline personality disorder: Prevalence and clinical management. *Current Opinion in Psychiatry*, *26*, 113–119.

Silk, K. R. (2000). Borderline personality disorder. Overview of biologic factors. *Psychiatric Clinical North America*, *23*(1), 61–75.

Silk, K. R. & Feurino III, L. (2012). Psychopharmacology of personality disorders. In T. Widiger (Ed.), *The Oxford handbook of personality disorders* (pp. 713–726). Oxford, UK: Oxford University Press.

Soderstrom, H., Blennow, K., Sjodin, A. K., & Forsman, A. (2003). New evidence for an association between the CSF HVA: 5-HIAA ratio and psychopathic traits. *Journal of Neurology, Neurosurgery and Psychiatry*, *74*(7), 918–921.

Soloff, P., Lis, J., Kelly, T., Cornelius, J., & Ulrich, R. (2004). Risk factors for suicidal behavior in borderline personality disorder. *American Journal of Psychiatry*, *151*(9), 1316–1323.

Stern, A. (1938). A psychoanalytic investigation and therapy in the borderline group of neuroses. *Psychoanalytic Quarterly*, *7*, 467–489.

Stepp, S. D., Scott, L. N., Morse, J. Q., Nolf, K. A., Hallquist, M. N., & Pilkonis, P. A. (2014). Emotion dysregulation as a maintenance factor of borderline personality disorder features. *Comprehensive Psychiatry*, *55*(3):657–666. doi: 10.1016/j.comppsych.2013.11.006 (online ahead of print).

Strike, C., Rhodes, A. E., Bergmans, Y., & Links, P. (2006). Fragmented pathways to care: The experiences of suicidal men. *Crisis*, *27*(1), 31–38.

Torgersen, S. (2012). Epidemiology. In Widiger, T. A. (Ed.), *The Oxford handbook of personality disorders* (pp. 186–205). Oxford, UK: Oxford University Press.

van den Bosch, L. M., Verheul, R., Schippers, G. M., & van den Brink, W. (2002). Dialectical behavior therapy of borderline patients with and without substance use problems: Implementation and long-term effects. *Addictive Behaviors*, *27*(6), 911–923.

Van Wel, B., Kockmann, I., Blum, N., Pfohl, B., Black, D., & Heesterman, W. (2006). STEPPS group treatment for borderline personality disorder in the Netherlands. *Annals of Clinical Psychiatry*, *18*(1), 63–67.

Verheul, R., Berghout, C. D., Busschbach, J. J. V., Bateman, A. W., Andrea, H., Dolan, C., … Fonagy, P. (2008). Severity Indices of Personality Problems (SIPP-118): Development, factor structure, reliability, and validity. *Psychological Assessment*, *20*(1), 23–34.

Voglmaier, M. M., Seidman, L. J., Niznikiewicz, M. A., Dickey, C. C., Shenton, M. E., & McCarley, R. W. (2000). Verbal and nonverbal neuropsychological test performance in subjects with schizotypal personality disorder. *American Journal of Psychiatry*, *157*(5), 787–793.

Waldeck, T. L. & Miller, L. S. (2000). Social skills deficits in schizotypal personality disorder. *Psychiatry Research*, *93*(3), 237–246.

Waldman, I. D. & Slutske, W. S. (2000). Antisocial behavior and alcoholism: A behavioral genetic perspective on comorbidity. *Clinical Psychological Review*, *20*(2), 255–287.

Ward, R. K. (2004). Assessment and management of personality disorders. *American Family Physician*, *70*(8), 1505–1512.

Widiger, T. (Ed.). (2012). *The Oxford handbook of personality disorders*. Oxford, UK: Oxford University Press.

Weston, D. Beton, E., & Defife, J. A. (2011). Identity disturbance in adolescence: Associations with borderline personality disorder. *Development and Psychopathology*, *23*(1), 305–313.

Yen, S., Shea, M. T., Battle, C. L., Johnson, D. M., Zlotnick, C., Dolan-Sewell, R., … McGlashan, T. H. (2002). Traumatic exposure and posttraumatic stress disorder in borderline, schizotypal, avoidant and obsessive-compulsive personality disorders: Findings from the Collaborative Longitudinal Personality Disorders Study. *Journal of Nervous and Mental Disease*, *190*, 510–518.

Yeomans, F., Hull, J., & Clarkin, J. (1994). Risk factors for self-damaging acts in a borderline population. *Journal of Personality Disorders*, *8*(1), 10–16.

Young, J. E. (1999). *Cognitive therapy for personality disorders: A schema-focused approach* (3rd ed.). Sarasota, FL: Professional Resource Press.

Zanarini, M. C., Frankenburg, F. R., Reich, D. B., Silk, K. R., Hudson, J. I., & McSweeney, L. B. (2007). The subsyndromal phenomenology of borderline personality disorder: A 10-year follow-up study. *American Journal of Psychiatry*, *164*(6), 929–935.

Zanarini, M. C., Ruser, T., Frankenburg, F. R., & Hennen, J. (2000). The dissociative experiences of borderline patients. *Comprehensive Psychiatry*, *41*(3), 223–227.

Zanarini, M. C., Williams, A. A., Lewis, R. E., Reich, R. B., Vera, S. C., Marino, M. F., … Frankenburg, F. R. (1997). Reported pathological childhood experiences associated with the development of borderline personality disorder. *American Journal of Psychiatry*, *154*(8), 1101–1106.

Zweig-Frank, F., Paris, J., & Guzder, J. (1994a). Dissociation in female patients with borderline and non-borderline personality disorders. *Journal of Personality Disorders*, *8*(3), 203–209.

Zweig-Frank, F., Paris, J., & Guzder, J. (1994b). Psychological risk factors for dissociation and self-mutilation in female patients with borderline personality disorder. *Canadian Journal of Psychiatry*, *39*(5), 259–264.

28 Sleep–Wake Disorders

Anne Marie Creamer

After studying this chapter, you will be able to:

- Describe the phases of sleep and physiologic changes that occur during sleep.
- Discuss the bio/psycho/social/spiritual factors that impact sleep.
- Identify strategies used to assess sleep and sleep disturbances.
- List the sleep–wake diagnoses described in the *Diagnostic and Statistical Manual of Mental Disorders* (5th edition).
- Explain the impact of medications and other substances on the stages of sleep.
- Discuss the interaction between mental illness and sleep.
- Describe the role nurses play in the assessment and management of sleep problems and sleep disorders.

KEY CONCEPTS

- insomnia
- sleep

KEY TERMS

- circadian • electroencephalogram (EEG) • electromyogram (EMG) • electrooculogram (EOG) • narcolepsy • obstructive sleep apnea • polysomnography • sleep architecture • sleep efficiency • sleep hygiene • sleep hypnogram • sleep latency • sleep phases • Zeitgeber

Nurses need to understand sleep. Knowledge of sleep and of the role sleep plays in healthy living is necessary across all areas of nursing practice. It is necessary to nurses' own health, given that the majority of nurses are shift workers. Poor sleep is associated with higher death rates; even when health status, age, gender, alcohol use, social network size, smoking, and obesity are considered, death rates remain higher (Motivala, 2011). Chronic insomnia symptoms are associated with hypertension and cardiovascular disease, including myocardial infarction. Sleep duration and quality are intimately linked with metabolic functions through a number of factors including insulin sensitivity and secretion, inflammatory processes, hormones such as ghrelin and leptin that impact satiety, and appetite and energy homeostasis (Morselli, Guyon, & Spiegel, 2012). Obesity is linked with obstructive sleep apnea (OSA), and those who are obese without apnea experience more waking in the night and daytime sleepiness. Short or long

(≥9 hours) sleep duration and poor sleep quality predict higher incidence of diabetes. In this chapter, the question "What is sleep?" is answered, the phases of sleep are explained, and sleep patterns over the life span are described. Sleep–wake disorders and ways to assess them are identified and common circadian rhythm disorders discussed. A bio/psycho/social/spiritual approach to nursing interventions for the disorders of insomnia and OSA is delineated.

HISTORICAL PERSPECTIVES ON SLEEP AND DREAMS

In ancient times, the Egyptians and Mesopotamians thought that dreams were the means by which the gods communicated their wishes to mortals (Palagini & Rosenlicht, 2011). Joseph was the most famous dream interpreter in the Bible. The Egyptians wrote the earliest known document of dream interpretation around 1275

BCE; this papyrus is found in the British Museum today. In Greek mythology, Oneiros, the god of dreams, and Hypnos, the god of sleep, helped reduce human suffering. The Greek philosopher Plato ascribed the site of dream prophecy to the liver and felt that humans express their bestial desires while dreaming. However, Aristotle rejected the idea that dreams were prophecies and posited that dreams were residual perceptions travelling through the bloodstream and activating the heart. In the second century, an Asian "diviner" named Artemidorus Daldianus described more than 30,000 different types of dreams.

The 18th-century German philosopher Leibniz posited that dreams were a product of the mind. This concept was developed further in the late 19th century when Freud described dreams as expressions of man's emotions and attempts by the unconscious to reconcile psychological conflicts. Freud also hypothesized a mind/brain model that included neurobiologic aspects of psychological activities (Palagini & Rosenlicht, 2011).

When Hans Berger, a German psychiatrist, recorded electrical activity in the human brain in 1928, he demonstrated that different rhythms occurred during sleep and waking times (Roehrs, 2011). These brain signal recordings were called **electroencephalograms** (EEG), and they allowed scientists to conduct more detailed studies of sleep without waking the person. By the late 1930s, all the major elements of sleep brain wave patterns were described. However, it was not until the 1950s that the cyclical variation of EEG patterns during sleep was identified. With the discovery of the rapid eye movement (REM) stage and its characteristic features, it was realized that sleep consists of two very different states: REM and non-REM or NREM. These states are as different from each other as each is from the wake state. Since then, a tremendous amount of research has explained much of what happens during sleep; among the many important questions that remain is *why* we sleep.

▬ WHAT IS SLEEP?

Until recently, it was thought that sleep was a resting period for the brain; with the decrease of sensory input, brain activities diminished and sleep occurred (Roehrs, 2011). However, several other theories have been suggested (Harrison, 2012). For example, sleep is thought to have an important relationship with visual processes. Compared with the other senses, vision requires a very large amount of processing capacity in the brain; with sleep, visual input to the brain is reduced. Another theory is that sleep is necessary for the maintenance and enhancement of memory, with its two stages playing different roles. However, it is known that because humans can go for extended periods of time without REM sleep, as is seen when individuals take different medications like tricyclic antidepressants, NREM can play a role, albeit less efficiently, in memory processing. The function of sleep remains little understood.

Sleep has two distinct phases, rapid eye movement (REM) and non-rapid eye movement (NREM). The NREM stage is further subdivided into three stages according to depth:

- Intermediate stage 1 (drowsiness and sleep onset)
- Light stage 2
- Deep stage 3 or slow-wave sleep (SWS). Until recently, there were four stages of NREM sleep, but stages 3 and 4 have been consolidated.

The amount and distribution of the sleep stages is called **sleep architecture**. In healthy young people, sleep progresses fairly consistently each night through stages NREM 1 to 3 within 45 to 60 minutes. NREM sleep always precedes REM sleep unless there are certain pathologies (e.g., narcolepsy). **Sleep latency** is the length of time it takes to fall asleep once the person tries to sleep. Although differences in individual sleepers exist, when asked how long it takes them to fall asleep, normal sleepers will report 15 to 30 minutes. This suggests that stage 2 is related to when the person believes he or she fell asleep. The first REM sleep episode occurs during the 2nd hour of sleep; more rapid onset of REM sleep may suggest a problem like depression or narcolepsy. It normally takes 70 to 100 minutes for a young healthy person to move from stage 1 through to REM sleep. The sleeper may complete up to five cycles in a regular 8-hour night. A **sleep hypnogram** is a graphic display of the individual's experience of moving through the stages of sleep during a sleep period (Fig. 28-1). **Sleep efficiency** is the ratio of the time spent sleeping to the total amount of time spent in bed.

The duration of the NREM–REM cycle usually stays the same, but as the night progresses, the REM episodes become longer and the NREM episodes become shorter. During the period of drowsiness as the person transitions from wakefulness to sleep, things that happen within the few minutes before dropping into phase 1 are often forgotten. The first REM cycle of the night is usually very short, lasting 1 to 5 minutes. As the sleep session progresses through the night, the REM cycles become longer and the SWS phase that occupied much of NREM during the first third of the night, occupies less time as the night progresses. These differences are thought to be related to different processes at work. The circadian oscillator (see below) is thought to influence REM sleep so that there is more REM sleep later in the night while more SWS at the beginning at the night is related to the homeostatic sleep system (see below). A good sleeper may return to wakefulness several times a night, with many of these occurrences taking place when the brain is moving between REM and NREM sleep and with changes in body position. However, these awakenings are usually only 30 to 60 seconds long and are not remembered in

FIGURE 28-1. Top: Brain wave patterns during a normal sleep cycle. Sleep cycles are divided into REM (rapid eye movement) and NREM (nonrapid eye movement) sleep. NREM is further divided into three stages: N1, N2, and N3. **Bottom:** Normal hypnogram: The various stages of sleep are represented by levels on the vertical axis; time of night is shown on the horizontal axis. In this patient, there were four sleep cycles, each composed of a segment of NREM sleep followed by REM sleep. The length of REM sleep increased toward morning. Conversely, most of the stage N3 sleep was in the early portion of the night. In recent research, stages 3 and 4 have been consolidated. (Sources: Rhoades, R. A. & Bell, D. R. (Eds.). (2012). *Medical physiology: Principles for clinical medicine* (4th ed.). Philadelphia, PA: Lippincott Williams & Wilkins; Carney, P. R., Berry, R. B., & Geyer, J. D. (2012). *Clinical sleep disorders* (2nd ed.). Philadelphia, PA: Lippincott Williams & Wilkins.)

the morning. When asked, the sleeper may report waking one to three times in the night.

A person's usual length of sleep is dependent on several factors including personal choice, genetics, and the length of time one has been awake since the last sleep.

Most young adults report sleeping about 7.5 hours on a weekday night and 8.5 hours on a weekend night. Several changes in sleep patterns occur over the person's lifetime (see below, special populations). Some people are "short sleepers." They may require less than the usual amount of

Table 28-1		Stages of Sleep		

Stage	Percentage of Sleep Time During the Night	Physical Signs	Behavioural and Brain Activity
N1	2%–5%	Decrease in muscular activity; slow eye movement; pupils become smaller	Begin to fail to respond to auditory stimuli but easily awakened Awakened person reports not having been asleep
N2 Light NREM sleep	45%–55%	Eye movements stop; heart rate and respiration slow; body temperature, cerebral blood flow, and metabolism decrease	Less likely to react to light or noise unless it is very bright or loud
N3 Slow-wave sleep (SWS); deepest stage of NREM sleep	13%–23%	Brain's temperature at its lowest; heart rate, respiration, and blood pressure decrease	Harder to wake; possible confusion or disorientation after waking Will wake if the stimulus has strong personal meaning (e.g., mother hears her baby crying)
REM sleep	20%–25%	Rapid eye movements; general muscle tone is very low or absent; increased variability in pulse rate, blood pressure, and respiration Upper respiratory airway resistance increases; muscle tone in muscles associated with breathing is more flaccid Body temperature is not regulated, no shivering or sweating Partial or full penile erection	EEG waves look similar to waves seen in wakefulness Waking is more likely to occur toward the end of REM sleep period Cerebral blood flow and metabolism are restored to waking-state level Dreaming occurs High level of brain activity

sleep. In comparison with those with insomnia, they have no difficulty falling or staying asleep and are not troubled by daytime symptoms of insufficient sleep. Similarly, some individuals require longer than usual sleep time.

Different things are occurring in the body during the NREM and REM phases (see Table 28-1). For example, during NREM sleep, the body can move and mental activity is usually associated with little or fragmented activity. In contrast, during REM sleep, the body is almost paralyzed, except for episodes of rapid eye movement and muscle twitches, and the brain is activated (Fig. 28-2). Therefore, someone walking about while dreaming is a sign of altered brain function.

KEY CONCEPT   Sleep is a behavioural and physiologic state of temporary disconnection from the environment, characterized by
- Physical stillness characterized by no or few movements
- Stereotypical body postures (closed eyes, usually lying down)
- Reduced responsiveness to external stimulation
- Rapid reversibility between states, as compared with other states of altered vigilance like coma, hypothermia, or being anaesthetized (Landis, 2011; Peigneux, Urbain, & Schmitz, 2012)

DREAMING

Initially, it was believed that dreaming occurred only during REM sleep, but now it is believed that about 20% of dreams occur during NREM sleep (Ropper & Samuels, 2009). The purpose of dreams is not yet known. Several theories have been suggested, some significantly different from others (Dubuc, n.d.). For example, Freud thought that our dreams are manifestations of our desires and motivation. In the 1970s, Hobson and McCarley proposed a model suggesting that the cortex is subjected to random stimulation by meaningless signals from the pons. However, we know that people who have injuries to two areas of the brain that are not involved in REM sleep report not dreaming. One area is where the occipital, temporal, and parietal cortices meet; this area is involved in spatial imagery (Fig. 28-3). The other area is located in the frontal cortex, which receives neural pathways from the mesolimbic system. This system is involved in positive reinforcement and motivation. Dream therapy is practised today as a form of psychotherapy that helps the dreamer increase self-awareness. However, "dream symbols" found in popular books do not have a scientific basis.

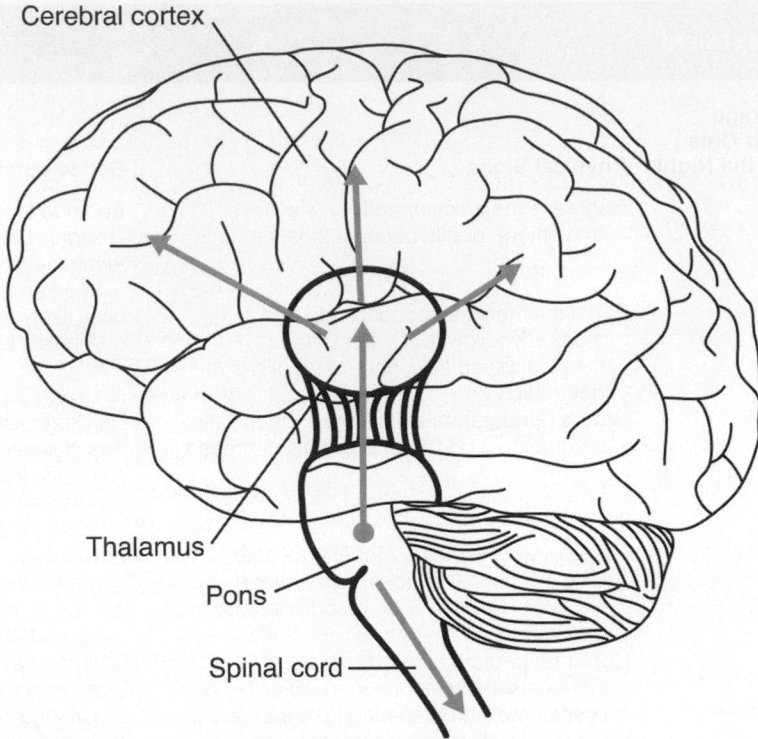

FIGURE 28-2. Pathways of brain activity during REM sleep. (Source: BSCS. (2003). *Sleep, sleep disorders, & biological rhythms.* NIH publication No. 04–4984. Bethesda, MD: National Institutes of Health. Copyright © 2003 by BSCS. All rights reserved. Used with permission.)

FIGURE 28-3. Areas of the brain active during REM sleep. (Source: BSCS. (2003). *Sleep, sleep disorders, & biological rhythms.* NIH publication No. 04–4984. Bethesda, MD: National Institutes of Health. Copyright © 2003 by BSCS. All rights reserved. Used with permission.)

BIOLOGIC PROCESSES
Process C and Process S

A two-process model provides a broad perspective on the sleep–wake cycle. These two processes oppose each other, enabling us to be awake during the daylight hours and sleep during the night. Process S, or homeostatic factor, represents sleep need. It drives how intensely we sleep, rising over the wake period and declining during sleep; the longer a person is awake, the stronger the drive to sleep. Additionally, loss of a specific phase of sleep results in a stronger drive to recover the lost phase. Adenosine may be a sleep-promoting substance that affects process S. Caffeine and theophylline, which is found in tea, act as antagonists at adenosine receptors and counter the effects of sleep deprivation.

Process C denotes **circadian** timing of the sleep–wake cycles in the day; the word "circadian" means "about the day." Circadian rhythms are biochemical, physiologic, and behavioural cycles in the body, lasting between 24.2 and 25.5 hours. While the difference between a 24-hour day and 24.2- to 25.5-hour day does not seem significant, if the brain is unable to keep a consistent schedule, over a 3-week period, things that were done in the daytime would end up being done at night. Therefore, the body's ability to make adjustments to suit the environment is essential.

Circadian rhythms are thought to be coordinated by the molecular oscillations of neurons in the suprachiasmatic nuclei (SCN), two small areas in the hypothalamus. In order to maintain accuracy, these molecular oscillations are synchronized every day with external cues, also called **Zeitgebers**. Examples of these cues include ambient temperature and noise, meal consumption, and the body's activity level. The strongest cue is the intensity of ambient light. These SCN neurons receive stimuli from specialized light-sensitive ganglion cells in the retina. Timing information from the SCN is transmitted to the sleep–wake centres in the brain (Fig. 28-4).

FIGURE 28-4. The biologic clock is located within the suprachiasmatic nucleus of the brain. (Source: BSCS. (2003). *Sleep, sleep disorders, & biological rhythms.* NIH publication No. 04–4984. Bethesda, MD: National Institutes of Health. Copyright © 2003 by BSCS. All rights reserved. Used with permission.)

The sleep–wake cycle is divided into two shorter cycles, each about 12 hours long. The longest period of sleepiness occurs when we normally go to bed in the evening and is deepest between 3:00 and 6:00 AM. This is also when body temperature is at its lowest. A second period of sleepiness usually occurs between 2:00 and 4:00 PM. Of note, if a person is exposed to bright light in the hours prior to the occurrence of minimum temperature, the internal clock is reset to a later time. Alternatively, exposure to bright light after the body's lowest temperature is reached will move the clock earlier.

Several hormones fluctuate over the day, including melatonin, cortisol, and growth hormone. Melatonin is produced in the pineal gland under the control of signals from the SCN. Melatonin is released into the bloodstream, beginning in the mid-evening, 1 to 2 hours before the usual bedtime and peaks between 2:00 and 4:00 AM. The melatonin level begins to fall in the early morning because daylight inhibits the pineal gland's activity. As the level of melatonin rises, the need for sleep increases. Melatonin is thought to mediate dark signals and to stabilize and reinforce circadian rhythms. While melatonin has a hypnotic effect, it is more involved in the circadian rhythm of sleep–wake regulation.

The hormone *cortisol* is synthesized and released by the adrenal gland. Its levels are very low at evening bedtime but will rise while we are asleep, reaching the peak at our usual wake time. Cortisol levels are minimally affected by whether we sleep during that time. Additionally, at the beginning of sleep and especially during SWS, the anterior pituitary releases a surge of *growth hormone*. The release of growth hormone will not occur if the person is not asleep. Other hormones that are released when the person is asleep or resting are prolactin, thyroid-stimulating hormone, and ghrelin and leptin, which are appetite-regulating hormones.

From a neurologic perspective, animal studies suggest that the medullary reticular formation, the thalamus, and the basal forebrain are involved in generating sleep, whereas the brain stem reticular formation, the midbrain, brain stem, thalamus, and the subthalamus are involved in generating wakefulness. Wakefulness is essential to survival and involves maintaining activation of the cortex. A complex network of neurons involving about 10 structures arising from the brain stem and progressing to the basal telencephalon supports the wake-promoting structures. Acetylcholine plays a key role in the executive networks. Alzheimer's disease is associated with a loss of cholinergic neurons and sleep disturbances.

The neurons associated with wakefulness and the phases of sleep are like switches: as neurons for one phase become active, another set ceases activity. When the wakefulness circuits are inhibited, the brain can transition through alternating periods of NREM and REM sleep. Different neuronal systems drive the different phases of sleep. Additionally, different neurotransmitters involving

the neural circuits are at work. The neurochemicals involved in sleep–wakefulness neural transmission include acetylcholine, histamine, norepinephrine, serotonin, hypocretin/orexin, dopamine, and glutamate (see Table 28-2). Other molecules that are involved in the sleep–wake process include adenosine, prostaglandin, cytokine, and GABAergic cells.

Normal sleep and several sleep disorders have been found to have genetic underpinnings, but a specific "sleep gene" has not been identified. Genome-wide association studies (see Epigenetics section in Chapter 9) have found 14 different areas linked with sleep disorders such as **narcolepsy** and night terrors (Sehgal & Mignot, 2011).

Sleep Pattern Changes Across the Life Span

Adolescents

A delay in the circadian rhythm system and a slower build-up of homeostatic sleep pressure are seen during puberty. Other environmental influences such as school and homework, social and extracurricular activities, employment, and increased electronic media exposure (screen time) impact the total sleep time adolescents are getting. Healthy adolescents need 8.5 to 9.5 hours of sleep in a 24-hour day (Weiss & Corkum, 2012). Recent studies have shown that the more time adolescents spend in computer use and television viewing, the shorter the sleep duration and later the sleep times (Nuutinen, Ray, & Roos, 2013). Consequences of poor or insufficient sleep in adolescents include increased risk of anxiety, depression, suicidal ideation, school absence, and decreased cognitive function and school behaviour (Colrain & Baker, 2011). Other increased risks associated with poor sleep include obesity, alcohol, cigarette and other substance use, and motor vehicle accidents caused by driving while drowsy.

Women

Compared with men, women generally have more difficulty getting to sleep and staying asleep (Driver, 2012). Women tend to sleep 15 to 20 minutes longer than men (7 hours versus 6 hours and 42 minutes); they may awaken more easily and have more difficulty falling back to sleep. Additionally, women tend to use hypnotics more frequently than do men, especially among the elderly. Hormonal changes seen with the menstrual cycle, pregnancy, and menopause can all negatively affect sleep. Some menopausal women find that hormone replacement therapy can help sleep problems. Insomnia symptoms are a known predictor for depression, especially among women.

Children

In the developing foetus, electrical patterns that can be associated with different sleep phases are seen at about 28-week gestation (Graven & Browne, 2008). REM sleep,

Table 28-2   Neurobiology of Sleep

Neurochemical	Site of Synthesis	Wake (+) or Sleep (–)	Action
Acetylcholine (Ach)	Brain stem and anterior hypothalamus of the basal forebrain	+	Ach has high activity during wakefulness (especially the basal forebrain) and REM sleep and significantly lower activity during NREM sleep. Specific Ach-releasing neurons in the brain stem are selectively active during REM sleep to decrease muscle tone, thereby preventing motor activity during sleep. Basal forebrain Ach cells are involved in promoting wakefulness behaviours, especially attention, sensory processing, and learning.
Histamine (HA)	HA cells in the posterior hypothalamus project into wake-promoting areas in the brain stem and basal forebrain	+	Neurons from this region are most active, and HA release is highest during periods of wakefulness; less so during NREM sleep and least so during REM sleep. HA improves attention and psychomotor performance. Lesions in this area of the brain produce a coma-like sleepiness.
Norepinephrine (NE)	Locus coeruleus of the pons. NE-producing neurons extend into the cerebral cortex, hippocampus, amygdala	+	NE neurons fire regularly during wakefulness, slow down during SWS, and are inactive during REM sleep. During REM sleep, their inactivity seems to be related to loss of muscle tone. NE may be in promoting arousal in stressful situations, while excess NE may contribute to insomnia.
Serotonin (5-HT)	The raphe nuclei in the brain stem	+ (?)	There are many sources of 5-HT in the body, with at least 15 different receptors to bind to, influencing various behaviours in the body. Its impact on brain arousal is unclear, but it is thought that 5-HT cells are very active during wakefulness and decreased in SWS. 5-HT is not active during, and may even suppress, REM sleep. 5-HT may play a role in regulating muscle tone during sleep.
Hypocretin/orexin	Lateral hypothalamus between sleep-initiating GABA cells in the anterior hypothalamus and the wake-initiating histamine cells in the posterior hypothalamus	+	Wakefulness is sustained by projections of these neurons into many of the primary wake-promoting systems in the brain. Loss of these cells is associated with narcolepsy. Orexin also increases arousal in motivating situations such as seeking food.
Dopamine	Substantia nigra compacta and ventral tegmental area in the midbrain	+	Extracellular concentrations of dopamine are increased during wake periods.
Glutamate	Mesencephalic reticular formation in the midbrain	+	Imaging techniques have shown that these cells are more active during wakefulness, supporting the proposal that they are important in maintaining wakefulness. Lesions in this region may cause a coma-like state of sleepiness.
GABA	Hypothalamus	–	GABA neurons are most active during NREM sleep; less so during REM sleep and least so during wake periods. They are the most powerful sleep promoters in the brain. Bursts of GABA blocks transmission of signals into the cortex by inhibiting the histamine and cholinergic systems and serotonin and norepinephrine activity in the brain stem. Growth hormone–releasing hormone facilitates GABA.
Ghrelin and neuropeptide Y (NPY)	Hypothalamus	+	A hypothalamic NPY–orexin–ghrelin network is involved in integrating circadian, visual, and metabolic signals. The effects of ghrelin are less well understood. Sleep restriction to 4 hours a night is associated with increased plasma ghrelin levels and increased hunger.

Adapted from Peigneux, P., Urbain, C., & Schmitz, R. (2012). Sleep and the brain. In C. Morin & C. Espie (Eds.), *The Oxford handbook of sleep and sleep disorders* (pp. 11–37). New York, NY: Oxford University Press.

which takes up most of the sleep cycle at this early phase, is thought to be associated with the development of sensory systems, including touch, motion, position, smell, taste, and hearing. At full term, the REM and NREM phases comprise equal parts of sleep (50:50). The ratio of REM to NREM sleep time changes over the next year, with REM sleep making up 20% of total sleep time by 12 months of age. REM to NREM sleep time will remain at that proportion for the rest of the life span. The sleep cycle of a newborn lasts approximately 60 minutes and with age it lengthens to 90 minutes. As the child ages, the need for sleep decreases from 16 to 20 hours a day in newborns to 10 to 11 hours a day in preschool and school-aged children. It is estimated that up to 25% of children have difficulty settling, falling asleep, and staying asleep; this increases to more than 50% of children with physical and mental health needs (Weiss & Corkum, 2012).

Older Adults

Sleep gradually changes as we age. Sleep becomes lighter; there is less slow-wave sleep and more superficial sleep. Additionally, there are more awakenings, especially in the latter part of the night (Carrier, Lafortune, & Drapeau, 2012). Normal circadian changes result in earlier bedtimes, earlier morning awakenings, and more difficulty adjusting to challenges to circadian rhythm such as jet lag. Moreover, older adults are more vulnerable to sleeping medications, because of slower drug absorption and elimination. Noteworthy changes in polysomnography studies (see below) have found that the percentage of lighter sleep increases with age while the percentage of REM and SWS sleep decreases. Awakenings in the night tend to last longer and occur more frequently during the latter part of the night. The decrease in SWS is thought to reflect age-related neuronal loss in the brain. However, compared with younger adults, tests of alertness and attention in older adults who have been sleep-deprived found that the older adults did better.

Compared with matched controls, older people with sleep disorders have more problems with memory encoding and retrieval and attention span. Some describe visuoperceptual and orientation difficulties. The prevalence of some sleep disorders, such as obstructive sleep apnea, periodic leg movement, REM sleep behaviour disorder, and advanced sleep phase disorder, start to increase from about the age of 40 years. As many as 50% of older adults report difficulty initiating or maintaining sleep (Crowley, 2011).

The most common primary sleep disorders in older adults are insomnia, sleep disordered breathing, REM sleep behaviour disorder, and restless legs syndrome/periodic limb movements during sleep. Other causes include medical or psychiatric illnesses, psychosocial factors, and medications. The number of medications used by older adults correlates well with the severity of sleep problems.

Cultural and Racial Factors

Much of what is discussed in the literature about racial and cultural differences comes from American sources. Research into the impact race plays on sleep is in the early phases. Researchers have looked at several aspects of sleep, including sleep duration, sleep architecture, and specific sleep disorders among people of different races. However, for nurse researchers, areas that may be of particular interest include how sleep and sleep disorders are perceived, which sleep measurement tools are culturally and linguistically appropriate, and what sleep health promotion interventions are effective.

Consequences of Inadequate Sleep

Inadequate sleep can result in a number of cognitive and psychological deficits (Caruso & Hitchcock, 2010). These include impaired performance of tasks requiring intense or prolonged attention, as well as cognitive slowing. Inadequate sleep impairs information processing and learning, cognitive flexibility, and imagination. Further, it decreases insight and ability to assess risks. Mood may be impaired; the person may experience depression, irritability, and anxiety. Chronically disturbed sleep both increases the risk for developing a mental illness and impedes recovery from one. For example, alcohol is linked with poor sleep quality, and insomnia is associated with an increased risk for alcohol dependence. Sleep loss is linked with increased risk of motor vehicle accidents and non–motor vehicle accidents. For example, errors associated with sleep loss were linked with the *Exxon Valdez* oil tanker spill in 1989 (*Exxon Valdez* Oil Spill Trustee Council, 1990) and the Chernobyl nuclear reactor disaster in 1986 (Mitler et al., 1988).

■ EPIDEMIOLOGY: CANADIAN SLEEP HABITS

A 2005 survey of Canadians found that men sleep on average 11 minutes less than women but women experience more disturbed sleep because they wake more easily (Hurst, 2008). Women also have more trouble falling asleep. Men who work full-time sleep on average 14 minutes less each night than do women who work full-time. Those 14 minutes a night translate to approximately 85 hours less sleep per year. Those not in the labour force have about 24 minutes more sleep each night than those who work full-time. Canadians who sleep with a partner sleep about 24 minutes less each night than those who sleep alone; those with two or more children get about 25 minutes less sleep each night. Another survey of 2,000 Canadians between 18 and 99 years of age found that 19.8% were dissatisfied with their sleep and 40.2% had one insomnia symptom at least three nights a week (Morin et al., 2011). More than a third of those surveyed did not feel rested after sleeping.

OVERVIEW OF SLEEP–WAKE DISORDERS

It is important to remember that occasionally having a disturbed sleep is a normal life experience, especially during times of stress. In order for a mental disorder diagnosis to be applied, the sleep issue must cause clinically significant disturbances in a number of areas, and these disturbances must be attributed to dysfunctional processes that underlie mental functioning (American Psychiatric Association [APA], 2013). The *Diagnostic and Statistical Manual of Mental Disorders* (5th ed.) (APA, 2013) lists 10 sleep–wake disorders. In addition to sleep problems, sleep–wake disorders include problems with staying awake when required. The 10 disorders include: insomnia disorder, hypersomnolence disorder, narcolepsy, breathing-related sleep disorders, circadian rhythm sleep–wake disorders, NREM sleep arousal disorders, REM sleep behaviour disorder, restless legs syndrome, and substance/medication-induced disorder. See Table 28-3 for a description of the prevalence and features associated with these disorders.

Sleep–wake disorders accompany mental disorders such as anxiety and depression, but, as previously noted, persistent sleep disturbances are also risk factors for the development of substance use and mental disorders. Furthermore, they may represent an early expression of an episode of a mental illness. For example, a person with bipolar disorder may identify changes in sleep patterns as something that precedes an episode of mania. The nurse who is aware of this and intervenes early may prevent this person's hospitalization, in addition to many other consequences of a manic episode. Figure 28-5 demonstrates the links between impaired sleep substance use, morbidity, and impaired function (Fleming, 2013).

Other clinical disorders are seen very commonly with sleep–wake disorders; in particular, breathing-related sleep disorders, heart and lung disorders, neurodegenerative disorders (e.g., Alzheimer's disease), and musculoskeletal disorders (e.g., osteoarthritis). How a person sleeps can affect how they are able to manage their other conditions. For example, people who sleep poorly have more difficulty coping with pain (Smith, Nasir, Campbell,

Table 28-3   *DSM-5* Sleep–Wake Disorders, Significant Statistics, and Essential Features

Sleep–Wake Disorder	Significant Statistics	Essential Feature(s)
Insomnia disorder	Population studies: 6%–10% prevalence Female-to-male ratio is 1.44:1 40%–50% of those with insomnia have a comorbid mental disorder	Dissatisfaction with sleep quantity or quality Difficulty initiating (sleep latency is greater than 20–30 minutes) or maintaining sleep (awake greater than 20–30 minutes after having been asleep).
Hypersomnolence disorder	At sleep disorder clinics: 5%–10% of those with complaints of daytime sleepiness Female-to-male ratio is 1:1	Excessive sleepiness (extended nighttime or involuntary daytime sleeping) Deteriorated quality of wakefulness (difficulty awakening or inability to remain awake when necessary) Sleep inertia is a highly specific feature
Narcolepsy	0.02%–0.04% of the general population May be slightly more common in men than in women	Recurrent daytime naps Generally produces cataplexy, which is triggered by laughter or joking. Cataplexy can present atypically in children or those within rapid onset Hypocretin deficiency (as measured using cerebrospinal fluid testing) Specific polysomnography sleep study and MSLT abnormalities
Breathing-Related Sleep Disorders		
Obstructive sleep apnea or hypopnoea	1%–2% of children 2%–15% of middle-aged adults Greater than 20% of older adults Male-to-female ratio is 2.4:1, but difference declines in older age	Repeated episodes of upper airway obstruction during sleep as noted by polysomnography testing Key features are daytime sleepiness and snoring
Central sleep apnea	Prevalence increases with age; most patients are greater than 60 years old Significantly more males than females Thirty percent of those taking chronic opioids for nonmalignant pain and those receiving methadone maintenance therapy can have central sleep apnea	Several episodes of apneas and hypopnoeas during sleep, caused by variations in respiratory effort These episodes are noted by polysomnography Cheyne-Stokes breathing is a type of central sleep apnea

(Continued)

Table 28-3   *DSM-5* Sleep–Wake Disorders, Significant Statistics, and Essential Features (*Continued*)

Sleep–Wake Disorder	Significant Statistics	Essential Feature(s)
Sleep-related hypoventilation	Seen in sleep-related hypoventilation, where the person has a condition such as chronic obstructive pulmonary disease Other causes are much less common	Decreased respiration associated with increased carbon dioxide levels during sleep as noted by polysomnography
Circadian Rhythm Sleep–Wake Disorders		
Delayed sleep phase type	0.17% in the general population but more than 7% in adolescents	A delay by usually more than 2 hours for the typical desired major sleeping–waking period Symptoms of insomnia and excessive sleepiness
Advanced sleep phase type	Thought to be inherited Approximately 1% in middle-aged adults	Sleep–wake times are significantly earlier (usually greater than 2 hours) than typically desired
Irregular sleep–wake type	Unknown	Insomnia at night and excessive sleepiness in the day, with no main sleep period The sleep–wake circadian rhythm is not evident
Shift work type	Estimated at 5%–10% of night workers Increasing frequency with aging	Work is outside the normal 8:00 AM to 6:00 PM period Excessive sleepiness at work and impaired sleep at home
Parasomnias		
Nonrapid eye movement sleep arousal disorder	Single episodes are common in the general population Ten percent to thirty percent of children have had at least one episode of sleepwalking Prevalence of sleepwalking disorder is 1%–5% Prevalence of sleep terror episodes among 18-month-olds is approximately 37%; decreases with age	Repeated episodes of incomplete awakenings, usually in the first third of main sleep period Person usually does not remember the event Varying degrees of wakefulness and NREM sleep possible Eyes usually open during the event
Nightmare disorder	Nightmares often begin in the preschool years, peaking in late adolescence and early adulthood	Recurring nightmares that cause distress or impairment in important areas of functioning Occur almost always during REM sleep, more often later in the main sleep period
Rapid eye movement sleep behaviour disorder	0.38%–0.5% of the general population	Recurring arousals during sleep, often accompanied by verbalizations and/or movements in response to dreams occurring during REM sleep Can be dangerous for the person or others Upon awakening the person is often able to remember the dream Eyes usually closed during the event
Restless legs syndrome	Prevalence of 2%–7.2% Female-to-male ratio 1.5:2 Increases with age	Uncomfortable feelings in the arms or legs (e.g., creeping, crawling, tingling, burning, itching) usually accompanied by wanting to move the arms or legs Worse in the evening or night
Substance/ medication-induced sleep disorder	Not available	Sleep disturbance associated with effects of a substance Four types reported (depending on substance): insomnia type, daytime sleepiness, parasomnia type, mixed type

Source: American Psychiatric Association. (2013). *Diagnostic and statistical manual of mental disorders* (5th ed.). Washington, DC: Author.

& Okonkwo, 2011). For this reason, it is essential to rule out and address contributors to sleep disturbances before assuming the issue can be addressed by a treatment for sleep complaints alone. Nurses can play an important role in identifying factors that affect sleep behaviours.

Assessment based on a bio/psycho/social/spiritual framework will provide a systematic approach.

As with most mental disorder diagnoses, many of the sleep–wake disorders are further categorized in the *DSM-5* by how long the symptoms have been

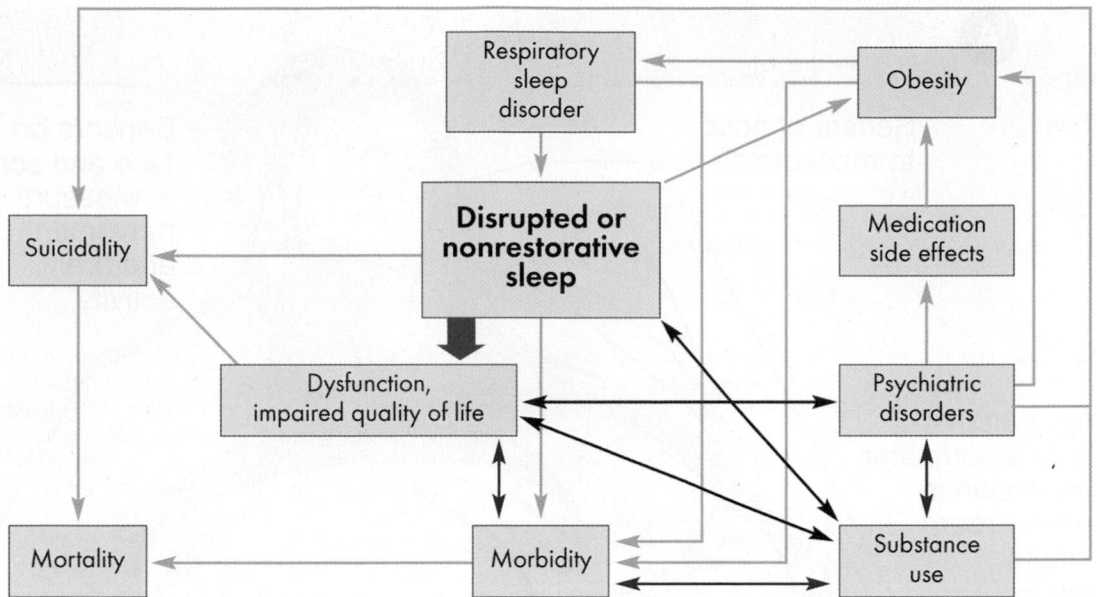

The primary effect of acute insomnia is daytime dysfunction, but when it is chronic, it is associated with psychiatric disorders that have a bidirectional relationship (coloured arrows) with sleep disturbance, substance use, dysfunction, and morbidity. Sleep deprivation, psychiatric disorders, and medication side effects can cause obesity that may cause or worsen a respiratory sleep disorder and directly or indirectly affect morbidity.

FIGURE 28-5. Interrelationship between disturbed sleep and dysfunction. (Source: Fleming, J. (2013). Psychiatric disorders and insomnia: Managing the vicious cycle. *Insomnia Rounds*, *2*(1). Copyright © 2013 by the Canadian Sleep Society. Used with permission.)

present, the degree of severity, and whether another disorder or factor is playing a prominent role. In some cases, the diagnosis of a sleep disorder is based on the symptoms the person has (e.g., insomnia), and specific testing may or may not be a component of diagnosis. Additionally, the *DSM-5* has "Other Specified" and "Unspecified" categories that allow for diagnoses of conditions that have symptoms characteristic of a particular sleep–wake disorder but do not meet full criteria for the condition.

Sleep–Wake Assessments

Polysomnography is a sleep study that measures several variables associated with sleep (see Fig. 28-6). A sleep study can include an electroencephalogram (EEG), electrooculogram (EOG), electromyogram (EMG), and a video recording of the person sleeping. Other measures include oxygen saturation, electrocardiography, air flow, and respiratory effort. Based on the level of assessment required, different techniques are used. There are four levels of testing. A level 4 study involves recording one or two variables, including oxyhaemoglobin saturation. The patient can do this at home with a small piece of equipment. A level 1 study includes many of the above measurements in a sleep lab, attended by a technician. A level 2 study records seven

or more measures in a home sleep study. Level 3 sleep studies are frequently completed in primary care settings. A level 3 study records four to seven variables, including airflow and effort, pulse or ECG, and oxyhaemoglobin saturation. Several factors can impact the results of these tests, including fever, drugs, electrolyte imbalance, and hypoxaemia.

EEGs measure electrical activity in the brain and record brainwave patterns. Electrodes are stuck to the scalp using a paste, and pick up and record electrical signals produced by postsynaptic potentials in brain neurons. In some settings, a cap with electrodes is worn instead. The signals are amplified, digitalized, and filtered; the artefact is removed, and then the result is examined for rhythms and transient events. The EEG plays a vital role in capturing the state of vigilance in the brain.

EEG patterns show waveforms that are specific to brain activity (Dubuc, n.d.). For example, delta waves are seen in deep sleep and coma. Theta waves are seen when limbic system activity is noted; this would suggest that the emotions and memory are involved. Alpha waves occur when the person is alert but the eyes are closed and he or she is not actively processing information. Beta waves are seen when the person is alert and actively processing information; gamma waves may be related to communication between various parts of the brain when concepts are being formed. In NREM sleep, other waveforms called

FIGURE 28-6. Standard setup for a polysomnogram: (**A**) the patient lies in a bed with sensors attached to the body; (**B**) the polysomnogram recording shows blood oxygen level, breathing event, and REM sleep stage over time. (Source: National Heart, Lung, and Blood Institute, U.S. Department of Health & Human Services. (2012). What to expect during a sleep study. www.nhlbi.nih.gov/. Used with permission.)

sleep spindles, K-complexes, and high voltage waves are seen. Paradoxically, the EEG waves of REM sleep are similar to those seen in someone who is awake.

Patients who are scheduled for an EEG should wash their hair with shampoo the night before the test but refrain from using other hair products like conditioners and gels. They should not eat or drink anything containing caffeine for 8 hours prior to the test. Depending on the test's requirements, patients may or may not take their medications before the test. They may be asked to do certain things during the test, like look at a flashing light or breathe in and out deeply and quickly.

Eye movement in any direction generates electrical volt changes, and these changes are recorded with **electrooculogram** (EOG) testing. In essence, the moving eyeball acts like a small battery, and an electrode placed beside each eye records horizontal eye movements while an electrode placed above and below one of the eyes records vertical movements. Recorded eye movements will show when the person is in REM sleep.

An **electromyogram** (EMG) records electrical activity generated with muscle activity. Electrodes are usually placed under the chin, where muscle tone changes associated with **sleep phases** are most apparent. The electrodes can also be placed on the limbs, most commonly the lower legs. As sleep approaches, muscles relax, and this change in activity is recorded. However, this test cannot show when sleep begins because, if the person is completely relaxed, there is no difference in the recording between sleep and being relaxed.

Respiratory and Cardiac Assessment

The person's efforts to breathe, and whether air is getting into the body, are assessed by different methods. Sensors pick up electrical or pressure changes, and measure and record abdominal and/or chest movements. A sensor is placed in front of the person's nose and mouth to pick up changes in air temperature and pressure. Some sensors also pick up vibrations that occur with snoring. Measuring pulse oximetry using a sensor that fits over a finger or an earlobe provides information about respiratory functioning. Fingernail polish and acrylic nails can cause problems for recording for pulse oximetry. Sometimes carbon dioxide levels in the exhaled air are also measured (Dondelinger, 2009). Chest electrodes may be used to monitor the person's heart rate and cardiac rhythm.

Other Physiologic Measures

Orexin is a neural peptide that stimulates waking and inhibits sleep-promoting neurons. A deficiency in cerebrospinal fluid levels is seen in narcolepsy. Melatonin level and minimum core-body temperature measures are more likely to be used in research than in clinical practice.

Other Tests

Multiple Sleep Latency Test

The multiple sleep latency test (MSLT) measures the types (REM or NREM) and phases of sleep a person has during the day. It is used to diagnose sleep disorders such as narcolepsy and idiopathic insomnia. In this test, the person is provided an opportunity to fall asleep in a dark, quiet room, four or five times over the course of a day. Brain activity and eye movements are recorded. In adults, average *sleep latency* (i.e., length of time it takes to fall asleep) is calculated. An average latency of less than 5 minutes indicates pathologic daytime sleepiness. An average latency of more than 10 minutes is normal. An MSLT demonstrating average sleep latency of less than or equal to 8 minutes is one element in the diagnosis of narcolepsy.

Maintenance of Wakefulness Test

The maintenance of wakefulness test (MWT) is another daytime test that measures the person's ability to stay awake in a quiet setting for a period of time. It can be used to test for narcolepsy, response to medications, or the ability to stay awake for work or safety issues. In this test, the person sits quietly on a chair and is asked to stay awake for 40 minutes. These sessions are scheduled every 2 hours throughout the day.

Actigraphy

Actigraphy measures sleep–wake behaviour over several days and nights. The actigraph is a motion detector commonly worn on the wrist. It provides an indirect measure of several sleep–wake variables. The device is usually worn for about 1 week. This measurement tool can be helpful for populations that would be more difficult to assess using polysomnography, such as children and those with agitation or dementia. However, in some cases, it can overestimate sleep time, especially if the person is awake but not moving much.

Sleep Diary

A person can use a sleep diary to record information related to sleep over time. Several details are collected including waking time and time in bed, sleep latency, waking during sleep time, naps, lights-out time, medications, and caffeine intake. A sleep diary is a helpful tool in the assessment of sleep–wake patterns.

Sleep Questionnaires

There are several questionnaires available for assessing sleep–wake disturbances for children and adults, including the Epworth Sleepiness Scale, Pediatric Sleep Questionnaire (PSQ), Children's Sleep Habits

Questionnaire (CSHQ), Pittsburgh Sleep Quality Index, and Dysfunctional Beliefs and Attitudes about Sleep Scale (DBAS).

COMORBID MENTAL ILLNESSES AND MENTAL HEALTH PROBLEMS

Insomnia can be a symptom of mental disorders, but when it is severe enough that it requires focused attention, it is classified as a comorbid illness. Sleep disturbances are commonly seen in the presentation of many psychiatric illnesses (Fleming, 2013). One of the criteria of posttraumatic stress disorder is sleep disturbance, with 65% of people with this diagnosis experiencing significant problems such as insomnia and dreams and/or nightmares about the trauma. Those with generalized anxiety disorder (GAD) frequently experience difficulty falling

or staying asleep, as well as a restless, unsatisfying sleep. In depression, the length of time to REM sleep is often shortened, but it remains normal in those diagnosed with GAD alone. Up to 70% of those with panic disorder can be awakened from sleep with a panic attack. Individuals with schizophrenia experience decreased latency to REM sleep onset, more wake time in the night, less total sleep time, less SWS sleep, and it takes longer to fall asleep. Disturbances noted in mood disorders include disruptions in sleep continuity, deficits in SWS, and REM sleep changes (Fleming, 2013). Approximately 80% of those with depression have insufficient sleep, while the other 20% sleep too much (Saleh, Ahmadi, & Shapiro, 2010). Many of the medications commonly used to treat psychiatric illnesses also affect sleep. See Table 28-4 for a list of medications used to treat other mental disorders and their impact on sleep.

Table 28-4   Effects of Commonly Used Psychiatric Drugs on Sleep and Waking

Drug Type	Examples	Pharmacologic Effect	Clinical Effects
Selective serotonin reuptake inhibitors (SSRIs)	Fluoxetine Fluvoxamine Citalopram	Increases extracellular levels of 5-HT, which inhibit REM sleep–producing cells	Decreased REM sleep Several SSRIs decrease sleep continuity; increase dreaming, nightmares, and sexual dreams
Norepinephrine–dopamine reuptake inhibitors (NDRIs)	Bupropion	Inhibits reuptake of NE and DA into presynaptic neurons	Decreased REM latency and increased REM sleep; decreased slow-wave sleep
Serotonin–norepinephrine reuptake inhibitors (SNRIs)	Venlafaxine Duloxetine	Inhibits 5-HT and NE	Decreased sleep continuity and the percentage of REM sleep, vivid nightmares
Tricyclic antidepressants (TCAs)	Amitriptyline Nortriptyline Clomipramine Desipramine	Increases extracellular levels of 5-HT and NE, thereby inhibiting REM sleep–producing cells	Decreased REM sleep Some TCAs will increase slow-wave sleep
Traditional amphetamine-like stimulants	Amphetamine Dextroamphetamine Methylphenidate	Increases extracellular levels of DA and NE	Increased wakefulness
Wake-promoting, nontraditional stimulants	Modafinil Armodafinil	Increases extracellular levels of DA	Increased wakefulness
Benzodiazepines	Diazepam Clonazepam Lorazepam Triazolam	Enhance GABA signalling via GABA$_A$ receptors	Shortened sleep latency, decreased nocturnal wake times, increased total sleep; decreased REM possible
Nonbenzodiazepine sedative–hypnotics	Zolpidem Zopiclone	Enhance GABA signalling via GABA$_A$ receptors, inhibiting the arousal systems	Increased sleep
Classic antihistamines	Diphenhydramine Triprolidine	Block HA H$_1$ receptors, reducing HA signalling	Increased NREM and REM sleep
Typical antipsychotics	Haloperidol Chlorpromazine	Block DA receptors, reducing DA signalling	Data inconclusive and inconsistent
Atypical antipsychotics	Clozapine Olanzapine Quetiapine Risperidone	See Chapter 12 for description of receptor-binding profile	Shortening of sleep onset latency (SOL), increases in sleep efficiency and total sleep time Olanzapine enhances slow-wave sleep and REM sleep

| Table 28-4 | | Effects of Commonly Used Psychiatric Drugs on Sleep and Waking *(Continued)* | |

Drug Type	Examples	Pharmacologic Effect	Clinical Effects
Mood stabilizers	Lithium	Exact mechanism unknown but may strengthen GABA inhibitory and reinforce serotonergic neurotransmission	Slowed circadian rhythms, increased slow-wave sleep and wake time after sleep onset, decreased REM sleep, increased sleep continuity
	Carbamazepine	Reinforces GABA and blocks excitatory glutamatergic neurotransmission	Increased sleep efficiency, decreased SOL, decreased wake time after sleep onset, increased slow-wave sleep
	Valproic acid	Similar to carbamazepine	Increased total sleep time and slow-wave sleep
	Lamotrigine	Similar to carbamazepine	Less well studied
Other mechanisms of action	Clonidine	Via α2-agonists, norepinephrine inactivates neurons in the locus coeruleus	Increased NREM sleep
	Mirtazapine		Increased sleep continuity
	Trazodone		Increased slow-wave sleep and sleep continuity, suppressed REM sleep

Sources: España, R. & Scammell, T. (2011). Sleep neurobiology from a clinical perspective. *Sleep, 34*, 845–58; Mayers, A. & Baldwin, D. (2005). Antidepressants and their effect on sleep. *Human Psychopharmacology, 20*, 533–559; Riemann, D. & Nissen, C. (2012). Sleep and psychotropic drugs. In C. Morin & C. Espie (Eds.), *The Oxford handbook of sleep and sleep disorders* (pp. 190–220). New York, NY: Oxford University Press.

INSOMNIA

The fundamental characteristics of insomnia are being dissatisfied with sleep quantity or quality and having difficulty initiating and/or maintaining sleep. The *DSM-5* identifies several specific features of insomnia in addition to time and severity descriptors. Insomnia is more common among women and middle-aged and older people (Morin et al., 2011). Approximately 40% of people with insomnia also have a mental illness. Insomnia carries significant psychosocial, occupational, economic, and safety risks (Morin, 2012), and it has a profound impact on the economy: in Québec, for instance, the annual cost to the province has been estimated at $6.5 billion (Daley, Morin, LeBlanc, Grégoire, & Savard, 2009). Numerous studies have demonstrated that nondepressed individuals with insomnia have double the risk of developing depression compared with those without insomnia. Nurses can play an important role in assessing and supporting treatment. Additionally, they can play critical roles as educators and participate in research and policy development.

Several factors and conditions are known to be linked with insomnia. Medical conditions include psychiatric disorders, other sleep disorders, chronic pain, cardiovascular, respiratory, neurologic, and urinary problems, to name a few. Frequently prescribed medications such as corticosteroids (e.g., prednisone), calcium channel blockers and beta-blockers (which are common antihypertensive medications), and decongestants are associated with insomnia. Examples of psychosocial stressors that are associated with insomnia include grief, job pressures, and the birth of a child.

Some behaviours perpetuate insomnia, such as drinking alcohol before bed, using the bed for tasks other than sleep and intimacy (e.g., eating, watching television), and having dysfunctional beliefs, such as focusing on potential catastrophic outcomes of insomnia (being fired, having an accident). **Sleep hygiene** is a term used to describe behaviours that promote healthy sleep habits. Box 28-1 reviews elements of sleep hygiene that nurses can include in educational programs.

> **KEY CONCEPT** **Insomnia** is "a subjective complaint of difficulty falling or staying asleep or poor sleep quality" (APA, 2013, p. 823).

Nursing Management: Insomnia Nursing

Nursing diagnoses specific to sleep–wake disorders include insomnia and disturbed sleep pattern. When making a nursing diagnosis, several questions will help develop an understanding of what "normal" is for the patient and identify aspects of his or her sleep problem. The BEARS framework is a mnemonic that is helpful in guiding questions involved in assessing sleep (see Table 28-5). The person's medical and psychiatric history and collateral information from bed partners and family members need to be included in a comprehensive sleep assessment. See Figure 28-7 for the bio/psycho/social/spiritual outcomes of sleep loss.

Hospital inpatient units are often guided by rigid routines that are directed by care providers' schedules.

BOX 28-1 Sleep Hygiene

Identify and break habits that disturb sleep:
- Have a set bedtime and waking time. The brain will adapt to a fixed sleeping and waking time.
- Avoid daytime napping. Sleeping during the day will disrupt nighttime sleep. If a nap is necessary, limit it to 30 to 45 minutes.
- Avoid alcohol 4 to 6 hours prior to bedtime. While alcohol will induce sleep in the immediate term, sleep will be disrupted as the blood alcohol level decreases.
- Develop a bedtime routine. This may include a warm bath or shower, or consuming warm milk, which contains tryptophan, a protein thought to promote relaxation.
- Set aside time to relax prior to bedtime. This can consist of a formal activity, such as breathing or deep relaxation exercises, or more informal activities, such as listening to calming music or reading.
- Relaxation techniques can be helpful (see Box 28-3 for an example).
- Maintain a healthy diet. Eat moderately and at regular times throughout the day rather than eating a large meal in the evening. A light carbohydrate snack at bedtime might be helpful. Avoid greasy foods.
- Caffeine consumed later in the day or in the evening may disturb sleep.
- For those who wake hungry in the early morning, adding a snack at bedtime may promote a later sleep. Avoid sugary snacks and greasy foods at bedtime; consume food containing tryptophan or high in protein, which will take some time to digest and therefore maintain a more constant blood sugar level.
- Exercise regularly but avoid vigorous exercise at bedtime; exercise late in the evening can be stimulating rather than relaxing.
- Go to bed and get up the same time every day, regardless of how much sleep is obtained. This will help set the biologic clock.
- Keep the bed only for sleep and intimacy time. Maintaining that space as an exclusive place strengthens the association between lying on the bed and sleeping. Using the bed for other daily activities, such as eating or surfing the Internet, weakens the association between the bed and sleep.
- Keep a notepad and pen at the bedside to write down worries, thoughts, and plans that come to mind once in bed.
- Do not "try" to fall asleep or watch the clock if unable to sleep. This may make the problem worse. If unable to go to sleep, get up, leave the room, and do something boring.
- Ensure that the bedroom is comfortable (e.g., temperature, level of darkness, noise).
- Limit exposure to electronics before bedtime, and consider eliminating electronics from the bedroom.

Someone who normally eats a snack, takes a shower, and then reads quietly in bed until he or she is tired enough to fall asleep will struggle settling to sleep when the routine is disrupted by being on a noisy, active unit with lights being turned on and off, doors opening and closing, alarms and phones ringing. Quieter, personalized settings are more conducive to promoting healthy sleep patterns. See Box 28-2 for nursing management strategies for hospitalized and institutionalized individuals.

IN A LIFE

Charles Dickens (1812–1870)

Public Persona

Charles Dickens experienced significant episodes of insomnia during his lifetime (Horne, 2008). When he couldn't sleep, he walked the streets of London, drawing inspiration from what he encountered for many of his 15 major novels. He would return home to sleep exactly in the middle of his northward-pointed bed with his arms out and his hands equidistant from the bed's edges.

Realities

The term "insomniac" did not appear until 38 years after Dickens' time (Horne, 2008). In Victorian Britain, the usual remedies for sleeplessness were either alcohol (whiskey or brandy for the more affluent, and gin for the poor) or opium. Laudanum, a solution of alcohol and morphine, was the most common form of opium consumed. It could be purchased easily and was so popular that Britain went to war with China to secure the free trade of opium. Another Victorian treatment for insomnia included embedding pillows with pieces of iron ore with magnetic polarity (called lodestones).

Biologic Domain

Insomnia is thought to be the result of an imbalance in the sleep–wake-promoting systems of the brain, which causes a state of hyperarousal. The consequence is an increase in body and brain metabolism, manifested by an increased heart rate and temperature and elevated cortisol, norepinephrine, and epinephrine levels. Factors that predispose an individual to chronic insomnia include genetic factors and biologic traits such as hyperactivity, hypervigilance, increased metabolic rate, and chronically elevated cortisol or reduced melatonin levels. Not only are sleep disorders linked to an increased risk of developing other physical illnesses, but physical illnesses such as congestive heart failure, neurologic diseases, breathing problems, and diabetes can precipitate or worsen insomnia.

Many nonpharmacologic approaches are very helpful in the treatment of insomnia. These include acupuncture, exercise (including Tai Chi and yoga), massage, heat (sauna and hot tub), cooling (in hot environments), music and art therapy, and body and skin manipulations. Transcranial magnetic stimulation (TMS), which involves application of an electromagnetic field to the brain, thereby impacting nerve function, has been used to treat depression. The use of this treatment for insomnia is being investigated.

Pharmacologic Approaches to Insomnia

Historical Perspective

Over the ages, mankind has used many different substances to improve sleep (Riemann & Nissen, 2012). Alcohol and opium products have long been used by some people to promote sleep. However, these substances are known to have highs risks of abuse, dependence, and overdose. Bromides were used in the early 20th century,

Table 28-5	BEARS Sleep Screening Questionnaire

Bedtime problems	Do you have any problems going to bed or falling asleep?
Excessive daytime sleepiness	Do you feel sleepy during the day? at work or school? driving? Do you take naps during the day? when and for how long?
Awakenings during the night	Do you wake up during the night? What wakes you up? Do you have trouble getting back to sleep?
Regularity and duration of sleep	What time do you usually go to bed during the week? on weekends? How much sleep do you typically get?
Snoring and sleep-related breathing problems	Have you ever been told that you snore or seem to stop breathing in your sleep?

Adapted from *BEARS sleep screening questionnaire: Examples of developmentally appropriate trigger questions.* See Weiss, S. & Corkum, P. (2012). Pediatric behavioural insomnia—"Good night, sleep tight" for child and parent. *Insomnia Rounds, 1*(5). Retrieved from http://www.insomniarounds.ca/crus/150-005%20English.pdf.

but these medications carried the risk of poisoning, nausea, rash, ataxia, and psychotic symptoms. Barbiturates began to be used in 1903 and were initially thought to be harmless, but they too were found to have a high risk of abuse, dependence, and overdose. Thalidomide was used mainly in Germany as an over-the-counter (OTC) product for sleep, but it was found to be highly teratogenic, and many babies were born with malformed limbs. In the 1960s, benzodiazepines were introduced. Initially, they were thought to be effective and without risk of abuse, but mounting evidence suggests that there is a risk of developing tolerance, rebound insomnia, and falls during the night. When Zopiclone was introduced to Canada, it was claimed to carry less risk of falls, tolerance, and abuse. However, it has been found to have some risk of abuse and dependence. Recently, Zolpidem has been approved for use in Canada. Future medical treatments may include products aimed at orexin receptors.

Present-Day Pharmacotherapy

Herbal drugs sold over the counter (OTC) for sleep include humulus, passiflora, melissa, extractum cava, and valerian. Research on these products has not been comprehensive. Valerenic acid, thought to be the active

FIGURE 28-7. Bio/psycho/social/spiritual outcomes of sleep loss.

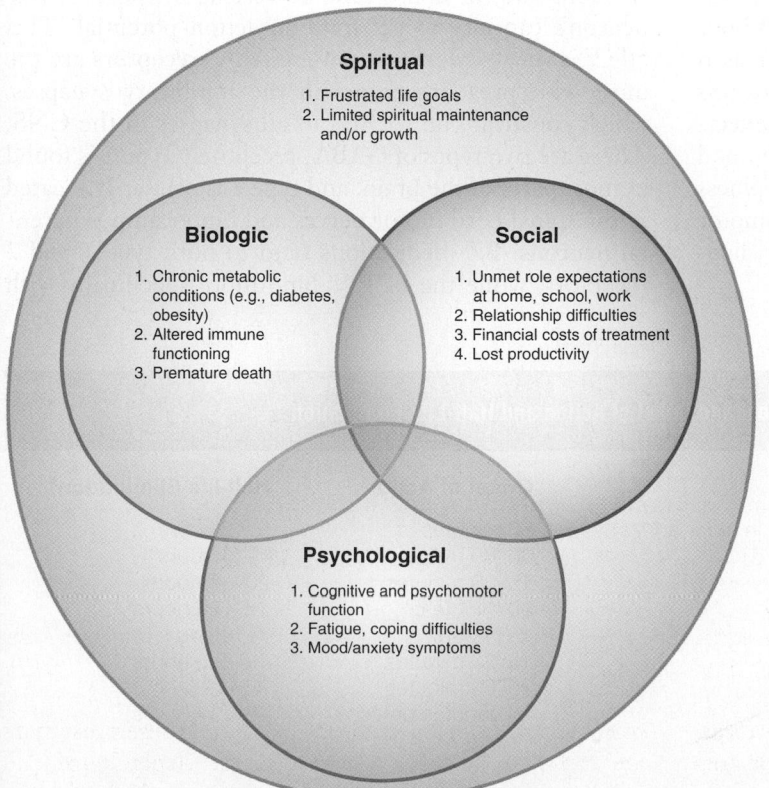

Spiritual
1. Frustrated life goals
2. Limited spiritual maintenance and/or growth

Biologic
1. Chronic metabolic conditions (e.g., diabetes, obesity)
2. Altered immune functioning
3. Premature death

Social
1. Unmet role expectations at home, school, work
2. Relationship difficulties
3. Financial costs of treatment
4. Lost productivity

Psychological
1. Cognitive and psychomotor function
2. Fatigue, coping difficulties
3. Mood/anxiety symptoms

BOX 28-2 Nursing Management Strategies for Hospitalized and Institutionalized Patients

- Nursing and medical staff need to work together to minimize interruptions to patients' sleep at night.
- Nursing stations are usually not soundproofed; nurses need to protect patient privacy and sleep.
- Identify the patient's normal sleep routines and facilitate maintaining them where possible.
- Examine the medications the patient is taking to see if any might be affecting sleep; assess to see if any usual home medications have not been provided since admission.
- Identify and manage barriers to sleep (e.g., pain, excessive fluid and caffeine intake) where possible.
- Examine the environment for sources of possible disturbances: reduce alarm levels on equipment where possible; offer earplugs or headphones.
- Offer light therapy, relaxation techniques, sleep education, back rubs, bedtime snacks.

Adapted from Gilsenan, I. (2012). Nursing interventions to alleviate insomnia. *Nursing Older People*, 24, 14–18.

ingredient of valerian, may be related to benzodiazepine-like activity on the GABA receptors. The use of this product is not recommended near conception, during pregnancy, or during lactation, because of possible mutagenic effects. Overall, no clear evidence supports the use of herbal products for insomnia (Riemann & Nissen, 2012).

A list of commonly used medications, their dosages, onset of action, and half-life elimination is found in Table 28-6. First-generation antihistamines such as diphenhydramine and hydroxyzine are commonly used in OTC products for insomnia. These medications have a 3- to 9-hour half-life, and CNS effects include sedation, decreased alertness, and slowed reaction times. Most drugs of this class also have some anticholinergic effects. The effects of these drugs on sleep have not been well studied and long-term use is not recommended. Besides sleepiness and grogginess, other side effects include psychomotor impairment, dizziness, tinnitus, decreased appetite, nausea and vomiting, constipation, and weight gain.

Chloral hydrate has been used in the past for insomnia but is no longer recommended. It is converted in the liver to trichloroethanol, which acts on the barbiturate binding site on $GABA_A$ receptors in the CNS. It has been found to reduce sleep latency and improve sleep continuity without significant effect on REM or SWS. A serious potential side effect is a liver lesion. Because the range between therapeutic and toxic effect is narrow, overdosing can be fatal. Difficulties with tolerance, loss of effectiveness, and severe withdrawal syndromes on discontinuation have been reported.

Melatonin has been found to help with the symptoms of jet lag and have a mild reduction on sleep latency, particularly in those with delayed sleep-phase syndrome. In the short term (less than 4 weeks), the side effect profile is low, but caution is needed for those with liver impairment. There is minimal risk of abuse or tolerance. The recommended dose for OTC melatonin is 3 to 5 mg. L-Tryptophan, an essential amino acid in the human diet, is a precursor of serotonin and is thought to be metabolized to serotonin in the brain. It has been found to decrease sleep latency without affecting SWS or REM sleep. The recommended dose is 500 to 1,000 mg, and the half-life is 1 to 2 hours.

Benzodiazepines (BZ), such as lorazepam, and benzodiazepine receptor agonists (BZRAs) like zopiclone are probably the most commonly used medications for the treatment of insomnia (Riemann & Nissen, 2012). These medications work by binding to the GABA receptor site, thereby enhancing the flow of negatively charged chloride ions into the neuron and decreasing the postsynaptic neuron's capacity to generate an action potential. This effect is very powerful because $GABA_A$ receptors are the most widespread receptors in the inhibitory synapses, which constitute up to 30% of all synapses in the CNS. There are two types of $GABA_A$ receptors: Type 1 is found in most parts of the brain, and type 2 is primarily located in the spinal cord motor nerves and hippocampus parental neurons. BZ medications bind to both type 1 and 2 receptors, while the BZRAs bind more specifically with

Table 28-6 Commonly Used Hypnotics, Dosages, and Onset of Action and Half-Life Elimination

Medication	Dosage	Onset of Action	Half-life Elimination*
Zopiclone (Imovane)	5.0–7.5 mg (lower in older adults)	30 minutes	5–12 hours
Diphenhydramine (Benadryl)	12.5–50 mg	60–80 minutes	4–18 hours
Hydroxyzine (Atarax)	50–100 mg	15–30 minutes	20–37 hours
Zolpidem (Ambien)	5–10 mg	30 minutes	1.5–4.5 hours
Trazodone (Desyrel)	25–100 mg	1–3 hours	7–10 hours
Triazolam (Halcion)	0.125–0.25 mg	15–30 minutes	1.5–5.5 hours
Temazepam (Restoril)	7.5–30 mg	30–60 minutes	9.5–12.5 hours
Flurazepam (Dalmane)	15–30 mg	15 minutes or less	40–114 hours

*Elimination can be affected by age and metabolic function.

type 1 receptors. This may explain why BZs have muscle relaxant, anxiolytic, and anticonvulsant effects and can cause nighttime falls that result from muscle relaxation. Other side effects of both the BZs and BZRAs include next-morning hangovers, next-day performance deficits, amnesia, sleepwalking, and nocturnal eating. Difficulty driving a car, attention problems, and hangover effects occur primarily with longer-acting BZs. Some researchers advise that the risks outweigh the benefits of using these hypnotics in persons over 60 years of age (Glass, Lanctôt, Herrmann, Sproule, & Busto, 2005).

The use of other psychotropic medications such as antidepressants and atypical antipsychotics as first-line treatment for insomnia has not been thoroughly studied, and most cannot be recommended for general use. The serious side effect profile for many of these medications will place patients at risk. However, other medications used to treat specific psychiatric conditions can impact sleep as a side effect, and indeed, this side effect should be considered when selecting a drug. For example, a side effect of mirtazapine, which is an antidepressant, is somnolence. This medication may be used for someone who has depression and insomnia.

Caffeine taken orally is absorbed rapidly; peak blood levels are reached after 30 to 75 minutes. The half-life of one dose of caffeine is 3 to 7 hours. With increasing amounts of caffeine intake, the duration of action is longer because the renal clearance of caffeine is delayed and paraxanthine, one of its metabolites, accumulates. Caffeine blocks adenosine receptors, which are found throughout the brain, blood vessels, kidneys, heart, and gastrointestinal tract. Adenosine is thought to promote sleep by inhibiting cholinergic neurons in the basal forebrain that normally mediate arousal. Anxiety, insomnia, and mood changes can occur with high doses of caffeine in addition to high blood pressure, cardiac arrhythmias, a racing heart, and gastrointestinal effects. Taken 1 hour before sleep time, 77 to 322 mg of caffeine delays sleep onset, reduces total sleep time, and decreases SWS. No effect on REM sleep has been observed. One small cup of Tim Hortons coffee contains 80 mg of caffeine (Tim Hortons Research and Development, 2008). Caffeine has been found to improve vigilance, attention, reaction times, and several aspects of memory.

Psychological Domain

Cognitive–behavioural models of insomnia posit that insomnia results from conditioning. Individuals with insomnia develop misperceptions and dysfunctional ideas about their sleep that affect their ability to initiate and maintain sleep. For example, a person can develop and retain an idea that they "will never sleep well," thereby perpetuating poor sleep. Some people with insomnia will complain of not sleeping at all, but polysomnography testing may show that they do sleep. This is called a "sleep-state misperception"; it is thought to be caused by high-frequency EEG activity at sleep onset that may alter the person's perceptions of sleep and wake (Jungquist, 2011).

Several psychological and behavioural approaches can be used to treat insomnia and other sleep–wake disorders. These include sleep hygiene education, stimulus control therapy, sleep restriction, cognitive–behavioural therapy, and relaxation training. Nurses have been involved in education for implementing several of these therapies.

Stimulus Control Therapy

Stimulus control therapy involves implementing several behavioural strategies that promote conditioning the brain to associate the sleep environment with sleepiness. Strategies include using the bed for sleep and intimacy only (not watching TV or eating), maintaining a regular wake-up time and bedtime, and avoiding napping.

Sleep Restriction Therapy

Some people who are awake for long periods in the night will try to deal with poor sleep by sleeping later into the morning. This may lead to more difficulty falling asleep and, subsequently, later sleep-ins. Sleep restriction helps to reset the sleep–wake cycle. It involves restricting the total time in bed at night to the average amount of time the person would sleep, as long as it is not less than 4 hours. The person is advised to maintain a consistent bedtime and waking schedule and avoid daytime naps. This will cause a partial sleep deprivation, making it easier to fall asleep the next night. Increasing daytime activity will help deal with any daytime sleepiness.

Relaxation Training

Relaxation training involves learning and practising several relaxation techniques that counteract muscle tension and cognitive arousal. Examples of these include guided imagery, progressive muscle relaxation, and mindfulness. The 5-4-3-2-1 exercise is an example of a relaxation strategy that nurses can teach (see Box 28-3).

BOX 28-3 The 5-4-3-2-1 Relaxation Technique

While lying in bed with eyes closed:
- Think of **5** things that you could see in your bedroom if your eyes were open. Then listen for **5** things that you can hear. Once you have heard **5** things, identify **5** things that you can physically feel (e.g., your head on the pillow, one leg touching the other).
- Next, think of **4** things you can see, **4** you can hear, **4** you can feel.
- Then think of **3** things…
- Then **2**…
- **1**…
- If you are still awake, begin again at **5**.

Adapted from Ericksonian.Info. (n.d.). Self hypnosis: The Betty Erickson special. Retrieved from http://www.ericksonian.info/BETTY.html

Social Domain

Social factors that predispose someone to chronic insomnia may include societal or bed partner demands that disrupt the person's sleep schedule. Low income, inadequate family support, and family and/or work stressors are all associated with insomnia. The estimated $6.5 billion attributed to the cost of insomnia in Québec are accounted for by health care visits ($191.2 million), prescription medications ($16.5 million), alcohol used as a sleep aid ($339.8 million), insomnia-related absenteeism ($970.6 million), and insomnia-related productivity losses ($5.0 billion) (Daley et al., 2009).

Spiritual Domain

For some, spiritual distress can lead to insomnia. Conversely, insomnia can affect a person's capacity to address their personal spirituality. One research study in Saskatchewan showed that Aboriginal individuals who engage in traditional spirituality sessions with healing elders as an approach to reduce domestic violence experienced a significant reduction in the incidence of violence, sleep problems, and other symptoms of distress by the end of their sessions (Puchala, Paul, Kennedy, & Mehl-Madrona, 2010). A nursing study in Thailand, which examined the effectiveness of using Buddhist doctrine-based programs to enhance spiritual well-being, coping, and sleep quality among Thai seniors, found that practising either meditation or chanting resulted in significant improvements in sleep quality (Wiriyasombat, Pothiban, Panuthai, Sucamvang, & Saengthong, 2011).

■■■ OBSTRUCTIVE SLEEP APNEA

Obstructive sleep apnea (OSA) is the most common sleep-related breathing disorder. A 2009 survey of Canadians by Statistics Canada found that approximately 3% of Canadian adults have been told by a health professional that they have sleep apnea; three-quarters of these were 45 years of age and older, and men were almost twice as likely as women to have the disorder (Public Health Agency of Canada, 2009). Nurses can play an important role in helping identify people at risk for OSA in addition to educating about and advocating for assessment and treatment. Nurses can help individuals identify factors that promote adherence to treatment and intercede.

Signs and symptoms of untreated OSA include snoring, witnessed apneas, and restless sleep. A physical assessment may reveal an overweight or obese person (although not always) and specific oronasopharyngeal characteristics such as a large tongue with or without a scalloping pattern on the lateral aspects and/or crowding in the posterior aspect of the pharynx, which may be erythematous and/or oedematous. Nurses can identify patients at risk for OSA by asking questions using the STOP and BANG mnemonics (see Table 28-7). Positive responses to at least three of the eight questions suggest the need for a sleep assessment. Polysomnography is the best tool for assessing OSA but is not always available; portable home sleep studies are also used. Nurses can play an important role in helping to identify people at risk, advocating for assessment and treatment, and educating about the disorder.

Nursing Management: Obstructive Sleep Apnea

Biologic Domain

In OSA, the person has partial and/or complete upper pharyngeal airway closure accompanied by on-going efforts to breathe, resulting in sporadic oxyhaemoglobin desaturation and broken sleep. Mixed apneas, which are apneas associated with and without respiratory efforts, are also common. Respiratory events are seen more frequently during phases 1 and 2 of NREM sleep and REM sleep as opposed to SWS. When the person has a respiratory event, he or she will arouse from sleep, thereby ending the respiratory event. A diagnosis is applied when there are more than five episodes in an hour of partial and/or complete airway obstruction, each resulting in at least 10 seconds of hypopnoea or apnea. Daytime symptoms include sleepiness and fatigue, impaired cognition and daily function, and significant morbidity and mortality.

Risk factors for developing OSA include increased body mass index (BMI), genetics, race, and age (Sawyer, Deatrick, Kuna, & Weaver, 2010). Other risk factors include smoking cigarettes, consuming alcohol, and sedative and hypnotic medication use. Links have been found between OSA and specific medical conditions such as diabetes, polycystic ovary syndrome, hypertension, coronary artery disease, heart failure, and stroke. However, it is not known if the conditions are caused by OSA or contribute to its development.

Treatments for OSA include continuous positive airway pressure therapy (CPAP), surgical treatments, oral appliances, and weight loss. CPAP is most commonly used for treating OSA. It involves delivering a positive pressure into the person's airway through a nasal or full facemask. This pressure will help maintain the patency of the airway. The use of CPAP therapy has been shown to reduce respiratory events and oxyhaemoglobin desaturation, but its impact on daytime outcomes is not consistent. Improvements have been found in subjective sleepiness (especially among those with severe OSA), blood pressure, vigilance, OSA symptoms (e.g., snoring, dry mouth, morning headaches), and productivity after instituting CPAP treatment. Improvements in quality of life and neurobehavioural function have not been found consistently. Adherence to CPAP is a significant limitation to effective treatment; rates of adherence range from 30% to 60% (Sawyer et al., 2010). Early experiences

Table 28-7	BANG and STOP Mnemonics for Assessment of Sleep Apnea

BANG	**STOP**
Body mass index greater than 35	Do you **S**nore?
Age greater than 50	Do you feel **T**ired, fatigued, or sleepy during the day?
Neck size greater than 40 cm	Has anyone **O**bserved your stopping breathing in your sleep?
Gender is male	Do you have high blood **P**ressure?

Adapted from Driver, H., Gottschalk, R., Hussain, M., Morin, C., Shapiro, C., & Van Zyl, L. (2012). Insomnia in adults and children (p. 35). Retrieved from http://www.canadiansleepsociety.ca/Map/www/pdf/brochure/Insomnia_Adult_Child.pdf

with CPAP, the individual's perceptions and beliefs about CPAP and OSA, and social and situational variables can negatively impact adherence.

Psychological Domain

Two of the main consequences of OSA are impaired cognitive performance and mood disturbance. Impaired executive function, including memory, mental flexibility, planning, organization, behavioural inhibition, and problem solving can negatively impact work, school, and everyday life. The relationship between depression and OSA is complex; it varies depending on age, gender, and other health characteristics. The risk of depression depends on the severity of the OSA; as the OSA becomes more serious, the risk of depression rises.

Social cognitive theory has been used as a framework for understanding adherence to CPAP treatment (Sawyer et al., 2010). Commitment to long-term use of CPAP has been found to be determined by the person's experience with the treatment within the 1st week of starting treatment; a positive experience correlated with commitment to using CPAP. Understanding that specific signs and symptoms are because of OSA is an important motivator for seeking assessment and treatment. Other beliefs and perceptions that affected commitment to CPAP included outcome expectations, treatment goals, self-efficacy, and treatment barriers/facilitators.

Social Domain

OSA has been associated with decreased work productivity, marital problems, and motor vehicle and work incidents. The risk of a motor vehicle incident for those with untreated OSA is twice as likely as for those without. Nurses should ask individuals being assessed for OSA about their driving habits and occupational requirements. Questions should include the number of hours and days the person drives, history of vehicle incidents and near misses caused by sleepiness, and history of single-vehicle incidents. Those suspected to have severe OSA should avoid driving or operating heavy equipment until their OSA is treated. Those who live alone and have had a recent traumatic life event have been shown to have decreased adherence to

CPAP; attending support groups and having an immediate social support person are promoting factors.

Spiritual Domain

While research that looks at the link between spirituality and OSA was not found in the literature, OSA has been found to be associated with a decreased quality of life (Sampaio, Pereira, & Winck, 2012). Understandably, it would be difficult to develop and participate in spiritual experiences if the person is dealing with impaired executive functioning, mood disturbance, sleepiness, and other related physical complaints in addition to social difficulties.

COMMON CIRCADIAN RHYTHM SLEEP–WAKE DISORDERS

Shift Workers

Approximately 15% to 20% of workers in industrialized countries are engaged in shift work, and intolerance of being awake during the night hours is not uncommon (Stokowski, 2012). For those trying to sleep during the day, typically the duration is shorter and the quality is less consolidated than nighttime sleep. Health and safety problems associated with managing shift work may include an increased risk of gastrointestinal and cardiovascular disorders, depression, some cancers, and accidents and injuries due to decreased alertness (Rosenberg & Doghramji, 2011).

Among nurses, nightshift work has been associated with more work-related injuries (Hopcia et al., 2012). A national survey of 6,312 Canadian nurses found that more than 25% had observed unsafe practice related to health professional fatigue and had considered resigning because of feelings of fatigue (Canadian Nurses Association, 2010a). The rate of needle sticks and laceration from sharp instruments among medical residents is twice as high during the night as the day (Barger, Lockley, Rajaratnam, & Landrigan, 2009). Several strategies can be used to help cope with sleepiness associated with shift work (see Box 28-4).

In 2010, the Canadian Nurses Association (CNA) released a position statement on nurse fatigue, which

---

BOX 28-4 Behavioural Strategies to Manage Effects of Shift Work

- If working 8-hour rotating shifts, rotate the shifts clockwise, from days to evenings to nights.
- Avoid switching to different shifts rapidly within a short time period.
- Follow a regular sleep schedule regardless of the shift you are working.
- Keep your bedroom as dark as possible when you are sleeping.
- When awake, spend as much time as possible in brightly lit rooms.
- Wear sunglasses to block blue light on the way home from work in the morning.
- Avoid scheduling appointments during your daytime sleep hours.
- After the last night shift, sleep 4 hours and then get up.
- Avoid eating large meals within 4 hours of going to bed.
- Avoid caffeine and nicotine before sleep.

A short nap (15 to 20 minutes) during the night shift may reduce sleepiness and increase alertness.

Adapted from Rosenberg, R. & Doghramji, P. (2011). Is shift work making your patient sick? Emerging theories and therapies for treating shift work disorder. *Postgraduate Medicine, 123*(5), 106–115.

BOX 28-5 Canadian Nurses Association Position Statement: Taking Action on Nurse Fatigue

Individual-level responsibilities for nurses managing fatigue:
1. Nurses learn to be aware of and recognize signs, symptoms, and responses to personal fatigue.
2. Nurses understand and work within the policies related to safe patient care within their organizations and within professional practice expectations.
3. Nurses take responsibility for mitigating and managing fatigue while at work, including professional approaches to decline work assignments. When deciding to work extra shifts, nurses act on their ethical obligation to maintain fitness to practise.
4. Nurses act on their ethical obligation to maintain fitness to practise when planning non–work-related activities
5. Nurses work through their professional associations and nursing unions to advocate for safe patient care through safe scheduling practices in the work environment.

Nurses support policies, procedures, and health promotion initiatives that manage fatigue in the workplace.

Source: Canadian Nurses Association. (2010). *Position statement: Taking action on nurse fatigue.* Retrieved from http://www.cna-aiic.ca/~/media/cna/page%20content/pdf%20en/2013/07/26/10/39/ps112_nurse_fatigue_2010_e.pdf. Reprinted with permission.

---

they defined as a "subjective feeling of tiredness (experienced by nurses) that is physically and mentally penetrative" (Canadian Nurses Association, 2010b, p. 1). This fatigue could not be "slept off" and so it is more than sleep deprivation, but circadian rhythm disturbances, sleepiness, and sleep habits were identified as contributing factors. The CNA has identified several systemic, organizational, and individual responsibilities to manage nurse fatigue. See Box 28-5 for the individual responsibilities of nurses.

Jet Lag

Jet lag occurs when a person travels by air across several time zones in a short period of time, and the person's internal clock is out of phase with the light–dark cycle of the destination. Symptoms of jet lag include poor sleep at night and feeling groggy during the day. Additionally, some travellers experience gastrointestinal upset and general malaise. Flying westbound is generally less challenging to adapt to than flying eastward. Because our internal clocks are a little longer than 24 hours, a person can move his or her internal clock *later* by approximately 2 hours a day but *earlier* by only 1 to 1½ hours a day. Other factors that can contribute to jet lag include sleep deprivation, the discomfort of airplane travel, and in-flight caffeine and/or alcohol intake.

Treatments of circadian rhythm disorders include melatonin, strategic avoidance or exposure to light and napping, BZRA medications (e.g., zopiclone), strategically consumed stimulants such as caffeine and modafinil, and bright light therapy. Bright light therapy is used to treat circadian rhythm disorders, including jet lag and shift work. Its effectiveness is dependent on the part of the circadian cycle during which it is used. This therapy works through the action of the light on the eyes and retina; the person does not need to look directly at the light in order to benefit. The usual "dose" of light is 5,000 lux shortly after waking in the morning, typically obtained through exposure to a 10,000-lux light box for 30 minutes every day. A benefit can be felt within days. Eye damage due to this therapy has not been found, but nausea, headache, and nervousness can occur.

SUMMARY OF KEY POINTS

■ The brain has three different naturally occurring states: wakefulness, REM sleep, and NREM sleep. Coma and anaesthesia are other physiologic brain states not discussed in this chapter.

■ Physical, psychological, social, and/or spiritual disturbances can cause sleep problems and vice versa. Any assessment of sleep complaints needs to include a review of these possible influences.

■ Sleep disorders are common comorbidities of many mental disorders. However, sleep disturbances can be risk factors as well as early or prodromal symptoms for mental disorders.

■ Nurses have an important role to play in assessing and helping people manage sleep difficulties.

■ Many nurses are also at risk for sleep-related problems because of the nature of their work. It is important that nurses understand the risks and manifestations of these problems and develop strategies to prevent and manage the issues.

CRITICAL THINKING CHALLENGES

1 What theory of "why we sleep" is captured in these poetic lines from William Shakespeare's *Henry IV, Part II*: "O sleep, O gentle sleep,/ Nature's soft nurse, how have I frighted thee,/ That thou no more wilt weigh my eyelids down/ And steep my sense in forgetfulness?"

2 Describe the link between mental health and illness and the sleep problems that you have seen in your practice.

3 A large number of nurses perform shift work. Does your work schedule involve or will it involve alternating shift work, including switching from day to night shifts? How does shift work affect sleep quality? How can nurses manage the fatigue that frequently comes with shift work?

4 Choose a patient that you have cared for who has struggled with a sleep disorder and review the links between the medications used and neurotransmitters involved, and how they may be impacting his or her sleep architecture.

5 At a family party, Myrtle, an older family member, mentions that for the last month she has been sleeping poorly. What are the things that need to be assessed when investigating the complaint of poor sleep? She tells you that her husband died recently and she is finding it difficult to rest, but she also mentions that she feels short of breath when she lies down. What would you advise her to do?

6 What role does bright light play in sleep and wakefulness? What other internal processes have a role in sleep and wakefulness?

7 What role do you see nurses playing in applying their knowledge about sleep in the health care system? For example, how can nurses working in public health, intensive care, neonatal, or psychiatry use their understanding of sleep?

8 Prolonged sleep deprivation is used as a strategy for eliciting information from individuals thought to be involved in terrorist behaviour. What are your thoughts on this? How does one balance ethical responsibilities with maintaining national security?

9 Think of some patients that you have worked with recently. What were the factors that affected their sleep and wake periods? For those living in the community, what resources are available to help manage the sleep-related effects of their illness and treatments (e.g., boredom, anxiety, motivation levels, and medication side effects)?

REFERENCES

American Psychiatric Association (APA). (2013). *Diagnostic and statistical manual of mental disorders* (5th ed.). Washington, DC: Author.

Barger, L. K., Lockley, S. W., Rajaratnam, S. W., & Landrigan, C. P. (2009). Neurobehavioral, health and safety consequences associated with shift work in safety sensitive professions. *Current Neurology and Neuroscience Reports, 9*(2), 155–164.

Canadian Nurses Association. (2010a). Nurse fatigue and patient safety: Research report. Retrieved from http://www.cna-aiic.ca/sitecore-modules/web/on-the-issues/better-care/patient-safety/nurse-fatigue-and-patient-safety?sc_lang=en

Canadian Nurses Association. (2010b). *Position statement: Taking action on nurse fatigue.* Retrieved from http://www2.cna-aiic.ca/CNA/documents/pdf/publications/PS112_Nurse_Fatigue_2010_e.pdf

Carrier, J., Lafortune, M., & Drapeau, C. (2012). Sleep in the elderly : When to reassure, when to intervene. Retrieved from http://www.insomnia-rounds.ca/crus/150-004%20English.pdf

Caruso, C. & Hitchcock, E. (2010). Strategies for nurses to prevent sleep-related injuries and errors. *Rehabilitation Nursing, 35,* 192–197.

Colrain, I. & Baker, F. (2011). Changes in sleep as a function of adolescent development. *Neuropsychology Review, 21,* 5–21.

Crowley, K. (2011). Sleep and sleep disorders in older adults. *Neuropsychology Review, 21,* 41–53.

Daley, M., Morin, C., LeBlanc, M., Grégoire, J. -P., & Savard, J. (2009). The economic burden of insomnia: Direct and indirect costs for individuals with insomnia syndrome, insomnia symptoms, and good sleepers. *Sleep, 32,* 55–64.

Dondelinger, R. (2009). Sleep studies. *Biomedical Instrumentation and Technology, 43,* 458–462.

Driver, H. (2012). Sleepless women: Insomnia from the female perspective. *Insomnia Rounds, 1*(6). Retrieved from http://www.canadiansleepsociety.ca/images/150-006_Eng.pdf

Driver, H., Gottschalk, R., Hussain, M., Morin, C., Shapiro, C., & Van Zyl, L. (2012). Insomnia in adults and children (p. 35). Retrieved from http://www.canadiansleepsociety.ca/Map/www/pdf/brochure/Insomnia_Adult_Child.pdf

Dubuc, B. (n.d.). The different types of sleep. Retrieved from McGill University, The Brain from Top to Bottom website. http://thebrain.mcgill.ca/flash/a/a_11/a_11_p/a_11_p_cyc/a_11_p_cyc.html

Ericksonian. (n.d.). Self hypnosis: The Betty Erickson special. Retrieved from http://www.ericksonian.info/BETTY.html

España, R. & Scammell, T. (2011). Sleep neurobiology from a clinical perspective. *Sleep, 34,* 845–58.

Exxon Valdez Oil Spill Trustee Council. (1990). Details about the accident. Retrieved from http://www.evostc.state.ak.us/index.cfm?FA=facts.details

Fleming, J. (2013). Psychiatric disorders and insomnia: Managing the vicious cycle. *Insomnia Rounds, 2*(1). Retrieved from http://www.canadiansleepsociety.ca/images/150-007_Eng.pdf

Gilsenan, I. (2012). Nursing interventions to alleviate insomnia. *Nursing Older People, 24,* 14–18.

Glass, J., Lanctôt, K., Herrmann, N., Sproule, B., & Busto, U. (2005). Sedative hypnotics in older people with insomnia: Meta-analysis of risks and benefits. *British Medical Journal, 19,* 1169–1173.

Graven, S. & Browne, J. (2008). Sleep and brain development: The critical role of sleep in fetal and early neonatal brain development. *Newborn and Infant Nursing Reviews, 8,* 173–79.

Harrison, Y. (2012). The functions of sleep. In C. Morin & C. Espie (Eds.), *The Oxford handbook of sleep and sleep disorders* (pp. 61–74). New York, NY: Oxford University Press.

Hopcia, K., Dennerlein, J., Hashimoto, D., Stoddard, A., Orechia, T., & Sorensen, G. (2012). A case–control study of occupational injuries for consecutive and cumulative shifts in hospital registered nurses and patient care associates. *Workplace Health and Safety, 60*(11), 437–444.

Horne, J. (2008). Insomnia—Victorian style. *The Psychologist, 21* (10), 910–911.

Hurst, M. (2008). Who gets any sleep these days? Sleep patterns of Canadians. Statistics Canada Catalogue No. 11-008-X Canadian Social Trends. Retrieved from http://www.statcan.gc.ca/pub/11-008-x/2008001/article/10553-eng.htm

Jungquist, C. (2011). Insomnia. In N. Redeker & G. McEnany (Eds.), *Sleep disorders and sleep promotion in nursing practice* (pp. 71–93). New York, NY: Springer.

Landis, C. (2011). Physiological and behavioral aspects of sleep. In N. Redeker & G. McEnany (Eds.), *Sleep disorders and sleep promotion in nursing practice* (pp. 1–18). New York, NY: Springer.

Mayers, A. & Baldwin, D. (2005). Antidepressants and their effect on sleep. *Human psychopharmacology, 20,* 533–559.

Mitler, M. M., Carskadon, M. A., Czeisler, C. A., Dement, W. C., Dinges, D. F., & Graeber, R. C. (1988). Catastrophes, sleep, and public policy: Consensus report. *Sleep, 11*(1), 100–109.

Morin, C. (2012). Insomnia: Prevalence, burden, and consequences. *Insomnia Rounds, 1*(1), Retrieved from www.insomniarounds.ca

Morin, C., LeBlanc, M., Bélanger, L., Ivers, H., Mérette, C., & Savard, J. (2011). Prevalence of insomnia and its treatment in Canada. *Canadian Journal of Psychiatry, 56,* 540–548.

Morselli, L., Guyon, A., & Spiegel, K. (2012). Sleep and metabolic function. *Pflügers Archiv: European Journal of Physiology, 463*, 139–160.

Motivala, S. (2011). Sleep and inflammation: Psychoneuroimmunology in the context of cardiovascular disease. *Annals of Behavioral Medicine, 42*, 141–152.

Nuutinen, T., Ray, C., & Roos, E. (2013). Do computer use, TV viewing, and the presence of the media in the bedroom predict school-aged children's sleep habits in a longitudinal study? *BMC Public Health, 13*, 684. doi: 10.1186/1471-2458-13-684

Palagini, L. & Rosenlicht, N. (2011). Sleep, dreaming, and mental health: A review of historical and neurobiological perspectives. *Sleep Medicine Reviews, 15*, 179–186.

Peigneux, P., Urbain, C., & Schmitz, R. (2012). Sleep and the brain. In C. Morin & C. Espie (Eds.), *The Oxford handbook of sleep and sleep disorders* (pp. 11–37). New York, NY: Oxford University Press.

Public Health Agency of Canada. (2009). What is the impact of sleep apnea on Canadians? Retrieved from http://www.phac-aspc.gc.ca/cd-mc/slee-papnea-apneesommeil/pdf/sleep-apnea.pdf

Puchala, C., Paul, S., Kennedy, C., & Mehl-Madrona, L. (2010). Using traditional spirituality to reduce domestic violence within aboriginal communities. *The Journal of Alternative and Complementary Medicine, 16*, 89–96.

Riemann, D. & Nissen, C. (2012). Sleep and psychotropic drugs. In C. Morin & C. Espie (Eds.), *The Oxford handbook of sleep and sleep disorders* (pp. 190–220). New York, NY: Oxford University Press.

Roehrs, T. (2011). Normal sleep and its variations. In M. Kryger, T. Roth, & W. Dement. (Eds.), *Principles and practice of sleep medicine* (5th ed., pp. 1–100). St. Louis, MO: Elsevier Saunders.

Ropper, A. H. & Samuels, M. A. (2009). Sleep and its abnormalities. In A. H. Ropper & M. A. Samuels (Eds.), *Adams and Victor's principles of neurology* (9th ed.). Retrieved from http://www.accessmedicine.com/content.aspx?aID=3633173.

Rosenberg, R. & Doghramji, P. (2011). Is shift work making your patient sick? Emerging theories and therapies for treating shift work disorder. *Postgraduate Medicine, 123*(5), 106–115.

Saleh, P., Ahmadi, N., & Shapiro, C. (2010). Sleep and psychiatric disease. In M. Kryger (Ed.), *Atlas of clinical sleep medicine* (pp. 254–260). Philadelphia, PA: Saunders Elsevier.

Sampaio, R., Pereira, M. G., & Winck, J. C. (2012). Psychological morbidity, illness representations, and quality of life in female and male patients with obstructive sleep apnea syndrome. *Psychology, Health and Medicine, 17*, 136–149.

Sawyer, A., Deatrick, J., Kuna, S., & Weaver, T. (2010). Differences in perceptions of the diagnosis and treatment of obstructive sleep apnea and continuous positive airway pressure therapy among adherers and nonadherers. *Qualitative Health Research, 20*(7), 873–892.

Sehgal, A. & Mignot, E. (2011). Genetics of sleep and sleep disorders. *Cell, 146*, 194–207.

Smith, M., Nasir, A., Campbell, C., & Okonkwo, R. (2011). Sleep disturbance and chronic pain: Behavioral interactions. In C. Morin & C. Espie (Eds.), *The Oxford handbook of sleep and sleep disorders* (pp. 846–863). New York, NY: Oxford University Press.

Stokowski, L. (2012). Help me make it through the night (shift). *Ohio Nurses Review, 87*, 12–16.

Tim Hortons Research and Development. (2008). Tim Hortons caffeine content. Retrieved from http://www.timhortons.com/ca/pdf/caffeine-canada-en.pdf

Weiss, S. & Corkum, P. (2012). Pediatric behavioral insomnia— "Good night, sleep tight" for child and parent. *Insomnia Rounds, 1*(5). Retrieved from http://www.insomniarounds.ca/crus/150-005%20English.pdf

Wiriyasombat, R., Pothiban, L., Panuthai, S., Sucamvang, K., & Saengthong, S. (2011). Effectiveness of Buddhist doctrine practice-based programs in enhancing spiritual well-being, coping and sleep quality of Thai elders. *Pacific Rim International Journal of Nursing Research, 15*, 203–219.

Mental Health
Across the
Lifespan

29 Mental Health Promotion With Children and Adolescents

Lorelei Faulkner-Gibson and Kimberly Wong
Adapted from the chapters "Mental Health Promotion With Children and Adolescents" by Wendy Austin and by Jean Robinson Hughes, Catherine Gray Deering, Lawrence Scahill, Nazilla Khanlou, and Freida Chavez

KEY CONCEPTS

- grief
- personal fable

LEARNING OBJECTIVES

After reading this chapter, you will be able to:

- Describe the protective factors in the mental health promotion of children and adolescents.
- Identify the risk factors for the development of psychopathology in childhood and adolescence.
- Analyze the role of the nurse in mental health promotion with children and families.

KEY TERMS

- attachment • bibliotherapy • child abuse/neglect • developmental delays • early intervention programs • formal operations
- normalization • protective factors • psychoeducational programs
- resilience • risk factors • social skills training • support groups

C hildren and adolescents respond to the stresses of life in different ways according to their developmental levels. This chapter examines the importance of childhood and adolescent mental health, identifies core prevention strategies, discusses the effects of common childhood stressors, identifies stressors that create risk for psychopathology, and provides guidelines for mental health promotion and risk reduction. By virtue of their close contact with families in health care settings and their role as educators, nurses are in a key position to identify and intervene with children and adolescents at risk for psychopathology. Knowing the difference between normal child development and psychopathology is crucial in helping parents to view their children's behaviour realistically and respond appropriately.

CHILDHOOD AND ADOLESCENT MENTAL HEALTH

The Child and Youth Advisory Committee of the Mental Health Commission of Canada has identified strategic directions for promotion, prevention, intervention and ongoing care, research, and evaluation to address the mental health needs of children and youth. The Committee's *Evergreen* framework (Kutcher & McLuckie, 2010) upholds the values of human rights; dignity, respect, and diversity; best available evidence; choice, opportunity, and responsibility; collaboration, continuity, and community; and access to information, programs, and services for all children, youth, and families. The framework is available to guide service providers, policy makers, and officials to create mental health programs and services for children, youth, and families.

The health of Canada's young people: A mental health focus (Freeman et al., 2010) reported on views of youth about health and well-being, and health behaviours of young people aged 11 to 15 years. The report indicated that there are youth mental health issues specific to age and gender and that positive adult relationships, supportive home, school, and community environments, and general health in the form of nutrition, safety, and security are all critical in the mental health of youth. In 2000, the Federal-Provincial-Territorial Council of Ministers on Social Policy Renewal outlined a national children's agenda, identifying basic needs of children as physical and emotional health, safety and security, success at learning, and social engagement and responsibility. Supportive social networks and positive childhood and adolescent experiences maximize the mental health of children and adolescents.

Children are more likely to be mentally healthy if they have normal physical and psychosocial development, an easy temperament (e.g., adaptable, low intensity, positive mood), and a secure attachment at an early age. These three areas are considered in the mental health assessment of children (see Chapter 30). **Attachment** is the emotional bond between a child and parent (or parental figure); a secure attachment helps the child test the world without fear of rejection. Parents, in particular, play a critical role in preventing adverse outcomes in their children and, if needed, can be assisted to learn ways of being optimally responsive to their children. Families transmit and interpret values to their children and teach them how to make connections with, and get along in, the larger world—particularly during the early years of life (Schor & the American Academy of Pediatrics Task Force on the Family, 2003). It is therefore important to consider the role of the family. The family environment provides a child's largest share of human contact. Families (or primary caregivers) mediate a child's contact with the broader environment. Young children need the opportunity to explore their world, to play, and to learn how to speak and listen to others. Families want to provide these opportunities for their children, but they may need support from their community and health care providers (Siddiqi, Irwin, & Hertman, 2007).

● **STUDY NOTE**

Attachment and temperament are important elements in the behaviour of children and adolescents in any health care setting. Consider how you would apply these concepts to the care of any paediatric patient.

■ **COMMON CHILDHOOD STRESSORS**

Stress is an inevitable part of life and may occur in one or a number of spheres of influence in a child's life (Siddiqi et al., 2007). Stressors in each sphere of influence can include the following:

- Child: difficult temperament, birth difficulties (e.g., genetic anomalies, prematurity, developmental delay, failure to thrive), extreme sensitivity to sensory experiences, suspected abuse/neglect, loss of a significant caregiver, withdrawal, extreme activity level, aggressive behaviour and emotional dysregulation/reactivity, substance abuse.

- Family: Primary caregivers may lack parenting knowledge, skills, and education. They may be experiencing unresolved loss/trauma, developmental delay, financial and marital stress, chronic health problems, and/or substance abuse resulting in negative attributions to the child. They may show insensitivity or responses of rejection, angry or harsh discipline, frightened behaviour, and a failure to protect the child. Ultimately, parent–child attachment may be negatively affected (Infant Mental Health Promotion, 2005, p. 2).

- Residential community: Neighbourhoods with a lower socioeconomic status may be exposed to toxic or hazardous wastes, residential overcrowding, and poor housing quality. They may also have limited access to services such as facilities for learning and recreation, child care, medical facilities, access to transportation, and opportunities for employment.

Regardless of the origin, stress often causes conflict and difficulty within family relationships. These responses to stress can disrupt parenting as well as the interactions between the parent and the child and can lead to short-term or lasting poor outcomes. The earlier these events begin and the longer that the disruption lasts, the worse the outcomes for children (Schor & the American Academy of Pediatrics Task Force on the Family, 2003).

Grief and Loss

It is important for nurses to recognize that grief and loss are universally experienced by children and therefore are the most common stresses encountered. It is of paramount importance for nurses to understand that children do not respond in the same way as adults. The most common losses experienced are death of a grandparent, parental divorce, family separation (parents who work away or are ill for periods of time), death of a pet, and loss of friends through moving or changing schools. Learning to mourn losses can lead to a renewed appreciation of the precious value of life and close relationships. Vast research shows that both children and adults who experience major losses are at risk for mental health problems, particularly if the natural grieving process is impeded. The grieving process differs somewhat between children and adults (see Table 29-1).

| Table 29-1 | Grieving in Childhood, Adolescence, and Adulthood | |

Children	Adolescents	Adults
• View death as reversible: do not understand that death is permanent until about age 7 years	• Understand that death is permanent but may flirt with death (e.g., reckless driving, unprotected sex) due to omnipotent feelings	• Understand that death is permanent: may struggle with spiritual beliefs about death
• Experiment with ideas about death by killing bugs, staging funerals, acting out death in play	• May be fascinated by death, enjoy morbid books and movies, listen to rock music about death and suicide	• May try not to think about death, depending on cultural background
• Mourn through activities (e.g., mock funerals, playing with things owned by the loved one); may not cry	• Mourn by talking about the loss, crying, and reflecting on it, sometimes becoming dramatic (e.g., overidentifying with the lost person, developing poetic or romantic ideas about death)	• Mourn through talking about the loss, crying, reviewing memories, and thinking privately about it
• May not discuss the loss openly, but express grief through regression, somatic complaints, behaviour problems, or withdrawal	• Often withdraw when mourning or seek comfort through peer groups; may feel parents do not understand their feelings	• Usually discuss loss openly, depending on the level of support available; may feel there is a "time limit" on how long it is socially acceptable to grieve
• Need repeated explanations to fully understand the loss; it may be helpful to read children's books that explain death	• Need permission to grieve openly because they may believe they should act strong or take care of the adults involved; need acceptance of their sometimes extreme reactions	• Need friends, family, and other supportive people to listen and allow them to mourn for however long it takes; need opportunities to review their feelings and memories

KEY CONCEPT Grief is the subjective experience (i.e., the thoughts, feelings, body sensations, and behaviours) that accompanies the perception of a loss. Children grieve in stages, similar to adults, but children's grief is shaped by developmental stages as well as experiences.

Children's responses to loss reflect their developmental level, as well as their previous experience. As early as age 3 years, children can have some concept of death. For example, the death of a pet goldfish provides an opportunity for the child to grasp the idea that the fish will never swim again. However, it is not until about age 7 that most children understand the permanence of death. Before this age, they may verbalize that someone has "died" but in the next sentence ask when the dead person will be "coming back." Even though the finality of death is understood by early adolescence (Brown, 2009), adolescents sometimes flirt with death by engaging in risky behaviours, such as driving dangerously, as if they believe that they are immune to death. This phenomenon is a result of the *personal fable* (Elkind, 1967) whereby adolescents view themselves in an egocentric way and as unique and invulnerable to the consequences experienced by others.

The concept of death is difficult to grasp, and adults should be sensitive to the child's struggle to understand and cope with it. Most children closely watch their parents' response to grief and loss and use fantasy to fill the gaps in their understanding. In many cases, family members take turns grieving, and some children may sense that their parents are so overwhelmed by their own emotional pain that they cannot bear the children's grief. Adults may attribute certain responses or reactions to the child that may not be accurate. It is important for the nurse to be aware of this when working with families and with differing familial and cultural norms and to be able to assess and respond to their needs accordingly.

It has been recognized that children and adolescents may experience complicated grief. *Complicated grief* is a form of bereavement-related distress that can include such symptoms as being preoccupied with thoughts of the deceased, including difficulty accepting the death, and numbness, bitterness, or a sense of futility (Dillen, Fontaine, & Verhofstadt-Denève, 2009; Melhem, Moritz, Walker, Shear, & Brent, 2007). An indication that bereaved children may need mental health services is related to such things as level of functioning (e.g., grief responses), coping, self-esteem, and aspects of their family environment (e.g., stressors, parenting) (Brown, Sandler, Tein, Liu, & Haine, 2007).

Grief in childhood is shaped by developmental stages and life experiences (Pfund, 2006). Similar to the experience of adults, children's grief is experienced in stages. Children's grief usually begins without understanding the full effects of the loss, and they experience some numbness or dulling of emotional pain. This stage progresses to a greater acceptance of the reality of the loss, which leads to more intense psychological pain. Finally, they

KEY CONCEPT **Personal fable** is an aspect of egocentric thinking in adolescence, characterized by the belief that one is unique and invulnerable to harm. This belief often leads to risk-taking behaviours such as unprotected sex, fast driving, and drug abuse.

undergo a reorganization of identity to incorporate the loved person, which may involve engaging in new activities and interests.

Loss and Preschool-Aged Children

The preschool-aged child may react more to a parent's distress about a death than to the death itself. Young children who depend totally on their parents may be frightened when they see their parents upset. Anything the parent can do to alleviate the child's anxiety, such as reassuring him or her that the parent will be okay and continuing the child's normal routine (e.g., regular bedtimes, snacks, play times), will help the child to feel secure. Because preschool-aged children have limited ability to verbalize their feelings, they may need to express them through fantasy play and activities, such as mock funerals. Books that explain death, such as *Charlotte's Web* by E. B. White, may also be helpful. Parents should take care not to use euphemisms that could fuel misconceptions of death, such as "He went to sleep" or "Jesus took him." Young children may interpret these messages literally and fear going to sleep (because they might die) or focus their natural, grief-related anger on the irrational idea that the person deliberately has not returned. The best approach is to explain honestly that the person has died and is not coming back, to elicit the child's understanding and questions about what has happened, and then to repeat this process continually as the child gradually begins to grasp the reality of the situation. The decision whether to take a small child to a funeral may be particularly complex.

Loss and School-Aged Children

School-aged children understand the permanence of death more clearly than do preschoolers, but they may be unable to express their feelings similarly to adults. Children in this age group may express their grief through somatic complaints; finding comfort in behaviours engaged in during earlier developmental stages, also known as regression; behavioural reactions; withdrawal; and even hostility towards parents. They may think that others expect them to cry and react with immediate emotional intensity to the death; when they do not react this way, they may feel guilty.

Loss and Adolescents

Adolescents who are in Piaget's stage of formal operations can better understand death as an abstract concept. **Formal operations** is the period of cognitive development characterized by the ability to use abstract reasoning to conceptualize and solve problems. Because adolescents tend to be idealistic and to think in extremes, they may even have poetic or romantic notions about death. Some teenagers may become fascinated with morbid rock music, movies, and books. Although they may be able to express their thoughts and feelings about death more clearly than younger children, they often are reluctant to do so for fear of being viewed as childish. Some adolescents assume a parental role in the family after a death, denying their own needs. School settings may be particularly helpful in providing group and individual support for grieving adolescents, particularly as a preventive intervention (Van Epps, Oppie, & Goodwin, 1997).

Families

The Canadian family is a diverse form. There are traditional families of mother and father, same-sex marriages, common-law relationships, coparenting relationships: the nurse must clarify with the child/youth and care provider who is *the family* of reference in varying circumstances. There are also a number of families where parents may not cohabitate but do care for the children together (i.e., couple has separated or divorced but with one partner sleeping in a separate bedroom or living in a basement suite, in order to provide parental consistency and/or financial support). Yet, many parents or care providers live separately for many reasons.

Separation and/or Divorce

Separation

Separation of families may occur for a variety of reasons: marital/partner discord, parental mental/physical illness, work circumstances, ill extended family, or immigration. Many Canadian couples live in a variety of complex situations in order to cope with financial, professional, and life circumstances. This can include "living apart together," that is, being in an intimate relationship with someone living in another dwelling. It is estimated that in 2011 about 1.9 million Canadians aged 20 years and over were in a "living apart together" relationship (Statistics Canada, 2011a). According to this national census, the reasons individuals gave for living apart were due to studying for school (26%) and financial circumstances (25%), primarily for those under age 30. Individuals aged 40 to 49 identified "work circumstances" (32%). Regardless of the reason, many couples are living separately yet *together*. As this becomes more common in our society, the impact on children and youth must be attended to in order for them to feel safe and secure regardless of the circumstances.

One agency that is much attuned to this phenomenon is the Canadian Armed Forces. There are many support resources available for families in which parents are deployed away from home (see Web Links on the thePoint). The developmental age of children in military families will need to be taken into consideration as regards their understanding of where and what the parent may experience or how they may be upon return from a military mission. The child may also need support if there are events publicized in the media.

Divorce

Divorce can be one of the most stressful life events for both children and parents. Predivorce disruption and conflict may contribute to the overall functioning of the child/youth, so that when the actual divorce or separation occurs, it may or may not be perceived as a negative event (Strohschein, 2012). During times of stress, the child/youth's ability to cope is determined by factors of resilience and overall family/parental coping and support.

In Canada, married couples are still the predominant family structure, with an increase of 5.5% from 2006 to 2011 (Statistics Canada, 2011b). Married couples with children account for 43% of Canadian families and common-law couples with children 9% of families. Married-couple families accounted for 67.0% of all census families in 2011, down from 70.5% in 2001. The number of common-law families increased 13.9% in 2011. Stepfamilies consisted of 12.7% of couples with children. The number of lone-parent families rose from 15.7% to 16.3%, with male lone-parent families (+16.2%) compared with female lone-parent families (+6.0%). About 8 in 10 lone-parent families were female lone-parent families.

Divorce rates in Canada are difficult to obtain; the last year such data were collected by Statistics Canada was 2008. Although many families adapt to separation and divorce without long-term negative effects for the children, research indicates that youth often show at least temporary difficulties dealing with this common stressor in our society (Pruett, Williams, Insabella, & Little, 2003). Parental separation and divorce create changes in the family structure, which can result in a substantial reduction in the contact that children have with one of their parents. The child's response to divorce can be similar to the response to death. In some ways, divorce may be harder for the child to understand because the noncustodial parent is gone but still alive, and the parents have made a conscious choice to separate. Research shows that children of divorce are at increased risk for emotional, behavioural, and academic problems. However, the analysis of data from Canada's Longitudinal Survey of Children and Youth shows that children who grow up in a married biologic-parent household do not have better short-term behavioural outcomes than those who do not

(Wu, Hou, & Schimmele, 2008). Rather, behavioural outcomes are related to such things as income, family dysfunction, and parental nurturance. The response to the loss that divorce imposes varies depending on the child's predivorce experience (Kelly, 2003); the child's temperament; the parents' interventions; and the level of stress, change, and conflict surrounding the divorce (Hetherington & Kelly, 2002). Major changes in socioeconomic status, such as moving from a dual-earner status to a single-parent family status, may account for much of the variation in levels of distress among divorcing families (Jeynes, 2002; Sun & Li, 2002).

The first 2 or 3 years after the couple's breakup tend to be the most difficult. Typical childhood reactions include confusion, guilt, depression, regression, somatic symptoms, acting-out behaviours (e.g., stealing, disobedience), fantasies that the parents will reunite, fear of losing the custodial parent, and alignment with one parent against the other. After an initial adjustment period, children usually accept the reality of the situation and begin coping adaptively. If the divorced parents remarry new partners, this often imposes another period of coping difficulties for the children. Children with stepparents and stepsiblings are at renewed risk for emotional and behavioural problems as they struggle to cope with the new relationships (Reifman, Villa, Amans, Rethinam, & Telesca, 2001).

Protective factors against emotional and behavioural problems in children of divorce include parental nurturance, parents' mental health, joint custody, and low parental conflict (Kelly, 2003). For children of divorce and remarriage, protective factors also include a structured home and school environment with reasonable and consistent limit setting and a warm, supportive relationship with stepparents (Hetherington & Kelly, 2002). Helpful interventions for children of divorce include education regarding children's reactions; promotion of regular and predictable visitation; reduction of conflict between the parents through counselling, mediation, and clear visitation policies; continuance of usual routines; and family counselling to facilitate adjustment after remarriage (Table 29-2). Some evidence shows that it is not the divorce itself but rather the continuing conflict between the parents that is most damaging to the child. Parents manage divorce better if they can remember that children naturally idealize and identify with both parents and need to view both of them positively. Therefore, it is helpful for parents to reinforce each other's good qualities and focus on evidence of their former partner's love and respect for the child.

Sibling Relationships

The family often consists of various constellations of parents, children, and others. The family is whoever they define themselves to be. Within many families,

Table 29-2	Play Therapy With a 4-Year-Old Child Whose Parents Are Divorcing	

Child Statement	Nurse Response	Analysis and Rationale
(The child smashes two cars together and makes loud, crashing sound.)	That's a loud crash. They really hit hard.	The child may be expressing anger and frustration nonverbally through play. The nurse attempts to establish rapport with the child by relating at the child's level, using age-appropriate vocabulary.
Crrrash!	I know a boy who gets so mad sometimes that he feels like smashing something.	The child is engrossed in fantasy play, typical of preschoolers. Children often use toys as symbols of human figures. The nurse uses an indirect method of eliciting the child's feelings, because preschoolers often do not express feelings directly. Reference to another child's anger helps to normalize this child's feelings.
Yeah!	Sounds like you feel angry too sometimes … the same way the other boy feels.	The child is beginning to relate to the nurse and senses her empathy. The nurse reflects the child's feelings to facilitate further communication.
Yeah, when my mom and dad fight.	It's tough to listen to parents fighting. Sometimes it's scary. You wonder what's going to happen.	The child is experiencing frustration and helplessness related to family conflict. The nurse expresses empathy and attempts to articulate the child's feelings, because preschool children have a limited ability to identify and label feelings.
My mom and dad are getting a divorce.	That's too bad. Children often feel mixed up when their parents get divorced. What's going to happen when they get the divorce?	The child has a basic awareness of the reality of the parents' divorce but may not understand this concept. The nurse expresses empathy and attempts to assess the child's level of understanding of the divorce.
Dad's not going to live in our house.	Oh, I guess you'll miss having him there all the time. It would be nice if you all could live together, but I guess that's not going to happen.	The preschool child focuses on the effects the divorce will have on him (egocentrism). The child seems to have a clear understanding of the consequences of the divorce. The nurse articulates the child's perspective and reinforces the reality of the divorce to avoid fuelling the child's possible denial and reconciliation fantasies.
(Silently moves cars across the floor.)	What do you think is the reason your parents decided to get a divorce?	The child expresses sadness nonverbally. The nurse further attempts to assess the child's understanding of the circumstances surrounding the divorce.
Because I did it.	What do you mean—you did it? How?	The child provides a clue that he may be feeling responsible. The nurse uses clarification to fully assess the child's understanding.
I made them mad because I left my bike in the driveway and dad ran over it.	Do you think that's why they're getting the divorce?	The child uses egocentric thinking to draw a conclusion that his actions caused the divorce. The nurse continues to clarify the child's thinking. The goal is to elicit the child's perceptions so that misperceptions can be corrected.
Yeah, they had a big fight.	They may have been upset about the bike, but I don't think that's why they're getting a divorce.	The nurse goes on to explain why parents get divorced and to provide opportunities for the child to ask questions.
Why?	Because parents get divorced when they're upset with *each other*— when they can't get along—not when they're upset with their children.	

siblings are an integral part of that constellation. Some parents prefer not to have the siblings present if they have brought one child in for a mental health assessment. It is important for the nurse to encourage the parents/care providers to include the siblings in the process, as they often add information of which the parents may be unaware. Nurses also need to be aware of siblings who may also be mentally unwell or experiencing distress due to an unwell sibling or parent. Wright and Leahey (2013) encourage nurses to consider the sibling "rank order—the position of children in the family in respect to age and gender" (p. 60). Depending on parental functioning (e.g., mental or physical illness), or cultural and ethnic background, sibling position may have a positive or negative effect on children's functioning. For example, older children may be put in the position of care provider if both parents work outside the home. This may create added stress with respect to their ability to manage sibling care, domestic chores, and school work (or employment in the case of an adolescent).

Until recently, the role of siblings in a child's development was underemphasized. There are a number of theoretical perspectives in viewing relational development between siblings. Whiteman, McHale, and Soli (2011) present four perspectives within sibling research literature: psychoanalytic–evolutionary, social psychological, social learning, family–ecological systems. No one theory is emphasized; however, because families function as a system and within the context of relationships, it would stand to reason that sibling relationships would be multidimensional and affected by numerous variables based on the context of their development. A growing body of research shows that sibling relationships significantly influence personality development. Positive sibling relationships can be protective factors against the development of psychopathology, particularly in troubled families in which the parents are emotionally unavailable. A Canadian longitudinal study revealed that sibling affection moderated the effects of stressful life events on "internalized symptomatology" (e.g., being anxious, depressive, overcontrolled) (Gass, Jenkis, & Dunn, 2007). Nurses working with families need to pay attention not only to the parent–child dynamic but also to the sibling dynamic with regards to whether positive or negative behaviours are being modelled. "Children learn social competencies in their interactions with parents and siblings and by observing their family members' interactions with others" (Whiteman et al., 2011, p. 9). Nurses working with families should therefore support parents to model effective problem solving and engage with their children in the same process to minimize sibling rivalry and maximize cooperative behaviour benefiting their children's social and emotional development throughout life. Sibling rivalry can begin with the birth of the second child. It is a natural experience, and some

sibling rivalry is inevitable. The birth of a sibling can be a surprise for the first child who, up until then, was the sole focus of the parents' attention. The older sibling may react with anger and reveal not-so-subtle fantasies of getting rid of the new sibling (e.g., "I dreamed that the new baby died"). Parents should pay attention to these comments and observe behaviours while also recognizing that these reactions are natural. The child should be allowed to express feelings, both positive and negative, about the baby while being reassured of his or her special place in the family. Allowing the older child opportunities to care for the baby and reinforcing any nurturing or affectionate behaviour will promote positive bonding.

Physical Illness

Many children experience a major physical illness or injury at some point during development. The experience of hospitalization and intrusive medical procedures can have a lasting and possibly acutely traumatic impact on many children. The likelihood of lasting psychological problems resulting from physical illness depends on the child's experiences during hospitalization; their developmental level and coping mechanisms; the family's level of functioning before, during, and after the illness; and the nature and severity of the illness. As with any major stressor, the perception of the event (i.e., meaning of the illness) will influence the family's ability to cope.

Common childhood reactions to physical illness include developmental regression (e.g., in toilet training, social maturity, autonomous behaviour), sleep and feeding difficulties, behavioural reactions (e.g., negativism, tantrums, withdrawal), somatic complaints that mask attempts at emotional expression (e.g., headaches, stomachaches), and depression. Infants and children younger than school age are particularly vulnerable to separation anxiety during illness and may regress to earlier levels of anxiety about strangers, becoming fearful of health care providers. Young children often have magical thinking about the illness, and their tendency to process information in concrete terms may lead to misperceptions about the illness and treatment procedures (e.g., dye = die; stretcher = stretch her) (Deering & Cody, 2002). Adolescents may be concerned about their body image and maintaining their sense of independence and control.

Nurses must remember that parents are the primary resource to the child and the experts who know the child's needs and reactions. Thus, nurses must maintain a collaborative approach in working with parents of both physically and/or mentally ill children. If the child is a sick infant, nurses should take care to allow the normal attachment process between parents and the infant to unfold, despite health care professionals' efforts to assume some parenting functions. Parents who view their children as physically and emotionally fragile will feel disempowered in decision making and boundary setting and may develop helpless or overprotective styles of dealing with their children.

Many parents react with fear and anxiety that can lead to feelings of guilt about their child's illness or injury, especially if the illness is genetically based or partially the result of their own behaviour (e.g., drug or alcohol abuse during pregnancy). Parents may project their feelings onto each other or health care professionals, lashing out in anger and blame. Nurses should view these responses as part of the grieving process and help parents to move forward confidently in caring for their children. Teaching parents how to care for their children's health needs and reinforcing their successes in doing so will help. For example, rather than reacting to what may appear to be an abdication of parenting responsibilities, nurses can instead use empathy to acknowledge the parent's feelings and discuss ways to help the parent regain a sense of control with comments such as the following:

> It's pretty confusing to know how best to respond to your child's behaviour. Before receiving her diagnosis, you felt comfortable setting reasonable limits on her behaviour, but now that seems to have changed. Sometimes parents feel guilty and are even afraid of setting limits because they know how sick their child is…. It may seem odd, but children actually feel safer and more secure when their parents let them know what the boundaries for their behaviour are…. Let's talk about some of the boundaries that you might feel most comfortable setting up for your daughter to help her feel safe and secure while she is so ill?

Chronic physical illness in childhood presents a unique set of challenges, with survival rates of previously fatal diseases at an all-time high (Martinez & Ercikan, 2009). Although studies show that most children with chronic illnesses and their families are remarkably resilient and adjust to the stressors and regimens involved in their care (LeBlanc, Goldsmith, & Patel, 2003), research shows that children with chronic health conditions are at higher risk for developing anxiety-related disorders, academic problems, and learning disabilities (Martinez & Ercikan, 2009). Children with chronic health conditions are also three to four times more likely to experience psychiatric symptoms than are their healthy peers (Lewis & Vitulano, 2003). Conditions that affect the central nervous system (CNS) (e.g., infections, metabolic diseases, CNS malformations, brain and spinal cord trauma) are particularly likely to result in psychiatric difficulties. Nurses who understand pathophysiologic processes are in a unique position to assess the interaction between biologic and psychological factors that contribute to mental health problems in chronically ill children (e.g., lethargy

from high blood sugar levels or respiratory problems; mood swings from steroid use). Inactivity and a lack of sensory stimulation from hospitalization or bed rest may contribute to neurologic deficits and **developmental delays**. The major challenge for a chronically ill child is to remain active despite the limitations of the illness and to become fully integrated into school and social activities. Children who view themselves as different or defective will experience low self-esteem and be more at risk for depression, anxiety, and behaviour problems. Studies show that parental perceptions of the child's vulnerability predict greater adjustment problems, even after controlling for age and disease severity (Anthony, Gil, & Schanberg, 2003). Educating parents about these facts and helping them to foster maximum independence within the limitations of the child's health problem is the key. For example, nurses might comment,

> Having kidney disease is certainly no fun … and it would be wonderful if wrapping your son in a cocoon would ensure that he came to no harm. Unfortunately, there is no such way of protecting him completely…. But we know that children seem to manage better with their illness when their parents believe that they have possibilities. Even with all the limitations, what are the best things your son has going for him?

Physical and Developmental Challenges in Adolescence

Adolescence is a time of growing independence and, consequently, experimentation. Emotional extremes prevail. To adolescents, the world seems great one day and terrible the next; people are either for them or against them. Adolescents are struggling to consolidate their abilities to control their impulses and react to the many "crises" that may seem trivial to adults but are very important to teens. Biologic changes (e.g., the onset of puberty, height and weight changes, hormonal changes), psychological changes (e.g., increased ability for abstract thinking), and social changes (e.g., dating, driving, increased autonomy) are all significant. The primary developmental task of identity formation leads teenagers to test different roles and struggle to define who they are. This process may include testing various peer groups to find one that fits their unfolding self-image.

Adolescence often is a time of exploring social and personal boundaries. This can involve experimentation, which can increase the risk of poor physical health, mental health problems, substance use including tobacco, high-risk behaviours including driving at excessive speeds, high-intensity sports, and exploration of sexuality that may lead to unsafe sexual behaviours and psychological distress (Canadian Population Health Initiative, 2005). According to the Sexual Information and Education

Council of Canada, the overall Canadian teen pregnancy rate decreased by 20.3% from 2001 to 2010 (McKay, 2013). However, from 2006 to 2010, the national teen pregnancy rate increased by 1.1%, and in four provinces, the rate increased by 15.1% or more (New Brunswick, Newfoundland, Nova Scotia, Manitoba). Trends in teen pregnancy reflect sexual and reproductive health and overall well-being of young women in Canada, which is important for educators, policy makers, and especially nurses to pay attention to, as nurses are often the first contact many young women have in relation to their pregnancy.

Nurses will also be in the position to provide assessments, education, and, in some circumstances, intervention in relation to sexually transmitted infections (STIs). According to the Public Health Agency of Canada (2010b), the most common infections are chlamydia (15- to 24-year-old women, slightly older for young men); gonorrhoea (same age groups); infectious syphilis (older HIV-positive men and sex trade workers); human papillomavirus, which is more common at 70% of adult population (true numbers unknown); genital herpes (HSV1 and 2) (exact numbers unknown); and HIV (exact numbers unknown).

Among youth in later adolescence, approximately one in five reports symptoms associated with a major mental disorder, and nearly 1 in 10 reports substance dependence (Centre for Addiction and Mental Health, 2012; Statistics Canada, 2004). Although most youths eventually become more conventional in their behaviour, some develop harmful behaviour patterns and addictions that endanger their mental and physical health. Adolescents whose psychiatric problems are developing are particularly vulnerable to engaging in risky behaviours because they may have limited coping skills, may attempt to self-medicate their symptoms, and may feel an increased pressure to fit in with other teens. Moreover, high-risk behaviours tend to be interrelated (Eggert, Thompson, Randell, & Pike, 2002).

Enhanced life skills and supportive school and family environments can mediate the effect of stressful life events (Burns, Andrews, & Szabo, 2002). Programs that enhance the school environment are associated with improved behaviour and well-being. Interventions that teach cognitive skills are associated with a reduction in one of the most prevalent mental health problems affecting adolescents—depression (Puskar, Sereika, & Tusaie-Mumford, 2003). Current evidence suggests that for an intervention to be sustainable, it must encompass multiple components across several levels, including the classroom, curriculum, whole school, and school–community boundaries. Several approaches to mental health promotion with adolescents are recommended. First, intervening at the peer group level through educational programs, alternative recreational activities, and peer counselling are most successful.

Adolescents are sceptical of authority figures and tend to take cues from one another. Nurses working with teenagers find it helpful to use a discussion approach that encourages questioning and argument, as opposed to talking down to or "talking at" teenagers (Deering & Cody, 2002).

Second, training in values clarification, decision making, problem solving, social skills, and assertiveness helps give adolescents the skills to cope with situations in which they are pressured by their peers (Botvin, 2000). Social psychological research shows that if just one person can find the strength to express an unpopular viewpoint in a group and decline to participate in a destructive activity, others will quickly follow. It takes enormous courage, as well as concrete knowledge and practise with assertiveness, to speak up in these situations.

A third type of intervention is a program that uses team efforts by teachers, parents, community leaders, and teen role models. These programs help at-risk youth by building self-esteem, setting positive examples, and working to involve the youth in community activities. It is important to note that teaching interpersonal skills, including cognitive and problem-solving skills, should be coupled with the promotion of positive school and family environments to prevent mental health problems in young people, notably depression (Burns et al., 2002).

It is also important to consider the use of social media and other digital forms of communication by which to reach adolescents. Program staff and youth perceive these forms of communication as credible and essential methods of communication in the context of public health programs. Public health interventions must continue to evolve and integrate new technologies in order to reach young people (Vyas, Landry, Schnider, Rojas, & Wood, 2012).

Approaches that have not proved effective include more education and information about dangerous activities without the supplemental behaviour training, as well as programs that provide inadequate training and support for the professionals implementing them.

DEVELOPMENT OF CHILD PSYCHOPATHOLOGY

The factors that affect the development of child psychopathology are also the factors that protect children. The issues presented are not independent components but are intertwined and interdependent, thus indicating that the care provided must be collaborative, holistic, and socially/culturally relevant to those involved. Creating a structure to describe the context in which child psychopathology develops is difficult, and one must remember that this is not a black and white process but that all aspects are systemically interwoven and affect the whole.

Protective Factors

Protective factors that have been identified for several decades focus on the child/youth's ability to develop self-confidence, positive relationships, competencies (skills/strengths), self-regulation, and community involvement (Blaustein & Kinniburgh, 2010; Brendtro, 2004; Canadian Council on Learning, 2008; Eriksson, Cater, Andershed, & Andershed, 2010; Foster, O'Brien, & Korhonen, 2012; Unger, 2013; Waddell, McEwan, Sheperd, Offord, & Hua, 2005; Zolkoski & Bullock, 2012). In the family, low stress, stable employment, adequate child care resources, and higher socioeconomic status can serve as protective factors. In the community, protective factors include positive and cohesive families, schools, and neighbourhoods. All of the protective factors intertwine to create a context in which the child/youth thrives. The research on resilience provides insight and direction to focus attention and care when working with children/youth and families (Eriksson et al., 2010).

Resilience

Nurses will work with a variety of children/youth and families throughout their career, but the majority will not have psychopathology. Many children/youth and families come from life circumstances that often lead to severe consequences, yet they function at or above what would be expected. These individuals have what is referred to as **resilience**. Resilience is the ability to overcome or rise above adversity, learn from the experience, and apply strategies and cope with other life events even when the situation dictates otherwise. "In the context of exposure to significant adversity, resilience is both the capacity of individuals to navigate their way to the psychological, social, cultural, and physical resources that sustain their well-being, and their capacity individually and collectively to negotiate for these resources to be provided in culturally meaningful ways" (Unger, 2013, p. 1). Therefore, resilience is not limited to the individual but can apply to a group's or society's ability to move beyond negative circumstances.

Risk Factors

Impact of Social Determinants of Health

The World Health Organization (see, for example, Currie et al., 2011) has brought attention to the broad social factors that influence the health and well-being of children. The health of young people and their families is generally determined less by lifestyle choices or application of medical knowledge than by the complex interaction of living conditions that often transcend the capacities of the individual, such as income and distribution of wealth; employment and working conditions; quality of food and housing and of health care and other social services; and equitable access to education. In short, communities and institutions, and economic and social circumstances shape much of a child's development, pose as greater **risk factors** in his or her well-being, and have health impacts with short- and long-term implications for individuals and society.

Poverty

According to the United Nations Children's Fund (UNICEF) (2012), an estimated 14% of children in Canada live in poverty, a rate higher than that of the general population (12%). The low-income rates for children vary significantly according to their type of family. For instance, in 2008, 6.5% of children in two-parent families were in a low-income environment, while almost one in four children (23.4%) in female lone-parent families faced this reality. Children in certain populations can be more at risk of low income. For example, it is known that in 2005, recent immigrant families had a low-income rate of 39.3% (Canada Parliament, 2010). Children/youth and families living in poverty are at increased risk of exposure to additional factors that will contribute to childhood psychopathology.

The effects of poverty on child development and family functioning are numerous and pervasive. The obstacles to overcoming the effects of poverty can seem insurmountable to young people. Lack of proper nutrition and lack of access to prenatal and mother–infant care can place children from impoverished families at risk for physical and mental health problems. Children from impoverished rural areas often lack access to educational and other community support resources. Children living in poverty-stricken inner-city neighbourhoods are vulnerable to violent crimes, crowded living conditions, and an increased access to drugs (Leventhal & Brooks-Gunn, 2000). Although crime, drug abuse, gang activity, and teenage pregnancy are seen in adolescents from all socioeconomic backgrounds, children living in poverty are more vulnerable to these problems because they may have limited opportunities for change (Kelly & Caputo, 2007).

A major focus of preventive nursing interventions for disadvantaged families involves simply forming a relationship that conveys respect and willingness to work as an advocate to assist clients' seeking out and accessing resources. In terms of Maslow's need hierarchy, families living in poverty may be more focused on survival needs (e.g., food, shelter) than on self-actualization needs (e.g., insight-oriented psychotherapy for themselves or their children). Unless the nurse can work as a partner with the family and address the issues most pressing for the family with an active problem-solving approach, other types of intervention may be fruitless. At the same time, it is inappropriate to assume that poor families will be resistant to or unable to benefit from psychotherapies or other mental health interventions.

Homelessness

Homelessness is a very complex phenomenon that reveals the failure of a society to ensure that systems and support are in place so that everyone has access to housing (Gaetz, Donaldson, Richter, & Gulliver, 2013). The homeless are not a homogenous population but include women, children, youth, families, new immigrants, people with mental illness, ethnic minorities, and Aboriginal people. The number of children staying in shelters in Canada increased by over 50% between 2005 (6,205) and 2009 (9,459) (Segaert, 2012). A national study found that, in 2009, an estimated 29,964 youth (ages 16 to 24 years) and 9,459 children (under the age of 16 years) stayed in emergency shelters across the country (Employment and Social Development Canada, 2012). Youth homelessness refers to youth who are homeless, at-risk of homelessness, or caught in a cycle of homelessness for whatever reason. This includes the many homeless youth (some say as high as 80%) who don't live on the street and who are among the hidden homeless, living in temporary shelter, or unsafe or crowded conditions (Hulchanski, Campsie, Chau, Hwang, & Paradis, 2009). Youth cite parental drug and alcohol use as a reason for leaving home, as it is often associated with parental abandonment, family violence (sexual, physical, and psychological abuse), and neglect. Particularly, at-risk populations for becoming homeless or street involved are youth in foster care and lesbian, gay, bisexual, and transgender youth (Edidin, Ganim, Hunter, & Karnik, 2012).

There is an increased risk for physical health problems (e.g., nutritional deficiencies, infections, chronic illnesses, injuries as a result of violence, STIs), mental health problems (particularly developmental delays in language, fine or gross motor coordination, and social development; depression, anxiety, posttraumatic stress disorder, and psychotic symptoms; disruptive behaviour disorders; substance abuse), and educational underachievement in homeless youth. Many homeless youth have been physically or sexually abused, leading to elevated rates of externalizing disorders for boys and internalizing disorders for girls (Cauce et al., 2000).

Though a heterogeneous population, typically street youth have experienced extreme stress in the course of their lives even before they run away, with most fleeing temporary living arrangements (e.g., foster homes, friends, relatives) (Kelly & Caputo, 2007). Their runaway experience thus serves only to compound an already chronic history of trauma and disruption. The key is to prevent the conditions that preceded the runaway behaviour.

Unfortunately, responses to homelessness too often result only in greater social control measures (e.g., rendering panhandling illegal, excluding the homeless from the community) rather than the development of strategies to address underlying causes. Street nurses are often one of the few resources available to marginalized populations who face a variety of barriers to accessing traditional health care services, such as mental health problems, criminal involvement, lack of transportation, lack of ability to pay for prescriptions, lack of specialized or knowledgeable providers, and provider discrimination (Self & Peters, 2005). Street services are effective because they are delivered wherever the person feels comfortable: a school, youth centre, drop-in centre, mall, or simply the street.

The living conditions of many shelters place children at risk for irregular patterns of sleep, feeding, play, and bathing, all of which are important for normal development. Nurses working with homeless youth and families need to be aware of the effects of this lifestyle on children, because they have a limited ability to speak for themselves and because their needs are often overlooked. As well, transition services for women and children who are victims of abuse are available across the country; however, depending on the community and the ability of the women to access these resources, support may be limited. Nurturing one's children while living in homeless shelters is highly challenging.

While there is no evidence that Canada's efforts to date to reduce homelessness have had an overall positive effect, there are reasons to be optimistic. Meaningful collaboration at the national, provincial, municipal, and community levels to address this major social problem is occurring (e.g., Homeless Partnering Strategy; Housing First) (see Chapter 2).

The Traumatic Effects of Child Abuse and Neglect

The experience of trauma, specifically in **childhood abuse/neglect** and violence, affects the overall growth and development of the individual and impacts health and well-being, even when the individual is resilient (Blaustein & Kinniburgh, 2010; Perry, 2004). The 2008 Canadian Incidence Study of reported child abuse and neglect indicated that less than 4% of children are investigated for maltreatment (Trocmé et al., 2010). The types of maltreatment identified during investigation were 34% neglect, 34% exposure to intimate partner violence, 20% physical abuse, 9% emotional maltreatment, and 3% sexual abuse (Trocmé et al., 2010). The majority of children were documented to have received diagnoses other than posttraumatic stress disorder or chronic paediatric stress disorder. It therefore raises questions as to whether a trauma diagnosis such as developmental or complex trauma disorder was even considered (Kinniburgh, Blaustein, & Spinazzola, 2005; van der Kolk, 2005).

In Canada, in 2011, police reported nearly 70,000 child victims of violence or a rate of 1,014 victims per 100,000 under the age of 18. This rate was 9% lower than the rate for adults. While the overall prevalence of violence against children and youth was lower than violence directed at adults, this was not consistently seen across all types of violent offences. Children and youth

Table 29-3	Types and Rates of Abuse in Canada	
Type	**Description**	**Rate**
Neglect	Is often chronic and usually involves repeated incidents of failing to provide what a child needs for his or her physical, psychological, or emotional development and well-being	4.81 confirmed cases per 1,000 children
Physical abuse	May consist of just one incident or happen repeatedly. It involves deliberately using force against a child in such a way that the child either is injured or is at risk for being injured. Injuries may include bruises, lacerations, burns, and fractures caused by another person or object (e.g., belt, cords, cigarette) *Note:* Many injuries do not represent child abuse; therefore, when abuse is suspected, bruising must be assessed in the context of medical, social, and developmental histories; the explanation given; and the patterns of nonabusive bruising (Maguire, Mann, Sibert, & Kemp, 2005)	2.86 confirmed cases per 1,000 children
Emotional abuse	Involves harming a child's sense of self. It includes acts (or omissions) that result in, or place a child at risk for, serious behavioural, cognitive, emotional, or mental health problems	1.23 confirmed cases per 1,000 children
Sexual abuse and exploitation	Involves using a child for sexual purposes, resulting in physical wounds such as bruises or bleeding of the genitals or rectum, STIs, sore throat, enuresis/encopresis, pregnancy, and foreign objects in the vagina or rectum. The child may also display sophisticated knowledge/behaviour/preoccupation with sexual activities, withdrawal, hypervigilance, or sleep difficulties	0.43 confirmed cases per 1,000 children

From Public Health Agency of Canada. (2010a). *Canadian Incidence Study of reported child abuse and neglect—2008: Major findings.* Ottawa, ON: Author.

are far more likely to be victims of sexual offences, with police-reported rates five times higher than among adults (207 victims per 100,000 versus 41 victims per 100,000). This was true for all types of sexual assaults, as well other sexual offences. A family member (parent or stepparent) is the perpetrator of these offences in 68% of children under 1 year of age, 69% of children aged 1 to 3 years, and 67% of children aged 4, while percentages decline with further increase in age. Gender also plays a role: Rates of family violence towards girls were 56% higher, and they were four times as likely to be sexually assaulted (Sinha, 2011). Table 29-3 lists types and rates of abuse of children in Canada.

Trauma is often not factored out from the various diagnoses such as anxiety disorder or conduct disorder; it is therefore difficult, if not impossible, to determine the causation of some of the applied diagnostic labels. It has been noted that in research of childhood psychiatric disorders, the trauma experience is often an afterthought (Brendtro, 2004; Perry, 2004; van der Kolk, 2009). "Young children often lack words to express themselves, relying instead on a range of adaptive and maladaptive behaviors to communicate their needs, including crying, tantrums, facial expressions, running away, and other demonstrations of urgency or demand" (Arvidson et al., 2011, p. 42).

Adults with mental illness are more likely than not to have a trauma history of abuse and/or neglect—upwards of 95% (McKenna, 2007). Many individuals develop

chronic illnesses as the result of childhood trauma (Bynum et al., 2010). The importance of recognizing the impact of trauma in children and families and the subsequent long-term effects is well established (Bloom, 1994). The importance of this literature points to the effects of childhood trauma on relationships and possibly the impact of psychiatric hospitalization, later in life.

Child and Family Services: Protection

Nurses must be aware that they are legally mandated to report any reasonable suspicion of abuse and neglect to the appropriate provincial and child protection systems. Mandated reporting laws are designed to allow the provinces and child protection systems to investigate the possibility of abuse, provide protection to children, and link families with the support and services that they need to reduce the risk for further abuse. Nurses are ethically and legally responsible for reporting abuse. The Canadian Child Welfare Research Portal (2011) reports:

> There were an estimated number of 235,315 child investigations for abuse and neglect in 2003, of which almost 50% were fully confirmed and led to further inquiry. Canada has an estimated child abuse and neglect rate of 22 cases of substantiated maltreatment (i.e., maltreatment confirmed by investigations) per 1,000 children. The actual rate of maltreatment is thought to be much higher due to underreporting.

The decision to report abuse sometimes poses an ethical dilemma for nurses as they try to balance the need to maintain the family's trust against the need to protect the child. This decision is further complicated by the knowledge that, if temporary out-of-home placement is necessary, the effect of the placement may also contribute to the child's and family's suffering.

Experts recommend that, when possible, nurses report abuse in the presence of the parents, preferably with the parent initiating the telephone call, and that the professional should explain the reporting as necessary to provide safety for the child and to obtain services for the family. If the parents cannot be present when the report is made, the nurse should, at minimum, notify the family that the report was made and explain the reasons. A major protective factor against psychopathology stemming from abuse and neglect is the establishment of a supportive relationship with at least one adult who can provide empathy, consistency, and caring for the child (Taussig, 2002).

The prevention of child abuse and neglect can occur with interventions that support and attend to the parents with physical, financial, mental health (with respect to parents' own trauma history), and medical resources that will reduce stress within the family system. Early intervention and family support programs are considered the cornerstones of preventive efforts. Nurses working with traumatized children should resist the temptation to view the child as the only victim. It will help the nurse maintain empathy towards the parents if it is acknowledged that most parents were themselves traumatized as children and may therefore have limited coping mechanisms or little access to positive parental role models. Once agencies intervene to establish the child's safety, a family system approach that is supportive of the whole family unit is most effective.

Children in Care

The adjustment to an out-of-home placement can be viewed through the conceptual framework of Bowlby's stages of coping with parental separation. According to Bowlby (1960), the child initially responds to separation from parents with protest (crying, kicking, screaming, pleading, and attempting to elicit the parent's return). The child then moves to a state of despair (listlessness, apathy, and withdrawal, which lead to some acceptance of caregiving by others, but with reluctance to reattach fully). Finally, the child experiences detachment if the child and the new parent cannot manage to form an emotional bond. Because children often experience multiple placements, the potential for a disrupted attachment may be great by the time the child faces the prospect of a permanent family. After repeatedly undergoing separation and mourning, the child learns that rejection is inevitable and may automatically maintain distance from a new caregiver.

The trauma elicited, not only from the reason for children's placement but from their being exposed to multiple placements, can include detachment, diffuse rage, chronic depression, low self-esteem, and emotional dependency or insatiable need for nurturing and support. Sometimes, these symptoms develop into attachment disorders that can be challenging to treat (O'Connor, Bredenkamp, & Rutter, 1999) (see Box 29-1). It takes

---

BOX 29-1 | **Research for Best Practice**

THE MEANING OF REACTIVE ATTACHMENT DISORDER

From Kay, C., & Green, J. (2013). Reactive attachment disorder following early maltreatment: Systematic evidence beyond the institution. Journal of Abnormal Child Psychology, 41(4), 571–581.

The Question: Reactive attachment disorder is one of the least evidence-based diagnoses in both the *DSM* and the World Health Organization's International Classification of Diseases. This study examined the effects of a systemic study of reactive attachment disorder (RAD) in maltreated, noninstitutionalized adolescents from a high-income country.

Methods: The following were assessed for RAD behaviours: 153 high-risk adolescents residing in foster or group residential care (mean age 14.5 years, 52% male) and 42 low-risk community controls (mean age 14 years, 38% male). Detailed histories were gathered of maltreatment and care placements (age of entry to care, evidence or not of maltreatment, numbers of placements). An unpublished 24-item questionnaire was used, the Development and Wellbeing Assessment—Reactive Attachment Disorder (DAWBA-RAD). A Child Behaviour Checklist (CBCL) was completed by the care providers of the high-risk group and by parents of the low-risk group. The UK Health of the Nation Outcome Scales for Children and Adolescents and the Child Global Assessment Scale (C-GAS) were used to assess adaptive functioning.

Findings: Both groups were comparable for age, gender, and ethnicity. In the high-risk group, 97% had experienced at least one form of maltreatment. Using regression analysis and adjusting for age, gender, and ethnicity, the high-risk group demonstrated higher scores on the DAWBA-RAD and 63% met criteria of total RAD symptoms. All DAWBA-RAD scales were highly associated with increased symptoms on the CBCL subscales and more impairment noted in the C-GAS. Factor analysis identified four symptom groups: *disinhibited indiscriminate*, *attention seeking*, *superficial relationships*, and *unpredictability*. RAD was associated with increased experiences of maltreatment, earlier age of entry into care, and increased rates of psychopathology. This study indicates that a high number of youth in care struggle with RAD. Fifty-eight percent were assessed *disinhibited indiscriminate* (overly friendly, poor boundaries, e.g., asking personal questions, hugging strangers, wandering away from care providers) and 52% *attention seeking* (demanding, possessive).

Implications for Nursing Practice: Nurses need to be in tune and aware of the boundary challenges that children and adolescents with these concerns may present within the various care settings. Appropriate strategies of nursing care, including parental teaching, are critical to working with this population. Further research is needed to ascertain more specific strategies in working with various age groups of children in care.

knowledgeable, committed, and resilient care providers to work with a child who is challenged by these significant emotional and behavioural problems and struggles to reciprocate caring.

It is estimated that, in 2007, there were 67,000 children in out-of-home care across Canada (Mulcahy & Trocmé, 2010). The difficulty with identifying and tracking the numbers of children in care is that child welfare services fall under the jurisdiction of provincial and territorial authorities. The various provincial legislation directives make it difficult to compare rates of children in out-of-home care across provinces. The most recent report from the Canadian Incidence Study of Reported Child Abuse and Neglect (2008) is unable to be compared directly with previous reports due to changes in policy, public awareness of the problem, CIS criteria, and rates of maltreatment (Fig. 29-1).

The National Household Survey indicates that, of the approximately 30,000 children in care in Canada in 2011, 14,225 were Aboriginal. Overall, 4% of Aboriginal (First Nations, Métis, and Inuit) children were in care, compared with 0.3% of non-Aboriginal children, or 15,345 children (Statistics Canada, 2011b). The over-representation of Aboriginal children in care is of significant concern; however, research-based explanations for its occurrence are lacking (Fluke, Chabot, Fallon, MacLaurin, & Blackstock, 2010). There are several studies from the United States, Australia, and Canada that imply worker ethnicity, education, gender, political ideology, worker age, and agency policies play a role, yet there is

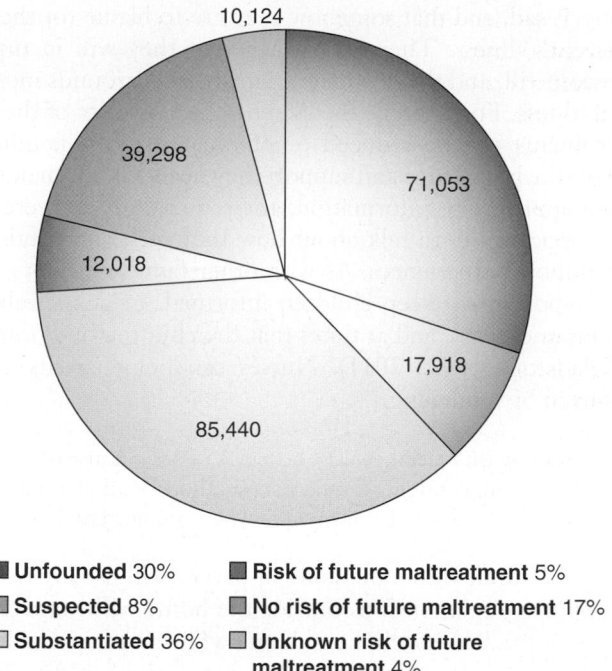

■ **Unfounded** 30%   ■ **Risk of future maltreatment** 5%
■ **Suspected** 8%   ■ **No risk of future maltreatment** 17%
☐ **Substantiated** 36%   ☐ **Unknown risk of future**
                               maltreatment 4%

FIGURE 29-1. Child maltreatment investigations and level of substantiation in Canada in 2008. (Source: Public Health Agency of Canada. (2008). *Canadian Incidence Study of reported child abuse and neglect—2008* (p. 2). Ottawa, ON: Author.)

limited information to this effect. Overall, Aboriginal children "receive less funding per child for federal child welfare services, and families living on reserve have been found to receive minor support from the voluntary sector" (Fluke et al., 2010, p. 67). More work needs to be done with Aboriginal communities in order to address the "social, economic, and cultural risk factors" that affect these communities (Fluke et al., 2010, p. 67).

Parents With Mental Illness

A parent with mental illness can have a number of profound effects on a child, directly through genetics, the intrauterine environment and antenatal stressors, and experience of the illness itself, or indirectly due to socioeconomic issues such as poverty, marital conflict, or addiction (Manning & Gregoire, 2006). Approximately 10% of pregnant women will develop postpartum depression, with a 50% to 62% chance of future depressions (Bernard-Bonnin, 2004; Public Health Agency of Canada, 2012). Postpartum depression can affect the mother–child bond and impact the attachment process for children. Therefore, it is important for nurses to assess the child presented to them and to gather a parental history of stressors and physical and mental illness throughout the pregnancy and during the child's development.

Many children know that something is wrong when a parent has a mental illness, but they may not be able to identify the problem specifically (Gladstone, Boydell, Seeman, & McKeever, 2011). They feel alone, left out, distanced, and powerless to participate in decisions. They report feeling

---

IN A LIFE

Evelyn Lau (1971–)

Evelyn Lau is a noted poet, novelist, and short story writer. She was born in Vancouver, British Columbia, and wanted to pursue a career in the arts; however, this was not the desire of her traditional Chinese parents. Evelyn challenged her traditional family upbringing and left home when she was 14 years old. She spent much of the next 2 years living on the streets as a prostitute and drug addict, resulting in suicide attempts. She has portrayed her experiences through her art, creating *Runaway: Diary of a Street Kid* (1989), which was later made into a CBC movie called *The Diary of Evelyn Lau*. Subsequently, her first collection of poetry, *You Are Not Who You Claim* (1990), reflected much of that same time, and Evelyn was the recipient of the Milton Acorn People's Poetry Award. A second memoir, *Inside Out*, was published in 2001.

She was the youngest poet to receive a nomination for the Governor General's Award for *Oedipal Dreams*. She won the Air Canada Award in 1990 for Most Promising Writer under 30 and the Vantage Woman of Originality Award in 1999. *Living Under Plastic*, her most recent work, won the Pat Lowther Award for best book of poetry by a woman in Canada. Evelyn Lau is Vancouver's Poet Laureate.

Evelyn has spoken and written about her experiences and how this has created the work and person she has become. She does not make excuses for her choices and shares openly her feelings on various topics. Her story is one of how rigid traditional values can clash with youths' desires and dreams and of how she was fortunate that, for her, it resulted in a successful career. Unfortunately, this is not the case for many youth who find themselves living on the street in a life of drugs and prostitution.

angry, sad, and that somehow they are to blame for their parent's illness. They also worry that they will in turn become ill, and they fear the stigma that surrounds mental illness. Fortunately, the likelihood or severity of these problems can be reduced or eliminated when families have the knowledge and support they need. Children need age-appropriate information, their questions answered, an opportunity to talk about how they feel, and routine childhood experiences. As with other family stressors, it is important to keep children informed, in manageable ways and doses, and at times that the children determine (Gladstone et al., 2011). Nurses can help parents get started by modelling.

> Mommy isn't feeling well. She feels sad, it's because of an illness and it's not her fault. It is a sad time for all of us but I'm here to talk with you about it when you need to do so.

Children with a mentally ill parent will usually need supportive relationships outside the home with someone (e.g., a teacher, coach, neighbour) who can provide a listening ear, extra support, and a measure of respite for the family. Children need to know that their routine in life will continue, including the fun times, and that their relationship with both parents is valued by the parents. Parents worry about how their mental illness will affect their child. Support and education need to be provided to all during these challenging times (Costea, 2011; Gladstone et al., 2011). Evidence shows that when children and their families are given information about the affected parent's mental illness, they show improved knowledge and long-standing positive effects in how they problem solve (a resilience-related quality) around parental illness (Beardslee, Gladstone, Wright, & Cooper, 2003; Gladstone et al., 2011).

Parent With a Substance Abuse Problem

Exposure to parental addiction in childhood is fairly common in Canada: 16% among men and 20% among women (Langlois & Garner, 2013). Children whose parents are dependent on alcohol live in an unpredictable family environment, coping with stress that may disrupt their ability to perform in school and lead to other emotional problems (Casa-Gil & Navarro-Guzman, 2002). A study that examined the course of psychological distress among a nationally representative sample of Canadians (aged 18 to 74) revealed that those who experienced parental addictions had consistently higher distress scores than those who did not (Langlois & Garner, 2013).

Such experience appears associated, as well, with other childhood adversities, parental comorbidities, and a negative family environment; thus, understanding the effects of exposure to parental addiction on children requires further study (Langlois & Garner, 2013). The integrated role of biologic–genetic mechanisms and environmental mechanisms in creating an increased risk for

psychological problems among children of those who abuse substances must be considered (see Chapter 26).

Biologic factors affecting children of those who abuse substances include foetal alcohol spectrum disorder, nutritional deficits stemming from neglect, and neuropsychiatric dysfunction. Genetic factors are at least partly responsible for the well-documented increased risk for substance abuse. Studies are beginning to link a family history of mental disorders and alcoholism with genetically transmitted mental disorders, which may be a precursor to alcohol abuse. The precise mechanism of family transmission of alcoholism remains unknown. Children of those who abuse substances may inherit a predisposition to a nonspecific form of biologic dysregulation that may be expressed phenotypically, either as alcoholism or as some other psychiatric disorder (e.g., hyperactivity, conduct disorder, depression), depending on the individual's developmental history.

Children of persons who abuse substances are at high risk for both substance abuse and behaviour disorders (Mylant, Ide, Cuevas, & Meehan, 2002). Moreover, some evidence shows that other factors related to addiction, such as family stress, violence, divorce, dysfunction, and other concurrent parental psychiatric disorders (e.g., depression, anxiety), are as important as the alcoholism itself in increasing this risk (Ritter, Stewart, Bernet, Coe, & Brown, 2002). The experience of growing up in a substance-abusing family is marked by unpredictability, fear, and helplessness because of the cyclic nature of addictive patterns.

The literature on children of parents who have alcoholism has described several typical roles that children assume, including the "hero" (overly responsible children who may ignore their own needs to take care of parents and other children), "scapegoat" (problem children who divert the attention away from the parent), "mascot" (family clowns who relieve tension and mask feelings through joking), and "lost child" (children who suffer in silence but may exhibit difficulties at school or in later life) (Veronie & Freuhstorfer, 2001). These roles, combined with the enabling behaviours of other family members who attempt to cover up and minimize the effects of the addiction, may become so rigid and effective in masking the problem that children of substance abusers may not come to the attention of mental health professionals until after the parent stops drinking and family roles are disrupted.

The experience of growing up in a substance-abusing family can lead to poor self-concept if children feel responsible for their parents' behaviour. The child becomes isolated and learns to mistrust his or her own perceptions as the family denies the reality of the addiction. There is, however, no uniform pattern of outcomes, and many children demonstrate resilience (Harter, 2000). Resilience is the phenomenon by which some children at risk for psychopathology—because of genetic or experiential circumstances—attain good mental health, maintain hope, and achieve healthy outcomes (Masten, 2001). Again, individual protective factors and preventive interventions are paramount.

MENTAL ILLNESS AMONG CHILDREN AND ADOLESCENTS

The Mental Health Commission of Canada (MHCC) estimates that 1.2 million children and youth are affected by mental illness in our country. Over 800,000 Canadian children and youth experience significant mental health issues (School-Based Mental Health and Substance Abuse [SBMHSA] Consortium, 2013). It is highly relevant that two thirds of adults living with mental illness report experiencing first symptoms in their youth (SBMHSA Consortium, 2013). As well, suicide is the leading nonaccidental cause of death among youth (23%) (Navaneelan, 2012), and the rates are two to seven times higher among Aboriginal populations (Federal-Provincial-Territorial Advisory Committee on Population Health, 2000). Most children and youth will not receive appropriate treatment, due to factors such as social stigma and problems with access and availability (SBMHSA Consortium, 2013). Fortunately, strategies endorsed by the MHCC, such as those of the Evergreen Framework (Kutcher & McLuckie, 2010), are allowing such service challenges to be addressed and, hopefully, overcome.

APPROACHES TO ADDRESSING CHILDHOOD TRAUMA

Considering the impact of trauma on the developing brain, nurses need to become aware of and use strategies to intervene and alter the trajectory of the child's overall functioning. The neurodevelopment of children exposed to traumatic events affects their cognitive and emotional development (Brendtro, 2004, 2009; Glaser, 2000; Hodas, 2004; Kinniburgh et al., 2005; McEwen, 2004, 2007; Porges, 2004; van der Kolk, 2005, 2006, 2009). "These children may demonstrate hypervigilance, intrusive thoughts, nightmares, bed-wetting, excessive clinginess, inconsolable crying, and severe tantrums" (Arvidson et al., 2011, p. 41). Programs that emphasize establishing self-regulation strategies and attachment attunement and that work towards development or repair of cognitive skills have been shown to shift affected children towards better success and reduced psychopathology (Abramovitz & Bloom, 2003; Arvidson et al., 2011; Blaustein & Kinniburgh, 2010; Bloom, 1994; Brendtro, 2004; Harris & Morrison, 1995; Mulvihill, 2005; Murphy & Bennington-Davis, 2005, 2006; Kinniburgh et al., 2005; van der Kolk, 2009). An example is the Attachment, Self-regulation and Competency program that works towards teaching both the health care provider and parent how to modulate their own emotional responses, attune to the

child, and assist with their self-regulation. "Caregivers and clinicians play an essential role in restoring a sense of safety and security to traumatized children by developing predictable routines and rituals in their lives" (Arvidson et al., 2011, p. 42). Once the child is better able to self-regulate, they are more open to learning and experiencing the world from a safer perspective (Blaustein & Kinniburgh, 2010). A trauma-informed approach has been shown to benefit children attending inpatient settings and outpatient settings, as well as schools and residential care homes (Arvidson et al., 2011).

Mental health promotion with children, adolescents, and their families encompasses the full range of preventive efforts discussed in Chapter 30. Current thinking argues that a mix of psychological and social determinants affects health overall and mental health in particular.

> At the individual level, such factors as secure attachment, good parenting, friendship and social support, meaningful employment and social roles, adequate income, physical activity, and internal locus of control will strengthen mental health and, indirectly, reduce the impact or incidence of some mental health problems. (Health Canada, 2002, p. 23)

At a system level, strategies that create supportive environments, strengthen community actions, develop personal skills, and orient health services can help to ensure that the population has some control over the psychological and social determinants of mental health.

Professional nursing emphasizes an interdisciplinary approach in which the nurse acts as the collaborator, coordinator, case manager, and advocate to establish linkages with physicians and nurse practitioners, teachers, speech and language specialists, social workers, and other professionals to develop and implement comprehensive preventative interventions (Box 29-2). A view of parents as partners should be foremost. In the past, parents have been too often viewed as the culprits in creating children's mental health problems. Recent insights into the biologic and genetic origins of psychiatric disorders have contributed to a shift from blaming parents to seeking their collaboration in treatment. Promotion and prevention programs incorporate a range of techniques to provide reassurance and education, skills training, or direct intervention. The programs may use face-to-face techniques (e.g., home visits, educational groups), literature (e.g., pamphlets, books), phone (e.g., crisis lines), or electronic mechanisms (e.g., Internet, telehealth).

Psychoeducational programs are a particularly effective form of mental health promotion and intervention. These programs are designed to teach parents and children basic coping skills for dealing with various stressors. Among other techniques, they use the process of **normalization** (i.e., teaching families what are normal behaviours and expected responses) and provide families with information about normal child development and expected reactions to various stressors so that the families

BOX 29-2 Clinical Vignette

PREVENTIVE INTERVENTIONS WITH AN ADOLESCENT IN CRISIS

- Having been removed from their mother's care when she relapsed on cocaine and left them unattended, Aiden and Jenna have now been transferred to a second foster home. The plan is for the two children to return to their mother's home after she completes a 30-day drug treatment program. Aiden, who is in the 10th grade, is in the school nurse's office asking for aspirin for another headache.
- The nurse notices that Aiden's nose looks inflamed, he is sniffling, and he seems more "hyper" than usual. In a concerned tone of voice, she asks him if he has been using cocaine. "Just because my mother's a cokehead," he snaps, "doesn't give you the right to suspect me!" When the nurse gently says, "I'm sorry, I had no idea. Would you like to tell me about what's been happening with your mother?" Aiden responds less defensively and explains the situation about the foster home and his mother's drug problem. He says that if it were not for Jenna, his younger sister, he would have run away by now. His foster parents are "making him" go to school, but he is going to drop out as soon as he returns to live with his mother. The only thing he likes about school is playing basketball; the basketball coach, who is his gym teacher, wants him on the team.
- After a lengthy talk with Aiden, the nurse finishes the assessment interview and concludes that he is at risk for

drug abuse, running away, and dropping out of school. He is also showing symptoms of depression, which he may be attempting to medicate with cocaine. Protective factors for Aiden include his strong attachment to his sister, his ability and willingness to express his thoughts and feelings, his interest in basketball, and a positive relationship with the basketball coach.
- The nurse discusses with Aiden what to do next. Using motivational interviewing strategies and over several weeks, the nurse develops a plan with Aiden to attend the school's weekly drug and alcohol discussion group, so that he can talk with other teens from substance-abusing families and learn coping skills to prevent addiction. The nurse contacts the basketball coach, who agrees to find a student mentor who can shoot hoops with Aiden and help him come up with a plan to stay in school, maybe find a part-time job, and join the basketball team. Aiden agrees to check in regularly with the nurse to report how the plan is working, and they can revise it if needed. The nurse feels optimistic that with support from his peers, coach, mentor, and herself, Aiden can reduce his risk for depression and addiction. Aiden shows signs of resilience. He is motivated to "keep his act together for Jenna," capable of forming positive attachments, and willing to seek help when he knows where to find it.

---

will feel less isolated, know what to expect, and put their reactions into perspective. For example, if families learn that anger is a natural part of grieving, they will be less likely to view it as abnormal and more likely to accept and cope with it constructively.

An excellent example is *Transitions* (2013), a downloadable resource for teenagers and their families that is one aspect of the Teen Mental Health Web site developed by a Canadian expert in adolescent mental health, Stanley Kutcher at Dalhousie University and his colleagues. *Transitions* is focused on helping youth make the transition from high school to university and covers topics ranging from study tips, time management, and exams to sexuality and dating to mental illness, unhealthy behaviours (e.g., violence), substance use, and suicide. Psychoeducational approaches that utilize parallel curricula, established with concurrent psychoeducational groups for adults and children, are helpful. Most foster care agencies now provide a program of education and training for prospective foster parents to help them know what to expect and how to help the child adjust to placement.

Social skills training is one psychoeducational approach that has been useful with youth who have low self-esteem, aggressive behaviour, or a high risk for substance abuse (Cavell, Ennett, & Meehan, 2001). Social skills training involves instruction, feedback, support, and practise with learning behaviours that help children to interact more effectively with peers and adults. When combined with assertiveness training, social skills

training can be particularly helpful in providing children with coping skills to resist engaging in addictive or anti-social behaviours and to prevent social withdrawal under stress. Social skills training may be particularly helpful for children who are bullies or who are rejected by their peers (Fopma-Loy, 2000).

Bibliotherapy is the therapeutic use of books, stories, and other reading materials. It can be used to help children, adolescents, and families to gain information and understanding about life stressors, illness, and recovery. It is a particularly potent form of intervention because it empowers families to learn and develop coping mechanisms on their own. A wide variety of books are available to help children understand issues such as death, divorce, chronic illness, stepfamilies, adoption, and the birth of a sibling. For instance, Baker (2007) describes the way stories about being in foster care can help foster children, parents, and caseworkers in discussing their own situation. By using eight stories to reveal the themes found in accounts of foster care (e.g., the fear of foster children in developing attachments; the way siblings can play a powerfully supportive role; the importance of recognizing the humanity of the biologic parents), Baker highlights the benefits of this therapeutic approach. Children and adolescents can find comfort and increased understanding through stories that reflect their own experience. Parents can use stories as a way to learn about their children's concerns: the adventures and/or tribulations of a story's characters can be a means to discover their child's thoughts and feelings about an experience. Some health centres and hospitals have patient library services available (Anglin, 2008). Many mental health organizations such as the Canadian Mental Health Association, public health agencies, and Health Canada have pamphlets or Web site information designed for parents or children and youth about various physical and psychological problems. In addition to providing concrete information and advice, these reading materials help to reduce anxiety by pointing out common reactions to the various stressors so that families do not feel alone.

Support groups are available for just about every kind of stressor that a family can experience, including substance abuse, death, divorce, and coping with a chronic illness. Both parents and children in groups can experience Yalom's (1985) healing effects of group therapy, including group cohesiveness, universality (awareness of the normalcy and commonality of one's reactions), catharsis, hope, and altruism (being able to help others).

Early intervention programs, possibly the most important form of primary prevention available to children and families, offer regular home visits, support, education, and concrete services to those in need. Research supports the effectiveness of these programs, which may be the key to preventing the placement of children outside the home (Gimpel & Holland, 2003; Tomlin & Viehweg, 2003). The assumption underlying these programs is that parents are the most consistent and important figures in children's lives, and they should be afforded the opportunity to define their own needs and priorities. With support and education, parents will be empowered to respond more effectively to their children.

Canada invests in early intervention to promote healthy child development by enhancing such programs as paid parental leave (now 1 year), child care, family resource centres, and early learning (Waddell et al., 2005). A number of jurisdictions have introduced promotion and prevention programs aimed at high-risk families (low income, lone parents) around the birth of a newborn (e.g., Better Beginnings Better Futures in Ontario; Healthy Beginnings: Enhanced Home Visiting in Nova Scotia). Many of these programs involve nurse home visitation. There is growing evidence that intensive postpartum support (more than antenatal support) provided by a health care professional prevents postpartum depression (Dennis, 2005) and that early interventions are effective in preventing child maltreatment among disadvantaged first-time mothers (MacMillan & Canadian Task Force on Preventive Health Care, 2000). Other population-based early intervention initiatives are aimed at older children in socioeconomically disadvantaged communities. These universal programs are directed towards the child (e.g., classroom enrichment, quality child care), parent (e.g., home visiting, parent help/information/crisis phone lines, parent–child play groups), and neighbourhood

(information that engages families and connects them to community supports), with an emphasis on providing intensive services to children directly. They have demonstrated improvements in children's emotional problems, behavioural problems, social skills, and a decreased need for special education during the early years (ages 4 to 8) (Peters, Petrunka, & Arnold, 2003).

Prevention and promotion programs designed for adolescent mental health should support and educate youth (e.g., through peer mentoring in community organizations and schools); enhance self-help and self-responsibility, coping skills, self-esteem, and skill development in ways that foster mental health; and teach youth when and how to seek assistance for problems (Federal-Provincial-Territorial Advisory Committee on Population Health, 2000). Particular emphasis has been given to ways of creating healthy images related to gender, body image, and empowerment.

Historically, nurses have been underused in school-based mental health efforts, although schools are good locations for other early intervention programs because they are physically near the families they serve and are less intimidating than mental health centres. Programs can be targeted for very young children before symptoms have time to develop. Studies show that by fourth grade, a large number of young children already use some kind of substance (e.g., inhalants, which are toxic); therefore, prevention efforts may be crucial in the early grades (Finke et al., 2002). In numerous schools throughout Canada, Youth Health Centres have become familiar resources.

The number of promotion and early intervention mental health services provided through electronic media (e.g., Internet, telehealth) is growing. Targeted support groups are increasingly available through the Internet. Dedicated Web sites providing both universal mental health information and confidential intervention services by e-mail are also available through some school systems. Similar services around specific mental health issues are also being tested with high-risk populations. Telehealth, which involves telephone and video support to rural and remote Canada (see Chapter 6), is increasingly offered both to practitioners and to children or their parents (Urness, Hailey, Delday, Callanan, & Orlik, 2004). The full capacity of these approaches is largely unknown, and contrary to professional fears, the users are generally more than satisfied with the services (Williams, May, & Esmail, 2001). Some users even prefer the anonymity of electronic media.

Although a number of children's mental health promotion and prevention programs have proven effective on their own, less understood are the effects of programs that include an array of comprehensive health care services, parent education, and support on the mental health of children and youth (Breton, 1999; Peters et al., 2003). Best thinking to date suggests that the most effective strategies for reducing the burden of suffering from child psychiatric disorders are those that consist of a number of concurrent steps (Offord, Kraemer, Kazdin, Jensen, & Harrington, 1998). First, effective universal programs should be in place. Targeted programs should follow for those not helped sufficiently by the universal programs. Finally, for those unaffected by the targeted programs, clinical services should be available. To be effective, prevention programs need to start early, continue long term, and involve multiple domains in a child's life (Offord & Bennett, 2002).

In conclusion, undertaking interventions to promote the mental health of children and adolescents is time and effort well spent. Many adult mental health problems can be prevented, coped with more effectively, or at least reduced in their scope and severity through focused intervention with children, youth, and families. Children and youth lack the power and voice to fight for their own needs, making them one of the most vulnerable groups in society. By virtue of their close interaction with families, nurses are in a key position to identify the mental health needs of children and youth and to intervene, particularly in times of crisis.

NEW DIRECTIONS IN COMMUNITY-BASED MENTAL HEALTH PROMOTION

Mental health promotion with children and youth can occur at individual, familial, community, and global levels. There is growing recognition that multiple factors affect mental well-being, that mental health does not equate to a lack of mental illness, that mental health is also affected by the social determinants of mental well-being, and that health promotion efforts need to span across systems (Khanlou, 2003; Khanlou et al., 2002). Mental health promotion initiatives need to be individualized to the circumstances of the children and youth with whom we work (including their familial and social resources), must be sensitive to context (e.g., rural setting or urban multicultural setting), and must incorporate the latest empirical and theoretical developments (see Box 29-3). Among children and youth, in addition to the health and social services systems, the education system can be among the sites where mental health promotion initiatives take place.

The School-Based Mental Health in Canada project (SBMHSA Consortium, 2013), commissioned by MHCC, discovered in a survey of the research that universal programs can be effective in promoting the well-being of children and youth and that social skills training or social emotional learning increases coping and problem-solving abilities, as well as increases academic achievement. The programs that are taught systematically at a classroom level and that involve the entire school for more than 1 year were most effective (SBMHSA Consortium, 2013).

BOX 29-3 Research for Best Practice

RESULTS OF THE IMPLEMENTATION OF TRAUMA-INFORMED CARE

From Muskett, C. (2013). Trauma-informed care in inpatient mental health settings: A review of the literature. International Journal of Mental Health Nursing, 23(1), 51–59.

The Question: This study conducted a literature review of studies of specific individual actions taken by nurses in order to fulfill a trauma-informed care practice.

Methods: A literature review was conducted examining electronic databases of nursing, psychology, and behavioural sciences and allied health comprehensive and biomedical collections. A total of 116 articles were identified; abstracts were screened to identify quantitative and qualitative studies that met criteria related to trauma-informed approaches or special care provided in inpatient adult, youth, or forensic mental health settings.

Findings: A total of 13 articles met the criteria. What became evident was a focus on seclusion and restraint practices as key outcome measures. There was also a focus on the U.S. National Association of State Mental Health Program Directors' six core strategies for reducing use of seclusion and restraint. It appears that leadership practices are associated with successful trauma-informed care implementation. The inclusion of direct care providers such as nurses in the data collection related to trauma-informed care practices is also important. The creation of a culture that values trauma-informed care is a critical factor. Inclusive in this culture is the physical environment in which care is delivered to create a space that is warm, inviting, and home-like. Inclusion of service users is also a critical factor in the implementation of a trauma-informed care environment.

Implications for Nursing Practice: This study is an example of a literature review. Trauma-informed care is an established framework or philosophy in which many health care agencies have begun to practise. This review highlights the need for more in-depth research into the specific nursing care practices that support a trauma-informed care environment. The inclusion of service users and families, especially in a child and/or youth mental health setting, would be beneficial to the literature in this field.

SUMMARY OF KEY POINTS

■ Nurses working with children and adolescents are in a key position to identify risk and protective factors for psychopathology and to intervene to reduce risk.

■ Nurses who are aware of normal developmental processes can educate parents about their children's behaviours, help them better understand their children's reactions to stress, and decide when intervention may be warranted.

■ If the process of normal biologic maturation in childhood is disrupted through trauma or neglect, developmental delays and disorders can occur, some of which may have irreversible effects.

■ From early infancy, children exhibit different kinds of temperaments that are at least partially biologically determined.

■ Studies of attachment show that the quality of the emotional bond between the child and the parental figure is an important determinant of the success of later relationships.

■ Research shows that children who experience major losses, such as death or divorce, are at risk for developing mental health problems.

■ Sibling relationships have significant effects on personality development. Positive sibling relationships can be protective factors against the development of mental health problems.

■ Medical problems in childhood and adolescence may cause psychological problems when illness leads to behaviours common to an earlier developmental stage (regression) or lack of full participation in family, school, and social activities.

■ Striving for identity and independence may lead adolescents to participate in high-risk activities (e.g., substance use, including tobacco; unprotected sex; delinquent behaviours) that may lead to mental health problems.

■ Poverty, homelessness, abuse, neglect, and parental alcoholism all create conditions that undermine a child's ability to make normal developmental gains and contribute to the child's vulnerability for various emotional and behavioural problems.

■ Children who experience disrupted attachments because of out-of-home placements may have difficulty forming close relationships with their new parents and trusting others.

■ Family support services and early intervention programs are designed to prevent the removal of the child from the family as a result of abuse or neglect and to maintain a strong, nurturing family system.

CRITICAL THINKING CHALLENGES

1 Analyze a case of a family that is grieving a loss and compare the parents' and children's reactions. Include an evaluation of how each child's reactions differ, depending on his or her developmental level.

2 Watch a movie or read a book that provides a child's view of death, divorce, or some other loss and consider how adults may be insensitive to the child's reactions.

3 Examine your own developmental history and pinpoint periods when stressful life events might have increased the risk for emotional problems for you or other family members. What protective factors in your own personality and coping skills, as well as in the environment around you, helped you to maintain your good mental health?

4 What aspects of life are more stressful for children than for adults (i.e., how is it different to experience life as a child)?

5 Examine how your own social and cultural background may either facilitate or create barriers to your ability to interact with families from other ethnic backgrounds or those who are poor or homeless.

6 Allow yourself to reflect on how your own attitudes might interfere with your ability to communicate effectively with families who have abused or neglected their children.

7 Why is the process of normalization of feelings such a powerful intervention with children and families? What kinds of mental health issues, developmental processes, or both would benefit from teaching related to normal reactions? How can nurses incorporate this kind of intervention into their practice roles?

8 How can nurses expand their roles to have maximal effects on primary, secondary, and tertiary mental health interventions with children, youth, and families?

REFERENCES

Abramovitz, R. & Bloom, S. (2003). Creating sanctuary in residential treatment for youth: From the "well-ordered asylum" to a "living-learning environment". *Psychiatric Quarterly*, 74(2), 119–135.

Anglin, C. (2008). Providing pediatric psychosocial support through patient library services in an outpatient hematology/oncology clinic. *Primary Psychiatry*, 15(7), 78–83.

Anthony, K. K., Gil, K. M., & Schanberg, L. E. (2003). Parental perceptions of child vulnerability in children with chronic illness. *Journal of Pediatric Psychology*, 28(3), 185–190.

Arvidson, J., Kinniburgh, K., Howard, K., Spinazzola, J., Strothers, H., Evans, M., ... Blaustein, M. (2011). Treatment of complex trauma in young children: Developmental and cultural considerations in application of the ARC intervention model. *Journal of Child and Adolescent Trauma*, 4, 34–51.

Baker, A. (2007). Fostering stories: Why caseworkers, foster parents, and foster children should read stories about being in foster care. *American Journal of Family Therapy*, 35, 151–165.

Beardslee, W. R., Gladstone T. R., Wright, E. J., & Cooper, A. B. (2003) A family-based approach to the prevention of depressive symptoms in children at risk: Evidence of parental and child change. *Pediatrics*, 112(2), e119–e131.

Bernard-Bonnin, A. -C. (2004). Maternal depression and child development. *Pediatric Child Health*, 9(8), 575–583.

Blaustein, M. E. & Kinniburgh, K. M. (2010). *Treating traumatic stress in children and adolescents: How to foster resilience through attachment, self-regulation, and competency*. New York, NY: Guilford Press.

Bloom, S. (1994). The Sanctuary Model: Developing generic inpatient programs for the treatment of psychological trauma. In M. B. Williams & J. F. Sommer, Jr. (Eds.), *Handbook of post-traumatic therapy: A practical guide to intervention, treatment, and research* (pp. 471–491). West Port, CT: Greenwood Publishing.

Botvin, G. J. (2000). Preventing drug abuse in schools: Social and competence enhancement approaches targeting individual-level etiologic factors. *Addictive Behaviors*, 25(6), 887–897.

Bowlby, J. (1960). Grief and mourning in infancy and early childhood. *Psychoanalytic Study of the Child*, 15, 9–52.

Brendtro, L. (2004). *From coercive to strength-based intervention: Responding to the needs of children in pain*. Retrieved from http://nospank.net/brendtro.pdf

Brendtro, L. (2009). Developmental audit. *Reclaiming Youth: Circle of Courage* workshop series. Victoria, BC.

Breton, J. J. (1999). Complementary development of prevention and mental health promotion programs for Canadian children based on contemporary scientific paradigms. *Canadian Journal of Psychiatry*, 44(3), 227–234.

Brown, E. (2009). Helping bereaved children and young people. *British Journal of School Nursing*, 4(2), 69–73.

Brown, A., Sandler, I., Tein, J., Liu, X., & Haine, R. (2007). Implications of parental suicide and violent death for promotion of resilience of parentally-bereaved children. *Death Studies, 31*, 301–335.

Burns, J. M., Andrews, G., & Szabo, M. (2002). Depression in young people: What causes it and can we prevent it? *Medical Journal of Australia, 177*(Suppl.), S93–S96.

Bynum, L., Griffin, T., Ridings, D. L., Wynkoop, K. S., Anda, R. F., Edwards, V. J., ... McKnight-Eily, L. R. (2010). Adverse childhood experiences reported by adults—five states, 2009. *Centers for Disease Control and Prevention, Weekly MMWR, 59*(49), 1609–1613.

Canadian Child Welfare Research Portal. (2011). *Frequently asked questions.* Retrieved from http://cwrp.ca/faqs

Canadian Council on Learning. (2008). *Evaluation of the Ontario Ministry of Education's Student Success/Learning to 18 strategy—final report.* Toronto, ON: Ontario Ministry of Education.

Canada Parliament. House of Commons. Standing Committee on Human Resources, Skills and Social Development and the Status of Persons with Disabilities. (2010). *Federal poverty reduction plan: Working in partnership towards reducing poverty in Canada. Report of the Standing Committee on Human Resources, Skills and Social Development and the Status of Persons with Disabilities, 40th Parliament, 3rd Session.* Retrieved from http://www.parl.gc.ca/HousePublications/Publication.aspx?DocId=4770921&File=27&Mode=1&Parl=40&Ses=3&Language=E

Canadian Population Health Initiative. (2005). *Improving the health of young Canadians.* Ottawa, ON: Canadian Institutes for Health Information.

Cauce, A. M., Paradise, M., Ginzler, J. A., Embry, L., Morgan, C. J., Lohr, Y., & Theofelis, J. (2000). The characteristics and mental health of homeless adolescents: Age and gender differences. *Journal of Emotional and Behavioral Disorders, 8*(4), 230–239.

Casa-Gil, M. J. & Navarro-Guzman, J. I. (2002). School characteristics among children of alcoholic parents. *Psychological Reports, 90*(1), 341–348.

Cavell, T., Ennett, S. T., & Meehan, B. T. (2001). Preventing alcohol and substance abuse. In J. N. Hughes, A. M. LaGreca, & J. C. Conoley (Eds.), *Handbook of psychological services for children and adolescents* (pp. 133–160). Oxford, UK: Oxford University Press.

Centre for Addiction and Mental Health. (2012). *Mental health and addiction statistics.* Retrieved from http://www.camh.ca/en/hospital/about_camh/newsroom/for_reporters/Pages/addictionmentalhealthstatistics.aspx

Child Support Team. (2000). *Selected statistics on Canadian families and family law* (2nd ed.). Ottawa, ON: Department of Justice Canada.

Costea, G. O. (2011). Considering the children of parents with mental illness: Impact on behavioral and social functioning. *Brown University Child and Adolescent Behavior Letter, 27*(4), 1–6.

Currie, C., Zanotti, C., Morgan, A., Currie, D., de Looze, M., Roberts, C., ... Barkenow, V. (Eds.) (2011). *Social determinants of health and well-being among young people. Health Behaviour in School-aged Children (HBSC) study: International report from the 2009/2010 survey.* Copenhagen, Denmark: World Health Organization Regional Office for Europe.

Deering, C. G., & Cody, D. J. (2002). Communicating effectively with children and adolescents. *American Journal of Nursing, 102*(3), 34–42.

Dennis, C. L. (2005). Psychosocial and psychological interventions for prevention of postnatal depression: Systematic review. *British Medical Journal, 331*(7507), 15–24.

Dillen, L., Fontaine, J., & Verhofstadt-Denève, L. (2009). Confirming the distinctiveness of complicated grief from depression and anxiety among adolescents. *Death Studies, 33*, 437–461.

Edidin, J. P., Ganim, Z., Hunter, S. J., & Karnik, N. S. (2012). The mental and physical health of homeless youth: A literature review. *Child Psychiatry and Human Development, 43*(3), 354–375.

Eggert, L. L., Thompson, E. A., Randell, B. P., & Pike, K. (2002). Preliminary effects of brief school-based prevention approaches for reducing youth suicide: Risk behaviors, depression, and drug involvement. *Journal of Child and Adolescent Psychiatric Nursing, 15*(2), 48–64.

Elkind, D. (1967). Egocentrism in adolescence. *Child Development, 38*, 1025–1034.

Employment and Social Development Canada. (2012). *The National Shelter Study 2009–2009.* Available at http://www.hrsdc.gc.ca/eng/communities/homelessness/reports/shelter_study.html

Eriksson, I., Cater, A., Andershed, A-K., & Andershed, H. (2010). Protection against externalizing and internalizing behavior among children at risk. *Paper presented at the annual meeting of the ASC Annual Meeting,* San Francisco, California.

Federal-Provincial-Territorial Advisory Committee on Population Health. (2000). *The opportunity of adolescence: The health sector contribution.* Cat. N(o): H39–548/200E. Ottawa, ON: Author.

Federal-Provincial-Territorial Council of Ministers on Social Policy Renewal. (2000). *Public report: Dialogue on the national children's agenda—developing a shared vision.* Ottawa, ON: Author.

Finke, L., Williams, J., Ritter, M., Kemper, D., Kersey, S., Nightenhauser, J., ... Hail, A. (2002). Survival against drugs: Education for school-age children. *Journal of Child and Adolescent Psychiatric Nursing, 15*(4), 163–169.

Fluke, J., Chabot, M., Fallon, B., MacLaurin, B., & Blackstock, C. (2010). Placement decisions and disparities among Aboriginal groups: An application of the decision-making ecology through multi-level analysis. *Child Abuse and Neglect, 34*(1), 57–69.

Fopma-Loy, J. (2000). Peer rejection and neglect of latency age children: Pathways and group psychotherapy model. *Journal of Child and Adolescent Psychiatric Nursing, 13*, 29–38.

Foster, K., O'Brien, L., & Korhonen, T. (2012). Developing resilient children and families when parents have mental illness: A family-focused approach. *International Journal of Mental Health Nursing, 21*(1), 3–11.

Freeman, J. G., King, M., Pickett, W., Craig, W., Elgar, F., Janssen, I., & Klinger, D. (2010). *The health of Canada's young people: A Mental health focus.* Retrieved from http://www.phac-aspc.gc.ca/hp-ps/dca-dea/publications/hbsc-mental-mentale/assets/pdf/hbsc-mental-mentale-eng.pdf

Gaetz, S., Donaldson, J., Richter, T., & Gulliver, T. (2013). *The state of homelessness in Canada.* Toronto, ON: Canadian Homelessness Research Network Press.

Gass, K., Jenkins, J., & Dunn, J. (2007). Are sibling relationships protective? A longitudinal study. *Journal of Child Psychology and Psychiatry, 48*(2), 167–175.

Gimpel, G. & Holland, M. (2003). *Emotional and behavioral problems of young children: Effective interventions in the preschool and kindergarten years.* New York, NY: Guilford Press.

Gladstone, B. M., Boydell, K. M., Seeman, M. V., & McKeever, P. D. (2011). Children's experiences of parental mental illness: A literature review. *Early Intervention in Psychiatry, 5*(4), 271–289.

Glaser, D. (2000). Child abuse and neglect and the brain: A review. *Journal of Child Psychology and Psychiatry, 41*(1), 97–116.

Harris, D. & Morrison, E. F. (1995). Managing violence without coercion. *Archives of Psychiatric Nursing, 9*(4), 203–210.

Harter, S. (2000). Psychosocial adjustment of adult children of alcoholics: A review of recent empirical literature. *Clinical Psychology Review, 20*(3), 311–337.

Health Canada. (2002). *A report on mental illness in Canada.* Cat. N(o): 0–662–32817–5. Ottawa, ON: Author.

Hetherington, E. M. & Kelly, J. (2002). *For better or for worse: Divorce reconsidered.* New York, NY: WW Norton.

Hodas, G. (2004). Restraint and seclusion are therapeutic failures. *Residential Group Care Quarterly, 1*, 12–13.

Hulchanski, J. D., Campsie, P., Chau, S. B. Y., Hwang, S. H., & Paradis, E. (Eds.) (2009). *Finding home: Policy options for addressing homelessness in Canada.* Retrieved from http://www.homelesshub.ca/library/finding-home-policy-options-for-addressing-homelessness-in-canada-45761.aspx

Infant Mental Health Promotion. (2005). *Core prevention and intervention for the early years.* Retrieved from http://www.imhpromotion.ca/Portals/0/IMHP%20PDFs/Core%20Prevention_Supporting%20References.pdf

Jeynes, W. (2002). *Divorce, family structure, and the academic success of children.* New York, NY: Haworth Press.

Kay, C. & Green, J. (2012). Reactive attachment disorder following early maltreatment: Systemic evidence beyond the institution. *Journal of Abnormal Child Psychology, 41*, 571–581.

Kelly, J. (2003). Changing perspectives on children's adjustment following divorce: A view from the United States. *Childhood, 10*(3), 237–254.

Kelly, K. & Caputo, T. (2007). Health and street/homeless youth. *Journal of Health Psychology, 12*(5), 726–736.

Khanlou, N. (2003). Mental health promotion education in multicultural settings. *Nurse Education Today, 23*, 96–103.

Khanlou, N., Beiser, M., Cole, E., Freire, M., Hyman, I., & Kilbride, K. M. (2002). Mental health promotion among newcomer female youth: Post-migration experiences and self-esteem. Available at http://dsp-psd.communication.gc.ca

Kinniburgh, K. J., Blaustein, M., & Spinazzola, J. (2005). Attachment, self-regulation, and competency: A comprehensive intervention framework for children with complex trauma. *Psychiatric Annals, 35*(5), 424–430.

Kutcher, S. & McLuckie, A. (2010). *Evergreen: A child and youth mental health framework for Canada.* Calgary, AB: Mental Health Commission of Canada.

Langlois, K. A. & Garner, R. (2013). Trajectories of psychological distress among Canadian adults who experienced parental addiction in childhood. *Health Reports, 24*(3), 14–21.

LeBlanc, L. A., Goldsmith, T., & Patel, D. R. (2003). Behavioral aspects of chronic illness in children and adolescents. *Pediatric Clinics of North America, 50*(4), 859–878.

Leventhal, T. & Brooks-Gunn, J. (2000). The neighborhoods they live in: The effects of neighborhood residence on child and adolescent outcomes. *Psychological Bulletin, 126*, 309–337.

Lewis, M. & Vitulano, L. A. (2003). Biopsychosocial issues and risk factors in the family when the child has a chronic illness. *Child and Adolescent Psychiatric Clinics of North America, 12*(3), 389–399.

MacMillan, H. L. & Canadian Task Force on Preventive Health Care. (2000). Preventive health care, 2000 update: Prevention of child maltreatment. *Canadian Medical Association Journal, 163*(11), 1451–1458.

Maguire, S., Mann, M. K., Sibert, J., & Kemp, A. (2005). Are there patterns of bruising in childhood which are diagnostic or suggestive of abuse? A systematic review. *Archives of Disease in Childhood, 90*(2), 182–186.

Manning, C. & Gregoire, A. (2006). Effects of parental mental illness on children. *Psychiatry, 8*(1) 7–9.

Manser, L. (2001). *Enhancing academic success of youth in care—a research brief.* Ottawa, ON: National Youth in Care Network.

Martinez, Y., & Ercikan, K. (2009). Chronic illnesses in Canadian children: What is the effect of illness on academic achievement, and anxiety and emotional disorders? *Child: Care, Health and Development, 35*(3), 391–401.

Masten, A. S. (2001). Ordinary magic: Resilience processes in development. *American Psychologist, 56*(3), 227–238.

McEwen, B. S. (2004). Protection and damage from acute and chronic stress: Allostasis and allostatic overload and relevance to the pathophysiology of psychiatric disorders. *Annals of the New York Academy of Sciences, 1032*, 1–7.

McEwen, B. S. (2007). Physiology and neurobiology of stress and adaptation: Central role of the brain. *Physiological Review, 87*, 873–904.

McKay, A. (2013). *Trends in Canadian national and provincial/territorial teen pregnancy rates: 2001–2010.* Retrieved from http://www.sieccan.org/pdf/TeenPregancy.pdf

McKenna, K. (2007). Training 'who' to do 'what': Reappraising the role function and purpose of training in the management of aggression and violence within clinical settings. *5th European Congress on Clinical Violence in Psychiatry*, October 25–27, Amsterdam.

Melhem, N., Moritz, G., Walker, M., Shear, M. K., & Brent, D. (2007). Phenomenology and correlates of complicated grief in children and adolescents. *Journal of the American Academy of Child and Adolescent Psychiatry, 46*(4), 493–499.

Mulcahy, M. & Trocmé, N. (2010). *Children and youth in out-of-home care in Canada.* Retrieved from http://cwrp.ca/sites/default/files/publications/en/ChildrenInCare78E.pdf

Mulvihill, D. (2005). The health impact of childhood trauma: An interdisciplinary review, 1997–2003. *Issues in Comprehensive Pediatric Nursing, 28*(2), 115–136.

Murphy, T. & Bennington-Davis, M. (2005). *Restraint and seclusion: The model for eliminating their use in health care.* Marblehead, MA: HCPro, Inc.

Murphy, T. & Bennington-Davis, M. (2006). Engagement model and trauma-informed care. Presentation to Child and Youth Mental Health Programs, University of British Columbia, Vancouver, BC.

Muskett, C. (2013). Trauma-informed care in inpatient mental health settings: A review of the literature. *International Journal of Mental Health Nursing, 23*(1), 51–59.

Mylant, M. L., Ide, B., Cuevas, E., & Meehan, M. (2002). Adolescent children of alcoholics: Vulnerable or resilient? *Journal of the American Psychiatric Nurses Association, 8*(2), 57–64.

Navaneelan, T. (2012). *Suicide rates: An overview.* Statistics Canada, Catalogue no. 82-624-X.

O'Connor, T. G., Bredenkamp, D., & Rutter, M. (1999). Attachment disturbances and disorders in children exposed to early severe deprivation. *Infant Mental Health Journal, 20*(1), 10–29.

Offord, D. R. & Bennett, K. J. (2002). Prevention. In M. Rutter & E. Taylor (Eds.), *Child and adolescent psychiatry* (4th ed.). Oxford, UK: Blackwell Science.

Offord, D. R., Kraemer, H. C., Kazdin, A. E., Jensen, P. S., & Harrington, R. (1998). Lowering the burden of suffering from child psychiatric disorder: Trade-offs among clinical, targeted, and universal interventions. *Journal of the American Academy of Child and Adolescent Psychiatry, 37*(7), 686–694.

Perry, B. D. (2004). *Maltreatment and the developing child: How early childhood experience shapes child and culture.* Retrieved from http://www.lfcc.on.ca/mccain/perry.pdf

Peters, R., Petrunka, K., & Arnold, R. (2003). The Better Beginnings, Brighter Futures Project: A universal, comprehensive, community-based prevention approach for primary school children and their families. *Journal of Clinical Child and Adolescent Psychology, 32*, 215–227.

Pfund, R. (2006). *Palliative care nursing for children and young people.* Oxford, UK: Radcliffe.

Porges, S. (2004). Neuroception: A subconscious system for detecting threats and safety. *Zero to Three*, 19–24.

Pruett, M. K., Williams, T. Y., Insabella, G., & Little, T. D. (2003). Family and legal indicators of child adjustment to divorce among families with young children. *Journal of Family Psychology, 17*(2), 169–180.

Public Health Agency of Canada. (2010a). *Canadian Incidence Study of reported child abuse and neglect—2008: Major findings.* Ottawa, ON: Author.

Public Health Agency of Canada. (2010b). *Canadian guidelines on sexually transmitted infections.* Available at http://www.phac-aspc.gc.ca/std-mts/sti-its/cgsti-ldcits/section-5-1-eng.php

Public Health Agency of Canada. (2012). Depression in pregnancy. Retrieved from http://www.phac-aspc.gc.ca/mh-sm/preg_dep-eng.php

Puskar, K. R., Sereika, S., & Tusaie-Mumford, K. (2003). Effect of the Teaching Kids to Cope (TKC) program on outcomes of depression and coping among rural adolescents. *Journal of Child and Adolescent Psychiatric Nursing, 16*(2), 71–80.

Reifman, A., Villa, L. C., Amans, J. A., Rethinam, V., & Telesca, T. Y. (2001). Children of divorce in the 1990's: A meta-analysis. *Journal of Divorce and Remarriage, 35*(1–2), 27–36.

Ritter, J., Stewart, M., Bernet, C., Coe, M., & Brown, S. A. (2002). Effects of childhood exposure to familial alcoholism and family violence on adolescent substance use, conduct problems, and self-esteem. *Journal of Traumatic Stress, 15*(2), 113–122.

School-Based Mental Health and Substance Abuse (SBMHSA) Consortium. (2013). *School-based mental health in Canada: A Final Report.* Mental Health Commission of Canada. Available at www.mentalhealthcommission.ca

Schor, E. L., & the American Academy of Pediatrics Task Force on the Family. (2003). Family pediatrics: Report of the task force on the family. *Pediatrics, 111*(6 Pt 2), 1541–1571.

Segaert, A. (2012). *The national shelter study: Emergency shelter use in Canada 2004–2009.* Ottawa, ON: Homelessness Partnering Secretariat, Human Resources and Skills Development Canada.

Self, B. & Peters, H. (2005). Street outreach with no streets. *Canadian Nurse, 101*(1), 20–24.

Siddiqi, A., Irwin, L. G., & Hertzman, C. (2007). *Total environment assessment model for early child development: Evidence report for the World Health Organization's Commission on the Social Determinants of Health.* Retrieved from www.who.int/social_determinants/resources/ecd_kn_evidence_report_2007.pdf

Sinha, M. (Ed.) (2011). *Measuring violence against women: Statistical trends.* Retrieved from http://www.statcan.gc.ca/pub/85-002-x/2013001/article/11766-eng.pdf

Statistics Canada. (2004). *Canadian community health survey: Mental health and well-being.* Ottawa, ON: Author.

Statistics Canada. (2011a). Living apart together. Retrieved from http://www.statcan.gc.ca/pub/75-006-x/2013001/article/11771-eng.htm

Statistics Canada. (2011b). *National household survey.* Retrieved from http://www5.statcan.gc.ca/researchers-chercheurs/result-resultat

Strohschein, L. (2012). Parental divorce and child mental health: Understanding predisruption effects. *Journal of Divorce and Remarriage, 53*(6), 489–502.

Sun, U. & Li, Y. (2002). Children's well-being during parents' marital disruption process: A pooled time-series analysis. *Journal of Marriage and the Family, 64*(2), 472–488.

Taussig, H. N. (2002). Risk behaviors in maltreated youth placed in foster care: A longitudinal study of protective and vulnerability factors. *Child Abuse and Neglect, 26*(11), 1179–1199.

Tomlin, A. M. & Viehweg, S. A. (2003). Infant mental health: Making a difference. *Professional Psychology: Research and Practice, 34*(6), 617–625.

Trocmé, N., Fallon, B., MacLaurin, B., Sinha, V., Black, T., Fast, E., … Holroyd, J. (2010). *Canadian Incidence Study of reported child abuse and neglect—2008: Major findings.* Ottawa, ON: Public Health Agency of Canada.

Unger, A. (2013). Children's health in slum settings. *Archives of Disease in Childhood, 98*(10), 799–805.

United Nations Children's Fund. (2012). UNICEF report card 10. Retrieved from http://www.unicef.ca/en/discover/article/unicef-report-card-10#Report%20Card

Urness, D., Hailey, D., Delday, L., Callanan, T., & Orlik, H. (2004). The status of telepsychiatry services in Canada: A national survey. *Journal of Telemedicine and Telecare, 10*(3), 160–164.

van der Kolk, B. (2005). Developmental trauma disorder. *Psychiatric Annals, 35*(5), 401–408.

van der Kolk, B. (2006). Clinical implications for neuroscience in research in PTSD. *Annals of the New York Academy of Sciences, 1071*, 277–293.

van der Kolk, B. (2009). *New frontiers in trauma treatment.* Presentation at Coquitlam, BC.

Van Epps, J., Opie, N. D., & Goodwin, T. (1997). Themes in the bereavement experience of inner city adolescents. *Journal of Child and Adolescent Psychiatric Nursing, 10,* 25–36.

Veronie, L. & Freuhstorfer, D. B. (2001). Gender, birth order and family role identification among children of alcoholics. *Current Psychology: Developmental, Learning, Personality, Social, 20*(1), 53–67.

Vyas, A., Landry, M., Schnider, M., Rojas, A. M., & Wood, S. F. (2012). Public health interventions: Reaching Latino adolescents via short message service and social media. *Journal of Medical Internet Research, 14*(4), 31–40.

Waddell, C., McEwan, K., Shepherd, C. A., Offord, D. R., & Hua, J. M. (2005). A public health strategy to improve the mental health of Canadian children. *Canadian Journal of Psychiatry, 50*(4), 226–233.

Whiteman, S. D., McHale, S. M., & Soli, A. (2011). Theoretical perspectives on sibling relationships. *Journal of Family Theory and Review, 3,* 124–139.

Williams, T. L., May, C. R., & Esmail, A. (2001). Limitations of patient satisfaction studies in telehealthcare: A systematic review of the literature. *Telemedicine Journal and E-Health, 7*(4), 293–316.

Wu, Z., Hou, F., & Schimmele, C. (2008). Family structure and children's psychosocial outcomes. *Journal of Family Issues, 29*(12), 1600–1624.

Wright, L. M. & Leahey, M. (2013). *Nurses and families: A guide to family assessment and intervention* (6th ed.). Philadelphia, PA: F. A. Davis.

Yalom, I. D. (1985). *The theory and practice of group psychotherapy* (2nd ed.). New York, NY: Basic Books.

Zolkoski, S. M. & Bullock, L. M. (2012). Resilience in children and youth: A review. *Children and Youth Services Review, 34*(1), 2295–2303.

CHAPTER 30

Mental Health Assessment of Children and Adolescents

Lorelei Faulkner-Gibson and Kimberly Wong
Adapted from the chapters "Mental Health Assessment of Children and Adolescents" by Wendy Austin and by Jean Robinson Hughes, Vanya Hamrin, Catherine Gray Deering, and Lawrence Scahill

KEY CONCEPT

• attachment

LEARNING OBJECTIVES

After studying this chapter, you will be able to:

• Define the assessment process for children and adolescents.

• Discuss the techniques of assessment data collection used with children and adolescents.

• Discuss the synthesis of bio/psycho/social/spiritual assessment data for children and adolescents.

• Delineate the important bio/psycho/social/spiritual areas of assessment for children and adolescents.

KEY TERMS

• developmental delays • disorganized attachment • egocentrism

• genogram • maturation • self-concept

The mental health assessment of children and adolescents is challenging. At any given time, 14% of children aged 4 to 17 years (over 800,000 in Canada) experience mental disorders that cause significant distress and impairment at home, at school, and in the community (School-Based Mental Health and Substance Abuse [SBMHSA] Consortium, 2013; Waddell, McEwan, Shepherd, Offord, & Hua, 2005). Yet, fewer than 25% of these children receive specialized treatment services. There are a number of reasons for this situation. First, mental health services are woefully inadequate in many regions of Canada and often are limited to urban areas (e.g., Breton, Plante, & St-Georges, 2005). Second, evidence from large studies using national survey data shows that differences in government policies and health care system characteristics cause variances in service use (Sturm, Ringel, & Andreyeva, 2003). Third, some children do not get help when those who serve as gatekeepers to treatment (parents, teachers, and physicians) either fear the stigma that children will carry

with mental illness (Jellnick, Patel, & Froehle, 2003) or fail to recognize mental illness as a childhood problem or the impact of early emotional experience on a child's capacity to develop relationships and to learn (Carter, Briggs-Gowan, & Davis, 2004). Given the evidence that the largest determinants of service provision to youth are provider assessment of mental health problems and provider knowledge of service resources (Stiffman et al., 2000), it is crucial that health professionals be knowledgeable and proficient in these areas.

The assessment of children and adolescents is a specialized process that considers their unique problems and responses within the context of their development. The Canadian Federation of Mental Health Nurses' (CFMHN) *Standards of Psychiatric-Mental Health Nursing* (CFMHN, 2014) serves as a guide for this process. These standards argue that effective diagnosis and monitoring are dependent on a client-centred approach, one that incorporates both theory and an understanding of the meaning of the health or illness experience from the perspective of the client. The nurse acknowledges clients as valued and respected partners throughout the decision-making process and supports them in drawing on their own assets and resources for self-care and mental health promotion. The nurse also incorporates knowledge of family dynamics as well as knowledge of cultural values and beliefs about families in the assessment.

■ ASSESSING THE MENTAL HEALTH OF CHILDREN AND ADOLESCENTS

The assessment of children and adolescents generally follows the same format as that for adults (see Chapter 10), but there are significant differences. In working with children/youth and families, "we embrace the notion that there are multiple realities in and of the 'world,' that each family member and nurse see a world that he/she brings forth through interacting with themselves and with others in language" (Wright & Leahey, 2005, p. 4). Children think in more concrete terms; the nurse therefore needs to ask more specific and fewer open-ended questions than would typically be asked of adults. The nurse should use simple phrasing because children have a narrower vocabulary than do adults. Examples include saying "sad" instead of "depressed" or "nervous" or "worried" instead of "anxious." The nurse needs to corroborate information that children offer with more sources (e.g., parents, teachers) than the nurse might with adults. The nurse may want to use artistic and play media (e.g., puppets, family drawings) to engage children and evaluate their perceptions, inner worlds, fine motor skills, and intellectual functions. Children have a less specific sense of time and a less developed memory than do adults. When children are asked about a sequence of events or specific times when events occurred, they may not be able to provide accurate information.

Adolescents must be assessed within their cognitive and developmental range of functioning. Adolescents may or may not be willing participants in the assessment process, depending on why they have been referred and who has referred them. It is always important to meet with clients separately from their care providers, and this is especially true with adolescents. It is critical for the nurse to ensure what level of confidentiality s/he is able to provide to the youth in the context of an individual interview. For example, issues of safety, such as suicidality, would need to be revealed to care providers, whereas issues of sexual identity are less immediately urgent. There is usually time to determine when or if this issue should be shared collaboratively with the child/youth's care providers. Mental health assessment involves much more than completing assessment tools and considers far more than the individual. A conceptual framework used as a guide can assist in planning the goals of the assessment, as well as identify the factors, types of information and sources, and the elements within the environment to be considered. Frameworks that shape the mental health assessment of children and youth in Canada are identified and described below.

The Canadian Mental Health Association's (CMHA) Framework for Support

The CMHA's Framework for Support (Trainor, Pomeroy, & Pape, 2004) identifies three resource bases important to mental health assessment: the Person Resource Base, the Knowledge Resource Base, and the Community Resource Base. By focusing on the *Person Resource Base*, the nurse acknowledges that the child/youth is far more than a repository of illness and symptoms and that positive change builds on existing strengths. Hence, when approaching assessment, the nurse considers their understanding of their mental health problem/illness as well as their self-esteem, sense of belonging (within their family and community), and sense of purpose and meaning in the world. The nurse also assesses the child/youth's skills and capacities (sense of personal control, confidence, resilience, hope) to confront illness. By focusing on the *Knowledge Resource Base*, the nurse takes into consideration not only medical–clinical and social science knowledge but also experiential (firsthand experience) and traditional knowledge (cultural ways). The nurse's assessment considers how children experience mental illness and how the family and community (public attitudes and conventional wisdom) accept it. A critical analysis of such information assists the nurse in building a rich understanding of children and guards against drawing inaccurate assumptions. It can also identify inaccuracies and misconceptions that may be held within the family or community about mental illness. By focusing on the *Community Resource Base*, the nurse gains an understanding of the many factors and social determinants (housing, education, income, meaningful work) that affect the everyday life of children and youth (Trainor et al., 2004, pp. 8–10). The Community Resource Base also acknowledges the importance of both formal services (mental health services, generic community services) and the network of natural supports (family and friends, self-help and consumer organizations) available to promote mental health and recovery. Equally important, it recognizes the person (child or youth) as having the power (age-appropriate) to make choices about resources to use, if any, and to participate fully in decision making.

The Framework for Support helps the nurse focus assessment on outcomes and, in particular, on those outcomes that play a critical role in recovery from mental illness. Specifically, it supports assessment of whether a child has access to the social determinants of good mental health (housing, school, family, friends, a sense of purpose), feels well and has a sense of personal control, and has various personal resources in place and ways to connect with the formal service system if needed. Finally, the framework assesses how the individual's age (child or youth) and life circumstances (e.g., breakup or death in family, being cut from a sport team) have challenged the child.

Evergreen: A Child and Youth Mental Health Framework for Canada

The Mental Health Commission of Canada's (MHCC) Evergreen Framework provides values and strategic directions for child and youth mental health care in Canada (Kutcher & McLuckie for MHCC, 2010). The values identified are

- Human rights
- Dignity, respect, and diversity
- Best available evidence
- Choice, opportunity, and responsibility
- Collaboration, continuity, and community
- Access to information, programs, and services

Health professionals should be cognizant of human rights documents in a way that informs their practice. These documents include United Nation's (UN) *Convention on the Rights of the Child* and the *Convention on the Rights of Persons with Disabilities*, as well as *A Canada Fit for Children* that is Canada's response to the UN's *A World Fit for Child*ren. Valuing dignity, respect, and diversity involves striving for equal access to services and programs for all children and their families in Canada. Ongoing commitment is necessary for best evidence-based programs to evolve; children and families need to be able to make informed choices about what best fits their needs. Collaboration among all those who have a significant role in a child's life allows for meaningful networks of support. Publically accessible mental health information, along with the promotion of access to programs and services, is crucial to an equitable health care system. These explicitly stated values contribute to a common vision for the evolution of child and adolescent mental health in Canada.

Four categories of strategic directions are identified in the Evergreen Framework, envisioned as separate but overlapping categories: *promotion*; *prevention*; *intervention and ongoing care*; and *research and evaluation*. The first three categories are part of the continuum of mental health care (see Chapter 4), while the fourth, research and evaluation, is an essential component to each of them, as well as being a component in itself. Within the Evergreen Framework, specific strategies for each category are identified.

The Bio/Psycho/Social/Spiritual Model

The holistic, integrated approach of the bio/psycho/social/spiritual model of health that is used to frame nursing practice in this textbook is applicable to child and adolescent care. Thus, a comprehensive evaluation includes a bio/psycho/social/spiritual history, mental status examination, additional testing (e.g., cognitive or neuropsychological), and, if necessary, records of the child's school performance and medical–physical history, and information from other agencies that may be providing services (e.g., department of child and family services, juvenile court). The nurse may use various assessment tools, including the Child Attention Profile and the Devereux Early Childhood Assessment (DECA), the Behaviour Assessment System for Children (BASC), the Child Behaviour Checklist (CBCL), or the Children's Depression Inventory (CDI).

> ● **STUDY NOTE**
> Whenever assessing children or adolescents, cognitive and developmental level will frame the assessment and the design and implementation of the management plan.

■ COLLECTION OF ASSESSMENT DATA

Comprehensive collection of meaningful data is crucial to an accurate, holistic assessment of the mental health of a child or youth. Components of assessment data and the nursing skills necessary to them are addressed here. (Note: where appropriate, "child" will be the term used to refer to both children and adolescents).

The Clinical Interview

The clinical interview is the primary assessment tool used in child and adolescent psychiatry. A unique set of skills is necessary for interviewing children and adolescents. How the nurse obtains mental health information depends on the developmental level of each child, specifically considering the child's language and cognitive, social, and emotional skills. For example, the nurse should simplify questions for young children or children with developmental delays or communication issues (e.g., autism spectrum disorder, hearing impairment, English as a second language) so that these children can understand and respond accordingly.

The assessment interview may be the initial contact between the child and parent/guardian and the nurse. The first step is to establish a relationship, and the second is to assess the interactions between the child and his or her caregivers. It is important to understand that children cannot be considered apart from their caregivers and the context in which they live. However, defining the caregiving context is sometimes a challenge (Carter et al., 2004). The nurse needs to identify the child's primary caregivers, the patterns of current caregiving relationships (e.g., how often the child goes to other caregivers), and the history of these relationships (e.g., multiple transitions, abrupt losses) (Carter et al., 2004, p. 114). The nurse should also explore the family's definition of *family* and identify those included in the family constellation (Carter et al., 2004, pp. 114–115). This would include biologic, psychosocial, and spiritual relationships (e.g., uncle, Big Brother/Big Sister volunteer, friends, neighbours, godmother).

Building Rapport

To reduce anxiety and establish trust during the assessment, the nurse strives to develop rapport with the family members. The nurse can establish the relationship with the child/youth and family by recognizing the child's individuality and showing respect and concern for that child. The nurse should demonstrate sensitivity, objectivity, and confidentiality. The child will be more forthcoming if he or she believes that the nurse is listening carefully and is interested in what he or she has to say. Establishing rapport can be facilitated by making and maintaining eye contact (as culturally relevant); speaking slowly, clearly, and calmly, with friendliness and acceptance; using a warm and expressive tone; reacting to communications objectively; showing interest in what families are saying; and making the interview a joint undertaking (Sattler, 1998).

Building rapport, which can be challenging, is fundamental to any mental health assessment of children and youth. The developmental transitions throughout childhood and adolescence are rapid, and there are few guidelines about how information from many sectors should be integrated, how impairment levels should be determined, or how assessing function that may be specific to context (relational or cultural) or caregiver (e.g., parents, relatives, day care staff, teachers) can be achieved practically (Carter et al., 2004).

The information in Box 30-1 can serve as a guide to asking specific questions during a comprehensive assessment of the child. The Community Resource Base of the Framework for Support (Trainor et al., 2004) provides a useful guide for identifying a range of stakeholders from the child's daily living activities (e.g., parent, school, day care, recreation, arts) as well as services (formal or informal) that might be consulted (with family permission) for related information about the various contexts in which the child interacts. These stakeholders can provide complementary information (formal or informal) about how the child is functioning in critical developmental domains (language and literacy, physical, cognitive, social, and emotional). They also provide an understanding of how the child is treated within, and copes with, various peer environments involving diverse cultures (e.g., ethnic, socioeconomic, language) and activities (e.g., scholastic, recreational, artistic). This information can assist the nurse in formulating a well-balanced and integrated mental health assessment (strengths and limitations from multiple contexts) of the child.

Child and Parent Observation

Because the child's primary environment is most often with the parent, child–parent interactions provide important data about the child–parent attachment and parenting practices. Attachment is the term used to name the emotional bonds between a child and parent (or parental figure) that begin in infancy (see "Attachment: The Caregiving Context"). The nurse's observations focus on both the child alone and the child within the family. The nurse can make some of these observations while the family is in the waiting area, noting behaviours (Barnard, 1994):

- Sensitivity/clarity/responsiveness to cues
- How the child and parent get each other's attention
- How parent and child interact with and talk to each other (clarity of cues)
- How frequently each initiates conversation and how promptly each responds
- How the child and parent separate
- Whether the parent and child play together
- How responsive the parent is to the child's attention-seeking initiatives
- How the parent and child show affection to each other
- How attached the parent and the child appear
- Response to distress
- Whether the parent starts/stops/notes the distress/changes in activity
- How the parent consoles the child
- How the parent disciplines the child (clear directive voice, yells, hits)
- Social–emotional growth fostering
- Use of talking, smiling, laughing, singing, touching (praising or criticizing)
- Cognitive growth fostering
- Parent talks about/describes objects/ideas using developmentally appropriate and stimulating language
- Parent provides child with/points out objects of interest
- Parent encourages and/or allows the child to explore

KEY CONCEPT Attachment is the emotional bond between an infant and his or her parental figure. Attachment behaviours of an infant include crying, clinging, calling, following, and protesting.

Interview Techniques

To get an accurate picture of the child, the nurse should interview the child and parent individually for some part of the session because each can provide unique, meaningful information. Often disagreement between child and parent regarding signs and symptoms relevant to diagnostic criteria emerges in separate interviews. Generally,

BOX 30-1 Semistructured Interview With School-Aged Children

This guide identifies a range of areas and sample questions that can be addressed during an interview with a school-aged or adolescent child. The nurse should note that children generally prefer to be engaged in a conversation rather than peppered with questions. The interview should be tailored in a way that is comfortable and relevant for the child. Although some direct questions are inevitable, open-ended questions are preferable. Similarly, phrasing questions to get at what a child is thinking (e.g., "I can see you are trying to tell me something" or "tell me more") is preferable to asking "why" questions that tend to put people on the defensive. Finally, trying to match the child's emotional state (unless hostile) helps people feel understood (Forgatch & Patterson, 1989). The interview can begin with a simple greeting, such as the following: "Hi, I am (your name and title). You must be Tom Brown. Come in."

For All School-Aged Children
Presenting Concern
Thank you for coming to talk with me today. To begin, it would help me if I knew what, if anything, you have been told about why you are here or what will go on today…. Can you tell me *your* story of how you came to be here today? (If necessary, probe with specific questions below. Let the child take the lead and explore issues as he or she raises them. If the child raises a problem, explore it in detail.

Demographic Information
I'd like to know you better. Could you tell me about yourself?

Probes
1. How old are you?
2. When is your birthday?
3. Where do you live? (address)
4. And your telephone number is…?

School
Tell me about your school.

Probes
5. Which school do you go to? Is it close to your home? How do you get there each day?
6. Where do you go after school (home, sitter, etc.)… and who is there (parent/relative, sitter, no one)?
7. What do most kids think about your school?… What is it like for you?
8. What grade are you in? What do most kids think about it?… What is it like for you?
9. What subjects do you like the best?… Like least?
10. What subjects give you the least trouble?… Most trouble?
11. How well do you do in school—about the same as, better than, or not as well as other kids in your class?
12. On the whole, would you say that you are doing better or worse than last year?
13. What activities do you participate in at school?
14. How well do you get along with your classmates?
15. How well do you get along with your teachers?
16. Tell me how you spend a usual day at school.

Home and Family
To help me understand your family, can you name each of the people who live with you … and then other important family members who live somewhere else … and I'll put them into a picture…. Now, using the picture, tell me a little about your family.

(A **genogram** [Wright & Leahey, 2005] provides a useful diagram of family relationships. It resembles a family tree but includes additional relationships among individuals. It permits the nurse and the child to quickly see patterns in family history. It maps relationships and traits that may otherwise be missed and includes basic information about number of families, number of children in each family, birth order, and deaths. Some genograms include information on disorders running in the family such as alcoholism, depression, diseases, alliances, and living situations. Older children

can provide additional information [e.g., about separation/divorce, death] for understanding family dynamics.) (See Chapter 15.)

Probes
17. Tell me a little about each of them.
    - Who makes you happy and who makes you sad/angry/worried? Explain.
    - Do you have a favourite photo of you and your family? Tell me about it… and why you like it.
18. What does your father do during the day—does he work? (other activities at home/with friends)?
19. What does your mother do during the day—does she work? (other activities at home/with friends)?
20. Tell me what your home is like.
21. Tell me about your room at home.
22. What chores do you do at home?
23. How do you get along with your father?
24. What does he do that you like?… Don't like?
25. How do you get along with your mother?
26. What does she do that you like?… Don't like?
27. (Where relevant) Some brothers and sisters get along well, whereas others don't get along at all… How do you get along with your brothers and sisters?
28. What do (does) they (he/she) do that you like?… That you don't like?
29. Who handles the discipline at home?
30. Tell me about how they (he/she) handle (handles) it.
    - When you do something good, what happens and who is involved?
    - When you get in trouble, what happens and who is involved?
    - If you want to do something different from the rest of your family, would that be okay? Explain… Who would support you?
    - If you need help, what would you do? Would someone support you? Explain.
    - Are there other relatives who are important to you? Tell me about who they are and how they connect with you (if not already discussed with the genogram).
    - Would you say that your family is like most other families in your school/neighbourhood or different? Explain. Does that make it easy or difficult for you/your family… and in what ways and in what types of situations? This question gets at culture (ethnicity, socioeconomic status, language, beliefs/values, etc.) in a broad way.

Interests
Now let's talk about the things you like to do?

Probes
31. What hobbies and interests do you have?
32. What do you do in the afternoons/evenings after school?
33. Tell me what you usually do on Saturdays and Sundays.
    - What do you do on special holidays? Tell me about the best holiday you ever had.
    - When you are having fun, what are you doing, who are you with? Tell me about a time when you were really having a good time.

Friends
Tell me about your friends.

Probes
34. What do you like to do with your friends?
    - Any best friends?
    - If you needed help, could you count on them to support you? Give an example.
    - If you wanted to do something different from them, would that be okay?

Moods and Feelings
Probes
35. Everybody feels happy at times. What things make you feel happiest?

(Continued)

36. What are you most likely to get sad about?
37. What do you do when you are sad?
38. Everybody gets angry at times. What things make you angriest?
39. What do you do when you are angry?

Fears and Worries
Probes
40. All children get scared sometimes about some things. What things make you feel scared?
41. What do you do when you are scared?... What takes away the fear?
    - How well does that work?
42. Tell me what you worry about... What takes away the worry?
    - How well does that work?
43. Any other things?

Self-Concerns
Probes
44. What do you like best about yourself?... Anything else?
45. What do you like least about yourself?... Anything else?
46. Tell me about the best thing that ever happened to you.
47. Tell me about the worst thing that ever happened to you.
    - What did you do about this situation?
    - How well does that work?
    - Overall, how much would you say you believe in yourself?

Somatic Concerns
Probes
48. Do you ever get headaches?
49. (If yes) Tell me about them. (How often? What do you usually do?)
50. Do you get stomachaches?
51. (If yes) Tell me about them. (How often? What do you usually do?)
52. Do you get any other kinds of body pains?
53. (If yes) Tell me about them.
    - What do you do to ease these problems?
    - How well does that work?

Thought Disorder
Probes
54. Do you ever hear things that seem funny or unusual?
55. (If yes) Tell me about them. (How often? How do you feel about them? What do you usually do?)
56. Do you ever see things that seem funny or unreal?
57. (If yes) Tell me about them. (How often? How do you feel about them? What do you usually do?)

Help-Seeking
Probes
58. Tell me about a time when you have needed help. What did you do? Whom did you ask for help? What kind of help did you get? How did things work out?
59. Have you ever gone to see a counsellor before? Explain. Did it help?

Memories and Fantasy
Probes
60. What is the first thing you can remember from the time when you were a very little baby?
61. Tell me about your dreams.
62. Which dreams come back again?
63. Who are your favourite television characters?
64. Tell me about them.
65. What animals do you like best?
66. Tell me about these animals.
67. What animals do you like least?
68. Tell me about these animals.
69. What is your happiest memory?
70. What is your saddest memory?
71. If you could change places with anyone in the whole world, who would it be?

72. Tell me about that.
73. If you could go anywhere you wanted to right now, where would you go?
74. Tell me about that.
75. If you could have three wishes, what would they be?
76. What things do you think you might need to take with you if you were to go to the moon and stay there for 6 months?

Aspirations
77. What do you plan on doing when you become an adult?
78. What things will help you be successful? Is there anything standing in the way of you being successful?
    - How hopeful are you that you might be successful? (suggestion—using a visual analogue with a series of faces on a line [sad face to very happy face] ask child to choose the face that best describes their hopefulness)
79. If you could do anything you wanted when you become an adult, what would it be?

Concluding Questions
80. Do you have anything else that you would like to tell me about yourself?
81. Do you have any questions that you would like to ask me?
    - What are you hoping will happen as a result of our talking today?

For Adolescents
These questions can be inserted after number 57 (the help-seeking section).

Sexual Relations
Adolescence is a very confusing time emotionally. Our bodies change as we begin to look more like adults. Our relationships also change. While our sexual relationships are new and exciting, they can also be puzzling, frustrating, or even frightening.
1. Do you have any romantic feelings or relationship(s) with guys or girls? Do you feel comfortable talking about them? With girls/guys/or both?
2. What makes you feel good about it/them?
3. What makes you feel not so good about them?
4. Do you have any special girlfriend (boyfriend)?
5. (If yes) Tell me about her (him). Most people have lots of questions about their sexual relationships and yet are not sure whom to trust to talk openly...
6. What kind of sexual concerns do you have?
7. (If present) Tell me about them.
8. (If applicable) What do you think might be helpful to do about your concerns? (getting information, talking to someone, getting a checkup/some medication)
9. Are you interested in getting help? Would you like me to help you make the right connections?

Drug and Alcohol Use
10. Do your parents/sister/brothers drink?
11. (If yes) Tell me about their drinking. (How much, how frequently, and where?)
12. Do your friends drink alcohol?
13. (If yes) Tell me about their drinking.
14. Do you drink alcohol?
15. (If yes) Tell me about your drinking.
16. Do your parents use drugs?
17. (If yes) Tell me about the drugs they use. (How much, how frequently, and for what reasons?)
18. Do your friends use drugs?
19. (If yes) Tell me about the drugs they use.
20. Do you use drugs?
21. (If yes) Tell me about the drugs you use. (Sattler, 1998)
22. Are you worried about the way your parents/siblings/friends use alcohol or drugs?
23. Are you worried about the way you use alcohol/drugs?
24. (If yes) Are you interested in getting help?
25. (If applicable) What do you think might be helpful to do regarding your concerns?

children provide better information about internalizing symptoms (e.g., mood, sleep, suicide ideation), and parents provide better information about externalizing symptoms (e.g., behaviour disturbances, oppositionality, relationship with parents).

Discussion With the Child

After talking with the parent and child together, the nurse should ask to speak with the child alone for a while. Young children may fear separating from their parents. The nurse can reassure children by showing them where the waiting area is and telling them, "Mommy and Daddy are going to be waiting right here for you. You and I are going to be in a room close by. But if you get worried, we can come back out here to check on them." Introducing a toy or game or giving the child a transitional object to hold may help. For example, young children often like holding the family house or car keys, knowing that their parents cannot go anywhere without them. Remember that observing how the child separates from the parent is part of the data needed to complete the assessment.

Adolescents may act indifferent or even hostile when the nurse asks to speak with them alone. Remember that this can be a pose to cover anxiety and fear. Teens tend to be sceptical that adults can really understand their experience, suspicious that they will be blamed for their problems, and fearful that their thoughts and feelings are abnormal. The nurse should be patient with adolescents and show empathy for their concerns through comments such as, "I can see that you're pretty angry about being here. There might be a way that I can help…. But in order to help, I need to know from *you* what is going on that is making you so angry. I want to assure you that I am not here to judge or blame. I can also promise you that if you tell me anything that I think needs to be shared with your parents, then I will tell you first." If the youth is particularly silent, the nurse might comment, "You've been pretty quiet during the last few minutes…. I'm not sure if that means you're having trouble expressing yourself…". The nurse should allow the adolescent time to respond and then offer other prompts. "That can be really frustrating. If that is the case, then, maybe if you just start talking, we can try to find some words together to express your ideas…." "You may be wondering if it is safe to tell me what you're thinking. It can be frightening to trust a stranger with your most private thoughts…." "You may be wondering whether I really meant what I said about confidentiality/keeping things private…. or about not judging you…. I guess the dilemma/problem is whether it is safer to keep troubling thoughts and feelings to oneself or to take a chance that someone might be able to help."

To begin the initial assessment of a child, the nurse introduces himself or herself and explains briefly what they will be doing together. For children younger than 11 years of age, the nurse should explain that he or she helps worried or upset children by talking, playing, and together with his or her parents, thinking of ways to make things better. The nurse should then ask about the child's understanding of why he or she is there. This question often helps to identify children's misconceptions (e.g., believing the nurse is going to give them an injection, thinking that they have done something bad) that could create barriers to working with them. When conducting the child interview, the nurse will need to get several releases of information from the child's guardian to obtain corroborating reports, such as the child's physical assessment from the paediatrician or paediatric nurse practitioner; the school's report about the child's academic (report card) and behavioural performance (interactions with peers and adults); and records of diagnosis and treatment from any previous psychiatric provider. Youth are often very sensitive when reports are requested from school. They worry about repercussions if they have had prior difficulties (e.g., disciplinary problems). It is important that the nurse explain how these reports will be used, whether the school will be involved in the development of treatment plans, and how the youth and family will participate.

The nurse must adapt communication to the child's age level (Box 30-2). The challenge is to avoid using overly complex vocabulary or talking down to children. Young children often express themselves more easily in

---

BOX 30-2 Strategies for Interviewing Children

- Use a simple vocabulary and short sentences tailored to the child's developmental and cognitive levels.
- Be sure that the child understands the questions and that you do not lead the child to give a particular response. Presenting polar opposite choices (never … or all the time) or scaled questions (1–10) is helpful. For example, "Some people feel angry all the time, some only feel angry at certain times, and others don't seem to feel angry at all. On a scale of 1–10, where 1 means never and 10 means all the time, how often do you feel angry?" If the child chooses a number greater than 1, she can be asked to describe times when she is angry.
- Select the questions for your interview on an individual basis, using judgement and discretion and considering the child's age and developmental level.
- Be sure that the manner and tone of your voice do not reveal any personal biases.
- Speak slowly and quietly, and try to allow the interview to unfold, using the child's verbalizations and behaviour as guides.
- Use simple terms (e.g., "sad" for "depressed") in exploring affective reactions, and ask the child to give examples of how he or she behaves or how other people behave when emotionally aroused.
- Assume an accepting and neutral attitude towards the child's communications.
- Learn about children's current interests (e.g., by looking at Saturday morning television programs, talking with parents, visiting toy stores) (Sattler, 1998).

the context of play than through adult-like conversation. For example, a child may use puppets to reenact a conversation that he or she had with a sibling or parent. Children respond well to third-person conversation prompts, such as "Some kids don't like being compared to their brothers and sisters," or "I know a kid who was so sad when he lost his dog that he thought he would never be happy again."

Early in the interview, the goal is to explain the nurse's purpose, elicit any concerns the child may have about what is happening, and establish rapport with the child by engaging in unthreatening discussion. Many adults rarely ask children about things that truly interest them, but expect children to respond readily to adult conversation. The nurse can establish a high degree of credibility simply by taking note of and asking about things that are obviously important to children (e.g., a sport that they participate in, a rock group displayed on a shirt, a toy they have brought with them). However, children have uncanny natural "radar" for dishonest adult behaviour. Attempts to establish rapport work only when the nurse is genuinely interested in the child's life.

Discussion With the Parents

After meeting alone with the child, the nurse should discuss with the child that s/he would now like to talk with the parents alone, just as s/he did with the child. The nurse should be careful to reiterate that s/he wants to help and will not judge anyone in the family. The nurse should ensure that the child has a safe place to wait and is given age-appropriate activities. When the nurse meets with the parents, s/he should review the expectations and provide similar reassurances around confidentiality, building trust, and being nonjudgemental as those given to the child. The nurse then proceeds to ask parents to describe their view of the problem. When alone, parents often feel more comfortable discussing their children in depth and sharing their frustrations. Parents need this opportunity to speak freely, without being constrained by concern for the child's feelings. Although children often have a pretty good sense about their parents' reactions, it may not be constructive for them to hear the full force of the parents' complaints and feelings, such as their sense of helplessness, anger, or disappointment. Parents sometimes feel guilty and need permission to express their negative feelings without feeling judged. This session is the nurse's opportunity to enlist the help of parents as partners in understanding and addressing the child's problem. This time is also good for filling in any gaps in the history and clarifying the data obtained from the interview with the child.

Parents need the chance to describe the presenting problem in their own words. The nurse can encourage them by asking general questions, such as, "It is not easy for parents to recognize that childhood is sometimes unhappy and that their child needs help. A child's emotions and behaviour can be pretty confusing, even frightening, and many parents hope that, with time, the problems will disappear on their own. Unfortunately, that is sometimes not the case, and if left unattended over time, the problems can worsen. It takes great courage to seek help, and you took a big step in coming here today. I hope that by working together with your child, we will find some ways of assisting. I am interested in *your* story. Tell me what brings *you* here *today*." The nurse should then reflect his or her understanding of the problem, showing empathy and respect for both parent and child.

Asking any other family members about their view of the problem is always a good idea to clarify discrepancies, obtain additional data, and communicate awareness that different family members experience the same problem in different ways.

Child and Adolescent Rating Scales

There are a number of instruments available for conducting bio/psycho/social/spiritual assessments. They vary according to age and target areas of interest as well as purpose. Observational assessment and parent-report questionnaires are generally used for screening, whereas in-depth surveys and interviews help formulate diagnoses of psychopathology. Evidence shows that *screening* for early problems is both feasible and effective in improving rates of referral for mental health services (Murphy et al., 1996). Screening can be administered in stages starting with short screens of groups of children (e.g., in clinics, day care, school) followed by more in-depth screens involving parents and observations of those identified to be at elevated risk. Most effective screening methods involve brief standardized measures that are easy to administer, score, and interpret (Carter et al., 2004). The Ages and Stages Questionnaire–Social–Emotional Version (Squires, Bricker, & Twombly, 2002) is a parent-report screen for measuring social–emotional and behavioural problems and competencies from birth to 5 years. The 6-item Kutcher Adolescent Depression Scale (KADS) is a screening tool for youth at risk for depression that can be used in such institutional settings as schools. It evolved from the 11-item KADS that can be used for monitoring an adolescent's response to (psychopharmacologic) treatment (Brooks, 2004).

It is important to remember that screening measures have proved most effective in evaluating the level of risk for children with socioemotional problems within a population (e.g., a community, school) and are less effective in identifying with certainty an individual at risk (Costello, Egger, & Angold, 2005). This means that the nurse should not rely on one source of evidence but, instead, use multiple sources of data to understand a child's emotional well-being.

The BASC, developed by Reynolds and Kamphouse (1998), is a tool to measure behaviours and emotions in children aged 2 to 18 years. The scales include a teacher rating scale, parent rating scale, and 180-item self-report of personality. The scale evaluates several dimensions, including attitude towards school, attitude towards teachers, sensation seeking, atypicality, locus of control, somatization, social stress, anxiety, depression, sense of inadequacy, relations with parents, interpersonal relations, self-esteem, and self-reliance. The CBCL developed by Achenbach and Edelbrock (1983) is a 113-item self-report tool to identify forms of psychopathology and competencies that occur in children ages 4 to 16 years. This instrument provides scores on internalizing and externalizing behaviours.

Several scales are useful for diagnosing specific problems in children and adolescents. The CDI developed by Kovacs (1982) is a 27-item self-rated symptom orientation scale for children aged 7 to 17 years that is useful for diagnosing physical symptoms, harm avoidance, social anxiety, and separation or panic disorder. The Multidimensional Anxiety Scale for Children developed by March (1997) is a 39-item self-rating scale that assesses severity of anxiety in children and adolescents. The paediatric anxiety rating scale developed by the RUPP Anxiety Study Group (2002) is a clinician-administered, 50-item semi-structured interview to assess the severity of anxiety in children aged 6 to 17 years. The Kutcher Generalized Social Anxiety Disorder Scale for Adolescents has four subscale scores (fear and anxiety, avoidance, affective distress and somatic distress) plus a total score (Brooks and Kutcher, 2004).

The SNAP-IV developed by Swanson (1983) is a 90-item teacher and parent rating scale containing items from the Conners' questionnaire for measuring inattention and overactivity; it is useful for diagnosing attention deficit hyperactivity disorder (ADHD—inattentive and impulsive types) and oppositional defiant disorder. The Children's Yale-Brown Obsessive Compulsive Scale developed by Goodman et al. (1989) is a 19-item scale that can help diagnose childhood obsessive–compulsive disorder in children aged 6 to 17 years.

Assessments performed for *diagnostic* purposes most often require trained administrators and interpreters; they take more time to complete and score and are more rigorous to administer than screens. However, evidence shows that they are very useful because they highlight both positive and negative aspects of the child and identify delays, evaluate the relative degree of impairment associated with extant problem behaviours, and facilitate the design of interventions that capitalize on children's strengths (Carter et al., 2004).

Assessment Within Age Groups

Preschool-Aged Children

When interviewing preschool-aged children, the nurse should understand that these children may have difficulty putting feelings into words and provide assistance (e.g., "When I see your face all wrinkled up, it tells me that you are mixed up—confused"). The nurse should also understand that young children think in very concrete terms. For example, when talking to a young boy (3 to 6 years) about the death of his father, the nurse needs to recognize that, although children can acknowledge physical death, they consider it as temporary or gradual and not fully separate from life. The young boy may believe that his father continues to live (in the ground where he was buried) and ask questions about his activities (e.g., how is Dad eating, going to the toilet, breathing, playing?) (National Cancer Institute, 2005). The child may also believe that something the child thought or did actually caused the father's illness and subsequent death. In response to death, children younger than 5 years will often exhibit disturbances in eating, sleeping, and bladder or bowel control that may result in a parent's seeking help (Grollman, 1990). The nurse should keep language simple and tailored to the child's developmental level. Any discussion about death should include concrete terms (e.g., cancer, died, death) and avoid euphemisms (e.g., "he passed away," "he is sleeping," "we lost him"), because they can confuse children and lead to misinterpretations (Wass & Corr, 1984).

The nurse can achieve rapport with preschool-aged children by joining their world of play. Play is an activity by which the child transforms an experience from real life into a symbolic, nonliteral representation. Play encourages verbalizations, promotes manual strength, teaches rules and problem solving, and helps children master control over their environment (Taylor, Menarchek-Fetkovich, & Day, 2000). With children younger than 5 years of age, the nurse may conduct the assessment in a playroom. Useful materials are paper, pencils, crayons, paints, paintbrushes, easels, clay, blocks, balls, dolls, dollhouses, puppets, animals, dress-up clothes, and a water supply. The nurse must inform preschool-aged children about any rules for the play. For example, the nurse must tell the child that the nurse must ensure safety so that there will be no hitting in the playroom.

When observing the child in a free play setting, the nurse should pay attention to initiation of play, energy level, manipulative actions, tempo, body movements, tone, integration, creativity, products, age appropriateness, and attitudes towards adults. In addition, themes of play, expression of emotions, and temperament are important to observe. The nurse must allow children to direct and initiate these themes. When evaluating the young child's peer relationships through play therapy in a play group or school setting, observe play settings and themes, initiation of play, response to peer initiations of play, integration of affect and action during play, resolution of conflicts, responses to suggestions of others during play, and the ability to engage in role taking and role reversals (Howes & Matheson, 1992).

The nurse's roles are to be a good listener; to use appropriate vocabulary; to tolerate a child's anxious, angry, or sad behaviour; and to use reflective comments about the child's play. Through play, the nurse can assess the child's sensorimotor skills, cognitive style, adaptability, language functioning, emotional and behavioural responsiveness, social level, moral development, coping styles, problem-solving techniques, and approaches to perceiving and interpreting the surrounding world. For example, when assessing a child's problem-solving skills, the nurse might say to a preschooler, "I can see that you've noticed the tent in the corner and would like to check it out. Yes, the tent does look interesting … but I can also see that you have a problem … the tent looks a little scary to you … and you do not want to check it out alone. Hmm… can you think of someone whom you would like to take with you?" Then, in response to the child's answer, the nurse says, "Mr. Bear … because he protects you…. Oh, then Mr. Bear is a great choice. You chose a friend who would be sure to keep you safe…. You made a good decision."

In any assessment, the nurse should be careful to assess both strengths and limitations and then build on the strengths to address the child's problem areas. For example, the nurse might engage a preschooler with the comment, "Sara, you are a great storyteller; I wonder if you could tell me a story about this doll, Jane, who is afraid at day care just like you."

Lidz (2003) developed a tool that the clinician can use to assess preschoolers' play (Box 30-3). Analyzing children's perceptions of fairy tales can provide the clinician with clues to culture, problems, solutions, and elements of mental functioning (LeBuffe & Naglieri, 1999; Trad, 1989).

Drawings are also used in child assessment to illuminate the child's intellect, creative talents, neuropsychological deficits, body image difficulties, and perceptions of family life (Fig. 30-1). Types of drawings used in child assessments are free drawings; self-portraits; the kinetic family drawing; tree, person, house drawing; and a picture of someone of the opposite sex (Cepeda, 2000). The DECA (LeBuffe & Naglieri, 2003) screening instrument measures protective factors of attachment, self-control, and initiative in children 2 to 5 years of age. The DECA tool is used in the preschool classroom setting with the goal of promoting positive resilience in children.

School-Aged Children

Unlike preschool-aged children, school-aged (5 to 11 years) children can use more constructs, provide longer descriptions and make better inferences of others, and acquire more complete conceptions of various social roles. Children in middle school are more capable of verbal exchange and can tolerate limited periods of direct questioning (Box 30-4). The nurse can establish rapport with school-aged children by using competitive board games, such as checkers, and playing cards. A therapeutic game helpful in assessing the child's perceptions, cognition, and emotions and in establishing rapport between clinician and child is the thinking–feeling–doing game. In this game, the clinician and the child take turns drawing cards that pose hypothetical situations and ask what a person might think, feel, or do in such scenarios. For example, one card might say, "A boy has something on his mind that he is afraid to tell his father. What is he scared to talk about?" Another

---

BOX 30-3 Lidz Assessment Tool

Child's Name: _____ Birth Date: _____ Age: _____
Assessor: _____ Date of Assessment: _____

Describe typical play style/sequence.

Describe range of levels of play from lowest to highest level with age estimates and within contexts of independent/facilitated, familiar/unfamiliar, single/multiple toys.

Describe language and evidence of self-talk and internalized speech.

Describe interpersonal interactions with assessor and facilitator (if not assessor).

Describe content of any play themes.

What held the child's attention the longest? (For how long?) And what were the child's toy/play preferences?

Describe the child's affective state during play.

Implications of above for intervention: _____

From Lidz, C. S. (2003). *Early childhood assessment.* Hoboken, NJ: Wiley & Sons, Inc., Copyright 2003, John Wiley & Sons. Used with permission.

FIGURE 30-1. Me and my mom going for ice cream. Drawing and writing by a 5-year-old girl.

BOX 30-4 Bio/psycho/social/spiritual Psychiatric Nursing Assessment of Children and Adolescents

1. **Identifying information**
   Name
   Sex
   Date of birth
   Age
   Birth order
   Grade
   Ethnic background
   Religious preference
   List of others living in household

2. **Major reason for seeking help**
   Description of presenting problems or symptoms
   When did the problems (symptoms) start?
   Describe both the child's and the parent's perspectives.

3. **Psychiatric history**
   Previous mental health contacts (inpatient and outpatient)
   Other mental health problems or psychiatric diagnosis (besides those described currently)
   Previous medications and compliance
   Family history of depression, substance abuse, psychosis, etc., and treatment

4. **Current and past health status**
   Medical problems
   Current medications
   Surgery and hospitalizations
   Allergies
   Diet and eating habits
   Sleeping habits
   Height and weight
   Hearing and vision
   Menstrual history
   Immunizations
   If sexually active, birth control method used
   Date of last physical examination
   Paediatrician or nurse practitioner's name and telephone number

5. **Medications**
   Prescription (dosage, side effects)
   OTC drugs

6. **Neurologic history**
   Right handed, left handed, or ambidextrous
   Headaches, dizziness, fainting
   Seizures
   Unusual movement (tics, tremors)
   Hyperactivity
   Episodes of weakness or paralysis
   Slurred speech, pronunciation problems
   Fine motor skills (eating with utensils, using crayon or pencil, fastening buttons and zippers, tying shoes)
   Gross motor skills and coordination (walking, running, hopping)

7. **Responses to mental health problems**
   What makes problems (symptoms) worse or better?
   Feelings about those experiences (what helped and did not help)
   What interventions have been tried so far?
   Major losses or changes in the past year
   Fears, including punishment

8. **Mental status examination**
   Appearance, gait, posture, dress, nutrition, gestures
   Motor/motility
   Interaction with nurse, eye contact
   Psychosis, hallucinations, delusions
   Mood, affect, anxiety
   Speech (clarity, speed, volume), language (articulation, tone, modulation, coherence).

Writing/reading (comprehension), content
Thought patterns (organization, thought content)
Intellectual ability, judgement, insight, general knowledge, orientation to date, time, person
Activity level, stereotypes, mannerisms, obsessions or compulsions, attention, phobia

9. **Developmental assessment**
   Mother's pregnancy, delivery
   Child's Apgar score, whether preterm or full-term, weight at birth
   Physical maturation
   Psychosocial
   Language
   Developmental milestones: walking, talking, toileting

10. **Attachment, temperament/significant behaviour patterns**
    Attachment
    Concentration, distractibility
    Eating and sleeping patterns
    Ability to adjust to new situations and changes in routine
    Usual mood and fluctuations
    Excitability
    Ability to wait, tendency to interrupt
    Responses to discipline
    Lying, stealing, fighting, cruelty to animals, fire-setting

11. **Self-concept**
    Beliefs about self
    Body image
    Self-esteem
    Personal identity

12. **Risk assessment**
    History of suicidal thoughts, previous attempts
    Suicide ideation, plan, lethality of plan, accessibility of plan
    History of violent, aggressive behaviour
    Homicidal ideation

13. **Family relationships**
    Relationship with parents
    Deaths/losses
    Family strengths and conflicts (nature and content)
    Nurturing and disciplinary methods
    Quality of sibling relationship
    Sleeping arrangements
    Who does the child relate to or trust in the family?
    Relationships with extended family

14. **School and peer adjustment**
    Learning difficulties and strengths
    Behaviour problems and strengths at school
    School attendance
    Relationship with teachers
    Special classes
    Best friend
    Relationships with peers
    Dating
    Drug and alcohol use
    Participation in sports, clubs, other activities
    After-school routine

15. **Community resources**
    Professionals or agencies working with child or family
    Day care resources

16. **Functional status**
    See Functional Status section of this chapter.

17. **Stresses and coping behaviours**
    Psychosocial stresses
    Coping behaviours (strengths)

18. **Summary of significant data**

might read, "A girl heard her parents fighting. What were they fighting about? What was the girl thinking while she listened to her parents?"

Adolescents

Adolescents have an increased command of language concepts and have developed the capacity for abstract and formal operations thinking. Their social world is also more complex. "Identity" is a core psychosocial developmental task of this phase of life (Erikson, 1968). Some early adolescents may assume that their subjective experiences are real and congruent with objective reality, which can lead to egocentrism (Shave & Shave, 1989). **Egocentrism** is a preoccupation with one's own appearance, behaviour, thoughts, and feelings. For example, a preteen may think that he caused his parents to divorce because he fought with his father the day before the parents announced their decision to separate. Because teenagers have a new, heightened sense of self-consciousness, they may be preoccupied during the interview with applying makeup or other self-grooming tasks.

During early adolescence, cognitive changes include increased self-consciousness, fear of being shamed, and demands for privacy and secrecy. An adolescent's willingness to talk to a nurse will depend partly on his or her perception of the degree of rapport between them. The nurse's ability to communicate respect, cooperation, honesty, and genuineness is important. Rejection by the adolescent, even outright hostility, during the first few interactions is not uncommon, especially if the teen is having behaviour problems at home, at school, or in the community. The nurse should be patient and avoid jumping to conclusions. Hostility or defiance may be a test of how much the teen can trust the nurse, a defence against anxiety, or a transference phenomenon (see Chapter 8).

Adolescents are likely to be defensive in front of their parents and concerned with confidentiality. At the start of the interview, the nurse should clearly convey to the adolescent what information will and will not be shared with parents. Adolescents generally prefer a straightforward, candid approach to the interview because they often distrust those in authority. Making a commitment to adolescents that they do not have to discuss anything they are not ready to reveal is important so that they will feel in control while they gradually build trust.

■ BIO/PSYCHO/SOCIAL/SPIRITUAL PSYCHIATRIC NURSING ASSESSMENT OF CHILDREN AND ADOLESCENTS

As discussed, the comprehensive assessment of the child or adolescent includes interviews with the child and parents, child alone, and parents alone. After completing these components, the nurse should bring the child and parents back together to summarize his or her view of their concerns and to ask for feedback regarding whether these perceptions agree with theirs. The nurse must give the family a chance to share additional information and ask questions. The nurse should then thank them for their willingness to talk and give them some idea of the next steps. The use of an assessment tool is helpful in organizing data for mental health planning and intervention. The nurse should also ask for feedback on the suggested next steps of both child and parents and discuss any areas of disagreement to find a plan with which all can live.

When interviewing both child and parents, directly asking the child as many questions as possible is generally the best way for the nurse to get accurate, firsthand information and to reinforce interest in the child's viewpoint. Asking the child questions about the history of the current problem, previous psychiatric experiences (both good and bad), family psychiatric history, medical problems, developmental history (to get an idea of what the child has been told), school adjustment, peer relationships, and family functioning is particularly important. If necessary, the nurse can ask some or all of these same questions of the parents to get consensus or another opinion about the matter, attain supplemental information, or both. Keep in mind that developmental research shows moderate to low correlation between parent and child reports of family behaviour. It is helpful to discuss openly with the family the fact that different perspectives exist and to note that the nurse's role is not to judge or side with one view, but rather to understand the different perspectives and how they might be affecting the family.

Biologic Domain

Nurses should include a thorough history of psychiatric and medical problems in any comprehensive assessment. A physical assessment is necessary to rule out any medical problems that could be mistaken for psychiatric symptoms (e.g., weight loss resulting from diabetes, not depression; drug-induced psychosis). Pharmacologic assessment should include prescription and over-the-counter (OTC) medications. Nurses should ask about any allergies to food, medications, or environmental triggers.

Genetic Vulnerability

The line between nature and nurture is not always clear. Characteristics that appear to be inborn may influence parents and teachers to respond differently towards different children, thus creating problems in the family environment. A phenomenon called *assortative mating*—the tendency for individuals to select mates who are similar in genetically linked traits such as intelligence and personality style—may contribute to the genetic transmission of psychiatric disorders. Research increasingly shows that major psychiatric disorders (e.g., depression, anxiety disorder, schizophrenia, bipolar disorder, substance abuse) run in families. Thus, having a parent or sibling with a psychiatric disorder usually indicates an increased risk for the same or another closely related disorder in a child or adolescent. In addition, many psychiatric disorders appearing in childhood, such as autism spectrum disorder, intellectual developmental disorder, some language disorders, ADHD, Tourette's syndrome, enuresis (bed wetting), and trisomy disorders (e.g., Down's syndrome), have genetic factors associated with their aetiology (American Psychiatric Association, 2013). Certain disorders (e.g., ADHD, enuresis, stuttering) are more common in boys than in girls.

Neurologic Examination

A full neurologic evaluation is beyond the scope of practice for a baccalaureate-level or master's-level nurse without specific neuropsychiatric training. However, a screening of neurologic soft signs can help establish a database that will clarify the need for further neurologic consultation. The nurse should ask the child directly the brief neurologic screening questions suggested in Box 30-4 and also should note any soft signs of neurologic dysfunction, such as slurred speech, unusual movements (e.g., tics, tremors), hyperactivity, and coordination problems. The nurse can ask young children to hop on one foot, skip, or walk from toe to heel to assess their gross motor coordination and to draw with a crayon or pencil or to play pick-up sticks or jacks to assess their fine motor coordination.

Psychological Domain

Children can usually identify and discuss what improves or worsens their problems. The assessment may be the first time that someone has asked the child to explain his or her view of the problem. It is also a perfect opportunity to discuss any life changes or losses (e.g., death of grandparents or pets, parental divorce) and fears.

Mental Status Examination

The mental status examination combines observation and a clinical interview. The exam is conducted taking into account the child or youth's age and developmental level and presenting problems. The establishment of therapeutic rapport and the nurse's observational skills are the foundations of the assessment. The nurse should note the child's general appearance, including age (actual and apparent), self-care/hygiene, and dress. The nurse also should note the child's nonverbal behaviour, including posture, tone of voice, eye contact, and affect. What is the child or youth's attitude towards the interviewer, others involved, and the interview process itself? How active is the child? Does he or she seem to have difficulty focusing on the interview, sitting still, refraining from impulsive behaviour, and listening without interrupting? Does the child seem underactive, lethargic, distant, or hopeless?

The nurse should observe the child's sentence structure and vocabulary for a general sense of his or her intellectual functioning. Speech patterns, such as rate (overly fast or slow), clarity, and volume, and any speech dysfluencies (e.g., stuttering, halting) are important in screening for mood disorders (e.g., depression, mania), language disorders, psychotic processes, and anxiety disorders.

Asking children general questions about their everyday lives and observing the content and process of their play (e.g., ability to focus on an activity, play themes, boundaries between themselves and others) help to reveal the level of organization and content of their thinking. The nurse should also note the level of speech organization. Young children normally shift subjects rather abruptly, but adolescents should continue with one train of thought before moving to another. The nurse should note any morbid or eccentric thoughts, violent fantasies, and self-deprecating statements that could reflect a poor self-concept. Assessment of preteens and adolescents should address substance use and sexual activity, because responses may provide useful information about high-risk behaviour or harmful substance use. In addition, the nurse should inquire about any obsessions or compulsions (e.g., worries about germs, severe hand-washing).

Developmental Assessment

A developmental assessment is one of the core components of any psychiatric evaluation. Determining psychopathology involves evaluating the extent to which behaviours and experiences are appropriate for a child's age and stage of development. Developmental disorders are commonly associated with psychiatric and behavioural disorders.

Disorders characterized by intellectual disabilities (mild, moderate, severe, and profound forms) are distinguished from disorders that affect specific functional domains (communication disorders, specific learning disorders, attention deficit/hyperactivity disorder, or motor disorders), as well as from an autism spectrum disorder that exhibits a distinctive pattern of deviation from the normal developmental trajectory. The conditions are not mutually exclusive, and comorbidity is common. Therefore, it is necessary to evaluate both the extent to which development is progressing at the right rate and the extent to which it is following the correct path.

It is best to obtain information from a variety of sources (parents, teachers, other professionals) and to use a number of different methods of gauging progress (developmental history, current functioning by report and on specific tests) to ensure an accurate developmental picture. A comprehensive assessment may require input from a range of professionals (psychiatrists, psychologists, speech/

language and occupational therapists, physiotherapists) and entail some form of multidisciplinary evaluation (Bolton, 2001). The key areas for assessment include maturation, psychosocial development, and language.

Maturation

Healthy development of the brain and nervous system during childhood and adolescence provides the foundation for successful functioning throughout life. Such development, called **maturation**, unfolds through sequential and orderly growth processes. These processes are biologically and genetically based but depend on constant interactions with a stimulating and nurturing environment.

If trauma impairs the process of normal biologic maturation, **developmental delays** and disorders that may not be fully reversible can result. Trauma is defined as experiences that overwhelm an individual's capacity to cope. Trauma early in life, including child abuse, neglect, witnessing violence, and disrupted attachment, as well as later traumatic experiences such as violence, accidents, natural disaster, war, sudden unexpected loss, and other life events that are out of one's control can be devastating. There are a number of dimensions of trauma, including magnitude, complexity, frequency, duration, and whether it occurs from an interpersonal or external source (BC Provincial Mental Health and Substance Use Planning Council, 2013).

The nurse can assess for developmental delays by asking questions from specific sections of the mental status examination:

- *Intellectual functioning*: Evaluate the child's creativity, spontaneity, ability to count money and tell time, academic performance, memory, attention, frustration tolerance, and organization.
- *Gross motor functioning*: Ask the child to hop on one foot, throw a ball, walk up and down the hall, and run.
- *Fine motor functioning*: Ask the child to draw a picture or play pick-up sticks.
- *Cognition*: The nurse can evaluate the child's general level of cognition by assessing the child's vocabulary, level of comprehension, drawing ability, and responsiveness to questions. Testing, such as the Wechsler Intelligence Scale for Children (WISC-III), provides measures of intelligence quotient. A psychologist usually performs such tests. The nurse can request cognitive testing if he or she has concerns about developmental delays or learning disabilities.
- *Thinking and perception*: Evaluate level of consciousness; orientation to date, time, and person; thought content; thought process; and judgement.
- *Social interactions and play*: Assess the child's organization, creativity, drawing capacity, and ability to follow rules. Children experiencing developmental delays may remain engaged solely in parallel play instead of moving to reciprocal play. They may consistently play with toys designed for younger children, draw crude body pictures, or display receptive (understanding) or expressive (communicative) language problems.

Psychosocial Development

Assessment of psychosocial development is very important for children with mental health problems. Various theoretical models are available from which to choose; the most commonly used model is Erikson's stages of development (see Chapter 8). When considering this model, the nurse should examine the child's gender and cultural background for appropriateness.

Language

At birth, infants can emit sounds of all languages. Maturation of language skills begins with babbling, or the utterance of simple, spontaneous sounds. By the end of the 1st year, children can make one-word statements, usually naming objects or people in the environment. By age 2 years, they should speak in short, telegraphic sentences consisting of a verb and noun (e.g., "want cookie"). Between ages 2 and 4, vocabulary and sentence structure develop rapidly. In fact, the preschooler's ability to produce language often surpasses motor development, sometimes causing temporary stuttering when the child's mind literally works faster than the mouth.

Language development depends on the complex interaction of physical maturation of the nerves, development of head and neck musculature, hearing abilities, cognitive abilities, exposure to language, educational stimulation, and emotional well-being. Social needs create a natural inclination towards communication, but the child needs reinforcement to develop correct pronunciation, vocabulary, and grammar.

Before a diagnosis of a communication disorder (i.e., impairment in language expression, comprehension, or both) can be made, the child must be tested to rule out hearing, visual, or other neurologic problems. Brain damage, especially to the left hemisphere (dominant for language in most individuals), can seriously impair the development of communication abilities in children. Any child who has experienced brain damage from anoxia at birth, congenital trauma, head injury, infection, tumour, or drug exposure should be closely monitored for signs of a communication disorder. Before the age of 5 years, the brain has amazing plasticity, and sometimes other intact areas of the brain can take over functions of damaged areas, especially with immediate speech therapy. Genetically based disorders such as autism can cause language delays that are sometimes permanent and severe. Children with language delays need particular encouragement to communicate in a way that others can understand, because they tend to compensate by using nonverbal signals (Tanguay, 2000).

The nurse must recognize normal variations in child development and assess lags in the development of vocabulary and sentence structure during the critical preschool years (Table 30-1). Delays in this area can seriously affect other areas, such as cognitive, educational, and social development. Many children who receive psychiatric treatment have speech and language disorders that are sometimes undetected, either leading to or compounding their emotional problems. Cantwell and Baker (1991) studied 600 consecutive child referrals to an urban community clinic for speech and language disorders and found that the psychiatric prevalence was 50% for any diagnosis, 26% for behaviour disorders, and 20% for emotional disorders. The most common individual psychiatric diagnoses were ADHD (19%), oppositional defiant disorder (7%), and anxiety disorders (10%). Beitchman, Cohen, Konstantareas, and Tannock (1996) found that children with receptive language disorders also had a high prevalence of ADHD (59%).

By the time a child is 4.5 years old, he or she will have a vocabulary of approximately 2,000 words and will be able to listen well, and 90% to 100% of his or her speech will be understandable. Most English-speaking children will have mastered all English speech sounds by the age of seven or eight. By school age, a child should be able to speak in complete sentences with minor grammatical errors. A child's language skills continue to develop through the school years. From about age 9 to 19, most language growth occurs in the area of written language (Canadian Association of Speech-Language Pathologists and Audiologists, 2000).

Attachment: The Caregiving Context

Current thinking among researchers and clinicians who assess early emerging social–emotional and behavioural problems holds that children must be evaluated in

Table 30-1	Milestones for Normal Language Development in the Preschool Years
Birth to 3 months	Makes cooing sounds Has different cries for different needs Startles to loud sounds Soothed by calm, gentle voices
4–6 months	Babbles and makes different sounds Makes sounds back when you talk Turns his/her eyes towards a sound source Responds to music or toys that make noise
7–12 months	Waves hi/bye Responds to his/her name Lets you know what he/she wants using sounds and/or actions like pointing Begins to follow simple directions (e.g., Where is your nose?) Localizes correctly to sound by turning his/her head towards it Pays attention when spoken to
By 12–18 months	Uses common words and starts to put words together Enjoys listening to storybooks Points to body parts or pictures in a book when asked Looks at your face when talking to you
By 18–24 months	Understands more words than he/she can say Says two words together (e.g., More juice) Asks simple questions (e.g., What's that?) Takes turns in a conversation
2–3 years	Uses sentences of three or more words most of the time Understands different concepts (e.g., in/on, up/down) Follows two-part directions (e.g., Take the book and put it on the table) Answers simple questions (e.g., Where is the car?) Participates in short conversations
3–4 years	Tells a short story or talks about daily activities Talks in sentences with adult-like grammar Generally speaks clearly so people understand Hears you when you call from another room Listens to TV at the same volume as others Answers a variety of questions

Source: Speech-Language & Audiology Canada. (2014). Speech, language and hearing milestones. Retrieved from www.sac-oac.ca

relation to their primary caregivers (Carter et al., 2004). Although parents usually serve as the primary caregivers, in today's world, other family members (biologically or psychologically related), babysitters, day care, and club activity staff, to name a few, often play a significant role in the development of child attachment and should be assessed. In addition, recognizing that children respond differently in different situations, the routine environments in which the child interacts need to be evaluated. Finally, the nurse considers the contexts of culture, class, ethnicity, language, stigma, and social exclusion on the therapeutic process and negotiates care that is sensitive to these influences as suggested in the CFMHN's *Standards of Psychiatric-Mental Health Nursing* (CFMHN, 2014).

Studies of attachment show that the quality of the emotional bond between the infant and parental or caregiver figures provides the groundwork for future relationships. The need to touch and be close to a parental figure appears biologically driven and has been demonstrated in classic studies of monkeys who bonded with a terrycloth surrogate mother (Harlow, Harlow, & Suomi, 1971). A secure attachment is based on the caretaker's consistent, appropriate response to the infant's attachment behaviours (e.g., crying, clinging, calling, following, protesting). Children who have developed a secure attachment protest when their parents leave them (beginning at about age 6 to 8 months), seek comfort from their parents in unfamiliar situations, and playfully explore the environment in the parent's presence. When parents are unresponsive to a child's attachment behaviours, the child may develop an insecure attachment, evidenced by clinging and lack of exploratory play when the parent is present, intense protest when the parent leaves, and indifference or even hostility (Thompson, 2002) when the parent returns (Ainsworth, 1989).

Secure attachments in early childhood produce cooperative, harmonious parent–child relationships in which the child is responsive to the parents' socialization efforts and likely to adopt the parents' viewpoints, values, and goals. Securely attached young children also socialize competently, are popular with well-acquainted peers during the preschool years, and have warm relationships with important adults in their lives. Securely attached children see themselves and others constructively and have relatively sophisticated emotional and moral understanding (Thompson, 2002).

Although the importance of the parent's responsiveness is unquestionable in determining the development of a secure attachment, the process works both ways. Some babies seem to encourage attachment naturally with their parents by responding positively to holding, cuddling, and comforting behaviours. Others, such as those with developmental delays or autistic disorders, may respond less readily and even reject parental attempts at connecting. The interrelatedness of child behaviour and the

parenting context is not only reciprocal but also extends over time (Sameroff, 2000). The goodness of fit of the caregiving relationship is, at least in part, dependent on infant temperament, parental perceptions, and the parenting style used, which either lessens or heightens the risk for later psychopathology (Seifer, 2000).

Attachment Theories

Bowlby's early studies (Bowlby, 1969) of maternal deprivation formed the initial framework for attachment theory, based on the notion that the infant tends to bond to one primary parental figure, usually the mother. Contemporary nursing theories, such as Barnard's parent–child interaction model (1994), have stressed the importance of the interaction between the child's spontaneous behaviour and biologic rhythms and the mother's ability to respond to cues that signal distress (Baker et al., 1998). The model provides the foundation for the development of several scales measuring dimensions of attachment. These standardized, observational assessment scales use routine parent–child interaction activities involving feeding (the Nursing Child Assessment of Feeding Scale, or NCAFS—76 items, birth to 1 year) and teaching (NCATS scale—73 items, birth to 3 years) to assess a dyad's strengths and limitations during the early years. Areas assessed include contingency (reciprocal communication patterns between caregiver and child), positioning (caregiver's sensitivity to child developmental stage and needs), verbalness (ability to stimulate language development), sensitivity (psychological availability and responsivity to the child), affect (positive or negative quality of communication patterns), and attention regulation (engaging and disengaging behaviours). Such measures can provide informed assessments to nurses in a variety of settings, such as postpartum hospital care, the home (e.g., public health newborn visits), or primary care settings (e.g., mental health nurse in community health centre). Doyle and colleagues (2000) studied 216 parents' attachment style and marital adjustment and found that mothers having an anxious attachment style uniquely predicted that children's attachment to both mother and father would be insecure. Child–mother attachment was associated uniquely with perceived global self-worth and physical appearance for both younger and older children, whereas child–father attachment was associated uniquely with child-perceived school competence and, only for older children, with global self-worth. Although most attachment research has been done with mothers, the father's role in child development has become better understood through research done over the past few decades. Grossman, Grossman, Kindler, and Zimmerman (2008) found that mothers and fathers foster security of attachment and exploration and thus provide psychological security for the child. Security of attachment involves tender loving care, comfort and consolation, and external help with emotion regulation. Security of exploration, based on sensitive support from both mother and father, allows a child to explore to gain knowledge and skills.

Fathers play an important role in children's play, which affects the quality of the child's attachment. Playful interactions involving emotional arousal provide an especially good opportunity to learn how to get along with peers, with fathers' modelling and reinforcing turn-taking, affect regulation, and acceptable ways of competing, as well as the sports skills that facilitate acceptance into peer groups. Fathers are also important as role models who assist in their sons' identity formation and serve as models of gender-appropriate behaviour, particularly around aggressive behaviour (DeKlyen, Speltz, & Greenberg, 1998). Children who have active, committed, and involved fathers generally perform better cognitively, academically, athletically, and socially than do children who do not benefit from such involvement (Biller & Lopez-Kimpton, 1997). It is important that the father is included in the mental health assessment of his child.

Disrupted Attachments

Disrupted attachments resulting from deficits in infant attachment behaviours, lack of responsiveness by caregivers to the child's cues, or both may lead to a diagnosis of reactive attachment disorder, feeding disorder, failure to thrive, or anxiety disorder. A reactive attachment disorder may exist when a child, before the age of 5 years, demonstrates a pattern of markedly disturbed and developmentally inappropriate attachment behaviours in which he or she rarely or minimally turns preferentially to an attachment figure for comfort, support, protection, and nurturance (APA, 2013). O'Connor and Rutter (2000) studied 163 adopted children with early severe deprivation at 4 years of age and again at 6. Longitudinal findings showed that attachment disorder behaviours were correlated with attention and conduct problems. Attachment theory describes a **disorganized attachment** as a consequence of extreme insecurity that results from a disrupted attachment from the primary caregiver (Solomon & George, 1999). Emotional or physical separation can result from parental mental health problems, such as substance use or depression, or from frequently changing caregivers such as may be experienced by a child in foster care. Infants with disorganized attachment appear to be unable to maintain the strategic adjustments in attachment behaviour, represented by organized avoidant or ambivalent attachment strategies, with the result that an alteration in both behavioural and physiologic behaviour occurs. Preschoolers with disorganized attachment manifest behaviours of fear, contradictory behaviour, or disorientation or disassociation in the caregivers' presence.

Temperament and Behaviour

Temperament, as defined in Chapter 27, is a recognizable and distinctive pattern of behaviour, evident during the first few months of life that is believed to be neurobiologically determined.

Temperament traits are early-emerging basic dispositions in the domains of activity, affectivity, attention, and self-regulation (Shiner et al., 2012). Thomas, Chess, and Birch (1968) classified children's temperaments into three broad types. Approximately 40% of the children in the total sample were deemed to be "easy children" who are generally cheerful and adapt quickly to new foods and new people, 10% were "difficult children" who tend to be easily frustrated and contribute to negative social interactions, and 15% were "fearful children" who have relatively low activity levels and tend to withdraw on their first exposure to new stimuli. The remaining 35% did not seem easily classifiable into one of these groups. There have been numerous other investigations to characterize the structure of temperament. Among the currently most widely accepted are Rothbart and Bates' (2006) three dimensions of extraversion/surgency, negative affectivity, and effortful self-control and Kagan and Fox's (2006) two basic dimensions of uninhibited and inhibited, with intermediate phenotype.

Temperamental differences can be observed early in life, suggesting that they are at least partly biologically determined, and patterns of temperament can be correlated with emotional and behavioural problems (Kagan, 1999). One basic aspect of temperament, the tendency to approach or avoid unfamiliar events, appears moderately stable over time and has been associated with distinct, apparently genetically based, physiologic profiles in 2-year-old children (Caspi & Silva, 1995; Schwartz, Snidman, & Kagan, 1999; Snidman, Kagan, Riordan, & Shannon, 1995). When looking at the cerebral asymmetry of the brain in children with inhibited compared with uninhibited temperaments, Davidson (1994) found that inhibited children in the 3rd year of life showed greater electroencephalographic activation on the right frontal area under resting conditions.

An easy temperament can serve as a protective factor against the development of psychopathology. Children with easy temperaments can adapt to change without intense emotional reactions. Difficult temperament places children at high risk for adjustment problems, such as with adjustment to school or bonding with parents.

Temperament has a major influence on the chances that a child may experience psychological problems;

however, temperament is not unchangeable, and environmental influences can change or modify a child's emotional style. Kerr and Mcgehee (1964) found that temperament remained stable from childhood to adulthood only in those children who were extremely inhibited or uninhibited.

The concept of temperament provides an excellent example of the interaction between biologic–genetic factors and environmental factors in producing child psychopathology. Although a child may be born with a particular temperament, longitudinal studies show that the temperament itself is less influential than the "goodness of fit" (Chess & Thomas, 2002) between the child's temperament and the reactions of parents and significant others. Difficult children in particular may evoke negative reactions in parents and teachers, thereby creating environments that exacerbate their biologically based behaviour problems and initiating a vicious cycle. Vanden Boom and Hoeksma (1994) found that infants with difficult temperaments received less sensitive caring than did other children, and parents of 2-year-old children with difficult temperaments often resorted to angry, punitive discipline.

Most research in temperament has focused on the child with a difficult temperament. Studies show that the difficult temperament is correlated with the development of child psychopathology, but only if such temperament persists beyond 3 years of age. Furthermore, the effects of a difficult temperament are more significant in psychiatric populations than in nonpsychiatric populations (Tubman, Lerner, Lerner, & Von Eye, 1992). Extremely difficult temperament shows an association with the development of oppositional and conduct disorders as well as ADHD (Dulcan & Martini, 1999; McClowry, 1995). McClowry developed a school-age temperament inventory for parental report of children 8 to 11 years old. Four empirically derived dimensions were proposed: task persistence, negative reactivity, approach/withdrawal, and energy.

The nurses working with parents of young children need to understand temperament so that they can educate families about this concept, particularly because many parents of children with difficult temperaments blame themselves for their children's behaviour. Parents may compare the child with a difficult temperament to children with easier temperaments and wonder what they have done wrong or attribute negative motives to the child. The nurse can help parents accept biologically based differences in their children and learn to adapt their behaviour to each child's needs to improve "fit." Linder (1993) developed a worksheet to assist the clinician in evaluating the child's temperament during play that is divided into measures of activity level, adaptability, and reactivity (Box 30-5).

Self-Concept

Self-concept is a child's knowledge about her or his own self. For young children, eliciting their view of themselves and the world through projective techniques is helpful. For example, the nurse should ask them what they would wish for if they had three wishes. Answers can be revealing. An inability to wish for anything beyond a nice meal or place to live may reflect hopelessness,

---

BOX 30-5 Social–Emotional Observation Worksheet

Name of child: _____   Date of birth: _____   Age: _____

Name of observer: _____   Discipline or job title: _____   Date of assessment: _____

On the following pages, note specific behaviours that document the child's abilities in the social–emotional categories. Qualitative comments should also be made. The format provided here follows that of the Observation Guidelines for Social–Emotional Development in Transdisciplinary Play-Based Assessment. It may be helpful to refer to the guidelines while completing this form.

1. Temperament
   A. Activity level
      1. Motor activity
      2. Specific times that are particularly active
         a. Beginning, middle, or end
         b. During specific activities
   B. Adaptability
      1. Initial response to stimuli
         a. Persons
         b. Situations
         c. Toys
      2. Demonstration of interest or withdrawal (*circle one*)
         a. Smiling, verbalizing, touching
         b. Crying, ignoring or moving away, seeking security

3. Adjustment time
4. Adjustment time after initially shy or fearful response (*circle one*)
   a. Self-initiation
   b. Adult as base of security
   c. Resists; stays uninvolved
C. Reactivity
   1. Intensity of stimuli for discernible response
   2. Type of stimulation needed to interest child (circle those that apply)
      a. Visual, vocal, tactile, combination
      b. Object, social
   3. Level of affect and energy
   4. Common response mode
   5. Response to frustration

From Linder, T. W. (1993). *Transdisciplinary play-based assessment: A functional approach to working with young children* (Revised ed.). Baltimore, MD: Paul H. Brookes Publishing Co., Inc. Copyright © 1993 by Paul H. Brookes Publishing Co., Inc. Used with permission.

whereas wishes to conquer the world or put one's teacher in jail may indicate feelings of grandiosity. Another technique is to tell a story and ask the child to make up an ending for it. For example, a baby bird fell out of a nest—what happened to it?… or, a little girl went to the mall with her mother but got lost—what happened to her? The nurse may design stories to elicit particular fears or concerns that he or she suspects may be relevant for the individual child.

Drawings also provide an excellent window into the child's internal world (Fig. 30-2). Asking the child to draw a picture of a person can provide data about the child's self-concept, sexual identity, body image, and developmental level. By age 3 years, children should be able to draw some facial features and limbs, but their drawings may have an "x-ray" quality, in which clothing is transparent and the body can be seen underneath. Older children should produce more sophisticated drawings, unless they are resistant to the task. After the child has finished the drawing, the nurse can ask what the person in the drawing is thinking and feeling, using this device to assess the child's mental processes. For example, one adolescent with school phobia drew a person fully dressed, in great detail, but with no feet. When asked about the drawing, he said that the boy could not go anywhere because his mother was afraid to let him leave home.

FIGURE 30-2. Self-portrait of a girl, age 5.

Other ways to assess children's self-concepts include asking them what they want to do when they grow up, what their best subjects are in school, what things they are really good at, and how well-liked they are at school. Before concluding the individual interview with a child, the nurse should always ask whether the child has any other information to share and whether he or she has any questions.

Nurses need to recognize the difference between self-concept and self-esteem. Self-esteem is a child's general attitude about himself. Self-concept and self-esteem have a lot in common and can be similarly assessed. Both are reflective processes that are also influenced by comparison with others around you and how others respond to you. The main difference in self-esteem is the addition of feelings.

Nurses need to be aware that, though relatively rare, some children's sense of self is affected by gender dysphoria, that is, they strongly feel that there is a discrepancy between the sex they were assigned at birth and their own sense of gender. For instance, a girl may feel she is a boy, even though her body is female. This gender confusion can be temporary, but if it causes significant distress for the child or youth, parents may wish for an assessment from a paediatric endocrinologist or from a nurse clinician, psychiatrist or psychologist with expertise in this area.

Risk Assessment

The nurse must ask the child about any suicidal or violent thoughts. The best way to assess these areas is to ask straightforward questions, such as, "Have you ever thought about hurting yourself? Have you ever thought about hurting someone else? Have you ever acted on these thoughts? Have you thought about how you would do it? What did you think would happen if you hurt yourself? Have you ever done anything to hurt yourself before?" Contrary to popular belief, talking about suicide with someone who can help can provide great relief to a child or youth. Further, no age should be exempt from assessment because even young children attempt suicide, and they are capable of violent acts towards other children, adults, and animals. An assessment of lethality and access to means must also be assessed to determine risk. Questions such as "Do you have a plan to hurt yourself (or others)? How would you go about hurting yourself (or others)?" and "Do you have access to guns, knives, pills… (or whatever means the child has identified)?"

The TASR-A or Tool for Assessment of Suicide Risk for Adolescents is a clinical tool that assists in the evaluation of adolescents at imminent risk for suicide. A semi-structured measure, it helps clinicians ensure that in their evaluation of an adolescent the most common risks factors are assessed. It was derived from the adult TASR that was developed for use in emergency room, hospitals, and outpatient settings (Chehil & Kutcher, 2012).

When a child shares the intent to commit a suicidal or violent act, the nurse must remind him or her that the nurse will have to discuss this concern with the parent to keep the child and others safe. It is helpful to ask the child if he or she wants anything in particular to be said to the parent and if he or she wants to be present when the nurse talks with the parents. Although painful, such conversations can serve as an abrupt halt to the charade of happiness that the child may feel forced to portray to the outside world, and often open honest dialogue within a family in which none has occurred for some time. Alternatively, the conversation can sometimes give words to what the family feared but were without the

skills or courage to break the silence. The nurse provides a safe environment for the family to begin to face the issues.

Substance use disorders across the life span account for more deaths, illness, and disabilities than any other preventable health condition. Screening for potential use and abuse of substances is becoming a priority in mental health assessment of adolescents. An interview guide has been adapted from questions on substance use developed by Adlaf (Adlaf & Zdanowicz, 1999) to serve as a useful screen for identifying substance use problems in youth. Other screening tools for clinicians include the SACS: Substances and Choices Scale (Christie et al., 2010) and the CAGE questionnaire for alcohol use (Ewing, 1984). Given that many younger children engage in substance use (see Chapter 26), the nurse should consider assessing younger children as well (Box 30-6).

BOX 30-6 Practice Note 0.1: An Interview Protocol for Reviewing Chemical Use in Youths

As with other topics, questions about substance use are interactive—the answers given determine, to some extent, the subsequent questions. The questions can be used for investigating the use of tobacco, alcohol, and drugs.

Tobacco
- Many youth smoke; do you?
- Do you ever feel you should smoke less?
- Do you wish you could smoke less than you do now?
- Have others bothered you by complaining about your smoking?
- Have you felt bad or guilty because of your smoking?
- Have you thought you had a problem because of your smoking?
- Have you ever had a medical problem as a result of your smoking?
- Have you been in hospital because of your smoking?
- Have you gone to anyone for help for a smoking problem?
- How many of your friends smoke occasionally/regularly?
- How many of your family smoke occasionally/regularly?

Alcohol
- Many youth drink; do you?
- Are you always able to stop drinking when you want?
- Have you felt you should drink less?
- Have others bothered you by complaining about your drinking?
- Have you felt bad or guilty because of your drinking?
- Have you been arrested or warned by police because of your drinking?
- Have you ever had "blackouts" or "flashbacks" due to your drinking?
- Have you drunk in the early morning or drunk to get rid of a hangover?
- Have you ever had any medical problem as a result of your drinking?
- Have you been in hospital because of your drinking?
- Have you gone to anyone for help for a drinking problem?
- How many of your friends drink occasionally/regularly?
- How many of your family drink occasionally/regularly?

Drugs
- Many youth use drugs; do you?
- Do you ever feel concerned about your drug use?
- Are you always able to stop using drugs when you want?
- Have you been arrested or warned by police because of your drug use?
- Have you ever had "blackouts" or "flashbacks" due to your drug use?
- Do you wish you could use fewer drugs than you do now?
- Have you ever had any medical problems as a result of your drug use?
- Have you gone to anyone for help for a drug problem?
- Have you ever seen a doctor or been in the hospital because of your drug use?
- How many of your friends use drugs occasionally/regularly?
- How many of your family use drugs occasionally/regularly?

Adapted from Adlaf, E. M. & Zdanowicz, Y. M. (1999). A cluster-analytic study of substance problems and mental health among street youths. *American Journal of Drug and Alcohol Abuse, 25*(4), 639–660.

Social Domain

Family Relationship

Children depend on adults to create a safe, nurturing, and appropriate environment to support their development. The nurse should assess the quality of the home in terms of its ability to provide appropriate physical space (living space, sleeping arrangements, safety, cleanliness), child care arrangements (age-appropriate supervision), and stimulation (activities or resources), either through a home visit or by discussing these issues with the family. The Home Observation for Measurement of the Environment scale (Caldwell & Bradley, 1984) is a widely used standardized measure to assess the quality of the home environment for fostering child development at any age according to cognitive, social, and emotional growth. It is a 45-item binary (yes/no) scale and best administered in the home through parent interview and observation. The scale addresses six areas: emotional and verbal responsivity of caregiver, avoidance of restriction and punishment, organization of the environment, provision of appropriate play material, caretaker involvement with child, and opportunities for variety in daily stimulation.

When gathering a family history, a genogram and timeline are also useful tools to map family members according to birth order and medical and psychiatric histories; family roles, norms, boundaries, strengths, and subgroups; birth dates, deaths, and relationships; stage in the family cycle; and critical events. To understand fully the family's values, goals, and beliefs, the nurse must consider the family's ethnic, cultural, and economic background throughout the assessment (Carter & McGoldrick, 1999). A comprehensive family assessment should be considered (see Chapter 15).

School Functioning

The child's adjustment to school is also significant. Often, children are referred for a mental health assessment as a result of changes in behaviour at school. Falling grades, loss of interest in normal activities, decreased concentration, or withdrawal from or aggression towards peers may indicate that the child is experiencing emotional problems. It is very important that the nurse obtain signed permission from the parents to talk to the child's teacher for his or her observations of the child. The nurse may want to observe the child in school, if feasible, to see how the child functions there. The parent can request a treatment planning conference in which the teacher, parent, and nurse discuss the child's school performance and plan ways to promote the child's emotional, cognitive, and social functioning in school. For older children, and in particular youth, the nurse should include the child, if even for only a portion of the meeting. It is critically important that children feel that they are consulted and have an opportunity to participate in the planning processes. Although such involvement is not always comfortable or even desired by all parties, it provides formal recognition of each participant involved in the change process. Suggestions emanating from such planning sessions may range from having the child tested (e.g., for learning disabilities) to designing strategies for addressing predictable situations that routinely dissolve into chaos, in which rewards result for each party (e.g., extra computer time for the child, quiet time for the parent) for improved functioning.

Community

Assessing the child's economic status, access (psychologically, geographically, economically) to health and other services, housing and home environment, exposure to environmental toxins (e.g., lead), neighbourhood safety, and exposure to violence is important in understanding the social context of children and families. Such assessment is also important given the evidence from large, longitudinal population-based studies that have demonstrated the links between social disadvantage (socioeconomic, residential stability, community efficacy, and willingness to help neighbours) and mental illness in children (Xue, Levanthal, Brooks-Gunn, & Earls, 2005) and adults (Fryers, Melzer, Jenkins, & Brugha, 2005).

Children and adolescents function better if they are linked to community supports, such as churches, recreational programs, park district programming, and after-school programming. A number of voluntary organizations such as the YWCA or Big Brothers and Big Sisters offer mentoring relationship programs for children in communities. Before making a commitment, a family should visit the organization and talk with staff to ensure that the programs are well organized and monitored by trained staff. The mentor may perform a wide range of services, from taking a child to community events, helping with homework, or talking about how the child can achieve his or her dreams and goals. Some towns offer community-based juvenile justice programs to rehabilitate children who have had an altercation with the legal system. Juvenile justice programs provide support, such as individual and family counselling and pro-social recreational activities; teach children how to make positive choices about spending free time; and closely monitor their behaviours.

Functional Status

Functional status can be evaluated in children and adolescents using various scales. The Global Assessment of Functioning (GAF) scale (APA, 2000), which tallied behaviours related to school, peers, activity level, mood, speech, family relationships, behavioural problems, self-care skills, and self-concept on a scale of 0 to 100, is no longer recommended by the American Psychiatric Association because of a lack of clarity, questionable psychometrics in routine practice, and concerns about inter-rater reliability (APA, 2013). Instead, in its 5th edition of the *Diagnostic and Statistical Manual of Mental Disorders (DSM-5)*, the American Psychiatric Association (APA) (2013) recommends the use of the World Health Organization Disability Assessment Scale Version 2.0 (WHODAS 2.0; WHO, 2011). The WHODAS 2.0 is a generic assessment instrument for health and disability used across all diseases, including mental, neurologic, and addictive disorders. It is a 36-item self-reporting scale that is applicable in both clinical and general population settings. It produces standardized disability levels and profiles and is applicable across cultures, in all *adult* populations. There is a direct conceptual link to the International Classification of Functioning, Disability and Health. The WHODAS 2.0 covers six domains: cognition, mobility, self-care, getting along, life activities, and participation. The WHODAS for Children and Adolescents has been developed and field tested (Canino, Fisher, Alegria, & Bird, 2013) but, as this textbook goes to press, is not yet available. Until it is, the GAF will probably be the preferred scale of functioning of mental health clinicians.

Stresses and Coping Behaviours

Biologic, behavioural, and personality predispositions, family, and community environment may affect a child's ability to cope with stressful life events. Stressful experiences for children include the death of a loved person or pet, parental divorce, violence, physical illness (especially chronic illness), mental illness, social isolation, racial discrimination, neglect, and physical and sexual abuse. The Difficult Life Circumstances scale (Barnard, 1989) is a 28-item self-report measure, administered in interview format to a parent, to identify the existence of chronic family problems in a variety of activities of daily life (e.g., partner in jail, financial problems, partner or child abuse).

Spiritual Domain

Nurses and other health professionals are increasingly aware that spiritual assessment is an important aspect of the assessment of children and adolescents. Although adult spiritual assessment tools exist, to date no validated instrument exists for use with children and adolescents. Rubin and colleagues (2009) assessed the applicability of two adult scales (the Spiritual Involvement and Beliefs Scale; the Spirituality Well-Being Scale) with chronically ill and healthy adolescents and their parents. The conclusion made was that there is a need to develop a specific spirituality scale for adolescents, as

less than half the adolescents in the study considered either scale as an effective measure of their spiritual well-being. Parents, too, did not feel the scales to be adequate measures of their own spirituality. Measuring spirituality, even with adults, continues to have its challenges and limits.

Spiritual beliefs (the way spirituality is understood by an individual) are shaped by experience, family, friends, community, culture, and religious affiliation. With children and adolescents, in particular, developmental level is a significant factor. This can be seen in children's response to loss, for instance (see Chapter 29). In addressing the spiritual domain with children and adolescents, openness and receptivity to their questions and concerns, as well as sensitivity to their level of understanding, are important. Nurses can use stories to open discussion about the way a child or an adolescent understands and gives meaning to their experiences. There is a wide range of classic and contemporary literature (across levels of development) that address spiritual concerns such as loneliness, illness, injury, disability, and death. For instance, *Charlotte's Web* by White (1952) and *The Ten Good Things about Barney* by Viorst (1972) are stories about the death of beloved animals that can help young children to express themselves about death and dying. Adolescents may be particularly hesitant to raise their spiritual concerns unless "an open, acceptable attitude and atmosphere" is available, and they feel safe and comfortable in revealing their feelings and beliefs (Callaghan, 2005, p. 115). Importantly, paediatric nurses describe approaching the spiritual domain primarily at the family level (Whitehead, 2008). There is recognition that establishing a relationship with the family, as well as the child, is foundational to understanding spiritual beliefs, values, and needs (see Chapter 5).

Spiritual assessment, including the expressed values and beliefs of children, youth, and families, should be appropriately documented so that other health professionals can be involved in spiritual care (Callaghan, 2005). Pastoral care services are a resource in many health services, and representatives of the family's religious or cultural community may be utilized as a resource under the family's direction. For example, Aboriginal elders and/or cultural workers have been described by paediatric nurses as being very helpful in the provision of spiritual care to Aboriginal families (Whitehead, 2008).

Evaluation of Child Abuse

Thousands of Canadian children suffer maltreatment (intentional physical or emotional abuse, neglect, or sexual exploitation) each year as the result of their parents' action or inaction (Trocmé, McPhee, & Tam, 1995;

Wolfe, 1998). The 2008 Canadian Incidence Study of Reported Child Abuse and Neglect (Trocmé, McPhee, Tam, 2010) revealed an incidence rate of 16.19 substantiated investigations per 1,000 children in 2008. The three most common categories of substantiated maltreatment were exposure to domestic violence (31%), neglect (28%), and physical abuse (15%). Emotional maltreatment accounted for another 6% of cases, whereas sexual abuse cases represented only 2% of all substantiated investigations. Most referrals (68%) came from professionals (e.g., police and school). Nevertheless, as a Senate report on the sexual exploitation of children in Canada (i.e., prostitution, child pornography, luring of children over the Internet, and any sexual abuse) noted: "The sexual exploitation of children is a deeply rooted reality in too many Canadian homes, families and communities" (Jaffer & Brazeau, 2011, p. vi).

The effects of family-engendered maltreatment can result in a lifetime of debilitating bio/psycho/social/spiritual problems. A maltreated child may have difficulty managing emotions (Campbell, 1995), communicating effectively (Browne & Saqi, 1988), developing satisfying relationships with others (Crittenden, 1996), and learning in productive ways (Aber, Allen, Carlson, & Cicchetti, 1989; Doherty, 1997). Attention must be paid to ways of building child competence, resilience, and health potential (i.e., autonomous self-regulation) (Wolfe, 1998) than simply on issues of protection and deviance.

Although the cause of child abuse is not absolutely clear, best thinking suggests that an ecologic model better captures the influencing factors of child abuse and neglect, because it understands the child within the context of the family and the larger community (Wachtel, 1999). Such a model uses a broad multifactorial approach for assessment. Such assessment takes into consideration the child's current developmental level and understands that compromises to his or her early development may continue in various ways through all the developmental stages that follow. It is child-centred (child welfare is critical), family-focused (most child abuse occurs within the family), has a community context (forms a key part of the child's environment), and is culturally sensitive (the nurse must be culturally competent). It also involves gathering information from a number of stakeholders and ensures that information is gathered in a coordinated way to maximize the integrity of the data collection.

Although a number of assessment tools exist, three general areas should be addressed in any assessment (English, 1996):

1. Are the child's immediate circumstances unsafe? Does the child have to be taken into care or removed to a safe place?

2. For current cases, what is the assessed risk of repeat abuse? What are the issues that merit intervention on a priority basis?

3. For ongoing cases, to what extent are interventions working? What is the current situation of the child, the family, and any substitute care arrangement?

Nurses need to understand the forensic implications of an assessment of a child for abuse. As these implications begin when the child is first asked about abuse, immediate referral to or consultation with a nurse or physician trained in this area is recommended. Nursing professionals who regularly interview children who have been abused may have special training in the use of anatomically correct dolls to obtain information about the abuse. They know to use the same language and vocabulary that the child uses to describe the abuse or anatomical terms and to ask nonleading questions.

If a child reports abuse, the nurse has a legal and ethical responsibility to report the abuse to the child protection agencies and to follow their organizational policies and procedures. The laws governing such reporting are at the provincial level and need to be known by nurses. The CFMHN's *Standards of Psychiatric-Mental Health Nursing* (CFMHN, 2014) identifies a nurse's role in assessing clients for the risk of victim violence and abuse.

In the case of family-perpetrated child abuse, the nurse should consider very carefully whether the report will be made *with* or *without* the knowledge of the child's family. The nurse should consider factors such as whether she or he has developed a relationship with the family, the degree of imminent risk to the child, and whether she or he is likely to continue working with the family. The reality is that maltreatment is a complex phenomenon, and families tend to stay connected with services for long periods. Finding ways to build a positive working relationship with families becomes a crucial, yet challenging, goal for nurses. When nurses are open, honest, and direct, families know what to expect. If nurses have an established working relationship with families, they can often share their specific observations about parenting practices and the need to involve child protection services. Nurses might also invite the family to make the call themselves with the nurse's support. For example, the nurse might say, "I know that you love your child but your actions are causing harm … I don't think your child is safe…. He needs help…. I need to call child protection services to get some help for your family. I know this is scary for you … but you could take an important step in the right direction by making the first call and asking for help for your child and you. I would be happy to support you while you make that call right now… before I make my call." See Chapter 37 for further understanding of caring for abused persons.

Resilience

Resilience refers to achieving positive outcomes despite challenging or threatening circumstances, coping successfully with traumatic experiences, and avoiding negative paths linked with risks (Zolkoski & Bullock, 2012). Risk factors inhibit resilience while protective factors promote it. The number of stresses that a child experiences, the supports that the child has in place, and the child's developmental stage influences his or her ability to cope with stressors. Nurses can assess for biologic and environmental risk factors. These include congenital defects, low birth weights, poverty, education level of parents, negative life experiences such as abuse or neglect, minority status, and racial discrimination (Zolkoski & Bullock, 2012). Protective factors identified include the following:

- Individual attributes, such as problem-solving skills, sense of self-efficacy, accurate processing of interpersonal cues, positive social orientation, and self-regulation
- A supportive family environment, including attachment with adults in the family, low family conflict, and supportive relationships
- Environmental supports, including those that reinforce and support coping efforts and recognize and reward competence

Children who show resilience in the face of adversity typically have good intellectual functioning, positive and easygoing temperament, positive social orientation, strong self-efficacy, achievement orientation with high expectations, positive self-concept, faith, high rate of involvement in productive activities, close affective relationship with at least one caregiver, effective parenting, access to positive extrafamilial models, and strong connections with prosocial institutions (Doll & Lyon, 1998). A longitudinal study of the determinants and processes of mental disorders in adolescence identified that self-esteem, active coping, parental warmth, and peer acceptance, in different combinations, acted as protective factors against internalizing and externalizing mental disorders (Steinhausen, 2006).

SUMMARY OF KEY POINTS

■ Mental health assessment of children and adolescents includes evaluating the child's biologic, psychological, social, and spiritual factors.

■ Assessment of children and adolescents differs from assessment of adults in that the nurse must consider the child's developmental level, specifically addressing the child's language, cognitive, social, and emotional skills. Establishing a treatment alliance and building rapport are essential to obtaining a good mental health history.

■ The mental status examination includes observations and questions about the child's appearance, speech, language, vocabulary, orientation, knowledge base (including reading, writing, and math skills), attention level, activity level, memory, social skills, peer relationships, relationship to interviewer, mood, affect, suicidal or homicidal tendencies, thinking (presence or absence of hallucinations or delusions), substance use, and behaviours.

■ Assessment of the child and caregiver together provides important information regarding child–parent attachment and parenting practices.

■ The three main types of temperament include the easy temperament, difficult temperament, and slow-to-warm-up temperament. Temperament can be evaluated by assessing the child's sleep and eating habits, mood, emotional intensity, and responses to new stimuli.

■ A child's self-concept can be evaluated using tools such as play, stories, asking three wishes, and asking the child to draw a picture of himself or herself.

■ If a child reveals suicidal ideation in the interview, the nurse must determine whether the child has a plan, let the parent know the child is suicidal, and make a plan to keep the child safe, including consideration of inpatient hospitalization.

■ If a child reports to the nurse neglect or physical or sexual abuse, the nurse must by law report the child's disclosure to Child Protection Services.

■ Protective factors that promote resiliency in children are active coping and the ability to solve problems, a sense of self-efficacy, self-esteem, accurate processing of social cues, supportive family environment, peer acceptance, and environmental supports that promote coping efforts and recognize and reward competence.

CRITICAL THINKING CHALLENGES

1 An adolescent is hostile and refuses to talk in an interview. How would you respond?
2 What are some strategies for building rapport with children?
3 A child reports that he or she is suicidal. What would be your next question? What measures would you take next?
4 What are some techniques and media for obtaining information about a child's inner world, such as self-concept, sexual identity, body image, and developmental level?
5 Explain why it may be detrimental to interview a child in front of his or her parent. Why may it be detrimental to interview a parent in front of his or her child? Why is it useful, in most cases, to ensure that both parent and child are also interviewed together?

6 Why is obtaining the mental health histories of parents relevant to the child's mental health assessment?

7 What are useful tools in obtaining a family history from the child and parent?

8 Anatomically correct dolls are used in what specific type of child assessment?

9 Describe five characteristics of the resilient child.

REFERENCES

Aber, J. L., Allen, J. P., Carlson, V., & Cicchetti, D. (1989). The effects of maltreatment on development during early childhood: Recent studies and their theoretical, clinical, and policy implications. In D. Cicchetti & V. Carlson (Eds.), *Child maltreatment: Theory and research on the causes and consequences of child abuse and neglect* (pp. 570–619). New York, NY: Cambridge University Press.

Achenbach, T. M. & Edelbrock, C. (1983). *The child behavior checklist: Manual for the child behavior checklist and revised child behavior profile*. Burlington, VT: Queen City Printers.

Adlaf, E. M. & Zdanowicz, Y. M. (1999). A cluster-analytic study of substance problems and mental health among street youths. *American Journal of Drug and Alcohol Abuse, 25*(4), 639–660.

Ainsworth, M. D. S. (1989). Attachments beyond infancy. *American Psychologist, 44*, 709–716.

American Psychiatric Association. (2000). *Diagnostic and statistical manual of mental disorders* (4th ed., Text revision). Washington, DC: Author.

American Psychiatric Association (APA). (2013). *Diagnostic and statistical manual of mental disorders* (5th ed.). Washington, DC: Author.

Baker J. K., Borchers, D. A., Cochran, D. T., Kaltofen, K. G., Orcutt, N., Peacock, J. A., et al. (1998). Kathryn E. Barnard: Parent–child interaction model. In A. Marriner-Tomey (Ed.), *Nursing theorists and their work* (4th ed.), (pp. 423–438). St. Louis, MO: Mosby.

Barnard, K. E. (1989). *Difficult life circumstances manual*. Seattle, WA: NCAST Publications, University of Washington, School of Nursing.

Barnard, K. E. (1994). The Barnard model. In G. Sumner & A. Spitz (Eds.), *NCAST caregiver/parent–child interaction feeding manual* (pp. 6–14). Seattle, WA: NCAST Publications, University of Washington, School of Nursing.

BC Provincial Mental Health and Substance Use Planning Council. (2013). Trauma-informed practice guide. Retrieved from http://bccewh.bc.ca/publications-resources/documents/TIP-Guide-May2013.pdf

Beitchman, J. H., Cohen, N. J., Konstantareas, M. M., & Tannock, R. (Eds.). (1996). *Language, learning, and behavior disorders: Developmental, biological, and clinical perspectives*. New York, NY: Cambridge University Press.

Biller, H. & Lopez-Kimpton, J. (1997). The father and the school-aged child. In M. Lamb (Ed.), *The role of the father in child development* (3rd ed., pp. 143–161). New York, NY: Wiley & Sons.

Bolton, P. (2001). Developmental assessment. *Advances in Psychiatric Treatment, 7*, 32–40.

Bowlby, J. (1969). *Attachment (Vol. 1 of Attachment and loss)*. New York, NY: Basic Books.

Breton, J. J., Plante, M. A., & St-Georges, M. (2005). Challenges facing child psychiatry in Quebec at the dawn of the 21st century. *Canadian Journal of Psychiatry, 50*(4), 203–212.

Brooks, S. (2004). The Kutcher adolescent depression scale. *Child and Adolescent Psychopharmacology News, 9*(5), 4–6.

Brooks, S. & Kutcher, S. (2004). The Kutcher generalized anxiety disorder scale for adolescents: Assessment of its evaluative properties over the course of a 16-week pediatric psychopharmacotherapy trial. *Journal of Child and Adolescent Psychopharmacology, 14*(2), 273–286.

Browne, K. & Saqi, S. (1988). Approaches to screening for child abuse and neglect. In K. Browne, C. Davies, & P. Stratton (Eds.), *Early prediction and prevention of child abuse* (pp. 57–85). Toronto, ON: John Wiley & Sons.

Caldwell, B. & Bradley, R. (1984). *Home observation for measurement of the environment*. Little Rock, AK: University of Little Rock at Arkansas.

Callaghan, D. M. (2005). The influence of spiritual growth on adolescents' initiative and responsibility for self-care. *Pediatric Nursing, 31*(2), 91–115.

Campbell, S. (1995). Behaviour problems in pre-school children: A review of recent research. *Journal of Child Psychology and Psychiatry, 36*, 113–149.

Canadian Association of Speech-Language Pathologists and Audiologists. (2000). School age speech & language development fact sheet. Retrieved from http://www.saslpa.ca/school_age_speech_and_language.pdf

Canadian Federation of Mental Health Nurses. (2014). *The Canadian standards for psychiatric-mental health nursing* (4th ed.). Toronto, ON: Author.

Canino, G.J., Fisher, P.W., Alegria, M. & Bird, H. R. (2013). Assessing child impairment in functioning in different contexts: Implications for use of services and the classification of psychiatric disorders. *Open Journal of Medical Psychology, 2*, 29–34.

Cantwell, D. P. & Baker, L. (1991). *Psychiatric and developmental disorders in children with communication disorders*. Washington, DC: American Psychiatric Press.

Carter, B. & McGoldrick, M. (1999). *The expanded family life cycle: Individual, family, and social perspectives* (3rd ed.). Needham Heights, MA: Allyn & Bacon.

Carter, A. S., Briggs-Gowan, M. J., & Davis, N. O. (2004). Assessment of young children's social-emotional development and psychopathology: Recent advances and recommendations for practice. *Journal of Child Psychology and Psychiatry, 45*(1), 109–134.

Caspi, A. & Silva, P. A. (1995). Temperamental qualities at age 3 predict personality traits in young adulthood: Longitudinal evidence from a birth cohort. *Child Development, 66*, 486–498.

Cepeda, C. (2000). *The concise guide to the psychiatric interview of children and adolescents*. Washington, DC: American Psychiatric Press.

Chess, S. & Thomas, A. (2002). Temperament and its clinical applications. In M. Lewis (Ed.), *Child and adolescent psychiatry: A comprehensive textbook* (3rd ed.). Philadelphia, PA: Lippincott Williams & Wilkins.

Chehil, S. & Kutcher, S. (2012). *Suicide risk management: A manual for health professionals* (2nd ed.). Oxford, MS: Wiley-Blackwell.

Christie, G., Marsh, R., Sheridan, J., Wheeler, A., Suaalii-Sauni, T., Black, S., & Butler, R. (2010). The substances and choices scale manual. Retrieved from http://www.sacsinfo.com/docs/SACSusermanual2010.pdf

Costello, E. J., Egger, H., & Angold, A. (2005). Ten-year research update review: The epidemiology of child and adolescent psychiatric disorders. I. Methods and public health burden. *Journal of American Academy of Child and Adolescent Psychiatry, 44*(10), 972–986.

Crittenden, P. M. (1996). Research on maltreating families: Implications for intervention. In J. Briere, L. Berliner, A. Bulkey, C. Jenny, & T. Reid (Eds.), *The APSAC handbook on child maltreatment* (pp. 158–174). Thousand Oaks, CA: Sage.

Davidson, R. J. (1994). Asymmetric brain function, affective style, and psychopathology. *Development and Psychopathology, 6*, 741–758.

DeKlyen, M., Speltz, M., & Greenberg, M. (1998). Fathering and early onset conduct problems: Positive and negative parenting, father–son attachment, and the marital context. *Clinical Child and Family Psychology Review, 1*, 3–21.

Doherty, G. (1997). *Zero to six: The basis for school readiness*. Ottawa, ON: Human Resources Development Canada, Applied Research Branch, Strategic Policy.

Doll, B. & Lyon, M. A. (1998). Risk and resilience: Implications for delivery of educational and mental health services in the schools. *School Psychology Review, 27*(3), 348–363.

Doyle, A., Markiewicz, D., Brendgen, M., Lieberman, M., & Voss, K. (2000). Child attachment security and self-concept: Associations with mother and father attachment style and marital quality. *Merrill-Palmer Quarterly, 46*(3), 514–539.

Dulcan, M. & Martini, D. R. (1999). *Child and adolescent psychiatry*. Washington, DC: American Psychiatric Press.

English, D. T. (1996). *The promise and reality of risk assessment: Protecting children*. Ottawa, ON: Public Health Agency of Canada. Retrieved from http://www.phac-aspc.gc.ca/ncfv-cnivf/familyviolence/html/nfntsptprevention_e.html

Erikson, E. (1968). *Identity, youth and crisis*. New York, NY: Norton.

Ewing, J. A. (1984). Detecting alcoholism: The CAGE questionnaire. *Journal of the American Medical Association, 252*(14), 1905–1907.

Forgatch, M. & Patterson, G. (1989). *Parents and adolescents: Living together (Part 2: Family problem-solving)*. Eugene, OR: Castalia Publishing Company.

Fryers, T., Melzer, D., Jenkins, R., & Brugha T. (2005). The distribution of the common mental disorders: Social inequalities in Europe. *Clinical Practice in Epidemiology and Mental Health, 1*, 14.

Goodman, W. K., Price, L. H., Rasmussen, S. A., Mazure, J. C., Fleischmann, R. L., Hill, C. L., ... Charney, D. S. (1989). The Children's Yale-Brown Obsessive Compulsive Scale (CYBOCS). I. Development, use, and reliability. *Archives of General Psychiatry, 46*, 1006–1011.

Grollman, E. A. (1990). *Talking about death: A dialogue between parent and child* (3rd ed.). Boston, MA: Beacon Press.

Grossman, K., Grossman, K. E., Kindler, H., & Zimmerman, P. (2008). A wider view of attachment and exploration: The influence of mothers and fathers on the development of psychological security from infancy to young adulthood. In J. Cassidy & P. Shaver (Eds.), *Handbook of attachment: Theory, research, and clinical applications* (2nd ed.), (pp. 857–879). New York, NY: Guilford Press.

Harlow, H. F., Harlow, M. K., & Suomi, S. J. (1971). From thought to therapy: Lessons from a private laboratory. *American Scientist*, *59*(5), 538–549.

Howes, C. & Matheson, C. (1992). Sequences in the development of competent play with peers: Social and social pretend play. *Developmental Psychology*, *28*(5), 961–974.

Jaffer, M. S. B. & Brazeau, P. (2011). *The sexual exploitation of children in Canada: The Need for national action.* Retrieved from Parliament of Canada website: http://www.parl.gc.ca/content/SEN/Committee/411/ridr/rep03nov11-e.pdf

Jellnick, M., Patel, B. P., & Froehle, M. C. (2003). Bright futures in practice: Mental health (Vol. 1, practice guide and Vol. 2, tool kit). *Journal of the American Academy of Child and Adolescent Psychiatry*, *1–2*, 507–508.

Kagan, J. (1999). The concept of behavioral inhibition. In L. Schmidt & J. Schulkin (Eds.), *Extreme fear, shyness, and social phobia: Origins, biological mechanisms, and clinical outcomes. Series in affective science.* New York, NY: Oxford University Press.

Kagan, J. & Fox, N. A. (2006). Biology, culture, and temperamental biases. In W. Damon & N. Lerner (Eds.), *Social, emotional, and personality development* (6th ed.), (pp. 167–255). New York, NY: Wiley.

Kerr W. A. & Mcgehee, E. M. (1964). Creative temperament as related to aspects of strategy and intelligence. *Journal of Social Psychology*, *62*, 211–216.

Kovacs, M. (1982). *Children's depression inventory*. North Tonawanda, NY: Multi-Health Systems.

Kutcher, S. & McLuckie, A.; for the Child and Youth Advisory Committee, Mental Health Commission of Canada. (2010). *Evergreen: A child and youth mental health framework for Canada*. Calgary, AB: Mental Health Commission of Canada.

LeBuffe, P. A. & Naglieri, J. A. (1999). *Devereux early childhood assessment. The Devereux Foundation*. Lewisville, NC: Kaplan Press.

LeBuffe, P. A. & Naglieri, J. A. (2003). *The Devereux early childhood assessment clinical form (DECA)*. Lewisville, NC: Kaplan Press.

Lidz, C. S. (2003). *Early childhood assessment*. Hoboken, NJ: Wiley & Sons.

Linder, T. W. (1993). *Transdisciplinary play-based assessment: A functional approach to working with young children* (Rev ed.). Baltimore, MD: Paul H. Brookes Publishing.

March, J. (1997). *Multidimensional anxiety scale for children*. North Tonawanda, NY: Multi-Health Systems.

McClowry, S. G. (1995). The development of the School-Age Temperament Inventory. *Merrill-Palmer Quarterly*, *41*(3), 271–285.

Murphy, J. M., Ichinose, C., Hicks, R. C., Kingdon, D., Crist-Whitzel, J., Jordan, P., ... Jellinek, M. S. (1996). Utility of the pediatric symptom checklist as a psychosocial screen to meet the federal Early and Periodic Screening, Diagnosis, and Treatment (EPSDT) standards: A pilot study. *Journal of Pediatrics*, *129*, 864–869.

National Cancer Institute, US National Institutes of Health. (2005). *Grief, bereavement, and coping with loss*. Retrieved from http://www.cancer.gov/cancertopics/pdq/supportivecare/bereavement/Patient/page1/AllPages

O'Connor, T. & Rutter, M. (2000). Attachment disorder behavior following early severe deprivation: Extension and longitudinal follow-up. *Journal of the American Academy of Child and Adolescent Psychiatry*, *39*(6), 709–712.

Research Unit on Pediatric Psychopharmacology (RUPP) Anxiety Study Group (2002). The pediatric anxiety rating scale (PARS): Development and psychometric properties. *Journal of the American Academy of Child and Adolescent Psychiatry*, *41*, 1061–1069.

Reynolds, C. R. & Kamphouse, R. W. (1998). *Behavior assessment system for children (BASC)*. Circle Pines, MN: American Guidance Service.

Rothbart, M. K. & Bates, J. E. (2006). Temperament. In W. Damon & N. Lerner (Eds.), *Social, emotional, and personality development* (6th ed.), (pp. 99–166). New York, NY: Wiley.

Rubin, D., Dodd, M., Desai, N., Pollock, B., & Graham-Pole, J. (2009). Spirituality in well and ill adolescents and their parents: The use of two assessment scales. *Pediatric Nursing*, *35*(1), 37–42.

Sameroff, A. J. (2000). Dialectical processes in developmental psychopathology. In A. J. Sameroff, M. L. Lewis, & S. M. Miller (Eds.), *Handbook of developmental psychopathology* (2nd ed.), (pp. 23–40). New York, NY: Kluwer Academic.

Sattler, J. (1998). *Clinical and forensic interviewing of children and families*. San Diego, CA: Jerome Sattler Publisher.

School-Based Mental Health and Substance Abuse (SBMHSA) Consortium. (2013). *School-based mental health in Canada: A Final Report.* Mental Health Commission of Canada. Calgary, AB: Author. Available at www.mentalhealthcommission.ca

Schwartz, C., Snidman, N., & Kagan, J. (1999). Adolescent social anxiety as an outcome of inhibited temperament in childhood. *Journal of the American Academy of Child and Adolescent Psychiatry*, *38*(8), 1008–1015.

Seifer, R. (2000). Temperament and goodness of fit: Implications for developmental psychopathology. In A. J. Sameroff, M. L. Lewis, & S. M. Miller (Eds.), *Handbook of developmental psychopathology* (2nd ed.), (pp. 257–276). New York, NY: Kluwer Academic.

Shave, D. & Shave, B. (1989). *Early adolescence and search for self: A developmental perspective*. New York, NY: Praeger Publishers.

Shiner, R. L., Buss, K. A., McClowry, S. G., Putnam, S. P., Saudino, K. J., & Zentner, M. (2012). What is temperament *now*? Assessing the progress in temperament research on the twenty-fifth anniversary of Goldsmith et al. *Child Development Perspectives*, *6*(4), 436–444.

Snidman, N., Kagan, J., Riordan, L., & Shannon, D. C. (1995). Cardiac function and behavioural reactivity. *Psychopathology*, *32*, 199–207.

Solomon, J. & George, C. (1999). *Attachment disorganization*. New York, NY: Guilford Press.

Speech-Language & Audiology Canada. (2014). Speech, language and hearing milestones. Retrieved from www.sac-oac.ca

Squires, J., Bricker, D., & Twombly, E. (2002). *The ASQ: SE user's guide*. Baltimore, MD: Paul H. Brookes Publishing.

Steinhausen, H. C. (2006). Developmental psychopathology in adolescence: Findings from a Swiss study–the NAPE Lecture 2005. *Acta Psychiatrica Scandinavica*, *113*(1), 6–12.

Stiffman, A. R., Hadley-Ives, E., Dore, P., Polgar, M., Horvath, V. E., Striley, C., & Elze, D. (2000). Youths' access to mental health services: The role of providers' training, resource connectivity, and assessment of need. *Mental Health Services Research*, *2*(3), 141–154.

Sturm, R., Ringel, J. S., & Andreyeva, T. (2003). Geographic disparities in children's mental health care. *Pediatrics*, *112*(4), e308.

Swanson, J. M. (1983). *The SNAP-IV*. Irvine, CA: University of California, Irvine.

Tanguay, P. (2000). Pervasive developmental disorders: A 10-year review. *Journal of the American Academy of Child and Adolescent Psychiatry*, *39*, 1079–1095.

Taylor, K. M., Menarchek-Fetkovich, M., & Day, C. (2000). The play history interview. In K. Gitlin-Weiner, A. Sandgrund, & C. Scafer (Eds.), *Play diagnosis and assessment* (2nd ed.). New York, NY: Wiley.

Thomas, A., Chess, S., & Birch, H. G. (1968). *Temperament and behavior disorders in childhood*. New York, NY: New York University Press.

Thompson, R. (2002). Attachment theory and research. In M. Lewis (Ed.), *Child and adolescent psychiatry: A comprehensive textbook* (3rd ed.). Philadelphia, PA: Lippincott Williams & Wilkins.

Trad, P. (1989). *The pre-school child assessment, diagnosis and treatment*. New York, NY: Wiley.

Trainor, J., Pomeroy, E., & Pape, B. (2004). *A framework for support* (3rd ed.). Toronto, ON: Canadian Mental Health Association.

Trocmé, N., McPhee, D., & Tam, K. K. (1995). Child abuse and neglect in Ontario: Incidence and characteristics. *Child Welfare*, *74*, 563–586.

Trocmé, N., Fallon, B., MacLaurin, B., Sinha, V., Black, T., Fast, E., ... Holroyd, J. (2010). *Canadian Incidence Study of reported child abuse and neglect—2008: Major findings*. Ottawa, ON: Public Health Agency of Canada.

Tubman, J. G., Lerner, R. M., Lerner, J. V., & Von Eye, A. (1992). Temperament and adjustment in young adulthood: A 15-year longitudinal analysis. *American Journal of Orthopsychiatry*, *62*, 564–574.

Vanden Boom, D. C. & Hoeksma, J. B. (1994). The effect of infant irritability on mother–infant interaction: A growth curve analysis. *Developmental Psychology*, *30*, 581–590.

Viorst, J. (1972). *The ten good things about Barney*. New York, NY: Simon & Schuster.

Wachtel, A. (1999). *"State of the art" in child abuse prevention*. Prepared for the Family Violence Prevention Unit, Health Canada. Cat. H72–21/151–1997E. Ottawa, ON: Minister of Public Works and Government Services Canada, National Clearing House on Family Violence.

Waddell, C., McEwan, K., Shepherd, C. A., Offord, D. R., & Hua, J. M. (2005). A public health strategy to improve the mental health of Canadian children. *Canadian Journal of Psychiatry*, *50*(4), 226–233.

Wass, H. & Corr, C. A. (1984). *Childhood and death*. Washington, DC: Hemisphere Publishing.

White, E. B. (1952). *Charlotte's web*. New York, NY: HarperCollins.

Whitehead, M. (2008). *Pediatric nurses' perspectives of spirituality and spiritual care within nurse-patient relationships: An interpretive description.* University of Alberta, Canada: Unpublished Master Thesis.

Wolfe, D. A. (1998). *Prevention of child abuse and neglect.* Ottawa, ON: Health Canada.

World Health Organization. (2011). WHO disability assessment schedule 2.0. Retrieved from http://www.who.int/classifications/icf/whodasii/en/index.html

Wright, L. M. & Leahey, M. (2005). The three most common errors in family nursing: How to avoid or sidestep. *Journal of Family Nursing, 11*(2), 90–101.

Xue, Y., Leventhal, T., Brooks-Gunn, J., & Earls, F. J. (2005). Neighborhood residence and mental health problems of 5- to 11-year-olds. *Archives of General Psychiatry, 62*(5), 554–563.

Zolkoski, S. M. & Bullock, L. M. (2012). Resilience in children and youth: A review. *Children and Youth Services Review, 34*(12), 2295–2303.

31 Psychiatric Disorders Diagnosed in Children and Adolescents

Lorelei Faulkner-Gibson, Kimberly Wong, and Wendy Austin
Adapted from the chapters "Psychiatric Disorders Diagnosed in Children and Adolescents" by Julia Gajewski-Noel and by Lawrence Scahill, Vanya Hamrin, and Catherine Gray Deering

KEY CONCEPTS

- attention
- autism spectrum disorder
- developmental delay
- hyperactivity
- impulsiveness

LEARNING OBJECTIVES

After studying this chapter, you will be able to:

- Identify the disorders usually first diagnosed in infancy, childhood, or adolescence, according to the *Diagnostic and Statistical Manual of Mental Disorders*, 5th ed. (*DSM-5*).
- Identify the bio/psycho/social/spiritual dimensions of the neurodevelopmental disorders of childhood.
- Discuss the epidemiology, aetiology, psychopharmacologic interventions, and nursing care of children with disorders of mood and anxiety, including trauma disorders (e.g., posttraumatic stress disorder).
- Relate the assessment data of children with attention deficit hyperactivity disorder to the development of nursing diagnoses, interventions, and evaluation of outcomes.
- Compare the disruptive, impulse control, and conduct disorders: oppositional defiant disorder and conduct disorder.
- Discuss the epidemiology, aetiology, psychopharmacologic interventions, and nursing care of children with disorders of mood and anxiety, including trauma disorders (e.g., posttraumatic stress disorder).
- Discuss the behavioural intervention strategies for the treatment of enuresis and encopresis.

KEY TERMS

- communication disorders • compulsions • concordant • dyslexia
- encopresis • enuresis • externalizing disorders • habit reversal therapy • internalizing disorders • learning disorders • obsessions
- school phobia • stereotypic behaviour • tic

C hild and adolescent mental health is a relatively new phenomenon in the field of psychiatry. It therefore stands to reason that as research into the neurobiology and genetics of human development advances, the various categories and diagnoses identified will change. The understanding of child psychiatric disorders has benefited from advances in several related fields, including developmental biology, neuroanatomy, psychopharmacology, genetics, and epidemiology.

The American Psychiatric Association (APA) has incorporated those findings over the decades, moving from the *Diagnostic and Statistical Manual of Mental Disorders* (DSM-III) in 1980, through the *DSM IV-TR* (2000), to the most recent version, the *DSM-5* (2013). These changes will have an impact on future research as well as the interventions nurses will use in working with children and families. The changes to *DSM-5* have been brought into this chapter with a focus on transition to new and more evidence-based interventions.

Child and adolescent psychiatric disorders are impacted by the *DSM-5* in relation to reclassification and diagnostic category changes in the areas of neurodevelopmental disorders; depressive disorders; anxiety disorders; obsessive–compulsive and related disorders; trauma and stressor-related disorders; feeding and eating disorders; sleep–wake disorders; gender dysphoria; disruptive, impulse control, and conduct disorders; and substance-related and addictive disorders. Attention in this chapter is focused on the neurodevelopmental disorders, trauma, and stressor-related disorders.

The prevalence of child psychiatric disorders varies across these categories. For example, although childhood schizophrenia is rare, first onset of psychosis is typically in mid–late adolescence. Attention deficit hyperactivity disorder (ADHD) is a relatively common diagnosis in children; however, over the last 20 years, there has been recognition that ADHD continues into adulthood (Canadian ADHD Resource Alliance [CADDRA], 2013a). Prevalence is impacted by these changes to diagnostic classification and therefore will evolve over time. Gender ratios may also vary with some disorders according to age and genetics. For example, ADHD is more prevalent in boys than girls in childhood (3:1); however, that discrepancy evens out in adulthood (CADDRA). The Canadian Pediatric Society (2006) contends that mental health problems among children and youth have increased in recent years and are predicted to increase by 50% by the year 2020.

A Mental Health Commission of Canada study (2011) projected that by 2041 there would be 8.9 million people in Canada living with mental health problems or illness. Based on demographic changes alone, this represents a slight increase to 20.5% of the projected population. An estimated 2.2 million more people in Canada will be living with mental health problems and illnesses in 30 years compared with those today. This represents a 31% increase compared with a 26% projected growth in the population. Specifically, over 1 million children and adolescents aged 9 to 19 years are expected to be living with mental illness by 2041.

Fewer than 25% of the approximately 800,000 Canadian children aged 4 to 17 years who experience mental disorders causing significant distress and impairment at home, at school, and in the community receive specialized treatment (Waddell, McEwan, Shepherd, Offord, & Hua, 2005). This discrepancy appears to be the result of limited access to treatment facilities, either because of financial constraints or because appropriate mental health services for children are simply unavailable. Psychiatric problems are less easily diagnosed in children than they are in adults. One factor contributing to this difference is that sometimes the symptoms of disorders are difficult to distinguish from the turbulence of normal growth and development. For example, a 4-year-old child who has an invisible imaginary friend is normal; however, an adolescent with an invisible friend might be experiencing a hallucination. The certainty of current estimates for the frequency of the various psychiatric disorders is also inconsistent, partly because of changing definitions of these disorders.

This chapter presents an overview of the childhood disorders that a nurse may encounter and discusses the nursing care of children with these challenges. It is beyond the scope of this text to present all child and adolescent psychiatric disorders in detail. Each category will be reviewed briefly with respect to the bio/psycho/social and spiritual aspects of the child's care. Nursing management will be embedded within each category as pertinent. A more in-depth look at ADHD with respect to assessment, management, and follow-up is provided. The various aspects of the family dynamics are incorporated within this overview.

● **STUDY NOTE**

All of the psychiatric disorders of childhood and adolescence should be viewed within the context of growth and development models (Box 31-1). Safety and self-esteem are priority considerations.

BOX 31-1 History and Hallmarks of Childhood and Adolescent Disorders

- Maternal age and health status during pregnancy
- Exposure to medication, alcohol, or other substances during pregnancy
- Course of pregnancy, labour, and delivery
- Infant's health at birth
- Eating, sleeping, and growth in 1st year
- Health status in first year
- Interest in others in first 2 years
- Motor development
- Mastery of bowel and bladder control
- Speech and language development
- Activity level
- Response to separation (e.g., school entry)
- Regulation of mood and anxiety
- Medical history in early childhood
- Social development
- Interests

SCHIZOPHRENIA SPECTRUM AND OTHER PSYCHOTIC DISORDERS

The symptoms of psychotic disorders cluster into five common domains: delusions, hallucinations, disorganized thinking (speech), grossly disorganized or abnormal motor behaviour (including catatonia), and negative symptoms. Negative symptoms typically are deficits of normal emotional responses or of other thought processes, and they respond less well to medication. They commonly include flat or blunted affect and emotion, poverty of speech (alogia), inability to experience pleasure (anhedonia), lack of desire to form relationships (asociality), and lack of motivation (avolition). Research suggests that negative symptoms contribute more to poor quality of life, functional disability, and the burden on others than do positive symptoms (see Chapter 20).

Brief Psychotic Disorder

In children and youth, what is commonly observed and diagnosed is either *brief psychotic disorder* or *substance/medication-induced psychotic disorder*, prior to a confirmed diagnosis of schizophrenia or other related psychotic disorder. Although psychosis can occur in children under 13 years, it is rare.

Nursing Management: Human Response to Psychotic Disorders

The management priority for a child or youth with a diagnosis of psychosis is to ensure safety. Altered perceptions affect the individual's organization and thus affect adequate intake, output, and general hygiene and health. Education of the child/youth and family as to signs and symptoms of relapse is important. Encouragement of daily exercise, healthy nutrition, and the maintenance of social connections will assist the youth in prevention of illness relapse. Monitoring of medication adherence and follow-up are critical for patients and families. Engaging families in support programs also alleviates the stigma associated with psychotic illnesses.

Biologic Domain

It is well established that schizophrenia spectrum disorders typically have a neurologic basis with some linkages to genetics. No definitive cause has been identified to date. There is strong evidence that first-degree relatives of individuals with schizophrenia are at higher risk. In relation to brief psychotic disorder, there may be evidence of a marked stressor, or postpartum onset, or it may be related to catatonia (APA, 2013). The incidence is approximately 9% of first onset psychosis. The symptoms typically dissipate within 1 month; however, if the duration is longer, the diagnosis may be altered. See Box 31-2 for early warning signs of psychosis.

BOX 31-2 Early Warning Signs of Psychosis

Withdrawal from activities and social contacts
　Irrational, angry, or fearful responses to friends and family
　Sleep disturbances
　Deterioration in studies or work
　Inappropriate use of language—words that do not make sense
　Sudden excesses, such as extreme religiosity, extreme activity
　Deterioration in personal hygiene
　Difficulty controlling thoughts, difficulty concentrating
　Hearing voices or sounds others don't hear
　Seeing people or things others don't see
　A constant feeling of being watched
　Inability to turn off the imagination, delusions, off-the-wall ideas
　Mood swings, increased anxiety
　Somatic symptoms: weakness, pains, bizarre body sensations

Most psychoses, including schizophrenia are treated with medications called antipsychotics/neuroleptics. These medications often cause unpleasant side effects that contribute to clients' stopping or being inconsistent in adhering to their medication regimen. This affects the duration and prognosis of the illness. For example, with the advent of the second-generation antipsychotic medications, the increase in metabolic illnesses has increased. Many youth gain substantial amounts of weight, which can further contribute to stigma and illness (Panagiotopoulos, Ronsley, Kuzeljevic, & Davidson, 2012). Nurses working with clients need to provide support and work to mitigate these side effects.

Psychosocial Domain

Youth do not usually recognize that they are ill or, if they do, they often do not tell their families or friends out of fear of stigma. Many families may not be aware of symptoms until they become overtly severe. The earlier symptoms are identified and treated, the more likely the illness will move into remission. The better the medical and psychosocial management are, the better chance of remission and/or recovery. Family education and support are critical to prognosis and remission. Early psychosis intervention (EPI) programs are available in most provinces to provide support, education, and group or individual support (see Web Links on the thePoint for examples).

Spiritual Domain

With psychosis, it is important to understand the cultural and spiritual beliefs of cultures. Within some cultures, psychosis is the sign of a spiritual inhabitation that may be perceived to be positive or negative, or a curse. Some cultures may wish to conduct interventions that are different from Western cultural beliefs and practices. The agency and treatment team will determine how they wish to work with the family in this circumstance in order to protect the child and maintain a therapeutic relationship with the family.

DISORDERS OF MOOD AND ANXIETY

Bipolar and Related Disorders

Bipolar disorder often first presents in youth. Symptoms include periods of mania (extreme optimism, euphoria, and feelings of grandeur; rapid, racing thoughts and hyperactivity; a decreased need for sleep; increased irritability; impulsiveness and possibly reckless behaviour; and alternate periods of depression) (Canadian Mental Health Association [CMHA], 2013a). This can be a very difficult experience for youth and their family, as the youth may engage in behaviours that contribute to ongoing stigma about mental illness. Bipolar disorder is rare in children, and the observed symptoms may fall into a diagnosis of attention deficit hyperactivity disorder, oppositional defiant disorder, or disruptive mood regulation disorder (see section "Disruptive Mood Regulation Disorder" below for details).

Nursing Management: Human Response to Bipolar Disorder

Biologic Domain

A family history of bipolar disorder is correlated with a "10-fold increased risk among adult relatives" (APA, 2013, p. 130). Females tend to have an increased incidence of rapid cycling phases in this disorder (National Institute of Mental Health, 2013). Various mood stabilizer medications are used, with the majority of clients requiring daily or weekly blood tests to assess for therapeutic levels until stable.

Psychosocial Domain

The risk of suicide among the population of individuals with bipolar disorder is 15 times the general population. With suicide being the leading cause of nonaccidental death in individuals 15 to 24 years of age (CMHA, 2013b), it is critical to assess for risk and intent with this group. Bipolar illness can affect various relationships in the individual's life. Education for friends and school assists the youth.

Spiritual Domain

As with all mental illness, it is important for the nurse to assess the client's and family's beliefs and support them as best as possible.

ANXIETY DISORDERS

Anxiety disorders are the most prevalent mental illness in Canadian children between 4 and 17 years of age. Approximately 6 in 100 children have severe problems with worries and fears warranting a clinical diagnosis (Children's Health Policy Centre, Simon Fraser University, 2007; Waddell, Godderis, Hua, McEwan, & Wong, 2004). Many childhood fears are developmentally normal: it is common for toddlers to fear the dark, for school-aged children to fear animals, and for teenagers to worry about relationship with peers. These typical anxiety experiences do not usually interfere with the child's development and functioning (Children's Health Policy Centre, Simon Fraser University, 2007). Children with anxiety disorders, however, experience excessive, prolonged, or recurrent fears or symptoms of anxiety, with accompanying impairment in age-appropriate functioning at home, at school, and with peers (Manassis, 2004).

To screen quickly for one or more anxiety disorders in children, the following questions may be useful:

- Does the child worry or ask for parental reassurance every day?
- Does the child consistently avoid age-appropriate situations or activities or avoid doing them without a parent?
- Does the child have frequent episodes of stomachaches, headaches, or hyperventilation?
- Does the child have daily repetitive rituals?

These four questions address the main thoughts, behaviours, and feelings related to anxiety seen in children (Manassis, 2004). This section focuses on separation anxiety, a disorder diagnosed in childhood, and obsessive–compulsive disorder (OCD), a disorder that occurs in both adults and children (see Chapter 23).

Separation Anxiety Disorder

Separation anxiety disorder is excessive anxiety on separation from home or major attachment figure before the age of 18 years. It is manifested by acute distress, frequent nightmares about separation, and reluctance or refusal to separate. It lasts for at least 1 month and causes clinically significant impairment in social or academic functioning. Some have suggested that separation anxiety disorder is the childhood equivalent of panic disorder in adults. Although many children experience some discomfort on separation from their mothers or major attachment figures, children with separation anxiety disorder suffer great distress when faced with ordinary separations, such as going to school. In most cases, the mother is the focus of the child's concern, but this may not be so, especially if the mother is not the primary caregiver. The child may exhibit extraordinary reluctance or even refusal to separate from the primary caregiver. When asked, most children with separation anxiety disorder will express worry about harm or permanent loss of their major attachment figure. Other children may express worry about their own safety.

A common manifestation of anxiety is **school phobia**, in which the child refuses to attend school, preferring to stay at home with the primary attachment figure. However, it should be noted that school phobia is a common presenting complaint in child psychiatric clinics and may be part of separation anxiety disorder, general anxiety disorder, social phobia, OCD, depression, or conduct disorder. In rare cases, school phobia can be a side effect of antipsychotic medication (Scahill, Leckman, Schultz, Katsovich, & Peterson, 2003). When another disorder such as depression is identified, it becomes the focus of treatment. In some cases, the school phobia may resolve when the primary disorder is successfully treated.

Epidemiology and Aetiology

The prevalence of separation anxiety disorder is estimated at 4% of school-aged children; thus, it is relatively common. Anxiety disorders run in families, and it appears that both environmental and genetic factors affect the risk for separation anxiety disorder. For example, it may emerge after a move, change to a new school, or death of a family member or pet. By contrast, recent evidence suggests that traits such as shyness and behavioural inhibition (reluctance in new situations) are inherited (Rapee & Spence, 2004). Furthermore, not only are children with an enduring "inhibited" temperament at greater risk for anxiety disorders themselves, but their immediate family members are also at greater risk for anxiety disorders compared with a psychiatric control group. Others have argued in favour of environmental determinants of separation anxiety, contending that anxious parents communicate to the child that the world is inhospitable and menacing in order to keep the child near. Available data suggest that the long-term outcome of childhood disorders is favourable in many cases but may evolve and take other forms in adulthood. For example, separation anxiety in childhood may reemerge as panic disorder in adults (Koda, Charney, & Pine, 2003).

Psychopharmacologic Interventions

Selective serotonin reuptake inhibitors (SSRIs) are currently considered first-line medications for treating children with anxiety disorders. All SSRIs have been used for children, and no clear evidence suggests that one is superior to another. Findings suggesting increased suicidal ideations in children taking paroxetine have resulted in a Health Canada warning to avoid this medication in children. All SSRIs can result in nausea or changes in sleep patterns early in treatment, but these usually resolve within a week. In the past, tricyclic antidepressants were used for treating anxiety disorders in children but are currently considered second-line medications due to the risk of cardiac conduction disturbances (Manassis, 2004). If tricyclic antidepressants are used, baseline and follow-up electrocardiograms are recommended (King, Scahill, Lombroso, & Leckman, 2003).

Nursing Management

School phobia is often what prompts the family to seek consultation for the child. The onset of school refusal may be gradual or acute. Because school phobia can be a behavioural manifestation of several different child psychiatric disorders, it requires careful assessment. Issues to consider are whether the parents have been aware that the child is avoiding school (separation versus truancy); what efforts the family has made to return the child to school; the presence of significant subjective distress in the child with anticipation of going to school; and whether school refusal occurs in the context of other behavioural, social, or emotional problems. The nurse should also review the purpose and dose of current medications.

The child's developmental history and response to new situations and prior separations provide essential background information for understanding the child's current separation anxiety. The assessment should also include a review of recent life events and the methods the family has used to promote the child's return to school. Finally, the family history with respect to anxiety, panic attacks, or phobias is also informative.

Most clinicians agree that the child should return to school as soon as possible because resistance to attending school invariably mounts the longer the child remains absent. Several therapeutic approaches are used in treating separation anxiety disorder, including individual psychotherapy, behavioural treatment, and pharmacotherapy. Although individual psychotherapy is a common treatment, data to support this approach are sparse. By contrast, evidence suggests that behavioural techniques can be effective in reducing separation anxiety. These techniques include flooding (rapid and forcible return to school) and desensitization, in which the child is gradually returned to school (Labellarte & Ginsberg, 2003). To be successful, these techniques require close collaboration with the family and the school and may also include medication (Labellarte & Ginsberg, 2003).

Obsessive–Compulsive Disorder

Obsessive–compulsive disorder (OCD) is characterized by intrusive thoughts that are difficult to dislodge (**obsessions**, i.e., unwanted persistent, intrusive thoughts, impulses, or images related to anxiety) or by ritualized behaviours that the child feels driven to perform (**compulsions**, i.e., unwanted behavioural acts or patterns) to prevent or reduce anxiety. The most common obsessions in children are fears of contamination. Worries about personal and family safety are also frequent. The most common compulsions are excessive washing, cleaning, and checking actions. Historically, OCD was regarded as a neurosis, and the primary symptoms were viewed as the expression of unresolved sexual and aggressive impulses. Recent evidence from family genetic studies, pharmacologic trials, and neuroimaging studies has dramatically shifted the conceptualization of OCD (see Chapter 23). The notion that OCD is the manifestation of internal conflicts concerning sexual and aggressive impulses has given way to a more biologic model (Stewart et al., 2007).

Epidemiology and Aetiology

OCD was once considered uncommon in adults and even rarer in children, but research over the last two decades has identified OCD as one of the most common psychiatric illnesses in both children and adults. Prevalence in the paediatric population has been reported to be in the range of 1% to 3% (Stewart et al., 2004). OCD can affect the child or adolescent's physical, psychological, social, and emotional well-being.

Family studies and twin studies indicate that genetic determinants play a significant role in the aetiology of OCD, as well as anxiety disorders, and recur with a greater than expected frequency in the families of clients with OCD or Tourette disorder (Van Grootheest, Cath, Beekman, & Boomsma, 2005). Many biologic theories of OCD hypothesize that abnormalities in serotonin metabolism and frontal–striatal circuitry operation are responsible for the creation of OCD symptomatology. The serotonin hypothesis is based on the observation that, in most cases, individuals with OCD respond to SSRIs as opposed to nonserotonergic medications or placebos (Cameron, 2007). Neuroimaging studies and neurosurgical evidence suggest that OCD is associated with hyperactive operation in the frontal–striatal circuitry of the brain, which includes the orbital frontal cortex, anterior cingulated cortex, caudate nucleus, and thalamus (Leonard, Ale, & Freeman, 2005). Despite advances in the genetics, diagnosis, and treatment of OCD in children and adolescents, little is known about the disorder's long-term outcome (Stewart et al., 2004).

Psychopharmacologic Interventions

Current and past studies suggest that psychotropic medications can be introduced to supplement psychosocial interventions in the treatment of OCD but should never be used as the sole form of intervention (Cameron, 2007). The tricyclic antidepressant clomipramine was the first drug reported to be effective for treating OCD (Clomipramine Collaborative Study Group, 1991). In recent years, SSRIs have become the pharmacologic intervention of choice for OCD. Effective SSRIs include fluoxetine, sertraline, and fluvoxamine. These SSRIs have demonstrated effectiveness in older children and adolescents, although little is known about their efficacy with preschool or younger school-aged children (Leonard et al., 2005). Parental education regarding SSRI treatment should include a discussion of the medication's action and potential side effects and a realistic assessment of potential outcomes (Cameron, 2007).

Nursing Management

Recurrent worries and ritualistic behaviour can occur normally in children at particular stages of development. The first step in the assessment of OCD in children is to distinguish between normal childhood rituals and worries and pathologic rituals and obsessional thoughts (Cameron, 2007). Obsessional thoughts are recurrent, nagging, and bothersome. Although children may describe obsessions as occurring "out of the blue," external events may trigger obsessions. For example, a child may fear contamination whenever he or she is in contact with a certain person or object. Likewise, compulsions waste time, cause distress, and interfere with daily living (Box 31-3).

The severity of the child's and family's response to OCD will determine the appropriate nursing diagnoses. When the obsessions and compulsions emerge, these children or adolescents are in distress because of the disturbing and relentless nature of the symptoms.

BOX 31-3   Clinical Vignette

KIMBERLY AND OCD

Kimberly, an 11-year-old fifth grader, comes for evaluation because her mother and teacher have become increasingly concerned about her repetitive behaviours. In retrospect, Kim's mother recalls first noticing repetitive rituals about 2 years ago, but she did not become alarmed about these behaviours until recently when they began to interfere with daily living. At the time of referral, Kim exhibits complicated jumping rituals that involve a specific number of jumps and a particular manner of jumping. She also turns light switches off and on and performs complex movements, such as blinking in patterns and thrusting her arms back and forth a certain number of times. Her mother also reports Kim's near-constant request for reassurance about her own safety. In recent months, her incessant demands for reassurance have been more frequent and elaborate. For example, Kim's mother has to answer three times that everything is all right and then say, "I swear to it."

At the evaluation, Kim expresses fears that some ill fate, such as catastrophic illness or injury, will befall her. This fear is triggered by contact with any individual who seems sick, chance exposures to foul smells or dirt, or minor scrapes or bumps. Once the fear is triggered, she becomes increasingly anxious and consumed with the fear that she will develop an illness and die. Sometimes her fears are specific, such as cancer or AIDS; other times, her fears are more ambiguous, as evidenced by statements that "something bad will happen" if she doesn't complete the ritual. Kim acknowledges that the ritual is probably not related to the feared event, but she is reluctant to take a chance. If the ritual does not reduce her anxiety, she seeks reassurance from her mother.

Kim's medical history was negative for serious illness or injury; she was born after an uncomplicated pregnancy, labour, and delivery and achieved developmental milestones at appropriate times. Indeed, her mother could recall no unusual problems in the first few years of life except that Kim was typically anxious in new situations. Kim's mother reports a prior history of panic attacks, but the family history is otherwise negative for anxiety disorders, including OCD.

What distinguishes OCD families from families of children with other mental disorders is the inextricable way that they are brought into the illness. Parents may be pulled into the child's rituals. The term *family accommodation* is often used to refer to family responses that are direct (e.g., participation in or assistance with the ritual) or indirect (e.g., modification in the family's lifestyle around the OCD symptomatology) (Cameron, 2007). Ineffective coping, compromised family coping, and ineffective role performance are likely nursing diagnoses for these families.

Treatment goals focus on reducing the obsessions and compulsions and their effects on the child's development. Cognitive–behavioural therapy, particularly exposure and response prevention (ERP), was found to be an effective intervention in children with OCD (Bolton & Perrin, 2008). Exposure consists of gradual confrontation with events or situations that trigger obsessions and cause the urge to ritualize. According to the theory behind ERP therapy, repeated exposure works because the client learns that the immediate anxiety will subside even if he or she does not complete the ritual. Response prevention complements exposure and consists of instructing the client to delay the execution of the ritual. When exposure and response prevention are combined, the client is confronted with a triggering stimulus such as dirt (exposure) but agrees not to do the hand washing for a brief period (response prevention) and tracks the anxiety level during the exercise. Successful cognitive–behavioural treatment of children with OCD includes parents, both to include them in the treatment plan and to reduce their involvement in the ritualized behaviour. For example, the child may demand that the parent participate in a washing and checking ritual (Bolton & Perrin, 2008). Because of the dynamic impact OCD in children and adolescents has on families, they should be involved in psychosocial interventions whenever possible (Cameron, 2007).

Depressive Disorders

Major Depressive Disorder

Depressive disorders have prevalence rates of up to 3% in children and 8% in adolescents, with a lifetime prevalence of 25% by the end of adolescence (Zinck, Bagnell, Bond, & Newton, 2009). According to Statistics Canada (2012), in 2009, 202 Canadian individuals aged 15 to 19 committed suicide. Suicide is second only to accidental death as the leading cause of death in this age group (Statistics Canada, 2012).

Nursing Management: Human Response to Depressive Disorder

Nurses need to develop comfort and confidence in assessing children and youth about suicidal thoughts and intention. Various tools are available to assist the nurse with those assessments. Education and support are needed for parents and caregivers to understand that asking about suicide does not increase the risk of suicide.

Biologic Domain

Depression has been demonstrated to have a familial or genetic link. Depression can also be caused by stressful events or experiences, medical illness, or medications. Regardless of the cause, depression can look very different in children and youth than it does in adults. Young children may become withdrawn, have trouble sleeping, regress in certain behaviours (e.g., bed wetting), or become irritable. Older children may start to report headaches and stomachaches or withdraw from activities and friends. Adolescents may be better able to articulate what is happening for them, but they may not necessarily report directly to parents. They may experience sadness and become withdrawn and may exhibit increases or decreases in sleep and appetite (HealthLinkBC, 2012).

Psychosocial Domain

Depression has been linked with life stressors (Box 31-4). Stressors for children can include the death or loss of a pet, parental separation or divorce, or household relocation. There is also evidence that depression and anxiety are higher in children who have suffered maltreatment, specifically their own "substance abuse, emotional maltreatment, primary caregivers' mental illness, sexual abuse, and numerous moves in a year" (Tonmyr, Williams, Hovdestad, & Draca, 2011, p. 497). The most serious concern of children/youth with depression is the risk of suicide. Suicide screening and assessment need to start with children as young as 10 years and increase over adolescence (see Chapter 30). Children report feeling relieved when finally asked about their feelings.

Spiritual Domain

For many youth, the issues surrounding their mental illness may have a context within their spiritual or cultural beliefs or family of origin. Specifically, when assessing for suicide risk, it is important to know the child/youth/families' cultural or spiritual beliefs about what would happen to them if they did kill themselves. What are their beliefs about death: that they would go to a better place, or enlightenment, or be punished? (Preet, 2007). A child/youth may be fearful of repercussions of sharing information with family if he or she has experienced conflict between traditional belief systems and his or her own beliefs.

Disruptive Mood Dysregulation Disorder

This diagnostic category is new for the *DSM-5* and especially for the assessment of children. The category was

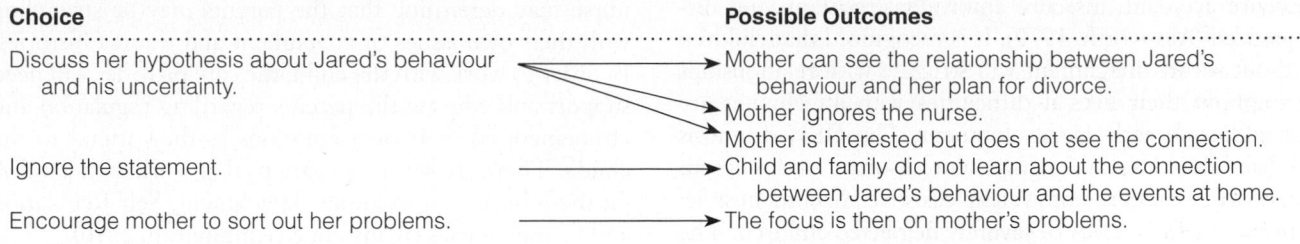

BOX 31-4 Questions, Choices, and Outcomes

Mrs. S has just returned with her son Jared to the child psychiatric inpatient services following an overnight pass. She reports that the visit did not go well due to Jared's anger and defiance. She remarked that this behaviour was distressingly similar to his behaviour before the hospitalization. She expressed additional concern because of the upcoming discharge from the hospital. After saying goodbye to Jared, she pulled the nurse aside and stated that she had decided to file for divorce.

Mrs. S indicated that she had not told her husband or the family therapist. When asked whether Jared knew about her decision, Mrs. S suddenly realized that he may have overheard her discussing the matter with her sister on the telephone during this home visit.

How should the nurse approach this situation?

Choice	Possible Outcomes
Discuss her hypothesis about Jared's behaviour and his uncertainty.	Mother can see the relationship between Jared's behaviour and her plan for divorce.
	Mother ignores the nurse.
	Mother is interested but does not see the connection.
Ignore the statement.	Child and family did not learn about the connection between Jared's behaviour and the events at home.
Encourage mother to sort out her problems.	The focus is then on mother's problems.

Analysis

The best response is focusing on the possible relationship between Jared's recent behavioural deterioration and his uncertainty of his family's future. If the nurse ignores the statement or focuses on the mother's interpretation of Jared's behaviour, the mother is less likely to appreciate the connection between pending divorce and Jared's behaviour. The nurse should also emphasize the importance of discussing the matter in family therapy.

---

developed to better distinguish bipolar disorder in children from other related disorders. The incidence of this disorder is estimated to be 2% to 5% of children, who demonstrate a chronically irritable temperament, and the majority of whom are male (APA, 2013; Axelrod, 2013). "In severe mood dysregulation, irritability is defined as having two components: (1) temper outbursts that are developmentally inappropriate, frequent, and extreme; and (2) negatively valenced mood (anger or sadness) between outbursts" (Leibenluft, 2011, p. 4). According to a study review by Copeland and colleagues (2013), there appears to be an overlap with childhood diagnoses of depression and/or oppositional defiant disorder. As this new category for children unfolds, it will be important that nurses work closely with children and families to ensure they access the best and most appropriate interventions.

■ TRAUMA- AND STRESSOR-RELATED DISORDERS

It is well documented that early chronic stress or trauma affects how the developing brain grows and evolves (Gunnar & Quevedo, 2007; National Scientific Council on the Developing Child, 2012; Perry, 2004; Porges, 2004; van der Kolk, 2009). Childhood trauma can be the result of a physically or emotionally absent parent; erratic or inconsistent caregiving; abuse (verbal, sexual, or emotional); neglect; violence in the home or community; and war or disasters. The brain of a child/youth with a trauma history prepares him or her to live in a state of neurologic hyperarousal in order to be alert and safe in his or her environment. Traumatized individuals often do not come out of this hyperaroused state and are "hypervigilant and focused on nonverbal cues" even when they are in a situation that is perceived to be safe (Perry, 2002a, p. 6; Mulvihill, 2005). Traumatized individuals often have difficulty with verbal interactions or therapy when memories evoke "trauma-related physical sensations and physiologic hyper- or hypoarousal, which evoke emotions" (van der Kolk, 2006, p. 284). There are many triggers—loud noises, tone of voice, nonverbal behaviours, gender, the environment, the gender, stance, intonation, or touch of other—that can initiate a hyperarousal response. The reactivity is in the form of automatic fight-or-flight system and can take the form of overt aggression or internal withdrawal (Gunnar & Quevedo, 2007; Perry, 2001, 2002b, 2002c; van der Kolk, 2006). When nurses work with children/youth or families in these circumstances, they need to be aware of what the triggers may be, how to mitigate them, and how to access the families' coping strategies when possible.

Trauma in early childhood interferes with the child's ability to seek safety, especially if the trauma is directly related to the primary attachment/care provider. Young children learn that emotions are scary and that the related body arousal can be dangerous. Children in these circumstances are less likely to explore and learn from their environment and thus may not develop relationships as needed. Older children may have impairments in school achievement, emotional reactivity, frustration tolerance, and overall self-esteem. These children may be diagnosed with ADHD or ODD or other pathology. Adolescents may rely on less sophisticated coping strategies and engage in substance use, cutting, sensory-seeking behaviours, or sexual behaviours. Self-esteem and self-awareness are affected, leaving the individual without a positive sense of self-identity (Blaustein & Kinniburgh, 2010).

With the advent of the *DSM-5*, there have been some changes to the categories within the trauma section that have direct impact on children and youth.

Reactive Attachment Disorder

Attachment disorders are typically identified prior to the age of 5 years. Previously, Mary Ainsworth's work (Cornell & Hamrin, 2008) on attachment described four types: secure; insecure avoidant; insecure ambivalent/resistant; and disorganized (Ainsworth, 1979). It is recognized that children without secure attachment will struggle with relationships throughout their lives if difficulties with attachment are not addressed early in development. The *DSM* diagnosis of disinhibited social engagement disorder is similar to Ainsworth's insecure-ambivalent–resistive attachment style; it occurs in about 20% of severely neglected children. The behaviours seen with this disorder include a lack of social or cultural boundaries and overfamiliarity with strangers (APA, 2013). The *DSM* diagnosis of reactive attachment disorder (RAD) is most similar to Ainsworth's disorganized attachment style, the style most likely to develop into later psychopathology without early intervention (Holmes, 2004; Main, 1996). The focus here will be on RAD.

Nursing Management: Human Response to Reactive Attachment Disorder

Some of the interventions used for treating RAD are relevant for posttraumatic stress disorder (PTSD) and acute traumatic stress response, depending on the context and situation. Care for a family with a child/youth with RAD is complex. The first component of intervention is the provision of psychoeducation about the disorder, context, and strategies of therapy. Interventions will depend on the age of the child/youth, symptoms being expressed, and severity of the attachment dysfunction at the time. Relational therapy between the therapist and child is paramount to establish trust and rapport, as well as with the family. Some interventions will include specific behavioural management components such as the Incredible Years by Webster-Stratton and Reid (see for example Webster-Stratton, 2011), or Parent–Child Interaction Therapy by Eyberg and Boggs (see Buckner, Lopez, Dunkel, & Joiner, 2008). The use of these programs will depend greatly on the caregivers' ability to participate and the overall issues facing for the child. Holding therapies are not considered safe or evidence based. Family or individual therapy is recommended; pharmacotherapy is used only if required for a coexisting diagnosis (Mayo Clinic, 2013).

The first component of intervention is to explore the rationale for the various behaviours being expressed by the child/youth and that the caregivers are experiencing. The nurse works with the caregivers to learn the child's language of emotional expression (verbal and nonverbal). The caregiver begins to attune to the child's expressions of need

and reciprocate to meet that need; the pattern of coregulation begins. The caregiver then develops a consistent response to the child that is predictable. From this point, the caregiver and child learn self-regulation strategies to calm or arouse the child as reflective of the circumstance at hand. As the child and caregiver develop competence in these areas, the child will be increasingly free to develop and to learn new skills. This is not a "quick-fix" process and may take several months to years for some families. The nurse may determine that the parents may be struggling with their own issues of attachment and trauma histories. In order to work with the child, the care provider will need support and educate the parents regarding regulation and attunement of their own emotions as they attend to the child's. There are several programs that work with families on these issues, for example, Attachment, Self-Regulation and Competencies (Blaustein & Kinniburgh, 2010).

Biologic Domain

There do not appear to be specific biologic factors attributed to the development of RAD; however, parents who may be compromised neurologically or psychologically may create an environment in which RAD would develop.

Psychosocial Domain

The prevalence is unknown, but environmental factors that create severe neglect have a significant impact. RAD can also develop from unpredictable care providers who create a sense of fear in the child to the extent that they are unsure of where their safety net may be (Cornell & Hamrin, 2008). Children with RAD do not typically turn to their primary attachment figure for "comfort, support, protection, or nurturance" (American Psychiatric Association, 2013, p. 266). The nurse may suspect potential for attachment concerns if the primary caregiver is being seen because the child has nonorganic failure to thrive or if the primary caregiver has an active psychiatric illness such as postpartum depression (Cornell & Hamrin, 2008).

Spiritual Domain

It will be important for the nurse to explore the cultural and spiritual context of the child's care and to work with the caregivers to support the interventions needed. Belief systems are very important in working with children and youth with trauma histories, especially if that history involves an agency or religious institution.

Posttraumatic Stress Disorder and Acute Stress Disorder

These two diagnoses are separated based on duration of symptom presentation. Children are exposed to multiple events in their lives that can lead to a trauma response or PTSD. The National Child Traumatic Stress Network (NCTSN, 2013) identifies that one in four children will be exposed to trauma prior to the age of 16 years. A child may have been exposed to domestic violence, community violence, war, natural disasters, or various forms of abuse and neglect. All of these events put a child/youth and family at risk of developing PTSD. Children experience and express their symptoms of PTSD differently from adults. For example, expression of recurrent involuntary distressing memories may manifest in repetitive play themes, as nightmares or reenactment of the event in a dissociative space or in play, or in regression of otherwise acquired skills (e.g., bedwetting) (APA, 2013; NCTSN, 2013; Public Health Agency of Canada, 2005). The same *DSM-5* criteria for PTSD apply to adults, adolescents, and children over 6 years, with notations regarding children's symptom expression. For instance, the symptom of reoccurring distressing dreams may appear in children as "frightening dreams without recognizable content" (APA, 2013, p. 271). There are separate PTSD criteria for children 6 years and younger. *DSM-5* criteria for acute stress disorder apply to adults, adolescents, and children, with notations regarding children's symptom expression (APA, 2013).

Nursing Management: Human Response to Traumatic Stress

Creating safety, support, guidance, and education for the child/youth and family, regardless of the cause of the trauma, will be the primary focus for the nurse. Cognitive–behavioural therapy has been shown to be most effective in treating PTSD. It would include stress management and relaxation strategies; creating a story or narrative to assist with understanding events; correcting misinformation or distorted beliefs; deflecting self-blame; and engaging parents or primary care providers in the process (Kelty Mental Health Resource Centre, 2013; NCTSN, 2013) (see also Chapter 13).

In the event of a natural disaster where the family home may no longer exist, it will be important for the parent/primary caregivers to create an atmosphere of as much normalcy as possible. Supporting the child/youth's and family's return to regular routines as much as possible will help with recovery and general wellness. Activities such as regular exercise, relaxation, a balanced diet, positive relationships, stress management, adequate sleep, community involvement, and social support are very important in managing anxiety in relation to PTSD or acute stress response, and for general wellness (see Box 31-5). Children or youth may need the assistance of medication during this time; however, that is a collaborative conversation between the family, child/youth, and therapist and physician involved.

Biologic Domain

Over the past 20 years, research regarding the neurodevelopmental effects of trauma and neglect on the developing brain has been evolving (Blaustein & Kinniburgh, 2010;

BOX 31-5 Tips for Caregivers Managing a Child's Symptoms of PTSD

Maintain a calm, structured home environment (e.g., practice relaxation, develop routines)
  Keep your routines the same (morning, school, homework, bedtime)
    Provide clear expectations, limits, and consequences
    Help your child learn about and identify feelings
    Pay attention to your child's feelings
    Remain calm when your child is anxious
    Hold realistic expectations for your child's age—change them if you need to
    Plan for transitions (e.g., getting to school)
    Focus on the here and now—use the sense to notice what is going on in the moment (e.g., your child describes what he or she hears, see), PTSD anxiety forces children to be focused on the future
    Show your child the way you identify and accept your feelings
    Show your child how to solve problems
    Take care of your own needs—parenting an anxious child can be challenging
    Talk to others for support, and ask for help when you need it
    Be aware of and manage your own reactions. Seek help if you are struggling with this
    Praise effort and provide rewards for effort

Source: Kelty Mental Health Resource Centre. (2013). *Post-traumatic stress disorder.* Retrieved from http://keltymentalhealth.ca/mental-health/disorders/post-traumatic-stress-disorder.

Gunnar & Quevedo, 2007; Mulvihill, 2005; Perry, 1994, 2004; Porges, 2004; Siegel, 2001; van der Kolk, 2005, 2006). Although there may not be an overt genetic pathway, the environmental exposures that create a brain sensitive and receptive to developing PTSD are clear. Gender plays a role: risk is increased for females. Risk negatively correlates with age: the younger the age of exposure, the greater the risk of developing PTSD (APA, 2013). Temperament and preexisting psychopathology may also increase the risk for anxiety or panic disorders and depression.

Psychosocial Domain

Children exposed to various life stressors, who live in communities where violence and/or war exist, and those who are deprived of the basic determinants of health (nutrition, housing, safety) are at risk. Resilience may be a protective factor, however, depending on the circumstance/event, is not absolute.

Spiritual Domain

Religion or culture may affect the development or severity of PTSD in relation to the meaning attributed to the event(s), ongoing exposure, and development of coping strategies. If a particular group is singled out or persecuted in some way, the interventions may need to focus on a larger group rather than just the child or family.

■ GENDER DYSPHORIA

Gender dysphoria (previously known as gender identity disorder) in children is a controversial and highly debated subject. There are clinics around the world, with varying approaches, where children and youth go for assessment, including in Canada and Holland (de Vries & Cohen-Kettenis, 2012; Zucker, Wood, Singh, & Bradley, 2012). See Zucker et al. (2012) for a description of a developmental bio/psycho/social therapeutic model and approach used in a Canadian gender identity service. Gender confusion can be temporary, and the identification or labelling of children with gender dysphoria brings multiple challenges for the child, family, and the community in which the child lives. The challenges include stigma, as much of society remains uninformed or judgmental about transgendered identity. Questions such as "Transgendered kids: Have we gone too far?" are being raised and debated in the media (Wente, 2014). There are political, medical, social, moral, and ethical questions that contribute to the issue (Reiner & Reiner, 2012). Some nurses argued against the inclusion of a diagnosis of gender dysphoria for children and adolescents in the *DSM-5* on the basis that it is not in the best interests of a child. They perceive it as a stigmatizing diagnosis that can exclude the child from health insurance in nations where health care is not publically funded, as well being concerned that some treatments for it have been associated with later suicidality (Hein & Berger, 2012). Children and youth with gender dysphoria and their families need knowledgeable support from nurses and other health professionals as they make life-altering decisions regarding the various options open to them and their child. They will need to be provided with information about evidence-based treatment options and be able to get informed answers to their questions.

Nursing Management: Human Response to Gender Dysphoria

Assessment and evaluation of the child/youth's health, cross-gender feelings, the history of the gender dysphoria, school functioning, and peer relationships provide the basis for care management and treatment. The parents' and family's feelings, beliefs, and concerns about what is happening for the child/youth must be explored, as well. There are structured assessments and questionnaires for the parents and child/youth regarding gender identity, such as the Gender Identity Interview for Children and the Gender Identity Questionnaire for Children (Zucker et al., 2012). Full psychiatric and family assessments are also part of the evaluation. For adolescents, a determination is required of whether the youth is truly experiencing gender dysphoria or whether she or he is questioning his or her sexual identity. General cognitive and psychological functioning is assessed to attend to possible contributing factors.

An important factor that must be considered prior to moving into a treatment phase is the support system of the child/youth. Is it satisfactory and sufficient? Barriers to going forward with treatment can include parental role in the maintenance of the gender dysphoria, their inability to engage with the child in relation to the disorder, or psychopathology of the parent.

Treatment with a younger child includes psychotherapy, often in the form of play therapy, to ascertain an understanding of the child's reasoning for wanting to be the other gender. Most clinicians take a wait-and-observe approach with young children to ascertain if the desire to be the other gender persists into the prepubertal phase of development (de Vries & Cohen-Kettenis, 2012). The nurse may be asked to provide education and supportive guidance during this time for parents. Children may need encouragement to maintain friendships to aid in clarification of desires to be the other gender.

Once a diagnosis is confirmed, further psychoeducation for parents, children, and youth will occur. Expectations regarding living as the other gender will begin. Hormonal treatment may be initiated in the initial stages of puberty as a diagnostic assessment. The rationale is that if the dysphoria persists even when one's own puberty has begun, then it is validated (de Vries & Cohen-Kettenis, 2012). Parents and youth will need significant counselling and support during this phase and evaluation if this is what they wish to pursue. Gender reassignment may be much later in the youth's adult life depending on the circumstances.

Biologic Domain

Assessment for gender dysphoria should include a full genetic screening for disorders of sexual development (a.k.a. intersex) used to describe developmental anomalies that affect the development of genitalia and that may impact hormonal release during foetal development (Reiner & Reiner, 2012). Although these tests neither confirm nor deny a diagnosis of gender dysphoria, it is important rule out. There may also be indications of temperamental differences as well as other factors yet to be determined (Zucker et al., 2012).

Psychosocial Domain

A child's self is shaped, in part, by the perceptions and attitudes of significant others. A component of assessment and intervention for the nurse will include evaluating parental understanding and of the child's disposition. The nurse will need to ascertain the parental belief system for the child's behaviours (e.g., cross-dressing), as well as whether their responses are neutral, encouraging, or discouraging. The social context in which the child resides will also have an impact on whether he or he are ostracized, or if there exists psychopathology within the family that is contributory. Many children and youth with gender dysphoria suffer with anxiety and depression, as well as other mental health issues. There has been some indication that children with gender dysphoria also show signs of autism spectrum disorder (ASD) (De Vries, Noens, Cohen-Kettenis, van Berckelaer-Onnes, & Doerleijers, 2010; Zucker et al., 2012). Children and youth presenting with any issues related to gender or sexual identity need to be taken seriously and their behaviour explored to alleviate any related tension and stress the child/youth may be experiencing.

Spiritual Domain

The context of a family's beliefs and religious practices can have a significant impact on the child/youth's disclosure of gender dysphoria or sexual preference. Children and youth may have set beliefs about what will happen to them within their family, culture, and religious circle if anyone were to find out. Anxiety, fear, depression, and perhaps suicidal ideation may be prevalent factors as symptoms of the child/youth's secret.

NEURODEVELOPMENTAL DISORDERS OF CHILDHOOD

Under the primary influences of genes and environment, development may be said to proceed along several pathways, such as attention, cognition, language, affect, and social and moral behaviours. The neurodevelopmental disorders' common feature is significant developmental delays or deficits in one or more lines of development that impair functioning (personal, social, academic, and occupational) (APA, 2013). These deficits can be closely interwoven. For example, a language delay can interfere with a child's social development and contribute to behaviour problems (Russell & Grizzle, 2008).

Neurodevelopmental disorders are classified in the *DSM-5* in several categories: intellectual disability, communication disorders (e.g., childhood-onset fluency disorder [stuttering]), ASD, ADHD, specific learning disorder, and motor disorders (e.g., tic disorders) (APA). Disorders that were once classified as pervasive developmental disorders in the *DSM-IV-TR* now receive the diagnosis of ASD, which places autism-related deficits along a mild to severe continuum.

> **KEY CONCEPT** **Developmental delay** means that the child's development is outside the norm, including delayed socialization, communication, peculiar mannerisms, and idiosyncratic interests.

Autism Spectrum Disorder

Children with ASD may or may not have an intellectual disability, but they commonly show an uneven pattern of intellectual strengths and weaknesses. They can show a lifelong pattern of being rigid in style, intolerant of change, and be prone to behavioural outbursts in response to environmental demands or changes in routine. ASD is diagnosed with a severity level requiring support (level 1), substantial support (level 2), or very substantial support (level 3) in the areas of social communication and restricted, repetitive behaviours. Other specifiers include with or without accompanying intellectual impairment; language impairment; association with a known medical or genetic condition or environmental factor; association with another neurodevelopmental, mental, or behavioural disorder; and with catatonia.

Autism has been a subject of considerable interest and research effort since its original description more than 50 years ago, when Leo Kanner (1943) described the profound isolation of these children and their extreme desire for sameness. These children appear aloof and indifferent to others and often seem to prefer inanimate objects.

The impairment in communication is severe and affects both verbal and nonverbal communication (APA, 2000). Children with autism manifest delayed and deviant language development, as evidenced by *echolalia* (repetition of words or phrases spoken by others), and a tendency to be extremely concrete in the interpretation of language. Pronoun reversals and abnormal intonation are also common. Other common features of severe autism categorized as **stereotypic behaviour** include repetitive rocking, hand flapping, and an extraordinary insistence on sameness. The child may also engage in self-injurious behaviour, such as hitting, head banging, or biting. For some children, their unusual interests may evolve into fascination with specific objects, such as fans or air conditioners, or a particular topic, such as Prime Ministers of Canada.

> **KEY CONCEPT** An **autism spectrum disorder** is a marked impairment of development in social interaction and communication with a restrictive repertoire of activity and interest.

Epidemiology and Aetiology

There has been a dramatic rise in the incidence of ASD, from 6.4 per 1,000 children aged 8 years in 2002 to 11.4 per 1,000 in 2008 for the 13 sites that provided data for both surveillance years in the United States (Centers for Disease Control and Prevention, 2012). The use of broader diagnostic criteria, more systematic assessment practices, and increased awareness and attention by health care professionals are factors that may be contributing to this apparent increase (Persico & Bourgeron, 2006).

ASD occurs more often in boys than in girls, with the ratio ranging from 2:1 to 5:1. However, when girls are affected, they tend to be more severely impaired and have poorer outcomes (Volkmar, Klin, & Paul, 2004). About half of children with ASD are intellectually disabled, and about 25% have seizure disorders.

The aetiology of ASD remains elusive, though research continues in the areas of genetics, neurology, and metabolic disorders. Numerous theories suggest various causes for autism, including genetics, perinatal insult, and impaired parent–child interactions (Volkmar et al., 2004). It was fashionable in the 1950s and 1960s to believe that the "indifference" of parents was a contributing cause of autism. This explanation is no longer seriously considered. It represents a failure to recognize that the child's disability may have contributed to disturbed parent-child interactions, rather than being an effect of these interactions.

Low IQ and autism recur at a higher than expected rate in the siblings of children with autism, and monozygotic twins are more likely to be **concordant** (mutually affected) than are dizygotic twins, suggesting that genetic factors play a role in the disorder. Other proposed causes include perinatal complications, such as exposure to infectious agents or medications during gestation; prematurity; and gestational bleeding. The role of environment in autistic disorder has been conclusively demonstrated only for prenatal or perinatal exposure to viral agents, such as rubella and cytomegalovirus, and prenatal exposure to thalidomide and valproic acid. Vaccinations have also drawn attention as possible causative factors due to their high content of thimerosal, a preservative containing mercury, and due to the proposed causal link between autism and the measles–mumps–rubella vaccine. However, recent epidemiologic studies have excluded a widespread causal role for vaccines in autism (Persico & Bourgeron, 2006). The specific cause remains unknown and may result from multiple factors. Studies of genetic, epigenetic, and environmental factors are finally beginning to provide some insights into solving the complexities of autistic disorder. Structural and functional imaging studies also provide intriguing leads for future inquiry (Fig. 31-1).

The literature quite clearly supports the need for early screening and referral programs to promote early diagnosis and treatment (Pinto-Martin, Souders, Giarelli, & Levy, 2005). Some early developmental indicators that suggest that a child should be referred for a full assessment include lack of babbling or gestures at 12 months, lack of single words by 16 months, lack of two-word combinations by 18 months, and any regression or loss of words or skills. Other developmental indicators include lack of joint attention (pointing to show), lack of response to name, and unusual or absent eye contact and use of facial expression (Perry & Condillac, 2003). Parents who report concerns about their child's development should be taken seriously. Early identification through screening followed by psychosocial support

FIGURE 31-1. The client with autism (right) may have decreased metabolic rates in the cingulate gyrus and other associated areas; however, wide heterogeneity in brain metabolic patterns is seen in clients with autism. (Courtesy of Monte S. Buchsbaum, MD, Mount Sinai Medical Centre and School of Medicine, New York, NY.)

and education about the disorder and treatment options can help families to adjust and cope (Pinto-Martin et al., 2005). Nursing has a pivotal role to play in all these areas.

Psychopharmacologic Interventions

No medication has proved effective at changing the core social and language deficits of autism. However, numerous psychiatric medications have been used to treat the associated coexisting challenges that can arise in ASD (Palermo & Curatolo, 2004; Witwer & Lecavalier, 2005). Medications can reduce the frequency and intensity of behavioural disturbances, including hyperactivity, agitation, mood instability, aggression, self-injury, and stereotypic behaviour, if they are causing trouble for the child/youth. Antipsychotic medications may be used to reduce aggression, but they may cause other serious side effects. Their use must be carefully reviewed. For example, studies have documented in a variety of clinical domains of autism the efficacy of several atypical antipsychotics, including risperidone, olanzapine, quetiapine, and clozapine. Risperidone, however, appears to be the most effective in treating core social–cognitive symptoms and other domains (stereotyped and repetitive behaviours) that are compromised in autism. Furthermore, its efficacy in improving working memory, executive function, and attention in schizophrenia, in addition to the clinical improvements in conditions that share certain clinical features with autism, such as obsessive–compulsive spectrum disorder, further strengthens evidence for its use. Due to the possible side effects of hyperprolactinemia and severe weight gain, children and adolescents on risperidone should be monitored closely, as the long-term consequences of elevated serum prolactin are not clear (Shea et al., 2004). Although considerable research has been conducted on the use of risperidone in treating autism, the long-term risks of use in children needs further study (Anderson et al., 2007).

The serotonin reuptake inhibitors, both selective (fluoxetine, sertraline, and paroxetine) and nonselective (clomipramine), also have a role in the treatment of interfering behaviours of autism, specifically repetitive and aggressive ones, and have been found to improve social relatedness in autistic children, more so in the presence of a positive family history for affective disorders (Palermo & Curatolo, 2004). Although no medication studies have been conducted on children with ASD, approaches to the treatment of depression and anxiety disorders would be the same as those used in typically developing young children.

Continuum of Care

ASD is chronic and usually requires long-term care at various levels of intensity. Children and adolescents with autism are a heterogeneous group, and as such, they have diverse needs. It is essential that intervention treatment plans be based on individual patterns of strengths and limitations (Perry & Condillac, 2003). Intervention treatment consists of designing academic, interpersonal, and social experiences that support the child's development. Children with autism, even those who are severely affected, may be able to live at home and attend a special school for children with autism that uses behaviour modification. Other outpatient services may include family counselling, home care, and medication. As the child moves towards adulthood, living at home may become more difficult, given the appropriate need for greater independence. The level of structure required depends primarily on IQ and adaptive functioning. Ongoing support and respite for the family are critical and an essential part of the intervention treatment plan in which nursing plays an integral role.

Nursing Management: Human Response to Autistic Spectrum Disorder

The nursing assessment is an ongoing process in which attention is given to establishing a positive relationship with the child and the family. The assessment should include a review of the child's capacity for self-care and maladaptive behaviours (Pinto-Martin et al., 2005; Sherer & Schreibman, 2005). Self-injury and aggression are sometimes present, and children may need to be protected from hurting themselves and others. Inquiry should also include the presence of perseverative behaviours and preoccupation with restricted interests. These odd behaviours may not necessarily cause a problem, but they often interfere with the child's relationships.

Another important domain to consider in the nursing assessment is the effect of the child's developmental delays on the family. Having a child with ASD is bound to influence family interaction, and responding to the child's needs may adversely affect family functioning. For example, sleep disruption in family members who care for these children may increase family stress.

Assessment data generate a variety of potential nursing diagnoses, including social isolation. The family may be grieving the loss of the normal child it had expected and is trying to cope with the multitude of problems inherent in raising a child with a disability. Because of the long-term nature of these disorders, the aims of treatment may change with time. However, throughout childhood, the focus should be on the development of age-appropriate adaptive and social skills.

Biologic Domain

The assessment of children with ASD is a complex endeavour (Pinto-Martin et al., 2005; Sherer & Schreibman, 2005). Biologic assessment should include a review of physical health and neurologic status, giving particular attention to coordination, childhood illnesses, injuries, and hospitalizations. The nurse should assess sleep, appetite, and activity patterns because they may be disturbed in these children. Lack of adequate sleep can increase irritability. Sleep problems are common in children with ASD. Comorbid seizure disorders are common in autism, and depression may be seen concurrently. The nurse should therefore also consider these conditions in his or her assessment of the child.

Youngsters with additional psychiatric disorders or seizures may be receiving multiple medications and require the care of several clinicians. Therefore, the assessment should include a careful review of current medications by treating clinicians. Assessment data generate a variety of potential nursing diagnoses, including self-care deficits, impaired verbal communication, disturbed sensory perceptions, delayed growth and development, and disturbed sleep patterns. Treatment outcomes need to be individualized to the child, family, and social environment.

Psychosocial Domain

Planning interventions for youngsters with severe developmental problems considers the child, family, and community supports, such as schools, rehabilitation centres, mental health centres, or group homes and available respite services. First and foremost, the various clinicians involved in the child's treatment should collaborate with the family to promote reaching the same general goals. As the number of clinicians and educators involved increases, the chance of fragmentation in treatment planning also increases. The nurse can serve as a case coordinator to ensure that the plan of care is both comprehensive and appropriate in meeting the needs of both the child and the family.

Promoting Interaction

Many of the core deficits in ASD fall within the domain of social development, regardless of the level of cognitive functioning of the particular child or youth. The goal of intervention in the social domain is to increase meaningful relationships by teaching skills that support the development of social interest, social initiation, social responsiveness, empathy, and understanding of the other's perspective. It is critical that intervention treatment plans include strategies to enhance social understanding, social relating, and play skills, and that these strategies take into account the individual's cognitive, learning, linguistic, and developmental abilities (Perry & Condillac, 2003). Interventions fostering nonverbal social interactions may sometimes be more useful than those based on speech. For higher-functioning children, activities such as getting the mail, passing out snacks, or taking turns in the context of simple games can engage them in social activities without requiring the use of their limited language skills. Structuring social interactions so that the child has to share a task with another (e.g., carrying a load of books) may help to boost confidence in relating to others.

Ensuring Predictability and Safety

When children with ASD are hospitalized, milieu management—a consistent, structured environment with predictable routines for activities, mealtimes, and bedtimes—is necessary for successful treatment. Changes in routine may provoke disorganization in the child with ASD, leading to emotional disequilibrium and explosive behaviour. The safety of the inpatient unit offers an opportunity to try behavioural strategies, such as rewards for managing transitions. Health care professionals can explore with family the strategies that have been successful for managing behaviours in the past and can also share new successful strategies with parents or primary caregivers.

Self-Care

In teaching self-care skills, the nurse needs to consider the child's current adaptive skills and language limitations. Developing a list of activities for the child to post in his or her bedroom may be effective for some children. Drawings or symbols may be useful for nonverbal children. Physical safety is an important concern for children who are cognitively delayed and may have impaired judgment.

As noted earlier, children with ASD may be treated with multiple medications in novel combinations (Martin, Van Hoof, Stubbe, Sherwin, & Scahill, 2003).

In some cases, these unusual combinations are the result of careful management; in other cases, the combinations are the result of clinical mismanagement, perhaps because of poor coordination among treating prescribers. Consequently, the nurse should carefully review the target symptoms for each drug treatment with the parents. This review includes possible drug interactions that are especially important for this clinical population.

Managing Behaviour

Because children with ASD have difficulty relating to others, they should spend most of their time within the therapeutic environment of the unit. These children can learn social and communication skills, such as taking turns in conversation and warning the listener before changing the subject in the context of milieu. If a child requires a break from the milieu to reduce stimulation and regain control of aggressive or assaultive behaviour, a brief break away followed by prompt reentry into unit activities is optimum.

Managing the repetitive behaviours of these children will depend on the specific behaviour and its effects on others or the environment. If the behaviour, such as rocking, has no negative effects, ignoring it may be the best approach. If the behaviour, such as head banging, is unacceptable, redirecting the child and using positive reinforcement are recommended. In some cases, especially in severely delayed children, these strategies may not work, and environmental alterations and perhaps protective headgear are needed.

Supporting Family

Autism and related disorders are chronic conditions that call for extraordinary patience and determination. Unfortunately, lack of integration of medical, psychiatric, social, and educational services can add to the family's burden. Family stress research has repeatedly demonstrated that parents (especially mothers) of children with ASDs experience greater stress, depression, and mental health difficulties than parents of children with other types of disability (Perry & Condillac, 2003). Parents may manifest feelings of denial, grief, guilt, anger, and sorrow at various points as they adjust to their child's disability. The nurse can offer parents the opportunity to express their frustrations and disappointments and can be alert for indications that parents are in need of additional assistance, such as parent support groups or respite care. Residential and respite care may be necessary in some cases. After making the decision to place a child into someone else's care, family members may experience guilt, loss, and a sense of failure concerning their inability to care for the child at home.

Family interventions include support, education, counselling, and referral to self-help groups. Whenever possible, the nurse provides education to help parents determine appropriate expectations for their child with

ASD and to meet the child's special needs. The following are examples of potentially useful nursing interventions focusing on the family:

- Interpreting the treatment plan for parents and the child
- Modelling appropriate behaviour modification techniques
- Including the parents as cotherapists for the implementation of the care plan
- Assisting the family members in identifying and resolving their sense of loss related to the diagnosis
- Coordinating support systems for parents, siblings, and family members
- Maintaining interdisciplinary collaboration
- Facilitating access to and encouraging families to use formal support services such as respite care
- Assisting parents to advocate/lobby on behalf of their child and children with disabilities

There are a number of support services in Canada and throughout the provinces; however, it is best that parents access services through legitimate agencies and organizations. For examples of these, see the Web Links on the thePoint.

Evaluation of client and family outcomes is an ongoing process. Short-term outcomes might consist of discrete behavioural improvements, such as reducing self-injurious behaviour by 50%. The long-term goal is for the client to achieve the highest level of functioning. The prognosis depends on the severity of the impairments, the interventions available, and the cognitive ability of the child. The use of standardized rating scales before and after the treatment can improve the precision of outcome measurement (Perry & Condillac, 2003).

Spiritual Domain

As spirituality is about who we are and our connections with one another and the sacred, it shapes our lives (see Chapter 5). Children with ASD may face particular challenges in terms of evolving and sustaining their spirituality. Children understand themselves and the world around them based on their level of development and experience (Smith & McSherry, 2004). Children with ASD will need spiritual support (e.g., help to express their spiritual needs) based on their individual capacity for understanding and interacting with others. A major challenge, however, is that the spiritual lives of children with special needs or disabilities can be devalued or ignored. A study of parents/caregivers of such children revealed that they were disillusioned or alienated from potential spiritual support when, for instance, they found their children to be unwelcome at their church or synagogue (Speraw, 2006). No participant in this study perceived nurses as being aware of or interested in their family's spiritual needs. Yet, this is where spiritual care must begin: with an explicit regards for the

---

IN A LIFE

Temple Grandin (1949–)
Scientist and a Person With Autism

Public Persona
Dr. Temple Grandin is a gifted scientist and world-renowned expert on cattle. Her book *Thinking in Pictures and Other Reports of My Life With Autism* (1996) is an astonishing examination of the profoundly different way in which a person with autism conceives and experiences the world. Her story shows the extraordinary way in which she uses her visual thinking ability to develop her field of animal science. It gives us a view of her world and helps us understand the reason she identifies with Data, the android in *Star Trek*. In 2010, her story appeared as a movie, *Temple Grandin*, starring Claire Danes.

Personal Realities
As a child, Temple experienced life as chaotic, full of engulfing sensations of sound, smell, and touch. She would scream, rock, or spin continually and shut the world out by fixing for hours on one object. At first thought to be deaf when she did not learn to speak, she was taken to a neurologist and labelled "brain damaged." Although she gained a sense of language and speech, connecting with others was affected by her inability to understand them or them, her. She dreamed of a magic machine that could give her safe "hugging." Her mother's dedication to her and the guidance of a gifted science teacher enabled her to create a life as a scientist.

---

importance of this domain to one's clients (see Chapter 30 for ways to address children's spiritual domain).

Specific Learning Disorders

Specific **learning disorders** (also called learning disabilities) are among the most common neurodevelopmental disorders in children and are defined as difficulties in learning and using academic skills. They are important causes of poor school performance. For this diagnosis to be given, a child must have at least one of the following symptoms for over 6 months:

- Inaccurate or slow, effortful word reading
- Difficulty understanding meaning of what is read
- Difficulties with spelling
- Difficulties with written expression
- Difficulties mastering number sense, number facts, or calculation
- Difficulties with mathematical reasoning

The affected academic skills must be begin during school-age years, not be better accounted for by another disorder/adversity (e.g., visual or auditory impairment; lack of language proficiency), be significantly below expected for age, and interfere with academic or occupational performance. (Note: For an individual >17 years, a documented history of learning impairment can be used for assessment.) **Dyslexia** is a term that has been used for a specific learning disorder involving reading impairment and "dyscalculia" for impairment in mathematical abilities.

For children with learning disabilities, the negative effects of low achievement or failure may be manifested in low self-esteem and reduced academic effort. Some children and adolescents may also exhibit difficulties in age-appropriate social interactions. Postsecondary students with learning disabilities have been observed to exhibit poor self-concepts, have problems with interpersonal skills, and have deficits in processing and study skills (Ransby & Swanson, 2003). Research also suggests that children and adolescents with learning disorders experience more feelings of loneliness, depression, stress, and suicidal ideations than their peers without learning disabilities (Buysse, Goldman, & Skinner, 2003). For the child/adolescent with learning disabilities, nurses can focus on building self-confidence and helping the family connect with guidance and educational resources that support his or her ongoing development.

Communication Disorders

Communication disorders involve deficits in speech, language, and communication. *Speech* refers to the motor aspects of making sounds and includes "articulation, fluency, voice, and resonance quality" (APA, 2013, p. 41). *Language* consists of higher-order aspects of formulating and comprehending a conventional system of symbols (e.g., spoken words, sign language, pictures) (APA). *Communication* involves verbal and/or nonverbal behaviour (whether or not intentional) that influences another person (APA). Communication disorder in the *DSM-5* includes "language disorder, speech sound disorder, childhood-onset fluency disorder (stuttering), social (pragmatic) communication disorder, and other specified and nonspecified communication disorders" (APA, 2013, p. 41).

Communication disorders are an area in which assessments must be absolutely relevant to the cultural and linguistic background of the individual, if they are to be valid. Speech pathologists conduct the diagnostic assessment. Services such as speech therapy (directed at the motor aspects of speaking) or social skills groups (directed at the social and interpersonal aspects of language) may be available in some school districts and can be obtained if a speech or language disorder has been identified. For some children with communication disorders, the services offered by the school may be insufficient. In such cases, the nurse can help the family locate resources that can provide these needed services.

For the child with a communication disorder, interventions focus on fostering social and communication skills, identifying and addressing low self-esteem, and making referrals for specific speech or language therapy. Modelling appropriate communication in spontaneous situations with the child can be a useful intervention for some children. As with other neurodevelopmental disorders, education and support of the parents are a key intervention.

■ DISRUPTIVE IMPULSE CONTROL AND CONDUCT DISORDERS

The disruptive behaviour disorders within the *DSM-5* include oppositional defiant disorder, conduct disorder, intermittent explosive disorder, kleptomania, and pyromania. For purposes of this text, we will focus on oppositional defiant disorder (ODD) and conduct disorder, syndromes marked by significant problems of conduct. These **externalizing disorders** are in contrast to disorders of mood (e.g., anxiety, depression), which are referred to as internalizing disorders because the symptoms tend to be within the child.

Oppositional Defiant Disorder

Unfortunately, some children are labelled oppositional if they challenge authority or have temper tantrums. The diagnostic criteria for ODD, however, require that the symptoms be persistent, consistent, and exceed what is normative for age, development, gender, and culture. They must be exhibited with at least one individual who is not a sibling (APA, 2013). The pattern of angry/irritable mood, argumentative defiant behaviour, and/or vindictiveness must have occurred for at least 6 months for this diagnosis to be ascribed. It is the persistence and frequency of the behaviours that distinguish them as disordered; these behaviours cannot occur exclusively in the presence of "a psychotic, substance use, depressive, or bipolar disorder" (APA, 2013, p. 462).

Nursing Management: Human Response to Oppositional Defiant Disorder

Nurses working with families of children who have ODD may be frustrated and focused on the negative behaviour challenges of the child. The nurse's primary task, however, is to assist the family to refocus and find the child's strengths and skills, as well as learn to respond to negative behaviours in ways that promote positive change. Similar to working with the child with a trauma history, the caregivers work to develop strategies to attune to their child and understand the child's emotional triggers. The family is taught to work with the child to recognize those feelings and develop new coping skills that allow the child to socialize with others in a more positive manner (Boston Children's Hospital, 2013). Depending on the child's age and family circumstances, some programs take a behavioural modification approach. The evidence for successful outcomes with this approach is inconsistent. Mindfulness is being used in some programs as a strategy; others are incorporating technology, such as computer games, to teach children emotional regulation (Boston Children's Hospital, 2013).

The nurse will need to work with the child and family to attend to coexisting conditions such as ADHD, anxiety disorder, or depression. Specific interventions to support the child coping with anxiety may alleviate some of the oppositional traits. Similarly, if the ADHD is treated medically or structurally, the symptoms of ODD may be alleviated. The nurse will need to provide additional teaching and direction regarding ODD to support groups and agencies primarily focused on working with children with ADHD and mood and anxiety disorders.

Biologic Domain

The aetiology of ODD is complex; however, there is growing evidence that indicates both genetic and environmental components (Bornovalova, Hicks, Iacono, & McGue, 2010). Complicating a diagnosis of ODD is often a coexisting condition such as ADHD, a learning disability, internalizing disorder, and/or trauma disorder.

Psychosocial Domain

Children with ODD that persists across their development struggle socially: they experience frequent conflicts with peers, teachers, siblings, and caregivers. The child may have experienced negative parenting (e.g., neglectful, punitive, erratic), perhaps due to parental frustration or a parent's own oppositional traits. The child may have experienced bullying, or may be the bully. If the challenges are significant, the family will need to consider if the child's recovery will be better supported in a new school environment. The nurse will need to work closely with those involved with the child to create an environment where the child learns new communication strategies and others learn ways to respond to the child that are helpful and supportive of change. Evaluation for secondary contributing disorders such as ADHD, anxiety, or depression will need to occur (Boylan, Vaillancourt, Boyle, & Szatmari, 2007).

Spiritual Domain

The nurse works closely with caregivers to assist with cultural understanding and access community supports. Families may struggle with participation in religious, cultural, or community-based organizations if the child has been identified as causing trouble or parents are identified in some way as not "parenting effectively." Again, this strongly depends on context and belief systems. A proactive strategy may be to offer to help the family provide their community with information about ODD.

Conduct Disorder

Conduct disorder has been identified as having three potential onsets: childhood before the age of 10 years; adolescence after 10 years; and unspecified, wherein no information is available to determine the age of onset. Childhood-onset conduct disorder may have a poorer prognosis than adolescent onset. The disorder typically occurs in males and may or may not have precursor conditions such as ODD, ADHD, or internalizing disorders. There is some indication that a traumatic childhood or poor attachment may also lead to the development of conduct disorder symptoms.

Nursing Management: Human Response to Conduct Disorder

Determining what the child/youth and family are ready to address is critical with this population. There are several family-based treatments that have demonstrated success over time. The challenge for the nurse is engaging the child/youth and family in the process (Box 31-6). For example, multisystem therapy is an intensive family- and community-based treatment program that focuses on addressing all environmental systems—home, school, neighbourhood—and works towards affecting change in all domains. The primary focus is developing the child/youth's relationships; identifying and building on

---

BOX 31-6   Clinical Vignette

LEON (CONDUCT DISORDER)

Leon, a 14-year-old boy, was admitted to the child psychiatric inpatient service from the emergency department after a fight with his mother. His mother reported that she and Leon had argued earlier in the evening and that he stormed out of the house screaming and vowing that he would never return. Several hours later, Leon came back, yelling and demanding entry into the apartment. Leon's father was working. While his mother was getting up to open the door, Leon continued to yell and scream, waking the neighbours. This led to further arguing between Leon and his mother. Before long, the police were called, and Leon was taken to the emergency department.

The admission interview revealed that Leon had run away on several occasions and had even stayed away overnight. Although he strongly denied drug use, he had gotten drunk on several occasions. He had also been in several fights, the latest of which resulted in an expulsion from school. Three months before admission, he was caught trying to steal a CD from a music store. More recently, he boasted that he and his friends had snatched a purse at an outdoor concert and had broken into a car to steal its contents. Leon's school performance has been declining; he was truant on several occasions and will probably have to repeat ninth grade.

Leon was born in Cape Breton, N.S., and is the oldest of three children. His family moved to Toronto shortly after his birth. His father is employed as a janitor and is illiterate. His mother works as a secretary and has recently completed a BA in English. There is much marital discord at home. Leon has received no treatment except for consultation with the school social worker.

What Do You Think?
- When conducting a nursing assessment, what would you want to learn about Leon's school performance?
- What information could you provide Leon's parents about pharmacotherapy? About behaviour management?
- How would you present the material so it meets the learning needs of both parents?

strengths; developing responsibility and accountability; and promoting success (Henggeler & Sheidow, 2012).

Biologic Domain

There is evidence of genetic contribution that is complicated by environmental factors. For instance, the risk for conduct disorder is increased in the offspring of individuals with conduct disorder. The effects of a traumatic home environment that includes family disruption, parental mental illness, poverty, community violence, and abuse also increase the risk for conduct disorder in biologic or adopted children (Bornovalova et al., 2010; Kim-Cohen et al., 2005). Recent studies have been examining the neurodevelopment of children with conduct disorder. There is exploratory research indicating some evidence that there may be a reduction in grey matter in the brain in areas that govern social–emotional functioning; the cause, however, remains unclear (Fairchild et al., 2011). Lower than average intelligence, verbal IQ in particular, may be contributory to the diagnosis. Males with conduct disorder often exhibit more overt aggression, whereas females tend to be more subversive in their aggression (APA, 2013).

Psychosocial Domain

Children/youth with conduct disorder are often in trouble with the law, school authorities, and family. They often experience rejection from caregivers, school, and their community. They may also be exposed to abusive home environments if parents also have conduct traits or there are environmental contributors such as poverty or violence. The context in which a diagnosis is applied needs to be taken into account if it is considered normative for the community and general survival. Coexisting disorders that are often associated with conduct disorder are ODD, ADHD, learning and/or communication disorders, as well as internalizing disorders such as anxiety, depression, and likely PTSD.

Spiritual Domain

The nurse works closely with caregivers to assist with cultural understanding and access community supports. Families may struggle with participation in religious, cultural, or community-based organizations if the child has been identified as causing trouble or parents are identified in some way as not "parenting effectively." Again, this strongly depends on context and belief systems (see Box 31-7).

Attention Deficit Hyperactivity Disorder

All children have occasional experiences with inattention and high energy levels. For most children, these occurrences do not interfere with daily life. According to the Canadian ADHD Resource Alliance (CADDRA),

---

BOX 31-7   Research for Best Practice

CHANGE IN FATHERS' PERCEPTIONS OF MENTAL HEALTH WHEN HIS CHILD IS DIAGNOSED WITH A MENTAL ILLNESS

Morris, M. (2014). Diagnosis in young children: How a father's perceptions of mental health change. Journal of Child and Adolescent Psychiatric Nursing, 27(2), 52–60.

Questions: How does diagnosing mental illness in a young child (<10 years) affect a parent's perception of mental health?

Methods: Case study method was used, guided by Denzin's interpretive interactionism, in which "epiphanies" or pivotal life experiences that deeply affect one's sense of self and the world are explored. "Joe," the father in this case study, has a son, "Billy," who struggled behaviourally when he attended kindergarten in a charter school. Joe was asked to come with Billy to help him adjust. When, on the advice of the school counsellor, this ended, Billy reacted violently, destroying part of his classroom and hurting teachers and classmates. Diagnoses proposed for Billy, now 7 years old, include attachment disorder, ADHD, mood disorder, bipolar disorder, and low-grade autism. Billy's parents have sought help for him from a play therapist with a specialty in attachment; an occupational therapist; a psychotherapist; an alternative school psychologist; and a neurologist. Joe and his wife have reached out to other parents with similar experiences.

Findings: Themes that emerged for Joe were "alienation from peers, ambivalence, shifting orientation to mental illness, school system stigmatization/conflict with mental health care, and discovery of mental health care specialists and new peers." Joe stated, "It has been this progression of acceptance." "… I even started to see going to play therapy, it was partly just for me as much as for [Billy] … I actually was looking forward to going because … I was getting as much out of it as he was in a lot of ways. I wasn't exactly expecting that, I guess.…"

Implications for Nursing Practice: The researcher notes that the loss of self-agency experienced by this parent in his interactions with school and health care systems was notable. This points to the need for active promotion of a meaningful sense of agency and hope in working with parents, in addition to offering medical and technologic interventions.

---

attention deficit hyperactivity disorder (ADHD) is a neuropsychiatric developmental disorder affecting 5% to 12% of school-aged children, 8% to 10% of males under the age of 18, and 3% to 4% of females under 18 (CADDRA, 2013b). It is associated with functional impairments such as school dysfunction, peer problems, and family conflicts. Children and youth with ADHD can struggle in a multitude of domains at different times throughout their development. It is likely that, at some point in their career, nurses will work with children/youth and adults with ADHD.

ADHD is a persistent pattern of inattention, hyperactivity, and impulsiveness that interferes with functioning or development (APA, 2013). Parents and teachers describe children with ADHD as restless, always on the go, highly distractible, unable to wait their turn, heedless, and frequently disruptive. Often it is their disruptive behaviour that brings these children into treatment. The historical debate concerning the nature of ADHD is reflected in the labels once used to describe it: organic brain syndrome, hyperkinetic impulse disorder, minimal brain dysfunction, hyperkinetic reaction of childhood, hyperkinesis, attention deficit disorder, and, most recently in the *DSM-5*, ADHD. Despite the historical shifts in terminology that reflect various proposals for aetiology, the accumulated consensus during the past several decades is that three core symptoms define the disorder: inattention, impulsiveness, and hyperactivity.

The *DSM-5* defines ADHD as predominantly hyperactive/impulsive presentation, predominantly inattentive presentation, or combined presentation. To be diagnosed with ASD, a child must show a persistent pattern of inattention and/or hyperactivity–impulsivity that interferes with his or her development (APA, 2013). Attention is a complex mental process that involves the ability to concentrate on one activity to the exclusion of others, as well as the ability to sustain focus. Children with ADHD are easily distracted and lack persistence in the performance of age-appropriate tasks, reflecting an inability to filter stimuli, sustain attention, or both. The inability to screen stimuli leaves the child unable to identify salient stimuli. The child may then treat all incoming stimuli with equal regards and respond to multiple incoming stimuli. An alternate argument holds that the distractibility seen in ADHD is the result of stimulus-seeking behaviour. Given the heterogeneity of ADHD, either of these models may be true for subgroups of affected children.

Both clinical observations and laboratory studies support the conclusion that children with ADHD can be prone to impulsiveness and risk-taking behaviours (Biederman & Faraone, 2005). In behavioural terms, children with ADHD often fail to consider the consequences of their actions, exercise poor judgement, and tend to have more than the usual lumps, bumps, and bruises because of their risk-taking behaviour. They often require a high degree of structure and supervision. In many cases, it is the hyperactivity that prompts the search for treatment. Parents typically report that the child's hyperactivity was manifest early in life and evident in most situations. These behaviours, although challenging, were not deemed problematic until the child entered a more structured environment such as daycare, kindergarten, or school.

The diagnosis of ADHD is based upon the ability to observe symptoms that seem to occur consistently in at least two different environments, such as home and school. For the diagnosis to be given, there must be at least some symptoms present before the age of 12 years and they must be present for at least 6 months. A physical exam should be performed, as well as a hearing and eyesight test, to rule out any physical reasons for the symptoms. A psychoeducational assessment is recommended to determine whether other learning disabilities coexist with the ADHD or cause the symptoms (CADDRA, 2013b).

Gender distribution of ADHD is approximately three males to one female in a community population; however, this almost triples in a clinical sample, with boys to girls at 9:1 (Ramtekkar, Reiersen, Todorov, & Todd, 2010). Longitudinal studies that followed groups of children with ADHD into adulthood have shown the persistence of symptoms (Biederman & Faraone, 2005). There is change in symptom presentation as an individual grows and develops and perhaps acquires compensatory strategies; however, even when symptoms are not prominent, they remain associated with clinically significant impairments (Centre for ADHD Awareness, Canada [CADDAC], 2013). Older adolescents and young adults with a history of ADHD may struggle with staying in school and keeping a job, maintaining relationships and have more traffic violations and accidents than individuals without the diagnosis of ADHD (CADDAC).

KEY CONCEPT **Attention** is a complex process that involves the ability to concentrate on one activity to the exclusion of others and the ability to sustain that focus.

KEY CONCEPT **Impulsiveness** refers to hasty actions that occur in the moment, without forethought, and that are potentially highly harmful to the individual (APA, 2013).

KEY CONCEPT **Hyperactivity** refers to excessive motor activity when it is not appropriate, or to excessive fidgeting, tapping, or talkativeness (APA, 2013).

Aetiologic Factors

ADHD emerged as the first psychiatric disorder to be diagnosed and treated in children, with studies of stimulant treatment beginning in 1937 and regulatory approval for it occurring in the 1960s (Doyle, 2004). ADHD has emerged from the 20th century with a good deal of scientific investigation of its validity and clarification of clinical controversies. Nevertheless, the aetiology of ADHD remains unclear. Risk factors for the development of the disorder include genetic predisposition, as well as biologic, environmental, and psychosocial factors. No one causal factor is necessary or sufficient to trigger the disorder, and risk factors are interchangeable. What is critical is the total number of risk factors (Biederman & Faraone, 2005).

Brain imaging studies have revealed that, in youth with ADHD, the brain matures in a normal pattern but is delayed, on average, by about 3 years (Shaw et al., 2007).

The delay is most pronounced in brain regions involved in thinking, paying attention, and planning. More recent studies have found that the outermost layer of the brain, the cortex, shows delayed maturation overall (Shaw et al., 2012), and a brain structure, important for proper communication between the two hemispheres of the brain, shows an abnormal growth pattern. These delays and abnormalities may underlie the hallmark symptoms of ADHD and help to explain the disorder's development (Gilliam et al., 2011). It is with this understanding that ADHD has been reclassified most recently in the *DSM-5* under neurodevelopmental disorders.

Biologic Factors

There have been various theories regarding the neurobiologic site of presumed dysfunction in ADHD. One such theory is that the pattern of neuropsychological deficit in individuals with ADHD is caused by the dysregulation of the frontal–subcortical circuits. That finding has now been confirmed by structural and functional neuroimaging studies showing those individuals to have small volume reductions in these regions (Faraone & Bierderman, 2004). Other findings suggest that aberrant frontal–subcortical circuitry is not sufficient to explain the pathophysiology of the disorder. One study has revealed widespread but small volume reductions throughout the brain; another has shown widespread cortical abnormalities (Sowell et al., 2003). A later study implicated structures such as the cerebellum and the corpus callosum, which are outside the frontal–subcortical circuits (Seidman, Valera, & Bush, 2004). Molecular imaging studies suggest that abnormalities of the dopamine transporter lead to impaired neurotransmission (Durston et al., 2003). A study using MRI scans of the putamen in 44 males (25 recruited from a residential treatment centre and having comorbid ADHD and psychopathic traits and 19 healthy community controls) found no differences in the total left or right volume of the putamen. The study did however find a reversal of symmetry in the ADHD group compared with the control group. The ADHD children's group generally had a larger right putamen than left, whereas control children's group had a larger left putamen than right (McMahon-Wellington, Semrud-Clikeman, Gregory, Murphy, & Lancaster, 2006).

For many decades, studies have shown that ADHD is transmitted in families (Faraone, 2004). According to twin and adoption studies carried out in Australia, Sweden, the United Kingdom, and the United States, genes have a substantial role in familial transmission. The data from this study also suggest that estimates of heritability have not changed from 1973 to 2004. Adoptive studies also implicate genetic causes. Adoptive relatives of children with ADHD are less likely than biologic relatives to have the disorder or associated syndrome (Biederman & Faraone, 2005).

Molecular genetic studies are beginning to unravel the complex genetics of ADHD. Genome scans of individuals with ADHD have used the method of linkage analysis to screen the genome for regions that might include disease-related susceptibility genes (Bakker et al., 2003). Candidate gene studies of ADHD have produced substantial evidence implicating several genes in the aetiology of the disorder (Faraone et al., 2005).

Numerous environmental exposures, including food sensitivity, food additives, and lead poisoning, have been examined as potential causes of ADHD and generally have been found to be false (Biederman & Faraone, 2005). A balanced diet and regular activity and exercise are a good strategy for everyone. There is increasing evidence, however, that a relative lack of omega-3 fatty acids may contribute to many psychiatric and neurodevelopmental disorders, including ADHD (Richardson, 2006). A positive correlation has been found between obstetrical complications and ADHD and learning disorders. A Quebec study of 64 children aged 6 to 12 diagnosed with ADHD was conducted to assess for a history of obstetrical complications using the Kinney Medical and Gynecological Questionnaire. Children with ADHD and a learning disability in mathematics or reading had a higher rate of neonatal complications than children with ADHD and no disability (Bhat, Grizenko, Ben-Amor, & Joober, 2005). These results further support what has already been shown for ADHD and learning disorders individually: that the events in the early life of a child are critical to brain development.

Psychosocial Factors

Although genetic endowment clearly plays a fundamental role in the aetiology of ADHD, psychosocial factors are also important. Children with ADHD live in families with a host of problems that both affect and are affected by the child. Parents of children with ADHD report more frequent and severe interparental discord and child-rearing disagreements, more negative parenting practices, greater caregiver strain, and more psychopathology themselves. Children with ADHD (impulsive/hyperactive) can be bossy, intrusive, immature, boisterous, aggressive, and less aware of social cues. Such behaviours affect social function, making and keeping friends, and can contribute to parental unwillingness to take their ADHD child on social outings or vacations. These children are also often rejected from sports teams and other recreational and social groups (Pelham, Fabiano, & Massetti, 2005).

Nursing Management: Human Response to Attention Deficit Hyperactivity Disorder

In the school setting, the primary focus of the assessment is the impact of ADHD symptoms on academic and social functioning. In a hospital setting, the nurse tries to determine the contribution of ADHD to the acute psychiatric problem. In both cases, the nurse collects assessment data through direct interview, observation of the child and parent, and teacher ratings. Because children with ADHD may have difficulty sitting through long sessions, interviews are typically brief. Parents and teachers are extremely important sources for assessment data. To this end, the nurse can make use of several standardized instruments (Box 31-8) including those outlined in the *Canadian ADHD Practice Guidelines* (revised 3rd edition), available for download at the CADDRA Web site (see Web Links on the thePoint).

As with other psychiatric disorders with onset in childhood, the nursing assessment of children with ADHD begins with the identification and exploration of the presenting problem. This typically entails a review of the child's developmental course, the onset and pattern of the current symptoms, factors that have worsened or improved the child's problems, and prior treatment or self-initiated efforts to remedy the situation. The association of ADHD and communication disorders suggests a need for careful consideration of language development and current language functioning. Medical history is also essential, consisting of perinatal course, childhood illnesses, hospital admissions, injuries, seizures, tics, physical growth, general health status, and timing of the child's last physical examination. Family history is also an important part of assessment data.

BOX 31-8 Standardized Tools for ADHD Diagnosis

The Conners Parent Questionnaire is a 48-item scale that a parent completes about his or her child. Each item is a statement that the parent rates on a four-point scale from 0 (not at all) to 3 (very much). The Conners Teacher Questionnaire is a 28-item questionnaire that the child's teacher completes according to the same four-point scale as the Parent Questionnaire. Both questionnaires have been standardized by age and gender for a mean of 50 and a standard deviation of 10 (Conners, 1989; Goyette, Conners, & Ulrich, 1978).

The ADHD Rating Scale is a recently developed measure that asks parents or teachers to respond directly to 18 items in the *DSM-IV-TR* criteria (see Barkley, 1998, for a description of this scale). A similar scale called the SNAP-IV is available online for free at www.adhd.net. The SNAP-IV was used as the primary outcome measure in the MTA Cooperative Group Study (1999).

The Child Behaviour Checklist (CBCL) is a 118-item questionnaire that a parent completes. In addition to the 118 questions about specific behaviours and psychiatric symptoms, the CBCL also includes questions concerning the child's competence in social and academic spheres as well as age-appropriate activities. Normative data are available allowing the conversion of raw scores to standard scores for age and gender. There is also a teacher version of this scale.

Note that the diagnosis of ADHD is not made on the basis of questionnaires alone. Data from these rating scales augment the information gathered through interview and observation. These questionnaires can be especially useful before and after initiating a treatment plan to measure the change.

Children with ADHD can be very active; they struggle to sit still and often fidget or bounce their leg to keep moving. They may be more active during sleep than normal children. A careful assessment of eating, sleeping, and activity patterns is therefore essential. Assessing daily food intake, typical diet, and frequency of eating will help identify any nutrition problems. Caffeinated products can contribute to hyperactivity. Sleep is often disturbed for children with ADHD and, consequently, the family. A detailed sleep assessment can provide points for interventions and help the interpretation of drug effects.

Depending on the severity of the responses, family situation, and school environment, several nursing diagnoses could be generated from the assessment data, including self-care deficit, risk for imbalanced nutrition, risk for injury, and disturbed sleep pattern. The outcomes should be individualized to the child (Fig. 31-2).

Treatment of ADHD typically is conducted in community clinic settings. Optimal treatment is multimodal (includes several types of interventions), encompassing five main areas: psychoeducation for the child and family, behavioural and/or occupational interventions for the child, individual and family support, counselling and therapy, school accommodations, and medication management. Well-managed medication is an important intervention for the core symptoms of ADHD to facilitate the other areas of intervention (CADDRA, 2011). Parent training and social skills training also help diminish disruptive and defiant behaviours (see Nursing Care Plan 31-1). Treatment plans need regular upgrading to address important social, cognitive, psychological, and physical changes that occur as the child ages (Children's Health Policy Centre, Simon Fraser University, 2007).

The planning of nursing interventions must be done within the context of the family, treatment setting, and school environment. With the parents, clinical team members, and school personnel, the nurse participates in designing a plan of care that fits the child's and family's needs.

FIGURE 31-2. Long-term outcomes of optimal treatment for clients with attention deficit hyperactivity disorder.

Nursing Care Plan 31-1

Attention Deficit Hyperactivity Disorder

Jamie, age 6 years, comes to the mental health clinic with his mother Lillian because of motor restlessness, distractibility, and disruptive behaviour in the classroom. According to Lillian, Jamie had a reasonably good year in kindergarten, but early in the first grade, the teacher began to report disruptive behaviour such as not waiting his turn and interrupting his peers. On reflection, Lillian recalls that kindergarten was a half-day program with more activity. By contrast, Jamie is expected to sit in his seat and pay attention for longer periods in first grade.

Jamie's medical history is unremarkable. Lillian's pregnancy with Jamie was her first and unplanned. Although there were no complications during the pregnancy, the period was marked by significant marital discord, culminating in divorce before Jamie's first birthday. Jamie was born by caesarean section after a long, unproductive labour. He was healthy at birth and grew normally, with no develop-

mental delays. Despite genuine interest in other children, his intrusive style and inability to wait his turn resulted in frequent conflicts with them. The family history is positive for substance abuse in his father. In addition, Lillian reports that her ex-husband was disruptive in school, had trouble concentrating, and was highly impulsive. These problems have continued into adulthood and the father is inconsistent in his visits with Jamie.

During the two evaluation sessions, Jamie is active but cooperative. His speech is fluent and normal in tone and tempo, but somewhat loud. His discourse is coherent, but at times, he makes rather abrupt changes in conversation without warning his listeners. Psychological testing done at the school revealed average to above-average intelligence. Parent and teacher questionnaires concurred that Jamie was overactive, impulsive, inattentive, and quarrelsome, but not defiant.

Setting: Mental Health Centre—Child and Adolescent Services

Baseline Assessment: Jamie is a 6-year-old boy with prominent hyperactivity and disruptive behaviour. These problems interfere with his interpersonal relationships and academic progress. He lives with Lillian, his single mother. Lillian is discouraged and feels unable to manage Jamie's behaviour.

Associated Psychiatric Diagnosis

Attention deficit hyperactivity disorder
Other issues of note:
Parent–child relational problem (mother exhausted/father absent)
Educational problems (peer conflict)
Low income (mother in entry-level job
Disruption of family by separation (father inconsistent in visitation routine)
GAF = 52*
*Although the *DSM-5* does not endorse the Global Assessment of Functioning Score, it may still be seen on a diagnostic report.

Medications

Methylphenidate 5 mg at breakfast and lunch (i.e., at 8 AM and 12 noon), then adding 5 mg at 4 PM. The likely dose would be 7.5 mg at 8 AM and 12 noon and 5 mg at 7 PM.

Nursing Diagnosis 1: Impaired Social Interaction

Defining Characteristics

Cannot establish and maintain developmentally appropriate social relationships
Has interpersonal difficulties at school
Is not well accepted by peers
Is easily distracted
Interrupts others
Cannot wait his turn in games
Speaks out of turn in the classroom

Related Factors

Impulsive behaviour
Overactive
Inattentive
Risk-taking behaviour (tried to climb out the window to get away from Lillian)
Failure to recognize the effects of his behaviour on others

(Continued)

Outcomes

Initial	Discharge
1. Decrease hyperactivity and disruptive behaviour.	4. Improve capacity to identify alternative responses in conflicts with peers.
2. Improve attention and decrease distractibility.	5. Improve capacity to interpret behaviour of age-mates.
3. Decrease the frequency of acting without forethought.	

Interventions

Interventions	Rationale	Ongoing Assessment
Educate the mother and teach her about ADHD and the use of stimulant medication.	Better understanding helps to ensure adherence; parents and teachers often miscast children with ADHD as "troublemakers."	Determine the extent to which the parent or teacher "blames" Jamie for his problems.
Monitor adherence to medication schedule.	Inconsistent use may contribute to a failed trial of medication.	Administer parent and teacher questionnaires; inquire re: behaviour across the day.
Ensure that the medication is both effective and well tolerated.	Stimulants can affect appetite and sleep and can cause irritability when wearing off (called "rebound") (Biederman & Faraone, 2005).	Administer parent and teacher questionnaires; check weight; ask about sleep and appetite.

Evaluation

Outcomes	Revised Outcomes	Interventions
Jamie shows decreased hyperactivity and less disruption in the classroom.	Improve the ability to identify disruptive classroom behaviour.	Initiate a point system to reward appropriate behaviour.
Jamie shows improved attention and decreased distractibility.	Improve school performance.	Move to the front of the classroom as an aid to attention.

Evaluation

Outcomes	Revised Outcomes	Interventions
Mother and teacher attest to Jamie's decreased impulsive behaviour.	Increase Jamie's capacity to recognize the effects of his behaviour on others.	Encourage participation in structured activities.
Jamie identifies alternative responses such as walking away until it is his turn.	Increase the frequency of acting on these alternative approaches.	Inquire about friendship groups (work on socialization strategies) at school, if available.
Jamie improves interpretation of motives and behaviours of others.	Improve acceptance by peers.	Encourage participation in community activities.

Nursing Diagnosis 2: Parent–Child Relational Problem—Ineffective Coping (Lillian)

Defining Characteristics	Related Factors
Verbalizes discouragement and inability to handle the situation with Jamie	Chronicity of ADHD
Expresses frustration in her parenting abilities, admits to "giving in"	More than average child-rearing problems

Outcomes

Initial	Discharge
1. Verbalize frustration at trying to raise a child with ADHD alone.	3. Identify coping patterns that decrease the sense of frustration and increase parental competence.

Nursing Care Plan 31-1 (*Continued*)

Outcomes

Initial	Discharge
2. Identify positive methods of interacting with and managing Jamie that will support the parent–child relationship as well as meet Jamie's developmental needs.	4. Initiate a collaborative relationship with the teacher. 5. Identify sources of support in the community and begin to access these resources.

Interventions

Interventions	Rationale	Ongoing Assessment
Assess the mother's discouragement and feelings about parenting, identifying specific problem areas.	Helping the mother verbalize her feelings and identify problem areas helps in formulating problem-solving strategies.	Assess the severity of the problems with which she is living.
Refer the mother to a community health centre for free parenting class.	Parent training based on clear directives and rewards can be effective for decreasing impulsive and disruptive behaviours.	Monitor the mother's level of confidence and perceived change in Jamie's behaviour.
Refer the mother to a self-help organization.	Parent groups such as Children and Adults with Attention Deficit Disorder (CHADD) can be sources of support and information.	Determine whether contact was made and whether it was helpful.
Make contact with school to enhance collaboration with the mother.	Assess the effectiveness of medication and other interventions, need feedback from teachers.	Determine whether the mother has been able to contact the teacher.

Evaluation

Outcomes	Revised Outcomes	Interventions
After four sessions, Lillian expresses her frustrations, but she has begun to identify different ways of relating to Jamie and his developmental needs.	None.	None.
Through attending the parenting class and joining a support group, Lillian begins to change her coping patterns, decrease her frustrations, and increase parental competence.	Complete the parenting class; attend at least two support group meetings each month.	If necessary, refer for additional parent counselling.
Lillian initiates a collaborative relationship with Jamie's teacher.	Lillian and Jamie's teacher mutually develop and implement behaviour plans for home and school.	Have the mother observe in the classroom; have the mother visit highly structured classroom.

Biologic Domain

A combined behavioural–psychosocial and medication approach allows for significantly lower doses of medication than a medication-only approach in achieving treatment outcomes and decreasing the risk of side effects (Chronis, Jones, & Raggi, 2006). Behavioural programs focus on creating success and achievement for the child/youth. The system should be based on acknowledgement for positive behaviour, such as waiting, or completing chores. Interventions may also include specific cognitive behavioural techniques in which the child learns to "stop, look, and listen" before doing.

Medication can help the hyperactivity, impulsiveness, and inattention; therefore, teaching the parent, child, and school personnel about the importance of the medication in ADHD and the potential side effects is a place to begin. Explaining to the child that the medication improves concentration and the ability to sit still can help strengthen motivation and adherence to treatment; however, nonadherence is typically more a matter of forgetting than one of deliberate avoidance.

For 40 years, the main treatment for ADHD has been the stimulant medications (Table 31-1). Although each of these medications has demonstrated efficacy in controlled studies, methylphenidate has received considerably more research effort and has emerged as the first-line effective therapy to treat ADHD (Flapper & Schoemaker, 2008). It should be noted that stimulants are not effective in all cases; alternatives have been created such as norepinephrine reuptake inhibitor and atomoxetine. Occasionally the use of antidepressants may be beneficial. The overuse of medication to treat ADHD is an ongoing concern of parents and others. Careful assessment and education for child/youth and family will determine the individual need and areas of concern. As with most mental health disorders in children, the aim of treatment for ADHD is to decrease symptoms, enhance functionality, and improve well-being for the child and his or her close contacts.

Psychosocial Domain

Hyperactivity, impulsivity, and inattention are typically pervasive problems evident both at school and at home. Management of symptoms is frequently an issue because parents may have difficulty controlling their child's behaviour, which is disruptive and occasionally destructive. Assessment of the psychological domain may generate several diagnoses, including anxiety and defensive coping. The outcomes should be individualized to the child.

Dysfunctional interactions can develop within the family. Reviewing the problematic behaviours and the situations in which they occur is a way to identify negative interaction patterns. These children are often behind in their work at school because of poor organization, off-task behaviour, and impulsive responses. They can exhaust their parents, aggravate teachers, and annoy siblings with their intrusive and disruptive behaviours. Because ADHD often occurs in the context of psychosocial adversity, it is important to review the family situation, including parenting style, stability of household membership, consistency of rules and routines, and life events, such as divorce, moves, deaths, and job loss. Identification of these factors can be useful in shaping a care plan that builds on potential strengths and mitigates the effects of environmental factors that may perpetuate the child's disruptive behaviour. Data regarding school performance, behaviour at home, and comorbid psychiatric disorders are essential for developing school interventions and behaviour plans and establishing the baseline severity for medication.

Depending on the severity of the child's responses, family situation, and school environment, several nursing diagnoses could be generated from the assessment data, including impaired social interaction, ineffective role performance, and compromised family coping. Short-term outcomes, such as decreasing the number of classroom ejections within a 2-week period, may be useful for one child, whereas reducing the frequency and amplitude of angry outbursts at home may be relevant to another child.

Parents, caregivers, and educators often require information about what ADHD is and what it is not. There are many misconceptions, myths, and falsehoods about ADHD and its management. The nurse will therefore be called on to have accurate information.

Family treatment is nearly always a component of cognitive–behavioural treatment approaches with the child. This may involve parent training that focuses on the principles of creating a home environment that has increased predictability and structure. This may prove to be a challenge for parents who have ADHD themselves.

Table 31-1	Stimulant Medications Used in Treating ADHD	
Medication	**Total Daily Dosage***	**Common Side Effects**
Methylphenidate	10–60 mg in two or three divided doses	Loss of appetite, insomnia, rebound activation, increase in tics or compulsive behaviour, psychotic reaction
Metadate CD	Once-daily capsule in children 6 and over. 18 mg daily	
Concerta	Maximum dose 54 mg daily. Once daily capsule 18 mg daily. Maximum 72 mg daily. Dosage not to exceed 2 mg/kg daily	
D-Amphetamine	5–40 mg in two divided doses	Similar to methylphenidate
D, L-Amphetamine	5–40 mg in two divided doses	Similar to methylphenidate

*Dosage ranges are similar for long-acting products Concerta, Metadate, and Adderall.

At times, the institution of more formal behaviour management may be required, such as boundary setting and the use of reward systems, as well as revised expectations about the child's behaviour. School programming often involves increasing structure in the child's school day to offset the child's tendency to act without forethought and to be easily distracted by extraneous stimuli. Specific remediation is required for the child with comorbid deficits in learning or language. Some children may require specialized self-contained classrooms; however, they typically have coexisting challenges such as learning disabilities and oppositional defiant or conduct disorder.

Children with ADHD, a learning disability, or a language deficit may frequently encounter failure and acquire a bitter and hostile attitude. Appropriate treatment focused on the child's strengths will foster more positive interactions and promote success at school. Success in these areas may lead to more positive behaviour in some cases.

Spiritual Domain

There needs to be concerted effort on the part of nurses and other health care professionals to address the spiritual domain of children with ADHD. Their environment must be, in addition to being calm and predictable, one in which they have the opportunity to express their questions, fears, and hopes about life, death, and the sacred. The expression of their spiritual needs should not be dismissed but rather encouraged appropriately and understood in terms of stage of development and life experience. There needs to be openness to families' spiritual needs as well. ADHD symptoms in a child can overwhelm a family and disconnect them from sources of spiritual support when such symptoms are not tolerated by others.

Motor Disorders: Tourette's Disorder

Motor disorders include developmental coordination disorder, stereotypic movement disorder, and tic disorders (American Psychiatric Association, 2013). Tic disorders, specifically Tourette's disorder, will be the focus here. A tic "is a sudden, rapid, recurrent, nonrhythmic motor movement or vocalization" (APA, 2013, p. 81). Tourette's disorder is diagnosed when "multiple motor and one or more vocal tics" (not necessarily appearing concurrently) have been present in a child prior to 18 years of age, and have persisted for more than 1 year after onset of the first tic (APA, 2013, p. 81). The movements and vocalizations must not be attributable to effects of a substance, such as cocaine, or to another medical condition, such as Huntington's disease (APA). Simple motor tics include eye blinking, shoulder shrugging, extension of limbs; simple vocal tics include throat clearing, sniffing, grunting. Tics are usually experienced as voluntary, but can be

suppressed for variable lengths of time (APA). Tics have different degrees of severity, and no two children have the same pattern (Singer, 2005). The typical age of onset for tics is between 4 and 6 years (APA, 2013); motor tics generally precede vocal tics. Tourette's disorder exhibits a waxing and waning course. Regarding prognosis, by late adolescence/early adulthood, the disorder will have disappeared for one third of those diagnosed with it, improved for another one third, and continue to fluctuate for the remaining third (Singer, 2013).

Tourette's disorder is undetectable in CAT, PET, and MRI scans (Murray, 2008), and there are no diagnostic laboratory tests for it. The Yale Global Tic Severity Scale has been found to be a reliable and valid instrument for the assessment of paediatric Tourette syndrome (Storch et al., 2005).

Epidemiology

The prevalence of Tourette's disorder is estimated to be from 3 to 8 per 1,000 in school-aged children, with boys being affected more than girls at a 2:1 to 4:1 ratio (APA, 2013). Tourette's disorder is common in children with ASD (Singer, 2005).

Aetiology

Named after George Gilles de la Tourette, a French neurologist who described "Maladie des tics" in the late 1880s, Tourette's syndrome was originally deemed psychological in origin—Freud considered it a form of hysteria—with treatment thus being psychoanalytic therapy and/or hypnosis (Bennett, Keller, & Walkup, 2013). In the 1960s, a biologic aetiology became the preferred causal explanation, supported by the efficacy (although limited) of treatment with antipsychotics (e.g., chlorpromazine and haloperidol). Today, innovations in neuroscience and genetics have moved understanding of this disorder further: it is viewed as the result of an interplay of brain, behaviour, and environment. The individual with tic disorder is seen as having a biologic (genetic) vulnerability that is affected by physiologic arousal related to stress (personal, environmental) (Bennett et al., 2013).

The neurologic abnormality related to tic disorder likely involves several genes, but which ones remain unknown. Direct and indirect evidence has found that corticostriatal–thalamocortical pathways are involved in the expression of this disorder. The possibility of dopaminergic abnormality continues to receive attention because of the therapeutic response to neuroleptics in vocal and motor tics (Singer, 2005). Many approaches are being used to search for a genetic site, including cytogenetics, candidate gene studies, and molecular genetic studies. Linkage analyses have suggested several chromosomal locations, without a clear reproducible locus or convergence of findings (Singer, 2005, 2013). It is recognized that "Obstetrical complications, older parental age, lower birth weight, and maternal smoking during pregnancy are associated with worse tic severity" (APA, 2013, p. 83).

Nursing Management

A major focus of the nursing care of a child or adolescent with Tourette's disorder is the careful exploration of the way that tics are affecting the child's physical, psychological, social, and academic well-being. The way the family members are dealing with the child's symptoms is important information, as well. A completion of a family history of tic disorder may also provide critical assessment data.

To get a clear understanding of an individual child's manifestation of the disorder, a functional assessment is required. Specific information is needed regarding when tics occur and when their severity decreases (usually when the child is calm, asleep, concentrating, or focused on an activity) and when severity increases (usually when the child is excited, emotionally upset, fatigued) (Bennett et al., 2013). As the child can suppress the tics for brief periods, it is not uncommon to learn that the child has more frequent tics at home than at school. It is helpful to explore, however, the times in class that are associated with increased severity of the tics. For instance, is it when new material is being taught or when the child is called upon to speak? Older children and adults may describe a "premonitory urge" or a physical sensation before having a tic and a sense of tension reduction afterwards (APA). This cycle of tension-tic-tension reduction makes it possible to envision tics as goal-directed behaviours (Singer, 2013). This is an important perspective for treatment of the disorder.

A Canadian review of evidence-based treatment of tic disorders that made recommendations regarding pharmacotherapy concluded that behaviour therapy and the alpha-2-adrenergic antagonists are the firstline of therapy for children with tic disorders (Pringsheim et al., 2012). A similar review but focused on behavioural and other therapies (e.g., brain stimulation), strongly recommended habit reversal therapy with accompanying psychoeducation, and with or without pharmacotherapy (Steeves et al., 2012). Comprehensive Behavioural Intervention for Tics (CBIT) is a treatment whose efficacy has been measured in randomized control trials. This behavioural approach is based on the assumption that, while tics are neurologic in origin, their expression is determined by the interplay of biologic and environmental factors (Bennett et al., 2013). It has three elements: psychoeducation, functional assessment and intervention, and habit reversal therapy (HRT) (Bennett et al., 2013).

The *psychoeducation* component involves providing the child and her or his family general information about Tourette's disorder that includes its prevalence, course, and aetiology. The behavioural model of treatment should be explained. They will need to learn about

the role context and consequences in the expression and maintenance of the child's tics. It is in the modification of these, targeting internal and external reinforcements of the tics that forms the basis of the functional intervention. The *functional assessment*, described above, allows for the identification of tic triggers and consequences specific to the child and for *functional interventions* to reduce or eliminate them to be developed (Bennett et al., 2013).

In CBIT, the child with Tourette's disorder is coached in HRT. This is based on the fact that a premonitory urge occurs prior to tic expression and then the expression of the tic relieves the tension. This positively reinforces the tic behaviour. HRT involves using a competing response (i.e., one that is incompatible with tic expression) to diminish the habitual undesired behaviour (tic). Deep breathing is one such competing behaviour (Bennett et al., 2013). The child can be taught how to deep breathe when s/he feels tic expression is imminent. Using HRT to manage symptoms and to maintain his or her everyday routine despite tic expression can bring rewards for the child (positive reinforcement) in the form of a sense of achievement and self-efficacy, as well as increased opportunities to stay active and engaged with others (Bennett et al., 2013).

CBIT also involves recognizing the positive consequences or secondary gains of tics for the child, such as no chores when tics occur; mom giving massages and sympathy; or teacher excusing homework. Such positive consequences reinforce the tic "behaviour" and thus the severity and frequency of tics can increase (Bennett et al., 2013). It is important to ensure that parents do not misinterpret behavioural interventions as indicating that tics are voluntary; this could create inappropriate expectations of the child. Nurses need to be knowledgeable about CBIT in order to assist and support the child and family in enacting this treatment and to appropriately monitor changes in the frequency, intensity, complexity, and interference of the tics as they occur. They may serve as consultants with the child's school.

Pharmacotherapy for Tourette's disorder has good-to-moderate efficacy for reduction of the expression and severity of tics. Atypical antipsychotics ziprasidone, risperidone (the most studied), quetiapine, and olanzapine can be used (Singer, 2005), but due to their side effect profile, they are recommended only when tics are severe and/or debilitating (Pringsheim et al., 2012). Recommended, in a consensus review by clinical experts, as a potential part of the first-line of therapy for tics, are the alpha-2-adrenergic antagonists, clonidine and guanfacine, which have moderate efficacy. A withdrawal phenomenon (rebound hypertension) can be experienced with clonidine, so it is important for parents to know that it cannot be stopped abruptly. Currently, guanfacine requires approval from Health Canada's Special Access Program to be prescribed (Pringsheim et al., 2012).

Teachers, guidance counsellors, and school nurses will need current information about Tourette's disorder and related problems. Discussions with school personnel often include issues such as how to deal with tic behaviours if they are disruptive in the classroom (Box 31-9), how to manage teasing from other children, and how to deal with medication side effects. In some situations, a brief presentation about Tourette's disorder to the class/school can reduce teasing and help both teachers and classmates tolerate the tic symptoms (Prestia, 2003). There are videos and information pamphlets available to use as resources (see Tourette's Syndrome Foundation in Web Links on the thePoint). Informative presentations foster openness and understanding and help students with this disorder feel included. Before initiating these interventions, it is essential to identify the child's needs and to pursue these strategies in collaboration with the family and other clinical team members. If evidence shows that Tourette's disorder is hindering academic progress, the nurse can help families negotiate with the school to obtain appropriate services.

BOX 31-9   Therapeutic Dialogue

TICS AND DISRUPTIVE BEHAVIOURS
....

Ineffective Approach
Teacher: I see the tics. He jerks his head, makes faces, and flicks his hands.

Nurse: What do you do about them?

Teacher: What can I do? If he isn't disrupting the class, I leave him alone. Even when he is throwing spitballs.

Nurse: Spitballs! He shouldn't be allowed to throw spitballs.

Teacher: Oh, I thought that was a part of his problem.

Nurse: Well, throwing spitballs has nothing to do with tics.

Effective Approach
Teacher: I see the tics. He jerks his head, makes faces, and flicks his hands.

Nurse: He cannot help the tics that you are seeing. Tic disorders can exhibit a wide range of severity, from mild to severe and from simple to complex. Some complex tics may be difficult to distinguish from habits or rituals.

Teacher: What about things like throwing spitballs? When he does things like that, I try to ignore that behaviour.

Nurse: Sounds like you give him the benefit of the doubt. (Validation) However, throwing a spitball is not a tic behaviour.

Teacher: What should I do?

Nurse: How do you usually handle that type of behaviour? (A modification of reflection)

Teacher: I'd ask him to stop and sometimes go into the hall.

Nurse: Disruptive behaviour that is voluntary in a student with a tic disorder should be handled as you would handle any other child.

Critical Thinking Challenge
• Compare the responses of the nurse in these scenarios. What made the difference in the teacher's responsiveness to the nurse?

Nursing diagnoses may include ineffective coping, chronic low self-esteem, impaired social interaction, anxiety, and compromised family coping. Children with Tourette's disorder typically have normal intelligence, although clinical samples may show a higher frequency of learning problems. These learning problems may include subtle problems of organization and planning or more severe problems with reading (Burd, Freeman, Klug, & Kerbeshian, 2005). Handwriting, including both speed and legibility, is another common problem for these youngsters. The use of a computer in some cases can obviate difficulties with handwriting.

■■■ ELIMINATION DISORDERS
Enuresis

Enuresis means involuntary or intentional voiding of urine in inappropriate places. It may occur at night (nocturnal) or during the day (diurnal) or both. The *DSM-5* diagnostic criteria specify that bedwetting occurs at least twice per week for a duration of 3 months and that the child is at least 5 years of age; moreover, the behaviour cannot be attributed to a medication side effect or to another medical condition. Even without treatment, 50% of these children can achieve dryness by the age of 10 years.

Epidemiology and Aetiology

The prevalence of nocturnal enuresis varies with age and gender, being most common in young boys—an estimated 15% to 20% of 5-year-old boys, 7% of boys aged 7 to 9 years, and 1% of 14-year-old boys have nocturnal enuresis. The frequency in girls is about half that of boys in each age group. The aetiology of enuresis is unknown, with probably no single cause. Most children with nocturnal enuresis are urologically normal. The prevalence of nocturnal enuresis decreases from early childhood to adolescence, and time is the cure for bedwetting in the majority of cases (Nield & Kamat, 2004).

Nursing Management

The nursing assessment should include the child's developmental history, the onset and course of enuresis, prior treatment, presence of emotional problems, medical history, and family history of enuresis, diabetes, or kidney disease. Psychosocial issues such as a change in living arrangements, a new child in the family, or a death should also be documented because stress can be a contributing factor to the problem (Nield & Kamat, 2004). The nurse should also explore the family's home environment and family attitudes about the child's enuresis. Routine laboratory tests such as urinalysis and a urine culture are used to determine the presence of infection. The nurse should obtain baseline data regarding toileting habits, including daytime incontinence, urinary frequency, and constipation. He or she should refer children with persistent daytime enuresis for consultation with a urologist (Reiner, 2003).

The nurse can explore and dispel myths and misconceptions that parents may have about bedwetting, such as that the child is lazy, defiant, attention seeking or misbehaving (Schlomer, Rodriguez, Weiss, & Copp, 2013). In addition, education about bedwetting and its causes may help to alleviate parents' feelings of frustration and the child's feelings of humiliation and shame. The nurse can also encourage parents to limit fluid intake in the evening and treat constipation (if present).

Interventions

Treatment for enuresis encompasses both behavioural interventions and pharmacotherapy.

Simple behavioural interventions are undemanding strategies that the child may achieve with help from his or her parents. They include reward for "staying dry" such as receiving a sticker on a chart; being wakened to urinate at night, retention control training to enlarge the bladder and fluid restriction. A Cochrane systematic review of the literature found evidence that these simple interventions are superior to no active treatment, but inferior to more complex behavioural interventions such as alarms, and to some pharmacotherapy (Caldwell, Nankivell, & Sureshkumar, 2013). Alarms are devices that children wear or lie upon while sleeping which are activated by moisture. Imipramine (Tofranil) and amitriptyline (Elavil), tricyclic antidepressants, have shown efficacy in the treatment of nocturnal enuresis when given once daily an hour prior to bedtime. They have the multiple systemic side effects of anticholinergics (see Chapter 12). The majority of children will relapse once the medication is stopped (Nield & Kamat, 2004). This can cause recurrence of parental frustration, and shame and humiliation in addition to feelings of failure in the child. A study of treatment response to outpatient training using such interventions found that after 4 months, 46% of children (*n* = 66) had a full response, 15%, good response, and 21% only partial response. After 16 months, 53% of children (*n* = 34) had a full response, 6%, good response, and 25% partial; use of pharmacotherapy declined over time (Cobussen-Boekhorst, van Genugten, Postma, Feitz, & Kortmann, 2012).

Behavioural Interventions

The most effective nonpharmacologic treatment is the bedwetting alarm. In this form of behavioural treatment, the bed is equipped with a pad that sets off a buzzer if the child wets. The buzzer then wakes up the child, thereby reminding the child to void. Six to 16 weeks of alarm treatment may be necessary for the majority of children to experience 2 consecutive weeks of dry night.

Encopresis

Encopresis involves soiling clothing with feces or depositing feces in inappropriate places, whether involuntarily or intentionally. Additional diagnostic criteria include that the child is older than 4 years, that the soiling occurs at least once per month for at least 3 months, and that the soiling is not the result of a medical disorder, such as aganglionic megacolon (Hirschsprung's disease). The most common form of encopresis is fecal impaction accompanied by leakage around the hardened mass of stool. Because of the loss of muscle tone in the lower bowel, the child loses the usual urge to defecate and may not feel the leakage. Surprisingly, the child may not detect the smell of the stool because the olfactory apparatus becomes accustomed to the odour. If left untreated, this problem generally resolves independently by middle adolescence (North American Society for Pediatric Gastroenterology, Hepatology and Nutrition, 2006). Encopresis can affect the lives of children in the following areas: physical, psychological, educational, social, emotional, and in the area of self-esteem.

Epidemiology and Aetiology

The problem of encopresis has received less attention in paediatric literature compared with enuresis. As with enuresis, encopresis is more common in boys, and the frequency of the condition declines with age. Recorded prevalence of encopresis varied between studies from 1% to 4% in children older than 4 years of age, 1% to 2% in children 7 years of age, and 1.6% in those 10 to 11 years of age, with boys three to four times more likely to have encopresis than girls (Bongers, Tabbers, & Benninga, 2007). Fecal incontinence is reported to be responsible for 3% of referrals to health care professionals.

The diagnosis of encopresis includes both retentive fecal incontinence and nonretentive fecal incontinence, which present as a single symptom without any organic cause or signs of constipation (Bongers et al., 2007). The reasons for withholding stool and starting the cycle of fecal impaction are unclear but are usually not the result of physical causes. However, as noted, once the fecal impaction occurs, there is a loss of tone in the bowel and leakage.

Nursing Management

The assessment includes a detailed interview with the child and parent regarding the pattern of the encopresis. A calm, matter-of-fact approach can help to reduce the child's embarrassment. A physical examination is also necessary; collaboration with the child's family physician or consulting paediatrician is therefore essential. The presence of encopresis does not necessarily signal severe emotional or behavioural disturbances, but the nurse should inquire about other psychiatric disorders. The diagnosis of encopresis is presumed given a history of intermittent constipation and soiling. Collaboration with the family physician and paediatrician often is helpful to rule out rare medical conditions, such as Hirschsprung's disease.

 TEACHING POINTS

Effective intervention begins with educating the parents and the child about normal bowel function and the self-perpetuating cycle of fecal impaction and leakage of stool around the hardened mass of feces. The short-term goal of this educational effort is to decrease the anger and recrimination that often complicate the picture in these families. It is important for parents to understand that soiling from overflow incontinence is not a willful and defiant manoeuvre. Parents are encouraged to maintain a consistent, positive, and supportive attitude in all aspects of treatment (North American Society for Pediatric Gastroenterology, Hepatology and Nutrition, 2006). Because encopresis often results in a loss of bowel tone, it may help to motivate children by emphasizing the need to strengthen their muscles. In many cases, cleaning out the bowel is necessary before initiating behavioural treatment. Disimpaction may be accomplished with the use of oral cathartics such as polyethylene glycol. Once the colon has been evacuated, long-term laxative use is often continued during the bowel retraining program. A high-fibre diet is also recommended.

The behavioural treatment program involves daily sitting on the toilet after each meal for a predetermined period (e.g., 5 to 10 minutes). The child and parents can measure the time with an ordinary kitchen timer, and the parents can encourage the child to read or look at picture books while sitting. They can give the child rewards in the form of stars, stickers, or points for complying with the retraining program and add bonuses for successful defecation. The family can tally stickers or points on a calendar, and the child can "cash in" collected points for small prizes (Reiner, 2003). Children with nonretentive fecal incontinence should not be treated with laxatives. After the exclusion of underlying organic diseases, the treatment is based on the following aspects: education, toilet training, a daily bowel diary with a reward system, and medication. Loperamide has been found effective in the short-term treatment of nonretentive fecal incontinence (Bongers et al., 2007).

SUMMARY OF KEY POINTS

■ Improved methods of assessing and defining psychiatric disorders have enhanced appreciation for the frequency of psychiatric disorders in children and adolescents.

■ An estimated 14% of children 4 to 17 years of age (more than 800,000) in Canada experience mental disorders that cause significant distress and impairment at home, at school, and in the community.

■ The developmental disorders include intellectual disability, ASDs, and specific developmental disorders. Assessment findings should guide nursing management. Specific developmental disorders include communication disorders and learning disorders. These disorders are fairly common in the general population, but they are more common in children with other primary psychiatric disorders.

■ Child psychiatric disorders can be divided into externalizing and internalizing disorders. Externalizing disorders include the disruptive behaviour disorders: ODD and conduct disorder. Internalizing disorders include depression and anxiety disorders.

■ ADHD is defined by the presence of inattention, impulsiveness, and, in most cases, hyperactivity. This heterogeneous disorder affects boys more often than girls.

■ Effective treatment of ADHD often involves multiple approaches, including medication and parent teaching.

■ Assessment of children involves securing data from multiple sources, including the child, parents, and school personnel.

■ Standardized rating instruments can assist data collection from multiple informants.

■ Separation anxiety and OCD are relatively common anxiety disorders in school-aged children. (OCD becomes more common in adolescents.)

■ Treatment of separation anxiety and OCD may include medication, behavioural therapy, or a combination of these treatments.

■ Major depression in children/youth is believed to be similar to major depression in adults; however, it may be expressed differently.

■ The efficacy of antidepressant medications is less well established in children and adolescents than in adults.

■ Childhood schizophrenia is a rare disorder.

■ Elimination disorders include encopresis and enuresis. Behavioural therapy approaches are the most effective treatment for these disorders. Medication may also be used.

CRITICAL THINKING CHALLENGES

1 Analyze how genetic and environmental factors may interact in the aetiology of child psychiatric disorders.

2 Learning disabilities and communication disorders are more common in children with psychiatric disorders than in the general population. How might a learning disability or a communication disorder complicate a psychiatric illness in a school-aged child?

3 Compare and contrast nursing approaches for a child with ADHD with those used for a child with an autism spectrum disorder. How are they different? How are they similar?

4 Many children have imaginary playmates. What are the benefits to the child? At what age level is this considered developmentally normal? When is it not?

5 Children and youth who arrive as new immigrants or as refugees may have experienced significant community violence or lived through war. Discuss how this may impact their integration into Canadian society. What factors might serve as protective factors to these previously traumatized children?

6 How would you help parents differentiate between normal adolescent mood and behaviour and depression?

REFERENCES

Ainsworth, M. D. S. (1979). Infant–mother attachment. *American Psychologist*, *34*, 932–937.

American Psychiatric Association. (2000). *Diagnostic and statistical manual of mental disorders* (4th ed., Text revision) (*DSM-IV-TR*). Washington, DC: Author.

American Psychiatric Association. (2013). *Diagnostic and statistical manual of mental disorders* (5th ed.) (*DSM-5*). Washington, DC: Author.

Anderson, G., Scahill, L., McCracken, J., McDougle, C., Aman, M., Tierney, E. ... Vitiello, B. (2007). Effects of short- and long-term risperidone treatment on prolactin levels in children with autism. *Biological Psychiatry*, *61*(4), 545–550.

Axelrod, D. (2013). Taking disruptive mood dysregulation disorder out for a test drive. *American Journal of Psychiatry*, *170*(2), 136–139.

Bakker, S. C., van der Meulen, E. M., Buitelaar, J. K., Sandkuijl, L. A., Pauls, D. L., Monsuur, A. J., ... Sinke, R. J. (2003). A whole-genome scan in 164 Dutch sib pairs with attention-deficit/hyperactivity disorder: Suggestive evidence for linkage on chromosomes 7p and 15q. *American Journal of Human Genetics*, *72*(5), 1251–1260.

Barkley, R. A. (1998). *Attention deficit hyperactivity disorder: A handbook for diagnosis and treatment* (2nd ed.). New York, NY: Guilford.

Bennett, S. M., Keller, A. E., & Walkup, J. T. (2013). The future of tic disorder treatment. *Annals of the New York Academy of Sciences*, *1304*(1), 32–39.

Bhat, M., Grizenko, N., Ben-Amor, L., & Joober, R. (2005). Obstetric complications in children with attention deficit/hyperactivity disorder and learning disability. *McGill Journal of Medicine*, *8*(2), 109–113.

Biederman, J. & Faraone, S. (2005). Attention-deficit hyperactivity disorder. *Lancet*, *366*(7), 237–248.

Blaustein, M. & Kinniburgh, K. (2010). *Treating traumatic stress in children and adolescents: How to foster resilience through attachment, self-regulation, and competency.* New York, NY: Guilford Press.

Bolton, D. & Perrin, S. (2008). Evaluation of exposure with response-prevention for obsessive compulsive disorder in children and adolescents. *Journal of Behavior Therapy and Experimental Psychiatry*, *39*(1), 11–22.

Bongers, M., Tabbers, M., & Benninga, M. (2007). Functional nonretentive fecal incontinence in children. *Journal of Pediatric Gastroenterology and Nutrition*, *44*(1), 5–13.

Bornovalova, M., Hicks, B., Iacono, W., & McGue, M. (2010). Familial transmission and heritability of childhood disruptive disorders. *American Journal of Psychiatry*, *167*, 1066–1074.

Boston Children's Hospital. (2013). *Disruptive behavior disorders*. Retrieved from http://www.childrenshospital.org/health-topics/conditions/disruptive-behavior-disorders

Boylan, K., Vaillancourt, T., Boyle, M., & Szatmari, P. (2007). Comorbidity of internalizing disorders in children with oppositional defiant disorder. *European Child and Adolescent Psychiatry*, *16*(8), 484–494.

Buckner, J., Lopez, C., Dunkel, S., & Joiner, T. (2008). Behaviour management training for the treatment of reactive attachment disorder. *Child Maltreatment*, *13*(3), 289–297.

Burd, L., Freeman, R., Klug, M., & Kerbeshian, J. (2005). Tourette syndrome and learning disabilities. *BMC Pediatrics*, *5*(34). Retrieved from http://www.biomedcentral.com/1471-2431/5/34

Buysse, V., Goldman, B. D., & Skinner, M. L. (2003). Seeing effects on friendship formation among young children with and without disabilities. *Exceptional Children*, *68*(4), 503–517.

Caldwell, P. H., Nankivell, G., & Sureshkumar, P. (2013). Simple behavioral interventions for nocturnal enuresis in children (Review). *Cochrane Database of Systematic Reviews*, Art no. jCD003637. doi: 10.1002/14651858.CD003637.pub3

Cameron, C. L. (2007). Obsessive-compulsive disorder in children and adolescents. *Journal of Psychiatric and Mental Health Nursing*, *14*(7), 696–704.

Canadian ADHD Resource Alliance (CADDRA). (2011). *Canadian ADHD practice guidelines (CAP-guidelines)* (3rd ed). Toronto, ON: Author.

Canadian ADHD Resource Alliance (CADDRA). (2013a). *Adult ADHD. Does it exist?* Retrieved from http://www.caddra.ca/public-information/adults

Canadian ADHD Resource Alliance (CADDRA). (2013b). *Information for educators: ADHD in the classroom.* Retrieved from http://www.caddra.ca/public-information/educators

Canadian Mental Health Association (CMHA). (2013a). *Bipolar disorder*. Retrieved from http://www.cmha.ca/mental-health/understanding-mental-illness/bipolar-disorder/

Canadian Mental Health Association (CMHA). (2013b). *Fast facts about mental illness*. Retrieved from http://www.cmha.ca/media/fast-facts-about-mental-illness/#.UubdVrRlC70

Canadian Pediatric Society. (2006). *Mental health of children and adolescents*. Retrieved from http://www.cps.ca/english/Advocacy/MentalHealth.htm

Centre for ADHD Awareness, Canada (CADDAC). (2013). *Adult attention deficit hyperactivity disorder*. Retrieved from http://www.caddac.ca/cms/page.php?82%29

Centers for Disease Control and Prevention. (2012). Prevalence of autism spectrum disorders—Autism and Developmental Disabilities Monitoring Network, 14 sites, United States, 2008. *MMWR Surveillance Summaries*, *61*(SS03), 1–19.

Children's Health Policy Centre, Simon Fraser University. (2007). *Addressing attention problems in children. Children's Mental Health Research Quarterly, Fall.* Retrieved from http://www.childhealthpolicy.sfu.ca/research_quarterly_08/rq-pdf/RQ-4-07-Fall.pdf

Chronis, A. M., Jones, H., & Raggi, V. (2006). Evidence-based psychosocial treatments for children and adolescents with attention deficit/hyperactivity disorder. *Clinical Psychology Review*, *26*(4), 486–502.

Clomipramine Collaborative Study Group. (1991). Clomipramine in the treatment of patients with obsessive compulsive disorder. *Archives of General Psychiatry*, *48*(8), 730–738.

Cobussen-Boekhorst, H. J., van Genugten, L. J., Postma, J., Feitz, W. F., & Kortmann, B. B. (2012). Treatment responses of outpatient training for children with enuresis in a tertiary healthcare setting. *Journal of Pediatric Urology*, *9*, 516–520.

Conners, C. K. (1989). *Conners' rating scales manual*. North Tonawanda, NY: Multi-Health Systems.

Copeland, W., Angold, A., Costello, E. J., & Egger, H. (2013). Prevalence, comorbidity, and correlates of *DSM-5* proposed disruptive mood dysregulation disorder. *American Journal of Psychiatry*, *170*(2), 173–179.

Cornell, T. & Hamrin, V. (2008). Clinical interventions with children with attachment problems. *Journal of Child and Adolescent Psychiatric Nursing*, *21*(1), 35–37.

de Vries, A. L. & Cohen-Kettenis, P. T. (2012). Clinical management of gender dysphoria in children and adolescents: The Dutch approach. *Journal of Homosexuality*, *59*(3), 301–320.

De Vries, A. L. C., Noens, I., Cohen-Kettenis, P., van Berckelaer-Onnes, I., & Doerleijers, T. (2010). Autism spectrum disorders in gender dysphoric children and adolescents. *Journal of Autism and Developmental Disorders*, *40*, 930–936.

Doyle, R. (2004). The history of attention deficit/hyperactivity disorder. *Psychiatric Clinics of North America*, *27*(2), 203–214.

Durston, S., Tottenham, N. T., Thomas, K. M., Davidson, M. C., Eigsti, I., Yang, Y., ... Casey, B. J. (2003). Differential patterns of striatal activation in young children with and without ADHD. *Biological Psychiatry*, *53*, 871–878.

Fairchild, G., Passamonti, L., Hurford, G., Hagan, C. C., von dem Hagen, E. A., van Goozen, S., ... Calder, A. J. (2011). Brain structure abnormalities in early-onset and adolescent-onset conduct disorder. *American Journal of Psychiatry*, *168*(6), 624–633.

Faraone, S. V. (2004), Genetics of adult attention deficit hyperactivity disorder. In T. Spencer (Ed.), *Psychiatric clinics of North America* (pp. 303–321). Philadelphia, PA: Saunders Press.

Faraone, S. V. & Bierderman, J. (2004). The neurobiology of attention deficit hyperactivity disorder. In D. S. Charney, E. J. Nestler, & B. S. Bunney (Eds.), *Neurobiology of mental illness* (2nd ed., pp. 979–999). New York, NY: Oxford University Press.

Faraone, S. V., Perlis, R. H., Doyle, A. E., Smoller, J. W., Goralnick, J. J., Holmgren, M. A., & Sklar, P. (2005). Molecular genetics of attention-deficit/hyperactivity disorder. *Biological Psychiatry, 57*(11), 1313–1323.

Flapper, B. & Schoemaker, M. (2008). Effects of methylphenidate on quality of life in children with both developmental coordination disorder and ADHD. *Developmental Medicine and Child Neurology, 50*(4), 294–299.

Gilliam, M., Stockman, M., Malek, M., Sharp, W., Greenstein, D., Lalonde, F., … Shaw, P. (2011). Developmental trajectories of the corpus callosum in attention-deficit/hyperactivity disorder. *Biological Psychiatry, 69*(9), 839–846.

Goyette, G. H., Conners, C. K., & Ulrich, R. F. (1978). Normative data on the revised Connors parent and teacher rating scales. *Journal of Abnormal Child Psychology, 6,* 221–236.

Gunnar, M. & Quevedo, K. (2007). The neurobiology of stress and development. *Annual Review of Psychology, 58,* 145–173.

HealthLinkBC. (2012). Depression in children and teens. Retrieved from http://www.healthlinkbc.ca/kb/content/major/ty4640.html

Hein, L. C. & Berger, K. C. (2012). Commentary: Gender dysphoria in children: Let's think this through. *Journal of Child and Adolescent Psychiatric Nursing, 25*(4), 237–240.

Henggeler, S. W. & Sheidow, A. J. (2012). Empirically supported family-based treatments for conduct disorder and delinquency in adolescents. *Journal of Marital and Family Therapy, 38*(1), 30–58.

Holmes, J. (2004). Disorganized attachment and borderline personality disorder. A clinical perspective. *Attachment and Human Development, 6,* 181–190.

Kanner, L. (1943). Autistic disturbances of affective contact. *Nervous Child, 2,* 217–250.

Kelty Mental Health Resource Centre. (2013). Post-traumatic stress disorder. Retrieved from http://keltymentalhealth.ca/mental-health/disorders/post-traumatic-stress-disorder

Kim-Cohen, J., Arsenault, L., Caspi, A., Tomás, M. P., Taylor, A., & Moffitt, T. (2005). Validity of *DSM-IV* conduct disorder in 4½-5-year-old children: A longitudinal epidemiological study. *American Journal of Psychiatry, 162*(6), 1108–1117.

King, R. A., Scahill, L., Lombroso, P. J., & Leckman, J. F. (2003). Tourette's syndrome and other tic disorders. In A. Martin, L. Scahill, D. S. Charney, & J. F. Leckman (Eds.), *Pediatric psychopharmacology: Principles and practice* (1st ed., pp. 526–542). New York, NY: Oxford University Press.

Koda, V. H., Charney, D. S., & Pine, D. S. (2003). Neurobiology of early-onset anxiety disorders. In A. Martin, L. Scahill, D. S. Charney, J. F. Leckman (Eds.), *Pediatric psychopharmacology: Principles and practice* (1st ed., pp. 138–149). New York, NY: Oxford University Press.

Labellarte, M. J. & Ginsberg, G. S. (2003). Anxiety disorders. In A. Martin, L. Scahill, D. S. Charney, J. F. Leckman (Eds.), *Pediatric psychopharmacology: Principles and practice* (1st ed., pp. 497–510). New York, NY: Oxford University Press.

Leibenluft, E. (2011). Severe mood dysregulation, irritability, and the diagnostic boundaries of bipolar disorder in youths. *American Journal of Psychiatry, 162*(2), 129–142.

Leonard, H. L., Ale, C. M., & Freeman, J. B. (2005). Obsessive-compulsive disorder. *Child and Adolescent Psychiatric Clinics of North America, 14,* 727–743.

Main, M. (1996). Introduction to the special section on attachment and psychopathology: Overview of the field of attachment. *Journal of Consulting and Clinical Psychology, 64*(2), 237–243.

Manassis, K. (2004). Childhood anxiety disorders: Approach to interventions. *Canadian Family Physician, 50,* 379–384.

Martin, A., Van Hoof, T., Stubbe, D., Sherwin, T., & Scahill, L. (2003). Multiple psychotropic pharmacotherapy in children and adolescents: A study of Connecticut Medicaid managed care recipients. *Psychiatric Services, 54,* 72–77.

Mayo Clinic. (2013). *Reactive attachment disorder.* Retrieved from http://www.mayoclinic.org/diseases-conditions/reactive-attachment-disorder/basics/definition/CON-20032126

McMahon-Wellington, T., Semrud-Clikeman, M., Gregory, A. L., Murphy, J. M., & Lancaster, J. L. (2006). Magnetic resonance imaging volumetric analysis of the putamen in children with ADHD: Combined type versus control. *Journal of Attention Disorders, 10*(2), 171–180.

Mental Health Commission of Canada. (2011). *Making the case for investing in mental health in Canada.* Retrieved from http://www.mentalhealthcommission.ca/English/node/5020?terminitial=41

Morris, M. (2014). Diagnosis in young children: How a father's perceptions of mental health change. *Journal of Child and Adolescent Psychiatric Nursing, 27*(2), 52–60.

MTA Cooperative Group. (1999). A 14-month randomized clinical trial of treatment strategies for attention-deficit/hyperactivity disorder. Multimodal treatment study of children with ADHA. *Archives of General Psychiatry, 56*(12), 1073–1086.

Mulvihill, D. (2005). The health impact of childhood trauma: An interdisciplinary review, 1997–2003. *Issues in Comprehensive Pediatric Nursing, 28*(2), 115–136.

Murray, B. (2008). Disorders diagnosed in infancy, childhood or adolescence. In P. O'Brien, W. Kennedy, & K. Ballard (Eds.), *Psychiatric mental health nursing: An introduction to theory and practice* (pp. 207–234). Boston, MA: Jones and Bartlett Publishers.

National Child Traumatic Stress Network (NCTSN). (2013). Effective treatments for youth trauma. Retrieved from http://www.nctsn.org/resources/audiences/parents-caregivers/treatments-that-work

National Institute of Mental Health (NIMH). (2013). Bipolar disorder. Retrieved from http://www.nimh.nih.gov/health/topics/bipolar-disorder/index.shtml

National Scientific Council on the Developing Child. (2012). The science of neglect: The persistent absence of responsive care disrupts the developing brain: Working Paper 12. Retrieved from http://www.developingchild.harvard.edu

Nield, L. & Kamat, D. (2004). Enuresis: How to evaluate and treat. *Clinical Pediatrics, 43*(5), 409–415.

North American Society for Pediatric Gastroenterology, Hepatology and Nutrition. (2006). Evaluation and treatment of constipation in infants: Clinical practice guidelines. *Journal of Pediatric Gastroenterology and Nutrition, 43*(3), 1–13.

Palermo, M. & Curatolo, P. (2004). Pharmacologic treatment of autism. *Journal of Child Neurology, 19*(3), 155–164.

Panagiotopoulos, C., Ronsley, R., Kuzeljevic, B., & Davidson, J. (2012). Waist circumference is a sensitive screening tool for assessment of metabolic syndrome risk in children treated with second-generation antipsychotics. *Canadian Journal of Psychiatry, 57*(1), 34–44.

Pelham, W., Fabiano, G., & Massetti, G. (2005). Evidence-based assessment of attention deficit hyperactivity disorder in children and adolescents. *Journal of Clinical Child and Adolescent Psychology, 34*(3), 449–476.

Perry, A. & Condillac, R. (2003). *Evidence-based practices for children and adolescents with autism spectrum disorders: Review of the literature and practice guide.* Toronto, ON: Children's Mental Health.

Perry, B. D. (1994). Neurobiological sequelae of childhood trauma: Post traumatic stress disorders in children. In M. Murburg (Ed.) *Catecholamine function in post-traumatic stress disorder: Emerging concepts.* Washington, DC: American Psychiatric Press.

Perry, B. D. (2001). The neurodevelopmental impact of violence in childhood. In D. Schekty & E. Benedek (Eds.), *Textbook of child and adolescent forensic psychiatry* (pp. 221–238). Washington, DC: American Psychiatric Association.

Perry, B. D. (2002a). *The vortex of violence: How children adapt and survive in a violent world.* Available at www.childtrauma.org.

Perry, B. D. (2002b). *Brain structure and function I: Basics of organization.* Retrieved from http://www.childtrauma.org/ctamaterials/brain_I.asp.

Perry, B. D. (2002c). *Brain structure and function II: Special topics information work with maltreated children.* Retrieved from http://www.childtrauma.org/ctamaterials/brain_II.asp

Perry, B. D. (2004). *Maltreatment and the developing child: How early childhood experience shapes child and culture.* Retrieved from http://www.lfcc.on.ca/mccain/perry.pdf

Persico, A. & Bourgeron, T. (2006). Searching for ways out of the autism maze: Genetic, epigenetic and environmental clues. *Trends in Neurosciences, 29*(7), 349–358.

Pinto-Martin, J., Souders, M., Giarelli, E., & Levy, S. (2005). The role of the nurse in screening for autistic spectrum disorder in pediatric primary care. *Journal of Pediatric Nursing, 20*(3), 163–169.

Porges, S. (2004). Neuroception: A subconscious system for detecting threats and safety. *Zero to Three, 24*(5), 19–24.

Preet, J. (2007). Suicide and spirituality: A clinical perspective. *Southern Medical Journal, 100*(7), 752–755.

Prestia, K. (2003). Tourette's syndrome: Characteristics and interventions. *Intervention in School and Clinic, 39*(2), 67–71.

Pringsheim, T., Doja, A., Gorman, D., McKinlay, D., Day, L., Billinghurst, L., … Sandor, P. (2012). Canadian Guidelines for evidence-based treatment of tic disorders: Pharmacotherapy. *Canadian Journal of Psychiatry, 57*(3), 133–143.

Public Health Agency of Canada (PHAC). (2005). *Responding to stressful events: Helping children cope.* Ottawa, ON: Author.

Ramtekkar, U. P., Reiersen, A. M., Todorov, A. A., & Todd, R. D. (2010). Sex and age differences in attention-deficit/hyperactivity disorder symptoms and diagnoses: Implications for DSM-V and ICD-11.

Journal of the American Academy of Child and Adolescent Psychiatry, 49(3), 217–228.

Ransby, M. & Swanson, H. L. (2003). Reading comprehension skills of young adults with childhood diagnosis of dyslexia. *Journal of Learning Disabilities, 36*(6), 538–555.

Rapee, R. & Spence, S. (2004). The etiology of social phobia: Empirical evidence and an initial model. *Clinical Psychology Review, 24,* 737–767.

Reiner, W. & Reiner, D. T. (2012). Thoughts on the nature of identity: How disorders of sex development inform clinical research about gender identity disorders. *Journal of Homosexuality, 59*(3), 434–449.

Reiner, W. G. (2003). Elimination disorders: Enuresis and encopresis. In A. Martin, L. Scahill, D. S. Charney, & J. F. Leckman (Eds.), *Pediatric psychopharmacology: Principles and practice* (1st ed., pp. 686–698). New York, NY: Oxford University Press.

Richardson, A. J. (2006). Omega-3 fatty acids in ADHD and related neurodevelopmental disorders. *International Review of Psychiatry, 18*(2), 155–172.

Russell, R. & Grizzle, K. (2008). Assessing child and adolescent pragmatic language competencies: Toward evidence-based assessments. *Clinical Child and Family Psychology Review, 11*(1), 59–73.

Scahill, L., Leckman, J. F., Schultz, R. T., Katsovich, L., & Peterson, B. S. (2003). A placebo-controlled trial of risperidone in Tourette syndrome. *Neurology, 60,* 1130–1135.

Schlomer, B., Rodriguez, E., Weiss, D., & Copp, H. (2013). Parents' beliefs about nocturnal enuresis causes, treatments and the need to seek professional medical care. *Journal of Pediatric Urology, 9,* 1043–1048.

Seidman, L. J., Valera, E. M., & Bush, G. (2004). Brain function and structure in adults with attention-deficit/hyperactivity disorder. *Psychiatric Clinics of North America, 27*(2), 323–347.

Shaw, P., Eckstrand, K., Sharp, W., Blumenthal, J., Lerch, J. P., Greenstein, D., ... Rapoport, J. L. (2007). Attention-deficit/hyperactivity disorder is characterized by a delay in cortical maturation. *Proceedings of the National Academy of Sciences of the United States of America, 104*(49), 19649–19654.

Shaw, P., Malek, M., Watson, B., Sharp, W., Evans, A., & Greenstein, D. (2012). Development of cortical surface area and gyrification in attention-deficit/hyperactivity disorder. *Biological Psychiatry, 72*(3), 191–197.

Shea, S., Turgay, A., Carroll, A., Schulz, M., Orlik, H., Smith, I., & Dunbar, F. (2004). Risperidone in the treatment of disruptive behavioral symptoms in children with autistic and other pervasive developmental disorders. *Pediatrics, 114*(5), e634–e641.

Sherer, M. R. & Schreibman, L. (2005). Individual behavioral profiles and predictors of treatment effectiveness for children with autism. *Journal of Consulting and Clinical Psychology, 75,* 525–538.

Siegel, D. (2001). Toward an interpersonal neurobiology of the developing mind: Attachment relationships, "mindset," and neural integration. *Infant Mental Health Journal, 22*(1–2), 67–94.

Singer, H. S. (2005). Tourette's syndrome: From behaviour to biology. *Lancet Neurology, 4*(3), 149–159.

Singer, H. S. (2013). Motor control, habits, complex motor stereotypies, and Tourette Syndrome. *Annals of the New York Academy of Sciences, 1304*(1), 22–31.

Smith, J. & McSherry, W. (2004). Spirituality and child development: A concept analysis. *Journal of Advanced Nursing, 45*(3), 307–315.

Sowell, E. R., Thompson, P. M., Welcome, S. E., Henkenius, A. L., Toga, A. W., & Peterson, B. S. (2003). Cortical abnormalities in children and adolescents with attention-deficit hyperactivity disorder. *Lancet, 362*(9397), 1699–1707.

Speraw, S. (2006). Spiritual experiences of parents and caregivers who have children with disabilities or special needs. *Issues in Mental Health Nursing, 27,* 213–230.

Statistics Canada. (2012). *Suicide rates: An overview.* Retrieved from http://www.statcan.gc.ca/pub/82-624-x/2012001/article/11696-eng.htm

Steeves, T., Mckinlay, B. D., Gorman, D. Billingshurst, L., Day, L., Carroll, A. ... Pringsheim, T. (2012). Canadian guidelines for evidence-based treatment of tic disorders: Behavioural therapy, deep brain stimulation, and transcranial magnetic stimulation. *Canadian Journal of Psychiatry, 57*(3), 144–151.

Stewart, S. E., Geller, D. A., Jenike, M., Pauls, D., Shaw, D., Mullin, B., & Faraone, S. V. (2004). Long-term outcome of pediatric obsessive-compulsive disorder: A meta-analysis and qualitative review of the literature. *Acta Psychiatrica Scandinavica, 110*(1), 4–13.

Stewart, S. E., Rosario, M. C., Brown, T. A., Carter, A. S., Leckman, J. F., Sukhodolsky, D., ... Pauls, D. L. (2007). Principal components analysis of obsessive-compulsive disorder symptoms in children and adolescents. *Biological Psychiatry, 61,* 285–291.

Storch, E. A., Murphy, T. K., Geffken, G. R., Sajid, M., Allen, P., Roberti, J. W., & Goodman, W. K. (2005). Reliability and validity of the Yale Global Tic Severity Scale. *Psychological Assessment, 17*(4), 486–491.

Tonmyr, L., Williams, G., Hovdestad, W., & Draca, J. (2011). Anxiety and/or depression in 10–15-year-olds investigated by child welfare in Canada. *Journal of Adolescent Health, 48,* 493–498.

van der Kolk, B. (2005). Developmental trauma disorder. *Psychiatric Annals, 35*(5), 401–408.

van der Kolk, B. (2006). Clinical implications for neuroscience in research in PTSD. *Annals of the New York Academy of Sciences, 1071,* 277–293.

van der Kolk, B. (2009). *New frontiers in trauma treatment.* Presentation at Coquitlam, BC.

Van Grootheest, D., Cath, D., Beekman, A., & Boomsma, D. (2005). Twin studies on obsessive compulsive disorder: A review. *Twin Research and Human Genetics, 8*(5), 450–458.

Volkmar, F. R., Klin, A., & Paul, R. (2004). *Handbook of autism and pervasive developmental disorders* (3rd ed) New York, NY: Wiley.

Waddell, C., Godderis, R., Hua, J., McEwan, K., & Wong, W. (2004). Preventing and treating anxiety disorders in children and youth. In *Children's Mental Health Policy Research Program.* Vancouver, BC: British Columbia Ministry of Children and Family Development.

Waddell, C., McEwan, K., Shepherd, C., Offord, D., & Hua, J. M. (2005). A public health strategy to improve the mental health of Canadian children. *Canadian Journal of Psychiatry, 50*(4), 226–233.

Webster-Stratton, C. (2011). *The incredible years: Parents, teachers and children's training series. Program content, methods, research and dissemination 1980–2011.* Seattle, WA: Incredible Years, Inc.

Wente, M. (2014). *Globe Debate: Transgendered kids: Have we gone too far? The Globe and Mail.* Retrieved from http://www.theglobeandmail.com/globe-debate/transgender-kids-have-we-gone-too-far/article16897043/

Witwer, A. & Lecavalier, L. (2005). Treatment incidence and patterns in children and adolescents with autism spectrum disorder. *Journal of Child and Adolescent Psychopharmacology, 15*(4), 671–681.

Zinck, S., Bagnell, A., Bond, K., & Newton, A. S. (2009). The Cochrane library and the treatment of major depression in children and youth: An overview of reviews. *Evidence-Based Child Health: A Cochrane Review Journal, 4*(4), 1336–1350.

Zucker, K. J., Wood, H., Singh, D., & Bradley, S. (2012). A developmental, biopsychosocial model for the treatment of children with gender identity disorder. *Journal of Homosexuality, 59,* 369–397.

32 Mental Health Promotion With Older Persons

Sharon L. Moore

Adapted from the chapter "Mental Health Promotion with the Older Adult" by Mary Ann Boyd

KEY CONCEPT

- late adulthood

KEY TERMS

- gerotranscendence • middle-old • old-old • young-old

Global aging is occurring at an unprecedented rate, and Canada, like many other countries, is experiencing a boom in population growth of seniors (Sciegaj & Behr, 2010; World Health Organization, 2012). Currently the population in Canada is 34.3 million, and it is estimated to reach almost 48 million by 2036. In 2010, persons over the age of 65 accounted for 14% of the population, a proportion predicted to rise to 25% by 2036 (Public Health Agency of Canada [PHAC], 2010; Statistics Canada, 2010). With the increase in aging population, there is a concomitant increase in the number of older adults with mental health issues. "Canadians are living longer, healthier lives—but as the population grows, so does the number of people at risk of experiencing mental health issues. One in four seniors lives with a mental health problem (e.g., depression, anxiety, or dementia) or illness" (Mental Health Commission of Canada, 2013).

These disorders can substantially impair functioning and can result in unnecessary hospitalizations and nursing home placement, poorer health outcomes, and increased rates of mortality. For example, older persons who suffer from depression have worse outcomes after medical events such as hip fractures, heart attacks, or cancer, and individuals who are aged 75 and older have the highest suicide rate of any age group (National Alliance on Mental Illness, 2001, p. 1). It is also well documented that, for older adults, it takes less alcohol to exacerbate medical and mental problems, and, in turn, medical and emotional problems may contribute to further alcohol use (PHAC, 2002; Sattar, Petty, & Burke, 2003).

Nurses need to understand and respond well to the unique needs of this population. Older adults' mental health needs are not easily addressed within generic treatment programs, because older adults have "unique attributes that distinguish their mental health needs from those of other groups" (Standing Senate Committee on Social Affairs, Science and Technology, 2006, p. 158). Mental health promotion and mental illness prevention efforts, targeted at older adults' needs, are key to helping older adults live healthy lives with purpose and meaning. Healthy aging has become a mantra for living well in the 21st century (Bryant et al., 2012; Lezwijn, Vaandrager, Naaldenberg, Wagemakers, & van Woerkum, 2011). This chapter explains the effect of aging on mental health and identifies risk factors related to geriatric psychopathology. Concepts related to the promotion of mental health are identified.

MENTAL HEALTH OF THE OLDER ADULT

Adults 85 years and older are the most rapidly growing segment of the Canadian population. From 1921 through 1998, the population of **old-old** adults had increased

20 times (Lindsay & Almay, 1999). The transition from **young-old** to old-old is more than a series of birthdays; it is a gradual bio/psycho/social/spiritual process that may be viewed as both positive and negative. From a positive perspective, the later years provide time for personal growth and development, providing an opportunity to do all the things that were impossible when work and family responsibilities took precedence. Travelling, visiting friends, and engaging in neglected hobbies enhance quality of life and improve well-being.

In late adulthood, changes in health status can lead to negative outcomes. A loss in physical functioning can lead to a loss in independence, which can result in an unplanned change in residence. Family relationships change, as once-dependent children grow into adulthood and become parents themselves. Friendships change, and losses occur. Many older adults retire from meaningful lifelong work and are faced with establishing new meaning in life. To have a sense of meaning and purpose is a critical factor in older adults' mental health and is one of the factors that serves as a protection against suicide and despair in later life (Moore, 2005; Moore, Metcalf, & Schow, 2000).

In all health care settings, communication is an integral factor in nursing care. Recent studies have shown the importance of nurse–patient interactions in helping older adults have hope and meaning in life (Haugan, 2013). Communication with older adults requires special attention to verbal interactions and environmental influences. Box 32-1 highlights some necessary considerations.

BOX 32-1 Communicating with Older Adults

- Focus the person's attention on the exchange of communication; the older adult may need extra time to begin to process information.
- Face the person when speaking to him or her.
- Minimize distractions in the room, including other people, objects in your hands, noise, and other activities.
- Reduce glare from room lighting by dimming too-bright lights. Conversely, avoid sitting in shadows.
- Speak slowly and clearly. Older adults may depend on lip reading, so ensure that the individual can see you. Speak loudly, but do not shout. It is not necessary to over enunciate with exaggerated lip movements.
- Use short, simple sentences and be prepared to repeat or revise what you have said.
- Limit the number of topics discussed at one time to prevent information overload.
- Ask one question at a time to minimize confusion. Allow plenty of time for the person to answer and express ideas.
- Frequently summarize the important points of the conversation to improve understanding and comprehension.
- Avoid the urge to finish sentences.
- If the communication exchange is going poorly, postpone it for another time.
- Greet the older person by name.
- Invest time in a caring and respectful interaction.
- Encourage connectedness with like-minded persons.

KEY CONCEPT Late adulthood can be divided into three chronologic groups: *young-old* (ages 65 to 74 years), **middle-old** (ages 75 to 84 years), and *old-old* (age 85 years and older).

Biologic Domain

The human life span encompasses the stages of embryogenesis, growth and development, and senescence or growing old (Panno, 2010). During senescence, there is a natural, gradual deterioration of the body: aging affects the cells of every major bodily organ (National Institute on Aging [NIA], 2011/updated 2013). During aging, arteries will become more rigid; body fat will increase; some brain neurons will be lost without affecting basic functioning; ventricular walls of the heart will thicken; high-frequency sounds will not be easily heard; some hormones (e.g., oestrogen, testosterone) will decrease while others (e.g., insulin, vasopressin) increase; night vision will decline; mild arthritis will affect joints; and vital capacity of the lungs will decline (Panno, 2010).

The immune system's effectiveness in its function to defend the body from pathogens decreases over time, leaving the body more vulnerable. This is known as *immunosenescence*. With age, innate immune system cells seem to have less ability to communicate with each other, affecting the adequacy of the immune response (NIA, 2011/updated 2013). Inflammation, which plays a key role in resisting disease, may over time initiate a chronic inflammatory state; researchers note that older adults without chronic inflammation recover more efficiently from infection (NIA, 2011/updated 2013). Part of the adaptive immune system, "naive" T cells (i.e., those not programmed as yet for a specific pathogen) decrease in number with aging. This causes the older adult to be less resistant to new threats and less responsive to vaccines (NIA, 2011/updated 2013).

The metabolic activities that sustain human life also create stress that ultimately damages the body. For example, when oxygen is used by cells to convert food into energy, there are by-products created called *free radicals*. These are also created by environmental factors, like tobacco smoke and sun exposure. Some free radicals cause damage to components of cells, including DNA. The role of such oxidation (free radical) damage in aging is being explored. Free radicals have been connected to cancer and neurodegeneration, Alzheimer's and Parkinson's diseases, and arthritis (Moody & Sasser, 2011; NIA, 2011). Although consuming antioxidants (such as vitamins A, C, and E) seems to have only minimal effects on aging (as evident in animal studies), some individuals strive to increase them in their diet (Moody & Sasser, 2011).

The study of aging is focused on examining both life span (number of years in an individual's life) and health span (number of years of good health and functioning) (NIA, 2011). The complex role genetics plays in aging is a key area. For instance, in the New England Centenarian Study, researchers found 281 genetic markers that were 61% accurate in predicting who was 100 years old, 73% accurate in predicting who was 102 years old or older, and 85% accurate in predicting who was 105 years old or older. The genetic component of longevity seems to increase with exceptional age (Sebastiani et al., 2012). Exceptionally long-lived individuals appear to delay health problems until late in life (NIA, 2011/updated 2013). Senescence occurs, of course, at the cellular as well as the organism level. Epigenetic studies are finding that senescent cells undergo changes in their chromatin (see Chapter 9); similar changes are found in prematurely aging cells (Berger, 2013).

The 21st century has seen rapid advances in the knowledge of human biology related to aging. In the Canadian Longitudinal Study on Aging, which involves 30,000 to 50,000 Canadians over 40, biologic and other aspects of aging are being further explored. Nurses will be able to use this and other research to enrich their knowledge of aging and to improve health promotion of the older adult (Carstairs & Keon, 2009).

Psychological Domain

Cognitive Function

Changes in cognition are most likely accounted for by structural and functional changes in the brain (Rosenzweig & Barnes, 2003). These alterations are probably highly specific because aspects of cognitive decline are very specific (e.g., secondary memory), and many abilities are preserved. Moreover, external factors, including activity levels, socioeconomic status, education, and personality, may modify the development or the expression of age-related changes in cognition (see Chapter 34). Normal aging does not impair consciousness. Alertness is required for attention, but the alert patient may not necessarily be able to attend. Attention has two aspects: sustained attention (vigilance) and selective attention (ability to extract relevant from irrelevant information). Numerous studies indicate that older adults perform well on tests of sustained and selective attention (Ebersole, Touhy, Hess, & Jett, 2007; Yevchak, Loeb, & Fick, 2008). Earlier findings of poor performance on tests of selective attention have been attributed to lack of control for perceptual difficulties (e.g., vision and hearing deficits).

Slower reaction time may affect how quickly an older adult responds to questions. Hurrying older adults to answer questions may interfere with their ability to provide the correct answer. This has been labelled the *speed–accuracy shift*, by which the older adult focuses more on accuracy than on speed in responding. Caution tends to increase, whereas risk-taking behaviour tends to decrease; older adults are more likely to make errors of omission

(leaving the answer out) than errors of commission (making a guess) (Zimprich, 2002).

Recent studies have shown that there are several factors that contribute to cognitive health in later years (Evers, Klusmann, Schwarzer, & Heuser, 2011; Lee & Hung, 2011; Newberg, 2011). Meditation, prayer, and other spiritual practices have a positive effect on the aging brain such that memory, mood and cognition, and overall mental health are improved (Newberg, 2011). Lifestyle interventions have been found to enhance cognitive functioning and brain reserve (Lam & Cheng, 2012). Reminiscence is recognized as a key strategy to "foster identity and self-continuity, and to achieve a sense of coherence and meaning in life" for older persons (O'Rourke, Cappeliez, & Claxton, 2011, p. 272) with autobiographical memory appearing "to exert both direct and indirect effects on well-being" (p. 279). Available for health care professionals is a "life story toolkit" that focused on the use of life review to develop life storybooks with older adults (Moya & Arnold, 2012).

A key psychosocial resource for older adults' physical and mental health is hope (Duggleby et al., 2010; Duggleby et al., 2012; Hammer, Mogensen, & Hall, 2009; Moore, 2012). While there are many definitions of hope, its positive role in living and facilitating meaning and life is well documented (Duggleby et al., 2012; Hammer, Mogensen, & Hall, 2009; Haugan, 2013; Moore, 2012). Hope provides a reason to live and allows one to see the smallest ray of light when the world looks dark. Hope allows the older person to go on in the face of adverse circumstances and to be "okay" regardless of the outcome.

Learning

Intelligence and personality are stable across the life span in the absence of disease; however, the learning abilities of older adults may be more selective, requiring motivation ("How important is this information?"), meaningful content ("Why do I need to know this?"), and familiarity with the idea or content. Although age causes no differences in the ability to process knowledge to learn a skill, younger people are more likely to employ strategies to learn tasks. Level of education needs to be considered in evaluating responses on mental status examinations because it may represent socioeconomic status and occupation.

Memory

Other than overall intelligence, age-related memory alterations have been more widely studied than any other aspect of cognition. Contrary to popular belief, memory loss is not a normal part of aging. To remember events, individuals must first attend to information and process it. Older adults may well dismiss information that is not important to them. Memory problems in later life are believed to result from encoding problems or "getting" the information in the first place. This problem may be related to sensory problems, not paying attention, or a general failure to link the "to-be-remembered" information to existing knowledge through association or to strengthen the memory through repetition. However, it is important not to confuse decline with deficit. Although a decline in memory ability may be frustrating for the older individual, it does not necessarily hamper his or her ability to function daily. Threats to memory include medications, depression (impairs concentration and attention), poor nutrition, infection, heart and lung disease (lack of oxygen), thyroid problems (can cause symptoms of depression or confusion that mimic memory loss), alcohol use, and sensory loss (interferes with perception).

Development

The psychologist Erik Erikson identified "integrity versus despair" as a developmental task specific to late adulthood. An extension of his theory published by Joan Serson Erikson, his wife, included old age as a ninth stage, **gerotranscendence** (Erikson & Erikson, 1997). Gerotranscendence, developed further by Tornstam (1989), is a psychosocial theory that regards aging as the final stage in a "possible natural progression towards maturation and wisdom" (Tornstam, 2005, p. 1), which generally results in increased satisfaction and meaning in life. Rather than emphasizing decrements in physical capacity for function, gerotranscendence theory provides for continued growth in dimensions such as spirituality and inner strength (Wadensten & Carlsson, 2007a; Wadensten & Carlsson, 2007b). There is growing evidence to support the effects of gerotranscendence in the promotion of mental health and well-being of institutionalized older adults (Wang, Lin, & Hsieh, 2011). Duggleby and colleagues (2012), in their metasynthesis of hope, older adults, and chronic illness, found that transcendence beyond current difficulties was a major theme in how older persons coped and hoped. They described transcendence as "a process that involved the subprocesses of reaching inwardly and outwardly finding meaning and purpose" (p. 1218). This process of transcending occurred through positive reappraisal and "included the sub processes of reevaluating hope and seeing positive possibilities" (p. 1218).

The concept of gerotranscendence may be used in establishing health promotion interventions. Research suggests that the following guidelines may help the staff support older adults in their process towards gerotranscendence:

- Accept the possibility that behaviours resembling the signs of gerotranscendence are normal signs of aging.
- Foster strategies to find and maintain hope.
- Foster the older persons' ability to imagine other perspectives.
- Respond to the older person's thoughts and conversation about death.

- Introduce topics of conversation that may facilitate older adults' personal growth.
- Accept, create, and introduce new types of activities.
- Create opportunities for older persons to connect with one another and to engage in conversations that facilitate reminiscence and life review.
- Facilitate opportunities for older persons to come together and talk about existential issues such as hope, spirituality, and transcending.

Relationship Strains

As family relationships change, interpersonal relationship strains can develop. Disappointments with lifestyles of adult children and changes in caregiving responsibilities may affect the quality of a longtime family relationship. In some instances, young-old adults assume caregiving responsibilities for their old-old relatives. It is also common for grandparents to assume some caregiving responsibilities for their grandchildren. A change in work status of grandparents (the fact that many of them work today) has drastically changed the "face" of grandparenting in Canada.

With Canadians living longer and healthier lives, grandparents are playing a larger part in the lives of their families. A century ago, grandparents could expect to have only 10 years with their grandchildren; that statistic has doubled to 20 years today. As most Canadian women can expect to live to be at least 86 years of age, many will spend nearly half of their lives as grandmothers. As well, many more Canadians can expect to become great-grandparents than those in the past (Martin-Matthews, 2007). While relationship strains can occur, "families are our most valuable resources, providing not only caregiving but also a sense of worth, emotional ties, and human dignity in approaching life's end" (Walsh, 2012, p. 170). Irrespective of the varied family structures, "what remains constant is the centrality of relatedness" (p. 170). Nurses must strive to understand and support families and to encourage the development of meaning and purpose not just individually, but collectively. They must recognize the potential for aging to achieve personal, relational, and spiritual growth and possibility.

Social Domain

Functional Status

Functional status (i.e., the extent to which a person can independently carry out personal care, home management, and social functions in everyday life in a way that has meaning and purpose) often changes during the later years (see Chapter 33). Estimates of the prevalence of functional dependency vary, but, in general, studies show that difficulty in performing activities of daily living (ADLs) increases with advancing age and that rates of dependency are significantly higher for women than for men, particularly for women who live alone (von Strauss, Aguero-Torres, Kareholt, Winblad, & Fratiglioni, 2003).

Although older women and men have similar paths to life satisfaction, a Canadian study conducted by Bourque, Pushkar, Bonneville, and Beland (2005) reported that there are important differences. Men's greater independence allows them to be less dependent on environmental and social factors for life satisfaction; women's greater social embeddedness enables them to be as satisfied as men with life in general, even though their life circumstances may be poorer.

Retirement

While in previous years, there has been a trend towards early retirement in Canada, legislated changes in the Canada Pension Plan provide incentives for workers to delay their retirement (Sheets & Gallagher, 2013). Canadians, regardless of their education, are working later and delaying retirement (Statistics Canada, 2012). The transition from a paid work role to a potentially less structured and purposeful pattern of living can lead to alterations in self-concept. While retirement is often chosen, it is frequently characterized as a stressful life event that may bring psychological, social, and economic uncertainty. It affects social roles, income, use of health services, and participation in leisure activities. Although these changes are often associated with negative myths and stereotypes, most people do very well in retirement. Adequate pensions, savings/investments, and social assistance contribute to its success.

Cultural Impact

As the population ages in Canadian society, it is also becoming more culturally diverse, and diversity is changing the landscape of aging populations. The senior population of Canada is heterogenous, composed of many groups whose similarities and differences intersect (e.g., First Nations, lesbian gay bisexual transgendered [LGBT], employed, immigrants, refugees, ethnocultural and racialized groups) (Mental Health Commission of Canada, 2011). Our North American communities are increasingly a reflection of multiple ethnic histories and values. Before the 1960s, immigrants to Canada were mostly from Europe; since the late 1980s, immigrants are increasingly from Asia, Central and South America, and Africa (Tam, Fletcher, & Chi, 2004). Wide cultural variations exist in family expectations of and responsibilities for the older adult. Some groups, such as First Nations and Asian cultures, tend to value highly the experience and wisdom of their older family members, and younger family members feel a responsibility for their care. This cultural belief can create additional pressures for younger family members who may not have the resources to fulfill these expectations.

Immigrants and refugees who come to Canada frequently experience loneliness, uprootedness, "brokenness," and "woundedness." Older adults, in addition to facing such problems, often do not speak the language, become further isolated, and have difficulty expressing mental health needs (Standing Senate Committee on Social Affairs, Science and Technology, 2006).

Further research is needed to understand and address the relationships between cultural issues related to aging, health, and health care delivery. We do know that treatment and intervention are most effective when patients, families, and the health care team can work together to integrate patients' beliefs and cultural values into the plan of care.

Social Activities

While the majority of older adults acknowledge that their health is good, there are health conditions that may prevent participation in home maintenance and leisure activities such as walking, gardening, and active sports. However, there has been increasing support for the importance of physical and social activity in successful aging. Wilson, Harris, Hollis, and Mohankumar (2010) note that social isolation poses serious health risks for older persons and suggest that nurses have key roles to play in minimizing social isolation for seniors. They suggest "upstream solutions" involving primary intervention strategies to address this problem. Nurses can identify the potential for social isolation and build strategies to mitigate against this. Interestingly, in a study of older adults volunteering for Habitat for Humanity, it was found that these volunteers were not physically healthier than their community counterparts but were mentally healthier (Brown, Mefford, Chen, & Brown, 2009). Positive attitudes around notions of "everyone contributes" and "adjusting to limitations" were displayed.

Impacts of Aging on Housing and Communities

The aging of the Canadian population is requiring a reshaping of the pattern of housing needs, the demand for services, and the ways in which communities are being structured to make them more responsive to individuals with disabilities (Canada Mortgage and Housing Corporation [CMHC], 2008). The CMHC further reports that while life expectancy for men is increasing, women in their 80s outnumber men by almost 50% and by more than 50% among older adults in their 90s. These trends are placing additional demands for a variety of services responsive to the needs of this population.

Most older adults prefer to "age in place" in surroundings that are familiar to them until their health prohibits them from doing so. The CMHC (2008) reported that, in a survey, 85% of individuals over 55 said they planned to remain in their own homes as long as possible, even if health challenges required additional support for home maintenance or personal care from government and private service providers. Implications for health promotion are such that nurses need to be vigilant in their assessment skills, providing ongoing support and facilitating early intervention when needed.

The types of facilities and supports to assist older adults to age in place vary across the country and seem to depend in large part on provincial funding. All provinces will need to address the changing demographics that require a variety of community and residential housing options.

The rapid growth in numbers of older seniors who live alone, are frail, or have disabilities will necessitate considerable expansion of supportive housing choices that enable them to stay in the community rather than in long-term health facilities, such as nursing homes (CMHC, 2008, p. 5).

Residential Care

Various residential care models are in part a response to the medical model emphasized in most long-term care facilities and the need to develop alternatives to nursing home care. Residential care models include a spectrum of residential living environments, such as foster care homes, family homes, personal care homes, residential care facilities, and assisted living arrangements.

Approximately 7% of seniors live in nursing homes and health care facilities, and "the proportion of seniors who enter those facilities rises steadily with age, to 13% of those 75 and older" (CMHC, 2008, p. 5). Residential facilities are seeing increased numbers of older adults with mental and physical health challenges, presenting both opportunities and challenges to supporting these individuals. As the population ages, it stands to reason that more older people will be living in long-term care environments.

It is important to recognize the role that transcendence plays as a developmental resource in old age. Research investigating living with chronic illness into old age found themes based on strengths of adaptation and adjusting; many older persons demonstrated inner strength despite age and physical or mental challenges (Moe, Hellzen, Ekker, & Enmarker, 2013). Even though the oldest old women and men were vulnerable, they had inner strength. The researchers concluded that "encouraging participation using the inner strength of even the oldest old can contribute to strengthen their experiences of independence, integrity, and enjoying life" (Moe et al., 2013, p. 189).

Assisted Living

The assisted living concept has emerged as an important long-term care alternative for older adults who are mentally and physically frail. Assisted living provides community-based residential services for older adults and adults with physical disabilities who need help with ADLs. Assisted living services combine housing, personal services, and light medical or nursing care. Perhaps the most important feature of these assisted living facilities is the orientation towards the older resident that empowers the frail older adult by sharing responsibilities for care and ADLs, enhancing their choices, and managing risks.

Spiritual Domain

Humanists suggest that the main purpose of life is to find meaning and that this can be accomplished through creations (or accomplishments), experiences in the world, and attitude towards suffering (Frankl, 1963). In the past decade, there is a growing recognition of the important role that spirituality plays in aging successfully. Likewise, successful aging is broadening our understanding of what constitutes spirituality. In nursing, spirituality is recognized as a basic quality, inherent in all humans. The spiritual perspective includes critical attributes such as

- Connectedness (with other humans, nature, universal forces, or God)
- Beliefs in powers or forces beyond the self and a faith that affirms life
- A creative energy
- Hope

The spiritual perspective also can provide a path for the quest for the meaning of life and can organize and guide human values and motivations.

▬ HEALTHY AGING: THE EXAMPLE OF SEXUAL HEALTH

Cross-cultural research confirms that healthy aging is an ongoing process of adaptation across the four primary bio/psycho/social/spiritual domains (Scharlach & Hoshino, 2013). Sexual health, an important aspect of overall well-being at any age, serves as a good illustration of this necessary adaptation. As one ages, the desire for intimacy does not go away. Many older adults continue to have an active and fulfilling sex life (Mayo Clinic, 2011). Practicing safe sex is as important for older persons as for younger persons. There are physical changes that can affect ones' ability to have and enjoy sex (e.g., vaginal dryness in women, often relieved by using a lubricant, and in men impotence or erectile dysfunction, often relieved by medication) (NIA, 2009). In both these instances, encouraging consultation with a family physician may be useful, while the nurse reassures that these issues are common and can most often be remedied. There are some physical illnesses, disabilities, and medications that can cause sexual problems (NIA, 2009). Conditions such as arthritis, chronic pain, dementia, diabetes, heart disease, incontinence, surgery, mastectomy, prostatectomy, and certain medications can affect sexual desire and performance.

There are some strategies for each of these conditions that may help alleviate worrisome symptoms and increase pleasure, performance, and desire. Communication with one's partner is a key strategy. Problems in the relationship can create problems in the bedroom (NIA, 2009).

The sustaining of sexual health in older adulthood illustrates well the developmental tasks of healthy aging. These have been identified across sociocultural contexts (USA, Japan, & Sweden) as continuity (maintenance of roles and activities), compensation (accommodation and social support), connection (meaningful relationships), contribution (generativity and engagement), and challenge (stimulation and growth) (Scharlach & Hoshino, 2013).

■ RISK FACTORS FOR GERIATRIC PSYCHOPATHOLOGY

Chronic Illnesses

Although the frequency of acute conditions declines with advancing age, about 90% of older adults have chronic medical conditions that can adversely affect function. Poor physical health is a well-established risk factor for mental disorders. The major chronic conditions experienced by older adults are ischemic heart disease, hypertension, vision impairment, hearing impairment, osteo- and rheumatoid arthritis, dementia, cerebrovascular disease, chronic obstructive pulmonary disease, and depression (World Health Organization, 2012). More than 120,000 older Canadians die of cancer, cardiovascular disease, or respiratory distress every year (Statistics Canada, 2010). Chronic illnesses can reduce physiologic capacity and consequently increase functional dependency. In addition, during acute episodes of illness, many older adults lose functional ability because they have limited reserves or cannot mobilize reserves to regain their premorbid performance levels.

Polypharmacy

Polypharmacy, the use of several medications, is often associated with chronic illness and long-term drug therapy (see Chapter 33). The Canadian Broadcasting Corporation (CBC, 2007) reports that seniors in Canada take more prescription drugs than the general population and account for almost 40% of all prescription medications. In 2005, through an analysis of Health Canada data, the CBC estimated that "3,330 seniors die every year due to adverse drug reactions," a number that probably underestimates the actual number of deaths. In addition, many more older adults are impacted by adverse drug reactions. The Canadian Institute for Health Information (CIHI) notes that "seniors are at greater risk for adverse effects due to complex drug therapies and age-related changes to the body" (Canadian Institute for Health Information, 2007, p. 19). Adverse drug reactions create a significant economic burden on the health care system.

The Beers criteria is an internationally recognized list of drugs, developed by Dr. Mark Beers, that identifies potentially inappropriate drugs to prescribe to seniors due to a heightened risk of adverse effects. Updated in 2012 by a panel of experts of the American Geriatric Society (AGS), the Beers criteria aid prescribers in avoiding the use of inappropriate and high-risk drugs. Such avoidance reduces drug-related complications in older persons.

The CBC reported, however, that in 2004, almost 1.5 million—more than a third of Canadian seniors—were prescribed such drugs, even though safer alternatives were available (CBC, 2005). According to a study carried out by the CIHI (2007), the percentage of Canada's older adults taking potentially harmful drugs dropped from 34% in 2000–2001 to 17% in 2005–2006 based on an analysis of drug claims in four Canadian provinces. While this is encouraging, the study also noted an increase in the use of other drugs, such as the antidepressant amitriptyline.

Serious problems result when coordination of the care delivery and treatment regimen specific to prescribed medications is lacking. These problems are compounded when the patient uses over-the-counter drugs, herbal remedies, and home or folk remedies without considering their potential interaction with prescribed drugs. Nurses can follow the principles delineated in Box 32-2 to improve drug therapy with older adults.

Bereavement and Loss

Older adults experience many losses—friends and family members die, physical health compromises, and social status diminishes. Loss of one's spouse, particularly when the relationship has been long and satisfying, constitutes a major life event. Women are more likely to lose their spouses and tend to be widowed at a younger age than are men. Consequently, women have more time to adjust and develop substitute social relationships to replace the spouse. Conversely, men tend to lose their wives at an older age, have fewer social networks to replace the spouse, and express feelings of loneliness and abandonment. Because of differences in longevity, men and women usually experience life events at different ages.

Regardless of gender differences, survivors are at higher risk for depression and may face financial issues after the death of a loved one. Health care professionals should work closely with grieving survivors to help them understand that their lives will be displaced for some time. Support sessions on the grief process, facilitating meaningful engagement and connectedness, can help older persons feel supported and understand that they are not alone.

Poverty

Because retirement and losing a spouse are common events in later life, older adults (particularly women) can be at higher risk for poverty than other age groups. Two

BOX 32-2 Drug Therapy Interventions

- Administer priority/life essential medications first.
- Minimize the number of drugs that the person uses, keeping only those drugs that are essential.
- Always consider alternatives among different drug classifications or dosage forms that are more suitable for older adults. Monitor the claim trends for Beers drugs.
- Implement preventive measures to reduce the need for certain medications. Such prevention includes health promotion through proper nutrition, exercise, and stress reduction.
- Most age-dependent pharmacokinetic changes lead to potential accumulation of the drug; therefore, medication dosage should start low and go slow.
- Exercise caution when administering medication with a long half-life or in an older adult with impaired renal or liver function. Under these conditions, the time may be extended between doses.
- Be knowledgeable of each drug's properties, including such factors as half-life, excretion, and adverse effects. For example, venlafaxine HCl (Effexor), a structurally novel antidepressant that inhibits the reuptake of serotonin and norepinephrine, requires regular monitoring of the older person's blood pressure.
- Assess the individual's clinical history for physical problems that may affect excretion of medications to assess for orthostatic hypotension and the potential for falls.
- Monitor laboratory values (e.g., creatinine clearance) and urinary output in patients receiving medications eliminated by the kidneys.
- Monitor plasma albumin levels in patients receiving drugs that have high binding affinity to protein.
- Regularly monitor the older person's reaction to all medications to ensure a therapeutic response.
- Look for potential drug interactions that may complicate therapy. Antacids lower gastric acidity and may decrease the rate at which other medications are dissolved and absorbed.
- Remind older adults to consult with their health care provider before taking any over-the-counter medications.

groups of poor older adults include those who have lived in poverty all their lives and those who become impoverished in late life. Poverty may result from inadequate retirement income, illness, discrimination against women in pension plans, and financial exploitation of older individuals. Poverty has significant effects on this population, including higher mortality rates, poorer health, lower health-related quality of life, lower likelihood of participating in health screening programs, and higher likelihood of using the emergency department for acute illness (Fleming, Evans, & Chutka, 2003).

Suicide and the Lack of Social Support

Suicide is a leading cause of preventable death in Canada and worldwide. The Canadian Association for Suicide Prevention (CASP) reports that more than 400,000 Canadians engage in some type of self-harm behaviour every year and that in the past 30 years, many of the 100,000 people who have died by suicide in Canada have been older adults (CASP, 2009). The highest rate of suicide in Canada (deaths per 100,000) in 2009 was highest among men aged

85 to 89 years of age (Monette, 2012). Older adults tend to use more lethal methods than younger people in their suicide attempts. Firearms are the most common method of suicide for men, while women tend to use self-poisoning or suffocation (Moore, Grek, Heisel, & Jackson, 2006). The general population engages in suicidal behaviour approximately 20 times for every death to suicide; older adults, in contrast, may do so fewer than four times (Canadian Coalition for Seniors' Mental Health, 2006). "The lethality of suicidal behaviour and related likelihood of death among older adults are especially disturbing in light of large estimated increases in the older Canadian population in coming years" (Statistics Canada, 2005, p. 1).

A lack of social support has been linked to the rate of suicide in older adults (Heisel, 2004; Heisel & Duberstein, 2005), the highest rates being for divorced or widowed men. Risk factors for suicide in older adults include being white, male, widowed or divorced, retired or unemployed, living alone in an urban area, in poor health (including poor mental health), or lonely, and having a history of poor interpersonal relationships (Waern, Rubenowitz, & Wilhelmson, 2003).

MENTAL ILLNESS PREVENTION AND MENTAL HEALTH PROMOTION

"Rates of mental illness for adults between the ages of 70 and 89, including but not limited to dementia, are projected to be higher than for any other age group by 2041" (Mental Health Commission of Canada [MHCC], 2012). This fact alone calls for urgent action to look for ways to promote mental health and to prevent mental health issues. There is growing evidence of the cumulative benefits of regular physical activity when sustained over time (Evers et al., 2011; Lee & Hung, 2011; MHCC, 2009; Shields & Martel, 2006). An improvement in mental health and psychological well-being has been noted, and there is some early, promising evidence that links participation in regular physical activity with a decreased likelihood of developing dementia (Larson et al., 2006; Wang, Larson, Bowen, & van Belle, 2006). While these benefits are widely known, there are also a large number of older Canadians who do not participate in enough activity to maintain or promote their health and well-being. Further, there is growing evidence about the relationship between attitudes, aging, and physical and mental health. As successful aging is gaining further prominence, research studies are pointing to powerful effects of attitudes and beliefs in relation to overall well-being (Bryant et al., 2012).

Mental health promotion efforts of nurses should include facilitating appropriate levels and types of increased physical activity for older adults. There is substantial evidence to show the positive benefits and improvements not only in physical well-being but also in mental and emotional well-being (Ministry of Healthy Living and Support, 2008; Shields & Martel, 2006).

Mental Illness

Preventing Depression and Suicide

Mental illness prevention is aimed at addressing the risk factors associated with mental illness and "enhancing the protective factors that inhibit its onset or shorten its duration" (Mental Health Commission of Canada, 2012; Standing Senate Committee on Social Affairs, Science and Technology, 2006, p. 515). Depression is one of the most common mental disorders in older adults (see Chapter 22). Recognition and early intervention are the keys to preventing ongoing depressive episodes. Early indications of symptomatology can be identified in primary care settings. Several preventive interventions, such as grief counselling for widows and widowers, self-help groups, and social activities, are helpful. Community-based projects have been effective in significantly reducing suicide rates in older adults (Heisel & Duberstein, 2005). By assessing and addressing cognitive and social–cognitive vulnerability factors and by focusing on the promotion of life satisfaction, nurses can help not only to prevent suicide but also to assist the older adult in achieving a healthier and more meaningful life (Grek, 2007; Heisel, 2004; Heisel, 2006). Increasingly, studies are exploring concepts such as meaning and hope and the role that these play in helping older adults live well (Heisel & Duberstein, 2005).

Reducing the Stigma of Mental Health Treatment

The stigma of mental illness continues to interfere with the willingness of older adults to seek treatment. Today's older Canadians grew up during a time when institutionalization in asylums, electroconvulsive treatments, and other treatment approaches were regarded with fear. This fear can lead to denial of problems. The work of the MHCC has recognized the critical importance of combating stigma and discrimination. The commission has launched a 10-year antistigma campaign, recognizing that combating stigma requires a multipronged effort sustained over a long period of time and includes ongoing community-based education and action, media campaigns, and forums of exchange between affected individuals and other Canadians to enhance public awareness, and professional awareness campaigns to reduce structural discrimination in the health care system and in the mental health system itself (MHCC, 2012; Standing Senate Committee on Social Affairs, Science and Technology, 2006, p. 25).

Nurses are in a primary position to participate in these initiatives at local and national levels. They can also assist older adults in understanding mental health concerns when they arise and encourage them to access appropriate services. They can reassure older adults that many of the issues they experience are common and very amenable to intervention. Nurses must realize that the therapeutic nurse–patient interaction is a key strategy that they can develop and, by so doing, foster hope, transcendence, and meaning in life in the older adults they work with (Haugan, 2013) (see Box 32-3).

BOX 32.3 **Research for Best Practice**

THE POWER OF THE NURSE–PATIENT RELATIONSHIP

Haugan, G. (2013). Nurse–patient interaction is a resource for hope, meaning in life and self-transcendence in nursing home patients. Scandinavian Journal of Caring Sciences, 1–15. doi: 10.1111/scs.12028.

Question: Does the nurse–patient interaction affect hope, self-transcendence, and meaning together in cognitively intact nursing home patients?

Method: The relationship between nurse–patient interaction, hope, meaning, and self-transcendence among cognitively intact nursing home patients was investigated using a cross-sectional design and structural equation modelling. The sample consisted of 202 long-term nursing home residents across 44 nursing homes. "Hope" was assessed using the HHI (Herth Hope Index). "Meaning in life" was assessed using the PIL (Purpose in Life) tool, and "self-transcendence" was assessed using the STS (self-transcendence scale). The Nurse–Patient Interaction Scale (NPIS) was used to measure nursing home residents' experiences of "being understood, respected, and recognized as a person, as well as being listened to and feeling good as a result of nurse–patient interaction" (Haugan, 2013, p. 5).

Findings: Findings suggest that it is possible to enhance residents' hope, self-transcendence, and meaning in life (aspects crucial to positive mental health). There was a significant impact of nurse–resident interaction on hope, self-transcendence, and meaning.

Implications for Practice: Hope, meaning in life, and transcendence are all believed to be life sustaining for older persons. This study suggests that the nurse–resident interaction in long-term care provides the opportunity to foster these concepts, thus contributing to an overall sense of physical and mental well-being. Nurses have the opportunity to develop creative strategies through their therapeutic use of self. "Nurses have to be aware that their attitude, appearance, and behaviour are interpreted as a confirmation of the patient's worthiness or worthlessness" (Haugan, 2013, p. 8). Confirming the residents' self worth and value through a caring, compassionate, and respectful encounter can lead to positive outcomes and is very meaningful for both the resident and nurse.

● **STUDY NOTE**

Safety concerns are a priority. Carefully explore any suicidal ideation and develop a plan for intervention and prevention. Recognize that older persons may not always say outright that they are thinking about suicide. Consider other cues (e.g., behavioural, mood) that may suggest they are having thoughts of suicide.

Use of Medications

With the approval of new medications, older adults will be able to treat health problems with pharmacologic agents that were not previously available. Side effects and drug interactions should be carefully monitored to detect untoward symptoms and delirium (see Chapter 34).

Education of older adults and their families regarding a medication regimen is crucial to ensure adherence and to minimize untoward effects. Basic principles regarding neurobiologic changes in normal aging (as previously discussed) should be applied when designing teaching strategies. The nurse must consider the older adult's pace of learning as well as any visual and hearing deficits. Education should include the reason for administering the drug and important side effects of the drug. The nurse should provide instructional aids, large-print labelling, and devices such as medication calendars that encourage adherence to the treatment plan. Patients should be aware that they can reject childproof containers for their medications if they have trouble opening them.

Avoiding Premature Institutionalization

In Canada, as in many countries around the world, health care reform has drastically affected how health care is delivered. Such reform has focused on a move from institutional care to home care. Research has demonstrated that there is significant potential for home care to support the mental health and well-being of seniors in the community (Ontario Home Care Association, 2010). Supportive community-based services can help to avoid premature institutionalization in seniors. There is evidence that governments are increasingly recognizing the impacts of population aging and looking to make necessary changes. These include appropriate adaptations to "facilitate mobility, improve safety and security and to permit ADL without strain or injury"; improved access to transportation and to location of services; proper housing management practices; and newer housing and infrastructures that include a wider range of housing choices, accessible community facilities, and opportunities for active living and volunteer involvement (Canada Mortgage and Housing Corporation, 2008, p. 14). There are housing initiatives across Canada with alternate levels of care to facilitate increased access to health services for seniors. There are innovative trends in housing design that combine assisted living with programs such as active living and creative arts. Other programs across Canada (e.g., The Meanderthals hiking groups and elder hostels) are also directed at promoting active lifestyles and the physical and mental well-being of seniors.

Mental Health

Social Support Transitions

Older adults may compensate for loss of family by expanding friendship networks, and employment may become an important method of establishing a network in later life. The older adult can be prepared for the transition by receiving information about internal developmental processes, sources of social support, and opportunities for personal growth. Nurses can foster opportunities for connectedness among older adults and initiate strategies to foster hope and meaning in life through life transitions.

Lifestyle Support

Lifestyle interventions, such as exercise promotion and nutrition counselling, are particularly important in later life because a tendency to slow down and to become more sedentary usually accompanies aging. For many, retirement provides an opportunity to restructure the time that was previously spent working. Developing regular exercise habits can help maintain physical and psychological well-being. Self-help programs generally include components of exercise, nutrition, health screening, and health habits.

Spiritual Support

Supporting contact with spiritual leaders important to the patient is an ongoing mental health promotion

IN A LIFE

Verna Splane (1914–) and
Dr. Helen Mussallem (1915–2012)
Outstanding Canadian Nurses Acknowledged
at Dr. Mussallem's Birthday Party, 2005

Dr. Helen Mussallem
(*right*) celebrated her 90th birthday in 2005. She passed away in November 2012 in Ottawa. She was a trailblazer, her storied career a microcosm of the evolution of modern nursing. And, along the way, "she helped to reshape health care in Canada and nursing education around the world" (Picard, 2012). She was a former chairperson of the Board of the Victorian Order of Nurses, a Companion of the Order of Canada, and Canada's most decorated nurse. She held seven Honorary Doctorates and was a recipient of the Florence Nightingale Medal of the International Red Cross. Beginning her career in 1937, she dedicated her life to nursing and was, in the words of Public Health Reporter Andre Picard, "a decorated, celebrated, altruistic activist."

Verna Splane
(*left*) celebrated her 99th birthday in 2013; that year she became the first Honorary Life Member of the Association of Registered Nurses of British Columbia in recognition of her contribution to nursing. She was Chief Nursing Officer in National Health and Welfare and worked with the World Health Organization in International Nursing and Public Health. She served also as Vice President of the International Council of Nurses (ICN). She received the Order of Canada in 1996 and the Centennial Award of the Canadian Nurses Association in 2008. She is an Honorary Professor at the University of British Columbia.

intervention. The nurse can also support a patient's spiritual growth by exploring the meanings that a particular life change has for the elder. In later life, existential issues such as experiencing losses, redefining meanings in existence, and finding and nurturing hope become the standard, replacing the performance and future orientation that characterize earlier adulthood.

Community Services

More emphasis should be placed on community care options, services that provide both sustenance and growth. Examples of supportive services that foster independent community living include information and referral services; transportation and nutrition services; legal and protective services; comprehensive senior centres; homemaker and handyman services; matching of older with younger individuals to share housing; and use of the supports available through churches, community groups, or mental health and other community agencies (e.g., area agencies on aging) to maintain elderly individuals in the community for as long as possible. The availability and accessibility of these services vary greatly, and eligibility requirements may exist. A Canadian Mental Health Association project, funded by the Population Health in Canada, examined seniors' mental health and home care using mental health promotion principles. A variety of methods grounded in the principle of participation explored the perspectives of seniors, family caregivers, and home care providers. A policy guide was developed (in 2004 and updated in 2008) as an outcome of the project to provide direction for a holistic model of care, incorporating both medical and psychosocial supports to meet the needs of seniors (MacCourt, 2008).

Summary

Home care can contribute to a holistic approach to the health and well-being of older adults (Ontario Home Care Association, 2010). For older adults who suffer from mental health issues or mental illness, "the negative impacts are far reaching" (PHAC, 2010). While recognizing that effective mental health promotion requires a comprehensive, interdisciplinary, and cross-sectoral approach, nurses in particular are well situated in institutions, in home care, and in community settings to provide important interventions, guidance, and support for seniors in Canada. Given the demographic shifts in Canada (and globally), aging is one of the most significant social forces shaping our society over the next 20 to 30 years (Martin-Matthews, 2007). Nurses have an important opportunity to influence and advance knowledge in this field. Responding to this opportunity, nurses have key roles in contributing to the mental health promotion of older adults and supporting them and their families to live their lives with hope, meaning, and purpose.

SUMMARY OF KEY POINTS

■ The aging of the Canadian population is a significant force shaping our society.

■ Late adulthood is conceived as having three chronological groups: young-old (65 to 74 years), middle-old (75 to 84 years), and old-old (85 years and older).

■ Studies of aging, such as the Canadian Longitudinal Study of Aging, focus on life span (years of life) and health span (years of good health and functioning). The role of genetics is a key area of interest.

■ All human senses decline with age. Cognitive changes with aging are, for the most part, accounted for by structural and functional changes in the brain, with external factors (e.g., activity levels; socioeconomic status) also having an effect.

■ Threats to memory in older persons include medications, depression, poor nutrition, infection, heart and lung disease, thyroid problems, alcohol use, and sensory loss.

■ Nurses need to recognize that older persons may need time to process information and that they tend to focus on accuracy in their answers rather than on giving a prompt reply.

■ Aging affects pharmacokinetics, including drug absorption, distribution, metabolism, and excretion, and nurses need to know the drug therapy implications of such changes.

■ Gerotranscendence is a concept related to aging in which spiritual growth and the development of inner strength is emphasized over decrements in functioning.

■ The majority of Canadian seniors wish to "age in place" and need adequate support to do so.

■ Risks to health during this phase of the life span include chronic illness, polypharmacy, loss and bereavement, poverty, and lack of social support. The latter has been associated with suicide.

■ Older persons experience many physical changes, but they can remain sexually active.

■ Nurses can play a significant role in the mental health promotion of older persons and in supporting them and their families in living meaningful, hopeful lives.

CRITICAL THINKING CHALLENGES

1 Describe key strategies for communicating with older persons. Take some time to talk with a few older persons (at a variety of ages—young-old and old-old) about their views of mental health. Observe similarities and differences in their points of view.

2 Describe strategies that might facilitate older adults finding hope and renewing a sense of purpose and meaning in their lives.

3 Hypothesize why IQ tests and personality do not change with time.

4 Use the concept of *gerotranscendence* to explain differences between the young-old and the old-old. How does this concept help nurses understand meaning at the end of life?

5 Identify positive and negative perspectives of retirement.

6 Explain why chronic illnesses, polypharmacy, and poverty are all risk factors for mental health problems in later life.

7 Describe mental health promotion interventions that relate to social support transitions, lifestyle support, and self-care.

REFERENCES

American Geriatrics Society. (2012). American Geriatrics Society updated Beers Criteria for potentially inappropriate medication use in older adults. *Journal of the American Geriatric Society*, 60(4), 616–13. Doi:10.1111/j.1532-5415.2012.03923.x

Berger, S. (2013). Balancing act: cell senescence, aging related to epigenetic changes: Penn study links epigenetics, aging, mutations in nuclear proteins to better understand cancer, rare disorders. *Penn Medicine News Release*. Retrieved from http://www.uphs.upenn.edu/news/News_Releases/2013/08/berger/

Bourque, P., Pushkar, D., Bonneville, L., & Beland, F. (2005). Contextual effects on life satisfaction of older men and women. *Canadian Journal on Aging*, 24(1), 31–44.

Brown, J. W., Mefford, L., Chen, S., & Brown, A. (2009). Health and function of older persons volunteering for Habitat for Humanity. *Southern Online Journal of Nursing Research*, 9(3). Retrieved from http://www.resourcenter.net/images/SNRS/Files/SOJNR_articles2/Vol09Num03Art02.html

Bryant, C., Bei, B., Gilson, B., Komiti, A., Jackson, H., & Judd, F. (2012). The relationship between attitudes to aging and physical and mental health in older adults. *International Psychogeriatrics*, 24(10), 1674–83. doi: 10.1017/S1041610212000774

Canada Mortgage and Housing Corporation. (2008). *Impacts of the aging of the Canadian population on housing and communities: Research highlights*. Retrieved from http://www.cmhc-schl.gc.ca/odpub/pdf/65913.pdf

Canadian Association for Suicide Prevention. (2009). *CASP: Blueprint for a Canadian national suicide prevention strategy*. Retrieved from http://suicideprevention.ca/wp-content/uploads/2009/12/SuicidePreventionBlueprint0909.pdf

Canadian Broadcasting Corporation. (2005). *CBC news in depth: Seniors and drugs: Prescribed to death*. Retrieved from http://www.cbc.ca/news/background/seniorsdrugs/prescribed-to-death.html

Canadian Broadcasting Corporation. (2007). *Drugs seniors should avoid—The Beers criteria*. Retrieved from http://www.cbc.ca/news2/background/seniorsdrugs/beers_table_more.html

Canadian Coalition for Seniors' Mental Health (CCSMH). (2006). *National guidelines for seniors' mental health: The assessment and treatment of depression*. Retrieved from: www.ccsmh.ca

Canadian Institute for Health Information. (2007). *Drug claims by seniors: An analysis focusing on potentially inappropriate medication use, 2000 to 2006*. Retrieved from http://secure.cihi.ca/cihiweb/en/downloads/Potentially_Inappropriate_Medications_EN.pdf

Carstairs, S. & Keon, J. (2009). *Special Senate Committee on Aging Final report: Canada's aging population: Seizing the opportunity*. Retrieved from www.senate-senat.ca/org.asp

Duggleby, W., Hicks, D., Nekolaichuk, C., Holtslander, L., Williams, A., Chambers, T., & Eby, J. (2012). Hope, older adults, and chronic illness: A metasynthesis of qualitative research. *Journal of Advanced Nursing*, 68(6), 1211–1223.

Duggleby, W., Holtslander, L., Kylma, J., Duncan, V., Hammond, C., & Williams, A. (2010). Metasynthesis of the hope experience of family caregivers of persons with chronic illness. *Qualitative Health Research*, 20(2), 148–158.

Ebersole, P., Touhy, T. A., Hess, P., & Jett, K. (2007). *Toward healthy aging: Human needs and nursing response*. Philadelphia, PA: Mosby.

Erikson, E. H. & Erikson, J. M. (1997). *The lifecycle completed, extended version*. New York, NY: WW Norton.

Evers, A., Klusmann, V., Schwarzer, R., & Heuser, I. (2011). Improving cognition by adherence to physical or mental exercise: A moderated mediation analysis. *Aging and Mental Health*, 15(4), 446–455. doi: 10.1080/13607863.2010.543657

Fleming, K. C., Evans, J. M., & Chutka, D. S. (2003). A cultural and economic history of old age in America. *Mayo Clinic Proceedings*, 78(7), 914–921.

Frankl, V. (1963). *Man's search for meaning: An introduction to logotherapy*. New York, NY: Pocket Books.

Grek, A. (2007). Clinical management of suicidality in the elderly: An opportunity for involvement in the lives of older patients. *The Canadian Journal of Psychiatry*, 56(Suppl. 1), 47S–57S.

Hammer, K., Mogensen, O., & Hall, E.O.C. (2009). The meaning of hope in nursing research: A metasynthesis. *Scandinavian Journal of Caring Sciences*, 23, 549–557.

Haugan, G. (2013). Nurse–patient interaction is a resource for hope, meaning in life and self-transcendence in nursing home patients. *Scandinavian Journal of Caring Sciences*, 1–15. doi: 10.1111/scs.12028

Heisel, M. J. (2004). Suicide ideation in the elderly. *Psychiatric Times*, XXI(3). 1–2. Retrieved from http://www.psychiatrictimes.com/display/article/10168/48656?pageNumber=2

Heisel, M. J. (2006). Suicide and its prevention among older adults. *Canadian Journal of Psychiatry*, 51(3), 143–154. Retrieved from https://ww1.cpa-apc.org/Publications/Archives/CJP/2006/march1/heisel-IR.asp

Heisel, M. J. & Duberstein, P. R. (2005). Suicide prevention in older adults. *Clinical Psychology: Science and Practice*, 12(3), 242–59. doi:10.1093/clipsy/bpi030

Lam, L. C. & Cheng, S. T. (2012). Maintaining long-term adherence to lifestyle interventions for cognitive health in late life. *International Psychogeriatrics*, 25(2), 171–73.

Larson, E. B., Wang, L., Bowen, J. D., McCormick, W. C., Teri, L., Crane, P., & Kukull, W. (2006). Exercise is associated with reduced risk for incident dementia among persons 65 years of age and older. *Annals of Internal Medicine*, 144(2), 73–81.

Lee, Y. J. & Hung, W. L. (2011). The relationship between exercise participation and well-being of the retired elderly. *Aging and Mental Health*, 15(7), 873–881.

Lezwijn, J., Vaandrager, L., Naaldenberg, J., Wagemakers, A., & van Woerkum, C. (2011). Healthy ageing in a salutogenic way: Building the HP 2.0 framework. *Health and Social Care in the Community*, 19(1), 43–51.

Lindsay, C. & Almay, M. (1999). *A portrait of seniors in Canada*. Ottawa, ON: Statistics Canada.

MacCourt, P. (2008). *Promoting seniors' well-being: A seniors' mental health policy lens toolkit*. Victoria, BC: British Columbia Psychogeriatric Association.

Martin-Matthews, A. (2007). *The future is aging. Institute of Aging strategic plan 2007–2012*. Canadian Institute for Health Research. Retrieved from http://www.cihr-irsc.gc.ca/e/34013.html

Mayo Clinic. (2011). *Sexual health and aging: Keep the passion alive*. Rochester, NY: Author. Retrieved from: http://www.mayoclinic.com/health/sexual-health/HA00035

Mental Health Commission of Canada. (2009). *Toward recovery and well-being. A framework for a mental health strategy for Canada (draft)*. Retrieved from http://www.mentalhealthcommission.ca/SiteCollectionDocuments/Key_Documents/en/2009/Mental_Health_ENG.pdf

Mental Health Commission of Canada. (2011). *Guidelines for comprehensive mental health services for older adults in Canada*. Retrieved from http://www.mentalhealthcommission.ca/English/document/279/mental-health-commission-canada-seniors-guidelines-print

Mental Health Commission of Canada. (2012). *Changing directions: Changing lives: The mental health strategy for Canada*. Retrieved from http://www.mentalhealthcommission.ca/English/node/721

Mental Health Commission of Canada. (2013). *Issue: Seniors*. Retrieved from http://www.mentalhealthcommission.ca/English/issues/seniors?routetoken=506cfdc903b5867d6ed9f3a14a42971e&terminitial=27

Ministry of Healthy Living and Support. (2008). *Seniors in British Columbia: A healthy living framework*. Retrieved from http://www.hls.gov.bc.ca/seniors/PDFs/seniors_framework_web.pdf

Moe, A., Hellzen, O., Ekker, K., & Enmarker, I. (2013). Inner strength in relation to perceived physical and mental health among the oldest old people with chronic illness. *Aging and Mental Health*, 17(2), 189–196. doi: 10.1080/13607863.2012.717257

Monette, M. (2012). Senior suicide: An overlooked problem. *CMAJ News*. Retrieved from http://www.cmaj.ca/site/earlyreleases/15oct12_senior_suicide.xhtml

Moody, H. & Sasser, J. R. (2011). *Aging: Concepts and controversies*. Los Angeles, CA: Sage.

Moore, S. L. (2005). Hope makes a difference. *Journal of Psychiatric and Mental Health Nursing*, 12(1), 100–105. doi : 10.1111/j.1365-2850.2004.00802.x

Moore, S. L. (2012). The experience of hope and aging: A hermeneutic photography study. *Journal of Gerontological Nursing*, 38(10), 28–36.

Moore, S. L., Grek, A., Heisel, M., & Jackson, F. (2006). *Canadian Coalition for Seniors Mental Health: National guidelines initiative. Suicide assessment and prevention*. Toronto: Canadian Coalition for Seniors Mental Health.

Moore, S. L., Metcalf, B., & Schow, E. (2000). Meaning in life: Examining the concept. *Geriatric Nursing, 21*(1), 27–29. doi: //0-dx.doi.org.aupac.lib.athabascau.ca/10.1067/mgn.2000.105790

Moya H., & Arnold, P. (2012). A life story toolkit to support recovery from mental distress. *Mental Health Practice, 16*(1), 14–18.

National Alliance on Mental Illness. (2001). *Mental illness, healthy aging: A NH guide for older adults and caregivers*. Retrieved from http://www.nami.org/Content/ContentGroups/Home4/Home_Page_Spotlights/Spotlight_1/Guidebook.pdf

National Institute on Aging (NIA). (2009). *Sexuality in later life*. UAS: US Department of Health and Human Services. Retrieved from http://www.nia.nih.gov/health/publicaiton/sexuality-later-life

National Institute on Aging (NIA). (2011; updated 2013). *Biology of aging: Research today for a better tomorrow*. US Department of Health and Human Services. Retrieved from http://www.nia.nih.gov/health/publication/biology-aging

Newberg, A.B. (2011). Spirituality and the aging brain. *Generations-Journal of the American Society on Aging, 35*(2), 83–91.

O'Rourke, N., Cappeliez, P., & Claxton, A. (2011). Functions of reminiscence and the psychological well-being of young-old and older adults over time. *Aging and Mental Health, 15*(2), 272–281.

Ontario Home Care Association. (2010). *Home care in 2010—Essential for an aging population*. Retrieved from http://www.homecareontario.ca/public/docs/publications/position%20papers/2010/home-care-essential-for-an-aging-population.pdf

Panno, J. (2010). *Aging: Modern theories and therapies* (2nd ed.). New York, NY: Facts on File.

Picard, A. (2012). Nurse 98: Helen Mussallem was a decorated, celebrated, altruistic activist. *Globe and Mail*. Retrieved from http://www.theglobeandmail.com/news/national/helen-mussallem-was-a-decorated-celebrated-altruistic-activist/article5633553/

Public Health Agency of Canada (PHAC). (2002). *A report on mental illnesses in Canada*. Retrieved from http://www.phac-aspc.gc.ca/publicat/miic-mmac/

Public Health Agency of Canada (PHAC). (2010). *The Chief Public Health Officer's report on the state of public health in Canada 2010*. Ottawa, ON: Author.

Rosenzweig, E. S. & Barnes, C. A. (2003). Impact of aging on hippocampal function: Plasticity, network dynamics and cognition. *Progress in Neurobiology, 69*(3), 143–179. doi:10.1016/S0301-0082(02)00126-0

Sattar, S. P., Petty, F., & Burke, W. J. (2003). Diagnosis and treatment of alcohol dependence in older alcoholics. *Clinics in Geriatric Medicine, 19*, 743–764.

Scharlach, A.E. & Hoshino, K. (2013). Conclusion. In Scharlach, A.E. & Hoshino, K., (Eds.) *Healthy aging in sociocultural context* (pp. 97–105). New York, NY: Routledge.

Sciegaj, M. & Behr, R. A. (2010). Lessons for the United States from countries adapting to the consequences of aging populations. *Technology and Disability, 22*, 83–88. doi: 10.3233/TAD-2010-0283

Sebastiani, P., Solovieff, N., De Wan, A., Walsh, K. M., Puce, A., Hartley, S. W., & Perls, T. T. (2012). Genetic signatures of exceptional longevity in humans. *PLoS One, 7*(1) e29848. doi:10.1371/journalpone.00229848

Sheets, D. J. & Gallagher, E. M. (2013). Aging in Canada: State of the art and science. *The Gerontologist, 53*(1), 1–8. doi: 10.1093/geront/gns150

Shields, M. & Martel, L. (2006). Healthy living among seniors. *Supplement to Health Reports, 16*, 7–20. Retrieved from http://www.statcan.ca/english/freepub/82–003-SIE/2005000/pdf/82–003-SIE20050007445.pdf

Standing Senate Committee on Social Affairs, Science and Technology. (2006). *Out of the shadows at last: Transforming mental health, mental illness and addictions in Canada*. Retrieved from http://www.parl.gc.ca/content/sen/committee/391/soci/rep/pdf/rep02may06part1-e.pdf

Statistics Canada. (2005). *Population projections, 2005 to 2031*. Retrieved from http://www.statcan.ca/Daily/English/051215/d051215b.htm

Statistics Canada. (2010). *Statistics Canada population estimates 1971–2010*. Ottawa, ON: Statistics Canada. Retrieved from http://www.statcan.gc.ca/daily-quotidien/100628/dq100628a-eng.htm

Statistics Canada. (2012). *Years to retirement, 1998 to 2009. Insights on Canadian Society* (75-006-X): Author. Retrieved from http://www.statcan.gc.ca/daily-quotidien/121204/dq121204b-eng.pdf

Tam, E. Y., Fletcher, P. C., & Chi, I. (2004). Cultural and gender diversity in health. *STRIDE, 1*. Retrieved from http://www.stridemagazine.com

Tornstam, L. (1989). Gero-transcendence: A theoretical and empirical reformulation of the disengagement theory. *Aging: Clinical and Experimental Research, 1*, 55–63.

Tornstam, L. (2005). *Gerotranscendence: A developmental theory of positive aging*. New York, NY: Springer.

von Strauss, E., Aguero-Torres, H., Kareholt, I., Winblad, B., & Fratiglioni, L. (2003). Women are more disabled in basic activities of daily living than men only in very advanced ages: A study on disability, morbidity, and mortality from the Kungsholmen Project. *Journal of Clinical Epidemiology, 56*(7), 669–677.

Wadensten, B. (2007). The theory of gerotranscendence as applied to gerontological nursing-Part I. *International Journal of Older People Nursing, 2*, 289–294.

Wadensten, B. & Carlsson, M. (2007a). Adoption of an innovation based on the theory of gerotranscendence by staff in a nursing home–Part III. *International Journal of Older People Nursing, 2*, 302–14. doi: 10.1111/j.1748-3743.2007a.00087.x

Wadensten, B. & Carlsson, M. (2007b). The theory of gerotranscendence in practice: Guidelines for nursing–Part II. *International Journal of Older People Nursing, 2*, 295–301. doi: 10.1111/j.1748-3743.2007b.00085.x

Waern, M., Rubenowitz, E., & Wilhelmson, K. (2003). Predictors of suicide in the old elderly. *Gerontology, 49*(5), 328–334.

Walsh, F. (2012). Successful aging and family resilience. *Annual Review of Gerontology and Geriatrics, 32*(1), 151–72. doi: 10.1891/0198-8794.32.153

Wang, L., Larson, E. B., Bowen, J. D., & van Belle, G. (2006). Performance-based physical function and future dementia in older people. *Archives of Internal Medicine, 166*, 1115–1120.

Wang, J. J., Lin, Y. H., & Hsieh, L. Y. (2011). Effects of gerotranscendence support group on gerotranscendence perspective, depression, and life satisfaction of institutionalized elders. *Aging and Mental Health, 15*(5), 580–86. doi: 10.1080/13607863.2010.543663

Wilson, D. M., Harris, A., Hollis, V., & Mohankumar, D. (2010). Upstream thinking and health promotion planning for older adults at risk of social isolation. *International Journal of Older People Nursing, 6*(4), 282–288.

World Health Organization. (2012). *Good health adds years to life. Global brief for World Health Day 2012*. Geneva: Author.

Yevchak, A. M., Loeb, S. J., & Fick, D. M. (2008). Promoting cognitive health and vitality: A review of clinical implications. *Geriatric Nursing, 29*(5), 302–310.

Zimprich, D. (2002). Cross-sectionally and longitudinally balanced effects of processing speed on intellectual abilities. *Experimental Aging Research, 28*(3), 231–251. doi: 10.1080/03610730290080290

33 Mental Health Assessment of Older Persons

Sharon L. Moore

Adapted from the chapters on "Mental Health Assessment of the Older Adult" by Annette M. Lane and by Mary Ann Boyd and Mickey Stanley

KEY CONCEPTS

- bio/psycho/social/spiritual geriatric mental health nursing assessment
- normal aging

LEARNING OBJECTIVES

After studying this chapter, you will be able to:

- Compare changes in normal aging with those associated with mental health problems in older adults.
- Select various techniques in assessing older adults who have mental health problems.
- Delineate the important areas of assessment for the biologic domain in completing the geriatric mental health nursing assessment.
- Delineate the important areas of assessment for the psychological domain in completing the geriatric mental health nursing assessment.
- Delineate the important areas of assessment for the social domain in completing the geriatric mental health nursing assessment.

KEY TERMS

- dysphagia • functional activities • insomnia • polypharmacy
- xerostomia

I n 1920, the average life span in Canada was 60 years (Statistics Canada, 2005). By 2009, this life span increased to 78.8 years for men and 83.3 years for women (Human Resources and Skills Development Canada, 2012a). Health care providers will face new and increased challenges as the generation known as "the baby boomers" (born 1946 to 1964) moves into the rank of older adults. Over the 5-year period from 2006 to 2011, the number of people aged 60 to 64 rose by 29.1%; the number of people aged 65 or older rose by 14.1%, and the number of people aged 100 or older rose by 25.7% (CIHR-IA, 2013). By the year 2036, projections are that there will be almost 10.4 million older adults (65 years of age and older); this group is expected to compose 25% of the Canadian population by 2051. The fastest growing segment of the older population is the group 85 years of age and older (Human Resources and Skills Development Canada, 2012b).

Normal aging is associated with some physical decline, such as decreased sensory abilities and decreased pulmonary and immune functions, but many important functions do not change. Intellectual function, capacity for change, and productive engagement with life remain stable. Many myths exist about normal aging. Some people believe that "senility" is normal or that depression or hopelessness is natural for older individuals. If older adults and family members believe these myths, they will be less likely to seek treatment for themselves or their elders with real problems. Even if they seek help for themselves or their older adults, health care providers may fail to identify depression or simply attribute symptoms to normal aging (Gregg, Fiske, & Gatz, 2013). As the population ages, there will be increased numbers of seniors with mental health illnesses and problems (Mental Health Commission of Canada, 2013). Older adults with mental health problems comprise different population groups. One group consists of those with long-term mental illnesses who have reached the ranks of the older adult population. These individuals usually understand their disorders and treatments. Unfortunately, the changes associated with aging can affect a client's control of his or her chronic mental illness. Symptoms may reappear, and medications may need to be adjusted. Another group includes individuals who are relatively free of mental health problems until their later years. These individuals, who may already have other health problems, develop late-onset mental disorders, such as depression, psychotic symptoms, or dementia. For these individuals and their family members, the development of a mental disorder can be very traumatic. Research that examined the relationship between age and depression in older adults in Canada found that "there is a linear increase in depressive symptoms after age 65, but this occurs in the context of medical comorbidity and is not an independent effect of aging" (Wu, Schimmele, & Chappell, 2012, p. 3).

Mental health problems in older adults can be especially complex because of coexisting medical problems and treatments. Many symptoms of somatic disorders mimic or mask psychiatric disorders. For example, fatigue may be related to anaemia, but it also may be symptomatic of depression. In addition, older individuals are more likely to report somatic symptoms than psychological ones, making identification of a mental disorder even more difficult.

The purpose of this chapter is to present a comprehensive geriatric mental health nursing assessment process that serves as the basis of care for older individuals (discussed in Chapters 32 and 34). A mental health assessment is necessary when psychiatric or mental health issues are identified or when clients with mental illnesses reach their later years (usually about age 65 years). The assessment generally follows the same format as described in Chapter 10. However, the overall health care issues for older adults can be very complex, so it follows that certain components of the geriatric mental health nursing assessment are unique. The geriatric assessment emphasizes some areas that are less critical to the standard adult assessment.

KEY CONCEPT **Normal aging** is associated with some physical decline, such as decreased sensory abilities and decreased pulmonary and immune functions, but many important functions do not change.

TECHNIQUES OF DATA COLLECTION

The nurse assesses the older client using an interview format that may take a few sessions to complete. She or he also may rely on self-report standardized tests, such as depression and cognitive functioning tools. A wide variety of physiologic disorders may cause changes in mental

BOX 33-1 Changes That Affect Mental Status

- Acid–base imbalance
- Dehydration
- Drugs (prescribed and over the counter)
- Electrolyte changes
- Hypothyroidism
- Hypothermia and hyperthermia
- Hypoxia
- Infection and sepsis

status for older adults; thus, results of laboratory tests often are significant. For example, urinalysis can detect a urinary tract infection that has affected a client's cognitive status. Box 33-1 contains a representative listing of common physiologic causes of changes in mental status. In addition, medical records from other health care providers are useful in developing a complete picture of the client's health status.

An important source of client data is family members, who often notice changes that the older individual overlooks or fails to recognize. A client with memory impairment may be unable to give an accurate history. By interviewing family members, the nurse expands the scope of the client assessment. Moreover, the nurse has an opportunity to evaluate the caregivers themselves to determine whether they can care for the older individual adequately and how they are coping with the situation. For example, a husband may be unable to care for his wife but is unwilling to admit it. If the nurse can establish rapport with the husband, the nurse may use the assessment interview as an opportunity to help the husband to examine his wife's care requirements realistically. The nurse may be able to explain to the husband the impact of caregiving on his health. For instance, it is not uncommon for the caregiving spouse to experience significant physical and mental health decline because of extreme and prolonged stresses.

BIO/PSYCHO/SOCIAL/SPIRITUAL GERIATRIC MENTAL HEALTH NURSING ASSESSMENT

At the beginning of the assessment, the nurse should determine the client's ability to participate. For example, if a client is using a wheelchair, he or she may have physical limitations that prevent full participation in the assessment. The older client must be able to hear the nurse. For a client with compromised hearing, the nurse must attend to voice projection and volume. Shouting at the older individual is unnecessary. The nurse should remember to lower the pitch of her or his voice because higher-pitched sounds are often lost with presbycusis (loss of hearing sensitivity associated with aging). The nurse should eliminate distracting noises, such as from a television or radio, and ensure that the client's hearing aid is in place and turned on. Facing the client and using distinct enunciation will help lip-reading clients understand what is being said. Sometimes, deafness is mistaken for cognitive dysfunction. If a client's hearing is questionable, the nurse should examine the client for buildup of cerumen. If this is not believed to be contributing to hearing loss, the nurse can enlist the help of a speech and language specialist. Generally, the pace of the interview should mirror the older adult's ability to move through the assessment. Usually, the pace will be slower than the nurse uses with younger populations.

> **KEY CONCEPT** A **bio/psycho/social/spiritual geriatric mental health nursing assessment** is the comprehensive, deliberate, and systematic collection and interpretation of bio/psycho/social/spiritual data that are based on the special needs and problems of older adults to determine current and past health, functional status, and human responses to mental health problems, both actual and potential (Box 33-2).

Biologic Domain

Collecting and analyzing data for the assessment of the biologic domain include areas similar to those discussed in Chapter 10. The assessment components include present and past health status, physical examination results, physical functioning, and a pharmacology review. When focusing on the biologic domain, the nurse pays special attention to the client's general physical appearance as well as any observable manifestations of illness. The nurse should assess how all physical problems affect the client's mental well-being. For example, pain and immobility are physical problems that can negatively affect mental health. Low energy level may be immediately apparent. Women with obvious osteoporosis are experiencing pain most of the time. Men undergoing radiation for prostate cancer worry about sexual functioning and urinary incontinence.

Present and Past Health Status

A review of the older adult's current health status includes examining health records and collecting information from the client and family members. The nurse must identify chronic health problems that could affect mental health care. For example, the client's management of diabetes mellitus could provide clues to the likelihood of complications such as retinopathy or neuropathy, which in turn will affect the individual's ability to follow a mental health treatment regimen. The nurse must document a history of psychiatric treatment.

Physical Examination

The psychiatric and mental health (PMH) nurse reviews the physical examination findings, paying special attention to recent laboratory values, such as urinalysis, white

and red blood cell counts, and fasting blood glucose data (see Chapter 10). Results of neurologic tests could indicate compromise of the neuromuscular systems. Many psychiatric medications lower the seizure threshold, making a history of seizures, which can cause behavioural changes, an important assessment component. The nurse should note any evidence of movement disorders, such as tremors, abnormal movements, or shuffling. If a client has been taking conventional antipsychotics, the nurse should consider assessment for symptoms of tardive dyskinesia, using one of the appropriate assessment tools (see Chapter 12 for additional discussion of tardive dyskinesia).

The nurse should take routine vital signs during the assessment. She or he should note any abnormalities in blood pressure (i.e., hypertension or hypotension) because many psychiatric medications affect blood pressure. Generally, these medications may cause orthostatic hypotension, which can lead to dizziness, unsteady gait, and falls. A baseline blood pressure is needed for future monitoring of medication side effects. Lying, sitting, and standing blood pressures are especially useful in assessing for orthostatic hypotension.

Physical Functions

The nurse must consider the older client's physical functioning within the context of the normal changes that accompany aging and the presence of any chronic disorders. The nurse should note the client's use of any personal devices, such as canes, walkers, wheelchairs, or oxygen, or environmental devices, such as grab bars, shower benches, or hospital beds. Specific areas to consider are nutrition and eating, elimination, and sleep patterns.

Nutrition and Eating

There is growing evidence about the importance of nutrition and physical activity in fostering successful aging (Wilcox, 2012). An assessment of the type, amount, and frequency of food eaten is standard in any assessment of the older adult. The nurse should note any unintentional weight loss of more than 4.5 kg. She or he must consider such nutrition changes in light of mental health problems. For example, is a client's weight loss related to an underlying physical problem or to the client's belief that she is being poisoned, which makes her afraid to eat? Or, is the older adult not eating because of an active wish to die?

Eating is often difficult for older adults, who may experience a lack of appetite. The nurse must assess eating and appetite patterns because many psychiatric medications can affect digestion and may impair an already compromised gastrointestinal tract. A common problem of older individuals who live in long-term care facilities is **dysphagia**, or difficulty swallowing. Dysphagia can lead to dehydration, malnutrition, pneumonia, or asphyxiation. People

BOX 33-2 Bio/Psycho/Social/Spiritual Geriatric Mental Health Nursing Assessment

I.   Major reason for seeking help _____
II. Initial information
     Name _____
     Age _____ Current marital status _____
     Gender_____ Caregiver's name _____
     Living arrangements _____
III. Level of independence:
     High (needs no help) _____
     Moderate (lives independently, but needs some help with instrumental activities) _____
     Low (relies on others for help in meeting functional and instrumental activities) _____
     Physical limitations _____
     Level of education completed_____

	Normal	Treated	Untreated
Physical functions: system review	☐	☐	☐
Activity/exercise	☐	☐	☐
Sleep patterns	☐	☐	☐
Appetite and nutrition	☐	☐	☐
Hydration	☐	☐	☐
Elimination	☐	☐	☐
Existing physical illnesses	☐	☐	☐

     List any chronic illnesses
     Presence of pain (Use standardized instrument if pain is present.) No _____Yes _____
     Score _____Treatment of pain _____

Medication (prescription and over the counter)	Dosage	Side Effects	Frequency of Side Effects

Significant Laboratory Tests	Values	Normal Range

IV. Responses to mental health problems
     Major concerns regarding mental health problem _____
     Major loss/change in past year: No _____ Yes _____
     Fear of violence: No _____ Yes _____
     If yes, type of violence _____
     Strategies for managing problems/disorder _____
V.   Mental status examination _____
     General observation (appearance, psychomotor activity, attitude) _____
     Orientation (time, place, person)
     Mood, affect, emotions (Geriatric Depression Scale should be used if evidence of depression)
     Speech (verbal ability, speed, use of words correctly) _____
     Thought processes (hallucinations, delusions, tangential, logic, repetition, rhyming of words, loose connections, disorganized) (*Describe the content of hallucinations, delusions.*)
     Cognition and intellectual performance (*Use standardized test scores as well as observations.*)
     Attention and concentration _____
     Abstract reasoning and concentration _____
     Memory (recall, short term, long term) _____
     Judgement and insight _____
     (MMSE, CASI scores)_____
VI. Significant behaviours (psychomotor, agitation, aggression, withdrawn) (*Use standardized test if behaviours are problematic.*) _____
     When did problem behaviour begin? Has it gotten worse?

BOX 33-2 Bio/Psycho/Social/Spiritual Geriatric Mental Health Nursing Assessment *(Continued)*

VII. Self-concept (beliefs about self: body image, self-esteem, personal identity)
VIII. Risk assessment
 Suicide: High _____ Moderate _____ Low _____ Assault/homicide: High _____
 Low _____

 Suicide thoughts or ideation: No _____ Yes _____
 Current thoughts of harming self _____ Plan _____
 Means _____
 Means available
 Assault/homicide thoughts: No _____ Yes _____
 What do you do when angry with a stranger? _____
 What do you do when angry with family or partner? _____
 Have you ever hit or pushed anyone? No _____ Yes _____
 Have you ever been arrested for assault? No _____ Yes _____
 Current thoughts of harming others _____
IX. Functional status (*Use standardized test such as FAQ.*) _____
X. Cultural assessment
 Cultural group _____
 Cultural group's view of health and mental illness _____
 By what cultural rules do you try to live? _____
 Special, cultural foods that are important to you _____
XI. Stresses and coping behaviours
 Social support _____
 Family members _____
 Which members are important to you? _____
 On whom can you rely? _____
 Community resources _____
XII. Spiritual assessment _____
XIII. Economic status _____
XIV. Legal status _____
XV. Quality of life _____
Summary of significant data that can be used in formulating a nursing diagnosis:

SIGNATURE/TITLE _____ Date _____

who have been exposed to conventional antipsychotics (e.g., haloperidol, chlorpromazine) may have symptoms of tardive dyskinesia, which can make swallowing difficult. Thus, the nurse should evaluate any client who has been exposed to the older psychiatric medications for symptoms of tardive dyskinesia.

Xerostomia, or dry mouth, which is common in older adults, also may impair eating. The nurse should pay particular attention to those who are currently receiving treatment for mental illnesses, particularly with medications that have anticholinergic properties. Dry mouth is also a side effect of many other anticholinergic medications, such as cimetidine, digoxin, and furosemide. Frequent rinsing with a non–alcohol-based mouthwash will help to correct the dry condition. Decreased taste or smell is common among older adults and may reduce the pleasure of eating so that the client may eat less. Making meal times social and relaxing experiences can help the older individual compensate for some of the loss of pleasure associated with decreased taste or smell. Preparing favourite foods will also enhance the quality of meals and meal times.

The nurse also must determine the client's use of alcohol. Alcoholism is a growing problem in the older adult population. According to the Canadian Addiction

Survey (Adlaf, Begin, & Sawka, 2005), just over 20% of older adults aged 65 to 74 years and 24% of individuals over 75 years of age admit to consuming alcohol four or more times per week. The incidence of drinking frequency is approximately double that of younger adults. There is a substantially increased mortality risk for heavy drinkers and a slightly reduced risk for lighter drinkers. Other studies show that substance use is increasing among older adults (Wu & Blazer, 2011) and those older adults frequently use alcohol as a means of managing pain (Brennan & Soohoo, 2013). The use of the CAGE questionnaire (see Chapter 26, Box 26-6) or the SMAST-G (Short Michigan Alcoholism Screening Test—Geriatric Version) (University of Michigan Alcohol Research Centre, 1991) may be helpful in this area. If an older adult screens negatively for problem drinking using one of these scales, yet the nurse believes that he or she may have an alcohol problem, the nurse might choose to retest the older adult using the other instrument. According to one study (Moore, Seeman, Morgenstern, Beck, & Reuben, 2002) that compared the CAGE instrument with the SMAST-G, less than half of the older individuals who tested positive on one screening tool did so on the other. They concluded that each instrument may target different facets of problem drinking. Given that physical and mental health problems are associated with increased substance use at older ages, it is important for nurses to be able to assess when substance use and/or abuse might be contributing to problems that older persons are experiencing (Koechl, Unger, & Fischer, 2012).

Elimination

The nurse must assess the client's urinary and bowel functions. Older individuals are more likely to experience constipation because the peristaltic movement of the bowel slows. Medications with anticholinergic properties can cause constipation, leading to faecal impaction. Abuse of laxatives is common among older adults and requires evaluation. Although the addition of fibre is recommended for constipation, such measures may cause bloating and excessive gas production. Older clients are also more likely to experience urinary frequency because the strength of the sphincter muscle decreases. Because many older adults drink fewer fluids to manage urinary incontinence, fluid intake also becomes an important factor in assessing urinary functioning and constipation. The nurse should remember that urinary incontinence is a symptom of a disorder that requires follow-up and treatment.

Sleep

During the normal aging process, sleep patterns change, and clients often sleep less than they did when younger. The nurse must assess any recent changes in sleep patterns and evaluate whether they are related to normal aging or are symptomatic of an underlying disorder. **Insomnia**, the inability to fall or remain asleep throughout the night, can be related to depression (Box 33-3) and lead to the regular use of sleep medications. Clients with insomnia report that they cannot sleep at night and do not feel rested in the morning. Approximately 57% of older adults complain of sleep disturbances of some kind (e.g., insomnia, early morning wakening, or the inability to fall asleep) (Brandt & Piechocki, 2013). It is also noted that sleep problems tend to increase with age and occur more frequently in women (Morin & Benca, 2012). Montgomery and Shepard (2010) note that more than 50% of older adults report problems with sleep. Sleep problems are also often linked to the use of alcohol. If an older individual reports sleep problems, the nurse should ask about his or her use of alcohol, over-the-counter medications, and prescription drugs (see Chapter 28).

BOX 33-3 Therapeutic Dialogue

ASSESSMENT INTERVIEW

Tom, 79 years old, is being seen for the first time in a geriatric mental health clinic because of recent changes in his behaviour and his accusations that family members are trying to steal his house and car. He locked his wife out of the house, accusing her of being unfaithful. When Susan, the PMH nurse assigned to his case, is conducting the assessment interview, Tom cooperates and is very pleasant until the nurse begins to assess the psychological domain.

Ineffective Approach

Nurse: Have there been times when you have had problems with any members of your family?

Client: No. (Silence)

Nurse: Have you noticed that lately you have been getting more upset than usual?

Client: No. Who has been talking to you?

Nurse: Your wife seems to think that you may be getting a little more upset than usual.

Client: You are just like her. She keeps telling me something is wrong with me. (Getting very agitated)

Nurse: Please, I'm trying to help you. I understand that you locked your wife out of the house last week.

Client: Leave me alone. (Gets up and leaves)

Effective Approach

Nurse: How have things been going at home?

Client: All right.

Nurse: (Silence)

Client: Well, my wife and I sometimes argue.

Nurse: Oh. Most husbands and wives argue. Any special arguments?

Client: No. Just the usual. I don't pick up after myself enough. I don't dress right to suit her. But, lately, she's gone a lot.

Nurse: She is gone a lot?

Client: Yeah! A lot.

Nurse: The way you say that, it sounds like you have some feelings about her being gone.

Client: You're damned right I do—and you would, too.

Nurse: I'm missing something.

Client: Well, if you must know, I think she's having an affair with the man next door.

Nurse: Really? That must upset you to think your wife is having an affair.

Client: I am devastated. I feel so bad.

Nurse: Would you say that you are depressed?

Client: Well, wouldn't you be? Yes, I'm feeling pretty low.

Critical Thinking Challenge

- How do the very first questions differ in the two interviews?
- What therapeutic techniques did the nurse use in the second interview to avoid the pitfalls the nurse encountered in the first scenario?
- How did the nurse in the second scenario elicit the client's delusion about his wife's affair?
- From the data that the second nurse gathered, how many of the client's problems can be identified?

Pain

Older adults are more likely to experience pain than younger adults because they are at increased risk for chronic illness and may be suffering from the consequences of a lifetime of injuries. For a number of older individuals, pain is a constant companion; for instance, in 1999, 27% of home-dwelling older adults admitted to living with chronic pain (Public Health Agency of Canada, 2005). The experience of chronic pain often contributes to unexplained behaviour and personality changes. To assess pain, the nurse can use many pain instruments. One of the most popular instruments is the Wong-Baker FACES Pain Rating Scale, initially developed for children but now used for all age groups (Fig. 33-1). This scale is especially useful in communicating with people from different cultures and languages than the nurse's. See Chapter 36 for further discussion of pain.

The assessment of pain is especially critical for those older adults who are cognitively impaired and living in long-term care institutions. In one study, researchers utilized interviews and focus groups to examine attitudes and beliefs of physicians and nurses about administering pain medications to cognitively impaired residents in four long-term care facilities in Ontario (Kaasalainen et al., 2007). They found that physicians and nurses expressed uncertainty about assessing pain in cognitively impaired individuals, admitted reluctance to administer opioids, and voiced concerns about overmedicating these residents. These results suggest that pain may be underrecognized and undertreated in older adults with cognitive impairment. Kaasalainen and her colleagues are developing a tool for pain assessment in the cognitively impaired (Kaasalainen et al., 2011a, 2011b).

Pharmacologic Assessment

One of the most important areas of the biologic domain is the pharmacologic assessment. **Polypharmacy**, the concurrent use of several different medications, is common in older individuals. The nurse must ask the client and family to list all medications and times that the client takes them. Asking family members to bring in all the medications that the client is taking, including over-the-counter medications, vitamins, and herbal supplements, is a good idea. Because older adults are more sensitive than younger people to medications, the possibility of drug–drug interactions is greater. Adverse drug interactions may cause delirium in older adults and constitute a medical emergency that may result in death (see Chapter 12). Also, when considering potential drug interactions, the nurse should ask the older individual about his or her consumption of grapefruit juice, which contains naringin, a compound that inhibits the CYP3A4 enzyme involved in the metabolism of many medications (e.g., antidepressants, antiarrhythmics, erythromycin, several statins). The American Geriatrics Society (AGS) updated the Beers criteria, the most highly used information source for prescribing medications in older adults, which may provide a useful resource when examining pharmacologic interventions (American Geriatrics Society, 2012). Comprehensive geriatric assessment has proven effective for addressing many problems associated with polypharmacy (Sergi, De Rui, Sarti, & Manzato, 2011).

Psychological Domain

The assessment of the psychological domain provides the nurse with the opportunity to identify limitations, behavioural symptoms, and reactions to illness. The

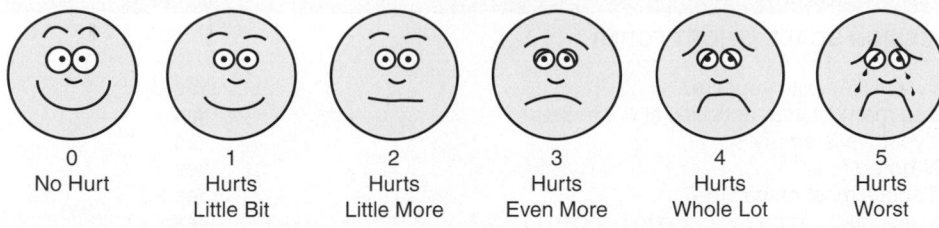

Wong-Baker FACES Pain Rating Scale

Each face represents a person who is happy or sad depending on how much or how little pain he/she has:

0	"a person who is very happy because he/she doesn't hurt at all"
1	"it hurts just a little bit"
2	"it hurts a little more"
3	"it hurts even more"
4	"it hurts a whole lot"
5	"it hurts as much as you can imagine, but you don't have to be crying to feel this bad"

Subject ID #:_____ Date:___/___/___ Visit #_____

Pt. name:_____

RA:_____

FIGURE 33-1. Wong-Baker FACES Pain Rating Scale.

nurse assesses many of the same areas as in other adult assessments, but again, the emphasis may be different. The following discussion focuses on the responses of older adults to mental health problems, mental status examinations, behavioural changes, stress and coping patterns, and risk assessments.

Responses to Mental Health Problems

Many older clients are reluctant to admit that they have psychiatric symptoms, particularly if their culture stigmatizes mental illness, and may deny having mental or emotional problems. They may also fear that if they admit to any symptoms, they may be placed outside their home. Clients who do not recognize or admit to having psychiatric symptoms are increasingly vulnerable to being taken advantage of or injured.

Throughout the assessment, the nurse evaluates the client's verbal reports, obvious symptoms, and family reports. If a client flatly denies any psychiatric symptoms (e.g., depression, mood swings, outbursts of anger, memory problems), the nurse should respectfully accept the older adult's answer and avoid arguments or confrontation (Box 33-4). If the client's family members contradict the client's report or symptoms are obvious during the interview, the nurse can approach the issue while planning care. Nurses may need to use conflict resolution strategies in helping families and clients obtain appropriate care despite disagreement about symptoms experienced by the older adults.

Mental Status Examination

The areas of special interest in the mental status examination are mood and affect, thought processes, and cognitive functioning. The nurse should interpret the results in light of any accompanying physical problems, such as chronic pain, or life changes, such as loss of a spouse.

Mood and Affect

Depression is the most common mental disorder in older adults (Skoog, 2011) and associated with the following risk factors: loss of spouse, physical illness, education below high school, impaired functional status, and heavy alcohol consumption. In older people, other disorders may mask depression. When symptoms are present, they may be attributed to normal aging or atherosclerosis or other age-related problems. Older clients are less likely to report feeling sad or worthless than are younger clients. As a result, family members and primary care providers often overlook depression in older adults (Gregg et al., 2013). Depressive symptoms are much more common than a full-fledged depressive disorder, as characterized by the *Diagnostic and Statistical Manual of Mental Disorders-5* (American Psychiatric Association, 2013). Between 10% and 15% of older adults living in the community experience depressive symptoms (Mental Health Commission of Canada, 2012). Approximately 50% of older adults living in long-term care facilities show signs of depression (MHCC, 2012). Research suggests that untreated depression in older adults may result in the overuse of health care

BOX 33-4 Research for Best Practice

GERIATRIC DEPRESSION SCALE (SHORT FORM)

1. Are you basically satisfied with your life?	Yes	No
2. Have you dropped many of your activities and interests?	Yes	No
3. Do you feel that your life is empty?	Yes	No
4. Do you often get bored?	Yes	No
5. Are you in good spirits most of the time?	Yes	No
6. Are you afraid that something bad is going to happen to you?	Yes	No
7. Do you feel happy most of the time?	Yes	No
8. Do you often feel helpless?	Yes	No
9. Do you prefer to stay at home rather than go out and do new things?	Yes	No
10. Do you feel you have more problems with memory than most?	Yes	No
11. Do you think it is wonderful to be alive now?	Yes	No
12. Do you feel pretty worthless the way you are now?	Yes	No
13. Do you feel full of energy?	Yes	No
14. Do you feel that your situation is hopeless?	Yes	No
15. Do you think that most people are better off than you are?	Yes	No

Score: ____/15 One point for "No" to questions 1, 5, 7, 11, 13

One point for "Yes" to other questions

Normal	3 ± 2
Mildly depressed	7 ± 3
Very depressed	12 ± 2

services, longer hospital stays, decreased treatment compliance, and increased morbidity and mortality (Skoog, 2011).

The Geriatric Depression Scale (GDS) is a useful screening tool with demonstrated validity and reliability (Hyer & Blount, 1984). The GDS was designed as a self-administered test, although it also has been used in observer-administered formats. One advantage of the test is its "yes/no" format, which may be easier for older adults than the Hamilton Rating Scale for Depression, which uses a scale from 0 to 4 (see Appendix E). This tool is easy to administer and provides valuable information about the possibility of depression (Box 33-5). If results are positive, the nurse should refer the client to a psychiatrist or advanced practice nurse for further evaluation.

Among residents in long-term care facilities, the usefulness of the GDS depends on the degree of cognitive impairment. Residents who are mildly impaired may be able to answer yes/no questions; however, moderately to severely impaired older adults will be unable to do the same. The best validated scale for individuals with dementia is the Cornell Scale for Depression in Dementia (CSDD) (Alexopoulos, Abrams, Young, &

BOX 33-5 Loneliness in Older Adults: An Embodied Experience

The Question: How do older adults living in the community experience loneliness in their everyday lives? How do they cope with loneliness? How do older adults perceive loneliness and its effect on their health and well-being?

Methods: This study used a qualitative approach (interpretive phenomenology) to study the meaning of loneliness in older adults, the way they coped with loneliness, and how loneliness was manifested in their day-to-day lives. Twelve older adults, who responded positively to the question "Have you experienced loneliness in the past 6 months?" described their experience. The 20-item UCLA Loneliness Scale was used as a baseline descriptor of the participants, with descriptive data collected through in-depth interviews using three interview guides (History Interview, Loneliness Coping Interview, and the Daily Life Interview).

Findings: Findings revealed that loneliness frequently occurred as a result of declining health and mobility challenges, which disrupted meaningful opportunities for engaging with others. Retirement, widowhood, and giving up driving were also factors that decreased opportunities for meaningful engagement with others. Loneliness was experienced (embodied) physically and emotionally. This phenomenologic perspective can help nurses gain insight into the experience and significance of loneliness and its impact on the physical and psychological well-being of older adults.

Implications for Nursing
Loneliness is a frequently overlooked and unassessed phenomenon in older adults, despite being a significant risk factor affecting physical and psychological well-being. Nurses are in key positions to assess for people at risk and to advocate for interventions and programs that foster meaningful engagement.

Smith, J. M. (2012). Loneliness in older adults: An embodied experience. *Journal of Gerontological Nursing, 38*(8), 45–53.

Shamoian, 1998). The CSDD is an interview-administered scale that uses information from both the client and an outside informant.

Anxiety is another important mood for nurses to assess in older adults because it can interfere with normal functioning. In dementia, anxiety is common (Skoog, 2011). The Rating Anxiety in Dementia (RAID) scale was developed as a global scale to assess anxiety in clients with dementia (Shankar, Walker, Frost, & Orrell, 1999). The domains that the RAID scale assesses include worry, apprehension and vigilance, motor tension, autonomic hyperactivity, and phobias and panic attacks.

Thought Processes

Thought processes and content are critical in the assessment of older adults. Can the client express ideas and thoughts logically? Can the client understand questions and follow the conversation of others? If the older adult shows any indication of hallucinations or delusions, the nurse should explore the content of the hallucination or delusion. If the client has a history of mental illness, such as schizophrenia, these symptoms may be familiar to family members, who can validate whether they are old or new problems. If this is the first time the client has experienced these abnormal thought processes, the nurse should further evaluate the content. Suspicious and delusional thoughts that characterize dementia often include some of the following beliefs:

- People are stealing my things.
- My spouse is having an affair.
- My relative is an impostor.

If a client shares any such thoughts, the nurse can complete further assessment by using the Behavioural Pathology in Alzheimer's Disease rating scale (BEHAVE-AD). This 25-item scale is based on caregivers' reports within the previous 2 weeks (Reisberg & Ferris, 1985). The BEHAVE-AD measures thought and behavioural disturbances in seven major categories, with each item scored on a four-point scale of severity (0 to 3), including delusions, hallucinations, activity disturbances, aggressiveness, diurnal rhythm disturbances, mood disturbances, and anxieties and phobias. The BEHAVE-AD also contains a four-point global assessment of the overall magnitude of the behaviour symptoms in terms of disturbance to the caregiver, dangerousness to the client, or both. The reliability of the BEHAVE-AD (0.95 and 0.96; $p < 0.01$) is comparable to that of the Mini-Mental State Examination (MMSE) (Reisberg, Auer, & Monteiro, 1996).

Cognition and Intellectual Performance

Cognitive functioning includes such parameters as orientation, attention, short- and long-term memories, consciousness, and executive functioning. Intellectual functioning, also considered a cognitive measure, is rarely formally assessed with a standardized intelligence test in older adults. Considerable variability among individuals depends on lifestyle and psychosocial factors. Some changes in cognitive capacity accompany aging, but important functions are spared. Normal cognitive changes during aging include a slowing of information processing and memory retrieval. Abnormalities of consciousness, orientation, judgement, speech, or language are not related to age but to underlying neuropathologic changes. Cognitive changes in older adults are associated with delirium or dementia (see Chapter 34) or with schizophrenia (see Chapter 20).

The assessment includes the number of years of education. An inverse relationship between Alzheimer's disease and the number of years of education exists. When assessing cognitive functioning, the nurse should use standardized instruments in combination with their assessment skills to assess for cognitive impairment in older adults residing in hospitals and long-term care facilities. Of such instruments, the MMSE, discussed in Chapter 10, is recommended for use in screening for cognitive functioning related to dementia (Leifer, 2009). Various studies suggest that an MMSE score below 24 of 30 has a reasonable sensitivity (80% to 90%) and specificity (80%) for discriminating between those with dementia and those without. Studies suggest that education has a protective effect against cognitive decline in early-stage mild cognitive impairment but that this effect disappears in late-stage mild cognitive impairment (Ye et al., 2013). Assessment should always take into account not only an individual's educational background but also his/her cultural background as these can influence scores.

Evidence suggests that severe cognitive deterioration may occur in older individuals with schizophrenia. In assessing the cognitive status of this population, the Cognitive Abilities Screening Instrument (CASI) demonstrates greater specificity than does the MMSE (Sherrell, Buckwalter, Bode, & Strozdas, 1999). The CASI is a 25-item test developed as a research instrument and piloted in Japan and the United States (Teng et al., 1994). The total score ranges from 0 (poor) to 100 (good), with a suggested cutoff of 74 for classifying dementia. The CASI provides quantitative assessment of nine domains: attention, concentration, orientation, long-term memory, short-term memory, language, visual construction (copying pentagons), fluency (naming four-legged animals), and abstraction and judgement. Because it determines the level of cognitive impairment, the CASI could be used in establishing individualized care plans.

In 2012, the diagnostic approach to Alzheimer's disease was revised at the fourth Canadian Consensus Conference on the Diagnosis and Treatment of Dementia, based in part on recommendations by the International Working Group and workgroups of the National Institute on Aging/Alzheimer Association. These recommendations can be found in Gauthier et al. (2012).

Behaviour Changes

Behaviour changes in older adults can indicate neuropathologic processes and thus require nursing assessment. If such changes occur, it is most likely that family members will notice them before the client does. Apraxia (the inability to execute a voluntary movement despite normal muscle function) is not attributed to age but indicates an underlying disease process, such as Alzheimer's disease, Parkinson's disease, or other disorders. Various other behaviour problems are associated with psychiatric disorders in older individuals, including irritability, agitation, apathy, and euphoria. Other behaviours in older adults who are experiencing psychiatric problems include wandering and aggressive behaviours. The BEHAVE-AD identifies these behaviours.

The Neuropsychiatric Inventory (NPI) was developed in 1994 to assess behaviour problems associated with dementia. The scale assesses 10 behaviour problems: delusions, hallucinations, dysphoria, anxiety, agitation/aggression, euphoria, disinhibition, irritability/lability, apathy, and aberrant motor behaviour (Cummings et al., 1994). The NPI was subsequently refined to include two more behavioural problems: nighttime behavioural disturbances such as difficulties with sleep and changes in eating patterns. The NPI also added a component to assess for caregiver distress (Cummings, 1997). This very popular tool is used in many medication clinical trials. There are two versions. The standard version is used when the client is still at home, whereas a different version is used when the client is in a long-term care facility.

Stress and Coping Patterns

Identifying stresses and coping patterns is just as important for older individuals as it is for younger adults. Unique stresses for older clients include living on a fixed income, handling declining health, losing partners and friends, and ultimately confronting death. Coping ability varies, depending on clients' unique circumstances. For example, some older adults respond to stressful events with amazing adaptability, whereas others become depressed and suicidal.

Loss of a spouse is common in late life, especially for women in older age groups. Forty-five percent of women and fifteen percent of men over the age of 65 have lost a spouse (Itzhar-Nabarro & Smoski, 2012). Bereavement, a natural response to the death of a loved one, includes crying and sorrow, anxiety and agitation, insomnia, and loss of appetite. These symptoms of grief may cause much suffering, but they do not lead to a major depressive disorder except, perhaps, when the person is vulnerable to depressive disorders (APA, 2013). Although bereavement is a normal response, the nurse must identify it and develop interventions to help the individual successfully resolve the loss. Bereavement is an important and well-established risk factor for depression. Factors such as previous mental or physical health conditions in the surviving spouse, high levels of caregiver strain before the death of the spouse, and a lack of social support increase the likelihood of depression postbereavement (Itzhar-Nabarro & Smoski, 2012; Stahl & Schulz, 2013).

Loneliness is another concern in older adults that significantly impacts health and well-being. It is also an issue that nurses can positively influence by assessing for it. "Similar to pain and suffering, loneliness is part of human beings' embodied condition … and what it means to be human" (Smith, 2012, p. 52) (see Box 33-5).

Risk Assessment

Suicide is a major mental health risk for older adults. Men 85 years of age and older have the highest suicide rate of all age groupings in Canada (Government of Canada, 2006). Most older individuals who die by suicide have visited their family physician within the month of their death (Gregg et al., 2013; Juurlink, Herrmann, Szalai, Kopp, & Redelmeier, 2004).

When caring for the older client with mental health problems, the nurse always should consider the individual's potential to die by suicide. Depression is the greatest risk factor for suicide. In assessing an older client, the nurse should consider the following characteristics as indications of high risk for committing suicide:

- Depression
- Previous suicide attempts
- Family history of suicide
- Firearms in the home
- Abuse of alcohol or other substances
- Unusual stress
- Chronic medical condition (e.g., cancer, neuromuscular disorders)
- Feelings of helplessness and hopelessness
- Feelings of being a burden to others
- Social isolation

● **STUDY NOTE**

Current mental health policy's focus on community-based care and integration aims at moving away from older, more stigmatizing approaches of long-term institutionalization and custodial care.

Social Domain

An assessment of the social domain includes determining the client's interactions with others in his or her family and community. The nurse targets social support because it is so important to the well-being of older adults, functional status because of the potential physical changes that can affect this area, and social systems, which encompass all community resources.

Social Support

Remaining active throughout one's life is one of the best predictors of mental health and wellness in an older individual. People obtain their sense of self-worth through their interactions with others in their environment. A sense of "who one is" is closely tied to the roles that a person plays in life. When older adults relinquish such roles because of physical disabilities, become isolated from friends and family, or begin to sense that they are a burden to those around them rather than contributing members of society, a sense of hopelessness and helplessness may follow.

The role of social support is critical to assess in this age group. Social support is a reciprocal concept, meaning that simply receiving assistance increases the person's sense of being a burden. Those older individuals who also believe that they contribute to the welfare of others are most likely to remain mentally healthy. For this reason, pets are often "life savers" for older adults who live alone. Nothing can be more understanding and accepting of an older adult's behaviour or disabilities than a beloved pet.

The nurse should assess the client's number of formal and informal social contacts. The nurse should ask about the frequency of contacts with others (in person and through telephone calls, letters, and cards) that the older adult has. Research has shown that social support and the quality of relationships are significant in contributing to quality of life for older persons (Merz & Huxhold, 2010). The amount of social support currently experienced should be compared with the amount and kinds of support the client received in the past. Determining whether these contacts are actually satisfying and supporting to the client is essential. If family members are important to the client's well-being, the nurse should complete a more in-depth family assessment (see Chapter 15).

The nurse can use the following questions to focus on social support (Kane, 1995):

- In the past 2 weeks, how often would you say that others let you know that they care about you?
- In the past 2 weeks, how often has someone provided you with help, such as giving you a ride somewhere or helping around the house?
- Do you have any one special person you could call or contact if you needed help? Who?
- In general, other than your children, how many relatives do you feel close to and have contact with at least once a month?

Other important questions for assessing social support include questions regarding the quality of relationships with family and others. For older clients who are isolated with few social contacts, the nurse can develop interventions to improve social support.

Functional Status

As part of a complete assessment, the nurse will need to assess the older adult's functional status. **Functional activities** or activities of daily living (ADLs) are the activities necessary for self-care (i.e., bathing, toileting, dressing, transferring). Instrumental ADLs (IADLs) include those that facilitate or enhance the performance of ADLs (i.e., shopping, using the telephone, using transportation). These aspects are critical to consider for any older adult living alone. When possible, the older adult should be observed for his or her ability to complete ADLs, rather than relying on self-report or report of the family. Common tools used to assess functional status include the Index of Independence in ADLs and the IADLs (Katz & Akpom, 1976). The Functional Activities Questionnaire (FAQ) measures an adult's functional abilities based on the information from family members and caregivers. The older person is rated on 10 complex, higher-order activities, such as writing cheques, assembling tax records, and driving (Pfeffer, Kursaki, Harrah, Chance, & Filos, 1982). The Functional Autonomy Measuring System (Hebert, Guilbeault, & Pinsonnault, 2002; McKye, Naglie, Tierney, & Jaglal, 2009) is designed for use in a community setting and measures a person's actual performance on a task (e.g., performs task alone; with cueing or help; total help needed). Client and family reports can be used in completing it.

Social Systems

Community resources are essential to an older adult's ability to maintain mental health and wellness, as well as to his or her ability to remain at home throughout the later years. Senior centres are federally or provincially funded community resources that provide a wide array of services to Canada's older population. They may provide daily balanced meals at a nominal cost. In addition, they provide opportunities for socialization, which is key to combating loneliness and social isolation. Many senior centres provide annual influenza and pneumonia vaccination clinics and education on such topics as fall prevention and the recognition and prevention of elder abuse. Additional community resources that are specific to older individuals include geriatric assessment clinics and adult day programs.

During the assessment, the nurse must determine which community resources are available and if the older client uses them. Lack of transportation to and from these community resources may be a barrier to use. Most communities have buses available for older or handicapped individuals. As more communities are recognizing the importance of being "age friendly," more resources are being made available and accessible for older persons. Nurses may need to assist the older adult in accessing these important resources.

While Canada does fairly well with respect to poverty rates among seniors (6.7%) in comparison with other countries, the poverty rates for the elderly rose between the mid-1990s and late 2000s; there are still many seniors who are classified as low-income (Conference Board of Canada, 2013). Low income is particularly prevalent among older women living on their own (Government of Canada, 2008). A number of older adults rely on Canada Pension Plan (or for older adults living in Quebec, the Quebec Pension Plan), Old Age Security, and Guaranteed Income Supplement for their monthly income. For these older individuals, this financial support, although less than adequate in most instances, is their only source of income. The nurse should assess a client's sources of financial support. Nurses are sometimes uncomfortable asking for financial information, fearing that they are invading the client's privacy. However, such data are important for the nurse to determine whether an older individual's resources adequately meet his or her needs. The source of financial support is also important. For example, a client whose income is adequate and comes from personal resources is more likely to be independent than is a client who depends on family members for income.

The nurse should ask the client about accessible health care facilities; available transportation to and from health care facilities; formal supports such as physicians, nurses, and other health care professionals; and the client's ability to pay for medications and health aids. Information about available health care resources beyond standard provincial health care (e.g., plans to pay for additional services such as medications or foot care) will alert the nurse to what services the client currently can and cannot access. In urban areas that are likely to have adequate health care resources, cultural and language barriers may prohibit access. People who live in rural areas where health care resources are limited are less likely to enjoy the full range of health care resources than are those in urban areas. For instance, older adults in Canadian rural settings have greater difficulty accessing geriatric mental health services than those in urban sites (Conn, 2003). Even in centres with geriatric mental health services, however, many older adults are reluctant to access services because of a lack of awareness of available help, stigma, or cultural issues (Sadavoy, Meier, & Ong, 2004). Initiatives of the Mental Health Commission of Canada (MHCC) and its Seniors Advisory Committee have involved strategies aimed at reducing the stigma of mental illness and aging (MHCC, 2011, 2012).

Legal Status

A growing trend in Canada and the United States is to view older adults as a special population whose rights deserve increased attention. Instances of elder abuse are far too common. Every nurse must consider herself or himself a client advocate and be vigilant in recognizing the signs of neglect or abuse, such as unexplained injuries. At times, abuse can take the form of another individual (sometimes an adult child) usurping the rights of the older person. Unless the older person is medically and legally determined to be incompetent, he or she has the same rights to personal decision making as any other adult, including the right to refuse treatment.

Spiritual Domain

Spiritual needs are basic for all age groups and are requirements for establishing meaning and purpose, love and relatedness, and forgiveness. There is growing evidence of the significance that spirituality plays in successful aging (Haugan, 2013; Lavretsky, 2010). Spirituality is sometimes expressed through commitment to organized religion, while other times it is expressed differently. Aging is a process that can bring individuals closer to understanding the finite nature of existence and evokes an awareness of their spiritual needs. With advanced age, many people begin to reflect on their successes and failures. During such reflection, many seek out God or a higher being to make sense of the past and establish hope for the future.

The process of spiritual assessment involves active listening, thoughtful observing, and sensitive questioning. The nurse may simply ask if the older adult would find comfort from a visit from a minister or a spiritual leader. Many forms of religion use various rituals that are important to the older individual's daily routine. The nurse should explore and honour these aspects to the extent possible (see Chapters 5 and 11).

A sense of quality of life is closely tied to values and beliefs about life's meaning. For many older individuals, quality of life is not reflected in material possessions or physical health but more by contentment over how the person has lived life and the extent to which his or her life has had meaning and purpose. Keeping close personal contacts with friends and family and having the opportunity to share stories of lifetime experiences are important to mental health and spiritual well-being. For older individuals, physical illnesses may affect the quality of life more than psychiatric disorders. The assessment of quality of life becomes especially important when assessing a client living in a continuing care facility or isolated in his or her own home. The assessment of quality of life of older adults is similar to that for younger adults (see Chapter 10).

SUMMARY OF KEY POINTS

■ Normal aging is associated with some physical decline, but most functions do not change. Intellectual functioning, capacity for change, and productive engagement with life remain stable.

■ Mental health assessments are necessary when older clients face psychiatric or mental health issues. The bio/psycho/social/spiritual geriatric mental health nursing assessment examines many sources of data, including self-reports, laboratory test results, and reports from family members.

■ The bio/psycho/social/spiritual geriatric mental health nursing assessment is based on the special needs and problems of older individuals. This assessment examines current and past health, functional status, and human responses to mental health problems.

■ The assessment of the biologic domain involves collecting data about the past and present health status, physical examination findings, physical functions (i.e., nutrition and eating, elimination patterns, sleep), pain, exercise, and pharmacologic information.

■ The assessment of the psychological domain includes the client's responses to mental health problems, mental status examination, behavioural changes, stress and coping patterns, and risk assessment.

■ When conducting an assessment, the nurse may find several tools useful. For clients with possible depression, the GDS may be helpful. For clients with anxiety, nurses can use the RAID scale. In addition to a careful interview, the nurse can use the BEHAVE-AD scale to determine delusions, hallucinations, activity disturbances, aggressiveness, diurnal rhythm disturbances, mood disturbances, anxieties, or phobias. It is important to remember that all assessment tools should be used in conjunction with the nurse's clinical assessment skills and judgement.

■ The nurse can conduct cognitive assessments using the MMSE or the CASI.

■ Coping with the stresses of aging varies among clients. Determining stresses and coping skills for dealing with stresses is important.

■ Social support is critical to clients in this age group and requires assessment.

■ Determination of the client's ability to perform functional and instrumental ADLs is critical in the assessment of older adults. The FAQ measures the functional abilities based on information from others.

■ Social systems, spiritual assessment, legal information, and the quality of life are components within the social domain that the nurse should consider.

■ Remember that assessment should always occur within a climate of respect for the older adult, recognizing his/her life history and ability to participate in the process.

CRITICAL THINKING CHALLENGES

1 The director of your church's senior centre has asked you to be the guest speaker at the monthly meeting of the Retired Active Citizens' group. The subject is to be "Maintaining Your Mental Health After Retirement." What key points will you touch on in your presentation? What activities or handouts will you use to highlight your talk?

2 When asking about current illnesses, a client begins telling you her whole life story. What approach would you take to elicit the most important information needed to develop an individualized plan of care for your older client?

3 A caregiver tells you that her mother has become suspicious of the neighbours and other family members. How would you assess this perceptual experience? What other data should you gather from this client?

4 A caregiver brings a bag of medications to the client's assessment interview. What information should you obtain from the caregiver regarding the older individual's use of these medications?

5 A woman brings her father, who has a long history of frequent psychiatric hospitalizations for depression, to the clinic. The client's wife recently died, and the daughter fears that her father is becoming depressed again. What approach would you use in assessing for changes in mood?

6 Obtain a listing of the social services available in your community. Examine the list for areas of duplication and omission of services needed by an older adult living alone in his or her own home.

REFERENCES

Adlaf, E. M., Begin, P., & Sawka, E. (Eds.). (2005). *Canadian Addiction Survey (CAS): A national survey of Canadians' use of alcohol and other drugs: Prevalence of use and related harms: Detailed report*. Ottawa, ON: Canadian Centre on Substance Abuse.

Alexopoulos, G. S., Abrams, R. C., Young, R. C., & Shamoian, C. (1998). Cornell scale for depression in dementia. *Biological Psychiatry, 23*, 271–284.

American Geriatrics Society. (2012). AGS updated Beers Criteria for potentially inappropriate medication use in older adults. *Journal of the American Geriatrics Society, 60*, 616–631.

American Psychiatric Association. (2013). *Diagnostic and statistical manual of mental disorders* (5th ed.). Washington, DC: Author.

Brandt, N. J. & Piechocki, J. M. (2013). Treatment of insomnia in older adults. Re-evaluating the benefits and risks of sedative hypnotics. *Journal of Gerontological Nursing, 39*(4), 48–54.

Brennan, P. L. & Soohoo, S. (2013). Pain and use of alcohol in later life: Prospective evidence from the health and retirement study. *Journal of Aging and Health, 25*(4), 656–677.

CIHR-IA (Canadian Institute for Health Research-Institute of Aging). (2013). *Living longer, living better. Canadian Institutes of Health Research Institute of Aging 2013–18 strategic plan*. Ottawa, ON: Author. Retrieved from http://www.cihr-irsc.gc.ca/e/47179.html

Conference Board of Canada. (2013). *Elderly poverty*. Retrieved from http://www.conferenceboard.ca/hcp/details/society/elderly-poverty.aspx

Conn, D. K. (2003). Oral presentation to the Standing Senate Committee on Social Affairs, Science and Technology. *Bulletin of the Canadian Academy of Geriatric Psychiatry, 10*(3), 5–8.

Cummings, J. L. (1997). The neuropsychiatric inventory: Assessing psychopathology in dementia patients. *Neurology, 48*(5)(Suppl. 6), S10–S16.

Cummings, J. L., Mega, M., Gray, K., Rosenberg-Thompson, S., Carusi, D. A., & Gornbein, J. (1994). The Neuropsychiatric inventory: Comprehensive assessment of psychopathology in dementia. *Neurology, 44*(12), 2308–2314.

Gauthier, S., Patterson, C., Chertkow, H., Gordon, M., Herrmann, N., Rockwood, K., ... Soucy, J. P. (2012). Recommendations of the 4th Canadian consensus conference on the diagnosis and treatment of dementia (CCCDTD4). *Canadian Geriatrics Journal, 15*(4), 120–126.

Gregg, J. J., Fiske, A., & Gatz, M. (2013). Physician's detection of late-life depression: The roles of dysphoria and cognitive impairment. *Aging and Mental Health, 13*(45), 1–11.

Government of Canada. (2006). *The human face of mental health and mental illness in Canada—2006* (Cat. No. HP5-19/2006E). Ottawa, ON: Minister of Public Works and Government Services Canada.

Government of Canada. (2008). *Reducing poverty among older women: The potential of retirement income policies*. Retrieved from www.swc-cfc.gc.ca/pubs/pubspr/0662659271/200008_0662659271_9_e.html

Haugan, G. (2014). Nurse-patient interaction is a resource for hope, meaning in life and self-transcendence in nursing home patients. *Scandinavian Journal of Caring Sciences, 28*(1):74–88. doi: 10.1111/scs.12028

Hebert, R., Guilbeault, J., & Pinsonnault, E. (2002). *Functional autonomy measuring system user guide*. Sherbrooke, QC: Centre d'expertise de l'Institut universitaire de geriatrie de Sherbrooke.

HRSDC (Human Resources and Skills Development Canada). (2012a). *Indicators of well-being in Canada. Health-life expectancy at birth*. Ottawa, ON: Author. Retrieved from http://www4.hrsdc.gc.ca/.3ndic.1t.4r@-eng.jsp?iid=3#M_1

HRSDC (Human Resources and Skills Development Canada). (2012b). *Indicators of well-being in Canada. Canadians in context-aging population*. Ottawa, ON: Author. Retrieved from http://www4.hrsdc.gc.ca/.3ndic.1t.4r@-eng.jsp?iid=33

Hyer, L. & Blount, J. (1984). Concurrent and discriminant validities of the geriatric depression scale with older psychiatric inpatients. *Psychological Reports, 54*, 611–616.

Itzhar-Nabarro, Z. & Smoski, M. J. (2012). A review of theoretical and empirical perspectives on marital satisfaction and bereavement outcomes: Implications for working with older adults. *Clin Gerontol, 35*, 257–269.

Juurlink, D. N., Herrmann, N., Szalai, J. P., Kopp, A., & Redelmeier, D. A. (2004). Medical illness and the risk of suicide in the elderly. *Archives of Internal Medicine, 164*(11), 1179–1184.

Kaasalainen, S., Coker, E., Dolovich, L., Papaioannou, A., Hadjstavropoulous, T., Emili, A. & Ploeg, J. (2007). Pain management decision making among long-term care physicians and nurses. *Western Journal of Nursing Research, 29*(5), 561–580.

Kaasalainen, S., Stewart, N., Middleton, J., Knezacek, S., Hartley, T., Ife, C., & Robinson, L. (2011a). Pain assessment in the communicatively impaired (PACI) tool: part 1. *International Journal of Palliative Nursing, 17*(8), 387–391.

Kaasalainen, S., Stewart, N., Middleton, J., Knezacek, S., Hartley, T., Ife, C., & Robinson, L. (2011b). Pain assessment in the communicatively impaired (PACI) tool: part 2. *International Journal of Palliative Nursing, 17*(9), 431–438.

Kane, R. A. (1995). Assessment of social functioning: Recommendations for comprehensive geriatric assessment. In Z. Rubenstein, D. Wieland, & R. Bernabei (Eds.), *Geriatric assessment technology: The state of the art* (pp. 91–110). New York, NY: Springer.

Katz, S. & Akpom, A. (1976). A measure of primary sociobiological functions. *International Journal of Health Science, 6*, 493.

Koechl, B., Unger, A., & Fischer, G. (2012). Age-related aspects of addiction. *Gerontology, 58*, 540–544.

Lavretsky, H. (2010). Spirituality and aging. *Aging Health, 6*(6), 749–769.

Leifer, B. (2009). Alzheimer's disease: Seeing the signs early. *Journal of the Academy of Nurse Practitioners, 21*, 588–595.

McKye, K. A., Naglie, G., Tierney, M., & Jaglal, S. (2009). Comparison of older adults' and occupational therapists' awareness of functional abilities at discharge from rehabilitation with actual performance in the home. *Physical & Occupational Therapy in Geriatrics, 27*(3), 229–244.

Mental Health Commission of Canada. (2011). *Guidelines for comprehensive mental health services for older adults in Canada*. Ottawa, ON: Author. Retrieved from http://www.mentalhealthcommission.ca/English/document/279/mental-health-commission-canada-seniors-guidelines-print

Mental Health Commission of Canada. (2012). *Changing directions, changing lives: The mental health strategy for Canada*. Ottawa, ON: Author. Retrieved from http://www.mentalhealthcommission.ca/English/node/721

Mental Health Commission of Canada. (2013). *Municipalities and the aging population*. Ottawa, ON: Author. Retrieved from http://www.mentalhealthcommission.ca/English/document/7176/fact-sheet-municipalities-and-aging-population

Merz, E. M. & Huxhold, O. (2010). Wellbeing depends on social relationship characteristics : Comparing different types and providers of support to older adults. *Ageing and Society, 30*(5), 843–857.

Montgomery, P. & Shepard, L. D. (2010). Insomnia in older people. *Reviews in Clinical Gerontology, 20*, 205–218.

Moore, A. A., Seeman, T., Morgenstern, H., Beck, J. C., & Reuben, D. B. (2002). Are there differences between older persons who screen positive on the CAGE questionnaire and the Short Michigan Alcoholism Screening Test—Geriatric Version? *Journal of the American Geriatrics Society, 50*(5), 858–862.

Morin, C. M. & Benca, R. (2012). Chronic insomnia. *Lancet, 379*, 1129–1141.

Pfeffer, R., Kurosaki, T., Harrah, C., Chance, J., & Filos, S. (1982). Measurement of functional activities in older adults in the community. *Journal of Gerontology, 37*(3), 323–329.

Public Health Agency of Canada. (2005). *Seniors experiencing chronic pain: Statistical snapshot # 34.* Statistics Canada. Retrieved from http://www.phac.aspc.gc.ca/seniors-aines

Reisberg, B., Auer, S., & Monteiro, I. (1996). Behavioural Pathology in Alzheimer's Disease (BEHAVE-AD) rating scale. *International Psychogeriatrics, 8*(3), 301–308.

Reisberg, B. & Ferris, S. (1985). A clinical rating scale for symptoms of psychosis in Alzheimer's disease. *Psychopharmacology Bulletin, 21,* 101–104.

Sadavoy, J., Meier, R., & Ong, A. Y. M. (2004). Barriers to access to mental health services for ethnic seniors: The Toronto study. *Canadian Journal of Psychiatry, 49*(3), 192–199.

Stahl, S. T. & Schulz, R. (2013). Changes in routine health behaviors following late-life bereavement: A systematic review. *Journal of Behavioral Medicine* [online ahead of print]. doi: 10.1007/s10865-013-9524-7

Sergi, G., De Rui, M., Sarti, S., & Manzato, E. (2011). Polypharmacy in the elderly: Can comprehensive geriatric assessment reduce inappropriate medication use? *Drugs and Aging, 28*(7), 509–518.

Shankar, K. K., Walker, M., Frost, D., & Orrell, M. W. (1999). The development of a valid and reliable scale for rating anxiety in dementia (RAID). *Aging & Mental Health, 3*(1), 39–49.

Sheikh, J. I. & Yesavage, J. A. (1986). Geriatric Depression Scale (GDS): Recent evidence and development of a shorter version. In T. L. Brink (Ed.), *Clinical gerontology: A guide to assessment and interventions* (pp. 165–177). Binghamton, NY: Haworth Press.

Sherrell, K., Buckwalter, K., Bode, R., & Strozdas, L. (1999). Use of the cognitive abilities screen instrument to assess elderly persons with schizophrenia in long-term care settings. *Issues in Mental Health Nursing, 20,* 541–558.

Skoog, I. (2011). Psychiatric disorders in the elderly. *Canadian Journal of Psychiatry, 56*(7), 387–397.

Smith, J. M. (2012). Loneliness in older adults: An embodied experience. *Journal of Gerontology Nursing, 38*(8), 45–53.

Statistics Canada. (2005). Life expectancy at birth, by sex, by provinces. Retrieved from http://www.40.statcan.ca/101/cst01/health26.htm

Teng, E., Kazuo Hasegawa, K., Homma, A., Imai, Y., Larson, E., Graves, A., et al. (1994). The cognitive abilities screen instrument (CASI): A practical test for cross-cultural epidemiological studies of dementia. *International Psychogeriatrics, 6*(1), 45–58.

University of Michigan Alcohol Research Centre. (1991). Short Michigan Alcoholism Screening Test—Geriatric Version (SMAST-G). Retrieved from http://www.hartfordign.org/publications/trythis/issue17.pdf

Wilcox, B. (2012). Successful aging: Is there hope? *Can Med Assoc J, 184*(18), 1973–1974.

Wu, L. T. & Blazer, D. G. (2011). Illicit and nonmedical drug use among older adults: A review. *Journal of Aging and Health, 23*(3), 481–504.

Wu, Z., Schimmele, C. M., & Chappell, N. L. (2012). Aging and late-life depression. *Journal of Aging and Health, 24*(1), 3–28.

Ye, B. S., Seo, S. W., Cho, H., Kim, S. Y., Lee, J. S., Kim, E. J., ... Na, D. L. (2013). Effects of education on the progression of early versus late-stage mild cognitive impairment. *International Psychogeriatrics, 25*(4), 597–606.

34 Neurocognitive Disorders: Delirium and Dementia

Dorothy Forbes and Wendy Austin
Adapted from chapters "Delirium, Dementia, and Related Disorders" by Mary Haase (2010) and Mary Ann Boyd, Linda Garand, Linda A. Gerdner, Bonnie J. Wakefield, and Kathleen Buckwalter (2008)

KEY CONCEPTS

- cognition
- delirium
- dementia
- memory

LEARNING OBJECTIVES

After studying this chapter, you will be able to:

- Distinguish the clinical characteristics, onset, and course of the neurocognitive disorders (NCDs), delirium, and dementia.
- Describe the biologic, psychological, social, and spiritual factors that relate to NCDs in older adults.
- Discuss the emotional impact of dementia for the patient, family, and caregiver.
- Formulate nursing diagnoses based on a bio/psycho/social/spiritual assessment of patients with impaired cognitive function.
- Identify the expected outcomes and nursing interventions and provide an evaluation for patients with impaired cognition.

KEY TERMS

- agnosia • aphasia • apraxia • beta-amyloid plaques • bradykinesia
- catastrophic reactions • cortical dementias • disinhibition
- hyperactive delirium • hypoactive delirium • illusions
- neurofibrillary tangles • mixed delirium • oxidative stress
- postoperative delirium • subcortical dementia

C ognition and memory are important in many psychiatric disorders, but in this chapter on neurocognitive disorders (NCDs), they are the key concepts (American Psychiatric Association [APA], 2013). Cognition is the ability to think and know. The definition is further refined to be understood as a relatively high level of intellectual processing in which perceptions and information are acquired, used, or manipulated.

Specific functions include the acquisition and use of language, the ability to be oriented in time and space, judgement, reasoning, attention, comprehension, concept formation, planning, and the use of symbols, such as numbers and letters used in mathematics and writing. Cognition and behaviour are so closely linked that even mild cognitive impairment (MCI) can affect a person's ability to function effectively on a daily basis (Wadley, Okonkwo, Crowe, & Ross-Meadows, 2008).

In relation to social wellness, research evidence shows that adults who lived without a partner at midlife experienced nearly twice the risk of cognitive impairment in older age compared with the adults who live with a partner (Strout & Howard, 2012). The neuropsychologic literature generally describes MCI as cognitive test performance that falls one to two standard deviations below the expected normative performance (Bauer, Johnson, &

Pozehl, 2011) or such as related to expected functional abilities.

Memory, a facet of cognition, refers to the ability to recall or reproduce what has been learned or experienced. It is more than simple storage and retrieval; it is a complex cognitive mental function that includes most areas of the brain, especially the hippocampus, which is believed to be essential to the transfer of some memories from short-term to long-term storage. Defects of memory are an essential feature of many cognitive disorders, particularly dementia. In relation to cognition, it is important to note that memory loss increases with age, and this reality poses challenges to the older adult.

The NCDs discussed in this chapter, delirium and dementia, are characterized by deficits in cognition or memory that represent a clear-cut deterioration from a previous level of functioning. Delirium is a disorder of acute cognitive impairment and can be caused by a medical condition (e.g., infection) or substance abuse, or it may have multiple aetiologies. Dementia is characterized by chronic cognitive impairments and is differentiated by the underlying cause, not by symptom patterns, which are often similar. Some dementias are irreversible and progressive. Some organic compounds and chemicals, such as lead, manganese, and toluene (one of the toxins in glue and paint), may produce the symptoms of dementia. Once a person with chemically-induced symptoms is evaluated and treated, the symptoms of dementia may resolve.

Delirium's essential features are fluctuating alterations in attention or awareness along with a change in baseline cognition that cannot be explained by a preexisting or evolving NCD (APA, 2013, p. 599). The trigger is a somatic factor that can involve diverse illnesses, surgery, or substance (medication) intoxication or withdrawal (van Munster, de Rooij, & Korevaar, 2009).

Cortical dementias such as Alzheimer's disease (AD) and prion disease result from a disease process that globally afflicts the cortex. **Subcortical dementia** is caused by dysfunction or deterioration of deep grey- or white-matter structures inside the brain and brain stem. Symptoms of subcortical dementia may be more localized and tend to disrupt arousal, attention, and motivation, but they can produce a variety of clinical behavioural manifestations. Examples of subcortical dementias include those

> **KEY CONCEPT Cognition** involves multiple brain processes that enable an individual to perceive, learn, and recall specific information for the purpose of reasoning or problem solving. It is based on a system of complex interrelated abilities, such as perception, reasoning, judgement, intuition, and memory that allow one to be aware of oneself and one's surroundings. Impairments in these abilities can result in a failure of the afflicted person to recognize that he or she is not well and is in need of treatment.

due to Huntington's disease, Parkinson's disease, and HIV infection. In this chapter, AD is highlighted because it is the most prevalent form of dementia in Canada.

> **KEY CONCEPT Memory** is a facet of cognition concerned with retaining and recalling past experiences, whether they occurred in the physical environment or internally as cognitive events.

> **KEY CONCEPT Delirium** is a temporary disorder of physical origin with an abrupt onset characterized by fluctuating consciousness and attention.

> **KEY CONCEPT Dementia** is characterized by chronic, progressive neurocognitive impairment and is differentiated by affected areas in the brain, underlying cause, and by symptom patterns.

DELIRIUM
Clinical Course of the Disorder

Delirium is an acute disorder of physical origin that develops over a short period of time, and it is characterized by fluctuating consciousness and attention. The individual with delirium has reduced ability to focus, sustain, or shift attention, which is marked by a decline in cognitive function (memory, orientation, speech, thinking), perceptual abnormalities, circadian disruption, and psychomotor disturbances (Ansaloni et al., 2010). Delirium is usually reversible if treated promptly, but it is a serious disorder associated with high morbidity and mortality. Research evidence shows that delirium is related with longer duration of hospitalization and is independently associated with increased intensive care unit mortality and hospital mortality (Salluh et al., 2010). In spite of the benefits of genetic studies in pathophysiologic research of psychiatric disorders such

EMERGENCY !

"Delirium is an acute, complex disorder that requires immediate interventions to prevent permanent brain damage and death" (Registered Nurses Association of Ontario [RNAO], 2004). A systematic review conducted by Zhang, Pan, and Ni (2013) revealed that delirious patients were three times more likely to die than were nondelirious patients during a follow-up period. The pathophysiologic mechanisms leading to delirium are still largely unknown in spite of its immense impact and life-threatening nature (Maclullich, Ferguson, Miller, de Rooij, & Cunningham, 2008). It is associated with mortality rates of 25% to 33% (Inouye, 2000).

as dementia, schizophrenia, and depression (Beck, 2008; Maier, 2008), research related to delirium is scarce, probably due to the characteristics and aetiology of the syndrome (van Munster et al., 2009).

Diagnostic Criteria

The lack of familiarity with valid and reliable delirium measurement or screening tools has been a contributing factor to either missed diagnosis or underdiagnosis (Balas et al., 2012). It is therefore important to identify a diagnostic strategy that specifically reveals patients at higher risk of adverse outcomes, independent of other clinical features that signal disease severity (Reade, Guenther, Gesin, & Devlin, 2012). Unstructured subjective assessments may be used to diagnose delirium (Patel & Kress, 2011) and identify patients with poor outcomes; however, no single method has proved to be more effective or efficient than the other (Reade et al., 2012). Delirium is likely to be underdiagnosed in terminally ill patients and may be confused with dementia, which can also present with impaired memory and disorientation (Candy et al., 2012). It is possible to have a delirium superimposed on a dementia.

Impaired consciousness is the key diagnostic criterion of delirium. The patient becomes less aware of his or her environment and loses the ability to focus, sustain, and shift attention. Associated cognitive changes typically include problems in memory, orientation, and language. The patient may not know where he or she is, may not recognize familiar objects, or may be unable to carry on a conversation. An assessment of MCI requires interpretation of neuropsychological test scores and validation of the scores against functional measures within a given population (Bauer et al., 2011). An important diagnostic indicator is that delirium develops rapidly, usually over hours or days. Table 34-1 presents the diagnostic criteria of delirium caused by a general medical condition. Figure 34-1 shows the kaleidoscope of care strategies of delirium, dementia, and depression. Nurses are in a unique position to plan, implement, and coordinate services for these patients and evaluate care aimed at improving patients' health outcomes.

> ● STUDY NOTE
> Delirium can be life threatening; identifying potential underlying causes of symptoms is a priority.

Delirium in Special Populations

Children

Delirium can occur in children and may be related to medications (anticholinergic agents) or fever. In children and adolescents, delirium is commonly associated

| Table 34-1 | Diagnostic Criteria for Delirium |

A. A disturbance in attention (i.e., reduced ability to direct, focus, sustain, and shift attention) and awareness (reduced orientation in the environment).

B. The disturbance develops over a short period of time (usually hours to a few days), represents a change from baseline attention and awareness, and tends to fluctuate in severity during the course of a day.

C. An additional disturbance in cognition (e.g., memory deficit, disorientation, language, visuospatial ability, or perception).

D. The disturbances in criteria A and C are not better explained by another preexisting, established, or evolving NCD and do not occur in the context of a severely reduced level of arousal, such as coma.

E. There is evidence from the history, physical examination, or laboratory findings that the disturbance is a direct physiologic consequences of another medical condition, substance intoxication or withdrawal (i.e., due to a drug of abuse or to a medication), or exposure to a toxin, or is due to multiple aetiologies.

From American Psychiatric Association. (2013). *Diagnostic and statistical manual of mental disorders* (5th ed., p. 596). Washington, DC: Author.

with sepsis and/or endocrine–metabolic disturbances; patients must therefore be closely monitored to ensure early detection (Grover et al., 2012). Children seem especially susceptible to this disorder, likely because of their immature brain. However, delirium may be hard to diagnose and may be mistaken for uncooperative behaviour. A systematic review revealed that delirium in children has been a neglected area of research, and unanswered questions remain as to which interventions reduce the incidence, severity, and duration of paediatric delirium (Hatherill & Flisher, 2010).

Older Adults

Although delirium may occur in any age group, it is most common among the older adults. Older adults often present with multiple medical comorbidities and higher risk for postoperative complications (Flinn, Diehl, Seyfried, & Malani, 2009). Older age (85 years) is associated with undetected delirium (Voyer et al., 2012). Nurses must therefore recognize that delirium, dementia, and depression present with overlapping clinical features and may coexist in the older adult (RNAO, 2003). **Postoperative delirium** is associated with increased length of hospital stay, higher patient care costs, rise in morbidity rates, decline in function, and greater risk of death in the older population (Ansaloni et al., 2010; Flinn et al., 2009; Leslie, Marcantonio, Zhang, Leo-Summers, & Inouye, 2008). Early diagnosis and resolution therefore remain critical to achieving favourable outcomes (Leslie et al., 2008; van Munster et al., 2009). Screening

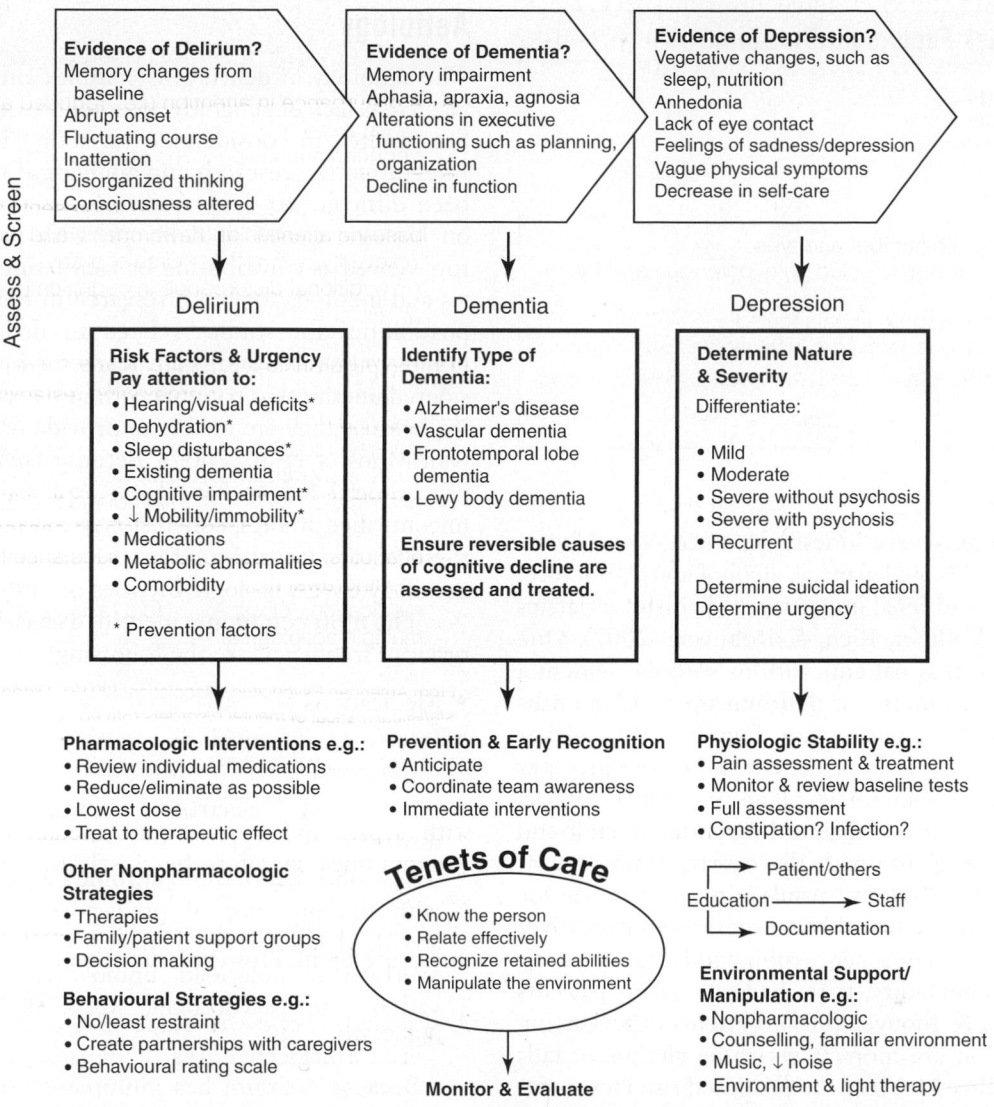

Assess & Screen

Evidence of Delirium?
Memory changes from
 baseline
Abrupt onset
Fluctuating course
Inattention
Disorganized thinking
Consciousness altered

Evidence of Dementia?
Memory impairment
Aphasia, apraxia, agnosia
Alterations in executive
 functioning such as planning,
 organization
Decline in function

Evidence of Depression?
Vegetative changes, such as
 sleep, nutrition
Anhedonia
Lack of eye contact
Feelings of sadness/depression
Vague physical symptoms
Decrease in self-care

Delirium

Dementia

Depression

**Risk Factors & Urgency
Pay attention to:**
• Hearing/visual deficits*
• Dehydration*
• Sleep disturbances*
• Existing dementia
• Cognitive impairment*
• ↓ Mobility/immobility*
• Medications
• Metabolic abnormalities
• Comorbidity

* Prevention factors

**Identify Type of
Dementia:**
• Alzheimer's disease
• Vascular dementia
• Frontotemporal lobe
 dementia
• Lewy body dementia

**Ensure reversible causes
of cognitive decline are
assessed and treated.**

**Determine Nature
& Severity**

Differentiate:

• Mild
• Moderate
• Severe without psychosis
• Severe with psychosis
• Recurrent

Determine suicidal ideation
Determine urgency

Pharmacologic Interventions e.g.:
• Review individual medications
• Reduce/eliminate as possible
• Lowest dose
• Treat to therapeutic effect

**Other Nonpharmacologic
Strategies**
• Therapies
• Family/patient support groups
• Decision making

Behavioural Strategies e.g.:
• No/least restraint
• Create partnerships with caregivers
• Behavioural rating scale

Prevention & Early Recognition
• Anticipate
• Coordinate team awareness
• Immediate interventions

Tenets of Care
• Know the person
• Relate effectively
• Recognize retained abilities
• Manipulate the environment

Monitor & Evaluate

Physiologic Stability e.g.:
• Pain assessment & treatment
• Monitor & review baseline tests
• Full assessment
• Constipation? Infection?

Patient/others
Education ——→ Staff
Documentation

**Environmental Support/
Manipulation e.g.:**
• Nonpharmacologic
• Counselling, familiar environment
• Music, ↓ noise
• Environment & light therapy

Adapted with permission from Dianne Rossy, RN, MScN, GNC(C), Advanced Practice Nurse, Geriatrics, The Ottawa Hospital
Note: The above Kaleidoscope does not contain all the caregiving strategies for delirium, dementia and depression.

FIGURE 34-1. Kaleidoscope of care strategies for delirium, dementia, and depression. (From Registered Nurses Association of Ontario. (2004). *Caregiving strategies for older adults with delirium, dementia, and depression* (p. 19). Toronto, ON: Author.)

for delirium should be considered as part of the clinical routine for older adults in their first postoperative days (Popp & Arlt, 2012). Delirium in older adults is associated with poor outcomes, including increased length of stay, higher costs, greater use of physical restraints, continuous sedation, increased unintended removal of catheters, and higher mortality rates (Balas et al., 2012; van Munster et al., 2009).

Epidemiology and Risk Factors

Statistics concerning the prevalence of delirium are based primarily on older individuals in acute care settings. Estimated prevalence rates range from 10% to 30% of patients. In nursing homes, the prevalence is much higher, approaching 60% of those older than the age of 75 years. The use of opioid analgesics in the management of postoperative pain has been found to correlate with the development of respiratory depression and postoperative delirium (Leung et al., 2009). Delirium occurs in as many as 30% of patients hospitalized for cancer and in 30% to 40% of those hospitalized with acquired immunodeficiency syndrome (AIDS). It has been estimated that 80% of terminally ill patients nearing death experience delirium (APA, 2000). Ansaloni et al. (2010) indicate that the incidence of postoperative delirium in patients who underwent emergency surgery was significantly higher (17.9%) than those operated under elective conditions (6.7%). The most powerful risks for developing delirium are present before admission: for

BOX 34-1   Risk Factors for Delirium

- Advanced age
- Preexisting dementia
- Functional dependence
- Preexisting illness
- Bone fracture
- Infection
- Medications (both number and type)
- Changes in vital signs (including hypotension and hyper- or hypothermia)
- Electrolyte or metabolic imbalance
- Admission to a long-term care institution
- Postcardiotomy
- AIDS
- Pain

example, old age, severe illness, dementia, visual/hearing impairments, polypharmacy, alcohol abuse, fracture, infection, pain, and renal impairment (British Geriatrics Society, 2006; Vollmer, Rich, & Robinson, 2007). One study concluded that patients with or without dementia had persistent symptoms of delirium up to 12 months after diagnosis. The same study found that a quicker in-hospital recovery is associated with better outcomes (McCusker, Cole, Dendukuri, Han, & Belzile, 2003). Analysis of data from a Delirium Prevention Trial found that patients (aged 70+) with the overlap syndrome of delirium and dementia had resided in a nursing home prior to hospitalization and had experienced cognitive/functional impairment, depression, and higher levels of medical comorbidity than had all other patients (Givens, Jones, & Inouye, 2009). Patients experiencing mental confusion are more likely to be victims of falls and fractures. Box 34-1 lists the proposed risk factors for delirium, and Box 34-2 presents a vignette of an individual who experienced delirium after using an over-the-counter (OTC) sleeping medication.

Aetiology

The aetiology of delirium is complex and usually multifaceted. A lack of generally accepted theories of causation has resulted in considerable variability in the research. Integrating the research and applying it to practice have been difficult. To date, studies focus almost exclusively on biologic causes of delirium, with psychosocial factors viewed as contributing or facilitating. Genetic studies and methods for brain research in humans offer new possibilities for studies related to delirium; however, lumbar punctures and brain scans for research are considered unethical in patients with impaired mental capacity, because they are unable to provide informed consent (van Munster et al., 2009). Because environmental and psychosocial factors have been explored only in small, uncontrolled studies, conclusions cannot be drawn about these factors. For this reason, the following discussion of aetiology covers biologic theories of cause.

The most commonly identified causes of delirium, in order of frequency, are the following:

- Medications
- Infections (particularly urinary tract and upper respiratory)
- Fluid and electrolyte imbalance; metabolic disturbances
- The probability of the syndrome's developing increases with the presence of predisposing factors such as advanced age, brain damage, or dementia. Sensory overload or underload, immobilization, sleep deprivation, and psychosocial stress also contribute to delirium.

Because delirium has multiple causes, a wide variety of brain alterations may also be responsible for its development. In certain cases, delirium may be the only manifestation of an underlying medical problem

BOX 34-2   Clinical Vignette

DELIRIUM

Mrs. Campbell, a widowed 72-year-old woman living in her own home, has been having trouble sleeping. Her daughter visits her and suggests that she try an OTC sleeping medication. Mrs. Campbell has also been taking antihistamines for allergies and the antidepressant amitriptyline. Three nights later, a neighbour calls the daughter, concerned because she encountered Mrs. Campbell wandering the streets, unable to find her home. When the neighbour approached Mrs. Campbell to help her home, she began to scream and strike out at the neighbour.

The daughter visits immediately and discovers that her mother does not know who she is, does not know what time it is, appears dishevelled, and is suspicious that people have been in her home stealing the things she cannot find. Mrs. Campbell does not recall taking any medication, but when her daughter investigates she finds that 10 pills of the

new sleeping aid have already been used. Mrs. Campbell is irritable and refuses to go to the hospital, but over the course of a few hours, she appears to calm down, and the following morning her daughter is able to take her to see her physician. After hearing the history, the physician hospitalizes Mrs. Campbell, withholds all medication, and provides intravenous hydration. Within 3 days, she is again able to recognize her daughter, and her mental status appears to be greatly improved.

What Do You Think?

- Identify risk factors that may have contributed to Mrs. Campbell's experiencing delirium.
- How could the addition of an OTC sleeping medication interact with the antihistamine and antidepressant to be responsible for her delirium?

needing immediate attention, as seen in cases of sepsis or myocardial infarction (Voyer et al., 2012). Even though the most widely propagated theory centres on the neurotransmitter system, several theories have identified that the causes relate to brain disturbances such as inflammation, physiologic stress, oxygen supply, and sleep–wake cycle. The burden of proof for such diverse hypotheses varies from the role of melatonin to imbalance between dopamine and acetylcholine activity in the brain (van Munster et al., 2009). Major theories of causation are

- A general reduction in brain functioning, which can result from a decrease in the supply, uptake, or use of substances for metabolic activity
- Damage of enzyme systems, the blood–brain barrier, or cell membranes
- Reduced brain metabolism resulting in decreased acetylcholine synthesis
- Imbalance of neurotransmitters such as acetylcholine, norepinephrine, and dopamine
- Increased plasma cortisol level in response to acute stress, which affects attention and information processing
- Involvement of the white matter, especially in the thalamocortical projections (Tune, 2000)
- Direct brain insults that reflect dysfunction or damage of the brain, resulting from mainly indiscriminate effects such as hypoxia or metabolic disturbance (Maclullich et al., 2008)

Interdisciplinary Treatment and Priority Care

Delirium may be recognized and diagnosed in any health care setting, and the interdisciplinary team needs to act promptly to reverse the symptoms (Heidrich, 2007). The management of delirium includes four key steps: (1) elimination or correction of the underlying cause(s), (2) management of behavioural disturbances, (3) anticipation and prevention of complications of delirium, and (4) support and restoration of functional needs (White & Bayer, 2007). A current challenge to the potential use of nondrug therapy interventions is the lack of controlled trials that evaluate drug therapy, dosing schedules, or combination regimens (Candy et al., 2012).

When developing a treatment plan for a patient in whom delirium is suspected, close attention must be paid to correcting any organic or disease-related factors. Initially, life-threatening illnesses must be ruled out or corrected, such as cerebral hypoxia, hypertensive encephalopathy, intracranial haemorrhage, meningitis, severe electrolyte and metabolic imbalances, hypoglycaemia, and intoxication. If possible, the use of all suspected medications should be stopped and vital signs monitored at least every 2 hours. Many patients with delirium are seriously ill, thus necessitating close or constant nursing care. An observational study over a 6-month period found a low rate of detection of delirium (13%) and individual delirium

symptoms (32% to 58%) by nurses (Voyer et al., 2012). The plan of care requires close observation for changes in vital signs, behaviour, and mental status. Patients are monitored until the delirium subsides. If the delirium still exists at discharge, it is critical that referrals be implemented for postdischarge follow-up assessment and care.

Nursing Management: Human Response to Delirium

By definition, a biologic insult must be present for delirium to occur, but psychological and environmental factors are often involved. Because delirium develops in a matter of hours or days and has been associated with increased mortality, nurses should be particularly vigilant in assessing patients who are at increased risk for this syndrome. (If the patient is a child, the assessment process presented in Chapter 30 should be used.) If the patient is an older person, the assessment that follows will serve as a guide. Special efforts should be made to include family members in the nursing process.

> ● **STUDY NOTE**
>
> Nurses need to be able to differentiate between the characteristics of dementia and those of delirium. Particular attention should be paid to the scores of items appearing on both scales for delirium and dementia. Remember it is possible to have delirium superimposed on dementia (DSD); therefore, if agitation and a sudden change in mental status occur, assess the person for delirium.

Biologic Domain

Biologic Assessment

The onset of symptoms is typically signalled by a rapid or acute change in behaviour. To assess the symptoms, the nurse needs to know what is normal for the individual. Caregivers, family members, or significant others may be the only resource for accurate information and should be interviewed.

Current and Past Health Status

History should include a description of the onset, duration, range, and intensity of associated symptoms. Chronic physical illness, dementia, depression, other psychiatric illnesses, referrals, and any past hospitalizations should be identified. Sorting out historical information may be particularly problematic when delirium accompanies acute illness, recent surgery, or infection.

Physical Examination and Review of Systems

In an attempt to discover the underlying cause of suspected delirium, monitoring of vital signs is crucial. An examination of body systems needs to be conducted. Laboratory data are gathered, including complete blood count, blood/urine glucose, blood urea nitrogen, creatinine, serum electrolyte analyses, liver function, and oxygen saturation levels. Fluid balance and bowel action disturbances relating to constipation or a recent history of diarrhoea should be assessed.

Physical Functions

A functional assessment includes physical functional status (activities of daily living [ADL]), the use of sensory aids (eyeglasses, contact lenses, and hearing aids), mobility aids, dentures/braces, sleep pattern, usual activity level and any recent changes, and pain assessment. Sleep disturbances are a symptom of delirium and may precipitate confusion. Often, the sleep–wake cycle of the patient becomes reversed, with the individual attempting to sleep during the day and be awake at night. Restoration of a normal sleep cycle is extremely important.

Pharmacologic Assessment

A substance use history (including alcohol intake and smoking) should be obtained (see Chapters 26 and 35). Information regarding medication use must be obtained, with particular attention given to new medications or changes in the dose or strength of current medications. Table 34-2 lists some of the drugs that can cause an acute change in mental status. Special attention should be given to combinations of medications because drug interactions can cause delirium.

Information regarding OTC medications should be included in this assessment. OTC medications are often thought of as harmless, but several medications, such as cold medications, taken in sufficient quantities may produce restlessness and confusion, especially in children and older individuals.

Findings from the medication and physical assessments are integrated and analyzed with a focus on improving health outcomes. Chronic pain may lead an individual to use more medication than has been intended. The increase in medication then results in delirium. Careful monitoring of the effectiveness of pain medications may be supportive in the order of a more effective medication that results in less potential misuse. Because many classes of medications have been associated with delirium, the focus is on changes in the type and number of medications and how medications relate to other findings in the history and physical assessment.

Nursing Diagnoses for the Biologic Domain

The nursing diagnoses typically generated from assessment data are acute confusion, impaired memory, disturbed thought processes, impaired environmental interpretation syndrome, or disturbed sensory perception (visual or auditory) (North American Nursing Diagnosis Association [NANDA], 2012). However, an astute nurse

Table 34-2   Categories of Drugs That Can Cause "Acute Change in Mental Status"*

Mnemonic: ACUTE CHANGE IN MS

Drug Category	Examples of Drugs
Antiparkinsonian drugs	Trihexyphenidyl, benzatropine, bromocriptine, levodopa, selegiline (deprenyl)
Corticosteroids	Prednisolone
Urinary incontinence drugs	Oxybutynin (Ditropan), flavoxate (Urispas)
Theophylline	Theophylline
Emptying drugs (motility drugs)	Metoclopramide (Reglan), cisapride (Propulsid)
Cardiovascular drugs (including antihypertensives)	Digoxin, quinidine, methyldopa, reserpine, beta blockers (propranolol—to a less amount), diuretics, ACE inhibitors (captopril, enalapril), calcium channel antagonists (nifedipine, verapamil, diltiazem)
H$_2$ blockers	Cimetidine (uncommon on its own but increased risk with renal impairment)
Antimicrobials	Cephalosporins, penicillin, quinolones, others
NSAIDs	Indomethacin, ibuprofen, naproxen, salicylate compounds
Geropsychiatry drugs	1. Tricyclic antidepressants (e.g., amitriptyline, desipramine—to a lesser extent, imipramine, nortriptyline)
	2. SSRIs—safer but watch if hyponatraemia present
	3. Benzodiazepines (e.g., diazepam)
	4. Antipsychotics (e.g., haloperidol [Haldol], chlorpromazine, risperidone)
ENT drugs	Antihistamines, decongestants, cough syrups in OTC preparations
Insomnia	Nitrazepam, flurazepam, diazepam, temazepam
Narcotics	Meperidine, pentazocine (risky)
Muscle relaxants	Cyclobenzaprine (Flexeril), methocarbamol (Robaxin)
Seizure drugs	Phenytoin, primidone

*This table notes some examples of possible medications that can contribute to delirium. It is the physiologic status of the older adult and the combination of medications, among other factors, that increase risk. Therefore: "Watch and Beware."
Reprinted from Flaherty, J. H. (1998). Commonly prescribed and over the counter medications: Causes of confusion. *Clinics in Geriatric Medicine, 14*(1), 101–125, copyright (1998), with permission from Elsevier.

will also use nursing diagnoses based on her or his observations linked to indicators such as hyperthermia, dehydration, cyanosis, acute pain, risk for infection, and disturbed sleep pattern. Observation skills are most needful in critically ill/lethargic patients who are voiceless due to the effects of intubation and mechanical ventilation.

Interventions for the Biologic Domain

Important interventions for a patient experiencing acute confusional state include providing a safe, calm, and therapeutic environment; removing the stressor (if possible); and maintaining fluid and electrolyte balance. Nurses are often involved in the assessment of vital signs, blood glucose levels, pulse oximetry monitoring, and interpretation of laboratory or diagnostic profiles related to chemistry studies, drug levels, urinalysis, and arterial blood gas analysis. Other interventions include ensuring adequate nutrition, preventing aspiration and decubitus ulcers, and those related to a particular nursing diagnosis that focus on individual symptoms and underlying causes—for example, for patients with disturbed sleep patterns. Protocols to enhance sleep with an emphasis on noise reduction and appropriate timing of laboratory and/or X-ray tests (if any) have been delineated (Humphries, 2008; Cmiel, Karr, Gasser, Oliphant, & Neveau, 2004) (see Chapter 28). Interventions to prevent delirium can reduce the length of stay in health facilities (Ansaloni et al., 2010; White & Bayer, 2007).

Safety Interventions

Behaviours exhibited by the delirious patient, such as hallucinations, delusions, illusions, aggression, or agitation (restlessness or excitability), may pose safety problems. The patient must be protected from physical harm through the use of low beds, padded guardrails (use with caution when putting up both bedrails, as a confused person may try to climb over the rail), bed alarms, and careful supervision. Risk for injury is a high-priority diagnosis because individuals with delirium are more likely to fall or injure themselves during a confused state (Carpenito-Moyet, 2004). "Prevention of Falls and Fall Injuries in the Older Adult" (RNAO, 2005, updated 2011) is a good resource to use for assessment and response to risk for falls.

Pharmacologic Interventions

There is a lack of research to support the use of drugs in the management of delirium; in fact, they may worsen symptoms (White & Bayer, 2007). Pharmacologic treatment of delirium, however, is commonly directed at decreasing agitation and related psychotic symptoms (Balas et al., 2012). The goal of psychopharmacologic management is typically focused on treatment of the behaviours associated with delirium, such as agitation, inattention, sleep disorder, and psychosis, with the aim of making the patient comfortable. The decision to use medications should be based on the specific symptoms. Dosages are usually kept very low. Medications should be chosen with reference to potential side effects (particularly anticholinergic effects, over-sedative effects, hypotension, and respiratory suppression) (see Box 34-3 for research on best practices with respect to use of sedatives). The use of antipsychotic agents in older individuals is discussed in greater detail later in the chapter. To avoid worsening the

---

BOX 34-3 Research for Best Practice

SEDATING MEDICATIONS AND DELIRIUM IN OLDER INPATIENTS

From Rothberg, M., Herzig, S., Pekow, P., Avrunin, J. Lagu, T., & Lindauer, P. (2013). Association between sedating medications and delirium in older inpatients. Journal of the American Geriatrics Society, 61(6), 923–930.

The Objective: To examine the association between sedative medication, identified in the Beers criteria of potentially inappropriate medications (PIM) for older adults, and delirium in a large cohort of hospitalized older patients with common medical conditions.

Methods: A retrospective cohort study was conducted that involved patients at 374 American hospitals (N = 225,028) who were 65+ years of age and admitted over a 22-month period with one of six diagnoses: acute myocardial infarction, chronic pulmonary disease, community-acquired pneumonia, congestive heart failure, ischemic stroke, or urinary tract infection. Hospital-acquired delirium was defined as initiation of an antipsychotic medication or restraints on hospital day 3 or later. Chi-square and t-tests were carried out to assess associations between delirium, participant characteristics, and sedative use. Regression analysis was used to model the association between sedation and delirium. A second "nested case–control" study was conducted with matched controls (matched on hospital, primary diagnosis, sex, and

age within 3 years) identified for each delirium case. The controls had a length of stay at least as long as the time when treatment for delirium began in their matched case. Cases and controls were assessed for treatment with the sedatives of interest to the study (i.e., identified in Beers criteria).

Findings: The median age of the sample was 82 years with 17% (38,883 patients) receiving one or more sedative medications. Four percent of participants were identified as having hospitalized delirium. In the cohort study, diphenhydramine and short-acting benzodiazepines were associated with greater risk of subsequent delirium. In the case–control study, both short- and long-acting benzodiazepines, diphenhydramine, and promethazine were associated with delirium. Amitriptyline and muscle relaxants were not associated with delirium in either study. Patients with delirium had longer length of stay, higher costs, and higher mortality than patients who did not experience delirium.

Implications for Nursing: The prevalence of sedation use in older hospitalized adults and the associated risk for delirium warrants a high level of vigilance by nurses. It appears that sedative medications identified as PIM are commonly prescribed and that some are associated with more risk for delirium than others are. Further investigation is needed.

patient's condition, benzodiazepines should be used only when the delirium is related to alcohol withdrawal, but polypharmacy is not encouraged at this point. In some patients, the sedation effect may further impair cognition or a paradoxic agitation may develop (Gleason, 2003).

Administering and Monitoring Medications

Patients experiencing delirium may resist taking medications because of their confusion. If a medication is given, ideally it should be oral. Medications should *not* be hidden in food.

Monitoring and Managing Side Effects.

Monitoring drug action and side effects is especially important because the cause of the delirium may not be known, and the patient may inadvertently be affected by the medication. Both aripiprazole and haloperidol have been shown to be effective in providing relief from delirium symptoms, but aripiprazole was found to be more tolerable due to lack of extrapyramidal side effects (Boettger, Friedlander, Breitbart, & Passik, 2011, p. 481). Patients should be monitored for sedation, hypotension, or extrapyramidal symptoms such as dystonia, repetitive, involuntary muscle movements (e.g., lip smacking), and/or an extreme urge to be moving constantly. Although mental status often fluctuates during delirium, it may also be influenced by these medications, and any changes or worsening of mental status after the administration of the medication should be reported immediately to the prescriber. Some side effects may also be confused with the symptoms of delirium. For example, akathisia (see Chapter 12) may appear to be agitation or restlessness. The patient's physical condition and concurrent medication regimen may also influence the bioavailability, metabolism, distribution, and elimination of these medications. Adequate hydration and nutrition must be maintained. When using antipsychotic medications, closely monitor the patient for symptoms of neuroleptic malignant syndrome (see Chapter 12). The appearance of these symptoms may be confused with those related to delirium and therefore missed.

The use of medications for treating symptoms related to delirium should be discontinued as soon as possible, but these medications should be withdrawn gradually during a period of several days or weeks.

Identifying Drug Interactions.

The aetiology of delirium is often a drug–drug interaction. OTC sleeping, cold, or allergy medication may be the cause. It is the nurse's responsibility to critically review each patient's medication record and discuss findings with the attending physician/nurse practitioner to avoid drug over-dosage and intoxication, which can worsen symptoms. If medication is the underlying cause, it is important to identify accurately which medications are involved before administering any other drugs. Consultation with a clinical pharmacist may also be helpful, but exploring a patient's medication history in a physical assessment allows access

to relevant data for guiding the care plan. Many of the medications used to treat symptoms of delirium (e.g., restlessness, altered sleep cycle) may in fact have potential side effects that worsen symptoms (Balas et al., 2012).

Teaching Points

To prevent future occurrences, the nurse needs to educate the patient, family, and caregivers about the underlying causes and predisposing factors related to delirium. If the delirium is not resolved before discharge, caregivers need to know how to care for the patient at home and offer information on where to receive additional community or social welfare support.

Psychological Domain

Assessment

The psychological assessment of the individual with delirium focuses on cognitive changes revealed through the mental status examination as well as the resulting behavioural manifestations. Since nurses are with patients around the clock, they are often the key interdisciplinary team members who first notice that the patient is experiencing a change in mental status or other indications of distress such as pain, anxiety, and behavioural changes. A needs-based care plan can then be implemented to promote the patient's comfort and safety. Changes in mental status must be monitored frequently for an early detection of delirium, especially in older individuals. In addition, other factors such as stressors and environmental changes may contribute to the symptoms.

Mental Status

Rapid onset of global cognitive impairment that affects multiple aspects of intellectual functioning is the hallmark of delirium. An essential nonpharmacologic nursing intervention for a patient experiencing delirium is to identify and help correct any unstable physiologic and haemodynamic conditions that evoke an acute change in mental status, such as sepsis, poisoning, or drug intoxication. Mental status evaluation usually reveals several changes such as:

- Fluctuations in the level of consciousness with a reduced awareness of the environment
- Difficulty focusing and sustaining or shifting attention
- Severely impaired memory, especially immediate and recent memory

Patients may be disoriented to time and place but rarely to person. Environmental perceptions are often disturbed. The patient may believe that shadows in the room are really people. Thought content is often illogical, and speech may be incoherent or inappropriate to context. Each variation in mental status tends to fluctuate over the course of the day. On any given day, an individual with delirium may appear confused and uncooperative but later may be lucid and able to follow instructions.

BOX 34-4 Rating Scales for Use With Delirium

The Confusion Assessment Method (CAM)
Inouye, S. K., van Dyck, C. H., Alessi, C. A., Balkin, S., Siegal, A. P., & Horwitz, R. I. (1990). Clarifying confusion: The confusion assessment method. *Annals of Internal Medicine, 113*, 941–948.

Delirium Rating Scale (DRS)-R-98
Trzepacz, P. T., Mittal D., Torres, R., Kanary, K., Norton, J., & Jimerson, N. (2001). Validation of the Delirium Rating Scale-revised-98: Comparison with the delirium rating scale and the cognitive test for delirium. *Journal of Neuropsychiatry and Clinical Neurosciences, 13*, 229–242.

Neecham Confusion Scale
Registered Nurses Association of Ontario. (2003). Neecham confusion scale. *Screening for delirium, dementia and depression in older adults*, Appendix G, pp. 66–71. Available at www.rnao.org/bestpractices

Nurses must assess and document the cognitive status of the individual throughout the day so that interventions can be modified accordingly.

Calculations, orientation (especially to time), and recall are most affected in delirium, whereas naming and registration are relatively preserved. Several rating scales are available for use in assessing the cognitive and behavioural fluctuations of delirium (Box 34-4).

Behaviour

Delirious patients exhibit a wide range of behaviours, complicating the process of making a diagnosis and planning interventions. At times, the individual may be restless or agitated, and at other times, lethargic and slow to respond. Precautions to prevent falls, aspiration, and accidental self-inflicted injuries should be established to ensure patient safety. Delirium can be categorized into three types:

- **Hyperactive delirium** involves behaviours such as being overly alert, exhibiting disturbing episodes of psychomotor hyperactivity, and marked excitability (may hallucinate). The patient may scream out in fear, describe hallucinations, pull at tubes, attempt to climb out of bed, and may attempt to hit staff (Balas et al., 2012).

- **Hypoactive delirium** is marked by lethargy, sleepiness, apathy, and psychomotor slowing; this is the "quiet" patient for whom the diagnosis of delirium often is missed (especially in seriously ill patients), as such patients often remain withdrawn or lie quietly in bed.

- **Mixed delirium** involves behaviour that fluctuates between the hyperactive and the hypoactive states over brief or long periods.

Nursing Diagnoses for the Psychological Domain

The nursing diagnosis of acute confusion is also associated with impaired cognitive functioning. Although the underlying cause of confusion is physiologic, nursing care should focus on the psychological domain, as well as the physical. Other typical nursing diagnoses related to the psychological domain include risk for acute confusion, disturbed thought process, ineffective coping, disturbed personal identity, and deficient knowledge (specify).

Interventions for the Psychological Domain

Staff members should have frequent interactions with patients and support them with institutional and community resources if they are confused, experiencing illusions, or hallucinating. Patients should be encouraged to express their fears and discomforts that result from frightening or disconcerting psychotic experiences. Adequate lighting, easy-to-read calendars and clocks, a quiet noise level, and frequent verbal orientation may reduce this frightening experience. If the patient wears eyeglasses or uses a hearing aid, these devices should be used. Including familiar personal possessions such as favourite clothing and footwear, or wall paintings in the environment, may also help. Interventions that may be useful for these individuals are discussed in detail later in the chapter (see the section on dementia).

Social Domain

Assessment

Discussions should be initiated with the family to determine whether the patient's behaviours are new. An assessment of living arrangements may provide information about sensory stimulation or social isolation. Cultural and educational background must be considered when the patient's mental capacity is evaluated. Individuals from certain ethnic backgrounds may not be familiar with the information used in tests of general knowledge (e.g., names of prime ministers, geographic knowledge), memory (e.g., date of birth in cultures that do not routinely celebrate birthdays), and orientation (e.g., sense of placement and location may be conceptualized differently in some cultures) (APA, 2000). Some cultural practices may involve using substances such as elixirs that contain chemicals that may exacerbate delirium. The assessment should be language specific and must address such practices, as well as exploring other relevant culture-specific practices.

Family Roles

Delirium is a burden not only for the patient but also for the patient's family caregivers (Balas et al., 2012). Family support for the individual and understanding of the disorder must therefore be assessed. The behaviours exhibited by the person experiencing delirium may be frightening or at least confusing for family members and significant others. Some family members may actually contribute to the patient's increased agitation. Observing and assessing family interactions and family members' ability to understand delirium is important. If feasible, family presence may help to calm and reassure the patient.

Behavioural interventions related to repeated orientation of patients and encouragement of the presence of relatives known to the patient may potentially reduce psychological stress with its associated cortisol levels (Maclullich et al., 2008, p. 235).

Nursing Diagnoses for the Social Domain

Among the several nursing diagnoses associated with the social domain, the most typical are interrupted family processes, ineffective protection, ineffective role performance, ineffective community coping, and risk for injury.

Interventions for the Social Domain

The environment needs to be safe to protect the patient from injuries. A predictable, orienting environment will help to reestablish order to the patient's life. That is, a calendar, clock, music, and other items may be provided to help orient the patient to time, place, and person. If the patient is agitated, de-escalation techniques should be used (see Chapter 11). Physical restraint should be avoided as much as possible.

Support for Families

Families can be encouraged to work with staff members to reorient the patient and provide a supportive environment. Families need to understand that important decisions requiring the patient's input should be delayed if possible until the patient has fully recovered. Although patients may be able to participate in decision making, they may not remember the decision later; it is therefore important to have several witnesses present and to document and keep record of any images and information in an ethical manner.

Spiritual Domain

Because delirium involves global cognitive impairment, including fluctuations in the level of consciousness and severely impaired memory, and may include agitation or lethargy, persons with delirium are very dependent on others for their comfort, dignity, and spiritual well-being. Communication and connection with others is often seriously affected, and the nurse will need to enact well the critical qualities of spiritual care: receptivity, humanity, competency, and positivity (see Chapter 11). Patients experiencing hallucinations, delusions, and/or illusions in delirium may understand them as having a spiritual cause or ancestral connection or purpose. This can make them more or less frightening at the time, depending on the meaning attributed to them, particularly if a family member had undergone a similar experience ending in a poor outcome. The patient may benefit from a visit offered by his or her spiritual leader. Once the delirium passes, the person may want to discuss such experiences (if remembered). The confusion of delirium necessitates, for the most part, that spiritual care of the patient is intensively "in the moment," as the nurse strives to sustain the person through the episode with family and religious support.

Evaluation and Treatment Outcomes

The primary treatment goal is the prevention or resolution of the delirious episode with return to previous cognitive status. Outcome measures include

- Correction of the underlying physiologic alteration
- Resolution of confusion
- Family member verbalization of understanding of confusion
- Prevention of injury

Resolution of confusion is the primary goal; however, the nurse makes important contributions to all four of these outcomes. The end result of delirium is full recovery, incomplete recovery, incomplete recovery with some residual cognitive impairment, or a downward course leading to death.

Continuum of Care

The nurse may encounter patients with delirium in a number of management settings (e.g., home, nursing home, ambulatory care, day treatment, outpatient setting, hospital). Patients usually are admitted to an acute care setting for rapid evaluation and treatment of the underlying aetiology. An abrupt change in cognitive status can also occur while the patient is hospitalized for another reason. Delirium often persists beyond discharge from the hospital. Discharge planning should routinely include family education and referrals to community health care providers and social welfare facilities. If the patient will return to a residential long-term care setting, communication with facility staff about the patient's hospital stay, family support, and treatment regimen is crucial. Education of family members of persons with delirium (reversible or irreversible) in palliative care settings is also important (Irwin, Pirrello, Hirst, Buckholz, & Ferris, 2013). For a checklist of psychoeducational topics to guide teaching of caregivers of individuals with delirium, see Box 34-5.

BOX 34-5 Psychoeducation Checklist: Delirium

When caring for the patient with delirium, be sure to include the caregivers, as appropriate, and address the following topic areas in the teaching plan:
- Psychopharmacologic agents, if used, including drug action, dosage, frequency, and possible adverse effects
- Underlying cause of delirium
- Mental status changes
- Safety measures
- Hydration and nutrition
- Avoidance of restraints
- Decision-making guidelines

DSD occurs when a patient with dementia develops a delirium (Fick, Hodo, Lawrence, & Inouye, 2007). The co-occurrence of delirium and dementia (overlap syndrome) substantially impairs functional recovery from acute illness and hospitalization, as compared with those affected by depression or delirium alone. This suggests that depression and delirium act in an additive and independent fashion to produce higher rates of adverse outcomes (Givens et al., 2009). The overlap syndrome carries significant risk for functional decline and nursing home placement, as well as increased incidence of death in the following year; research is needed to elucidate specific mechanisms underlying this increased risk (Givens et al., 2009).

DSD is often poorly identified or misdiagnosed. Fick et al. (2007) used case vignettes to assess experienced nurses' recognition of DSD. The researchers found that nurses were more able to recognize dementia and hyperactive delirium than dementia and hypoactive delirium (or hypoactive delirium alone). These case vignettes can be used as a learning tool for nurses.

DEMENTIA

Dementia is an irreversible syndrome characterized by ongoing decline in intellectual functioning sufficient to disrupt physical, social, and/or occupational functioning. Dementia falls within three categories: early-onset familial AD; rapidly progressive dementia such as Creutzfeldt-Jakob disease (CJD), which is a mandatory reportable condition in Canada; and later-onset dementia, which includes four primary types of dementia: AD, vascular dementia, dementia with Lewy bodies (DLB), and frontotemporal dementia (FTD).

ALZHEIMER'S DISEASE

In 1901, Alois Alzheimer observed Auguste Deter, a 51-year-old patient at the Frankfurt Asylum who exhibited strange behavioural symptoms and memory disturbance. The patient died 5 years later, but the neuropathology results revealed neuritic plaques and neurofibrillary tangles; over the years, this discovery became consistent and was named AD (Kaiser et al., 2012). Statistics Canada (2013) reports that 12.8 individuals out of every 100,000 Canadians died of AD in 2008.

Clinical Course of Disorder

AD is a progressive neurodegenerative disorder characterized by memory loss, irreversible cognitive deficits, and behavioural changes (Carter, Resnick, Mallampalli, & Kalbarczyk, 2012). It is typified by forgetfulness and is sometimes referred to as "the dotage" (Tasci, Kartin, Ceyhan, Sungur, & Göris, 2012). The person's ability to function gradually declines, although physical status often remains intact until late in the disease. AD is a terminal illness.

Generally seen at age 50, AD's prevalence doubles every 5 years after the age of 60; at 65 years, it is seen in 6% to 10% of the population and by 85 years and above in 30% to 47% (California Workgroup on Guidelines for Alzheimer's Disease Management, 2008). Two subtypes have been identified: the less common early-onset AD (familial symptoms of dementia starting before age 65) and late-onset AD (older than 65 years). AD is also routinely conceptualized in terms of three stages: early, middle, and late. Signs and symptoms of AD change as the patient passes from one stage of the illness to another (Table 34-3). Persons with AD tend to pass through a specific sequence of deterioration and symptoms (Forbes et al., 2012). Staging (i.e., identifying the stage the patient

Table 34-3	Stages of Dementia

Early Stages
Forgetfulness
Problems with orientation (e.g., cannot follow directions)
Communication difficulties
Limited attention span
Difficulty learning new things
Changes in mood and behaviour
May understand how they are changing and may wish to help plan and direct future care

Middle Stages
Memory problems are obvious (e.g., does not know address, own history)
Restlessness (e.g., wandering, pacing)
Spatial problems that may affect mobility
Confused, difficulty following a topic of conversation
Problems understanding verbal and written language
Changes in wake–sleep patterns; lack of appetite
Apprehensive and/or withdrawn
Uninhibited behaviour
Delusions and hallucinations

Late Stage
Severe cognitive impairment (memory, information processing, orientation)
Closes capacity for recognizable speech
Needs help with eating, toileting; may be incontinent
Loses ability to walk without assistance, to sit without support, to smile, hold head up
May have impaired swallowing and loss of weight

End of Life
Changes in blood circulation; skin breakdown
No longer accepting food and drink
Increased sleepiness; changes in breathing
Agitation
May have buildup of secretions; fever
Still experiences and senses emotion
Spiritual experience may be important

Adapted from Alzheimer Society of Canada. (2013a). Stages of Alzheimer's disease (what happens). Available at http://www.alzheimer.ca/en/About-dementia/Alzheimer-s-disease/Stages-of-Alzheimer-s-disease. Refer to this site to see strategies for responding to the symptoms of each stage.

Table 34-4	Key Diagnostic Characteristics of Alzheimer's Disease

Diagnostic Criteria	Symptoms
Impaired ability to acquire and remember information	Repetitive questions or conversations, misplacing personal belongings, forgetting events or appointments, getting lost on a familiar route.
Impaired reasoning and handling of complex tasks, poor judgement	Poor understanding of safety risks, inability to manage finances, poor decision-making ability, inability to plan complex or sequential activities.
Impaired visuospatial abilities	Inability to recognize faces or common objects or to find objects in direct view despite good visual acuity, inability to operate simple implements, or orient clothing to the body.
Impaired language functions (speaking, reading, writing)	Difficulty thinking of common words while speaking, hesitations; speech, spelling, and writing errors.
Changes in personality, behaviour, or comportment	Uncharacteristic mood fluctuations such as agitation; impaired motivation, initiative, apathy; loss of drive; social withdrawal; decreased interest in previous activities; loss of empathy; compulsive or obsessive behaviours; socially unacceptable behaviours.

Source: Canadian Dementia Knowledge Translation Network (CDKTN). (2012). Recommendations for the diagnosis and treatment of dementia 2012: Based on the Canadian Consensus Conference on the Diagnosis and Treatment of Dementia 2012 (CCCDTD4). Retrieved from http://www.slideboom.com/presentations/702016/Canadian-Consensus-Conference-2012-Dementia-Diagnosis-and-Treatment-Recommendations

is experiencing) is a useful technique for determining the person's current cognitive status and provides a sound basis for decisions in clinical management. People with AD live an average of 8 years with the disease, but some people may survive up to 20 years. The course of the disease depends in part on age at diagnosis and whether a person has other health conditions (see Alzheimer's Association, 2013a).

Diagnostic Criteria

The Canadian diagnostic criteria for dementia were reevaluated in 2012 by the fourth Canadian Consensus Conference on the Diagnosis and Treatment of Dementia (CCCDTD4). The new criteria are based on those of the National Institute on Aging (NIA) and the Alzheimer's Association, both based in the United States. The criteria for AD include cognitive and/or behavioural symptoms that (1) interfere with the ability to function at work or at usual activities; (2) represent a decline from previous levels of functioning and performing; and (3) are not related to delirium or a major psychiatric disorder. Cognitive impairment is detected and diagnosed through a combination of history taking from the person and a knowledgeable informant and an objective cognitive assessment, such as a mental status examination. Neuropsychologic testing should only be performed when the routine history and mental status examination cannot provide a confident diagnosis (Canadian Dementia Knowledge Translation Network [CDKTN], 2012).

The cognitive and/or behavioural impairment must involve a minimum of two of the following domains: (1) impaired ability to acquire and remember new and retained information; (2) impaired reasoning and handling of complex tasks, poor judgement; (3) impaired visuospatial abilities; (4) impaired language functions (speaking, reading,

writing); and (5) changes in personality, behaviour, or comportment (CDKTN, 2012). Table 34-4 lists the presenting symptoms related to each of these criteria. Box 34-6 lists 10 warning signs of AD. Clinical diagnosis is therefore based on the patient's detailed history, a comprehensive physical and neurologic examination, and the application of established diagnostic criteria that are reliable and valid. Diagnosis may be supported through neuropsychological testing and diagnostic investigations, such as neuroimaging of the brain to detect and monitor progressive atrophy. Cerebrospinal fluid (CSF) examination is not routinely performed to detect biomarkers, but it would be expected to be acellular with no signs of oligoclonal band (Schott & Warren, 2012). Where possible, testing for CSF β-amyloid (Aβ) 1–42 (low) and tau or phosphorylated tau (raised) would support a diagnosis of AD (Blennow, Hampel, Weiner, & Zetterburg, 2010).

Table 34-4 lists essential symptoms of dementia, along with other possible behavioural and psychological changes that may or may not be present. Both delirium

BOX 34-6 Ten Warning Signs of AD

To help the public know the warning signs of AD, the Alzheimer Society of Canada lists the following:
1. Memory loss that affects day-to-day function
2. Difficulty performing familiar tasks
3. Problems with language
4. Disorientation of time and place
5. Poor or decreased judgement
6. Problems with abstract thinking
7. Misplacing things
8. Changes in mood and behaviour
9. Changes in personality
10. Loss of initiative

See http://www.alzheimer.ca for more information.

and dementia are characterized by global cognitive impairment and may present diagnostic challenges in differentiation, but DSD may show a prolonged and refractory course (Boettger, Passik, & Breitbart, 2011).

Mild Cognitive Impairment

According to the Alzheimer's Association (2013b), long-term studies suggest that 10% to 20% of those aged 65 years and older may have MCI. The diagnostic criteria for MCI include a change in cognition over time in comparison with the person's previous level of performance. In addition, the cognitive performance is lower than expected for the person's age and education level. This change can occur in a variety of cognitive domains, including memory, executive function, attention, language, and visuospatial skills. An impairment in episodic memory (i.e., the ability to learn and retain new information) is seen most commonly in MCI patients who subsequently progress to a diagnosis of AD dementia. Persons with MCI commonly have mild problems performing complex functional tasks such as paying bills, preparing a meal, or shopping. They may take more time, be less efficient, and make more errors at performing such activities than in the past. Nevertheless, they generally maintain their independence of function in daily life, with minimal aids or assistance (CDKTN, 2012). It is not yet possible to tell for certain what the outcome of MCI will be for a specific person or to determine the underlying cause of MCI from a person's symptoms (Alzheimer's Association, 2013b).

Epidemiology and Risk Factors

In 2011, 15% of Canadians aged 65 years and older (roughly 747,000 people) were living with cognitive impairment including dementia. By 2031, at the current rate, this figure will increase to 1.4 million. The economic impact of dementia, in both direct costs (e.g., medical) and indirect costs (e.g., lost salary), totals $33 billion per year. If nothing changes, this number will by 2040 climb to $293 billion (Alzheimer Society of Canada [ASC], 2012).

Age is the most acknowledged risk factor for developing AD. It is estimated that dementia affects 1 in 14 people over the age of 65 and 1 in 6 over the age of 80. Females are at higher risk, even discounting the fact that they tend to live longer. A gene called apolipoprotein E (ApoE) has been shown to play a small part in the development of AD and vascular dementia. Specifically, the ApoE4 variant somehow preferentially promotes the production of the A-beta protein, constituting a significant risk. It is also possible to inherit genes that cause dementia such as familial early-onset AD and Huntington's disease. Conditions that affect the heart, arteries, or blood circulation all significantly affect a person's chances of developing dementia, particularly vascular dementia.

These conditions include diabetes, midlife high blood pressure, high blood cholesterol levels, midlife obesity, heart problems, and stroke. Indeed, a history of stroke doubles the risk of dementia in older adults. People who experience severe or repeated head injuries are at increased risk of dementia. On the other hand, there is evidence that lifestyle factors such as a Mediterranean diet, regular physical activity, moderate (250 to 500 mL/day) amounts of alcohol, and social and mental activities may reduce the risk of dementia (Alzheimer Society UK, 2013; van den Berg & Splaine, 2012).

The controversy over aluminium exposure and brain toxicity has not disappeared. Research suggests that aluminium is linked to neurotoxicity and even dementia (Shaw & Tomljenovic, 2013). Aluminium is found in higher concentrations in the brains of Alzheimer's patients (Walton, 2013), and there is growing concern that aluminium is involved in the development of AD (De Sole et al., 2013). A preliminary study found that drinking silicon-rich mineral water helps remove aluminium from the body and may improve cognition (Zhang, Sheng, & Qin, 2013).

Aetiology

Researchers have yet to identify a definitive cause of AD. In the brain of a person with AD, the cortex shrivels up, damaging areas involved in thinking, planning, and remembering. Shrinkage is especially severe in the hippocampus that plays a key role in formation of new memories. Ventricles (fluid-filled spaces within the brain) grow larger (Fig. 34-2).

Magnetic resonance imaging and CSF and/or amyloid positron emission tomography (see Chapter 9) have

FIGURE 34-2. Healthy brain and advanced AD brain. (Courtesy of National Institute on Aging.)

been found supportive in identifying or ruling out the presence of AD pathology; these potentially offer opportunities for improving diagnostic sensitivity and specificity (Schott & Warren, 2012).

Beta-Amyloid Plaques

Following Alois Alzheimer's discovery of neuritic plaques and **neurofibrillary tangles**, accumulations of two separate proteins in the brain—beta-amyloid peptide and tau proteins—have been associated with AD (Casey, 2012). Jack Diamond (2011), Scientific Director Emeritus of the Alzheimer Society of Canada, explains that plaques are made largely of a protein called beta amyloid (A-beta). In low concentrations, A-beta may be part of the body's defences against invading bacteria and other microbes. However, in AD, A-beta accumulates in the brain to a level that overwhelms the enzymes and other molecules that clear away A-beta and the plaques. Both the production of A-beta and, especially, the processes that clear it away appear to be defective, at least in part because the impaired blood vessels in the brain cannot adequately pick up and remove the A-beta. There is evidence that these fine blood vessels proliferate and become leaky, possibly allowing hazardous substances to get into the brain. The accumulating individual A-beta molecules begin to clump together to form small aggregates called oligomers. Their continuing aggregation eventually leads to the formation of the amyloid plaques. However, it is the oligomers, not the plaques, that are the real problem; they appear to be toxic to the brain's nerve cells and, by the time enough A-beta molecules have stuck together to form the plaques, the damage has already been done (Fig. 34-3).

Alpha-synuclein, a protein found in neurons, is thought to play a key role in the remodelling of synapses and in microtubule transport and found to be associated with **beta-amyloid plaques** in AD (Casey, 2012).

FIGURE 34-3. Plaques and tangles. (Courtesy of National Institute on Aging.)

Antibodies to beta amyloid, such as bapineuzumab and solanezumab, are undergoing phase III clinical trials; they are known to reduce the amount of beta-amyloid plaques in the brain, but there is, as yet, little evidence that they improve cognitive function (Casey, 2012).

Neurofibrillary Tangles

Neurofibrillary tangles are made of a protein called tau (Diamond, 2011). Tau is present in normal nerve cells, but in AD, it becomes chemically altered (phosphorylated) and tends to pile up as thread-like tangles, preventing its normal functions. A critical function is to provide a kind of railroad track system inside the nerve cells and along the nerve fibres that are spun off from the cell body. The tau pathways are inside the nerve cells and fibres. Their main role in fibres is to convey essential nutrient and instructional chemicals and tiny organelles (structures) up and down the fibres in both directions. Interruption in this internal transport does not stop the nerve messages, but the tangles choke the cells to death. The first casualties of the compromised internal transport system are the distant nerve endings, which are especially vulnerable. The synapses deteriorate, impairing the transmission of messages to the next cell. The first symptoms of AD appear. Synapses are now a prime focus of researchers to find curative therapies. Another important function of the tau protein, which suffers in AD, is its role in nerve sprouting. Sprouting of new branches leads to new connections between nerve cells; not only do more connections help the nerve cells keep communicating with one another as the disease progresses but new sprouts can also help compensate for lost connections. Consequently, a new interest in the cure for AD is towards developing therapies that promote nerve sprouting, including ways to normalize the altered tau protein.

Inflammation

An inflammatory response is normal whenever and wherever the body suffers trauma or is attacked by some kind of potentially threatening influence, such as an infection or a toxin. Neuroinflammation is the inflammatory response that occurs in the brain of the person with AD. Unfortunately, with AD, this inflammatory immune response can become excessive; the brain's immune cells (microglia) become overactive and instead of helping, they actually worsen the situation by overproducing substances that can promote the death of cells and possibly also contribute the formation of tangles. As well, although not yet proven to result from the inflammation, AD appears to cause both proliferation and impairments of the brain's blood vessels, changes that exacerbate the progression of the disease (Diamond, 2011).

Oxidative Stress and the Role of Antioxidants

Oxidative stress refers to the threatening situation created when reactive oxygen species (ROS) begin to accumulate faster than the body can get rid of them. ROS are normal products of metabolism. However, if ROS are allowed to build up, they become damaging, poisoning the cells of the body, including those of the brain. Normally, this is prevented by the body's antioxidants. Natural antioxidants also occur in food, such as vitamins C and E.

Unfortunately, as AD progresses, the production of ROS increases to levels that overwhelm the available antioxidants, which themselves are reduced by a number of factors, including stress. Probably most of the risk factors for AD contribute to this stress, as does the accumulating A-beta protein. Somewhat paradoxically, in the earlier stages, before the accumulation reaches toxic levels, the A-beta acts as an antioxidant and could represent the body's early protective response to the disease. Oxidative stress is becoming one of the key targets of AD treatments (Diamond, 2011).

Many scientists now believe that oxidative stress is the primary event in AD responsible for the impairment of both mitochondria and calcium regulation. Mitochondria are tiny organelles found in all cells, and their role is critically important in satisfying the cell's energy needs. Mitochondrial impairment in AD is a key factor contributing to the impairment of the brain's nerve cells and the glial cells. There are about 10 glial cells for every nerve cell in the brain, and they have a huge caregiving role in maintaining the health and connectivity of the brain cells. It seems highly likely that many or most of the features of AD are primarily due to direct actions of the disease, not on the nerve cells, but on the glial cells. Sick glial cells lose their ability to maintain the normal healthy functioning of the nerve cells (Diamond, 2011).

In nerve cells, calcium is involved in the creation of nerve messages and their transfer across the synapses to other nerve cells. The concentrations of calcium inside cells have to be rigorously regulated. In AD, calcium regulation is disturbed and nerve cell functions are impaired, eventually affecting cognition and memory storage. One player in the dysregulation of calcium in AD is a gene that has mutated over time; the abnormal genes, and in this instance the consequent impaired calcium regulation, enhance the accumulation of the threatening A-beta protein (Diamond, 2011).

Genetic Factors

The rare familial AD (FAD) is almost totally attributable to genes that have mutated to an extent that makes them function abnormally, and the abnormal functions are responsible for the disease. This form of AD can result from mutations in one of three genes, *APP, PSEN1, or PSEN2* (Genetica Home Reference, 2013). The abnormal genes are passed from generation to generation (Ringman, 2011). Genetic mutations account for only 5% of Alzheimer's cases where the onset is early middle age (Casey, 2012). Genetic forms of AD including trisomy 21 typically involve mutations related to beta-amyloid (Casey, 2012).

Interdisciplinary Treatment

In designing services and interventions, the interdisciplinary team must keep in mind that AD has a progressively deteriorating clinical course and that the anatomic and neurochemical changes that occur in the brain are accompanied by impairments in cognition, affect, behaviour, and psychosocial functioning. The nature and range of information and services needed by patients and families throughout their journey with dementia can vary dramatically at different stages. Pharmacologic intervention modestly improves cognitive symptoms and may subsequently decrease the rate of disease progression, typically at the early stage of AD (Forbes et al., 2012).

For a variety of reasons (e.g., stigma, reluctance of family physicians to make a diagnosis as they believe little can be done), many persons with dementia never receive a diagnosis of dementia, which limits their ability to receive appropriate treatment and services. Heightening awareness of the importance of receiving an informed diagnosis, possibly from a neurologist or geriatrician, is strongly recommended. Initial assessment of the person suspected of having dementia has three main objectives: (1) confirmation of the diagnosis through neuropsychological testing and diagnostic investigations, such as neuroimaging of the brain type and severity of dementia; (2) establishment of baseline levels in a number of functional spheres; and (3) establishment of a therapeutic relationship with the patient and family that will continue through subsequent phases of the disease. Treatment efforts currently focus on managing the cognitive symptoms, delaying the cognitive decline (e.g., memory loss, confusion, and problems with learning, speech, and reasoning), treating the noncognitive symptoms (e.g., psychosis, mood symptoms, agitation), and supporting the caregivers as a means of improving the quality of life for both patients and their family and friend caregivers. Patients with both delirium and dementia (overlapping syndrome) may require more intensive rehabilitation services at home or in postacute facilities since they have a higher likelihood of functional decline in ADL 1 month postdischarge (Givens et al., 2009).

Priority Care Issues

The priority of care for AD will change throughout its course. There appears to be four phases of health care experience for persons with dementia and their caregivers, each with health service implications, a meta-analysis of studies has determined (Prorok, Horgan, & Seitz, 2013). In the first phase, *seeking information and understanding*, there is distress regarding the changes in the individual and uncertainty about what is happening, a situation which public awareness and education could, at least in part, relieve. *Identifying the problem* comes with the formal diagnosis of dementia, bringing anxiety but also relief as understanding of the changes is achieved. The *role transition* phase sees both the person with dementia and his or her caregivers beginning to prepare for coping with the illness. It is important that informed support is available to them and goals and treatments wishes are discussed. The final phase, *living with change*, evolves as current and future care needs are focused upon (Prorok et al., 2013).

What may living with such changes be like? A person with dementia usually experiences difficulties remembering the last meal taken or how to use a knife and fork, and confuses names of even close relations, house address, or significant dates. Impaired self-care (loss of ability to perform routine household chores, bathing, dressing, and eating) becomes prominent as the disease progresses. Often, she or he may ask the same questions repetitively, despite answers being previously given. The disease places the person at an increased risk of getting lost, even inside the home. Close observation is necessary outside the home. As the disease progresses, the person becomes highly dependent due to deterioration in physiologic functions (e.g., enuresis) added to the existing cognitive challenges. Initially, the priority is delaying cognitive decline and supporting family members. Later, the priority changes to protecting the person from injury. Near the end, the physical and emotional needs of the person are the focus of care.

Family Response to Disorder

Families are often the first to be aware of the cognitive problems of a loved one. The patient may be unaware of the extent of memory impairment. A diagnosis of AD means long-term care responsibilities, while the essence of the patient diminishes day by day. Nurses need to support patients and their families with education about treatment and choices (Casey, 2012) as well as healthy coping strategies. Most families wish to keep their relative at home as long as possible to maintain contact and to avoid costly nursing home placement. The symptoms that often result in nursing home placement are incontinence that cannot be managed and behavioural problems, such as wandering, especially at night, and aggression.

The needs of family members should also be considered. Caring for a family member with dementia takes its toll. Caregivers' health is often compromised, and normal family functioning is threatened. Caregiver distress is a major health risk for the family, and "caregiver burnout" is a common cause of the institutionalization of patients with dementia.

Nursing Management: Human Response to Alzheimer's Disease

The development and implementation of appropriate, effective, and safe nursing care and services that support patients with dementia and their families are a particular challenge because of the complex nature of the illness. Although AD is caused by biologic changes, the psychological and social domains are seriously affected by this disorder (see Box 34-6). The assessment of the person with AD needs to follow the geriatric mental health nursing assessment in Chapter 33.

Biologic Domain

Assessment

Nursing assessment provides a foundation for the creation of a needs-specific patient care plan since the gathered data serve as evidence for appropriate interventions. Beta-amyloid protein "plaques" in the brain are one of the defining features of AD. However, the effects of beta amyloid on a person's brain and cognitive abilities are not straightforward. Research has shown that up to a third of older people without cognitive problems also have beta-amyloid accumulation in their brains (Rowe et al., 2010). The beta amyloid can be present for years before symptoms of dementia become apparent (Villemagne et al., 2011), and the proportion of those with beta amyloid in their brains who go on to develop AD remains unknown. Thus, at the CCCDTD4, it was recommended that if amyloid imaging technology becomes available in Canada, amyloid imaging must only ever be used in conjunction with a thorough and detailed clinical exam and in consultation with specialists (Gauthier et al., 2012a, 2012b). Further, since it is unknown what proportion of people with positive amyloid scans will go on to develop AD, amyloid imaging should not be used for screening people without symptoms of dementia, as the potential harms outweigh the benefits (ASC, 2013a; CDKTN, 2012).

The nursing assessment should include a medical history, current medication profile (prescription and OTC medications or home and traditional remedies), substance use history (including alcohol intake and smoking history), chronic physical or psychiatric illness, and a description of the onset, duration, range, and intensity of symptoms associated with dementia. Past history of hospitalization and its respective reasons must be noted. The onset of AD symptoms is typically gradual, with insidious changes in behaviour. To conduct a thorough assessment of the patient, the nurse needs to know what is typical for the individual; therefore, caregivers, family members, or significant others can be sources of valuable information.

Physical Examination and a Review of Body Systems

A review of body systems must be conducted on each person suspected of experiencing having AD. Specific biologic assessment parameters include vital signs, neuromuscular status, nutritional and weight status, bladder and bowel function, hygiene, skin integrity, rest and activity level, sleep patterns, and fluid and electrolyte balance. The neurologic function is usually preserved through the early and middle stages of AD, although seizures, gait disturbances, and tremors may occur at any time. Gait issues have long been associated with dementia, but GAITRite can be used as a feasible instrument to assess and predict short-term fall risk in patients with a diagnosis of moderate to severe dementia (Sterke, van Beeck, Looman, Kressig, & van der Cammen, 2012). In the later stages of the disease, neurologic signs such as flexion contractures and primitive reflexes are prominent features.

Physical Functions

At first, limitations may primarily involve instrumental activities, such as shopping, preparing meals, and performing other household chores. Later in the disease process, basic physical dysfunctions occur, such as incontinence, ataxia, dysphagia, and contractures. Incontinence can be a major source of stress and a considerable burden to family caregivers.

Assessment of physical functions includes ADL, recent changes in functional abilities (dressing, toileting, and feeding), use of sensory aids (eyeglasses and hearing aids), activity level, and assessment of pain.

Self-Care

Alterations in the central nervous system (CNS) associated with AD impair the patient's ability to collect information from the environment, retrieve memories, retain new information, and give meaning to current situations. Therefore, patients with dementia often neglect self-care activities such as bathing, eating, and oral and skin care.

Sleep–Wake Disturbances

About one-quarter to a half of older adults with AD and other dementias experience some form of sleep disruption. Diverse nonpharmacologic options are available to support affected persons in the regulation of sleep–wake rhythms (Rose & Lorenz, 2010). The sleep–wake disturbances that commonly occur in persons with dementia are hypersomnia, insomnia, and reversal of the sleep–wake cycle. The disruptions in sleep at night are particularly difficult for family caregivers. The neurobiologic basis of these sleep disorders is related to degenerative changes in the suprachiasmatic nucleus of the hypothalamus that result in the loss of the expression of vasopressin (AVP) mRNA (Liu et al., 2000).

Patients with dementia have frequent daytime napping. Their nighttime periods of wakefulness mean that they have reduced rapid eye movement sleep. Sleep disturbances often increase as dementia advances. Where the patient is unable to provide a reliable sleep history, the nurse must obtain the information from the patient's caregiver. Such history usually encompasses sleep hygiene measures, use of sleep-promoting medications, and history of any sleep difficulties or underlying medical conditions. Increasing daylight exposure, engaging in daytime activities and exercises, and adhering to basic sleep hygiene measures can enhance nighttime sleep.

Activity and Exercise

Despite being physically capable, a person in the early phase of AD will often withdraw from normal activities due to the developing symptoms of memory loss, decrease in self-motivation, and, possibly, depression.

Nutrition

Eating can become a problem for persons with dementia as they may have difficulty chewing and swallowing. As the disease progresses, they may lose the ability to feed themselves or recognize what is offered as food. The hyperactive patient requires frequent feedings of a high-protein, high-carbohydrate diet in the form of finger foods (which they can carry while on the go). Most persons with dementia prefer to feed themselves with their fingers when appropriate rather than have someone feed them. Weight loss is a common consequence. It is important to monitor persons with altered appetites for hydration and electrolyte imbalances.

Pain

Assessment and documentation of any physical discomfort or pain the patient may be experiencing are a part of any psychogeriatric nursing assessment (see Chapter 33). Although AD is not usually thought of as a physically painful disorder, patients often have other comorbid physical diseases. In the early stages of AD, the patient can usually respond to verbal questions regarding pain. Later, it may be difficult to assess the comfort level objectively, especially if the person cannot communicate.

Pain can be assessed through physical examination and use of a pain assessment scale (see http://www.hartfordign.org/ for resources for pain assessment) and through asking the right questions of both the patient and family caregivers (see video by Dr. Romayne Gallager, http://www.alzheimer.ca/en/Living-with-dementia/Caring-for-someone/Late-stage-and-end-of-life).

Nursing Diagnoses for the Biologic Domain

The unique and changing needs of persons with dementia present a challenge for nurses in all settings. A sample of common nursing diagnoses include imbalanced nutrition: less (or more) than body requirements, feeding self-care deficit, impaired swallowing, bathing/hygiene self-care deficit, dressing/grooming self-care deficit, toileting self-care deficit, constipation (or perceived constipation), bowel incontinence, impaired urinary elimination, functional incontinence, total incontinence, deficient fluid volume, risk for impaired skin integrity, impaired physical mobility, activity intolerance, fatigue, disturbed sleep pattern, pain, chronic pain, ineffective health maintenance, and impaired home maintenance.

Interventions for the Biologic Domain

The numerous interventions for the biologic domain vary throughout the course of the disease. Initially, the patient requires simple directions for self-care activities and initiation of psychopharmacologic treatment. At the end of the disorder, total patient care is required.

Self-Care Interventions

Promotion of self-care supports cognitive functioning and a sense of independence. In the early stages, the nurse should maximize normal perceptual experiences by making sure that the patient and family have appropriate eyeglasses and working hearing aids. If eyeglasses and hearing aids are needed, but not used, patients are more likely to have false perceptual experiences. Ongoing monitoring of self-care is necessary throughout the course of AD. Oral hygiene can be a problem and, although this may be difficult, requires excellent basic nursing care (see http://www.marep.uwaterloo.ca/ for resource materials). Aging and many medications reduce salivary flow, leading to a painfully dry and cracking oral mucosa. Drugs that have xerostomia (dry mouth) as a side effect and are commonly prescribed for persons with progressive dementia include antidepressant, antispasmodic, antihypertensive, bronchodilator, and some antipsychotic agents. For patients with xerostomia, hard candy or chewing gum may stimulate salivary flow, or modification of the drug regimen may be necessary. Glycerol mouthwash may also provide some relief from xerostomia.

Nutritional Interventions

Maintenance of nutrition and hydration are essential nursing interventions. The patient's weight, oral intake, and hydration status should be monitored carefully. Patients need to eat well-balanced meals that are appropriate to their activity level and eating abilities, with special attention given to electrolyte balance and fluid intake.

The dining environment should be calm and food presentation appealing. If the person eats only a small portion of food at one meal, reduce the presentation of food in terms of the amount and number of choices. One-dish meals (e.g., a casserole) are ideal. If the person is distressed, delay feeding because eating, chewing, and swallowing difficulties are accentuated and choking becomes a risk.

Patients should be presented food that is appropriate for their individual needs (see http://www.hartfordign.org/ for publication on nutrition). When swallowing is a problem, thick liquids or semisoft foods are more effective than traditionally prepared foods. If the patient is likely to choke or aspirate food, semisolid foods should be offered, because liquids flow into the pharyngeal cavity more quickly and may cause choking. In the later stages, some patients hoard food in their mouths; others swallow too rapidly or fail to chew their food sufficiently before attempting to swallow. The nurse needs to watch for swallowing difficulties that place the person at risk for aspiration and asphyxiation. Swallowing difficulties may result from changes in oesophageal motility and decreased secretion of saliva.

As dementia progresses, and food intake is low, oral assisted feedings are encouraged and vitamin and mineral supplements may be indicated. Percutaneous feeding tubes in persons with advanced dementia are not recommended. Careful hand-feeding is at least as good as tube-feeding for the outcomes of death, aspiration pneumonia, functional status, and patient comfort. Tube-feeding is associated with agitation, increased use of physical and chemical restraints, and worsening pressure ulcers (American Geriatrics Society, 2013).

Supporting Bowel and Bladder Function

Urinary or bowel incontinence affects many persons with dementia. During middle stage of the disease, incontinence may be caused by the person's apathy or inability to communicate the need to use the toilet or locate a toilet quickly, undress appropriately to use the toilet, or recognize the sensation of fullness signalling the need to urinate or defecate.

For the person who is incontinent because of an inability to locate the toilet, reorientation may be helpful. Displaying pictures or signs on bathroom doors provides visual cues while verbal prompts promote reorientation to the environment.

Getting to know the person's habits and moods can help the nurse identify signals that indicate a need to void. The patient can then be assisted to reach the bathroom in time. Positioning the patient near the toilet or placing a portable commode nearby may help if the person cannot reach a toilet quickly. If the person demonstrates dressing **apraxia** (cannot undress appropriately), clothing can be modified with easy-to-open fasteners in place of zippers or buttons. For nocturnal incontinence, limiting the amount of fluid consumed after the evening meal and taking the person to the toilet just before going to bed or upon awakening during the night should reduce or eliminate nocturia.

Indwelling urinary catheters are contraindicated in persons with dementia, because they are generally not well tolerated and because hand restraints are often needed to prevent them from removing the catheter. Indwelling urinary catheters foster the development of urinary tract infections and may compromise the person's dignity and comfort. Urinary incontinence can be managed with the use of disposable incontinent products.

Persons with dementia often experience constipation, although they may not be able to tell the nurse about this change. Therefore, subtle signs such as lethargy, reduced appetite, and abdominal distension need to be assessed frequently. Medications, decreased food and liquid intake, lack of motor activity, and decreased intestinal motility contribute to developing constipation. The patient's diet should be rich in fibre, including bran or whole grains, vegetables, and fruit. Adequate oral intake (minimum of 1,500 to 2,000 mL per day) helps to prevent constipation. A gentle laxative such as milk of magnesia (1 to 2 tablespoons every other evening) is commonly used to promote bowel elimination. Enemas and harsher chemical cathartics should be avoided because they may increase pain or discomfort.

Sleep Interventions

Disturbed sleep cycles are particularly stressful to both family caregivers and nursing staff. Disturbed sleep is difficult to manage from a behavioural perspective, and the person's overall level of health may suffer because sleep serves a restorative function. Bright light therapy such as Brite-light boxes and ceiling-mounted light fixtures have shown promise in improving sleep in persons with dementia by regulating the sleep–wake cycle (Forbes, Blake, Thiessen, Peacock, & Hawranik, 2014). However, the best source of bright light is natural daylight. Physical activity such as walking and socializing outdoors has been shown to improve nighttime sleep (Brown et al., 2013).

Other sleep hygiene interventions that are helpful include having a fixed bedtime and awakening time that are the same every day; having certain activities that are always associated with going to bed (e.g., a particular piece of music or putting on a specific body lotion); avoiding napping during the day; avoiding alcohol 4 to 6 hours before bedtime; and having lots of fluids during the day but not a few hours before going to bed (Brown et al., 2011). In addition, rest periods (in reclining chairs) in the morning and afternoon may help to eliminate late-day confusion (sundowning) and nighttime awakenings.

Benzodiazepines or other sedative–hypnotics should be the last choice for insomnia (American Geriatrics Society, 2013). These may be prescribed for a short time for restlessness or insomnia, but they may also cause a paradoxic reaction of agitation and insomnia.

Activity and Exercise Interventions

Activity and exercise programmes appear to have a significant impact on improving cognitive functioning and ability to perform ADL (Forbes, Thiessen, Blake, Forbes, & Forbes, 2013). To promote a feeling of success, any activity or exercise plan must be culturally sensitive and adapted to the person's functional ability and interests. The activity or exercise must be designed to prevent excess stress (both physical and psychological). If the programme of rest, activity, and exercise is truly individualized, the resultant feelings of value and competency may enhance the person's functional ability, cognition, and sleep pattern.

Pain and Comfort Management

Nursing care of noncommunicative patients with dementia and pain can be challenging. Common behaviours associated with pain may be difficult to interpret or absent. Signs to watch for that may indicate pain include body language and nonverbal signs that may indicate the person is uncomfortable; changes in behaviour (especially anxiety, agitation, shouting, and sleep disturbances); pale or flushed skin tone; dry, pale gums; mouth sores; vomiting; feverish skin; and swelling of any part of the body. Because of the difficulty in identifying and monitoring pain, persons with dementia are often undertreated. Undertreatment of pain may result in further cognitive and behavioural problems.

Relaxation

Approaching the patient in a calm, confident, unhurried manner; maintaining a soothing, quiet environment; avoiding unnecessary noise or chatter around them and lowering vocal tone and rate when addressing them; maintaining eye contact; and using touch judiciously are likely to promote a sense of security conducive to relaxation and comfort. Simple relaxation exercises can be used by the patient to reduce stress.

Administering and Monitoring Medications

Due to the potential side effects of many medications, nonpharmacologic interventions should be the first approach used to address behavioural and psychiatric symptoms of dementia. Because no medication can cure AD, psychopharmacologic interventions have two goals: restoration or maintenance of cognitive function, and treatment of related psychiatric and behavioural disturbances that cause discomfort for the individual, interfere with treatment or worsen the individual's functional and/or cognitive status. However, medications for AD must be used with caution. Doses must be kept extremely low, and individuals should be monitored closely for any side effects or worsening of cognitive status. "Start low and go slow" is the principle guiding the administration of psychopharmacologic agents to older adults.

Often, convincing the person with dementia to take the medication is one of the biggest nursing challenges. They may be unwilling, even though they previously agreed to take the drugs. The nurse will need to investigate and hypothesize the reason(s) for their reluctance to take medication. It may be because of difficulty swallowing pills, paranoid ideas, or lack of understanding. The underlying reason(s) for medication refusal will determine the strategy. If the person has difficulty swallowing, most medications come in concentrate liquid form and can be easily swallowed. Medications should never be mixed in food without the person being made aware. If suspicion or paranoia is the reason, the nurse will need to try to identify the conditions under which the person feels safe to take the medication, such as in the presence of a favourite nurse or relative.

Cholinesterase Inhibitors. In Canada, three cholinesterase inhibitors (CIs) are approved: Aricept (donepezil), Exelon (rivastigmine), and Reminyl (galantamine). They help preserve the ability of sick nerve endings in the brain to transmit the nerve messages to the next cell in the chain. However, over time (usually 2 to 3 years or more), the sick nerve endings degenerate to the point where no transmitter is released at all, and the drugs are then totally ineffective. All three CIs are recommended as a treatment option for mild to severe AD with cerebrovascular disease and for dementia associated with Parkinson's disease. The research is inconsistent related to the use of CIs for the treatment of vascular dementia.

Some people are affected by the side effects from CIs, which include diarrhoea, insomnia, nausea, infection, and bladder problems. To avoid side effects, CIs are now contained in a skin patch, allowing the drug to be absorbed directly into the body.

N-Methyl-D-Aspartate Antagonists. Overstimulation of the N-methyl-D-aspartate receptor by glutamate (excitatory neurotransmitter) is considered to have a role in AD. When cells get sick, especially nerve cells, glutamate leaks out, and its concentrations outside the sick nerve cells can be so high that the increased amount taken back by way of the glutamate receptors is toxic and leads to the death of the nerve cells. The drug Ebixa (memantine hydrochloride) acts by blocking the glutamate receptors and preventing the reuptake of toxic amounts of the glutamate into the nerve endings. Since the glutamate threat develops late in AD, memantine is effective at moderate to advanced stages of the disease (Diamond, 2011). Insufficient research evidence exists to recommend for or against combining memantine with CIs (Gauthier et al., 2012a, 2012b).

Antipsychotic Agents. Antipsychotic drugs have historically been used to treat the severe distortions in thought,

perception, and emotion that characterize psychosis and have increasingly been used to treat the behavioural and psychological symptoms (e.g., delusion, aggression, and agitation) in persons with dementia. The adverse effects include sedation, higher risks of falls and hip fractures, Parkinson's disease–type symptoms, cardiovascular events (stroke and heart attack), and the greater risk of death. In 2005, Health Canada issued a statement that treatment with atypical antipsychotic medication of behavioural disorders in persons with dementia is associated with an increased risk for all-cause mortality and is not approved for use. Policy and practice quality initiatives are being implemented to discontinue the use of these medications. For example, the Ontario Ministry of Health and Long-Term Care aim was to significantly increase the number of health care workers provincewide to provide better care for aggressive and "difficult" patients with dementia, a strategy that should help keep more people at home and out of long-term care facilities as long as possible and to reduce the use of medications and restraints for institutionalized patients with dementia. The American Geriatrics Society (2013) has stated that the use of antipsychotic drugs should be limited to cases where nonpharmacologic measures have failed and the person poses an imminent threat to self or others. The CCCDTD4 has recommends that risperidone, olanzapine, and aripiprazole be used for severe agitation, aggression, and psychosis associated with dementia where there is risk to the person and/or others (Gauthier et al., 2012a, 2012b). However, identifying and addressing the causes of behaviour change can make drug treatment unnecessary. The Beers Criteria for PIM use in older adults (Campanelli, 2012) is an excellent resource.

Antidepressant Agents and Mood Stabilizers. A depressed mood is common in persons with dementia, but they often respond with improved mood to physical activity such as a walk outdoors, engagement in a group activity, and psychotherapeutic intervention (individual or group therapy), if necessary, in combination with pharmacotherapy. Low doses of the selective serotonin reuptake inhibitors and other antidepressive agents should be considered.

Antianxiety Medications (Sedative–Hypnotics). Antianxiety medications, also known as benzodiazepines, should only be used as a last resort for insomnia, agitation, or delirium (American Geriatrics Society, 2013). Large-scale studies consistently show that the risk of motor vehicle accidents, falls, and hip fractures leading to hospitalization and death can more than double in older adults taking benzodiazepines and other sedative–hypnotics. Sedative–hypnotic agents may be prescribed for a short time for restlessness or insomnia, but they may also cause a paradoxic reaction of agitation and insomnia (especially in older adults).

BOX 34-7 Medications With Strong Anticholinergic Properties

Antihistamines	Antiparkinson Agents	Skeletal Muscle Relaxants
Brompheniramine	Benztropine	Carisoprodol
Carbinoxamine	Trihexyphenidyl	Cyclobenzaprine
Chlorpheniramine		Orphenadrine
Clemastine		Tizanidine
Cyproheptadine		
Dimenhydrinate		
Diphenhydramine		
Hydroxyzine		
Loratadine		
Meclizine		

Antidepressants	Antipsychotics
Amitriptyline	Chlorpromazine
Amoxapine	Clozapine
Clomipramine	Fluphenazine
Desipramine	Loxapine
Doxepin	Olanzapine
Imipramine	Perphenazine
Nortriptyline	Pimozide
Paroxetine	Prochlorperazine
Protriptyline	Promethazine
Trimipramine	Thioridazine
	Thiothixene
	Trifluoperazine

Antimuscarinics (urinary incontinence)	Antispasmodics
Darifenacin	Atropine products
Fesoterodine	Belladonna alkaloids
Flavoxate	Dicyclomine
Oxybutynin	Homatropine
Solifenacin	Hyoscyamine products
Tolterodine	Propantheline
Trospium	Scopolamine

From Campanelli, C. M. (2012). American Geriatrics Society updated Beers Criteria for potentially inappropriate medication use in older adults. *Journal of the American Geriatrics Society*, 60(4), 616–631.

Other Medications. Clinical observations indicate that persons with dementia are more vulnerable to the effects of anticholinergic drugs that can cause confusion and amnesia. Anticholinergic medications should be avoided for them if at all possible due to the CNS effects. See Box 34-7 for examples of medications that are commonly prescribed to older adults, all of which have anticholinergic receptor activity.

Psychological Domain

Psychological Assessment

As the disease progresses, personality changes can take the form of either an accentuation or a marked alteration from a person's previous lifelong character traits.

The neural substrates underlying personality change in AD are not understood, but researchers have identified two contrasting patterns. One is marked by apathy, lack of spontaneity, and passivity. The other involves growing irritability, sarcasm, self-preoccupation, and intolerance of and lack of concern for others.

Cognitive Status

Cognitive disturbance is the clinical hallmark of dementia. The most commonly used cognitive assessment instrument is the Mini-Mental State Examination (MMSE; Box 35-8). If cognitive deterioration occurs rapidly, delirium should be suspected. The patient should be quickly evaluated by a physician because delirium calls for immediate attention to diagnose and treat the underlying cause.

Memory. The most dramatic and consistent cognitive impairment is in memory. Persons with early-stage dementia appear mildly forgetful and repetitive in conversation. They misplace objects, miss appointments, and forget what they were just doing. They may lose track of a conversation or television story. Initially, they may complain of memory problems, but in the course of the illness, insight is lost and they become unaware of what is lost. Sometimes, they may confabulate, making what appears to be an appropriate explanation of why the information or object is missing. Eventually, all aspects of memory are impaired. Short-term memory loss is usually readily evident by the patient's inability to recall three or four words given to him or her at the beginning of an assessment. Often, the earliest symptom of AD is the inability to retain new information.

Language. Language is progressively impaired. Individuals with AD may initially have **agnosia**, difficulty finding a word in a sentence or in naming an object. They may be able to talk around it, but the loss is noticeable. Later, fluent **aphasia** develops, comprehension diminishes, and, finally, they become mute and unresponsive to directions or information.

Visuospatial Impairment. Deficits in visuospatial tasks that require sensory and motor coordination develop early, drawing is abnormal, and the ability to write may change. Inaccurate drawings on the MMSE or clock drawings (see RNAO, 2003, *Screening for delirium, dementia and depression in older adults*) are diagnostic of impairment. Sequencing tasks, such as cooking or other self-care skills, become impaired. The individual becomes unable to complete complex tasks that require calculations, such as balancing a chequebook.

Executive Functioning. Judgement, reasoning, and the ability to problem solve or make decisions are also impaired in the late stage of AD. It is hypothesized that as the disease progresses, the degeneration of neurons is spread diffusely throughout the neocortex.

BOX 34-8 Cognitive Assessment Tools for Use With Dementia

Mental Status Questionnaires
Mini-Mental State Examination
Folstein, M. F., Folstein, S. E., & McHugh, P. R. (1975). Mini-mental state: A practical method for grading the cognitive state of patients for the clinician. *Journal of Psychiatric Research, 12,* 189–198. See Chapter 10 for components of the mental status examination.

Cognitive Abilities Screening Instrument
Teng, E. L., Hasegawa, K., Homma, A., Imai, Y., Larson, E., Graves, A., … Chiu, D. (1994). The Cognitive Abilities Screening Instrument (CASI): A practical test for cross-cultural epidemiological studies of dementia. *International Psychogeriatrics, 6,* 45–58.

Montreal Cognitive Assessment
Nasreddine, Z. S., Phillips, N. A., Bedirian, V., Charbonneau, S., Whitehead, V., Collin, I, …Chertkow, H. (2005). The Montreal Cognitive Assessment, MoCA: A brief screening tool for mild cognitive impairment. *Journal of the American Geriatrics Society, 53*(4), 695–699. See www.mocatest.org for more details.

Combination of Cognitive and Functional Assessment
Brief Cognitive Rating Scale
Reisberg, B., Schneck, M. K., & Ferris, S. H. (1983). The Brief Cognitive Rating Scale (BCRS): Findings in primary degenerative dementia. *Psychopharmacology Bulletin, 19,* 47–50.

Includes five scales: concentration, recent memory, remote memory, orientation, and functioning and self-care.
Agitation Scale
Rosen, J., Burgio, L., Kollar, M., Cain, M., Allison, M., Fogleman, M., … Zubenko, G. S. (1994). The Pittsburgh agitation scale: User-friendly instrument for rating agitation in dementia patients. *The American Journal of Geriatric Psychiatry, 2*(1), 52–59.

Rating Scales of Activities of Daily Living
Progressive Deterioration Scale
DeJong, R., Osterlund, O. W., & Roy, G. W. (1989). Measurement of quality-of-life changes in patients with Alzheimer's disease. *Clinical Therapeutics, 11,* 545–554.

Dependence Scale
Stern, Y., Albert, S. M., Sano, M., Richards, M., Miller, L., Folstein, M., … Lafleche, G. (1994). Assessing patient dependence in Alzheimer's disease. *Journal of Gerontology, 49,* M216–M222.

Ratings Scales for Relatives
Geriatric Evaluation by Relatives Rating Scale Instrument
Schwartz, G. E. (1983). Development and validation of the Geriatric Evaluation by Relatives Rating Instrument (GERRI). *Psychological Reports, 53,* 478–488.

Psychotic Symptoms
Suspiciousness, Delusion, and Illusions

During the early and middle stages of dementia, many patients are aware of their cognitive losses and compensate with hyperalertness. In a hyperalert state, one becomes aware of many environmental stimuli one does not readily understand. **Illusions** (mistaken perceptions) are common with dementia. These experiences can be very frightening for the patient and family. A kind, caring approach is needed.

As the disease progresses, delusions develop in 34% to 50% of people with dementia. These characteristic delusions are different from those discussed in the psychotic disorders. Common delusional beliefs include the following:

- Belief that his or her partner is engaging in marital infidelity
- Belief that other patients or staff are trying to hurt him or her
- Belief that staff or family members are impersonators
- Belief that people are stealing his or her belongings
- Belief that strangers are living in his or her home
- Belief that people on television are real

Hallucinations Hallucinations occur frequently in dementia and are usually visual or tactile (they can also be auditory, gustatory, or olfactory). A frequent concern is that children, adults, or strange creatures are entering the house or the person's room. These hallucinations may not seem unusual to the person. If possible, the content and form of hallucination should be ascertained because this information may suggest a treatable disorder. For example, an auditory hallucination commanding the person to commit suicide may be caused by a treatable depression, not dementia.

Mood Changes

Recognition of coexisting (and often treatable) psychiatric disorders in persons with dementia is often missed. One of the challenges of caring for them is when there is the coexistence of depression. Depression is characterized by alterations in sleep, lack of eye contact, feelings of sadness, expression of somatic concerns, and decrease in self-care. A recent meta-analysis (Graham, 2013) revealed a correlation between depression and subsequent vascular dementia and AD, as depressed older adults were more than twice as likely to develop vascular dementia and 65% more likely to develop AD compared with older adults who were not depressed. A person with dementia may experience one or more depressive episodes with symptoms such as psychomotor retardation, anxiety, feelings of guilt and worthlessness, sadness, frequent crying, insomnia, loss of appetite, weight loss, and suicidal rumination. Depressive symptoms are most prevalent in the early stages of dementia, which may be attributed to the person's awareness of cognitive changes, memory loss, and functional decline. However, dysphoric symptoms can occur at any stage, even in the most disoriented older person. In more advanced stages of dementia, an assessment of depression depends more on changes in behaviour than on the verbal expression of concerns.

Anxiety It is common to observe symptoms of anxiety with depression; therefore, it is important to assess for depression when signs of anxiety appear. Moderate anxiety is a natural reaction to the fear engendered by gradual deterioration of intellectual function and the realization of impending loss of control over one's life. Becoming unsure of one's surroundings and the expectations of others and failing to complete a task once regarded as simple creates a source of anxiety in a person. It is thought that anxious behaviour occurs when the patient is pressed to perform beyond his or her ability.

Catastrophic Reactions.

Catastrophic reactions are overreactions or extreme anxiety reactions to everyday situations. Catastrophic responses occur when environmental stressors are allowed to continue or increase beyond the person's threshold of stress tolerance. Behaviours indicative of catastrophic reactions typically include verbal or physical aggression, violence, agitated or anxious behaviour, emotional outbursts, noisy behaviour, compulsive or repetitive behaviour, agitated night awakening, and other behaviours in which the person is cognitively or socially inaccessible. Factors that contribute to catastrophic responses in persons with progressive cognitive decline include fatigue, change in routine (pace or caregiver), demands beyond the person's ability, overwhelming sensory stimuli, and physical stressors, such as pain or hunger.

Behavioural Responses
Apathy and Withdrawal

Apathy, the inability or unwillingness to become involved with one's environment, is common in AD, especially in moderate to late stages. Apathy leads to withdrawal from the environment and a gradual loss of empathy for others. The lack of empathy is very difficult for families and friends to understand.

Restlessness, Agitation, and Aggression.

Restlessness, agitation, and aggression become more prominent in the middle to late stages of dementia. Restlessness should be further evaluated to determine its underlying cause. If the restlessness occurs during medication change or adjustment, side effects should be suspected.

Agitation and aggressive physical contacts are among the most dangerous behaviour management problems encountered in any setting. They often result in the placement of the person with dementia in a nursing home. Careful evaluation of the antecedents of the behaviour enables the nurse to plan nursing care that prevents future occurrences.

Aberrant Motor Behaviour.

Symptoms such as fidgeting, picking at clothing, wringing hands, loud vocalizations, and wandering may all be signs of underlying conditions such as dehydration, medication reaction, pain, or infection (suggesting delirium). One of the most difficult behaviours for which to determine an underlying cause is hypervocalization; the screams, curses, moans, groans, and verbal repetitiveness that are common in

the later stages of dementia. In the assessment of these hypervocalizations, it is important to identify when the behaviour is occurring and any antecedents to the behaviour.

Disinhibition.

One of the most frustrating symptoms of AD is **disinhibition**, acting on thoughts and feelings without exercising appropriate social judgement. The patient may decide that he or she is more comfortable naked than with clothes. Or the person may not be able to find his or her clothes and may walk into a room of people without any clothes on. This behaviour is extremely disconcerting to family.

Hypersexuality.

A closely related symptom is hypersexuality, inappropriate and socially unacceptable sexual behaviour. The person may begin talking and behaving in ways that are uncharacteristic of premorbid behaviour.

Stress and Coping Skills.

Persons with dementia seem extremely sensitive to stressful situations and often do not have the coping abilities to deal with the situation. A careful assessment of the triggers that precede stressful situations will help in understanding a provoking event.

Nursing Diagnoses for the Psychological Domain

A multitude of potential nursing diagnoses can be identified for the psychological domain of this population. A sample of common nursing diagnoses can include chronic confusion, impaired environmental interpretation syndrome, risk for violence: self-directed or directed at others, risk for loneliness, risk for caregiver role strain, ineffective individual coping, hopelessness, and powerlessness (Carpenito-Moyet, 2013).

Interventions for the Psychological Domain

The therapeutic relationship is the basis for assessing and recommending interventions for the person with dementia and their family members. Care entails a long-term relationship, much support, and expert nursing care.

Cognitive Impairment
Validation Therapy

Validation therapy emerged in the 1970s as a method for communicating with patients with AD. It was developed as a contrast to reality therapy, which attempted to provide a here-and-now, factual focus to the interaction. Validation therapy focuses on the emotions and subjective reality of the patients using an empathic approach. In validation therapy, individuals with cognitive impairment are viewed on one of four stages of a continuum: malorientation, time confusion, repetitive motion, and vegetation. The benefits of validation therapy for patients are reported as restoration of self-worth, less withdrawal from the outside world, communication and interaction with other people, reduction of stress and anxiety, help in resolving unfinished life tasks, and facilitation of independent living for as long as possible. These outcomes are highly desirable, but no substantive research supports its effectiveness (Neal & Barton Wright, 2009). Validation therapy is a useful model for nursing care of persons with dementia. The nurse does not try to reorient the person but rather respects the individual's sense of reality.

Memory Enhancement. Interventions for progressive memory impairment should always be a part of the treatment plan. The sooner patients begin taking CI, the slower the cognitive decline. However, pharmacologic agents are only a small part of the intervention picture. The nursing goal is to maintain memory functioning as long as possible. The nurse should make a concerted effort to reinforce short- and long-term memory. For example, reminding patients what they had for breakfast, which activity was just completed, or who their visitors were a few hours ago will reinforce short-term memory. Encouraging individuals to tell the stories of their earlier years will help bring long-term memories into focus. In the earlier stages of AD, there is considerable frustration when the person realizes that he or she has short-term memory loss. In a matter-of-fact manner, the nurse should "fill in the blanks" and then redirect to another activity. Pictures of familiar people, places, and activities are also important tools in memory retrieval. Using scents (perfume, shaving lotions, spices, different foods) to stimulate memory retrieval and asking patients to relate memories are also useful. Formalized reminiscence groups also help them relive their earlier experiences and support long-term memories.

Orientation Interventions. To enhance cognitive functioning, attempts should be made to remind patients of the day, time, and location. However, if the person begins to argue that he or she is really at home or that it is really 1992, the person need not be confronted by facts. Any confrontation could easily escalate into an argument. Instead, the nurse should either redirect the person or focus on the topic at hand (see Box 34-9).

BOX 34-9 — **Therapeutic Dialogue**

THE PERSON WITH ALZHEIMER'S DISEASE

Lois's daughter has told the home care nurse that on several occasions, Lois has been found cowering and fearful under the kitchen table, saying she was hiding from voices. The nurse also knows that Lois denies having any difficulty with her memory or her ability to care for herself.

Ineffective Approach
Nurse: I'm here to see you about your health problems.

Patient: I have no problems. Why are you here?

Nurse: I'm here to help you.

Patient: I do not need any help. I think there is a mistake.

Nurse: Oh, there is no mistake. Your name is Ms. W, isn't it?

Patient: Yes, but I don't know who you are or why you are here. I'm very tired, please excuse me.

Nurse: OK. I will return another day.

Effective Approach
Nurse: Hello, my name is Susan Miller. I'm the home health nurse and I will be spending some time with you.

Patient: Oh, alright. Come in. Sit here.

Nurse: Thank you.

Patient: There is nothing wrong with me, you know.

Nurse: Are you wondering why I am here? Tell me what is on your mind (open-ended statement).

Patient: I know why you are here. My children think that I cannot take care of myself.

Nurse: You're feeling concerned and perhaps a little worried your family seems to think you need more help at home?

Patient: Of course I can care for myself. When people get older they slow down. I'm just a little slower now and that upsets my children.

Nurse: You are a little slower and that's what you think is concerning your children.

Patient: I sometimes forget things.

Nurse: Such as… (open-ended statement)

Patient: Sometimes, I cannot remember a telephone number or a name of a food.

Nurse: ….and that causes problems.

Patient: According to my children, it does!

Nurse: What about you? What causes problems for you?

Patient: Sometimes the radio says terrible things to me.

Nurse: That must be frightening to experience while listening to the radio.

Patient: It's terrifying. Then, my daughter looks at me as if I am crazy. Am I?

Nurse: Some people, when they become older, experience challenges with their memory. Also for some people, the daily living tasks which used to be carried out easily become more challenging. For you it seems doubly scary because you doubt yourself and you're afraid your daughter doesn't understand.

Patient: Oh, OK. Will you tell my daughter that I am not crazy?

Nurse: Sure, I would be happy to meet with both you and your daughter if you would like (acceptance).

Critical Thinking Challenge
- How did the nurse's underlying assumption that the patient would welcome the nurse in the first scenario lead to the nurse's rejection by the patient?
- What communication techniques did the nurse use in the second scenario to open communication and set the stage for the development of a sense of trust?

Maintaining Language. Losing the ability to name an object (agnosia) is frustrating. For example, the patient may describe a flower in terms of colour, size, and fragrance but never be able to name it a flower. When this happens, the nurse should immediately say the name of the item. This reinforces cognitive functioning and prevents disruption in the interaction. Referral to speech therapists may also be useful if the language impairment impedes communication.

Supporting Visuospatial Functioning. The patient with visuospatial impairments loses the ability to sequence automatic behaviours, such as getting dressed or eating with silverware. For example, patients often put their clothes on backward, inside out, or with undergarments over outer garments. Once dressed, they become confused as to how they arrived at their current state. If this happens, the nurse should begin to place clothes for dressing in a sequence so that the person can move from one article to the next in the correct sequence. This same technique can be used in other situations, such as eating, bathing, and toileting.

Managing Suspicions, Illusions, and Delusions. Patients' suspiciousness and delusional thinking must be addressed to be certain that they do not endanger themselves or others. Often, delusions are verbalized when patients are placed in a situation they cannot master cognitively. The principle of nonconfrontation is most important in dealing with suspiciousness and delusion formation. No efforts should be made to ease the person's suspicions directly or to correct delusions. Efforts should be directed at determining the circumstances that trigger suspicion or delusion formation and creating a means of avoiding these situations.

Frequent causes of suspicion are changes in daily routine and strangers. The common accusations that "Someone has entered my room," or "Someone has changed my room," can be managed by asking, "Do you want to see if anything is missing?" Such accusations usually arise when the person cannot remember what the room looked like or when the room was rearranged or cleaned.

Persons with dementia often hide or misplace their belongings and later complain that the item is missing. It is helpful if the nurse and other caregivers pay attention to the person's favourite hiding places and communicate this so that objects can be more easily retrieved. An outburst of delusional accusations after a social outing or other activity may indicate that the activity was too long, the setting was too stimulating, there was too much activity, or the pace was too fast for the person. All these elements can be modified, or it may be necessary to engage the person in quieter activities.

Persons with dementia may have delusions that a spouse, child, or other significant person is an impostor.

If this situation occurs, it is important to assert in a matter-of-fact manner, "This is your wife Barbara" or "I am your daughter Jenny." More vigorous assertions, such as offering various types of proof, tend to increase puzzlement as to why a person would go so far to impersonate the spouse or child.

When persons experience illusions, the nurse needs to find the source of the illusion and remove it from the environment if possible. For example, if a patient is watching a television programme featuring animals and then verbalizes that the animal is in the room, switch the channel and redirect the conversation. Some patients may no longer recognize the reflection in the mirror as self and become agitated, thinking that a stranger is staring at them. Potentially misleading or disturbing stimuli, such as mirrors or art work, can be easily covered or removed from the environment.

Managing Hallucinations. Reassurance and distraction may be helpful for the patient who is hallucinating. For example, an 89-year-old patient with AD in a residential care facility would get up each night, walk to the nursing station, and whisper to the nurses, "There's a man in my bed who won't let me sleep. You should patrol this place better!" If the hallucination is not too disturbing for the person, it can often be dismissed calmly with diversion or distraction. Because this person did not seem too concerned by the man in her bed, the nurse may gently respond by saying, "I'm sorry you have to put up with so much. Just wait here (or come with me) and I'll make sure your room is ready for you." The nurse should then take the person back to her room and help her into bed.

Frightening hallucinations and delusions should be first dealt with by decreasing the perceptual cues (cover mirrors or turn off the television) and by encouraging patients to stay physically close to their caregivers. For example, one person complained to her visiting nurse that she was being poisoned by deadly bugs that crawled up and down her arms and legs while she tried to sleep at night. Reassurance and protection should be provided. Patients often benefit if nurses give them a specific distracting intervention to alleviate anxiety and to help diminish the hallucination, such as applying moisturizing lotion to her legs and arms to repel the bugs at night. The nurse does not agree with the person's hallucination or delusion but lets the person know that the feelings are justified based on his or her perception of the threat. If these strategies are not effective, as a last resort antipsychotic medication may help this person sleep at night.

Interventions for Mood Changes
Managing Depression
Psychotherapeutic nursing interventions for depression that accompanies dementia are similar to interventions for any depression. It is important to spend time alone with patients and to personalize their care as a

way of communicating the person's value. Encouraging the expression of negative emotions is helpful because patients can talk honestly to a nonjudgemental person about their feelings. Depressed patients, especially in the early stage of dementia, may attempt and commit suicide. It is wise to remove potentially harmful objects from the environment.

Do not force depressed persons to interact with others or participate in activities, but encourage activity and exercise. One of the psychogenic aspects of depression is a sense of lowered worth related to the person's actual decreased competence to work and to deal with the problems of daily living. Therefore, it may be helpful to involve the person in a simple repetitive task or project (such as folding linens or setting the table), especially one that involves helping someone else. Assist the person to meet self-care needs while encouraging independence when possible.

Managing Anxiety. Cognitively impaired persons are particularly vulnerable to anxiety. As patients with dementia become increasingly unsure of their surroundings or what is expected of them, they tend to react with fear and distress. They may feel lost, insecure, and left out. Failure to complete a task once regarded as simple creates anxiety and agitation. Often, they cannot explain the source of their anxiety. The difficulty in developing interventions for the anxious patient with dementia is that the symptoms may also be a sign of underlying illnesses, such as depression, pain, infection, or other physical illnesses.

In many cases, lowering the demands, or perceived demands, on the person will be conducive to promoting comfort. Although maintaining autonomy in any remaining function is a high priority in nursing care of the patient, it may decrease the person's anxiety or stress level to have things done for him or her at certain points along the illness continuum. Frequently, as the day progresses and the person becomes more fatigued, his or her ability to cope with stressors is increasingly challenged. Many patients with dementia experience "sundowning" where they have an increased restlessness and agitation as the day draws to a close. In addition, being sensitive to the pronounced startle reflexes and potential hypersensitivity to touch also helps reduce stress.

The threshold for stress is progressively lowered in AD and other progressive dementias. A healthy person frequently uses cognitive coping strategies when under stress, whereas the person with dementia can no longer use many of these strategies. Effective nursing interventions include simplifying routines, making routines as consistent and predictable as possible, reducing the number of choices the person must make, identifying areas in which control can be maintained, and creating an environment in which the person feels safe. With any of the therapeutic interventions discussed, the nurse is reminded that each person has relative strengths and weaknesses and that sound nursing judgement must be used in each situation.

Commonly used therapeutic approaches may exacerbate anxiety in a patient with dementia. For example, reality orientation is contraindicated in the later stages of dementia because it is possible that the person's disoriented behaviour or language has inherent meaning. If the disoriented behaviour or language is continuously neglected or corrected by the nurse, the person's sense of isolation and anxiety may increase.

Another therapeutic intervention that may (or may not) be contraindicated in patients with dementia is providing the person with information before a difficult or painful procedure. Anticipatory preparation for nonroutine events may produce anxiety because the person is unable to retain information, use reasoning skills, or make sound judgements. Telling the person that he or she is scheduled for an upcoming diagnostic test only communicates, on an emotional level, that something distressing is about to happen. A simple explanation immediately before the event may be more helpful.

Managing Catastrophic Reactions. If a person reacts catastrophically, the nurse needs to remain calm, minimize environmental distractions (quiet the environment), get the person's attention, and softly assure the person that he or she is safe. Give information slowly, clearly, and simply, one step at a time. Let the person know that you understand the fear or other emotional response, such as anger or anxiety.

As the nurse becomes skilled at identifying antecedents to the person's catastrophic reactions, it becomes possible to avoid situations that provoke such reactions. Patients with AD respond poorly to change and respond well to structure. Attempts to argue or reason with them only escalate their dysfunctional responses.

Interventions for Behaviour Problems
Managing Apathy and Withdrawal

As the patient withdraws and becomes more apathetic, the nurse is challenged to engage the person in meaningful activities and interactions. To provide this level of care, the nurse must know the premorbid functioning of the person. Close contact with family helps give the nurse ideas about meaningful activities. For example, the use of a multi-sensory room (Snoezelen therapy; Staal et al., 2007) and involvement with music, art therapy, and a psychomotor activity (Ferrero-Arias et al., 2011) have been shown to reduce apathy.

Managing Restlessness and Wandering. Restlessness and wandering are major concerns for caregivers, especially in the community (home) and long-term care setting. The principal means of dealing with restless patients who wander into other patient's rooms or out the door is to have an adequate number of staff or caregivers, in

A NURSE'S DILEMMA

It is 8 AM and you are working as a nurse on an inpatient general medical unit of a large urban hospital. A 72-year-old man is admitted to your unit with symptoms of disorientation to time and place, and he is intermittently exhibiting signs of agitation. He thinks you are his child, and he falls asleep while you ask him questions about his symptoms. When you ask him to sign a consent form and hand him a pen, he looks at you as if he didn't understand your request.

The patient's wife tells you that he has had trouble with his memory for the past 3 or 4 years but that her husband has been "acting strange for the past 4 days." The patient's wife denies any history of substance abuse or head injury but states that her husband has been recently diagnosed as having dementia of the Alzheimer's type.

The patient's physician gives a verbal order to restrain the patient "as needed" while writing orders for lab work.

What Do You Think?
- What assessment techniques would you use to determine whether this patient has dementia, delirium, or both?
- What nursing diagnosis would be included in the patient's plan of care?
- What nursing interventions would promote comfort and safety for this patient?
- Is this patient able to give consent?
- What would be the possible outcomes of physically restraining this patient (e.g., would restraints be helpful or harmful for the patient)?

the home setting, to provide supervision, as well as electronically controlled exits. For example, a home security system and a bed occupancy sensor provided information to the family caregiver regarding the whereabouts of the person that resulted in participants being 85% less likely to sustain an injury caused by nighttime activities than those in the control group and possibly delayed admission to nursing homes (Rowe et al., 2009).

Wandering behaviour may be interrupted in more cognitively intact persons by distracting them verbally or visually. Persons who are beyond verbal distraction can be distracted by physically joining them on their walk and then interrupting their course of action and gently redirecting them back to the house or facility. In a long-term care setting, colour and structure of the setting can serve as cues (Gibson, MacLean, Barrie, & Geiger, 2004), and window boxes that contain photographs of family, personal mementoes, or pieces of art may cue a patient to identify their room.

Managing Aberrant Behaviour. When patients are picking in the air or wringing their hands, simple distraction may work. Hypervocalizations have meaning to the person. The nurse should develop strategies to try to reduce the frequency of vocalizations such as offering comfort measures (change of position, a snack or drink, or warm face cloth to refresh the person's hands and face). Gotell, Brown, and Ekman (2009) revealed that caregiver singing and background music can enable the hypervocal patient to express positive emotions and moods.

Managing Agitated Behaviour. Omelan (2006) suggests the following strategies when dealing with an agitated patient with dementia:

- Examine person for any physical causes (pain or infection)
- Review medications (check for any anticholinergic drugs)

- Observe the environment for contributing factors (noise or activity)
- Assess for depression and/or anxiety
- Focus on one behaviour at a time (reduce confusion for the patient)
- Constantly be aware of safety issues for the person (see clinical vignette, Box 34-10).

Reducing Disinhibition. Anticipation of disinhibiting behaviour is the key to nursing interventions for this problem. Disinhibition can take many forms, from undressing in a public setting to touching someone inappropriately, to making cruel statements. With keen behavioural assessment of the patient, the nurse should be able to anticipate the likely socially inappropriate behaviour and redirect the person or change the context of the situation. If the person starts undressing in the dining room, offering a robe and gently escorting him or her to another part of the room might be all that is needed. If the person is trying to fondle a staff member or another patient, having the person leave the immediate area or redirecting the patient may alleviate the situation.

Social Domain

Social Assessment

Dementia interferes with a person's ability to interact socially as much as it disrupts intellectual functioning. The social domain assessment should include those areas explained in Chapter 33, including functional status, social systems, legal status, and quality of life.

The person's whole social network is affected by dementia, and the primary caregiver of the person is often considered a coclient. It is important to assess the family caregiver's health status and willingness to use supportive resources to maintain his or her own health throughout the dementia journey.

The extent of the primary caregiver's personal, informal, and formal support systems must also be assessed, as well as personal resources, skills, and stressors. The assessment of the social domain provides objective data on the person's social circumstances and impressions of his or her family structure, sociocultural beliefs, attitudes towards health and disease, myths about dementia, patterns of communication, and degree of psychopathology (such as potential for abuse). If the person with dementia resides in the community, a home visit will prove useful because it gives the nurse information about the person in his or her own environment. From this assessment, the nurse can identify the situational and psychosocial stressors that affect the family and patient and can begin to develop relationships and interventions to strengthen coping strategies.

Nursing Diagnoses for the Social Domain

Typical nursing diagnoses for the social domain are deficient diversional activity, impaired social interaction, social isolation, risk for loneliness, caregiver role strain, ineffective coping, hopelessness, and powerlessness (Carpenito-Moyet, 2013). Outcomes are determined according to nursing diagnoses.

Interventions for the Social Domain

Safety Interventions

One of the primary concerns of the nurse should be safety for the patient. In the early stages of the illness, safety may not seem to be a prime concern. However, early behaviours suggesting dementia are often related to safety, such as the person getting lost while driving or going the wrong way on a highway. Determining the ability of a person with dementia to drive and taking away his or her driving licence are recognized as challenges for family caregivers and health care providers. Safety may be an issue in the home when the person engages in unsupervised cooking, cleaning, or household tasks. Day care centres provide a safe and structured environment for these individuals. Family members should be encouraged to continually assess the abilities of the person to live at home safely and to implement appropriate responses and safety strategies.

In hospital and long-term care settings, the safety issues are different. By the time persons with dementia are admitted to a facility, they are in the middle to late stage of their illness. Cognitive impairments are more pronounced, and safety is of greater concern. Most psychogeriatric units are locked, and in a dementia unit, there often is an electronic alarm system to alert the staff of persons attempting to leave the secured floor. Staff and visitors need to be vigilant of unsafe situations.

Environmental Interventions

The need for stimulation varies from individual to individual and can change, depending on many factors, including cognitive intactness, alertness, emotional state,

and physical state. The amount of stimulation received also influences each person's behaviour. Lack of stimulation or intense stimulation may cause emotional distress and aggression. Generally speaking, the more severe the dementia, the less stimulation can be integrated. The nurse should attempt to determine each person's optimal level of stimulation at various times of the day. Music and hand massage are effective in reducing agitation in patients with dementia (Hicks-Moore & Robinson, 2008).

Socialization Activities

Overlearned social skills are rarely lost in dementia. It is not unusual for the person to respond appropriately to a handshake or smile well into the disease process. Even persons who are no longer able to communicate coherently will carry on long discussions with people who are willing to listen and respond. There is a strong risk for social isolation because of communication difficulties. Reinforcing social remarks and gestures, such as eye contact, smiling, greetings, and farewells, can promote a sense of competency and self-esteem (Box 34-11). Pet therapy may enhance social interaction in cognitively impaired individuals. It is important to remember that the ability to laugh and play is not lost, and the psychosocial benefits of humour are well known.

The nurse who engages a patient with dementia in an activity is encouraged to (1) avoid confrontation, (2) allow the level of autonomy best tolerated by the person, (3) simplify activities and directions to the point that they can be mastered, (4) provide adequate structure, and (5) recognize that instructions may not be carried out correctly. It is important to monitor the length of time, crowding, and noise level when the person participates in a group activity because all these factors may increase his or her stress level.

Activities that elicit pleasant memories from an earlier time in the person's life (reminiscence) may produce a soothing effect. Eliciting pleasant memories may be enhanced by gentle stimulation of the person's senses, for example, viewing and discussing photo albums, looking at personal memorabilia, providing a favourite food item,

---

BOX 34-11 Psychoeducation Checklist: Tips for Caregivers of Persons With Dementia

When caring for the patient with dementia, be sure to include the caregivers, as appropriate, and address the following topic areas in the teaching plan:
- Psychopharmacologic agents, if used, including drug action, dosage, frequency, and possible adverse effects
- Rest and activity
- Consistency in routines
- Nutrition and hydration
- Sleep and comfort measures
- Protective environment
- Communication and social interaction
- Diversional measures
- Community resources

playing a musical instrument, or listening to music the person preferred in younger years.

It may be useful to incorporate movement or dance along with a singing exercise. If the patient resists structured exercise, it may be because of a fear of falling or injury or of demonstrating to others that his or her health is failing. Patients often forget how to move or how to coordinate their movements in relation to objects. Therefore, exercise should be light and enjoyable. Encourage the person to participate and to take rest periods at intervals throughout the activity in an effort to minimize stress (see Power of Music video, http://www.alzheimer.ca/en/We-can-help/Resources/Multimedia).

Home Visits

Recognizing the importance of supporting persons with dementia to remain at home for as long as possible and support their family caregivers in sustaining their role, cost-effective in-home– and community-based long-term care services are expanding. Their goals are to maintain such persons in a self-determining environment that provides the most home-like atmosphere possible, allows maximum personal choice for care recipients and caregivers, and encourages optimal family caregiving involvement without overwhelming the resources of the family network. All services for these patients and their families are provided within a context of continuity of care, a concept that mandates access to a variety of health and supportive services over an unpredictable and changing clinical course.

Community Actions

Home care nurses and community public health nurses working with persons with dementia are especially knowledgeable about all aspect of the illness and care. These nurses often consult with local organizations, such as the Alzheimer Society of Canada, and participate on interdisciplinary teams. Issues of care, safety, and access to services often require professional expertise and influence.

Family Interventions

Family caregivers are faced with extreme challenges. Caregivers are either spouses of the person or children, usually a daughter, who also have other responsibilities, such as children and a job. The caregiver often feels isolated, frustrated, and trapped. The potential for abuse of the person with dementia is significant, especially if agitated and aggressive behaviours are present. The use of home care services may assist in decreasing the burden and depression in family caregivers.

As family caregivers provide up to 80% of the care needed and make up 4 million Canadians (Canadian Caregiver Coalition, 2008), it is important that the nurse recognize and assess the needs of the caregivers for support and relief from the 24-hour responsibility. Determining the availability of family members or friends to assist with personal care of the person with dementia should be included in the assessment (see Box 34-11). If they are not available, home care may assist with personal care needs of the person and provide respite for the caregiver. Caregivers should be encouraged to attend support groups and carve out personal time. Educational and training programmes may help in understanding the complex nature of the disorder. Community resources, such as day care centres, home care agencies, and other community services, can be an important aspect of nursing care for the person and their family caregivers (see Box 34-12).

BOX 34-12   Research for Best Practice

EMERGENCE OF DEMENTIA AS A FIRST NATIONS' HEALTH CONCERN

From Jacklink, K., Walker, J., & Shawande, M. (2013). The emergence of dementia as a health concern among First Nations populations in Alberta, Canada. Canadian Journal of Public Health, 104(1), e39–e44.

The Questions: Dementia is predicted to increase as a health challenge for Canadian health care systems, yet there is little data available concerning the prevalence of dementia in First Nations communities. The questions asked in this study were: Are rates for dementia increasing more rapidly among First Nations (FN) populations than Non-First Nation (NFN) populations? Are FN populations experiencing dementia at a younger age than NFN populations? Does the sex distribution of dementia differ between these populations?

Methods: Population-level data from Alberta Health and Wellness were analyzed. Physician-treated prevalence rates for dementia were calculated for FN and NFN populations seeking treatment between 1998 and 2009. Using linear regression models, trends in age-adjusted rates over time were compared; age and sex effects were examined.

Findings: The age-standardized prevalence of dementia rose higher for FN populations (7.5/1,000) than NFN populations

(5.6/1,000). The prevalence also rose more quickly for FNs (p = 0.032). Dementia appears to disproportionately affect younger age groups (60 to 69; 70 to 79) and males in FN populations when FN and NFN data are compared. The researchers note that the increase in prevalence may be driven by trends among FN populations, such as demographic transitions (the rate of FN population increase; the number of those over 60 is predicted to increase 3.4 times by 2031), factors related to social determinates of health (e.g., lower income and lower educational attainment), and higher rates of conditions/factors associated with dementia (e.g., diabetes, heart disease, smoking, and obesity). Research associating increased risk of dementia with posttraumatic stress disorder may also play a role, given the traumatic legacy of residential school experiences.

Implications for Nursing: Nurses need to be cognizant of the increased risk for dementia among FN populations and to work to identify and help address preventable factors contributing to it. As well, population-level health databases need to have data elements that allow identification of disease prevalence among First Nations, Inuit, and Métis populations.

Spiritual Domain

The changes in cognition and ability to communicate that occur in dementia may discourage some nurses from attempting to provide individualized spiritual care. Yet, despite communication impairment, the need to be respected, to have hope, and to connect with others and, perhaps, a higher power does not diminish. If the spiritual domain is neglected in care, the person with dementia may be denied important comforting and supportive measures. It is important to understand the person's spiritual beliefs as early as possible in the progression of dementia when they may be better able to explain what has spiritual importance for them. Their religious beliefs, rituals, and their participation in a religious community can be explored at this time. The diagnosis of dementia may have brought despair that challenged the person's existing spiritual beliefs. This needs to be recognized, and opportunities for the person to express spiritual distress should be created.

Béphage (2009) has outlined strategies for spiritual care with persons with dementia under three categories: communication, religious interventions, and nonreligious interventions. Communication is the foundation for identifying the person's spiritual disposition. A key action is to look for positive efforts to communicate by the person. Nurses can be sensitive to the spirituality-related verbal and nonverbal cues from the person and to the presence of spiritually meaningful items or artefacts (e.g., Bible, Koran, prayer wheel). Helping the person remain connected with religious activities can be accomplished by support from the family and/the person's religious community and from pastoral care workers. If the person can no longer attend religious services, alternative forms of attendance may be possible, such as via radio or television. The person may want to share past memories of faith and practices or listen to hymns or spiritual music. Being able to see and touch meaningful symbols may be comforting. Nonreligious interventions that support spiritual well-being include art therapy (e.g., drawing or simply looking at paintings), outdoor activities, meditation, pet therapy, and reminiscence therapy. As well, active efforts to fulfil the person's need for companionship may relieve the loneliness and social isolation that dementia brings.

For patients with dementia, Procedural and Emotional Religious Activity Therapy (PERAT) is an approach that may provide some spiritual support (Vance, Moore, Farr, & Struzick, 2008). Based on matching the cognitive ability of the person with the cognitive demands of an emotionally meaningful activity, such as a religious or spiritual activity, PERAT involves an assessment of the person's religious and spiritual history and of their cognitive status. Tasks are selected for their procedural memory capability and emotional salience to the person. Materials (i.e., items that have an emotional attachment) for the activities are obtained, usually from family members. Making family photographs, religious pictures, and books available within the person's setting can be helpful and soothing. Activities can include reciting favourite scripture, engaging in prayer, holding a religious icon, or maintaining a shrine. This is a counterproductive approach if the activities are not spirituality appropriate to the individual person, and more research is required to develop this approach (Vance et al., 2008).

Evaluation and Treatment Outcomes

The objectives of nursing interventions are to help the person living with dementia remain as independent as possible and to function at the highest cognitive, physical, emotional, spiritual, and social levels. The maximum level of functional ability can be promoted when nursing care is related to and based on the remaining abilities of the person. Those who receive diagnoses of AD or other types of dementia still have a wide and varying range of functional abilities. As cognitive decline progresses, there is a tendency for caregivers to perform more and more tasks for the person. It is essential to assess for strengths and to assist in the maintenance of existing skills. Adaptive and appropriate behaviours continue to some degree, even in the presence of increasing cognitive decline. It is important for nursing interventions to focus on more than the maintenance of optimal physical functional ability; interventions also must focus on meeting psychological, social, and spiritual needs of the person.

Nurses can maintain quality of life if they protect a person's overall well-being by balancing physical, mental, social, and spiritual health. Figure 34-4 illustrates the truly bio/psycho/social/spiritual aspects of the treatment of individuals with dementia by summarizing potential outcomes of nursing care.

Forbes et al. (2008) and Jansen et al. (2009) studied the role of home care and other agencies in meeting the needs of Canadians with dementia and their family and friend caregivers. Service *availability* and *acceptability* were the overarching themes of the study findings. Family caregivers desired an integrated continuing care model that includes the person with dementia and family as partners in care, addresses all the determinants of health, and encompasses sensitivity, flexibility, and diversity. Home care providers described challenges to service availability as including service waitlists, lack of home care provider training, lack of community-based dementia care, lack of service infrastructure, and sociocultural and geographical barriers. Agency partnerships, however, facilitated availability. Key to the acceptability of services was comprehensive personal care with adequate service time for such care, as well as for support of the family caregivers. A difficulty family caregivers specifically identified was navigating the health care system. This type of research, focused on the voices of those directly affected by and

FIGURE 34-4. Bio/psycho/social/spiritual interventions for patients with dementia.

involved with dementia care, has direct implications for the evolution of services.

Continuum of Care

Community Care

In 2011, 1.4 million Canadians received home care, of whom 61% were older adults. This translates into one in every six seniors in Canada were receiving publically funded home care (Canadian Home Care Association [CHCA], 2013). Service delivery models vary across the country, with services provided through the public sector and/or contracted with private sector providers. Most home care programmes provide case management, nursing, and personal care. There is a wide variation in the provision of therapies such as physiotherapy, occupational therapy, speech and language pathology, respiratory therapy, dietetic care, and social work. Similarly, home care programmes vary in the range of and access to homemaking services such as cleaning, laundry, meal preparation and, very rarely, assistance with transportation, shopping, and banking (CHCA, 2013). Collaboration among health care providers of different disciplines and in various settings is needed to meet the highly individualized needs of persons with dementia and their family caregivers

(Forbes et al., 2012). For more information on caring for the patient with dementia, see Nursing Care Plan 34-1.

Acute Care Setting

Although admission to an acute care setting is not likely related to dementia, older adults with other conditions may have symptoms of dementia. A comprehensive admission assessment that encompasses dementia, followed by the development of an individualized (and constantly updated) care plan that involves the patient, significant others, and a variety of health care professionals, is the foundation of an effective and efficient predischarge plan. Attention to all aspects of this process is necessary to continuity of care. The hospital-based nurse may initiate family education and counselling as part of discharge planning.

Nursing Home Care

As dementia progresses, most family members can no longer manage the symptoms, such as wandering at night and incontinence. A nursing care home may be necessary. Here, nursing care is usually provided by nurses' aides, who need support and direction from other health care professionals. Persons with dementia require complex nursing care, yet the skill level of people providing

Nursing Care Plan 34-1

Patient With Dementia

LW is a 76-year-old widow who lives with her oldest son. He is with her during the evening and night. Recently, her children have noticed that she is becoming more forgetful and seems to have periods of confusion. LW refuses to see a health care provider but did agree to go in for a routine checkup. Her daughter helped her get dressed and took her to the primary health care clinic.

Setting: Primary Health Care Clinic

Baseline Assessment: A well-groomed woman is accompanied by her daughter. LW says there is nothing wrong, but her daughter disagrees. A review of body systems reveals poor hearing and vision but is otherwise unremarkable. MMSE score is 19. Daughter reports that LW has become very suspicious of neighbours and has changed her locks several times.

Associated Diagnoses	Medications
Probable dementia of the Alzheimer's type (some memory problems) History of breast cancer, unilateral mastectomy, arthritis Other relevant factors: Social problems (suspiciousness)	Galantamine (Reminyl) 4 mg bid, titrate to 8 mg bid over 4 weeks.

Nursing Diagnosis 1: Impaired Memory

Defining Characteristics	Related Factors
Inability to recall information Inability to recall past events Observed instances of forgetfulness Forgets to perform daily activities—grooming	Neurocognitive changes associated with dementia

Outcomes

Initial	Long Term
Maintain or improve current memory	Delay cognitive decline associated with dementia

Interventions	Rationale	Ongoing Assessment
Develop memory cues in home. Have clocks and calendars well displayed. Make lists for patients. Teach the patient and family about taking an acetylcholinesterase inhibitor. Review expected effects, side effects, and adverse effects. Develop a titration schedule with family to decrease the appearance of side effects. Observe the patient for visuospatial impairment. If present, sequence habitual activities, such as eating, dressing, bathing, etc.	Maintaining current level of memory involves providing cues that will help patient recall information. Confidence and self-esteem improve when a person looks well groomed. Visuospatial impairment is one of the symptoms of dementia.	Contact family members for the patient's ability to use memory cues. Monitor response to suggestions. Observe for appropriate dress, bathing, eating, etc.

Evaluation

Outcomes	Revised Outcomes	Interventions
LW did have some improvement in memory. Suspiciousness and grooming improved.	Continue maintaining memory.	Continue with memory cues and galantamine.

the direct care is often minimal, making education and support of the care providers a significant focus for nursing homes.

OTHER MAJOR NCDS (DEMENTIAS)

Dementia symptoms may occur as a result of a number of NCDs and underlying aetiologies. The subsequent sections provide a brief description of some of the aetiologic subtypes identified in the *Diagnostic and Statistical Manual of Mental Disorders* (5th edition) (APA, 2013). In each case, significant cognitive decline must be evident in one or more cognitive domains (e.g., language, learning and memory, social cognition); the cognitive deficits affect independence in everyday life, and they do not occur exclusively with delirium (APA, 2013, p. 602). Nursing interventions for the subtypes of major NCDs are similar to those described for individuals with AD.

Vascular Neurocognitive Disorder

Vascular dementia, also called multi-infarct dementia, is the second most common form of dementia following AD. More than 20% of all those who have dementia have vascular dementia. When AD and vascular dementia occur at the same time, the condition is called mixed dementia. Vascular dementia occurs from multiple cerebral infarctions (transient ischemic attacks [TIAs]) or a stroke. These occur when blood flow in the brain is blocked or a blood vessel bleeds, preventing the blood from flowing properly through the vessel. Certain medical conditions such as type II diabetes, high blood pressure, and an unhealthy lifestyle are all contributory factors to developing vascular dementia. It is essential that anyone who demonstrates symptoms of dementia or who has a history of stroke should have a complete physical examination that includes diet, smoking, medication history, review of recent stressors, and an array of laboratory tests.

The behaviour changes that result from vascular dementia are similar to those found in AD, such as loss of memory, judgement and reasoning, depression, emotional lability, wandering or getting lost in familiar places, bladder or bowel incontinence, difficulty in following instructions, gait changes, and problems handling daily activities. However, these symptoms usually begin more suddenly, rather than developing slowly, as is the case in AD. Often, the neurologic symptoms associated with a TIA are minimal (slight weakness in an extremity, dizziness, or slurred speech) and may last only a few days. Thus, the clinical progression is often described as step-like deterioration, with the person's cognitive and functional status plateauing for a period of time, followed by a rapid decline in function after another series of small strokes. Treatment aims to reduce the primary risk factors for vascular dementia, including hypertension, diabetes, and additional strokes. Interventions that reduce the tendency of the blood to clot and of platelets to aggregate include lifestyle changes (diet, exercise, and smoking cessation) and using appropriate medications. Increasingly, physicians are recommending anticoagulants and medication to control hypertension, elevated levels of cholesterol, and glucose. There is insufficient and inconsistent evidence on which to make a recommendation either for or against the use of the currently available CIs for the treatment of vascular dementia (Gauthier et al., 2012a, 2012b).

NCD (Dementia) With Lewy Bodies

The clinical features of DLB and Parkinson's disease dementia (PDD; see below) often overlap. DLB should be diagnosed when this pattern of dementia occurs before or concurrently with parkinsonism. In addition, AD and DLB frequently coexist. Persons with DLB may have symptoms much like those of both Parkinson's disease and AD, making it impossible to offer guidelines that could separate the diagnoses with a high specificity (CDKTN, 2012).

DLB usually progresses quickly. Symptoms include a progressive loss of memory, language, reasoning, and other higher mental functions, and occasionally depression, anxiety, and apathy. Obvious changes in alertness may also happen. The person may be sleepy during the day but wide awake at night, unable to sleep. Visual hallucinations are common and can be worse during times of increased confusion. The visual hallucinations often come back repeatedly, and typically are of people, children, or animals. People with the disease may also make errors in perception, for example, seeing faces in a carpet pattern. Some features of DLB that resemble those in Parkinson's disease include rigidity (stiffness of muscles), tremors (shaking), stooped posture, and slow, shuffling movements. Sensitivity to medication, especially some sedatives, may make these symptoms worse (see Masellis, 2012).

NCD (Dementia) Due to Parkinson's Disease

PDD can be diagnosed when there is well-established Parkinson's disease followed by gradual onset of cognitive decline. Parkinson's disease is a neurodegenerative disease. The most common symptoms affect movement such as **bradykinesia** (the slowing of body movements), rigidity, resting tremor, and postural changes. The person's gait is unstable, resulting in frequent falls. Approximately 20% of people with Parkinson's disease will develop PDD, usually 10 to 15 years following a diagnosis of Parkinson's disease. The hallmark abnormality in Parkinson's disease is Lewy bodies, deposits of a protein called alpha-synuclein, in a specific brain region critical for control of movement. People can live with Parkinson's for years, although currently there is no cure. Medical treatment of Parkinson's disease typically is with anticholinergics and dopamine agonists. However, anticholinergic medications may cause adverse mental effects (e.g., confusion, memory problems, restlessness, and hallucinations) (Katzenschlager, Sampaio, Costa, & Lees, 2003).

Frontotemporal NCD (Dementia)

FTD tends to occur at a younger age than AD, accounting for approximately 2% to 5% of all dementia. FTD is an umbrella term for a group of rare disorders that primarily affect the frontal and temporal lobes of the brain, the areas generally associated with personality and behaviour. With this form of dementia, a person may have symptoms such as sudden onset of memory loss, behaviour changes, or difficulties with speech and movement. In some cases, brain cells in these areas shrink or die. In other cases, the brain cells in these areas get larger, containing round, silver "Pick's bodies." Pick's disease refers to a subtype of FTD that has these specific abnormalities.

Since the frontal and temporal areas of the brain are affected, early symptoms of FTD often involve behaviour and/or speech. Changes in behaviour may include becoming either withdrawn and apathetic or disinhibited and impulsive. The person may lose interest in personal hygiene, become easily distracted, or repeat the same action over and over again. Overeating or compulsively putting objects in the mouth may occur. Sometimes incontinence is an early symptom of FTD. There may be significant decline in language ability (e.g., "speech production, word finding, object naming, grammar, or word comprehension") (APA, 2013).

A person with FTD may have changes in personality but continue to manage the running of a home and manage all the psychomotor and spatial skills needed to maintain employment. However, the person often loses his or her position due to changes in personality. The individual may become easily irritated, loud, and argumentative. This is particularly distressing to a family if they do not understand that these are symptoms of FTD.

Dementia Caused by Other General Medical Conditions

People of any age, race, or gender are at risk for dementia caused by a medical condition known to cause cerebral pathology. Older adults are particularly vulnerable to the development of dementia caused by general medical conditions because so many are affected by one or more of these illnesses. Strong relationships have been reported between the following chronic medical illness and the development of dementia.

NCD (Dementia) Caused by HIV Infection

Dementia associated with HIV infection has been called AIDS dementia complex (ADC). ADC has been observed in nearly two thirds of all patients with AIDS. AIDS is caused by human immunodeficiency virus 1 (HIV-1), which infects and destroys T lymphocytes as well as the CNS. HIV-1 directly invades the CNS and allows opportunistic infections of the CNS and other organ systems. Although there has been a proportional increase in ADC at AIDS diagnosis, survival has improved markedly in the era of highly active antiretroviral therapy (HAART) (Dore et al., 2003). The essential features of ADC are disabling cognitive impairment accompanied by motor dysfunction, speech problems, and behavioural change. Dementia only exists when neurocognitive impairment in the person is severe enough to interfere markedly with day-to-day function.

NCD (Dementia) Due to Traumatic Brain Injury

When head trauma occurs in the context of a single traumatic injury, the resulting dementia is usually not progressive, but repeated head injury (e.g., from the sport of boxing) may lead to a progressive dementia. When the nurse observes progressive decline in intellectual functioning after a single incident of head trauma, the possibility of another superimposed process must be considered. Head injury associated with a prolonged loss of consciousness (days to months) may be followed by delirium, dementia, or a profound alteration in personality. Falls are a common cause of head injury in the older adult. Subarachnoid haemorrhage is often a result of an unwitnessed fall and often gets missed, leading to the potential for permanent brain damage and/or death. Subarachnoid haemorrhage is treatable if caught early.

The degree and type of cognitive impairment or behavioural disturbances demonstrated by a person with head trauma depend on the location and extent of the brain injury (as with other forms of dementia). Repeated head injuries, such as those sustained by young, healthy boxers, may lead to *dementia pugilistica* or "punchdrunk syndrome." Symptoms and signs of dementia pugilistica develop progressively over a long latent period sometimes amounting to decades, with the average time of onset being about 12 to 16 years after the start of a career in boxing. The condition is thought to affect around 15% to 20% of professional boxers.

NCD (Dementia) Due to Huntington's Disease

Huntington's disease is a progressive, genetically transmitted autosomal dominant disorder. Anyone with a parent with Huntington's has a 50% chance of inheriting the gene. People are born with the defective gene, but symptoms usually do not appear until middle age. Symptoms include the following: involuntary movements such as twitches and muscle spasms, balance problems, personality changes such as irritability, depression and mood swings, difficulties with memory, concentration, learning new things, or making decisions, and in late stage difficulty concentrating, eating independently, or swallowing. Research on potential treatments is moving forward since scientists have identified the gene involved (ASC, 2013b).

NCD (Dementia) Due to Prion Disease

Prion disease (including CJD) is a rare form of deadly dementia that is caused by infectious proteins known as *prions*. When prions are abnormally shaped, they can attack the brain, kill cells, and create gaps or holes in brain tissue. Prion diseases affect both humans and animals. The best-known prion disease in humans is CJD. It affects about one to two persons per million worldwide each year, with about 35 new cases being diagnosed in Canada every year (ASC, 2013c).

There are two types of CJD: classic CJD and variant CJD (vCJD). Classic CJD is primarily composed of the sporadic type of CJD, which accounts for 90% of cases in Canada. It affects people between 45 and 75 years old. The cause of sporadic CJD is not known. The disease appears without warning and most people die within 1 year. vCJD affects younger people with an average age of 28 years. This form of CJD can develop from eating beef that was infected with bovine spongiform encephalopathy (BSE), and a recent case was reported to be transmitted by a blood transfusion from a person with vCJD in the United Kingdom.

At present, there is no effective treatment for the disease, and nothing has been found to slow progression of the illness. Because of its rapid clinical course, an important nursing role is assisting family members to understand and come to terms with the illness and to make decisions related to treatment setting and life-sustaining treatments.

Substance/Medication-Induced NCD (Dementia)

If dementia results from the persisting effects of a substance (e.g., drugs of abuse, a medication, or exposure to toxins), substance/medication-induced NCD (dementia) is diagnosed. Other causes of dementia (e.g., dementia caused by a general medical condition) must always be considered, even in a person with a dependence on or exposure to a substance. For example, head injuries often result from substance use and may be the underlying cause of the NCD.

Drugs of abuse are the most common toxins in young adults, and prescription drugs are the most common toxins in older people. In older patients, dementia results from the use of long-acting benzodiazepines, barbiturates, meprobamate, and a host of other drugs, depending on their dose and the length of time they have been used. Drugs such as flurazepam (Dalmane), with a half-life of more than 120 hours, accumulate rapidly in a person's body. Other drugs accumulate more slowly or require relatively high doses for toxicity to develop.

A toxic aetiology should be suspected in every patient with a probable diagnosis of dementia. The nurse should inquire about exposure to drugs and toxins (exposure to toxins at work sites, medication use, and recreational drug use) for each patient with dementia, and any substances known to be potentially injurious to the nervous system should be withdrawn if possible.

Most of the dementias in this category are related to chronic alcohol abuse. Understanding the cognitive deficits associated with chronic alcohol consumption is complicated. Alcoholic dementia is directly related to the toxic effects of alcohol, although the vitamin deficiencies associated with alcoholism (thiamine and niacin) are also known to be aetiologically related to dementia. Individuals with alcoholism also have a high incidence of systemic illnesses that can affect cognition (e.g., cirrhosis, cardiomyopathy), and they are susceptible to repeated head injuries, which carry cognitive consequences of their own.

Much of our knowledge about cognitive deficits in individuals with alcoholism comes from the study of patients with Korsakoff's syndrome, which is a profound deficit in the ability to form new memories and is associated with a variable deficit in the recall of old memories, despite a clear sensorium. Further careful examination reveals a flattening of drives, unconcern about incapacity, and profound apathy. Nonetheless, Korsakoff's syndrome does not qualify as a dementia; rather, it is considered an amnestic syndrome (or restricted deficit of memory). In alcohol-induced dementia, the cognitive deficits span a wider range of functioning than with Korsakoff's syndrome (see Chapter 26).

Chemicals and organic compounds that impair functioning of the CNS usually have their primary effects on other body systems: the gastrointestinal, renal, hepatic, blood-forming, and peripheral nervous systems. For example, metal poisonings generally produce gastrointestinal symptoms and peripheral neuropathy. Cognitive changes with poisoning tend to be more characteristic of delirium than dementia, with altered levels of consciousness a prominent feature. Many adolescents and indigent adults engage in the act of "huffing" because the cost of purchasing spray paint, hair spray, glue, and other aerosol products is relatively inexpensive (compared with illicit street drugs). The nurse is reminded to evaluate people who abuse drugs for signs of cognitive impairment because neural and cognitive symptoms tend to appear before permanent brain damage occurs. It is also important to realize that the patient's cognitive status may not immediately improve after discontinuation of use of the offending agent. The effects of drugs taken for a long period may be long lasting, and improvement may be slow following discontinuation of drug use. For example, in dementia associated with chronic alcoholism, cognition may improve only after many months of abstinence.

SUMMARY OF KEY POINTS

■ NCDs, such as delirium and dementia, are characterized clinically by significant deficits in cognition or memory that represent a clear-cut change from a previous level of functioning. In some disorders, the loss of cognitive function is progressive, such as in AD.

■ Two major syndromes of cognitive impairment in older adults are delirium and chronic cognitive impairments, such as dementia. It is crucial to recognize the differences because the interventions and expected outcomes of the two syndromes differ.

■ The symptoms of depression can overlap with the symptoms of both delirium and dementia. One individual may have one, two, or three of the conditions in the triad of delirium, dementia, and depression simultaneously.

■ Delirium is characterized by a disturbance in attention (e.g., ability to focus) and awareness (reduced orientation to environment) that develops over a short period of time. It requires rapid detection and treatment because in 25% of cases, it is a sign of impending death.

■ Usually, delirium is caused by a combination of precipitating factors. The most commonly identified causes are medications, infections (particularly urinary tract and upper respiratory tract infections), fluid and electrolyte imbalance, and metabolic disturbances such as electrolyte imbalance or poor nutrition. Other important predisposing factors include advanced age, brain damage, preexisting dementia, and bio/psycho/social/spiritual stressors.

■ The primary goal of treatment of delirium is prevention or resolution of the acute confusional episode with return to previous cognitive status and interventions focusing on (1) elimination or correction of the underlying cause and (2) symptomatic and safety and supportive measures.

■ Dementia is characterized by the gradual onset of decline in cognitive function, especially memory, usually accompanied by changes in behaviour and personality. Neurologic changes and damage in the brain may be present for many years before symptoms present. Although there are many proposed reasons for these changes, they are not entirely understood. Thus, cures for specific types of dementia have not been discovered.

■ AD is an example of a progressive, degenerative dementia. Treatment efforts currently focus on the reduction of cognitive symptoms (e.g., memory loss, confusion, and problems with learning, speech, and reasoning) in attempts to improve the quality of life for both the patient and their family caregivers.

■ Several potential explanations for the presentation of AD symptoms are currently being explored: the build-up of beta-amyloid plaques, neurofibrillary tangles that become chemically altered, excessive neuroinflammatory responses, and oxidative stress that many researchers believe may be the primary event in AD as oxidative stress is responsible for the impairment of both mitochondria and calcium regulation. In addition, there is a rare FAD that is almost totally attributable to genes that have mutated to an extent that makes them function abnormally resulting in a form of AD.

■ Symptoms of NCD (dementia) may occur as a result of a number of other types of NCDs including vascular dementia, DLB, Parkinson's disease dementia, and FTD. Symptoms of dementia may also be related to other conditions such as HIV infection, traumatic brain injury, Huntington's disease, and prion disease.

■ Educating families and caregivers about what to expect related to the progressive cognitive decline and behaviour changes, safety issues, and available community resources is essential to ensuring appropriate and adequate care.

CRITICAL THINKING CHALLENGES

1 Compare the defining characteristics and related risk factors of acute confusion with those for the NANDA diagnoses of impaired thought processes and sensory/perceptual disturbances. What are the differences and similarities between the recommended nursing interventions for delirium and dementia? What is the theoretic base for these similarities and differences?

2 What are some of the explanations for the presentation of AD symptoms and what remains unknown?

3 What factors should the nurse consider in differentiating AD from vascular dementia?

4 Suggest reasons that older adults are particularly vulnerable to the development of dementia.

5 In what ways can culture and education influence mental status test scores?

6 The physical environment is particularly important to the person with dementia. Every effort should be made to modify the physical environment to compensate for the cognitive and functional impairment associated with AD and related disorders, including safety measures and the avoidance of misleading stimuli. Visualize your last experience in a care setting (hospital, nursing home, day care programme, or home care setting). Identify environmental factors that could be misleading or stress producing to a person with impaired cognition (dementia), and identify ways to modify this environment to alleviate some of the stressors or misleading stimuli.

REFERENCES

Alzheimer Society of Canada. (2012). A new way of looking at the impact of dementia in Canada. Retrieved from http://www.alzheimer.ca/on/~/media/Files/national/Media-eleases/asc_factsheet_new_data_09272012_en.ashx

Alzheimer Society of Canada. (2013a). Stages of Alzheimer's disease (what happens). Available at http://www.alzheimer.ca/en/About-dementia/Alzheimer-s-disease/Stages-of-Alzheimer-s-disease

Alzheimer Society of Canada. (2013b). Treatment of Huntington's. Retrieved from http://www.alzheimer.ca/en/About-dementia/Dementias/Huntington-s-Disease

Alzheimer Society of Canada. (2013c). Creutzfeldt-Jakob disease. Retrieved from http://www.alzheimer.ca/en/About-dementia/Dementias/Creutzfeld-Jakob-Disease

Alzheimer Society UK. (2013). Be head strong: A guide to help you reduce your risk of developing dementia. Retrieved from http://www.warwickshire.gov.uk/Web/corporate/wccweb.nsf/Links/80FFFB1BCC5BB75580257A8C0032E156/$file/Be_head_strong_booklet_web_17-05-12[1].pdf

Alzheimer's Association. (2013a). Inside the brain: Alzheimer's brain tour. Available at http://www.alz.org/research/science/alzheimers_brain_tour.asp

Alzheimer's Association. (2013b). Mild cognitive impairment. Retrieved from http://www.alz.org/dementia/mild-cognitive-impairment-mci.asp

American Geriatrics Society. (2013). Choosing wisely: Five things that physicians and patients should question. Retrieved from http://www.americangeriatrics.org/files/documents/jgs12226.pdf

American Psychiatric Association. (2000). Practice guideline for the treatment of patients with delirium. Available at http://psycho.silverchair.com/pracGuide/pracGuideTopic_2.aspx

American Psychiatric Association. (2013). Diagnostic and statistical manual of mental disorders (5th ed.). Washington, DC: Author.

Ansaloni, L., Catena, F., Chattat, R., Fortuna, D., Franceschi, C., Mascitti, P., & Melotti, R. M. (2010). Risk factors and incidence of postoperative delirium in elderly patients after elective and emergency surgery. British Journal of Surgery, 97(2), 273–280.

Balas, M. C., Rice, M., Chaperon, C., Smith, H., Disbot, M., & Fuchs, B. (2012). Management of delirium in critically ill older adults. Critical Care Nurse, 32(4), 15–26.

Bauer, L. C., Johnson, J. K., & Pozehl, B. J. (2011). Cognition in heart failure: An overview of the concepts and their measures. Journal of the American Academy of Nurse Practitioners, 23(11), 577–585.

Beck, A. T. (2008). The evolution of the cognitive model of depression and its neurobiological correlates. American Journal of Psychiatry, 165(8), 969–977.

Béphage, G. (2009). Care approaches to dementia. British Journal of Healthcare Assistants, 3(1), 43–46.

Blennow, K., Hampel, H., Weiner, M., & Zetterburg, H. (2010). Cerebrospinal fluid and plasma biomarkers in Alzheimer disease. Nature Reviews, Neurology, 6(3), 131–144.

Boettger, S., Friedlander, M., Breitbart, W., & Passik, S. (2011). Aripiprazole and haloperidol in the treatment of delirium. Australian and New Zealand Journal of Psychiatry, 45(6), 477–482.

Boettger, S., Passik, S., & Breitbart, W. (2011). Treatment characteristics of delirium superimposed on dementia. International Psychogeriatrics, 23(10), 1671–1676.

British Geriatrics Society and Royal College of Physicians Guidelines for the prevention, diagnosis and management of delirium in older people. (2006) Diagnosis and management of delirium in older people. London, UK: RCP.

Brown, C. A., Berry, R., Tan, M., Khoshia, A., Turlapati, L., & Swedlove, F. (2013). A critique of the evidence base for non-pharmacological sleep interventions for persons with dementia. Dementia, 12(2), 174–201.

California Workgroup on Guidelines for Alzheimer's Disease Management. (2008). Guideline for Alzheimer's disease management: Final report. California Council of the Alzheimer's Association. Retrieved from http://www.caalz.org/PDF_files/Guideline-FullReport-CA.pdf

Campanelli, C. M. (2012). American Geriatrics Society updated Beers Criteria for potentially inappropriate medication use in older adults. Journal of the American Geriatrics Society, 60(4), 616–631.

Canadian Caregiver Coalition (2008). A framework for a Canadian caregiver strategy. Retrieved from http://www.ccc-ccan.ca/

Canadian Dementia Knowledge Translation Network (CDKTN). (2012). Recommendations for the diagnosis and treatment of dementia 2012: Based on the Canadian Consensus Conference on the Diagnosis and Treatment of Dementia 2012 (CCCDTD4). Retrieved from http://www.slideboom.com/presentations/702016/Canadian-Consensus-Conference-2012-Dementia-Diagnosis-and-Treatment-Recommendations

Canadian Home Care Association (CHCA) (2013). Portraits of home care in Canada. Ottawa, ON: Author.

Candy, B., Jackson, K. C., Jones, L., Leurent, B., Tookman, A., & King, M. (2012). Drug therapy for delirium in terminally ill adult patients. Cochrane Database of Systematic Reviews, 11. Art. no. CD004770. doi: 10.1002/14651858.CD004770.pub2

Carpenito-Moyet, L. (2013). Handbook of Nursing Diagnoses (14th ed.). Philadelphia, PA: Wolters Kluwer.

Carter, C. L., Resnick, E. M., Mallampalli, M., & Kalbarczyk, A. (2012). Sex and gender differences in Alzheimer's disease: Recommendations for future research. Journal of Women's Health, 21(10), 1018–1023.

Casey, G. (2012). Alzheimer's and other dementias. Kai Tiaki Nursing New Zealand, 18(6), 20–24.

Cmiel, C. A., Karr, D. M., Gasser, D. M., Oliphant, L. M., & Neveau, A. J. (2004). Noise control: A nursing team's approach to sleep promotion. American Journal of Nursing, 104(2), 40–48.

DeJong, R., Osterlund, O. W., & Roy, G. W. (1989). Measurement of quality-of-life changes in patients with Alzheimer's disease. Clinical Therapeutics, 11, 545–554.

De Sole, P., Rossi, C., Chiarpotto, M., Ciasca, G., Bocca, B., Alimonti, A., … Masullo, C. (2013). Possible relationship between Al/ferritin complex and Alzheimer's disease. Clinical Biochemistry, 46(1–2), 89–93.

Diamond, J. (2011, May 12). Alzheimer's disease: What's it all about? Where do we stand in the search for a cure? Hope, courage, progress. Toronto, ON: Alzheimer Society of Canada. Retrieved from http://www.alzheimer.ca/~/media/Files/national/Research/Research_Lay_Report_2011_e.ashx

Dore, G. J., McDonald, A., Li, Y., Kaldor, J. M., Brew, B. J.; National HIV Surveillance Committee. (2003). Marked improvement in survival following AIDS dementia complex in the era of highly active antiretroviral therapy. AIDS, 17(10), 1539–1545.

Ferrero-Arias, J., Goñi-Imízcoz, M., González-Bernal, J., Lara-Ortega, F., da Silva-González, A., & Díez-Lopez, M. (2011). The efficacy of nonpharmacological treatment for dementia-related apathy. Alzheimer Disease and Associated Disorders, 25(3), 213–119.

Fick, D. M., Hodo, D. M., Lawrence, F., & Inouye, S. K. (2007). Recognizing delirium superimposed on dementia. Journal of Gerontological Nursing, 33(2), 40–47.

Flaherty, J. H. (1998). Commonly prescribed and over the counter medications: Causes of confusion. Clinics in Geriatric Medicine, 14(1), 101–125.

Flinn, D. R., Diehl, K. M., Seyfried, S. L., & Malani, N. P. (2009). Prevention, diagnosis and management of postoperative delirium in older adults. Journal of the American College of Surgeons, 209(2), 261–268.

Folstein, M. F., Folstein, S. E., & McHugh, P. R. (1975). Mini-mental state: A practical method for grading the cognitive state of patients for the clinician. Journal of Psychiatric Research, 12, 189–198.

Forbes, D. A., Finkelstein, S., Blake, C., Gibson, M., Morgan, D. G., Markle-Reid, M., … Thiessen, E. J. (2012). Knowledge exchange throughout the dementia care journey by rural community-based health care practitioners, persons with dementia, and their care partners: A qualitative interpretive descriptive study. Journal of Rural and Remote Health, 12, 2201.

Forbes, D. A., Markle-Reid, M., Hawranik, P., Peacock, S., Kingston, D., Morgan, D., …Jansen, S. L. (2008). Availability and acceptability of Canadian home and community-based services: Perspectives of family caregivers of persons with dementia. Home Health Care Services Quarterly, 27(1), 75–99.

Forbes, D., Blake, C., Thiessen, E., Finkelstein, S., Gibson, M., Morgan, D., …Culum, I. (2013). "I couldn't be in a better place": Dementia care knowledge sharing within a First Nations community. Canadian Journal on Aging (online ahead of print)

Forbes, D., Blake, C., Thiessen, E. J., Peacock, S., & Hawranik, P. (2014). Light therapy for improving cognition, activities of daily living, sleep, challenging behaviour, and psychiatric disturbances in dementia. Cochrane Database of Systematic Reviews, 2, CD003946.

Forbes, D., Thiessen, E. J., Blake, C. M., Forbes, S. C., & Forbes, S. (2013). Physical activity programs for persons with dementia. Cochrane Database of Systematic Reviews, 2013(12), CD006489.

Gauthier, S., Patterson, C., Chertkow, H., Gordon, M., Herrmann, N., Rockwood, K., … Soucy, J. P. (2012a). 4th Canadian Consensus Conference on the Diagnosis and Treatment of Dementia. Canadian Journal of Neurological Sciences, 39(Supp. 5), S1–S8.

Gauthier, S., Patterson, C., Chertkow, H., Gordon, M., Herrmann, N., Rockwood, K., … Soucy, J. P. (2012b). Recommendations of the 4th Canadian Consensus Conference on the Diagnosis and Treatment of Dementia (CCCDTD4). Canadian Geriatric Journal, 15(4), 120–126.

Genetica Home Reference. (2013). Alzheimer disease. Retrieved from http://ghr.nlm.nih.gov/condition/alzheimer-disease

Gibson, M., MacLean, J., Barrie, M., & Geiger, J. (2004). Orientation behaviors in residents relocated to a redesigned dementia care unit. American Journal of Alzheimer's Disease, 19(1), 45–49.

Givens, J., Jones, R., & Inouye, S. (2009). The overlap syndrome of depression and delirium in older hospitalized patients. *Journal of the American Geriatrics Society, 57*(8), 1347–1353.

Gleason, O. C. (2003). Delirium. *American Family Physician, 67*(5), 1027–1034.

Gotell, E., Brown, S., & Ekman, S-L. (2009). The influence of caregiver singing and background music on vocally expressed emotions and moods in dementia care: A qualitative analysis. *International Journal of Nursing Studies, 46*(4), 422–430.

Graham, J. (2013). Does depression contribute to dementia? *New York Times, Old Age: Caring and Coping*. Retrieved from http://newoldage.blogs.nytimes.com/2013/05/01/does-depression-contribute-to-dementia/

Grover, S., Kate, N., Malhotra, S., Chakrabarti, S., Mattoo, S., & Avasthi, A. (2012). Symptom profile of delirium in children and adolescents—does it differ from adults and elderly? *General Hospital Psychiatry, 34*(6), 626–632.

Hatherill, S. & Flisher, A. J. (2010). Delirium in children and adolescents: A systematic review of the literature. *Journal of Psychosomatic Research, 67*, 337–344.

Heidrich, D. E. (2007). Delirium: An under-recognized problem. *Clinical Journal of Oncology Nursing, 11*(6), 805–807.

Hicks-Moore, S. L. & Robinson, B. A. (2008). Favorite music and hand massage: Two interventions to decrease agitation in residents with dementia. *Dementia, 7*(1), 95–108.

Humphries, J. D. (2008). Sleep disruption in hospitalized adults. *Nursing, 17*(6), 391–395.

Inouye, S. K. (2000). Prevention of delirium in hospitalized older patients: Risk factors and targeted intervention strategies. *Annals of Medicine, 32*(4), 257–263.

Inouye, S. K., van Dyck, C. H., Alessi, C. A., Balkin, S., Siegal, A. P., & Horwitz, R. I. (1990). Clarifying confusion: The confusion assessment method. *Annals of Internal Medicine, 113*, 941–948.

Irwin, S. A., Pirrello, R. D., Hirst, J. M., Buckholz, G. T., & Ferris, F. D. (2013). Clarifying delirium management: Practical, evidence-based, expert recommendations for clinical practice. *Journal of Palliative Care Medicine, 16*(4), 423–435.

Jacklink, K., Walker, J., & Shawande, M. (2013). The emergence of dementia as a health concern among First Nations populations in Alberta, Canada. *Canadian Journal of Public Health, 104*(1), e39–e44.

Jansen, L., Forbes, D. A., Markle-Reid, M., Hawranik, P., Kingston, D., Peacock, S ... Leipert, B. (2009). Formal care providers' perceptions of home and community-based services: Informing dementia care quality. *Home Health Care Services Quarterly, 28*(1), 1–23.

Kaiser, N. C., Melrose, R. J., Liu, C., Sultzer, D. L., Jiminez, E., Su, M., Monserratt, L., & Mendez, M. F. (2012). Neuropsychological and neuroimaging markers in early versus late-onset Alzheimer's disease. *American Journal of Alzheimer's Disease and Other Dementias, 27*(7), 520–529.

Katzenschlager, R., Sampaio, C., Costa, J., & Lees, A. (2003). Anticholinergics for symptomatic management of Parkinson's disease. *Cochrane Database of Systematic Reviews, 2003*(2), CD003735.

Leslie, L. D., Marcantonio, R. E., Zhang, Y., Leo-Summers, L., & Inouye, K. S. (2008). One-year health care costs associated with delirium in the elderly population. *Archives of Internal Medicine, 168*(1), 27–32.

Leung, M. J., Sands, P. L., Paul, S., Joseph, T., Kinjo, S., & Tsai, T. (2009). Does postoperative delirium limit the use of patient-controlled analgesia in older surgical patients? *Anesthesiology, 111*(3), 625–631.

Liu, R. Y., Zhou, J. N., Hoogendijk, W. J. G., van Heerikhuize, J., Kamphorst, W., Unmehopa, U. A., ... Swaab, D. F. (2000). Decreased vasopressin gene expression in the biological clock of Alzheimer disease patients with and without depression. *Journal of Neuropathology and Experimental Neurology, 59*(4), 314–322.

Maclullich, A. M., Ferguson, K. J., Miller, T., de Rooij, S. E., & Cunningham, C. (2008). Unravelling the pathophysiology of delirium: A focus on the role of aberrant stress responses. *Journal of Psychosomatic Research, 65*(3), 229–238.

Maier, W. (2008). Common risk genes for affective and schizophrenic psychoses. *European Archives of Psychiatry and Clinical Neurosciences, 258*(suppl 2), 37–40.

Masellis, M. (2012). Dementia with Lewy bodies (DLB), diagnosis, Parkinson's disease dementia (PDD) webinar. Retrieved from http://www.dementiaknowledgebroker.ca/events/webinar/spectrum-lewy-body-disease-dementia-lewy-bodies-and-parkinson%E2%80%99s-disease-dementia

McCusker, J., Cole, M., Dendukuri, N., Han, L., & Belzile, E. (2003). The course of delirium in older medical inpatients: A prospective study. *Journal of General Internal Medicine, 18*, 696–704.

Nasreddine, Z. S., Phillips, N. A., Bedirian, V., Charbonneau, S., Whitehead, V., Collin, I, ...Chertkow, H. (2005). The Montreal Cognitive Assessment, MoCA: A brief screening tool for mild cognitive impairment. *Journal of the American Geriatrics Society, 53*(4), 695–699.

Neal, M. & Barton Wright, P. (2009). Validation therapy for dementia. *Cochrane Database of Systematic Reviews*, Issue 3, Art. No. CD001394. doi: 10.1002/14651858.CD001394

North American Nursing Diagnosis Association (NANDA). (2012). *Nursing diagnoses: Definition and classification* 2012–2014. Philadelphia, PA: NANDA International.

Omelan, C. (2006). Approach to managing behavioural disturbances in dementia. *Canadian Family Physician, 52*, 191–199.

Patel, S. B. & Kress, J. P. (2011). Accurate identification of delirium in the ICU: Problems with translating the evidence in the real life setting. *American Journal of Respiratory Critical Care Medicine, 184*, 287–288.

Popp, J. & Arlt, S. (2012). Prevention and treatment options for postoperative delirium in the elderly. *Current Opinion in Psychiatry, 25*(6), 515–521.

Prorok, J. C., Horgan, S., & Seitz, D. P. (2013). Health care experiences of people with dementia and their caregivers: A meta-ethnographic analysis of qualitative studies. *Canadian Medical Association Journal, 185*(14), E669–E680.

Reade, M., Guenther, U., Gesin, G., & Devlin, J. W. (2012). Delirium diagnosis: What you do with the information matters most. Implications of objective vs subjective delirium assessment in surgical intensive care patients. *American Journal of Critical Care, 21*, e12–e20.

Registered Nurses Association of Ontario. (2003). *Screening for delirium, dementia and depression in older adults*. Toronto, ON: Author.

Registered Nurses Association of Ontario. (2004). *Caregiving strategies for older adults with delirium, dementia, and depression*. Toronto, ON: Author.

Registered Nurses Association of Ontario. (2005). *Prevention of falls and fall injuries in the older adult*. Toronto, ON: Author.

Reisberg, B., Schneck, M. K., & Ferris, S. H. (1983). The Brief Cognitive Rating Scale (BCRS): Findings in primary degenerative dementia. *Psychopharmacology Bulletin, 19*, 47.

Ringman, J. M., (2011). Setting the stage for prevention of familial Alzheimer's disease. *Lancet Neurology, 10*(3), 200–201.

Rose, K. M. & Lorenz, R. (2010). Sleep disturbances in dementia. *Journal of Gerontological Nursing, 35*(5), 9–14.

Rosen, J., Burgio, L., Kollar, M., Cain, M., Allison, M., Fogleman, M., ... Zubenko, G. S. (1994). The Pittsburgh agitation scale: User-friendly instrument for rating agitation in dementia patients. *The American Journal of Geriatric Psychiatry, 2*(1), 52–59.

Rothberg, M., Herzig, S., Pekow, P., Avrunin, J. Lagu, T., & Lindauer, P. (2013). Association between sedating medications and delirium in older inpatients. *Journal of the American Geriatrics Society, 61*(6), 923–930.

Rowe, M. A., Kelly, A., Horne, C., Lane, S., Campbell, J., Lehman, B., .. . Benito, A. P. (2009). Reducing dangerous nighttime events in persons with dementia by using a nighttime monitoring system. *Alzheimer's and Dementia, 5*(5), 419–426.

Rowe, C. C., Ellis, K. A., Rimajova, M., Bourgeat, P., Pike, K., Jones, G., ... Villemagne, V. L. (2010). Amyloid imaging results from the Australian Imaging, Biomarkers and Lifestyle (AIBL) study of aging. *Neurobiology of Aging 31*(8), 1275–1283.

Salluh, J. I., Soares, M., Teles, J. M., Ceraso, D., Raimondi, N., Nava, V. S., ... Rocha, M. G. (2010). Delirium epidemiology in critical care (DECCA): An international study. *Critical Care, 14*(6), R210. doi: 10.1186/cc9333

Schott, J. M. & Warren, J. D. (2012). Alzheimer's disease: Mimics and chameleons. *Practical Neurology, 12*(6), 358–366.

Schwartz, G. E. (1983). Development and validation of the Geriatric Evaluation by Relatives Rating Instrument (GERRI). *Psychological Reports, 53*, 478–488.

Shaw, C. A. & Tomljenovic, L. (2013). Aluminum in the central nervous system: Toxicity in humans and animals, vaccine adjuvants, and autoimmunity. *Immunologic Research, 56*(2–3), 304–316.

Staal, J. A., Sacks, A., Matheis, R., Collier, L., Calia, T., Hanif, H., & Kofman, E. S. (2007). The effects of Snoezelen (multi-sensory behavior therapy) and psychiatric care on agitation, apathy, and activities of daily living in dementia patients on a short term geriatric psychiatric inpatient unit. *The International Journal of Psychiatry in Medicine, 37*(4), 357–370.

Statistics Canada. (2013). *Health Trends*. Statistics Canada Catalogue 82-213-XWE. Retrieved from http://www12.statcan.gc.ca/health-sante/82-213/index.cfm?Lang=ENG

Sterke, C. S., van Beeck, E. F., Looman, C. W., Kressig, R. W., & van der Cammen, T. J. (2012). An electronic walkway can predict short-term fall risk in nursing home residents with dementia. *Gait and Posture, 36*(1), 95–101.

Stern, Y., Albert, S. M., Sano, M., Richards, M., Miller, L., Folstein, M., ... Lafleche, G. (1994). Assessing patient dependence in Alzheimer's disease. *Journal of Gerontology, 49*, M216–M222.

Strout, K. A. & Howard, E. P. (2012). The six dimensions of wellness and cognition in aging adults. *Journal of Holistic Nursing, 30*(3), 195–204.

Tasci, S., Kartin, P., Ceyhan, Ö., Sungur, G., & Göris, S. (2012). Living with an Alzheimer patient in Turkey. *Journal of Neuroscience Nursing, 44*(4), 228–234.

Teng, E. L., Hasegawa, K., Homma, A., Imai, Y., Larson, E., Graves, A., … Chiu, D. (1994). The Cognitive Abilities Screening Instrument (CASI): A practical test for cross-cultural epidemiological studies of dementia. *International Psychogeriatrics, 6,* 45–58.

Trzepacz, P. T., Mittal D., Torres, R., Kanary, K., Norton, J., & Jimerson, N. (2001). Validation of the Delirium Rating Scale-revised-98: Comparison with the delirium rating scale and the cognitive test for delirium. *Journal of Neuropsychiatry and Clinical Neurosciences, 13,* 229–242.

Tune, L. (2000). Delirium. In C. E. Coffey & J. L. Cummings (Eds.), *American Psychiatric Press textbook of geriatric neuropsychiatry* (2nd ed., pp. 441–462). Washington, DC: American Psychiatric Press.

van den Berg, S. & Splaine, M. (2012). *Policy brief: Risk factors for dementia. Policy recommendations by Alzheimer's Disease International.* Retrieved from http://www.alz.co.uk/sites/default/files/policy-brief-risk-factors-for-dementia.pdf

van Munster, B. C., de Rooij, S. E., & Korevaar, J. C. (2009). The role of genetics in delirium in the elderly patient. *Dementia and Geriatric Cognitive Disorders, 28*(3), 187–195.

Vance, D., Moore, B., Farr, K., & Struzick, T. (2008). Procedural memory and emotional attachment in Alzheimer disease: Implications for meaningful and engaging activities. *Journal of Neuroscience Nursing, 40*(2), 96–102.

Villemagne, V. L., Pike, K. E., Chetelat, G., Ellis, K. A., Mulligan, R. S., Bourgeat, P., … Rowe, C. C. (2011). Longitudinal assessment of Aβ and cognition in aging and Alzheimer disease. *Annals of Neurology, 69*(1), 181–192.

Vollmer, C., Rich, C., & Robinson, S. (2007). How to prevent delirium: A practical protocol. *Nursing, 37*(8), 26–28.

Voyer, P., Richard, S., McCusker, J., Cole, M. G., Monette, J., Champoux, N., … Belzile, E. (2012). Detection of delirium and its symptoms by nurses working in a long term care facility. *Journal of the American Medical Directors Association, 13*(3), 264–271.

Wadley, V. G., Okonkwo, O., Crowe, M., & Ross-Meadows, L. A. (2008). Mild cognitive impairment and everyday function: Evidence of reduced speed in performing instrumental activities of daily living. *American Journal of Geriatric Psychiatry, 16,* 416–424.

Walton, J. R. (2013). Aluminum involvement in the progression of Alzheimer's disease. *Journal of Alzheimer's disease, 35*(1), 7–43.

White, S. & Bayer, A. (2007). Delirium—a clinical overview. *Reviews in Clinical Gerontology, 17,* 45–62.

Zhang, Z., Pan, L., & Ni, H. (2013). Impact of delirium on clinical outcome in critically ill patients: A meta-analysis. *General Hospital Psychiatry, 35*(2), 105–111.

Zhang, L., Sheng, S., & Qin, C. (2013). The role of HDAC6 in Alzheimer's disease. *Journal of Alzheimer's Disease, 33*(2), 283–295.

UNIT 7

Care of Persons With Additional Vulnerabilities

CHAPTER 35

Care of Persons With Concurrent Substance-Related, Addictive, and Other Mental Disorders

Charl Els and Diane Kunyk

KEY CONCEPT

- concurrent disorders

LEARNING OBJECTIVES

After studying this chapter, you will be able to:

- Define the term *concurrent disorders*.
- Discuss the epidemiology of concurrent disorders.
- Understand the aetiologic theories of the development of concurrent disorders.
- Describe the effects of alcohol, tobacco, and other substances on other mental disorders.
- Describe the most common co-occurring conditions.
- Outline the assessment approaches specific to concurrent disorders.
- Outline care and treatment approaches specific to concurrent disorders.
- Appreciate the opportunities and barriers to the care and treatment of persons with concurrent disorders.
- Identify some future directions for research and care in the field of concurrent disorders.

KEY TERMS

- anxiety disorders • attention deficit hyperactivity disorder
- coordinated/parallel care • impulsivity • integrated care • mood disorders • personality disorders • prevention • psychotic disorders • serial treatment • simultaneous/parallel care • stress • substance-related/addictive disorder • trauma

The term *concurrent disorders* is used to describe the situation when an individual suffers from at least one **substance-related/addictive disorder** as well as at least one *other* mental disorder. The *Diagnostic and Statistical Manual of Mental Disorders* (5th ed.) *(DSM-5)* (American Psychiatric Association [APA], 2013) lists the symptoms of more than 300 psychiatric maladies. With more than 1,000 different street drugs available (along with tobacco, alcohol, and prescription drugs), the number of possible combinations between one or more substance-related/addictive disorders and one or more other mental disorders is enormous. Concurrent disorders are highly heterogeneous: neither a prototypical patient nor typical scenario can be described. Although varying degrees of empirical evidence exist for the different categories, the most salient examples of combinations of substance-related/addictive disorders with other mental disorders in the literature include the following:

- Mood disorders and substance-related/addictive disorders
- Eating disorders and substance-related/addictive disorders

- Anxiety disorders and substance-related/addictive disorders
- Attention deficit hyperactivity disorder and substance-related/addictive disorders
- Psychotic disorders and substance-related/addictive disorders
- Personality disorders and substance-related/addictive disorders
- Posttraumatic stress disorder and substance-related/addictive disorders

Concurrent disorders have also been called *dual disorders*, *comorbidity*, *co-occurring substance use and mental health problems*, *mentally ill chemical abuser*, and *dual diagnosis*. In many jurisdictions, however, the term *dual diagnosis* is reserved for persons with an intellectual disability and a mental health problem. For this reason, the term "dual diagnosis" is avoided when referring to the concurrent substance-related/addictive disorders and other mental disorders.

Concurrent disorders are a ubiquitous and urgent health issue. They are among the most complex, intractable, and difficult clinical scenarios in health care. Persons with concurrent disorders typically have many severe life problems and issues related to their disorders. They often experience behavioural health problems, physical health problems, traumatic brain injuries, trauma histories, developmental problems, education problems, housing problems, family problems, employment problems, economic problems, and legal problems (Drake & Green, 2013). Persons with concurrent disorders are more likely to be stigmatized, are socially marginalized, experience high degrees of relational problems, and are more likely to become involved in the criminal justice system. Per capita, they are less likely to continue with their care, likely to require crisis services more often, are more frequently hospitalized, and overall use more health care resources.

The knowledge and practice related to the care and treatment of concurrent disorders are a dynamic, complex, and constantly evolving area in health care. One of the most salient negative challenges to date has been that health care systems tend to be organized for the care and treatment delivery of single disorders. As is the case in many countries, Canada's mental health and addiction care systems are largely independent from each other and compartmentalized. Persons with concurrent disorders can find themselves not fitting well into either the mental health or the addiction treatment systems. This too often results in them "falling through the cracks" and not obtaining access to appropriate levels of safe, effective evidence-based care and treatment. Increased knowledge and skills in caring for persons with concurrent disorders will improve outcomes for this vulnerable population. It is important that nurses recognize that, despite the adverse short-term consequences of co-occurring disorders, many people do recover.

This chapter outlines the concept of **concurrent disorders** and the aetiologic models for co-occurrence of mental illness and addiction. The general principles of care and treatment for persons with concurrent disorders are outlined and nursing strategies and interventions specific to this population recommended. Given the vast number of possible combinations of mental illness and addiction, only the most salient and clinically meaningful examples of such disorders will be discussed. This chapter focuses on an integrated approach aimed at the **prevention** of these disorders and reduction of the severity and progression of existing conditions. See Chapter 26 for a comprehensive presentation of substance-related and addictive disorders.

EPIDEMIOLOGY OF CONCURRENT DISORDERS

It is broadly estimated that approximately 50% of persons seeking help for addiction also suffer from a mental disorder, while 15% to 20% of persons with mental illness also suffer from a substance-related/addictive disorder. Concurrent disorders affect young people, old people, those in the early phases of mental illness, and those with long-term illnesses. People who live in poverty, those who are particularly disenfranchised, and those from minority backgrounds are more likely to be affected.

Canada's first national assessment of the prevalence of concurrent disorders (Rush et al., 2008) suggests that Canadian rates are at the lower end of the range reported internationally. The actual numbers, however, may be much higher as the Canadian studies excluded certain populations who are known to be at high risk for concurrent disorders. A secondary analysis of data from the 2002 Canadian Community Health Survey ($n = 36,984$) reports the 12-month prevalence to be 1.7%, with no significant gender and age differences found. Rates were highest in British Columbia and lowest in Quebec. A second Canadian study (Rush & Koegl, 2008) examined the prevalence and profile of people with concurrent disorders, collecting data on 9,839 cases from specialty tertiary inpatient, specialty outpatient, and community-based mental health programs. Their findings suggest that the overall prevalence of concurrent disorders is 18.5% and that rates are highest in the inpatient settings and within selected populations (i.e., younger adults, persons with personality disorders). The researchers noted that the co-occurrence was strongly associated with antisocial and challenging behaviour, legal involvement, and risk of suicide or self-harm. Lifetime substance use is particularly high in persons suffering from **psychotic disorders** (Margolese et al., 2004), confirming international estimates of lifetime prevalence for individuals with schizophrenia, which is around 50% (Mueser, Bennet, & Kushner, 1995; Regier et al., 1990).

> **KEY CONCEPT Concurrent disorders** is the term used when an individual has at least one substance-related or addictive disorder co-occurring with at least one other mental disorder. Nurses must be attentive to the possibility that patients presenting with either a substance-related disorder or a mental illness may have a concurrent disorder. It is established that about half of persons presenting with a substance-related/addictive disorder also suffer from a mental disorder; one in five persons presenting with a mental disorder also suffers from a substance-related/addictive disorder. Screening for a concurrent mental illness or substance-related/addictive disorder is recommended with the presentation of either condition.

AETIOLOGIC THEORIES: DEVELOPMENT OF CONCURRENT DISORDERS

Despite its high prevalence and established negative consequences, an explanation for the aetiology of co-occurrence of substance-related/addictive disorders and other mental disorders remains largely unclear. Four general models have emerged with varying degrees of empirical support for each model's validity (Mueser, Drake, & Wallach, 1998). These models are: (1) common factor models, (2) secondary substance use disorder models (including supersensitivity and self-medication models), (3) secondary psychiatric disorder models, and (4) bidirectional models.

The *common factor model* suggests that the same set of variables may contribute to an increased risk for the development of substance-related/addictive and other mental health problems. The cited risk factors may be biologic, psychological (including temperamental), social, or environmental. There is some degree of support in this theory that antisocial personality disorder accounts for at least some increased comorbidity.

The *secondary substance use disorder model* proposes that mental health conditions increase the relative risks of developing a substance use disorder. This model includes the *supersensitivity model*, which proposes that there is an existing vulnerability in persons suffering from psychiatric disorders that results in their sensitivity to even small amounts of substances. There is also the *self-medication* model, which suggests that people use substances to relieve subjective distress related to their mental illness. Despite its intuitive appeal, there is minimal empirical support for this theory; it may be more applicable to anxiety and mood disorders than to psychotic disorders. It has, however, been suggested that the accumulation of multiple risk factors related to mental illness, including subjective distress, may indeed increase the relative risk of a substance-related/addictive disorder.

The *secondary psychiatric disorder model* suggests that the use of substances may precipitate mental health conditions in persons who would not otherwise have developed them. It should be noted that substance use is associated with the development of certain psychiatric symptoms. For example, amphetamines can cause psychotic symptoms and alcohol may cause depressive symptoms. However, the evidence to suggest that substance use is causally linked to the development of a bona fide psychiatric disorder is limited. One notable exception is the link between cannabis (smoking marijuana) and schizophrenia. Andréasson, Engström, Allebeck, & Rydberg (1987) studied the association between cannabis and the development of schizophrenia during a 15-year follow-up in a cohort of 45,570 Swedish conscripts and concluded that cannabis is an independent risk factor for schizophrenia.

The *bidirectional model* posits a two-way aetiologic process whereby substance-related/addictive disorders and other mental illnesses increase the risk for the development of the other condition. It holds that a problem in one domain increases the individual's vulnerability to developing challenges in the other area. The link between **stress** and/or **trauma** and the development of substance-related/addictive disorders has been empirically validated. Individuals who have been exposed to traumatic events may increase substance use, which can in turn lead to new traumatic exposures, which may perpetuate the stress–substance use cycle. Both acute stress and chronic stress lead to changes in the natural neurochemical homeostasis, modulated by numerous factors, which may increase the risk of the development of substance-related/addictive disorders. Impulsivity, which may be a feature of some psychiatric conditions, has also been linked with an increased risk of developing substance-related/addictive disorders.

IN A LIFE

Drew Barrymore (1975–)
Actor, Producer, Director, and Model

Public Persona

Drew Blyth Barrymore is a granddaughter of film legend John Barrymore. She first started modelling when she was 11 months old, and her film breakout role was as Gertie in *E.T. the Extra-Terrestrial*. She made the transition from child star to film actress with a number of films (e.g., *The Wedding Singer* and *50 First Dates*). She appeared on the cover of the 2007 *People* magazine's Most Beautiful People issue; is the Ambassador Against Hunger for the UN World Food Programme; and has been awarded the Screen Actors Guild Award and the Golden Globe Award for Best Actress in a Miniseries or Television Film.

Personal Realities

Barrymore endured a notoriously troubled childhood. She started smoking cigarettes at age 9, drinking alcohol at 11, smoking marijuana at 12, snorting cocaine at 13, and entered residential treatment for the first time at age 15. She shares her experience with alcoholism and substance abuse, and her struggle with bipolar illness in the book *Beyond Crazy* (2004).

Source: Simmie, S. & Nunes, J. (2004). *Beyond Crazy*. Toronto, ON: McClelland & Stewart.

THE EFFECTS OF ALCOHOL, TOBACCO, AND OTHER SUBSTANCES ON MENTAL HEALTH

Apart from co-occurring, the use of substances (even in the absence of a diagnosed substance-related/addictive disorder) may negatively impact on the natural course, care/treatment, and prognosis of mental illness. It has been established that

- Alcohol use may induce liver enzymes, leading to more rapid metabolism of medication to treat mental illness. This may worsen symptoms of the mental illness. Apart from this, the use of alcohol may also exacerbate psychosis, bipolar disorder, anxiety disorders, sleep disorders, sexual function, delirium, and neurocognitive disorders.

- Caffeine may worsen anxiety disorders and sleep disorders.

- Cannabis may amplify symptoms of psychosis and anxiety disorders, as well as sleep disorders. It is also associated with worsening of delirium.

- The hallucinogens are associated with worsening of psychotic symptoms, bipolar disorder, depressive conditions, anxiety disorders, and delirium.

- The inhalants may worsen psychotic conditions, depressive conditions, anxiety disorders, and delirium.

- The use of opioids may worsen depressive conditions, anxiety disorders, sleep disorders, sexual dysfunctions, and delirium.

- Sedatives, hypnotics, or anxiolytics may also be associated with an increased risk of worsening symptoms of psychotic disorders, bipolar disorder, depressive disorders, anxiety disorders, sleep disorders, sexual dysfunctions, delirium, and neurocognitive disorders.

- The stimulants (e.g., cocaine, amphetamine, "crystal meth") are associated with worsening of symptoms of psychotic disorders, bipolar disorder, depressive disorders, anxiety disorders, obsessive–compulsive disorder (OCD), sleep disorders, sexual dysfunctions, and delirium.

- Tobacco smoke contains polynuclear aromatic hydrocarbons, which can induce liver enzymes, leading to the liver's capacity to metabolize certain antipsychotics more rapidly. As almost 90% of persons with schizophrenia smoke, this is a clinically relevant interaction. Induction of liver enzymes results in lower bioavailable levels of medications and an increased risk of relapse to the condition in those who smoke. Smoking also induces the metabolism of certain antidepressants, with a similar positive effect on mood. Smoking tobacco can worsen sleep disorders as well.

ASSESSMENT APPROACHES SPECIFIC TO CONCURRENT DISORDERS

Assessment of persons with concurrent disorders follows the principles of assessment for each category of the mental disorder encountered. Screening for tobacco use, illicit substance use, substance use disorders, at-risk drinking, and alcohol use disorders is discussed in Chapter 26.

To allow for adequate treatment planning and appropriate utilization of resources in those with concurrent disorders, assessment of the following six domains is recommended: (1) acute intoxication and/or withdrawal potential; (2) biomedical conditions and complications; (3) emotional/behavioural/cognitive conditions and complications; (4) readiness to change; (5) relapse/continued use/continued problem potential; and (6) recovery environment.

CARE AND TREATMENT APPROACHES SPECIFIC TO CONCURRENT DISORDERS

Care and treatment for concurrent disorders should include screening for both substance-related/addictive disorders and other mental health disorders, a comprehensive assessment of both, psychosocial and pharmacologic interventions, and a plan for coordinated care. As this population is highly heterogeneous, there is no single approach or set of interventions that is proven to be effective for all persons with concurrent disorders (Kavanagh, Mueser, & Baker, 2003).

Different models of care and treatment exist for persons with concurrent disorders: **serial treatment** (whereby care is received in sequential treatment episodes in separate systems of care), **simultaneous/parallel care** (accessed for all disorders simultaneously, but in different and uncoordinated systems), or **coordinated/parallel care** (where all conditions are treated in separate but well-coordinated and linked systems, with seamless collaboration), and **integrated care** (where care is provided by the same cross-trained team members in the same program, resulting in an integration of services). Improving care and treatment for persons suffering from concurrent disorders requires changes to the health care delivery system to allow for simultaneous and coordinated care or integrated care of conditions. Despite the obvious disadvantages of treating mental health disorders separately from addictions in those suffering from both disorders, it is still not common to find truly integrated care and treatment systems in Canada. The optimal degree of integration should ensure that evidence-based safe and effective care is available, accessible, and affordable to each person suffering from a concurrent disorder. Early detection of the disorders, as well as primary, secondary, and tertiary prevention, warrants special attention. Box 35-1 outlines

Source: Minkoff, K. (2001). Developing standards of care for individuals with co-occurring psychiatric and substance disorders. *Psychiatric Services*, 52(5), 597–599.

BOX 35-1 General Treatment Principles for Concurrent Disorders

1. All good treatment proceeds from an empathic, hopeful nurse–patient relationship.
2. Consequently, the nurse should promote opportunities to initiate and maintain continuing empathic, hopeful relationships whenever possible.
3. Care should be taken to remove arbitrary barriers to initial assessment and evaluation including initial psychopharmacology evaluation (e.g., length of sobriety, alcohol level, etc.)
4. As a general principle, medication for a known serious mental illness should not be discontinued because a patient is using substances.
5. A substance disorder evaluation and/or treatment should not be denied because a patient is on a prescribed non-addictive psychotropic medication.
6. When mental illness and substance disorder coexist, both disorders require specific and appropriately intensive primary treatment.
7. The specific content of dual primary treatment for each person must be individualized according to diagnosis, phase of treatment, level of functioning and/or disability, and assessment of level of care based on acuity, severity, medical safety, motivation, and availability of recovery support.

general treatment principles for individuals with concurrent disorders.

Treatment Matching

The overarching principle in matching persons to the right level of care is to provide treatment at the least restrictive level of care that will be effective and safe. The concept of treatment matching has been formalized and is available through a systematic approach called Patient Placement Criteria (PPC). PPC provide separate placement criteria for individualized treatment plans through a multidimensional assessment that evaluates acute intoxication/withdrawal; biomedical conditions/complications; emotional, behavioural, or cognitive conditions/complications; readiness to change; relapse, continued use, or continued problem potential; and recovery environment. Based on this multidimensional assessment, treatment placement on one of five levels is recommended: Level 0.5 (early intervention), Level I (outpatient services), Level II (intensive outpatient/partial hospitalization services), Level III (residential/inpatient services), or Level IV (medically managed intensive inpatient services).

Indications for Hospitalization

Substance use and mental illness are both risk factors for thoughts of death, dying, and suicide. The potential risk of harm has to be carefully assessed (and repeated serially) in those with both conditions. Attention should be given to detecting other risk factors, which include previous attempts, history of violence and/or trauma, lack of social support systems, and physical illness. Those at imminent and substantial risk of harm to self should be hospitalized to ensure safety. Other indications for hospitalization may include complicated withdrawal syndromes, or where interventions on a less restrictive level of care have failed to yield the necessary outcomes. Individual approaches should incorporate engagement, persuasion, active treatment, and relapse prevention (RP). Psychoeducation and support for treatment adherence will be important. Multimodal and integrated pharmacotherapy and behavioural approaches are key treatment options.

IMPLEMENTING INTERVENTIONS FOR SPECIFIC CONCURRENT DISORDERS

There is no standardized intervention that will work for every individual with a concurrent disorder, because each may differ greatly with respect to severity, substance of abuse, mental illness, and the individual's unique biologic, psychological, social, and spiritual considerations. Often several approaches can work together while others are deemed inappropriate. Treatment programs usually combine psychosocial interventions with other different approaches to provide a comprehensive plan based on the individual's needs. Nursing interventions vary depending on the nature of the current problems, the status and severity of the illnesses, and the individual's situation. Continuity of treatment is clearly important, but even more critical is the need to develop specific evidence-based treatments—pharmacologic and psychosocial interventions—for specific situations and specific individuals. A summary of evidence-based nursing approaches for patients with concurrent disorders is found in Box 35-2. The following section discusses the most salient examples of concurrent disorders that the nurse will encounter during his or her practice.

Mood Disorders and Substance-Related/Addictive Disorders

Mood disorders are among the most common psychiatric disorders in the general population, and approximately 15% to 50% of those presenting for treatment for substance use disorders also have a lifetime diagnosis of a depressive disorder. This is one example of a putative common vulnerability as a result of genetic and/or environmental factors. Individuals with mood disorders tend to be more likely to use substances, with the highest rates found among persons with bipolar disorder.

It is often difficult to distinguish between substance-induced mood symptoms and those associated with a bona fide mood disorder. To distinguish, it is useful to examine the onset of the conditions and to determine which condition preceded which or to investigate the persistence of mood symptoms during periods of sobriety and abstinence. It is often necessary to wait for a period of 4 weeks of sobriety/abstinence before diagnosing an independent mood disorder versus a substance-induced mood disorder. This poses obvious clinical concerns in terms of having to wait for weeks prior to intervening. Suffering from a mood disorder and substance-related/addictive disorder may increase the risk of suicide and shorten life expectancy, and it may also adversely impact the clinical course of either or both disorders.

Treatment of co-occurring depression with antidepressant medication is helpful in reducing both substance abuse and depressive symptomatology. It should, however, not be considered stand-alone treatment and will unlikely resolve the substance-related/addictive disorder, hence necessitating concurrent treatment of both conditions. Similar to other studies of mood disorders, the placebo response rate is high. The selective serotonin reuptake inhibitors (SSRIs) are among the most favourable first-line options due to their tolerability and safety profile. The tricyclic antidepressants are problematic in this population due to the sedating effects, the risk of overdose, and the risk of seizures. If SSRIs fail, alternative options include compounds like duloxetine, mirtazapine, venlafaxine, desvenlafaxine (serotonin and norepinephrine reuptake inhibitor, or SNRI), or bupropion. Bupropion should not be used in persons with a history of seizures or those in alcohol withdrawal (see Chapters 12 and 22). Cognitive–behavioural therapy (CBT) and community reinforcement approaches have demonstrated benefits in depression and substance use,

while integrated group therapy, which is based on CBT, has shown benefit in those with bipolar disorder and substance use (see Chapters 13 and 14).

Anxiety Disorders and Substance-Related/Addictive Disorders

Persons with **anxiety disorders** are two to five times more likely to have a substance-related/addictive problem when compared with the general population. In the short term, selected substances may relieve symptoms of anxiety, but in the medium and long term, such substances may worsen symptoms. Of the range of anxiety disorders, panic disorder is the single anxiety disorder most closely associated with addiction to alcohol, while generalized anxiety disorder (GAD) is the one most closely associated with dependence on substances other than alcohol. The presence of GAD is also associated with a more rapid progression from first drink to addiction as compared with individuals without anxiety disorder. For most persons with anxiety and substance-related/addictive disorder, it has been determined that the anxiety disorder generally preceded the development of the substance-related/addictive disorder. The association between substance-related conditions and OCD is considered the least robust of all the anxiety disorders.

CBT is considered the most effective treatment for anxiety co-occurring with substance-related/addictive disorder, and some benefits may be yielded from pharmacotherapy. In general, the use of benzodiazepines should be avoided due to the potential for abuse. There is a dearth of evidence to guide treatment, but in general, the SSRIs or SNRIs may be considered helpful (see Chapter 23).

Attention Deficit Hyperactivity Disorder and Substance-Related/Addictive Disorders

Attention-deficit hyperactivity disorder (ADHD) is the most common behavioural disorder of childhood, and those with ADHD are more prone to develop substance-related/addictive disorders, especially if ADHD remains untreated in the early stages. This is particularly the case for those with concurrent conduct disorder. The majority of children with ADHD continue to have symptoms in adulthood even though they may not meet the criteria for the disorder as an adult. The diagnosis of ADHD is complicated in persons who are already using substances as their use may mimic symptoms of ADHD, and the latter is often underdiagnosed in clinical populations. Major depressive disorder (MDD), bipolar disorder, or psychotic disorders may also co-occur in those with ADHD and substance-related/addictive disorders, further complicating diagnostic uncertainty.

Attention placed on prevention, early identification, and care/treatment strategies can diminish the adverse consequences of ADHD. These include the trait of **impulsivity** and one of its most damaging consequences, namely that of substance use and addiction. Stimulant medications (dextroamphetamine or methylphenidate) are the mainstay of treatment, and, despite the abuse potential of these drugs, clinical evidence suggests that such treatment can be conducted safely and effectively. Nonstimulant medications like atomoxetine, clonidine, and modafinil are also considered reasonable options. Precautions should be taken to avoid abuse when using medications that are associated with risk of abuse. Psychosocial interventions that are proven to yield benefits include contingency management and CBT.

Psychotic Disorders and Substance-Related/ Addictive Disorders

The rates of substance-related/addictive disorders are substantially elevated in those with psychotic disorder when compared with persons in the general population. Substance use may expedite the onset of a psychotic disorder, and cannabis has been determined to be an independent risk factor in the development of schizophrenia. The most obvious psychotic symptoms related to alcohol use occur during alcohol withdrawal. Symptoms typically emerge within 2 days from stopping consumption and often present with command hallucinations and/or agitation. Cannabis use may be associated with suspiciousness, confusion, and memory impairment, while the psychosis associated with cocaine use is typically associated with transient paranoia. Substance use may also worsen the symptoms and complicate the diagnostic certainty, course, and treatment of the illness.

A wide range of substances may mimic psychotic symptoms, both during intoxication and withdrawal. Evidence suggests that, because of genetic factors or brain abnormalities shared by the two disorders, the risk of schizophrenia or psychosis is higher in those who use drugs than those who do not. Almost 90% of persons with schizophrenia smoke cigarettes, and persons with mental illness consume an estimated 44% of all cigarettes smoked in North America. Smoking is the leading preventable cause of death and disease in persons with schizophrenia, and they die 25 years younger than persons in the general population.

The first step in management is to ensure adequate safety. Following this, the concurrent treatment of psychotic symptoms and substance use is indicated. Special attention should be given to medication adherence, and the use of depot antipsychotics may have a special utility in ensuring such. The use of atypical antipsychotics appears to be superior to the use of typical/conventional antipsychotics in this regard, as the former appear to better target negative symptoms and are less prone to be associated with dysphoria. Atypical antipsychotics are also associated with greater success in smoking cessation in persons with schizophrenia. Psychosocial approaches

that have demonstrated effectiveness are motivational enhancement therapy, RP, and 12-step facilitation (see Chapters 20 and 21).

Personality and Substance-Related/Addictive Disorders

Although antisocial personality disorder is the most commonly associated **personality disorder** with substance-related/addictive disorders, the most challenging is likely borderline personality disorder. Both the addiction and the personality disorder are likely to result in complex and serious behavioural problems, often with an associated risk of harm to self. It is also often associated with the co-occurrence of other mental disorders, for example, MDD, an eating disorder, or OCD. The category of concurrent personality disorders and substance-related/addictive disorders pose some of the most vexing problems in care of this population.

Attention should first be paid to ensuring safety to self and to others. General principles of treatment include offering pharmacotherapy for comorbid conditions like MDD, OCD, or an eating disorder. No medication is indicated for any specific personality disorder. Behavioural interventions form the mainstay of treatment, specifically dialectical behavioural therapy (DBT). Applying the principles of DBT for the population of concurrent disordered individuals has demonstrated significant benefit by teaching patients cognitive self-control techniques that allow for turning themselves to abstinence. Principles that have been found beneficial in this context include the following: Do not give lethal drugs to lethal people; combine pharmacotherapy with a psychosocial treatment; do not reinforce dysfunctional, ineffective behaviour; catch the patient "being good" (e.g., acting skillfully); and validate appropriate behaviour (see Chapter 27).

● **STUDY NOTE**

The best approach in caring for patients with concurrent disorders is to address both illnesses simultaneously. Intervention for only one disorder has not been shown to be effective. The intervention into one disorder alone does not mean that the other one will no longer be expressed.

■■ NURSING MANAGEMENT: SUMMARY

Nurses working in nonpsychiatric inpatient and community settings may be the first health care contact made by the individual with a concurrent disorder. It is important to recognize that the stigma associated with both substance use and mental disorders can affect the person's readiness to address his or her illnesses. A helpful, knowledgeable, and nonjudgemental approach to the person may open a "window of opportunity" for seeking care and treatment. As persons with concurrent disorders may have difficulty relating openly with others and with trusting those in "authority positions," engaging the person in a way that concretely addresses presenting issues (e.g., acquiring social services; getting relief from psychiatric symptoms) can be particularly helpful. Note that assessment procedures that are protracted, are complicated, and involve intimate personal questions may be discouraging to the individual. As well, it may take some time and further engagement for the individual to be willing and able to provide an accurate history of substance use, severity of symptoms, and problems in living. Denial to oneself regarding these issues is a common defensive mechanism for persons with concurrent disorders; it may therefore be particularly difficult for them to be a reliable historian. Medical records, other health care professionals, family members, and significant others may be of assistance to the person and the nurse in developing an accurate health history.

Families of the individual with a concurrent disorder will need education about concurrent disorders and guidance as to the best way to support their family member in recovery. Developing and sustaining a healthy lifestyle is an important aspect of recovery, and families can be particularly helpful in this area. Nurses can provide information at a level appropriate to the family, as well as the individual, on diet, exercise, sleep routine, stress management, and leisure activities. These are essential to a lifestyle that supports sobriety and prevents relapse. At times, families of persons with a concurrent disorder are no longer involved in their lives or are also living with addiction and/or mental health problems. Nurses need to assess the existing support system of the individual, as finding alternative supports and/or social services may need to be an immediate goal.

Psychoeducation regarding goal setting can give the individual a core strategy for making positive change. Access to crisis counselling is important, as is housing that allows for a situation supportive of recovery. Opportunities for a social network that reinforces sobriety and the maintenance of treatment plans for psychiatric symptoms will be important. Nurses can assist by referrals to local groups (e.g., Alcoholics Anonymous; mental health drop-in clubs; partnership with volunteers) that aim to facilitate the development of such social networks. At an appropriate point in recovery, referral to vocational and employment guidance will be a priority.

Relapse prevention is crucial to the care of the person in recovery from a concurrent disorder; patient education, whether offered on a one-to-one basis or in a group setting, is a key strategy. See Box 35-3 for recommended psychoeducational topics.

> **BOX 35-3 Psychoeducational Topics for Relapse Prevention**
>
> - Understanding addiction
> - Effects and interaction of tobacco, alcohol, and other drugs in the body
> - What is my relationship with tobacco, alcohol, and other drugs?
> - How to live in a healthy way
> - Leisure and relaxation
> - Coping with stress
> - Coping with anger
> - Communicating with others
> - Problem-solving strategies
> - The relapse cycle
> - Strategies for preventing relapse
> - My plan for avoiding relapse
> - My personal cues that relapse is imminent
> - Dealing with crisis

WHERE DO WE GO FROM HERE?

Canada's mental health and addiction systems continue to be largely independent and compartmentalized. As a result, the focus of treatment for people with concurrent disorders tends to be on one component of their concurrent disorder but not the other. This challenge is likely as intractable as concurrent disorders themselves. Apart from research into the effectiveness of different treatment approaches, research into systems' approaches is also direly needed. Universal education and training are needed for the workforce responsible for the care and treatment of those with concurrent disorders.

The only viable solution to prevent those with concurrent disorders from "falling through the cracks" is to merge the national agendas for mental health and addiction. The national mental health strategy established by the Mental Health Commission of Canada Commission (2012) fails to do so, leaving Canadians with separate strategies for mental health and for addiction. This is the case, even though addiction is recognized as a bona fide mental illness. Unless we have a unified approach to all components of concurrent disorders, our patients will not be able to reach their potential and thrive.

SUMMARY OF KEY POINTS

■ *Concurrent disorders* is the term used when individuals suffer from at least *one* substance-related or addictive disorder as well as one or more *other* mental disorder. When these conditions co-occur, treatment should address both (or all) at the same time (integrated or parallel treatment).

■ Many individuals with co-occurring disorders, despite the adverse short-term consequences, do recover.

■ An important reason why persons with addiction relapse to drug use is the presence of untreated mental illness. An important reason why persons with mental illness relapse to mental illness is untreated addiction issues.

■ When mental illness and substance disorder coexist, both disorders require specific and appropriate primary treatment.

■ All types of disorders are considered "primary" in that there is not a disorder or approach to treatment that is considered more important than another.

■ The specific content of primary treatment for each person with concurrent disorders must be individualized according to diagnosis, phase of treatment, level of functioning and/or disability, and assessment of level of care based on acuity, severity, medical safety, motivation, and availability of recovery support.

■ The most effective approach for patients is to have health care professionals, programs, and resources colocated and such services offered on a long-term basis with continuity of care across programs and time. Patients benefit from a chronic care approach rather than episodic care.

■ Psychoeducation regarding the effects of tobacco, alcohol, and other drug use, a healthy lifestyle, and relapse prevention is a key element of nursing care for persons with concurrent disorders, in addition to health education regarding their co-occurring mental disorder.

CRITICAL THINKING CHALLENGES

1 What is your understanding of the aetiology of concurrent disorders? Based on this understanding, how does this influence the scope of your nursing assessment?

2 Nellie G. is being treated for a MDD in a psychiatric hospital. She asks you whether she should try to quit smoking at the same time. What do you think would be the most appropriate response?

3 John M. has sought treatment for a psychotic disorder. He came to your psychiatric assessment unit smelling of cannabis. He explains that smoking marijuana helps him to cope. How would this change your assessment approach?

4 You were selected to be on a committee responsible for reducing duplication of resources. One of the key recommendations brought forward is to offer addiction services at one treatment centre and psychiatric services at another. Presently, they are both offered at each site, and it was suggested that splitting the services would be more efficient for management. What evidence would you provide that would not support this recommendation?

5 How would you respond to Cheryl P., a patient with MDD and alcohol use disorder, who states, "Once my medication is stable, I will be able to drink again."

REFERENCES

American Psychiatric Association. (2013). *Diagnostic and statistical manual of mental disorders* (5th ed.). Washington, DC: Author.

Andréasson, S., Engström, A., Allebeck, P., & Rydberg, U. (1987). Cannabis and schizophrenia: A longitudinal study of Swedish conscripts. *Lancet*, *2*(8574), 1483–1486.

Cleary, M., Walter, G., Hunt, G. E., Clancy, R., & Horsfall, J. (2008). Promoting dual diagnosis awareness in everyday clinical practice. *Journal of Psychosocial Nursing*, *46*(12), 43–49.

Drake, R. E. & Green, A. I. (2013). The challenge of heterogeneity and complexity in dual diagnosis. *Journal of Dual Diagnosis*, *9*(2), 105–106.

Kavanagh, D. J., Mueser, K. T., & Baker, A. (2003). Management of comorbidity. In M. Teesson & H. Proudfoot (Eds.), *Comorbid mental disorders and substance use disorders: Epidemiology, prevention and treatment* (pp. 78–120). Sydney, Australia: National Drug and Alcohol Research Centre.

Margolese, H. C., Malchy, L., Carlos Negrete, J., Tempier, R., & Gill, K. (2004). Drug and alcohol use among patients with schizophrenia and related psychoses: Levels and consequences. *Schizophrenia Research*, *67*, 157–166.

Mental Health Commission of Canada. (2012). *Changing directions, changing lives: The mental health strategy for Canada*. Calgary, AB: Author.

Minkoff, K. (2001). Developing standards of care for individuals with co-occurring psychiatric and substance disorders. *Psychiatric Services*, *52*(5), 597–599.

Mueser, K. T., Bennet, M., & Kushner, M. G. (1995). Epidemiology of substance use disorders among persons with chronic mental illnesses. In A. F. Lehman & L. B. Dixon (Eds.), *Double-jeopardy: Chronic mental illness and substance use disorders* (Vol. 3, pp. 9–25). Longhorne, PA: Harwood Academic.

Mueser, K. T., Drake, R. E., & Wallach, M. A. (1998). Dual diagnosis: A review of etiological theories. *Addictive Behaviours*, *23*(6), 717–734.

Regier, D. A., Farmer, M. E., Rae, D. S., Locke, B. Z., Keith, S. J., Judd, L. L., & Goodwin, F. K. (1990). Comorbidity of mental disorders with alcohol and other drug abuse: Results from the epidemiologic catchment area (ECA) study. *JAMA*, *264*(19), 2511–2518.

Rush, B. & Koegl, C. J. (2008). Prevalence and profile of people with co-occurring mental and substance use disorders within a comprehensive mental health system. *Canadian Journal of Psychiatry*, *53*(12), 810–821.

Rush, B., Urbanoski, K., Bassani, D., Castel, S., Wild, T. C., Strike, C., & Somers, J. (2008). Prevalence of co-occurring substance use and other mental disorders in the Canadian population. *Canadian Journal of Psychiatry*, *53*(12), 800–809.

Simmie, S. & Nunes, J. (2004). *Beyond crazy*. Toronto, ON: McClelland & Stewart.

36 Care of Medically Compromised Persons

Michel A. Tarko

Adapted from the chapter "Psychosocial Aspects of Medically
Compromised Persons" by Gail L. Kongable

LEARNING OBJECTIVES

After studying this chapter, you will be able to:

- Identify medically ill populations at risk for secondary mental illness.
- Analyze the effect on clients and their families of mental illness associated with the medical illness.
- Discuss neurobiologic and psychological disturbances associated with specific medical illnesses and the medications used to treat them.
- Discuss comorbid psychosocial and biologic disorders seen in psychiatric settings and their treatments.
- Develop a plan of care for clients who are experiencing mental illness associated with medical illness.
- Discuss bio/psycho/social/spiritual interventions that promote clients' mental health in physical illness.

KEY TERMS

- acute pain • allodynia • chronic pain • comorbidity • endorphins
- gate-control model • HIV-1–associated cognitive–motor complex
- hyperalgia • hyperesthesia • hypothalamic–pituitary–adrenal
(HPA) axis • ischaemic cascade • kindling • neurotransmitters
- nociception • plasticity • self-efficacy • serotonin • substance P

Mental health problems or illness often accompanies medical illness and is a significant health care problem in the medically ill population. People who have chronic medical illnesses have a nearly 41% higher rate of psychiatric disorders than do people without chronic medical illness. In addition, the chronically medically ill have a 28% higher lifetime prevalence of psychiatric disorders than do people without psychiatric disorders. Studies spanning decades indicate that diabetes mellitus, cardiac disease, and associated metabolic disorders are more common among clients with psychiatric disorders than among the general population (De Hert et al., 2009; Joffe, Brasche, & MacQueen, 2003). As many as 70% to 80% of chronically mentally ill clients have significant medical illness (Jones, Marcias, & Harding, 2004) that may or may not be related to psychopharmacologic therapy (Dixon, Postrado, Delahanty, Fischer, & Lehman, 1999; Goldsmith, 1999). Mood, anxiety, and substance use disorders are the most prevalent psychiatric conditions of clients with chronic or terminal illnesses, such as chronic pain, acquired immunodeficiency syndrome (AIDS), acute trauma, stroke, and cancer (Ford, Trestman, Steinberg, Tennen, & Allen, 2004). Because most medically ill people are older adults, biologic, psychological, social, and spiritual changes may place them at greater risk for mental illness and increased potential morbidity and mortality.

PSYCHOLOGICAL ILLNESS RELATED TO SPECIFIC PHYSIOLOGIC DISORDERS

The biologic basis of mental disorders that are preceded by comorbid medical disorders is thought to be similar to the biologic basis of primary psychiatric disorders, in which neurochemical changes occur in the process of catecholamine metabolism (Arnsten, 1997, 2011; Arnsten & Pliszka, 2011). The neurochemicals (transmitters) that orchestrate thinking, learning, speaking, and motor responses also influence mood, perception, and emotional interpretation. Neurochemical modulation maintains a balance in the essential levels of these transmitters. When modulation is disrupted, either mechanically or chemically, disorder occurs.

Unfortunately, mental illness is not commonly recognized or treated in general medical settings. Psychiatric symptoms may be masked by medical symptoms or misdiagnosed as somatoform disorders. The treatment regimen may contribute to psychosocial dysfunction because many medications prescribed for chronic illness alter affect (Goldsmith, 1999; Neese, 1991). Generally, health care providers expect clients to exhibit depressed mood and anxiety as a normal response to illness. In fact, it is considered abnormal if a client does not grieve over the loss of health or does not express discouragement or anxiety about treatment and the possibility of death.

When psychosocial dysfunction remains unexamined and untreated, the course and outcome of associated medical illness may be affected. Mental illness may weaken the motivation for self-care, impair symptom reporting, and delay the search for treatment (Cooper, Corrigan, & Watson, 2003). These symptoms may precede or occur during acute hospitalization and continue after discharge and apparent physical recovery. As a result, hospitalization may be prolonged and recovery delayed, or impaired, at increased emotional and financial cost to the client and the family (Levenson, 1992). In severe cases, mood disorders associated with medical illness increase morbidity and mortality (Eriksson et al., 2004; Hill, Kelleher, & Shumaker, 1992; Paten, 1999; Polsky et al., 2005). Careful assessment to identify and evaluate symptoms of concomitant mental illness separately from those of medical illness is required, together with appropriate treatment, to achieve the client's best psychological and medical outcome. Evidence is emerging in the literature that there is substantially reduced psychological and physical quality of life in medically ill patients with comorbid mental disorders and that there is need for psychiatric treatment in medically oriented contexts of care (Baumeister, Hutter, Bengel, & Harter, 2011).

Another aspect of psychiatric disorders and medical illness is the common **comorbidity** of physical disorders among people who require primary psychiatric care. Factors associated with increased hospital stays of psychiatric clients include physical disability and concomitant medical illness (Bressi, Marcus, & Solomon, 2006; Cohen & Cosimer, 1989; Collins, 1991). Mental health care professionals must carefully evaluate and monitor changes in coexisting medical conditions to prevent their exacerbation or serious complications that would necessitate acute medical treatment or prolonged hospital stay.

This chapter reviews issues related to mental illness in the medically ill population and common comorbid medical disorders in the psychiatric population. The psychosocial disturbances associated with chronic pain, human immunodeficiency virus (HIV), trauma, neurologic disorders, stroke, and chronic medical illnesses such as heart disease and cancer are presented. Suggestions for diagnostic appraisal and appropriate intervention are given. These medical conditions were chosen because they are responsible for most hospital admissions and frequently are associated with psychiatric comorbidity. The content of this chapter underscores the need for all nurses to have adequate preparation and support in attending to the mental health needs of clients and for effective collaboration between primary care clinicians and clinicians practising in psychiatric and mental health settings (World Health Organization & World Organization of Family Doctors, 2008).

> **KEY CONCEPT** **Neurochemical modulation**
> maintains a balance in the essential levels of the neurotransmitters that influence mood, perceptions, and emotional interpretation.

PSYCHOLOGICAL IMPACT OF PAIN

Physiologic pain is a protective response to noxious stimuli that serves as a warning of injury. Clinical pain related to inflammation and pathologic processes is characterized by low-threshold sensitization. Despite major advances in treatments that lessen its force, pain remains one of the most powerful and complex human experiences. Assessing and treating pain are difficult because the pain response is subjective and a client's degree of pain cannot be observed directly. A client's complaints may be difficult to localize. Moreover, the person's discomfort may seem out of proportion to the observed conditions or influenced by disordered emotions, personality, or environmental conditioning. Severe or chronic pain may affect mentally healthy people in adverse ways. The prevalence and impact of pain have led to numerous approaches to therapy, including the use of antipsychotic drugs, antidepressants, antianxiety agents, and stimulants. Considerable evidence suggests that psychiatric medications and interventions can be effective in treating acute and chronic pain.

The **gate-control model** of pain response, based on physiologic evidence that pain perception (**nociception**) involves pathways in the dorsal horn of the spinal cord that relay noxious stimuli to the brain, was first published in 1965 and stands the test of time (Dickerson, 2002). In addition, certain other nerve fibres function as an antagonistic "gate" to augment or dampen the subjective experience of pain (Melzack, 1993; Robinson, 2003). The cognitive–biobehavioural model (see Chapter 13) considers not only the client's emotive and cognitive perception of pain but also the interaction of environmental influences, physical factors, and pain perceptions over time. From this perspective, clients' interpretation of pain, their coping resources, and their emotive psychological processes interact with the experience of pain and can influence the physiologic activities that characterize pain (Turk, 2004). Some pain theorists believe that the gate-control theory has been largely discredited (McCaffery & Pasero, 1999); others are working to refine the theory as more knowledge of pain becomes available.

> **KEY CONCEPT** The **cognitive–behavioural model** is the model of perception that includes emotion, cognition, environment, and physical and psychological factors.

Biologic Basis of the Pain Response

Pain is transmitted through specific neural pathways that carry information about touch and temperature (Fig. 36-1). Recent physiologic evidence obtained from magnetic resonance imaging and positron emission tomography has demonstrated that painful stimuli also cause significant activation in areas of the brain responsible for memory, emotion, and personality (Talbot

FIGURE 36-1. Pain stimuli activate regions of the brain that influence memory, emotion, and personality.

& Marrett, 1991) (Fig. 36-2). Pain receptors may be activated by mechanical, thermal, or chemical stimuli. **Neurotransmitters** are chemicals circulating in the synaptic areas of neurons. They serve to initiate, block, or modulate nerve signal transmission and ultimately control neural function. Several neurotransmitters within primary pain pathways are involved in pain transmission (Box 36-1). When these neurochemicals are released, they initiate local inflammatory reactions and sensitize and stimulate central pain receptors. **Substance P** and prostaglandins are the most common nociceptive transmitters that are released and transported along the central and peripheral pain synapses in the presence of noxious stimuli. **Endorphins**, neurotransmitters that have opiate-like behaviour, produce an inhibitory effect at opiate receptor sites and probably are responsible for pain tolerance. The release of endorphins is centrally mediated by serotonin (Zangen, Nakash, & Yadid, 1999). Serotonin, histamine, and bradykinin sensitize and stimulate the pain receptors to generate the experienced pain. Direct demonstrations of changes in endorphin levels during pain and relief from pain are being reported (Ren, 1994; Sosnowski, 1994). The role of endorphins may go beyond pain modulation to include mood enhancement behaviour modification and influence the development of tolerance or dependence on narcotics.

Acute pain, one of the most common symptoms of clients in emergency and acute care settings, can result from a variety of physiologic abnormalities and trauma. It is characterized by sudden, severe onset and generally subsides as the injury heals. Postoperative incisional pain is an iatrogenic (physician-induced) tissue injury most often seen in medical settings. Careful assessment and treatment of pain in these settings have a great impact on healing and recovery.

Chronic pain, defined as pain on a daily basis or pain that is constant for more than 6 months (Atkinson & Slater, 1989), can be related to various pathologies and takes the form of syndromes such as headache, temporomandibular pain disorders, back pain, and arthritis and can further be conceptualized multidimensionally in terms of future pain course and outcomes (Von Korff & Dunn, 2008). Clinical syndromes with chronic pain symptoms include neoplasia (cancer), thalamic stroke (central pain), neuropathies (diabetes), and reflex sympathetic dystrophy (Box 36-2). Nervous tissue injury leads to neuropathic pain that may be described as burning, aching, pricking, or lancinating. This central or neuropathic pain is the underlying mechanism for most chronic pain and leads to **hyperalgia** (increased sensation of pain), **allodynia** (lowered pain threshold), and **hyperesthesia** (increased nociceptor sensitivity). Permanent change in central pain interpretation frequently results in abnormal physiologic, biochemical, cellular, and molecular responses that misinterpret nonpainful sensations as painful (**plasticity**; Melzack, Coderre, Katz, & Vaccarino,

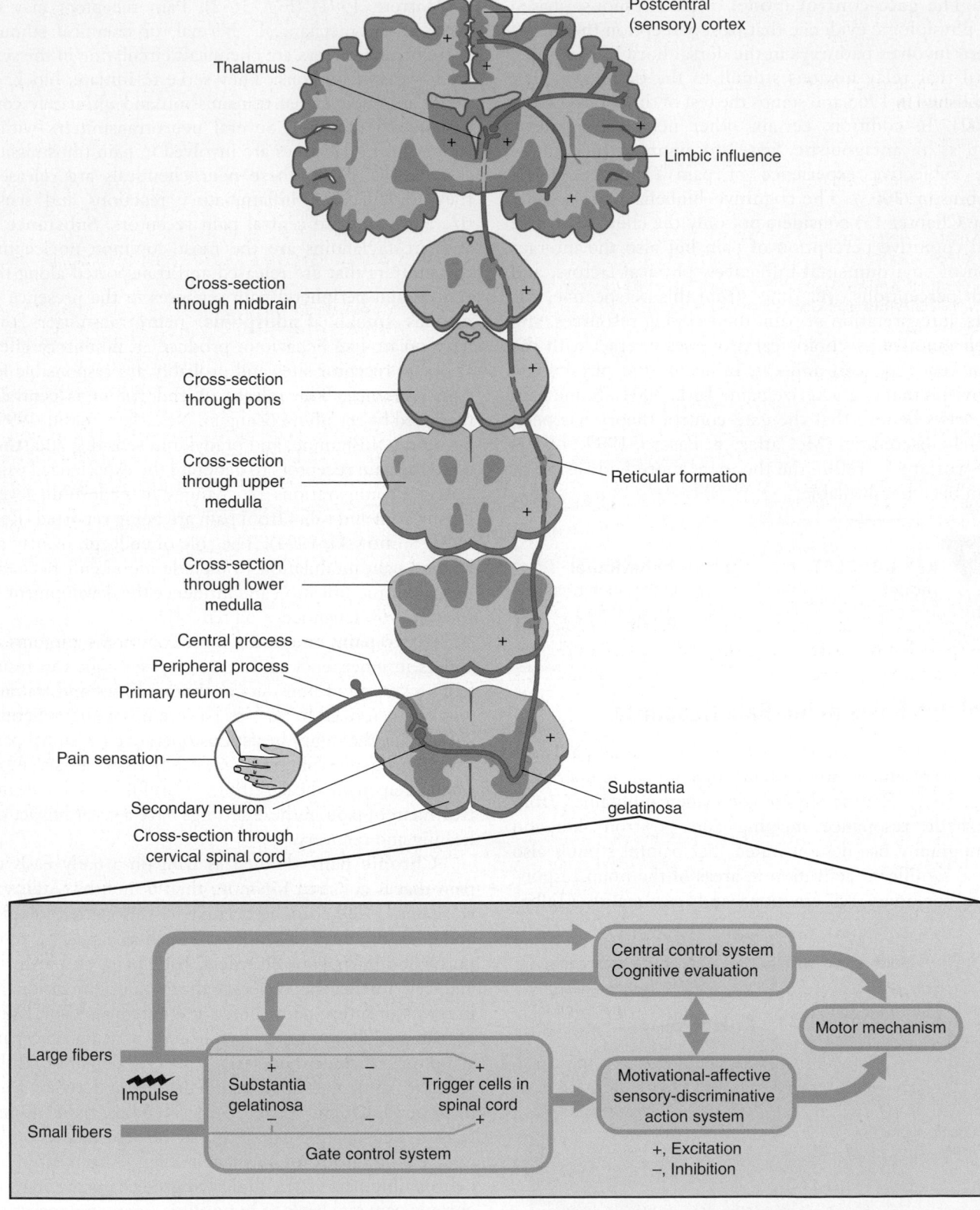

FIGURE 36-2. Ascending sensory pathways: anterior spinothalamic tract with a schematic diagram of the gate-control theory of pain mechanism.

BOX 36-1 Neurotransmitters Active in Pain Sensation and Induced Plasticity

C-Fibre Neuropeptides Released by Noxious Stimulation Peripherally
Substance P
Neurokinin A
Somatostatin
Calcitonin gene–related peptide
Prostaglandins
Galanin
Vasoactive intestinal polypeptide
Cholecystokinin

Excitatory Amino Acids With Widespread Activity in the CNS (Thalamus and Somatosensory Cortices)
L-Glutamate
N-methyl-D-aspartate (NMDA)

Pain-Modulating Neurotransmitters
Endorphins
Enkephalin
Serotonin

Note: Many of these same neurotransmitters are released in large amounts during brain injury and contribute to neuronal cell death in a variety of neurologic and psychological disease processes.

BOX 36-2 Pain Syndromes Seen in the Primary Care Setting

Migraine Headache: a cerebrovasomotor disorder in which a focal reduction of cerebral blood flow initiates an ischaemic headache. May be preceded by a visual aura and followed by nausea, vomiting, and incapacitating head pain

Low Back Pain: pain arising from the vertebral column or surrounding muscles, tendons, ligaments, or fascia. Causes range from simple muscle strain to arthritis, fracture, or nerve compression from a ruptured disk

Chronic Benign Orofacial Pain: temporomandibular joint pain

Rheumatoid Arthritis: more than 100 different types of joint disease produce inflammation of the joints. Associated with varying degrees of pain and stiffness and eventual loss of use of the affected joints

Reflex Sympathetic Dystrophy: causalgia. A painful burning syndrome that occurs after peripheral nerve injury. Associated with hyperesthesia, vasomotor disturbances, and dystrophic changes due to sympathetic hyperactivity

Cancer Pain: pain from malignant tumours that is caused by local infiltration or metastatic spread involving specific organs, bones, peripheral or cranial nerves, or the spinal cord. Pain therapy aimed at providing sufficient relief to allow maximum possible daily functioning and a relatively pain-free death

Neuropathic Pain

Polyneuropathy: neuropathy involving multiple peripheral nerves

Diabetic Neuropathy: neuropathy due to diabetes mellitus; marked by diminished sensation secondary to vascular changes

Inflammatory Neuropathy: neuropathy related to the presence of chemical or microorganic pathogens

Traumatic Neuropathy: neuropathy caused by avulsion or compression

Plexopathy: neuropathy involving a peripheral nerve plexus

Peripheral or Central Neuralgia: abrupt, intense, paroxysmal pain due to intrinsic nerve injury or extrinsic nerve compression

Herpetic Neuralgia: pain associated with the dermatomal rash of acute herpes zoster

Radiculopathy: pain radiating along a peripheral nerve tract, such as sciatica

Vasoocclusive Pain: thrombotic crisis of sickle cell anaemia in joints and peripheral muscles that is caused by ischaemia

Myofascial Pain: pain in palpable bands (trigger points) of muscle. Associated with stiffness, limitation of motion, and weakness

2001). This neural plasticity contributes to the development of errant firing and the pain syndromes of referred pain (pain felt in a part other than where it was produced) and phantom pain (pain that feels as though its source is a missing [amputated] limb).

Psychological Aspects of the Pain Response

Pain is not only a sensation but also a perceptual phenomenon with an important affective component. When a client's pain persists for an extended period, a range of psychosocial and spiritual influences, such as the client's mood, fears, expectancies, coping efforts, and financial, social, and spiritual resources, and the responses of significant others begin to influence the client's perception of the pain. Affective and anxiety disorders are prevalent among people with chronic pain. They may be a symptom of or a defence against psychological stress caused by continuous nociceptive input (Koob, 1999). Bio/psycho/social/spiritual stimuli and responses may cause the client with chronic pain to become preoccupied with the pain and can contribute to depression. In addition, the presence of persistent noxious sensations contributes to neurochemical and neurohormonal imbalances that lead to depressed mood and anxiety. Whether the psychological pain is primary or secondary may be difficult to determine because the neurovegetative symptoms of depression may resemble the client's attempts to control the pain or the concomitant medical–physical conditions. Anorexia, sleep disturbance, and agitation or psychomotor retardation may be present. In addition, affective disturbances, such as sadness, loss of interest in life, feelings of worthlessness,

self-reproach, excessive guilt, indecisiveness, and suicidal ideation, are all symptoms reported by clients with chronic pain (Turk, 2004). Substance use disorder may arise from the client's search for relief through overuse of drugs that lessen the pain sensation. A formal psychiatric assessment is essential when these symptoms exist.

IN A LIFE

Sue Rodriguez (1950 to 1994),
Gloria Taylor (1948 to 2012) and
Susan Griffith (1941 to 2013):

Aid-In-Dying

Sue Rodriguez and Gloria Taylor were Canadian women diagnosed with amyotrophic lateral sclerosis (ALS) who, separately, challenged Canadian laws that make aiding a person in dying illegal. Susan Griffith, diagnosed with multiple system atrophy, chose to go to Switzerland for a legally assisted death through the organization Dignitas. She went public with her decision in support of changes to the same Canadian laws. Under the Canadian Criminal Code, while suicide is not illegal, assisting a person in committing suicide is, as is euthanasia (i.e., deliberately ending the life of a suffering person).

Sue Rodriguez, diagnosed in 1991 with ALS, challenged the law against assisted suicide all the way to the Canadian Supreme Court but failed to change them. Ultimately, she defied the law in 1994 by deciding the time and the method of her death. She had an unnamed physician and a friend, Svend Robinson (who was a Member of Parliament at the time), by her side.

Gloria Taylor appealed to the BC Supreme Court to be allowed aid-in-dying. She wrote in her affidavit, "I live in apprehension that my death will be slow, difficult, unpleasant, painful, undignified and inconsistent with the values and principles I have tried to live by." While Justice Lynn Smith suspended for 1 year her decision that the law against assisted suicide was unconstitutional, infringing on the rights of persons like Gloria, to give Parliament time to change the law, she granted Gloria an exception that would make her the first person in Canada to have a legally assisted death. Gloria, however, died on October 4, 2012, before the physician-assisted processed occurred. The federal government appealed the BC ruling.

Susan Griffith died on April 25, 2013, in Switzerland at a Dignitas clinic with some of her family present. The day before her death she told a reporter: "It's very important that people feel in the future that they have control of their life and their death. And I have not felt that control in the last year or so, and it's been very distressing for me." She gave a last message: "Just please, members of Parliament, get going on discussing making the end of people's lives a lot easier than mine has been."

The Canadian Medical Association policy is against both assisted suicide and euthanasia. Persons requesting aid-in-dying are often in psychological distress. It is argued that improving the end of life for Canadians means responsive, more accessible palliative care rather than assisted death.

Sources: British Columbia Civil Liberties Association. (2013). *Right to die: Gloria Taylor's family heads to Court of Appeal for death with dignity case.* Retrieved from http://bccla.org/news/2013/03/right-to-die-gloria-taylors-family-heads-to-court-of-appeal-for-death-with-dignity-case-2/

Canadian Medical Association. (2007). *Euthanasia and assisted suicide (update 2007).* Retrieved from http://policybase.cma.ca/dbtw-wpd/Policypdf/PD07-01.pdf

CBC Digital Archives. (2013). *Sue Rodriguez and the right-to-die debate.* Retrieved from http://www.cbc.ca/archives/categories/politics/rights-freedoms/sue-rodriguez-and-the-right-to-die-debate/topic-sue-rodriguez-and-the-right-to-die-debate.html

CBC News. (2013). *Winnipeg's Susan Griffiths dies by assisted suicide in Zurich.* Retrieved from http://www.cbc.ca/news/canada/manitoba/winnipeg-s-susan-griffiths-dies-by-assisted-suicide-in-zurich-1.1315114

Assessment of the Client With Chronic Pain

Appropriate diagnosis and treatment of pain as a primary presenting symptom must begin with a comprehensive history and physical examination. In talking with the nurse about the pain, a client will not only describe its characteristics, location, and severity but may also provide information about possible psychosocial and behavioural factors that are influencing the pain experience. No direct relationship may be evident between the severity or extent of detectable disease and the intensity of the client's pain.

A number of assessment instruments have been developed to aid in evaluation. While nurses' clinical judgement remains foundational to pain assessment, such tools can enhance early identification of clients' needs and response to pain and improve the quality of documentation (Wølen & Bjørk, 2013). A fundamental approach is necessary to determine the impact of pain on

BOX 36-3 Assessing Clients Who Report Pain

A. What is the extent of the client's disease or injury (physical impairment)?
B. What is the magnitude of the illness? That is, to what extent is the client suffering, disabled, and unable to enjoy usual activities?
C. Does the client's behaviour seem appropriate to the disease or injury, or is there any evidence of amplification of symptoms for any of a variety of psychological or social reasons or purposes?
D. How often and for how long does the client perform specific behaviours, such as reclining, sitting, standing, and walking?
E. How often does the client seek health care and take analgesic medication (frequency and quantity)?

The Multiaxial Assessment of Pain (Rudy & Turk, 1991) includes evaluation of three axes: biomedical, psychosocial, and behavioural.

Pain Behaviour Checklist
Pain behaviours have been characterized as interpersonal communications of pain, distress, or suffering. Pain behaviour may be a more accurate indication of intensity and tolerance than verbal reports. Check the box of each behaviour you observe or infer from the client's comments.
• Facial grimacing, clenched teeth
• Holding or supporting of affected body area
• Questions such as, "Why did this happen to me?"
• Distorted gait, limping
• Frequent shifting of posture or position
• Requests to be excused from tasks or activities; avoidance of physical activity
• Taking of medication as often as possible
• Moving extremely slowly
• Sitting with rigid posture
• Moving in a guarded or protective fashion
• Moaning or sighing
• Using a cane, cervical collar, or other prosthetic device
• Requesting help in ambulation; frequent stopping while walking
• Lying down during the day
• Irritability

the client's life. All systems must be examined in the client to determine the degree to which biomedical, psychosocial, and behavioural factors interact to influence the nature, severity, and persistence of the client's pain and disability. Box 36-3 presents a pain assessment tool. An excellent resource for both pain assessment and management is offered by the Registered Nurses Association of Ontario (2007) as a Best Practice Guideline.

Table 36-1 Treatment Approaches to Pain

Principles of Pain Treatment

- Establish the correct diagnosis
- Recognize that pain reduction, rather than complete pain control, is a reasonable goal
- Control other symptoms besides pain. This includes treating the symptoms that were present before treatment (such as depression and anxiety) and the adverse effects associated with the pain therapy
- Treat physical conditions that may initiate or exacerbate the pain

First Step

Analgesics for treatment of pain and
Nonsteroidal anti-inflammatory drugs (NSAIDs)
  Acetaminophen
  Acetylsalicylic acid
  Ibuprofen
Oral local anaesthetics
  Flecainide
  Mexiletine
  Tocainide
Topical agents
  Capsaicin
  EMLA
  Lidocaine gel
  Baclofen
  Neuroleptics
  Pimozide
  Corticosteroids
  Calcitonin
  Benzodiazepines
  Clonazepam
Drugs for sympathetically maintained pain
  Nifedipine
  Phenoxybenzamine
  Prazosin
  Propranolol

Second Step

Antidepressants, TENS, and psychosocial support, and/or
Tricyclic and tetracyclic antidepressants
  Amitriptyline
  Clomipramine
  Desipramine
  Doxepin
  Imipramine
  Maprotiline
  Nortriptyline
  Mirtazapine
Selective and nonselective serotonin reuptake inhibitors
  Buproprion
  Fluoxetine
  Fluvoxamine
  Nefazodone
  Olanzapine
  Paroxetine
  Sertraline
  Trazodone
  Venlafaxine
Anticonvulsants
  Carbamazepine
  Neurontin
  Phenytoin
Opioid analgesics
  Codeine
  Meperidine
  Morphine
Monoamine oxidase inhibitors
  Isocarboxazid
  Phenelzine sulphate
  Tranylcypromine
Herbal and alternative medicine
  SamE
  Ginseng
  Swedish massage
  Acupressure
  Acupuncture
  Zero balancing
  Refloxology
  Meditation
  Prayer
Note: Treat the adverse effects of all the agents used

Third Step

Adrenergic agents, TENS, and psychosocial support, and/or
Clonidine
Naloxone infusion, and/or
Other agents (mexiletine, diphenhydramine)
Note: Add the third-step agents to partially helpful agents used in first step, or use alone and treat the adverse effects of all the agents used

Fourth Step

Psychiatric intervention
Psychotherapy with pain clients

Cognitive
- Explain the nature of the pain sensation
- Describe realistic expectations about the degree and course of pain
- Describe realistic expectations of treatment and side effects
- Use the placebo effect by supporting the treatment efficacy
- Relieve anxiety

Behavioural
- Make the initial doses large rather than small, to effect some relief
- Reassure that medication will be available, not contingent on proof of need
- Reinforce healthy behaviour/adaptation; do not reinforce obsession with pain
- Assure of regular evaluation not contingent on presence of pain

Ablative Procedure for Selected Clients
Neuroblockade
- Trigger point injection (TPI)
- Epidural steroid injection
- Facet joint injection
- Nerve root blocks
- Medical branch blocks
- Peripheral nerve block
- Sympathetic nerve block

Spinal Cord Stimulation
- Neurostimulator implants
- TENS
- Thalamic stimulation

Note: If the client has failed to experience response to all standard pharmacologic treatments, psychiatric evaluation for underlying problems (such as severe depression and risk for suicide) should be emphasized.

TENS, transcutaneous electrical nerve stimulation.

Sensory and Pharmacologic Modulation of Pain

Chronic pain occurs with a wide variety of medical illnesses. Proper diagnosis of the underlying condition determines primary treatment, which could eliminate or significantly reduce the need for analgesic drugs. Unsuspected medical conditions, such as alcoholism, autoimmune disease, or cancer, must be considered if pain develops in the absence of a known cause. Caregivers must know the mechanisms of action of analgesic drugs to administer them safely and monitor their effects. Clients' responses to individual drugs vary, and many agents at different doses may be tried before pain relief is achieved. Table 36-1 presents treatment approaches to pain. The use of physical and psychological modulation techniques, as well as pharmacotherapy or physical therapy, is more successful than the latter therapies alone (Turk, 2004). Combination treatment often affects mood and anxiety levels as well. Clients educated to use cognitive strategies such as biofeedback, a positive emotional state, relaxation, physical therapy or exercise, meditation, guided imagery, suggestion, hypnosis, placebos, and positive self-talk are able to tolerate higher levels of pain than are clients without specific coping strategies (Turk & Feldman, 1992). Most of these techniques involve redirecting the client's attention away from the pain and helping the client learn strategies of **self-efficacy** (self-effectiveness). Some of the bio/psycho/social/spiritual outcomes that can be measured to determine effectiveness of prescribed therapies include improvements in biologic, psychological, sociocultural, and spiritual well-being (Fig. 36-3). The biologic basis for the effectiveness of these strategies may be their ability to increase brain endorphin production (Bandura, O'Leary, & Taylor, 1987; Daley, 2002).

Many barriers exist to effective pain management (Boxes 36-4 and 36-5). Reluctance on the part of health professionals and the client may contribute to persistent pain, which ultimately can adversely affect the client's quality of life. Clients with chronic pain experience not only decreased functional capability but also diminished strength and endurance, nausea, poor appetite, and poor, interrupted sleep. The psychological impact includes diminished leisure and enjoyment, anxiety and fear, depression, somatic preoccupation, and difficulty concentrating. Social impairment may exist in the form of diminished social and sexual relationships, altered appearance, and increased dependence on others. While persons living with chronic pain can find that their suffering helps them to understand the "real value of life," they may wonder why they deserve such suffering (Dusŝová & Cseszárová, 2008, p. 29). All these contribute to the misery caused by the pain experience.

FIGURE 36-3. Bio/psycho/social/spiritual outcomes for clients with pain.

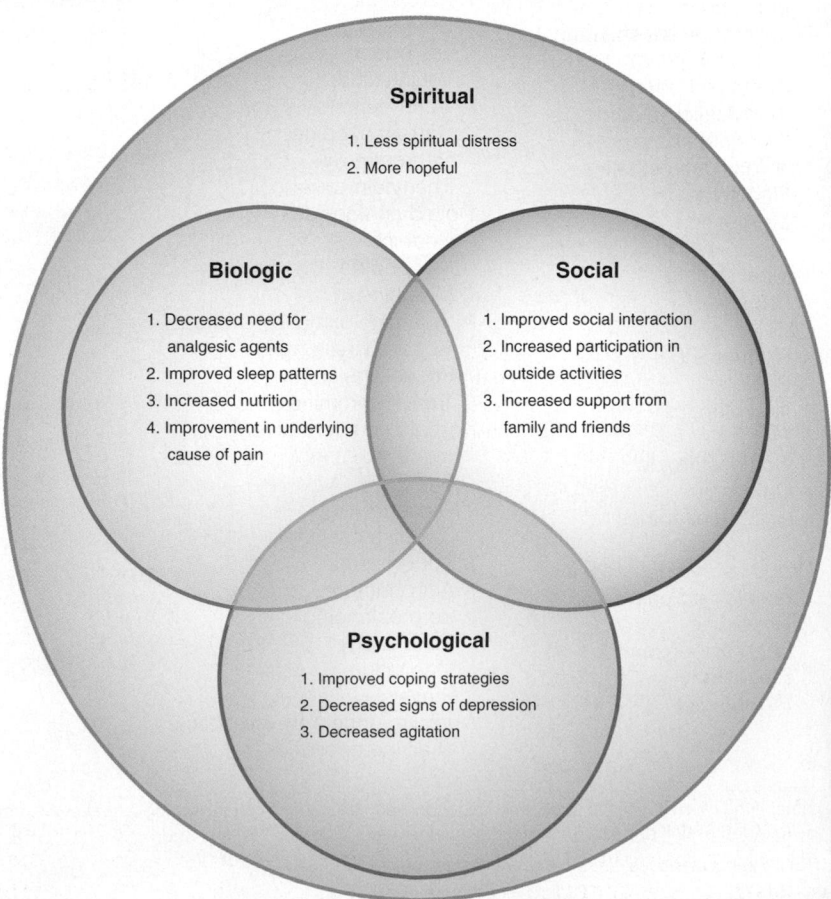

Shor, R. & Shalev, A. (2013). *Identifying barriers to improving wellness of persons with severe mental illness in community residential mental health facilities.* Social Work in Mental Health, 11, 334–48.

BOX 36-4 Research for Best Practice

BARRIERS TO IMPROVING WELLNESS OF PERSONS WITH SEVERE MENTAL ILLNESS LIVING IN A COMMUNITY RESIDENTIAL FACILITY

The Question: What difficulties and barriers do persons with severe mental illness (SMI) living in residential mental health facilities experience that prevent them from maintaining healthy nutritional practices and from involvement in physical activities?

Methods: Participants (*n* = 84) had a SMI, lived in a community residential facility, and were taking a 16-session health promotion course at a psychiatric hospital. Each participant was on antipsychotic medication and met at least two of the following criteria: overweight, not physically active, or had difficulty maintaining healthy nutrition habits. Data were gathered on participants' background and mental illness. Interviews, conducted before the health promotion course, focused on difficulties and barriers, as well as what participants expected of staff in their facility regarding the topics of nutrition and physical activity. The question of expectations was asked via questionnaire every 2 weeks across the course. The group sessions in the course were audiotaped and analyzed. Grounded theory guided data analysis.

Findings: Fifty-one percent of participants were male; 49% female; 86% single; 67% stated they had physical problems in addition to mental illness. The barriers identified fit a biopsychosocial framework. *Biologic barriers* were the impact of medications (increased appetite; decreased ability for activity) and comorbid health problems. The *psychological barrier* was relapse in mental illness (less able to be involved in activities and maintain good eating habits). The *social barrier* was lack of supporting companionship (no one with whom to dine, go for walks, etc.). *Organizational barriers* were lack of organizational support for physical activity (absent from facility routine and dialogue) and access to healthy food (menu items not always healthy; lack of choice). A *societal barrier* was being unable to understand food labelling.

Implications for Nursing: In promoting healthy behaviours and habits among persons with SMI, the focus is often on providing knowledge regarding healthy choices and supporting individual self-control. Recognition must be given to the social and organizational barriers that persons with SMI may face in institutional living. These need to be identified and addressed within a facility, including ways to increase opportunities for welcomed companionship.

BOX 36-5 Barriers to Pain Management

Problems of Health Care Professionals
- Inadequate knowledge and experience with pain management
- Poor assessment of pain
- Concern about regulation of controlled substances
- Fear of client tolerance and addiction
- Concern about side effects of analgesics

Problems of Clients
- Reluctance to report pain
- Concern about primary treatment of underlying disease
- Fear that pain means the disease is worse
- Concern about being a good client and not a complainer
- Reluctance to take pain medications
- Fear of tolerance and addiction, fear of "addict" label
- Fear of unmanageable side effects

Problems of Health Care System
- Restrictive regulation of controlled substances
- Problems with availability of treatment or access to it

The nurse can enhance adherence to the intervention plan by closely monitoring the therapeutic efficacy and untoward effects of the treatments being used, involving the client and family in treatment planning, educating the client and family about self-care, and instructing the client in noninvasive approaches to pain control. Effective communication with the client and family is of prime importance (Mackintosh & Elson, 2008).

● **STUDY NOTE**

In the assessment of a client's pain, it is important to determine a baseline measure of the person's experience of pain against which changes can be noted. Changes in the words used by a client to describe his or her pain (e.g., from "sharp" to "shooting") should alert the nurse to possible changes in client status.

Maladaptive coping by clients with chronic pain leads them to fear pain and to acquire a negative attitude about pain and how it affects their lives. These negative views can adversely influence biopsychological and physiologic processes, thereby sustaining or even exacerbating the pain. Nonadherence by these clients with sequential prescription changes and combined treatments also can be problematic. Strategies to assess adherence are regular self-report, assessment of behavioural change, biochemical assay, clinical improvement, and outcome assessment.

■ PSYCHOPATHOLOGIC COMPLICATIONS OF AIDS

The medical syndrome of AIDS is characterized by multiple opportunistic infections and is associated with malignancy. People with AIDS are often overwhelmed by devastating disorders that cause profound fatigue, insomnia, anorexia, emaciation, pain, and disfigurement. The psychological impact of AIDS is considerably worsened by the social stigma associated with the infection and the special affinity of HIV for brain and central nervous system (CNS) tissue.

Biologic Basis of Neurologic Manifestations of HIV

In as many as 60% of those who have AIDS, neurologic complications occur that are directly attributable to infection of the brain. Important clinical manifestations include impaired cognitive and motor functions. This aspect of the syndrome is referred to as the **HIV-1–associated cognitive–motor complex**. Neuronal injury and frank nerve cell loss probably contribute to the neurologic deficits (Manji & Miller, 2004). Other researchers are noting the term "asymptomatic neurocognitive impairment" to categorize individuals with subclinical impairment (Antinori et al., 2007). Evidence suggests that the presence of HIV stimulates brain cells to release neurotoxins and excitatory amino acids in excess. The resultant neurochemical changes and disrupted cell membrane integrity cause cell death similar to that which occurs with other types of brain injury. These neurochemical changes and eventual catecholamine depletion contribute to the cognitive, motor, and psychiatric manifestations of HIV infection.

Psychological Aspects of AIDS

The most common initial signs and symptoms of the AIDS–dementia complex are changes in mentation and personality, followed by delirium, dementia, organic mood disorder, and organic delusional disorder. The onset of major depression and uncomplicated bereavement soon after diagnosis is common. Comorbid neurologic infections such as encephalitis and meningitis can predispose the client with AIDS to delirium. The clinical picture reflects the areas of the brain invaded by HIV; however, physiologic conditions such as addiction to alcohol or drugs, brain damage, chronic illness, hypoxia related to pneumonia, infections, space-occupying brain lesions, and systemic reactions to medications may contribute to the progression of mental changes. Loss of normal cortical function may lead to abnormal social behaviour, depression, psychosis, and anxiety. The psychological influences of stress and sleep and sensory deprivation can further contribute to the altered perception and mentation.

Psychiatric disorders contribute to the course of AIDS in several ways. Mood disorder may be reflected in the client who has an initial substance use disorder or an antisocial personality that predisposes him or her to a lifestyle that increases his or her risk for exposure to HIV. The neuropathology associated with the presence of HIV then contributes to the progression of the disease and deterioration. AIDS-associated psychopathology frequently is unrecognized, misdiagnosed, and incorrectly treated. Diagnosis can be difficult when risk factors are not known or when cognitive or psychiatric symptoms precede the onset of other manifestations of HIV infection. Early CNS involvement is detected through neuropsychological testing and magnetic resonance imaging. The degree of cognitive dysfunction may not be a valid indication of the degree of organic involvement. In addition, diagnostic findings on computed tomography scans, such as cerebral atrophy and prominent basal ganglia calcification, may not correlate with the severity of the client's dementia (Gabuzda & Hirsch, 1987).

Assessment of the Client With AIDS

Early recognition of psychiatric disorders associated with AIDS is important to enhance our understanding of the behaviour of people with AIDS. Mental status changes and altered affect should be investigated through formal neurologic and psychological testing to determine the extent of impairment. Successful coping and cognitive adaptation are often further hindered by the presence of psychiatric disorders associated with HIV (Box 36-6). These mental illnesses include mood disorders, adjustment disorders, anxiety disorders, substance use disorders, and personality disorders. Organic mood disorder may be characterized by symptoms of a major depressive or manic episode. The depressed mood, feelings of guilt, anhedonia, and hopelessness can be accompanied by insomnia or hypersomnia, psychomotor retardation or agitation, and suicidal ideation. Low self-esteem, feelings of worthlessness and hopelessness, and impaired thinking or concentration are other likely findings. It is important

---

BOX 36-6 Psychiatric Disorders Associated With HIV Infection

ORGANIC MENTAL DISORDER
Dementia
  HIV dementia or AIDS–dementia complex
  Dementia associated with opportunistic infection
    Fungal
      Cryptococcoma
      Cryptococcal meningitis
      Candidal abscesses
    Protozoal
      Toxoplasmosis
    Bacterial
      Mycobacterium avium–intracellulare
    Viral
      Cytomegalovirus
      Herpesvirus
      Papovavirus progressive multifocal
        leukoencephalopathy
Dementia associated with cancer
  Primary cerebral lymphoma
  Disseminated Kaposi's sarcoma
  Delirium
  Organic delusional disorder

ORGANIC MOOD DISORDER
Depression
  Mania
  Mixed
Affective disorders
  Major depression
  Dysthymic disorder
Adjustment disorders
  Adjustment disorder with depressed mood
  Adjustment disorder with anxious mood
Substance abuse disorder
Borderline personality disorder
Antisocial personality disorder
Bereavement
Anxiety disorders
  Obsessive–compulsive disorder
  Panic

to differentiate between major depression and complicated or uncomplicated grieving over the loss of health or of significant others to premature death because of HIV. When a client receives a diagnosis of AIDS, he or she may face social isolation, severe life-threatening complications, unfamiliar and perhaps ineffective treatments, and the prospect of premature death. As with any life crisis, the client and family members experience severe anxiety, fear, and depression. They may develop obsessive–compulsive rituals to allay anxiety related to the infection. In addition, these clients may experience panic disorders.

People who do not engage in high-risk behaviour and who are unlikely to have been exposed to HIV may nevertheless report physical and psychological manifestations associated with HIV. Anxiety about the disease can produce symptoms not unlike those of HIV infection. Phobias, delusions, and factitious (Munchausen's syndrome) AIDS disorders have all been reported in uninfected people. In many cases, psychotherapy for the underlying psychological disorder is effective.

Bio/Psycho/Social/Spiritual Interventions

Treatment of AIDS should attempt to maintain normal hydration, electrolyte balance, and nutrition, as well as a safe, comfortable environment promoting a sense of peace, love, and creativity. Antiviral agents, such as zidovudine, ribavirin, phosphonoformate, maraviroc, raltegravir, and etravirine, cross the blood–brain barrier and achieve adequate anti-HIV concentrations in cerebrospinal fluid after systemic administration (Hammer et al., 2008).

In addition, it is important to provide the client and the client's family, friends, and caregivers with emotional and educational support. Their sense of competence and control in relation to living with AIDS should be promoted (Littrell, 1996; Mo & Coulson, 2008). Those close to the client may especially need psychotherapy if the client is young. Treatment of psychiatric disorders should include the individual and family, as well as psychotropic medications, in a manner similar to the treatment of primary psychiatric disorders.

Early diagnosis and treatment are imperative to maximize the client's adherence to risk reduction regimens and to prevent the transmission of infection. Treatment plans can often be tailored to meet the needs of the client and family. The consultation–liaison psychiatric professional can recommend appropriate multidisciplinary interventions to meet the challenge of AIDS with compassion and dignity.

PSYCHOLOGICAL ILLNESS RELATED TO TRAUMA

Physiologic trauma activates the overall stress response of the autonomic nervous system (see Chapter 17). Massive catecholamine release causes certain cardiovascular, muscular, gastrointestinal, and respiratory symptoms that release energy stores and support survival. Tissue destruction, musculoskeletal pain, physical disability, and body image changes all contribute to the physiologic and psychological stress response, which continues long after the injury is sustained. The overwhelming behavioural responses are hypervigilance, fear, and anxiety; psychological sequelae may include social isolation, agitation, personality disorders, posttraumatic stress disorder, and depression or, in extreme cases, dissociative identity disorders.

Biologic Basis of the Trauma Response

The neurotransmitters responsible for behavioural responses to fear and anxiety are usually held in balance to maintain a level of arousal appropriate for environmental threat. Information from the sensory processing areas in the thalamus and cortex alerts the amygdala (the lateral and central nucleus). Events that are interpreted as threatening activate the **hypothalamic–pituitary–adrenal (HPA) axis**, initiating the stress response. Adrenal steroids are released and trigger the physiologic reactions just described. Complex neurochemical processes involving norepinephrine, γ-aminobutyric acid, and serotonin are overwhelmed by the catecholamine release. For example, norepinephrine receptors adjust to the increased level of hyperstimulation. Then, as the catecholamines are depleted, the norepinephrine receptors react to the relative catecholamine shortage. This response alters cognitive and affective functions similar to the altered function that occurs in anxiety disorders. Persistent, severe distress leads to a general dysregulation of the HPA axis and inappropriate and prolonged secretion of high levels of catecholamines. This chronic stress disorder has been linked to increased susceptibility to immunosuppressive medical illness, such as certain cancers, as well as to infection, myocardial disease, and neurologic degenerative disorders (Radley et al., 2004).

Adaptation to trauma is related to such factors as the severity of the trauma, the person's maturity and age when the trauma occurs, available social support, and the person's ability to mobilize coping strategies (Heim, Newport, Mletzko, Miller, & Nemeroff, 2008). During adaptation to prolonged stress, the client's cognitive thought processes and coping behaviours cause dopamine to be released in the prefrontal cortex of the brain. These dopaminergic systems are presumed to play a major role in physiologic and emotional coping responses, storage of the trauma experience into memory, and possibly the development of posttraumatic stress disorder (McAllister, Flashman, Sparling, & Saykin, 2004). **Serotonin** is also thought to influence adaptation and mobilize coping strategies.

Psychological Aspects of the Trauma Response

Individual behaviour and perception are essential components of the stress reaction. Response to the challenge depends on prior experience, developmental history, and

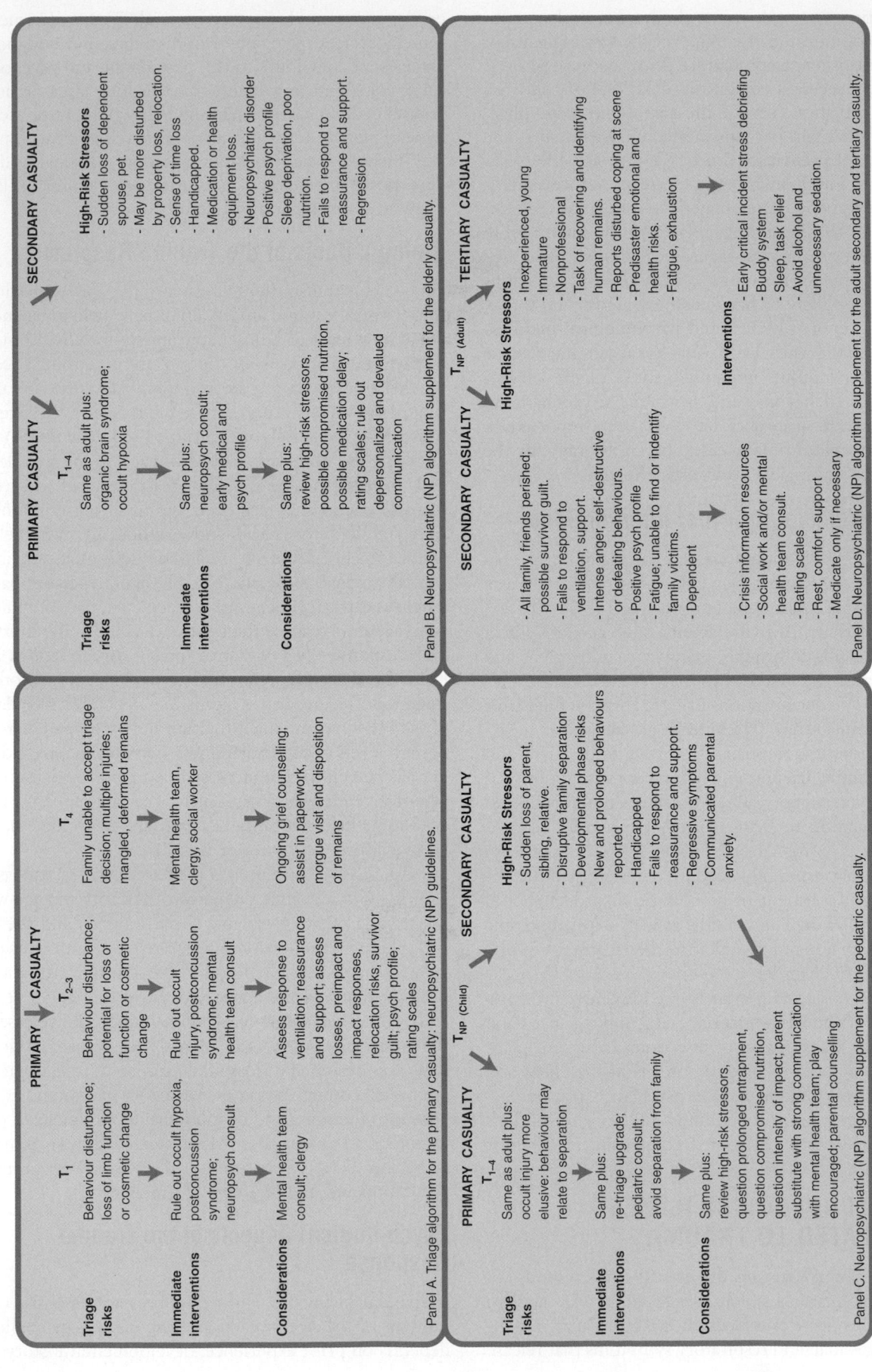

FIGURE 36-4. Triage algorithm for the primary casualty: neuropsychiatric guidelines (Adapted from Burkle, F. M. Jr. (1991). Triage of disaster-related neuropsychiatric casualties. *Psychiatric Aspects of Emergency Medicine, 9*(1), 87–105.).

PRIMARY CASUALTY

T₁

Triage risks
Behaviour disturbance; loss of limb function or cosmetic change

Immediate interventions
Rule out occult hypoxia, postconcussion syndrome; neuropsych consult

Considerations
Mental health team consult; clergy

T₂₋₃
Behaviour disturbance; potential for loss of function or cosmetic change

Rule out occult injury, postconcussion syndrome; mental health team consult

Assess response to ventilation; reassurance and support; assess losses, preimpact and impact responses, relocation risks, survivor guilt; psych profile; rating scales

T₄
Family unable to accept triage decision; multiple injuries; mangled, deformed remains

Mental health team, clergy, social worker

Ongoing grief counselling; assist in paperwork, morgue visit and disposition of remains

Panel A. Triage algorithm for the primary casualty: neuropsychiatric (NP) guidelines.

SECONDARY CASUALTY

T_NP (Child)

PRIMARY CASUALTY
T₁₋₄

Triage risks
Same as adult plus: occult injury more elusive: behaviour may relate to separation

Immediate interventions
Same plus: re-triage upgrade; pediatric consult; avoid separation from family

Considerations
Same plus: review high-risk stressors, question prolonged entrapment, question compromised nutrition, question intensity of impact; parent substitute with strong communication with mental health team; play encouraged; parental counselling

High-Risk Stressors
- Sudden loss of parent, sibling, relative.
- Disruptive family separation
- Developmental phase risks
- New and prolonged behaviours reported.
- Handicapped
- Fails to respond to reassurance and support.
- Regressive symptoms
- Communicated parental anxiety.

Panel C. Neuropsychiatric (NP) algorithm supplement for the pediatric casualty.

SECONDARY CASUALTY

High-Risk Stressors
- Sudden loss of dependent spouse, pet.
- May be more disturbed by property loss, relocation.
- Sense of time loss
- Handicapped.
- Medication or health equipment loss.
- Neuropsychiatric disorder
- Positive psych profile
- Sleep deprivation, poor nutrition.
- Fails to respond to reassurance and support.
- Regression

PRIMARY CASUALTY
T₁₋₄

Triage risks
Same as adult plus: organic brain syndrome; occult hypoxia

Immediate interventions
Same plus: neuropsych consult; early medical and psych profile

Considerations
Same plus: review high-risk stressors, possible compromised nutrition, possible medication delay; rating scales; rule out depersonalized and devalued communication

Panel B. Neuropsychiatric (NP) algorithm supplement for the elderly casualty.

SECONDARY CASUALTY

T_NP (Adult)

TERTIARY CASUALTY

High-Risk Stressors
- All family, friends perished; possible survivor guilt.
- Fails to respond to ventilation; support.
- Intense anger, self-destructive or defeating behaviours.
- Positive psych profile
- Fatigue; unable to find or indentify family victims.
- Dependent

Interventions
- Crisis information resources
- Social work and/or mental health team consult.
- Rating scales
- Rest, comfort, support
- Medicate only if necessary

High-Risk Stressors
- Inexperienced, young
- Immature
- Nonprofessional
- Task of recovering and identifying human remains.
- Reports disturbed coping at scene
- Predisaster emotional and health risks.
- Fatigue, exhaustion

Interventions
- Early critical incident stress debriefing
- Buddy system
- Sleep, task relief
- Avoid alcohol and unnecessary sedation.

Panel D. Neuropsychiatric (NP) algorithm supplement for the adult secondary and tertiary casualty.

physical status. Individual differences in the extent of endocrine and autonomic activity also occur during stress. Psychological sequelae of sustained stress and trauma may be manifested as flashbacks, intrusive recurring thoughts, panic or anxiety attacks, paranoia, inappropriate startle reactions, nightmares, or the extreme of posttraumatic stress disorder. Catecholamine depletion and activation of the dopamine pathways may contribute to deterioration in social and intellectual functioning after severe physical or emotional trauma. The client may become so withdrawn and depressed that he or she stops participating in activities of daily living (ADLs). Towards the other extreme, the client may become agitated and combative, perceiving any treatment as a continued threat.

Extreme forms of maladaptation are manifested in kindling and dissociative identity disorder. **Kindling** is thought to be responsible for the spontaneous recurrence of depressive illness that is associated with loss and trauma at an early age. Permanent biochemical changes from the early trauma response precipitate the sudden onset of affective disorder in the absence of any present stressor (Nemeroff, 2004). Dissociation disorders are rare but take the form of somatization (physical symptoms), agnosia, multiple personalities, or amnestic fugue states in which the client escapes the stressor by subconscious loss of identity or adoption of a new identity. Although these disorders are not common, mood and anxiety disorders may occur after a trauma event. They are associated with slowed rehabilitation and deterioration in social functioning and ADLs after the trauma period has passed (Jorge et al., 2004).

Assessment of the Traumatized Client

Complete physical assessment after physical traumatic injury is imperative in life-threatening circumstances. Multiple trauma and head injury are the major causes of death and disability in young adults. Emergency care and intensive care providers are highly trained to recognize signs and symptoms of physiologic injury and to intervene to stabilize primary and secondary trauma in the general medical setting. Trauma scales and triage models have been developed to assist in immediate assessment and to measure neurologic and physical conditions (Fig. 36-4) (Burkle, 1991). They have also been used to predict long-term outcome in clients for whom permanent cognitive and physical disability may limit recovery and challenge adaptive responses.

Psychological injury must be evaluated thoroughly through observation and interview to determine prevalent signs and symptoms of accompanying psychological disorders. This process includes evaluating the client's adjustment and coping skills, personal way of dealing with the trauma, social circumstances, and environmental and life stressors. Assessment must be ongoing to help the client deal with disfigurement, sudden disability,

and changes in self-care. The evaluation should include assessment of the client's perception of experienced stress, feelings related to the stress, dominant mood, cognitive functioning, defence and coping mechanisms, and available support systems. In addition, assessment of the risk for self-inflicted injury or suicide is critical.

Bio/Psycho/Social/Spiritual Interventions

Psychiatric clinicians provide an important aspect of emergency care. Interventions that establish trust, reduce anxiety, promote adaptive coping, and cultivate a sense of control help the client to begin recovery and maintain emotional health. Crisis intervention methods, stress management, cognitive–behavioural therapies, psychotherapy, and psychotropic medications, alone or in combination, may be useful in achieving the best possible outcome.

When trauma causes the client's death, the family must be informed of the death and allowed to grieve, to prevent the development of a pathologic or prolonged grief response. Traumatic death is sudden and unexpected, and often the victim is young. Surviving family members usually have a severe emotional reaction to the death. Dysfunctional family dynamics may become evident during this period. The psychiatric liaison nurse can use family intervention strategies to enhance or improve relationships, while the family's motivation to do all that is possible is high.

■ PSYCHOLOGICAL ILLNESS RELATED TO CNS DISORDERS

Neurologic impairment is most often related to brain cell (neuron) destruction. The primary causes of neuronal damage are traumatic injury, ischaemia, infarction (cerebrovascular accident), abnormal neuron growth (brain tumour), and metabolic poisoning associated with systemic disease. Brain cell loss may also be the result of degenerative processes, such as those that occur in Alzheimer's or Parkinson's disease. Psychological illness often is a complication of organic neurologic disease and may be difficult to distinguish from the neuropathology itself. Therefore, appropriate intervention depends on skilled assessment to discriminate and detect mental status changes related to organic brain injury, as well as disorders of mood and thought.

Biologic Basis of Neurologic Impairment

All mechanisms of brain cell injury destroy brain cells directly or initiate a cascade of cell breakdown from ischaemia. This **ischaemic cascade** begins with hypoxia and is followed by paralysis of the ion exchange across the cell membrane, oedema, calcium influx, free radical production, and lipid peroxidation. The severity of brain injury is related to the degree and duration of ischaemia.

Complete ischaemia results in brain infarction, commonly known as stroke. The resulting neurologic impairment is related to the size and location of the affected brain area (Fig. 36-5). More eloquent areas of the brain, such as the internal capsule, are extremely sensitive to ischaemia. They are typically injured first and contribute to more generalized impairment, such as memory loss or altered judgment.

The primary psychological disorder experienced by people with traumatic brain injury is depression (Schwarzbold, Diaz, & Walz, 2008). In a study of 559 clients at a Level 1 trauma centre, over 53% met the criteria for major depressive disorder (MDD) within a year of the trauma; MDD was an independent predictor of lower health-related quality of life (Bombardier et al., 2010). Depressive symptoms related to organic brain injury are generated by altered biochemical neurotransmitter systems. Hyperactivity and dysregulation of the HPA axis probably contribute to the elevated cortisol and catecholamine levels after a cerebral insult. In addition, changes in the metabolism of biogenic amines after brain cell death and ischaemia may mediate both mood disturbances and cognitive dysfunction in clients who have had stroke (Luis, Vanderploeg, & Curtiss, 2003).

In cognitive brain function, dopamine is essential for normal neurotransmission of motor messages, motivation, and level of anxiety and mood; epinephrine establishes learning and memory; and serotonin regulates the level of alertness, the categorization of information, and the perception of well-being. These neurotransmitter pathways are temporarily interrupted or permanently disrupted during the acute injury. Secondary injury caused by swelling and compression may further compromise neurons in the surrounding areas, causing marginal neurotransmitter function. In addition, circulating catecholamines can lead to oversecretion of dopamine or serotonin, which disrupts the necessary balance in production and uptake of the transmitters.

Psychological Aspects of Neurologic Impairment

Depressive disorder is a common complication of brain injury, particularly ischaemic stroke. About 20% of clients with acute stroke have the symptom cluster of the (*Diagnostic and Statistical Manual of Mental Disorders*, 5th ed.; American Psychiatric Association, 2013) criteria for major depression (see Chapter 22). Other symptoms, such as sleep disturbances, cognitive dysfunction, poor concentration, difficulty making decisions, somatic discomfort, poor appetite, social withdrawal, and fatigue or agitation, often accompany the mood disturbance. The high-risk period extends for 2 years after the stroke and, left untreated, the depression generally lasts for at least 6 months (Verdelko, Henon, Lebert, Pasquiere, & Leys, 2004). There are challenges to assessing mood after stroke that are related to the complexity of clients' poststroke impairments and their premorbid sensory condition (Gurr, 2011).

Mild and moderate levels of depression may go unrecognized and undiagnosed when clients who have had a stroke describe somatic symptoms and demonstrate lack of motivation in ADLs. Depression is more likely to develop in such clients if they have altered speech or

FIGURE 36-5. Functional cerebral anatomy and stroke.

aphasia, severe hemiparesis, or both. However, clients who have had a stroke experience depression more frequently than do other disabled and chronically ill clients, although the level of functional disability is the same (Verdelko et al., 2004). This phenomenon is thought to possibly be related to the combination of permanent disability and altered neurotransmitter systems that persist after cerebral infarction.

Although the mechanism of neuronal injury is one of degeneration in Parkinson's disease and other neuromuscular diseases, the neurochemical changes in the brain are similar with respect to the loss of dopamine secretion and receptor sites in the internal capsule motor pathways. It is noted that approximately 40% of clients with Parkinson's disease experience depression (Rojo et al., 2003), although as much as a 50% incidence has been reported (Rejinders, Ehrt, Weber, Aarsland, & Leentjens, 2008). Although major depression may occur, most have less severe forms that may contribute as much to impairment in daily functioning as does the underlying disease. Depression is the main factor negatively affecting the quality of life and is a source of distress for the client and the family and caregivers. There is evidence suggesting that altered serotonergic function may be responsible, at least in part, for the depressive symptoms in Parkinson's disease and that altered noradrenergic function may underlie some of the associated anxiety symptoms. Clinical trials have demonstrated that selective serotonin reuptake inhibitors (SSRIs) and combined selective serotonin and norepinephrine reuptake inhibitors (SNRIs) are more effective than traditional tricyclic antidepressants in reducing or relieving depression and anxiety in clients with neurologic disease (Murai et al., 2001). In addition, the serotonergic system is disrupted as the neuronal synapses are destroyed or injured. This generalized loss of dopaminergic activity and decreasing functional ability also probably contribute to depressed mood in clients who have had a stroke.

Mental illness related to organic brain injury is consistently dependent on the degree of functional impairment, particularly loss of the ability to communicate and administer self-care. Depressed mood may become evident in the acute recovery phase or during rehabilitation. Depression often negatively affects survival and recovery. It impedes progress throughout the rehabilitation process and ultimately prevents an optimal outcome. Early evaluation assists in the detection of mental illness after brain injury.

Assessment of the Client With Neurologic Problems

A thorough neurologic examination is important in determining the location and degree of disability but is even more critical in establishing the locus of the retained function. Many scales exist that accurately assess

neurologic function and that are easy to administer and generally accepted as reliable tools to detect the degree and limitations of disability. Cognition and mentation can be more discretely measured by the Folstein Mini-Mental State examination (Folstein, Folstein, & McHugh, 1975), and functionability for self-care can be measured using the Barthel Index (Mahoney & Barthel, 1965). The evaluation of mood using the Center for Epidemiological Studies Depression Scale (CES-D) or the Beck Depression Inventory (Beck, Ward, Mendelson, Mock, & Erbaugh, 1961) provides important information for designing intervention strategies for the at-risk client who has had a stroke. Findings of depressive symptoms indicate the need for a more definitive neuropsychological referral. The dexamethasone suppression test (DST) has also been used to diagnose clinical depression. However, it is not completely reliable, and frequent false-positive test results limit its clinical utility (Carroll et al., 1981). Ribeiro et al. (1993) in their meta-analysis of the literature contend that baseline DST results are not reliable for any prognosis, while nonsupression of cortisol on the DST is strongly related with poor outcomes. Their findings underscore the need to investigate biologic measures as factors impacting psychiatric illness.

Bio/Psycho/Social/Spiritual Interventions

Isolation, lack of companionship, bereavement, and poverty are associated with depressive symptoms in the general population and compound the relative risk of depression developing after brain damage. In addition, a personal or family history of major depression increases the risk for depressed mood. Prevention strategies should be used as early as possible for clients known to have these risks. These strategies include the assessment and provision of social support resources while the client is hospitalized as an important component of discharge planning to rehabilitation services; the prescription of therapies to enhance competence in the performance of ADLs, with a focus on the use of retained function, rather than on adaptation to disabilities only; and formal psychosocial testing and psychopharmacologic treatment when appropriate (Palomäki et al., 1999; Robinson, 2003; Robinson et al., 2000). Assessment and support of the client's own spiritual resources should be addressed, particularly related to change in life meaning for the client that may have occurred due to the neurologic impairment. There needs to be education of the client and family to increase their awareness of signs and symptoms of depressed mood so that they will know when to seek medical attention and treatment to avert major depression, if possible. In addition, the presence of depressed mood and other symptoms of the depressive cluster indicates the need for cognitive, behavioural, biologic, social, and spiritual interventions to support appropriate psychopharmacologic treatment.

PSYCHOLOGICAL ILLNESS RELATED TO ACUTE AND CHRONIC MENTAL ILLNESS

Systemic medical illness is associated with a higher prevalence of concurrent psychiatric disorders. Disorders such as cancer, heart disease, endocrine abnormalities, and organ failure are often associated with more functional disabilities than most chronic medical illnesses and may be the basis of medically unexplained somatic symptoms. Among the psychiatric disorders, substance use disorder, anxiety, and depressive disorder occur most frequently in clients with chronic medical illnesses. Within the anxiety disorders, phobias are most common, with panic disorder and obsessive–compulsive disorder less common (Härter, Conway, & Merikangas, 2003). There is a positive relationship between and anxiety and physical disorders, yielding higher levels of being physically compromised (Sareen, Cox, Clara, & Asmundson, 2005). Table 36-2 compares the prevalence rates of depressive and anxiety disorders in people who are medically ill with the rates in people who are not.

Biologic Aspects of Mental Illness Related to Medical Disease

The nervous, endocrine, and immune systems and their components are designed to communicate and interact through biochemical means. The cerebral cortex and limbic system initiate neuroendocrine HPA axis activity by thought processes in response to environmental stimuli. Various hormonal messengers travel between the hypothalamic, pituitary, and adrenal systems to initiate secondary peripheral responses. The immune system responds to signals from the HPA axis and returns messages as well. Its protective activities rely on neurochemicals to initiate the infection defence and stress response. At all levels, the circulating hormone levels serve as feedback messengers to inhibit HPA activity after sufficient response has occurred.

Dysregulation of the hypothalamic, pituitary, and adrenal systems at all levels leads to malfunction of the other systems. Abnormal nervous system firing in the hippocampus alerts the adrenal and immune systems unnecessarily and vice versa. The principal neurochemical messengers in this regulation are thought to be norepinephrine, endorphins, cortisol, and dopamine. This trio of systems detects metabolic and cellular disease processes that eventually cause signs and symptoms of medical diseases, and body resources are activated to stop these pathologic processes. Psychiatric conditions occur during the course of these medical illnesses and, in some instances, may contribute to the genesis of the physiologic disease.

A psychiatric disorder may be the first manifestation of a primary disease, such as depressive syndrome in Huntington's chorea, multiple sclerosis, Parkinson's disease, HIV, Cushing's disease, and systemic lupus erythematosus. Depressive symptoms are an intrinsic part of the primary pathophysiology of endocrine disorders, metabolic disturbances, malignancies, viral infections, inflammatory disorders, and cardiopulmonary conditions. Tables 36-3 and 36-4 list medical conditions associated with anxiety disorders and depression, respectively.

Endocrine system pathologic processes involve abnormal HPA axis function, which affects neurotransmitter balance (Stratakis & Chrousos, 1995). Depression and anxiety are often present in clients with hyperthyroidism

Table 36-2	Prevalence of Psychiatric Disorders in Medically Ill Compared With People Who Are Not Medically Ill	
Prevalence of Psychiatric Disorders*	**Medically Ill (%)**	**Not Medically Ill (%)**
6-month prevalence	24.7	17.5
Substance abuse	8.5	
Anxiety	11.9	
Affective disorder	9.4	
Lifetime prevalence	42.4	37.0
Substance use	26.2	
Anxiety	18.2	
Phobias	12.1	
Panic disorder	1.5	
Obsessive–compulsive disorder	2.4	
Affective disorder	12.9	

*Prevalence rates are sex and age adjusted.

Adapted from National Institute of Mental Health Epidemiologic Catchment Area Program & Burkle, F. M. Jr. (1991). Triage of disaster-related neuropsychiatric casualties. *Psychiatric Aspects of Emergency Medicine, 9*(1), 87–104.

Table 36-3	Medical Conditions Associated With Anxiety Disorders
Psychiatric Disorder	**Medical Illness**
Panic disorder	Parkinson's disease
	Primary biliary cirrhosis
	Chronic obstructive pulmonary diseases
	Cardiomyopathy
	Post-MI
	Chronic pain
	Focal seizures
Social phobia	Parkinson's disease
Obsessive–compulsive disorder	Sydenham's chorea
Phobia	Multiple sclerosis
Generalized anxiety	Primary biliary cirrhosis
	Graves' disease

Table 36-4	Medical Illnesses Associated With Symptoms of Depression
Endocrinopathies	Hypothyroidism and hyperthyroidism
	Hypoparathyroidism and hyperparathyroidism
	Cushing's syndrome (steroid excess)
	Adrenal insufficiency (Addison's disease)
	Hyperaldosteronism
Malignancies	Abdominal carcinomas, especially pancreatic
	Brain tumours (temporal lobe)
	Breast cancer
	Gastrointestinal cancer
	Lung cancer
	Prostate cancer
	Metastases
Neurologic disorders	Ischaemic stroke
	Subarachnoid haemorrhage
	Parkinson's disease
	Normal-pressure hydrocephalus
	Multiple sclerosis
	Closed head injury
	Epilepsy
Metabolic imbalance	Serum sodium and potassium reductions
	Vitamin B_{12}, niacin, vitamin C deficiencies; iron deficiency (anemias)
	Metal intoxication (thallium and mercury)
	Uraemia
Viral/bacterial infection	Infectious hepatitis
	Encephalitis
	Tuberculosis
	AIDS
Hormonal imbalance	Premenstrual, premenopausal, postpartum periods
Cardiopulmonary	Acute MI
	Post–cardiac arrest
	Post–coronary artery bypass graft
	Post–heart transplantation
	Cardiomyopathy
Inflammatory disorders	Rheumatoid arthritis

and hypothyroidism, Cushing's disease (hyperadrenalism), and Addison's disease (hypoadrenalism).

Malignancies have also been associated with anxiety and depression. Depressive syndromes have been associated with cancer, and biologic relationships between the two disorders may exist such that the onset of depression may herald undetected carcinoma. Diagnoses range from major depression to adjustment disorder with depressed mood.

Systemic infections and generalized inflammatory disorders such as rheumatoid arthritis that acutely and chronically stress the immune system or that may be the result of immune dysfunction are associated with psychological disorders. In addition, renal, pancreatic, and

hepatic transplant recipients, who are artificially immunosuppressed because of treatment with prophylactic anti-infectious agents, experience primary neuropsychiatric symptoms related to metabolic imbalances and neuropsychiatric side effects from treatment.

Cardiac disease deserves special attention because it has been associated with precipitated depressive syndromes and anxiety disorders. The fact that more than 70% of clients who have an acute myocardial infarction (MI) remain depressed for as long as 1 year after the event indicates that the mental illness may not be simply an adjustment disorder. Gender differences in risk for anxiety and depression after MI have been found. In a 5-year prospective study, women had increased risk for both anxiety and depression in the first 2 years after MI, whereas men had increased risk for depression that began 2 years after MI (Bjerkeset, Nordahl, Mykletun, Holmen, & Dahl, 2005). The incidence of depression is also high in cardiac transplant recipients (54%) but is much lower in clients who undergo cardiac bypass surgery (6% to 15%). In a study of clients with coronary heart disease and elevated depressive symptoms, the majority of the sample size ($n = 101$) experienced reductions in their depressive symptoms when engaged in regular exercise and antidepressant medication treatment (Blumenthal et al., 2012); in an earlier study, 75% of cardiac clients who received therapy for their depression experienced response to treatment (Hill et al., 1992).

In addition to the disease process contributing to psychological complications, the drugs used to treat chronic disease may induce mental illness. Psychotropic and nonpsychotropic medications can be potent generators of depression and anxiety (Table 36-5). The indications and pharmacologic activity of these medications often have bio/psycho/social/spiritual implications. In addition, medically ill elderly clients are particularly susceptible to medication effects at lower doses. Depressive and anxiety-related symptoms may in fact have an additive effect on client function, well-being, and recovery when combined with medical illness. When a drug is suspected of causing mental changes, the recommended course of action is to withdraw the drug and find an effective alternative. When an alternative is not available, the dosage should be decreased to an effective level at which symptoms resolve.

Psychological Aspects of Medical Illness

In all cases of medical illness, it is natural for clients to respond to the loss of health with hopelessness, particularly when the illness is demoralizing, life threatening, and without a clear prognosis. People who are chronically ill are distressed by loss of function and limitations on their daily activities. They are often forced to comply with treatments that add discomfort but no apparent benefit. Medical clients commonly experience weight

Table 36-5	Medications Associated With Mental Illness in Medically Ill Clients
Analgesics and NSAIDs	Ibuprofen
	Indomethacin
	Opiates
	Pentazocine
	Phenacetin
	Phenylbutazone
Antihypertensives	Clonidine
	Hydralazine
	Methyldopa
	Propranolol
	Reserpine
Antimicrobials	Ampicillin (gram-negative agents)
	Clotrimazole
	Cycloserine
	Griseofulvin
	Metronidazole
	Nitrofurantoin
	Streptomycin
	Sulfamethoxazole (sulphonamides)
Neurologic agents	l-Dopa
	Levodopa
Antiparkinsonian drugs	Amantadine
Anticonvulsants	Carbamazepine
	Phenytoin
Antispasmodics	Baclofen
	Bromocriptine
Cardiac drugs	Digitalis
	Guanethidine
	Lidocaine
	Oxprenolol
	Procainamide
Psychotropic drugs	Benzodiazepines
Stimulants/sedatives	Amphetamines
	Barbiturates
	Chloral hydrate
	Clorazepate
	Diethylpropion
	Ethanol
	Fenfluramine
	Haloperidol
Steroids and hormones	Adrenocorticotropic hormone
	Corticosteroids
	Estrogen
	Oral contraceptives
	Prednisone
	Progesterone
	Triamcinolone
Antineoplastic drugs	Bleomycin
	C-Asparaginase
	Trimethoprim
	Vincristine
Other miscellaneous drugs	Anticholinesterases
	Cimetidine
	Diuretics
	Metoclopramide

loss, insomnia, and motor retardation but perhaps not to the degree of "conspicuous" psychiatric illness. In addition, chronic life stress and mental illness may have set in motion a series of biologic processes ultimately resulting in the medical disorder, which may be further exacerbated by the stress of hospital admittance. A vicious cycle of medical and mental disorders may arise.

Mental illness in medically ill people is potentially lethal because normal affects and cognitive functioning may be essential to recovery and adherence to the medical treatment plan. In addition, the use of excessive analgesics and reluctance to perform self-care and rehabilitative activities hinder recovery and expose the person to other potential complications. The detection and diagnosis of any secondary mental illnesses in clients with medical illnesses are critical. The physiologic and pharmacologic factors that contribute to the mental illness must be explored and ruled out before effective intervention can begin.

Assessment of the Client With Medical Illness

Unfortunately, it may be very difficult for the clinician, evaluating a medically ill client in whom psychiatric symptoms develop, to ascertain whether these symptoms are the result of direct psychobiologic changes brought about by the illness. The psychosocial impact of the medical illness can influence the illness experience in such ways as frustration, fear, loss, fatigue, isolation, and confusion about the future (Costello & Boblin, 2004). People at obvious risk have a family history or personal history of mental illness or were experiencing psychological problems before symptoms of the medical illness were present. The main problem for the clinician is to determine which signs and symptoms are part of the medical illness and its treatment and which signify the presence of a psychological disorder. A complete health assessment and physical examination, including a psychological examination and a cognitive–affective assessment, will help determine the priority and severity of symptoms and interventions. In some instances, the primary diagnosis may be depression, although the symptoms may be similar to those of medical illness in the absence of diagnostic findings. Factors to be considered in diagnosing mental illness in medical clients are outlined in Box 36-7.

Several important cognitive–affective symptoms best differentiate the effects of depression from those of medical illness. These include feelings of failure, low self-esteem, guilt feelings, loss of interest in people, feelings of being punished, suicidal ideation, dissatisfaction, difficulty with decisions, and crying (Neese, 1991). The severity of the vegetative symptoms generally increases with the severity of the depressive disorder as well as the severity of the medical illness. Decreased appetite, sleep disturbances, and loss of energy are not considered indicators of depression in the medically ill client because these symptoms are

BOX 36-7 Factors to Consider in Diagnosing Depression in Medical Clients

- One or more specific medical illnesses
- Defining criteria for one of the depressive syndromes
- Family psychiatric history
- Past psychiatric history of the client
- Client's response to treatment, if any, for any prior depressive episode
- Sex of the client
- Client's age at onset of depression
- Depression that preceded the medical illness
- Psychosocial precipitants before onset of depression
- Duration of depressive illness
- Biologic markers of depression
- Relative frequency in the population of diagnoses under consideration
- Diagnosis by commission, not omission

common in medical illness as well. The Beck Depression Inventory and the CES-D are easy to administer and may indicate the need for a psychiatric referral.

Clinical Features of Special Significance

Two problems of special significance, psychosis and suicidal thoughts, are related in that clients with delusions or hallucinations tend to be at greater risk for suicide attempts or more likely to resist treatment (e.g., to refuse to eat or take medication) for their medical condition. It is important to distinguish between a mentally competent client's right to refuse life-saving medical treatment and a depressed client's desire to die. A clinical evaluation of the effect of depression on the client's capacity to make competent decisions is imperative. If optimal medical and psychiatric treatments have been provided and the client has been found competent enough to make decisions about further medical care, it may be appropriate to honour the client's desire to die.

Clients with chronic medical illness and clients with primary mental illness may pose similar problems in psychiatric hospitals when their medical condition fails. The use of advance directives helps in addressing these problems.

Bio/Psycho/Social/Spiritual Interventions

It is essential to provide optimal treatment of clients' medical illnesses without neglecting their mental distress. Most reports suggest that clinicians should be more aggressive in the pharmacologic treatment of mental illness in the medically ill. The basic rules for medicating clients include using the minimum dose initially, advancing the dose slowly, and performing frequent blood level monitoring. The doses required to achieve therapeutic blood levels may be lower or even half the usual therapeutic dose and take longer to titrate. It is important to understand the pharmacokinetics (absorption, distribution, metabolism, and elimination) of the treatment of

choice, to prevent further systemic effects. SSRIs and SNRIs are used equally as the treatment for depression in the medically ill client population. Because the side effects of psychopharmacologic agents can be especially troublesome in medically ill people, treatment must be changed or stopped if drug or illness interactions occur or if treatment of the mental illness appears to be unsuccessful. SSRIs are increasingly popular in treating medically ill clients because their side effect profile is more tolerable within a wider therapeutic range. Most clients experience response to antidepressant therapy with a decrease in the severity of their vegetative symptoms in 4 to 8 days.

Both supportive individual psychotherapy and family therapy are helpful. Assisting the client and family in understanding the nature and relationship of the medical and psychiatric diagnoses may strengthen the support system, alter the perception of caregiver burden, and identify appropriate coping strategies. Mutually agreed-upon goals and therapy actively involve the client in progress towards recovery. At some point, the clinician may need to help the client identify psychodynamic conflicts, maladaptive coping strategies, and, perhaps, spiritual concerns related to being ill that may be contributing to his or her distress. Cognitive intervention should address those areas of the client's life that can be controlled, despite major lifestyle changes, to reinforce a feeling of competence. It also is important to convey the fact that although medical and mental illnesses are difficult to prevent, they are often treatable.

INTERVENING IN MENTAL AND MEDICAL ILLNESSES

The relationship between stress and illness is becoming more apparent as studies increasingly disclose the effects of stress on the body. Chronic illness is viewed as a stressor and is associated with increased psychological distress, and interventions can minimize that distress. Nurses are committed to preventing illness and promoting healthy living. Thus, it is essential that they be aware of the physiologic and psychological impact of chronic stress, understand the coping process, and know appropriate alternative strategies for coping with illness. In addition, nurses can evaluate the effectiveness of strategies being used and revise care plans to improve outcomes for the client.

Clients with primary mental illness in need of medical care are at particular risk when somatic complaints are viewed as part of the primary process. Undiagnosed pathophysiologic processes may become advanced while being attributed to somatization. As well, comorbid medical conditions can affect the psychiatric illness. For instance, a study of depressed geriatric inpatients found that 62% reported chronic pain; those with chronic pain were more likely to report suicidal ideation (Meeks et al., 2008). A thorough medical history and physical examination are standard practice for clients in all settings. Ideally, a multidisciplinary team of care providers that includes a psychiatric and mental health liaison nurse should work together to deliver optimum treatment of complex medical and mental illnesses. All clients with chronic medical illnesses are at risk for psychological distress and should be approached with this understanding. Clinicians should include a general cognitive–affective status evaluation in their assessment of all medically ill clients and make appropriate psychiatric liaison consultation to offset the negative impact of mental illness on recovery.

A psychosocial review of systems is useful in admission assessment to detect psychosocial stress or risk. This review provides the minimum information needed for each client—neglect of even one area could compromise client care. The review obtains information on substance use, stressful life events, expectations, fears, meanings, social support, sexual concerns, work, finances, education, psychiatric history, mood, cognition, culture, and functional status. This information is useful in determining relevant nursing diagnoses and developing the plan of care.

Stress management training, systematic relaxation, supportive education, and stress monitoring should be built into the plan of care, regardless of the medical diagnosis. Assessment of anxiety and depression is ongoing, and crisis intervention with psychotherapy may be necessary to reduce the severity of mental distress. Physiologic stress factors, such as increased heart rate, blood pressure, and respiration, and signs of restlessness and sadness can be measured to determine the effectiveness of the intervention. Secondary mental illness can be approached using the same strategies that are effective for primary mental dysfunction. Interventions overlap across criteria, and all interventions provide some element of supportive therapy or social support.

Mental health can and should be monitored in clients who have physical illnesses. This monitoring may need to be long term. Research is suggesting that survivors of a life-threatening illness can have psychological problems or distress that persist over time (Mitka, 2009). Certain kinds of pathologic processes place clients at greater risk for mental illness. These processes can be identified and interventions prescribed to prevent psychiatric disorders from developing or to minimize their severity. Cognitive and behavioural strategies have a place in the treatment regimen and offer the practitioner an opportunity to expand the boundaries of traditional client-oriented practice in effective ways.

Alternatives to traditional medical intervention are increasingly employed as adjunct therapy in clients with pain related to cancer, neuropathy, or degenerative disorders. Natural and herbal therapies, therapeutic massage, zero balancing, thought field therapy, imaging, prayer, and meditation have all been found to be useful in easing the mental and physical discomfort of the client with medical illness. In addition, these therapies are more satisfying to clients who otherwise must receive toxic medication as part of their conventional medical treatment (see Table 36-1).

SUMMARY OF KEY POINTS

■ Psychiatric disorders are more common in people with systemic or chronic medical illnesses than in other people. Comorbid depression is common in certain medical diseases, such as endocrine and metabolic disturbances, viral infections, inflammatory disorders, and cardiopulmonary diseases. Specific anxiety disorders are associated with other medical conditions, such as Parkinson's disease, focal seizures, primary binary cirrhosis, and chronic pain.

■ Psychiatric illness that accompanies medical illness is seldom recognized and treated. Psychiatric symptoms may precede the onset of disease symptoms, and it may be difficult to distinguish between the symptoms of the two conditions.

■ The biologic basis of mental illness associated with medical illness (e.g., catecholamine depletion, disorders in metabolism or production of neurotransmitters) is similar to that of primary psychiatric illness, and bio/psycho/social/spiritual interventions are effective.

■ Mental illness in medically ill people is potentially lethal because normal affective–cognitive function may be critical to recovery and adherence to the medical treatment plan. Therefore, it is imperative that mental health is included in the standard health assessment of all medically ill people and that appropriate referrals be made.

CRITICAL THINKING CHALLENGES

1 You are caring for a client who has had a stroke and who refuses breakfast and a morning bath. Applying what you know about the neurologic damage caused by stroke and the frequency of depression in such clients, develop a care plan addressing the client's bio/psycho/social/spiritual needs.

2 As you care for a client with AIDS, you notice that his partner is pacing and hyperventilating. Using your knowledge of relationships, systems, and the interconnectedness of physical and psychological illness, how would you approach him?

3 A client is being seen for chronic pain. Discuss how you would go about assessing barriers to pain management with this client.

4 What is your own worst pain experience? What is the worst pain you can imagine like? To compare your answer with that of other nursing students, refer to Bergh, Jakobsson and Sjöström (2008).

5 You are a psychiatric and mental health liaison nurse and have been asked to prepare a program for the

medical–surgical nursing staff on psychiatric aspects of medical illnesses. What topics would you include, and what would be your rationale for including each?

REFERENCES

American Psychiatric Association. (2013). *Diagnostic and statistical manual of mental disorders* (5th ed). Washington, DC: Author.

Antinori, A., Arendt, G., Becker, J. T., Brew, B. J., Byrd, D. A., Cherner, M., ... Wojna, V. E. (2007). Updated research nosology for HIV-associated neurocognitive disorders. *Neurology, 69*(18), 1789–1799.

Arnsten, A. F. (1997). Catecholamine regulation of the pre-frontal cortex. *Journal of Psychopharmacology, 11,* 151–162.

Arnsten, A. F. (2011). Catecholamine influences on dorsolateral prefrontal cortical networks. *Biological Psychiatry, 69*(12), 89–99.

Arnsten, A. F. & Pliszka, S. R. (2011). Catecholamine influences on pre-frontal cortical function: Relevance to treatment of attention deficit/hyperactivity disorder and related disorders. *Pharmacology, Biochemistry, and Behavior, 8*(99), 211–216.

Atkinson, J. H. Jr & Slater, M. A. (1989). Psychiatric medications and pain management in emergency medicine. *Topics in Emergency Medicine, 11*(3), 1–110.

Bandura, A., O'Leary, A., & Taylor, C. B. (1987). Perceived self-efficacy and pain control-opioid and nonopioid mechanisms. *Journal of Personality and Social Psychology, 53,* 563–571.

Baumeister, H., Hutter, N., Bengel, J., & Harter, M. (2011). Quality of life in medically ill persons with comorbid mental disorders: a systematic review and meta-analysis. *Psychotherapy and psychosomatics, 80*(5), 275–286.

Beck, A. T., Ward, C. H., Mendelson, M., Mock, J., & Erbaugh, J. (1961). An inventory for measuring depression. *Archives of General Psychiatry, 4,* 561–571.

Bergh, I., Jakobsson, E., & Sjöström, B. (2008). Worst experiences of pain and conceptions of worst pain imaginable among student nurses. *Journal of Advanced Nursing, 61*(5), 484–491.

Bjerkeset, O., Nordahl, H., Mykletun, A., Holmen, J., & Dahl, A. (2005). Anxiety and depression following myocardial infarction: Gender differences in a 5-year prospective study. *Journal of Psychosomatic Research, 58,* 153–161.

Blumenthal, J. A., Sherwood, A., Babyak, M. A., Watkins, L. L., Smith, P. J., Hoffman, B. M., ... Hinderliter, A. L. (2012). Exercise and pharmacological treatment of depressive symptoms in patients with coronary heart disease: Results from the UPBEAT (Understanding the Prognostic Benefits of Exercise and Antidepressant Therapy) study. *Journal of the American College of Cardiology, 60*(12), 1053–1063.

Bombardier, C., Fann, J., Temkin, M., Esselman, P., Barber, J., & Dikmen, S. (2010). Rates of major depressive disorder and clinical outcomes following traumatic brain injury. *Journal of the American Medical Association, 303*(19), 1938–1945.

Bressi, S., Marcus, S., & Solomon, P. (2006). The impact of psychiatric comorbidity on general hospital length of stay. *Psychiatric Quarterly, 77*(3), 203–209.

British Columbia Civil Liberties Association. (2013). *Right to die: Gloria Taylor's family heads to Court of Appeal for death with dignity case.* Retrieved from http://bccla.org/news/2013/03/right-to-die-gloria-taylors-family-heads-to-court-of-appeal-for-death-with-dignity-case-2/

Burkle, F. M. Jr. (1991). Triage of disaster-related neuropsychiatric casualties. *Emergency Medicine Clinics of North America, 9*(1), 87–105.

Canadian Medical Association. (2007). Euthanasia and assisted suicide (update 2007). Retrieved from http://policybase.cma.ca/dbtw-wpd/Policypdf/PD07-01.pdf

Carroll, B. J., Feinberg, M., Greden, J. F., Tarika, J., Albala, A. A., Haskett, R., ... Young, E. (1981). A specific laboratory test for the diagnosis of melancholia: Standardization, validation and clinical utility. *Archives of General Psychiatry, 38,* 15–22.

CBC Digital Archives. (2013). *Sue Rodriguez and the right-to-die debate.* Retrieved from http://www.cbc.ca/archives/categories/politics/rights-freedoms/sue-rodriguez-and-the-right-to-die-debate/topic-sue-rodriguez-and-the-right-to-die-debate.html

CBC News. *Winnipeg's Susan Griffiths dies by assisted suicide in Zurich.* (2013). Retrieved from http://www.cbc.ca/news/canada/manitoba/winnipeg-s-susan-griffiths-dies-by-assisted-suicide-in-zurich-1.1315114

Cohen, C. & Cosimer, G. (1989). Factors associated with increased hospital stay by elderly psychiatric patients. *Hospital and Community Psychiatry, 40*(7), 741–743.

Collins, J. G. (1991). Acute pain management. *International Anesthesiology Clinics, 29*(1), 23–36.

Cooper, A. E., Corrigan, P. W., & Watson, A. C. (2003). Mental illness, stigma and care seeking. *Journal of Nervous and Mental Disease, 191*(5), 339–341.

Costello, J. & Boblin, S. (2004). What is the experience of men and women with congestive heart failure? *Canadian Journal of Cardiovascular Nursing, 14*(3), 9–20.

Daley, A. J. (2002). Exercise therapy and mental health in clinical populations: Is exercise therapy a worthwhile intervention? *Advances in Psychiatric Treatment, 8,* 262–270.

De Hert, M., Dekker, J. M., Wood, D., Kahl, D., Kahl, K., Holt, R., & Moller, M. (2009). Cardiovascular disease and diabetes in people with severe mental illness position statement from the European Psychiatric Association, supported by the European Association for the study of diabetes and European society of cardiology. *European Psychiatry, 24,* 412–424.

Dickerson, A. H. (2002). Gate control theory of pain stands the test of time. *British Journal of Anaesthesia, 88*(6), 755–757.

Dixon, L., Postrado, L., Delahanty, J., Fischer, P. J., & Lehman, A. (1999). The association of medical comorbidity in schizophrenia with poor physical and mental health. *Journal of Nervous and Mental Disease, 187*(8), 496–502.

Dussová, B. & Cseszárová, M. (2008). An overview of the quality of life of clients with chronic pain. *Primary Health Care, 18*(1), 25–29.

Eriksson, M., Asplund, K., Glader, E. L., Norrving, B., Stegmayr, B., Terént, A.,... Riks-Stroke Collaboration. (2004). Self-reported depression and use of antidepressants after stroke: A national survey. *Stroke: A Journal of Cerebral Circulation, 35*(4), 936–941.

Folstein, M. F., Folstein, S. E., & McHugh, P. R. (1975). Mini-Mental state: A practical method for grading the cognitive state of patients for the clinician. *Journal of Psychiatric Research, 12,* 189–198.

Ford, J. D., Trestman R. L., Steinberg, K., Tennen, H., & Allen, S. (2004). Prospective association of anxiety, depressive, and addictive disorders with high utilization of primary, specialty and emergency medical care. *Social Science and Medicine, 58*(11), 2145–2148.

Gabuzda, D. H. & Hirsch, M. S. (1987). Neurologic manifestations of infection with human immunodeficiency virus: Clinical features and pathogenesis. *Annals of Internal Medicine, 107,* 383–391.

Goldsmith, R. J. (1999). Overview of psychiatric comorbidity: Practical and theoretical considerations. *Psychiatric Clinics of North America, 22*(2), 331–349.

Gurr, B. (2011). Stroke mood screening on an inpatient stroke unit. *British Journal of Nursing, 20*(2), 94–100.

Hammer, S. M., Eron, J. J., Reiss, P., Schooley, R. T., Thompson, M. A., Walmsley, S., ... International AIDS Society-USA. (2008). Antiretroviral treatment of adult HIV infection: 2008 recommendations of the International AIDS Society-USA panel. *Journal of the American Medical Association, 300*(5), 555–570.

Härter, M. C., Conway, K. P., & Merikangas, K. R. (2003). Associations between anxiety disorders and physical illness. *European Archives of Psychiatry and Clinical Neuroscience, 253*(6), 313–320.

Heim, C., Newport, D. J., Mletzko, T., Miller, A. H., & Nemeroff, C. B. (2008). The link between childhood trauma and depression: Insights from HPA axis studies in humans. *Psychoneuroendocrinology, 33,* 693–710.

Hill, D. R., Kelleher, K., & Shumaker, S. A. (1992). Psychosocial interventions in adult patients with coronary heart disease and cancer: A literature review. *General Hospital Psychiatry, 14*(6 Suppl.), 28S–42S.

Joffe, R. T., Brasche, J. S., & MacQueen, G. M. (2003). Psychiatric aspects of endocrine disorders in women. *Psychiatric Clinics of North America, 261*(3), 683–691.

Jones, D. H., Marcias, C., & Harding, C. (2004). Prevalence, severity, and co-occurrence of chronic physical health problems of persons with serious mental illness. *Psychiatric Services, 55*(11), 1250–1257.

Jorge, R. E., Robinson, R. G., Moser, D., Tateno, A., Crespo-Facorro, B., & Arndt, S. (2004). Major depression following traumatic brain injury. *Archives of General Psychiatry, 61*(1), 42–50.

Koob, G. F. (1999). Corticotrophin-releasing factor, norepinephrine and stress. *Biological Psychiatry, 46,* 1167–1180.

Levenson, J. L. (1992). Psychosocial interventions in chronic medical illness: An overview of outcome research. *General Hospital Psychiatry, 14*(6 Suppl.), 43S–49S.

Littrell, J. (1996). How psychological states affect the immune system: Implications for interventions in the context of HIV. *Health and Social Work, 21*(1), 287–296.

Luis, C. A., Vanderploeg, R. D., & Curtiss, G. (2003). Predictors of postconcussion symptom complex in community dwelling male veterans. *Journal of the International Neuropsychological Society, 9*(7), 1001–1015.

Mackintosh, C. & Elson, S. (2008). Chronic pain: Clinical features, assessment and treatment. *Nursing Standard, 23*(5), 48–56.

Mahoney, F. T. & Barthel, D. W. (1965). Functional evaluation: Barthel index. *Maryland Medical Journal, 14,* 61–65.

Manji, H. & Miller, R. (2004). The neurology of HIV infection. *Journal of Neurology, Neurosurgery, and Psychiatry, 75*(Suppl.), 29–38.

McAllister, J. W., Flashman, L. A., Sparling, M. B., & Saykin, A. J. (2004). Working memory deficits after traumatic brain injury: Catecholaminergic mechanisms and prospects for treatment. *Brain Injury, 18*(4), 331–350.

McCaffery, M. & Pasero, C. (1999). *Pain clinical manual* (2nd ed). St. Louis, MO: Mosby.

Meeks, T., Dunn, L., Kim, D., Golshan, S., Sewell, D., Atkinson, J., & Lebowitz, B. D. (2008). Chronic pain and depression among geriatric psychiatry inpatients. *International Journal of Geriatric Psychiatry, 23,* 637–642.

Melzack, R. (1993). Pain: Past, present and future. *Canadian Journal of Experimental Psychology, 47*(4), 615–629.

Melzack, R., Coderre, T. J., Katz, J., & Vaccarino, A. L. (2001). Central neuroplasticity and pathological pain. *Annals of the New York Academy of Sciences, 933,* 157–174.

Mitka, M. (2009). New focus on long-term mental health of patients who survive serious illness. *Journal of the American Medical Association, 302*(13), 1408–1409.

Mo, P. K. & Coulson, N. S. (2008). Exploring the communication of social support within virtual communities: A content analysis of messages posted to an online HIV/AIDS support group. *Cyberpsychology and Behavior: The Impact of the Internet, Multimedia and Virtual Reality On Behavior and Society, 11*(3), 371–374.

Murai, T., Muller, U., Werheid, K., Sorger, D., Reuter, M., Becker, T., von Cramon, D. Y., & Barthel, H. (2001). In vivo evidence for differential association of striatal dopamine and midbrain serotonin systems with neuropsychiatric symptoms in Parkinson's disease. *Journal of Clinical Neuroscience, 13,* 222–228.

Neese, J. B. (1991). Depression in the general hospital. *Nursing Clinics of North America, 26*(3), 613–622.

Nemeroff, C. B. (2004). Neurobiological consequences of childhood trauma. *Journal of Clinical Psychiatry, 65*(Suppl. 1), 18–28.

Palomäki, H., Kaste, M., Berg, A., Lonnqvist, R., Lonnqvist, J., Lehtihalmes, M., & Hares, J. (1999). Prevention of poststroke depression: 1 Year randomised placebo controlled double blind trial of mianserin with 6 month follow up after therapy. *Journal of Neurology, Neurosurgery and Psychiatry, 66,* 490–494.

Paten, S. B. (1999). Long-term medical conditions and major depression in the Canadian population. *Canadian Journal of Psychiatry, 44*(2), 151–157.

Polsky, D., Doshi, J. A., Marcus, S., Oslin, D., Rothbard, A., Thomas, N., & Thompson, C. L. (2005). Long-term risk for depressive symptoms after a medical diagnosis. *Archives of Internal Medicine, 165*(11), 1260–1266.

Radley, J. J., Sisti, H. M., Has, J., Rocker, A. B., McCall, T., Hof, P. R., McEwen, B. S., & Morrison, J. H. (2004). Chronic behaviour stress induces apical dendritic reorganization in pyramidal neurons of the medial prefrontal cortex. *Neuroscience, 125*(1), 1–6.

Registered Nurses Association of Ontario. (2007). *Nursing best practice guideline: Assessment and management of pain.* Retrieved from http://rnao.ca/bpg/guidelines/assessment-and-management-pain

Rejinders, J. S., Ehrt, U., Weber, W. E., Aarsland, D., & Leentjens, A. F. (2008). A systematic review of prevalence of depression in Parkinson's disease. *Movement Disorders, 23*(2), 183–189.

Ren, K. (1994). Wind-up and the NMDA receptor: From animal studies to human pain. *Pain, 59,* 157–158.

Ribeiro, S. C., Tandon, R., Grunhaus, L., & Greden, J. F. (1993). The DST as a predictor of outcome in depression: A meta-analysis. *American Journal of Psychiatry, 150*(11), 1618–1629.

Robinson, R., Schultz, S., Castillo, C., Kopel, T., Kosier, J. T., Newman, M., … Starkstein, S. E. (2000). Nortriptyline versus fluoxetine in the treatment of depression and in short-term recovery after stroke: A placebo controlled, double-blind study. *American Journal of Psychiatry, 157,* 351–359.

Robinson, R. G. (2003). Poststroke depression: Prevalence, diagnosis, treatment, and disease progression. *Biological Psychiatry, 54*(3), 376–387.

Rojo, A., Aguilar, M., Garolera, M. T., Cubo, E., Navas, I., & Quintano, S. (2003). Depression in Parkinson's disease: Clinical correlates and outcomes. *Parkinsonism and Related Disorders, 10*(1), 23–28.

Rudy, T. E. & Turk, D. C. (1991). Psychological aspects of pain. *International Anesthesiology Clinics, 29*(1), 9–21.

Sareen, J., Cox, B. J., Clara, I., & Asmundson, G. J. (2005). The relationship between anxiety disorders and physical disorders in the U.S. national comorbidity survey. *Depression and Anxiety, 21*(4), 193–202.

Schwarzbold, M., Diaz, A., & Walz, R. (2008). Psychiatric disorders and traumatic brain injury. *Journal of Neuropsychiatric Disorder Treatment, 4*(4), 797–816.

Shor, R. & Shalev, A. (2013). Identifying barriers to improving wellness of persons with severe mental illness in community residential mental health facilities. *Social Work in Mental Health, 11,* 334–348.

Sosnowski, M. (1994). Pathophysiology of acute pain. *Pain Digest, 4,* 100–105.

Stratakis, C. & Chrousos, G. (1995). Neuro-endocrinology and pathophysiology of the stress system. *Annals of the New York Academy of Sciences, 771,* 1–18.

Talbot, J. D. & Marrett, S. (1991). Multiple representations of pain in human cerebral cortex. *Science, 251*(4999), 1355–1358.

Turk, D. C. (2004). Understanding pain sufferers: The role of cognitive successes. *Spine Journal, 4*(1), 1–7.

Turk, D. C. & Feldman, C. S. (1992). Facilitating the use of non-invasive pain management strategies with the terminally ill. *Hospice Journal, 8*(1–12), 193–214.

Verdelko, A., Henon, H., Lebert, F., Pasquiere, F., & Leys, D. (2004). Depressive symptoms after stroke and relationship with dementia: A three year follow-up study. *Neurology, 62*(6), 905–911.

Von Korff, M. & Dunn, K. M. (2008). Chronic pain reconsidered. *Pain, 138*(2), 267–276.

Wølen, H. & Bjørk, I. T. (2013). Intensive care pain and sedation: Nurses' experience of the conflict between clinical judgement and standardized care: an explorative study. *Intensive and Critical Care Nursing, 29,* 128–136.

World Health Organization, & World Organization of Family Doctors (2008). *Integrating mental health into primary care: a global perspective.* Geneva, Switzerland: World Health Organization.

Zangen, A., Nakash, R., & Yadid, G. (1999). Serotonin-mediated increases in the extracellular levels of beta-endorphins in the arcuate nucleus and nucleus accumbens: A microdialysis study. *Journal of Neurochemistry, 73*(6), 2569–2574.

37 Care of Persons With a History of Abuse

Elizabeth A. McCay

Adapted from the chapter "Caring for Abused Persons" by
Mary R. Boyd

KEY CONCEPTS

- resilience
- self-esteem

LEARNING OBJECTIVES

After studying this chapter, you will be able to:

- Describe the bio/psycho/social/spiritual theories of abuse.
- Discuss theories explaining why some persons become abusive and why some persons remain in violent relationships.
- Describe the bio/psycho/social/spiritual consequences of abuse.
- Describe the diagnostic criteria for posttraumatic stress disorder (PTSD).
- Discuss the three major symptom categories found in PTSD and their associated aetiologic factors.
- Describe the diagnostic criteria for dissociative identity disorder (DID).
- Integrate bio/psycho/social/spiritual theories into the analysis of human responses to abuse.
- Formulate nursing care plans for survivors of abuse.

KEY TERMS

- abuse • acute stress disorder (ASD) • alexithymia • behavioural sensitization • complex posttraumatic stress disorder (C-PTSD) • cycle of violence • dissociation • dissociative identity disorder (DID) • emotional abuse • extinction • fear conditioning • intergenerational transmission • neglect • physical abuse • posttraumatic stress disorder (PTSD) • sexual abuse • traumatic bonding

Violence demonstrated in the **abuse** of women, men, children, and elders is a national health problem that causes significant harm in survivors. Abuse of any type permanently changes the survivor's construction of reality and the meaning of his or her life. It wounds deeply, endangering core beliefs about self, others, and the world. It usually devastates the survivor's self-esteem.

Nurses encounter survivors of abuse in all health care settings. For this reason, they must be knowledgeable about abuse. They must understand its indicators, causes, assessment techniques, and effective nursing interventions. The importance of assessing for abuse in health care settings is being increasingly recognized (Gallop, McCay, Austin, Bayer, & Peternelji-Taylor, 1998; Hollingsworth & Ford-Gilboe, 2006). It requires nurses to possess the necessary educational background to ask questions about abuse that will ultimately prevent further abuse (Yonaka, Yoder, Darrow, & Sherck, 2007) and facilitate recovery. Adopting the Routine Universal Comprehensive Screening Protocol was found to be an effective strategy that increased public health nurses' knowledge and comfort to inquire about domestic abuse within a maternal–child visiting program (Vanderburg,

Wright, Boston, & Zimmerman, 2010). Failure to assess for abuse communicates a powerfully disturbing message: that the most traumatic event of a patient's life is too upsetting for others to hear. Protection and recovery from abuse require survivors to remember and discuss terrible events. Secrecy and silence may protect perpetrators and seriously endanger survivors. If nurses do not allow and encourage survivors to tell their stories, the abuse experiences will continue to haunt patients as symptoms of mental disorders.

This chapter focuses on the nursing process with women, men, children, and elders who are survivors of abuse. It provides basic nursing information needed to address the multiple, complex problems of these patients.

> ▼ **KEY CONCEPT** **Self-esteem** is how one
> feels about oneself. Its components are self-
> acceptance, self-worth, self-love, and self-nurturing.

▬▬ TYPES OF ABUSE

Most abuse that women, men, children, and elders experience is intimate violence; that is, the perpetrator is a loved and trusted partner or family member. As a result, the world and home may no longer be safe, people seem dangerous, and life may become a tortured existence of warding off ever-present threats. However, for some resilient individuals, healthy relationships across the life span appear to be protective, such that minimal psychological sequelae occur in adult life in spite of childhood abuse (Collishaw et al., 2007). A recent study provides evidence that resilience offered protection for First Nation's youth who were exposed to emotional, physical, and/or sexual abuse; specifically, the presence of community and family resilience significantly reduced symptoms of posttraumatic stress disorder (PTSD) (Zahradnik et al., 2010).

> ▼ **KEY CONCEPT** **Resilience** is the capacity to
> overcome adversity in spite of extreme stress
> and involves the balancing of risk and protective
> factors.

Woman Abuse

Woman abuse, domestic violence, spousal abuse, partner abuse, and battered wives are terms used interchangeably to denote violence directed towards women. However, some of these terms do not specifically refer to the abuse of a woman by an intimate partner. For example, the term *domestic violence* may be used in cases in which one person directs abuse against an entire family. The terms *spouse abuse* and *partner abuse* could indicate that the couple in whom abuse occurs, either heterosexual or homosexual,

lives together, but is unmarried. For these reasons, *woman abuse* has been chosen as the most appropriate term to use in this chapter in designating violence, including rape, directed towards a woman by an intimate partner.

Woman abuse is a significant health problem that crosses all ethnic, racial, and socioeconomic lines. Estimates of the annual prevalence of woman abuse range from 2 million to approximately 4 million cases (Brady and Dansky, 2002). According to Statistics Canada, men account for 83% of violence that is committed against women (Canadian Centre for Justice Statistics, 2013). Specific rates of victimization were assessed in the 2004 General Social Survey (GSS) on Victimization of 25,000 women and men. Survey results indicated that women and men report similar levels of spousal violence; however, women are more likely than are men to experience serious injury, as well as multiple assaults (Canadian Centre for Justice Statistics, 2013). It is possible that these figures may be low since underreporting may contribute to conservative estimates. Many women are afraid or reluctant to identify their abusers. In some cases, they fear retaliation against themselves or their children. In other cases, they continue to hold strong feelings for their partners, despite the abuse. On the other hand, men, given the societal expectation of male strength, may not want to admit to being victims of violence. A recent critique of the Canadian literature regarding violence against women underscores the importance of considering the context in which the violence occurs (Dragiewicz and DeKeseredy, 2012). For example, violent responses in women are frequently in self-defence (DeKeseredy, 2007), whereas men may use violence to exert control over their partner (DeKeseredy & Dragiewicz, 2007). An additional analysis of the 2004 Canadian General Social Survey on Victimization adds further evidence that intimate partner violence (IPV) is more chronic and severe for women than for men (Ansara & Hindin, 2010, 2011).

It is important to recognize that women of all ages and sociocultural backgrounds may experience abuse. Regardless, certain factors have been found to be associated with increased risk for violence in women. Specifically, police-reported and self-reported victimization data indicate that women who are at higher risk of violence are younger (15 to 24 years of age), with the risk of victimization decreasing with age (Canadian Centre for Justice Statistics, 2013). Women living with disabilities, such as a physical or mental health challenge that restricts activity, or who are young and/or experience emotional and financial abuse may be at increased risk of spousal abuse (Canadian Centre for Justice Statistics, 2013). Further, evidence suggests that single, divorced, and separated women may be at greater risk for abuse than are married women (Fishwick, Campbell, & Taylor, 2004; Romans, Forte, Cohen, Du Mont, & Hyman, 2007). Moreover, this group is at particularly high risk for severe violence. Danger assessments show that abusive ex-partners often exhibit obsessive threatening behaviour after their relationships end and pose significant dangers to women. Forty-three percent of women seen in emergency departments (EDs) attributed their abuse to a past partner. These findings emphasize that ending a relationship often does not end violence (Fishwick et al., 2004; Stewart, MacMillan, & Wathen, 2013). This information is important for health care providers, who frequently pressure women to end abusive relationships. Rates of woman abuse vary among women of different racial backgrounds. Research supports that Aboriginal women are at high risk for violence in their intimate relationships. Specifically, the results of the 2009 GSS data indicate that Aboriginal women in Canada are two to four times more likely than are non-Aboriginal women to experience IPV by a male partner (Canadian Centre for Justice Statistics, 2011). Even higher rates of woman abuse have been reported for Aboriginal women by other studies. For example, a study in Ontario documents that 8 of 10 Aboriginal women experienced violence in their intimate relationships (Health Canada, 2009), with 87% reporting physical abuse and 57% reporting sexual abuse. Further, physical abuse of women in Northern Aboriginal communities is thought to be pervasive, with estimates ranging from 75% to 90% (Health Canada, 2009) (see Box 37-1).

The perpetuation of violence begins early in dating relationships. The prevalence of dating violence is on the rise in Canada with rates of police-reported dating violence steadily increasing from 2004 to 2008 for women and men (Statistics Canada, 2011). A report examining the prevalence of police-reported incidents of dating violence in Canada documents that in 2008, dating violence constituted approximately one quarter of all IPV (Mahoney, 2010). The majority of victims were female, and those most at risk for dating violence were between the ages of 30 to 39, with risk declining as age increased (Mahoney, 2010). Dating violence can also occur in same-sex relationships. Police-reported incidents of dating violence in 2008 indicated that 10% of male victims reported dating violence involving same-sex relationships, whereas only 1% of females reported dating violence in same-sex relationships (Mahoney, 2010). Several recent Canadian studies have focused on the underlying factors that influence dating violence in youth populations.

A qualitative study of 40 adolescent girls aged 15 and 16 years provides some insight into factors associated with high rates of dating violence (Banister, Jakubec, & Stein, 2003). Specifically, the study findings highlight the tremendous power imbalance that exists in dating relationships for adolescent girls, which frequently gives rise to a tolerance of violence simply to maintain the relationship (Banister et al., 2003). A related study demonstrates that higher levels of affiliation with deviant peers are associated with high-risk lifestyles, as well as increased levels of dating violence amongst a community sample of adolescent girls ($N = 550$) in Québec (Vézina et al., 2011).

BOX 37-1 Research for Best Practice

UNDERSTANDING STRATEGIES USED BY RURAL WOMEN TO STOP, AVOID, OR ESCAPE FROM IPV

Riddell, T., Ford-Gilboe, M., & Leipert, B. (2009). Strategies used by rural women to stop, avoid or escape from intimate partner violence. Health Care for Women International, 30, 134–159.

The Question: What are the strategies used by rural women to stop, avoid, or escape from violence in a relationship with an abusive partner?

Methods: The researchers used a mixed-methods approach employing two quantitative measures, as well as qualitative interviews to identify the frequency and helpfulness of strategies used to cope with IPV. Forty-three rural Canadian women (13 from Ontario and 30 from New Brunswick) enrolled in an ongoing longitudinal study were included in the analysis. In order to gain further understanding of the quantitative findings, interactive collaborative qualitative interviews were conducted with 9 of the 43 participants. Audiotaped interviews were transcribed verbatim, and the data were analyzed initially using a line-by-line approach to identify strategies used by women to deal with IPV. Conceptual-based patterns and themes were developed and integrated with the quantitative findings.

Findings: Quantitative findings revealed that placating and resistance strategies were used most frequently by the women in the study to deal with IPV, even though these strategies were rated as least helpful. On the other hand, only half of the women in the study identified that they used safety planning, seeking legal counsel, and seeking help from networks (formal and informal) even though these strategies were rated as most effective in dealing with IPV. The qualitative findings further explicated the quantitative findings. Specifically, the women in the study deliberately used placating and resistance strategies to keep their children and themselves safe while planning ultimately to leave the abusive relationship. Further, numerous barriers exist in rural settings to seeking help for IPV, including physical and social isolation, limited resources, and patriarchal attitudes. The integration of the quantitative and qualitative findings revealed the critical role of safety planning in living with IPV.

Implications for Nursing: Nurses providing care for women in rural communities need to be cognizant of the many factors that may impede women from seeking help for IPV. These factors include physical and social isolation, limited economic resources, controlling patriarchal attitudes, and limited access to services. The researchers suggest that nurses create opportunities to speak privately with women living in rural settings in an open and direct manner to facilitate disclosure and access to much needed help. Nurses practising in rural communities are in an ideal position to advocate for social change and to enhance existing resources in rural communities for women dealing with IPV.

Further, peer group relational aggression was found to predict dating violence amongst both male and female adolescents (Ellis, Chung-Hall, & Dumas, 2013). The importance of familial factors for adolescent boys in dating violence is highlighted in a longitudinal study of dating violence in adolescent boys residing in Montreal (LaVoie et al., 2002). Specifically, harsh parenting and antisocial behaviour were found to be predictive of dating violence in 717 boys aged 16 to 17 years living in a less affluent area of Montreal (LaVoie et al., 2002). In the 2004 GSS, dating violence accounted for 28% of nonfamilial violence. It is also noteworthy that dating violence was found to be more prevalent than was spousal abuse. Research suggests that supporting youth in the context of early dating relationships is important since future patterns of violence and assault are frequently established in early relationships (Wolfe, 2006).

Battering

Battering is the single greatest cause of serious injury to women. Battering can be defined as repeated physical or sexual violence with the intent of coercive control (Humphreys & Campbell, 2011). Estimates of injury related to battering seen in EDs range from 14% to 50% (Campbell, Torres, McKenna, Sheridan, & Landenburger, 2004). In 2010, there were 593 shelters in Canada specifically for women who have experienced abuse (Burczycka & Cotter, 2011). Sixty-seven percent of women who were residing in shelters were seeking a secure setting away from an abusive partner (Burczycka & Cotter, 2011). Accordingly, women are about three times more likely to be victims of homicide by a spouse than are men (Canadian Centre for Justice Statistics, 2011) and also experience repeated victimizations (Health Canada, 2009). Indeed, the realistic fear of being killed is one factor that keeps many women from leaving abusive partners, even after years of severe abuse. IPV against women is more likely to be consistent with battering, such that it is severe, repetitive, and likely to result in injury and has been found to be associated with a wide range of poor mental health outcomes, such as increased anxiety and suicidal ideation (Afifi, Boman, Fleisher, & Sareen, 2009). Moreover, many women who experience abuse also live with PTSD (Stewart et al., 2013). In a study of 65 women receiving treatment from three Canadian urban mental health centres, women reporting early-onset sexual abuse were more likely to meet the criteria for complex PTSD than were women reporting late-onset PTSD (McLean & Gallop, 2003). In addition, based on an analysis of the Canadian Community Health Survey, PTSD was determined to be associated with severe physical health problems such as cardiovascular disease, chronic pain, and cancer amongst others, as well as increased suicide attempts, poor quality of life, and increased disability (Sareen et al., 2007).

Battering also poses a significant danger to unborn children. The literature suggests that there is an increased risk of violence for women who are pregnant, although this observation may be related to increased opportunities for detection of abuse at health clinics during pregnancy (Cook & Dickens, 2009). According to a 2009 Canadian GSS, 11% of women who reported being victims of IPV also reported being pregnant (Sinha, 2013). Abuse during pregnancy is a significant risk factor for several foetal and maternal complications, including low birth weight, low maternal weight gain, infections, and anaemia (Sinha, 2013). Moreover, abuse of women often results in their use of alcohol and other drugs (AOD), which, in turn, may harm unborn children (Parker, Bullock, Bohn, & Curry, 2004).

Rape and Sexual Assault

Rape and sexual assault are common in Canada. Sexual assault includes any form of nonconsenting sexual activity, ranging from fondling to penetration. According to the 2004 GSS, there were 512,000 incidents of sexual assault reported in the Canadian population aged 15 years and older (Brennan & Taylor-Butts, 2008). Also based on the 2004 GSS, rates of sexual victimization for women were found to be five times higher than for men. Overall, age is a risk for sexual assault with the rate of sexual assault for youth ages 15 to 24 being 18 times higher than for Canadians age 55 years and older, with 81% of young victims being female (Brennan & Taylor-Butts, 2008). Most sexual assaults are underreported for the same reason that domestic violence is underreported—women may feel embarrassed and ashamed and fear being blamed for the assault (Ansara & Hindin, 2010).

Sex and Increased Risk for Human Immunodeficiency Virus

Woman abuse is also a risk factor for human immunodeficiency virus (HIV) infection among women. In one study where screening for domestic violence was part of ongoing care for an HIV population in Alberta, a strong association was found between domestic violence victimization and HIV infection (Siemieniuk, Krentz, Gish, & Gill, 2010). Of those individuals with HIV who were screened, 34% reported having experienced abuse, and among these, more than half were abused as children (Siemieniuk et al., 2010). Further, women were 1.6 times more likely than were men and over twice as likely as heterosexual men to have experienced IPV. An association was also found between a history of domestic violence and delayed access to care, missed appointments, and an increased use of clinic resources such as social work. An abusive partner may increase the risk for HIV infection in several ways. Women who have abusive partners may not be able to avoid sexual contact. Fear of a partner's violent behaviour may prevent women from insisting on the use of condoms. A woman's insistence on condom use can imply that either partner is being unfaithful and can result in abuse. Victimized women are also four times more likely to have sex with a risky partner than are women who have not been abused (Morrill, Kasten, Urato, & Larson, 2001).

It is noteworthy that Aboriginal peoples are overrepresented among HIV and AIDS cases in Canada. In 2008, Aboriginal persons living with HIV represented 8% of all prevalent HIV infections (Public Health Agency of Canada, 2010a). In the same year (2008), the HIV infection rate among Aboriginal persons was about 3.6 times higher than among non-Aboriginal persons (PHAC). A qualitative study of 18 HIV-positive Aboriginal women indicates that these women endured abusive childhood experiences that lead to the adoption of high-risk life on the street, which frequently included running away from home, involvement in the sex trade, intravenous drug use, and incarceration in jail, increasing the risk for HIV infection (McKeown, Reid, & Orr, 2004). Further, high rates of sexual abuse documented among Aboriginal youth (48% of 543 surveyed) are clearly linked to an increased risk for HIV infection through injection drug use and/or ongoing sexual contact (Cedar Project Partnership, 2008).

Stalking

Stalking is a crime of intimidation. In legal terms, stalking is referred to as criminal harassment and involves behaviour that occurs over a period of time and which causes individuals to experience significant distress or fear for their safety or that of someone they know (Department of Justice, Canada, 2003a). Examples include following or communicating with another person, repeatedly watching someone's house or workplace, or directly threatening another person or their family member (Milligan, 2011). Criminal harassment legislation was introduced in 1993 to deal with harassment and prevent escalation into serious physical harm primarily against women. The legislation applies to all victims of harassment (Department of Justice, Canada, 2003a). In 2009, however, females accounted for three quarters of all individuals experiencing criminal harassment with almost half of these incidents by a former intimate partner. Those who were stalked by an ex-spouse were pursued for well over a year (Canadian Centre for Justice Statistics, 2005). In contrast, males were more often harassed by a casual acquaintance (37%) than by a former (21%) or current (2%) intimate partner (Milligan, 2011).

Probation was the most common sentence imposed for those found guilty of criminal harassment in 2008/2009 (Canadian Centre for Justice Statistics, 2011). Over the years, the Criminal Code has been amended to put in place procedural protections for the victim when an individual is accused and convicted of criminal harassment such as prohibiting possession of weapons (Department of Justice, Canada, 2012a).

Abuse of Men

Although sexual assault and violence have typically focused on women, the literature is now indicating that the rate of violence and sexual assault is now higher in men than traditionally believed (Romans et al., 2007; Stermac, Del Bove, & Addison, 2004). As noted earlier, the GSS data indicated that men and women experience similar levels of spousal violence, with 6% of men being victims of IPV, only 1% less than the rate of IPV reported for women (Brzozowski & Brazeau, 2008; Department of Justice, Canada, 2013). Police-reported victimization data indicate that men were more likely than were women to be physically assaulted in a public place such as a parking lot or on public transit (Canadian Centre for Justice Statistics, 2010). Males were also more likely to be victims of more serious assaults than were women and have a weapon used against them (Canadian Centre for Justice Statistics, 2010). The consequences of violence and sexual assault can also be devastating for men. Hopton and Huta (2013) evaluated an intervention designed specifically for men who had experienced childhood abuse (sexual, physical, and/or emotional). Their findings suggest that male survivors who seek services are suffering from high rates of self-reported posttraumatic stress and symptoms of depression. Men are less likely than are women to seek help despite significant levels of functional distress. The authors suggest that factors such as stigma, underrecognition and underreporting of male sexual abuse, and the lack of services tailored to the needs of men are barriers to seeking treatment. A recent study examined 141 cases from a sexual assault database located in a large urban Ontario city (Stermac et al., 2004). The data suggest that male victims of sexual assault are more likely to be young, street involved, with an increased vulnerability such as either a cognitive or a physical disability (Stermac et al., 2004). The authors suggest that future research is needed to understand better this previously unrecognized vulnerable group.

Child Abuse

All forms of child abuse deprive children of the rights and protection to which they are entitled. These rights are clearly set out in the United Nations Convention of the Rights of the Child (United Nations, 1989) and include basic rights to the provision of an adequate standard of living, to be protected from harm and abuse, and to participate in children's programs and services (Canadian Child Care Federation, 2012).

The prevalence of child abuse is far reaching. The 2008 Canadian Incidence Study of Reported Child Abuse and Neglect estimated that there were 235,842 child maltreatment investigations that year (Public Health Agency of Canada, 2010b). Of course, this figure does not include cases that were unreported. The most common forms of child maltreatment included witnessing IPV (34%), neglect (34%), physical violence (20%), and emotional neglect (9%) (Public Health Agency of Canada, 2010b). Maltreatment investigations were examined specifically with regard to Aboriginal children, given their high rate of involvement with the child welfare system. Data from 2008 indicate that 22% of all substantiated cases of maltreatment involved children of Aboriginal heritage. It is also extremely important to acknowledge the child abuse that occurred in the residential schools for Aboriginal children within the last century (Law Commission of Canada, 2000). The Law Commission of Canada noted that Aboriginal children were the only children who were designated to live in an institution, away from their families and communities, because of their race. Frequently, these children were prohibited from speaking their mother tongue and were deliberately deprived of all connections with their culture and identity, placing this group of children at high risk for abuse (Law Commission of Canada, 2000). The report acknowledges the profound level of harm to the children, families, and communities that occurred as a result of these children being displaced and mistreated. A recent study by Bombay, Matheson, and Anisman (2011) examined the relationship between the intergenerational experience of residential schools and depressive symptomatology amongst First Nation adults. First Nation adults who had a parent who attended a residential school were compared with First Nation adults who had a parent who did not attend a residential school. Second-generation adults whose parents attended residential schools demonstrated significantly greater levels of depression than did those adults whose parents did not attend residential schools. The study results suggest that the residential school experience evoked intergenerational trauma most likely through experiences of childhood adversity, trauma, and perceived discrimination (Bombay et al., 2011).

Child Neglect

Child **neglect** is the most common form of child abuse reported (Allin, Wathen, & MacMillan, 2005) and frequently is chronic (Department of Justice, Canada, 2003b). Physical neglect occurs when a parent or guardian does not meet a child's needs such as food, clothing, shelter, cleanliness, health care, or emotional needs (Department of Justice, Canada, 2012b). Neglect can be as harmful as physical abuse. In some instances, such as child abandonment, neglect is a crime in Canada (Department of Justice, Canada, 2012b). Indicators of physical neglect may include diaper dermatitis, lice, scabies, dirty appearance, clothes inappropriate for the weather, and unclean and unsafe living environment. Just how to respond to neglected children and their families is relatively unknown. A systematic literature review highlights the dramatic need for effective interventions to neglected children and their families (Allin et al., 2005).

Physical Abuse

Physical abuse is the deliberate use of force against a child and may include hitting, slapping, punching, biting, burning, kicking, pushing, shoving, choking, or any other type of physical action directed towards the child that results in nonaccidental injury (Department of Justice, Canada, 2012b). Injuries to children caused by physical abuse range from mild to severe and life threatening. Types of injuries include cutaneous injuries (e.g., contusions, abrasions, burns, bite marks), abusive head trauma (e.g., direct trauma, vigorous shaking), ocular injuries (e.g., retinal haemorrhage), ear injuries (e.g., contusions, swelling), and abdominal trauma (e.g., blunt abdominal trauma from punching or kicking) (Gary & Humphreys, 2004; Kelley, 2011). The leading cause of death in children who have been maltreated is head trauma, followed by abdominal trauma (Kelley, 2011). Often, clothing hides these injuries, and practitioners must look for other signs of abuse, such as fear, aggressive or withdrawn behaviour, poor social relations, learning problems, delinquent behaviour, and wearing clothing that is meant to cover injuries but is inappropriate for the weather. In addition, when treating a child with such injuries, professionals should suspect abuse when explanations are implausible and inconsistent with injuries, when involved parties give different versions of the incident, or when treatment seeking is delayed (Kelley, 2011).

Sexual Abuse

Any sexual behaviour towards a child under the age of 16 in Canada constitutes a crime (Department of Justice, Canada, 2012b). Child **sexual abuse** can range from mild, covert behaviours to overt sexual acts and can include exhibitionism; voyeurism; touching the child's sexual organs; and oral, anal, and vaginal sex (Department of Justice, Canada, 2003b; Draughon & Urbancic, 2011; Gary, Campbell, & Humphreys, 2004; Gary & Humphreys, 2004). Childhood sexual exploitation is also included with the discussion of childhood sexual abuse, specifically, using children for the purpose of pornography or prostitution (Department of Justice, Canada, 2012b). There are three categories of sexual abuse: incest, sexual abuse perpetrated by a nonfamily member, and paedophilia. Incest is defined in the Criminal Code of Canada (1985) in this way: Everyone commits incest who, "Knowing that another person by blood relationship is his or her parent, child, brother, sister, grandparent, or grandchild, as the case may be, has sexual intercourse with that person" (5.155). This definition limits the illegal sexual activity to sexual intercourse; it does not include fondling, oral sex, and masturbation. These acts, when committed against children, are covered under other laws not restricted to blood relatives. Paedophilia describes those who have a sexual fixation on young children that usually translates into sexual acts with the victims. Police-reported data in Canada in 2007 indicated that 58% of sexual assault victims were under the age of 18, with 25% of all sexual assault victims in the same year being under the age of 12 (Brennan & Taylor-Butts, 2008). Further, police-reported data from 2003 reveal that the largest percentage (48%) of sexual assaults against children were committed by individuals known to the victimized children, while 32%

of sexual assaults against children were committed by family members (AuCoin, 2005).

Several factors may mediate the effects of child sexual abuse. In general, younger children with a history of emotional difficulties may be more traumatized than will be older and more stable children. Repeated abuse for long periods with more violence and bodily penetration results in greater traumatization. Sexual abuse by someone whom the child knows and trusts causes more severe trauma. The child abused by a family member experiences a devastating breach of trust, loss of a safe home, and threats to fundamental survival requirements (Boyd & Mackey, 2000a), which for some may last a lifetime (Draughon & Urbancic, 2011).

Emotional Abuse

Emotional abuse includes acts or omissions that psychologically damage the child (Gary et al., 2004), such as humiliating a child, constantly yelling, and criticizing or threatening a child (Department of Justice, Canada, 2012b). The emotionally abused child does not have visible injuries to alert others, but it severely disturbs the child's sense of security. Consequently, emotional abuse severely affects a child's self-esteem and often leaves permanent emotional scars, which can take a prolonged time to heal (Department of Justice, Canada, 2012b). In Canada, various forms of emotional abuse against children constitute a crime and may include serious forms of harmful threats or threats to a child's personal property, such as a pet (Department of Justice, Canada, 2012b). According to Canadian child welfare statistics, an estimated 3.6 children out of 1,000 experience emotional or psychological abuse, a figure that is readily acknowledged to be underestimated (Trocmé, Fallon, MacLaurin, Black, & Roy, 2005). It is also recognized that children who experience emotional abuse are more likely than are children who are not emotionally abused to have increased psychological difficulties, such as depression, and increased risk-taking behaviour (Chamberland, Laporte, Lavergne, & Baraldi, 2003). Children who witness domestic violence are also thought to be victims of emotional abuse, and they demonstrate increased anxiety and insecurity compared with children who do not witness domestic violence (Chamberland et al., 2003). Frequently, emotional abuse occurs within the context of other forms of abuse or maltreatment, underlining the complexity and urgent need for responsive and innovative interventions for this serious problem.

Factitious Disorder by Proxy: Munchausen's Syndrome by Proxy

Factitious disorder by proxy is another form of child abuse (see Chapter 24). This disorder includes "the intentional production or feigning of physical or psychological signs or symptoms in another person who is under the individual's care for the purpose of indirectly assuming the sick role" (American Psychiatric Association [APA], 2000, p. 781) and is listed as factitious disorder imposed on another in the current *Diagnostic and Statistical Manual of Mental Disorders* (*DSM-5*) (American Psychiatric Association, 2013). The signs of this disorder include repeated hospitalizations and medical evaluations of the child without definitive diagnosis; symptoms or medical signs that are inappropriate or inconsistent; symptoms that disappear when the child is away from the parent; a parent who encourages medical tests for the child; parental uneasiness as the child recovers; and a parent who is less concerned with the child's health than with spending time with caregivers (Bartsch, Risse, Schutz, Weigand, & Weiler, 2003). This disorder was once thought to be relatively rare; however, it is now recognized as more common and with serious outcomes, such as the death of a child (Truman & Ayoub, 2002).

Secondary Abuse: Children of Battered Women

Exposure to violence is a serious stressor for children (Zahradnik et al., 2010). Research on children of battered women has become more evident over the past 25 years (Clements, Oxtoby, & Ogle, 2008). Children may witness their mother being choked, threatened with a weapon, or threatened with death (Berman, Hardesty, Lewis O'Connor, & Humphreys, 2004; Boyd & Mackey, 2000a; Campbell & Lewandowski, 1997). These children fear for both their mother's safety and their own (Boyd & Mackey, 2000a). Children who grow up in violent families experience living with secrecy, relocations as the mother leaves home to seek safety, economic hardship, maternal depression that may reduce her ability to nurture, and frightening interactions with the police and court systems (Berman et al., 2004; Boyd & Mackey, 2000a; Campbell & Lewandowski, 1997). According to the 2009 GSS, children are more likely to observe IPV if the victim is female or separated from a partner. Furthermore, findings from the 2009 GSS on victimization indicate that children witnessing violence has increased 43% between 2004 and 2009 (Sinha, 2012). Research has substantiated the traumatic long-term effects of witnessing violence and indicates that children who witness violence are more likely to experience negative outcomes throughout childhood, such as dropping out of school, PTSD, and/or problems with alcohol or illicit drug use (Zahradnik et al., 2010). A National Longitudinal Survey of Children and Youth in 1994–1995 found that children who witnessed violence in the home were at increased risk of being physically aggressive 2 to 4 years later (Statistics Canada, 2003). In addition, children who have witnessed violence in the home were also found to be more likely to demonstrate increased levels of depression, emotional problems, and delinquency (Fitzgerald, 2004, as cited in Canadian Centre for Justice Statistics, 2005). Emerging research has shed some light on the important role of resilience in moderating the relationship between youth exposure to violence and mental health for school age youth who had been exposed to violence (Zahradnik et al., 2010).

Elder Abuse

The population aged 65 years and older now represents one of the fastest-growing cohorts of the population, increasing from 9% in 1981 to 14% of the population in 2009 (Sinha, 2012). In the coming decades, it is projected that Canada's population will continue to age considerably, with the proportion of Canadians aged 55 years and older rising from 27% in 2011 to 35% in 2031 (Brennan, 2012). This is the result of the ageing of baby boomers, decreasing fertility rates, and increase in life expectancy (Turcotte & Schellenberg, 2007). Elder abuse, in the context of a growing ageing population, is increasingly recognized as a serious problem in Canada and other countries. Despite this observation, it has been reported that seniors aged 65 years and older have the lowest risk of experiencing violence compared with any other age groups, regardless of whether the abuse was by a family member or not (Sinha, 2012). Adult children (34 per 100,000) have been identified most often as responsible for family violence against older adults, with women being particularly vulnerable (Sinha, 2012). Specifically, senior women have been found to be more vulnerable to family violence, at a rate of 34% higher than men (Sinha, 2012). Based on the GSS 2009 survey, approximately 2% of Canadians aged 65 years or older reported that a child, relative, friend, or caregiver had been emotionally or financially abusive in the preceding 5 years (Brennan, 2012). Risk factors for elder abuse include older age, impairment in the activities of daily living (ADLs), cognitive disability or other mental illness, dependency on the caregiver, isolation, stressful events, and a history of intergenerational conflict between the elder and the caregiver (Sengstock, Ulrich, & Barrett, 2004).

■ THEORIES OF ABUSE

Many theories have attempted to explain violence between intimate partners and in the family. The theories reviewed here have been categorized as biologic, psychological, and social. In all likelihood, family violence is truly a bio/psycho/social/spiritual phenomenon that no one of these theories can fully explain (Fig. 37-1). Violent or aggressive behaviour therefore needs to be regarded in a broader context as a complex phenomenon that takes into account environmental as well as genetic or neurobiologic factors (Nelson & Trainor, 2007). A separate section presents additional theories that are more specific to the phenomenon of woman abuse.

FIGURE 37-1. Bio/psycho/social/spiritual aetiologies for violent behaviour.

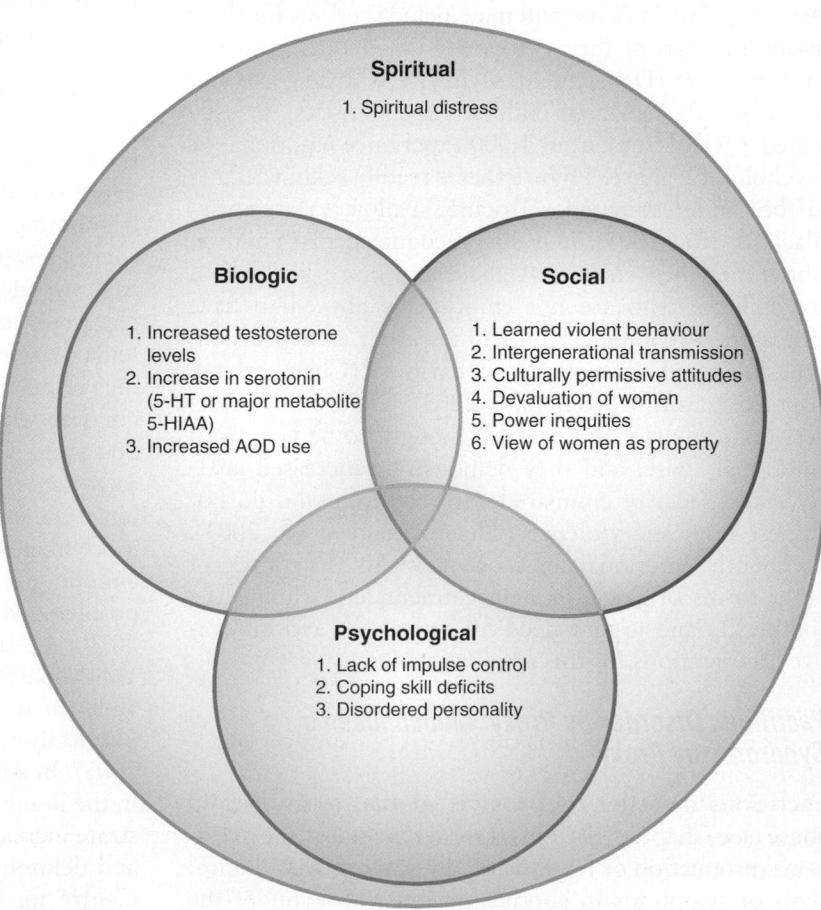

Biologic Theories

Neurologic Problems

Aggressive behaviour may be associated with several neurologic conditions, including traumatic brain injury, seizure disorder, and dementia (see Chapter 18). Neurodevelopmental factors and traumatic brain injury can produce seizure disorders, attentional dysfunction, or focal neurobehavioural syndromes, all of which are associated with aggressive behaviour. The most common association between seizures and aggressive behaviour occurs during the postictal period (the period immediately after the seizure), during which the individual may be confused.

Damage to the orbitofrontal cortex often causes impulsive, labile, irritable, and socially inappropriate behaviour. Individuals with such damage often respond aggressively to trivial stimuli. In addition, damage to the neocortex, limbic system, and hypothalamus may result in aggressive behaviour. These systems have hierarchic control over one another. Damage to higher centres may disinhibit aggression from lower centres. Aggressive behaviour also may be related to disruptions in neurotransmitter systems. Those with mental disorders are at an increased risk for developing aggressive behaviour. Disruption in serotonin, dopamine, and gamma-aminobutyric acid systems has been linked with several psychiatric disorders, including depression, schizophrenia, impulsive behaviour, suicide, and aggression (Comai, Tau, & Gobbi, 2012; Nelson & Trainor, 2007). Complex interactions among neurotransmitter systems and their respective receptors are thought to play a role in aggressive behaviour. Psychopharmacologic agents (e.g., atypical antipsychotics, anticonvulsants, and lithium) have changed the course of treatment for aggressive behaviour by effecting change at an intracellular level (Comai et al., 2012).

Links With Substance Abuse

The use of AOD is commonly associated with violent incidents. Alcohol has been found to be present in approximately one half to two thirds of sexual assaults (Ulman, 2003). Although AOD use alone is rarely sufficient to account for violence, the Ontario Mental Health Supplement indicated that parental substance use is significantly associated with an increased risk for childhood physical and sexual abuse (Walsh, MacMillan, & Jamieson, 2003). Other factors, such as low family income, stress, and abuse in the family of origin, are often more important (Stewart et al., 2013). The relationship of AOD to violence may result from three factors: (1) AOD-induced cognitive impairment, (2) the user's expectations that AOD increases the tendency towards aggression, and (3) socioculturally grounded beliefs that people are unaccountable for their behaviour while intoxicated (Abbey, Zawacki, Buck, Clinton, & McAuslan, 2003).

Studies have demonstrated that drinking alcohol may change perceptions about accountability for behaviour (Abbey et al., 2003). The belief that intoxicated behaviour will be judged less harshly may encourage and provide an excuse for those who abuse substances to engage in normally unacceptable behaviours. Research shows that people attempt to justify their criminal behaviour by blaming alcohol after the fact (Abbey et al., 2003), given the general belief that alcohol use is associated with aggression (Stewart et al., 2013). Alcohol use has also been associated with IPV both in terms of its occurrence and its severity through a biochemical effect that impacts cognitive and physical function and reduces self-control (Kelly, Gonzalez-Guarda, & Taylor, 2011; Stewart et al., 2013). For those individuals who are impulsive, alcohol use is a concern. There has been increasing concern about the growing number of drug-facilitated sexual assault. In particular, flunitrazepam has become known as the date rape drug (Du Mont et al., 2009). A recent Canadian study of primarily female sexual assault victims receiving care at hospital-based treatment centres found that 21% of the sample ($n = 882$) met the criteria for suspected drug-facilitated assault. The researchers conclude that treatment centres need to be prepared to respond to date rape victims, since it is a common problem (Du Mont et al., 2009).

Psychosocial Theories

Psychopathology Theory

Psychopathology theory seeks to understand violence by examining the characteristics of individual men and women (Wallace, 1999). Theorists from this perspective focus on personality traits, internal defence systems, and mental disorders. An outdated theory that was particularly damaging labelled women as masochistic, paranoid, or depressed (Bograd, 1999). One underlying assumption of this labelling was that some women enjoy abuse and deliberately provoke attacks because they need to suffer.

Research on batterers has shown that there is not a common profile or a typical batterer. Studies have found evidence of personality disorders, including antisocial, borderline, narcissistic, and dependent. A Canadian study of 997 men who were recruited from outpatient forensic settings and the community indicated that abusive or severely abusive men were more likely to have antisocial personality disorders, demonstrate impulsive behaviour, and have dysfunctional attitudes regarding spousal abuse compared with nonabusive men (Hanson, Cadsky, Harris, & Lalonde, 1997). Abusive men were also more likely to have a history of violence during childhood.

Although research has not consistently found one common mental disorder or set of characteristics in violent individuals, there is a typology of men who batter that shows promise (Emery & Laumann-Billings, 1998). Type I batterers are violent in many situations, have many victims, and display antisocial characteristics. Type II batterers abuse only their family, commit less severe violence, are generally less aggressive, and demonstrate remorse. These men tend to be dependent, jealous, and unlikely to have personality or other disorders. Type III batterers display dysphoric–borderline or schizoid characteristics, such as emotional volatility, depression, feelings of inadequacy, and social isolation (Emery & Laumann-Billings, 1998). Type III batterers also tend to be violent only within their families.

Social Learning Theory

Violent families create an atmosphere of tension, fear, intimidation, and tremendous confusion about intimate relationships (Boyd & Mackey, 2000a). Children in violent homes often learn violent behaviour as an approved and legitimate way to solve problems, especially within intimate relationships. Social learning theory posits that men who witness violence in their homes often perpetuate violent behaviour in their families as adults (Berman et al., 2011; Dewey, 2004). Moreover, women who grow up in violent homes learn to accept violence and expect it in their own adult relationships (Boyd & Mackey, 2000a). These concepts are often referred to as the **intergenerational transmission** of violence. Consistent with the theory of intergenerational transmission of violence, research findings from a telephone survey of 1,249 adults living in the city of Vancouver provide evidence that all forms of violence occurring in families of origin are predictive of relationship violence (Kwong, Bartholomew, Henderson, & Trinke, 2003). In another Canadian study of intergenerational violence, negative childhood experiences of family violence carried over into adolescence and intimate relationships (Laporte, Jiang, Pepler, & Chamberland, 2011). Further, female adolescents were found to be at greater risk for revictimization, whereas males who reported violence in childhood, particularly by their fathers, were more likely to be aggressive towards their girlfriends.

Findings of extreme violence in the parental homes of battered individuals and individuals who grew up witnessing violence are common and support the intergenerational transmission of violence theory (Dewey, 2004). Although violence in the home can have a serious and negative effect on children, it does not necessarily predict with certainty that violence will occur in future relationships. As Berman and colleagues (2011) point out, the relationship between exposure to violence and being violent towards others is a complex one associated with a range of factors.

Social Theories

Covering the many sociologic theories of violence is beyond the scope of this chapter. Sociologic theories posit that abuse occurs because of cultural norms that permit and even glamorize violent behaviour (Lucea, Glass, & Laughon, 2011). From a societal perspective, the acceptance of violence as normal appears widespread among young people. In one Canadian study of female university students, physical assaults by dating partners were both common and frequent among the women sampled (Brownridge, 2006). A study conducted by Ellis et al. (2013), among Canadian high school students, showed that aggressive adolescent peer groups influenced relationships and was predictive of later dating violence. In another study, dating violence was seen as unacceptable by adolescents; however, behaviours such as grabbing, hitting, and kicking within dating relationships were regarded as acceptable in certain situations such as when "joking around" (Sears et al., 2006). In keeping with these findings, a qualitative study by Canadian researchers revealed that young adolescent girls (15 and 16 years of age) were so eager to have a male dating partner that they were willing to tolerate physical violence and verbal abuse, just to "keep the guy" (Banister, Jakubec, & Stein, 2003).

Family violence is also related to qualities of the community in which the family is embedded. Poverty, absence of family services, social isolation, lack of cohesion in the community, and stress contribute to family violence (Schaefer-McDaniel, 2004). The relationship of poverty, social isolation, and child abuse has been well established (Coulton, Crampton, Irwin, Spilsbury, & Korbin, 2007; Health Canada, 2004; Leschied, Chiodo, Whitehead, Hurley, & Marshall, 2003). Economic disadvantage creates tremendous stress for families, increasing the risk for child abuse and maltreatment. It should be kept in mind that economically impoverished families may seek social services more frequently, and as such, the reporting of abuse may be increased in these families (Health Canada, 2004). However, not all poor families abuse their children. One difference between poor families who do and do not abuse their children lies in the degree of social cohesion and mutual caring found in their communities (Rothman, 2007). Neighbourhoods with high levels of child abuse frequently have severe social disorganization and lack of community identity. In addition, they have higher rates of juvenile delinquency, drug trafficking, and violent crime (O'Campo, Burke, Peak, McDonnell, & Gielen, 2005). Regardless, there is evidence that some neighbourhoods may provide a protective effect. For example, a recent study found that immigrant women who were living in low-income and high-immigrant neighbourhoods were less likely to experience abuse, notwithstanding the length of time that the women had spent in Canada (Daoud, O'Campo, Urquia, & Heaman, 2012).

One of the most accepted theories of elder abuse is the family stress theory. The theory hypothesizes that providing care for an elder induces stress within the family. Family stress includes economic hardship, loss of sleep, and intrusions into family activities and routines.

Moreover, caring for a dependent elder takes an enormous physical toll on the caregiver. If there is no relief, the caregiver may become overwhelmed, lose control, and abuse the elder (Norris, Fancey, Power, & Ross, 2013; Sengstock et al., 2004). With the ageing of the Canadian population, the demands on family members to provide care are rising, as are the associated stress of caregiving and the increased risk for elder abuse (Canadian Centre for Justice Statistics, 2005). Other characteristics of caregivers that may predispose them to abuse elderly parents include alcohol or drug abuse, dementia, restricted outside activities, unrealistic expectations, and a blaming, hypercritical personality.

Theoretic Dynamics Specific to Woman Abuse

Feminist Theories

Feminist theory focuses on issues of gender, inequality, power and privilege, patriarchy, and the subordination of women as explanations for woman abuse (Damant et al., 2008; Landenburger, Campbell, & Rodriguez, 2004; Yodanis, 2004). According to the feminist perspective, woman abuse results from a patriarchal society that perpetuates attitudes that support violence against women (Ford-Gilboe et al., 2005; Lloyd & Emery, 2000; Yodanis, 2004). Three major characteristics of such a patriarchal society are the devaluation of women, power inequities, and the view of women as property (Hunnicutt, 2009; Kelly et al., 2011).

Feminists also point to a power inequity in society as a contributing factor to woman abuse. Women have made many advances in recent years; however, men continue to control most institutions (Lloyd & Emery, 2000). Women continue to earn less than do men for paid work and are less likely to advance to positions of authority and power (Nolen-Hoeksema, 2002; Singh & Peng, 2010). Moreover, marriage often victimizes women in ways other than through violence. Although men now contribute to household work, most women who hold jobs outside the home continue to perform most household and childcare tasks (Lloyd & Emery, 2000). This power inequity is reflected in higher depression rates among married women than among married men (Nolen-Hoeksema, 2002). According to the Canadian Survey of Labour and Income Dynamics, one in five Canadian women experienced low income for at least a year following the breakup of their marriage, with women under the age of 40 being at higher risk of poverty (Gadalla, 2008). Further, findings from a feminist grounded theory study of 40 single mothers who recently left abusive partners in Ontario and New Brunswick reveal that the majority of participants continued to experience ongoing harassment, even though these single mothers had left their abusive partners (Ford-Gilboe, Wuest, & Merritt-Gray, 2005).

The central challenges faced by these women included decreased resources, persistent persecution, and ongoing chronic health problems that were, in fact, a consequence of leaving the abusive relationship (Ford-Gilboe et al., 2005).

Women are viewed as property in many parts of the world. As described in the seminal work of Kilbourne (1987, 1999), the entertainment and advertising industries perpetuate the image of women as property by depicting them as objects and often portraying the dismembering of women's bodies. Moreover, the explicit portrayal in the media of women in various states of undress and in seductive postures suggests that they are vulnerable and openly welcome sexual advances. Frequently, the message is, "Buy the product and get the woman" (Kilbourne, 1987).

The focus on women's body parts in advertising dehumanizes women, and that dehumanization is often the first step in making women acceptable targets of violence. For example, a 3-month study of newspaper coverage of disabled men and women in Canada and Israel indicated that women received less media coverage than did men, yet the media coverage of women demonstrated a higher level of victimization and violence, overall (Gold & Auslander, 1999). Recently, Hassouneh and Curry (2011) cite a number of studies demonstrating that women with disabilities experience more IPV than do those without disabilities.

Theories of Why Women Stay in Violent Relationships

A more appropriate question than "Why do women stay in violent relationships?" is "How does she ever manage to leave given all the strikes against her?" (Anderson & Saunders, 2003). There are many reasons why women stay in violent relationships. One of the strongest reasons is economic (Canadian Women's Foundation, 2013, November). Despite years of progress, women still earn less than do men for equal work. Many women lack the education or skills that would allow them to earn an adequate living outside the home. For these women, leaving their abusive partners means that they and their children would be homeless and without any source of support for even basic necessities. Furthermore, many shelters for battered women have long waiting lists and provide only temporary housing.

The socialization of women to assume major responsibility for marriages and child rearing is often another barrier to leaving abusive relationships. Society teaches women that their proper place is at home and their primary responsibility is caring for their husbands and children (Chodorow, 1974; Gilligan, 1982), although this trend is beginning to shift as reflected in household division of labour (Marshall, 2006). Many women believe that making their marriage a success is their responsibility. Therefore, when they are abused, they assume that it is their fault and that their duty is to remain and try harder for their children's sake (Boyd & Mackey, 2000a; Lloyd & Emery, 2000). Moreover, many women who were abused in childhood or witnessed abuse of their mothers think that abuse is part of a normal relationship (Boyd & Mackey, 2000a).

Research suggests that factors influencing women's decision to stay or leave a relationship are complex and varied. Alhalal, Ford-Gilboe, Kerr, and Davies (2012) examined indicators of intrusion (i.e., unwanted interference in everyday life) that predicted whether women remained separated from an abusive partner. Levels of depression and symptoms of PTSD were associated with an increased risk of returning to an abusive partner and being less likely to remain separated. Furthermore, in a study of help-seeking behaviour focused on the power dynamic between partners of women experiencing IPV, Kaukinen, Meyer, and Akers (2013) observed that women were more likely to seek support to deal with IPV if status incompatibilities between partners favour women.

Women also face political and legal obstacles in leaving abusive partners. If a man is arrested for assault and no action is taken to prevent future violence, he may be released shortly and retaliate against his partner. Fear for their lives and the lives of their children and other relatives often keeps women from attempting to leave abusive relationships (Anderson & Saunders, 2003; Boyd & Mackey, 2000a). Even more difficult to understand is why some women stay in violent dating relationships. Straus (2004) found the prevalence of violence in dating relationships among university students in 16 countries to range from 17% to 45%. This is similar to Brownridge's (2006) report on a number of Canadian studies that estimated dating violence to range from 25% to 45%. Understanding the phenomenon of dating violence is critical to preventing long-term violence in relationships. One factor is that dating violence often does not occur until the relationship has been sustained for a long time. Research has shown that the length of the relationship, as well as the level of commitment, is positively correlated with physical and sexual abuse. Women with strong emotional commitments and who have invested in the relationship in terms of time, money, or children may be more reluctant to leave (Hendy, Eggen, Gustitus, McLeod, & Ng, 2003).

Survivors may go through a process consisting of several phases in leaving an abusive relationship (Anderson & Saunders, 2003). Women may leave and return several times as they are learning new coping skills. The phases may involve cognitive and emotional "leaving" before actually leaving the relationship. The phases may include (1) enduring and managing the violence while disconnecting from self and others; (2) acknowledging the abuse, reframing it, and counteracting it; and (3) disengaging and focusing on her own needs (Anderson & Saunders, 2003). The phase immediately following separation from

an abusive partner is extremely important as the woman attempts to establish a new life. Based on the findings from a qualitative study of 15 women residing in eastern Canada, a four-stage process of "reclaiming the self" emerged as the main psychological process central to leaving an abusive partner (Wuest & Merritt-Gray, 2001), which is consistent with the stages described by Anderson and Saunders (2003).

Cycle of Violence

Many cases of woman abuse reflect a recognized **cycle of violence** (Walker, 1979, 1984). Walker's work is regarded as seminal and describes the cyclical nature of abusive relationships, as well as the behaviour of abused women within the context of the cycle. This cycle consists of three recurring phases that often increase in frequency and severity (Walker, 1979, 1984) and is fully described in Figure 37-2.

Traumatic Bonding

The formation of strong emotional bonds under conditions of intermittent maltreatment has been reported in several studies with human and animal subjects. For example, people taken hostage may show positive regard for their captors. Abused children often show strong attachment to their abusing parents. Cult members show strong loyalty to malevolent cult leaders (Dutton, 1995, 2008). Therefore, the relationship between battered women and their partners may be just one example of traumatic bonding—the development of strong emotional ties between two people, one of whom intermittently abuses the other. Dutton and Painter put forth the theory of traumatic bonding to describe the bonds women develop for their abusers. **Traumatic bonding** suggests that a power imbalance and intermittent abuse help to form extremely strong emotional attachments. Traumatic bonding theory (Dutton, 2008; Dutton & Painter, 1993) explains why the cycle of violence is so powerful in entrapping a woman in a violent relationship. Researchers from British Columbia generated hypotheses based on Dutton's theory of traumatic bonding and attachment theory to assess the relevance of attachment theory to 63 women who had recently left abusive relationships (Henderson, Bartholomew, & Dutton, 1997). As predicted, women who demonstrated attachment patterns consistent with a negative view of the self composed the majority of the sample (88%).

The woman in a power imbalance perceives herself to be in a powerless position in relation to her partner, whom she perceives as extremely powerful. As the power imbalance intensifies, she feels increasingly worthless, less capable of fending for herself, and, therefore, more in need of her partner. This cycle of dependency and lowered self-esteem is continually repeated, eventually creating a strong affective bond to the partner (Dutton, 1995, 2008).

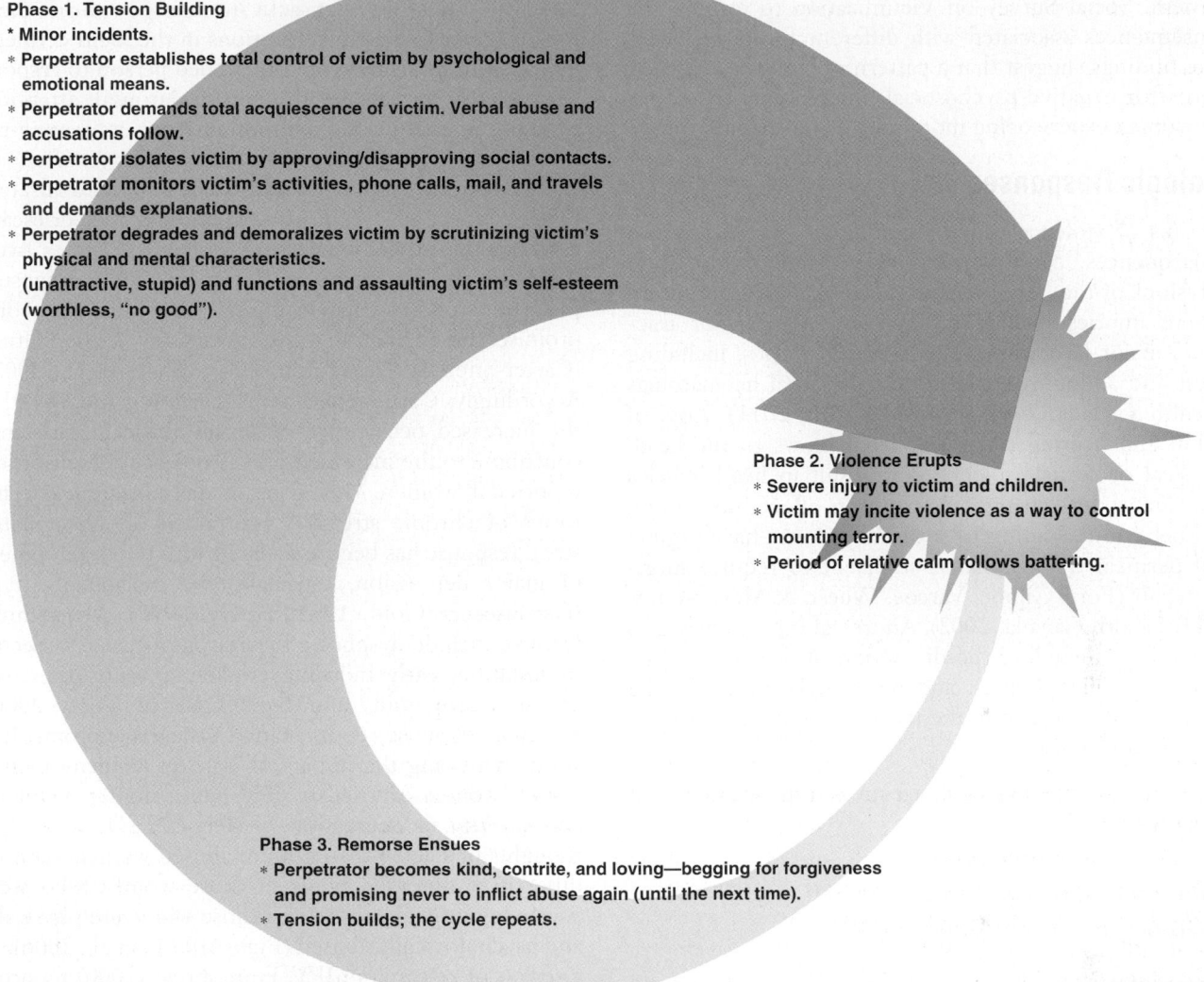

Phase 1. Tension Building
* Minor incidents.
* Perpetrator establishes total control of victim by psychological and emotional means.
* Perpetrator demands total acquiescence of victim. Verbal abuse and accusations follow.
* Perpetrator isolates victim by approving/disapproving social contacts.
* Perpetrator monitors victim's activities, phone calls, mail, and travels and demands explanations.
* Perpetrator degrades and demoralizes victim by scrutinizing victim's physical and mental characteristics.
(unattractive, stupid) and functions and assaulting victim's self-esteem (worthless, "no good").

Phase 2. Violence Erupts
* Severe injury to victim and children.
* Victim may incite violence as a way to control mounting terror.
* Period of relative calm follows battering.

Phase 3. Remorse Ensues
* Perpetrator becomes kind, contrite, and loving—begging for forgiveness and promising never to inflict abuse again (until the next time).
* Tension builds; the cycle repeats.

FIGURE 37-2. The cycle of violence. Adapted from Walker, 1979, 1984.

Intermittent reinforcement or punishment is one of the strongest learning paradigms in behavioural theory, especially in maintaining a particular behaviour (Dutton, 1995, 2008). An example that is often used to illustrate this concept is the gambler who persistently puts coins in a slot machine. Despite substantial losses, the gambler persists because the next time just might be the big payoff. Therefore, the gambler is not rewarded every time, but intermittently. To apply this to battered women, women may stay because this time the man may actually mean what he says and stop the abuse. After all, he has been kind and loving intermittently.

Research suggests that traumatic bonding is especially important when a woman attempts to leave her abusive partner (Dutton, 1995, 2008). When a woman leaves an abusive relationship, especially after a battering incident, she is emotionally drained and vulnerable. As time passes, her fear of her abuser diminishes, and needs

supplied by the partner become evident. At this time, she is particularly susceptible to the abuser's attempts to persuade her to return to the relationship (Dutton & Painter, 1993).

SURVIVORS OF ABUSE: HUMAN RESPONSES TO TRAUMA

The experience of violence and abuse is overwhelming for most survivors and often has devastating long-term consequences (Wilson, 2001; Wilson, Friedman, & Lindy, 2001). Victimization, such as IPV and childhood abuse, does not produce a single uniform syndrome or response. Research on the effects of abuse reflects the devastating long-term effects of trauma, which results in a range of responses that are characteristic for trauma survivors (Ansara & Hindin, 2011; Daigneault, Hébert, & McDuff, 2009; Hovsepian et al., 2010). Ansara and

Hindin (2011) analyzed data from the 2004 Canadian General Social Survey on Victimization to explore the consequences associated with different forms of abuse. The findings suggest that a pattern of violence is associated with negative psychosocial outcomes—particularly for women experiencing more severe and chronic abuse.

Biologic Responses

Victims of violence experience mild to severe physical consequences. Mild injuries may include bruises and abrasions of the head, neck, face, trunk, and extremities. Severe injuries include multiple traumas, major fractures, major lacerations, and internal injuries, including chest and abdominal injuries and subdural haematomas (Health Canada, 2002; Woods & Gill, 2011). Loss of vision and hearing can result from blows to the head. Physical or sexual violence may result in head injuries that can produce changes in cognition, affect, motivation, and behaviour. Victims of sexual abuse may have vaginal and perineal trauma that is sufficient to require surgical repair (Ford-Gilboe, Varcoe, Wuest, & Merrit-Gray, 2011; Health Canada, 2002). Anorectal injuries may also be present, including the disruption of anal sphincters, retained foreign bodies, and mucosal lacerations. The following section covers the most common responses to violence and abuse:

- Depression (the dysregulated stress response theory of depression)
- Acute stress disorder (ASD)
- Posttraumatic stress disorder (PTSD)
- Dissociative identity disorder (DID)

Depression

Depression, one of the most common responses to abuse, is a biologically based disorder that can result from the effects of chronic stress on neurotransmitter and neuroendocrine systems. The body's response to stress is a complex, integrated system of reactions, encompassing the body and mind. Threat or stress engages the stress system, which consists of the hypothalamic–pituitary–adrenal (HPA) axis and the sympathetic nervous system (Miller, Chen, & Zhou, 2007; Thase, Jindal, & Howland, 2002; Wong & Yehuda, 2002). Engagement of the HPA axis is associated with the release of corticotropin-releasing hormone (CRH) from the pituitary gland. CRH stimulates the pituitary gland to secrete adrenocorticotropic hormone (corticotropin), which stimulates the adrenal cortex to secrete cortisol. Stress also engages the sympathetic nervous system, causing the locus ceruleus and the adrenal medulla to release norepinephrine.

The CRH and locus ceruleus and norepinephrine systems participate in a mutually reinforcing feedback loop (Thase et al., 2002; Wong & Yehuda, 2002). That is, increases in CRH stimulate increased firing of the locus ceruleus and increased release of norepinephrine. Similarly, stressors that activate norepinephrine neurons increase CRH concentrations in the locus ceruleus. These systems prepare the threatened person to respond to danger by enhancing the person's arousal, attention, perception, energy, and emotion and by suppressing the immune response (Wong & Yehuda, 2002).

The stress response is meant to be of limited duration (Thase et al., 2002). However, when resistance or escape is impossible, the human stress system becomes overwhelmed and disorganized (Herman, 1997). Exposure to severe stressors early in life has been shown to compromise the regulation of HPA activity for a lifetime (Carter-Snell & Hegadoren, 2003; Thase et al., 2002). Accordingly, Carter-Snell and Hegadoren theorize that the increased occurrence of sexual abuse in girls may contribute to the increased prevalence of stress disorders reported in women. Most types of abuse result in extreme forms of chronic stress. A protracted or dysregulated stress response has been associated with the development of major depression, especially the melancholic type (Chrousos & Gold, 1992; Henry, 1992). Melancholic features include dysphoric hyperarousal that is reflected in agitation, early morning awakening, anorexia, anxiety, excessive guilt, and hypervigilance (APA, 2000). Survivors of abuse report many of these symptoms. In a study examining the impact of IPV on women's mental health, women exposed to IPV had a higher incidence and severity of depression, anxiety, PTSD, as well as thoughts of suicide than did nonabused women, with no differences observed between those women who were psychologically abused versus those who were physically and psychologically abused (Pico-Alfonso et al., 2006). In a review of research in IPV, Humphreys (2000) reported on the multiple health effects of violence against women, including depression and PTSD.

Acute Stress Disorder and Posttraumatic Stress Disorder

The experience of trauma exerts tremendous physical and psychological stress on survivors. The cluster of signs and symptoms that frequently occur after major trauma is now labelled **acute stress disorder** (ASD) and **posttraumatic stress disorder** (PTSD); for a comprehensive discussion of PTSD and ASD, see Chapter 17. Lasiuk and Hegadoren (2006a) in their historical overview of the PTSD concept describe the often-misunderstood link between the condition "hysteria" (as described in early-19th-century Europe), war trauma, and PTSD. Subsequent research has demonstrated that symptoms of ASD and PTSD occur not only after war but also after many types of severe trauma, including physical abuse, sexual abuse, and rape.

A comprehensive review of research on the epidemiology of PTSD suggests several gender differences

(Norris, Foster, & Weisshaar, 2002). Men have more exposure to traumatic events than do women. However, women are about twice as likely as men to experience PTSD, and the median time from onset to remission for women is 4 years, compared with 1 year for men (Lasiuk & Hegadoren, 2006b). Several factors may contribute to these differences. One factor is that men and women experience different types of traumatic events. More men report exposure to events such as fire or disaster, life-threatening accidents, physical assault, combat, being threatened with a weapon, and being held captive. More women report child abuse, sexual molestation, and sexual assault. Sexual violence is associated with a high risk for the development of PTSD. Other factors that may contribute to a higher prevalence of PTSD in women include higher rates of anxiety and depressive disorders and traumatic events before the age of 15 years (Carter-Snell & Hegadoren, 2003; Orsillo, Raja, & Hammond, 2002). One study of 1,698 urban young adults, focused on the impact of exposure to traumatic events, found that women's risk for PTSD varied according to the type of trauma (i.e., assaultive), as well as prior experience of trauma; whereas men's risk of PTSD was not related to the type of trauma or the experience of prior trauma (Breslau & Anthony, 2007).

PTSD may develop any time after the trauma. The delay may be as short as 1 week or as long as 30 years (Kaplan & Sadock, 2003). Symptoms may fluctuate in intensity with time and usually are worse during periods of stress. Some 30% of patients with PTSD recover completely, 40% continue to have mild symptoms, 20% continue to have moderate symptoms, and 10% remain unchanged or become worse (Kaplan & Sadock, 2003).

Young children and elderly people have special difficulty with traumatic events. Young children may not have developed adequate coping mechanisms to deal with severe stressors, and older people are likely to have rigid coping mechanisms, making successful coping with the trauma more difficult (Kaplan & Sadock, 2003).

Women with PTSD frequently have comorbid anxiety, depressive disorders, or both, and the association among childhood abuse, PTSD, and substance abuse is also becoming well established (Boyd, 2000, 2003; Boyd & Mackey, 2000b; Brady & Dansky, 2002; Stewart, Ouimette, & Brown, 2002).

Hyperarousal

After a traumatic experience, the stress system seems to go on permanent alert, as if the danger might return at any time (Rasmusson & Friedman, 2002; Wong & Yehuda, 2002). In this state of physiologic hyperarousal, the traumatized person is hypervigilant for signs of danger, startles easily, reacts irritably to small annoyances, and sleeps poorly. These symptoms are characteristic of increased noradrenergic function (O'Donnell, Hegadoren, & Coupland, 2004),

particularly in the locus ceruleus and limbic system (hypothalamus, hippocampus, and amygdala), and of increased dopamine activity, particularly in the prefrontal cortical dopamine system (Rasmusson & Friedman; Wong & Yehuda, 2002). Dopamine hyperactivity is associated with the hypervigilance seen in PTSD. Many people with PTSD do not return to their normal baseline level of alertness. Instead, they seem to have a new baseline of elevated arousal, as if their "thermostat" had been reset (Bremner, Southwick, & Charney, 1999). Based on advances in neuroscience, however, a sensorimotor approach to therapy is evolving that shows promise for helping persons with PTSD to restore normal arousal levels (Ogden, Minton, & Pain, 2006).

Behavioural sensitization may be one mechanism underlying the hyperarousal seen in PTSD. This phenomenon, sometimes referred to as *kindling*, occurs after an exposure to severe, uncontrollable stressors. The sensitized person reacts with a magnified stress response to later, milder stressors (Bremner et al., 1999; Monroe & Harkness, 2005).

Research shows that a single or repeated exposure to a severe stressor potentiates the capacity of a subsequent stressor to increase synaptic levels of norepinephrine and dopamine in the forebrain (Charney, Deutch, Krystal, & Southwick, 1993). This finding would account for the fact that some survivors with PTSD experience intense fear, anxiety, and panic in response to minor stimuli. One example of behavioural sensitization is that PTSD after combat exposure is more likely to develop in veterans who are survivors of childhood abuse than in those who have not experienced prior trauma (Southwick, Bremner, Krystal, & Charney, 1994).

The state of hyperarousal causes other problems for survivors. The loss of neuromodulation leads to a loss of affect regulation, so that the survivor is irritable and overreacts to others (van der Kolk & Fisler, 1993). This type of behaviour may cause others to avoid the survivor. The continual arousal may desensitize the survivor to real threat and decrease the probability that he or she will respond to perceived danger (Messman-Moore & Long, 2003). This development may cause the person to miss clues of danger and place himself or herself in situations that can lead to revictimization.

Intrusion

Long after abuse has stopped, survivors relive it as though it were continually recurring. Flashbacks and nightmares, which the survivor experiences with terrifying immediacy, are vivid and often include fragments of traumatic events exactly as they happened (Bremner et al., 1999; Courtis & Ford, 2009). Moreover, a wide variety of stimuli that may have been associated with the trauma can elicit flashbacks and dreams. Consequently, survivors avoid such stimuli (Bremner et al., 1999).

Three related but somewhat different explanations may account for the vivid, disturbing flashbacks and dreams that individuals with PTSD have: disturbances of memory, classic conditioning (fear conditioning), and extinction.

Memory function is altered in PTSD. Memory deficits include short-term memory and potentiation of recall of traumatic experiences and dissociative flashbacks. Human beings are bombarded constantly by sensory stimuli yet attend to and remember only a fraction of it (Bremner et al., 1999; Johnsen & Asbjørnsen, 2008; Southwick et al., 1994). People seem to remember best those events that have emotional effects and occur when they are alert, aroused, and responsive to their internal and external environments. Because noradrenergic activity is elevated in individuals with PTSD when exposed to emotional and traumatic stimuli, memory encoding may be improved, leading to intrusive thoughts and memories (O'Donnell et al., 2004).

During stress, there is a massive release of neurotransmitters, particularly norepinephrine, epinephrine, and opioid peptides. This flood of "stress hormones" may lead to structural changes in the brain that potentiate long-term memory. In most situations, this type of memory has survival value: remembering events that occur during danger may protect oneself during similar future situations. However, in PTSD, the memories occur when the individual is not in danger. Research supporting this hypothesis demonstrated that if norepinephrine is administered to animals immediately after training, long-term memory is enhanced. Epinephrine and endogenous opioids may influence memory consolidation (transforming short-term memory to long-term memory) by affecting norepinephrine (Bremner 1999; Southwick et al., 1994; van Stegeren, 2008).

The hippocampus and amygdala are involved in memory consolidation. The hippocampus is involved in object memory and placement of memory traces in space and time (Bremner et al., 1999; Cohen, Perel, DeBellis, Friedman, & Putnam, 2002; van Stegeren, 2008). High levels of stress have been shown to damage the hippocampus and decrease its volume, producing memory deficits such as amnesia and deficits in autobiographical memory (memory of one's life story; Bremner et al., 1999). The amygdala integrates sensory information for storage in and retrieval from memory. The amygdala also attaches emotional significance to sensory information and transmits this information to all the other systems involved in the stress response. Overreactivity of the amygdala might explain the recurrent and intrusive traumatic memories and the excessive fear associated with traumatic reminders characteristic of PTSD (Cohen et al., 2002). Moreover, electrical stimulation of the amygdala and hippocampal area has been associated with dream-like and memory-like hallucinations that are similar to flashbacks reported by patients with PTSD (Bremner, Narayan, et al., 1999).

Classic conditioning, or fear conditioning, occurs when a neutral stimulus (the conditioned stimulus [CS]) is paired with an aversive unconditioned stimulus that elicits an unconditioned fear response. After repeated pairing, the CS alone will elicit the fear response, which is now the conditioned response (CR). For example, certain sights, sounds, or smells that occurred in close proximity to the traumatic event may elicit a fear response in the future. The result of this process is that an individual becomes fearful and anxious in response to a wide variety of stimuli (Bremner et al., 1999; Shin et al, 2006; Southwick et al., 1994); therefore, a wide variety of stimuli can elicit symptoms of PTSD.

The amygdala and hippocampus also appear to be important players in fear conditioning (Bremner et al., 1999; O'Donnell et al., 2004; Shin et al., 2006; Southwick et al., 1994). Other important brain sites in PTSD in addition to the hippocampus and amygdala include the thalamus, locus ceruleus, and medial prefrontal cortex. Interaction between the cortex and the amygdala may be necessary for specific stimuli to elicit traumatic memories. Cortisol and norepinephrine are two neurochemical systems associated with the stress response (Bremner, 2006; Bremner et al., 1999; Charney et al., 1993).

Several neurochemical systems are involved in regulating fear conditioning, including norepinephrine, dopamine (DA), opiate, and corticotropin-releasing systems. In addition, N-methyl-D-aspartate (NMDA), one of the major excitatory neurotransmitters in the brain, appears necessary for this type of learning to occur. NMDA antagonists applied to the amygdala prevent the development of fear CRs (Bremner et al., 1999; Charney et al., 1993).

Extinction is the loss of a learned conditioned emotional response after repeated presentations of the conditioned fear stimulus without a contiguous traumatic event. In other words, the individual no longer responds with fear to the CR. For example, many children are afraid of the dark; however, after many uneventful nights, children gradually lose their fear. Failure of the neuronal mechanisms involved in extinction also may explain the continued ability of conditioned stimuli to elicit traumatic memories and flashbacks in PTSD (Bremner, 2006; Charney et al., 1993; Etkin & Wager 2007; Bremner et al., 1999). Recent research on brain dysfunction associated with PTSD resulting from childhood abuse of women has shown that damage to the medial prefrontal cortex interferes with extinguishing fear responses. In addition, individuals with damage to the medial prefrontal cortex show emotional dysfunction and an inability to relate in social situations that require correct interpretation of the emotional expressions of others. These findings suggest that dysfunction of this area of the brain may play a role in pathologic emotions that follow exposure to extreme stressors, such as childhood sexual abuse (Bremner,

Narayan, et al., 1999; Lanius, Frewen, Vermetten, & Yehuda, 2010).

Avoidance and Numbing (Dissociative Symptoms)

Survivors try to avoid people or situations that might provoke memories of the trauma. This restriction in their activities may interfere with normal functioning. Survivors also report anhedonia (loss of ability to sense pleasure) and may report that they feel as if parts of themselves have died. These disturbing symptoms may lead them to engage in acts of self-mutilation to feel alive or ultimately to suicide (Lanius et al., 2010; van der Kolk & Fisler, 1993).

A person who is completely powerless may go into a state of surrender. In that state, the person escapes the situation by altering his or her state of consciousness, that is, by dissociating (Herman, 1997). **Dissociation** is defined as a disruption in the normally occurring linkages between subjective awareness, feelings, thoughts, behaviours, and memories (APA, 2000; Briere & Elliott, 1994). It refers to changes in awareness in light of traumatic experience (Bryant, 2007).

Dissociation is a complex psychophysiologic process that produces alterations in sense of self, accessibility of memory and knowledge, and integration of behaviour (Briere, Weathers, & Runtz, 2005; Putnam, 1994; Rothschild, 1998). In simpler words, a person who dissociates is making himself or herself "disappear." That is, the person has the feeling of leaving his or her body and observing what happens to him or her from a distance. During trauma, dissociation enables a person to observe the event while experiencing no pain, or only limited pain, and to protect himself or herself from awareness of the full impact of the traumatic event. Following a review of relevant literature pertaining to the conceptualization and measurement of dissociation, Holmes and colleagues (2005) identify that dissociation consists of two domains: detachment (being an outside observer) and compartmentalization (phenomena such as amnesia), which offers promise regarding an improved understanding of dissociation and treatment choice. A study of Montreal school-aged girls indicates that sexual abuse was associated with eight times the level of dissociation and four times the level of PTSD in the girls who had been sexually abused compared with matched controls without sexual abuse (Collin-Vezina and Hebert, 2005). Examples of dissociation include (1) derealization and depersonalization (the experience of self or the environment as strange or unreal); (2) periods of disengagement from the immediate environment during stress, such as "spacing out"; (3) alterations in bodily perceptions; (4) emotional numbing; (5) out-of-body experiences; and (6) amnesia for abuse-related memories (Briere & Elliott, 1994; Holmes et al., 2005; Rothschild, 1998). Fear activates the endogenous opioid system, producing stress-induced analgesia (SIA) (Gueze et al., 2007; van der Kolk, 2005). SIA may be associated with avoidance and numbing. The purpose of SIA is to protect against pain in dangerous situations so that the individual (animal or human) can defend itself (fight) or escape the situation (flight). In severely stressed animals, opiate withdrawal symptoms can be produced by removing the stressor or by injecting naloxone, an opiate antagonist. In people with PTSD, SIA can become conditioned to stimuli resembling the original trauma. Excessive opioid and norepinephrine secretion can interfere with memory. Freezing or numbing responses may prevent animals from remembering situations of overwhelming stress. Trauma-related dissociative reactions after prolonged exposure to severe, uncontrollable stress may be analogous to this effect in animals (Hopper et al., 2007; van der Kolk, 2005).

Dissociative Identity Disorder

Dissociation exists on a continuum, with most people experiencing short, situation-specific episodes, such as daydreaming (Holmes et al., 2005; Putnam, 1994). Among survivors of abuse, dissociative symptoms may be part of the symptom picture of ASD and PTSD, or they may be the predominant symptom (Lasiuk & Hegadoren, 2006b). In such cases, the disorder is **dissociative identity disorder** (DID) (formerly multiple personality disorder) (Ross, 2009; Ross & Ness, 2010). The hallmarks of DID are two or more distinct identities with unique personality characteristics and an inability to recall important information about self or events that is too extensive to be explained by ordinary forgetfulness (APA, 2000). Other memory disturbances linked with dissociation include intermittent and disruptive intrusions of traumatic memories into awareness and difficulties in determining whether a given memory reflects an actual event or information acquired through another source (Putnam). The diagnostic criteria for DID are found in Table 37-1.

Two other dimensions of dissociation that are associated with DID include passive influence experiences and hallucinatory experiences. A passive influence experience is a situation in which a person feels as if he or she were controlled by a force from within. These experiences may include a sense that one is being made to do something against one's will that may be distasteful or harmful to self and others (Putnam, 1994; Vermetten, Schmahl, Lindner, Loewenstein, & Bremner, 2006).

Many survivors of abuse report dissociative perceptual disturbances, such as visual hallucinations, extrasensory perceptions, and peculiar time distortions (Anderson, Yasenik, & Ross, 1993; Hendricks-Matthews, 1993; Holmes et al., 2005; Vermetten et al., 2006). The hallucinatory experiences in dissociative disorders are distinct in several ways from those that occur in psychotic disorders. They are often experienced as internalized, rather than externalized, voices and may be associated with specific

| Table 37-1 | Key Diagnostic Characteristics for DID |

Diagnostic Criteria	Target Symptoms and Associated Findings
• Presence of two or more distinct personality states or identities • At least two identities or personality states recurrently take control of the person's behaviour • Inability to recall important information that is too extensive to be explained by ordinary forgetfulness • Not due to direct physiologic effects of substances or a general medical condition • In children, symptoms not attributable to imaginary playmates or other fantasy play	• Posttraumatic symptoms (nightmares, flashbacks, startle responses) • PTSD • Self-mutilation • Suicidal behaviour • Aggressive behaviour • Repetitive relationships characterized by physical and sexual abuse *Associated Physical Examination Findings* • Scars from self-inflicted injuries or physical abuse • Migraine and other types of headaches, irritable bowel syndrome, and asthma *Associated Laboratory Findings* • Physiologic functioning may vary across personality states • High scores on measures of hypnotizability and dissociative capacity

American Psychiatric Association. (2013). *Diagnostic and statistical manual of mental disorders* (5th ed.). Washington, DC: Author.

experiences or people. The affected person hears the voices distinctly; the voices often have particular attributes such as gender, age, and affect. The voices may be supportive and comforting or berating (Putnam, 1994). Hallucinatory experiences may also involve the appearance of "shadowy figures," ghosts or spirits, or rapidly moving objects. The person is generally aware that the voices or images are not real (Putnam, 1994).

The overall prevalence of DID is unknown. Estimates are that 1% of the American population may be affected and as many as 5% to 20% of people in psychiatric hospitals (National Women's Health Information Center, 2003). The cause of DID is unknown. However, the patient history invariably includes pathologic levels of stress such as a traumatic event in childhood (Kihlstrom, 2005). Causative factors that have been identified include a traumatic event, a psychological or genetic vulnerability to develop the disorder, formative environmental factors, and the absence of external support (Kaplan & Sadock, 2003). Examples of psychological vulnerability include being suggestible or easily hypnotized. Formative

environmental events may include a lack of role models who demonstrate healthy problem solving or practices to relieve anxiety or stress. Many who experience DID lack supportive others, such as parents, siblings, other relatives, and supportive people outside the family (e.g., teachers) (Kaplan & Sadock, 2003).

Complex Trauma

In her landmark book and seminal work, *Trauma and Recovery*, Herman (1997, p. 119) proposed a new diagnosis: **"complex posttraumatic stress disorder"** (C-PTSD). Her proposal was based on experience that none of the diagnostic categories in the APA's *Diagnostic and Statistical Manual* (3rd ed., Revision; APA, 1987) were appropriate for survivors of extreme, prolonged trauma, especially interpersonal trauma (i.e., severe, prolonged child abuse), including the diagnosis of PTSD. She noted that survivors of prolonged, repeated trauma experience characteristic personality changes, including problems of relatedness, identity, and vulnerability to repeated harm, inflicted by others or self. The symptoms of C-PTSD include impaired affect modulation (difficulty modulating anger or sexual behaviours; self-destructive and suicidal behaviours); impulsive/risk-taking behaviour; alterations in attention and consciousness (amnesia, dissociation); somatization; chronic characterologic changes, including alterations in relations with others (an inability to trust or maintain relationships, a tendency to be revictimized or to victimize others); and alterations in systems of meaning (e.g., despair, hopelessness, loss of previously sustaining beliefs) (Courtis & Ford, 2009; van der Kolk, 2005). Despite receiving considerable attention in the literature, C-PTSD is not included in the *DSM-5*, although there is now a dissociative subtype of PTSD, which enables some issues pertaining to C-PTSD to be addressed (American Psychiatric Association, 2013).

These symptoms are similar to those of borderline personality disorder (BPD). Many people with BPD were severely abused in childhood (Courtis & Ford, 2009). Splitting self and others into "all good" or "all bad" may result from a developmental arrest: a fragmentation of self, based on modes of organizing experience that were common in earlier developmental stages. Self-mutilation, often labelled as masochism or manipulative behaviour, may be a way of regulating psychological and biologic equilibrium when ordinary means of self-regulation have been disturbed by trauma. Psychotic episodes in patients with BPD are similar to flashbacks, intrusive recollections of traumatic memories that were stored on a somatosensory level (van der Kolk, 2005). Research findings demonstrate that the diagnoses of both BPD and C-PTSD were significantly higher in a group of women with early-onset sexual abuse compared with late-onset sexual abuse, suggesting that women with a history of childhood sexual abuse might be better understood within the rubric of C-PTSD (McLean & Gallop, 2003).

Substance Abuse and Dependence

Childhood abuse, PTSD, and substance abuse are known to be associated. Investigators have reported that as many as 84% of female inpatient substance abusers had a history of sexual or physical assault (Brady & Dansky, 2002; Stewart et al., 2002). High rates of abuse have also been found in samples of outpatient rural women (Boyd, 2000, 2003). The Vancouver Injection Drug User Study of sexual violence among intravenous drug users indicates that 68% of women and 19% of men had a lifetime history of sexual violence (Braitstein et al., 2003).

Survivors who experience PTSD, depression, and other forms of dysphoric hyperarousal or emotional distress often abuse substances, including alcohol and other sedative drugs, that lessen stress and reduce hyperarousal and distress by inhibiting noradrenergic activity (Brady & Dansky, 2002; Stewart et al., 2002). Increasing numbers of women reportedly abuse cocaine to wipe out dysphoric feelings caused by abuse. These women report that the intense high of cocaine totally obliterates painful feelings, if only for a short time (Boyd, 2000). A number of trauma-related responses can be seen in individuals with PTSD. These responses may include chronic interpersonal difficulties, somatization, and substance abuse. Since the outcomes of complex trauma can vary widely, a comprehensive assessment is essential (Courtis & Ford, 2009).

Psychological Responses

Low Self-Esteem

The consequences of abuse are devastating, and the term "low self-esteem" seems inadequate. Women who are abused as children often experience "alienation from self and others" (Boyd & Mackey, 2000a). Alienation from self includes painful feelings that go to the "core of a woman's being"—experiencing self as fundamentally flawed and having no purpose in life. Alienation from others, especially significant others, is associated with painful feelings of loneliness, depression, anger, shame, and guilt and with feeling hurt, unloved, and unwanted (Boyd & Mackey, 2000a). Women who experience alienation from self and others often turn to substance abuse to cope with their intense pain (Boyd & Mackey, 2000b).

Low self-esteem or alienation may be attributable to the direct effects of physical or sexual abuse or to the accompanying psychological abuse. One technique that perpetrators use to control and disempower women is to erode their sense of self-worth with a constant barrage of criticism. Perpetrators frequently tell women that they are stupid, ugly, inadequate wives and mothers, inadequate sexually, and incompetent. Other contributing factors include a sense of being different from other people, the need to maintain secrecy, lack of trust, and self-blame (Boyd & Mackey, 2000a).

Low self-esteem may be one factor contributing to a battered woman's reluctance to disclose her abuse. Because of low self-esteem, battered women, even many who are successful outside the home, underestimate their ability to do anything about the abuse (Boyd & Mackey, 2000a). As such, it is not surprising that "reclaiming the self" was identified as the main psychological process central to leaving an abusive partner in a qualitative study of women who had recently left abusive male partners (Wuest & Merritt-Gray, 2001).

Guilt and Shame

A history of abuse is often associated with excessive guilt and shame. These feelings stem from survivors' mistaken beliefs that they are somehow to blame for their abuse (Boyd & Mackey, 2000a; Campbell et al., 2004; Long & Smyth, 1998). Feelings of humiliation and shame may prevent women from seeking medical care and reporting abuse to authorities. The experience of being battered is so degrading and humiliating that women are often afraid to disclose it. Many women fear that they will not be taken seriously or will be blamed for inciting the abuse or for staying with their abusers (Boyd & Mackey, 2000a; Campbell et al., 2004; Long & Smyth, 1998). In keeping with this observation, research findings indicate that resilient women with a history of childhood sexual abuse and no history of substance abuse felt less blame and stigma associated with being sexually abused compared with women with a history of childhood sexual abuse who were currently receiving treatment for substance abuse (Dufour & Nadeau, 2001). A systematic review synthesizing research evidence concerning adults' disclosure of domestic violence when accessing health care services found that guilt, shame, and powerlessness were recurring themes, particularly for older women when accessing care (Robinson & Spilsbury, 2008).

Anger

Chronic irritability, unexpected or uncontrollable feelings of anger, and difficulties with the expression of anger are frequent experiences for survivors of abuse (Campbell et al., 2004). They may express anger towards the perpetrator, fate, those who have been spared the suffering, or someone whom the victim believes could have prevented the abuse (Barnett, Miller-Perrin, & Perrin, 1997). However, some incest survivors have difficulty expressing anger and may demonstrate helplessness or numbness or mask it with compliance and perfectionism (Campbell et al., 2004). Anger may surface at a later time and play a role in recovery that enables women to protect themselves from further abuse and "advocate for their children" (Thomas, Bannister, & Hall, 2012).

Social and Interpersonal Responses

Problems With Intimacy

The abused child experiences intrusion, abandonment, devaluation, or pain in the relationship with the abuser, instead of the closeness and nurturing that are normal for intimate relationships, such as those between the parent and the child (Briere & Elliott, 1994; Long & Smyth, 1998; Urbancic, 2004). As a result, many survivors have difficulty trusting and forming intimate relationships.

Sexual problems are common among survivors of abuse. Among the most common and chronic problems are fear of intimate sexual relationships, feelings of repulsion towards sex, lack of enjoyment of sex, dysfunctions of desire and arousal, and failure to achieve orgasm. Some survivors engage in compulsive promiscuity and prostitution, reflecting their internalization of the message that the only thing that they are good for is sex (Hendricks-Matthews, 1993; Long & Smyth, 1998; Urbancic, 2004).

Revictimization

Many women who have been sexually abused as children are revictimized on multiple occasions later in life. Among women with a history of sexual assault, rates of revictimization range from 15% to 79% (Arata, 2002; Breitenbecher, 2001; Messman-Moore & Long, 2003). In a study of women receiving treatment from three Canadian urban mental health centres, women who had experienced previous trauma in childhood were more likely to experience PTSD following IPV (Wuest et al., 2009). Numerous factors have been related to revictimization, including PTSD symptoms, dissociation, alexithymia, the use of AOD, boundary issues, and sexual behaviour (Breitenbecher, 2001; Messman-Moore & Long, 2003). Proneness to revictimization may result from a general vulnerability in dangerous situations that may be associated with dissociation. Dissociation makes women unaware of their environment and also may make them look confused or distracted. Shock and dissociation can also occur while the abuse is occurring and afterwards in order for the woman to avoid dealing with her immediate feelings (McCue, 2008).

Alexithymia may also add to a woman's risk for revictimization. Difficulty in labelling and communicating feelings may make it difficult for a woman to set limits on sexual advances. Moreover, these women may not be able to read accurately the emotional cues of others, which diminishes their ability to respond effectively in interpersonally dangerous situations (Cloitre, Scarvalone, & Difede, 1997; Ogden et al., 2006).

Women with abuse histories frequently have difficulty with boundaries. During childhood abuse, they experienced boundary violations as normal and connected with their expectations of intimate relationships. Confusion over boundaries may result in confusion about

appropriate behaviour in adult intimate relationships (Messman-Moore & Long, 2003).

The sexual behaviour pattern of survivors may place them at risk for revictimization. One effect of sexual victimization is that the child's sexuality is shaped by "traumatic sexualization." Traumatic sexualization occurs when a child is rewarded for sexual behaviour with affection, attention, privileges, and gifts. As a result, the child may learn that her self-worth is tied to her sexuality, and she may use sexual behaviour to manipulate others (Breitenbecher, 2001; Messman-Moore & Long, 2003).

■■■ NURSING MANAGEMENT: HUMAN RESPONSE TO ABUSE

Nurses encounter survivors of abuse in many health care settings. The percentage of ED visits that are attributed to domestic violence ranges from 4% to 18% (Campbell et al., 2004); however, reports have been as high as 80% (McGrath et al., 1997). In a Canadian study exploring the extent to which women disclosed IPV in EDs, it was found that only 2% reported abuse to a health professional (Catallo, Jack, Ciliska, & MacMillan, 2013). The principal reason for nondisclosure was fear of "being found out." The women's fears centred around such consequences as involvement of Children's Aid or violence associated with being exposed (Catallo et al., 2013). The findings have implications for nurses who are in a position to support women to disclose IPV by, for example, conducting the assessment in a private setting and reducing the number of professionals who interact with the client. A critical ethnographic study of 30 nurses working in the EDs of two urban hospitals in Canada also provides direction for the care of abused women in the ED (Varcoe, 2001). Specifically, issues that obscure the needs of abused women, such as the perceived need to focus on rapid processing of patients and stereotypical judgements, were identified (Varcoe, 2001). These findings were supported by Thurston and colleagues (2009), who identified barriers to nurses' screening for domestic violence including time constraints, ensuring privacy for clients, and uncertainty regarding how to ask clients about IPV within a busy clinical setting. In addition, the importance of supporting a sense of efficacy for nurses working in EDs has been identified by Canadian researchers (Hollingsworth & Ford-Gilboe, 2006). Other settings in which the nurse encounters battered women include primary care settings, obstetrics–gynaecology settings, paediatric units, well-child clinics, geriatric units, and nursing homes. Further, approximately 50% of female patients admitted to psychiatric facilities are victims of either child or adult abuse (Seeman, 2002).

The paediatric ED provides a unique opportunity to identify and respond to child survivors, as well as battered mothers (Campbell et al., 2004). As many as 59% of mothers of child abuse victims are battered women, and child abuse occurs disproportionately in homes with woman abuse (Wright, Wright, & Isaac, 1997). The negative effects of domestic violence on children have been well documented. Black, Trocmé, Fallon, and Maclaurin (2008) found in a secondary analysis of the data collected in the 2003 Canadian Incidence Study of Reported Child Abuse and Neglect that over one third of the child mistreatment investigations in Canada, excluding Quebec, involved exposure to domestic violence. Identifying battered mothers may be the most important means of identifying child abuse. Conversely, when a nurse suspects child abuse, he or she cannot ignore the possibility that the mother is also a victim. Recognizing children who are traumatized by witnessing the battering of their mothers also is essential. However, despite the opportunity the paediatric ED affords, disturbingly few battered women are identified there. Addressing the issue of family violence is critical given the potential for the cycle to continue across generations. Evidence points to a continuing cycle of violence with children who have witnessed family violence (Cunningham & Baker, 2004). Health care providers in paediatric EDs have reported several obstacles to identification, including lack of training, time constraints, powerlessness, lack of comfort, lack of control over the victim's circumstances, and fear of offending the patient (Beynon, Gutmanis, Tutty, Wathen, & Macmillan, 2012; Catallo et al., 2013; Thurston et al., 2009; Wright et al., 1997). Another important setting for an effective identification of battered women is in the postpartum setting. Researchers implemented a domestic violence assessment in two hospitals in the city of Vancouver and found that the screening rate for domestic violence increased from 42% to 60% for a period of 18 months (Janssen, Holt, & Sugg, 2002).

Nurses may encounter elder abuse in virtually any setting. Examples include EDs, medical–surgical units, psychiatric units, and homes during home care visits. In addition, nurses may encounter elder abuse in nursing homes. Events such as unnecessary chemical (medications) or physical restraints used to control an elder's behaviour may be abusive and should be investigated.

Although some aspects of care are specific to adult, child, or elderly survivors of abuse, many elements are common in the nursing care of all survivors, regardless of age or setting. The goals of all nursing interventions in cases of abuse are to stop the violence and to ensure the survivor's safety. Victimization removes all power and control from a woman, child, or elder. Therefore, as appropriate for age and ability, all nursing interventions should empower survivors to act on their own behalf and must be done in a collaborative partnership. To that end, nurses must be willing to offer support and information and not impose their own values on survivors by encouraging them to leave abusive relationships. Assessments need to be carried out in a thoughtful manner to minimize the number of times a woman must share her experiences with multiple health providers (Catallo et al., 2013). Strong psychological and economic bonds tie many women to their perpetrators. Moreover, adult survivors who are capable of making decisions are the experts on their situations. They are the best judges of how to deal with the abuse, and their life choices need to be respected (Registered Nurses' Association of Ontario, 2005).

However, removing children and elders from their families or caregivers often is necessary to ensure immediate safety. If the home of an abused or neglected child or elder cannot be made safe, the nurse must support other professionals involved in placing the child or elder in a foster or nursing home (Gary & Humphreys, 2004; Sengstock et al., 2004). However, intervening in cases of elder abuse is not a clear-cut issue. Nurses must allow elders whose decision making is not impaired (*competence* is a legal term) an appropriate degree of autonomy in deciding how to manage the problem, even if they choose to remain in the abusive situation (Killick & Taylor, 2009; Fulmer et al., 2011). Forcing an elder to do something against his or her wishes is itself a form of victimization.

Intervention strategies for elders depend on whether the elder accepts or refuses assistance and whether he or she can make decisions. If the elder refuses treatment, the nurse must remain nonjudgemental and provide information about available services and emergency numbers. The Canadian approach to adult protection legislation, concerned with preventing abuse and neglect, has been guided by reforms in adult guardianship and substitute decision making. There are four Canadian jurisdictions with adult protection legislation in place (Canadian Network for the Prevention of Elder Abuse, 2011).

Biologic Domain

Biologic Assessment

Research indicates that health care providers often fail to respond therapeutically to survivors of abuse. In many instances, they neglect to identify abuse as the cause of traumatic injuries or mental health problems (Blakeley & Ribeiro, 1997; Campbell et al., 2004; Henderson, 2001). Even more damaging, many health care professionals treat abuse survivors derogatorily, blaming them for the abuse or for staying in abusive situations. Unfortunately, nursing staff may revictimize survivors with BPD. Often, these women have been severely traumatized, and their behaviour is difficult and disruptive. In some cases, caregivers react negatively, labelling this behaviour as attention seeking and manipulative. When nurses react to the patient in a negative, punitive manner, they retraumatize these women (Gallop, McCay, Guha, & Khan, 1999). It is not uncommon to see this behaviour punished by staff avoidance, time in seclusion rooms, and overmedication. BPD symptoms or severe symptoms associated with trauma should be interpreted as ineffective coping strategies, developed in response to severe trauma, rather than as deliberate attempts to manipulate staff (Hattendorf & Tollerud, 1997; Huband & Tantam, 2000). Nurses may also make inaccurate assumptions about who experiences IPV (e.g., the poor) and may therefore respond in ways that not only do not help the woman but which contribute to victim blaming (Ford-Gilboe et al., 2011).

To improve providers' responses, the Canadian Nurses Association (CNA) recommends that students acquire the necessary knowledge and skill acquisition to prevent violence, as well as to detect and intervene with individuals who are survivors of abuse and violence. Wathen and colleagues (2009) surveyed postsecondary health science programs in Ontario to determine the extent to which program content in IPV was available to students. Significant variability was found among educational programs and gaps in IPV content that would support professional preparation. Nurses can play a significant role in addressing family violence because nurses are frequently the first professionals to interact with individuals affected by family violence. Nurses should assess everyone for violence—both women and men, no matter what age or presenting problem. An awareness of violence and a high index of suspicion are the most important elements in assessing the problem (Campbell et al., 2004). If suspected abuse is never assessed, it will never be uncovered.

Establishing a trusting nurse–patient relationship is one of the most important steps in assessing any type of abuse. Survivors are unlikely to disclose sensitive information unless they perceive the nurse to be trustworthy and nonjudgemental. Important considerations in establishing open communication are ensuring confidentiality and providing a quiet, private place in which to conduct assessment. The law mandates that nurses report child abuse to the authorities, and nurses must make that responsibility clear before beginning the assessment. Child abuse is usually reported to the children aid society.

Lethality Assessment

The most important assessment and the one to be done first is to assess safety and the level of risk (Ford-Gilboe et al., 2011). The nurse must ascertain whether the survivor is in danger for his or her life, either from homicide or suicide, and, if children are in the home, whether they are in danger (Campbell et al., 2004). The nurse should take immediate steps to ensure the survivor's safety. In the case of suspected child abuse assessed in a health care agency, an interdisciplinary team consisting of physicians, psychologists, nurses, and social workers usually makes this decision. In other settings, the nurse may be the person to make that decision. Nurses do not have to obtain proof of abuse, only a reasonable suspicion. The Danger Assessment Screen developed by Jacquelyn Campbell and colleagues is a useful tool for assessing the risk that

either the adult survivor or the perpetrator will commit homicide (Box 37-2).

Most survivors do not report abuse to health care workers without being asked specifically about it. Routine screening or asking about IPV by health care providers is low—approximately 5% to 25% in ED settings. Even among women who present at EDs with injuries likely resulting from IPV, the rate of inquiry is less than 80% (Gutmanis, Beynon, Tutty, Wathen, & MacMillan, 2007). A survey of the ED in 230 Canadian hospitals indicated that the implementation of domestic violence policies may be as low as 10% or 20% (Hotch, Grunfeld, Mackay, & Ritch, 1996). In a survey of 250 Canadian EDs (McClennan, Worster, & MacMillan, 2008), 31.9% reported having IPV policies and procedures in place. Remarkably, there had been no significant change over a 10-year period (1994 to 2004) in the existence of IPV polices in Canadian EDs, despite the call for recommendations for routine screening (Sprague et al., 2012).

Survivors may be reluctant to report abuse because of shame and fear of retaliation, especially if the victim depends on the abuser as caregiver. In addition, children may be afraid that they will not be believed. Care needs to be exercised in the use of language when assessing for IPV. For instance, a woman may not disclose her experiences

BOX 37-2 Danger Assessment

Several risk factors have been associated with homicides (murders) of both batterers and battered women in research that has been conducted after the killings have taken place. We cannot predict what will happen in your case, but we would like you to be aware of the danger of homicide in situations of severe battering and to see how many of the risk factors apply to your situation. (The "he" in the questions refers to your husband, partner, ex-husband, ex-partner, or whoever is currently physically hurting you.)

1. Has the physical violence increased in frequency during the past year?
2. Has the physical violence increased in severity during the past year, or has a weapon or threat with weapon been used?
3. Does he ever try to choke you?
4. Is there a gun in the house?
5. Has he ever forced you into sex when you did not wish to do so?
6. Does he use drugs? By drugs, I mean "uppers" or amphetamines, speed, angel dust, cocaine, "crack," street drugs, heroin, or mixtures.
7. Does he threaten to kill you, or do you believe he is capable of killing you?
8. Is he drunk every day or almost every day? (In terms of quantity of alcohol.)
9. Does he control most or all of your daily activities? For instance, does he tell you whom you can be friends with, how much money you can take with you shopping, or when you can take the car? (If he tries, but you do not let him, check here___.)
10. Has he ever beaten you while you were pregnant? (If never pregnant by him, check here___.)
11. Is he violently and constantly jealous of you? (For instance, does he say, "If I can't have you, no one can.")
12. Have you ever threatened or tried to commit suicide?
13. Has he ever threatened or tried to commit suicide?
14. Is he violent towards the children?
15. Is he violent outside the home?
TOTAL YES ANSWERS:___.

THANK YOU. PLEASE TALK TO YOUR NURSE, ADVOCATE, OR COUNSELLOR ABOUT WHAT THE DANGER ASSESSMENT MEANS IN TERMS OF YOUR SITUATION.

Adapted from Campbell, J. C., McKenna, L. S., Torres, S., Sheridan, D. & Landenburger, K. (1993). Nursing care of abused women. In Campbell, J. C. & Humphreys, J. (Eds.), *Nursing care of survivors of family violence* (p. 259). St. Louis, MO: Mosby.

comprehensive response to IPV (Ford-Gilboe et al., 2011). For that reason, nurses must develop a repertoire of age appropriate, culturally sensitive abuse-related questions using an approach that is trauma informed (Ford-Gilboe et al., 2011).

Appropriate questions to ask in assessing abuse in women are found in the Abuse Assessment Screen in Box 37-3. Other questions that might be useful in eliciting disclosure are "When there are fights at home, have you ever been hurt or afraid?" "It looks like someone has hurt you. Tell me about it." "Some women have described problems like yours and have told me that their partner has hurt them. Is that happening to you?" (Campbell et al., 2004). When survivors are disclosing abuse, they need privacy and time to tell their story. They need to know that the nurse is listening, believes them, and is concerned for their safety and well-being (Long & Smyth, 1998).

Most survivors are not offended when health care workers ask about abuse directly, as long as they conduct the interview nonjudgementally. Survivors may perceive failure to ask about abuse as evidence of lack of concern, adding to the feelings of entrapment and helplessness. The high prevalence of abuse and the reluctance of survivors to volunteer information about it mandate routine screening of every patient for abuse by explicit questioning. Perhaps even more important, the nurse must complete such screening in privacy, away from the woman's partner, the child's parents or legal guardians, or the elderly person's relative or companion (Campbell et al., 2004; Ford-Gilboe et al., 2011; Fulmer et al., 2011; Kelley, 2011). If a partner, parent, other relative, or companion accompanies the patient to the health care facility, protocols should be in place to separate the patient from these individuals until the assessment is completed. One approach is to ask the other person to wait in the reception area, explaining that assessments are always done in private.

BOX 37-3 Abuse Assessment Screen

1. Have you ever been emotionally or physically abused by your partner or someone important to you?
   YES _____
   NO _____
2. Within the past year, have you been hit, slapped, kicked, or otherwise physically hurt by someone?
   YES _____
   NO _____
   If YES, by whom: _____
   Number of times: _____
   Mark the area of injury on body map.
3. Within the past year, has anyone forced you to have sexual activities?
   If YES, who: _____
   Number of times: _____
4. Are you afraid of your partner or anyone you listed above?
   YES _____
   NO _____

as abusive, and a more useful approach may be to ask if she has experienced specific acts of abuse (Ford-Gilboe et al., 2011). The evidence to support routine screening is mixed. MacMillan and colleagues (2009) carried out a randomized control trial to determine the effectiveness of screening. The findings were not sufficiently conclusive to recommend routine screening. At this time, best practice is regarded as including routine universal screening, together with comprehensive staff education and ongoing agency and managerial support (Registered Nurses' Association of Ontario, 2005). Rather than simply focusing on screening, nurses should carry out an assessment in which the nurse seeks to identify and follow up with appropriate interventions in order to provide an effective and

After the assessment is completed in a health care agency, the nurse should offer the adult survivor use of the telephone. The agency appointment may be the only time that the survivor can make calls in private to family, who might offer support, or to the police, lawyers, or shelters. Scheduling future appointments may provide the survivor with a legitimate reason to leave the perpetrator temporarily and continue to explore her options.

History and Physical Examination

All survivors who report or for whom the nurse suspects abuse should receive a complete history and physical examination. Throughout, the nurse must remain nonjudgemental and communicate openly and honestly (Campbell et al., 2004; CNA, 1992; Ford-Gilboe et al., 2011). A Canadian grounded theory study of woman survivors of child sexual abuse indicates that feeling safe with a health care provider who is sensitive and willing to listen can facilitate disclosure (Schachter, Radomsky, Stalker, & Teram, 2004). It is not the nurse's responsibility to judge any situation, whether that is a woman's decision to remain in an abusive relationship, the abusive actions of children's parents, or abuse perpetrated by caregivers of the elderly. Therefore, nurses must continually monitor their own feelings towards the abuser and survivor, especially in cases of child abuse. Working with child survivors often causes distress and feelings of anger and inadequacy. Seeking supervision may prevent negative feelings from influencing the nurse–patient relationship in a nontherapeutic manner and perhaps retraumatizing the survivor (Long & Smyth, 1998). Nurses should reflect on their beliefs and values and how these may shape their practice including their interactions with women (Ford-Gilboe et al., 2011; Long & Smyth, 1998; Registered Nurses' Association of Ontario, 2005).

The history should include past and present medical histories, ADLs, and social and financial supports. The nurse should obtain a detailed history of how injuries occurred. As with any history, the nurse begins with the complaint that brought the patient to the health care agency. The nurse assesses whether the explanation for the injuries or symptoms is plausible, given their nature. Discrepancies between the history and the physical examination findings may suggest abuse or neglect. The nurse moves from safe to more sensitive topics, such as the nature of the injuries. Walker (1994) suggests using what she calls the "four-incident technique" to elicit a complete abuse history. The nurse asks the survivor to describe four battering incidents: the first incident that she remembers, the most recent incident, the worst incident, and a typical incident. This series of questions is designed to elicit a complete picture of the cycle of violence and its progression. If the child is too young or an elder is too impaired to give a history, the nurse should interview one or both parents of the child or the caregiver of the elder. If the

survivor is a child or dependent elder who cannot describe what happened or make decisions about personal safety and care, the health care team may take steps to place the survivor in protective custody and defer additional assessment to the appropriate agency. The physical examination should include a neurologic examination, radiographs to identify any old or new fractures, and an examination for sexual abuse. Nurses assessing the elderly need to be familiar with normal ageing and with the signs and symptoms of common illnesses in the elderly to distinguish those conditions from abuse (Allan, 1998; Fulmer et al., 2011). Similarly, nurses need to know healthy child development to detect deviations that abuse or neglect may cause. For children, assessing developmental milestones, school history, and relationships with siblings and friends is important (Kelley, 2011; Walker, 1994). Any discrepancies between the history and the physical examination and implausible explanations for injuries and other symptoms should alert the nurse to the possibility of abuse. Box 37-4 lists indicators of actual or potential abuse that need to be thoroughly assessed for all survivors.

The nurse should thoroughly document all findings. Injuries should be photographed if possible, but this can be done only with written permission from an adult survivor or one of the child's parents. If the survivor will not permit photographing, the nurse should document the injuries on a body map. Survivors may need assurance that their medical records will not be released to anyone without written permission and that documentation of injuries will be important if legal action is taken. If the survivor does not admit abuse, the nurse cannot note abuse in the record. However, the nurse can document that the description of injuries is inconsistent with the injury pattern.

Biologic indicators, such as elevated pulse and blood pressure, sleep and appetite disturbances, exaggerated startle responses, flashbacks, and nightmares, may suggest PTSD or depression. Signs and symptoms of dissociation include memory difficulties, a feeling of unreality about oneself or events, a feeling that a familiar place is strange and unfamiliar, auditory or visual hallucinations, and evidence of having done things without remembering them (Carlson & Putnam, 1993; Etkin & Wager, 2007). If any of these signs or symptoms is present, the survivor requires a thorough diagnostic workup for PTSD and DID. In a Canadian study of women survivors of IPV, only 7.1% of women had a formal diagnosis of PTSD although almost half met the diagnostic criteria for PTSD. Women who had experienced previous trauma in childhood such as severe abuse were more likely to demonstrate symptoms of PTSD following IPV (Wuest et al., 2009).

The nurse should assess every adult or adolescent who discloses victimization for substance abuse. The Michigan Alcoholism Screening Test (MAST; Selzer, 1971) and the Drug Abuse Screening Test (DAST; Skinner, 1982) are two screening instruments for use in any health assessment.

BOX 37-4 History and Physical Findings Suggestive of Abuse

Presenting Problem
- Vague information about the cause of the problem
- Delay between occurrence of injury and seeking of treatment
- Inappropriate reactions of significant other or family
- Denial or minimizing of seriousness of injury
- Discrepancy between the history and the physical examination findings

Family History
- Past family violence
- Physical punishment of children
- Children who are fearful of parent(s)
- Father and/or mother who demands unquestioning obedience
- Alcohol or drug abuse
- Violence outside the home
- Unemployment or underemployment
- Financial difficulties or poverty
- Use of elder's finances for other family members
- Finances rigidly controlled by one member

Health and Psychiatric History
- Fractures at various stages of healing
- Spontaneous abortions
- Injuries during pregnancy
- Multiple visits to the ED
- Elimination disturbances (e.g., constipation, diarrhoea)
- Multiple somatic complaints
- Eating disorders
- Substance abuse
- Depression
- PTSD
- Self-mutilation
- Suicide attempts
- Feelings of helplessness or hopelessness
- Low self-esteem
- Chronic fatigue
- Apathy
- Sleep disturbances (e.g., hypersomnia, hyposomnia)
- Psychiatric hospitalizations

Personal and Social History
- Feelings of powerlessness
- Feelings of being trapped
- Lack of trust
- Traditional values about home, partner, and children's behaviour
- Major decisions in family controlled by one person
- Few social supports (isolated from family, friends)
- Little activity outside the home
- Unwanted or unplanned pregnancy
- Dependency on caregivers
- Extreme jealousy by partner
- Difficulties at school or work
- Short attention span
- Running away
- Promiscuity
- Child who has knowledge of sexual matters beyond that appropriate for age
- Sexualized play with self, peers, dolls, toys
- Masturbation
- Excessive fears and clinging in children

Neurologic System
- Difficulty with speech or swallowing
- Hyperactive reflexes
- Developmental delays
- Areas of numbness
- Tremors

Mental Status
- Anxiety, fear
- Depression
- Suicidal ideation
- Difficulty concentrating
- Memory loss

- Verbal aggression
- Themes of violence in artwork and school work

Distorted Body Image
- History of chronic physical or psychological disability
- Inability to perform ADLs
- Delayed language development

Physical Examination Findings
General Appearance
- Fearful, anxious, hyperactive, hypoactive
- Watching partner, parent, or caregiver for approval of answers to questions
- Poor grooming or inappropriate dress
- Malnourishment
- Signs of stress or fatigue
- Flinching when approached or touched
- Inappropriate or anxious nonverbal behaviour
- Wearing clothing inappropriate to the season or occasion to cover body parts

Vital Statistics
- Elevated pulse or blood pressure
- Other signs of autonomic arousal (exaggerated startle response, excessive sweating)
- Underweight or overweight

Skin
- Bruises, welts, oedema, scars
- Burns (cigarette, immersion, friction from ropes, a pattern like electric iron or stove)
- Subdural haematoma
- Missing hair
- Poor skin integrity: dehydration, decubitus ulcers, untreated wounds, urine burns or excoriation

Eyes
- Orbital swelling
- Conjunctival haemorrhage
- Retinal haemorrhage
- Black eyes
- No glasses to accommodate poor eyesight

Ears
- Hearing loss
- No prosthetic device to accommodate poor hearing

Mouth
- Bruising
- Lacerations
- Missing or broken teeth
- Untreated dental problems

Abdomen
- Abdominal injuries during pregnancy
- Intra-abdominal injuries

Genitourinary System or Rectum
- Bruising, lacerations, bleeding, oedema, tenderness
- Untreated infections

Musculoskeletal System
- Fractures or old fractures in various stages of healing
- Dislocations
- Limited range of motion in extremities
- Contractures

Medications
- Medications not indicated by physical condition
- Overdose of drugs or medications (prescribed or over the counter)
- Medications not taken as prescribed

Communication Patterns/Relations
- Verbal hostility, arguments
- Negative nonverbal communication, lack of visible affection
- One person answers questions and looks to the other person for approval
- Extreme dependency of family members

An adolescent version of the MAST is also available (Snow, Thurber, & Hodgson, 2002). If the results of these tests or the answers to any alcohol-related or drug-related questions are positive, the nurse should evaluate the survivor further for an alcohol or drug disorder.

● STUDY NOTE

In accordance with the Canadian Standards of Psychiatric and Mental Health Nursing, people in abusive relationships have a right to self-determination. Care involves offering choice and respecting individual preference.

Nursing Diagnoses for the Biologic Domain

Selected nursing diagnoses focusing on the human responses that nurses manage in the biologic domain may include posttrauma syndrome, delayed growth and development, impaired memory, and rape trauma syndrome.

Interventions for the Biologic Domain

Restoring health is a primary concern for survivors of abuse. When injuries are severe and surgery is required, the survivor may require hospital admittance.

Treating Physical Symptoms

Treatment of trauma symptoms may include cleaning and dressing burns or other wounds and assisting with casting of broken bones (see Box 37-5 for more information). Malnourished and dehydrated children and elders may require nursing interventions such as intravenous therapy or nutritional supplements that alleviate the alteration in nutrition and fluid and electrolyte balance.

● STUDY NOTE

It is essential to assess the risk for danger to people who are experiencing abusive relationships. Remember that their basic needs must be met (safety, housing, food, child care) before their psychological traumas can be addressed.

Promoting Healthy Daily Activity

Teaching sleep hygiene and promoting exercise, leisure time, and nutrition will help battered survivors regain a healthy physical state and learn self-care. Taking care of oneself may be difficult, yet important, for survivors who have spent years trying to separate themselves from their bodies (dissociate) to survive years of abuse (Collin-Vézina, Cyr, Pauzé, & McDuff, 2005; Walker, 1994). A history of IPV threatens the physical and mental health of women and children in many ways (Ford-Gilboe et al., 2005). Techniques such as going to bed and

---

BOX 37-5   Special Concerns for Victims of Sexual Assault

Assessment Focus

The history and physical examination of the survivor of sexual assault differ significantly from other assessment routines because the evidence obtained may be used in prosecuting the perpetrator (Sheridan, 2004). Therefore, the purpose is twofold:

• To assess the patient for injuries
• To collect evidence for forensic evaluation and proceedings
  Usually, someone with special training, such as a nurse practitioner who has taken special courses, examines a rape or sexual assault victim. Generalist nurses may be involved in treating the injuries that result from the assault, including genital trauma, such as vaginal and anal lacerations, and extragenital trauma, such as injury to the mouth, throat, wrists, arms, breasts, and thighs (Sheridan, 2004).

Key Interventions

Nursing intervention to prevent short- or long-term psychopathology after sexual assault is crucial. Psychological trauma following rape and sexual assault includes immediate anxiety and distress and the development of PTSD, depression, panic, and substance abuse (Resnick, Acierno, Holmes, Kilpatrick, & Jager, 1999).
  Key interventions include:
• Early treatment because initial levels of distress are strongly related to later levels of PTSD, panic, and anxiety (Resnick et al., 1999).
• Supportive, caring, and nonjudgemental nursing interventions during the forensic rape examination are also crucial. This examination often increases survivors' immediate distress because they must recount the assault in detail and submit to an invasive pelvic or anal examination.
• Anxiety-reducing education, counselling, and emotional support, particularly in regard to unwanted pregnancies and sexually transmitted diseases, including HIV. All survivors should be tested for these possibilities. Treatment may include terminating a pregnancy; administering medications to treat gonorrhoea, chlamydia, trichomoniasis, and syphilis; and administering medications that may decrease the likelihood of contracting HIV infection.
• Interventions that are helpful for survivors of domestic violence; these also apply to the survivors of sexual assault.

---

rising at consistent times, avoiding naps and caffeine, and scheduling periods for relaxation just before retiring may be useful in promoting sleep. Aerobic exercise is a useful technique for relieving anxiety and depression and promoting sleep.

Administering and Monitoring Medications

Survivors with a comorbid mood or anxiety disorder including PTSD may require pharmacologic interventions. Although only nurses with advanced preparation and prescriptive authority may prescribe medications, all nurses must be familiar with medications used to treat mood and anxiety disorders and the side effects of these drugs. Medications may be contraindicated for young and elderly survivors.

  The autonomic nervous system is involved in many of the symptoms of depression and PTSD. Therefore, the use of agents that decrease its activity can help treat these symptoms (Friedman, 2001; Sutherland & Davidson, 1999). Tricyclics and other antidepressants are effective in treating depression and some symptoms of PTSD, such as nightmares, sleep disorders, and startle reactions. They are less effective in treating other PTSD symptoms, such as numbing (Friedman, 2001; Sutherland & Davidson, 1999). The benzodiazepines are useful in treating anxiety and sleep disturbances in PTSD, but because they can cause dependence, they are contraindicated in women who also have a substance abuse disorder.

Approved for treating PTSD, the selective serotonin reuptake inhibitor (SSRI) sertraline (Zoloft) has improved PTSD symptoms in women but not in men (Henney, 2000; see Chapters 21 and 22 for information on monitoring medications and their side effects).

Managing Care of Patients With Comorbid Substance Abuse

Survivors who have a comorbid substance abuse disorder need referral to a treatment centre for alcohol and drug disorders. The treatment centre should have programs that address the special needs of survivors. Alcohol-dependent and drug-dependent survivors frequently stop treatment and return to alcohol and drug abuse if their abuse-related problems are not addressed appropriately (Boyd, 2000; Ouimette, Moos, & Brown, 2003). As might be expected, research findings suggest that attitudes such as self-blame and stigmatization seem to be important variables related to substance abuse for women with a history of childhood sexual abuse (Dufour & Nadeau, 2001).

Survivors, especially those with substance abuse problems, are at high risk for HIV infection and AIDS. If women do not know their HIV status, they should be encouraged to get tested. Those with positive test results should receive counselling and begin taking appropriate medications. Those without HIV need to be taught about the high-risk behaviours for HIV infection and how to protect themselves from contracting HIV infection.

Psychological Domain

Psychological Assessment

A mental status evaluation should be part of every health assessment. Symptoms such as anhedonia, difficulties concentrating, feelings of worthlessness or guilt, and thoughts of death or suicide suggest depression or PTSD. A thorough assessment of suicidal intent is crucial.

Nursing Diagnoses for the Psychological Domain

Selected nursing diagnoses focusing on the human responses that nurses manage in the psychological domain may include ineffective coping, hopelessness, chronic low self-esteem, anxiety, risk for self-directed violence, and risk for other-directed violence.

Interventions for the Psychological Domain

Assisting With Psychotherapy for Counselling

Psychotherapy may include individual, group, family, or marital therapy. Only psychiatric nurse specialists at the master's or doctoral levels who have had training in these therapeutic methods may conduct psychotherapy. In addition, the nurse therapist should have training in conducting therapy specifically with survivors of abuse. That training should include care of PTSD, DID, depression, and substance abuse. The goals of the therapy are to integrate the patient's traumatic memories with the remainder of the patient's personal history and identity, manage painful affect, and restructure the meaning of the traumatic experiences (Wilson, 2001). The ultimate goal is for the survivor to integrate the trauma in memory as a past event that no longer has the power to terrorize.

Family or marital therapy may be unwise unless the perpetrator of abuse has obtained therapy for himself or herself and demonstrated change. Otherwise, survivors are placed in a very difficult situation. If they disclose abuse in family or marital therapy, perpetrators may retaliate with violence, but if they do not disclose the abuse, the crucial issue will not be addressed (Landenburger et al., 2004).

Several issues must be addressed for all survivors in psychotherapy or counselling (Campbell et al., 2004). All nurses can implement these interventions, using skills appropriate to their educational level and training. Nurses must address the guilt, shame, and stigmatization that survivors experience. They can approach these issues in several ways. Assisting survivors to verbalize their experience in an accepting, nonjudgemental atmosphere is the first step. Nurses must challenge directly attributions of self-blame for the abuse and feelings of being dirty and different. Helping survivors to identify their strengths and validating thoughts and feelings may help to increase self-esteem. An anonymous case report by a nursing student describes the importance of therapy for nurses who have a history of childhood sexual abuse in promoting their own healing journey and ultimately their capacity to help others (Anonymous, 1998).

Working With Children

Children may need to learn a "violence vocabulary" that allows them to talk about their abuse and assign responsibility for abusive behaviour. Children also need to learn that violence is not okay and it is not their fault (Berman et al., 2004). Allowing children to discuss their abuse in the safety of a supportive, caring relationship may alleviate anxiety and fear (Berman et al., 2004).

Reenacting the abuse through play is another technique that may be helpful in assisting children to express and work through their anxiety and fear. Play therapy uses dolls, human or animal figures, or puppets to work through anxieties or fears (Hill, 2003). Other techniques used with children to reduce fear include reading stories about recovery from abusive experiences (literal or metaphoric), using art or music to express feelings, and psychodrama. In addition, teaching strategies to manage fear and anxiety, such as relaxation techniques, coping skills, and imagery, may give the child an added sense of mastering his or her fear (Barnett et al., 1997; Draughon & Urbancic, 2011). In a comprehensive review of child maltreatment literature, MacMillan (2000) indicates that research supports the use of abuse-specific cognitive–behavioural therapy as a treatment to improve the outcome for school-aged children.

Managing Anger

Anger and rage are part of the healing process for survivors (Walker, 1994). Expression of intense anger is uncomfortable for many nurses. However, they should expect anger expression and develop comfortable ways to respond. Moreover, an important nursing intervention is teaching and modelling anger expression appropriately. Inappropriate expressions of anger might drive supportive people away. Anger management techniques include appropriately recognizing and labelling anger and expressing it assertively, rather than aggressively or passive aggressively. Assertive ways of expressing anger include owning the feeling by using "I feel" statements and avoiding blaming others. Teaching anger management and conflict resolution may be especially important for children who have seen nothing but violence to resolve problems (Lowenthal, 2001).

Teaching Skills and Clarifying Identity

Other nursing interventions include teaching self-protection skills, healthy relationship skills, and healthy sexuality. Again, this teaching may be especially important for children who have no role models for healthy relationships. Children also need to know what constitutes controlling and abusive behaviour and how to get help for abuse.

Children who have been sexually abused may become confused about their sexuality. They may regard sex as dirty and as something that can be used against other people. Discussions about healthy sexuality and feelings about sex may help these children regain a healthy perspective on sex-related matters (Kelley, 2011; Peled, Jaffe, & Edleson, 1995).

Group therapy with survivors offers a powerful method to counter self-denigrating beliefs and to confront issues of secrecy and stigmatization (Urbancic, 2004). Moreover, one of the therapeutic factors in group therapy—universality, or the discovery that others have had similar experiences—may be a tremendous relief, especially to child survivors.

Providing Education

Education is a key nursing intervention for survivors. As appropriate to age or condition, survivors must understand the cycle of violence and the danger of homicide

that increases as violence escalates or the survivor attempts to leave the relationship. Survivors also need information about resources, such as shelters for battered women, legal services, government benefits, and support networks (Registered Nurses' Association of Ontario, 2005; Walker, 1994). Before giving the survivor any written material, the nurse must discuss the possibility that if the perpetrator were to find the information in the survivor's possession, he or she might use it as an excuse for battering.

Survivors also need education appropriate for age and cognitive ability about the symptoms of anxiety, depression, dissociation, and PTSD. They must understand that these symptoms are common in anyone who has sustained significant stressors and are not signs of being "crazy" or weak. If survivors require medications for these symptoms, they must know how to monitor symptoms so that the effectiveness of pharmacologic management can be determined (Box 37-6).

One of the most important teaching goals is to help survivors develop a safety plan (Ford-Gilboe et al., 2011; Walker, 1994). The first step in developing such a plan is helping the survivor recognize the signs of danger. Changes in tone of voice, drinking and drug use, and increased criticism may indicate that the perpetrator is losing control. Detecting early warning signs helps survivors to escape before battering begins (Campbell et al., 2004; Urbancic, 2004; Walker, 1994).

The next step is to devise an escape route (Ford-Gilboe et al., 2011; Walker, 1994). This involves mapping the house and identifying where the battering usually occurs and what exits are available. The survivor needs to have a bag packed and hidden, but readily accessible, that has what is needed to get away. Important things to pack are clothes, a set of car and house keys, bank account numbers, birth certificate, insurance policies and numbers, marriage license, valuable jewellery, important telephone numbers, and money (Ford-Gilboe et al., 2011; Walker, 1994). The survivor must carefully hide the bag so that the perpetrator cannot find it and use it as an excuse for assault. If children are involved, the adult survivor should make arrangements to get them out

---

BOX 37-6 Psychoeducation Checklist: Abuse

When caring for the patient who has been abused, be sure to address the following topics in the teaching plan:

- Cycle of violence
- Access to shelters
- Legal services
- Government benefits
- Support network
- Symptoms of anxiety, dissociation, and PTSD
- Safety or escape plan
- Relaxation
- Adequate nutrition and exercise
- Sleep hygiene
- HIV testing/counselling

safely. That might include arranging a signal to indicate when it is safe for them to leave the house and to meet at a prearranged place (Walker, 1994). A safety plan for a child or dependent elder might include safe places to hide and important telephone numbers, including 911 and those of the police and fire departments and other family members and friends.

Finding Strength and Hope

Providing hope and a sense of control is important for survivors of trauma (Campbell et al., 2004). Nurses can help survivors find hope and view themselves as survivors by assisting them to identify specific strengths and aspects of their lives that are under their control. This type of intervention may empower women to find options to remaining in an abusive relationship. The research by Ford-Gilboe and colleagues (2005) indicates that women were able to promote the health of their families after leaving an abusive partner, offering hope and a means of understanding for nurses working with women who are struggling to find the strength to choose health.

Using Behavioural Interventions

Treatment for depression, anxiety, and PTSD symptoms can be divided into two categories: exposure therapy and anxiety management training (Rothbaum & Foa, 1996). Only professionals trained in exposure therapy techniques can use them; however, nurses need to be familiar with this approach. The goal of exposure therapy, which includes flooding and systematic desensitization, is to promote the processing of the traumatic memory by exposing the survivor to the traumatic event through memories or some cue that reactivates trauma memories. Through repeated exposure, the event loses its ability to cause intense anxiety (Coffey, Dansky, & Brady, 2003; Paunović, 2011).

Coping With Anxiety

Anxiety management is a crucial intervention for all survivors. There is a high comorbidity among trauma, PTSD, and anxiety disorders (Orsillo et al., 2002). During treatment, survivors will experience situations and memories that provoke intense anxiety and must know how to soothe themselves when they experience painful feelings. Moreover, most survivors struggle with control issues, especially involving their bodies. Anxiety management skills offer one way to maintain some control over their bodies (Lundberg-Love, 1997).

Anxiety management training may include progressive relaxation, deep breathing, imagery techniques, and cognitive restructuring. Progressive relaxation entails systematically tensing and then relaxing the major muscle groups. Visualization consists of imagining a scene that is especially relaxing (e.g., spending a day at the beach), while practising relaxation and deep breathing. Any interventions that reduce dysphoric symptoms can help survivors feel more in control of their situation.

Anxiety disorders, including PTSD and depression, are associated with cognitive distortions that cognitive therapy techniques can challenge (Zust, 2000). Self-defeating thoughts in anxiety disorders involve perceptions of threat and danger, and those in depression involve negative self-perceptions (Blackburn & Davidson, 1990). Nurses can teach survivors how to identify and challenge these self-defeating thought patterns. Cognitive therapy techniques may be especially useful in helping survivors to stop blaming themselves for their abuse.

Nurses must become accustomed to measuring gains in small steps when working with survivors. Making any changes in significant relationships has serious consequences, and it can be done only when the adult survivor is ready. Carter-Snell and Hegadoren (2003) point out that women are frequently the primary caregiver and, as such, may have limited resources to devout to therapy. Therefore, the context of each individual woman's life needs to be kept in mind. It is easy for nurses to become angry or discouraged, and they must be careful not to communicate these feelings to survivors (Campbell et al., 2004; Urbancic, 2004). Discussing such feelings with other staff provides a way of dealing with them appropriately. In such discussions with supervisors or other staff members, the nurse must protect the patient's confidentiality by discussing feelings around issues, not particular patients. The nurse should frame the discussion in such a way that individual patients cannot be identified.

Social Domain

Social Assessment

An evaluation of social networks and daily activities may provide additional clues of psychological abuse and controlling behaviour (Gary & Humphreys, 2004). When a nurse assesses social isolation, evaluating the reasons behind it is crucial. Many perpetrators isolate their family from all social contacts, including other relatives. Some survivors isolate themselves because they are ashamed of the abuse or fear nonsupportive responses. An evaluation of social support is important for other reasons. Having supportive family or friends is crucial in short-term planning for developing a safety plan and is also important to long-term recovery. A survivor cannot leave an abusive situation if she has nowhere to go. Supportive family and friends may be willing to provide shelter and safety.

Nurses can assess restrictions on freedom that may suggest abuse and control by asking such questions as "Are you free to go where you want?"; "Is staying home your choice?"; and "Is there anything that you would like to do that you cannot?"

The degree of dependency on the relationship is another important variable to assess. Women who have young children and are economically dependent on the perpetrator may feel that they cannot leave the abusive relationship. Those who are emotionally dependent on the perpetrator may experience an intense grief reaction that further complicates their leaving (Campbell et al., 2004; Wallace, 1999). Elders and children are often dependent on the abuser and cannot leave the abusive situation without alternatives.

Nursing Diagnoses for the Social Domain

Selected nursing diagnoses focusing on the human responses that nurses manage in the social domain may include hopelessness, powerlessness, and ineffective role performance.

Interventions for the Social Domain

Working With Abusive Families

Family interventions in cases of child abuse focus on behavioural approaches to improve parenting skills (Gary & Humphreys, 2004). A behavioural approach has multiple components. *Child management skills* help parents manage maladaptive behaviours and reward appropriate behaviours. *Parenting skills* teach parents how to be more effective and nurturing with their children. *Leisure skills* training is important to reduce stress in the houschold and promote healthy family time. *Household organization* training is another way to reduce stress by teaching effective ways to manage the multiple tasks that families have to perform. Such tasks include meal planning, cooking, shopping, keeping physician's appointments, and planning family activities (Gary & Humphreys, 2004).

Anger control and stress management skills are important parts of behavioural programs for families. Anger control programs teach parents to identify events that increase anger and stress and to replace anger-producing thoughts with more appropriate ones. Parents learn self-control skills to reduce the expression of uncontrolled anger. Stress-reduction techniques include relaxation techniques and methods for coping with stressful interactions with their children (Lowenthal, 2001). These skills may be especially important in families in which elder abuse is occurring. Both caregivers and abused elders may need to learn assertive ways to express their anger and healthy ways to manage their stress. Helping caregivers find ways to get some relief from their caregiving burdens may be crucial in reducing abuse that comes from exhaustion in trying to manage multiple roles. Examples might be to identify agencies that offer respite care or agencies that offer day care for elders and support groups in which caregivers can share experiences and gain support from others dealing with similar issues.

Working in the Community

Nurses may be involved in interventions to reduce violence at the community level. Many abusive parents and battered women are socially isolated. Assistance in developing support networks may help reduce stress and, therefore, reduce abuse. Community contacts vary for each survivor but might include crisis hotlines, support groups, and education classes (Gary & Humphreys, 2004).

Community health nurses (CHNs) may play a vital role in assessing for and preventing abuse as well as health promoting initiatives that help end violence. Malone (2012) identifies a number of strategies for CHNs to implement such as assessing for safety of the person; understanding the importance of and learning how to ask about abuse; making appropriate referrals for abused individuals; and working collaboratively with others to develop broad-based preventive approaches to family violence. Specifically, nurses may make home visits to abusive parents or to families whose children are at risk. Olds (2006) reports on a long-term study looking at the impact of nurses' home visits to low-income mothers and their infants to improve health and life outcomes for mother and child. Results demonstrated positive outcomes including fewer injuries associated with child neglect and better maternal life outcomes such as workforce participation and fewer subsequent pregnancies. Home visits provide support to families and provide them with knowledge about child development and management (Barnett et al., 1997). However, abuse of any kind is a volatile situation, and nurses may place themselves or the survivor in danger if they make home visits. Nurses should carefully assess this possibility before proceeding. If necessary, the nurse and the adult survivor may need to arrange a safe place to meet.

Spiritual Domain

Although abuse and violence can devastate one's understanding of life and one's relationship with the sacred, spirituality can be a source of great strength. It can be a significant personal coping resource (Humphreys, 2000). A spiritual response to violence and abuse begins with a sense of connection to a higher power (or with an attempt to connect) that allows a healing journey to begin (Knapik, Martsolf, & Draucker, 2008). Some individuals find that the struggle to recover and rebuild after abuse has made them stronger; it has helped them to grow spiritually, to have greater self-acceptance, and to express greater compassion towards others (Wright, Crawford, & Sebastian, 2007). For many individuals, however, abuse shatters any sense of a just, benevolent, and meaningful world. It becomes incredibly challenging for them to evolve a new sense of personal spirituality.

When abuse is perpetrated by a religious leader, it can be particularly devastating. The person is violated spiritually as well as physically (Guido, 2008). Women sexually abused by members of the clergy have described their survival as involving a reorientation away from structured traditional religious practice towards a form of spirituality that is more relationally grounded (Flynn, 2008).

Nurses and other health professionals have, in the past, tended to focus primarily on the bio/psycho/social domains of patients who have been abused. It is important to understand how spirituality affects both the impact of abuse and the healing from it (Pargament, Murray-Swank, & Mahoney, 2008). Such understanding can inform discussions with patients about spirituality and can point to ways of support for patients who want to explore spirituality as a means of healing (Knapik et al., 2008). Nurses can offer patients an environment in which spiritual concerns can be expressed and compassionate responses expected (Humphreys, 2000).

■ EVALUATION AND TREATMENT OUTCOMES

Evaluation and outcome criteria depend on the setting for interventions. For instance, if the nurse encounters a survivor in the ED, successful outcomes might be that injuries are appropriately managed and the patient's immediate safety is ensured. For long-term care, outcome criteria and evaluation might centre on ending abusive relationships. Examples of other outcome criteria that would indicate successful nursing intervention are recognizing that one is not to blame for the violence, demonstrating knowledge of strengths and coping skills, and reestablishing social networks.

The evaluation of nursing care for abused children depends on attaining goals mutually set with the parents. An end to all violence is the optimal outcome criterion; however, attainment of smaller goals indicates progress towards that end. Outcomes such as increased problem-solving and communication skills within the family, increased self-esteem in both children and parents, and increased use of nonphysical forms of discipline may all indicate progress towards the total elimination of child abuse.

Follow-up efforts are important in evaluating the outcomes of elder abuse. The optimal outcome is to end all abuse and keep the elderly person in his or her own living environment, if appropriate. Although the abuse may have been resolved temporarily, it may flare up again. Ongoing support for the caregiver and assistance with caregiving tasks may be necessary if the elder person is to remain at home. Nursing home or assisted living may be the most desirable option if the burden is too great for the family and the likelihood of ongoing abuse or neglect is high.

Another important outcome of nursing intervention with survivors is appropriate treatment of any disorder resulting from abuse (e.g., ASD, PTSD and other anxiety disorders, DID, major depression, substance abuse). Follow-up nursing assessments should monitor symptom reduction or exacerbation, adherence to any medication regimen, and side effects of medication. The ultimate outcome is to end violence and enable the survivor to return to a more productive, safe, and nurturing life without being continually haunted by memories of the abuse.

Treatment for the Batterer

Participants in programs that treat batterers are usually there because the court has mandated the treatment. Programs are often outpatient groups that meet weekly for an extended period of time, often 36 to 48 weeks. Some advocate longer programs, believing that chronic offenders require 1 to 5 years of treatment to change abusive behaviour.

Groups often use cognitive–behavioural techniques or a psychoeducational, skill-building approach (Glancy & Saini, 2005; Healey, Smith, & O'Sullivan, 1998). This approach offers the batterer tools that help him see that his violent acts are not uncontrollable outbursts but rather foreseeable behaviour patterns that he can learn to interrupt. Cognitive–behavioural interventions target three elements: (1) what the batterer thinks about just before a battering incident; (2) the batterer's physical and emotional responses to these thoughts; and (3) what the batterer does that progresses to violence (e.g., yelling, throwing things). The group teaches members to recognize and interrupt negative feelings about their partners and to reduce physiologic arousal through relaxation techniques.

Psychoeducational topics are often similar to those covered by the Duluth Curriculum, which is a model program. Topics may include nonviolence; nonthreatening behaviour; respect; support and trust; honesty and accountability; sexual respect; and partnership, negotiation, and fairness. Other programs also offer more in-depth counselling, arguing that psychoeducational approaches do not address the true problem (Healey et al., 1998; Pender, 2012). If the problem were simply a deficit in skills, the batterer would be dysfunctional in work or relationships outside the family. Batterers need resocialization that convinces them that they do not have the right to abuse their partners. Other programs add a moral aspect by taking a value-laden approach against violence and confronting the batterer's behaviour as unacceptable and illegal.

Accountability for violent acts is an important early goal in treating batterers (Healey et al., 1998; Lawson, 2003). Most batterers deny responsibility for their actions and refuse to look at battering as a choice. Therefore, it is important that batterers become accountable for their actions. Interventions aim at getting the batterer to acknowledge his violence across the full range of abusive acts that he has committed, for example, verbal abuse, intimidation, controlling behaviour, and sexual abuse. Batterers may use several tactics to avoid accountability, and all must be addressed. Those tactics include denying the abuse ever happened ("I never touched her"); minimizing the abuse by downplaying the violent acts or underestimating its effects ("It was just a slap" or "she bruises easily"); and blaming the abuse on the victim ("she pushed me too far"), alcohol or other drugs ("I was high"), or other life circumstances ("I had too many pressures at work").

A recent qualitative study conducted in Nova Scotia of six group facilitators engaged in providing programs to men who batter revealed the many complexities of providing effective treatment for these men (Augusta-Scott & Dankwort, 2002). Discussions with the group facilitators suggested that a form of narrative therapy, in which the men were invited to discover what would be personally meaningful about engaging in treatment, might be a necessary prerequisite to effective treatment (Augusta-Scott & Dankwort, 2002).

Because batterers typically minimize or deny their violent behaviour, it is often necessary to interview the survivor to gain a complete picture of the batterer's behaviour. A trained victim advocate usually contacts partners. There are other reasons for contacting partners. This may be the first contact the partner has had with professionals, and she may benefit by telling her story. Many partners do not know that services are available to them, and this is an opportunity to tell her what is available. In addition, advocates often explain the batterer program and emphasize that it takes a long time and requires the batterer to take responsibility for his violent behaviour. Partners need to hear that many batterers are not willing to change their behaviour. Another important point that partners need to know and discuss with professionals is that batterers often use entry into treatment as a justification for pressuring partners to remain in the relationship and seems to be a good indicator that abuse will continue. It is also noteworthy that women's perceptions of their risk of assault appears to be fairly accurate in predicting repeated assaults and should be taken into account when assessing risk factors (Heckert & Gondolf, 2004).

Batterer intervention must be culturally competent (Healey et al., 1998; Saunders, 2008). Many factors can affect violence against women, including socioeconomic status, racial or ethnic identity, country of origin, and sexual orientation, and those differences must be addressed. Another factor that must be addressed is AOD use. Intervention programs may require batterers to undergo substance abuse treatment concurrently, and batterers are required to remain sober and submit to random drug testing.

Treatment programs alone are not sufficient to stop many batterers (Healey et al., 1998; Lawson, 2003; Moe, 2007). To be effective, programs must operate within a comprehensive intervention effort that includes criminal justice support. The criminal justice response includes arrest, incarceration, adjudication, and probation supervision that includes issuing a warrant if the batterer does not attend the batterer program or supervision. The combination of criminal justice response and batterer treatment may convey a more powerful message to the batterer about the seriousness of his actions than a batterer program alone. Unfortunately, many offenders never show up for batterer intervention, and arrests for violation of probation may be rare because of overload and staffing shortages. Involvement of the criminal justice system is important in terms of fairness (Lawson, 2003). Inaction by the criminal justice system is serious; it sends the message that there is little concern for violence against women and that batterers can get away with it.

Anger management attributes battering to out-of-control anger and teaches anger management techniques. There are several arguments against this approach. It does not address the real issue—batterers' desire to control their partners. Batterers are able to control their behaviour in other difficult situations but choose anger and intimidation to control their partners. Anger management may merely teach batterers nonviolent methods to exert control. Couples counselling may endanger the survivor. Women will not be free to disclose, and any disclosures may give the batterer reason to retaliate. Self-help groups modelled on Alcoholics Anonymous are inappropriate for initial intervention for several reasons. Without trained facilitators who will confront denial and excuses, batterers may never accept accountability for their violence. On the other hand, an untrained facilitator may use an excessively confrontational approach that is abusive and models antagonistic behaviour.

How effective is batterer treatment? Results from an extended follow-up of court-ordered batterer intervention programs show that many men continue to be assaultive during or on completion of treatment. Based on partners' reports, 32% had reassaulted their partners by 15 months after treatment, 38% had done so by 30 months, and 42% had done so at 48 months. Twenty-five percent of the men repeatedly reassaulted their partners through 48 months of follow-up. However, the results did show that reassaults de-escalated somewhat with time (Gondolf, 2001).

SUMMARY OF KEY POINTS

■ The abuse of women, men, children, and elders is a national health problem that requires awareness and sensitivity from nurses.

■ The abuse of women may be physical, emotional and psychological, or social.

■ Child abuse may be neglectful, physical, sexual, or emotional. Other forms of child abuse include Munchausen's syndrome by proxy and witnessing abuse of their mothers or significant caregivers.

■ The abuse of Aboriginal children in residential schools was particularly harmful because these children were segregated from their families and communities, frequently for years at a time.

■ Elder abuse may be physical, emotional, neglectful, or financial.

■ Among the many theories that have been proposed to explain abuse are psychopathology, social learning, sociologic, feminist, neurobiologic, borderline personality disorder, and substance abuse.

■ A well-documented cycle of violence consists of three phases of increasing frequency and severity.

■ Child abuse leaves many scars that can lead to such problems in adulthood as depression, anxiety, self-destructive behaviour, poor self-esteem, and lack of trust.

■ Responses to abuse include depression, acute stress disorder, posttraumatic stress disorder, and dissociative identity disorder.

■ Nurses need to be familiar with the signs and symptoms of abuse and be vigilant when assessing patients.

■ Nurses can help victims of abuse to view themselves as survivors.

CRITICAL THINKING CHALLENGES

1 Abuse is a pervasive problem, and anyone can be a victim (women, men, children, elders, gays, lesbians). Why do so few nursing units and nurses make it a routine to ask questions about abuse?

2 Abuse is not just a "women's issue." The prevalence of abuse might decrease if men make it a "men's issue" as well. What is preventing this from happening?

3 What are your thoughts and feelings about women who are victims of abuse in which both partners (victim and perpetrator) abuse AOD?

4 What are your thoughts and feelings about women who will not leave an abusive relationship?

5 What are some reasons that women remain in abusive relationships?

6 Why do some women become involved in more than one abusive relationship?

7 How do you handle your feelings towards abusive parents or relatives who abuse elders?

8 What are the issues in mandatory reporting of violence towards women, particularly violence that occurs in the home?

REFERENCES

Abbey, A., Zawacki, T., Buck, P., Clinton, A., & McAuslan, P. (2003). Sexual assault and alcohol consumption. What do we know about their relationship and what types of research are needed? *Aggression and Violent Behavior, 277*, 1–33.

Afifi, T. O., Boman, J., Fleisher, W., & Sareen, J. (2009). The relationship between child abuse, parental divorce, and lifetime mental disorders and suicidality in a nationally representative adult sample. *Child Abuse & Neglect, 33*(3), 139–147.

Alhalal, E. A., Ford-Gilboe, M., Kerr, M., & Davies, L. (2012). Identifying factors that predict women's inability to maintain separation from an abusive partner. *Issues in Mental Health Nursing, 33*(12), 838–850.

Allan, M. A. (1998). Elder abuse: A challenge for home care nurses. *Home Health Care Nurse, 16*(2), 103–110.

Allin, H., Wathen, C. N., & MacMillan, H. (2005). Treatment of child neglect: A systematic review. *Canadian Journal of Psychiatry. Revue Canadienne De Psychiatrie, 50*(8), 497.

American Psychiatric Association. (2000). *Diagnostic and statistical manual of mental disorders* (4th ed., Text revision). Washington, DC: Author.

American Psychiatric Association. (2013). *Diagnostic and statistical manual of mental disorders* (5th ed.). Washington, DC: Author.

Anderson, D. K. & Saunders, D. G. (2003). Leaving an abusive partner: An empirical review of predictors, the process of leaving, and psychological well-being. *Trauma, Violence & Abuse, 4*(2), 163–191.

Anderson, G., Yasenik, L., & Ross, C. A. (1993). Dissociative experiences and disorders among women who identify themselves as sexual abuse survivors. *Child Abuse & Neglect, 17*(5), 677–686.

Anonymous. (1998). Battling back from childhood sexual abuse and surviving the journey. *Journal of Psychosocial Nursing & Mental Health Services, 36*(12), 13–17.

Ansara, D. L. & Hindin, M. J. (2010). Formal and informal help-seeking associated with women's and men's experiences of intimate partner violence in Canada. *Social Science & Medicine, 70*(7), 1011–1018.

Ansara, D. L. & Hindin, M. J. (2011). Psychosocial consequences of intimate partner violence for women and men in Canada. *Journal of Interpersonal Violence, 26*(8), 1628–1645.

Arata, C. M. (2002). Child sexual abuse and sexual revictimization. *Clinical Psychological: Science and Practice, 9*, 135–164.

AuCoin, K. (2005). *Family violence in Canada: A statistical profile 2005*. Catalogue no. 85-224-XIE. Ottawa, ON: Canadian Centre for Justice Statistics.

Augusta-Scott, T. & Dankwort, J. (2002). Partner abuse groups interventions: Lessons from educational and narrative therapy approaches. *Journal of Interpersonal Violence, 17*(7), 783–805.

Banister, E. M., Jakubec, S. L., & Stein, J. A. (2003). "Like what am I supposed to do?" Adolescent girls' health concerns in their dating relationships. *Canadian Journal of Nursing Research, 35*(2), 16–33.

Barnett, O. W., Miller-Perrin, C. L., & Perrin, R. D. (1997). *Family violence across the lifespan: An introduction*. Thousand Oaks, CA: Sage.

Bartsch, C., Risse, M., Schutz, H., Weigand, N., & Weiler, G. (2003). Munchausen syndrome by proxy (MSBP): An extreme form of child abuse with a special forensic challenge. *Forensic Science International, 137*(2–3), 147–151.

Berman, H., Hardesty, J., & Humphreys, J. C. (2004). Children of abused women. In J. C. Campbell & J. C. Humphreys (Eds.), *Family violence and nursing practice* (pp. 160–185). Philadelphia, PA: Lippincott Williams & Wilkins.

Berman, H., Hardesty, J., Lewis-O'Connor, A., & Humphreys, J. C. (2011). Childhood exposure to intimate partner violence. In J. Humphreys & J. C. Campbell (Eds.), *Family violence and nursing practice* (pp. 279–318). New York, NY: Springer.

Beynon, C. E., Gutmanis, I. A., Tutty, L. M., Wathen, C. N., & MacMillan, H. L. (2012). Why physicians and nurses ask (or don't) about partner violence: A qualitative analysis. *BMC Public Health, 12*(1), 473.

Black, T., Trocmé, N., Fallon, B., & Maclaurin, B. (2008). The Canadian child welfare system response to exposure to domestic violence investigations. *Child Abuse & Neglect, 32*(3), 393–404.

Blackburn, I. & Davidson, K. (1990). *Cognitive therapy for depression and anxiety*. Boston, MA: Blackwell Scientific Publications.

Blakeley, J. & Ribeiro, V. (1997). Community health and pediatric nurses' knowledge, attitudes, and behaviors regarding child sexual abuse. *Public Health Nursing, 14*(6), 339–345.

Bograd, M. (1999). Strengthening domestic violence theories: Intersections of race, class, sexual orientation, and gender. *Journal of Marital and Family Therapy, 25*(3), 275–289.

Bombay, A., Matheson, K., & Anisman, H. (2011). The impact of stressors on second generation Indian residential school survivors. *Transcultural Psychiatry, 48*(4), 367–391.

Boyd, M. R. (2000). Predicting substance abuse and comorbidity in rural women. *Archives of Psychiatric Nursing, 14*(2), 64–72.

Boyd, M. R. (2003). Vulnerability to alcohol and other drug disorders in rural women. *Archives of Psychiatric Nursing, 17*(1), 33–41.

Boyd, M. R. & Mackey, M. (2000a). Alienation from self and others: The psychosocial problem of rural alcoholic women. *Archives of Psychiatric Nursing, 14*(3), 134–141.

Boyd, M. R. & Mackey, M. (2000b). Running away to nowhere: Rural women's experience of becoming alcohol dependent. *Archives of Psychiatric Nursing, 14*(3), 142–149.

Brady, K. T. & Dansky, B. S. (2002). Effects of victimization and posttraumatic stress disorder on substance use disorders in women. In F. L. Hall, T. S. Williams, J. A. Panetta, & J. M. Herrera (Eds.), *Psychiatric illnesses in women* (pp. 449–466). Washington, DC: American Psychiatric Publishing.

Braitstein, P., Li, K., Tyndall, M., Spittal, P., O'Shaughnessy, M., Schilder, A., ... Schechfer, M. T. (2003). Sexual violence among a cohort of injection drug users. *Social Science & Medicine, 57*(3), 561–570.

Breitenbecher, K. H. (2001). Sexual victimization among women: A review of the literature focusing on empirical investigations. *Aggression and Violent Behavior, 6,* 415–432.

Bremner, J. D. (2006). Traumatic stress: Effects on the brain. *Dialogues in Clinical Neuroscience, 8*(4), 445–461.

Bremner, J. D., Narayan, M., Staib, L. H., Southwick, S. M., McGlashan, T., & Charney, D. S. (1999). Neural correlates of memories of childhood sexual abuse in women with and without posttraumatic stress disorder. *American Journal of Psychiatry, 156,* 1787–1795.

Bremner, J. D., Southwick, S. M., & Charney, D. S. (1999). The neurobiology of posttraumatic stress disorder: An integration of animal and human research. In P. A. Saigh & J. D. Bremner (Eds.), *Posttraumatic stress disorder: A comprehensive text.* Boston, MA: Allyn and Bacon.

Brennan, S. (2012). *Victimization of older Canadians, 2009.* Juristat article, Catalogue no. 85-002-x. Ottawa, ON: Statistics Canada.

Brennan, S. & Taylor-Butts, A. (2008). *Sexual assault in Canada.* Catalogue no. 85F0033M. Ottawa, ON: Statistics Canada.

Breslau, N. & Anthony, J. C. (2007). Gender differences in the sensitivity to posttraumatic stress disorder: An epidemiological study of urban young adults. *Journal of Abnormal Psychology, 116*(3), 607–611.

Briere, J. N. & Elliott, D. M. (1994). Immediate and long-term impacts of child sexual abuse. *The Future of Children, 4*(2), 54–69.

Briere, J., Weathers, F. W., & Runtz, M. (2005). Is dissociation a multidimensional construct? Data from the multiscale dissociation inventory. *Journal of Traumatic Stress, 18*(3), 221–231.

Brownridge, D. A. (2006). Intergenerational transmission and dating violence victimization: Evidence from a sample of female university students in Manitoba. *Canadian Journal of Community Mental Health, 25*(1), 75–93.

Bryant, R. A. (2007). Does dissociation further our understanding of PTSD? *Journal of Anxiety Disorders, 21*(2), 183–191.

Brzozowski, J. A. & Brazeau, R. (2008). *What are the trends in self-reported spousal violence in Canada.* Catalogue no. 89-630-X. Ottawa, ON: Statistics Canada.

Burczycka, M. & Cotter, A. (2011). *Shelters for abused women in Canada, 2010.* Juristat article, Catalogue no. 85-002-x. Ottawa, ON: Statistics Canada.

Campbell, J. C. & Lewandowski, L. A. (1997). Mental and physical effects of intimate partner violence on women and children. *Psychiatric Clinics of North America, 20*(2), 353–354.

Campbell, J. C., McKenna, L. S., Torres, S., Sheridan, D., & Landenburger, K. (1993). Nursing care of abused women. In J. C. Campbell & J. C. Humphreys (Eds.), *Nursing care of survivors of family violence* (pp. 248–289). St. Louis, MO: Mosby.

Campbell, J. C., Torres, S., McKenna, L. S., Sheridan, D. J., & Landenburger, K. (2004). Nursing care of survivors of intimate partner violence. In J. C. Campbell & J. C. Humphreys (Eds.), *Family violence and nursing practice* (pp. 307–360). Philadelphia, PA: Lippincott Williams & Wilkins.

Canadian Centre for Justice Statistics. (2005). *Family violence in Canada: A statistical profile 2005.* Ottawa, ON: Statistics Canada.

Canadian Centre for Justice Statistics. (2010). Gender differences in police-reported violent crime in Canada, 2008. Ottawa, ON: Statistics Canada.

Canadian Centre for Justice Statistics. (2011). *Family violence in Canada: A statistical profile.* Ottawa, ON: Statistics Canada.

Canadian Centre for Justice Statistics. (2013). *Measuring violence against women: Statistical trends.* Catalogue no. 85-002-X. Ottawa, ON: Statistics Canada.

Canadian Child Care Federation. (2012). *Respecting children's rights at home.* Ottawa, ON: Author.

Canadian Network for the Prevention of Elder Abuse. (2011). Canadian laws on abuse and neglect. Retrieved from http://www.cnpea.ca/canadian_laws_on_abuse_and_negle.htm

Canadian Nurses Association. (1992). *Family violence clinical guidelines for nurses.* Ottawa, ON: National Clearing House on Family Violence.

Canadian Women's Foundation. (2013, November). Fact sheet: Moving women out of violence. Retrieved from www.canadianwomen.org/sites/canadianwomen.org/files/FACT%20SHEET%20-%20Stop%20the%20Violence%20-%20June%2019%202012.pdf

Carlson, E. B. & Putnam, F. W. (1993). An update on the Dissociative Experiences Scale. *Dissociation, 6*(1), 16–27.

Carter-Snell C. & Hegadoren, K. (2003). Stress disorders and gender: Implications for theory and research. *Canadian Journal of Nursing Research, 35*(2), 34–55.

Catallo, C., Jack, S. M., Ciliska, D., & MacMillan, H. L. (2013). Minimizing the risk of intrusion: A grounded theory of intimate partner violence disclosure in emergency departments. *Journal of Advanced Nursing, 69*(6), 1366–1376.

Cedar Project Partnership, Pearce, M. E., Christian, W. M., Patterson, K., Norris, K., Moniruzzaman, A., ... & Spittal, P. M. (2008). The Cedar Project: Historical trauma, sexual abuse and HIV risk among young Aboriginal people who use injection and non-injection drugs in two Canadian cities. *Social Science & Medicine, 66*(11), 2185–2194.

Chamberland, C., Laporte, L., Lavergne, C., & Baraldi, R. (2003). Psychological abuse: Children's invisible suffering (CECW Information Sheet #5E). Retrieved from Canadian Child Welfare Research Portal, Université de Montréal: http://cwrp.ca/sites/default/files/publications/en/PsycAbuse5E.pdf

Charney, D. S., Deutch, A. Y., Krystal, J. H., & Southwick, M. (1993). Psychobiologic mechanisms of posttraumatic stress disorder. *Archives of General Psychiatry, 50*(4), 294–305.

Chodorow, N. (1974). Family structure and feminine personality. In M. R. Rosaldo & L. Lamphere (Eds.), *Woman, culture, and society* (pp. 43–66). Stanford, CA: Stanford University Press.

Chrousos, G. P. & Gold, P. W. (1992). The concepts of stress and stress system disorders. *Journal of the American Medical Association, 267*(9), 1244–1252.

Clements, M., Oxtoby, C., & Ogle, R. L. (2008). Methodological issues in assessing psychological adjustment in child witnesses of intimate partner violence. *Trauma, Violence & Abuse, 9*(2), 114–127.

Cloitre, M., Scarvalone, P., & Difede, J. (1997). Posttraumatic stress disorder, self and interpersonal dysfunction among sexually retraumatized women. *Journal of Traumatic Stress, 10*(3), 437–452.

Coffey, S. F., Dansky, B. S., & Brady, K. T. (2003). Exposure-based, trauma-focused therapy for comorbid posttraumatic stress disorder-substance use disorder. In P. Ouimette & P. J. Brown (Eds.), *Trauma and substance abuse: Causes, consequences, and treatment of comorbid disorders* (pp. 127–146). Washington, DC: American Psychiatric Association.

Cohen, J. A., Perel, J. M., DeBellis, M. D., Friedman, M. J., & Putnam, F. W. (2002). Treating traumatized children: Clinical implications of the psychobiology of posttraumatic stress disorder. *Trauma, Violence & Abuse, 3*(2), 91–108.

Collin-Vézina, D., Cyr, M., Pauzé, R., & McDuff, P. (2005). The role of depression and dissociation in the link between childhood sexual abuse and later parental practices. *Journal of Trauma & Dissociation, 6,* 71–97.

Collin-Vezina, D. & Hebert, M. (2005). Comparing dissociation and PTSD in sexually abused school-aged girls. *Journal of Nervous & Mental Disease, 193*(1), 47–52.

Collishaw, S., Pickles, A., Messer, J., Rutter, M., Shearer, C., & Maughan, B. (2007). Resilience to adult psychopathology following childhood maltreatment: Evidence from a community sample. *Child Abuse & Neglect, 31*(3), 211–229.

Comai, S., Tau, M., & Gobbi, G. (2012). The psychopharmacology of aggressive behavior: A translational approach: Part 1: Neurobiology. *Journal of Clinical Psychopharmacology, 32*(1), 83–94.

Cook, R. & Dickens, B. (2009). Dilemmas in intimate partner violence. *International Journal of Gynecology & Obstetrics, 106*(1), 72–75.

Coulton, C. J., Crampton, D. S., Irwin, M., Spilsbury, J. C., & Korbin, J. E. (2007). How neighborhoods influence child maltreatment: A review of the literature and alternative pathways. *Child Abuse & Neglect, 31*(11–12), 1117–1142.

Courtis, C. A. & Ford, J. D. (Eds.) (2009). *Treating complex traumatic stress disorders: An evidence-based guide.* New York, NY: Guilford Press.

Criminal Code of Canada. (1985). Criminal Code of Canada, Part V, Section 155. Retrieved from http://laws-lois.justice.gc.ca/PDF/C-46.pdf

Cunningham, A. & Baker, L. (2004). *What about me! Seeking to understand the child's view of violence in the family.* London, ON: Centre for Children & Families in the Justice System.

Daigneault, I., Hébert, M., & McDuff, P. (2009). Men's and women's childhood sexual abuse and victimization in adult partner relationships: A study of risk factors. *Child Abuse & Neglect, 33*(9), 638–647.

Damant, D., Lapierre, S., Kouraga, A., Fortin, A., Hamelin-Brabant, L., Lavergne, C., ... Lessard, G. (2008). Taking child abuse and mothering into account: Intersectional feminism as an alternative for the study of domestic violence. *Affilia, 23*(2), 123–133.

Daoud, N., O'Campo, P., Urquia, M. L., & Heaman, M. (2012). Neighbourhood context and abuse among immigrant and non-immigrant women in Canada: Findings from the maternity experiences survey. *International Journal of Public Health, 57*(4), 679–689.

DeKeseredy, W. S. (2007). Factoids that challenge efforts to curb violence against women. *Domestic Violence Report, 12,* 81–82.

DeKeseredy, W. S. & Dragiewicz, M. (2007). Understanding the complexities of feminist perspectives on woman abuse. *Violence Against Women, 13*(8), 874–884.

Department of Justice, Canada. (2003a). *Stalking is a crime called criminal harassment.* Ottawa, ON: Government of Canada.

Department of Justice, Canada. (2003b). *Child abuse: A fact sheet from the Department of Justice.* Ottawa, ON: Government of Canada.

Department of Justice, Canada. (2012a). *A handbook for police and Crown prosecutors on criminal harassment.* Ottawa, ON: Government of Canada.

Department of Justice, Canada. (2012b). *Family violence initiative: Child abuse is wrong: What can I do?* Ottawa, ON: Government of Canada.

Department of Justice, Canada. (2013). *Male survivors of sexual abuse and assault: Their experiences.* Ottawa, ON: Government of Canada.

Dewey, J. (2004). Theories of aggression and family violence. In J. C. Campbell & J. C. Humphreys (Eds.), *Family violence and nursing practice* (pp. 3–28). Philadelphia, PA: Lippincott Williams & Wilkins.

Dragiewicz, M. & DeKeseredy, W. S. (2012). Claims about women's use of non-fatal force in intimate relationships: A contextual review of Canadian research. *Violence Against Women, 18*(9), 1008–1026.

Draughon, J. E. & Urbancic, J. C. (2011). Childhood sexual abuse. In J. Humphreys & J. C. Campbell (Eds.), *Family violence and nursing practice* (pp. 319–346). New York, NY: Springer.

Du Mont, J., Macdonald, S., Rotbard, N., Asllani, E., Bainbridge, D., & Cohen, M. M. (2009). Factors associated with suspected drug-facilitated sexual assault. *Canadian Medical Association Journal, 180*(5), 513–519.

Dufour, M. H. & Nadeau, L. (2001). Sexual abuse: A comparison between resilient victims and drug-addicted victims. *Violence and Victim, 16*(6), 655–672.

Dutton, D. G. (1995). *The domestic assault of women.* Vancouver, BC: UBC Press.

Dutton, D. G. (2008). My back pages: Reflections on thirty years of domestic violence research. *Trauma, Violence & Abuse, 9*(3), 131–143.

Dutton, D. G. & Painter, S. (1993). Emotional attachments in abusive relationships: A test of traumatic bonding theory. *Violence and Victims, 8*(2), 105–120.

Emery, R. E. & Laumann-Billings, L. (1998). An overview of the nature, causes, and consequences of abusive family relationships: Toward differentiating maltreatment and violence. *American Psychologist, 53*(2), 121–135.

Ellis, W. E., Chung-Hall, J., & Dumas, T. M. (2013). The role of peer group aggression in predicting adolescent dating violence and relationship quality. *Journal of Youth and Adolescence, 42*(4), 487–99.

Etkin, A. & Wager, T. D. (2007). Functional neuroimaging of anxiety: A meta-analysis of emotional processing in PTSD, social anxiety disorder, and specific phobia. *The American Journal of Psychiatry, 164*(10), 1476–88.

Fishwick, N. J., Campbell, J. C., & Taylor, J. Y. (2004). Theories of intimate partner violence. In J. C. Campbell & J. C. Humphreys (Eds.), *Family violence and nursing practice* (pp. 29–57). Philadelphia, PA: Lippincott Williams & Wilkins.

Fitzgerald, R. (2004). *Childhood aggression and exposure to violence in the home. Crime and Justice Research Paper Series.* Canadian Centre for Justice Statistics. Catalogue no. 85-561-MIE. No. 002. Ottawa, ON: Statistics Canada.

Flynn, K. (2008). In their own voices: Women who were sexually abused by members of the clergy. *Journal of Child Sexual Abuse, 17*(3–4), 216–37.

Ford-Gilboe, M., Wuest, J., & Merritt-Gray, M. (2005). Strengthening the capacity to limit intrusion: Theorizing family health promotion in the aftermath of women abuse. *Qualitative Health Research, 15*(4), 477–501.

Ford-Gilboe, M., Varcoe, C., Wuest, J., & Merritt-Gray, M. (2011). Intimate partner violence and nursing practice. In J. Humphreys & J. C. Campbell (Eds.), *Family violence and nursing practice* (pp. 115–154). New York, NY: Springer.

Friedman, M. J. (2001). Allostatic versus empirical perspective in pharmacotherapy for PTSD. In J. P. Wilson, M. J. Friedman, & J. Lindy (Eds.), *Treating psychological trauma and PTSD* (pp. 94–124). New York, NY: Guilford.

Fulmer, T., Sengstock, M. C., Blankenship, J., Caceres, B., Chandracomar, A., Ng, N., & Wopat, H. (2011). Elder mistreatment. In J. Humphreys & J. C. Campbell (Eds.), *Family violence and nursing practice* (pp. 347–366). New York, NY: Springer.

Gadalla, T. M. (2008). Gender differences in poverty rates after marital dissolution: A longitudinal study. *Journal of Divorce & Remarriage, 49*(3–4), 225–238.

Gallop, R., McCay, E., Austin, W., Bayer, M., & Peternelji-Taylor, C. (1998). Working with psychiatric clients who have been sexually abused. *Journal of the American Psychiatric Nursing Association, 4*, 9–17.

Gallop, R., McCay, E., Guha, M., & Khan, P. (1999). The experience of hospitalization and restraint of women who have a history of childhood sexual abuse. *Health Care Women International, 20*(4), 401–16.

Gary, F. A., Campbell, D. W., & Humphreys, J. (2004). Theories of child abuse. In J. C. Campbell & J. C. Humphreys (Eds.), *Family violence and nursing practice* (pp. 58–73). Philadelphia, PA: Lippincott Williams & Wilkins.

Gary, F. A. & Humphreys, J. C. (2004). Nursing care of abused children. In J. C. Campbell & J. C. Humphreys (Eds.), *Family violence and nursing practice* (pp. 252–287). Philadelphia, PA: Lippincott Williams & Wilkins.

Gueze, E., Westenberg, H. G. M., Jochims, A., de Kloet, C. S., Bohus, M., Vermetten, E., & Schmahl, C. (2007). Altered pain processing in veterans with posttraumatic stress disorder. *Archives of General Psychiatry, 64*, 76–85.

Gilligan, C. (1982). *In a different voice: Psychological theory and women's development.* Cambridge, MA: Harvard University Press.

Glancy, G. & Saini, M. A. (2005). An evidenced-based review of psychological treatments of anger and aggression. *Brief Treatment and Crisis Intervention, 5*(2), 229–48.

Gold, N. & Auslander, G. (1999). Gender issues in newspaper coverage of people with disabilities: A Canada-Israel comparison. *Women and Health, 29*(4), 75–96.

Gondolf, E. W. (2001). *An extended follow-up of batterers and their partners.* Atlanta, GA: Centers for Disease Control and Prevention.

Guido, J. (2008). A unique betrayal: Clergy sexual abuse in the context of the Catholic religious tradition. *Journal of Child Sexual Abuse, 17*(3–4), 255–269.

Gutmanis, I., Beynon, C., Tutty, L., Wathen, C. N., & MacMillan, H. L. (2007). Factors influencing identification of and response to intimate partner violence: A survey of physicians and nurses. *BMC Public Health, 7*(1), 12.

Hanson, R. K., Cadsky, O., Harris A., & Lalonde, C. (1997). Correlates of battering among 997 men: Family history, adjustment and attitudinal differences. *Violence and Victims, 12*(3), 191–208.

Hassouneh, D. & Curry, M. A. (2011). Nursing care of women with disabilities who experience abuse. In J. Humphreys & J. C. Campbell (Eds.), *Family violence and nursing practice* (pp. 181–206). New York, NY: Springer.

Hattendorf, J. & Tollerud, T. R. (1997). Domestic violence: Counseling strategies that minimize the impact of secondary victimization. *Perspectives in Psychiatric Care, 33*(1), 14–23.

Health Canada. (2002). *Woman abuse: Information from the National Clearing House on family violence.* Ottawa, ON: Author.

Health Canada. (2004). *Child maltreatment: A public health issue.* Ottawa, ON: Author.

Health Canada. (2009). *Woman abuse: Overview paper.* Ottawa, ON: Author.

Healey, K., Smith, C., & O'Sullivan, C. (1998). *Batterer intervention: Program approaches and criminal justice strategies.* Washington, DC: U.S. Department of Justice, National Institute of Justice.

Heckert, A. D. & Gondolf, E. W. (2004). Battered women's perceptions of risk versus risk factors and instruments in predicting repeat reassault. *Journal of Interpersonal Violence, 19*(7), 778–800.

Henderson, A. (2001). Factors influencing nurses' responses to abused women: What they say they do and why they say they do it. *Journal of Interpersonal Violence, 16*(12), 1284–1306.

Henderson, A. J. Z., Bartholomew, K., & Dutton, D. G. (1997). He loves me; he loves me not: Attachment and separation resolution of abused women. *Journal of Family Violence, 12*(2), 169–91.

Hendricks-Matthews, M. K. (1993). Survivors of abuse: Health care issues. *Primary Care, 20*(2), 391–406.

Hendy, H. M., Eggen, D., Gustius, C., McLeod, K. C., & Ng, P. (2003). Decision to leave scale: Perceived reasons to stay in or leave violent relationships. *Psychology of Women Quarterly, 27*(2), 162–173.

Henney, J. E. (2000). Sertraline approved for posttraumatic stress disorder. *Journal of the American Medical Association, 283*(5), 596.

Henry, J. P. (1992). Biological basis of the stress response. *Integrative Physiological and Behavioral Science, 1*, 66–83.

Herman, J. (1997). *Trauma and recovery: The aftermath of violence—from domestic abuse to political terror.* New York, NY: Basic Books.

Hill, A. (2003). Issues facing brothers of sexually abused children: Implication for professional practice. *Child & Family Social Work, 8*(4), 281–91.

Hollingsworth, E. & Ford-Gilboe, M. (2006). Registered nurses' self-efficacy for assessing and responding to woman abuse in emergency department settings. *Canadian Journal of Nursing Research, 38*(4), 54–77.

Holmes, E. A., Brown, R. J., Mansell, W., Fearon, R. P., Hunter, E. C. M., Frasquilho, F., … Oakley, D. A. (2005). Are there two qualitatively distinct forms of dissociation? A review and some clinical implications. *Clinical Psychology Review, 25*(1), 1–23.

Hopper L. M., Spiteri A., Lambeth S. P., Schapiro S. J., Horner V., & Whiten A. (2007). Experimental studies of traditions and underlying transmission processes in chimpanzees. *Animal Behavior, 73*, 1021–32.

Hopton, J. L. & Huta, V. (2013). Evaluation of an intervention designed for men who were abused in childhood and are experiencing symptoms of posttraumatic stress disorder. *Psychology of Men & Masculinity, 14*(3), 300–313.

Hotch, D., Grunfeld, A., Mackay, K., & Ritch, L. (1996). Policy and procedures for domestic violence patients in Canadian emergency departments: A national survey. *Journal of Emergency Nursing, 22*(4), 278–82.

Hovsepian, S. L., Blais, M., Manseau, H., Otis, J., & Girard, M. (2010). Prior victimization and sexual and contraceptive self-efficacy among adolescent females under child protective services care. *Health Education & Behavior*, *37*(1), 65–83.

Huband, N. & Tantam, D. (2000). Attitudes to self-injury within a group of mental health staff. *The British Journal of Medical Psychology*, *73*, 495–504.

Humphreys, J. (2000). Spirituality and distress in sheltered battered women. *Journal of Nursing Scholarship*, *32*(3), 273–78.

Humphreys, J. & Campbell, J. C. (2011). *Family violence and nursing practice*. New York, NY: Springer.

Hunnicutt, G. (2009). Varieties of patriarchy and violence against women: Resurrecting "patriarchy" as a theoretical tool. *Violence Against Women*, *15*(5), 553–573.

Janssen, P. A., Holt, V. L., & Sugg, N. K. (2002). Introducing domestic violence assessment in a postpartum clinical setting. *Maternal Child Health Journal*, *6*(3), 195–203.

Johnsen, G. E. & Asbjørnsen, A. E. (2008). Consistent impaired verbal memory in PTSD: A meta-analysis. *Journal of Affective Disorders*, *111*(1), 74–82.

Kaplan, H. I. & Sadock, B. J. (2003). *Kaplan and Sadock's synopsis of psychiatry: Behavioral sciences/clinical psychiatry*. Philadelphia, PA: Lippincott Williams & Wilkins.

Kaukinen, C. E., Meyer, S., & Akers, C. (2013). Status compatibility and help-seeking behaviors among female intimate partner violence victims. *Journal of Interpersonal Violence*, *28*(3), 577–601.

Kelley, S. J. (2011). Theories and research on child maltreatment. In J. Humphreys & J. C. Campbell (Eds.), *Family violence and nursing practice* (pp. 91–114). New York, NY: Springer.

Kelly, U. A., Gonzalez-Guarda, R. M., & Taylor, J. (2011). Theories of intimate partner violence. In J. Humphreys & J. C. Campbell (Eds.), *Family violence and nursing practice* (pp. 51–90). New York, NY: Springer.

Kihlstrom, J. F. (2005). Dissociative disorders. *Annual Review of Clinical Psychology*, *1*(1), 227–253.

Kilbourne, J. (1987). *Still killing us softly*. Cambridge, MA: Cambridge Documentary Films.

Kilbourne, J. (1999). *Can't buy my love: How advertising changes the way we think and feel*. New York, NY: Simon & Schuster.

Killick, C. & Taylor, B. J. (2009). Professional decision-making on elder abuse: Systematic narrative review. *Journal of Elder Abuse and Neglect*, *21*(3), 211–238.

Knapik, G., Martsolf, D., & Draucker, C. (2008). Being delivered: Spirituality in survivors of sexual violence. *Issues in Mental Health Nursing*, *29*, 335–50.

Kwong, M. J., Bartholomew, K., Henderson, A. J. Z., & Trinke, S. J. (2003). The intergenerational transmission of relationship violence. *Journal of Family Psychology*, *17*(3), 288–301.

Landenburger, K., Campbell, D. W., & Rodriguez, R. (2004). Nursing care of families using violence. In J. C. Campbell & J. C. Humphreys (Eds.), *Family violence and nursing practice* (pp. 220–251). Philadelphia, PA: Lippincott Williams & Wilkins.

Lanius, R. A., Frewen, P. A., Vermetten, E., & Yehuda, R. (2010). Fear conditioning and early life vulnerabilities: Two distinct pathways of emotional dysregulation and brain dysfunction in PTSD. *European Journal of Psychotraumatology*, *1*, 1–10.

Laporte, L., Jiang, D., Pepler, D. J., & Chamberland, C. (2011). The relationship between adolescents' experience of family violence and dating violence. *Youth & Society*, *43*(1), 3–27.

Lasiuk, G. & Hegadoren, K. (2006a). Posttraumatic stress disorder. Part 1: Historical development of the concept. *Perspectives in Psychiatric Care*, *42*(1), 13–20.

Lasiuk, G. & Hegadoren, K. (2006b). Posttraumatic stress disorder. Part 2: Development of the construct within the North American Psychiatric Taxonomy. *Perspectives in Psychiatric Care*, *42*(2), 72–81.

LaVoie, F., Herbert, M., Tremblay, R., Vitaro, F., Vezina, L., & McDuff, P. (2002). History of family dysfunction and perpetuation of dating violence by adolescent boys: A longitudinal study. *Journal of Adolescent Health*, *30*, 375–83.

Law Commission of Canada. (2000). *Restoring dignity: Responding to child abuse in Canadian institutions*. Ottawa, ON: Minister of Public Works and Government Services.

Lawson, D. M. (2003). Incidence, explanations, and treatment of partner violence. *Journal of Counseling and Development*, *81*(1), 19–32.

Leschied, A. W., Chiodo, D., Whitehead, P. C., Hurley, D., & Marshall, L. (2003). The empirical basis of risk assessment in child welfare: The accuracy of risk assessment and clinical judgment. *Child Welfare*, *82*(5), 527–540.

Lloyd, S. A. & Emery, B. C. (2000). The context and dynamics of intimate aggression against women. *Journal of Social and Personal Relationships*, *17*(4–5), 503–521.

Long, A. & Smyth, A. (1998). The role of mental health nursing in the prevention of child sexual abuse and the therapeutic care of survivors. *Journal of Psychiatric and Mental Health Nursing*, *5*, 129–136.

Lowenthal, B. (2001). Teaching resilience to maltreated children. *Reclaiming Children and Youth*, *3*, 169–173.

Lucea, M. B., Glass, N., & Laughon, K. (2011). Theories of aggression and family violence. In J. Humphreys & J. C. Campbell (Eds.), *Family violence and nursing practice* (pp. 1–28). New York, NY: Springer.

Lundberg-Love, P. K. (1997). Current treatment strategies of adult incest survivors and their partners. In R. Geffner, S. B. Sorenson, & P. K. Lundberg-Love (Eds.), *Violence and sexual abuse at home: Current issues in spousal battering and child maltreatment* (pp. 293–311). New York, NY: Haworth Maltreatment & Trauma Press.

MacMillan, R. (2000). Adolescent victimization and income deficits in adulthood: Rethinking the costs of criminal violence from a life-course perspective. *Criminology*, *38*, 553–588.

MacMillan, H. L., Wathen, C. N., Jamieson, E., Boyle, M. H., Shannon, H. S., Ford-Gilboe, M., … McNutt, L. A. (2009). Screening for intimate partner violence in health care settings: A randomized trial. *Journal of the American Medical Association*, *302*, 493–501.

Mahoney, T. H. (2010). *Police-reported dating violence in Canada, 2008*. Juristat article, Catalogue no. 85-002-x. Ottawa, ON: Statistics Canada.

Malone, M. (2012). Violence in society. In L. Stamler & L. Yiu (Eds.), *Community health nursing*. Toronto, ON: Pearson.

Marshall, K. (2006). *Converging gender roles*. Catalogue no. 75-001-XPE. Ottawa, ON: Statistics Canada.

McClennan, S., Worster, A., & MacMillan, H. (2008). Caring for victims of intimate partner violence: A survey of Canadian emergency departments. *Canadian Journal of Emergency Medicine*, *10*(4), 325.

McCue, M. L. (2008). *Domestic violence: A reference handbook*. Santa Barbara, CA: ABC-CLIO.

McGrath, M. E., Bettacchi, A., Duffy, S. J., Peipert, J. F., Becker, B. M. & St. Angelo, L. (1997). Violence against women: Provider barriers to intervention in emergency departments. *Academic Emergency Medicine*, *4*, 297–300.

McKeown, I., Reid, S., & Orr, P. (2004). Experiences of sexual violence and relocation in the lives of HIV infected Canadian women. *International Journal of Circumpolar Health*, *63*(Suppl. 2), 399–404.

McLean, L. M. & Gallop, R. (2003). Implications of childhood sexual abuse for adult borderline personality disorder and complex posttraumatic stress disorder. *American Journal of Psychiatry*, *160*(2), 369–371.

Messman-Moore, T. L. & Long, P. J. (2003). The role of childhood sexual abuse sequelae in the sexual revictimization of women: An empirical review and theoretical reformulation. *Clinical Psychology Review*, *23*, 537–571.

Miller, G. E., Chen, E., & Zhou, E. S. (2007). If it goes up, must it come down? Chronic stress and the hypothalamic-pituitary-adrenocortical axis in humans. *Psychological Bulletin*, *133*(1), 25–45.

Milligan, S. (2011). *Criminal harassment in Canada, 2009*. Juristat Bulletin Catalogue no. 85-005-x. Ottawa, ON: Statistics Canada.

Moe, M. A. (2007). Silenced voices and structured survival: Battered women's help-seeking. *Violence Against Women*, *13*, 676–99.

Monroe, S. M. & Harkness, K. L. (2005). Life stress, the "kindling" hypothesis, and the recurrence of depression: Considerations from a life stress perspective. *Psychological Review*, *112*(2), 417–45.

Morrill, A. C., Kasten, L., Urato, M., & Larson, M. J. (2001). Abuse, addiction, and depression as pathways to sexual risk in women and men with a history of substance abuse. *Journal of Substance Abuse*, *13*, 169–84.

National Women's Health Information Center. (2003). Women with disabilities: Dissociative disorders. Retrieved from http://www.4woman.gov

Nelson, R. J. & Trainor, B. C. (2007). Neural mechanisms of aggression. *Nature Reviews Neuroscience*, *8*(7), 536–46.

Nolen-Hoeksema, S. (2002). Gender differences in depression. In I. H. Gotlib & C. L. Hammen (Eds.), *Handbook of depression* (pp. 492–509). New York, NY: Guilford.

Norris, D., Fancey, P., Power, E., & Ross, P. (2013). The critical-ecological framework: Advancing knowledge, practice, and policy on older adult abuse. *Journal of Elder Abuse & Neglect*, *25*(1), 40–55.

Norris, F. H., Foster, J. D., & Weisshaar, D. L. (2002). The epidemiology of sex differences in PTSD across developmental, social, and research contexts. In R. Kimmerling, P. Ouimette, & J. Wolfe (Eds.), *Gender and PTSD* (pp. 3–42). New York, NY: Guilford.

O'Campo, P., Burke, J., Peak, G. L., McDonnell, K. A., & Gielen, A. C. (2005). Uncovering neighbourhood influences on intimate partner violence using concept mapping. *Journal of Epidemiology and Community Health*, *59*(7), 603–608.

O'Donnell, T., Hegadoren, K., & Coupland, N. (2004). Noradrenergic mechanisms in the pathophysiology of post-traumatic stress disorder. *Neuropsychobiology*, *50*(4), 273–283.

Ogden, P., Minton, K., & Pain, C. (2006). *Trauma and the body: A sensorimotor approach to psychotherapy*. New York, NY: W.W. Norton & Company.

Olds, D. L. (2006). The nurse–family partnership: An evidence-based preventive intervention. *Infant Mental Health Journal*, *27*(1), 5–25.

Orsillo, S. M., Raja, S., & Hammond, C. (2002). Gender issues in PTSD with comorbid mental health disorders. In R. Kimerling, P. Ouimette, & J. Wolfe (Eds.), *Gender and PTSD* (pp. 207–31). New York, NY: Guilford.

Ouimette, P., Moos, R. H., & Brown, P. J. (2003). Substance use disorder—posttraumatic stress disorder comorbidity: A survey of treatments and proposed practice guidelines. In P. Ouimette & P. J. Brown (Eds.), *Trauma and substance abuse: Causes, consequences, and treatment of comorbid disorders* (pp. 91–110). Washington, DC: American Psychiatric Association.

Pargament, K., Murray-Swank, N., & Mahoney, A. (2008). Problem and solution: The spiritual dimension of clergy sexual abuse and its impact on survivors. *Journal of Child Sexual Abuse*, 17(3–4), 397–420.

Parker, B., Bullock, L., Bohn, D., & Curry, M. A. (2004). In J. C. Campbell & J. C. Humphreys (Eds.), *Family violence and nursing practice* (pp. 77–96). Philadelphia, PA: Lippincott Williams & Wilkins.

Paunović, N. (2011). Exposure inhibition therapy as a treatment for chronic posttraumatic stress disorder: A controlled pilot study. *Psychology*, 2(6), 605–614.

Peled, E., Jaffe, P. G., & Edleson, J. L. (1995). *Ending the cycle of violence*. Thousand Oaks, CA: Sage.

Pender, R. L. (2012). ASGW best practice guidelines: An evaluation of the Duluth model. *Journal for Specialists in Group Work*, 37(3), 218–231.

Pico-Alfonso, M. A., Garcia-Linares, M. I., Celda-Navarro, N., Blasco-Ros, C., Echeburúúa, E., & Martinez, M. (2006). The impact of physical, psychological, and sexual intimate male partner violence on women's mental health: Depressive symptoms, posttraumatic stress disorder, state anxiety, and suicide. *Journal of Women's Health*, 15(5), 599–611.

Public Health Agency of Canada. (2010a). *Population-specific HIV/AIDS status report: Aboriginal Peoples*. Ottawa, ON: Author.

Public Health Agency of Canada. (2010b). *Canadian Incidence Study of Reported Child Abuse and Neglect 2008: Major findings*. Ottawa, ON: Author.

Putnam, F. W. (1994). Dissociative disorders in children and adolescents. In S. J. Lynn & J. W. Rhue (Eds.), *Dissociation: Clinical and theoretical perspectives* (pp. 175–189). New York, NY: Guilford.

Rasmusson. A. M. & Friedman, M. J. (2002). Gender issues in the neurobiology of PTSD. In R. Kimerling, P. Ouimette, & J. Wolfe (Eds.), *Gender and PTSD* (pp. 43–75). New York, NY: Guilford.

Registered Nurses' Association of Ontario. (2005). *Woman abuse: Screening, identification and initial response*. Toronto, ON: Author.

Resnick, H., Acierno, R., Holmes, M., Kilpatrick, D. G., & Jager, N. (1999). Prevention of post-rape psychopathology: Preliminary findings of a controlled acute rate treatment study. *Journal of Anxiety Disorders*, 13(4), 359–370.

Riddell, T., Ford-Gilboe, M. & Leipert, B. (2009). Strategies used by rural women to stop, avoid or escape from intimate partner violence. *Health Care for Women International*, 30(1), 134–159.

Robinson, L. & Spilsbury, K. (2008). Systematic review of the perceptions and experiences of accessing health services by adult victims of domestic violence. *Health & Social Care in the Community*, 16(1), 16–30.

Romans, S., Forte, T., Cohen, M. M., Du Mont, J., & Hyman, I. (2007). Who is most at risk for intimate partner violence?: A Canadian population-based study. *Journal of Interpersonal Violence*, 22(12), 1495–1514.

Ross, C. A. (2009). Errors of logic and scholarship concerning dissociative identity disorder. *Journal of Child Sexual Abuse*, 18(2), 221–231.

Ross, C. A. & Ness, L. (2010). Symptom patterns in dissociative identity disorder patients and the general population. *Journal of Trauma & Dissociation*, 11(4), 458–68.

Rothbaum, B. O. & Foa, E. B. (1996). Cognitive-behavioral therapy for posttraumatic stress disorder. In B. A. van der Kolk, A. C. McFarlane, & L. Weisaeth (Eds.), *Traumatic stress: The effects of overwhelming experience on mind, body, and society* (pp. 491–509). New York, NY: Guilford.

Rothschild, B. (1998). Post-traumatic stress disorder: Identification and diagnosis. *Swiss Journal of Social Work*. Available at: http://www.healing-arts.org

Rothman, L. (2007). Oh Canada! too many children in poverty for too long. *Paediatrics & Child Health*, 12(8), 661–665.

Sareen, J., Cox, B. J., Stein, M. B., Afifi, T. O., Fleet, C., & Asmundson, G. J. G. (2007). Physical and mental comorbidity, disability, and suicidal behavior associated with posttraumatic stress disorder in a large community sample. *Psychosomatic Medicine*, 69(3), 242–48.

Saunders, D. G. (2008). Group interventions for men who batter: A summary of program descriptions and research. *Violence and Victims*, 23(2), 156–172.

Schachter, C. L., Radomsky, N. A., Stalker, C. A., & Teram, E. (2004). Women survivors of child sexual abuse. How can health professionals promote healing? *Canadian Family Physician*, 50, 405–412.

Schaefer-McDaniel, N. J. (2004). Conceptualizing social capital among young people: Towards a new theory. *Children Youth and Environments*, 14(1), 153–172.

Sears, H. A., Byers, E. S., Whelan, J. J., & Saint-Pierre, M. (2006). If it hurts you, then it is not a joke: Adolescents' ideas about girls' and boys' use and experience of abusive behavior in dating relationships. *Journal of Interpersonal Violence*, 21(9), 1191–1207.

Seeman, M. V. (2002). Single-sex psychiatric services to protect women. *Medscape General Medicine*, 4(3) [formerly published in Medscape *Women's Health eJournal* 7(4), 2002]. Available at: http://www.medscape.com

Selzer, M. L. (1971). The Michigan Alcoholism Screening Test: The quest for a new diagnostic instrument. *American Journal of Psychiatry*, 127, 89–94.

Sengstock, M. C., Ulrich, Y. C., & Barrett, S. A. (2004). Abuse and neglect of the elderly. In J. C. Campbell & J. C. Humphreys (Eds.), *Family violence and nursing practice* (pp. 97–149). Philadelphia, PA: Lippincott Williams & Wilkins.

Sheridan, D. (2004). Legal and forensic nursing responses to family violence. In J. C. Campbell & J. C. Humphreys (Eds.), *Family violence and nursing practice* (pp. 386–406). Philadelphia, PA: Lippincott Williams & Wilkins.

Shin, L. M., Rauch, S. L., & Pitman, R. K. (2006). Amygdala, medial prefrontal cortex, and hippocampal function in PTSD. *Annals of the New York Academy of Sciences*, 1071(1), 67–79.

Siemieniuk, R. A. C., Krentz, H. B., Gish, J. A., & Gill, M. J. (2010). Domestic violence screening: Prevalence and outcomes in a Canadian HIV population. *AIDS Patient Care and STDs*, 24(12), 763–770.

Singh, P. & Peng, P. (2010). Canada's bold experiment with pay equity. *Gender in Management: An International Journal*, 25(7), 570–585.

Sinha, M. (2012). *Family violence in Canada: A statistical profile, 2010*. Juristat article, Catalogue no. 85-002-x. Ottawa, ON: Statistics Canada.

Sinha, M. (2013). *Family violence in Canada: A statistical profile, 2011*. Juristat article, Catalogue no. 85-002-x. Ottawa, ON: Statistics Canada.

Skinner, H. A. (1982). The drug abuse screening test. *Addictive Behavior*, 7, 363–371.

Snow, M., Thurber, S., & Hodgson, J. M. (2002). An adolescent version of the Michigan Alcoholism Screening Test. *Adolescence*, 37(148), 835.

Sprague, S., Madden, K., Simunovic, N., Godin, K., Pham, N. K., Bhandari, M., & Goslings, J. C. (2012). Barriers to screening for intimate partner violence. *Women & Health*, 52(6), 587–605.

Southwick, S. M., Bremner, D., Krystal, J. H., & Charney, D. S. (1994). Psychobiologic research in post-traumatic stress disorder. *Psychiatric Clinics of North America*, 17(2), 251–264.

Statistics Canada. (2003). *The Daily. Witnessing violence: Aggression & anxiety in young children*. Ottawa, ON: Health Reports, Statistics Canada.

Statistics Canada. (2011). *Canada year book 2011*. Catalogue no. 11-402-X. Ottawa, ON: Author.

Stermac, L., Del Bove, G., & Addison, M. (2004). Stranger and acquaintance sexual assault of adult males. *Journal of Interpersonal Violence*, 19(8), 901–915.

Stewart, D., MacMillan, H., & Wathen, N. (2013). Intimate partner violence/La violence entre partenaires intimes. *Canadian Journal of Psychiatry*, 58(6), S1–S15, SS1–SS17.

Stewart, S. H., Ouimette, P., & Brown, P. J. (2002). Gender and the comorbidity of PTSD with substance use disorders. In R. Kimerling, P. Ouimette, & J. Wolfe (Eds.), *Gender and PTSD* (pp. 232–270). New York, NY: Guilford.

Straus, M. A. (2004). Prevalence of violence against dating partners by male and female university students worldwide. *Violence Against Women*, 10(7), 790–811.

Sutherland, S. M. & Davidson, J. T. (1999). Pharmacological treatment of posttraumatic stress disorder. In P. A. Saigh & J. D. Bremner (Eds.), *Posttraumatic stress disorder: A comprehensive text* (pp. 327–353). Boston, MA: Allyn & Bacon.

Thase, M. E., Jindal, R., & Howland, R. H. (2002). Biological aspects of depression. In I. H. Gotlib & C. L. Hammen (Eds.), *Handbook of depression* (pp. 192–218). New York, NY: Guilford.

Thomas, S. P., Bannister, S. C., & Hall, J. M. (2012). Anger in the trajectory of healing from childhood maltreatment. *Archives of Psychiatric Nursing*, 26(3), 169–180.

Thurston, W. E., Tutty, L. M., Eisener, A. C., Lalonde, L., Belenky, C., & Osborne, B. (2009). Implementation of universal screening for domestic violence in an urgent care community health center. *Health Promotion Practice*, 10(4), 517–526.

Trocmé, N., Fallon, B., MacLaurin, B., Black, T., & Roy, C. (2005). Child emotional maltreatment in Canada. (CECW Information Sheet #29E). Retrieved from Canadian Child Welfare Research Portal, Université de Montréal: http://cwrp.ca/sites/default/files/publications/en/CISEmotionalMaltreatment29E.pdf

Truman, T. L. & Ayoub, C. C. (2002). Considering suffocatory abuse and Munchausen by proxy in the evaluation of children experiencing apparent life-threatening events and sudden infant death syndrome. *Child Maltreatment*, 7(2), 138–148.

Turcotte, M. & Schellenberg, G. (2007). *A portrait of seniors in Canada*. Catalogue no. 89-519-XIE. Ottawa, ON: Statistics Canada.

Ulman, S. E. (2003). A critical review of field studies on the link of alcohol and adult sexual assault in women. *Aggression and Violent Behavior*, *8*, 471–486.

United Nations. (1989). Convention on the rights of the child. Retrieved from http://www.ohchr.org/EN/ProfessionalInterest/Pages/CRC.aspx

Urbancic, J. C. (2004). Sexual abuse in families. In J. C. Campbell & J. C. Humphreys (Eds.), *Family violence and nursing practice* (pp. 186–219). Philadelphia, PA: Lippincott Williams & Wilkins.

van der Kolk, B. A. (2005). Developmental trauma disorder. *Psychiatric Annals*, *35*(5), 401.

van der Kolk, B. A. & Fisler, R. E. (1993). The biologic basis of posttraumatic stress. *Primary Care*, *20*(2), 417–432.

van Stegeren, A. H. (2008). The role of the noradrenergic system in emotional memory. *Acta Psychologica*, *127*(3), 532–541.

Vanderburg, S., Wright, L., Boston, S., & Zimmerman, G. (2010). Maternal child home visiting program involves nursing practice for screening of woman abuse. *Public Health Nursing*, *27*(4), 347–352.

Varcoe, C. (2001). Abuse obscured: An ethnographic account of emergency nursing in relation to violence against women. *Canadian Journal of Nursing Research*, *32*(4), 95–115.

Vermetten, E., Schmahl, C., Lindner, S., Loewenstein, R. J., & Bremner, J. D. (2006). Hippocampal and amygdalar volumes in dissociative identity disorder. *The American Journal of Psychiatry*, *163*(4), 630–636.

Vézina, J., Hébert, M., Poulin, F., Lavoie, F., Vitaro, F., & Tremblay, R. E. (2011). Risky lifestyle as a mediator of the relationship between deviant peer affiliation and dating violence victimization among adolescent girls. *Journal of Youth and Adolescence*, *40*(7), 814–824.

Walker, L. (1979). *The battered woman*. New York, NY: Harper & Row.

Walker, L. (1984). *The battered woman syndrome*. New York, NY: Springer Publishing Co.

Walker, L. (1994). The abused women: A survivor therapy approach [Film]. Available from Newbridge Communications, Inc., 333 East Street, New York, NY 10016.

Wallace, H. (1999). *Family violence: Legal, medical, and social perspectives* (2nd ed.). Boston, MA: Allyn & Bacon.

Walsh, C., MacMillan, H. L., & Jamieson, E. (2003). The relationship between parental substance abuse and child maltreatment: Findings from the Ontario Health Supplement. *Child Abuse & Neglect*, *27*(12), 1409–1425.

Wathen, C. N., MacMillan, H., Tanaka, M., Catallo, C., Lebner, A., Friedman, M. K., ... the McMaster IPV Education Research Team. (2009). Are clinicians being prepared to care for abused women? A survey of health professional education in Ontario, Canada. *BMC Medical Education*, *9*(1), 34.

Watson, J. M., Cascardi, M., Avery-Leaf, S., & O'Leary, K. D. (2001). High school students' responses to dating aggression. *Violence and Victims*, *16*, 339–348.

Wilson, J. P. (2001). An overview of clinical considerations and principles in the treatment of PTSD. In J. P. Wilson, M. J. Friedman, & J. Lindy (Eds.), *Treating psychological trauma and PTSD* (pp. 59–93). New York, NY: Guilford.

Wilson, J. P., Friedman, M. J., & Lindy, J. D. (2001). A holistic, organismic approach to healing trauma and PTSD. In J. P. Wilson, M. J. Friedman, & J. Lindy (Eds.), *Treating psychological trauma and PTSD* (pp. 28–56). New York, NY: Guilford.

Wolfe, D. A. (2006). Preventing violence in relationships: Psychological science addressing complex social issues. *Canadian Psychology*, *47*, 44–50.

Wong, C. M. & Yehuda, R. (2002). Sex differences in posttraumatic stress disorder. In F. Lewis-Hall, T. S. Williams, J. A. Panetta, & J. M. Herrera (Eds.), *Psychiatric illnesses in women* (pp. 57–96). Washington, DC: American Psychiatric Press.

Woods, S. J. & Gill, J. (2011). Family violence: Long-term health consequences of trauma. In J. Humphreys & J. C. Campbell (Eds.), *Family violence and nursing practice* (pp. 29–50). New York, NY: Springer.

Wright, M. O., Crawford, E., & Sebastian, K. (2007). Positive resolution of childhood sexual abuse experiences: The role of coping, benefit-finding and meaning-making. *Journal of Family Violence*, *22*, 597–608.

Wright, R. J., Wright, R. O., & Isaac, N. E. (1997). Response to battered mothers in the pediatric emergency department: A call for an interdisciplinary approach to family violence. *Pediatrics*, *99*(2), 186–192.

Wuest, J., Ford-Gilboe, M., Merritt-Gray, M., Varcoe, C., Lent, B., Wilk, P., & Campbell, J. (2009). Abuse-related injury and symptoms of posttraumatic stress disorder as mechanisms of chronic pain in survivors of intimate partner violence. *Pain Medicine (Malden, Mass.)*, *10*(4), 739.

Wuest, J., & Merritt-Gray, M. (2001). While leaving abusive male partners, women engaged in a 4 stage process of reclaiming self. *Canadian Journal of Nursing Research*, *32*, 79–94.

Yodanis, C. L. (2004). Gender inequality, violence against women, and fear: A cross-national test of the feminist theory of violence against women. *Journal of Interpersonal Violence*, *19*(6), 655–675.

Yonaka, L., Yoder, M. K., Darrow, J. B., & Sherck, J. P. (2007). Barriers to screening for domestic violence in the emergency department. *The Journal of Continuing Education in Nursing*, *38*(1), 37–46.

Zahradnik, M., Stewart, S. H., O'Connor, R. M., Stevens, D., Ungar, M., & Wekerle, C. (2010). Resilience moderates the relationship between exposure to violence and posttraumatic reexperiencing in Mi'kmaq youth. *International Journal of Mental Health and Addiction*, *8*(2), 408–420.

Zust, B. L. (2000). Effect of cognitive therapy on depression in rural battered women. *Archives of Psychiatric Nursing*, *14*(2), 51–63.

38 Care of Persons Under Forensic Purview

Cindy Peternelj-Taylor

LEARNING OBJECTIVES

After studying this chapter, you will be able to:

- Describe the complexity of mental health challenges experienced by persons under forensic purview.
- Examine the issues that are critical to the development of therapeutic relationships in forensic settings.
- Consider the challenges and opportunities that exist for nursing given the diversity of settings in which forensic nurses practise.
- Analyze the issues inherent in professional role development for nurses practising in the forensic milieu.
- Evaluate the societal norms that affect contemporary care and treatment of persons under forensic purview.
- Discuss the strategies for ongoing education, research, and practice development in forensic nursing.

KEY CONCEPTS

- criminalization of the mentally ill
- custody and caring
- manipulation
- othering
- recovery
- vulnerable

KEY TERMS

- boundary violations • compassionate release • dynamic security
- forensic nursing • static security

In Canada, as in many Western countries, large numbers of vulnerable and at-risk individuals find themselves seeking mental health care under the auspices of the criminal justice system. This chapter focuses on persons under forensic purview: those who have violated the law in some way, including those remanded in custody while awaiting trial (charged but not yet sentenced); those who have been remanded in a secure forensic facility for a psychiatric evaluation; those who are found unfit to stand trial (UST) or not criminally responsible on account of a mental disorder (NCRMD); as well as those individuals who have been charged, sentenced by the courts to community supervision, or incarcerated in provincial, territorial, or federal correctional facilities. Nurses practising where the domains of criminal justice and health care intersect are typically referred to as *forensic* nurses, and their ability to provide competent and ethical care is often compromised by social and political animosity towards crime, criminality, and mental disorder.

Forensic nurses are responsible for providing mental health care and treatment to persons under forensic purview in a variety of secure institutional facilities, including forensic psychiatric units within general hospitals, forensic mental health hospitals, jails, prisons, correctional facilities, and young offender institutions. They are also involved in community-based court diversion schemes and community treatment orders (CTOs), and they assist forensic clients with recovery and reintegration into the community. Practising "at the interface of justice and mental health where the patient population does not fit neatly into either department" (Martin et al., 2013, p. 172) can be particularly challenging for nurses. A variety of terms are used to refer to this evolving specialty area of practice, including forensic psychiatric nursing, forensic mental health nursing, community forensic mental health nursing, and correctional or prison nursing. For simplicity, **forensic nursing** is used throughout this chapter and refers to nurses who integrate psychiatric and mental health nursing "philosophy and practice within a sociocultural context that includes the criminal justice system to provide comprehensive care to clients, families, and communities" (Peternelj-Taylor & Hufft, 2006, p. 379).

CRIMINALIZATION OF THE MENTALLY ILL

Throughout Canada, jails, prisons, and custodial facilities for youth in conflict with the law have become, by default, repositories for individuals with mental illness. In the past decade alone, the number of individuals with significant mental health needs within the federal correctional system in Canada has more than doubled. When compared with the general Canadian population, mental health problems are up to three times more common among federal correctional populations. Mental health services within correctional facilities have not kept up with this dramatic increase, and in many facilities, treatment is often nonexistent or unsatisfactory when compared with the community standard (Dupuis, MacKay, & Nicol, 2013; Office of the Correctional Investigator [OCI], 2012, 2013a). Unfortunately, for many individuals experiencing mental health problems and/or illness, correctional facilities have become "defacto psychiatric institutions" with "access to psychiatric care only [occurring] after they have been criminalized" (Chaimowitz, 2012, p. 5). The criminalization of the mentally ill has frequently been attributed to the deinstitutionalization movement that occurred in the 1960s and the 1970s. Unfortunately, the ongoing failure of provincial and federal governments to provide sufficient mental health funding to fully realize the goals of deinstitutionalization (e.g., independent living within the community) has resulted in a fragmented mental health system with woefully inadequate community-based services (Canadian Institute for Health Information [CIHI], 2008; Chaimowitz, 2012; Ormston, 2010). Individuals who experience chronic mental illness are often well known by the police, the courts, mental health services, jails, and correctional facilities. Critics conclude that for many individuals caught up in this web, their only crime is that they are "guilty of mental illness" (Kanapaux, 2004).

As outlined in the *Mental Health Strategy for Canada*, the overrepresentation of people with mental health problems and illnesses in the criminal justice system (whether on remand, in correctional custody, or in a forensic facility) needs to be reduced (Mental Health Commission of Canada [MHCC], 2012). Furthermore, those who are in the system need to be able to access appropriate services, treatments, and supports that are "consistent with professionally accepted standards" (MHCC, 2012, p. 47). In collaboration with the MHCC, a Correctional Service Canada Federal–Provincial/Territorial partnership developed the *Mental Health Strategy for Corrections in Canada* (Correctional Service Canada [CSC] Federal–Provincial/Territorial Partnership, 2012) to meet the needs of youth and adults with mental health problems and illnesses enmeshed with the criminal justice system. Seven key components of this strategy are highlighted in Box 38-1. Forensic nurses are critical to the adoption, implementation, and evaluation of this strategy.

BOX 38-1 Mental Health Strategy for Corrections in Canada: Key Elements

1. Mental Health Promotion
2. Screening and Assessment
3. Treatment, Services, and Supports
4. Suicide and Self-Injury Prevention and Management
5. Transitional Services and Supports
6. Staff Education, Training, and Support
7. Community Supports and Partnerships

From Correctional Service Canada, Federal–Provincial/Territorial Partnership. (2012). *Mental health strategy for corrections in Canada.* Retrieved from http://www.csc-scc.gc.ca/health/092/MH-strategy-eng.pdf

KEY CONCEPT Mental health care resource shortages and a fragmented mental health system have led to correctional facilities becoming psychiatric institutions by default. **Criminalization of the mentally ill** occurs when persons with an untreated mental illness contravene the law and enter the justice system rather than the health care system.

THE PARADOX OF CUSTODY AND CARING

Forensic settings are controversial. They arouse strong convictions from various sectors who debate their proper place in society. Nursing practice within this domain is particularly complex because it brings together the "coupling of two contradictory socioprofessional mandates: to punish and to provide care" (Holmes, 2005, p. 3). This paradox is disconcerting because a clear distinction between these two mandates is not always easily demarcated. Forensic settings provide society with two fundamental services: social necessities and social goods. Social necessities are considered essential to a community's existence; conversely, social goods are perceived as kindnesses, and although not necessarily essential, they are of benefit to the community nonetheless. Forensic settings meet their social necessity mandate through social control of those in their care. The protection of the community at large is perceived as a direct consequence of the processes of confinement and control. Forensic settings also provide social goods in the form of health care to those who are confined. In essence, forensic nurses are charged with the predicament of providing social good (e.g., health care) within institutions dedicated to the provision of social necessities (e.g., confinement) (Osborne, 1995; Peternelj-Taylor, 2004; Peternelj-Taylor & Johnson, 1995).

This coexistence of social control and nursing care creates a paradox for nurses (Holmes, 2005, 2007), one that is laden with clinical issues and moral dilemmas not commonly encountered in more traditional health care settings. This paradox requires special attention and discernment because it permeates every aspect of forensic nursing. It is likely the single factor that differentiates

FIGURE 38-1. Custody and caring. (Courtesy of the Division of Media and Technology, University of Saskatchewan.)

forensic nursing from mental health nursing in a more general sense (Peternelj-Taylor, 2000). It is within this paradox, where the competing demands for custody and caring are embraced, that the moral climate of forensic institutions is shaped (Austin, 2001) (Fig. 38-1).

> **KEY CONCEPT** Nurses in forensic settings must meet the competing demands of **custody** (confinement and security) **and caring** (nursing care).

■ FORENSIC NURSING: A MODEL FOR CARE

Nurses working with clients under forensic purview will find a familiar psychiatric and mental health nursing role, one that is "like 'stepping through the looking glass'—everything is the same, yet different" (Smith, 2005, p. 54). To illustrate the uniqueness of caring for this population, a model of care is presented. It highlights the contextual and clinical practice issues affecting the articulation of a professional nursing role with persons under forensic purview, regardless of setting. The five components of this model are the forensic client, nurse–client relationship, professional role development, treatment setting, and societal norms. Although each component of the model is discussed separately, in reality the components are dynamic and interactive in nature. Peternelj-Taylor and Hufft (2006) conclude that health care goals must be consistent with the reality of the client's life circumstances, as well as with the realities and the limitations of the setting in which nursing practice takes place. It may well be that not all forensic nurses will engage fully with each component of the model of care presented. However, the model as presented herein reflects the nature and scope of contemporary forensic nursing in Canada (Fig. 38-2).

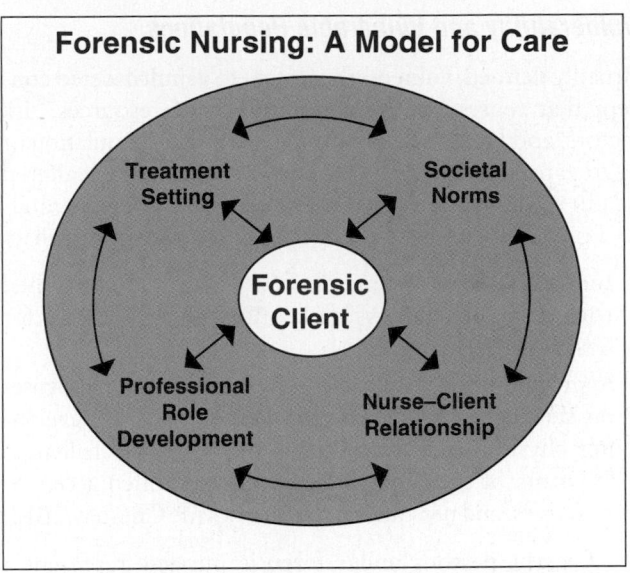

Forensic Nursing: A Model for Care

Treatment Setting · Societal Norms · Forensic Client · Professional Role Development · Nurse–Client Relationship

FIGURE 38-2. Forensic nursing: A model for care. (From Peternelj-Taylor, C. (2004). *NURS 486—Forensic nursing in secure environments* [Course material]. College of Nursing, University of Saskatchewan, Saskatoon, SK.)

Determinants of Health and the Forensic Client

As a group, persons under forensic purview present with a multitude of long-neglected physical and mental health care challenges, often complicated by significant substance abuse problems. The health and psychosocial issues that they experience are often complex and multifaceted, contributing to the challenges encountered in their attempts to engage in treatment, relapse prevention, recovery, and reintegration. Frequently, their lives have been marked by illiteracy, poverty, and homelessness. Cultural and ethnic minorities, in particular, are overrepresented in correctional institutions (Canadian Public Health Association [CPHA], 2004; OCI, 2013a). Morbidity and mortality data suggest that those who are incarcerated experience higher rates of disease and disability when compared with nonincarcerated populations, which highlights the need for nursing leadership in primary, secondary, and tertiary levels of intervention. Persons under forensic purview frequently experience discrimination, stigmatization, and marginalization, and they often lack supportive relationships commonly associated with emotional and mental well-being (MHCC, 2012). Moreover, they are totally dependent on the system (whether it is the correctional system or the health care system) to meet their health care needs. Given the magnitude of these commingling issues, many forensic clients are at risk for dual, multiple, and overlapping sources of vulnerability. Yet, referring to those who have committed crimes against society as "vulnerable" seems somewhat contrary to conventional wisdom (Peternelj-Taylor, 2005a).

Vulnerability and Vulnerable Populations

Broadly defined, vulnerability refers to a multifaceted concept that represents the commingling of resources, risk factors, and health status among a particular population or aggregate of people, which places them at risk for altered health status (de Chesnay, 2012). As a concept, vulnerability is generally understood in one of two ways, from an

- Individual focus (vulnerability)—which is concerned with such notions as "susceptibility" or "at risk for health problems"

- Aggregate view (vulnerable populations)—which focuses on those with a greater than average risk of developing physical, psychological, or social health challenges by virtue of their marginalized status, limited access to resources, and personal characteristics (de Chesnay, 2012)

Clearly, persons under forensic purview represent a significant portion of society's at-risk population. As such, understanding the concepts of vulnerability and vulnerable populations is essential to contemporary forensic nursing practice. Nurses are positioned at the interface of vulnerability and as such are challenged to engage in partnerships that encourage growth in their clients (Michaels & Moffett, 2008). Students and nurses alike can best work with vulnerable populations within forensic mental health settings by learning how to actualize respect (Rose, 2005; Rose, Peter, Gallop, Angus, & Liaschenko, 2011) (see Box 38-2).

> **KEY CONCEPT** Persons or populations are considered **vulnerable** when attributes, factors, or assigned status places them at greater risk for injury or poor health when compared with others.

Clients Experiencing Mental Illness

There is a great variation in the nature and severity of mental illnesses experienced by individuals who come into conflict with the law. In 1992, the Corrections and Conditional Release Act (Bill C-30) was proclaimed. This ended the Lieutenant Governor's Warrant system, whereby clients who were found "not guilty by reason of insanity" were held at the pleasure of the Lieutenant Governor for an unspecified period of time. It created review boards that are mandated to oversee the care and disposition of persons found UST or NCRMD (Statistics Canada, 2009). Under current Canadian law, an individual who comes into conflict with the law and is mentally ill can be found as follows:

- UST, when it is recognized that the accused is not fully capable of instructing legal counsel or not capable of understanding the nature and the consequences of a trial. In such situations, the judge has one of two choices: disposition for detention in hospital or a conditional

---

BOX 38-2 Research for Best Practice

RESPECT IN FORENSIC NURSE–PATIENT RELATIONSHIPS

Rose, D., Peter, E., Gallop, R., Angus, J. E., & Liaschenko, J. (2011). Respect in forensic psychiatric nurse-patient relationships: A practical compromise. Journal of Forensic Nursing, 7, 3–16.

Purpose: The purpose of this study was to explore the concept of respect as understood and enacted in discussion by forensic psychiatric nurses practising in a medium-security forensic unit.

Methods: Using a focused ethnography, research participants (13 registered nurses and 2 registered practical nurses) were invited to participate in two semistructured interviews. During the first interview, they engaged in a discussion of their perceptions of respect in their practice and were then invited to comment on one of four hypothetical clinical vignettes. In the second interview, participants were asked to elaborate and clarify themes that emerged from the first interview and to review the preliminary codes that emerged. Data were interpreted through a feminist philosophical lens.

Findings: Four major themes regarding respect emerged from the participants' narratives: (1) emotive–cognitive reactions, which included empathy, trust, and fear that either facilitated or impeded the enactment of respect; (2) nonjudgmental approach, which included moral culpability and likeableness; (3) social identity and power as seen in implied "oughts" and ideals and examples of others violating ideals related to respect; and (4) forensic psychiatric nursing context, including rewards and challenges. The tensions and contradictions that require a practical compromise when enacting respect underpinned all four themes. Respect was depicted in one of two ways: by describing normative expectations or by reporting contrary cases.

Implications for nursing: Respect as lived by forensic nurses in their practice is deeply complex, dynamic, and constrained by contextual factors. The researchers concluded that respect in forensic nursing is difficult to define. Practice implications include (1) engaging forensic nurses to help them understand how respect is developed and maintained; (2) teaching forensic nurses about the philosophy of respect to provide them with the vocabulary to articulate their observations of disrespect and respect to each other and other professionals; (3) providing an environment where forensic psychiatric nurses feel safe to discuss issues related to therapeutic relationships (i.e., moral distress, countertransference, and transference); and (4) providing the opportunity and permission for forensic nurses to recognize and express that not all patients are likeable and to be able to work respectfully with unlikable patients. This research contributes further to the significance of respect in developing and maintaining therapeutic relationships from a forensic psychiatric nursing perspective.

---

discharge (the person, however, can later be found "fit" and tried in court and convicted, or deemed NCRMD).

- NCRMD, based on the accused person's mental state at the time the offence was committed. Although it is not a finding of guilt, the court may give the following dispositions: detention in hospital, conditional discharge, or an absolute discharge. Individuals detained in a hospital are not required to submit to treatment; the disposition is meant to detain the person and make care available. If treatment is required, owing to the individual's deteriorating mental status, and the individual does not voluntarily agree to treatment, it is then provided as per provincial or territorial mental health policies.

- In some jurisdictions, instead of going to trial, CTOs and Court Diversion are options that may be exercised to treatment programs through community or provincial mechanisms (Dupuis et al., 2013; Statistics Canada, 2009).

In all cases, the mentally disordered offender challenges the collective wisdom of both the health care system and the criminal justice system, creating a "crossover" of sorts, particularly when the individual has been found responsible for his or her crimes despite the mental illness. The incarceration experience represents a significant stressful life event, even for those who do not have a mental disorder; separation from family and friends, limitations on privacy, overcrowding, and fear of assault severely affect the individual's quality of life. For those with mental illness, prisons are dangerous places; they are often victimized by other offenders; they are at greater risk for attempting suicide (including self-harming); and they are confined to segregation for their own protection. Unfortunately, such experiences can completely overwhelm the resources of individuals with mental illness. When compared with individuals in the community, offenders experience greater rates of schizophrenia, depression, bipolar disorder, anxiety disorders, and substance abuse disorders (CIHI, 2008; CPHA, 2004; Dupuis et al., 2013).

Suicide is the leading cause of death for persons under forensic purview, particularly those remanded or sentenced to a prison or correctional facility. Withdrawal from drugs or alcohol and the reality of incarceration/hospitalization, coupled with comorbid mental disorders, may exacerbate a client's risk for suicide and thus warrants ongoing assessment, intervention, and evaluation by forensic nurses. Recognizing factors that may contribute to a client's vulnerability is critical. High-risk periods are considered those immediately following hospitalization, incarceration, release, or the receipt of bad news (Olson, 2012; World Health Organization [WHO], 2007).

Recovery

Recovery is a major tenet of the MHCC's (2012) *Mental Health Strategy for Canada*, one that can be particularly challenging for persons under forensic purview, especially following a serious offence. Moreover, while detention, hospitalization, and incarceration are opportunities for recovery, the person has to be an active participant in the recovery journey, which can be especially trying when the person is not voluntarily seeking treatment (Drennan & Alred, 2012; McLoughlin, Geller, & Tolan, 2011). For persons under forensic purview, recovery is multifaceted and includes clinical recovery (symptom relief), functional recovery (life skills), social recovery (social inclusion), personal recovery (satisfying life living with illness), and offender recovery (redefinition of self). Of these, coming to terms with the offence clearly requires the active participation of the person (Drennan & Alred, 2012). Hope, empowerment, self-determination, and responsibility are considered the key principles of recovery (MHCC, 2012). Forensic nurses can foster recovery in a number of ways: through supporting hope, engaging in respectful dialogue, strengthening the working alliance, attending to personal strengths, bridging security and therapy, and supporting personal responsibility (Drennan & Alred, 2012; Simpson & Penney, 2011). Recovery is possible and needs to underpin the nursing care of persons under forensic purview.

KEY CONCEPT **Recovery** for persons under forensic purview includes clinical recovery through symptom relief, functional recovery through improving life-skills, social recovery through community reintegration, personal recovery through achieving life satisfaction despite illness, and offender recovery through a redefinition of self.

Special Populations in the Forensic Setting

Although it could be argued that all persons under forensic purview have special mental health needs requiring the attention of special services and interventions by forensic nurses, groups more likely to require unique approaches include women, older adults, youth, cultural minorities, and families.

The Female Forensic Client

The past decade has seen a marked increase in the number of women confined to forensic settings, and although they represent a small percentage of the overall forensic population, they currently account for its largest growth in Canada and other Western nations (Blanchette & Brown, 2006; CPHA, 2004). Of note, the Office of the Correctional Investigator (2013a) reports that between March 2003 and March 2013, the population of federally sentenced women in Canada increased by approximately 60%. Aboriginal women in particular are overrepresented within correctional systems. Nationally, one in three federally sentenced women is Aboriginal—an increase of 84% since 2003. Factors contributing to their overrepresentation include separation from family and community, isolation, violence, poverty, victimization, and discrimination (OCI, 2013a).

In general, women most likely to find themselves within forensic settings are those who have grown up in poor communities, have limited education and job skills, and are the primary caregivers for dependent children. For many women, the fear of losing custody of their children is ever present (Blanchard, 2004; Blanchette &

Brown, 2006; Harner, 2004; Maeve, 2003). Female forensic clients are frequently victims as well as perpetrators of crime, having experienced physical, emotional, and sexual abuse as children and as adults, at the hands of fathers, husbands, boyfriends, acquaintances, and strangers (Green, Miranda, Daroowalla, & Siddique, 2005; Maeve, 2003; Peternelj-Taylor, 2005b).

Common health concerns of incarcerated women include significant substance abuse problems; higher rates of blood-borne infections such as HIV/AIDS and hepatitis B and C viruses; significant mental health concerns including anxiety-related disorders (e.g., posttraumatic stress disorder), concerns related to personality disorders (e.g., poor interpersonal functioning and self-injurious behaviours), and serious mental illness (including depression and schizophrenia); pregnancy and gynaecologic problems; obesity; and chronic disorders such as diabetes, hypertension, epilepsy, and respiratory diseases (CPHA, 2004; de Sousa, 2013; Green et al., 2005; Maeve, 2003; Peternelj-Taylor, 2005b).

The management of self-injurious behaviour among women under forensic purview is particularly challenging for forensic nurses. Mangnall and Yurkovich (2010), in a study of deliberate self-harm in incarcerated women, reported that the most common method for self-harm was cutting, followed by carving arms, burning with an iron or with cigarettes, as well as swallowing glass shards, snipping veins with fingernail clippers, and punching walls or head-banging. In addition, although such behaviours typically result in immediate relief for the women, in practice, it is not uncommon for forensic nurses and correctional staff alike to be at odds with each other as they grapple to provide appropriate care for this group. In such cases, nursing typically assumes a therapeutic response, while correction adopts a more punitive or custodial stance (Mangnall & Yurkovich, 2010; OCI, 2013b).

In a comprehensive Canadian study addressing nonsuicidal self-injury (NSSI) in federally incarcerated women, Power, Brown, and Usher (2013) engaged participants in semistructured interviews focused on (1) reasons for self-injuring; (2) precipitating events; and (3) emotions experienced prior to, and after, the self-injury. While some common themes emerged in the data in relation to reasons (affect regulation), precipitating events (interpersonal conflict), emotions experienced prior to NSSI (anger and frustration), and emotions experienced after NSSI (relief), the researchers concluded that NSSI needs to be understood from a heterogeneous perspective, and that effective treatment approaches need to consider the unique experiences of each woman.

Finally, approaches to self-injurious behaviour ultimately need to address underlying motivations versus simply trying to stop the behaviour (as in the custodial response). Dialectical behavioural therapy has been found to be a useful approach when working with women who engage in NSSI, in both outpatient and inpatient settings (Power et al., 2013; Roth & Pressé, 2003).

The Older Forensic Client

For an increasing number of older Canadians, growing old in a prison or in a forensic psychiatric facility is a harsh reality. Forensic clients are considered to be "older" if aged 50 or more years. The transformation to being "older" is thought to be accelerated by 10 to 15 years within this group of clients (de Sousa, 2013; Hayes, Burns, Turnbull, & Shaw, 2012; Human Rights Watch, 2012). Since 2009, the CSC has seen a 33% increase in offenders over the age of 50 years, representing almost a quarter of the federal offender population (de Sousa, 2013).

Depending on the nature of imprisonment or hospitalization, persons under forensic purview may experience stressors related to general survival (particularly those who are incarcerated), coping with financial pressures, and withdrawal from drugs or alcohol, as well as the cumulative impact of high-risk behaviours, negative lifestyle practices, and inadequate health care, coupled with psychosocial issues related to confinement and isolation (Beckett, Peternelj-Taylor, & Johnson, 2003; de Sousa, 2013; Human Rights Watch, 2012). Older forensic clients experience both physical and mental health care needs that set them apart from their younger counterparts, as well as those typical age-related problems experienced by their nonincarcerated peers. Common concerns evident in this population include cardiovascular diseases, pulmonary disorders, diabetes, arthritis, and cancer. Common mental health risks include stress, social isolation, major depressive disorder, alcohol use disorder, suicide, and, increasingly, Alzheimer's disease and other dementias (Beckett et al., 2003; Hayes et al., 2012; Human Rights Watch, 2012; WHO, 2007). In short, those 50 years and older generally present with a high burden of disease. The Alzheimer Society Canada (2010) predicts a "rising tide" of dementia within the general Canadian population in the coming years, which will be felt by forensic and correctional authorities alike.

The health care needs of those under forensic purview clearly challenge traditional forensic and correctional resources and budgets, and questions related to the ability of these facilities to adequately care for older forensic clients are real (Beckett et al., 2003; Human Rights Watch, 2012). For increasing numbers of older and infirm forensic clients, the fear of dying while confined is a terse reality. Although **compassionate release** to community-based long-term care facilities, known in Canada as *parole by exception*, is allowed under the Corrections and Conditional Release Act, ongoing fears about community safety, bed shortages in long-term care facilities, and the stigma surrounding the circumstances of the forensic client's hospitalization or incarceration are considered on an individual basis. This option, however, is available to only a very few long-term and infirm forensic clients, and palliative care within forensic settings is a poignant reality (Beckett et al., 2003; Human Rights Watch, 2012).

Meeting the needs of terminally ill forensic clients within secure environments is a time-consuming, resource-intensive, exhaustive effort fraught with perplexing moral dilemmas not commonly encountered in traditional health care settings (Stone, Papadopoulos, & Kelly, 2012). In many secure environments, in the United States in particular, the implementation of palliative care programming is accomplished through the use of prisoner/inmate caregivers under the supervision of forensic nurses (Loeb et al., 2013). To date, this approach to palliative care within correctional environments has not been adopted in Canada.

Youth

The Youth Criminal Justice Act (YCJA), introduced in 2003, governs youth aged 12 to 17 who come into conflict with the law (Munch, 2012). As a group, youth under forensic purview are a vastly underserved population with greater than average health care needs, and because of this, they are particularly vulnerable to adverse outcomes. Studies consistently show that rates of anxiety disorders, attention deficit hyperactivity disorder (ADHD), depression, and substance abuse disorders are higher among youth in custody when compared with youth in the general population (CIHI, 2008). Frequently, their behavioural problems associated with their criminal charges mask their overall health care needs and thwart treatment efforts. It is not uncommon for youth who find themselves in custody to experience symptoms consistent with a wide array of mental health disorders, even though they may not have a formal diagnosis as such. Additionally, youth frequently demonstrate health patterns related to their family environments, as families commonly struggle with mental and physical health problems and substance abuse issues, and present with criminal histories and records (Shelton, 2000, 2001, 2004; Shelton & Pearson, 2005).

Since 2005–2006, the number of youth under correctional jurisdictions in Canada has declined by 12% (Department of Justice Canada, 2013). Ninety percent of these youth are engaged in community supervision, with the remainder detained in open or secure custody. However, Aboriginal youth continue to be disproportionately represented in the Canadian criminal justice system. When compared with their non-Aboriginal counterparts, Aboriginal youth represent 26% of youth in custody, which is particularly alarming when one considers that Aboriginal youth represent about 6% of the general Canadian youth population (Munch, 2012). The mental health care concerns of Aboriginal youth are equally alarming. High rates of foetal alcohol spectrum disorder (FASD), significant substance use issues, suicidal ideation, self-harm, histories of attempted suicide, and high rates of physical, sexual, and emotional abuse affect a large portion of the youth involved with a child protection agency at the time of their admission (Latimer & Foss, 2004). In a systematic literature review of FASD within correctional systems, Popova and colleagues (2011) concluded that individuals with FASD have 19 times greater risk of being incarcerated. Appropriate assessment and rehabilitative accommodations for this group are necessary, given the cognitive disabilities associated with FASD. Tragically, most forensic nurses will come into contact with youth through the criminal justice system because very few hospitals are set up to deal with the complexity of needs experienced by youth who come into conflict with the law. However, confinement in and of itself will not facilitate improvement in the mental health of this vulnerable group (Shelton, 2001). Efforts targeting prevention of mental health problems through the provision of services, treatments, and supports in the community are emphasized by the MHCC (2012), particularly when working with youth. Such initiatives, particularly early intervention approaches, are seen as an investment for the future and may prevent at-risk youth from involvement with the criminal justice system. Finally, intersectoral approaches that bring together justice, law, social services, education, and health care are necessary to address the complexity of issues facing at-risk youth. Forensic nurses are ideally situated to meet the needs of this group through engagement in interdisciplinary and intersectoral collaborations.

Culturally Diverse Clients

The ethnic diversity of Canada as a whole is reflected in the demographic profile of Canadian forensic facilities. However, as might be predicted, clients representing ethnic and racial minorities are disproportionately represented (CPHA, 2004), particularly in correctional facilities. The OCI (2013a) reports that the population of federally sentenced visible minorities increased by 40% in the last 5 years, with new growth seen in Aboriginal, Black, Asian, and other ethnic minorities. Of note, 25% of this group is represented by those who are foreign-born, which contributes to further challenges related to institutional adjustment and programming as well as transition to the community. Unfortunately, comparable figures for hospitalization in forensic settings operated by the health care system are unavailable.

Aboriginal people make up approximately 4% of Canada's adult population, but they represent about 21% of the federal incarcerated population (OCI, 2012). Overrepresentation of Aboriginal people within the criminal justice system is attributed to a number of complex factors related to the effects of rapid culture change, cultural oppression, and marginalization (Kirmayer, Brass, & Tait, 2000), resulting in high rates of poverty, substance abuse, and victimization within families and communities of origin (CSC, 2008; Latimer & Foss, 2004). There has been a growing awareness among the health care and criminal justice systems of the need to provide culturally sensitive and appropriate programming. In the past, programs were developed on the assumption of sameness; this approach not only negated the forensic client's ethnic identity and culture of origin but also created barriers in the formation of therapeutic relationships and treatment programs, which ultimately interfered with successful community rehabilitation (Hufft & Kite, 2003).

Families

In recent years, the needs of family members, the "forgotten clients" (Goldkuhle, 1999), have necessitated expanded roles for forensic nurses and community-based partnerships. Family members, children, and friends are a hidden forensic population; they are not accounted for and are rarely discussed by policy makers or health service providers. Incarceration has unintended consequences on families: higher rates of female-headed households, family disruption, family breakup, forced kinship care, and foster care (Freudenberg, Daniels, Crum, Perkins, & Richie, 2005). The legacy of family violence is profound. Family members have often experienced various types of violence (e.g., child abuse, domestic violence, elder abuse), and children in particular are more likely to experience physical, emotional, and cognitive problems and engage in self-destructive patterns that increase their likelihood of spending time within the forensic system (i.e., prisons) when compared with children of nonincarcerated parents.

All too often, forensic nurses assess their clients in isolation from their support systems, home environments, and daily routines, which is particularly problematic (Peternelj-Taylor, 2008). Creating a forensic family genogram is helpful when working with forensic clients (Kent-Wilkinson, 1999). A genogram is both an assessment and an intervention tool, one that can assist nurses in identifying individual and family patterns (e.g., mental health history, criminal behaviour, substance abuse) and contribute to more comprehensive assessments, interventions, and appropriate community referrals for family members (see Chapter 15 for information regarding genograms).

Collaborating with family members is critical to the safe reintegration of the forensic client into the community and is a role that is increasingly being embraced by forensic nurses, particularly those affiliated with community-based forensic mental health programs. For instance, family caregivers can play a vital role in the provision of community care of older offenders with dementia (Encinares, 2007). Many factors affect the forensic client's care in, and readjustment to, the community, including family dynamics, stress, and the family's degree of involvement. Family members can be profoundly impacted by the offence. They receive little support and frequently experience shame and stigma (Pierce, 2011), in addition to guilt and remorse regarding the forensic client's criminal acts (Encinares & Lorbergs, 2001). In some cases, the behaviours of family members can sabotage treatment and reintegration plans, and nursing staff members often bear the brunt of sarcasm and hostility (Encinares & Golea, 2005).

Nurse–Client Relationship

Nursing by its very nature is relational; it is through the nurse–client relationship that nurses gain a deeper understanding and appreciation of the human condition.

In fact, the ability to establish and maintain a therapeutic relationship with a forensic client is among the most important competencies required by forensic nurses (Peternelj-Taylor, 2002, 2004, 2012). In the forensic milieu, the emphasis of the therapeutic relationship as a primary intervention strategy is dependent on how the nurse's role is defined and on the context of the setting in which nursing practice takes place. For example, for forensic nurses practising in an inpatient forensic psychiatric unit, working in a sex offender treatment program, or counselling HIV-positive clients in a prison setting, the therapeutic relationship is fundamental to the identification and resolution of problems. In other areas of forensic nursing practice (e.g., an ambulatory care clinic in a correctional facility), the therapeutic relationship may be more in the background (Registered Nurses Association of Ontario, 2002, 2006). Regardless of the setting or the nature of the relationship, it cannot be assumed that a therapeutic relationship will be present simply by virtue of one's nursing role (Peternelj-Taylor, 2004; Schafer & Peternelj-Taylor, 2003).

Engagement in a therapeutic relationship can be especially difficult for nurses when the client is accused (or convicted) of committing a morally reprehensible act; such a client may "evoke feelings of disgust, repulsion, and fear" (Jacob, Gagnon, & Holmes, 2009, p. 153). They engage in threatening behaviours, they break rules and test boundaries, and they are unappreciative of nurses' efforts in providing health care (Austin, 2001; Schafer, 2002). In short, nurses, as members of society, are not immune to attitudes, beliefs, and stereotypes, and these may negatively colour their perceptions, therapeutic responses, and professional roles with forensic clients. The belief that every client has the potential to change and the right to treatment is one not shared by all forensic nurses (Peternelj-Taylor & Johnson, 1995; Rose, 2005). Martin (2001) warns that nurses "need to be cautious that their approach to patients does not reinforce the stigma and discrimination of the wider community" (p. 29).

To be successful, forensic nurses need to explore honestly and candidly their own preconceived ideas, attitudes, feelings, beliefs, and stereotypes regarding the forensic client. All too often, nurses can get caught up in the sensationalism that surrounds a particular forensic client (often fuelled by media hype), or the setting in which practice takes place, and ultimately they can lose sight of the person in need of care. Furthermore, it is not uncommon for nurses who are employed in forensic settings to experience additional stressors unique to their work, which ultimately affect their ability to establish and maintain therapeutic relationships with the clients in their care. Some examples are issues related to personal safety (i.e., threat of violence by forensic clients) (Jacob et al., 2009), ethical dilemmas (Peternelj-Taylor, 2004), understaffing

(Cyr & Paradis, 2012), secondary trauma and related posttraumatic stress disorder (Happell, Pinikahana, & Martin, 2003), and competing and conflicting expectations held between health care and correctional authorities (Lazzaretto-Green et al., 2011).

Common Relationship Issues Experienced by Forensic Nurses

Although barriers to therapeutic relationships can be found in all areas of nursing, it is the "special circumstance" (Austin, 2001) of forensic settings, where the moral climate is shaped by the divergent and competing demands for custody and caring, that contributes to forensic settings being described as "hotbeds" for potential problems. This is in part due to the complexity of health care needs experienced by forensic clients, the seductive pull of helping and the intensity of relationships that can develop, the professional isolation experienced by forensic nurses, and the cultural and philosophical differences that exist between forensic clients, forensic nurses, and other members of the treatment team (Lazzaretto-Green et al., 2011; Peternelj-Taylor, 2002, 2005a, 2012; Schafer & Peternelj-Taylor, 2003). Forensic nurses, like all nurses, are moral agents, and as such, they are responsible for practising ethically with the clients in their care, regardless of the setting in which care is provided (Canadian Nurses Association [CNA], 2008).

Othering

It is within these habitats of special circumstance that nurses meet forensic clients, and how the client is perceived is often illustrated by the language in which nurses frame their care. For example, are the clients seen as inmates, cons, psychopaths, murderers, psychos, or borderlines? Such labels not only evoke stereotypical images but also, more importantly, cast the individual into the role of the "other" (Peternelj-Taylor, 2004, 2005c). Mason, Hall, Caulfield, and Melling (2010) found that clients labelled personality disordered were perceived by forensic nurses as a management issue, as opposed to those labelled mentally ill who were considered from a clinical perspective. Such negative forms of engagement, known as *exclusionary othering*, can affect all aspects of nursing care and promote marginalization, stigmatization, and underinvolvement in a client's care. *Inclusionary othering*, on the other hand, is promoted as a way of learning about the other as an individual, and not simply as a crime or a label. One way of coming to know the forensic client is through role-taking and trying to understand the world from the client's perspective. Although this may be a tall order when working with forensic clients, nurses can learn about othering by gaining an appreciation for what it means to be othered (Canales, 2000, 2010).

KEY CONCEPT Othering is about the way one perceives and engages with another person. It can be exclusionary and negative (i.e., the other is different from and thus "less than" me) or inclusionary and tolerant or accepting (i.e., the other is different from me, so I need to learn about his or her worldview).

Boundary Violations

The complexities and uncertainties surrounding boundaries and **boundary violations** in practice can be difficult for forensic nurses to manage and lead to ongoing confusion in practice. The inability to differentiate the professional relationship from a social relationship by attempting to have one's personal needs met through the nurse–client relationship is consistently discussed as a precursor to boundary violations in the nursing literature (Peternelj-Taylor, 2012; Peternelj-Taylor & Schafer, 2008; Pilette, Berck, & Achber, 1995) (see Chapter 6). In forensic settings, nurses are often warned about getting "too close" to their patients, while at the same time painted as "victims of circumstances" when boundaries are transgressed with a forensic client. However, it is important to remember that, from an ethical perspective, the nurse is the one responsible for managing boundaries within the nurse–client relationship, not the client. Mixed messages regarding treatment boundaries can be especially disconcerting for forensic clients, who frequently have problems with boundaries in general. Forensic health care professionals, including nurses, are most vulnerable to transgressing boundaries when they are experiencing major life stressors in their personal lives, such as changing life circumstances, relationship problems, bereavement, or personal caregiving responsibilities. During such times, they are also at risk of being "targeted" by forensic clients who are looking to exploit the therapeutic relationship for personal gain (Faulkner & Regehr, 2011; Peternelj-Taylor, 2012).

Manipulation

The potential for manipulation is a very real factor in secure environments, one that requires thoughtful consideration by nurses in the provision of nursing care. As Austin (2001) notes, "cautioning, scepticism, and the questioning of patients' motives and actions are part of the daily experience of forensic nurses" (p. 13). Forensic clients can be powerful, dominant, intimidating, needy, charming, good-looking, and attentive, leading Gutheil and Brodsky (2008) to conclude that even the most ethical clinician can be tested by the manipulative behaviours of forensic clients. In some cases, individuals in forensic settings will attempt to manipulate health care services for some secondary gain (e.g., medication, escape from the prison environment, social diversion), and issues pertaining to safety cannot be ignored (Peternelj-Taylor, 2004; Schoenly, 2013).

Jacob (2014) notes that "the fact that patients are conceptualized as being con artists and manipulators inevitably affects the way care is delivered" (p. 50). When a forensic client is labelled a manipulator, nurses and others will generally respond more punitively and fail to engage the client in a therapeutic dialogue surrounding the meaning of his or her behaviours; in such cases, the opportunity for mutual problem-solving around the manipulative behaviours is lost in the relationship (Peternelj-Taylor, 2004; Schafer, 2002). To be successful, forensic nurses need to be astutely aware that there exists the potential for manipulation in all interactions with forensic clients, while simultaneously adhering to their professional responsibilities embedded within the therapeutic nurse–client relationship. In short, they have to negotiate the path between assuming the worst and recognizing that it can always happen (Schoenly, 2013; Smith, 2005).

> **KEY CONCEPT Manipulation** is a concern in secure environments because it can involve the use of deceit to reach a goal that could not be pursued openly (e.g., escape).

Professional Role Development

Historically, role development for forensic nurses has been difficult, owing to the myth that nurses who work with forensic clients are "second-class nurses" unable to secure employment elsewhere (Peternelj-Taylor & Johnson, 1995; Pullan & Lorbergs, 2001). In a recent study, Harris (2013) reported that the stigma experienced by forensic mental health nurses impacted negatively on their adaptation to their professional roles. During this time of a global nursing shortage, recruitment and retention of forensic nurses can be particularly challenging for both mental health care and correctional administrators (Cyr & Paradis, 2012; Pullan & Lorbergs, 2001). Given the breadth and scope of forensic nursing as illustrated within this chapter, it should be evident that forensic nurses are highly skilled and knowledgeable professionals, committed to the health and well-being of the clients in their charge, as well as the community at large.

Professional Nursing Identity

One of the greatest challenges that nurses experience when working in forensic environments is to remain true to their professional nursing roles and avoid being seduced or co-opted into assuming custodial roles, where expectations and responsibilities seem more clearly defined (Holmes, 2007; Maeve, 2003; Peternelj-Taylor & Johnson, 1995; Smith, 2005). Tensions that exist between custody and caring in forensic environments make it "difficult to maintain the therapeutic culture known to nurses" (Jacob, 2014, p. 48). In forensic settings operated by the criminal justice system, forensic nurses must have a strong nursing identity in order to maintain their professional authority and responsibility, without succumbing to the temptation to align themselves with the correctional staff. However, forensic nurses who work within the health care system should also heed this lesson, for they too can assume a more custodial stance, especially when they believe that CTOs or dispositions in hospital are lenient forms of punishment. Thus, even when the care of forensic clients is the responsibility of the health care system, incongruent attitudes among health care staff may prevail (Rose, 2005). Lawson (2005) states that when we "set ourselves up as judge and jury" (p. 149), we minimize our ability to be therapeutic.

Professional Development for Forensic Nurses

Petryshen (1981) published a classic paper entitled "Nursing the Mentally Disordered Offender." Since then, forensic nursing in Canada has undergone significant transformations in education, research, and practice developments related to the provision of nursing care to forensic clients.

Education

Forensic nursing content is slowly finding its way into undergraduate and graduate nursing curricula across the country, primarily through existing courses in psychiatric mental health or community health nursing. For example, the College of Nursing, University of Saskatchewan, offers an online elective nursing course entitled *Forensic Nursing in Secure Environments* in its undergraduate baccalaureate program. Furthermore, continuing professional development for nurses who practise in forensic settings is also critical as it reinforces the therapeutic identity of nurses, assists with nursing policy development (Smith, 2005), and contributes to recruitment and retention in this specialized area of practice (Thorpe, Moorhouse, & Antonello, 2009).

Research

Embracing a research agenda in forensic nursing will guide nursing practice in this highly specialized area; provide new insights into primary, secondary, and tertiary health care (including reintegration into the community); and contribute to nursing science through the advancement of nursing knowledge regarding vulnerable populations in general (Peternelj-Taylor, 2005a). Two research developments in this specialized area of practice include (1) the University of Ottawa's Research Chair in Forensic Nursing, established in 2009 to foster the development and dissemination of forensic nursing research and promote graduate student training; and (2) the Centre for Behavioural Science and Justice Studies, an interdisciplinary collaboration between the University of Saskatchewan, the Correctional Service Canada, and the Saskatchewan Ministry of Justice—Corrections and Policing (refer further to Web Links on thePoint). Such developments are fundamental to the advancement of forensic nursing as a specialty and will contribute to evidence-based care for those under forensic purview.

Practice Developments

Forensic nurses may find guidance in the Canadian Federation of Mental Health Nurses' (2014) *Canadian standards for psychiatric–mental health nursing*; however, standards to guide the unique needs of Canadian forensic mental health nurses are nonexistent. Recognizing the need to build upon traditional mental health standards when working with persons under forensic purview, Martin and colleagues (2013) developed 16 standards to guide education, practice, and research in forensic mental health nursing. Although written from an Australian perspective, these standards could easily cross international jurisdictions, as they capture the essence of forensic mental health nursing.

In July 2007, the Forensic Nurses Society of Canada (FNSC) was approved as an emerging special interest group by the CNA (see Web Links on thePoint). The mission of the Society is "to promote evidence-based comprehensive health care across the spectrum of forensic nursing with an aim to prevent violence or reduce its consequences on the individual" (FNSC, 2014). Such acknowledgment by the CNA is a formal recognition of forensic nursing as a specialty area; however, certification as a designated specialty remains uncertain (see Chapter 7).

Treatment Setting

Unlike more traditional practice settings, the interpersonal climate, organizational culture, and social context of forensic settings result in forensic environments being identified among the most severe and extreme environments known to society. Power, control, and implicit authority are manifested in the physical and interpersonal environments of both correctional systems and health care systems and can be incompatible with the achievement of treatment goals (Austin, 2001; Holmes, 2005).

Security Awareness

When working with forensic clients, issues surrounding safety and security are considered critical competencies, and nurses often struggle to find the right balance between their caring and custodial roles. The therapeutic treatment needs of their clients must always be considered within the context of maintaining security. Forensic settings (apart from community-based programs) are typically highly controlled environments, with the whereabouts of clients constantly monitored through a variety of institutional routines, mechanisms, rules, and regulations (Austin, 2001; Peternelj-Taylor & Johnson, 1995). Surveillance of staff and clients is deemed critical to the safe operation of all forensic facilities. Because of this, however, nursing staff members often experience additional stressors because they too are subject to the judgement of others: those who watch over are watched over in turn (Holmes, 2005).

Forensic nurses quickly become aware of two forms of security awareness: **static security** and **dynamic security**. Static security awareness includes such things as the structural or environmental artefacts common to secure environments, for example, the use of two-way radios, personal protection alarms, video monitoring, electronic door locks, internal barriers, and perimeter fences or walls. Dynamic security awareness, on the other hand, is concerned with institutional policies, staffing patterns, methods of operation, and relational security. Finding the right balance between the security needs of the forensic setting (and the community at large) and the client's treatment needs is a balancing act at best. Practical points for competent and safe practice are found in Box 38-3.

In forensic settings operated under the jurisdiction of the health care system (e.g., forensic psychiatric hospitals and forensic psychiatric units), forensic nurses assume

BOX 38-3 Tips for Security Awareness in Forensic Settings

- When working in institutional settings, never bring anything in or take anything out for a client, regardless of how insignificant the request may seem.
- Let coworkers know your whereabouts at all times; interview clients in designated interview rooms, or in places visible to other staff members. When working in the community, always leave your itinerary, the anticipated length of your visits, and how you can be reached.
- Observe policies and procedures related to security awareness specific to the forensic setting in which you are working. Ask questions in order to understand the rationale behind the policies.
- Do not share personal information about yourself, or other staff members, with clients.
- Clients will sometimes engage in sexually inappropriate banter or gestures. Report this immediately, no matter how embarrassed you may be.
- Be aware of the location of staff members in relation to clients. Use a buddy system (e.g., another staff member) when uncomfortable approaching a client, especially when entering the client's living space.
- In all cases, open communication is critical to safe and competent nursing practice. Report all suspicious behaviours as soon as possible.

broader roles in the maintenance of security. This can be particularly disconcerting because they may be expected to handcuff clients before a court visit or search them for contraband before and after personal visits (or absences from the unit), while at the same time engage them in a therapeutic nurse–client relationship. This overt attention to custodial roles can jeopardize the fragility of the developing therapeutic relationship, and systems often need to be in place that enable nurses from other units, or those not responsible for direct nursing care, to assist with these necessary custodial measures (Woods, 2004).

Risk Assessment and Management

Forensic nurses practising in forensic settings work with clients with a proven capacity for violence. In recent years, risk assessment and management have become increasingly important competencies required of forensic nurses. Risk assessment is critical because it guides intervention and treatment. Simply stated, the greater the assessed risk, the higher the levels of intervention and supervision that are required; conversely, the lower the assessed risk, the lower the levels of intervention and supervision that are required, regardless of whether the forensic client is seeking treatment within a secure environment or a community treatment program (Woods, 2004, 2013). Although a detailed discussion of risk assessment and management is beyond the scope of this chapter, it is mentioned here because increasingly, forensic nurses, with additional training and experience, are using actuarial (or statistical) tools and structured clinical judgement to formulate treatment plans that increasingly include risk assessment

and management (Encinares & Golea, 2005; Encinares & Lorbergs, 2001; Encinares, McMaster, & McNamee, 2005). In a review of the literature, Woods and Lasiuk (2008) concluded that forensic nurses should integrate the use of empirically guided approaches to risk, including actuarial measures and structured clinical approaches, along with their own subjective qualitative clinical assessments. However, reliance on clinical judgement alone, as noted in some settings, warrants further education and training in practice (Woods, 2013).

■■ SOCIETAL NORMS

Humane care is defined by society, including the public, politicians, and the media (Mason, Lovell, & Coyle, 2008). The continual expansion of correctional facilities, however, reveals society's failure to address complex health and social issues. The Canadian Association of Elizabeth Fry Societies has declared "Women don't belong in cages: Prisons are the real crime" (see Web Links on thePoint). There is a societal expectation that imprisonment will deter others from committing crimes, as well as contribute to community safety. This can mean that prisons are more readily funded than other strategies to deal with poverty, homelessness, and mental illness. The impact of interpersonal violence and illicit drug-related activities on individuals and communities is not sufficiently addressed, nor is the lack of health care services available to vulnerable and marginalized groups (Peternelj-Taylor, 2005b).

Understanding the comprehensive needs of individuals whose lives have become enmeshed within the criminal justice system requires an understanding of both the individual and the social determinants of health that are associated with mental health, mental illness and delinquency, and criminal activity. Such an understanding provides for greater opportunities for the development of interventions and policies that may be effective at promoting mental health, preventing crime, and reducing the risk of repeat offending among those with a mental illness (CIHI, 2008). "Nursing is uniquely positioned to intervene with the socially significant health issues associated with crime, incarceration, and release" (Maeve, 2003, p. 39). Such interventions must be grounded in the conviction that caring for forensic clients as vulnerable members of society is the appropriate and decent thing to do.

SUMMARY OF KEY POINTS

■ The provision of nursing care to persons under forensic purview is a challenging and rewarding psychiatric and mental health nursing experience, one that balances the conflicting convictions of custody and caring.

■ Components of care in forensic nursing include the forensic client, nurse–client relationship, professional role development, treatment setting, and societal norms.

■ The ability to engage the forensic client in a therapeutic relationship is critical to competent forensic nursing care. Relationship issues experienced by forensic nurses include othering, boundary violations, and manipulation.

■ Forensic nurses are uniquely situated to provide nursing care to forensic clients in a variety of community- and institution-based treatment settings.

■ Intersectoral approaches that bring together justice, law, social services, education, and health care are deemed necessary to address the multitude of issues facing forensic clients, their families, and their communities.

CRITICAL THINKING CHALLENGES

1 In recent years, correctional facilities have experienced great challenges in caring for older and infirm forensic clients, and on occasion, clients are transferred to community-based long-term care facilities for compassionate reasons. What challenges might accompany the implementation of such a policy?

2 Recovery is a major tenet of the Mental Health Commission of Canada's (2012) *Changing directions, changing lives: Mental health strategy for Canada*. What factors need to be taken into consideration when planning and implementing a recovery approach when working with clients under forensic purview?

3 The ability to engage the forensic client in a therapeutic relationship is a critical competency for forensic nurses. How might nurses overcome their negative reactions to a client who has committed a heinous crime?

4 The nursing profession as a whole has become more attuned to the importance of boundaries in the therapeutic relationship. How would you approach a colleague whom you suspected was struggling to maintain professional boundaries with a forensic client?

5 Suicide is the leading cause of death in forensic environments, particularly in prison environments. Forensic nurses are in key positions to assess those in their care and influence policy accordingly. Discuss.

REFERENCES

Alzheimer Society of Canada. (2010). *Rising tide: The impact of dementia on Canadian society*. Retrieved from http://www.alzheimer.ca/en/Get-involved/Raise-your-voice/Rising-Tide

Austin, W. (2001). Relational ethics in forensic psychiatric settings. *Journal of Psychosocial Nursing and Mental Health Services*, 39(9), 12–17.

Beckett, J., Peternelj-Taylor, C., & Johnson, R. (2003). Growing old in the correctional system. *Journal of Psychosocial Nursing and Mental Health Services*, 41(9), 12–18.

Blanchard, B. (2004). Incarcerated mothers and their children: A complex issue. *Forum on Correctional Research*, 16(1), 45–46.

Blanchette, K. & Brown, S. L. (2006). *The assessment and treatment of women offenders: An integrative perspective*. Chichester, UK: John Wiley & Sons.

Canadian Federation of Mental Health Nurses. (2014). *Canadian standards for psychiatric-mental health nursing* (4th ed.). Toronto, ON: Author.

Canadian Institute for Health Information (CIHI). (2008). *Improving the health of Canadians: Mental health, delinquency and criminal activity*. Ottawa, ON: Author.

Canadian Nurses Association (CNA). (2008). *Code of ethics for registered nurses*. Ottawa, ON: Author.

Canadian Public Health Association (CPHA). (2004). A health care needs assessment of federal inmates in Canada. *Canadian Journal of Public Health*, 95(Suppl. 1), S1–S63.

Canales, M. K. (2000). Othering: Toward an understanding of difference. *Advances in Nursing Science*, 22(4), 16–31.

Canales, M. K. (2010). Othering: Difference understood?: A 10 year analysis and critique of the nursing literature. *Advances in Nursing Science*, 33, 15–34.

Chaimowitz, G. (2012). Position paper: The criminalization of people with mental illness. *Canadian Journal of Psychiatry*, 57(2), Insert 1–6.

Correctional Service Canada (CSC). (2008). *Issues and challenges facing CSC*. Retrieved from http://www.csc-scc.gc.ca/text/pblct/sb-go/07-eng.shtml

Correctional Service Canada, Federal–Provincial/Territorial Partnership. (2012). *Mental health strategy for corrections in Canada*. Retrieved from http://www.csc-scc.gc.ca/health/092/MH-strategy-eng.pdf

Cyr, J. J., & Paradis, J. (2012). The forensic float nurse: A new concept in the effective management of service delivery in a forensic program. *Journal of Forensic Nursing*, 8(4), 188–194.

de Chesnay, M. (2012). Vulnerable populations: Vulnerable people. In M. de Chesnay & B. A. Anderson (Eds.), *Caring for the vulnerable: Perspectives in nursing theory, practice and research* (3rd ed., pp. 3–15). Burlington, MA: Jones & Bartlett.

de Sousa, H. (2013). Primary and specialized care, health promotion, disease prevention within the Correction Service Canada, and the challenges of an aging population. Paper presented at the *National Correctional Services Healthcare Conference*, Ottawa.

Department of Justice Canada. (2013). *Youth justice*. Retrieved from http://www.justice.gc.ca/eng/pi/yj-jj/ycja-lsjpa/why-pourq.html

Drennan, G. & Alred, D. (2012). Recovery in forensic mental health settings. In G. Drennan & D. Alred (Eds.), *Secure recovery: Approaches to recovery in forensic mental health settings* (pp. 1–22). Abingdon, UK: Routledge.

Dupuis, T., MacKay, R., & Nicol, J. (2013). *Current issues in mental health in Canada: Mental health and the criminal justice system*. Background Paper (Publication No. 2013-88-E). Ottawa, ON: Library of Parliament.

Encinares, M. (2007). Mental health forum: Community care of elderly offenders with dementia. *Journal of Chinese Clinical Medicine*, 2(1), 34–41.

Encinares, M. & Golea, G. (2005). Client centered-care for individuals with dual diagnoses in the justice system. *Journal of Psychosocial Nursing and Mental Health Services*, 43(9), 29–36.

Encinares, M. & Lorbergs, K. (2001). Framing nursing practice within a forensic outpatient service. *Journal of Psychosocial Nursing and Mental Health Services*, 39(9), 35–41.

Encinares, M., McMaster, J. J., & McNamee, J. (2005). Risk assessment of forensic patients: Nurses' role. *Journal of Psychosocial Nursing and Mental Health Services*, 43(3), 30–36.

Faulkner, C. & Regehr, C. (2011). Sexual boundary violations committed by female forensic workers. *Journal of the American Academy of Psychiatry and the Law*, 39, 154–163.

Forensic Nurses' Society of Canada. (2014). *Mission*. Retrieved from http://forensicnurse.ca/about/

Freudenberg, N., Daniels, J., Crum, M., Perkins, T., & Ritchie, B. E. (2005). Coming home from jail: The social and health consequences of community reentry for women, male adolescents, and their families. *American Journal of Public Health*, 95(10), 1725–1726.

Goldkuhle, U. (1999). Professional education for correctional nurses: A community-based partnership model. *Journal of Psychosocial Nursing and Mental Health Services*, 37(9), 38–44.

Green, B. L., Miranda, J., Daroowalla, A., & Siddique, J. (2005). Trauma exposure, mental health functioning, and program needs of women in jail. *Crime and Delinquency*, 51, 133–151.

Gutheil, T. G. & Brodsky, A. (2008). *Preventing boundary violations in clinical practice*. New York, NY: Guilford Press.

Happell, B., Pinikahana, J., & Martin, T. (2003). Stress and burnout in forensic psychiatric nursing. *Stress and Health*, 19(2), 63–68.

Harner, H. M. (2004). Relationships between incarcerated women: Moving beyond stereotypes. *Journal of Psychosocial Nursing and Mental Health Services*, 42(1), 38–46.

Harris, D. M. (2013). Working in forensic mental health. In P. Callaghan, N. Oud, J. H. Bjørngaard, H. Nijman, T. Palmstierna, R. Almvik, & B. Thomas (Eds.), *Proceedings of the 8th European Congress on Violence* in *Clinical Psychiatry* (pp. 395–398). Amsterdam, NL: Kavanah, Dwingeloo & Oud Consultancy.

Hayes, A. J., Burns, A., Turnbull, P., & Shaw, J. J. (2012). The health and social needs of older male prisoners. *International Journal of Geriatric Psychiatry, 27*, 1155–1162.

Holmes, D. (2005). Governing the captives: Forensic psychiatric nursing in corrections. *Perspectives in Psychiatric Care, 41*(1), 3–13.

Holmes, D. (2007). Nursing in corrections: Lessons from France. *Journal of Forensic Nursing, 3*(3–4), 126–131.

Hufft, A. & Kite, M. M. (2003). Vulnerable and cultural perspectives for nursing care in correctional systems. *Journal of Multicultural Nursing and Health, 9*(1), 18–26.

Human Rights Watch. (2012). *Old behind bars: The aging prison population in the United States.* Retrieved from http://www.hrw.org/reports/2012/01/27/old-behind-bars-0

Jacob, J. D. (2014). Understanding the domestic rupture in forensic psychiatric nursing practice. *Journal of Correctional Health Care, 20*(1), 45–58.

Jacob, J. D., Gagnon, M., & Holmes, D. (2009). Nursing so-called monsters: On the importance of abjection and fear in forensic psychiatric nursing. *Journal of Forensic Nursing, 5*(3), 153–161.

Kanapaux, W. (2004). Guilty of mental illness. *Psychiatric Times, XXI*(1). Retrieved from http://www.psychiatrictimes.com/p040101a.html

Kent-Wilkinson, A. (1999). Forensic family genogram: An assessment and intervention tool. *Journal of Psychosocial Nursing and Mental Health Services, 37*(9), 52–56.

Kirmayer, L. J., Brass, G. M., & Tait, C. L. (2000). The mental health of Aboriginal peoples: Transformations of identity and community. *Canadian Journal of Psychiatry, 45*(7), 607–616.

Latimer, J. & Foss, L. C. (2004). *A one-day snapshot of Aboriginal youth in custody across Canada: Phase II.* Ottawa, ON: Department of Justice Canada. Retrieved from http://www.justice.gc.ca/eng/rp-pr/cj-jp/yj-jj/yj2-jj2/index.html

Lawson, L. (2005). Furthering the search for truth and justice. *Journal of Forensic Nursing, 1*(4), 149–150.

Lazzaretto-Green, D., Austin, W., Goble, E., Buys, L., Gorman, T., & Rankel, M. (2011). Walking a fine line: Forensic mental health practitioners' experience of working with correctional officers. *Journal of Forensic Nursing, 7*(3), 109–119.

Loeb, S. J., Hollenbeak, C. S., Penrod, J., Smith, C. A., Kitt-Lewis, E., & Crouse, S. B. (2013). Care and companionship in an isolating environment: Inmates attending to dying peers. *Journal of Forensic Nursing, 6*, 35–44.

Maeve, K. M. (2003). Nursing care partnerships with women leaving jail: Effects on health and crime. *Journal of Psychosocial Nursing and Mental Health Services, 41*(9), 30–40.

Mangnall, J. & Yurkovich, E. (2010). A grounded theory exploration of deliberate self-harm in incarcerated women. *Journal of Forensic Nursing, 6*, 88–95.

Martin, T. (2001). Something special: Forensic psychiatric nursing. *Journal of Psychiatric and Mental Health Nursing, 8*, 25–32.

Martin, T., Maguire, T., Quinn, C., Ryan, J., Bawden, L., & Summers, M. (2013). Standards of practice for forensic mental health nurses: Identifying contemporary practice. *Journal of Forensic Nursing, 9*(3), 171–178.

Mason, T., Hall, R., Caulfield, M., & Melling, K. (2010). Forensic nurses' perceptions of labels of mental illness and personality disorder: Clinical versus management issues. *Journal of Psychiatric and Mental Health Nursing, 17*, 131–140.

Mason, T., Lovell, A., & Coyle, D. (2008). Forensic psychiatric nursing: Skills and competencies: I Role dimensions. *Journal of Psychiatric and Mental Health Nursing, 15*, 118–130.

McLoughlin, K. A., Geller, J. L., & Tolan, A. (2011). Is recovery possible in a forensic hospital setting? *Archives of Psychiatric Nursing, 25*(5), 390–391.

Mental Health Commission of Canada. (2012). *Changing directions, changing lives: The mental health strategy for Canada.* Retrieved from http://strategy.mentalhealthcommission.ca/pdf/strategy-text-en.pdf

Michaels, C. & Moffett, C. (2008). Rethinking vulnerability. In M. de Chesnay & B. A. Anderson (Eds.), *Caring for the vulnerable: Perspectives in nursing theory, practice and research* (2nd ed., pp. 15–24). Sudbury, MA: Jones & Bartlett.

Munch, C. (2012). *Youth correctional statistics in Canada, 2010/2011. Juristat* (Catalogue No. 85-002-X). Retrieved from http://www.statcan.gc.ca/pub/85-002-x/2012001/article/11716-eng.pdf

Office of the Correctional Investigator (OCI). (2012). *Annual report of the Office of the Correctional Investigator 2011–2012.* Retrieved from http://www.oci-bec.gc.ca/cnt/rpt/index-eng.aspx

Office of the Correctional Investigator (OCI). (2013a). *Annual report of the Office of the Correctional Investigator 2012–2013.* Retrieved from http://www.oci-bec.gc.ca/cnt/rpt/index-eng.aspx

Office of the Correctional Investigator (OCI). (2013b). *Risky business: An investigation of the treatment and management of chronic self-injury among federally sentenced women.* Retrieved from http://www.oci-bec.gc.ca/cnt/rpt/oth-aut/oth-aut20130930-eng.aspx

Olson, R. (2012). *Prison inmate suicide—Why it matters.* Centre for Suicide Prevention. Retrieved from http://suicideinfo.ca/Library/Resources/iEinfoExchange/iE8PrisonInmateSuicide.aspx

Ormston, E. F. (2010). The criminalization of the mentally ill. *Canadian Journal of Community Mental Health, 29*(2), 5–10.

Osborne, O. (1995). Public sector psychosocial nursing. *Journal of Psychosocial Nursing and Mental Health Services, 33*(8), 4–6.

Peternelj-Taylor, C. (2000). The role of the forensic nurse in Canada: An evolving specialty. In D. Robinson & A. Kettles (Eds.), *Forensic nursing and multidisciplinary care of the mentally disordered offender* (pp. 192–212). London, UK: Jessica Kingsley Publishers.

Peternelj-Taylor, C. (2002). Professional boundaries: A matter of therapeutic integrity. *Journal of Psychosocial Nursing and Mental Health Services, 40*(4), 22–29.

Peternelj-Taylor, C. (2004). An exploration of othering in forensic psychiatric and correctional nursing. *Canadian Journal of Nursing Research, 36*(4), 130–146.

Peternelj-Taylor, C. (2005a). Conceptualizing nursing research with offenders: Another look at vulnerability. *International Journal of Law and Psychiatry, 28*, 348–359.

Peternelj-Taylor, C. (2005b). "Ordinary" women, extraordinary life circumstances. *Journal of Forensic Nursing, 1*(2), 84–85.

Peternelj-Taylor, C. (2005c). Engaging the "other." *Journal of Forensic Nursing, 1*(4), 179, 191.

Peternelj-Taylor, C. (2008). Pregnancy, childbirth and mothering: A forensic nursing response. *Journal of Forensic Nursing, 4*(2), 53–54.

Peternelj-Taylor, C. (2012). Boundaries and desire in forensic mental health nursing. In A. Aiyegbusi & G. Kelly (Eds.), *Professional and therapeutic boundaries in forensic mental health practice* (pp. 124–136). London, UK: Jessica Kingsley Publishers.

Peternelj-Taylor, C. A. & Hufft, A. G. (2006). Forensic nursing. In W. K. Mohr (Ed.), *Psychiatric-mental health nursing* (6th ed., pp. 377–393). Philadelphia, PA: Lippincott Williams & Wilkins.

Peternelj-Taylor, C. & Johnson, R. (1995). Serving time: Psychiatric mental health nursing in corrections. *Journal of Psychosocial Nursing and Mental Health Services, 33*(8), 12–19.

Peternelj-Taylor, C. & Schafer, P. (2008). Management of therapeutic boundaries. In A. Kettles, P. Woods, & R. Byrt (Eds.), *Forensic mental health nursing: Capabilities, roles and responsibilities* (pp. 309–331). London, UK: Quay Books.

Petryshen, P. (1981). Nursing the mentally disordered offender. *Canadian Nurse, 77*(6), 26–28.

Pierce, S. (2011). The lived experience of parents of adolescents who have sexually offended: I am a survivor. *Journal of Forensic Nursing, 7*, 173–181.

Pilette, P. C., Berck, C. B., & Achber, L. C. (1995). Therapeutic management of helping boundaries. *Journal of Psychosocial Nursing and Mental Health Services, 33*(1), 40–47.

Popova, S., Lange, S., Bekmuradov, D., Mihic, A., & Rehm, J. (2011). Fetal alcohol spectrum disorder prevalence estimates in the correctional system: A systematic literature review. *Canadian Journal of Public Health, 102*(5), 336–340.

Power, J., Brown, S. L., & Usher, A. M. (2013). Non-suicidal self-injury in women offenders: Motivations, emotions, and precipitating events. *International Journal of Forensic Mental Health, 12*, 192–204.

Pullan, S. E. & Lorbergs, K. A. (2001). Recruitment and retention: A successful model in forensic psychiatric nursing. *Journal of Psychosocial Nursing and Mental Health Services, 39*(9), 18–25.

Registered Nurses Association of Ontario. (2002). *Establishing therapeutic relationships.* Toronto, ON: Author. Retrieved from http://rnao.ca/bpg/guidelines/establishing-therapeutic-relationships

Registered Nurses Association of Ontario. (2006). *Establishing therapeutic relationships: Supplement.* Toronto, ON: Author. Retrieved from http://rnao.ca/sites/rnao-ca/files/storage/related/943_BPG_TR_Supplement.pdf

Rose, D. (2005). Respect for patient autonomy. *Journal of Forensic Nursing, 1*(1), 23–27.

Rose, D. N., Peter, E., Gallop, R., Angus, J. E., & Liaschenko, J. (2011). Respect in forensic psychiatric nurse-patient relationships: A practical compromise. *Journal of Forensic Nursing, 7*, 3–16.

Roth, B. & Pressé, L. (2003). Nursing interventions for parasuicidal behaviors in female offenders. *Journal of Psychosocial Nursing and Mental Health Services, 41*(9), 20–29.

Schafer, P. E. (2002). Nursing interventions and future directions with patients who constantly break rules and test boundaries. In A. M. Kettles, P. Woods, & M. Collins (Eds.), *Therapeutic interventions for forensic mental health nurses* (pp. 56–71). London, UK: Jessica Kingsley Publishers.

Schafer, P. E. & Peternelj-Taylor, C. (2003). Therapeutic relationships and boundary maintenance: The perspective of forensic patients enrolled in a treatment program for violent offenders. *Issues in Mental Health Nursing, 24*, 605–625.

Schoenly, L. (2013). Safety for the nurse and the patient. In L. Schoenly & C. M. Knox (Eds.), *Essentials of correctional nursing* (pp. 55–79). New York: Springer.

Shelton, D. (2000). Health status of young offenders and their families. *Journal of Nursing Scholarship, 32*(2), 173–178.

Shelton, D. (2001). Emotional disorders in young offenders. *Journal of Nursing Scholarship, 33*(3), 259–263.

Shelton, D. (2004). Experiences of detained young offenders in need of mental health care. *Journal of Nursing Scholarship, 36*(2), 129–133.

Shelton, D. & Pearson, G. (2005). ADHD in juvenile offenders: Treatment issues nurses need to know. *Journal of Psychosocial Nursing and Mental Health Services, 43*(9), 38–46.

Simpson, A. I. F. & Penney, S. R. (2011). The recovery paradigm in forensic mental health services. *Criminal Behaviour and Mental Health, 21*, 299–306.

Smith, S. (2005). Stepping through the looking glass: Professional autonomy in correctional nursing. *Corrections Today, 54–56*, 70.

Statistics Canada. (2009). *Section A—Overview of issues: Mental health and the criminal justice system.* Retrieved from http://www.statcan.gc.ca/pub/85-561-m/2009016/section-a-eng.htm

Stone, K., Papadopoulos, I., & Kelly, D. (2012). Establishing hospice care for prison populations: An integrative review assessing the UK and the USA perspective. *Palliative Medicine, 26*, 969–978.

Thorpe, G., Moorhouse, P., & Antonello, C. (2009). Clinical coaching in forensic psychiatry: An innovative program to recruit and retain nurses. *Journal of Psychosocial Nursing and Mental Health Services, 47*(5), 43–47.

Woods, P. (2004). The person who uses forensic mental health services. In I. Norman & I. Ryrie (Eds.), *The art and science of mental health nursing: A textbook of principles and practice* (pp. 594–623). Maidenhead, UK: Open University Press.

Woods, P. (2013). Risk assessment and management approaches on mental health units. *Journal of Psychiatric and Mental Health Nursing, 20*, 807–813.

Woods, P. & Lasiuk, G. (2008). Risk prediction: A review of the literature. *Journal of Forensic Nursing, 4*(1), 1–11.

World Health Organization (WHO). (2007). *Preventing suicide in jails and prisons.* Retrieved from http://www.who.int/mental_health/prevention/suicide/resource_jails_prisons.pdf

Brief Psychiatric Rating Scale

DIRECTIONS: Place an X in the appropriate box to represent the level of severity of each symptom.

	Not Present	Very Mild	Mild	Moderate	Mod. Severe	Severe	Extremely Severe
SOMATIC CONCERN—preoccupation with physical health, fear of physical illness, hypochondriasis.	☐	☐	☐	☐	☐	☐	☐
ANXIETY—worry, fear, overconcern for present or future, uneasiness.	☐	☐	☐	☐	☐	☐	☐
EMOTIONAL WITHDRAWAL—lack of spontaneous interaction, isolation deficiency in relating to others.	☐	☐	☐	☐	☐	☐	☐
CONCEPTUAL DISORGANIZATION—thought processes confused, disconnected, disorganized, disrupted.	☐	☐	☐	☐	☐	☐	☐
GUILT FEELINGS—self-blame, shame, remorse for past behaviour.	☐	☐	☐	☐	☐	☐	☐
TENSION—physical and motor manifestations of nervousness, overactivation.	☐	☐	☐	☐	☐	☐	☐
MANNERISMS AND POSTURING—peculiar, bizarre unnatural motor behaviour (not including tic).	☐	☐	☐	☐	☐	☐	☐
GRANDIOSITY—exaggerated self-opinion, arrogance, conviction of unusual power or abilities.	☐	☐	☐	☐	☐	☐	☐
DEPRESSIVE MOOD—sorrow, sadness, despondency, pessimism.	☐	☐	☐	☐	☐	☐	☐
HOSTILITY—animosity, contempt, belligerence, disdain for others.	☐	☐	☐	☐	☐	☐	☐
SUSPICIOUSNESS—mistrust, belief that others harbour malicious or discriminatory intent.	☐	☐	☐	☐	☐	☐	☐
HALLUCINATORY BEHAVIOUR—perceptions without normal external stimulus correspondence.	☐	☐	☐	☐	☐	☐	☐
MOTOR RETARDATION—slowed, weakened movements or speech, reduced body tone.	☐	☐	☐	☐	☐	☐	☐
UNCOOPERATIVENESS—resistance, guardedness, rejection of authority.	☐	☐	☐	☐	☐	☐	☐
UNUSUAL THOUGHT CONTENT—unusual, odd, strange, bizarre thought content.	☐	☐	☐	☐	☐	☐	☐
BLUNTED AFFECT—reduced emotional tone, reduction in formal intensity of feelings, flatness.	☐	☐	☐	☐	☐	☐	☐
EXCITEMENT—heightened emotional tone, agitation, increased reactivity.	☐	☐	☐	☐	☐	☐	☐
DISORIENTATION—confusion or lack of proper association for person, place, or time.	☐	☐	☐	☐	☐	☐	☐
Global Assessment Scale (Range 1–100)	☐	☐	☐	☐	☐	☐	☐

Reprinted with permission from Overall, J. E. (1988). The Brief Psychiatric Rating Scale (BPRS): Recent developments in ascertainment and scaling. *Psychopharmacology Bulletin*, 24, 97–99.

APPENDIX B

Simpson-Angus Rating Scale

1. GAIT: The patient is examined as he walks into the examining room; his gait, the swing of his arms, and his general posture all form the basis for an overall score for this item. This is rated as follows:

   0 Normal
   1 Diminution in swing while the patient is walking
   2 Marked diminution in swing with obvious rigidity in the arm
   3 Stiff gait with arms held rigidly before the abdomen
   4 Stooped shuffling gait with propulsion and retropulsion

2. ARM DROPPING: The patient and the examiner both raise their arms to shoulder height and let them fall to their sides. In a normal subject, a stout slap is heard as the arms hit the sides. In the patient with extreme Parkinson's syndrome, the arms fall very slowly.

   0 Normal, free fall with loud slap and rebound
   1 Fall slowed slightly with less audible contact and little rebound
   2 Fall slowed, no rebound
   3 Marked slowing, no slap at all
   4 Arms fall as though against resistance, as though through glue

3. SHOULDER SHAKING: The subject's arms are bent at a right angle at the elbow and are taken one at a time by the examiner who grasps one hand and also clasps the other around the subject's elbow. The subject's upper arm is pushed to and fro, and the humerus is externally rotated. The degree of resistance from normal to extreme rigidity is scored as follows:

   0 Normal
   1 Slight stiffness and resistance
   2 Moderate stiffness and resistance
   3 Marked rigidity with difficulty in passive movement
   4 Extreme stiffness and rigidity with almost a frozen shoulder

4. ELBOW RIGIDITY: The elbow joints are separately bent at right angles and passively extended and flexed, with the subject's biceps observed and simultaneously palpated. The resistance to this procedure is rated. (The presence of cogwheel rigidity is noted separately.) Scoring is from 0 to 4, as in the Shoulder Shaking test.

   0 Normal
   1 Slight stiffness and resistance
   2 Moderate stiffness and resistance
   3 Marked rigidity with difficulty in passive movement
   4 Extreme stiffness and rigidity with almost a frozen shoulder

5. FIXATION OF POSITION OR WRIST RIGIDITY: The examiner holds the wrist in one hand and the fingers in the other hand, with the wrist moved to extension, flexion, and both ulnar and radial deviation. The resistance to this procedure is rated as in Items 3 and 4.

   0 Normal
   1 Slight stiffness and resistance
   2 Moderate stiffness and resistance
   3 Marked rigidity with difficulty in passive movement
   4 Extreme stiffness and rigidity with almost a frozen shoulder

6. LEG PENDULOUSNESS: The patient sits on a table with his legs hanging down and swinging free. The ankle is grasped by the examiner and raised until the knee is partially extended. It is then allowed to fall. The resistance to falling and the lack of swinging form the basis for the score on this item.

   0 The legs swing freely
   1 Slight diminution in the swing of the legs
   2 Moderate resistance to swing
   3 Marked resistance and damping of swing
   4 Complete absence of swing

7. HEAD DROPPING: The patient lies on a well-padded examining table, and his head is raised by the examiner's hand. The hand is then withdrawn, and the head is allowed to drop. In the normal subject, the head will fall upon the table. The movement

is delayed in extrapyramidal system disorder, and in extreme parkinsonism, it is absent. The neck muscles are rigid, and the head does not reach the examining table. Scoring is as follows:

    0 The head falls completely, with a good thump as it hits the table

    1 Slight slowing in fall, mainly noted by lack of slap as the head meets the table

    2 Moderate slowing in the fall, quite noticeable to the eye

    3 The head falls stiffly and slowly

    4 The head does not reach the examining table

8. GLABELLA TAP: The subject is told to open the eyes wide and not to blink. The glabella region is tapped at a steady, rapid speed. The number of times the patient blinks in succession is noted:

    0 0 to 5 blinks

    1 6 to 10 blinks

    2 11 to 15 blinks

    3 16 to 20 blinks

    4 21 or more blinks

9. TREMOR: The patient is observed walking into the examining room and then is reexamined for this item:

    0 Normal

    1 Mild finger tremor, obvious to sight and touch

    2 Tremor of hand or arm occurring spasmodically

    3 Persistent tremor of one or more limbs

    4 Whole body tremor

10. SALIVATION: The patient is observed while talking and then asked to open the mouth and elevate the tongue. The following ratings are given:

    0 Normal

    1 Excess salivation to the extent that pooling takes place if the mouth is open and the tongue raised

    2 When excess salivation is present and might occasionally result in difficulty in speaking

    3 Speaking with difficulty because of excess salivation

    4 Frank drooling

Scoring: Each item is rated on a 5-point scale, with 0 meaning the complete absence of the condition and 4 meaning the presence of the condition in extreme form. The score is obtained by adding the items and dividing by 10.

APPENDIX C

Abnormal Involuntary Movement Scale (AIMS)

	None	Minimal	Mild	Moderate	Severe
Facial and Oral Movements					
1: Muscles of facial expression (e.g., movements of forehead, eyebrows, periorbital area, cheeks, include frowning, blinking, smiling, grimacing)	0	1	2	3	4
2: Lips and perioral area (e.g., puckering, pouting, smacking)	0	1	2	3	4
3: Jaw (e.g., biting, clenching, chewing, mouth opening, lateral movement)	0	1	2	3	4
4: Tongue Rate only increase in movement both in and out of the mouth, NOT inability to sustain movement	0	1	2	3	4
Extremity Movements					
5: Upper (arms, wrists, hands, fingers) Include choreic movements (i.e., rapid, objectively purposeless, irregular, spontaneous), athetoid movements (i.e., slow, irregular, complex, serpentine) Do NOT include tremor (i.e., repetitive, regular, rhythmic)	0	1	2	3	4
6: Lower (legs, knees, ankles, toes) (e.g., lateral knee movement, foot tapping, heel dropping, foot squirming, inversion and eversion of the foot)	0	1	2	3	4
Trunk Movements					
7: Neck, shoulders, hips (e.g., rocking, twisting, squirming, pelvic gyrations)	0	1	2	3	4
8: Severity of abnormal movements	0	1	2	3	4
Global Judgment					
9: Incapacitation due to abnormal movements	0	1	2	3	4

10: Patient's awareness of abnormal movements
Rate only the patient's report

No awareness	0
Aware, no distress	1
Aware, mild distress	2
Aware, moderate distress	3
Aware, severe distress	4

Global Judgment

11: Current problems with teeth and/or dentures

No	0
Yes	1

12: Does the patient usually wear dentures?

No	0
Yes	1

Examination Procedures for AIMS

Either before or after completing the examination procedure, observe the patient unobtrusively, at rest (e.g., in the waiting room). The chair to be used in this examination should be a hard, firm one without arms.

  1: Ask the patient whether there is anything in his/her mouth (i.e., gum, candy, etc.) and if there is, to remove it.

  2: Ask the patient about the *current* condition of his/her teeth. Ask the patient if he/she wears dentures. Do teeth or dentures bother the patient *now?*

  3: Ask the patient whether he/she notices any movements in the mouth, face, hands, or feet. If yes, ask the patient to describe and to what extent they *currently* bother him/her or interfere with his/her activities.

  4: Have the patient sit in the chair with hands on knees, legs slightly apart, and feet flat on the floor. (Look at the entire body for movements while in this position.)

  5: Ask the patient to sit with his/her hands hanging unsupported. If male, between legs; if female and wearing a dress, hanging over knees. (Observe hands and other body areas.)

  6: Ask the patient to open his/her mouth. (Observe tongue at rest within the mouth.) Do this twice.

  7: Ask the patient to protrude the tongue. (Observe tongue at rest within the mouth.) Do this twice.

 *8: Ask the patient to tap the thumb, with each finger, as rapidly as possible for 10–15 seconds; separately with right hand, then with left hand. (Observe facial and leg movements.)

  9: Flex and extend the patient's left and right arms (one at a time). (Note any rigidity and rate on NOTES.)

10: Ask the patient to stand up. (Observe in profile. Observe all body areas again, hips included.)

*11: Ask the patient to extend both arms outstretched in front with palms down. (Observe trunk, legs, and mouth.)

*12: Have the patient walk a few paces, turn, and walk back to the chair. (Observe hand and gait.) Do this twice.

-----

*Activated movements.

Reprinted from Guy, W. (1976). *ECDEU: Assessment manual for psychopharmacology (DHEW Publication No. 76-338).* Washington, DC: Department of Health, Education, and Welfare, Psychopharmacology Research Branch.

APPENDIX D

Simplified Diagnoses for Tardive Dyskinesia (SD-TD)

PREREQUISITES—The three prerequisites are as follows. Exceptions may occur.

1. A history of at least 3 months' total cumulative neuroleptic exposure. Include amoxapine and metoclopramide in all categories below as well.
2. **SCORING/INTENSITY LEVEL.** The presence of a **TOTAL SCORE OF FIVE OR ABOVE.** Also, be alert for any change from baseline or scores below five that have at least a "moderate" (3) or "severe" (4) movement on any item or at least two "mild" (2) movements on two items located in different body areas.
3. Other conditions are not responsible for the abnormal involuntary movements.

DIAGNOSES—The diagnosis is based upon the current exam and its relation to the last exam. The diagnosis can shift depending upon (a) whether movements are present or not, (b) whether movements are present for 3 months or more (6 months if on a semiannual assessment schedule), and (c) whether neuroleptic dosage changes occur and effect movements.

- **NO TD**—Movements **are not** present on this exam **or** movements are present, but some other condition is responsible for them. The last diagnosis must be NO TD, PROBABLE TD, or WITHDRAWAL TD.
- **PROBABLE TD**—Movements **are** present on this exam. This is the first time they are present, **or** they have never been present for 3 months or more. The last diagnosis must be NO TD or PROBABLE TD.

- **PERSISTENT TD**—Movements **are** present on this exam, **and** they have been present for 3 months or more with this exam or at some point in the past. The last diagnosis can be any except NO TD.
- **MASKED TD**—Movements **are not** present on this exam, **but** this is due to a neuroleptic dosage increase or reinstitution after a prior exam when movements were present. Also, use this conclusion if movements are not present due to the addition of a nonneuroleptic medication to treat TD. The last diagnosis must be PROBABLE TD, PERSISTENT TD, WITHDRAWAL TD, or MASKED TD.
- **REMITTED TD**—Movements **are not** present on this exam, **but** PERSISTENT TD has been diagnosed **and** neuroleptic dosage increase or reinstitution has occurred. The last diagnosis must be PERSISTENT TD or REMITTED TD. If movements reemerge, the diagnosis shifts back to PERSISTENT TD.
- **WITHDRAWAL TD**—Movements **are not seen while** receiving neuroleptics or at the last dosage level **but are seen within** 8 weeks following a neuroleptic reduction or discontinuation. The last diagnosis must be NO TD or WITHDRAWAL TD. If movements continue for 3 months or more after the neuroleptic dosage reduction or discontinuation, the diagnosis shifts to PERSISTENT TD. If movements do not continue for 3 months or more after the reduction or discontinuation, the diagnosis shifts to NO TD.

Instructions	**Other Conditions (Partial List)**

Instructions

1. The rater completes the assessment according to the standardized exam procedure. If the rater also completes evaluation items 1–4, he or she must also sign the preparer box. The form is given to the physician. Alternatively, the physician may perform the assessment.

2. The physician completes the Evaluation section. The physician is responsible for the entire Evaluation section and its accuracy.

3. It is recommended that the physician examines any individual who meets the three prerequisites or who has movements not explained by other factors. Neurological assessments or differential diagnostic tests that may be necessary should be performed.

4. File form according to policy or procedure.

Other Conditions (Partial List)

1. Age
2. Blind
3. Cerebral Palsy
4. Contact Lenses
5. Dentures/No Teeth
6. Down's Syndrome
7. Drug Intoxication (specify)
8. Encephalitis
9. Extrapyramidal Side Effects (specify)
10. Fahr's Syndrome
11. Heavy Metal Intoxication (specify)
12. Huntington's Chorea
13. Hyperthyroidism
14. Hypoglycaemia
15. Hypoparathyroidism
16. Idiopathic Torsion Dystonia
17. Meige's Syndrome
18. Parkinson's Disease
19. Stereotypies
20. Sydenham's Chorea
21. Tourette's Syndrome
22. Wilson's Disease
23. Other (specify)

Sprague, R. L. & Kalachnik, J. E. (1991). Reliability, validity, and a total score cutoff for the Dyskinesia Identification System Condensed User Scale (DISCUS) with mentally ill and mentally retarded populations. *Psychopharmacology Bulletin*, *27*(1), 51–58.

Hamilton Rating Scale for Depression

Clinic No._____ Date_____ Rating No._____ Code Number_____

Sex_____ Age_____ Patient's Name_____

Patient's Address_____ Tel_____

Item	Range	Score
1. Depressed mood	0–4	
2. Guilt	0–4	
3. Suicide	0–4	
4. Insomnia initial	0–2	
5. Insomnia middle	0–2	
6. Insomnia delayed	0–2	
7. Work and interest	0–4	
8. Retardation	0–4	
9. Agitation	0–4	
10. Anxiety (psychic)	0–4	
11. Anxiety (somatic)	0–4	
12. Somatic gastrointestinal	0–2	
13. Somatic general	0–2	
14. Genital	0–2	
15. Hypochondriasis	0–2	
16. Insight	0–4	
17. Loss of weight	0–2	
Total score		
Diurnal variation (M.A.E.)	0–2	
Depersonalization	0–4	
Paranoid symptoms	0–4	
Obsessional symptoms	0–4	

The scale is designed to measure the severity of illness of patients already diagnosed as suffering from depressive illness. It is obviously not a diagnostic instrument because that requires much more information (e.g., previous history, family history, precipitating factors).

As far as possible, the scale should be used in the manner of a clinical interview. The first time, the interview should be conducted in a relaxed, free, and easy manner, giving the patients time to unburden themselves and giving them the opportunity to speak of their problems and ask whatever questions they wish. It may then be necessary to obtain further information by asking them questions. At subsequent assessments, the interview can be briefer and more to the point.

An observer rating scale is not a checklist in which each item is strictly defined. The raters must have sufficient clinical experience and judgment to be able to interpret the patients' statements and reticences about some symptoms and to compare them with other patients. They should use all sources of information (e.g., from relatives and nurses).

The scale consists of 17 items, the scores of which are summed to give a total score. These are four other items, one of which (diurnal variation) is excluded on the grounds that it is not an additional burden on the patient. The last three are excluded from the total score because they occur infrequently, although information on them may be useful for other purposes.

The method of assessment is simple. For some symptoms, it is difficult to elicit such information as will permit of full quantification. If present, score 2; if absent, score 0; and if doubtful or trivial, score 1. For those symptoms where more detailed information can be obtained, the score of 2 is expanded into 2 for mild, 3 for moderate, and 4 for severe. In case of difficulty, the raters should use their judgment as clinicians.

Hamilton, M. (1960). A rating scale for depression. *Journal of Neurology, Neurosurgery and Psychiatry, 23*, 56.

Clinical Institute Withdrawal Assessment of Alcohol Scale, Revised (CIWA-Ar)

Patient: _____ **Date:** _____ **Time:** _____ (24 hour clock, midnight = 00:00)

Pulse or heart rate, taken for 1 minute: _____ **Blood pressure:** _____

NAUSEA AND VOMITING—Ask "Do you feel sick to your stomach? Have you vomited?" Observation.
- 0 no nausea and no vomiting
- 1 mild nausea with no vomiting
- 2
- 3
- 4 intermittent nausea with dry heaves
- 5
- 6
- 7 constant nausea, frequent dry heaves and vomiting

TREMOR—Arms extended and fingers spread apart. Observation.
- 0 no tremor
- 1 not visible, but can be felt fingertip to fingertip
- 2
- 3
- 4 moderate, with patient's arms extended
- 5
- 6
- 7 severe, even with arms not extended

PAROXYSMAL SWEATS—Observation.
- 0 no sweat visible
- 1 barely perceptible sweating, palms moist
- 2
- 3
- 4 beads of sweat obvious on forehead
- 5
- 6
- 7 drenching sweats

TACTILE DISTURBANCES—Ask "Have you any itching, pins and needles sensations, any burning, any numbness, or do you feel bugs crawling on or under your skin?" Observation.
- 0 none
- 1 very mild itching, pins and needles, burning or numbness
- 2 mild itching, pins and needles, burning or numbness
- 3 moderate itching, pins and needles, burning or numbness
- 4 moderately severe hallucinations
- 5 severe hallucinations
- 6 extremely severe hallucinations
- 7 continuous hallucinations

AUDITORY DISTURBANCES—Ask "Are you more aware of sounds around you?" "Are they harsh?" "Do they frighten you?" "Are you hearing anything that is disturbing to you?" "Are you hearing things you know are not there?" Observation.
- 0 not present
- 1 very mild harshness or ability to frighten
- 2 mild harshness or ability to frighten
- 3 moderate harshness or ability to frighten
- 4 moderately severe hallucinations
- 5 severe hallucinations
- 6 extremely severe hallucinations
- 7 continuous hallucinations

VISUAL DISTURBANCES—Ask "Does the light appear to be too bright?" "Is its color different?" "Does it hurt your eyes?" "Are you seeing anything that is disturbing to you?" "Are you seeing things you know are not there?" Observation.
- 0 not present
- 1 very mild sensitivity
- 2 mild sensitivity
- 3 moderate sensitivity
- 4 moderately severe hallucinations
- 5 severe hallucinations
- 6 extremely severe hallucinations
- 7 continuous hallucinations

ANXIETY—Ask "Do you feel nervous?" Observation.
0 no anxiety, at ease
1 mild anxious
2
3
4 moderately anxious, or guarded, so anxiety is inferred
5
6
7 equivalent to acute panic states as seen in severe delirium or acute schizophrenic reactions

AGITATION—Observation.
0 normal activity
1 somewhat more than normal activity
2
3
4 moderately fidgety and restless
5
6
7 paces back and forth during most of the interview, or constantly thrashes about

HEADACHE, FULLNESS IN HEAD—Ask "Does your head feel different?" "Does it feel like there is a band around your head?" Do not rate for dizziness or light-headedness. Otherwise, rate severity.
0 not present
1 very mild
2 mild
3 moderate
4 moderately severe
5 severe
6 very severe
7 extremely severe

ORIENTATION AND CLOUDING OF SENSORIUM—Ask "What day is this?" "Where are you?" "Who am I?"
0 oriented and can do serial additions
1 cannot do serial additions or is uncertain about date
2 disoriented for date by no more than 2 calendar days
3 disoriented for date by more than 2 calendar days
4 disoriented for place/or person

Total **CIWA-Ar** Score _____
Rater's Initials _____
Maximum Possible Score 67

The CIWA-Ar is not copyrighted and may be reproduced freely. This assessment for monitoring withdrawal symptoms requires approximately 5 minutes to administer. The maximum score is 67 (see instrument). Patients scoring less than 10 do not usually need additional medication for withdrawal.

Sullivan, J. T., Sykora, K., Schneiderman, J., Naranjo, C. A., & Sellers, E. M. (1989). Assessment of alcohol withdrawal: The revised Clinical Institute Withdrawal Assessment for Alcohol scale (CIWA-Ar). *British Journal of Addiction, 84*, 1353–1357.

absorption Movement of drug from the site of administration into plasma.

acetylcholine (ACh) An important neurotransmitter associated with cognitive functioning, and disruption of cholinergic mechanisms damages memory in animals and humans.

acetylcholinesterase (AChE) Key enzyme that inactivates the neurotransmitter acetylcholine. AChE is found in high concentrations in the brain and is one of two cholinesterase enzymes capable of breaking down ACh.

acetylcholinesterase inhibitors (AChEIs) Mainstay of pharmacologic treatment of dementia; these drugs inhibit AChE, resulting in an enhancement of cholinergic activity. AChEIs have been shown to delay the decline in cognitive functioning but generally do not improve cognitive function once it has declined; therefore, it is important that this medication be started as soon as the diagnosis is made.

active listening Focusing on what the patient is saying in order to interpret and respond to the message in an objective manner, while using techniques such as open-ended statements, reflection, and questions that elicit additional responses from the patient.

acute stress disorder (ASD) A mental disorder characterized by persistent, distressing stress-related symptoms that last between 2 days and 1 month and that occur within 1 month after a traumatic experience.

adaptability Capacity of a person to survive and flourish.

adaptive inflexibility Rigidity in interactions with others, achievement of goals, and coping with stress.

addiction A chronic, relapsing brain disorder that results from the prolonged effects of exposure of the brain to drugs (substances or chemicals).

adherence A patient's maintenance of the therapeutic regimen, includes self-administering medications as prescribed, keeping appointments, and following other treatment suggestions; it exists on a continuum and can be conceived of as full, partial, or nil.

adverse reactions Unwanted medication effects that may have serious physiologic consequences.

affect An expression of mood manifest in a pattern of observable behaviours.

affective blunting Flat or blunted emotion.

affective instability Rapid and extreme shifts in mood, erratic emotional responses to situations, and intense sensitivity to criticism or perceived slights; one of the core characteristics of borderline personality disorder.

affective lability Abrupt, dramatic, unprovoked changes in the types of emotions expressed.

afferent Towards the central nervous system or a particular structure.

affinity Degree of attraction or strength of the bond between a drug and its receptor.

aggression Behaviours or attitudes that reflect rage, hostility, and the potential for physical or verbal destructiveness; usually occurs if the person believes someone is going to do him or her harm.

agitation Inability to sit still or attend to others, accompanied by heightened emotions and tension.

agnosia Failure to recognize or identify objects despite intact sensory function, or a disturbance in executive functioning (ability to think abstractly, plan, initiate, sequence, monitor, and stop complex behaviour).

agonists Chemicals producing the same biologic action as the neurotransmitter.

agoraphobia Anxiety about being in places from which escape might be difficult or embarrassing, or about being in places in which help may not be readily available if a panic attack should occur.

akathisia A medication-related, involuntary movement disorder characterized by the inability to sit still; may be experienced as "jitteriness" without obvious motor behaviour.

alexithymia Inability to experience and communicate feelings consciously.

allodynia Lowered pain threshold.

allostasis Adaptive processes that maintain homeostasis through the production of various brain and peripheral stress-related chemicals and promote adaptation to perceived threat or stress.

alogia Brief, empty verbal responses; often referred to as *poverty of speech*.

ambivalence Presence and expression of two opposing forces, leading to inaction.

amino acids Building blocks of proteins that have different roles. Amino acids function as neurotransmitters in as many as 60% to 70% of synaptic sites in the brain.

amygdala A bulb-like structure attached to the tail of the caudate and often considered part of the limbic system.

anger An affective state experienced as the motivation to act in ways that warn, intimidate, or attack those who are perceived as challenging or threatening.

anhedonia Inability to gain pleasure from activities.

anorexia nervosa A life-threatening eating disorder characterized by refusal to maintain body weight appropriate for age, intense fear of gaining weight or becoming fat, a severely distorted body image, and refusal to acknowledge the seriousness of weight loss.

antagonists Chemicals blocking the biologic response at a given receptor site.

anticholinergic crisis A potentially life-threatening medical emergency that occurs as a result of overdose or sensitivity to drugs with anticholinergic properties.

anxiety Apprehension or dread in response to internal or external stimuli that can be experienced in physical, emotional, cognitive, and/or behavioural ways.

anxiolytics Drugs that reverse or diminish anxiety.

apathy Reactions to stimuli that are decreased, along with a diminished interest and desire.

aphasia Alterations in language ability.

apraxia Impaired ability to execute motor activities despite intact motor functioning.

ascertainment bias Bias that occurs in research when the method of identifying cases creates a sample that differs from the population it purports to represent.

assertiveness A set of behaviours and a communication style that is open, honest, direct, and confident that enables the expression of emotions, including anger, in a manner that assumes responsibility.

assessment The purposeful and systematic collection, evaluation, and documentation of a client's health–illness information.

assortative mating Tendency for individuals to select mates who are similar in genetically linked traits such as intelligence and personality styles.

attachment Emotional bond between the infant and parental figure.

attention deficit hyperactivity disorder (ADHD) Neuropsychiatric developmental disorder associated with functional impairments such as school dysfunction and peer and family conflicts.

autism spectrum disorder A pervasive developmental disorder (PDD) that is distinguished from other PDDs by early age of onset (before age 30 months) and severe disturbance in social relatedness. Children with autism appear indifferent to others and to prefer inanimate objects.

automatic thoughts Spontaneous words and images generated in a particular situation that may be illogical and/or difficult to stop.

autonomic nervous system Part of the nervous system that regulates involuntary vital functions including cardiac muscle, smooth muscles, and glands. It is composed of the sympathetic and parasympathetic systems.

autonomy Concept that each person has the fundamental right of self-determination.

avolition Inability to complete projects, assignments, or work.

basal ganglia One set of structures in each hemisphere; areas of grey matter containing many cell bodies or nuclei.

behaviour modification A specific, systematized behaviour therapy technique that can be applied to individuals, groups, or systems.

behaviour therapy Interventions that reinforce or promote desirable behaviours or alter undesirable ones.

behaviourism A paradigm shift in understanding human behaviour that was initiated by Watson, who theorized that human behaviour is developed through a stimulus–response process rather than through unconscious drives or instincts.

beneficence The ethical principle of "try to do good"; promote benefit.

bereavement The objective event or occurrence of having suffered a loss.

best practice guidelines (BPGs) Clinical practice recommendations based on the best current evidence.

bibliotherapy The use of books and other reading materials to help individuals cope with various life stressors.

binge eating Episodes of uncontrollable, ravenous eating of large amounts of food within discrete periods of time, usually followed by feelings of guilt that result in purging.

bioavailability The amount of the drug that actually reaches systemic circulation; affected significantly by the route by which a drug is administered.

biogenic amines Small molecules manufactured in the neuron that contain an amine group. These include dopamine, norepinephrine, and epinephrine (all synthesized from the amino acid tyrosine); serotonin (from tryptophan); and histamine (from histidine).

biologic markers Physical indicators of disturbances within the central nervous system that differentiate one disease state from another.

biotransformation (metabolism) The process by which a drug is altered, often broken down into smaller substances known as *metabolites*.

body dissatisfaction The body becomes overvalued as a way of determining one's worth. Body dissatisfaction has been related to low self-esteem, depression, dieting, bingeing, and purging.

body image Self-perception of one's body. Extreme discrepancy between body image and others' perceptions of one's body indicates a *body image distortion*.

boundaries The defining limits of individuals, objects, or relationships.

boundary violation Behaviour by a professional that has violated the limits (what is and is not permitted) in a professional–client relationship.

bradykinesia An extrapyramidal condition characterized by a slowness of voluntary movement and speech.

brain stem Area of the brain containing the midbrain, pons, and medulla, which continues beneath the thalamus.

breach of confidentiality Release of patient information without the patient's consent in the absence of legal compulsion or authorization to release information.

Broca's area A section of the left frontal lobe of the brain thought to be responsible for the articulation of speech.

bulimia nervosa An eating disorder in which the individual engages in recurrent episodes of binge eating and compensatory behaviour to avoid weight gain through purging methods such as self-induced vomiting, or use of laxatives, diuretics, enemas, or emetics, or through nonpurging methods such as fasting or excessive exercise.

bullying Persistent physical or psychological harm that is intentionally inflicted on an individual who feels unable to avoid or stop the harm.

burnout Psychological exhaustion, detachment, and loss of sense of accomplishment related to chronic work-related stress.

butyrylcholinesterase (BuChE) A nonspecific cholinesterase found in the brain and especially in the glial cells. Both acetylcholinesterase and BuChE work in the gastrointestinal tract. If these enzymes are inhibited, the breakdown of acetylcholine will be delayed, resulting in an increase in acetylcholine activity.

case management Problem solving and coordinating services for the patient to ensure continuity of services and overcome system rigidity, fragmentation of services, misuse of facilities, and inaccessibility.

catatonic excitement Hyperactivity characterized by purposeless activity and abnormal movements like grimacing and posturing.

central sulcus Posterior boundary of the frontal lobe that separates it from the parietal lobe.

cerebellum Part of the brain that is responsible for controlling movement and postural adjustments; it receives information from all parts of the body.

cerebrospinal fluid Cushioning fluid that circulates around the brain beneath the arachnoid layer in the subarachnoid space; it is colourless and contains sodium chloride and other salts.

chemical restraints Use of medication to control patients or manage behaviour.

cholecystokinin A neuropeptide found in high levels in the cerebral cortex, hypothalamus, and amygdala; it is also excreted by the gastrointestinal system in response to food intake, which is believed to play a role in the control of eating and satiety by controlling the release of dopamine.

chronobiology Study and measure of time structures or biologic rhythms.

circadian rhythm (cycle) From the Latin *circa* and *dies*, meaning "about a day"; refers to a biologic system that fluctuates or oscillates in a pattern that repeats itself in about a day.

circumstantiality Occurs when an individual takes a long time to make a point because his or her conversation is indirect and contains excessive and unnecessary detail.

clang association Repetition of word phrases that are similar in sound but in no other way, for example, "right, light, sight, might."

classical conditioning A learning situation in which an unconditioned stimulus initially produces an unconditioned response; over time, a conditioned response is elicited for a specific stimulus (Pavlov).

clearance Total amount of blood, serum, or plasma from which a drug is completely removed per unit of time.

clinical domain outcome statements Statements that indicate a reduction in symptoms of illness or cure of a specific mental illness.

closed group A group in which all the members begin at one time. New members are not admitted after the first meeting.

cognition A system of interrelated abilities, such as perception, reasoning, judgement, intuition, and memory, that allow one to be aware of oneself and one's surroundings. Impairments in these abilities can result in a failure of the afflicted person to recognize that he or she is not well and is in need of treatment.

cognitive restructuring A process in which cognitions (automatic thoughts, intermediate and core beliefs) are identified, analyzed, and modified to effect positive change in mood and behaviour.

cognitive schema (core beliefs) Basic beliefs so fundamental that they are accepted as absolute truths; assist in evaluating and assigning meaning to events and influence subsequent affective and behavioural responses.

cognitive–behavioural model A model of perception that includes emotion, cognition, environment, and physical and psychological factors.

cognitive–behavioural therapy Psychotherapy focused on identifying, analyzing, and ultimately changing the habitually inflexible and negative cognitions about oneself, others, and the world that contribute to distress and problematic behaviours.

communication triad A technique used to provide a specific syntax and order for patients to identify and express their feelings and seek relief. The "sentence" consists of three parts: (1) an "I" statement to identify the prevailing feeling, (2) a nonjudgemental statement of the emotional trigger, and (3) a statement of what the person would like differently or what would restore comfort to the situation.

community treatment orders (CTOs) A type of mandatory outpatient treatment, usually initiated by a physician, that can require an individual with a mental illness who does not meet provincial involuntary admission criteria to comply with stipulated treatment.

comorbidity (comorbid) Disease that coexists with the primary disease.

compassion fatigue Disengagement on the part of caregiving professionals; frequently equated with burnout.

compassionate release *Parole by exception* for incarcerated offenders, allowed under the Corrections and Conditional Release Act, and considered on an individual basis (e.g., for palliative care due to a terminal illness).

competence The degree to which the patient is able to understand and appreciate the information given during the consent process; the patient's cognitive ability to process information at a specific time; the patient's ability to gather and interpret information and make reasonable judgements based on that information to participate fully as a partner in treatment.

compulsions Behaviours that are performed repeatedly, in a ritualistic fashion, with the goal of preventing or relieving anxiety and distress caused by obsessions.

concordant Used in genetics to indicate that both members of twins have same trait.

concrete thinking Lack of abstraction in thinking, in which people are unable to understand punch lines, metaphors, and analogies.

concurrent disorders The term used when an individual has at least one substance-related or addictive disorder co-occurring with at least one other mental disorder.

confabulation False memories, perceptions, or beliefs that are the consequence of neurologic dysfunction or damage.

confidentiality An ethical duty of nondisclosure; the patient has the right to disclose personal information without fear of it being revealed to others.

conflict resolution A specific type of counselling in which the nurse helps the patient resolve a disagreement or dispute.

conservation The child's awareness that a quantity remains the same despite its shape.

content themes Repetition of concerns or feelings that occur within the therapeutic relationship. Themes may emerge as symbolic representations of fears.

continuum of care The integrated health system of supports and services that is provided by professional health care clinicians (some who offer specialized services, such as psychiatric and mental health services), as well as by nonprofessional caregivers, designed to maximize people's health and well-being.

coping An individual's constantly changing cognitive and behavioural efforts to manage specific external or internal demands that are appraised as taxing or exceeding the individual's resources.

corpus callosum Functional link between the two hemispheres of the brain, made up of a thick band of fibres.

cortex Outer surface of the mature brain.

cortical dementia A type of dementia that is characterized by amnesia, aphasia, apraxia, and agnosia.

counselling interventions Specific time-limited interactions between a nurse and a patient, family, or group experiencing intermediate or ongoing difficulties related to their health or well-being.

countertransference The nurse's reactions to a patient that are based on the nurse's unconscious needs, conflicts, problems, and views of the world. It can significantly interfere with the nurse–patient relationship.

crisis A severely stressful experience for which coping mechanisms fail to provide any adaptation, whether the experience is positive or negative.

crisis intervention A specialized short-term (usually no longer than 6 hours) goal-directed therapy designed to assist patients in an immediate manner, after which they are usually transferred to an inpatient unit or an intensive outpatient setting.

crisis response Occurs when an individual encounters an obstacle or problem important to life goals that cannot be solved by customary problem-solving methods; acute, time-limited, and may be developmental, situational, or interpersonal in nature.

cultural brokering Act of bridging, linking, or mediating between groups or individuals of different cultural systems for the purpose of reducing conflict or producing change.

cultural competence The ability to give care and services appropriate to the cultural characteristics of the person, family, or community receiving them.

culture A way of life that is the totality of learned, socially transmitted beliefs, values, and behaviours emerging from interpersonal transactions of people who identify or associate with one another on the basis of a common purpose, need, or similarity of background.

cycle of violence A three-phase pattern of tension, abuse, and kindness in which the abuser engages first in abuse and then in seemingly sincere expressions of love, contrition, and remorse.

cyclothymic A term used to describe periods of hypomanic and depressive episodes that do not meet full criteria for a major depressive episode.

de-escalation An interactive process of calming and redirecting a patient who has an immediate potential for violence directed at others or self.

defence mechanisms Coping styles; the automatic psychological process protecting the individual against anxiety and creating awareness of internal or external dangers or stressors.

defining characteristics Key signs and symptoms that relate to each other and inform a nursing diagnosis.

deinstitutionalization Downsizing or elimination of psychiatric hospitals with a new orientation to community-based services.

delirium A disorder of physical origin that develops over a short period of time and is characterized by fluctuating consciousness and attention. *Hyperactive delirium* involves behaviours such as being overly alert, exhibiting psychomotor hyperactivity, and marked excitability (may hallucinate). *Hypoactive delirium* is marked by lethargy, sleepiness, apathy, and psychomotor slowing; *mixed delirium* involves behaviour that fluctuates between the hyperactive and hypoactive states over brief or long periods.

delirium tremens An acute syndrome related to alcohol withdrawal that is characterized by gross tremulousness, disorientation, delusions, hallucinations (auditory, visual or tactile), tachycardia, sweating, hypertension, irregular tremor, and severely agitated behaviour.

delusion A false, fixed belief, based on an incorrect inference about reality, not shared by others, inconsistent with the individual's intelligence or cultural background and which cannot be corrected by reasoning. *Delusions of control* are about one's thoughts, feelings, or will being controlled by outside forces; *delusions of grandeur*, one's importance or power; *paranoid delusions*, being the focus of others' harmful intent; *religious delusions*, being an agent of or favoured by a greater being; and *somatic delusions* involving the body or bodily functions.

delusional disorder A disorder in which there is the presence of nonbizarre delusions; includes several subtypes: erotomania, grandiose, jealous, somatic, mixed, and specified.

dementia A state characterized by chronic cognitive impairment; differentiated by underlying cause, not by symptom patterns, which are often similar; can be further classified as cortical or subcortical to denote the location of the underlying pathology.

denial Refusal to acknowledge some painful aspect of external reality or subjective experience that would be apparent to others. *Psychotic denial* is when there is gross impairment in reality testing.

deontology The approach to ethics that sets duty or obligation as the basis of doing right.

depersonalization A nonspecific experience in which the individual loses a sense of personal identity and feels strange or unreal.

depressive episode In a major depressive episode, either a depressed mood or a loss of interest or pleasure in nearly all activities must be present for at least 2 weeks. Four of seven additional symptoms must be present: disruption in sleep, appetite (or weight), concentration, energy; psychomotor agitation or retardation; excessive guilt or feelings of worthlessness; and suicidal ideation.

desensitization A rapid decrease in drug effects that may develop within a few minutes or over a period of days, months, years, or lifetime of exposure to a drug.

detoxification Process of safely and effectively withdrawing a person from an addictive substance, usually under medical supervision.

developmental delay The impairment of normal growth and development that may not be reversible.

diagnosis-specific outcomes Outcomes based on nursing diagnoses.

dialectical behaviour therapy (DBT) An important biosocial approach to treatment that combines numerous cognitive and behaviour therapy strategies. It requires patients to understand their disorder by actively participating in formulating treatment goals by collecting data about their own behaviour, identifying treatment targets in individual therapy, and working with the therapists in changing these target behaviours.

diathesis Constitutional predisposition or vulnerability to a disorder.

dichotomous thinking Tendency to view things as absolute, either black or white, good or bad, with no perception of compromise.

disaster A sudden, overwhelming, and catastrophic event that causes widespread damage, social disorganization, mass casualties, and human suffering.

discrimination The differential treatment of others because they are members of a particular group.

disinhibition A concept borrowed from physics and biology and based on the idea of a dynamic, self-regulatory model of equilibrium in which equilibrium is defined (Piaget) as compensation for external disturbance; a mechanism for providing the self-regulation by which intelligence adapts to internal and external changes.

disordered water balance A state of chronic fluid imbalance, vacillating between normal and hyponatremic, that commonly occurs in psychiatric patients with chronic illnesses.

disorganized symptoms Symptoms of schizophrenia that make it difficult for the person to understand and respond to the ordinary sights and sounds of daily living; include *confused speech and thinking* and *disorganized behaviour*.

dissociation A disruption in the normally occurring linkages among subjective awareness, feelings, thoughts, behaviour, and memories.

dissociative identity disorder (DID) A mental disorder characterized by the existence of two or more distinct identities with unique personality characteristics and the inability to recall important information about oneself or events.

dissupport Term for the opposite of support in a relationship, such as verbal, physical, or emotional abuse; discounting an individual's opinions, feelings, behaviours, or values; blocking access to resources; or consuming an individual's material resources.

distraction The purposeful focusing of attention away from undesirable sensations.

distribution The amount of a drug that may be found in various tissues at the site of the drug action for which it is intended.

disturbances of executive functioning Problems in the ability to think abstractly, plan, initiate, sequence, monitor, and stop complex behaviour.

dual diagnosis Presence of both substance-related disorder and mental illness.

dyad A group of only two people who are usually related, such as a married couple, siblings, or parent and child.

dynamic security Security awareness that is concerned with institutional policies, staffing patterns, methods of operation, and relational security.

dysfunctional family A family whose interactions, decisions, or behaviours interfere with the positive development of the family and its individual members.

dyslexia Significantly lower score for mental age on standardized test in reading that is not due to low intelligence or inadequate schooling.

dysphagia Difficulty swallowing.

dysthymic disorder A milder but more chronic form of major depressive disorder.

dystonia An impairment in muscle tone that is generally the first extrapyramidal symptom to occur, usually within a few days of initiating an antipsychotic. Dystonia is characterized by involuntary muscle spasms, especially of the head and neck muscles.

echolalia Parrot-like repetition of another's words; inappropriate choice of topics.

echopraxia Involuntary imitation of another person's movements and gestures; regressed behaviour that is child-like or immature.

efferent Away from the central nervous system or other particular structure.

efficacy Ability of a drug to produce a response as a result of the receptor or receptors being occupied.

egocentrism Tendency to view the world as revolving around oneself.

emotion The psychophysiologic reaction that shapes the individual's experience of a feeling state.

emotional circuit The interrelationship between the emotional processes of the limbic system and the neurocognitive processes of the frontal lobe and other parts of the cortex. It is hypothesized that the functioning of this system determines the meaning a person gives to a particular situation.

emotional dysregulation Inability to control emotion in social interactions.

emotional vulnerability Sensitivity and reactivity to environmental stress.

emotion-focused coping Coping strategies directed at managing one's emotional distress (e.g., through exercise, prayer/meditation, expressing emotions, talking to friends, etc.).

empathic linkage Ability to feel in oneself the feelings being expressed by another person or persons.

empathy The experience of putting oneself in another person's circumstances and imagining his or her feelings.

encopresis Soiling clothing with faeces or depositing faeces in inappropriate places.

endorphins Neurotransmitters that have opiate-like behaviour and produce an inhibitory effect at opiate receptor sites; probably responsible for pain tolerance.

enmeshment An extreme form of intensity in family interactions.

enuresis Involuntary excretion of urine after the age at which a child should have attained bladder control.

epidemiology The study of patterns of disease distribution in time and space that focuses on the health status of population groups or aggregates, rather than on individuals, and involves quantitative analysis of the occurrence of illnesses in population groups; basic science of public health.

epigenesis A concept borrowed from embryology: if a particular part does not manifest itself during the appropriate phase, it cannot reach full development because the moment for doing so has passed; each developmental stage must be completed at the appropriate time, or successful completion of the stage will not occur.

episode A period of a minimal duration of 2 weeks during which an individual experiences symptoms that meet the diagnostic criteria for that disorder.

equilibration Compensation for external disturbances; a mechanism for providing the self-regulation by which intelligence adapts to external and internal changes (Piaget).

erotomania The belief that someone (often a public figure) is in love with one or involved with one in a relationship when, in reality, one is a stranger to him or her.

ethnocentrism The notion that one's own culturally learned ideas and values are central and correct for everyone.

excretion The elimination of drugs from the body either unchanged or as metabolites. *Clearance* refers to the total volume of blood, serum, or plasma from which a drug is completely removed per unit of time.

exhibitionism A behaviour associated with paraphilias involving exposing one's genitals to strangers, with occasional masturbation.

existential anxiety The foreboding that arises from an awareness of human mortality. Also referred to as *angst*.

exposure therapy The treatment of choice for agoraphobia that puts the patient into contact with the feared situations until the stimuli no longer produce anxiety.

expressed emotion Family members' responses that include one or more of the following dynamics: critical comments, hostility, or emotional overinvolvement.

extended family Several nuclear families who may or may not live together and function as one group.

externalizing disorders Disorders that are characterized by acting-out behaviour.

extinction Elimination of a classically conditioned response by the repeated presentation of the conditioned stimulus without the unconditioned stimulus, or elimination of an operantly conditioned response by no longer presenting the reward after the response.

extrapyramidal motor system Collection of neuronal pathways that provides significant input in involuntary motor movements.

factitious disorder A type of psychiatric disorder characterized by somatization, in which the person intentionally causes an illness for the purpose of becoming a patient.

factitious disorder by proxy (Münchausen syndrome by proxy) The intentional production or feigning of physical or psychological signs or symptoms in one person by another who desires to indirectly assume the sick role.

family development A broad term that refers to all the processes connected with the growth of a family, including changes associated with work, geographic location, migration, acculturation, and serious illness.

family dynamics The patterned interpersonal and social interactions that occur within the family structure over the life of a family.

family life cycle A process of expansion, contraction, and realignment of relationship systems to support the entry, exit, and development of family members.

family structure According to Minuchin, the organized pattern within which family members interact.

first-pass effect Loss of orally administered drugs prior to entering the systemic circulation due to metabolism in the gastrointestinal wall.

fissures The grooves of the cerebrum.

flight of ideas Repeated and rapid changes in the topic of conversation, generally within just one sentence or phrase.

flooding A type of therapy for agoraphobia in which highly anxiety-provoking stimuli are presented to the patient in vivo or with imagery, with no relaxation until the anxiety dissipates.

foetal alcohol syndrome A group of noncurable growth, mental, and physical problems that may occur in a baby when a mother ingests alcohol during pregnancy.

forensic nursing Nursing practice in which psychiatric and mental health nursing philosophy and skills are integrated within a sociocultural context that includes the criminal justice system in order to provide comprehensive care to clients, families, and communities.

formal group roles The designated leader and members of a group.

formal operations The period of cognitive development, described by Piaget, characterized by the ability to use abstract reasoning to conceptualize and solve problems.

functional activities Activities of daily living necessary for self-care (i.e., bathing, toileting, dressing, and transferring).

functional status Extent to which a person has the ability to carry out independent personal care, home management, and social functions in everyday life that has meaning and purpose.

gate-control model Pain response based on the model that pain perception involves pathways in the dorsal horn of the spinal column that relay noxious stimuli to the brain and that certain other nerve fibres function as an antagonistic "gate" to augment or dampen the subjective experience of pain.

gender role How one functions and behaves as a male or a female in relation to others in society, also referred to as *sex role identity*.

genogram A multigenerational schematic diagram that lists family members and their relationships.

genome The complete set of human genes.

genomics The study of the complete DNA structure or genome.

gerotranscendence A psychosocial theory of aging that regards aging as the final stage in a natural progression towards maturation and wisdom that generally results in increased satisfaction and meaning in life.

glia (white matter) A fatty or lipid substance with a white appearance that surrounds the pathways of the cell body axons.

grey matter The cortex, with its grey-brown colour due to the capillary blood vessels.

grief The subjective experience (e.g., thoughts, feelings, behaviours, and body sensations) that accompanies the perception of a loss.

group An open or closed social system with structures, norms, and customary ways of acting.

group cohesion Forces that act on the members to stay in a group.

group dynamics Interactions within groups.

group process The "what is happening" in the group; how members are interacting and relating as individuals and as a whole group, including nonverbal communications.

groupthink The tendency of many groups to avoid conflict and adopt a normative pattern of thinking that is often consistent with the group leader's ideas.

guided imagery The purposeful use of imagination to achieve relaxation or direct attention away from undesirable sensations; especially useful in stress management.

gyri Bumps and convolutions in the brain.

half-life The time required for plasma concentrations of a drug to be reduced by 50%.

hallucinations Perceptual experiences that occur in the absence of actual external sensory stimuli and may be auditory, visual, tactile, gustatory, or olfactory.

hallucinogen A class of drug that produces euphoria or dysphoria, altered body image, distorted or sharpened visual and auditory perception, confusion, uncoordination, and impaired judgement and memory.

hallucinogen persisting perception disorder A transient and intermittent disorder associated with the long-term use of hallucinogens; includes depression, prolonged psychosis, and flashbacks.

harm reduction A community health intervention designed to reduce the harm (consequences) of substance use to the individual, the family, and society by reducing the risk for adverse consequences arising from substance use without necessarily reducing its use.

helplessness The perception of having limited ability or ambition to change one's current life situation; characterized by a sense of being unable to help oneself and a sense that there is a lack of support or protection.

hippocampus Subcortical grey matter embedded within each temporal lobe that may be involved in determining the best way to store information or memory; "time-dating" memory.

historical trauma The cumulative effect of maltreatment across the lifespan and over generations, resulting in maladaptive social and cultural behaviours.

HIV-1-associated cognitive–motor complex Neurologic complications that occur with HIV-1 that are directly attributable to infection of the brain and include impaired cognitive and motor function.

home visits Delivery of nursing care in a patient's living environment.

homeostasis The body's ability to maintain a stable internal environment despite changing environmental conditions.

hopelessness A perception of having no hope that one's life situation or circumstance will change or improve; characterized by feelings of inadequacy and an inability to act on one's own behalf.

hyperactivity Excessive motor activity, movement, and/or utterances that may be either purposeless or aimless.

hyperalgia Increased nociceptor sensitivity.

hyperesthesia Increased sensation of pain.

hypervigilance Sustained attention to external stimuli as if expecting something important or frightening to happen.

hypofrontality Reduced cerebral blood flow and glucose metabolism in the prefrontal cortex of people with schizophrenia.

hypomanic episode Mildly dysphoric mood that meets the same criteria as for a manic episode except that it lasts at least 4 days rather than 1 week and no marked impairment in social or occupational functioning is present.

hyponatraemia Decreased sodium concentration in the blood.

hypothalamic–pituitary–adrenal (HPA) axis Neurotransmitters responsible for behavioural responses to fear and anxiety that are usually held in balance until information from the sensory processing areas in the thalamus and cortex alerts the amygdala. If events are interpreted as threatening, this axis is activated, initiating the stress response.

hypothalamus Immediately ventral and slightly anterior to the thalamus, forming the floor and part of the walls of the third ventricle.

ideas of reference False belief that other people, objects, and events are related to or have a special significance for oneself (e.g., a person on television is sending one signals).

identity An integration of a person's social and occupational roles and affiliations, self-attributed personality traits, attitudes about gender roles, beliefs about sexuality and intimacy, long-term goals, political ideology, and religious beliefs.

identity diffusion Occurs when parts of a person's identity are absent or poorly developed; a lack of consistent sense of identity.

illogical thinking A thinking error that occurs when a person draws a faulty conclusion; for example, a university student equates failure on an examination with loss of future career.

illusions Disorganized perceptions that create an oversensitivity to colours, shapes, and background activities, which occur when the person misperceives or exaggerates stimuli in the external environment.

impulsivity Acting without considering the consequences of the act or alternative actions.

incidence A rate that includes only new cases that have occurred within a clearly defined time period.

indicators Representation of the dimension of outcome; data or information to answer the question of how close the patient is coming towards an outcome.

individual roles Group roles that either enhance or detract from the group's functioning but have nothing to do with either the group task or maintenance.

individual treatment plan A plan of care that identifies the patient's problems, outcomes, interventions, the individuals assigned to implement interventions, and evaluation criteria.

informal group roles Positions in the group with rights and duties directed towards other group members. These positions are not formally sanctioned.

informal support systems Family members, friends, and neighbours who can provide care and support to the individual.

informed consent Consent for treatment given by a competent adult after being provided the available information necessary for making an informed choice; based on the ethical principle of autonomy.

inhalants Organic solvents, also known as volatile substances, that are central nervous system depressants and when inhaled cause euphoria, sedation, emotional lability, and impaired judgement.

inhibited grieving Inability to fully experience and personally integrate or resolve significant traumatic events and loss.

insight The ability of the individual to be aware of his or her own thoughts and feelings and to compare them with the thoughts and feelings of others.

insomnia Inability to fall or remain asleep throughout the night.

instrumental activities Activities that facilitate or enhance the performance of activities of daily living (e.g., shopping, using the telephone, transportation). These aspects are critical to consider for any older adult living alone.

interdisciplinary approach Interventions from different disciplines integrated into the delivery of patient care.

interdisciplinary treatment plan A plan of care that identifies the patient's problems, outcomes, interventions, members of different disciplines assigned to implement interventions, and evaluation criteria.

intermediate beliefs Attitudes, rules or expectations, and assumptions that influence one's perceptions, affect, and behaviours; often take the form of "should" statements that are rigid and unrealistic.

internalizing disorders Anxiety disorders and depression in which the symptoms tend to be within the individual.

interoceptive awareness Term used to describe the sensory response to emotional and visceral cues, such as hunger.

intrinsic activity The ability of a drug to produce a biologic response when it becomes attached to its receptor.

invalidating environment A highly personal social situation that negates the individual's emotional responses and communication.

invincibility fable The egocentric phenomenon seen in adolescence where the individual views his or herself as unique, invulnerable, and immune to death.

ischaemic cascade Cell breakdown resulting from brain cell injury.

judgement The ability to reach a logical decision about a situation and to choose a course after looking at and analyzing various possibilities.

kindling Repetitive stimulation of certain tracts may facilitate conduction of impulses in the future and lead to enhancement of intense behaviours after even mild stimulation.

kleptomania A disorder in which the patient is unable to resist the urge to steal and independently steals items that he or she could easily afford. These items are not particularly useful or wanted. The underlying issue is the act of stealing.

Korsakoff's syndrome An amnestic syndrome in which there is a profound deficit in the ability to form new memories; associated with a variable deficit in recall of old memories despite a clear sensorium. Confabulation is a key feature.

lability of mood Rapid alternations of mood, usually between euphoria and irritability.

lateral ventricles The horn-shaped first and second ventricles that are the largest of the brain's ventricles.

learning disorder A discrepancy between actual achievement and expected achievement that is based on a person's age and intellectual ability.

least restrictive environment The patient has the right to treatment in an environment that restricts the exercise of free will to the least extent; an individual cannot be restricted to an institution when he or she can be successfully treated in the community.

level of consciousness An individual's level of arousal or wakefulness.

limbic system (limbic lobe) Structures including the septum and the fornix, as well as the amygdala, hippocampus, cingulate, parahippocampal gyrus, epithalamus, portions of the basal ganglia, parolfactory area, and the anterior nucleus of the thalamus.

longitudinal fissure The longest and deepest groove of the cerebrum, separating the right and left hemispheres.

loose associations Absence of the normal connectedness of thoughts and ideas; sudden shifts without apparent relationship to preceding topic.

magical thinking The belief that one's thought, words, or actions have the power to cause or prevent things happening; similar to Piaget's preoperational thinking in young children.

maintenance function A term used to describe the informal role of group members that encourages the group to stay together.

malingering The production of illness symptoms intentionally with an obvious self-serving goal such as being classified as disabled and avoiding work.

mandatory outpatient treatment (MOT) Legal provisions that can require an individual with a mental illness to comply with a treatment plan while living in the community.

mania A state characterized by an abnormally and persistently elevated, expansive, or irritable mood.

manic episode A distinct period during which there is an abnormally and persistently elevated, expansive, or irritable mood.

manipulation Influencing others or a situation for one's own benefit.

maturation The process of completing a state of development; a ripening.

memory A facet of cognition concerned with retaining and recalling past experiences, whether they occurred in the physical environment or internally as cognitive events.

meningeal layer The inner layer of dura mater that becomes continuous with the spinal dura mater and sends extensions into the brain for support and protection of the different lobes or structures.

mental disorder Health condition characterized by alterations in a variety of factors that include mood and affect, behaviour, thinking and cognition.

mental health act A law that gives certain powers, and sets the conditions (including time limits) for those powers, to stipulated health care professionals and designated institutions regarding the admission and treatment of individuals with a mental disorder.

mental health problem A term used when signs and symptoms of mental illnesses occur but do not meet specified criteria for a disorder.

mental illness A term used to mean all diagnosable mental disorders.

mental retardation Significantly below-average intelligence accompanied by impaired adaptive functioning.

mental status examination Systematic assessment of an individual's appearance, affect, behaviour, and cognitive processes, reflecting the examiner's observations and used in clinical settings to evaluate developmental, neurologic, and psychiatric disorders.

mesocortical Medial aspects of the cortex.

metabolism Biotransformation, or the process by which a drug is altered.

milieu therapy An approach using the total environment to provide a therapeutic community; a therapeutic environment.

misidentification Delusions in which the person believes that a familiar person is replaced by an impostor.

mixed episode Irritability or excitement and depression occurring at the same time.

mobbing Occurs when several people gang up and bully an individual.

mood A pervasive, sustained emotion that influences one's perception of the world and can be described as *euthymic* (normal), *euphoric* (elated), or dysphoric (depressed, disquieted, restless). Normal variations in mood (e.g., sadness, euphoria, anxiety) occur as responses to specific life experiences, are time limited, and are not associated with significant functional impairment.

mood disorder Recurrent disturbances or alterations in mood that cause psychological distress and behavioural impairment.

moral dilemma The need to make a morally relevant choice between conflicting options.

moral distress The anger, frustration, or anguish felt when one is unable to fulfil ethical obligations in the way one believes that one should.

moral treatment An approach to curing mental illness, popular in the 1800s, which was built on the principles of kindness, compassion, and a pleasant environment.

motivational interviewing (MI; motivational enhancement therapy) A directive, client-centred style of psychotherapy that helps clients to explore and resolve their ambivalence about changing.

mourning The external manifestation of grief, which is highly influenced by gender, ethnicity, culture, religion, and the cause of death.

multiaxial diagnostic system A diagnostic structure that includes more than one domain of information, such as the psychiatric diagnoses of the *DSM-IV-TR*.

multidisciplinary approach Several disciplines providing services to a patient at one time.

multigenerational transmission process The transmission of emotional processes from one generation to the next.

music therapy The controlled use of music to promote physiologic or psychological well-being.

myoclonus Twitching or clonic spasms of a muscle group.

myoglobinuria The presence of myohaemoglobin in the urine due to sustained muscular rigidity and necrosis.

negative symptoms Symptoms of schizophrenia that reflect a lessening or loss of normal functions, such as restriction or flattening in the range and intensity of emotion (*affective flattening* or *blunting*); reduced fluency and productivity of thought and speech (*alogia*); withdrawal and inability to initiate and persist in goal-directed activity (*avolition*); and inability to experience pleasure (*anhedonia*).

neglect Failure to protect from injury or to provide for the physical, psychological, and medical needs of a child or dependent elder.

neologisms Words that are made up that have no common meaning and are not recognized.

neuritic plaques Extracellular lesions consisting of β-amyloid protein and apolipoprotein A (apoA) cores that form in the nucleus basalis of Meynert, gradually increase in number, and are abnormally distributed throughout the cholinergic system.

neurochemical modulation Maintenance of a balance in the essential levels of the neurotransmitters that influence mood, perceptions, and emotional interpretation.

neurofibrillary tangles Fibrous proteins, or *tau proteins*, that are chemically altered and twisted together and spread throughout the brain, interfering with nerve functioning in cholinergic neurons. It is hypothesized that formation of these neurofibrillary tangles are related to the apolipoprotein E_4 (apoE$_4$).

neurohormones Hormones produced by cells within the nervous system, such as antidiuretic hormone (ADH).

neuroleptic malignant syndrome A syndrome caused by neuroleptic medications that are dopamine receptor blockers. The classic signs and symptoms include hyperthermia, lead-pipe rigidity, changes in mental status, and autonomic nervous system changes.

neuropeptide Y A recently discovered 36-amino-acid peptide that is a potent stimulator of feeding behaviour especially selective for foods heavy in carbohydrates.

neuropeptides Short chains of amino acids that exist in the central nervous system and have a number of important roles, including as neurotransmitters, neuromodulators, or neurohormones.

neurotransmitters Chemicals circulating in the synaptic areas of neurons that initiate, block, or modulate nerve signal transmission and ultimately control neural function.

nihilism A psychiatric term for the belief that one is dead or nonexistent.

nociceptive Pertaining to a neural receptor for painful stimuli.

nonmaleficence A principle of bioethics asserting the obligation to inflict no harm.

nonverbal communication The gestures, expressions, and body language used in communications between the nurse and the patient.

normalization Teaching individuals and families about normal development, behaviours, and responses that can be expected (e.g., child development, the grieving process).

no-suicide contract Written or verbal agreement between the health care professional and the patient that the patient will not engage in suicidal behaviour for a specific period of time.

nuclear family Two or more people related by blood, marriage, or adoption.

nurse–patient relationship A time-limited interpersonal process with definable phases during which the patient is able to consider alternative behaviours, try new health care strategies, and discuss complex health problems.

nursing diagnosis A clinical judgement about an identified problem/need that requires nursing interventions; based on nursing assessment.

nursing intervention Nursing activities that promote and foster health, assess dysfunction, assist patients to regain or improve their coping abilities, or prevent further disabilities.

nursing process Problem-solving method used by nurses that involves assessment, planning, implementation, and evaluation.

object relation The psychological attachment to another person or object.

observation Ongoing assessment of the patient's mental and health status to identify and subvert any potential problems.

obsessions Unwanted, intrusive, and persistent thoughts, impulses, or images that are incongruent with the patient's usual thought patterns.

obsessive–compulsive disorder (OCD) A disorder characterized by intrusive thoughts that are difficult to dislodge (obsessions) and ritualized behaviours that the person feels driven to perform (compulsions).

obstructive sleep apnea Repetitive pauses in breathing during sleep due to collapse of the upper airway; symptoms include snoring and restless sleep.

oculogyric crisis A medication side effect resulting from an imbalance of dopamine and acetylcholine, in which the muscles that control eye movements tense and pull the eyeball so that the patient is looking towards the ceiling; may be followed by torticollis or retrocollis.

open group A group in which new members can join at any time.

operant behaviour A type of learning that is a consequence of a particular behavioural response, not a specific stimulus.

opiate Any substance that binds to an opiate receptor in the brain to produce an agonist action, causing central nervous system depression, sleep or stupor, and analgesia.

orientation An individual's ability to perceive and grasp the significance of environmental information related to time, place, and person.

orientation phase The first phase of the nurse–patient relationship in which the nurse and the patient get to know each other. During this phase, the patient develops a sense of trust.

othering The way one perceives and engages with another person that can be exclusionary and negative (i.e., the other is different from and thus "less than" me) or inclusionary and tolerant or accepting (i.e., the other is different from me, so I need to learn about his or her world view).

outcomes Patient response to nursing care at a given point in time consisting of the patient's state, behaviour, or perception that is variable and can be measured.

panic A normal but extreme overwhelming form of anxiety often experienced when an individual is placed in a real or perceived life-threatening situation.

panic attacks Discrete periods of intense fear or discomfort that are accompanied by significant somatic or cognitive symptoms.

panic control treatment Systematic structured exposure to panic-invoking sensations such as dizziness, hyperventilation, tightness in chest, and sweating.

panicogenic Substances that produce panic attacks.

paranoia Suspiciousness and guardedness that is unrealistic and often accompanied by grandiosity.

parasomnia Disorders of abnormal physiologic or behavioural events that occur in relationship to sleep, specific sleep stages, or during transition from sleep to wakefulness.

parasuicidal behaviours Deliberate acts of self-injury.

parieto-occipital sulcus Separates the occipital lobe from the parietal lobe.

passive listening A nontherapeutic mode of interaction that involves sitting quietly and allowing the patient to talk without focusing on guiding the thought process; includes body language that communicates boredom, indifference, or hostility.

perceptions The awareness reached as a result of sensory inputs of real stimuli that are usually altered.

persecutory delusions Delusions in which the person believes that he or she is being conspired against, cheated, spied on, followed, poisoned, drugged, maligned, harassed, or obstructed in the pursuit of long-term goals.

personal fable Egocentric thinking in adolescence characterized by the belief that one is unique and invulnerable to harm, manifesting in risk-taking behaviours.

personality A complex pattern of characteristics, predominately outside the person's awareness, that compose a person's distinctive pattern of perceiving, feeling, thinking, and behaving.

personality disorder An enduring pattern of inner experience and behaviour that deviates markedly from the expectations of the individual's culture; is pervasive and inflexible; has an onset in adolescence or early adulthood; is stable over time; and leads to distress or impairment.

personality traits Prominent aspects of personality that are exhibited in a wide range of important social and personal contexts.

person–environment relationship The interaction between the individual and the environment that changes throughout the stress experience.

pet therapy The therapeutic use of animals as pets to promote physical, psychological, or social well-being.

pharmacodynamics The study of the biologic actions of drugs on living tissue and the human body in general.

pharmacogenomics The science of pharmacology combined with genetic knowledge.

pharmacokinetics The study of how the human body processes a drug, including absorption, distribution, metabolism, and elimination.

phobia Persistent, unrealistic fear of situations, objects, or activities that often leads to avoidance behaviours.

phonologic processing Thought to be the cause of reading disability; a process that involves the discrimination and interpretation of speech sounds. Reading disability is believed to be caused by some disturbance in the development of the left hemisphere.

phototherapy Also known as *light therapy*; involves exposing the patient to an artificial light source during winter months to relieve seasonal depression.

physical restraints The application of wrist, leg, and body straps made of leather or cloth for the purpose of controlling or managing behaviour.

pia mater The third layer of the central nervous system, in Latin, "soft mother."

pineal body Located in the epithalamus; contains secretory cells that emit the neurohormone melatonin (as well as other substances), which has been associated with sleep and emotional disorders and modulation of immune function.

plasticity Capability to change or adapt in form or physiology.

point prevalence Basic measure that refers to the proportion of individuals in a population who have a particular disorder at a specified point in time.

polydipsia Excessive thirst that can be chronic in patients with severe mental illness.

polypharmacy Use of several different medications at one time.

polysomnography A special procedure that involves the recording of the electroencephalogram throughout the night. This procedure is usually conducted in a sleep laboratory.

polyuria Excessive excretion of urine.

positive self-talk Countering fearful or negative thoughts by using preplanned and rehearsed positive coping statements.

positive symptoms Symptoms of schizophrenia that reflect an excess or distortion of normal functions, including delusions and hallucinations.

posttraumatic stress disorder A mental disorder characterized by persistent, distressing symptoms lasting longer than 1 month after exposure to an extreme traumatic stressor.

poverty The state when income and/or level of consumption are below what is necessary to meet basic needs; measured as absolute (comparison of total income against the cost of goods and services essential to daily life) or relative (comparison of total income and spending with the general population).

powerlessness The perception of having no power or control over one's life circumstance; feeling that the world will never be fair; feeling helpless and totally ineffectual; or feeling one lacks legal or other authority.

prejudice The preconceived, unreasonable judgement of others, usually negative, based solely on their membership in a particular group.

pressured speech A speech pattern in which the person is talkative due to a sense of pressure to speak; a symptom of manic episodes of bipolar disorder.

prevalence The total number of people who have a particular disorder within a given population at a specific time.

prevention Interventions used before the initial onset of a disorder that become distinct from the treatment.

principlism The approach to ethics that uses common principles or ethical norms as the basis for ethical decision making. In health ethics, the principles used include *nonmaleficence* (do no harm), *beneficence* (promote benefit), *respect for autonomy* (the right to make one's own decisions), and *justice* (fairness in the distribution of risks and benefits).

problem-focused coping Coping comprised of inner- or outer-directed coping strategies. Outer-directed strategies attempt to eliminate or alter a situation or another's behaviour, while inner-directed strategies aim at altering one's own beliefs, attitudes, skills, responses, etc.

process recording A verbatim transcript of a verbal interaction usually organized according to the nurse-patient interaction. It often includes analysis of the interaction.

projective identification A psychoanalytic term used to describe behaviour of people with borderline personality disorder when they falsely attribute to others their own unacceptable feelings, impulses, or thoughts.

pseudodementia Memory difficulties in older adults with major depression (may be mistaken for early signs of dementia).

pseudologia fantastica False stories of personal triumph that are a core symptom of factitious disorders.

pseudoneurologic symptoms Somatic symptoms of conversion disorders that pertain to neurologic conditions affecting voluntary motor or sensory function (e.g., impaired balance, paralysis, blindness, deafness). The symptoms do not follow neurologic paths, but rather follow the individual's conceptualization of the problem.

pseudoparkinsonism Sometimes referred to as *drug-induced parkinsonism*; presents identically as Parkinson's disease without the same destruction of dopaminergic cells.

psychoanalytic movement Freud's radical approach to psychiatric mental health care, which involved using a new technique called *psychoanalysis* based on unconscious motivations for behaviour, or drives.

psychodrama A group role-playing technique used to encourage expression of emotion and exploration of problems.

psychoeducation An educational approach used to enhance knowledge and shape behaviour so that coping skills are learned or enhanced.

psychoendocrinology The study of the relationships among the nervous system, endocrine system, and behaviour.

psychoimmunology The study of immunology as it relates to emotions and behaviour.

psychopathy Refers to individuals who behave impulsively and are interpersonally irresponsible, act hastily and spontaneously, are shortsighted, and fail to plan ahead or consider alternatives. Equated with antisocial personality disorder.

psychopharmacology A subspecialty of pharmacology that studies medications that affect the brain and behaviour and that are used to treat psychiatric and neurodegenerative disorders.

psychosis A state in which the individual is experiencing hallucinations, delusions, or disorganized thoughts, speech, or behaviour.

psychosomatic Conditions in which a psychological state contributes to the development of a physical illness.

purging A compensatory behaviour to rid oneself of food already eaten by means of self-induced vomiting or the use of laxatives, enemas, or diuretics.

pyromania An irresistible impulse to start fires.

rapidly cycling bipolar disorder The occurrence of four or more mood episodes during the past 12 months.

rapport Interpersonal harmony characterized by understanding and respect.

rate A proportion of the cases in the population compared to the total population.

reaction time The lapse of time between stimulus and response.

receptor Site where a substance can specifically interact with the cell membrane to produce a change; biologic action of a drug depends on how its structure interacts with a specific receptor.

recovery model An approach that supports individual potential for recovery, focusing on the personal journey involved, the upholding of human rights, a positive culture of healing, and recovery-oriented services.

regressed behaviour Behaving in the manner of a less mature life stage; childlike and immature.

relapse Return of symptoms after a period of remission.

relational ethics The approach to ethics that situates ethical action in relationship, recognizing that complexity, vulnerability, and the environment are important considerations.

relaxation A mental health intervention that promotes comfort, reduces anxiety, alleviates stress, reduces pain, and prevents aggressive behaviour.

religiosity A psychiatric symptom characterized by excessive or affected piety.

REM sleep A sleep cycle state of rapid eye movement.

reminiscence Thinking about or relating past experiences.

reminiscence therapy The healing process of looking back on specific times or events in one's life.

remission A period when the symptoms of a disease are abated.

resilience The capacity to overcome adversity in spite of extreme stress; involves the balancing of risk and protective factors.

resolution phase The termination phase of the nurse–patient relationship that lasts from the time the problems are resolved to the close of the relationship.

restraint The use of any manual, physical, or mechanical device or material, which when attached to the patient's body (usually the arms and legs) restricts the patient's movements.

retrocollis The neck muscles pull the head back.

risk factors Characteristics that do not cause the disorder or problem and are not symptoms of the illness, but rather are factors that have been shown to influence the likelihood of developing a disorder.

role An individual's social position and function within an environment.

ruminations Repetitive thoughts that are forced into a patient's consciousness even when unwanted; when a person goes over and over the same ideas endlessly; part of an obsessive style of thinking.

satiety Internal signals that indicate one has had enough to eat.

schema A cognitive structure that screens, codes, and evaluates the incoming stimuli through which the individual interprets events.

schizoaffective disorder An interrupted period of illness during which at some point there is a major depressive, manic, or mixed episode, along with two of the following symptoms of schizophrenia: delusions, hallucinations, disorganized speech, disorganized or catatonic behaviour, or negative symptoms (affective flattening, alogia, or avolition).

school phobia Anxiety in which the child refuses to attend school in order to stay at home and with the primary attachment figure. School phobia is a common presenting complaint in child psychiatric clinics and may be part of separation anxiety, general anxiety, social phobia, obsessive–compulsive disorder, depression, or conduct disorder.

seclusion The involuntary confinement of a person in a room which the person is physically prevented from leaving for the purposes of safety or behavioural management.

sedative–hypnotics Medications that induce sleep and reduce anxiety.

selectivity The ability of a drug to be specific for a particular receptor.

self-awareness Being cognizant of one's own beliefs, thought motivations, biases, physical and emotional limitations, and the impact one may have on others.

self-concept The sum of beliefs about oneself, which develops over time.

self-disclosure The act of revealing personal information about oneself.

self-efficacy Self-effectiveness.

self-esteem The way one feels about oneself; components are self-acceptance, self-worth, self-love, and self-nurturing.

self-identity Formed through the integration of social and occupational roles and affiliations, self-attributed personality traits, attitudes about gender roles, beliefs about sexuality and intimacy, long-term goals, political ideology, and religious beliefs. Without an adequately formed identity, goal-directed behaviour is impaired and interpersonal relationships are disrupted.

self-monitoring Observing and recording one's own information, usually behaviour, thoughts, or feelings.

separation–individuation A process during which the child develops a sense of self, a permanent sense of significant others (object constancy), and an integration of both bad and good as components of the self-concept.

serotonin Centrally mediates the release of endorphin. Along with histamine and bradykinin, serotonin stimulates the pain receptors to generate experienced pain. Serotonin is involved in inhibiting gastric secretion, stimulating smooth muscle, and serving as a central neurotransmitter.

serotonin syndrome A toxic side effect that occurs as a result of the newer serotonergic drugs; this syndrome is thought to be caused by hyperstimulation of the 5-HT receptor in the brain stem and spinal cord.

severe and persistent mental illness Mental disorders that are long term and have recurring periods of exacerbation and remission.

sexual abuse Sexual misconduct towards another person.

sexuality Basic dimension of every individual's personality, undergoing periods of growth and development, and influenced by biologic and psychosocial factors.

sibling position A child's place in the family based on birth order (e.g., first born, youngest).

side effects Unwanted or untoward effects of medications.

social change The structural and cultural evolution of society; is constant and, at times, erratic.

social distance Degree to which the values of a formal organization and its primary group members differ.

social functioning Performance of daily activities within the context of interpersonal relations and family and community roles.

social network Linkages among a defined set of people, among whom there are personal contacts.

social skills training A psychoeducational approach that involves instruction, feedback, support, and practice with learning behaviours, it helps people interact more effectively with peers, and also children with adults.

social support Resources provided to an individual by others that may moderate the adverse effects of stress.

somatization The manifestation of psychological distress as physical symptoms.

somatization disorder A polysymptomatic disorder that begins before age 30 years, extends over a period of years, and is characterized by a combination of pain and gastrointestinal, sexual, and psychoneurologic symptoms.

somatoform disorder One in which the patient experiences physical symptoms as a result of psychological stress.

speech The motor aspects of speaking.

spinal cord A long, cylindrical collection of neural fibres continuous with the brain stem, housed within the vertebral column.

spirituality A complex, even mysterious, concept related to one's connection to the sacred and to the beliefs and values that give meaning to one's life.

splitting A primitive defence mechanism involving the compartmentalization of opposite and conflicting affect states so that self, others, and events are understood as all one way or all another (e.g., viewing a particular person as being all good or all bad).

static security Security awareness focused on structural or environmental artefacts common to secure environments, for example, the use of two-way radios, personal protection alarms, video monitoring, electronic door locks, internal barriers, and perimeter fences or walls.

stereotypic behaviour Repetitive, driven, nonfunctional, and potentially self-injurious behaviour, such as head banging, rocking, and hand flapping, seen in autistic disorder, with an extraordinary insistence on sameness.

stereotyping The expectation that an individual will act in a characteristic manner that conforms to a perception, usually negative, of his or her cultural group.

stereotypy Repetitive, purposeless movements that are idiosyncratic to the individual and to some degree outside of the individual's control.

stigma The mark of a spoiled identity or disgrace.

stigmatization A process of assigning negative characteristics and identity to a person or group and causing that person or group to feel unaccepted, devalued, ostracized, and isolated from the larger society.

stress The relationship between the person and the environment that is appraised as exceeding the person's resources and endangering his or her well-being.

stressors Events that initiate a stress response; can be physical, psychological, or social; can be short-term (acute) or long-term (chronic).

stress–diathesis model An explanation about the relationship between stress and mental health illness that proposes that preexisting genetic, biologic, and psychological vulnerabilities interact with negative or stressful life events to cause illness; an inverse relationship between vulnerability and stress is predicted (i.e., the more vulnerable the individual, the less stress is required to cause illness).

structured interaction Purposeful interaction that allows patients to interact with others in a way that is useful to them.

subcortical Structures inside the hemispheres and beneath the cortex.

subcortical dementia Dementia that is caused by dysfunction or deterioration of deep grey- or white-matter structures inside the brain and brain stem.

substance abuse A maladaptive use of chemical substance(s) leading to clinically significant outcomes or distress (e.g., recurrent legal problems, failure to perform, engaging in physically hazardous behaviour). Criteria for abuse do not include tolerance, withdrawal, or compulsive use.

substance dependence Continued use of a substance despite significant substance-related problems, along with a pattern of repeated self-administration that can result in tolerance, withdrawal, and compulsive drug-taking behaviour.

substance P The most common nociceptive transmitter that is released and transported along the central and peripheral pain synapses in the presence of noxious stimuli.

substitute decision maker An individual appointed to make health care decisions on behalf of another who is unable to consent to treatment.

subsystems A systems term used by family theorists to describe subgroups of family members who join together for various activities.

suicidal contagion A social phenomenon seen among adolescents: when one teenager takes his or her life, others may follow.

suicidal ideation Thinking about and planning one's own death without actually engaging in self-harm.

suicide The act of killing oneself voluntarily.

symbolism The use of a word or a phrase to represent an object, event, or feeling.

symptom expression The behavioural symptoms of mental illness linked to their neurobiologic basis.

synapse The region across which nerve impulses are transmitted through the action of a neurotransmitter.

systematic desensitization A method used to desensitize patients to anxiety-provoking situations by exposing the patient to a hierarchy of feared situations. The patient is taught to use muscle relaxation as levels of anxiety increase through multisituational exposure.

tangentiality When the topic of conversation changes to an entirely different topic that is within a logical progression but causes a permanent detour from the original focus.

tardive dyskinesia A late-appearing extrapyramidal side effect of antipsychotic medication that includes abnormal involuntary movements of the mouth, tongue, and jaw such as lip smacking, sucking, puckering, tongue protrusion, the bon-bon sign, athetoid (worm-like) movements of the tongue, and chewing.

target symptoms Specific symptoms for which psychiatric medications are prescribed, such as hallucinations, delusions, paranoia, agitation, assaultive behaviour, bizarre ideation, social withdrawal, disorientation, catatonia, blunted affect, thought blocking, insomnia, and anorexia.

task function The group role that focuses on the task of the group.

telehealth The use of electronic information and communication technologies to support health care services over distance.

temperament A person's characteristic intensity, rhythmicity, adaptability, energy expenditure, and mood.

tenuous stability Fragile personality patterns that lack resiliency under subjective stress.

thalamus Thought to play a role in controlling electrical activity in the cortex; provides the relay mechanism for information to and from the cerebrum.

therapeutic communication The ongoing process of interaction, verbal and nonverbal, through which meaning emerges.

therapeutic index A ratio of the maximum nontoxic dose to the minimum effective dose.

thought broadcasting Belief that one's thoughts are open to others or are being broadcast to the world.

thought insertion Belief that thoughts or ideas are being inserted into one's mind by someone or something external to one's self.

thought stopping A practice in which a person identifies negative feelings and thoughts that exist together, says "stop," and then engages in a distracting activity.

thymoleptic Mood stabilizing.

tidal model A theory-based approach to mental health nursing that emphasizes empowering collaboration between the nurse and the person receiving nursing care.

token economy Applies behaviour modification techniques to multiple behaviours; clients are rewarded with tokens for selected desired behaviours.

tolerance Increased amounts of a substance are needed to achieve intoxication or desired effect, or there is diminished effect with the same amount of the substance.

torticollis The neck muscles pull the head to the side.

toxicity The point at which concentrations of a drug in the bloodstream become harmful or poisonous to the body.

transference The unconscious assignment to others of feelings and attitudes that were originally associated with important figures such as parents or siblings.

transition times A term used to describe times of addition, subtraction, or change in status of family members.

transitional object A symbolic attachment figure, such as a blanket or a stuffed animal, that a child may cling to when a parent is not available.

traumatic bonding A strong emotional attachment between an abused person and his or her abuser, formed as a result of the cycle of violence.

triad A group consisting of three people.

trichotillomania Chronic, self-destructive hair pulling that results in noticeable hair loss, usually in the crown, occipital, or parietal areas, though sometimes of the eyebrows and eyelashes.

unipolar A term used to describe depression where the affected person has never experienced a manic episode. When a manic episode has been experienced, the depression is termed *bipolar*.

universal preventive interventions Preventive interventions that are targeted to everyone within a general public or whole population group.

urine specific gravity A measure of the degree of concentration of solutes in urine.

utilitarianism The approach to ethics that sets what is right to do as being what gives the best consequences (happiness, pleasure, preference, satisfaction) for the greater number of people.

ventricles The four cavities of the brain.

verbal communication The use of the spoken word, including its underlying emotion, context, and connotation.

verbigeration Purposeless repetition of words or phrases.

vicious circles of behaviour A term used to describe the tendency to become trapped in rigid and inflexible patterns of behaviour that are self-defeating.

violence (violent behaviour) A physical act of force intended to cause harm to a person or an object and to convey the message that the perpetrator's, and not the victim's, point of view is correct.

voluntary admission The legal status of a patient who has consented to being admitted to the hospital for treatment, during which time he or she maintains all civil rights and is free to leave at any time, even if it is against medical advice.

water intoxication A severe state of fluid overload occurring when large amounts of water are ingested and serum sodium levels rapidly fall to a level below 120 mEq/L.

waxy flexibility Posture held in an odd or unusual fixed position for extended periods of time.

well-being The state of contentment and positive sense that one's existence is as it should be. It is connected with one's self-identity and relationships.

Wernicke's area An area in the left superior temporal gyrus of the brain thought to be responsible for comprehension of speech.

Wernicke's syndrome An alcohol-induced amnestic disorder caused by a thiamine-deficient diet and characterized by diplopia, hyperactivity, ataxia, and delirium.

withdrawal The adverse physical and psychological symptoms that occur when a person ceases to use a substance.

word salad A string of words that are not connected in any way.

working phase The second phase of the nurse–patient relationship, in which patients can examine specific problems and learn new ways of approaching them.

work–life balance Achieved when an individual finds a satisfactory interaction among all the domains of his or her life.

xerostomia Dry mouth.

zeitgebers Specific events that function as time givers or synchronizers and that result in the setting of biologic rhythms.

Page numbers followed by "b" indicate boxed materials; page numbers followed by "f" indicate figures; page numbers followed by "t" indicate tables.

A

A Mind That Found Itself (Beers), 6
Abnormal Involuntary Movement Scale
 (AIMS), 910–911
Aboriginal Community Wellness Strategies,
 345, 345b
Aboriginal peoples, 27–29, 28b
 assimilation, 28–29
 colonialism, 28–29
 cultural diversity, 28
 historical trauma, 28–29
 HIV infection, 856
 inhalant abuse, 590–591
 mental health, 12, 28
 protective factors, 345, 345b
 spirituality, 29
 substance-related disorders, 599
 suicide, 35, 344–345
Abuse
 batterer treatment, 883–884
 of children (*See* Child abuse and neglect)
 of elders, 860
 evaluation and treatment outcomes in,
  883–884
 of men, 857
 theories of, 860f
  biologic, 861
  psychosocial, 861–862
  social, 862–863
  specific to woman abuse, 863–865
 of women (*See* Woman abuse)
Abuse survivors
 assessment of
  in biologic domain, 873–878
  in psychological domain, 879
  in social domain, 881–882
 nursing diagnoses for
  for biologic domain, 878
  for psychological domain, 879–881
  for social domain, 882
 nursing interventions for
  for biologic domain, 878–879
  for psychological domain, 879–881
  for social domain, 882
  for spiritual domain, 882–883
 responses to abuse
  biologic, 866–871
  nursing and, 872–883
  psychological, 871

 revictimization of, 872
 social and interpersonal, 872
Acceptance, in therapeutic communication, 67t
Accommodation, workplace, mental health, 282
Acetylcholine (ACh), 134–135
 sleep-wake disorders, 649
Actigraphy, 655
Acting out, as defence mechanism, 74t
Active listening, 69
Activities of daily living (ADLs), 49
Activity interventions, 172
Acute extrapyramidal syndromes, 206
Acute inpatient care, 50
Acute pain, 833
Acute stress disorder (ASD), 726–727, 866
Adaptation, Roy's theory of, 101
Addiction treatment
 goals of, 579, 581, 581b
 principles of, 580b
Addictive disorders. *See* Substance-related
  disorders
ADHD Rating Scale, 739b
Adler, Alfred, 102t, 104
Adolescents. *See also* Youth
 anxiety disorders in
  obsessive-compulsive disorder, 722–724
  separation anxiety disorder, 722–723, 723b
 assessment, 701b, 702
  biologic domain, 702
  child abuse, 712–714
  psychological domain, 703–710
  social domain, 711–712
  spiritual domain, 712
 bipolar disorders in, 459
 disruptive behaviour disorders, 734–746
  attention deficit hyperactivity disorder,
   736–744
  conduct disorder, 735–736
  externalizing disorders, 734
  internalizing disorders, 734
  motor disorders, 744–746
  oppositional defiant disorder, 734
 grieving in, 670b
 mental health promotion (*See* Mental
   health promotion, in children and
   adolescents)
 mental illness among, 683
 physical and developmental challenges in,
  675–676

 sleep-wake disorders, 648
 substance-related disorders, 598
Adults
 grieving in, 669–671, 670t
 older (*See* Older adults)
Advice
 leading groups, 252t
 in therapeutic communication, 68b, 68t
Affect
 assessment of, in older adults, 772–773
 blunted, 159
 definition, 159
 in depressive disorders, assessment of, 451
 flat, 159
Affective instability, 612, 613
Affliation programs, 10
Ages and Stages Questionnaire-Social-
   Emotional Version, 698
Aggression and violence. *See also* Abuse; Anger
 analysis and outcome identification for, 326
 assessment of
  in biologic domain, 326–327
  in psychological domain, 327–329
  in social domain, 331
  in spiritual domain, 332–333
 characteristics and risk factors for, 324t
 clients etiologies for, 320f
 continuum of care for, 335–336, 336b
 definition of, 319
 evaluation and treatment outcomes in, 335
 interactional processes and, 333–334
 models of
  biologic, 320–321
  interactional, 323
  low serotonin syndrome, 321–322
  neurochemical model, 321–322
  psychological, 322–323
  sociocultural, 323
 nursing interventions for
  for biologic domain, 328
  planning and implementing, 326–327,
   327b, 327f
  for psychological domain, 329, 330b
  for social domain, 331–332
  for spiritual domain, 332–333
 predictors of, 325–326, 326t
 responding to assault and, 334–335, 335t
Agitation, 371
Agoraphobia, 486

Agreement, in therapeutic communication, 68t
AIDS
 bio/psycho/social/spiritual interventions, 841
 client assessment, 840–841
 psychological aspects, 840
 psychopathologic complications, 839–841
Akathisia, 207–208
Alanine aminotransferase (ALT; SGPT), serum level of, 157t
Alberta
 Alberta Hospital, 8, 10
 nurse education in, 10–11, 11f
 standard of practice in, 73t
 training in, 8
Alcohol. *See also* Substance use disorders
 addiction, 573
 aetiologic theories, 576–578
 withdrawal syndrome, 287–588
Alcoholics Anonymous (AA), 577b, 585
Allodynia, 833
Allostasis, 481
Altruistic suicide, 349
Alzheimer disease (AD)
 aetiology, 793–795
 assessment of
 biologic domain, 796–798
 psychological domain, 801–803
 social domain, 807–808
 spiritual domain, 810
 clinical course, 791–792, 791t
 continuum of care, 811, 813
 diagnostic criteria, 792–793, 792t
 epidemiology and risk factors for, 793
 evaluation, 810–811
 families, 796
 home visits and, 809
 interdisciplinary treatment, 795–796
 nursing care plan for, 811
 nursing diagnoses
 biologic domain, 798
 psychological domain, 803
 social domain, 808
 nursing home care, 811, 813
 nursing interventions
 biologic domain, 798–801
 psychological domain, 803–807
 social domain, 808–809
 priority care issues, 796
 treatment outcomes, 810–811
 warning signs of, 792
Ambivalence, schizophrenia, 370
American Psychiatric Association (APA), 719
Amygdala, 126–127
Amylase, serum level of, 157t
Anger. *See also* Aggression and violence
 continuum of care, 335–336, 336b
 definition, 318
 evaluation and treatment outcomes, 335
 experience of, 318, 318b
 expression, 318–319
 management groups, 256
 models of
 biologic theories, 320–321
 interactional theory, 323
 psychological theories, 322–323
 sociocultural theories, 323

physiologic and behavioural cues, 326t
 responding to assault, 334–335
 as response to abuse, 871
 spiritual domain, 332–333
Anhedonia, 593
Anomic suicide, 349
Anorexia nervosa (AN)
 aetiology, 530–534
 biologic theories, 531–629
 psychological theories, 530–531
 social theories, 532–533
 spiritual theories, 533–534
 assessment
 biologic domain, 538–539
 psychological domain, 543–544
 clinical course, 524–525
 continuum of care, 549
 diagnostic criteria, 525–526, 526t
 epidemiology, 527–530
 age of onset, 528
 comorbidity, 530
 ethnic and cultural difference, 529–530
 familial predisposition, 530
 gender differences, 528
 evaluation and treatment outcomes, 547b, 549
 interdisciplinary treatment, 536–537, 537t
 neurobiology and neurochemistry of, 526–527
 nurse spirituality, 546b
 nursing care plan
 clinical setting, 540
 disturbed body image/body experience, 541–542
 imbalanced nutrition, 540–541
 spiritual distress, 542–543
 nursing management
 biologic domain, 538–539
 psychological domain, 543–547
 social domain, 547–548
 spiritual domain, 548–549
 pharmacologic interventions, 537–538
 physiologic consequences of, 526–527, 527b
 priority care issues, 538
 psychoeducation, 547b
 risk factors
 biologic, 534–535
 psychological, 535
 sociocultural, 535–536
 spiritual, 536
Anticholinergic(s)
 crisis, 395
 side effects, nursing interventions, 390t
 signs and symptoms, 395
Anticonvulsants, bipolar disorders, 464
Antidepressants
 bipolar disorders, 466
 novel drug development, 219b
Antipsychotics
 anticholinergic side effects, 205
 for autistic disorder, 730
 for bipolar disorders, 466
 blood disorders, 205–206
 cardiovascular side effects, 205
 endocrine and sexual side effects, 205
 medication-related movement disorders
 acute extrapyramidal syndromes, 206

akathisia, 207–208
 chronic syndromes, 208
 dystonia, 206–207
 pseudoparkinsonism, 207
 tardive dyskinesia, 208–209
 nursing interventions, 376t
 schizophrenia, 376t
 side effects, 376t
 typical and atypical antipsychotics
 adverse reactions, 205–209
 chemical interactions, 203t
 drug formulations, 204
 indications and mechanisms of action, 201–202
 pharmacokinetics, 202–204, 203t
 side effects, 201t, 205–209
 toxicity, 205–209
 weight gain, 205
Antisocial personality disorder (ASPD)
 aetiology, 633
 clinical course, 629, 633
 comorbidity, 633
 nursing management, 633–634
 psychoeducation, 634b
Anxiety. *See also* Acute stress disorder (ASD); Generalized anxiety disorder (GAD); Obsessive-compulsive disorder (OCD); Panic disorder; Phobias; Posttraumatic stress disorder (PTSD)
 aetiologic theories
 genetic, 487
 neurobiology, 487
 neuroimaging techniques, 488–489
 neuropeptides, 488
 neurotransmitters, 488
 nursing management, 489
 psychodynamic, 489
 depressive disorders, 724–725
 Hamilton rating scale, 492t
 in interpersonal relations theory, 97
 normal *vs.* abnormal response, 481, 482t
 nursing interventions, 494t
 obsessive-compulsive disorder, 722
 epidemiology and aetiology, 723
 nursing management, 723–724
 psychopharmacologic interventions, 723
 in psychoanalytic theory, 102–103
 psychoeducation, 495b
 rating scales, 492b
 separation anxiety disorder
 epidemiology and aetiology, 722
 nursing management, 722, 723b
 psychopharmacologic interventions, 722
 spiritual domain of, 497
 substance-related disorders, 827
 symptoms, 482t
Anxiolytics, 491, 592
Appearance, in mental status examination, 158
Appetite, in depressive disorders, 445
Archetypes, 104
Aripiprazole (Abilify)
 dosage, half-life, and therapeutic blood level of, 203t
 side effects, 201t

Aspartate aminotransferase (AST), 157t
Assaultive ideation, 162
Assertiveness, 325
Assessment, 148–164. *See also* Bio/psycho/
        social/spiritual geriatric mental
        health nursing assessment;
        Bio/psycho/social/spiritual
        psychiatric and mental health
        assessment; specific disorders and
        conditions
    comprehensive assessment, 149
    definition of, 149
    of family systems, 269
    focused, 149
    as process, 148–149
    techniques for, 149, 152–154
        collaboration with colleagues, 154
        examination, 153
        interviewing, 153, 153b, 154b
        observation, 152–153
Assimilation, cultural, 28–29
Assisted living, for older adults, 757
Association
    clang, 160b
    cortex, 124
    loosening of, 160b
Asylum, early, 4–8
At Home/Chez Soi project, 22–23
Athletes, eating disorders among, 539
Attachment
    assessment of, in children and adolescents,
        705–707
    in children and adolescents, 669
    disorganization, 707
    disrupted, 707
    theories, 706–707
Attention
    definion, 737
    in mental status examination, 161
Attention deficit hyperactivity disorder
        (ADHD)
    aetiologic factors, 737–738
    biologic domain, 742–743
    biologic factors, 738
    nursing management, 738–744
    psychosocial domain, 743–744
    psychosocial factors, 738
    spiritual domain, 744
    substance-related disorders,
        827–828
Attitude toward interviewer, in mental status
        examination, 158
Atypical antipsychotics, 656t
Auditory hallucinations, schizophrenia, 370
Autism spectrum disorder (ASD)
    biologic domain, 731
    continuum of care, 731
    epidemiology and aetiology,
        729–730
    nursing management, 731–733
    psychopharmacologic interventions,
        730–731
    psychosocial domain, 731–733
    spiritual domain, 733
Automatic thoughts, of cognition, 177,
        234–235, 238–240
Avoidant personality disorder, 636

B
Bandura, Albert, 107
Barager, Charles A., 7
Barker, Philip, 99
Barnard's parent-child interaction model,
        694
Barrymore, Drew, 824
Basal ganglia, 124
Beck, Aaron T., 106t, 107–108
Bedlam, 2
Beers, Clifford, 6
Beginning stage of group development, 246
Behaviour Assessment System for Children
        (BASC), 693
Behaviour changes, assessment of, in older
        adults, 774
Behaviour modification, 177
Behaviour therapy, 177, 456
Behavioural experiments, 241–242, 242b
    modify symptoms, 241–242
    test beliefs, 241
Behavioural factors, in depressive disorders,
        443–444
Behavioural interventions
    for borderline personality disorder, 625
    enuresis, 746–747
Behavioural sensitization, 867
Behavioural theories
    applicability to psychiatric and mental
        health nursing, 108
    cognitive, 106t, 107
    reinforcement, 107
    stimulus-response, 105, 106t
Beliefs
    personal, understanding, 65
    religious, approaches to mental illness
        and, 29
Beneficence, 85
Benner, Patricia, 12, 99
Benzodiazepines, 656t
    adverse reactions, 220
    indications and mechanisms of
        action, 220
    panic disorder, 491
    pharmacokinetics, 220–221
    side effects, 221
    toxicity, 221
Benztropine mesylate (Cogentin), 391b
Bereavement, older adults, 758
Bibliotherapy, 684–685
Bicarbonate, serum level of, 157t
Bicetre, 3
Bidirectional model, concurrent disorders,
        824
Binge eating disorder (BED)
    aetiology
        biologic theories, 560
        psychological and social theories, 560
        spiritual theories, 560–561
    clinical course, 557–558
    continuum of care, 563
    diagnostic criteria, 558
    epidemiology
        age of onset, 558
        comorbidity, 559
        ethnic and cultural difference, 558
        familial difference, 558–559

    gender difference, 918
    medical complication, 559–560
    evaluation and treatment outcomes, 563
    interdisciplinary treatment, 561
    nursing management
        biologic domain, 561–562
        psychosocial domain, 562
        spiritual domain, 562–563
        therapeutic relationship, 561
    priority care issues, 561
    psychoeducation, 562b
    risk factors, 534f, 561
    special populations, 558
Biochemical theories
    bulimia nervosa, 552
    delusional, 430
    schizoaffective disorders, 418
Biogenic amines, 135
Biologic clock, 647f
Biologic domain
    assessment, 154–157 (*See also specific
        disorders and conditions*)
        in children and adolescents, 702
    attention deficit hyperactivity disorder,
        742–743
    autistic spectrum disorder, 731
    bipolar disorder, 721
    conduct disorder, 736
    depressive disorders, 445–451, 724
    family assessment, 264
    gender dysphoria, 728
    health history in, 150t–152t, 155–156
    insomnia, 658–661
    nursing diagnoses for (*See specific disorders
        and conditions*)
    nursing interventions, 171–175,
        356–357
        abuse survivors, 878–879
        bipolar disorders, 461–467
        delusional disorder, 431
        stress, 300
    obstructive sleep apnea, 662–663
    oppositional defiant disorder, 735
    physical examination in, 156,
        156t–157t
    psychotic disorders, 720
    reactive attachment disorder, 726
    schizoaffective disorder (SCA), 419,
        422–423
    schizophrenia, 386–395, 390t–391t, 394f
    stress, 300
    traumatic stress, 727
Biologic theories, 9, 101. *See also specific
        disorders and conditions*
Biological foundations
    behaviour
        epigenetics, 117
        genetics, 115–117
        population genetics, 116–117
        risk factors, 117
    central nervous system (CNS)
        neuroanatomy, 122–130
        neurophysiology, 130–138
    neuroimaging methods, 120t
        functional neuroimaging, 121
        structural neuroimaging, 119–121
        structure-function gap, 121–122

Biological treatment. *See also specific disorders and conditions*
  electroconvulsive therapy (ECT), 224–225
    for bipolar disorders, 467
    in depressive disorders, 451
  light therapy (phototherapy), 225
  nutritional therapies, 225–226
  psychosocial issues, 226–227, 227b
Bio/psycho/social/spiritual boundaries, 71–73
Bio/psycho/social/spiritual geriatric mental health nursing assessment
  biologic domain, 767, 769–771
    pain, 771
    pharmacologic assessment, 771
    physical examination, 767
    physical functions, 767, 769–770
    present and past health status, 767
  psychological domain, 771–775
    behaviour changes, 774
    mental status examination, 772–774
    responses to mental health problems, 772
    risk assessment, 775
    stress and coping patterns, 774–775
  social domain, 775–777
    functional status, 776
    legal status, 776–777
    social support, 775
    social systems, 776
    spiritual domain, 777
Bio/psycho/social/spiritual interventions, 166, 166f. *See also* Nursing interventions; *specific disorders and conditions*
Bio/psycho/social/spiritual nursing assessment. *See also* Bio/psycho/social/spiritual geriatric mental health nursing assessment; Bio/psycho/social/spiritual psychiatric and mental health assessment; *specific disorders and conditions*
  biologic domain, 702
  child abuse, 712–714
  psychological domain, 703–710
  social domain, 711–712
  spiritual domain, 712
Bio/psycho/social/spiritual psychiatric and mental health assessment, 9f, 154–163, 155f
  biologic domain and, 154–157
    health history in, 155–156
    physical examination in, 156–157
  documentation for, 155
  psychological domain and, 158–162
    mental status examination and, 158–161, 158b, 160b
    responses to mental health problems and, 158
    risk assessment and, 161–162, 162t
    stress and coping patterns and, 161
  social domain and
    functional status and, 163
    spiritual domain and, 163
  types and sources of information for, 154–155
Bio/psycho/social/spiritual self, 65
Biosocial theories, of borderline personality disorder, 615–617
Biperiden (Akineton), 207t

Bipolar disorders
  aetiology, 460
  biologic domain, 721
  clinical course, 457, 459
  continuum of care, 469
  diagnostic criteria, 457, 458t, 459b
  epidemiology, 459
  evaluation and treatment outcomes, 469
  family response to, 461
  interdisciplinary treatment of, 460–461
  medical comorbidity, 459–460
  nursing interventions for, 721
    biologic domain, 461–467
    nursing care plan for, 472–475
    psychological domain, 467–468
    social domain, 468–469
    spiritual domain, 469
  priority care issues, 461
  psychosocial domain, 721
  and related disorders, 721
  spiritual domain, 721
Bizarre delusions, 160b
Blood urea nitrogen (BUN), 157t
Blunted affect, 159
Borderline personality disorder (BPD), 870
  aetiology
    biosocial theories, 615–617
    genetic factors, 614–615
    maladaptive schemas, 615, 616t
    psychological theories, 615
    risk factors, 615
  behavioural patterns in, 616, 617b
  clinical course of disorder
    affective instability, 612–613
    cognitive dysfunctions, 613–614
    diagnostic characteristics of, 612, 612t
    dysfunctional behaviours, 614
    identity diffusion, 613
    unstable interpersonal relationships, 613
  continuum of care, 629
  evaluation and outcomes, 629
  family response, 618
  interdisciplinary treatment
    dialectical behaviour therapy, 617–618
    psychopharmacotherapy, 618
  nursing care plan, 630–632
  nursing management
    biologic domain, 619–621
    psychological domain, 621–23
    social domain, 627–629
    spiritual domain, 629
  response patterns, 619, 619b
Boundaries, in therapeutic communication, 71–73
Brain
  in attention deficit/hyperactivity disorder, 737
  in autism, 780f
Brain plasticity, 118, 119t
Breathing control, panic disorder, 490
Brief psychiatric rating scales, 907
Brief psychotic disorder, 434, 720
British Columbia, standard of practice in, 73t
British North America Act of 1867, 5
Bulimia nervosa (BN)
  aetiology
    biologic theories, 542–543

  psychological and social theories, 552–553
Binge-purge cycle, 550, 551f
clinical course, 549–550
continuum of care, 557
diagnostic criteria, 550–551
drug profile, 555b
epidemiology
  age of onset, 551
  comorbidity, 551
  ethnic and cultural difference, 551
  familial difference, 551
  gender difference, 551
evaluation and treatment outcomes, 557
interdisciplinary treatment, 553
nursing management
  biologic domain, 553–554
  psychosocial domain, 555–557
  spiritual domain, 557
  therapeutic relationship, 553
priority care issues, 553
psychoeducation, 556b
risk factors, 534f, 553
Bullying, workplace, mental health, 281, 281t
Burnout, workplace, mental health, 280, 283–284
Buspirone
  adverse reactions, 221
  indications, 220
  mechanisms of actions, 220
  pharmacokinetics, 220–221
  side effects, 221
  toxicity, 221

C
Caffeine, substance-related disorders, 589
Calgary Family Assessment Model (CFAM), 268
Calgary Family Intervention Model (CFIM), 268
Canada Disaster Database (CDC), 306, 308t
Canada Health Act (CHA), 3, 13
Canadian Alliance on Mental Illness and Mental Health (CAMIMH), 12, 13, 62
Canadian Collaborative Mental Health Initiative (CCMHI), 167
Canadian Index of Wellbeing (CIW), 18–19
Canadian Journal for Nursing Research, 12
Canadian Mental Health Acts, 37, 37b, 38b
Canadian Mental Health Association (CMHA), 10, 12, 693
Canadian National Committee for Mental Hygiene (CNCMH), 7
Canadian Nurses Association (CNA), 663–664
Canadian Psychiatric Association, 12
Canadian standards, 57, 58b–61b
Canadian Standards of Psychiatric-Mental Health Nursing, 12, 171
Cannabis, substance-related disorders, 589
Carbamazepine (Tegretol), 464, 466t
Caring
  custody and, paradox of, 892–893, 893f
  Watson's theory of, 99
Case management, 44, 44b
Casuistry, 84t, 86
Catapres (clonidine), for Tourette disorder, 745

Catatonic excitement, schizophrenia, 371
Catharsis, 319
Central nervous system (CNS)
  brain plasticity, 118, 119t
  chronobiology, 141
  diagnostic approaches
    biologic markers, 141
    electroencephalography, 141–142
    endocrine stimulation tests
    polysomnography, 143
  generalized anxiety disorder, etiologies, 142f, 143
  neuroimaging methods, 120t
    functional neuroimaging, 121
    structural neuroimaging, 119–121
    structure-function gap, 121–122
  neurophysiology (*See* Neurophysiology)
  psychoendocrinology, 139
  psychoimmunology, 140–141
Challenges, in therapeutic communication, 68t
Charter of Rights and Freedoms (1982), 37
Charting by exception, 155
Chemical messengers, in depressive disorders, 443
Chemical restraint, 180
Child abuse and neglect, 678–681, 679t, 680b, 712–714
  child and family services, 679–680
  children, 712–714
  emotional abuse, 679t, 859
  evaluation of, 712–714
  factitious disorder by proxy, 521, 859
  neglect, 679t, 858
  physical abuse, 679t, 858
  resilience, 714
  risk factors, 677–678
  secondary abuse, 859–860
  sexual abuse, 679t, 713, 858–859
Child and family services, 679–680
Child Attention Profile (CAP), 693
Child Behaviour Checklist (CBCL), 693, 699
Childhood psychopathology, risk factors
  child abuse and neglect, 678–681
  homelessness, 678
  parent with substance abuse problem, 682–683
  parents with mental illness, 681–682
  poverty, 677
Children. *See also* Youth
  with adolescents, 694–702
  anxiety disorders in
    nursing interventions, 494t
    obsessive-compulsive disorder, 722–724
    separation anxiety disorder, 722–723, 723b
  biopsychosocial nursing assessment of
    biologic domain, 702
    child abuse, 712–714
    psychological domain, 703–710
    social domain, 711–712
    spiritual domain, 712
  bipolar disorders in, 459
  depressive disorders in, 441
  disruptive behaviour disorders, 736–744
    (*See also* Conduct disorder; Oppositional defiant disorder)
    conduct disorder, 735–736

  motor disorders, 744–746
  oppositional defiant disorder, 734
  grieving in, 670b
  mental health assessment of, 691–714
  preschool-aged, 671, 699–700, 700b, 700f
  school-aged, 671, 700, 702
  sleep-wake disorders, 648, 650
  somatic symptom disorder, 506
Children's Depression Inventory (CDI), 693, 699
Children's Yale-Brown Obsessive Compulsive Scale (CY-BOCS), 699
Chloral hydrate, 660
Chloride, serum level of, 157t
Chlorpromazine (Thorazine), 9
Cholecystokinin (CCK), anxiety disorder, 488
Chronic illnesses, in older adults, 758
Chronic pain, 833, 835b
Chronobiologic theories, of bipolar disorders, 460
Chronobiology, 141
Circadian, 647
Circumstantiality, 160b
Clang association, 160b
Clarification, leading groups, 252t
Classic antihistamines, 656t
Classical conditioning, 105
Client/family education, 178, 178f, 627–629. *See also* Psychoeducation
Clinical decision making, 58
Clinical Institute Withdrawal Assessment of Alcohol Scale, Revised (CIWA-Ar), 915–916
Clinical interview, 693–702
  as assessment technique, 153, 153b, 154b
  barriers to, 154b
  with children and adolescents
    adolescents, 702
    Building Rapport, 694, 695b–696b
    child and parent observation, 694
    children's rating scales, 698–699
    discussion with child, 697–698, 697b
    discussion with parents, 698
    preschool-aged children, 699–700, 700b, 700f
  factors facilitating, 153b
Clomipramine (Anafranil), 447t
Clonidine(Catapres), for Tourette disorder, 745
Closed group, 245
Clozapine (Clozaril), 389b
CNS disorders. *See* Neurologic impairment
Codependency support groups, psychoeducational, 254, 254b
Cognition
  assessment of, in older adults, 773–774
  in bipolar disorders, assessment of, 467
  in depressive disorders, assessment of, 452
Cognitive dysfunction
  in borderline personality disorder, 613–614
  eating disorder, 547t
Cognitive function, 754
Cognitive interventions, 177. *See also* Cognitive therapy
Cognitive neuroassociation model, 321
Cognitive processes, maladaptive, in borderline personality disorder, 615, 616t

Cognitive restructuring, 238–241
  automatic thoughts
    core beliefs, 240–241
    evaluating, 238–239, 239b
    identifying, 238
    intermediate beliefs, 240, 240b
    modification of, 239–240
    thinking errors, 239b
Cognitive schemas, 234, 607
Cognitive theory, bulimia nervosa, 552–553
Cognitive therapy, 106t, 107
  for depressive disorders, 453
  substance-related disorders, 585
Cognitive-behavioural formulation, 236
Cognitive-behavioural model, 833
Cognitive-behavioural therapy (CBT)
  cognition levels
    automatic thoughts, 234–235
    core beliefs, 234
    intermediate beliefs, 234
    relationship, 235, 235f
  cognitive model, 233–234, 233f
  mindfulness, 242
  panic disorder, 495, 495b
  principles of
    cognitive-behavioural formulation, 236
    educative, 237
    goal oriented, problem focused, and change oriented, 236–237
    inductive reasoning, 237
    self-reflective exercises, 237–238
    Socratic questioning, 237
    structured and directive, 237
    therapeutic alliance, 236
    therapeutic collaboration, 237
    time limitation, 236
  research for, 242b
  substance-related disorders, 585
  thinking errors, 239, 239b
  treatment strategies
    behavioural techniques, 241–242, 242b
    cognitive techniques, 238–241, 239b, 240b
Collaboration, in assessment, 154
Collaborative care, 60–61
Collective unconscious, 104
Colonialism, 28–29
Command hallucinations, 159
Common factor model, concurrent disorders, 824
Communication, 64–80
  action, 182
  blocks, 75
  disorders, 734
  group, 247, 249
  nonverbal, 65, 69–70, 70f
    group, 249
  with older adults, 753b
  open, 179
  patterns, family assessment, 267–268
  self-awareness, 64–65
  therapeutic (*See* Nurse-client relationship; Therapeutic communication)
  triad, 625
  verbal, 66–69, 66f, 67t, 68b, 68t, 69b (*See also* Language; Speech)
    group, 247, 249

Community
  action, 182
  care, 410–411
  schizoaffective disorder, 426–427
  support, 49–50, 50b, 762
  treatment
    delusional disorder, 433
    obsessive-compulsive disorder, 500
    panic disorder, 499
    somatic symptom disorder, 517
Community assessment, with children and
    adolescents, 711
Community mental health nursing, 10
Community Resource Base, 692, 694
Community-based mental health promotion,
    new directions in, 686
Community-based residential services, 49
Comorbidity. *See specific disorders*
Compassion fatigue, 284
Competence
  apparent, in borderline personality
    disorder, 617b
  cultural, 32, 32b
  involuntary admission and, 37
Completed suicide, 340
Complex posttraumatic stress disorder
    (CPTSD), 870
Comprehensive assessment, 149
Compulsive personality disorder, 637
Computed axial tomography, 119
Concentration, in mental status examination,
    161
Concordant twins, 116
Concurrent disorders
  aetiologic theories, 824
  assessment, 825
  care and treatment, 825–826
  epidemiology of, 823
  interventions
    nursing for patients, 826, 827b
    substance-related disorders (*See*
      Substance-related disorders)
  nursing management, 828–829
Conditioning, classical (Pavlovian), 105
Conduct disorder, 637–638, 735–736
Confidentiality, 77, 91–92
Conflict resolution, 175–176
Confrontation
  leading groups, 252t
  in therapeutic communication, 67t
Conscientious objection, 83
Conscious mental processes, in
    psychoanalytic theory, 102–103
Consumer organizations, 12
Content themes, 75, 75b
Continuous positive airway pressure therapy
    (CPAP), 662–663
Continuum of care, 42–50. *See also specific
    disorders*
  acute inpatient care and, 50
  case management and, 44, 44b
  consumer self-help/survivor initiatives,
    46, 46b
  coordination of care and, 43–44
  crisis response systems and psychiatric
    emergency services, 46–47, 46b
  definition of, 43

housing and community support and, 49–50
in-home care and, 49
outpatient care, 48–49
supportive employment, 49–50
Control, delusions of, 160b
Conversion disorder, 517
Co-operative Commonwealth Federation, 11
Coordinated/parallel care, 825
Coordination of care, 43–44
Coping
  assessment of, 161
    in bipolar disorders, 467
    of children and adolescents, 712
    in older adults, 774–775
  principles, 296
  problem-focused *vs.* emotion focused, 296,
    298t
  reappraisal, 296
  skills, borderline personality disorder, 628
  social functioning, 296, 297f
  stress and health illness, 296, 298
  styles of (*See* Defence mechanisms)
Coping abilities, family assessment, 268
Coping mechanisms, 72
Core beliefs, of cognition, 234, 240–241
Corticotrophin-releasing hormone (CRH), 293
Cortisol, 648
Counselling, 175
Countertransference, 103
Craving, substance-related disorders, 574
Creatine phosphokinase (CPK), serum level
    of, 157t
Creatinine, serum level of, 157t
Criminalization, of the mentally ill, 892
Crisis
  balancing factors, 303, 303f
  community-based emergency housing, 305
  definition, 302
  developmental crisis, 303
  events, 304b
  intervention, 46
    early, 303
    facilitating, 304
    preventive, for adolescents, 684b
    problem focusing, 304
    Roberts' seven-stage, 306b
    self-reliance, 304
    stabilization, 304
  nursing care, 303–305
  response phases, 303f
  response systems, 46–47, 46b
  short-stay hospitalization, 305
  situational crisis, 303, 304b
  stabilization, 46–47, 46b
  telephone help lines, 305
Cultural assessment, 163
Cultural brokering, 176
Cultural competence, 32, 32b
Cultural diversity
  within Aboriginal peoples, 28
  diagnostic formulations and, 27
Cultural impact, in older adults, 756
Cultural safety, 32, 33b
Culture and ethnicity
  bipolar disorders and, 459
  delusional disorder, 429
  in depressive disorders, 442–443

eating disorder, 529–530, 551, 558
schizoaffective disorder, 417
somatization, 3
Culture-bound syndromes, 27
Cytokines in depressive disorders, 443

D

DAR method, 155
Day treatment, bipolar disorders, 456
Death, loss and
  in childhood, 669–671, 670t
  older adults and, 758–759
De-escalation, 180
Defence mechanisms, 72, 74t, 103
Deinstitutionalization, 10–12
Delirium
  aetiology, 784–785
  assessment of
    biologic domain, 785–786
    psychological domain, 788–789
    social domain, 789–790
    spiritual domain, 790
  in children, 782
  clinical course, 781–782
  continuum of care, 790–791, 790b
  diagnostic criteria, 782
  emergency care for, 781
  epidemiology, 783–784
  evaluation and treatment outcomes, 790
  hyperactive, 789
  hypoactive, 789
  interdisciplinary treatment, 785
  mixed variant, 789
  nursing diagnoses
    biologic domain, 786–787
    psychological domain, 789
    social domain, 790
  nursing interventions
    biologic domain, 787–788
    psychological domain, 789
    social domain, 790
  older adults, 782–783
  priority care, 785
  risk factors, 783–784
Delirium rating scale (DRS), 789b
Delusion(s), 160b, 329, 370, 397t, 398
Delusion of grandeur, 160b
Delusional disorder
  aetiology, 430
  assessment
    biologic domain, 430
    psychological domain, 432
    social domain, 433
    spiritual domain, 433
  biologic theories, 430
  clinical course, 427
  comorbidity, 430
  continuum of care, 433–434
  diagnostic criteria, 427–428, 427t
  epidemiology and risk factors, 429–430
  evaluation and treatment outcomes, 433
  interdisciplinary treatment, 430
  nursing diagnoses
    biologic domain, 431
    psychological domain, 432
    social domain, 433

nursing interventions
  biologic domain, 431
  psychological domain, 432
  social domain, 433
priority care issues, 430
psychoeducation, 432
subtypes
  erotomanic delusions, 428
  grandiose delusions, 428
  jealous delusions, 428
  somatic delusions, 429
  unspecified delusions, 429
Demara, Ferdinand Waldo, 607
Dementia, 791
  Alzheimer type (*See* Alzheimer disease
    (AD))
  definition of, 367
  HIV infection, 814
  Huntington's disease, 814–815
  prion disease, 815
  substance/medication-induced, 815
  traumatic brain injury, 814
Denial, as defence mechanism, 74t
Deontology, 85
Dependent personality disorder, 636
Depersonalization, 160b, 485t
Depression, 866
  schizophrenia, 373
Depressive disorders
  aetiology
    genetic factors, 443
    neurobiologic hypotheses, 443
    psychological theories, 443–444
    social theories, 444
  assessment
    biologic domain, 445–446
    psychological domain, 451
    social domain, 454
    spiritual domain, 455
  biologic domain, 724
  clinical course, 440–441
  continuum of care, 456
  disruptive mood dysregulation disorder,
    724–725
  epidemiology
    ethnic and cultural differences, 442–443
    risk factors, 443
  evaluation and treatment outcomes, 456
  family response to, 444
  interdisciplinary treatment, 444
  nursing diagnoses for
    biologic domain, 446
    psychological domain, 452
    social domain, 454
    spiritual domain, 455
  nursing management, 724–725
    biologic domain, 445–451
    psychological domain, 451–454
    social domain, 454–455
    spiritual domain, 455
  priority care issues, 444
  psychosocial domain, 724
  in special populations
    children and adolescents, 441
    older adults, 441–442
  spiritual domain, 724
Depressive episode, 440, 441t

Derealization, 485t
Destructive behaviour, in personality
    disorders, 608
Development
  depressive disorders and, 444
  in older adults, 755
Developmental assessment of children and
    adolescents, 703–704
Developmental delays, 669, 675, 678, 704
Developmental theories, 108–109
Devereux Early Childhood Assessment
    (DECA), 693
Dexamethasone suppression test (DST), 845
Diabetes mellitus, 373
*Diagnostic and Statistical Manual of Mental
    Disorders (DSM-III)*, 719
*Diagnostic and Statistical Manual of Mental
    Disorders*, 4th ed., Text revision
    (DSM-IV-TR), 74t, 416, 417t, 429
*Diagnostic and Statistical Manual of Mental
    Disorders*, 5th ed., Text revision
    (DSM-V-TR), 72, 154, 163, 369,
    440, 441, 441t, 442, 444, 445, 448,
    457, 458t, 481, 507, 517, 524, 525,
    527, 550, 551, 557, 558, 564, 564t,
    575, 576, 606, 651t–652t, 719, 822,
    870
Diagnostic assessments, 699
Dialectical behaviour therapy (DBT), 617–618
Dichotomous, in borderline personality
    disorder, 621
Diet, 496
Difficult temperament, 707–708
Diffusion Tensor Magnetic Resonance
    Imaging (DTI), 121
Disapproval, in therapeutic communication,
    68t
Disasters
  definition, 306
  mental health and illness in, 310–311
  phases of, 310, 311f
  preparedness and response
    government, role of, 307, 309
    individuals and families, role of,
      309–310
    nurses, role of, 309
  psychological first aid, 311
  public health principles for, 312t
  response to, 305–313
  vulnerable populations
    Aboriginal peoples, 313
    children and adolescents, 311–312
    disabled persons, 312–313
    ethnic minorities, 313
    persons with existing mental disorder,
      312
    relief workers, 313
  workplace mental health, 281
Discrimination, 62
Disinhibition, 107
Disliked member, groups, 254
Disordered water balance, schizophrenia,
    373–374
Disorganized symptoms, schizophrenia, 371
Displacement
  of Aboriginal people, 314
  as defence mechanism, 74t

Disruptive behaviour disorders, 734–746. *See
    also* Attention deficit/hyperactivity
    disorder (ADHD); Conduct
    disorder; Oppositional defiant
    disorder
Disruptive mood dysregulation disorder,
    724–725
Disruptive personality disorder, 637–638
Dissociation, 869
  in borderline personality disorder, 613,
    621–622
    management of, 624–625
  as defence mechanism, 74t
Dissociative identity disorder (DID),
    869–870, 870t
Distraction, 173, 174t, 493, 495
Divalproex sodium (Depakote; valproic acid),
    462, 462t, 463–464, 466b
Diversity, family assessment, 261, 265, 267,
    267b
Divorce, 672, 673t
Documentation, 155
Domains of practice, 57, 58b, 59b
Dopamine, 135–136, 136f
Dopamine hypothesis, schizophrenia, 378
Dorothea Lynde Dix, 6, 6f
Doubt, in therapeutic communication, 67t
Drug abuse. *See* Substance-related disorders
Dynamic Nurse-Patient Relationship, The
    (Orlando), 98
Dysfunctional thinking, in borderline
    personality disorder, addressing,
    626, 626b
Dyskinesia identification system, 386, 387t
Dyslexia, 733
Dysphagia, 767
Dysphoric mood, 159
Dysthymic disorder, 441
Dystonia, 206–207

E
Early intervention programs, mental health
    promotion with children and
    adolescents, 685
Easy temperament, 707
Eating. *See also* Diet; Nutrition; *Nutritional
    entries*
  in geriatric mental health assessment, 767,
    769–770
Eating disorders. *See also* Anorexia nervosa
    (AN); Binge eating disorder (BED);
    Bulimia nervosa (BN)
  assessment instruments, 545b
  boys and men, 529b
  cognitive distortion, 547t
  complications, 528t
  eating attitude test, 545b
  feminist ideology, 532b
  hospitalization criteria, 537t
  prevention, 563–564, 564t
  psychological characteristics, 527b
  recovery, 548b
  risk factors, 534–535, 534f
  therapeutic approach, 539b
Echolalia, 160b
Echopraxia, schizophrenia, 371

Education. *See also* Psychoeducation
nursing
early, 7
models of, 10–11
Egocentrism, 702
Egoistic suicide, 349
Elder abuse, 860
Electroconvulsive therapy (ECT), 224–225
for bipolar disorders, 467
for depressive disorders, 450–451
Electroencephalography (EEG), 141–142, 643
Electrolytes, serum level of, 157t
Electrooculogram (EOG) testing, 655
Elimination disorders
encopresis, 747–748
enuresis, 746–747
Elimination, in geriatric mental health assessment, 770
Emergency care. *See also* specific disorders and conditions; *specific disorders and conditions*
anorexia nervosa, 549
delusional disorder, 433
panic disorder, 497–498
schizoaffective disorder, 426
schizophrenia, 410
somatic symptom disorder, 517
Emotion(s). *See also* Feelings; specific emotions
abuse, of children, 679t
circuit, 321
definition of, 159, 607
Emotional dysregulation, in borderline personality disorder, 616
Emotional regulation, for borderline personality disorder, 625–626
Emotional vulnerability, in borderline personality disorder, 616
Empathic linkages, 65, 71
Empathic listening, 153
Empathy, 71
Employment, supportive, 49–50
Empowerment
encopresis, in children and adolescents, 747
epidemiology and aetiology, 747
nursing management, 747–748
recovery orientation and, 176
Endorphins, 833
Engagement, 262–263, 269
Enuresis
epidemiology and aetiology, 746
nursing management, 746–747
Epinephrine, 137
Erikson, Erik, 108
Erotomania, 160b
Erotomanic delusions, 428
Erythrocyte indices, 156t
Ethics
approaches, 84–88, 84t
of care, 84t, 86
case-based, 86
cause-based, 86
CNA code of, 83
definition of, 82
deontology and, 85

everyday, 83
feminist, 84t, 86
health, 83
human rights and, 84t, 87–88
issues in psychiatric and mental health settings
behaviour control and restraint as, 89–90
confidentiality and privacy as, 91–92
psychiatric advance directives (PADs), 90, 90b
relational engagement as, 90–91
research and, 93
social justice and, 92–93
Kantian, 85
legal domain as separate from, 82–83
moral dilemmas and, 88–89
moral distress and, 88
for nurses, 83
practice environments, 85
principlism and, 85
relational, 84t, 86–87
utilitarianism and, 84t, 85
virtue, 84–85
Ethics of care, 86
Ethnic assessment, 163
Euphoric mood, 159
Euthymic mood, 159
Everyday ethics, 83
Evoked potentials (EPs), 143
Examination, as assessment technique, 153
Exercise interventions, 172
Existential anxiety, 497
Existential theories, 98–100
Exposure therapy, 491, 495
Expressed emotion, 379
Extended family, 260
Externalizing disorders, 734
Extrapyramidal motor system, 127
Extrapyramidal side effects, 389–393, 391t

F

Factitious disorders. *See also* Somatic symptom disorder
diagnostic criteria, 520t
epidemiology, 520
imposed on another, 521
nursing interventions, 521
nursing management, 520–521
by proxy, 521
Families
access to services, 261
anorexia nervosa, 548, 548b
assessment
biologic domain, 264
ecomap, 263–264, 264f
engagement and, 262–263
genograms and, 262–263
mental health assessment, 262, 262b
psychological domain, 264–268
social domain, 268–269
spiritual domain, 269–270
bipolar disorders and, 461
bulimia nervosa, 553
Canadian families, 259–260
caregivers, 260–261

communication patterns, 267–268
concurrent disorder, 829
depressive disorders and, 444
development, 265
diversity of, 261
intervention
commendation, 272
individual strengths, 272
15-minute family interview, 270–271
therapeutic questions in, 271–272
life cycles, 265, 266t
meeting, 261
pyramid of family care framework, 270, 271f
separation and divorce, 671–672, 673t
stigma, 261
Family Care Framework, pyramid of, 270, 271f
Family dynamics, 109
Family education. *See* Client/family education; Psychoeducation
Family interventions. *See also* specific disorders and conditions
for bipolar disorders, 469
commendation, 272
delusional disorder, 433
for depressive disorders, 455
individual strengths, 272
15-minute family interview, 270–271
panic disorder, 498
schizoaffective disorder, 425–426
therapeutic questions in, 271–272
Family psychoeducation, 270
Family therapy, 270
applicability to psychiatric and mental health nursing, 109
substance-related disorders, 586
Fatalistic suicide, 349
Feelings
anorexia nervosa, 544, 546
personal, understanding, 65
Female forensic clients, 895–896
Feminism, eating disorders, 532b
Feminist ethics, 84t, 86
Feminist theories, eating disorders, 532, 532b
Fetal alcohol spectrum disorder, 682
Financial status, of families, 269. *See also* Poverty
First episode psychosis, schizophrenia, 368b
nursing care plan, 381–383
First-pass metabolism, 193
Fissures, 122
Flat affect, 159
Flight of ideas, 160b
in bipolar disorders, 457
Fluoxetine hydrochloride (Prozac), 555b
Focused assessment, 149
Folate deficiency, 156t
Forensic psychiatric and mental health nursing
client characteristics and
cultural diversity and, 897
experience of mental illness and, 894–895
families and, 898

female, 895–896
older forensic client, 896–897
recovery, 895
vulnerability, 894
youth, 897
criminalization of the mentally ill and, 892
model for care and, 893, 893f
nurse-client relationship and
issues experiences by nurses and, 899–900
professional development and, 900–901
professional nursing identity and, 900
paradox of custody and caring and, 892–893, 893f
security awareness and, 901–902, 902b
societal norms and, 902
Formal group roles, 247
Formal operations, 671
Formal support networks, 269
Framework for Support, 693
Frankl, Viktor, 110
Freud, Anna, 102t
Freud, Sigmund, 102
Frontal lobe(s), 123, 124b
Frontal lobe syndrome, 124b
Fry, Elizabeth, 6
Functional activities, of older adults, assessment of, 776
Functional neuroimaging, 120t, 121
Functional status, assessment of, 163
of children and adolescents, 711–712
of older adults, 776

G

Gabapentin (Neurontin), for bipolar disorders, 462
Gambling disorder, 595
Gamma-aminobutyric acid (GABA), 138, 649
Gate-control model, 833
Geel Lunatic Colony, 4
Gender
bipolar disorders and, 459
bulimia nervosa, 551
delusional disorder, 429
dysphoria, 728–729
schizoaffective disorder, 417
somatization, 507
substance-related disorders, 573
suicide, 344
General medical conditions. See Mental illness
Generalized anxiety disorder (GAD), 483
Generativity, 108
Genetic factors
bipolar disorders and, 460
bulimia nervosa, 552
eating disorder, 530, 552, 560
Genetic theories
anorexia nervosa, 530
bulimia nervosa, 552
delusional disorder, 430
schizoaffective disorders, 418
Genetic vulnerability, of children adolescents, assessment of, 702–703
Genograms, 695b, 711
family assessment, 263
Gestalt therapy, 105
Ghrelin, sleep-wake disorders, 649

Gilligan, Carol, 109
Glial cells, 130
Glutamate, 138
Grandiose delusions, 428
schizophrenia, 370
Grey matter, 122
Grieving
in childhood, adolescence, and adulthood, 669–671
inhibited, in borderline personality disorder, 617b
Gross National Happiness (GNH) index, 18
Group(s)
anger management, 256
closed, 245
cohesion, 250
communication, 247–249, 249f
definitions and concepts, 244–245
development, 246–247, 246t
groupthink and decision making, 250
interactive, 255
leadership
challenging behaviours, 253–254
member selection, 253
responsibilities and functions, 248t
seating arrangement, 253
styles, 251–253
techniques, 252t
medication, 255–256
member roles, 247, 248t
norms and standards, 249–250
nursing intervention, 255–256
open, 245
practices, 251b
psychoeducational, 254
psychotherapy, 255
reminiscence, 256
self-care, 256
self-help, 255
size, 245–246
structured, 254–255
supportive therapy, 255
symptom management, 256
Group cohesion, 250
Group conflict, 254
Group leadership, 247
Group themes, 249
Group therapy
bulimia nervosa, 557
for depressive disorders, 453
substance-related disorders, 586
Groupthink, 250
Guided imagery, 173
Guilt, as response to abuse, 871
Guns and suicide, 345–346
Gyri, 122, 123f

H

Hallucinations, 159
Hallucinogen, substance-related disorders, 590
Hamilton Rating Scale for Depression, 914
Harm reduction, substance-related disorders, 579, 583
Hazards, workplace, mental health, 276
Health care professionals, substance-related disorders, 578b

Health care reform, 12–13
Health ethics, 83
Health history, 150t–152t, 155–156
Health promotion, 44, 45
McGill model of nursing, 100
Health teaching. See Client/family education
Healthy workplaces, 277–280
psychosocial factors in, 277, 278t
unsafe workplaces, 279, 279b
work-life balance, 279–280
Helplessness, 342
Hematocrit (Hct), 156t
Hemoglobin (Hgb), 156t
Hierarchy of needs, 105
Highlighting, leading groups, 252t
Hippocampus, 126
Histamine, 137
History taking, for biologic domain assessment, 150t–152t, 155–156
Histrionic personality disorder, 635
Holistic nursing care, expansion of, 11–12
Home visits, 181–182
Homelessness, in childhood and adolescence, 677
Homicidal ideation, 162
Hope, 183
recovery orientation and, 176
Hopelessness, 342
Horney, Karen, 102t, 104
Hospitalization. See also Inpatient-focused care
admission criteria for, 38, 38b
dual disorders, 46–47
eating disorder, criteria, 537t
Housing services, 49
Human immunodeficiency virus (HIV) infection. See also AIDS
neurologic manifestations, 839–840
psychiatric disorders, 840b
psychological aspects, 840
Human rights, 84t, 87–88
Humane treatment, 3–4, 4f
Humanistic theories, 98–100, 102t, 104–105
Huntington's disease, 814–815
Hydration interventions, 174
Hydrotherapy, 9
Hyperactivity
ADHD, 737
definition, 737
Hyperalgia, 833
Hyperarousal, 867
Hyperesthesia, 833
Hypervigilance, schizophrenia, 371
Hypnagogic hallucinations, 159
Hypnotic, substance-related disorders, 592
Hypochondriasis, 517
Hypocretin, sleep-wake disorders, 649
Hypothalamic-pituitary-adrenal (HPA) axis, 841
Hypothalamus, 126

I

Idealization, as defence mechanism, 74t
Ideas
flight of, 160b
of reference, 160b

Ideation
    assaultive or homicidal, 162
    suicidal, 162
Identification, in psychoanalytic theory,
        102–103
Identity diffusion, in borderline personality
        disorder, 612, 613
Identity, in Erikson's theory, 108
Illogical thinking, 177
Illusions, 159
Imipramine (Tofranil), for enuresis, 747
Impulse-control disorders
    intermittent explosive disorder, 638
    kleptomania, 638
    pyromania, 638
Impulsivity
    in borderline personality disorder, 614
    personality disorder, 608, 610
Indian Residential School (IRS), 29
Individual placement and support (IPS),
        282–283
Individual role, group, 247
Informal group roles, 247
Informal support networks, 269
Information leading groups, 252t
Inhibited grieving, in borderline personality
        disorder, 617b, 621
Inpatient units, promotion of client safety on,
        179–181
Inpatient-focused care
    anorexia nervosa, 549
    for bipolar disorders, 468, 471, 475f
    delusional disorder, 433
    panic disorder, 497
    schizophrenia, 410
    somatic symptom disorder, 516
Insight, in mental status examination, 161
Insomnia, 770
    biologic domain, 658–661
    bio/psycho/social/spiritual outcomes, 657,
        659f
    psychological domain, 661
    sleep hygiene, 657, 658b
    social domain, 662
    spiritual domain, 662
Institutionalization. See also Hospitalization;
        Inpatient-focused care
    premature, avoiding, for older adults,
        760–761
Institution(s) early, 3–8, 5f, 5t
    life within, 6–7
Instrumental activities of daily living, older
        adults, assessment of, 776
Integration into psychosocial treatment, 9
Intellectual performance, assessment of,
        in older adults, 773–774
Intensive outpatient programs, 48
    for bipolar disorders, 469
Interdisciplinary approach, 60
    for bipolar disorders, 460–461
Intermediate beliefs, of cognition, 234, 240
Intermittent explosive disorder, 638
Internalizing disorders, 734
Interpersonal Relations in Nursing (Peplau), 76,
        97, 102t
Interpersonal relations theory, 98–100, 102t,
        104–105

Interpersonal relationships, unstable,
        borderline personality disorder, 613
Interpersonal skills, for borderline
        personality disorder, 628
Interpersonal therapy (IPT)
    anorexia nervosa, 546
    for depressive disorders, 453
Interpretation, in therapeutic
        communication, 67t
Intervention stage, of family systems, 269
Interventions. See specific disorders and
        conditions
Interviewing. See Clinical interview
Intimacy, fear of, in borderline personality
        disorder, 623
Invalidating environment, borderline
        personality disorder, 617
Involuntary hospitalization, admission
        criteria for, 38, 38b
Ischaemic cascade, 843

J
Jealous delusions, 428
Jet lag, 664
Job attitudes, workplace, mental health, 276
Job strain, workplace, mental health, 283–284
Journal(s), 11
Journal of Psychiatric Nursing, 11
Judgment, in mental status examination, 161
Jung, Carl Gustav, 102t, 104
Justice, 85

K
Kanner, Leo, 729
Kantian ethics, 85
King, Imogene M., 100
Kleptomania, 638
Knowledge development, dissemination, and
        application, 61
Knowledge Resource Base, 692

L
La Caridad y San Hipólito, order of, 3
Lactation, substance-related disorders, 599
Lamotrigine (Lamictal), for bipolar
        disorders, 462
Language. See also Speech; Verbal
        communication
    assessment of, in children and adolescents,
        704–705
Late adulthood, 753. See also Older adults
Leadership
    challenging behaviours, 253–254
    member selection, 253
    responsibilities and functions, 248t
    seating arrangement, 253
    styles, 251–253
    techniques, 252t
Learning disorders, 733
Learning, in older adults, 754
Least restrictive environment, 36
Legal issues
    basis for mental health treatment and,
        5–6, 5t
    context of mental health care and, 36–38

Legal status, of older adults, assessment of,
        775–776
Leininger, Madeleine, 110
Lethality, 344
Leukocyte count (WBC), 156t
Lewin, Kurt, 106t
Lidz assessment tool, 700b
Lifestyle support, for older adults, 761
Light therapy (phototherapy), 225
    for depressive disorders, 451
Limbic midbrain nuclei, 127
Limbic system
    amygdala, 126–127
    hippocampus, 126
    hypothalamus, 126
    limbic midbrain nuclei, 127
    pituitary, 124
    structures, 126f
    thalamus, 126
Locus caeruleus, 127, 127t–128t
Loosening, of association, 160b
Low-income families, 267

M
"Mad houses," 2
Magical thinking, 160b
Magnetic Resonance Imaging (MRI), 119–120
Maintenance functions, group, 247
Maintenance of Wakefulness Test (MWT), 655
Major depressive disorder. See also Mood
        disorders
    children and adolescents, 724
Males, eating disorder, 529b
Mandatory outpatient treatment (MOT), 38
Manic episodes, 457
Manic-depressive disorders. See Bipolar
        disorders
Manitoba, standard of practice in, 73t
MAPS theories, 111
Marital therapy, for depressive disorders, 453
Marriage. See also Remarriage
    separation and divorce and, 671–672, 673t
Maslow, Abraham, 102t, 105
Massachusetts State Hospital, 6
Maturation, assessment of, in children and
        adolescents, 704
Maximal mental disorder, 18
Medical illness
    anxiety disorders, 846t
    bio/psycho/social/spiritual interventions, 849
    client assessment, 848–849, 849b
    depression, 849t
    mental illness in
        biologic aspects, 846–847
        intervention, 849–850
        medications associated, 848t
        psychological aspects, 847–848
Medication groups, 255–256, 256b
Medication management, 175
Megavitamin therapy, 226
Melatonin, 660
Memory
    in depressive disorders, assessment of, 452
    in mental status examination, 161
    in older adults, 754–755
Men abuse, 857

Mental Disability Rights International (MDRI), 62
Mental disorders. *See also* Mental illness; *specific disorders*
  diagnosis of
    DSM-5, 19–20, 20b
    labelling, 21
  early explanations of, 3
  health states and, 21
  mental health literacy, 21
  responses to, 158
Mental health
  assessment
    of children and adolescents, 691–714
    data collection techniques for, 766
    family, 262, 262b
    of older adults, 765–777 (*See also* Bio/psycho/social/spiritual geriatric mental health nursing assessment)
  of Canadians, 22–23
  diagram of, 18
  At Home/Chez Soi, 22–23
  homelessness, 22–23
  mental illness
    diagnosis of, 19–21
    health states and, 21
    mental health literacy, 21
  recovery, 21
  socioeconomic influences, 34–35
  substance-related disorders, 825
  well-being
    canadian index of wellbeing, 18–19
    social progress index, 19
Mental Health Act, 6
Mental health care
  Aboriginal people, 27–29
  continuum of, 43–44
  coordination of, 43–44
  culture, 26, 26b, 32, 33b
  discrimination, 30
  legal basis, 5–6, 6t
  legal context of, 25–27, 36–39
  outpatients, 38, 38b
    mandatory, 38
  prejudice, 30
  primary care, 47–48, 47b
  recovery, 111
  research and context, 39
  socioeconomic context of, 33–35
  stereotyping, 5–6
  stigma of, 30–31
Mental Health Commission of Canada (MHCC), 260, 719
Mental Health for Canadians: Striking a Balance (p. 9), 18f
Mental health legislation, 36, 36b
Mental health literacy, 21
Mental health promotion, 45, 45b, 668–686
  in children and adolescents
    factors for psychopathology and, 676–683
    intervention approaches for, 683–686, 684b
    mental health in children and adolescents and, 668–669
    mental illness among children and adolescents, 683

    new directions in community-based mental health promotion, 686
    stressors and, 669–676
  in older adults
    biologic domain and, 753–754
    mental illness prevention and, 759–761
    psychological domain and, 754–755
    risk factors for psychopathology, 758–759
    social domain and, 755–757
    spiritual domain, 757
    schizophrenia, 411
    somatic symptom disorder, 517
Mental health services
  Aboriginal people's access, 35
  access to, 28, 35
Mental health treatment. *See also specific treatment approaches*
  legal basis for, 5–6, 6t
  reducing stigma of, 760
"Mental Hygiene," 7
Mental illness, 19–21. *See also specific disorders*
  among children and adolescents, 683
  biologic view, 8
  caregivers, 260
  causes of, 3, 9
  connection and assessment, 270
  consultation, 270
  cultural roots of, 27
  general education, 270
  human rights and, 36
  international agreements to protect people with, 36, 36b
  and interventions, 30–31
  life and economic impact of, 34
  parents, 681–683
  prevention of, among older adults, 759–761
  religious beliefs and approaches to, 29
  rights of persons with, 36, 36b
  stigma of, 30–31, 261
Mental status, 766, 766b
Mental status examination (MSE), 153, 158–161, 158b
  of children and adolescents, 703
  with older adults, 772–774
Mesolimbic pathway hyperactivity, schizophrenia, 376–378
Methylphenidate (Ritalin)
  adverse reactions, 223
  for attention deficit/hyperactivity disorder, 743t
  indications and mechanisms of action, 221
  off-label use, 221–222
  pharmacokinetics, 222–223
  side effects, 223
  toxicity, 223
Meyer, Adolf, 7
Middle-old, 753
Milieu therapy, 178–179, 454
Mindfulness, 242, 332–333
Mini-Mental Status Examination (MMSE), 160, 467
Mixed episode, in bipolar disorders, 458t
Modafinil (Alertec; Provigil)
  adverse reactions, 223
  indications and mechanisms of action, 221

  off-label use, 221–222
  pharmacokinetics, 222–223
  side effects, 223
  toxicity, 223
Modern thinking, scientific thought
  Meyer and psychiatric pluralism, 8
  psychoanalytic theory, 8–9
  psychosocial treatment, integration biologic theories, 9
Monoamine oxidase inhibitors (MAOIs)
  adverse reactions, 216–217
  indications and mechanisms of action, 215
  pharmacokinetics, 215–216
  side effects, 216–217
  toxicity, 216–217
Monopolizing group time, 253
Mood disorders
  assessment of, 159
    in older adults, 772–773
  bipolar disorder, 721
    aetiology, 460
    clinical course, 457, 459
    continuum of care, 469
    diagnostic criteria, 457, 458t
    epidemiology, 459
    evaluation and treatment outcomes, 469
    family response to disorder, 461
    interdisciplinary treatment of disorder, 460–461
    medical comorbidity, 459–460
    nursing care plan, 471–475
    nursing management, human response to, 461–469
    priority care issues, 461
  in children and adolescents, 721
  definition of, 159
  depressive disorders
    aetiology, 443–444
    children and adolescents, 441
    clinical course, 440–441
    continuum of care, 456
    diagnostic criteria, 441t
    epidemiology, 442–443
    evaluation and treatment outcomes, 456
    family response to disorder, 444
    interdisciplinary treatment, 444
    nursing management, 445–455
    in older adults, 441–442
    priority care issues, 444
    spiritual domain, 455
  secondary mania, 457
  substance-related disorders, 826–827
Mood stabilizers, 656t
  anticonvulsants
    adverse reactions, 213
    indications and mechanisms of action, 212
    pharmacokinetics, 212–213
    side effects, 213
    toxicity, 213
  lithium
    adverse reactions, 211
    indications, 210
    mechanisms of action, 210
    pharmacokinetics, 210–211
    side effects, 211
    toxicity, 211

Moral dilemmas, 88–89
Moral distress, 88
More for the Mind, 10
Motivational interviewing (MI), 583–586
Motor disorders
    aetiology, 744–745
    epidemiology, 744
    nursing management, 745–746
Multiple sleep latency test (MSLT), 655
Münchausen's syndrome by proxy, 859
Muscle relaxation, 490b
Mussallem, Helen, 761

N

Narcissistic personality disorder, 635–636
Nardil (phenelzine), 511, 512b
National Committee for Mental Hygiene, 7
National Mental Health Objectives, 13–14,
        13b
National, standard of practice in, 73t
Needs
    hierarchy of, 105
    in interpersonal relations theory, 97
Neglect, of children, 679t
Neo-Freudian models
    of Adler, 102t, 104
    of Horney, 102t, 104
    of Jung, 102t, 104
Neologisms, 160b
Neuman, Betty, 101
Neuman's theory of, 101
Neural connectivity, schizophrenia, 378
Neuroanatomy
    cerebrum, 122, 122f
    lobes of the brain, 123–124
    subcortical structures, 124–126, 125f
Neurochemical model, 321–322
Neurochemical modulation, 832
Neurocognitive disorders (NCDs)
    Alzheimer's disease
        aetiology, 793–795
        biologic domain, 796–801
        clinical course, 791–792, 791t
        continuum of care, 811, 813
        diagnostic criteria, 792–793, 792t
        epidemiology, 793
        evaluation, 810–811
        families, 796
        interdisciplinary treatment, 795–796
        priority care issues, 796
        psychological domain, 801–807
        risk factors, 793
        social domain, 807–809
        spiritual domain, 810
        treatment outcomes, 810–811
    delirium
        aetiology, 784–785
        biologic domain, 785–788, 786t, 787b
        in children, 782
        clinical course, 781–782
        continuum of care, 790–791, 790b
        diagnostic criteria, 782
        epidemiology, 783–784
        evaluation, 790
        interdisciplinary treatment, 785
        older adults, 782–783

        priority care, 785
        psychological domain, 788–789
        risk factors, 783–784
        social domain, 789–790
        spiritual domain, 790
        treatment outcomes, 790
    dementia, 791
        HIV infection, 814
        Huntington's disease, 814–815
        prion disease, 815
        substance/medication-induced, 815
        traumatic brain injury, 814
Neurodevelopmental disorders
    autism spectrum disorder
        biologic domain, 731
        continuum of care, 731
        epidemiology and aetiology, 729–730, 730f
        nursing management, 731–733
        psychopharmacologic interventions,
            730–731
        psychosocial domain, 731–733
        spiritual domain, 733
    communication disorders, 734
    specific learning disorders, 733–734
Neuroimaging
    functional, 120t, 121
    structural, 119–121
Neuroleptic malignant syndrome (NMS), 393
Neurologic examination, of children and
        adolescents, assessment of, 703
Neurologic impairment
    biologic basis, 843–844, 844f
    bio/psycho/social/spiritual interventions,
        845
    client assessment, 845
    functional cerebral anatomy and stroke, 844f
    ischemic cascade, 843
    psychological aspects, 844–845
Neuropathologic theories
    delusional disorder, 430
    schizoaffective disorders, 418
    somatic symptom disorder, 507–508
Neuropeptide Y (NPY), 649
Neuropeptides, 138
Neurophysiology
    categories, 134
    glial cells, 130
    neurons and nerve impulses, 130–132
    neurotransmitters, 134
        amino acids, 127t–128t, 138
        biogenic amines, 135–137
        cholinergic, 134–135, 135f
        neuropeptides, 138
        receptors, 134
        synaptic transmission, 132–134
Neuroplasticity, 118
Neurosis, 9
Neurotransmitters
    amino acids, 138
    biogenic amines
        dopamine, 135–136, 136f
        epinephrine, 137
        histamine, 137
        norepinephrine, 136, 137f
        serotonin, 137
    categories, 134
    cholinegeric, 134–135

    neuropeptides, 138
    psychosocial disturbances, 833
    synaptic transmission
        excitatory neurotransmitter, 132
        inhibitory neurotransmitter, 132
        lock-and-key analogy, 132
New Brunswick, standard of practice in, 73t
Newfoundland and Labrador, standard of
        practice in, 73t
Nicotine, 574–576, 578b, 582, 593–595, 594b
Nightingale, Florence, 97
Nihilism, 160b
Nihilistic delusions, schizophrenia, 370
Nonbenzodiazepine sedative-hypnotics, 656t
Nonmaleficence ethics, 85
Nontherapeutic relationships, 79
Nonverbal communication, 65, 69–70, 70f, 249
Norepinephrine (NE), 136, 136f, 137f, 488, 649
Norepinephrine- and serotonin-selective
        reuptake inhibitors (NSSRIs)
    panic disorder, 491
Norepinephrine-dopamine reuptake
        inhibitors (NDRIs), 656t
Normal aging, 765, 766
Normalization, mental health promotion
        with children and adolescents, 683
Norms, 249–250
North American Nursing Diagnosis
        Association (NANDA), 168
Northern areas, role of nurses in, 35
Northwest Territories and Nunavut, standard
        of practice in, 73t
Nova Scotia, standard of practice in, 73t
Nuclear families, 260, 265
Nurse-client relationship, 76–78. *See also*
        Therapeutic communication
    definition of, 76
    orientation phase, 76–77
    Orlando's theory of, 98
    resolution phase of, 78, 78b
    testing of, 77
    working phase of, 77–78
Nurses fatigue, 284
Nursing care plans. *See also* specific disorders
        conditions
    alcoholism, 596–598
    anorexia nervosa (AN), 540–543
    attention deficit/hyperactivity disorder,
        740–742
    bipolar disorder, 471
    BPD, 630–632
    ineffective individual coping, 474–475
    neurocognitive disorders, 812
    schizoaffective disorder, 419–421
    schizophrenia, 381–383
    self-harm, 472–473
    somatic symptom disorder, 518–519
Nursing diagnosis. *See also specific disorders
        and conditions*
    definition, 168
    deriving, 168
    evolution, 167–168
    and individual outcomes, 167–168
    RNAO, 167, 168b
Nursing education
    early, 7
    models of, 10–11

Nursing interventions. *See also specific disorders and conditions*
  for biologic domain, 171–175
    activity and exercise interventions, 172
    hydration interventions, 174
    medication management, 175
    nutrition interventions, 173
    pain management, 174–175
    promotion of self-care activities, 171
    relaxation interventions, 173–174
    sleep interventions, 173
    thermoregulation interventions, 174
  definition of, 172
  expected outcomes, 171t
  NIC, 171
  promotion of client safety on psychiatric units, 179–181
  for psychological domain
    behaviour therapy, 177
    cognitive, 177
    conflict resolution, 175–176
    counselling, 175
    health teaching, 178
    psychoeducation, 177–178
    recovery orientation, 176
    reminiscence, 176–177
  for social domain
    community action, 182
    home visits, 181–182
    Milieu therapy, 178–179
    psychiatric units, 179–181
  for spiritual domain, 182–183
Nursing Interventions Classification (NIC), 171, 172b
Nursing journals, 11
Nursing Mental Disease (Bailey), 8
Nursing outcomes
  depression, 169, 169t
  diagnosis and, 169, 171t
  diagnosis-specific, 169, 170t
  documentation of, 170
  purposes of, 170, 171t
  system-specific, 169, 170t
Nursing roles, 35
Nursing theories
  existential and humanistic theoretic perspectives, 98–100
  interpersonal relations models, 97
  of Nightingale, 97
  systems models, 100–101
Nutrition
  in geriatric mental health assessment, 767, 769–770
  regulation, somatic symptom disorder, 571
Nutritional balance, for borderline personality disorder, 620
Nutritional interventions, 173
Nutritional planning, panic disorder, 490
Nutritional therapies, 225–226

O

Object relations, in psychoanalytic theory, 102–103
Objective data, 154

Observation
  as assessment technique, 152–153
  promotion of client safety on, 179–180
  in therapeutic communication, 67t
Observation, in therapeutic communication, 67t
Obsession, 160b
Obsessive-compulsive disorder (OCD), 637
  assessment, 499
  clinical vignette, 499b
  cognitive restructuring interventions, 500
  community treatment, 500
  diagnostic criteria, 483
  epidemiology, 483
  exposure with response prevention, 500
  family response, 500
  lifetime prevalence, 484
  rating scales, 499b
  symptoms, 483
  Tourette syndrome, 484
  treatment, 500
Obstructive sleep apnea (OSA), 662–663
Occipital lobes, 123
Older adults
  bipolar disorders in, 459
  depressive disorders in, 441–442
  psychoeducational codependency support groups, 254, 254b
Old-old, 752
Ontario, standard of practice in, 73t
Open communication, 179
Open group, 245
Open-ended statements, in therapeutic communication, 67t
Operant behaviour, 107
Opioid, substance-related disorders, 591–592
Oppositional defiant disorder (ODD), 734–735
Optimal mental health, 18
Orem, Dorothea
Orexin, sleep-wake disorders, 649, 655
Orientation, in mental status examination, 160–161
Orientation phase of nurse-client relationship, 76–77
  confidentiality, 77
  first meeting, 77
  testing the relationship, 77
Orlando, Ida Jean, 98
Orthomolecular therapy, 226
Outcomes, individual development
  bio/psycho/social/spiritual, 169–170, 169t
  depression, 169t
  diagnosis-specific, 169, 170t
  discharge, 169
  documentation, 170
  evaluation, 170
  individual
    developing, 169–171
    evolution, 167–168
    purposes, 170–171
  initial, 169
  revised, 169
  system-specific, 170t
Outpatient care, 549
Overcoming stigma, 62

Overprotectiveness, anorexia nervosa, 533
Oxidative stress, 795

P

Paediatric anxiety rating scale (PARS), 699
Pain
  biologic basis
    acute pain, 833
    ascending sensory pathways, 834, 835f
    chronic pain, 833, 835b
    endorphins, 833
    neurotransmitters, 833, 835b
    pain stimuli activation, 833, 833f
  bio/psycho/social/spiritual outcomes, 838f
  gate-control model, 833
  in geriatric mental health assessment, 771
  management, 174–175
  pain management, barriers, 838–839
  psychological impact, 832–839
  sensory and pharmacologic modulation, 838–839
  treatment approaches, 837t
Panic attacks, 485–486, 485t
Panic disorder (PD), 485–486
  agoraphobia, 494b
  assessment
    biologic domain, 489–490
    occupational domains, 496–497
    psychological domain, 491–493
    social domains, 496–497
    spiritual domain, 497
  continuum of care, 497–499
  evaluation and treatment outcomes, 497
  interventions
    biologic domain, 490–491
    occupational domains, 496–497
    psychological domain, 493
    social domains, 496–497
  panic attacks, 485–486
Paranoid delusions, 160b
Paranoid personality disorder, 610
Paranoid schizophrenia, 375
Paraphrasing, leading groups, 252t
Parasuicidal behaviour, in borderline personality disorder, 614
Parasuicide, 340
Parent(s). *See also* Families
  interviewing, in mental health assessment of children and adolescents, 694
  mental illness, 681–682
  separation and divorce and, 671–672, 673t
  substance abuse, 682–683
Parent-child interaction model, 694
Paresthesias, 485t
Parietal lobes, 123, 123f
Parse, Rosemarie Rizzo, 98–99
Partial hospitalization programs (PHPs), 469
Passive listening, 69
Passivity, active, in borderline personality, 617b
Pathologic gambling, 638
Patient placement criteria (PPC), 826
Pavlov, Ivan P., 105, 106t
Pavlovian conditioning, 105
Peer relationships, assessment of, with children and adolescents, 701b

Pemoline (Cylert)
  adverse reactions, 223
  indications and mechanisms of action, 221
  off-label use, 221–222
  pharmacokinetics, 222–223
  side effects, 223
  toxicity, 223
Peplau, Hildegard, 11, 97–98
Perception, 159, 329
Perls, Frederick S., 102t, 105
Persecutory delusions, schizophrenia, 370
Perseveration, 160b
Person Resource Base, 692
Personal boundaries, 71–72
  establishing, in borderline personality
      disorder, 623–624
Personal fable, 671
Personality
  definition, 606
  psychoanalytic theory of, 102–103
Personality disorders (PD)
  cluster A
    continuum of care, 611
    paranoid, 610
    schizoid, 610–611
    schizotypal, 611
  cluster B
    antisocial, 629, 633–634
    borderline (See Borderline personality
        disorder (BPD))
    histrionic, 635
    narcissistic, 635–636
  cluster C
    avoidant, 636
    dependent, 636
    obsessive-compulsive, 637
  common features and diagnostic criteria
    affectivity and emotional instability, 607
    cognitive schemas, 607
    impulsivity and destructive behaviour,
        608
    self-identity and interpersonal
        functioning, 607
  severity, 608–609
  vs. traits, 607
Personality traits, personality disorder versus,
    607
Perspectives in Psychiatric Care, 11
Pharmacologic assessment
  for bipolar disorders, 461
  in borderline personality disorder, 620
  older adult, 771
Pharmacotherapy. See also specific disorders and
    conditions
  anorexia nervosa, 537–538
  for bipolar disorders
    antidepressants for, 466
    antipsychotics for, 466
    mood stabilizers for, 462–464, 462t
  bulimia nervosa, 554
  for depressive disorders
    medication administration for, 446,
        447b, 447t, 448
    monitoring medications and, 446, 447b,
        447t, 448
  for enuresis, 746–747
  medication groups, 255–256, 256b

medication management, 175
  polypharmacy among older adults and,
      758, 759b
  for separation anxiety disorder, 722
  substance-related disorders, 586
  for Tourette disorder, 745
Phenelzine (Nardil), 512b
Phobias, 160b, 481, 486, 492b
Phototherapy (light therapy), 225
Physical care, teaching
  in bipolar disorders, 462
  in depressive disorders, 446
Physical functioning
  in geriatric mental health assessment, 767,
      769–770
  somatic symptom disorder, 510
Physical restraint, 180–181
Piaget, Jean, 108–109
PIE method, 155
Pineal body, 127
Pituitary gland, 124
Platelet count, 156t
Polypharmacy, among older adults, 771
Polysomnography, 143, 653, 654f
Population genetics, 116–117
Positive self-talk, panic disorder, 495
Positron emission tomography
    (PET), 121
Postpartum onset specifier, of mood
    disorders, 440
Posttraumatic stress disorder (PTSD), 299,
    726–727, 727b, 866–867
Potassium, serum level of, 157t
Poverty, 33–34
  Aboriginal peoples, 28
  among older adults, 758–759
  in childhood and adolescence, 677
  federal action plan, 34
  investing cases, 34
  life and economic impact, 34
  mental health and, 34
Powerlessness, 342
Practical wisdom, 84
Preconscious, in psychoanalytic theory,
    102–103
Predictability, enduring, with autistic
    spectrum Disorder, 732
Pregnancy, substance-related disorders, 599
Prejudice, 29–31
Preschool-aged children
  clinical interview, 699–700, 700b, 700f
  loss and, 671
Pressured speech, 159, 160b
Primary health care, 42–43
Primary sources, 155
Prince Edward Island, standard of practice
    in, 73t
Principlism, 85
Prion disease, 815
Privacy Act, 91
Probing, leading groups, 252t
Problem solving, impaired, in borderline
    personality disorder, 614
Problem-oriented documentation, 155
Process recording, 74, 75b
Professional boundaries, 72, 73t
Projection, 74t

Projective
  in borderline personality disorder, 615
  identification, 615
Protective factors
  against childhood pathology, 672
  for children of divorce and remarriage,
      divorce and, 671–672, 673t
Provincial Lunatic Asylum (New Brunswick),
    4, 5f
Prozac (Fluoxetine hydrochloride), 555b
Pseudoparkinsonism, 207
Psychiatric advance directives (PADs), 90,
    90b
Psychiatric and mental health (PMH)
    nursing
  biologic domain, 55
  biologic theories of, 101
  Canadian Standards, 57, 58b
  challenges, 61–62
  collaborative care, 60–61
  continued evolution, 10–11, 11f
  development of, 7, 7b
    thought and, 8–9
  domains of practice, 57, 58b, 59b
  early views and, 7, 7b
  e-Mental Health, 62
  global community, 62
  humane treatment, 3–4
  institutional care, 2–3
  interdisciplinary approach, 60
  knowledge development, dissemination,
      and application, 61
  late 20th century, 11–12, 11f
  modern thinking, 8–11
  nursing theories of, 97
    existential and humanistic theoretic
        perspectives, 98–100
    interpersonal relations models, 97
    systems models, 100–101
  overcoming stigma and discrimination, 62
  practicing tools
    clinical decision making, 58
    critical pathways, 59
  psychological domain, 55–56
  psychological theories of, 101–109
    behavioural theories, 105–107, 106t
    cognitive theories, 107–108
    developmental theories, 108–109
    humanistic theories, 104–105
    psychodynamic theories, 101–104, 102t
  recovery, 60
  regional influences, 7–8
  RPN practice, 57–58
  scientific thought, 8–9
  social domain, 56
  social theories of, 109–110
    family dynamics, 109
    role theories, 109–110
    sociocultural perspectives, 110
  spiritual domain, 56–57
  spiritual theories of
    applicability to psychiatric and mental
        health nursing, 111
    of Frankl, 110–111
    of Yalom, 111
  standards, 57–58
  19th and early 20th centuries, 4–8

Psychiatric disorders, 9. *See also* Mental disorders; Mental illness
  anxiety disorders, 721–725
  disruptive behaviour disorders, 734–739, 742–746
  elimination disorders, 746–748
  gender dysphoria, 728–729
  mood disorders, 721
  neurodevelopmental disorders, 729–746
  schizophrenia, 720–721
  Tourette disorder, 744–746
Psychiatric hospitals, 7
Psychiatric nurse, tide of, 12
Psychiatric Nurses Association of Canada, 11
Psychiatric nursing textbooks, first, 8
Psychiatric pluralism, 8
Psychoanalysis, 102t, 103
Psychoanalytic movement, 8
Psychoanalytic theories, 322–323
  of borderline personality disorder, 615
  object relations and identification in, 103
  personality in, 103
  psychoanalysis and, 103
  sexuality in, 103
  transference and countertransference in, 103
  unconscious in, 102–103
Psychodynamic theories, 101–104, 102t. *See also* Neo-Freudian models; Psychoanalytic theories
  applicability to psychiatric and mental health nursing, 111
  humanistic, 102t, 104–105
  interpersonal, 105
Psychoeducation, 177–178
  anorexia nervosa, 547b
  for bipolar disorders, 468, 469t
  bulimia nervosa, 556, 556b
  delusional disorder, 432
  mental health promotion with children and adolescents, 683–684
  schizoaffective disorder, 423b
  schizophrenia, 404b
  somatic symptom disorder, 514b
Psychoeducational groups, 254
Psychoendocrinology, 139, 139f
Psychological domain
  assessment of, 158–162
    in children and adolescents, 703–710
    mental status examination, 158–161, 158b, 160b
    responses to mental health problems, 158
    risk assessment and, 161–162
    stress and coping patterns and, 161
  family assessment, 264–268
    communication patterns, 267–268
    diversity, 265, 267, 267b
    family development, 265
    family life cycles, 265, 266t
    low-income families, 267
    problem-solving skills, 268
    stress and coping abilities, 268
  insomnia, 661
  nursing interventions for (*See specific disorders and conditions*)
  obstructive sleep apnea, 663

Psychological first aid (PFA), 311
Psychological theories, 101–109
  anorexia nervosa, 531–532
  behavioural theories, 105–107, 106t
  of bipolar disorders, 460
  of borderline personality disorder, 615
  cognitive theories, 107–108
  of depressive disorders, 443–444
  developmental theories, 108–109
  humanistic theories, 104–105
  psychodynamic theories, 101–104, 102t
  schizoaffective disorder, 418
  substance-related disorders, 576–577
Psychomotor activity, in mental status examination, 158
Psychoneuroimmunology, 140–141
Psychopharmacologic drugs
  pharmacodynamics
    carrier proteins, 189, 189f
    efficacy and potency, 189–190, 191t–192t
    enzymes, 189
    ion channels, 189
    receptors, 188–189, 188f
    toxicity, 190–193
  pharmacokinetics
    absorption and routes of administration, 193, 194t
    distribution, 195, 195t
    excretion, 197
    individual variations in drug effects, 197–198
    metabolism, 195–197
  treatment phases
    discontinuation, 200
    initiation, 199
    maintenance, 200
    stabilization, 199–200
Psychosis. *See* Delusional disorder; Psychotic disorders; Schizoaffective disorder (SCA); Schizophrenia; Schizophreniform disorder
Psychosocial development
  assessment of, in children and adolescents, 704
  Erikson's theory of, 108
Psychosocial disturbances
  human immunodeficiency virus (HIV) infection
    neurologic manifestations, 839–840
    psychiatric disorders, 840b
    psychological aspects, 840
  medical illness
    anxiety disorders, 846t
    bio/psycho/social/spiritual interventions, 849
    client assessment, 848–849, 849b
    depression, 849t
    mental illness in, 846–847
    psychological aspects, 847–848
  pain response
    biologic basis, 833–835
    bio/psycho/social/spiritual outcomes, 838f
    gate-control model, 833
    pain management, barriers, 838–839
    psychological impact, 832–839

    sensory and pharmacologic modulation, 838–839
    treatment approaches, 837t
  trauma
    biologic basis, 841
    bio/psycho/social/spiritual interventions, 843
    client assessment, 843
    psychological aspects, 841, 843
Psychosocial domain
  attention deficit hyperactivity disorder, 743–744
  autistic spectrum disorder, 731–733
  bipolar disorder, 721
  conduct disorder, 736
  depressive disorders, 724
  gender dysphoria, 728–729
  oppositional defiant disorder, 735
  psychotic disorders, 720
  reactive attachment disorder, 726
  traumatic stress, 727
Psychosocial rehabilitation, 49
Psychosocial treatment, integration of biologic theories into, 9
Psychosocially oriented ideas, 8
Psychosurgery, 9
Psychotherapy. *See also specific types of psychotherapy*
  for bipolar disorders, 468
  transference and countertransference in, 103
Psychotherapy groups, 255
Psychotic disorders, 434. *See also* Delusional disorder; Schizoaffective disorder (SCA); Schizophrenia; Schizophreniform disorder
  substance-related disorders, 828
Psychotic episodes, in borderline personality disorder, 621–622
Pyromania, 638

Q

Quaker(s), 4
Quaker Friends Asylum, 4
Quality of life of older adults, assessment of, 777
Quebec, standard of practice in, 73t
Questioning, leading groups, 252t

R

Rapport, 71
  building with children and adolescents, 694, 695b–696b
Rating scales, for children, 698–699
Rationalization, as defence mechanism, 74t
Reaction formation, as defence mechanism, 74t
Reactive attachment disorder (RAD), 726
Reassurance, in therapeutic communication, 68t
Recovery orientation, 176
Red blood cell (RBC) count, 156t
Reflecting behaviour, leading groups, 252t
Reflecting feelings, leading groups, 252t
Reflection, in therapeutic communication, 67t

Registered nurse, title of, 10
Registered Nurses Association, 8
Registered Nurses Association of Ontario
    (RNAO), 167
Registered Psychiatric Nurses of Canada
    (RPNC), 83–84
Regressed behaviour, schizophrenia, 371
Rehabilitative services, 10
Reinforcement theories, 106t, 107
Reinier van Arkel asylum, 2
Reintegration, 48
Relapse, 46
Relapse prevention, 829
Relational ethics, 84t, 86–87
Relationship Strains, in older adults, 755
Relaxation techniques, 173–174, 174t,
    661b
    panic disorder, 490, 490b
    somatic symptom disorder, 511
Religion. See also Spiritual entries;
        Spirituality
    as cultural system, 29
Religious delusion, 160b
Religious orders, 3
Remarriage, children, 672
Reminiscence, 176–177, 256
Remote areas, role of nurses in, 35
Repeating, leading groups, 252t
Repetitive transcranial magnetic stimulation
    (rTMS), 226
Repression, as defence mechanism, 74t
Research ethics, 93
Residential services
    of older adults, 757
    respite, 45
Resilience, 677
Resolution phase of nurse-client relationship,
    78, 78b
Respect for autonomy, 85
Respondent behaviour, 107
Restatement, in therapeutic communication,
    67t
Restraints, 180–181, 332
Retirement, 756
Revictimization, 872
Rights, of persons with mental illness, 36,
    36b
Rigidity of families, anorexia nervosa, 533
Risk assessment
    in bipolar disorders, 467
    with children and adolescents, 709–710,
        710b
    with older adults, 775
Risk/rescue ratio, 344
Risperidone (Consta; Risperdal; Risperdal
        M-Tab), 389b, 462t
    for autistic disorder, 730
    for bipolar disorders, 462t
Riverview Hospital, 10, 11f
Roberts' seven-stage crisis intervention
        model, 306b, 307f
Rogers, Carl, 102t, 104
Rogers, Martha, 101
Role theories, 109–110
    applicability to psychiatric and mental
        health nursing, 110
Roy, Callista, 101
Rural areas, of persons with mental illness, 35

S
Safety interventions
    acute stress disorder, 732
    for safety promotion on inpatient units,
        179–181
Saint Dymphna Guesthouse, 4
Salpetrière, 4
San Hipólito, 3
Saskatchewan
    nurse education in, 11
    standard of practice in, 73t
Scale for the assessment of negative
        symptoms (SANS), 396, 398b
Scale for the assessment of positive
        symptoms (SAPS), 396, 397b
Schizoaffective disorder (SCA)
    aetiology, 418
    assessment
        biologic domain, 419
        clinical course, 415–416
        diagnostic criteria, 416, 417t
        epidemiology and risk factors, 416–417
        psychological domain, 423
        social domain, 424
    continuum of care, 425–427
    interdisciplinary treatment, 418
    nursing care plan, 419–421
    nursing diagnoses
        biologic domain, 419
        psychological domain, 423–424
        social domain, 424
    nursing interventions, 420f
        biologic domain, 419, 422–423
        psychological domain, 424
        social domain, 424–425
    priority care issues, 418
    psychoeducation, 423b
    spiritual domain, 425
Schizoid personality disorder, 610–611
Schizophrenia
    acute illness period, 367–368
    acute psychiatric wards, 406b
    aetiology
        biologic theories, 374
        bio/psycho/social/spiritual, 375f
        familial patterns, 374
        neuroanatomic findings, 374
        neurodevelopment, 374–375
        neurotransmitters, pathways, and
            receptors, 375–378, 376t,
            377f–378f
        psychological theories, 378–379
        social theories, 379
    assessment
        biologic domain, 383, 386, 387t
        psychological domain, 395–402
        social domain, 404–406
        spiritual domain, 406
    in children, 371
    continuum of care, 410
    diagnostic criteria, 369–371
    epidemiology
        age of onset, 372
        comorbidity, 373–374
        ethnic and cultural difference, 372
        familial difference, 373
        gender differences, 372
        risk factors, 372

evaluation and treatment outcomes, 410
family response to disorder, 380
fostering recovery, 369t
interdisciplinary treatment, 379–380,
    384–385
maintenance and recovery period, 368
negative symptoms, 370
neurocognitive impairment, 370–371
nursing care plan, 381–383, 407–410
nursing diagnoses
    biologic domain, 386
    psychological domain, 402
    social domain, 405
nursing interventions
    biologic domain, 386–395, 390t–391t,
        394f
    psychological domain, 402–404
    social domain, 405–406
in older adults, 371–372
paranoid, 375
positive symptoms, 370
priority care issues, 380
and psychotic disorders, 720–721
rating scales, 396b
recovery, 367b
relapses, 368–369
spiritual domain, 406
stabilization period, 368
subtypes, 369, 370t
Schizophrenia Society of Canada, 12
Schizophreniform disorder, 434
Schizotypal personality disorder, 611
Schneidman's common characteristics, 346,
    347b
School functioning, assessment of, 711
School phobia, 721–722
School-aged children
    loss and, 671
    semi-structured interview with,
        695b–696b
Scientific thought, evolution, 8–9
Scope and Standards of Psychiatric-Mental
        Health Nursing Practice, The, 53
Screening, 581–582, 698
Seasonal depression, of mood
        disorders, 440
Seating arrangement, groups, 253
Seclusion, 180, 181b, 332
Secondary psychiatric disorder model,
        concurrent disorders, 824
Secondary sources, 155
Secondary substance use disorder model,
        concurrent disorders, 824
Security awareness, forensic nursing,
        901–902, 902b
Selective serotonin reuptake inhibitors
        (SSRIs), 214t, 656t, 722
    adverse reactions, 216–217
    anorexia nervosa, 537
    concurrent disorders, 827
    panic disorder, 491
    pharmacokinetics, 216
    side effects, 216–217
    toxicity, 216–217
Self-awareness
    bio/psycho/social/spiritual self and, 65
    understanding personal feelings and beliefs
        and changing behaviour and, 65

Self-care
    groups, 256
    Orem's theory of, 171
    promotion of, 171
Self-concept, 708–709, 709f
Self-disclosure, 66, 67t
Self-efficacy, 107, 838
Self-esteem
    abuse, 871
    in borderline personality disorder, 628
Self-harm, suicidal behaviour, 341, 346
Self-help groups, 12, 255
Self-identity, impaired, in personality
        disorders, 607
Self-injurious behaviours, in borderline
        personality disorder, 614
Self-invalidation, in borderline personality
        disorder, 617b
Self-reflective exercises, of CBT, 237–238
Self-report scales, panic disorder, 491–492
Self-system, 97
Senate Standing Committee on Social
        Affairs, Science and Technology, 28
Sensitization, bipolar disorders and, 460
Sensorium, in mental status examination, 160
Separation anxiety disorder
    epidemiology and aetiology, 722
    nursing management, 722, 723b
    psychopharmacologic interventions, 722
Separation-individuation, in borderline
        personality disorder, 615
Serotonin (5-HT), 137, 649
Serotonin syndrome, low, 321–322
Serotonin-norepinephrine reuptake
        inhibitors (SNRIs), 656t
Serum creatinine, serum level of, 157t
Sexual abuse
    anorexia nervosa, 529b
    of children, 679t, 713
Sexuality, in psychoanalytic theory,
        102–103
Shadow, Jungian concept of, 104
Shame, as response to abuse, 871
Shared psychotic disorder, 436
Short term cognitive therapy Rating Scale
        (SRS), 236
Sibling relationships, 672, 674
Signs, 154
Silence, in therapeutic communication, 67t
Simple relaxation techniques, 173–174,
        174t
Simpson-Angus rating scale, 908–909
Simultaneous/parallel care, 825
Single photon emission computed
        tomography (SPECT), 121
Sisters of Mercy, 3
Skills groups, for borderline personality
        disorder, 618
Skinner, B.F., 106t, 107
Sleep, 770
    architecture, 643
    brain activity, 645, 646f
    definition, 645b
    efficiency, 643
    hygiene, 657, 658b
    hypnogram, 643, 644f
    latency, 643
    REM and NREM, 643, 645

restriction therapy, 661
    stages, 645t
Sleep disturbance, in depressive disorders, 460
Sleep interventions, 173
Sleep pattern, panic disorder, 489–490
Sleep restriction therapy, 661
Sleep-wake cycle, 648
Sleep-wake disorders
    actigraphy, 655
    assessments
        EEG, 653, 655
        orexin, 655
        polysomnography, 653
        respiratory and cardiac, 655
    common circadian rhythm
        jet lag, 664
        shift workers, 663–664, 664b
    comorbid mental illnesses and mental
            health problems, 656, 656t–657t
    consequences of inadequate sleep, 650
    dreaming, 645, 646f
    epidemiology, 650
    historical perspectives, 642–643
    impaired sleep substance use, 651, 653f
    insomnia (See Insomnia)
    maintenance of wakefulness test, 655
    morbidity and impaired function, 651, 653f
    multiple sleep latency test, 655
    obstructive sleep apnea, 662–663
    prevalence and features, 651t–652t
    process c and s
        biologic clock, 647f
        neurochemicals, 648t
    sleep, 655 (See also Sleep)
    sleep pattern changes
        adolescents, 648
        children, 648, 650
        cultural and racial factors, 650
        older adults, 650
        women, 648
    sleep questionnaires, 655–656
SNAP-IV, 699, 739b
SOAP method, 155
Social activities, of older adults, 756
Social change, 2–3
    Dix, Dorothea Lynde, 6, 6f
    during 19th and early 20th centuries,
            4–5, 5f
    during late 20th century, 11–12, 12f
    moral treatment, 2–3
    during pre-moral treatment era, 3–4
Social determinants of health, 33
Social domain, 163
    assessment of (See also specific disorders and
            conditions)
    in children and adolescents, 711–712
    family assessment, 268–269
        family systems, 268–269
        formal and informal support networks, 269
        perspectives on understanding families,
                269
        social and financial status, 269
    insomnia, 662
    nursing interventions for (See specific
            disorders and conditions)
    obstructive sleep apnea, 663
Social phobia, 484
Social Progress Index (SPI), 19

Social skills training, for mental health
        promotion, in children and
        adolescents, 684, 711
Social support
    in borderline personality disorder, 627–628
    of older adults, assessment of, 775
    transitions in, for older adults, 761
Social theories, 109–110
    anorexia nervosa, 532–533
    for bipolar disorders, 461
    of bipolar disorders, 460
    bulimia nervosa, 552–553
    of depressive disorders, 444
    eating disorders, 532–533
    family dynamics, 109
    role theories of, 109–110
    schizoaffective disorder, 418
    sociocultural perspectives, 110
    somatic symptom disorder, 508
    substance-related disorders, 577
Societal norms, forensic nursing, 902
Sociocultural risk factors, anorexia nervosa,
        535–536
Sociocultural theories, 110
Socratic questioning, of CBT, 237
Sodium, serum level of, 157t
Somatic delusions, 160b, 370, 429
Somatic symptom disorder
    aetiology
        biologic theories, 507–508
        psychological theories, 508
        social theories, 508, 508b
    age of onset, 507
    children, 506
    clinical course, 506
    comorbidity, 507
    continuum of care, 516–517
    conversion disorder, 517
    diagnostic characteristics, 507t
    diagnostic criteria, 506, 507b
    drug profile, 512b
    epidemiology, 507
    evaluation and treatment outcomes, 516, 516f
    gender, ethnic, and cultural differences, 507
    hypochondriasis, 517
    illness and anxiety disorder, 517
    interdisciplinary treatment, 508–509
    mental health promotion, 517
    nursing care plan
        chronic low self-esteem, 518b–519b
        clinical settings, 518b
        ineffective therapeutic regimen
                management, 519b
    nursing management
        biologic domain, 509–513
        characteristics, 515f
        interventions, 515, 515f
        psychological domain, 513–514
        social domain, 514–515
        spiritual domain, 515–516
        therapeutic approach, 514b
    older adults, 506–507
    psychoeducation, 514b
    risk factors, 508
    somatization
        Chinese culture, 508b
        cultural differences
            gender, 507

Source-oriented documentation, 155
Specific learning disorders, 733–734
Spectrum of care, for bipolar disorders, 469
Speech, 159
Spiritual assessment, 163, 777. *See also specific disorders and conditions*
Spiritual domain
  attention deficit hyperactivity disorder, 743–744
  autistic spectrum disorder, 733
  bipolar disorder, 721
  conduct disorder, 736
  depressive disorders, 724
  family assessment, 269–270
  gender dysphoria, 729
  insomnia, 662
  obstructive sleep apnea, 663
  oppositional defiant disorder, 735
  psychotic disorders, 720–721
  reactive attachment disorder, 726
  traumatic stress, 727
Spiritual interventions, 182–183
Spiritual support, for older adults, 761–762
Spiritual theories
  applicability to psychiatric and mental health nursing, 111
  eating disorders, 533–534
  of Frankl, 110–111
  of Yalom, 111
Spirituality. *See also specific disorders and conditions*
  among Aboriginal people, 29
  anorexia nervosa, 546b
  children and adolescents, 712
  definition, 56
  eating disorder, 533–534
  mood disorder, 455
  nurse, 546b
  older adults, 761–762, 777
  substance-related disorders, 577
Splane, Verna, 761
Splitting, as defence mechanism, 74t
Standards, 249–250
Standards of Psychiatric and Mental Health Nursing Practice, 691
Stereotypic behaviour, 729
Stereotyping, 30
Stereotypy, schizophrenia, 371
Stigma, 30–31
  of mental illness, 261
Stimulants, 221–223. *See also specific drugs*
Stimulus control therapy, 661
Stress
  assessment of individuals affected by, 161
    biologic, 300
    of children and adolescents, 712
    of older adults, 774–775
    psychological, 301
    social, 301
    spiritual, 301–302
  in bipolar disorders, assessment of, 467
  cognitive appraisal, 291, 291f
  coping (*See* Coping)
  emotional responses to, 295–298, 297f, 298b
  evaluation and treatment outcomes, 302
  family assessment, 268
  Neuman's theory of, 101
  nursing interventions for

biologic domain, 300
  psychological domain, 301
  social domain, 301
  spiritual domain, 301–302
person-environment transaction, 289–290
responses, 289
  allostasis, 291–292
  freeze-hide, 292
  physiological, 292–293, 293t
  tend and befriend, 292
social network and, 294–295
social support and, 293–294
spiritual domain, 301–302
as stimulus, 289
stressors, in childhood
  divorce, 672, 673t
  grief and loss, 669–671, 670b
  physical and developmental challenges, 675–676
  physical illness, 674–675
  separation and divorce, 671–672, 673t
  sibling relationships, 672, 674
traumatic stressor
  acute stress disorder, 298–299
  posttraumatic stress disorder, 299
workplace, mental health, 280
Structural neuroimaging, 119–121, 120t
Structured interaction, 179
Subjective data, 154
Substance P, 833
Substance use disorders (SUD), 573–574
Substance-induced psychotic disorder, 434–435, 435t
Substance-related disorders
  addiction treatment
    goals of, 579, 581, 581b
    principles of, 580b
  ADHD and, 827–828
  aetiologic theories
    biologic, 576
    psychological, 576–577
    public health model, 577–578, 578b
    social, 577
    spiritual, 577, 577b
  alcoholics anonymous, 577b
  anxiety disorders and, 827
  care, levels of, 581b
  diagnostic criteria
    clinical course, 574
    non-substance related disorders, 574–575
    substance classes, 574
  epidemiology
    alcohol, 575
    societal costs, 576
    tobacco, 575
  interdisciplinary treatment recommendations
    addiction treatment, 579–581
    brief intervention and referral, 581–582
    cognitive-behavioural therapy, 585
    family therapy, 586
    FRAMES, 585b
    group therapy, 586
    harm reduction, 579, 583
    intoxication and withdrawal, 583
    matching treatment principle, 581

motivational interviewing, 583–585, 584b
  multidimensional assessment, 582–583
  pharmacotherapy, 586
  psychosocial interventions, 583–586
  relapse prevention, 586
  screening, 581–582
  therapeutic alliance, 579
  toxicology testing/drug screening, 586
  twelve-step recovery programs, 585
on mental health, 825
mood disorders and, 826–827
neurobiology, 573
nurse, health advocate, 601
nursing care plan
  discomfort related to, tobacco withdrawal, 597–598
  risk related to, alcohol withdrawal, 596–597
  setting, 596
nursing for patients, 826, 827b
nursing interventions
  alcohol-related disorders, 587–588
  amphetamine, 592–593
  caffeine-related disorders, 589
  cannabis-related disorders, 589–590
  gambling disorder, 595
  hallucinogen-related disorders, 590
  hypnotic and anxiolytic-related disorders, 592
  inhalant-related disorders, 590–591
  opioid-related disorders, 591–592
  sedative-related disorders, 592
  stimulant-related disorders, 592–593
  tobacco-related disorders, 593–595
in parents, 682–683
personality disorders and, 828
psychotic disorders and, 828
special populations
  Aboriginal populations, 599
  college students, 598–599
  concurrent disorders, 600
  HIV/AIDS, 599–600
  mental illness and tobacco use, 600
  nurses, 600–601
  pregnancy and lactation, 599
  youth, 598
substance class
  alcohol, 825
  caffeine, 825
  cannabis, 825
  hallucinogens, 825
  sedatives, 825
  stimulants, 825
  tobacco, 825
Suggestions, leading groups, 252t
Suicidal behaviour
  aetiology
    biologic theories, 346–348
    psychological theories, 348–349
    Schneidman's common characteristics, 347b
    social theories, 349–351
    spiritual theories, 351
  among older adults, 759
  attempts, 162
  and Canadian military, 342, 342b

Canadian Suicide Statistics (2009), 346t
definition, 340
in depressive disorders, assessment of, 452
effects of, 351
epidemiology
    Aboriginal peoples, 344–345, 345b
    age, 342–344
    gender, 344
    guns and suicide, 345–346
    regional variations, 345, 346t
    sexual orientation, 345
    suicidal ideation and self-harm, 346
evaluation and treatment outcomes, 359–360
legal considerations
    confidentiality, 352–353
    documentation, 353
    informed consent, 353
    involuntary admission, 352
    Provincial Health Acts, 352
nursing assessment
    comprehensive assessment, 353, 354b
    contracting for safety, 355–356
    inpatient care and acute treatment, 356
    nursing diagnoses and outcome
        identification, 355
    planning and implementing nursing
        interventions, 355–356
    resources and support, 355
    self-harm assessment, 354
    tools, risk assessment, 353, 354b
nursing interventions
    biologic domain, 356–357
    planning and implementing, 355–356
    psychological domain
    social domain, 357–359
    spiritual domain, 359
physician-assisted suicide, 351, 351b
risk and protective factors for, 342, 343b
risk of
    in borderline personality disorder, 622
    risk assessment for, 162
    suicidal ideation, 162
Sulci, 122, 123f
Summarizing, leading groups, 252t
Superego, 103
Support groups, 685
Support, leading groups, 252t
Supported housing, 49
Supportive therapy groups, 255
Suppression, as defence mechanism, 74t
Suprachiasmatic nuclei (SCN), 647
Symbolism, 75
Symptom(s), 154
Symptom management groups, 256
Systematic desensitization, 495
Systems models, 100–101

T
Tangentiality, 160b
Tardive dyskinesia, 208–209, 378, 912–913
Task functions, group, 247, 248t
Teaching. See Client/family education
Telehealth, 80, 92
Temperament
    antisocial personality disorder and, 609
    in childhood, 707–708, 708b
Temporal lobes, 123

Termination stage
    of family systems, 269
    of group development, 247
Thalamus, 126
Therapeutic alliance. See also specific disorders
    and conditions
    anorexia nervosa, 538
    of CBT, 236
Therapeutic collaboration, of CBT, 237
Therapeutic communication, 65, 66b
    analyzing interactions and, 74–76, 75b
    defence mechanisms in, 72, 74t
    empathic linkages and, 65, 71
    empathy in, 71
    listening and, 69
    nonverbal, 65, 69–70, 70f
    personal boundaries in, 71–72
    professional boundaries in, 72, 73t
    rapport in, 71
    selecting techniques for, 70–71
    self-disclosure in, 66, 67t
    silence and, 68
    validation in, 70–71
    verbal, 66–69, 66f, 67t, 68b, 68t, 69b
Therapeutic index, 191
Therapeutic relationship. See also specific
    disorders and conditions
    in depressive disorders, assessment of,
        452–453
Thermoregulation interventions, 174
Thinking errors, in cognitive restructuring,
    239, 239b
Thinking in Pictures and Other Reports of My
    Life with Autism (Grandin), 733
Thorndike, Edward L., 106t, 107
Thought(s)
    assessment of, 160, 160b
    automatic, 177
    blocking, 160b
    broadcasting, 160b
    content of, 160, 160b, 451–452
    dichotomous, in borderline personality
        disorder, 621
    disturbances of, in bipolar disorders, 467
    dysfunctional, challenging, 626, 626b,
        627b
    illogical, 177
    insertion, 160b
    processes, 160, 160b, 773
    stopping, borderline personality disorder, 626
Threats of suicide, 162
Thyroid-stimulating hormone (TSH), 157t
Thyroxine (T_4), serum level of, 157t
Tidal model, 99–100, 99b
Tiredness, in depressive disorders, 445
Tobacco. See Nicotine
Token economy, 177
Tolerance, substance-related disorders, 576
Tolman, Edward Chace, 106t
Topiramate (Topamax), 462
Toronto Psychiatric Hospital (TPH), 6
Tourette syndrome (Tourette disorder).
    See also Motor disorders
    in children and adolescents
        aetiology, 744–745
        epidemiology, 744
        nursing management, 745–746
    obsessive-compulsive disorder and, 484

Toxicology testing, for substance-related
    disorders, 586
Training School for Nurses, 7
Training School model, 8
Transcultural health care, 110
Transition times, family assessment, 265
Trauma
    acute stress disorder, 726–727
    biologic basis, 841
    bio/psycho/social/spiritual interventions,
        843
    client assessment, 843
    nursing management, 727
    posttraumatic stress disorder, 726–727
    psychological aspects, 841, 843
    reactive attachment disorder, 726
Trauma, historical, 28–29
Travelbee, Joyce, 98
Tricyclic antidepressants (TCAs), 656t
    cardiotoxicity, 216
    indications, 215
    mechanisms of action, 216
    panic disorder, 491
    pharmacokinetics, 215–216
    side effects, 216–217
Triiodothyronine (T_3), serum level of, 157t
Typical antipsychotics, 656t
Tyramine-restricted diet, 218t
"Tyranny of the should," 104

U
Unconditional positive regard, 104
Unconscious
    collective, 104
    in psychoanalytic theory, 102–103
Unconscious mental processes, in
    psychoanalytic theory, 102–103
Undoing, as defence mechanism, 74t
Unemployment, 276–277
Unipolar disorders. See Depressive disorders
Unsafe workplace, 279, 279b
Unspecified delusions, 429
Utilitarianism, 84t, 85

V
Validation, 71, 179
    communication concepts, 71
    milieu therapy, 179
    in therapeutic communication, 67t
    verbal communication techniques, 67t
Verbal communication, 66–69, 66f, 67t,
    68b, 68t, 69b. See also Language;
    Speech
    group, 247, 249
Verbigeration, 160b
Vincent de Paul, 3
Violence. See also Aggression and violence
    workplace, mental health, 280, 284–285
Virtue ethics, 84–85, 84t
Visual hallucinations, schizophrenia, 370
Vitamin B_{12}, deficiency of, 157t
Vulnerability
    emotional, in borderline personality
        disorde, 617b
    forensic nursing, 894
    genetic, of children adolescents, 702–703
    schizophrenia, 374b

W

Wakefulness, 648
Walden II (Skinner), 107
Watson, Jean, 99
Watson, John B., 106t
Waxy flexibility, schizophrenia, 371
WBC differential, 156t
Weight gain
  antipsychotics, 205
  schizophrenia, 386, 392
  side effects
    antidepressant medications, 449t
    psychiatric medications, 192t
  substance-related disorders, 590
Wisdom, practical, 84
Woman abuse
  battering, 856
  dating violence, 855
  human immuno deficiency virus (HIV)
    infection, 856–857
  prevalence, 854
  racial backgrounds, 855
  rape and sexual assault, 856
  risk, 854
  secondary abuse of children and,
    859–860
  stalking, 857
  theories of
    cycle of violence, 864, 865f
    feminist theories, 863
    traumatic bonding, 864–865
    women remaining in abusive
      relationships, 863–864
Women
  incarcerated, 896
  living with schizophrenia, helping, 424b
  sleep-wake disorders, 648, 650

Wong-Baker Faces Pain Rating Scale, 771,
  771f
Word salad, 160b
Work culture, 277
Working phase of nurse-client relationship,
  77–78
Working stage of group development, 247
Work-life balance, 279–280
Work-life conflict, 279, 279b
Workplace, mental health
  health problems and disorders,
    281–283
    accommodation, 282
    symptoms, 282, 282t
    work and persons living, 282–283
  healthy workplaces, 277–280
    psychosocial factors in, 277, 278t
    unsafe workplaces, 279, 279b
    work-life balance, 279–280
  nurse
    burnout, 283–284
    compassion fatigue, 284
    fatigue, 284
    job strain, 283–284
    recommendations for, 283, 283t
    violence, 284–285
  threats
    bullying, 281, 281t
    burnout, 280
    emergencies/disasters, 281
    stress, 280
    violence, 280–281
  work
    changing nature of, 276–277
    and gender, 277
    unemployment, 276–277
Workplace violence, 280

World Federation for Mental Health
  (WFMH), 62
Worry, 480

X

Xenophobia, 486b
Xerostomia, 769

Y

Yale-Brown Obsessive Compulsive Scale
  (Y-BOCS), 499
Yale-Brown-Cornell Eating Disorder Scale
  (YBC-EDS), 545b
Yalom, Irving, 111
York Retreat, 4, 4f
Young-old, 753
Youth. *See also* Children, biopsychosocial
  nursing assessment of; Clinical
  interview
  forensic nursing, 897
  mental health assessment of, 691–714
Yukon, standard of practice in, 73t

Z

Zeitgebers, 141, 647
Ziprasidone (Geodon), 388, 392
Zolpidem (Ambien)
  adverse reactions, 221
  indications and mechanisms of
    action, 220
  pharmacokinetics, 220–221
  side effects, 221
  toxicity, 221
Zoophobia, 486b
Zyban, 217